Comprehensive Pediatric Hospital Medicine

Comprehensive Pediatric Hospital Medicine

Edited by

Lisa B. Zaoutis MD, FAAP

Assistant Professor of Pediatrics
University of Pennsylvania School of Medicine
Chief, Section of Inpatient Services
Division of General Pediatrics
The Children's Hospital of Philadelphia
Philadelphia, Pennsylvania

Vincent W. Chiang MD, FAAP

Assistant Professor of Pediatrics
Harvard Medical School
Chief, Inpatient Services
Children's Hospital Boston
Boston, Massachusetts

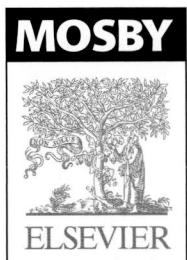

MOSBY

ELSEVIER

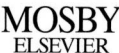

1600 John F. Kennedy Boulevard
Ste 1800
Philadelphia, Pennsylvania 19103-2899

COMPREHENSIVE PEDIATRIC HOSPITAL MEDICINE   ISBN: 978-0-323-03004-5

Library of Congress Cataloging-in-Publication Data

Comprehensive pediatric hospital medicine / [edited by] Lisa B. Zaoutis, Vincent W. Chiang.
   p. ; cm.
  ISBN 978-0-323-03004-5
  1. Pediatrics. 2. Hospital Care. I. Zaoutis, Lisa B. II. Chiang, Vincent W.
  [DNLM: 1. Pediatrics. 2. Child, Hospitalized. 3. Hospitalists. WS 100 C7368 2007]
RJ45.C6622 2007
618.92–dc22
                                           2006046688

Publishing Director: Judith Fletcher
Developmental Editor: Jean Nevius
Publishing Services Manager: Tina Rebane
Project Manager: Jodi Kaye

Printed in China

Last digit is the print number: 9 8 7 6 5 4 3 2 1

This book is dedicated to
  our mentors, whom we strive to emulate,
  our teachers, whom we hope to do proud,
  our colleagues, with whom we proudly persevere,
  our students, whom we dare to inspire,
  and our patients, whom we endeavor to serve.

LBZ and VWC

Thanks to Pat for her guidance, to Mr. Cairo and Dr. Bondoc for their early inspiration, and to Lou Bell for his support and encouragement.

Thanks to all my family, including my sons Mitch, Dan, Jake, and Sam; my parents; and most especially, my husband, Theo. Their love and support are my foundation.

LBZ

Deepest thanks to Gary Fleisher and Fred Lovejoy, both of whom I consider consummate clinician educators.

I also thank my family (Susanne, Molly, Grace, and Aidan) and my family (Edward, Alice, and Victor) for their love, support, and patience.

VWC

Section Editors:

Pamela J. Beasley MD
Assistant Professor of Psychiatry
Harvard Medical School
Director, Pediatric Psychiatry Service
Children's Hospital Boston
Boston, Massachusetts
Psychiatry

Patrick D. Brophy MD, FAAP, FRCPC
Assistant Professor
University of Michigan Medical School
Co-Director, Pediatric Lupus Clinic
Associate Director, Hemodialysis Unit—Acute Therapies
Pediatric Nephrology, Transplant and Dialysis
C.S. Mott Children's Hospital
Ann Arbor, Michigan
Nephrology

Manish J. Butte PhD, MD
Research Fellow in Pathology
Department of Pathology
Harvard Medical School
Boston, Massachusetts
Allergy and Immunology

Aaron S. Chidekel MD
Assistant Professor of Pediatrics
Jefferson Medical College of Thomas Jefferson University
Philadelphia, Pennsylvania
Attending Pulmonologist
Division of Pulmonology
Alfred I. duPont Hospital for Children
Wilmington, Delaware
Pulmonology

Jennifer A. Daru MD, FAAP
Clinical Associate Professor of Pediatrics
Northwestern University Feinberg School of Medicine
Director of Pediatrics and Education
Advocate Illlinois Masonic Hospital
Chicago, Illinois
Neonatology

Ralph Deberardinis MD, PhD
Instructor of Pediatrics
University of Pennsylvania School of Medicine
Attending Physician, Biochemical Genetics
The Children's Hospital of Philadelphia
Philadelphia, Pennsylvania
Genetics and Metabolism

John D'Orazio MD
Assistant Professor of Pediatrics
University of Kentucky College of Medicine
Attending Physician in Pediatric Hematology–Oncology
Markey Cancer Center
Albert Chandler University of Kentucky Medical Center
Lexington, Kentucky
Hematology

Robert L. Geggel MD
Associate Professor of Pediatrics
Harvard Medical School
Senior Associate in Cardiology
Director
Cardiology Consult Service
Children's Hospital Boston
Boston, Massachusetts
Cardiology

Mark H. Gorelick MD, MSCE
Associate Professor and Chief
Department of Pediatrics (Emergency Medicine)
Medical College of Wisconsin
Medical Director
Emergency Department
Children's Hospital of Wisconsin
Milwaukee, Wisconsin
Fluids and Electrolytes

Elizabeth A. Mullen MD
Instructor of Medicine
Harvard Medical School
Clinician
Department of Pediatric Oncology
Dana Farber Cancer Institute
Boston, Massachusetts
Oncology

Sharon E. Oberfield MD
Professor of Pediatrics
Columbia University
Director
Endocrinology, Diabetes, and Metabolism
Morgan Stanley Children's Hospital
Division of Pediatric Endocrinology
Children's Hospital of New York–Presbyterian
New York, New York
Endocrinology

Kevin C. Osterhoudt MD, MSCE, FAAP, FACMT
Associate Professor of Pediatrics
University of Pennsylvania School of Medicine
Medical Director
The Poison Control Center
Section of Medical Toxicology
Division of Emergency Medicine
The Children's Hospital of Philadelphia
Philadelphia, Pennsylvania
Toxicology, Substance Abuse, Environmental Exposure

Marc C. Patterson MD
Professor of Neurology and Pediatrics
Columbia University College of Physicians and Surgeons
Director, Pediatric Neurology Training Program
Morgan Stanley Children's Hospital of New York-Presbyterian
New York, New York
Neurology

Donald F. Schwarz MD, MPH
Associate Professor of Pediatrics
University of Pennsylvania School of Medicine
Vice-Chairman and Chief
Craig-Dalsimer Division of Adolescent Medicine
The Children's Hospital of Philadelphia
Philadelphia, Pennsylvania
Adolescent Medicine

Jordan Scott MD
Clinical Instructor, Allergy/Immunology
Harvard Medical School
Active Staff
Children's Hospital Boston
Boston, Massachusetts
Active Staff
UMass Memorial/Health Alliance
Leominster Campus
Leominster, Massachusetts
Allergy and Immunology

Samir S. Shah MD
Assistant Professor of Pediatrics and Epidemiology
University of Pennsylvania School of Medicine
Attending Physician
Divisions of Infectious Diseases and General Pediatrics
The Children's Hospital of Philadelphia
Philadelphia, Pennsylvania
Infectious Diseases

Rajendu Srivastava MD, FRCP(C), MPH, FAAP
Assistant Professor
Division of Pediatric Inpatient Medicine
Department of Pediatrics
University of Utah Health Sciences Center
Staff Hospitalist
Primary Children's Medical Center
Institute for Healthcare Delivery and Research
Intermountain Healthcare
Salt Lake City, Utah
Care of the Medically Complex Child

Robert Sundel MD
Associate Professor of Pediatrics
Harvard Medical School
Program Director
Department of Rheumatology
Division of Immunology
Children's Hospital Boston
Boston, Massachusetts
Rheumatology

Menno Verhave MD
Assistant Professor of Pediatrics
Harvard Medical School
Department of Gastroenterology
Division of Nutrition Medicine
Children's Hospital Boston
Boston, Massachusetts
Gastroenterology

Celeste R. Wilson MD
Instructor in Pediatrics
Harvard Medical School
Assistant in Medicine
Department of Medicine
Children's Hospital Boston
Boston, Massachusetts
Child Abuse and Neglect

Albert C. Yan MD
Assistant Professor of Pediatrics and Dermatology
University of Pennsylvania School of Medicine
Chief, Section of Pediatric Dermatology
The Children's Hospital of Philadelphia
Philadelphia, Pennsylvania
Dermatology

Theoklis Zaoutis MD, MSCE
Assistant Professor of Pediatrics and Epidemiology
University of Pennsylvania School of Medicine
Attending Physician
Division of Infectious Diseases
The Children's Hospital of Philadelphia
Philadelphia, Pennsylvania
Infectious Diseases

Contributors

David Adams, MD, PhD, DiplABP
Clinical Fellow in Biochemical and Clinical Genetics,
National Institutes of Health, Bethesda, Maryland
133: Metabolic Acidosis

Sherri L. Adams, MSN, RN, CPNP-AC/PC
Lecturer, Faculty of Nursing, and Associate Member,
School of Graduate Studies, University of Toronto; Clinical
Nurse Specialist–Nurse Practitioner, Division of Paediatric
Medicine, The Hospital for Sick Children, Toronto,
Ontario, Canada
192, 194: Introduction to the Medically Complex Child;
Common Reasons for Admission

Chhavi Agarwal, MD
Clinical Fellow, Division of Pediatric Endocrinology,
Children's Hospital of New York–Presbyterian Columbia
University Medical Center, New York, New York
91: Disorders of Calcium Metabolism

Elizabeth R. Alpern, MD, MSCE
Assistant Professor of Pediatrics, University of
Pennsylvania School of Medicine; Attending Physician,
Division of Emergency Medicine, The Children's Hospital
of Philadelphia, Philadelphia, Pennsylvania
60, 61: Fever; Prolonged Fever and Fever of Unknown
Origin

Armand H. Matheny Antommaria, MD, PhD
Assistant Professor of Pediatrics, Adjunct Assistant
Professor of Medical Ethics and Humanities, University of
Utah School of Medicine; Chair, Ethics Committee and
Ethics Consultation Service, Primary Children's Medical
Center, Salt Lake City, Utah
196: Do-Not-Resuscitate Orders

Megan H. Bair-Merritt, MD, MSCE
Assistant Professor of Pediatrics, Johns Hopkins School of
Medicine; Attending Physician, Division of General
Pediatrics and Adolescent Medicine, Johns Hopkins
Hospital, Baltimore, Maryland
64: Complications of Acute Otitis Media and Sinusitis

Lourival Baptista-Neto, MD
Instructor in Psychiatry, Harvard Medical School;
Assistant in Psychiatry and Director, Pediatric Psychiatry
Consultation Service, Children's Hospital Boston, Boston,
Massachusetts
168: Agitation

Jill Baren, MD, MBE, FACEP, FAAP
Associate Professor of Emergency Medicine and Pediatrics,
Associate, Center for Bioethics, Department of Medical
Ethics, University of Pennsylvania School of Medicine;
Attending Physician, Department of Emergency Medicine,
Hospital of the University of Pennsylvania; Attending
Physician, Division of Emergency Medicine, The
Children's Hospital of Philadelphia, Philadelphia,
Pennsylvania
210: Thoracentesis

Carl R. Baum, MD, FAAP, FACMT
Associate Professor of Pediatrics, Yale University
School of Medicine; Director, Medical Toxicology,
Director, Center for Children's Environmental Toxicology,
Yale–New Haven Children's Hospital, New Haven,
Connecticut
182: Drugs of Abuse

Eric D. Baum, MD
Connecticut Pediatric Otolaryngology, North Haven,
Madison, and New Haven, Connecticut
142: Ear, Nose, and Throat

Pamela J. Beasley, MD
Assistant Professor of Psychiatry, Harvard Medical School;
Director, Pediatric Psychiatry Service, Children's Hospital
Boston, Boston, Massachusetts
165, 167, 168, 169: Depression and Physical Illness;
Conversion and Pain Disorders; Agitation; New-Onset
Psychosis

Suzanne Beno, MD
Assistant Professor of Pediatrics and Emergency Medicine,
University of Alberta Faculty of Medicine and Dentistry;
Attending Physician, Division of Emergency Medicine, The
Stollery Children's Hospital, Edmonton, Alberta, Canada
204: Central Venous Access

Laurie A. Bernard, MD
Clinical Assistant Professor of Pediatrics, University of
California, San Diego, School of Medicine; Hospitalist,
Division of Pediatrics and Hospital Medicine, Rady
Children's Hospital, San Diego, California
159: Drug-Associated Rashes

Stacey E. Bernstein, MD, FRCPC
Assistant Professor of Pediatrics, Director of
Undergraduate Medical Education, University of Toronto
Faculty of Medicine; Pediatric Hospitalist, Division of
Pediatric Medicine, The Hospital for Sick Children,
Toronto, Ontario, Canada
107: Systemic Lupus Erythematosus

Chad K. Brands, MD
Assistant Professor of Medicine and Pediatrics, Mayo Clinic College of Medicine; Consultant, Mayo Clinic, Rochester, Minnesota
29: **Chest Pain**

Laura K. Brennan, MD
Instructor of Pediatrics, University of Pennsylvania School of Medicine; Attending Physician, Division of General Pediatrics, The Children's Hospital of Philadelphia, Philadelphia, Pennsylvania
94: **Constipation**

Marisa B. Brett-Fleegler, MD
Instructor in Pediatrics, Harvard Medical School; Attending Physician, Division of Emergency Medicine, Children's Hospital Boston, Boston, Massachusetts
146: **Burns and Other Skin Injuries**

Manish J. Butte, PhD, MD
Research Fellow in Pathology, Department of Pathology, Harvard Medical School, Boston, Massachusetts
137: **Intravenous Immunoglobulin**

Julie Story Byerley, MD, MPH
Assistant Professor, Department of General Pediatrics and Adolescent Medicine, University of North Carolina at Chapel Hill School of Medicine, Chapel Hill, North Carolina
138: **Gastrointestinal Obstruction: Pyloric Stenosis, Malrotation and Volvulus, and Intussusception**

Diane P. Calello, MD
Instructor of Pediatrics, University of Pennsylvania School of Medicine; Fellow, Pediatric Emergency Medicine and Medical Toxicology, Section of Clinical Toxicology, Division of Emergency Medicine, The Children's Hospital of Philadelphia, Philadelphia, Pennsylvania
180: **Hazardous Household Chemicals: Hydrocarbons, Alcohols, and Caustics**

Deirdre Caplin, PhD
Assistant Professor, University of Utah School of Medicine; Primary Children's Medical Center, Salt Lake City, Utah
215: **Child Development for Inpatient Medicine**

Rebecca G. Carlisle, MD
Assistant Professor, George Washington University School of Medicine and Health Sciences; Children's National Medical Center, Washington, DC
188: **Human and Animal Bites**

Douglas W. Carlson, MD
Associate Professor of Pediatrics, Chief, Pediatric Hospital Medicine, and Co-Course Master, Medical Student Education, Washington University at Saint Louis School of Medicine; Attending, St. Louis Children's Hospital, St. Louis, Missouri
197: **Procedural Sedation**

Jean Marie Carroll, BSN
Nurse Coordinator, Pediatric Advanced Care Team, The Children's Hospital of Philadelphia, Philadelphia, Pennsylvania
12: **Palliative, End-of-Life, and Bereavement Care**

Mary Wu Chang, MD
Associate Professor, Departments of Dermatology and Pediatrics, University of Connecticut School of Medicine; Chief of Pediatric Dermatology, Connecticut Children's Medical Center, Hartford, Connecticut
158: **Ecthyma Gangrenosum**

Grace M. Cheng, MD
Clinical Instructor of General Pediatrics, Stanford University School of Medicine; Clinical Instructor, Lucile Packard Children's Hospital, Palo Alto, California
9, 134: **The Approach to the Hospitalized Child and Family; Anaphylaxis**

Aaron S. Chidekel, MD
Assistant Professor of Pediatrics, Jefferson Medical College of Thomas Jefferson University, Philadelphia, Pensylvania; Attending Pulmonologist, Alfred I. duPont Hospital for Children, Nemours Children's Clinic, Wilmington, Delaware
74, 79: **Apparent Life-Threatening Event, Infant Apnea, and Pediatric Obstructive Sleep Apnea Syndrome; Choking and Foreign Body Aspiration**

Denesh K. Chitkara, MD
Assistant Professor of Pediatrics, Department of Pediatric Gastroenterology, University of North Carolina at Chapel Hill, Chapel Hill, North Carolina
95: **Dyspepsia**

Bill Chiu, MD
Resident in General Surgery, Department of Surgery, Children's Memorial Hospital, Chicago, Illinois
51: **Congenital Anomalies**

Christine S. Cho, MD, MPH
Instructor of Pediatrics, University of Pennsylvania School of Medicine; Fellow, Division of Emergency Medicine, The Children's Hospital of Philadelphia, Philadelphia, Pennsylvania
189, 206, 213, 214: **Envenomation; Phlebotomy; Cerebrospinal Fluid Shunt Assessment; Cerebrospinal Fluid Shunt Puncture**

Jeanne S. Chow, MD
Assistant Professor of Radiology, Harvard Medical School; Pediatric Radiologist, Children's Hospital Boston; Radiologist, Beth Israel Deaconess Medical Center; Associated Radiologist, Massachusetts General Hospital, Boston, Massachusetts
198: **Radiology for the Pediatric Hospitalist**

Bartley G. Cilento, Jr., MD, MPH
Assistant Professor in Surgery (Urology), Harvard Medical School; Staff Surgeon, Children's Hospital Boston, Boston, Massachusetts
148: **Urology**

Susan E. Coffin, MD, MPH
Associate Professor of Pediatrics, University of Pennsylvania School of Medicine; Medical Director, Infection Prevention and Control, Division of Infectious Diseases, The Children's Hospital of Philadelphia, Philadelphia, Pennsylvania
6: **Infection Control for Pediatric Hospitalists**

Bernard A. Cohen, MD
Professor of Pediatrics and Dermatology, Johns Hopkins University School of Medicine; Director of Pediatric Dermatology, Johns Hopkins Children's Center, Baltimore, Maryland
150: Purpura

Kristina A. Cole, MD, PhD
Fellow, Division of Hematology and Oncology, The Children's Hospital of Philadelphia, Philadelphia, Pennsylvania
121: Transfusion Medicine

Patrick H. Conway, MD
Instructor and Robert Wood Johnson Clinical Scholar, University of Pennsylvania School of Medicine; General Pediatrics Inpatient Attending, The Children's Hospital of Philadelphia, Philadelphia, Pennsylvania
13: Transitions in Care

Maura Cooper, MD
Assistant Professor of Pediatrics, George Washington University School of Medicine and Health Sciences; Hospitalist, Children's National Medical Center, Washington, DC; Pediatric Hospitalist, Department of Pediatric Education, Holy Cross Hospital, Silver Spring, Maryland
215: Child Development for Inpatient Medicine

Timothy Cornell, MD
Clinical Fellow, Department of Pediatrics, Division of Critical Medicine, University of Michigan Medical School and Mott Children's Hospital, Ann Arbor, Michigan
86: Pericarditis

Kate M. Cronan, MD
Associate Professor of Pediatrics, Jefferson Medical College of Thomas Jefferson University, Philadelphia, Pennsylvania; Division Chief, Department of Pediatrics, Division of Pediatric Emergency Medicine, Alfred I. DuPont Hospital for Children, Wilmington, Delaware
207: Replacing a Tracheostomy Tube

Catherine Cross, MD
Clinical Instructor in Pediatrics, Harvard Medical School; Hospitalist, Children's Hospital Boston, Boston, Massachusetts
41: Lymphadenitis

Bari B. Cunningham, MD
Assistant Clinical Professor of Pediatrics and Medicine (Dermatology), University of California, San Diego, School of Medicine; Children's Hospital and Health Center, San Diego, California
149: Lumps and Bumps: Benign and Malignant Tumors

Melody J. Cunningham, MD
Assistant Professor of Pediatrics, University of Tennessee College of Medicine; Assistant Member, Department of Hematology, St. Jude Children's Research Hospital, Memphis, Tennessee
121: Transfusion Medicine

Jennifer A. Daru, MD, FAAP
Clinical Associate Professor of Pediatrics, Northwestern University Feinberg School of Medicine; Executive Committee, AAP Section on Hospital Medicine; Director of Pediatrics and Education, Advocate Illinois Masonic Hospital, Chicago, Illinois
48: Delivery Room Medicine

Ian J. Davis, MD, PhD
Instructor in Pediatrics, Harvard Medical School; Attending Physician—Pediatric Oncology, Children's Hospital Boston and Dana Farber Cancer Institute, Boston, Massachusetts
116: Anemia

Matthew A. Deardorff, MD, PhD
Instructor in Pediatrics and Genetics, University of Pennsylvania School of Medicine; Fellow in Human Genetics, The Children's Hospital of Philadelphia, Philadelphia, Pennsylvania
130: Genetic Syndromes Caused by Chromosomal Abnormalities

Barbara Degar, MD
Instructor, Harvard Medical School; Attending Physician, Pediatric Oncology, Dana Farber Cancer Institute and Children's Hospital Boston, Boston, Massachusetts
123: Childhood Cancer

Michael DelVecchio, MD
Associate Professor of Pediatrics, Temple University School of Medicine; Director of Inpatient Pediatrics, Temple University Children's Medical Center, Philadelphia, Pennsylvania
190: Infant Botulism

David Ray DeMaso, MD
Professor of Psychiatry (Pediatrics), Harvard Medical School; Psychiatrist-in-Chief, Children's Hospital Boston, Boston, Massachusetts
167: Conversion and Pain Disorders

Marissa de Ungria, MD
Assistant Professor, Department of Pediatrics, Northwestern University Feinberg School of Medicine; Attending Neonatologist, Department of Neonatology, Children's Memorial Hospital; Attending Neonatologist, Department of Pediatrics, Prentice Women's Hospital, Chicago, Illinois
48: Delivery Room Medicine

Stephanie B. Dewar, MD
Associate Professor of Clinical Pediatrics, Northeastern Ohio Universities College of Medicine, Rootstown; Pediatric Residency Program Director; Director, Division of Diagnostic Referral Pediatrics; and Medical Director, Tri-County Child Advocacy Center, Forum Health, Tod Children's Hospital, Youngstown, Ohio
171: Sexually Transmitted Diseases

Craig C. DeWolfe, MD
Assistant Professor of Pediatrics, George Washington
University School of Medicine and Health Sciences;
Attending Hospitalist, Children's National Medical Center,
Washington, DC; Pediatric Hospitalist, Ann Arundee
Medical Center, Annapolis, Maryland
74: Apparent Life-Threatening Event, Infant Apnea, and
Pediatric Obstructive Sleep Apnea Syndrome

Martha Dimmers, MDiv, MSW
Manager of Pastoral and Spiritual Care, Children's Hospital
and Regional Medical Center, Seattle, Washington
11: Spiritual Care

James G. H. Dinulos, MD
Associate Professor of Medicine and Pediatrics
(Dermatology), Dartmouth Medical School; Dermatology
Section Chief (Interim) and Residency Program Director,
Dermatology, Dartmouth-Hitchcock Medical Center,
Lebanon, New Hampshire
152: Psoriasis

Ed Donovan, MD
Professor of Clinical Pediatrics and Obstetrics and
Gynecology, University of Cincinnati School of
Medicine; Director, Child Policy Research Center,
Cincinnati; Children's Hospital Medical Center,
Cincinnati, Ohio
8: Clinical Practices Guidelines

Kenneth J. Dooley, MD
Associate Professor of Pediatrics, Emory University School
of Medicine; Attending, Children's Healthcare of Atlanta,
Atlanta, Georgia
85: Myocarditis and Cardiomyopathy

Emmanuel Doyne, MD
Adjunct Professor of Pediatrics, University of Cincinnati
School of Medicine; Director, Section of Community
Pediatrics, Cincinnati Children's Hospital Medical Center,
Cincinnati, Ohio
8: Clinical Practice Guidelines

Christine N. Duncan, MD
Instructor in Pediatrics, Harvard Medical School;
Attending in Pediatric Hematology/Oncology, Dana Farber
Cancer Institute and Children's Hospital Boston, Boston,
Massachusetts
125: Stem Cell Transplants

Marie Egan, MD
Associate Professor, Departments of Pediatrics and Cellular
and Molecular Physiology, Yale University School of
Medicine; Director, Cystic Fibrosis Center Yale–New Haven
Medical Center, New Haven, Connecticut
78: Cystic Fibrosis

Lawrence F. Eichenfield, MD
Professor of Pediatrics and Medicine (Dermatology),
University of California, San Diego, School of Medicine;
Chief, Pediatric and Adolescent Dermatology, Rady
Children's Hospital, San Diego, California
159: Drug-Associated Rashes

Moussa El-hallak, MD
Research Fellow, Children's Hospital Boston, Boston,
Massachusetts
102: Kawasaki Disease

Scott A. Elisofon, MD
Instructor in Pediatrics, Harvard Medical School;
Attending Physician, Gastroenterology, Children's Hospital
Boston, Boston, Massachusetts
97: Liver Failure

Stephen C. Eppes, MD
Clinical Associate Professor of Pediatrics, Jefferson Medical
College of Thomas Jefferson University, Philadelphia,
Pennsylvania; Attending, Department of Pediatrics, Alfred
I. duPont Hospital for Children, Wilmington, Delaware
70: Bone, Joint, and Soft Tissue Infections

Michele Burns Ewald, MD
Assistant Professor of Pediatrics, Harvard Medical School;
Staff Physician, Division of Emergency Medicine; Medical
Director, Regional Center for Poison Control and
Prevention Serving MA/RI; Director, Harvard Medical
Toxicology Fellowship, Children's Hospital Boston, Boston,
Massachusetts
179, 185: Toxicity of Over-the-Counter and Oral
Hypoglycemic Agents; Heat Disorders

Mirna M. Farah, MD
Assistant Professor of Pediatrics, University of
Pennsylvania School of Medicine; Attending Physician, The
Children's Hospital of Philadelphia, Philadelphia,
Pennsylvania
201: Arterial Blood Gas

Chris Feudtner, MD, PhD, MPH
Assistant Professor of Pediatrics, University of
Pennsylvania School of Medicine; Attending Physician and
Director of Research for the Pediatric Advanced Care
Team, The Children's Hospital of Philadelphia,
Philadelphia, Pennsylvania
11, 12, 18: Spiritual Care; Palliative, End-of-Life, and
Bereavement Care; Ethical Issues in Pediatric Hospital
Practice

Andrew M. Fine, MD, MPH
Instructor in Pediatrics, Harvard Medical School; Assistant
in Medicine, Children's Hospital Boston, Boston,
Massachusetts
37: Shock

Susan Hetzel Frangiskakis, MD
Assistant Professor, Department of Pediatrics, University of
Pittsburgh School of Medicine; Attending Physician, Paul
C. Gaffney Diagnostic Referral Service, Children's Hospital
of Pittsburgh, Pittsburgh, Pennsylvania
44: Petechiae and Purpura

Gary Frank, MD, MS
Clinical Assistant Professor of Pediatrics, Emory University
School of Medicine; Pediatric Hospitalist, Scottish Rite
Hospital, Atlanta, Georgia
70: Bone, Joint, and Soft Tissue Infections

Eric Frehm, MD
Instructor, Department of Pediatrics, University of
Pennsylvania School of Medicine; Attending
Neonatologist, The Children's Hospital of Philadelphia,
Philadelphia, and the Chester County Hospital,
Westchester, Pennsylvania
53: **Congenital and Perinatal Infections**

Nicole R. Frei, MD
Adjunct Assistant Professor of Pediatrics, University of
Utah School of Medicine, Salt Lake City, Utah
43: **Neck Pain**

Ilona J. Frieden, MD
Professor of Dermatology and Pediatrics, University of
California, San Francisco, School of Medicine, San
Francisco, California
164: **Transplacentally Acquired Dermatoses of the
Newborn**

Eron Y. Friedlaender, MD, MPH
Assistant Professor of Pediatrics, University of
Pennsylvania School of Medicine; Attending Physician,
Division of Emergency Medicine, The Children's Hospital
of Philadelphia, Philadelphia, Pennsylvania
203, 212: **Intraosseous Catheters; Arthrocentesis**

Jeremy Friedman, MB, ChB, FRCPC, FAAP
Associate Professor, Department of Paediatrics,
University of Toronto Faculty of Medicine; Head,
Division of Paediatric Medicine, Department of
Paediatrics, The Hospital for Sick Children, Toronto,
Ontario, Canada
5, 195: **Patient Safety and Medical Errors; Technologic
Devices in the Medically Complex Child**

Robert Hugh Fryer, MD, PhD
Assistant Professor of Clinical Investigation, Department of
Developmental Neurobiology, Rockefeller University;
Clinical Assistant Professor, Department of Pediatric
Neurology, Weill Cornell Medical College; Assistant
Attending, Department of Pediatric Neurology, New York
Hospital, New York, New York
129: **Stroke and Aneurysms**

David R. Fulton, MD
Associate Professor, Department of Pediatrics, Harvard
Medical School; President, Physicians' Organization; Chief,
Cardiology Outpatient Services, Children's Hospital
Boston, Boston, Massachusetts
87: **Acute Rheumatic Fever**

Paul J. Galardy, MD
Assistant Professor of Pediatrics, Mayo Medical School;
Senior Associate Consultant, Division of Pediatric
Hematology/Oncology, Department of Pediatrics and
Adolescent Medicine, Mayo Clinic, Rochester,
Minnesota
120: **Disorders of Coagulation and Thrombosis**

Mirabai Galashan, BA
Chaplain, Pediatric Advanced Care Team, The Children's
Hospital of Philadelphia, Philadelphia, Pennsylvania
11: **Spiritual Care**

Mary Pat Gallagher, MD
Assistant Professor of Clinical Pediatrics, Columbia
University College of Physicians and Surgeons; Attending,
Morgan Stanley Children's Hospital of New
York–Presbyterian, New York, New York
88, 89, 90, 91, 92: **Diabetes Mellitus and Hyperglycemia;
Disorders of Thyroid Hormone; Disorders of Pituitary
Function; Disorders of Calcium Metabolism; Disorders of
the Adrenal Giand**

Beth D. Gamulka, MDCM
Adjunct Assistant Professor, Department of Pediatrics,
University of Toronto Faculty of Medicine; Pediatrician,
The Scarborough Hospital and The Hospital for Sick
Children, Toronto, Ontario, Canada
101: **Feeding Issues**

Rupali Gandhi, MD, JD
Clinical Fellow in Pediatrics, Harvard Medical School;
Resident in Pediatrics, Children's Hospital Boston, Boston,
Massachusetts
21: **Institutional Review Boards, Pharmaceutical Trials,
and the Protection of Research Subjects**

Mary B. Garza, MD
Clinical Associate in Pediatrics, University of Pennsylvania
School of Medicine, Philadelphia; Pediatric Hospitalist,
Abington Memorial Hospital, Abington, Pennsylvania
114, 115: **Renal Tubular Acidosis; Renal Venous
Thrombosis**

Maria C. Garzon, MD
Associate Professor of Clinical Dermatology and Clinical
Pediatrics, Columbia University College of Physicians and
Surgeons; Director, Department of Pediatric Dermatology,
Morgan Stanley Children's Hospital of
NewYork–Presbyterian, New York, New York
162: **Skin Disease in Immunosuppressed Hosts**

Robert L. Geggel, MD
Associate Professor of Pediatrics, Harvard Medical School;
Senior Associate in Cardiology and Director, Cardiology
Consult Service, Children's Hospital Boston, Boston,
Massachusetts
81: **The Cardiac Examination**

Michael H. Gewitz, MD
Professor and Vice Chairman, Department of Pediatrics,
New York Medical College; Executive Director/Physician-
in-Chief and Chief, Pediatric Cardiology, Maria Fareri
Children's Hospital at Westchester Medical Center, Valhalla,
New York
84: **Infective Endocarditis**

Timothy Gibson, MD
Assistant Professor of Pediatrics, University of
Massachusetts Medical School; Chief, Hanshaw Inpatient
Hospitalist Service, UMass Memorial Children's Medical
Center, Worcester, Massachusetts
26, 199, 208: **Abdominal Pain; Lumbar Puncture;
Intubation**

Amy E. Gilliam, MD
Assistant Professor of Dermatology and Pediatrics, University of California, San Francisco, School of Medicine, San Francisco, California
164: Transplacentally Acquired Dermatoses of the Newborn

Katherine B. Ginnis, MSW
Instructor, Harvard Medical School; Coordinator of Emergency Psychiatry, Children's Hospital Boston, Boston, Massachusetts
166: Assessment and Management of Suicidal Patients

Amy Goldberg, MD, FACS
Assistant Professor of Pediatrics, Brown University Medical School; Attending Physician, Child Protection Program, Hasbro Children's Hospital, Providence, Rhode Island
175: Injuries: Signs and Symptoms of Concern for Nonaccidental Trauma

Anna M. Golja, MD
Instructor of Radiology, Harvard Medical School; Attending, Division of Pediatric Neuroradiology, Children's Hospital Boston, Boston, Massachusetts
198: Radiology for the Pediatric Hospitalist

Melissa J. Gregory, MD
Physician, St. Joseph Mercy Hospital, Ypsilanti, Michigan
108, 109, 110, 113: Acute Renal Failure; Chronic Renal Failure; Glomerulonephritis; Nephrotic Syndrome

April A. Harper, MPH, MD
Clinical Fellow, Harvard Medical School; Pediatric Environmental Health Fellow, The Pediatric Environmental Health Center, Children's Hospital Boston, Boston, Massachusetts
181: Lead, Other Metals, and Chelation Therapy

Mary Catherine Harris, MD
Professor of Pediatrics, University of Pennsylvania School of Medicine; Senior Attending Physician, The Children's Hospital of Philadelphia and The Hospital of the University of Pennsylvania, Philadelphia, Pennsylvania
53: Congenital and Perinatal Infections

Natalie Hayes, DO
Post-Doctoral Fellow, Section of Respiratory Medicine, Department of Pediatrics, Yale University School of Medicine, New Haven, Connecticut
79: Choking and Foreign Body Aspiration

Matthew M. Heeney, MD
Instructor in Pediatrics, Harvard Medical School; Director, Sickle Cell Program, Children's Hospital Boston, Boston, Massachusetts
117: Sickle Cell Disease

Diana M. Heinzman, MD, FAAP
Assistant Professor, Department of Pediatrics, Paul C. Gaffney Diagnostic Referral Center, University of Pittsburgh School of Medicine; Attending, Children's Hospital of Pittsburgh, Pittsburgh, Pennsylvania
30: Cyanosis

Meredith Lee Heltzer, MD
Fellow in Allergy and Immunology, The Children's Hospital of Philadelphia, Philadelphia, Pennsylvania
75: Asthma

Keith D. Herzog, MD
Assistant Professor of Pediatrics, Drexel University College of Medicine; Director of Inpatient Services and Attending Physician, General Pediatrics and Section of Infectious Diseases, St. Christopher's Hospital for Children, Philadelphia, Pennsylvania
62: Fever and Rash

Malinda Ann Hill, MA
Bereavement Coordinator, The Children's Hospital of Philadelphia, Philadelphia, Pennsylvania
12: Palliative, End-of-Life, and Bereavement Care

Jessica L. Hills, MD
Clinical Associate, University of Pennsylvania School of Medicine; Pediatric Hospitalist, The Children's Hospital of Philadelphia, Philadelphia, Pennsylvania
154: Head Lice and Scabies

Alejandro Hoberman, MD
Chief, Division of General Academic Pediatrics, and Professor of Pediatrics and Jack L. Paradise Professor of Pediatric Research, University of Pittsburgh School of Medicine, Children's Hospital of Pittsburgh, Pittsburgh, Pennsylvania
69: Urinary Tract Infections in Childhood

K. Sarah Hoehn, MD, MBE
Assistant Professor of Pediatrics, University of Chicago Pritzker School of Medicine; Attending Physician, Pediatric Critical Care, Comer Children's Hospital, Chicago, Illinois
12, 18: Palliative, End-of-Life, and Bereavement Care; Ethical Issues in Pediatric Hospital Practice

Amber M. Hoffman, MD
Assistant Professor of Pediatrics, University of Pittsburgh School of Medicine; Pediatric Hospitalist, Diagnostic Referral Service, and Associate Residency Director, Children's Hospital of Pittsburgh, Pittsburgh, Pennsylvania
47: Vomiting

Robert J. Hoffman, MD
Assistant Professor of Emergency Medicine, Albert Einstein College of Medicine of Yeshiva University; Research Director, Department of Emergency Medicine, Beth Israel Medical Center, New York, New York
183: Withdrawal Syndromes

Amy P. Holst, MD
Assistant Professor of Pediatrics, Creighton University Medical School; Staff, Children's Hospital, Methodist Hospital, Bergen Mercy Hospital; Consultant, Nebraska Medical Center, Omaha, Nebraska
111: Hemolytic Uremic Syndrome

Charles J. Homer, MD, MPH
Associate Clinical Professor of Pediatrics, Harvard Medical School, Boston; President and CEO, National Initiative for Children's Healthcare Quality, Cambridge, Massachusetts
4: Quality of Care and Patient Satisfaction

Paul J. Honig, MD
Emeritus Professor of Pediatrics and Dermatology,
University of Pennsylvania School of Medicine; Attending
Physician, The Children's Hospital of Philadelphia,
Philadelphia, Pennsylvania
155, 163: Atopic Dermatitis; Epidermolysis Bullosa

Patricia M. Hopkins, MD
Assistant Professor, Department of Pediatrics, Albany
Medical College, Albany, New York
66: Middle Respiratory Tract Infections and
Bronchiolitis

Mark D. Hormann, MD
Assistant Professor and Director of Medical Student
Education, Department of Pediatrics, University of Texas
Medical School at Houston, Houston, Texas
50: Birth Injury

B. David Horn, MD
Assistant Professor of Orthopaedic Surgery, University of
Pennsylvania School of Medicine; Attending Surgeon, The
Children's Hospital of Philadelphia, Philadelphia,
Pennsylvania
145: Orthopedics

Michael S. Isakoff, MD
Assistant Professor of Pediatrics, University of
Connecticut School of Medicine, Farmington;
Attending Physician, Division of Hematology-Oncology,
Connecticut Children's Medical Center, Hartford,
Connecticut
123: Childhood Cancer

Katherine A. Janeway, MD
Fellow, Pediatric Hematology-Oncology, Dana Farber
Cancer Institute, Children's Hospital Boston, Boston,
Massachusetts
118: Neutropenia

Katherine Ahn Jin, MD
Instructor, Department of Pediatrics, Harvard
Medical School; Staff Physician, Department of
Medicine, Children's Hospital Boston, Boston,
Massachusetts
27: Acidosis

Maureen M. Jonas, MD
Associate Professor of Pediatrics, Harvard Medical School;
Associate in Gastroenterology, Children's Hospital Boston,
Boston, Massachusetts
97: Liver Failure

Tammy Kang, MD
Assistant Professor of Pediatrics, University of
Pennsylvania School of Medicine; Medical Director, The
Pediatric Advanced Care Team, The Children's Hospital of
Philadelphia, Philadelphia, Pennsylvania
12: Palliative, End-of-Life, and Bereavement Care

Krista Keilty, BN, MN
Associate Member, School of Graduate Studies, Faculty of
Nursing, University of Toronto; Clinical Nurse
Specialist–Nurse Practitioner, Division of Respiratory
Medicine, The Hospital for Sick Children, Toronto,
Ontario, Canada
77, 209: Bronchopulmonary Dysplasia and Chronic Lung
Disease of Infancy; Noninvasive Positive-Pressure
Ventilation

Ron Keren, MD, MPH
Assistant Professor, Department of Pediatrics, University of
Pennsylvania School of Medicine; Attending Physician, The
Children's Hospital of Philadelphia, Philadelphia,
Pennsylvania
55: Neonatal Hyperbilirubinemia

Anupam Kharbanda, MD
Assistant Clinical Professor of Pediatrics, Columbia
University College of Physicians and Surgeons; Attending,
Morgan Stanley Children's Hospital of
NewYork–Presbyterian, New York, New York
141: General Trauma

Marin Kiesau, MS, MD
Visiting Instructor, University of Pittsburgh School of
Medicine; Attending Physician, Children's Hospital of
Pittsburgh, Pittsburgh, Pennsylvania
31: Diarrhea

Caroline C. Kim, MD
Instructor of Pediatrics, Harvard Medical School; Director,
Pigmented Lesion Clinic, and Associate Director, BIDMC
Cutaneous Oncology Program, Beth Israel Deaconess
Medical Center and Children's Hospital Boston, Boston,
Massachusetts
153: Vascular Anomalies

Jason Y. Kim, MD
Attending Physician, Division of Infectious Diseases, The
Children's Hospital of Philadelphia, Philadelphia,
Pennsylvania
72: Human Immunodeficiency Virus

Juliann Lipps Kim, MD
Pediatric Hospitalist, Palo Alto Medical Foundation, Palo
Alto, California
45: Respiratory Distress

Nicola Klein, MD, PhD
Associate Director, Kaiser Permanente Vaccine Study
Center; Research Scientist, Division of Research, Kaiser
Permanente Northern California, Oakland, California
52: Respiratory Distress and Transient Tachypnea of the
Newborn

Paul K. Kleinman, MD
Professor of Radiology, Harvard Medical School; Children's
Hospital Boston, Boston, Massachusetts
174: Imaging of Child Abuse

Joel B. Korin, JD
Adjunct Professor, Rutgers School of Law, Camden;
Counsel, Ballard Spahr Andrews & Ingersoll, LLP,
Voorhees, New Jersey
19: Medicolegal Issues

Uma Kotagal, MBBS, MS
Professor of Pediatrics and Obstetrics and Gynecology, University of Cincinnati, College of Medicine; Vice President, Quality and Transformation, and Director, Health Policy and Clinical Effectiveness, Cincinnati Children's Hospital Medical Center, Cincinnati, Ohio
8: Clinical Practice Guidelines

Lisa K. Kresnicka, MD
Assistant Professor of Pediatrics, University of Florida College of Medicine–Jacksonville; Attending Physician, Division of Child Protection and Forensic Pediatrics, Wolfson Children's Hospital, Jacksonville, Florida
177: Legal Issues

Rana N. Kronfol, MD
Assistant Professor, Department of Pediatrics, Baylor College of Medicine, Houston, Texas
33: Fever

Cynthia L. Kuelbs, MD
Associate Clinical Professor of Pediatrics, Department of Pediatrics, University of California, San Diego, School of Medicine; Medical Director, Inpatient Services, Rady Children's Hospital and Health Center, San Diego, California
14: Medical Comanagement and Consultation

Subra Kugathasan, MD
Associate Professor of Pediatrics, Medical College of Wisconsin; Medical Director, Pediatric IBD Program, Children's Hospital of Wisconsin, Milwaukee, Wisconsin
98: Inflammatory Bowel Disease

Amethyst C. Kurbegov, MD, MPH
Assistant Professor of Pediatric Gastroenterology, University of Miami Miller School of Medicine, Miami, Florida
93: Pediatric Biliary Disease

Christopher P. Landrigan, MD, MPH
Assistant Professor of Pediatrics and Medicine, Harvard Medical School; Research Director, Fellowship Director, Inpatient Pediatrics Service, Children's Hospital Boston; Director, Sleep and Patient Safety Program, Brigham and Women's Hospital, Boston, Massachusetts
5, 20, 24: Patient Safety and Medical Errors; Clinical Research in the Pediatric Inpatient Setting; Pediatric Hospital Medicine: Future Directions

Miriam Laufer, MD
Assistant Professor of Pediatrics, Center for Vaccine Development, University of Maryland School of Medicine, Baltimore, Maryland
68: Gastrointestinal Diseases

Christine Lauren, MD
Resident Physician, Columbia University Pediatric Dermatology and Children's Hospital of New York, New York, New York
155: Atopic Dermatitis

Daniel J. Lebovitz, MD
Associate Professor, Department of Pediatrics, Case Western Reserve University School of Medicine; Pediatric Critical Care Physician, Rainbow Babies and Children's Hospital, Cleveland, Ohio
28: Altered Mental Status

Natasha Leibel, MD
Assistant Professor of Clinical Pediatrics, Columbia University College of Physicians and Surgeons; Staff Pediatrician, Morgan Stanley Children's Hospital of New York–Presbyterian, New York, New York
89: Disorders of Thyroid Hormone

Lucinda P. Leung, MD
Clinical Associate, University of Pennsylvania School of Medicine; Attending Physician, The Children's Hospital of Philadelphia, Philadelphia, Pennsylvania
67: Lower Respiratory Infections

Leonard J. Levine, MD
Assistant Professor of Pediatrics, Drexel University College of Medicine; Attending Physician, St. Christopher's Hospital for Children, Philadelphia, Pennsylvania
172: Dysfunctional Uterine Bleeding

Jason A. Levy, MD
Instructor in Pediatrics, Harvard Medical School; Faculty, Pediatric Emergency Medicine, Children's Hospital Boston, Boston, Massachusetts
144: Ocular Trauma

Phyllis A. Lewis, MD
Assistant Professor of Pediatrics, George Washington University School of Medicine and Health Sciences; Staff, Children's National Medical Center, Washington, DC
188: Human and Animal Bites

Marilyn G. Liang, MD
Assistant Professor, Department of Dermatology, Harvard Medical School; Pediatric Dermatologist, Children's Hospital Boston, Boston, Massachusetts
153: Vascular Anomalies

Daniel J. Licht, MD
Assistant Professor of Pediatrics and Neurology, University of Pennsylvania School of Medicine; Attending Physician, Pediatric Neurology, The Children's Hospital of Philadelphia, Philadelphia, Pennsylvania
12: Palliative, End-of-Life, and Bereavement Care

Carolyn M. Long, MSW
Social Worker, Pediatric Advanced Care Team, The Children's Hospital of Philadelphia, Philadelphia, Pennsylvania
12: Palliative, End-of-Life, and Bereavement Care

Jeffrey P. Louie, MD
Active Staff, Children's Hospital and Clinics of Minnesota, St. Paul, Minnesota
186: Hypothermia and Cold-Related Injuries

Barry A. Love, MD
Assistant Professor of Pediatrics and Medicine, Mount Sinai School of Medicine; Director, Congenital Cardiac Catheterization Laboratory, Mount Sinai Medical Center, New York, New York
83: **Congenital Heart Disease**

Patricia V. Lowery, MD
Fellow of Neonatology, Duke Endowment Fellow, MPH, The Brody School of Medicine, Pitt County Memorial Hospital, Greenville, North Carolina
100: **Pancreatitis**

Ian B. MacLusky, MBBS, FRCP(C), FAAP
Associate Professor of Paediatrics, University of Ottawa Faculty of Medicine; Director of Respiratory Medicine, Children's Hospital of Eastern Ontario, Ottawa, Ontario, Canada
77, 209: **Bronchopulmonary Dysplasia and Chronic Lung Disease of Infancy; Noninvasive Positive-Pressure Ventilation**

Katarzyna Madejczyk, MD
Clinical Assistant Professor of Pediatrics, UMDNJ–Robert Wood Johnson Medical School, New Brunswick; Pediatric Generalist, Jersey Shore University Medical Center, Neptune, New Jersey
49: **The Well Newborn**

Mary Beth Madonna, MD
Assistant Professor of Surgery, Northwestern University Feinberg School of Medicine; Attending Pediatric Surgeon, Children's Memorial Hospital, Chicago, Illinois
51: **Congenital Anomalies**

Sanjay Mahant, MD, FRCPC
Assistant Professor of Paediatrics, University of Toronto Faculty of Medicine; Staff Paediatrician, Division of Paediatric Medicine, Paediatric Outcomes Research Team, The Hospital for Sick Children, Toronto, Ontario, Canada
192: **Introduction to the Medically Complex Child**

Paul E. Manicone, MD, FAAP
Assistant Professor, Department of Pediatrics, George Washington University School of Medicine and Health Sciences; Faculty Fellow, Hospitalist Division, Children's National Medical Center, Washington, DC
126, 184: **Seizures; Fire-Related Inhalation Injury**

Jennifer Maniscalco, MD, MPH
Assistant Professor of Pediatrics, George Washington University School of Medicine and Health Sciences; Pediatric Hospitalist, Children's National Medical Center, Washington, DC
99: **Malnutrition**

Keith Mann, MD
Assistant Professor of Pediatrics, University of Missouri at Kansas City School of Medicine; Associate Director, Pediatric Residency Program, Children's Mercy Hospital, Kansas City, Missouri
73: **Infections in Special Hosts**

Rebekah Mannix, MD
Instructor in Pediatrics, Harvard Medical School; Staff Physician, Children's Hospital Boston, Boston, Massachusetts
179: **Toxicity of Over-the-Counter and Oral Hypoglycemic Agents**

Jonathan M. Mansbach, MD
Instructor in Pediatrics, Harvard Medical School; Inpatient Service, Children's Hospital Boston, Boston, Massachusetts
7: **Evidence-Based Medicine**

Peter Mattei, MD
Assistant Professor, Department of Surgery, University of Pennsylvania School of Medicine; Attending Physician, General, Thoracic, and Fetal Surgery, The Children's Hospital of Philadelphia, Philadelphia, Pennsylvania
140: **Hernias**

Oscar H. Mayer, MD
Assistant Professor of Pediatrics, University of Pennsylvania School of Medicine; Attending Physician, Pulmonary Medicine, The Children's Hospital of Philadelphia, Philadelphia, Pennsylvania
12: **Palliative, End-of-Life, and Bereavement Care**

Sarah C. McBride, MD
Instructor in Pediatrics, Harvard Medical School; Assistant in Medicine and Director of Resident Education, Inpatient Pediatric Service, Children's Hospital Boston, Boston, Massachusetts
20, 46: **Clinical Research in the Pediatric Inpatient Setting; Syncope**

Kevin D. McBryde, MD
Assistant Professor of Pediatrics, George Washington University School of Medicine and Health Sciences; Department of Nephrology, Children's National Medical Center, Washington, DC
112: **Interstitial Nephritis**

Michele R. McKee, MD
Assistant Professor of Pediatrics, Boston University School of Medicine; Pediatric Emergency Medicine Attending, Boston Medical Center, Boston, Massachusetts
191: **Biologic, Chemical, and Radiologic Terrorism**

William McNett, MD
Clinical Instructor, Jefferson Medical College of Thomas Jefferson University; Active Staff, Thomas Jefferson University Hospital, Philadelphia, Pennsylvania; Active Staff, Alfred I. duPont Hospital for Children, Wilmington, Delaware
56: **Neonatal Abstinence Syndrome**

Sanford M. Melzer, MD, MBA
Associate Professor of Pediatrics, University of Washington School of Medicine; Vice President, Strategic Planning and Business Development, Children's Hospital and Regional Medical Center, Seattle, Washington
16: **Financial Aspects of Pediatric Hospitalist Programs**

Talene A. Metjian, PharmD
Coordinator, Antimicrobial Stewardship Program, and
Clinical Specialist in Infectious Diseases and Pulmonary
Medicine, The Children's Hospital of Philadelphia,
Philadelphia, Pennsylvania
59: Empirical Treatment of Bacterial Infections

Denise W. Metry, MD
Associate Professor of Dermatology and Pediatrics, Baylor
College of Medicine; Chief, Pediatric Dermatology Clinic,
Texas Children's Hospital, Houston, Texas
161: Stevens-Johnson Syndrome and Toxic Epidermal
Necrolysis

Stephen E. Muething, MD
Associate Professor, University of Cincinnati School of
Medicine; Director, Clinical Services, Cincinnati Children's
Hospital Medical Center, Cincinnati, Ohio
13: Transitions in Care

Emily E. Milliken, MD
Assistant Professor of Pediatrics, University of
California, San Francisco, School of Medicine; Pediatric
Hospitalist, UCSF Children's Hospital, San Francisco,
California
36: Hypoglycemia

Laura J. Mirkinson, MD, FAAP
Associate Professor of Pediatrics, George Washington
University School of Medicine, Washington, DC; Adjunct
Associate Professor of Pediatrics, The Uniformed Services
University of the Health Sciences, Bethesda, Maryland;
Pediatric Hospitalist, Children's National Medical Center,
Washington, DC; Holy Cross Hospital, Silver Spring,
Maryland
54, 104, 106: Hypoglycemia and Infants of Diabetic
Mothers; Juvenile Dermatomyositis; Postinfectious
Arthritis

Manoj K. Mittal, MD, MRCP(UK)
Instructor of Pediatrics, University of Pennsylvania School
of Medicine; Fellow, Pediatric Emergency Medicine, The
Children's Hospital of Philadelphia, Philadelphia,
Pennsylvania
210: Thoracentesis

Angela C. Mix, DO
Assistant Professor of Pediatrics, University of Texas
Southwestern Medical School; Pediatric Hospitalist,
Children's Medical Center of Dallas and Parkland
Memorial Hospital, Dallas, Texas
63: Central Nervous System Infections

Debra Monzack, BS(ED)
Child Life Council, Lucile Packard Children's Hospital,
Palo Alto, California
9: The Approach to the Hospitalized Child and Family

Kimberly D. Morel, MD
Assistant Professor of Clinical Dermatology and
Clinical Pediatrics, Columbia University College of
Physicians and Surgeons; Active Staff, Morgan Stanley
Children's Hospital of New York–Presbyterian, New York,
New York
157: Staphylococcal Scalded Skin Syndrome

Douglas E. Moses, MD
Assistant Professor of Clinical Pediatrics, Northeastern
Ohio Universities College of Medicine, Rootstown; Staff,
Diagnostic Referral Service, Akron Children's Hospital,
Akron, Ohio
160: Erythema Multiforme

Eugene M. Mowad, MD
Assistant Professor of Clinical Pediatrics, Northeastern
Ohio Universities College of Medicine, Rootstown;
Pediatric Hospitalist, Akron Children's Hospital, Akron,
Ohio
82: Electrocardiogram Interpretation

Elizabeth A. Mullen, MD
Instructor of Medicine, Harvard Medical School; Clinician,
Department of Pediatric Oncology, Dana Farber Cancer
Institute, Boston, Massachusetts
122, 124: Oncologic Emergencies; Common
Complications of Chemotherapy and Radiation: Mucositis
and Febrile Neutropenia

John B. Mulliken, MD
Professor of Surgery, Harvard Medical School;
Director, Craniofacial Center; Co-Director, Vascular
Anomalies Center, Children's Hospital Boston, Boston,
Massachusetts
153: Vascular Anomalies

Sharon Muret-Wagstaff, PhD, MPA
Assistant Professor of Pediatrics, Harvard Medical School;
Associate Director, Harvard Pediatric Health Services
Research Fellowship Program, Children's Hospital Boston,
Boston, Massachusetts
4: Quality of Care and Patient Satisfaction

Nancy Murphy, MD, FAAP, FAAPMR
Assistant Professor of Pediatrics, University of
Utah School of Medicine; Pediatric Physiatrist,
Department of Pediatrics and Physical Medicine and
Rehabilitation, Primary Children's Medical Center;
Medical Director, Pediatric Home Care, Pediatric
Home and Hospice Services, Intermountain Healthcare
Home Care, Salt Lake City; Medical Director,
Pediatric Services, Pediatric Transitional Care
Program, South Davis Community Hospital, Bountiful,
Utah
193, 194: Acute Care of the Medically Complex Child;
Common Reasons for Admission

Frances M. Nadel, MD, MSCE
Assistant Professor of Pediatrics, University of
Pennsylvania School of Medicine; Attending
Physician, Division of Emergency Medicine, The
Children's Hospital of Philadelphia, Philadelphia,
Pennsylvania
187, 204: Near Drowning; Central Venous Access

Joshua Nagler, MD
Instructor in Pediatrics, Harvard Medical School; Staff
Physician in Pediatric Emergency Medicine, Children's
Hospital Boston, Boston, Massachusetts
147: Pneumothorax and Pneumomediastinum

James A. Nard, MD
Associate Professor of Clinical Pediatrics, Northeastern Ohio Universities College of Medicine, Rootstown; Director, Diagnostic Referral Service, Akron Children's Hospital, Akron, Ohio
106: Postinfectious Arthritis

Mark I. Neuman, MD, MPH
Instructor in Pediatrics, Harvard Medical School; Assistant in Medicine, Division of Emergency Medicine, Children's Hospital Boston, Boston, Massachusetts
76: Aspiration

Jason G. Newland, MD
Assistant Professor of Pediatrics, University of Missouri–Kansas City Medical School; Attending Physician, Section of Infectious Diseases, Children's Mercy Hospital, Kansas City, Missouri
66: Middle Respiratory Tract Infections and Bronchiolitis

Alice W. Newton, MD
Instructor in Pediatrics, Harvard Medical School; Medical Director, Child Protection Team, Children's Hospital Boston, and Medical Director, Child Protection Team, Massachusetts General Hospital, Boston, Massachusetts
173: Inflicted Traumatic Brain Injury

Peter F. Nichol, MD, PhD
Assistant Professor of Surgery and Clinician Scholar, University of Utah School of Medicine; Active Staff and Pediatric Surgeon, Primary Children's Medical Center, University of Utah Hospital and Clinics, Salt Lake City, Utah
140: Hernias

Lise E. Nigrovic, MD, MPH
Instructor in Pediatrics, Harvard Medical School; Assistant in Medicine, Children's Hospital Boston, Boston, Massachusetts
185: Heat Disorders

Richard J. Noel, MD, PhD
Assistant Professor of Pediatrics, Medical College of Wisconsin; Staff, Children's Hospital of Wisconsin, Milwaukee, Wisconsin
96: Disorders of Gastric Emptying

Sharon E. Oberfield, MD
Professor of Pediatrics, Columbia University; Director, Endocrinology, Diabetes, and Metabolism, Morgan Stanley Children's Hospital; Division of Pediatric Endocrinology, Children's Hospital of New York–Presbyterian, New York, New York
88, 90, 91, 92: Diabetes Mellitus and Hyperglycemia; Disorders of Pituitary Function; Disorders of Calcium Metabolism; Disorders of the Adrenal Gland

Maureen M. O'Brien, MD
Fellow, Pediatric Hematology and Oncology, Stanford School of Medicine, Lucile Packard Children's Hospital, Palo Alto, California
124: Common Complications of Chemotherapy and Radiation: Mucositis and Febrile Neutropenia

Karen J. O'Connell, MD
Assistant Professor of Pediatrics, George Washington University School of Medicine and Health Sciences; Attending Physician, Pediatric Emergency Medicine, Emergency Medicine and Trauna Center, Children's National Medical Center, Washington, DC
184, 211: Fire-Related Inhalation Injury; Paracentesis

Kevin C. Osterhoudt, MD, MSCE, FAAP, FACMT
Associate Professor of Pediatrics, University of Pennsylvania School of Medicine; Medical Director, The Poison Control Center, Section of Medical Toxicology, Division of Emergency Medicine, The Children's Hospital of Philadelphia, Philadelphia, Pennsylvania
178, 189: Stabilization and Hospitalization of the Poisoned Child; Envenomation

Mary Ottolini, MD, MPH
Professor of Pediatrics and Director, Pediatric Medical Student Education, George Washington University School of Medicine and Health Sciences; Hospitalist Division Chief, Children's National Medical Center, Washington, DC
22, 58: Medical Education; Fluid and Electrolyte Therapy

Raj Padman, MD
Clinical Associate Professor of Pediatrics, Jefferson Medical College of Thomas Jefferson University, Philadelphia, Pennsylvania; Chief, Division of Pulmonary Medicine, and Director, Cystic Fibrosis Program, Alfred I. duPont Hospital for Children, Wilmington, Delaware
209: Noninvasive Positive-Pressure Ventilation

Horacio M. Padua, MD
Instructor in Radiology, Harvard Medical School; Diagnostic and Interventional Radiologist, Children's Hospital Boston, Boston, Massachusetts
198: Radiology for the Pediatric Hospitalist

Alka Patel, MD, PhD
Physician, Veterans Affairs Hospital, Mather, California
9: The Approach to the Hospitalized Child and Family

Susmita Pati, MD, MPH
Assistant Professor of Pediatrics, University of Pennsylvania School of Medicine; Attending Physician, General Pediatrics, The Children's Hospital of Philadelphia, Philadelphia, Pennsylvania
10: Hospitalist as Patient Advocate

Jack M. Percelay, MD, MPH, FAAP
Director, Virtua Inpatient Pediatrics, and Chair, AAP Section on Hospital Care, Virtua Health Systems, Ridgewood, New Jersey
23: Pediatric Hospital Medicine Organizations

Jeannette M. Perez-Rossello, MD
Radiology Department, Children's Hospital Boston, Boston, Massachusetts
174: Imaging of Child Abuse

Kieran J. Phelan, MD, MSc
Assistant Professor of Pediatrics, University of Cincinnati
College of Medicine; Staff, Divisions of Health Policy and
Clinical Effectiveness and General and Community
Pediatrics, Department of Pediatrics, Cincinnati Children's
Hospital Medical Center, Cincinnati, Ohio
8: Clinical Practice Guidelines

Annapurna Poduri, MD
Instructor, Department of Neurology, Harvard Medical
School; Assistant in Neurology, Department of Neurology,
Children's Hospital Boston, Boston, Massachusetts
126, 127: Seizures; Headache

J. Rainer Poley, MD
Pediatric Gastroenterologist, Pitt County Memorial
Hospital, University Health Systems of Eastern Carolina,
Greenville, North Carolina
100: Pancreatitis

Jill C. Posner, MD, MSCE
Assistant Professor of Pediatrics, University of
Pennsylvania School of Medicine; Attending Physician,
Division of Pediatric Emergency Medicine, The
Children's Hospital of Philadelphia, Philadelphia,
Pennsylvania
206, 213, 214: Phlebotomy; CSF Shunt Assessment;
CSF Shunt Puncture

Sampath Prahalad, MD, MSc
Assistant Professor of Pediatrics, Division of Pediatric
Rheumatology and Immunology, University of Utah
School of Medicine, Salt Lake City, Utah
105: Juvenile Idiopathic Arthritis

Howard B. Pride, MD
Associate, Department of Dermatology, Geisinger Medical
Center, Danville, Pennsylvania
156: Cellulitis and Erysipelas

Daniel Rauch, MD
Associate Professor of Pediatrics and Director, Pediatric
Hospitalist Program, New York University School of
Medicine, New York, New York
17, 23, 25: Communication and Discharge Planning;
Pediatric Hospital Medicine Organizations; Abdominal
Mass

David J. Rawat, MD
Harvard Medical School; Children's Hospital Boston,
Boston, Massachusetts
95: Dyspepsia

Scott Reeves, MD
Assistant Professor of Clinical Pediatrics, University of
Cincinnati College of Medicine; Attending Physician,
Division of Emergency Medicine, Cincinnati Children's
Hospital Medical Center, Cincinnati, Ohio
8: Clinical Practice Guidelines

Daniel H. Reirden, MD
Instructor of Pediatrics, University of Pennsylvania School
of Medicine; Attending Physician, Craig-Dalsimer Division
of Adolescent Medicine, The Children's Hospital of
Philadelphia, Philadelphia, Pennsylvania
170: Eating Disorders

Brandie J. Roberts, MD
Assistant Clinical Professor of Pediatrics and Medicine
(Dermatology), University of California, San Diego, School
of Medicine; Attending, Children's Hospital of San Diego,
San Diego, California
149: Lumps and Bumps: Benign and Malignant Tumors

Jack Rodgers, MDiv, DMin
Chaplain Coordinator, Chaplaincy Service of Department
of Social Work and Family Services, The Children's
Hospital of Philadelphia, Philadelphia, Pennsylvania
11: Spiritual Care

José R. Romero, MD
Professor of Pediatrics, Pathology, and Microbiology,
University of Nebraska College of Medicine; Director,
Section of Pediatric Infectious Disease, University of
Nebraska Medical Center, Omaha, Nebraska
63: Central Nervous System Infections

Paul Rosen, MD, MPH, MMM
Assistant Professor of Pediatrics, University of Pittsburgh
School of Medicine; Clinical Director, Division of
Rheumatology, Children's Hospital of Pittsburgh,
Pittsburgh, Pennsylvania
103: Henoch-Schönlein Purpura

David M. Rubin, MD, MSCE
Assistant Professor, Department of Pediatrics, and Pediatric
Clerkship Director, University of Pennsylvania School of
Medicine; Director of Research and Policy, Safe Place:
Center for Child Protection and Health, The Children's
Hospital of Philadelphia, Philadelphia, Pennsylvania
22: Medical Education

Esther Maria Sampayo, MD
Clinical Instructor, University of Pennsylvania School of
Medicine; Fellow, The Children's Hospital of Philadelphia,
Philadelphia, Pennsylvania
201: Arterial Blood Gas

Lisa Samson-Fang, MD
Associate Professor, Department of Pediatrics, University
of Utah School of Medicine; Attending, Department of
Pediatrics, University of Utah Hospital, Salt Lake City,
Utah
193: Acute Care of the Medically Complex Child

Gina Santucci, MSN
Nurse Coordinator, The Pediatric Advanced Care Team,
The Children's Hospital of Philadelphia, Philadelphia,
Pennsylvania
12: Palliative, End-of-Life, and Bereavement Care

Julie V. Schaffer, MD
Assistant Professor of Dematology and Pediatrics, New
York University Medical Center; Director of Pediatric
Dermatology, Tisch Hospital and Bellevue Hospital Center,
New York, New York
158: Ecthyma Gangrenosum

Karen E. Schetzina, MD, MPH
Assistant Professor of Pediatrics, East Tennessee State
University James H. Quillen College of Medicine, Johnson
City, Tennessee
39: Irritability and Intractable Crying

Sandra Schwab, MD
Clinical Instructor, Pediatrics, University of Pennsylvania School of Medicine; Fellow, Pediatric Emergency Medicine, The Children's Hospital of Philadelphia, Philadelphia, Pennsylvania
200: Bladder Catheterization

Donald F. Schwarz, MD, MPH
Associate Professor of Pediatrics, University of Pennsylvania School of Medicine; Vice-Chairman and Chief, Craig-Dalsimer Division of Adolescent Medicine, The Children's Hospital of Philadelphia, Philadelphia, Pennsylvania
170, 172: Eating Disorders; Dysfunctional Uterine Bleeding

Jordan Scott, MD
Clinical Instructor, Allergy/Immunology, Harvard Medical School; Active Staff, Children's Hospital Boston, Boston; Active Staff, UMass Memorial/Health Alliance Leominster Campus, Leominster, Massachusetts
135: Drug Allergy

Steven M. Selbst, MD
Professor of Pediatrics, Jefferson Medical College of Thomas Jefferson University, Philadelphia, Pennsylvania; Vice-Chair for Education and Pediatric Residency Program Director, Alfred I. duPont Hospital for Children, Wilmington, Delaware
19: Medicolegal Issues

Kara N. Shah, MD, PhD
Pediatric Dermatology Fellow, University of Pennsylvania School of Medicine/The Children's Hospital of Philadelphia, Philadelphia, Pennsylvania
163: Epidermolysis Bullosa

Samir S. Shah, MD
Assistant Professor of Pediatrics and Epidemiology, University of Pennsylvania School of Medicine; Attending Physician, Divisions of Infectious Diseases and General Pediatrics, The Children's Hospital of Philadelphia, Philadelphia, Pennsylvania
59, 60, 61, 64, 66, 71: Empirical Treatment of Bacterial Infections; Fever; Prolonged Fever and Fever of Unknown Origin; Complications of Acute Otitis Media and Sinusitis; Middle Respiratory Tract Infections and Bronchiolitis; Device-Related Infections

Nader Shaikh, MD
Assistant Professor of Pediatrics, University of Pittsburgh School of Medicine; Attending, Children's Hospital of Pittsburgh, Pittsburgh, Pennsylvania
69: Urinary Tract Infections in Childhood

Michael W. Shannon, MD, MPH
Professor of Pediatrics, Harvard Medical School; Chief, Division of Emergency Medicine; Associate Director, The Pediatric Environmental Health Center, Children's Hospital Boston, Boston, Massachusetts
181: Lead, Other Metals, and Chelation Therapy

Adhi N. Sharma, MD
Associate Professor, New York College of Osteopathic Medicine, Old Westbury; Chairman, Department of Emergency Medicine, Good Samaritan Hospital Medical Center, West Islip, New York
183: Withdrawal Syndromes

George K. Siberry, MD, MPH
Assistant Professor of Pediatrics, Johns Hopkins University School of Medicine; Medical Director, Harriet Lane Clinic, Johns Hopkins Hospital, Baltimore, Maryland
68: Gastrointestinal Diseases

Karen Smith, MD, MA
Assistant Professor of Pediatrics, George Washington University School of Medicine and Health Sciences; Chief Medical Officer, HSC Pediatric Center; Pediatric Hospitalist, Children's National Medical Center, Washington, DC
131: Hyperammonemia

Michael J. Smith, MD
Instructor, Department of Pediatrics, University of Pennsylvania School of Medicine; Fellow, Division of Infectious Diseases, The Children's Hospital of Philadelphia, Philadelphia, Pennsylvania
71: Device-Related Infections

Michael J. G. Somers, MD
Assistant Professor of Pediatrics, Harvard Medical School; Director of Clinical Services, Division of Nephrology, Children's Hospital Boston, Boston, Massachusetts
35: Hypertension

Neal Sondheimer, MD, PhD
Instructor in Pediatrics, University of Pennsylvania School of Medicine; Attending Physician; Section of Biochemical Genetics, The Children's Hospital of Philadelphia, Philadephia, Pennsylvania
132: Hypoglycemia

Steven J. Spalding, MD
Senior Fellow, Children's Hospital of Pittsburgh, Pittsburgh, Pennsylvania
103: Henoch-Schönlein Purpura

Philip R. Spandorfer, MD, MSCE
Pediatric Emergency Medicine Attending Physician, Children's Healthcare of Atlanta at Scottish Rite, Atlanta, Georgia
57, 202: Dehydration; Peripheral Intravenous Access

Jonathan M. Spergel, MD, PhD
Associate Professor of Pediatrics and Allergy and Immunology, University of Pennsylvania School of Medicine; Assistant Physician and Chief, Allergy Section, and Director, Food Allergy Center and Center for Pediatric Eosinophilic Disorders, The Children's Hospital of Philadelphia, Philadelphia, Pennsylvania
75, 155: Asthma; Atopic Dermatitis

Jeffrey L. Sperring, MD
Assistant Professor of Clinical Pediatrics, Indiana University School of Medicine; Director, Pediatric Hospitalist Program, Riley Hospital for Children, Indianapolis, Indiana
65: Neck and Oral Cavity Infections

David A. Spiegel, MD
Assistant Professor of Orthopedic Surgery, University of Pennsylvania School of Medicine; Attending Surgeon, The Children's Hospital of Philadelphia, Philadelphia, Pennsylvania
145: Orthopedics

Rajendu Srivastava, MD, FRCP(C), MPH
Assistant Professor, Division of Pediatric Inpatient Medicine, Department of Pediatrics, University of Health Sciences Center; Staff Hospitalist, Primary Children's Medical Center, Institute for Healthcare Delivery and Research, Intermountain Healthcare, Salt Lake City, Utah
2, 194: Pediatric Hospitalists: Efficiency and Quality of Care; Common Reasons for Admission

Keith H. St. John, MT(ASCP), MS
Director, Infection Prevention and Control and Occupational Health, The Children's Hospital of Philadelphia, Philadelphia, Pennsylvania
6: Infection Control for Pediatric Hospitalists

Michael C. Stephens, MD
Assistant Professor of Pediatrics, Medical College of Wisconsin; Attending Pediatrician, Children's Hospital of Wisconsin, Milwaukee, Wisconsin
98: Inflammatory Bowel Disease

Christopher C. Stewart, MD
Assistant Professor of Pediatrics, University of California, San Francisco, School of Medicine; Director of Inpatient Pediatrics, San Francisco General Hospital, San Francisco, California
143: Neurosurgical Issues

Bryan L. Stone, MD
Assistant Professor, Department of Pediatrics, University of Utah School of Medicine; Inpatient Medicine, Primary Children's Medical Center, Salt Lake City, Utah
38: Hypoxemia

Erin R. Stucky, MD
Clinical Professor, Department of Pediatrics, University of California, San Diego, School of Medicine; Physician Advisor for Quality Management, Director of Graduate Medical Education, and Pediatric Hospitalist, Rady Children's Hospital, San Diego, California
14: Medical Comanagement and Consultation

Eric R. Sundel, MD
Chairman of Pediatrics and Director, Pediatric Hospitalist Program, BaltimoreWashington Medical Center, Glen Burnie, Maryland
139: Abdominal Pain and Acute Abdomen

Robert Sundel, MD
Associate Professor of Pediatrics, Harvard Medical School; Program Director, Department of Rheumatology, Division of Immunology, Children's Hospital Boston, Boston, Massachusetts
40: Limp

Suzanne Swanson, MD
Clincal Assistant Professor, Stanford University School of Medicine, Stanford; Pediatric Hospitalist, Santa Clara Valley Medical Center, San Jose, California
42: Oral Lesions

Lesli Taylor, MD
Professor of Pediatric Surgery, East Tennessee State University James H. Quillen College of Medicine, Johnson City, Tennessee
138: Gastrointestinal Obstruction: Pyloric Stenosis, Malrotation and Volvulus, and Intussusception

E. Douglas Thompson, MD
Assistant Professor of Pediatrics, Drexel University College of Medicine; Director, Pediatric Generalist Service; Member, Section of General Pediatrics, St. Christopher's Hospital for Children, Philadelphia, Pennsylvania
62: Fever and Rash

Avram Z. Traum, MD
Instructor in Pediatrics, Harvard Medical School; Pediatric Nephrology Unit, Massachusetts General Hospital, Boston, Massachusetts
35: Hypertension

Harsh K. Trivedi, MD
Clinical Assistant Professor of Psychiatry, Brown Medical School, Providence; Attending Psychiatrist, Adolescent Program/Safe Quest, Bradley Hospital, East Providence, Rhode Island
165: Depression and Physical Illness

Bryan D. Upham, MD
Instructor of Pediatrics, University of Pennsylvania School of Medicine; Fellow, Department of Emergency Medicine, The Children's Hospital of Philadelphia, Philadelphia, Pennsylvania
205: Umbilical Artery and Vein Catheterization

Andrea M. Vandeven, MD, MPH
Instructor in Pediatrics, Harvard Medical School; Assistant in Medicine and Medical Director, Child Protection Program, Children's Hospital Boston, Boston, Massachusetts
176: Munchausen by Proxy

Brigid L. Vaughan, MD
Assistant Professor of Psychiatry, Harvard Medical School; Senior Associate in Psychiatry and Medical Director, Psychopharmacology Program, Children's Hospital Boston, Boston, Massachusetts
169: New-Onset Psychosis

Charles P. Venditti, MD, PhD
Genetic Disease Research Branch, National Human Genome Research Institute, National Institutes of Health, Bethesda, Maryland
133: Metabolic Acidosis

Venus M. Villalva, MD
Adjunct Faculty, University of Utah School of Medicine; Active Staff, Primary Children's Medical Center, Salt Lake City, Utah
34: Gastrointestinal Bleeding

Robert N. Vincent, MD, CM
Professor of Pediatrics, Emory University School of
Medicine; Director, Cardiac Catheterization Laboratory,
and Medical Co-Director, Pediatric Heart Transplantation,
Children's Healthcare of Atlanta, Atlanta, Georgia
85: Myocarditis and Cardiomyopathy

Samuel Volchenboum, MD, PhD
Instructor in Pediatrics (Hematology/Oncology), Harvard
Medical School; Attending Physician, Dana Farber Cancer
Institute, Children's Hospital Boston, Boston,
Massachusetts
119: Thrombocytopenia

Michael T. Vossmeyer, MD
Assistant Professor of Clinical Pediatrics, University of
Cincinnati College of Medicine; Medical Director,
Generalist Inpatient Service, Cincinnati Children's Hospital
Medical Center, Cincinnati, Ohio
9: The Approach to the Hospitalized Child and Family

Robert M. Wachter, MD
Professor and Associate Chairman of Medicine, University
of California, San Francisco, School of Medicine; Chief,
Medical Service, UCSF Medical Center, San Francisco,
California
1: What Is a Hospitalist?

Daniel J. Weiner, MD
Assistant Professor of Pediatrics, University of Pittsburgh
School of Medicine; Attending Physician, Division of
Pulmonary Medicine; Associate Director, Antonio J. and
Janet Palumbo Cystic Fibrosis Center; Medical Director,
Pulmonary Function Laboratory, Children's Hospital of
Pittsburgh, Pittsburgh, Pennsylvania
80: Pulmonary Function Testing

Michael Weinstein, MD
Assistant Professor of Pediatrics, University of Toronto
Faculty of Medicine; Director, Paediatric Medicine
Inpatient Unit, The Hospital for Sick Children, Toronto,
Ontario, Canada
67: Lower Respiratory Tract Infections

Elizabeth A. Wharff, MSW, PhD
Instructor, Harvard Medical School; Director, Emergency
Psychiatry Service; Co-Director, Outpatient
Psychiatry Service, Children's Hospital Boston, Boston,
Massachusetts
166: Assessment and Management of Suicidal Patients

Stephen D. Wilson, MD, PhD
Associate Clinical Professor of Pediatrics, University of
California, San Francisco, School of Medicine; Director,
Pediatric Hospitalist Program, UCSF Children's Hospital,
San Francisco, California
32: Failure to Thrive

Jerry A. Winkelstein, MD
Professor of Pediatrics, Medicine, and Pathology, Johns
Hopkins University School of Medicine, Baltimore,
Maryland
136: Primary Immunodeficiency Diseases

Heidi Wolf, MD, FAAP
Johns Hopkins University School of Medicine; Director,
Pediatric Hospitalist Program, Johns Hopkins Hospital,
Baltimore, Maryland
128: Hypotonia and Weakness

George A. Woodward, MD, MBA
Professor of Pediatrics, University of Washington School of
Medicine; Chief, Division of Pediatric Emergency
Medicine, and Director, Emergency Services, Children's
Hospital and Regional Medical Center, Seattle, Washington
15: Transport Medicine

Albert C. Yan, MD
Assistant Professor of Pediatrics and Dermatology,
University of Pennsylvania School of Medicine; Chief,
Section of Pediatric Dermatology, The Children's Hospital
of Philadelphia, Philadelphia, Pennsylvania
154, 155, 163: Head Lice and Scabies; Atopic Dermatitis;
Epidermolysis Bullosa

Elaine H. Zackai, MD
Professor of Pediatrics, University of Pennsylvania School
of Medicine; Director of Clinical Genetics, The Children's
Hospital of Philadelphia, Philadelphia, Pennsylvania
130: Genetic Syndromes Caused by Chromosomal
Abnormalities

Andrea L. Zaenglein, MD
Assistant Professor of Dermatology and Pediatrics, Penn
State School of Medicine/Milton S. Hershey Medical
Center, Hershey, Pennsylvania
151: Vesicles and Bullae

Theoklis E. Zaoutis, MD
Assistant Professor of Pediatrics and Epidemiology,
University of Pennsylvania School of Medicine;
Attending Physician, Division of Infectious Diseases, The
Children's Hospital of Philadelphia, Philadelphia,
Pennsylvania
71: Device-Related Infections

David Zipes, MD
Director, Pediatric Hospitalist Program, and Director,
General Pediatric Unit, St. Vincent Children's Hospital,
Indianapolis, Indiana
3, 17, 23: Hospitalist Models of Care: Organization and
Compensation; Communication and Discharge Planning;
Pediatric Hospital Medicine Organizations

Preface

Pediatric hospital medicine is a dynamic and rapidly growing field. Attempts to define it are fraught with errors of perspective because it is so many things to so many different people. Yogi Berra is credited with saying "It is hard to make predictions, especially about the future." And so it is with pediatric hospital medicine. The term "hospitalist" itself was only coined just over 10 years ago by Doctors Wachter and Goldman. While we hope they will be pleased with our current effort to capture the field to date, it would not be surprising if 10 years from now the field will have evolved dramatically.

However, we are confident that future editions of this textbook will be able to capture these adaptive changes. We feel this way not because of *what* this book represents, but *who* this book represents. There are close to 300 contributing authors from up to 50 different institutions. Large and small children's hospitals, pediatric departments in academic medical centers, community hospitals, private practice, and everything in between are represented in this book. What brings this group of talented individuals together is their desire to provide the very best care for the infant, child, or adolescent in need of hospital care. As a result, we truly believe we have our collective fingers on the pulse of pediatric hospital medicine. In this way we hope this book serves as a resource to all those who are involved with hospital care of pediatric patients.

We would like to thank all of the individuals involved with this text for their valued contributions to this first edition. We would also like to recognize the fine efforts of our associate editors, Allison, Chris, and Laura. The folks at Elsevier have been so helpful throughout the process of publication for this textbook. Judy Fletcher, our Publishing Director at Elsevier, has been particularly supportive from the start. She has shown remarkable foresight in recognizing the growing field and the potential role for this textbook in pediatric hospital medicine.

Lisa B. Zaoutis, MD
Vincent W. Chiang, MD

Contents

PART I

General Issues of Inpatient Pediatric Medicine

CHAPTER *1*

What Is a Hospitalist?

Robert M. Wachter

Although hospital care has long been provided by specialists in inpatient medicine in Europe and Canada, the United States has only recently begun using dedicated inpatient physicians to care for hospitalized patients. There were rare examples of such specialists scattered across the country in the 1980s and early 1990s, but interest in the hospitalist model has accelerated in the past few years. In 1995 there were only a handful of hospitalists in the United States, whereas by 2006 there were about 15,000, a number projected to more than double in the coming decade.[1] The Society of Hospital Medicine, the professional association representing hospitalists, now has more than 6000 members.[2]

DEFINITIONS OF "HOSPITALIST"

In a 1996 article in the *New England Journal of Medicine*, Wachter and Goldman coined the term *hospitalist* and introduced the concept to the medical literature.[3] A few years later, I proposed a definition of hospitalists: "physicians who spend at least 25% of their professional time serving as the physicians-of-record for inpatients, during which time they accept 'hand-offs' of hospitalized patients from primary care providers, returning the patients back to the care of their primary care providers at the time of hospital discharge."[4] This definition has two key elements. The first is the handoff—a built-in and purposeful discontinuity in care between outpatient and inpatient providers. This discontinuity is responsible for one of the great strengths of the hospitalist model—the presence of a full-time physician in the hospital throughout the day who is able to coordinate inpatient care and react to clinical data in real time. However, this same discontinuity also leads to the two greatest potential liabilities of the hospitalist model: (1) loss of information (termed *voltage drop*) when moving from office to hospital ward and back to office again, and (2) potential patient dissatisfaction caused by the assignment of a new physician who is often a stranger. Studies have shown that although discontinuity remains a concern (and the subject of significant mitigating efforts by most hospitalists), patient dissatisfaction generally is not a major problem.[5]

The second key element in the definition is a temporal floor, here specified as at least 25% of time spent in the hospital. This minimum commitment allows the hospitalist to become expert in the care of common inpatient disorders, to recognize outliers and anticipate problems, to become familiar with all the key players in the hospital (e.g., medical and surgical consultants, discharge planners, nurses, clergy), to lead quality improvement efforts in this setting, and to become sufficiently invested in the hospital system to be accountable for its cost and quality.

In practice, the vast majority of community hospital–based hospitalists spend all their time caring for inpatients. The notion of a clinical hospitalist spending less than 100% of his or her time in the hospital is important, particularly in some academic programs, where many hospitalists combine clinical medicine with teaching and research. The Society of Hospital Medicine, in an attempt to capture the fact that some hospitalists mix clinical work with other inpatient-oriented activities, proposed the following definition: "Hospitalists are doctors whose primary professional focus is the general medical care of hospitalized patients. Their activities may include patient care, teaching, research, and leadership related to hospital care."[6]

Under either definition, a hospitalist is conceptually a site-defined generalist specialist: a specialist in the care of a wide array of diseases and organ system derangements in a given site of care (the hospital). This model distinguishes the hospitalist from organ-based specialists (e.g., cardiologists, nephrologists), disease-based specialists (oncologists), population-based specialists (pediatricians, geriatricians), or procedure-based specialists (electrophysiologists, radiologists). The hospitalist model is most akin to emergency medicine and critical care medicine, two site-based specialties that have emerged since the 1960s, when those venues became complex enough to require a constant physician presence, orchestration of care across multiple disciplines, and the acquisition of a discrete skill set and knowledge base.

UNIQUE SKILL SET OF HOSPITALISTS

One of the challenges faced by any generalist specialty is to define a unique skill set. Because so much of what hospitalists do involves coordination and overlap with other existing specialties, this undertaking is complex. Nevertheless, defining the skill set is crucial to delineating a core curriculum for the specialty, as well as the content of any postgraduate training programs, and ultimately the grounds for board certification and credentialing. A glance at the table of contents of this book or any other hospitalist book[7] demonstrates the editors' attempts to define the core knowledge base for the field. In this book, for example, one sees a mixture of traditional, disease-based chapters (e.g., asthma, inflammatory bowel disease), each described from an inpatient perspective; chapters based on signs and symptoms (e.g., headache, abdominal mass); and a distinctive array of systems-oriented (e.g., patient safety) and coordinative (e.g., transport) chapters. This breadth captures many of the issues inherent in defining a core skill set and some of the distinctiveness of the new field of hospital medicine. In many ways, the unique attributes of a hospitalist pertain to the fact that he or she is responsible for coordinating the care of individual patients in the hospital, managing the many complex transitions of such patients (both entering and leaving the hospital, as well as within the hospital itself), and helping to improve hospital systems of care.

To help define this skill set, in a 2001 survey we asked 389 hospitalists what they had learned in their training (most hospitalists in the sample dealt with adult patients, so their training was largely internal medicine) and what was most important in their daily practice (Table 1-1).[8] Interestingly, hospitalists felt that clinical skills (e.g., managing heart failure, inserting central lines, interpreting electrocardiograms) were very important and had been well taught during their training. Conversely, they cited major educational deficits in communication skills, end-of-life care, quality improvement and patient safety, medical economics, care of surgical patients, and postacute care. These topics are likely to form the core of future hospitalist curricula for both trainees and practicing physicians.

It is worth emphasizing the hospitalist's role in systems leadership. The emergence of the hospitalist movement coincided with an increasing appreciation of the importance of systems thinking in improving health care quality and efficiency. Hospitalists are well positioned to be natural leaders in this effort: they tend to be comfortable with interdisciplinary work and collaboration, are well versed in clinical computing, and, because their programs often receive financial support from their employer-institutions, are uniquely motivated to demonstrate their new field's value. It is no coincidence that hospitalists have already demonstrated leadership in several quality and safety arenas and are likely to continue to do so over the coming years.[9-11] The centrality of health services research and systems improvement efforts to the hospitalist field also argues for additional training in research methods, quality improvement, information technology, change management, and business skills.

NEW AREAS FOR HOSPITALISTS

Although the early years of hospital medicine saw hospitalists practicing mostly adult (and later pediatric) inpatient medicine, recent years have seen growth in new areas. For example, many hospitalists are taking increasingly active roles in managing the medical problems of surgical patients, moving from providing consultative advice to participating in true comanagement models. The degree to which such arrangements may improve quality or efficiency is not yet known, but I expect them to be major growth areas.

In adult medicine, many hospitalists follow patients into intensive care units (ICUs), either managing or comanaging (with intensivists) patients there. These models have some theoretical appeal, in that they may obviate the ICU-to-ward discontinuity and relieve some of the time pressure on intensivists (important because of a national shortage of these practitioners). Conversely, these models also raise questions regarding hospitalists' qualifications to manage ICU patients (particularly when compared with trained and certified intensivists). Here, too, there are few data to inform this debate, but many institutions, including my own, have found that collaborative intensivist-hospitalist models work quite well.[5]

Because of the limitations imposed on residents' on-duty hours in July 2003 by the Accreditation Council for Graduate Medical Education, services in teaching hospitals that were previously covered entirely by house officers now require increased hospital staffing. Hospitalists are stepping into this breach, creating nonteaching services and often supervising nonphysician providers. In addition, hospitalists are rapidly becoming the major teachers of inpatient medicine—both adult and pediatric—and new data suggest that such models are associated with improved education.[12,13]

However, the main impetus for the growth of hospitalist models is more traditional: research clearly demonstrates that hospitalists can improve the efficiency of inpatient care without compromising—and perhaps even improving—the quality of care.[5] Although most of these data have been generated by adult hospitalist programs, the findings appear to apply to pediatrics as well,[14,15] which may explain why the

Table 1-1   Mismatch between Hospitalists' Training and Practice Needs

Domain	Importance to Practice*	Emphasis in Residency Training*
Clinical skills (e.g., management of common diseases, performance of common procedures)	4.5	4.2
Health economics	4.0	2.1[†]
Quality assurance and quality improvement	4.1	2.1[†]
Subacute care	4.3	2.2[†]
Palliative care	4.5	3.2[†]
Communication skills	4.9	3.6[†]

*Scale for both measures is 1 to 5, where 5 is "very important" or "very adequate" and 1 is "very unimportant" or "very inadequate."
[†]*P* < .001.
From Plauth WH, Pantilat SZ, Wachter RM, Fenton CL: Hospitalists' perceptions of their residency training needs: Results of a national survey. Am J Med 2001;111:247-254.

model is growing so rapidly in children's services around the United States.

CONCLUSION

The emergence of the hospitalist model as the dominant organizational model for inpatient care has occurred with astonishing speed and has been accompanied—to a reassuring and unusual degree—by data indicating that the model improves the value (quality divided by cost) of inpatient care. One of the exciting attributes of this new field is its dynamism. "What is a hospitalist?" is a relatively easy question to answer today, but this definition is likely to change over time as new problems and challenges emerge and as hospitalists evolve to meet them. Defining a hospitalist may ultimately be as simple—and as complex—as saying that a hospitalist is a generalist physician focused on providing high-quality care and solving important clinical and systems problems in the inpatient setting.

REFERENCES

1. Lurie JD, Miller DP, Lindenauer PK, et al: The potential size of the hospitalist workforce in the United States. Am J Med 1999;106:441-445.
2. Wachter RM: Hospitalists in the United States—mission accomplished or work in progress? N Engl J Med 2004;350:1935-1936.
3. Wachter RM, Goldman L: The emerging role of "hospitalists" in the American health care system. N Engl J Med 1996;335:514-517.
4. Wachter RM: An introduction to the hospitalist model. Ann Intern Med 1999;130:338-342.
5. Wachter RM, Goldman L: The hospitalist movement 5 years later. JAMA 2002;287:487-494.
6. Society of Hospital Medicine website: available at *http://www.hospitalmedicine.org*
7. Wachter RM, Goldman L, Hollander H (eds): Hospital Medicine, 2nd ed. Philadelphia, Lippincott, Williams & Wilkins, 2005.
8. Plauth WH, Pantilat SZ, Wachter RM, Fenton CL: Hospitalists' perceptions of their residency training needs: Results of a national survey. Am J Med 2001;111:247-254.
9. Wachter RM, Shojania KG: Internal Bleeding: The Truth behind America's Terrifying Epidemic of Medical Mistakes. New York, Rugged Land, 2004.
10. Shojania KG, Duncan BW, McDonald KM, Wachter RM (eds): Making Health Care Safer: A Critical Analysis of Patient Safety Practices (AHRQ Publication No. 01-E058; Evidence Report/Technology Assessment No. 43). Rockville, Md, Agency for Healthcare Research and Quality; 2001, pp 111-116.
11. Fortescue EB, Kaushal R, Landrigan CP, et al: Prioritizing strategies for preventing medication errors and adverse drug events in pediatric inpatients. Pediatrics 2003;111:722-729.
12. Kripalani S, Pope AC, Rask K, et al: Hospitalists as teachers. J Gen Intern Med 2004;19:8-15.
13. Hunter AJ, Desai SS, Harrison RA, Chan BK: Medical student evaluation of the quality of hospitalist and nonhospitalist teaching faculty on inpatient medicine rotations. Acad Med 2004;79:78-82.
14. Tenner PA, Dibrell H, Taylor RP: Improved survival with hospitalists in a pediatric intensive care unit. Crit Care Med 2003;31:847-852.
15. Landrigan CP, Srivastava R, Muret-Wagstaff S, et al: Impact of a health maintenance organization hospitalist system in academic pediatrics. Pediatrics 2002;110:720-728.

Pediatric Hospitalists: Efficiency and Quality of Care

Rajendu Srivastava

CURRENT STATE OF AFFAIRS

The field of pediatric hospital medicine is evolving rapidly. Early studies have documented the high prevalence of hospitalists and defined a research agenda to study the value of pediatric hospitalist systems.[1,2] Studies have been conducted to identify the issues related to this new system for the delivery of inpatient care, including pediatric hospitalists' impact on resource utilization, medical students' and house staff's educational experiences and training needs, patient and provider experiences of care, quality of care, and specific populations cared for by pediatric hospitalists.

Concurrent with this research, the field has expanded dramatically and matured in certain fundamental respects. The number of hospitalists, including pediatric hospitalists, has increased exponentially since 2001 and is expected to keep growing.[3] Fellowship programs either have started or are slated to commence across the United States and Canada in several well-known centers. The first pediatric hospitalist conference, sponsored by the Ambulatory Pediatric Association, drew more than 120 participants from the United States and Canada. Pediatricians' organizations have expanded to meet the needs of hospitalists, and hospitalists' organizations have expanded to meet the needs of their pediatric contingent. The American Academy of Pediatrics has started the Section on Hospital Medicine, the Ambulatory Pediatric Association has the Special Interest Group on Pediatric Hospital Medicine, and the Society of Hospital Medicine (the largest hospitalist organization) has actively reached out to pediatric hospitalists and continues to add them as members. Important research collaboratives have begun. The Pediatric Research in Inpatient Settings (PRIS; pronounced *prize*) network has started a series of collaborative studies ultimately intended to improve the quality of inpatient care. Finally, pediatric hospitalists are continuing to expand their nonclinical responsibilities to include leadership roles in administration (as medical directors, quality improvement officers, and leaders in patient safety and informatics), research (developing health services research laboratories and training junior investigators to be competitive in obtaining grants), and education (as clerkship and residency directors).

A tremendous amount of knowledge has been gained from critical early work into the value of pediatric hospitalists in inpatient care delivery. This chapter outlines what we have learned from these early studies and what we still need to learn, and then proposes mechanisms to accomplish these next steps.

STUDIES ON EFFICIENCY

Several studies have been conducted on the efficiency of care delivered in pediatric hospitalist models. The general finding has been a reduced length of stay (LOS) and lower total costs (between 10% and 20%) for the cohort of children being cared for by pediatric hospitalists versus other models of care. In addition, specific studies have addressed unique aspects of the pediatric hospitalist model of care, thereby contributing details to the growing body of evidence regarding its efficiency.

Bellet and Whitaker's before-and-after study at the University of Cincinnati showed a decrease in mean LOS (11%, $P = .05$) and mean hospital charges (9%, $P = .01$) following the implementation of a pediatric hospitalist system in an academic children's hospital, compared with the traditional attending model (a mixture of academic generalists and community physicians) previously in place.[4] The study examined all inpatient pediatric conditions, with a subanalysis of children with bronchiolitis and asthma. Readmission rates were higher in the hospitalist group than in the traditional attending model (3% versus 1%, $P = .006$). Subspecialist consultation rates were similar.

Similarly, Landrigan and colleagues' study at Children's Hospital in Boston found a decrease in LOS (0.3 days, 12%, $P = .001$) and total costs ($217, 16%, $P = .004$) following the implementation of a hospitalist system in a managed care organization, when controlling for severity of illness.[5] Comparison groups (managed care and non–managed care groups that did not use hospitalists) experienced no change in LOS or costs over the same period. This study used time series analysis, a powerful study design that controls for secular trends and thus provides more evidence of causality than do simple before-and-after analyses. Children with all diagnoses were evaluated. Within the primary study group, readmission rates and follow-up after discharge were comparable before and after implementation of the hospitalist system, whereas patient satisfaction improved somewhat afterward.

In a before-and-after study, Dwight and coworkers at the Hospital for Sick Children in Toronto found a lower LOS (0.4 days, 14%, $P < .01$) for those patients cared for in an attending-only hospitalist model compared with an attending–house staff model, controlling for comorbidity and other demographic factors.[6] There were no significant differences between rates for subspecialty consultation, 7-day readmission, or mortality.

Srivastava and associates' study at Primary Children's Medical Center in Salt Lake City found that inpatient care efficiency was especially improved for a subpopulation of children with medically complex conditions (defined by high severity-of-illness scores, intensive care unit transfers, and parental responses to a tool that identifies children with special health care needs) cared for by hospitalists.[7] LOS and total costs for this subpopulation were significantly lower in a hospitalist system compared with a traditional system using academic attending physicians or community physicians.

Maggioni and Rolla conducted a before-and-after analysis at Miami Children's Hospital and found lower LOS (0.96 days, 20%) and total hospital charges ($4851, 31%) after implementation of a pediatric hospitalist service compared with a system of specialist attending physicians.[8] They examined the 20 most common diagnoses as defined by the All Patients Refined Diagnosis-Related Groups. No differences were found between groups in terms of mortality or 10-day readmission rates.

Wells and colleagues conducted a study on pediatric patients with some common conditions: asthma, bronchiolitis, gastroenteritis, and pneumonia.[9] LOS and total charges were lower only for children with asthma who were cared for by pediatric hospitalists rather than primary care physicians. Readmission rates and patient satisfaction scores were similar.

Only one study in the literature found no change in resource utilization after the institution of a pediatric hospitalist system. Seid and coworkers at San Diego Children's Hospital found no reduction in LOS and total costs for children with asthma and bronchiolitis who were cared for by pediatric hospitalists compared with a traditional attending model.[10] The authors cited the concurrent introduction of a clinical pathway as a potential confounder to explain the null findings.

In sum, six of seven studies found shorter LOS and reduced resource utilization (measured as charges or costs) in pediatric hospitalist systems. Each pediatric hospitalist service varied, but collectively, the studies included the following: academic and nonacademic pediatric hospitalist systems, managed care organization hospitalist systems, and attending-only hospitalist systems; one service that focused on medically complex cases, and another that focused on common conditions; and comparisons to community, general academic pediatric, and specialist attending physician systems. These findings, in conjunction with adult hospitalist studies (17 of 19) showing similar improvements in LOS and total costs and similar preservation of quality outcomes, indicate that the argument for the value of pediatric hospitalist systems is both strong and sound.[11] Research in this area will likely continue, and future studies should attempt to add new value rather than replicate well-established findings. For example, future studies might help answer questions about the advantages and disadvantages of specific types of pediatric hospitalist models, why they work, and which patient populations are most or least likely to benefit from such systems.

QUALITY

Only limited data have been collected on quality of care in pediatric hospitalist systems. The Institute of Medicine defines *quality care* as that which is effective, efficient, safe, patient centered, timely, and equitable[12] (see Chapter 4 for a further discussion). These aspects of care also include both processes and outcomes of care, as well as patient satisfaction. Some studies of adults cared for by hospitalists have focused on process measures. For example, one study of patients hospitalized with heart failure found similar rates of adherence to evidence-based care processes between hospitalists and nonhospitalists, with similar costs but shorter LOS for patients cared for by hospitalists.[13] Another adult study comparing processes and outcomes of pneumonia care found largely similar processes of care delivered by hospitalists and nonhospitalists, except for more rapid conversion from intravenous to oral antibiotics for those cared for by hospitalists, which helped reduce LOS and subsequent costs.[14] Although data are limited, these two studies suggest that the quality of the care processes used by hospitalist and nonhospitalist systems is similar, but that hospitalist systems reduce LOS and costs, yielding more efficient care. Further studies are needed.

Process measures are particularly challenging in inpatient pediatrics, because few diseases have well-defined quality measures or strong evidence to link particular processes of care with improved outcomes. A notable exception is asthma, for which evidence-based quality metrics have been developed (e.g., the percentage of asthmatic children discharged from the hospital with an inhaled steroid). To measure quality of care using such a process marker, a site would need to measure the frequency with which children are sent home with inhaled steroids, ideally controlling for severity of illness and potential confounders.

Beyond such limited, evidence-based measures of care processes, studies can evaluate other disease-dependent process measures, such as the use of inhaled ipratropium bromide on wards or the use of chest radiographs to rule out pneumonia. Unlike the example of postdischarge inhaled steroids, however, which has a strong evidence base to support it, these examples have a weaker evidence base and hence are subject to greater disagreement. For example, the clinical criteria to determine which hospitalized children with fever and respiratory symptoms, as well as a preexisting condition of asthma, should have chest radiographs have not been well studied; thus, it is difficult to define objectively what constitutes optimal care. Research is needed to identify such process measures across a range of conditions. Because most pediatric conditions do not have well-defined disease-dependent process measures, quality-of-care studies are challenging, particularly those assessing the quality of care in patients with uncommon conditions or complex diseases.

The development of disease-dependent measures has been extremely limited in pediatrics, for a number of reasons. One reason may be the fact that many pediatric diseases lead to hospitalization, whereas a relatively small number of acute conditions in adults (which have been more thoroughly studied) lead to hospitalization. Disease-independent process measures are one method of addressing quality of care in the face of such a large range of infrequent conditions. To take the discharge process as an example, one could operationalize, test, and validate measures of quality unrelated to a particular condition, such as patient or parental understanding of the discharge process; incidence of medical errors in discharge prescriptions; frequency of timely, accurate transmission of information from inpatient to outpatient providers before the follow-up visit; and timing and appropriateness of, and patient satisfaction with, follow-up visits with specialists involved in inpatient care.

Quality of care can also be measured by looking directly at outcomes. Two studies of hospitalist care for adults demonstrated decreased mortality in hospitalist systems.[15,16] In pediatrics, death is a rare outcome and is therefore an insensitive measure of quality of care. An elevated readmission rate may reflect inappropriate early discharge from the hospital or poor continuity between inpatient and outpatient care; the measure is complex, however, because an extremely low readmission rate might indicate a tendency to hospitalize patients for longer than necessary.

These outcomes of care—mortality and readmission rates—have been unchanged in most pediatric studies. The Cincinnati study found that the 10-day readmission rate increased from 1% to 3% ($P = .006$) with a hospitalist system, but no other study has replicated this finding.[4] One study comparing survival and LOS in a pediatric intensive care unit found that patients cared for by hospitalists had an odds ratio of 2.8 for survival and a 21.1-hour shorter LOS (both $P = .13$), when adjusted for severity of illness, compared with patients cared for by residents.[17]

Patient satisfaction and experience can also be measured. Studies of patients' and parents' experiences in hospitalist systems have found either no difference or occasionally improved satisfaction with care provided by hospitalists compared with nonhospitalist (general academic or community) attending physicians.[5,9]

EDUCATION

The experiences of both medical students and house staff in hospitalist systems have been studied. In general, medical students and residents gave hospitalists fairly high marks as educators, compared with either traditional academic attending physicians or subspecialists.[18,19] One potential downside of hospitalists' increasing role in the education of trainees is a decrease in students' exposure to subspecialists and community pediatricians in some medical centers. Strategies are being developed to give medical students exposure to faculty other than hospitalists during inpatient rotations. The professional development of hospitalist educators is an important area, and more research is needed on the educational impact of the hospitalist model.[20]

A pediatric study focusing on house staff experiences found that hospitalists received higher ratings as educators, and staff self-reported improved skills and knowledge in general pediatrics, compared with traditional academic attending systems. Less senior resident autonomy was discussed as a possible disadvantage of the hospitalist system. The following year's analysis, however, did not show that lack of autonomy was an ongoing issue.[21-23] (Medical education is discussed further in Chapter 22.)

PHYSICIAN ATTITUDES

Several studies have documented the experiences and attitudes of primary care physicians (those who refer patients to hospitalists) and subspecialists (those who serve as consultants to hospitalists) with regard to hospitalist models in adult medicine. These studies found that a substantial number of primary care physicians are concerned about the quality of care, teaching, and patient satisfaction provided by the hospitalist model.[24,25] One pediatric study found that community physicians and residents rated the hospitalist system as excellent, whereas subspecialty physicians rated it as average. The authors believed that the latter rating was related to subspecialists' perceived loss of control or income.[26] Another study of the initiation of a pediatric hospitalist service at a tertiary care children's hospital found that

community physicians were more ambivalent than specialty physicians; community physicians' specific concerns included impaired communication and the maintenance of long-term relationships with their patients.[27] As hospitalist models in pediatrics become more prevalent, and as studies on effective communication and collaboration between hospitalist and community physicians are conducted, it is likely that the acceptance of, and satisfaction with, hospitalist services will grow over time.[28]

VULNERABLE GROUPS

Some initial work has focused on patients with common conditions cared for by pediatric hospitalists. Although this is an important area, evaluating the care of children with chronic conditions (also known as technology-dependent children, children with special health care needs, and medically complex children) is also important, because they represent a growing proportion of hospitalized children. This heterogeneous group is difficult to identify explicitly and comprehensively, but most hospital-based physicians recognize these children when they see them. As a group, children with special health care needs are highly vulnerable, high resource users who are potentially susceptible to gaps in care coordination and communication, with resultant poor outcomes. Medically complex children are highly diverse, with several conditions or diseases accounting for their medical states. They may be dependent on technology (e.g., gastrostomy tubes, tracheostomies, ventriculoperitoneal shunts); many are neurologically impaired (from a variety of conditions); and as a group they share several comorbid conditions. One study found that medically complex children cared for in a hospitalist system had proportionally lower LOS and total costs compared with the already lower LOS and total costs of the cohort of all children cared for by hospitalists versus the traditional academic attending model or community physicians.[7] Further study is needed to determine how to measure the quality of care that medically complex children receive (process, outcome, and satisfaction) and to identify the needs of this special population. Measuring disease-dependent processes of care in this population is particularly challenging because many medically complex children have several conditions that lack a strong evidence base. For example, neurologically impaired children have various clinical presentations that may be responsible for their hospitalization, including seizures, aspiration pneumonia, or fever, but research into their care is sparse.

DIRECTIONS FOR THE FUTURE

There is still much work to be done. A study of office-based and hospital-based physicians with admitting privileges at one tertiary care children's hospital found that office-based physicians were less likely to believe that pediatric hospitalists would increase patient satisfaction or quality of care or provide more effective house staff education.[27] Divergent views on the value of hospitalists are likely to persist as this new field is adopted in a variety of inpatient settings. As inpatient systems are designed to ensure effective communication across all facets of inpatient and outpatient care, future studies should expand to include a new focus on how current inpatient care is being delivered (measuring the quality of inpatient pediatric care) and how this can be improved both for children with common conditions and for medically complex children who are frequent users of inpatient resources and highly susceptible to a fragmented delivery system.

One method of overcoming the challenges of studying vulnerable populations with small numbers or rare conditions has already begun. The Pediatric Research in Inpatient Settings (PRIS) collaborative was initiated to study unusual conditions, unusual outcomes of common pediatric illnesses, and variations in inpatient pediatric care across diverse hospital settings. An initial set of studies documented the practice patterns, training issues, and variations in clinical care of common conditions.[29] As this and other important endeavors gain momentum, two critical steps in research must occur to improve the current system of inpatient care. First, measures of inpatient processes of pediatric care must be explicitly defined, validated, and tested. Second, pediatric hospitalists must be studied in their natural laboratory (i.e., the hospital) to understand both the limitations and the possibilities of translating research findings into clinical practice using a variety of quality improvement techniques. As both these steps occur, the care delivered to each hospitalized child will undergo a paradigm shift, and we will be able to measure that care, compare it against high performers, and improve it so that we deliver care that is effective, efficient, safe, patient centered, timely, and equitable.

REFERENCES

1. Srivastava R, Landrigan C, Gidwani P, et al: Pediatric hospitalists in Canada and the United States: A survey of pediatric academic department chairs. Ambul Pediatr 2001;1:338-339.
2. Landrigan C, Srivastava R, Muret-Wagstaff S, et al: Pediatric hospitalists: What do we know, and where do we go from here? Ambul Pediatr 2001;1:340-345.
3. Lurie JD, Miller DP, Lindenauer PK, et al: The potential size of the hospitalist workforce in the United States. Am J Med 1999;106:441-445.
4. Bellet PS, Whitaker RC: Evaluation of a pediatric hospitalist service: Impact on length of stay and hospital charges. Pediatrics 2000;105:478-484.
5. Landrigan CP, Srivastava R, Muret-Wagstaff S, et al: Impact of a health maintenance organization hospitalist system in academic pediatrics. Pediatrics 2002;110:720-728.
6. Dwight P, MacArthur C, Friedman J, Parkin PC: Evaluation of a staff-only hospitalist system in a tertiary care academic children's hospital. Pediatrics 2004;114:1545-1549.
7. Srivastava R, Muret-Wagstaff S, Young P, James BC: Hospitalist care of medically complex children. Pediatr Res 2004;55:314A-315A.
8. Maggioni A, Rolla F: Comparison of hospitalist and pediatric subspecialist care on selected APR-DRGs: Length of stay and hospital charges. Pediatr Res 2004;55:315A.
9. Wells RD, Dahl B, Wilson SD: Pediatric hospitalists: Quality care for the underserved? Am J Med Qual 2001;16:174-180.
10. Seid M, Quinn K, Kuttin P: Hospital based and community pediatricians: Comparing outcomes for asthma and bronchiolitis. J Clin Outcomes Manage 1997;4:21-24.
11. Wachter RM, Goldman L: The hospitalist movement 5 years later. JAMA 2002;287:487-494.
12. Institute of Medicine (US) Committee on Quality of Health Care in America: Crossing the Quality Chasm: A New Health System for the 21st Century. Washington, DC, National Academy Press, 2001.
13. Lindenauer PK, Chehabeddine R, Pekow P, et al: Quality of care for patients hospitalized with heart failure: Assessing the impact of hospitalists. Arch Intern Med 2002;162:1251-1256.
14. Rifkin WD, Conner D, Silver A, Eichorn A: Comparison of processes and outcomes of pneumonia care between hospitalists and community-based primary care physicians. Mayo Clin Proc 2002;77:1053-1058.
15. Auerbach AD, Wachter RM, Katz P, et al: Implementation of a voluntary hospitalist service at a community teaching hospital: Improved clinical efficiency and patient outcomes. Ann Intern Med 2002;137:859-865.
16. Meltzer D, Shah M, Morrison J: Decreased length of stay, costs and mortality in a randomized trial of academic hospitalists. J Gen Intern Med 2001;16(Suppl):S208.
17. Tenner PA, Dibrell H, Taylor RP: Improved survival with hospitalists in a pediatric intensive care unit. Crit Care Med 2003;31:847-852.
18. Hunter AJ, Desai SS, Harrison RA, Chan BK: Medical student evaluation of the quality of hospitalist and nonhospitalist teaching faculty on inpatient medicine rotations. Acad Med 2004;79:78-82.
19. Kripalani S, Pope AC, Rask K, et al: Hospitalists as teachers. J Gen Intern Med 2004;19:8-15.
20. Hauer KE, Wachter RM: Implications of the hospitalist model for medical students' education. Acad Med 2001;76:324-330.
21. Landrigan CP, Muret-Wagstaff S, Chiang VW, et al: Effect of a pediatric hospitalist system on housestaff education and experience. Arch Pediatr Adolesc Med 2002;156:877-883.
22. Landrigan CP, Muret-Wagstaff S, Chiang VW, et al: Senior resident autonomy in a pediatric hospitalist system. Arch Pediatr Adolesc Med 2003;157:206-207.
23. Kemper AR, Freed GL: Hospitalists and residency medical education: Measured improvement. Arch Pediatr Adolesc Med 2002;156:858-859.
24. Auerbach AD, Nelson EA, Lindenauer PK, et al: Physician attitudes toward and prevalence of the hospitalist model of care: Results of a national survey. Am J Med 2000;109:648-653.
25. Auerbach AD, Davis RB, Phillips RS: Physician views on caring for hospitalized patients and the hospitalist model of inpatient care. J Gen Intern Med 2001;16:116-119.
26. Ponitz K, Mortimer J, Berman B: Establishing a pediatric hospitalist program at an academic medical center. Clin Pediatr (Phila) 2000;39:221-227.
27. Srivastava R, Norlin C, James BC, et al: Community and hospital-based physicians' attitudes regarding pediatric hospitalist systems. Pediatrics 2005;115:34-38.
28. Auerbach AD, Aronson MD, Davis RB, Phillips RS: How physicians perceive hospitalist services after implementation: Anticipation vs. reality. Arch Intern Med 2003;163:2330-2336.
29. Landrigan C, Stucky E, Chiang VW, Ottolini MC: Variation in inpatient management of common pediatric diseases: A study from the Pediatric Research in Inpatient Settings (PRIS) network. Pediatr Res 2004;55:315A.

CHAPTER 3

Hospitalist Models of Care: Organization and Compensation

David Zipes

Since Wachter and Goldman coined the term *hospitalist* in 1996,[1] the field has undergone tremendous growth and change. The National Association of Inpatient Physicians has evolved into the Society of Hospital Medicine (SHM), with more than 4000 members. The name change reflects the field's maturation as it begins to define a body of knowledge as opposed to a specific person (i.e., a hospitalist). The American Academy of Pediatrics Provisional Section on Hospital Care has become the Section on Hospital Medicine, and the Ambulatory Pediatric Association's special-interest group has shortened its designation from Inpatient Medicine/Hospitalist to simply Hospital Medicine. The field now boasts an estimated 12,000 hospitalists in the United States, with most statistics indicating that about 10% are pediatric hospitalists.

A 2002 survey by the American Academy of Pediatrics found that 40% of pediatricians are affiliated with hospitals that have full-time pediatric hospitalists, and these hospitalists provide care for about 45% of general pediatric inpatients.[2] Among the respondents who worked with pediatric hospitalists, 87% expressed satisfaction with the patient care the hospitalists provided. Reasons that pediatricians cited for using pediatric hospitalists included improved quality of care derived from the full-time hospital presence of hospitalists (61%) and greater efficiency, specifically, the decreased time pediatricians must spend away from the office (53%). More than 75% agreed that using pediatric hospitalists allowed their office practices to remain more predictable and manageable, and 57% said that the use of hospitalists increased their office productivity.

Although the term *hospitalist* is only 10 years old, the concept of an in-house physician is not new to the U.S. health care system or to health systems abroad. The traditional house physician has been around far longer than 10 years. Nonetheless, the growth of hospital medicine since the mid-1990s has been astronomical—it is one of the fastest growing health care specialties in the country. In the mid-1990s there were an estimated 800 hospitalists; today, hospital medicine is a larger specialty than gastroenterology, dermatology, pulmonology, and allergy.[3,4] This growth has been catalyzed by a constellation of forces, including changes in health insurance, decreased rates of admission, greater inpatient complexity, shifts in reimbursement for inpatient care, growing concerns about primary care providers' quality of life, and increased complexity of outpatient medicine. As the field of hospital medicine has evolved, specific models of care delivery have also evolved to address shifts in compensation and employer type and to optimize communication strategies to limit the loss of information (dubbed *voltage drop*) when patients transition from inpatient to outpatient settings and vice versa.

STAGES OF HOSPITAL MEDICINE

Wachter succinctly described four stages in the evolution of inpatient care,[1] ranging from the complete absence of hospitalists to their mandatory utilization (Table 3-1). The various modalities reflect both the need for different stages in different health care systems and the growth of hospital medicine. The numerical ranking of the stages is not meant to imply superiority of one over another, and the change from one model to another need not occur in an orderly progression or at all.

The first stage is the traditional model of care in which there are no hospitalists. Each primary care physician (PCP) cares for his or her own (usually uncomplicated) patients in both inpatient and outpatient settings. Typically, surgical and medical subspecialty patients are excluded because they are cared for by their respective specialists. In general, the PCP makes the rounds of his or her hospitalized patients once each morning and provides the remainder of care by telephone. Under this model, the average primary care pediatrician cares for one to two hospitalized patients in any given month. In the year 2000 there were 38,457 practicing pediatricians.[5] In the mid-1990s, before the explosive growth of hospitalists, stage 1 was the most common care model in nonacademic hospitals. This model thrived for many reasons and, like all the stages, has its advantages and disadvantages. For example, continuity of care during the hospitalization itself and from the inpatient to the outpatient setting ensures minimal loss of information or duplication of often costly diagnostic data. Patients may have long-standing relationships with their physicians, which can be comforting during the stress of hospitalization. The cost of hiring a hospitalist is avoided, which, according to the 2004 SHM survey,[4] averages an annual net cost of $60,000 per full-time employee (in other words, the average hospitalist generates enough revenue from professional fees to cover his or her salary minus $60,000). This stage was more practical when patients who were less sick were hospitalized, but it still thrives today, especially in a fee-for-service insurance environment and in areas where physicians' offices are located close to the hospital and there are a limited number of hospitals the physician must visit. This model also prevails where the number of pediatric beds at any given hospital may be too few to support pediatric hospitalists—much more common with pediatric than with adult care.

Although stage 1 is the most common model in many parts of the United States, its many disadvantages have, in part, catalyzed the tremendous growth of hospital medicine. Inpatients today are typically much more ill and often have multiple medical problems. They require frequent visits throughout the day, which is difficult for an office-based

Stage	Type	Description
		Table 3-1 Four Stages of Hospital Care
1	Traditional model	There are no hospitalists; each primary care physician cares for his or her own (usually uncomplicated) patients in both inpatient and outpatient settings
2	Primary care rotation	A group of primary care physicians rotates, each assuming the role of hospitalist for short periods, usually <25% of their total clinical time
3	Voluntary hospitalist	A hospitalist or group of hospitalists accepts other physicians' inpatients and cares for them during their hospitalization; at discharge, the patient's care reverts to the primary care physician
4	Mandatory hospitalist	Same as stage 3, except that the use of the hospitalist service is mandatory for all general inpatients; this is discouraged by most major medical organizations, including the Society of Hospital Medicine and the American Academy of Pediatrics Section on Hospital Medicine

patients—less ill, nonsubspecialty, and nonsurgical. These acting hospitalists do not care for the patients of PCPs outside their group. The model at academic hospitals, where physicians attend on the wards for 1 to 2 months per year and then do outpatient medicine or research for the remainder of the year, is a variant of this stage. This stage begins to reap some, though certainly not all, the advantages of the third stage, such as increased efficiency in caring for inpatients, increased physician availability for inpatients, and increased efficiency for primary practitioners; it also introduces many of the disadvantages, such as loss of information and discontinuity of care. The designated hospitalist's increased hospital presence and availability, with minimal to no outpatient responsibilities, allows that physician to care for more complex patients and to make multiple visits per day. Back at the office, the lack of interruptions from hospitalized patients enables the efficiency of outpatient care to be maintained. Time management is improved, decreasing travel time and office interruptions, and the designated hospitalist becomes familiar with the workings of the hospital. The lack of a full-time, dedicated hospitalist, however, limits the "practice makes perfect" benefit, as well as making it difficult for the hospitalist to become deeply entrenched with hospital systems issues—two major benefits of the third stage. Note that the physicians providing care in stages 1 and 2 do not typically meet the current SHM definition of a hospitalist: "Hospitalists are physicians whose primary professional focus is the general medical care of hospitalized patients. They may engage in clinical care, teaching, research, or leadership in the field of Hospital Medicine" (available at *www.hospitalmedicine.org*).

The third stage is the fastest growing and most prevalent of the models that use hospitalists in some fashion (stages 2, 3, and 4). This is the stage to which most individuals refer when they speak of hospitalists. In this model, a hospitalist or group of hospitalists accepts other physicians' patients on their service (the "handoff") when these patients require hospitalization, and they care for them during their hospital stay. At the end of the stay, the patient's care is handed back to the PCP. A recent survey in Massachusetts found that hospitalists are the care coordinators for about 42% of hospitalized patients,[7] and an American Academy of Pediatrics survey found that more than 40% of physicians have contact with hospitalists.[2] This stage reaps all the positives and, unfortunately, all the negatives of a hospitalist model. With stage 3, use of the hospitalist service is on a strictly voluntary basis, a stance favored by the SHM, the American Academy of Pediatrics Section on Hospital Medicine, and many other national medical organizations. The voluntary nature of the service encourages hospitalists to provide quality care to promote the use of their services and, just as important, creates a less threatening relationship between the hospitalist and the PCP. The hospitalist model is presented as an option for the PCP to use or not use at his or her discretion. The PCP's decision whether to use the hospitalist service is often complicated and multifactorial. Factors include, but are not necessarily limited to, the type of health insurance in the community, travel time to and from the hospital, patient acuity, number of inpatients, quality of life, job satisfaction, and personal preference. Stage 3 models can start at the request of the PCPs in the area, or they can be initiated by the hospital, insurance companies,

physician to accomplish. Insurance pressures make it impractical to keep a patient who is ready for discharge in the hospital overnight simply to wait for the attending physician to make rounds in the morning. At the same time, compared with the 1990s, the modern office-based pediatrician must see many more outpatients (often six patients or more an hour) to generate the same income and may be compelled to provide evening and weekend office hours as well. The time cost of caring for patients in the hospital is great, including driving to one or many hospitals, obtaining the necessary patient data (often computerized and difficult to access for those unfamiliar with the technology), examining the patient, and talking with the family. By seeing several office patients within the same time frame, the PCP can generate more revenue, maintain a smoother flow of patients, and potentially shorten his or her workday. In fact, one study showed that both the productivity and job satisfaction of PCPs increased with the availability of hospitalists.[6] In addition, with large call groups and weekend coverage schedules, the patient's actual PCP may not be the one to see him or her in the hospital, thus eliminating many of the advantages of stage 1.

Stage 2 represents the first step toward the use of hospitalists and involves the designation of a physician to function as a hospitalist for a short period. Typically, a large group (this model is difficult to implement with small groups) chooses one or more physicians to be the hospitalist for a predetermined period (usually 1 week to 1 month, accounting for less than 25% of the physician's time) and care for the group's inpatients. Although the patients may be more acutely ill, they are generally similar to stage 1 hospitalists themselves, or other means. The development of stage 3 models can be severely limited by the number of inpatient beds available; this is especially true of pediatric hospitalist models—the fewer the beds, the more difficult it is to support a hospitalist program.

Stage 4 is the same as stage 3, except that the use of the hospitalist service is mandatory for all general inpatients. Both the SHM and the American Academy of Pediatrics Section on Hospital Medicine, as well as many other professional medical societies (e.g., American Academy of Family Physicians, American College of Physicians), strongly oppose the implementation of a stage 4 model, promoting, instead, free choice. Typically, this model will develop and prosper only when a single entity, such as a managed care organization or large medical group, controls the hospital. It has all the advantages and all the disadvantages of the stage 3 model, plus the potential to greatly increase the animosity and hostility between hospitalists and PCPs. With the growth of hospital medicine, the loss of choice has become of increasing concern to PCPs; many compare it to the introduction and subsequent growth of neonatal intensivists, pediatric intensivists, and pediatric emergency physicians. Intensive care units and emergency departments were once the domain of the primary care pediatrician, whereas they are now, in general, closed units. By essentially creating a monopoly, the motivation to provide excellent care and to continually improve the service can be reduced.

As noted earlier, no model is necessarily superior to another, and no model fits every situation. Nonetheless, as the hospital medicine movement continues to expand, increasing evidence supports the efficiency and advantages of stage 3 and 4 hospitalist models. Stage 3 models, however, provide excellent cost-benefit ratios without alienating primary care providers.

EMPLOYMENT AND COMPENSATION MODELS

Just as there are different care models, there are different employment and compensation models for hospitalists (Table 3-2). Like care models, no one compensation model works for all situations, and each has different driving forces. At this time, there are six basic employment categories: self-employed hospitalist-only groups, multistate hospitalist-only groups, hospital or hospital corporations, academic

hospitals, multispecialty groups, and insurance industry groups (managed care organizations). Certainly, there are permutations of and variations on these schemes, and as hospital medicine grows and evolves, other models may emerge. According to the SHM's 2004 survey, most pediatric hospitalists are employed by academic institutions, with hospitals or hospital corporations running a close second (Table 3-2).

The financial implications and limitations of each employment model are the driving forces behind their development and utilization. According to the SHM survey, when professional fees are compared with the costs of providing services, 60% of groups are in the red. Most hospitalist programs therefore require external support to remain solvent. Although hospitalist systems yield cost savings to the system as a whole (usually more than accounting for their cost), largely owing to decreased lengths of stay and other benefits (e.g., system improvements, resident education), the decision of who should pay for these benefits has yet to be determined. Should it be the insurance companies, in the form of increased payments for inpatient care; the hospitals, in the form of bonuses, salaries, or subsidies; the PCPs; or the many other entities that benefit from a well-run hospitalist model? Currently, hospitals (academic and community) employ 68% of all pediatric hospitalists, according to the SHM survey. It is therefore not surprising that according to the Pediatric Research in Inpatient Settings (PRIS) survey, hospitals are also the most common source of external support for pediatric hospitalist programs.[8] Cost-sharing models for the beneficiaries of hospitalist programs must be developed. If increased reimbursement for hospitalized patients can be achieved, the employment models may shift, but for now, the trend of hospitals employing hospitalists will likely continue.

The basic compensation models include salary only, productivity only (i.e., professional fees), and mixed productivity and compensation. Again, permutations and variations may exist, and new models may emerge in the future. According to the 2004 SHM productivity and compensation survey, more than 60% of all hospitalist programs receive money beyond what their professional fees generate; 80% of academic models receive supplementation. Among individual hospitalists, 38% are purely salaried, 8% earn productivity-based income, and 45% receive a combination of the two. Bonuses can be a variable in any of the three compensation models, and according to the survey, 61% of hospitalists receive some sort of bonus.

Although bonuses can certainly be an effective motivational tool, one needs to be cognizant of the potential legal ramifications of incentive systems. The Stark laws, for example, prohibit the referral of Medicare and Medicaid patients to an entity for the provision of certain health services if the physician or a member of the physician's immediate family has a direct or indirect financial relationship with the entity. Bonuses can be interpreted as an indirect financial relationship. Consultation with legal counsel is strongly recommended during the development of incentive or bonus plans.

Type of insurance (e.g., Medicaid, private, health maintenance organization, self-pay), reimbursement strategy (e.g., fee for service, capitated), inpatient volume, and type of hospital (e.g., community, academic) all have an impact on the type of employment and compensation models imple-

Table 3-2 Employment Models		
Employer	Pediatric Hospitalists (%)	All Hospitalists (%)
Self-employed hospitalist-only group	5	20
Multistate hospitalist-only group	0	9
Hospital or hospital corporation	33	38
Academic hospital	35	16
Multispecialty group	13	17
Insurance industry (managed care organization)	NA	NA

NA, not applicable (not surveyed).
From Society of Hospital Medicine 2004 survey.

mented. Much like Charles Darwin's well-described Galapagos finches, the models that survive will be those that are well adapted to their particular environment. No one model works for every situation. Increased reimbursement for hospital care would likely affect compensation models as well as employment models.

SUBSPECIALTY HOSPITALIST MODELS

A growing field that does not fit neatly into any of the previously described models is that of the subspecialty hospitalist. At present, neonatal and pediatric intensive care units seem to be the biggest employers of general pediatric hospitalists in positions traditionally filled by subspecialists. These hospitalists may work exclusively in the intensive care unit or both in that unit and on the general pediatric floor. Additionally, urgent care centers and emergency departments may employ hospitalists. The phenomenon of using hospitalists in other subspecialties is burgeoning in adult patient care but is just beginning to occur in the pediatric hospitalist community. Adult subspecialties that commonly use hospitalists include cardiology, hematology-oncology, and pulmonology, with some growth seen in obstetrics and gynecology and orthopedics. These hospitalists can be trained in general pediatrics, internal medicine, or subspecialties. Any specialty with a large inpatient population can adopt this

model. The relatively small inpatient volumes of most pediatric subspecialties (excluding neonatal and pediatric intensive care units) may limit the cost-effectiveness of hiring hospitalists to care exclusively for patients of a particular subspecialty, although models in which general pediatric hospitalists care for subspecialty patients as part of their job may emerge.

REFERENCES

1. Wachter RM, Goldman L: The emerging role of "hospitalists" in the American health care system. N Engl J Med 1996;335:514.
2. Pediatrician attitudes toward and experiences with pediatric hospitalists: A national survey. Society of Hospital Medicine Sixth Annual Meeting Abstracts, 2003.
3. AMA Physician Characteristics and Distribution in the US, 2004.
4. AHA survey, 2004, submitted for publication.
5. Shipman SA, Lurie JD, Goodman DC: The general pediatrician: Projecting future workforce supply and requirements. Pediatrics 2004;113:435.
6. Wachter RM: The hospitalist movement: Ten issues to consider. Hosp Pract (Minneap) 1999;34:95-98, 104-106, 111.
7. Miller JA: The hospitalist movement: The quiet revolution in healthcare. HealthLeaders News, Jan 8, 2003.
8. Chiang VW, Landrigan CP, Stucky E, Ottolini MC: Financial health of pediatric hospitalist systems: A study from the Pediatric Research in Inpatient Settings (PRIS) network. Pediatr Res 2004;55:1794.

SECTION *B*

Improving the Quality of Care for Hospitalized Children

CHAPTER *4*

Quality of Care and Patient Satisfaction

Sharon Muret-Wagstaff and Charles J. Homer

Since the 1990s, quality of care has assumed its rightful place as a central focus of health care delivery and management. The increased attention to quality arose from abundant evidence that health care in the United States suffers from serious and pervasive quality-related problems that have staggering effects.

To assess the extent of the quality problem and develop ways to tackle it, the Institute of Medicine developed a definition of quality that remains a foundation for current thinking: "the degree to which health services for individuals and populations increase the likelihood of desired health outcomes and are consistent with current professional knowledge." This definition acknowledges the importance of outcomes, the key role of both individuals and the public in determining which outcomes matter, the essential role of probability (doing the right thing, even if the right result does not always occur), and the constraints imposed by the current state of knowledge.

In a later report, the Institute of Medicine refined this definition, viewing quality as an indicator of the extent to which the health care system fulfills its purpose (to continually improve the health of the American public).[1] More important, it defined six specific aims for the health care system, now widely conceived as the critical dimensions of quality. Health care should be:

1. Safe
2. Effective
3. Efficient
4. Patient centered
5. Timely
6. Equitable

The guiding principle of the health care system is to do no harm. The key insight emphasized by the Institute of Medicine is that safety is a system property, rather than a reflection of individual shortcomings, and system redesign is the necessary strategy to address problems in this area.[1,2] Chapters 5 and 6 address specific safety issues.

Effectiveness refers to the reliable delivery of care that is likely to achieve desired results (i.e., care consistent with evidence). Chapters 7 and 8 on evidence-based medicine and clinical practice guidelines, respectively, provide an orientation to the delivery of effective care. Guidelines must be coupled with effective strategies to incorporate evidence into clinical practice. This chapter addresses some strategies for initiating such an effort.

Efficiency refers to the judicious and appropriate use of resources or, more specifically, not delivering care known to be ineffective (eliminating overuse). Evidence-based medicine is the basis for determining what types of services are inappropriate; an analysis of variation in care also provides insight into potential areas of waste. Quality improvement tools can be used to identify and eliminate inefficiencies in care; some of these are reviewed in this chapter.

Patient centeredness is the core of health care. Recall that the fundamental definition of quality refers to *desired* outcomes—that is, outcomes desired by patients—as the key aim of care. The experience of care is one dimension of patient centeredness, and satisfaction with care is one component—a subjective assessment of how those experiences compare with expectations. This chapter touches on several aspects of satisfaction, experience, and patient centeredness. In pediatrics, patient centeredness is more appropriately reframed as family centeredness, or addressing the needs and desires of the child in the context of his or her family members and their needs.

Timeliness refers to the elimination of the waiting and delays omnipresent in health care; it is a dimension that clearly affects efficiency and patient centeredness. It also affects safety (e.g., delay in the administration of appropriate antibiotics) and effectiveness (e.g., delay in the scheduling of appropriate medical tests and therapies). Timeliness is receiving increasing attention in efforts to improve hospital quality through the use of sophisticated engineering models of flow and queuing theory. It is not specifically addressed in this chapter, but useful articles have been published.

Including equity in the definition of quality highlights that quality applies to the care of all patients, not simply subsets of those we care for. A 2002 Institute of Medicine report demonstrated that disparities exist throughout the health care system and called for widespread educational and improvement efforts to eliminate them.[3] Strategies to address disparities through the application of quality improvement methods are addressed briefly in this chapter.

Pediatric hospitalists are uniquely positioned to create dramatic improvements in the quality of care for hospitalized children by virtue of their extended presence, focused expertise, and familiarity with multidisciplinary team members and hospital systems.[4] Their position enables them to be leaders in transforming the quality of care that children and their families experience. Quality improvement provides an essential set of tools and techniques to accomplish this.

High-quality programs that meet the needs of children and families are characterized by excellence in all six aspects of quality. That is, programs that provide the best care deliver the right care (based on evidence and associated with the best outcomes) in a manner that is respectful of the family's needs and values, does not waste either resources or time, does not cause preventable harm, and is not biased.

ESTABLISHING PRIORITIES

Given the breadth and scope of quality and the substantial gaps in performance across the dimensions of quality, choosing where to begin can be daunting. The development of a "quality compass" or "balanced scorecard" can assist in determining where to set priorities. Such a compass might include measures of each aspect of quality: the proportion of patients with a particular condition receiving all evidence-based recommendations (effectiveness), length of stay or high-cost test use (efficiency), waiting times for consultations or radiologic procedures (timeliness), patient assessment of communication or discharge planning (patient centeredness), adverse drug events (safety), and differences in all of the above by insurance type or racial or ethnic group (equity). A balanced scorecard would combine these outcomes with additional performance metrics, such as financial performance and measures of staff satisfaction. Hospitalists developing such scorecards for a single hospital unit must consider overall institutional goals and take care not to harm performance elsewhere. For example, establishing rigid criteria for assessment and treatment before entry into a specific inpatient unit to address a safety concern may result in waits and delays in the emergency department or intensive care unit.

Although such a scientific approach to the setting of priorities is appealing, the multitude of quality deficiencies, the linked nature of many hospital processes, and the similar approach to tackling quality challenges bring other considerations to the fore. For example:

- Where can one gain an early success, building engagement and support?
- What initiative can bring widespread participation, laying the groundwork for future activities?
- What projects will further institutional aims, leading to institutional support and potentially long-term sustainability?

These tactical considerations are often at least as important as more technically based priorities.

UNDERTAKING AN IMPROVEMENT PROJECT

Regardless of the priority chosen, the fundamental approach to improving quality at the program, or microsystem, level is similar. The first step is creating a team to undertake improvement. Such a team should have a specific charge from leadership (which can be determined at the unit level), have its own leader, be multidisciplinary, and involve patients and families.

The first task of an improvement team is to establish an aim, which may be a refinement of the initial aim laid out by leadership. Aims for improvement programs should be based on data and should be sufficiently bold to engage the energies of team members. Similar to any research hypothesis, aims should be directional and specify magnitude; they should also be closely aligned with the mission and vision of the organization and, whenever possible, reflect the priorities of patients and families as the true organizational customers. A hypothetical aim statement might be: "Our project aim is to increase the proportion of children with gastroenteritis such that 95% receive perfect care while maintaining an average length of stay of 32 hours." In this case, perfect care must be precisely defined (e.g., assessment of dehydration, use of oral rehydration, and parental education about ongoing care).

This example clearly indicates the interrelatedness of the six quality aims. Although it is ostensibly focused on the effectiveness of care (giving evidence-based treatment for gastroenteritis), the project will necessarily involve issues of safety, efficiency (length of stay), timeliness (wait for initial assessment and treatment), patient and family engagement, and, given the increased rates of admission and death for poor and minority children due to gastroenteritis, equity.

The second step in an improvement program is to establish measures to assess performance and track gains. Generally, measurement of improvement should focus on the most important elements—"just enough" to undertake the work. Ideally, measures should be derived from data collected routinely in the course of care, such as electronic health records or ongoing patient surveys, but in most cases, it must be supplemented by project-specific data collection and analysis. Importantly, data should be plotted and tracked over time using simple tools such as run charts or more sophisticated tools such as control charts; they should not be kept hidden for evaluation-oriented before-and-after studies. A typical improvement project uses four to eight measures, including measures of the processes of care (was the right thing done?), the outcomes of care (did the right result occur?), and potential adverse outcomes (was there unintended harm?). In the previous example, measures of process might include whether a severity assessment was undertaken (or undertaken with specific components) and whether treatment was provided in the appropriate manner. Outcome measures might include the amount of time until the child returned to baseline weight or euvolemia, the length of stay, and the like. Balancing measures might include patient satisfaction, staff satisfaction (would administering oral rehydration be too much work?), or hours of sleep for resident staff.

The third step in an improvement initiative is to identify changes or innovations that are likely to accomplish the desired aims. Such changes can often be found in the medical literature, although one must realize that medical innovations often take 1 to 2 decades to achieve widespread use after being proved effective. Changes can also be found outside of health care; safety innovations, for example, are typically imported from high-reliability industries such as aviation, nuclear power, and high-speed transportation (e.g., trains). Patients and families, as well as health care staff, are other valuable sources of innovation. Generic change concepts from industry are another useful source of innovation that can be customized to the health care setting.

In a complex system such as a hospital, it is typically not possible to implement a new approach in a way that accounts for all the challenges accompanying such a change. A more effective approach to introducing change is to use repeated small tests of change; this is sometimes referred to as the Shewhart cycle, after the industrial engineer who developed the approach, or, more commonly, the plan-do-study-act (PDSA) cycle. The PDSA cycle starts with a question: What is the largest meaningful test of change that we can conduct by next Tuesday? That is, the priority for a PDSA cycle is to expeditiously try something out in a way that is planned and in a way that allows learning (study) and revision (acton). A typical health care PDSA cycle involves the care of one patient at one point in time by one provider, such as the use of a new dehydration assessment form or patient instruction diagram. A full cycle involves planning what will be done (including who, what, where, and when, if not why); doing the test; reflecting on what happened during the test (e.g., the patient did not understand the diagram, or it lengthened the interaction); and modifying the test for the next cycle. Effective improvement programs conduct numerous cycles, building on them and addressing different dimensions of the health care system with different series of tests.

This approach to improvement, the Model for Improvement developed by Associates in Process Improvement, is among the most widespread improvement frameworks in health care. Other approaches use different terminology and have somewhat different emphases but generally share the use of aims, measures, and repeated tests of change.

Six Sigma, for example, is another popular approach to process improvement that draws its name from the goal of reducing defects to the level of 6 standard deviations, or 3.4 defects per million opportunities.[5] Six Sigma relies on a rigorous cycle of steps known as DMAIC: define (the project's purpose and scope and the voice of the customer), measure (baseline data), analyze (to determine root causes), improve (test solutions aimed at the identified root cause), and control (maintain the gains by standardizing and then replicating the new process).

Lean production is generally associated with manufacturing and is based on eliminating waste. However, its proponents demonstrate that by streamlining services from a consumer's perspective, particularly with respect to waiting and delays, service organizations are able to work with consumers to save everyone time, increase satisfaction, and lower costs.[6] The application of such principles to hospital care shows promise in reducing frustration and wasted time for patients and families. Once again, this suggests that putting patients first can accelerate the achievement of not only patient satisfaction but also other quality aims, such as efficiency.

Because all these approaches entail learning from tests of change, it is advantageous for those using them to share their lessons with others. Moreover, the use of collaborative data allows individual organizations to better set priorities and identify settings that have better performance (also known as benchmarking). The benefits of collaborative learning have led to the formation of numerous collaborative improvement programs in children's health care. Many networks initially established for clinical and health services research, including the American Academy of Pediatrics' Pediatric Research in Office Settings (PROS), CORNET for academic primary care, the Cystic Fibrosis Foundation registry, and PECARN (for pediatric emergency departments), have the potential to serve this purpose, as does the Pediatric Research in Inpatient Settings (PRIS) network. Among these, the Cystic Fibrosis Foundation's program has achieved the greatest success in quality improvement, and numerous efforts are under way to extend this approach elsewhere in children's health care. Other programs that have been established specifically for quality improvement include the Vermont Oxford Network for neonatal intensive care and time-limited, topic-specific learning collaboratives conducted by the National Initiative for Children's Healthcare Quality (NICHQ) and other organizations. Participation in such external efforts typically accelerates learning and improvement.

ADDRESSING PROBLEMS IN PATIENT SATISFACTION

Addressing patients' and families' experience of care is often an excellent place to start when initiating improvement efforts. By listening, learning, and placing patients and families at the center of health care efforts, clinicians can accelerate improvements not only in satisfaction but also in safety, effectiveness, timeliness, efficiency, and equity of care.

Concerns expressed by children and families about the care they receive are remarkably consistent over time, age groups, and geographic locations. Coordination of care and discharge planning are the most common problematic areas; communication between clinicians and parents is the strongest determinant of the overall rating of quality of care by parents of hospitalized children.[7,8] Poor care coordination also emerged as one of the three most problematic aspects of care among adults in an international study.[9]

Pediatric hospitalists must pay particular attention to these concerns. Community-based physicians are more likely than their hospital-based counterparts to worry that the care of inpatients by hospitalists may impair communication with primary care physicians, adversely affect the physician-patient relationship, and hurt patient satisfaction.[10]

Several investigators have urged clinicians to go beyond satisfaction and make the effort to build confidence and trust and to treat families with respect and dignity. Joffe and colleagues, for example, found that these factors, along with staff courtesy and availability, continuity and transition, attention to physical comfort, and coordination of care, were highly associated with willingness to recommend a hospital.[11] Thom and associates noted that satisfaction looks backward, but trust looks forward and predicts adherence to and continuity of care.[12] Factors that promote trust include greater perceived mutual interests (e.g., the patient's health goal), clear communication, a history of fulfilled trust, less perceived difference in power, acceptance of personal disclosures, and expectation of a longer-term relationship.

Children who are minorities, whose preference is for a language other than English, and who come from resource-poor communities are known to experience lower levels of satisfaction, as well as higher rates of errors in inpatient

---

Opportunities to Engage Patients and Families and Improve Quality and Experiences of Care

- Patient and family perspectives in the mission statement
- Patient and family advisory council
- Hospital committees, searches, and decision-making bodies
- Facility design
- Improvement teams
- Family resource center
- Research agenda
- Patients and families as educators
- Peer-to-peer advising
- Open visiting and participation policies
- Self-management support
- Disclosure practices
- Information and technology access

Figure 4-1 Opportunities to improve the quality and experience of pediatric hospital care by engaging patients and families. (Adapted from Ahmann E, Johnson BH: New guidance materials promote family-centered change in health care institutions. Pediatr Nurs 2001;27:173–175.)

Elements of Culturally and Linguistically Appropriate Health Care Services

1. Effective, understandable, respectful care compatible with cultural health beliefs and practices and preferred language
2. Diverse staff representative of demographics of the hospital's service area
3. Training in culturally and linguistically appropriate service delivery for all staff
4. Timely bilingual staff and interpreter services at no cost at all points of contact during all hours
5. Verbal and written statements in families' preferred languages of their right to language assistance services
6. Competent language assistance
7. Materials and signs in common languages of the service area
8. Strategic plan includes provision of culturally and linguistically appropriate services
9. Organizational self-assessment of integrated, culturally and linguistically appropriate services
10. Current data on individual patient and family race, ethnicity, and language preferences in health records and information systems
11. Community cultural and epidemiologic profile and needs assessment
12. Participatory, collaborative partnerships with communities in design and implementation of CLAS-related activities
13. Culturally and linguistically sensitive conflict and grievance resolution processes
14. Public reporting of progress in implementing CLAS standards

Figure 4-2 Standards to ensure culturally and linguistically appropriate services (CLAS). (Adapted from US Department of Health and Human Services, Office of Minority Health: National Standards on Culturally and Linguistically Appropriate Services (CLAS) in Health Care: Final Report. Washington, DC, 2001.)

---

settings. For example, parents of Hispanic children are more likely than other parents to feel that health care providers do not listen carefully, explain things, show respect, or spend enough time with them. These same communication deficits are apparent with regard to lower income and insurance status.

ADDRESSING THE EXPERIENCE OF CARE

The general strategies referred to earlier can be applied to specific efforts to enhance the experience of care for patients and families. A wide variety of change concepts are readily available to be applied to any specific hospital setting. The American Academy of Pediatrics and the Institute for Family-Centered Care recently outlined core principles of family-centered care, reviewed the literature linking family-centered care to improved satisfaction and outcomes, and recommended ways that pediatricians can integrate these concepts into care systems.[13] For example, pediatric hospitalists can include families in patient rounds and discussions, promote the active participation of children in managing and directing their own care, facilitate family-to-family support and networking, create opportunities for children and families to serve as advisers and teachers, and guide facility design to promote family-centered care. The Institute for Family-Centered Care provides ideas, materials, guidance, and pediatric examples of best practices (Fig. 4-1).

Similarly, numerous change concepts have been developed to address the issue of disparities, particularly with respect to the care of individuals from racial and ethnic minorities. The Office of Minority Health developed the national standards for culturally and linguistically appropriate services in health care (the CLAS standards, summarized in Fig. 4-2) in 2001 to ensure that all people entering the health care system receive equitable and effective treatment in a culturally and linguistically appropriate manner. The standards address culturally competent care (standards 1 to 3); language access services (standards 4 to 7), mandated for all recipients of federal funds; and organizational support for cultural competence (standards 8 to 14). These standards

apply to all efforts to improve safety, effectiveness, patient centeredness, timeliness, and efficiency of care.

The NICHQ developed and pilot-tested a conceptual framework, a set of change concepts, and measures for cultural competency that await application in inpatient settings.[14] A measurement tool that specifically assesses the experience of inpatient care for individuals with limited English proficiency has been developed by the Child and Adolescent Health Measurement Initiative and the Florida Initiative for Children's Healthcare Quality. These measures and changes can be applied in the context of systematic improvement programs.

CONCLUSION

Widespread deficiencies exist in all six dimensions of health care quality. A systematic approach to monitoring quality can help set priorities for improvement, although the specific topics and initiatives to be undertaken must be customized to the institutional environment. Use of a quality improvement approach such as the Model for Improvement increases the likelihood of making positive changes in outcomes. Collaboration across institutions is a critical component of improvement efforts, as is building on established change concepts and frameworks. Such frameworks are readily available in the area of patient experience and cultural competency and should be incorporated into hospital improvement efforts. The pediatric hospitalist is uniquely positioned to lead this endeavor.

SUGGESTED READING

Agency for Healthcare Research and Quality: 2005 National Healthcare Disparities Report. Rockville, Md, Agency for Healthcare Research and Quality, 2006.

Baldrige National Quality Program, National Institute of Standards and Technology: 2006 Health Care Criteria for Performance Excellence. Gaithersburg, Md, Baldrige National Quality Program, 2006.

Dougherty D, Simpson LA: Measuring the quality of children's health care: A prerequisite to action. Pediatrics 2004;113:185-198.

Institute of Medicine: Performance Measurement: Accelerating Improvement. Washington, DC, National Academies Press, 2006.

Kaplan RS, Norton DP: Strategy Maps. Boston, Harvard Business School Press, 2004.

Langley GJ, Nolan KM, Nolan TW, et al: The Improvement Guide: A Practical Approach to Enhancing Organizational Performance. San Francisco, Jossey-Bass, 1996.

Leatherman S, McCarthy D: Quality of Health Care for Children and Adolescents: A Chartbook. New York, Commonwealth Fund, 2004.

Palmer RH, Miller MR: Methodologic challenges in developing and implementing measures of quality for child health care. Ambula Pediatr 2001;1:39-52.

US Department of Health and Human Services, Office of Minority Health: National Standards on Culturally and Linguistically Appropriate Services (CLAS) in Health Care: Final Report. Washington, DC, 2001.

REFERENCES

1. Institute of Medicine: Crossing the Quality Chasm: A New Health System for the 21st Century. Washington, DC, National Academy Press, 2001.

2. Institute of Medicine: To Err Is Human. Washington, DC, National Academies Press, 1999.

3. Institute of Medicine: Unequal Treatment: Confronting Racial and Ethnic Disparities in Health Care. Washington, DC, National Academy Press, 2002.

4. Lye PS, Rauch DA, Ottolini MC, et al: Pediatric hospitalists: Report of a leadership conference. Pediatrics 2006;117:1122-1130.

5. Breyfogle FW III: Implementing Six Sigma, 2nd ed. Hoboken, NJ, Wiley, 2003.

6. Womack JP, Jones DT: Lean consumption. Harvard Business Review 2005;83:58-68, 148.

7. Homer CJ, Marino B, Cleary PD, et al: Quality of care at a children's hospital: The parent's perspective. Arch Pediatr Adolesc Med 1999;153:1123-1129.

8. Co JPT, Ferris TG, Marino BL, et al: Are hospital characteristics associated with parental views of pediatric inpatient care quality? Pediatrics 2003;111:308-314.

9. Schoen C, Osborn R, Huynh PT, et al: Taking the pulse of health care systems: Experiences of patients with health problems in six countries. Health Aff (Millwood) 2005 (Epub ahead of print).

10. Srivastava R, Norlin C, James BC, et al: Community and hospital-based physicians' attitudes regarding pediatric hospitalist systems. Pediatrics 2005;115:34-38.

11. Joffe S, Manocchia M, Weeks JC, Cleary PD: What do patients value in their hospital care? An empirical perspective on autonomy centered bioethics. J Med Ethics 2004;30:610-612.

12. Thom DH, Hall MA, Pawlson LG: Measuring patients' trust in physicians when assessing quality of care. Health Aff 2004;23:124-132.

13. American Academy of Pediatrics, Committee on Hospital Care, Institute for Family-Centered Care: Family-centered care and the pediatrician's role. Pediatrics 2003;112:691-696.

14. National Initiative for Children's Healthcare Quality: Improving Cultural Competency in Children's Health Care. Cambridge, Mass, NICHQ, 2005.

CHAPTER 5

Patient Safety and Medical Errors

Christopher P. Landrigan and Jeremy Friedman

The Institute of Medicine (IOM) estimates that medical errors cause as many as 98,000 deaths each year in the United States,[1] which would make medical error the sixth leading cause of death nationally.[2] Such errors have been found to result predominantly from multiple subtle failures in complex systems rather than from single failures on the part of problematic providers. Improving safety in hospitals has become a priority of the U.S. government in recent years, but progress has been slow. Fundamental redesign of the health care system is required to improve patient safety, and many solutions are difficult to implement.[3]

Pediatric hospitalists are in a unique position to improve patient safety. Hospitalists are invested in the systems of delivering care in an unprecedented manner and are frequently in positions of leadership that facilitate education and change. This chapter reconsiders previously reviewed literature on the safety of hospitalized patients,[4] with an eye toward how hospitalists can implement safety improvements and educational initiatives to promote a culture of safety in their institutions.

ORIGINS OF MEDICAL ERROR

As the problem of patient safety has received increasing attention in recent years, it has become clear that errors are common and are closely tied to both our own thought processes and the current systems of care delivery. Adverse events due to health care providers' errors are reproducible products of working conditions and the environment, as well as the complexity of hospital systems. Human factors engineering, a discipline that combines an understanding of psychology with the study of the human–work setting interface, has cogently categorized the nature of human and systemic error across fields.[5-7] Effective systems can be designed that reduce the occurrence of errors as well as the harm that results from them.[5]

Human cognitive processes have inherent fallibilities that can be consistently unmasked under experimental conditions. Many of these fallibilities surround erroneous probabilistic thinking; failure to consistently recognize and actively focus on emerging problems when conducting routine, over-learned, largely automated activities; limitations of short-term memory; and misapplication of knowledge. For example, a hospitalist who recently admitted a child with mild, diffuse abdominal pain that unexpectedly turned out to be appendicitis may have an inappropriately increased probability of concluding that the next child who comes in with abdominal pain has appendicitis, rather than broadly considering all possibilities in the differential diagnosis (an

error referred to as the *availability heuristic*). He or she may ignore data to the contrary and focus only on data that support the initial supposition (confirmation bias). Similar errors in probabilistic thinking are common and well described elsewhere.[5-7]

System complexity likewise contributes to error. A medication delivery system, for example, has many individual steps (e.g., a physician writes an order, a nurse transcribes the order, a unit clerk faxes the order, and so on). With 25 serial steps in total, each of which is performed correctly 99% of the time, the net probability of a medication order making it through the system with no error is only 78% ($0.99^{25} = 0.78$).

Reason's model of how erroneous actions lead to harm may also be helpful in understanding how risks persist even in the face of systems established to prevent harm (Fig. 5-1).[8] When a "trigger," or error, occurs, multiple "shields" in place within the system may block the error from causing harm. For example, if a physician writes an erroneous order, a nurse, clerk, pharmacist, or parent of a patient may intercept it before it reaches the patient. All such shields are imperfect, however, and a small portion of errors will penetrate each defense and cause harm. Further, each of these shields may be capable of generating its own downstream errors, even when the initial action was error free (e.g., a nurse may make an error in transcribing an order or administering a drug). Better systems tend to have fewer triggers and fewer, more effective shields.

EPIDEMIOLOGY OF ADVERSE EVENTS

As indicated by the IOM report, serious errors and adverse events (AEs) in medicine are common (see Fig. 5-2 for definitions). In a review of 30,000 inpatient charts, the Harvard Medical Practice Study (HMPS) found that 3.7% of patients hospitalized in New York State experienced AEs.[9] Common AEs include nosocomial infections (see Chapter 6), medication errors, operative complications, and diagnostic mistakes. In this study, 71% of AEs caused short-term disability, 3% caused permanent disability, and 14% were fatal; 69% were judged to be due to an error.[5,10] In a similar study conducted in Utah and Colorado, Thomas and colleagues found that 2.9% of patients suffered AEs.[11] Using a more inclusive chart review methodology, the Quality in Australian Health Care Study found that 13% of all inpatients suffered AEs, half of which were preventable.[12]

AEs are expensive as well as harmful. The HMPS found the annual cost of AEs to New York State was $878 million. Looking at an important subset of AEs—adverse drug events (ADEs)—Bates and coworkers found that for a large teaching hospital, the annual costs of all ADEs and preventable ADEs were $5.6 million and $2.8 million, respectively.[13] Nationally, hospital ADEs may cost as much as $2 billion per year.[13,14]

Dr. Landrigan has conducted research on the incidence of adverse events and complications in patients with bronchiolitis that was supported by grants from Medimmune, Inc.

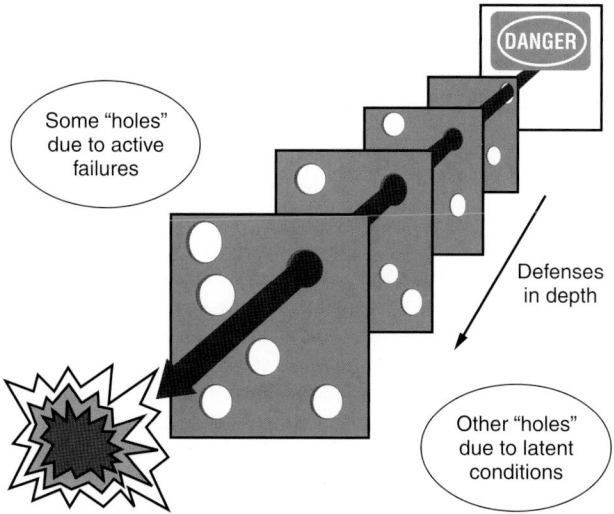

Figure 5-1 Reason's Swiss cheese model. (From Reason J: Managing the Risks of Organizational Accidents. Burlington, Vt, Ashgate, 2000.)

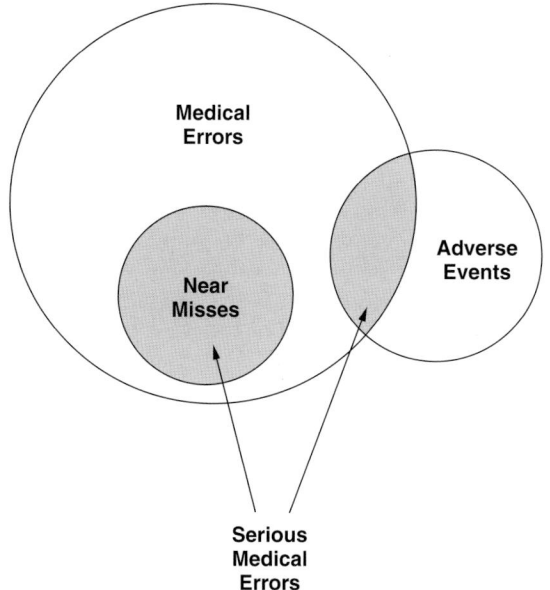

Figure 5-2 Relationship between adverse events and medical errors. An *adverse event* (AE) is any injury caused by medical management, whether due to an error (preventable AE) or not (nonpreventable AE). Injuries due to an underlying disease rather than medical management are not AEs. A *medical error* is any error in the delivery of care, whether it has the potential to cause harm or not. A *near miss* (or potential AE) is an error with significant potential to harm that does not do so, either because it is intercepted (intercepted near miss) or because the patient withstood the error without suffering detectable harm (nonintercepted near miss). Errors that cause harm or have the significant potential to cause harm are *serious medical errors* (i.e., near misses plus preventable AEs). Errors with little or no potential for harm are not serious medical errors, nor are nonpreventable AEs. (Adapted from Bates DW, Boyle DL, Vander Vliet MB, et al: Relationship between medication errors and adverse drug events. J Gen Intern Med 1995;10:205.)

The incidence of AEs among pediatric inpatients in particular has been examined in several ways. The HMPS included pediatric patients and found 12.9 AEs per 1000 discharges for patients aged 0 to 15 years.[15] Several recent studies have used the Agency for Healthcare Research and Quality's patient safety indicators (PSIs)—markers of possible AEs coded in administrative billing databases (e.g., foreign body left in after procedure, failure to rescue, iatrogenic pneumothorax, infection as a result of medical care)—to identify AEs.[16-18] These events are associated with significant and substantial increases in hospital charges, length of stay, and mortality. In 2000 PSI events led to charges of more than $1 billion in pediatric hospitals.[17] Because these events are identified from administrative databases, they represent only a fraction of all events, and not all events identified represent true AEs; nevertheless, the collection of such data can provide important high-level indicators of safety in an institution.

Some work has also been conducted to measure the incidence of complications and AEs in inpatients with bronchiolitis in particular, one of the most common diseases treated by pediatric hospitalists. Willson and associates analyzed clinical data from inpatients with bronchiolitis at 10 children's hospitals and found that 79% suffered a complication in care, although the proportion due to error was unclear.[19] McBride and colleagues, in a prospective study, found that 9 preventable AEs (i.e., those due to errors in care) occurred per 100 bronchiolitis admissions; among critically ill patients, 68 preventable AEs occurred per 100 admissions.[20] Studies evaluating AEs related to other common pediatric conditions should be a focus of future hospitalist research.

ADVERSE DRUG EVENTS AND MEDICATION ERRORS

ADEs are a common subtype of AE. Patients frequently suffer injuries secondary to medications,[21,22] many of which are preventable.[21,23] The ADE Prevention Study found that 6.5% of hospitalized adults suffered ADEs,[21,24] and of these, 28% were due to errors and thus were preventable.

Although preventable ADEs are common, medication errors that cause no harm are even more widespread. Only a fraction of all medication errors causes ADEs, because most are relatively minor, intercepted, or absorbed by a robust patient without causing any measurable damage. Studying noninjurious errors can be useful, however, because even minor errors can provide insights into latent systemic hazards that can lead to harm.

In some of the first studies of medication errors, Lesar and coworkers found that 3.1 errors occurred per 1000 orders, 58% of which were potentially harmful.[25] Folli and associates identified 4.7 errors per 1000 orders.[26,27] Both these studies included only those medication errors that were detected and prevented in the pharmacy, however, which represent only a fraction of all medication errors. In a more comprehensive study, Bates and colleagues found 5.3 errors per 100 orders,[28] a rate that is 10 times higher than that detected in the earlier pharmacist studies.

Hospitalized children are particularly vulnerable to medication errors. First, virtually all pediatric medications are weight based, which introduces the potential for serious errors due to miscalculations or misplaced decimal points. Moreover, many pediatric medications must be mixed by pharmacists or nurses at the time of use, providing a second opportunity for miscalculation. In addition, many pediatric medications come in multiple formulations (e.g., ibuprofen drops for infants and elixir for children), which can lead to over- or underdosing due to confusion regarding a medication's concentration. Finally, children are less likely than adults to detect errors or AEs in evolution.

In a study of the incidence of pediatric medication errors, Kaushal and coworkers found that total rates of medication errors and ADEs in pediatric settings were similar to adult hospital rates, but potential ADEs (near misses) were three times as common.[29] Of the 10,778 orders that were reviewed, 5.7% were found to contain errors. Of these, roughly 1 in 5 were serious errors, and a total of 5 erroneous orders went on to cause harm (1% of errors). Although 5 injuries per 10,000 orders (or 1 per 2000 admissions) initially sound reassuring, it is important to understand that these data were collected over only a handful of weeks in two hospitals. Extrapolated to a national level—in 2003 there were 36,610,535 admissions to 5,764 registered hospitals[30]—these data suggest a nationwide annual incidence of preventable ADEs similar to the number estimated by the IOM. Although medication errors can occur at any of the multiple steps in the medication delivery process, hospitalists should recognize that 74% of all errors in the Kaushal study, and 91% of near misses, were committed by physicians writing orders.

Additional studies of pediatric ADEs and medication errors have generally reinforced the finding that they are common.[31-33] In all these studies, decimal point errors and miscalculation of doses were important sources of serious error.

ADDRESSING AND IMPROVING PATIENT SAFETY

To date, efforts to improve pediatric patient safety have been hampered by the following factors:

- Failure to recognize the problem, exacerbated by a limited understanding among medical personnel of human factors and complexity theory.
- Inadequate reporting of errors, compounded by a justified fear of litigation.
- Limited number of interventions that have proved effective in pediatric settings, many of which are difficult to implement and have substantial up-front costs.

Many physicians continue to believe that injuries due to serious medical errors are uncommon and, when they do occur, inevitable. In part, this is a product of the epidemiology of errors: although serious errors leading to injury are quite common within a medical center, the number of errors in which any individual is involved (and of which he or she is aware) is typically quite small. When the uncommon experiences of many physicians nationwide are added together, however, the magnitude of the problem is substantial, as indicated by the IOM report.

Reporting of medical errors is particularly problematic. Most hospitals identify AEs primarily through the collection of formal incident reports.[34-36] This mechanism identifies only 6% of all AEs that could be captured with active surveillance, however, in pediatric as well as adult settings.[37-43] Physicians are typically loath to report any errors that they

recognize, out of fear that exposure could lead to malpractice litigation. Local and national initiatives are under way to promote anonymous reporting systems that will remove such concerns, but these efforts are in their infancy.

MEDICAL EDUCATION ON PATIENT SAFETY

In addition to these problems, the education of medical students, house officers, and practicing physicians regarding key topics in patient safety—teamwork training, medication safety, the effects of sleep deprivation, and the disclosure of medical errors, to name but a few—has been limited. Medical school and postgraduate training traditionally tend to focus on individual acquisition of pathophysiologic knowledge and case-based understanding of disease causes and management. Less training time is devoted to the individual physician-patient relationship. Many specialties remain rigidly hierarchical, and junior members of medical teams are discouraged from speaking up when safety concerns arise (sometimes referred to as hierarchical barriers).[44] The modern reality that hospital care involves large numbers of physicians, physicians-in-training, nurses, pharmacists, and ancillary clinical providers (each of whom thinks of the patient as his or her patient) is often largely ignored, and teamwork skills, shared responsibility, and systemic awareness are inadequately emphasized. Such education is essential if common sources of error, such as miscommunication, adverse working conditions, and hierarchical barriers, are to be overcome.

MORBIDITY AND MORTALITY REVIEWS

Although many mechanisms exist by which patient safety principles can be taught, one of the most effective may be the morbidity and mortality (M&M) review process. M&M review has been a part of hospital practice for generations, and it is a familiar forum in which to discuss adverse outcomes. In many institutions, however, it lacks a precise definition, a standard format, and consistently identified goals; as a result, it is less effective in providing a patient safety curriculum than it could be.

Most of the M&M literature pertains to surgery and anesthesia.[45] The Accreditation Council for Graduate Medical Education, the only North American organization that addresses when M&M reviews should occur and what should take place at them, requires that surgery programs discuss "all deaths and complications that occur on a weekly basis."[46] There is no similar requirement for medical specialties. It is generally accepted that all deaths that occur in the hospital require some level of review, but the process for doing so differs widely among institutions. There is even greater variability in dealing with morbidity reviews, because the definition of morbidity is more subjective and there are no uniform standards spelling out what type of morbidity requires review. The goals and objectives of M&M rounds are not uniform and are somewhat dependent on the individuals facilitating the reviews.

In setting up M&M rounds, it is important to establish both a goal for each individual session and goals for the M&M program as a whole. A comprehensive introductory patient safety curriculum, to be administered over the course of a year, can be introduced alongside case-based M&M

rounds. In a study of all university-affiliated pediatric hospitals in Canada, the primary purpose of M&M rounds was believed to be "education" and "improvement of patient care" as opposed to pure "peer review."[47] In a survey of staff surgeons and surgical house staff across the United States, both groups perceived "education" and "reduction of error" to be the primary focus.[48]

To achieve the goals of improving patient safety and effectively educating staff, relevant cases need to be presented and discussed in an appropriate manner. Often, minimal attempts are made to ensure the complete identification and reporting of complications. For instance, in a study of a large surgical program, there was a significant discrepancy in the number and types of adverse outcomes found in a prospective database of surgical complications and those actually presented at M&M reviews. Although the most severe complications were usually reported, a large proportion of less severe but more prevalent complications remained unreported.[49] It seems appropriate for morbidity cases to be selected for presentation based largely on the ability to learn from the case and make changes as a result of the lessons learned.

More than 90% of internal medicine programs in the United States report having M&M rounds, usually monthly, with mandatory attendance by trainees. Most cases are selected because of unexpected AEs or suspected errors, with the remainder being selected for teaching value.[45] In a prospective survey, however, it was noted that only 37% of internal medicine cases presented at M&M reviews included AEs (compared with 72% of surgical cases). Errors were attributed to a particular cause in only 38% of cases, and conference leaders seldom used explicit language signifying that an error was being discussed or acknowledged an error, thereby missing an opportunity to model the recognition and discussion of errors.[50] Some physicians believe that the give-and-take of the discussion constitutes effective peer review and that this provides an adequate means of changing practice patterns when needed. Often there is no documentation of conclusions and actions, however, so the ability to track the effectiveness of the actions or to detect trends is lost.

Barriers to performing appropriate M&M reviews include the anxiety of acknowledging individual error, potential loss of respect, and fear of legal action. Learning from one's errors is important, but confronting them is difficult, especially in front of a group of peers. Surgical residents across the United States believe that M&M reviews could be improved by decreasing defensiveness and blame.[48] Other barriers that have been identified are lack of time and resources. Only 11% of those responsible for running their divisional M&M reviews felt that they had received any training or guidance on how to conduct such reviews.[47]

There is no standard blueprint for the ideal pediatric M&M review process. One must take into account the size and type of hospital, the policies of the institution, the time and resources available, and the laws regarding confidentiality. As hospitalists, we are in an excellent position to deal with some of these issues. Studying the outcomes and effectiveness of M&M reviews is important and can serve as a vehicle for introducing house staff and faculty to core topics in patient safety. Box 5-1 contains a list of basic principles that can guide the M&M process.

Box 5-1   Principles of Effective Morbidity and Mortality Reviews

1. M&M reviews should be mandatory for all inpatient pediatric medicine units to ensure that the care provided was timely and appropriate, to learn from the event, and to develop new knowledge and improved systems of care. Reviews should emphasize learning and the prevention of similar occurrences.

2. Every mortality and significant morbidity should be reviewed in a timely manner. Morbidity can be defined as "an untoward event or complication, which under optimal conditions, is not a natural consequence of the patient's disease or treatment."[75]

3. Identification of cases varies among institutions, but a list of criteria should be developed (e.g., transfers to the ICU, respiratory or cardiac arrests on the unit, moderate and severe incident reports), and a number of key personnel should be designated to ensure that these cases are assessed regarding their suitability for presentation at rounds.

4. Cases should be selected both for their individual educational value and to expose attendees to a broad range of patient safety themes. In conjunction with case-based presentations, M&M can be an ideal forum to introduce monthly lectures on broader patient safety topics over the course of a year (see *http://www.rmf.harvard.edu/education-interventions/materials-for-instructors/patient-safety/instructors.aspx* for an example of a patient safety curriculum and some teaching materials).

5. M&M rounds should occur at least monthly and should be conducted in a multidisciplinary forum, with attendance expected by attending staff and trainees. When appropriate, members of other divisions should be invited to the review.

6. Confidentiality should be assured.

7. The moderator should be an experienced staff physician.

8. Reviews should include all the relevant information (including radiographs, pathology slides, and the like), and the presenters should review the applicable literature, if appropriate.

9. Minutes of the review should be recorded, including a brief summary of the relevant history, issues arising from the case, and recommendations and action plans. The individual or group responsible for carrying out the action plan should be named, and a timeline should be set. If a literature review was presented, one or two pertinent references can be included.

10. Recommendations for documentation include the following: names should not be used in the history and issue section, speculation and the language of blame should be avoided, reviews should emphasize "systems" rather than "individuals," and all pages should be numbered and marked "confidential."

11. Copies of the minutes should be sent to other divisions and individuals involved in the case for their review and comment.

12. The hospital should have an oversight committee with a broad-based membership that reviews the minutes from all divisional M&M reviews to identify hospital issues and trends, as well as to provide guidance and to act as a resource.

DISCLOSURE OF MEDICAL ERRORS

Historically, preventable AEs were disclosed in hospitals only when doing so was unavoidable. When disclosure occurred, it generally consisted of an unemotional statement of facts, perhaps out of fear that an apology would suggest legal liability. More recently, it has become clear that when a medical error occurs, patients want to be informed. They want to know what happened, why it happened, and what will be done to prevent a recurrence, and they want an apology.[51-53]

There are a number of ethical, moral, and professional principles underlying the physician's duty to inform patients of AEs. Respect for patient autonomy is a cornerstone of medical ethics and includes the patient's right to all the information necessary to make informed and educated decisions about his or her care. Honest communication promotes trust between the physician and patient, and open discussion of errors promotes patient safety by encouraging systems improvements. The main barriers to physician disclosure are difficulty admitting a mistake, fear of implicating others, and, most of all, concern about legal repercussions. This is compounded by the difficulty of communicating bad news and confusion about causation and responsibility.

One of the most controversial issues around the disclosure of AEs is the impact on possible litigation.[54] Disclosure may reduce the risks of lawsuits because some patients take legal action to find the answers they believe have been withheld by their physicians, to ensure that measures have been put in place to avoid a recurrence, or to have the responsible parties held accountable. Mock jury studies and empirical evidence suggest that disclosure can be helpful in limiting the amount of a settlement as well as moving the focus from the injury itself to the cause.[55] The Veteran Affairs Medical Center in Lexington, Kentucky, is an innovator in the area of disclosure, and empirical evidence from this center showed a favorable impact on the outcome of malpractice suits, with smaller payouts per claim.[56] The ability to generalize these findings to nonfederal medical centers is limited, however. In contrast, other studies have found that although full disclosure improved patient satisfaction, trust, and emotional response, it rarely abrogated the tendency for legal action.[51]

In the only pediatric study to date, almost all the parents wanted full and timely disclosure, regardless of the severity of the event.[57] It also found that the likelihood of parents taking legal action decreases with disclosure, versus learning of the error through other means. The question of whether or what to disclose to the child has not been studied.

Many institutions have begun to develop disclosure policies that deal with AEs due to medical errors. Such policies need to address what should be disclosed, by whom, and when and how to do it. The Harvard Hospitals consensus statement released in 2006 reflects current leading practices in the communication of this information and provides an excellent guide for hospital-based physicians.[58] Box 5-2 summarizes key recommendations from the consensus statement.

PREVENTING INJURY DUE TO ERROR

Once the presence of medical errors is acknowledged within an institution, and education regarding patient safety has been implemented, three types of strategies may be

---

Box 5-2 A Brief Guide to Disclosure

What and when?
  The patient, family, or both should be fully and promptly informed of any AE or serious error that reaches the patient.
  Disclosure should occur within 24 hours after the event is discovered.
  Provide an honest explanation of what happened (report the facts).
  Express regret.
  Explain that the cause of the event is being investigated.
  Explain what is being done to mitigate the effects of the injury.
  Explain what will be done to prevent future events.
  Provide clear documentation.
Who and how?
  Ideally, disclosure should be made by the attending physician or physician responsible for the treatment.
  The person responsible for the next steps in care should be present.
  Include the patient's primary nurse.
  Meet in a private, quiet, and nonintimidating environment.
  Conduct follow-up sessions promptly.
Support of the patient and family
  Inquire about their feelings related to the injury.
  Take these concerns seriously, and address them adequately.
  Maintain the therapeutic relationship.
  Provide the necessary information for clinical and financial counseling and support.
  Put billing on hold, pending an analysis of the event.
  Investigate ways to provide financial support for short-term expenses related to the event.
Follow-up care
  Schedule follow-up meetings and clinic visits.
  Provide psychological and social support.
  Ensure communication about the final results of investigations and remedial actions.
Support of caregivers
  Establish a program to provide support to caregivers involved in these events.
  Provide for structured debriefing and documentation.
  Coach caregivers in communication skills surrounding disclosure.
Teaching and education
  Provide educational and training programs for various levels of caregivers.
  Provide training in how to deal with personal feelings and how to support colleagues.
  Include disclosure training in general orientation as well as refresher courses.
  Provide contact numbers for expert assistance for staff after serious events.

Adapted from Massachusetts Coalition for the Prevention of Medical Errors: When Things Go Wrong: Responding to Adverse Events. A Consensus Statement of the Harvard Hospitals. March 2006.

---

used to take concrete steps to reduce medical error rates: (1) preventing errors from occurring in the first place; (2) intercepting errors early, before they reach the patient; and (3) ameliorating harm from errors that do reach the patient.

Studies conducted since the early 1990s have demonstrated the effectiveness of many such interventions. An evidence-based assessment of 79 interventions was published in 2001 by the Agency for Healthcare Research and Quality.[59] Selected interventions relevant to hospitalists are discussed briefly in this section.

Ensuring Medication Safety

Computerized physician order entry can effectively prevent and intercept serious medical errors. Bates and colleagues found that computerized physician order entry with decision support (e.g., automated checking for allergies and drug-drug interactions) led to an initial 55% decrease in the rate of serious medication errors and an ultimate 81% reduction following full implementation of iterative improvements.[60,61] ADEs due to antibiotics decreased 70% following implementation of another computerized system.[62] In pediatric hospitals, medication errors were reduced 40% or more after the introduction of such systems.[63,64]

Other technological tools also have the potential to improve safety. In one study, a structured computerized sign-out was found to reduce cross-coverage errors.[65] Computerized AE detection systems, bar coding, and smart intravenous pumps may also improve safety.[59]

Clinical pharmacists who monitor orders may also be able to improve safety. Leape and associates found that the presence of clinical pharmacists in intensive care units (ICUs) decreased preventable order-related ADE rates by 66%.[66] Introduction of ICU-based clinical pharmacists in pediatric hospitals was associated with a fivefold reduction in errors in another study, but no significant improvement in ward settings.[31,67]

Reducing Nosocomial Infections

Maximal sterile barriers (mask, cap, sterile gloves, gown, and large drape) and antiseptic-impregnated catheters significantly reduce nosocomial infections in adult settings. Nosocomial infections differ from noninfectious AEs, in that the precise timing of their origin (and thus the nature of any error that might have caused them) usually cannot be determined. Moreover, the percentage of nosocomial infections that may be preventable is unclear, because some occur despite perfect sterile techniques and catheter maintenance. Nevertheless, interventions to improve sterility have enhanced patient safety, indicating that many nosocomial infections are preventable. Raad and coworkers found that maximal sterile barriers decreased the number of catheter-related infections from 0.5 to 0.08 per 1000 catheter-days.[68] Antiseptic-coated catheters can lead to a twofold decrease in the odds of developing a catheter-related bloodstream infection in adults,[69] although their use in pediatrics has not been well studied (see Chapter 71).

Improving Working Conditions

Several recent studies have found that improving the working conditions of health care personnel can improve patient safety. The Harvard Work Hours, Health, and Safety Group found that eliminating traditional 24-hour-plus work shifts can substantially improve safety. Interns working traditional "q3" schedules with 30-hour shifts slept less, suffered twice as many attention-related failures on the job at night, and made 36% more serious medical errors, including more than five times as many serious diagnostic errors, than did those whose schedule was limited to 16 consecutive hours.[70,71] Interns themselves are placed at risk by traditional work schedules; those working 24 or more hours have twice the odds of being involved in a car crash while driving home from work.[72] Studies of nurses likewise suggest that workload and fatigue have substantial effects on error rates.[59,73]

CONCLUSION

Medical errors and AEs are common in hospitals and are just beginning to receive an appropriate level of attention in the medical community. Education regarding patient safety is essential for hospitalists and for their trainees and coworkers in inpatient settings; M&M conferences represent a powerful avenue for providing this education. Preventable AEs should be disclosed to families and patients, who universally expect an apology. Computerized order entry, clinical pharmacists, improved infection control, and amelioration of sleep deprivation and adverse working conditions have proved to be effective means of decreasing serious errors. Because recognition of patient safety hazards and adoption of solutions have been slow to date, the public has yet to experience the benefits from the extensive portfolio of patient safety research funded by the government since the mid-1990s.[3] Most Americans report dissatisfaction with the health care system, and half believe that it is unsafe.[74] Hospitalists are in a powerful position to study and improve the safety of pediatric inpatient care and translate research in patient safety into real improvements for hospitalized patients.

ACKNOWLEDGMENTS

Dr. Landrigan was the recipient of a career development award from the Agency for Healthcare Research and Quality (K08 HS13333).

REFERENCES

1. Institute of Medicine: To Err Is Human: Building a Safer Health System. Washington, DC, National Academy Press, 1999.
2. Kochanek KD, Murphy SL, Anderson RN, Scott C: Deaths: Final data for 2002. Natl Vital Stat Rep 2004;53:1-115.
3. Altman DE, Clancy C, Blendon RJ: Improving patient safety—five years after the IOM report. N Engl J Med 2004;351:2041-2043.
4. Landrigan CP: The safety of inpatient pediatrics: Preventing medical errors and injuries among hospitalized children. Pediatr Clin North Am 2005;52:979-993.
5. Leape LL: Error in medicine. JAMA 1994;272:1851-1857.
6. Reason J: Human Error. Cambridge, Cambridge University Press, 1990.
7. Rasmussen J, Jensen A: Mental procedures in real-life tasks: A case study of electronic trouble shooting. Ergonomics 1974;17:293-307.
8. Reason J: Managing the Risks of Organizational Accidents. Burlington, Vt, Ashgate, 2000.
9. Brennan TA, Leape LL, Laird N, et al: Incidence of adverse events and negligence in hospitalized patients: Results from the Harvard Medical Practice Study I. N Engl J Med 1991;1:370-376.
10. Leape LL, Lawthers AG, Brennan TA, Johnson WG: Preventing medical injury. QRB Qual Rev Bull 1993;19:144-149.

11. Thomas EJ, Studdert DM, Burstin HR, et al: Incidence and types of adverse events and negligent care in Utah and Colorado. Med Care 2000;38:271.

12. Wilson RM, Harrison BT, Gibberd RW, Hamilton JD: An analysis of the causes of adverse events from the Quality in Australian Health Care Study. Med J Aust 1999;170:411-415.

13. Bates DW, Spell N, Cullen DJ, et al: The costs of adverse drug events in hospitalized patients. Adverse Drug Events Prevention Study Group. JAMA 1997;227:307-311.

14. Classen DC, Pestotnik SL, Evans RS, et al: Adverse drug events in hospitalized patients: Excess length of stay, extra costs, and atttributable mortality. JAMA 1997;277:301-306.

15. Leape LL, Brennan TA, Laird N, et al: The nature of adverse events in hospitalized patients: Results of the Harvard Medical Practice Study II. N Engl J Med 1991;324:377-384.

16. Miller MR, Elixhauser A, Zhan C: Patient safety events during pediatric hospitalizations. Pediatrics 2003;111:1358-1366.

17. Miller MR, Zhan C: Pediatric patient safety in hospitals: A national picture in 2000. Pediatrics 2004;113:1741-1746.

18. Sedman A, Harris JM, Schulz K, et al: Relevance of the Agency for Healthcare Research and Quality patient safety indicators for children's hospitals. Pediatrics 2005;115:135-145.

19. Willson DF, Landrigan CP, Horn SD, Smout RJ: Complications in infants hospitalized for bronchiolitis or respiratory syncytial virus pneumonia. J Pediatr 2003;143(5 Suppl):S142-S149.

20. McBride SC, Chiang VW, Goldmann DA, Landrigan CP: Preventable adverse events in infants hospitalized with bronchiolitis. Pediatrics 2005;116:603-608.

21. Bates DW, Cullen D, Laird N, et al: Incidence of adverse drug events and potential adverse drug events: Implications for prevention. JAMA 1995;274:29-34.

22. Lazarou J, Pomeranz BH, Corey PN: Incidence of adverse drug reactions in hospitalized patients: A meta-analysis of prospective studies. JAMA 1998;279:1200-1205.

23. Bates DW, Leape LL, Petrycki S: Incidence and preventability of adverse drug events in hospitalized adults. J Gen Intern Med 1993;8:289-294.

24. Leape LL, Bates DW, Cullen DJ, et al: Systems analysis of adverse drug events. JAMA 1995;274:35-43.

25. Lesar TS, Briceland LL, Delcoure K, et al: Medication prescribing errors in a teaching hospital. JAMA 1990;263:2334.

26. Folli HL, Poole RL, Benitz WE, Russo JC: Medication error prevention by clinical pharmacists in two children's hospitals. Pediatrics 1987;79:718-722.

27. Institute of Medicine: Crossing the Quality Chasm: A New Health System for the 21st Century. Washington, DC, National Academy Press, 2001.

28. Bates DW, Boyle DL, Vander Vliet MB, et al: Relationship between medication errors and adverse drug events. J Gen Intern Med 1995;10:205.

29. Kaushal R, Bates DW, Landrigan C, et al: Medication errors and adverse drug events in pediatric inpatients. JAMA 2001;285:2114-2120.

30. American Hospital Association: Fast Facts on US Hospitals from AHA Hospital Statistics. *http://www.aha.org/aha/resource_center/fastfacts/fast_facts_US_hospitals.html.*

31. Kaushal R, Jaggi T, Walsh K, et al: Pediatric medication errors: What do we know? What gaps remain? Ambul Pediatr 2004;4:73-81.

32. Marino BL, Reinhardt K, Eichelberger WJ, Steingard R: Prevalence of errors in a pediatric hospital medication system: Implications for error proofing. Outcomes Manag Nurs Pract 2000;4:129-135.

33. Holdsworth MT, Fichtl RE, Behta M, et al: Incidence and impact of adverse drug events in pediatric inpatients. Arch Pediatr Adolesc Med 2003;157:60-65.

34. Berry LL, Segal R, Sherrin TP, Fudge KA: Sensitivity and specificity of three methods of detecting adverse drug reactions. Am J Hosp Pharmacy 1988;45:1534-1539.

35. Faich GA: National adverse drug reaction reporting: 1984-1989. Arch Intern Med 1991;151:1645-1647.

36. Rogers AS, Israel E, Smith CR, et al: Physician knowledge, attitudes, and behavior related to reporting adverse drug events. Arch Intern Med 1988;148:1600.

37. Cullen DJ, Bates DW, Small SD, et al: The incident reporting system does not detect adverse drug events: A problem for quality improvement. Jt Comm J Qual Improv 1995;21:541-548.

38. Scott HD, Thacher-Renshaw A, Rosenbaum SE, et al: Physician reporting of adverse drug reactions. Results of the Rhode Island Adverse Drug Reaction Reporting Project. JAMA 1990;263:1785-1788.

39. Classen DC, Pestotnik SL, Evans RS, Burke JP: Computerized surveillance of adverse drug events in hospital patients. JAMA 1991;266:2847-2851.

40. Bates DW, Makary MA, Teich JM, et al: Asking residents about adverse events in a computer dialogue: How accurate are they? Jt Comm J Qual Improv 1998;24:197-202.

41. Bates DW, O'Neil AC, Boyle D, et al: Potential identifiability and preventability of adverse events using information systems. J Am Med Inform Assoc 1994;1:404-411.

42. Bates DW, O'Neil AC, Petersen LA, et al: Evaluation of screening criteria for adverse events in medical patients. Med Care 1995;33:452-462.

43. Taylor JA, Brownstein D, Christakis DA, et al: Use of incident reports by physicians and nurses to document medical errors in pediatric patients. Pediatrics 2004;114:729-735.

44. Sexton JB, Thomas EJ, Helmreich RL: Error, stress and teamwork in medicine and aviation: Cross sectional surveys. BMJ 2003;320:745-749.

45. Orlander JD, Barber TW, Fincke BG: The morbidity and mortality conference: The delicate nature of learning from error. Acad Med 2002;77:1001-1006.

46. American Medical Association: Graduate Medical Education Directory 2002-2003. Chicago, AMA, 2002.

47. Friedman JN, Pinard MS, Laxer RM: The morbidity and mortality conference in university-affiliated pediatric departments in Canada. J Pediatr 2005;146:1-2.

48. Harbison SP, Regehr G: Faculty and resident opinions regarding the role of morbidity and mortality conference. Am J Surg 1999;177:136-139.

49. Feldman L, Barkun J, Barkun A, et al: Measuring postoperative complication in general surgery patients using an outcomes-based strategy: Comparison with complications presented at morbidity and mortality rounds. Surgery 1997;122:719.

50. Pierluissi E, Fischer MA, Campbell AR, Landefeld CS: Discussion of medical errors in morbidity and mortality conferences. JAMA 2003;290:2838-2842.

51. Mazor KM, Simon SR, Yood RA, et al: Health plan members' views about disclosure of medical errors. Ann Intern Med 2004;140:409-418.

52. Gallagher TH, Waterman AD, Ebers AG, et al: Patients' and physicians' attitudes regarding the disclosure of medical errors. JAMA 2003;289:1001-1007.

53. Mazor KM, Simon SR, Gurwitz JH: Communicating with patients about medical errors: A review of the literature. Arch Intern Med 2004;164:1690-1697.

54. Gallagher TH, Levinson W: Disclosing harmful medical errors to patients: A time for professional action. Arch Intern Med 2005;165:1819-1824.

55. Popp PL: How will disclosure affect future litigation? J Health Risk Manag 2003;23:5-9.

56. Kraman SS, Hamm G: Risk management: Extreme honesty may be the best policy. Ann Intern Med 1999;131:963-967.

57. Hobgood C, Tamayo-Sarver JH, Elms A, Weiner B: Parental preferences for error disclosure, reporting, and legal action after medical error in the care of their children. Pediatrics 2005;116:1276-1286.

58. Massachusetts Coalition for the Prevention of Medical Errors: When Things Go Wrong: Responding to Adverse Events. A Consensus Statement of the Harvard Hospitals. March 2006.

59. Making Health Care Safer: A Critical Analysis of Patient Safety Practices. AHRQ Publication No. 01-E058. Rockville, Md, Agency for Healthcare Research and Quality, 2001.

60. Bates DW, Teich J, Lee J, et al: The impact of computerized physician order entry on medication error prevention. J Am Med Inform Assoc 1999;6:321.

61. Bates DW, Leape LL, Cullen DJ, et al: Effect of computerized physician order entry and a team intervention on prevention of serious medication errors. JAMA 1998;280:1311-1316.

62. Evans RS, Pestotnik SL, Classen DC, et al: A computer-assisted management program for antibiotics and other antiinfective agents. N Engl J Med 1998;338:232-238.

63. King WJ, Paice N, Rangrej J, et al: The effect of computerized physician order entry on medication errors and adverse drug events in pediatric inpatients. Pediatrics 2003;112:506-509.

64. Potts AL, Barr FE, Gregory DF, et al: Computerized physician order entry and medication errors in a pediatric critical care unit. Pediatrics 2004;113:59-63.

65. Petersen LA, Orav EJ, Teich JM, O'Neil AC: Using a computerized sign-out program to improve continuity of inpatient care and prevent adverse events. Jt Comm J Qual Improv 1998;24:77-87.

66. Leape LL, Cullen DJ, Clapp MD, et al: Pharmacist participation on physician rounds and adverse drug events in the intensive care unit. JAMA 1999;282:267-270.

67. Kaushal R, Bates D, McKenna KJ, et al: Ward-based clinical pharmacists and serious medication errors in pediatric inpatients. In Proceedings of the Annual Meeting of the National Academy of Health, 2003.

68. Raad II, Hohn DC, Gilbreath BJ, et al: Prevention of central venous catheter-related infections by using maximal sterile barrier precautions during insertion. Infect Control Hosp Epidemiol 1994;15:231-238.

69. Veenstra DL, Saint S, Saha S, et al: Efficacy of antiseptic-impregnated central venous catheters in preventing catheter-related bloodstream infection: A meta-analysis. JAMA 1999;281:261-267.

70. Lockley SW, Cronin JW, Evans EE, et al: Effect of reducing interns' weekly work hours on sleep and attentional failures. N Engl J Med 2004;351: 1829-1837.

71. Landrigan CP, Rothschild JM, Cronin JW, et al: Effect of reducing interns' work hours on serious medical errors in intensive care units. N Engl J Med 2004;351:1838-1848.

72. Barger LK, Cade BE, Ayas NT, et al: Extended work shifts and the risk of motor vehicle crashes among interns. N Engl J Med 2005;352:125-134.

73. Rogers AE, Hwang WT, Scott LD, et al: The working hours of hospital staff nurses and patient safety. Health Aff (Millwood) 2004;23:202-212.

74. Kaiser Family Foundation, Agency for Healthcare Research and Quality, and Harvard School of Public Health: National Survey on Consumers' Experiences with Patient Safety and Quality Information, 2005.

75. Craddick JW, Bader BS: Medical Management Analysis: A Systematic Approach to Quality Assurance and Risk Management, vol 1. Auburn, Calif, JW Craddick, 1983.

CHAPTER 6

Infection Control for Pediatric Hospitalists

Susan E. Coffin and Keith H. St. John

INFECTION CONTROL: A PATIENT SAFETY ISSUE

Nosocomial infections are the single most common adverse event experienced by hospitalized children and adults. Recent data suggest that as many as 10% of patients develop nosocomial infections during admission to an acute care hospital.[1] Hospital-acquired infections increase morbidity, extend hospital stays, and raise hospital charges, and they are also associated with substantial increases of in-hospital mortality.

A recent analysis of discharge data from more than 5 million pediatric hospitalizations revealed that postoperative sepsis and infection as a result of medical care were common events among hospitalized children.[2] Children who developed nosocomial infections were found to have an increased median length of hospital stay, higher direct health care costs, and greater in-hospital mortality. These findings persisted even after adjustment for patient and hospital characteristics (Table 6-1).

Thus, the risk of hospital-acquired infections is significant, and the consequences are great. It is critical that all members of a health care team do everything they can to prevent their patients from acquiring nosocomial infections during hospitalization.

PREVENTING INFECTION

To prevent nosocomial infections, health care providers must understand how organisms are transmitted among individuals, how and when colonizing organisms (often referred to as commensal organisms) can become pathogenic, and how host and environmental factors modify the risk of nosocomial infection.

How Organisms Are Transmitted

Three basic mechanisms explain how most microorganisms are transmitted from one person to another: contact, either direct or indirect; droplet transmission; and airborne spread.

Contact is the most common route by which the vast majority of bacteria and viruses are spread among patients and health care workers. Viruses, such as respiratory syncytial virus, and bacteria, such as methicillin-resistant *Staphylococcus aureus* (MRSA), are typically spread directly from one person to another, particularly when infected or colonized children play together in hospital playrooms. Indirect contact or fomite transmission is another common way that organisms, especially those capable of surviving for long periods on inanimate objects, can spread within the hospital setting.

Respiratory droplets are responsible for the transmission of many common pediatric pathogens, including influenza viruses. Large respiratory droplets that contain viral particles are expelled from the nose and mouth during coughing, sneezing, and talking or during procedures such as suctioning, bronchoscopy, and cough induction by chest physiotherapy. These droplets can travel 3 to 6 feet in the air before settling. Transmission typically occurs when droplets come into contact with mucous membranes. Thus, face-to-face contact with an infected individual allows the transmission of many viral pathogens in the absence of direct physical contact.

Airborne transmission occurs by the dissemination of droplet nuclei (small particles ≤5 μm), which are evaporated droplets that contain infectious microorganisms. These droplet nuclei can remain suspended in the air for long periods, become airborne, and travel significant distances from their point of origin. Organisms such as *Mycobacterium tuberculosis* (MTB), varicella virus, and measles virus can survive desiccation and exist as droplet nuclei. The outbreak potential for these organisms is great.

Hand Hygiene and Standard Precautions

Hand hygiene is the most critical element in the prevention of nosocomial infections. Sadly, this practice is adhered to inconsistently by many individuals responsible for providing hands-on patient care.[3] Thus, health care workers are one of the most common sources of transmission of infection among patients. Hands should be washed with soap and water before and after eating, after using the bathroom, and when they are visibly soiled. At all other times, health care providers should use alcohol-based hand rubs. Alcohol hand rubs are more effective than soap and water at reducing microbial colonization of the hands.

In addition to performing hand hygiene before and after every patient contact, all health care workers should observe standard precautions with every patient. These are transmission-based precautions designed to protect health care workers from exposure to any known or unknown pathogens that might be transmitted by contact with blood or body fluids. Critical elements of standard precautions include (1) hand hygiene; (2) use of gloves when touching blood, body fluids, mucous membranes, or nonintact skin; and (3) mask, gown, and eye protection during procedures that might result in sprays of blood or body fluids.

Expanded Precautions and the Use of Personal Protective Equipment

In addition to standard precautions, expanded precautions markedly reduce the risk of transmission of many common agents of hospital-acquired infections (Table 6-2).[4] Because many community-acquired pediatric pathogens are easily spread in inpatient units, the use of expanded precautions is especially important for pediatric facilities.

Table 6-1 Impact of Nosocomial Infections in Hospitalized Children

	Mean Increase in Length of Stay (Days)	Mean Increase in Hospital Charges (US$)	Mean Increase in Hospital Mortality (OR)
Infection as a result of medical care	30	121,010	2.2
Postoperative sepsis	26	117,815	11

OR, Odds ratio.
Adapted from Miller MR, Zhan C: Pediatric patient safety in hospitals: A national picture in 2000. Pediatrics 2003;113:1741.

Some infections can be spread in multiple ways, necessitating the simultaneous use of multiple precautionary strategies (e.g., contact and airborne precautions for primary varicella infection). Special air handling and ventilation, as well as respiratory protection with a National Institute for Occupational Safety and Health–approved N-95 or higher respirator mask, are required to prevent airborne transmission of some microorganisms.

Health care workers must recognize the need for transmission-based precautions and be familiar with the appropriate use of personal protective equipment. For example, there is convincing evidence that the use of barrier precautions can reduce the transmission of MRSA. In an investigation that included weekly cultures of specimens from patients and personnel, molecular typing of isolates, and decolonization of organisms in some patients, investigators found that MRSA was spread to other patients at a rate of 0.14 transmission per day when patients who had been colonized or infected with MRSA were not cared for under contact isolation precautions. In contrast, when health care workers caring for patients with MRSA used gowns and gloves, the rate of MRSA transmission to other patients was 0.009 transmission per day. Thus, the risk of transmission was reduced nearly 16-fold when MRSA patients were cared for under contact isolation precautions.[5]

MINIMIZING THE RISK ASSOCIATED WITH MEDICAL DEVICES

Medical devices greatly increase the risk of nosocomial infection. Central venous catheters, urinary catheters, and endotracheal tubes all provide portals of entry that permit organisms to migrate from the skin and mucous membranes to sterile body sites. Implantable devices can also disrupt host defenses and provide a site sequestered from the surveillance of the immune system in which bacteria can flourish. Thus, strict adherence to aseptic technique when placing or manipulating a medical device is crucial to prevent device-related infection. The following sections outline additional strategies that reduce the risk of hospital-acquired infections in patients who require advanced medical technologies.

Table 6-2 Summary of Expanded Precautions for Selected Pathogens

Organism	Precautions*	Comments
Viruses		
Adenovirus	C + D	C only for patients with isolated conjunctivitis or gastroenteritis
Enterovirus	C	
Influenza virus	D	
Parainfluenza virus	C	
Respiratory syncytial virus	C	
Rotavirus	C	
Rubeola virus (measles)	A	
Varicella virus	C + A	Continue until all lesions are crusted; C only for immunocompetent patients with zoster
Bacteria		
Antibiotic-resistant organisms†	C	
Bordetella pertussis	D	Continue for 5 days after initiation of appropriate therapy
Clostridium difficile	C	
Mycobacterium tuberculosis	A	Only required for suspected cavitary, laryngeal, or miliary disease
Mycoplasma pneumoniae	D	
Neisseria meningitidis	D	Continue for 24 hr after initiation of appropriate therapy

*Specific recommendations for the proper use of personal protective equipment and patient placement can be found at
http://www.cdc.gov/ncidod/dhqp/gl_isolation.html.
†Including methicillin-resistant *Staphylococcus aureus*, vancomycin-resistant enterococci, and pan-resistant gram-negative organisms, including extended β-lactamase producers.
A, airborne precautions; C, contact precautions; D, droplet precautions.

Central Venous Catheters

Catheter-associated infections include localized infection at the site of catheter entry, phlebitis, and bloodstream infections. The latter is among the most common infection in hospitalized children, and the majority of these infections occur in patients with vascular catheters. Although the risk of bloodstream infection is greatest among patients with nontunneled central venous catheters, all vascular catheters, including peripheral intravenous catheters, are associated with an increased risk of infection.

Practices associated with a reduced risk of catheter-associated infection include (1) use of maximal sterile barrier precautions (e.g., cap, mask, sterile gown, sterile gloves, and large sterile drape) during catheter placement; (2) use of 2% to 3% chlorhexidine gluconate–70% isopropyl alcohol or other appropriate antiseptic agents to prepare the skin before placement and during routine catheter care; (3) prompt removal of catheters when they are no longer required; and (4) strict adherence to appropriate hand hygiene practices.[6] In studies performed in adult intensive care units, the use of antimicrobial-impregnated catheters led to reduced rates of central line–associated bloodstream infection. These catheters have not been adequately studied in children, however, and their role in the prevention of infection in pediatric patients remains unclear.[7]

Urinary Catheters

Similar to vascular catheters, the use of urinary catheters is associated with an increased risk of urinary tract infection. Experts estimate that catheter-associated urinary tract infections are the most common device-associated infection among hospitalized patients, although the burden of disease is likely greater in adult than in pediatric patients. Inappropriate and prolonged use of urinary catheters has been noted in as many as 50% of patients who develop catheter-associated urinary tract infections.

Guidelines have focused on several practices that can reduce the risk of these infections.[8] First, catheters should be placed in a sterile fashion. Second, a closed system for urine collection should always be maintained. Finally, the use of urinary catheters should be minimized by prompt removal whenever possible.

Ventilator–Associated Pneumonia

An endotracheal tube provides an ideal portal of entry for the numerous organisms that colonize the oropharynx, allowing their migration to the lower respiratory tract. An artificial airway also provides an ideal substrate for the formation of biofilm and inhibits host defenses, such as the gag reflex and cilia function. Pediatric patients appear to be at less risk of ventilator-associated pneumonia than adults, likely because they have fewer comorbid conditions such as chronic heart or lung disease or immunosuppressive conditions. However, pediatric intensive care physicians have developed strategies that reduce the risk of ventilator-associated pneumonia, including (1) use of noninvasive ventilation, (2) avoidance of nasotracheal intubation, (3) use of in-line suctioning to prevent the aspiration of pooled tracheal secretions, and (4) elevation of the head of the bed 45 degrees from horizontal, especially for patients receiving enteral nutrition.[9]

MANAGING PATIENTS WITH PROBLEM PATHOGENS

Antibiotic–Resistant Bacterial Organisms

Within 3 years of the introduction of penicillin, some strains of *Staphylococcus aureus* developed resistance to this drug. By the 1960s, some strains of *S. aureus* had become resistant to methicillin, a semisynthetic penicillin. Until recently, most infections due to MRSA species occurred in hospitalized patients, but MRSA has now emerged as a relatively common cause of infection among otherwise healthy children in the community, posing a challenge to infection control professionals. Hospital epidemiologists currently debate whether all patients admitted to the hospital should be screened to identify and isolate those colonized with MRSA.[10]

Contact precautions are commonly used to prevent patient-to-patient transmission of specific antibiotic-resistant bacteria. Because colonization with these organisms often persists for many months—even in the absence of ongoing exposure to antibiotics—precautions are typically continued indefinitely for patients known to harbor organisms such as vancomycin-resistant enterococci, extended-spectrum β-lactamase–producing gram-negative organisms, or pan-resistant enteric bacteria.

Mycobacterium tuberculosis

Unlike adults, many children infected with MTB are not considered contagious. Several factors explain the low rate of communicability associated with pediatric MTB infection.[11] First, most children infected with MTB have latent infections and small numbers of organisms that are well sequestered in granulomas. Second, children with active MTB infection rarely have endobronchial or cavitary lesions that communicate with the lower airways. Finally, young children typically do not generate sufficient intrathoracic pressure during coughing to raise MTB organisms into the oropharynx. Thus, expanded precautions are not routinely used for pediatric patients with MTB infection. Airborne precautions (including patient placement in a negative-pressure room and the use of N-95 respirator masks by health care providers) should be instituted for pediatric patients with suspected endobronchial or cavitary lesions or miliary disease. Precautions should be continued until the patient is demonstrated to have no acid-fast organisms visible on three consecutive induced sputum or gastric aspirates.

Viral Pathogens

During seasonal outbreaks, common pediatric viral pathogens can pose a significant risk to hospitalized children.[12] Transmission of organisms such as respiratory syncytial virus, influenza virus, or rotavirus is facilitated in inpatient pediatric units because of the relative concentration of susceptible subjects (i.e., the patients), ongoing introduction of virus from the community (by visitors, staff, and newly admitted patients), and environmental contamination with organisms that can live for hours on fomites. Hospital outbreaks of respiratory syncytial virus and rotavirus have been associated with insufficient staffing, suboptimal environmental cleaning, and illness among visitors and staff, as well as poor hand hygiene among health care workers.

CONCLUSION

Hospital-acquired infections are common and serious among pediatric patients. However, many of these infections can be prevented by the use of transmission-based standard and expanded precautions, uniform policies and procedures related to the use of medical devices, and scrupulous hand hygiene before and after patient care, between procedures, and when in contact with the patient's immediate environment.

REFERENCES

1. Burke JP: Infection control—a problem for patient safety. N Engl J Med 2003;348:651.
2. Miller MR, Zhan C: Pediatric patient safety in hospitals: A national picture in 2000. Pediatrics 2003;113:1741.
3. Boyce JM, Pittet D: Guideline for hand hygiene in health-care settings: Recommendations of the Healthcare Infection Control Practices Advisory Committee. MMWR Morb Mortal Wkly Rep 2002;51:1.
4. Huskins WC, Goldman DA: Prevention and control of nosocomial infections in health care facilities that serve children. In Feigin RD, Cherry J, Demmler G, Kaplan S (eds): Textbook of Pediatric Infectious Diseases. Philadelphia, WB Saunders, 2004, pp 2925-2941.
5. Jernigan JA, Titus MG, Groschel DH, et al: Effectiveness of contact isolation precautions during a hospital outbreak of methicillin-resistant *Staphylococcus aureus*. Am J Epidemiol 1996;143:496.
6. O'Grady NP, Alexander M, Dellinger EP, et al: Guidelines for the prevention of intravascular catheter-related infections. MMWR Recomm Rep 2002;51(RR-10):1.
7. McConnell SA, Gubbins PO, Anaissie EJ: Are antimicrobial-impregnated catheters effective? Clin Infect Dis 2004;39:1829.
8. Wong ES: Guideline for prevention of catheter-associated urinary tract infections. Available at *http://www.cdc.gov/ncidod/hip/GUIDE/uritract.htm.*
9. Tablan OC, Anderson LJ, Besser R, et al: Guidelines for preventing health-care–associated pneumonia, 2003: Recommendations of CDC and the Healthcare Infection Control Practices Advisory Committee. MMWR Recomm Rep 2004;53:1.
10. Muto CA, Jernigan JA, Ostrowsky BE, et al: SHEA guideline for preventing nosocomial transmission of multidrug-resistant strains of *Staphylococcus aureus* and *Enterococcus*. Infect Control Hosp Epidemiol 2003;24:362.
11. Diagnostic standards and classification of tuberculosis in adults and children. Am J Respir Crit Care Med 2000;161:1376.
12. Siegel JD: Controversies in isolation and general infection control practices in pediatrics. Semin Pediatr Infect Dis 2002;13:48.

CHAPTER 7

Evidence-Based Medicine

Jonathan M. Mansbach

Ideal clinical care integrates the health care professional's clinical experience, the individual patient's preferences and values, and the current best clinical evidence. Every hospitalist has his or her own set of clinical skills and experiences, and each patient has his or her own beliefs. The current best clinical evidence, however, is universal. How clinicians apply and explain this evidence to individual patients and integrate the evidence into care plans is the art of practicing evidence-based medicine (EBM). This chapter provides practical guidance on formulating questions and uses clinical examples to discuss how to efficiently and effectively search the medical literature.

FORMULATING QUESTIONS

Caring for patients frequently generates clinical questions. One study from 1985 found that general practitioners in office-based practices formulated two important clinical questions for every three patients examined.[1] Because there are millions of research articles in the world's literature, finding relevant articles and assessing their quality can be time-consuming and challenging. If a well-formulated clinical question is posed, the process of finding answers is easier.

There are four principal elements to consider when forming a focused clinical question: the patient population, the intervention being considered, the comparison group, and the measurable outcome. Including these four elements when formulating questions can help focus literature searches.[2]

The following example illustrates how a straightforward clinical question can be broken down into these four discrete elements. Suppose a 7-month-old with bronchiolitis is admitted to your service. You should consider the following elements:

1. Patient population (includes patient problem): children younger than 2 years with bronchiolitis
2. Intervention (diagnostic test or treatment), prognostic factor, or exposure: bronchodilators
3. Comparison group: placebo
4. Measurable outcome: reduce hospital length of stay

Often, developing one critical clinical question is sufficient, but a series of questions is sometimes required, especially when patients have complex medical problems. Clinical questions should be focused, but not overly narrow; a question that is too narrow may not have an answer, or the answer may not apply to the individual patient.

In pediatrics, defining the patient population is important. Many hospitalists care for patients ranging in age from infants to young adults, and they must often make judgments about whether studies that do not include a patient's specific age group are applicable. Frequently, a study in adults has been performed, and the hospitalist must decide whether the study applies to a particular pediatric or adolescent patient.

Sometimes the question may not have an intervention or a comparison group. For example, during morning rounds, you are informed that a 16-year-old girl with anorexia nervosa has been admitted for bradycardia. You then ask the question: In a female adolescent with a restrictive eating disorder and a heart rate of 35, what is the risk of sudden cardiac death? This question considers the prognosis of a specific population.

The measurable outcome chosen reflects the current clinical concerns, values, and preferences of the clinician and the patient. For example, when a child is admitted with right lower quadrant abdominal pain, the clinician may be most concerned about how to evaluate for appendicitis, but the patient and parent may be most concerned about pain control.

SEARCHING FOR INFORMATION

A solid comprehension of the disease process or syndrome is usually required before you can ask specific questions. Background information about pathophysiology, clinical presentation, treatment, complications, and outcomes may be found in print textbooks, review articles, or electronic textbooks. Print textbooks are valuable resources, particularly for well-established information. For example, if a patient presents with a parapneumonic effusion, reading a chapter in a textbook will help you understand the underlying disease process. A textbook chapter, however, may not contain up-to-date information on management; in this case, accessing electronic texts may be helpful.

You begin by reviewing the topic of parapneumonic effusions in children on UpToDate *(www.uptodate.com),* an easily accessible electronic textbook that is revised frequently and contains good references. If you enter "parapneumonic effusion" on the search line, there is one reference, "Pathogenesis and management of parapneumonic effusion and empyema." You click on the article and note when the review was most recently updated and when it is due to be revised. While reading the review, you remind yourself about the pathogenesis of pleural effusions and the differences among uncomplicated effusions, complicated effusions, and empyemas. There are more than 35 references, and each reference can be reviewed by clicking on the reference number. Other electronic texts are accessible via the Internet at Scientific American Medicine *(www.uic.edu/depts/lib/lhs/resources/guides/sam.pdf),* and an electronic version of the *Nelson Textbook of Pediatrics* and others textbooks are available through MD Consult *(www.mdconsult.com).* Some textbooks are also published electronically, such as *Oski's Pediatrics,* which comes with a CD-ROM.

Table 7-1 Suffixes

Suffix	Definition
.ab	Word in abstract
.au	Author
.jn	Journal
.ti	Word in title
.tw	Word in title or abstract
.yr	Year of publication

Table 7-2 Subheadings

Subheading	Definition
/ae	Adverse effects
/co	Complications
/di	Diagnosis
/dt	Drug therapy
/ep	Epidemiology
/hi	History
/th	Therapy

MEDLINE Searches

If you have more specific questions, MEDLINE is a good place to begin searching for answers. MEDLINE is a National Library of Medicine database derived from more than 4500 journals and includes over 10 million citations. PubMed, frequently used to access MEDLINE, contains additional basic science and life science articles. Ovid is another means of accessing MEDLINE and is the software referred to in this chapter.

Before you begin searching, it is helpful to understand how articles are indexed in MEDLINE. One method of limiting the number of articles you wade through is by attaching suffixes to the keyword. These suffixes allow you to search one journal, search by author, look for keywords in a title or abstract, or restrict the search by year of publication. Some useful suffixes are listed in Table 7-1. For example, if you search for articles related to bronchiolitis and type "bronchiolitis.tw", you will get 4000 hits. Typing "bronchiolitis.ti" generates 1900 hits. If you type "parapneumonic effusions.tw" and limit the search to review articles and English language, there are 32 hits. These articles include a consensus guideline published in *Chest* and Cochrane reviews. Note that a separate search must be conducted to find articles that specifically address the definition and management of empyema.

MEDLINE is also indexed using Medical Subject Headings, or MeSH terms. The keyword you type is automatically mapped to one of the subject headings. For example, if you search for the term *bronchiolitis*, it is automatically mapped to the MeSH terms *bronchiolitis*, *bronchiolitis obliterans*, *bronchiolitis viral*, and *bronchiolitis obliterans organizing pneumonia*. If you include *bronchiolitis* and *viral bronchiolitis*, there are 2100 hits and only 9 overlapping articles. To see the diagram of how bronchiolitis is mapped to the MeSH terms, type "tree bronchiolitis."

When there are too many articles to review, you can limit the search by using subheadings. Some helpful subheadings are listed in Table 7-2. For example, if you want to limit your search to 2003-2004 articles related to bronchiolitis therapy, you limit the publication years using the suffix ".yr" and type "bronchiolitis/dt" (generates 46 articles) and "viral bronchiolitis/dt" (generates 21 articles).

Other Web Resources

Other online resources include the National Guideline Clearinghouse. This site, accessed via *www.guidelines.gov,* is a database of evidence-based clinical practice guidelines and related documents originally developed by the Agency for Healthcare Research and Quality. A search for *bronchiolitis* will yield one clinical practice guideline from Cincinnati Children's Hospital Medical Center most recently updated in November 2001. Another site, *www.med.umich.edu/ pediatrics/ebm/Cat.htm,* from the University of Michigan, is a collection of critically appraised topics, many of which are applicable to inpatient medicine; these are short summaries and reviews of interesting articles in the literature. Another good site is *www.intensivecare.com.* This site has many EBM links and a searchable pediatric critical care evidence-based journal club. Although the reviews deal with critical care, many are relevant for hospitalists.

ASSESSING THE QUALITY OF INFORMATION

Once you find articles through MEDLINE, you still have to assess the quality of the studies and the validity of the conclusions. To bypass this time-consuming work, you can use Ovid to change the database searched from MEDLINE to EBM reviews. EBM reviews contain American College of Physicians (ACP) Journal Club, Database of Abstracts of Reviews of Effects (DARE), Cochrane Central Register of Controlled Trials, and Cochrane Database of Systematic Reviews. If you find an article on the topic of interest in one of these four databases, the quality of the article is assessed for you.

The editors of the ACP Journal Club collection identify clinically relevant, methodologically sound articles from top journals and provide commentary on the value of the article for clinical practice. If you search for *bronchiolitis* in the ACP, you will find one interesting article reviewing the use of dexamethasone for bronchiolitis.

DARE contains critical assessments of systematic reviews covering diagnosis, prevention, rehabilitation, screening, and treatment. DARE is produced by the National Health Services' Centre for Reviews and Dissemination at the University of York, England. If you search for *bronchiolitis* in DARE, you will find six articles.

The Cochrane Central Register of Controlled Trials is a database of definitive controlled trials in the literature; it is an unbiased source of data and information. The Cochrane group, the National Library of Medicine in Washington, DC, and Reed Elsevier of the Netherlands collaborate to identify relevant studies for inclusion in the database. The word *bronchiolitis* generates 239 articles.

Table 7-3	Validity
Parameter	Description
Prognosis	The patient population should be defined, and patients should be enrolled at a similar stage of illness. The follow-up rate should be high, and patients must be followed long enough to allow for the development of the chosen outcome. Better outcomes are objective and easily measured.
Treatment	The most valid treatment trials are randomized and blinded. The patients in each randomized group should be similar. An intention-to-treat analysis should be used; once a patient is randomized, he or she is included in the analysis. The chosen outcomes are relevant, objective, and measurable.
Diagnosis	The test being studied is explained in detail and compared to the best available standard. The cohort of patients tested is explained in detail and includes some measure of severity of illness.

The Cochrane Database of Systematic Reviews includes the Cochrane Collaboration's regularly updated systematic reviews about therapy, intervention, and prevention. The Cochrane Collaboration was developed in 1992 on the premise that interventions would be more effective if they were based on recent evidence. The reviews are presented as complete reviews or as protocols yet to be finished. The completed reviews have summary statements and graphs. There are 39 systematic reviews related to the word *bronchiolitis*.

ASSESSING VALIDITY

The aforementioned databases and websites cannot address all the problems a hospitalist will encounter. Therefore, having a basic understanding of how to assess an article's validity is helpful. Table 7-3 lists some basic parameters that can help evaluate the validity of an article investigating a prognostic factor, a treatment, or a diagnostic test.[2-4]

APPLYING INFORMATION TO PATIENTS

Integrating valid information into the care of individual patients is the art of practicing EBM. For example, a double-blind randomized, controlled trial has determined that when medicine Z is given to patients with bronchiolitis, it reduces the length of stay in the hospital. You determine that the study is valid but wonder whether it applies to your particular patient. For example, does the population in the trial sufficiently match the age, past medical history, severity of illness, and other characteristics of your patient? Is it possible that your patient with congenital heart disease is different enough from the otherwise healthy children in the trial that the risk of treatment increases? Does drug Z interact with other medications, altering the risk-benefit ratio? Are there other social factors (financial constraints, beliefs about medicine) that should be considered?

PUTTING IT ALL TOGETHER

During morning rounds, you are told about a 3-year-old child whose history, physical examination, and chest radiograph are all consistent with the diagnosis of pneumonia with an effusion. You begin considering antibiotic choices, the need for further diagnostic tests, and the merits of thoracentesis, video-assisted thoracoscopic surgery, and fibrinolytics. You decide that you need more information and want to review the most recent literature before making any decisions.

After reviewing background information on UpToDate, you pose the following question: In toddlers with parapneumonic effusions, does surgical management improve long-term lung function or shorten length of stay compared with nonsurgical management? You enter "parapneumonic effusion" into the EBM review database, which generates three articles. One Cochrane Database review investigates surgical (video-assisted thoracoscopic surgery) versus nonsurgical (chest tube drainage with streptokinase) management of pleural empyema. This topic review includes only one randomized trial of 20 adult patients.[5] Although it is problematic to make recommendations based on one small trial, the results of the trial demonstrated that the surgical group had a significantly shorter length of stay than the nonsurgical group. There is no mention in the study of long-term lung function. The possible benefits of shorter length of stay need to be weighed against the risks of general anesthesia and the necessity of one-lung ventilation. Additional risks and possible complications may not be apparent from such a small study. In addition, the hospitalist must decide whether this adult study is applicable to a pediatric patient.

The process described (using UpToDate and MEDLINE restricted to EBM reviews) likely takes less than 30 minutes. Yet this 30-minute search not only gives you a better understanding of background information but also reviews some of the most recent literature on the topic of interest. One of the drawbacks of EBM reviews, however, is the limited number of well-designed pediatric studies with large sample sizes that apply to general pediatric inpatient medicine. Further, the outcomes studied are not always relevant for an individual patient. Despite these drawbacks, searching for the most recent evidence always has merit. Even discovering that there are no studies adequately addressing the problem at hand is informative and can guide future research.

TEACHING EVIDENCE-BASED MEDICINE

One job of hospitalists who make rounds with medical students, residents, and fellows is teaching them how to practice EBM. Modeling your evidence-based approach to caring for patients is one method. Another interesting method presented by Sackett and Straus is having an "evidence cart" during rounds.[6] In their study, having quick and easy access to evidence altered patient care decisions and increased the incorporation of evidence into patient care. Effectively teaching specific evidence to fatigued residents and fellows is difficult. However, the results of an interesting ambulatory study suggest that the learner-focused "one-minute preceptor model" may be a quick, effective method of teaching.[7,8] As a group, hospitalists should not only continue to incorporate EBM into their practice but also to teach EBM to students, residents, fellows, and colleagues.

SUGGESTED READING

Feldman W: Evidence-Based Medicine. Hamilton, Ontario, BC Decker, 2000.

Moyer V, Elliott E, Davis R, et al (eds): Evidence Based Pediatrics and Child Health. London, BMJ Books, 2000.

Sackett D: Evidence Based Medicine: How to Practice and Teach EBM, 2nd ed. Philadelphia, Churchill Livingstone, 2000.

REFERENCES

1. Covell DG, Uman GC, Manning PR: Information needs in office practice: Are they being met? Ann Intern Med 1985;103:596-599.

2. Moyer V, Elliott E, Davis R, et al (eds): Evidence Based Pediatrics and Child Health. London, BMJ Books, 2000.

3. Richardson WS, Wilson MC, Guyatt GH, et al: Users' guides to the medical literature. XV. How to use an article about disease probability for differential diagnosis. Evidence-Based Medicine Working Group. JAMA 1999;281:1214-1219.

4. Richardson WS, Wilson MC, Williams JW Jr, et al: Users' guides to the medical literature. XXIV. How to use an article on the clinical manifestations of disease. Evidence-Based Medicine Working Group. JAMA 2000;284:869-875.

5. Wait MA, Sharma S, Hohn J, Dal Nogare A: A randomized trial of empyema therapy. Chest 1997;111:1548-1551.

6. Sackett DL, Straus SE: Finding and applying evidence during clinical rounds: The "evidence cart." JAMA 1998;280:1336-1338.

7. Irby DM, Aagaard E, Teherani A: Teaching points identified by preceptors observing one-minute preceptor and traditional preceptor encounters. Acad Med 2004;79:50-55.

8. Aagaard E, Teherani A, Irby DM: Effectiveness of the one-minute preceptor model for diagnosing the patient and the learner: Proof of concept. Acad Med 2004;79:42-49.

CHAPTER 8

Clinical Practice Guidelines

Kieran J. Phelan, Ed Donovan, Uma Kotagal, Emmanuel Doyne, and Scott Reeves

Clinical practice guidelines—systematically developed statements to assist practitioners and patients make decisions about appropriate health care for specific circumstances—are the cornerstone of efforts to improve the quality of inpatient pediatric care.[1,2] Since the Institute of Medicine's report on clinical practice guidelines in 1992 and its more recent *Crossing the Quality Chasm*, clinical practice guidelines have become widespread means of standardizing the care of patients with specific disorders.[1,3] Several national organizations and many regional and local health care organizations have developed such guidelines to assist practitioners in making management decisions.[4-6] The U.S. Agency for Healthcare Research and Quality has indexed thousands of adult and pediatric clinical practice guidelines and made them available electronically to the public through the National Guideline Clearinghouse *(http://www. guideline.gov/)*. Research on the development, evaluation, and dissemination of clinical practice guidelines and related process and patient outcomes has become more sophisticated.[7-11] Disseminating guidelines and changing physician behavior remain the challenges for institutions and individuals working toward more standardized, high-quality, evidence-based care.[12-15] When properly implemented, evidence-based clinical practice guidelines are a powerful method of reducing unnecessary variation in care and reliably delivering disease-specific best practices.[16-18]

WHY USE CLINICAL PRACTICE GUIDELINES?

Studies have shown that more than three quarters of the care provided on pediatric or medical inpatient services can be evidence based when the practitioner has the skills and resources available to efficiently access the best available evidence.[19,20] However, students, residents, physicians, patients, and families cannot help but be confused by the various opinions and management strategies employed by the different clinicians caring for children with seemingly common, well-understood disorders.[14,21,22] Experienced clinicians and clinical researchers seeking to develop and disseminate effective innovations in health care practice are often frustrated by the slow uptake and use of best evidence in the care of common pediatric conditions.[23] Clinical practice guidelines, when rigorously developed, implemented, and disseminated, are an attempt to bridge the gap between the best available research evidence and frontline practice. Guideline recommendations combine the best available evidence with clinical experience, patient biology, patient and family values regarding health care interventions, diagnostic testing, prognostication, cost-effectiveness, and other issues in the management of children with specific disorders.[11,24,25]

A critical issue for health care organizations and inpatient pediatric services in particular is reducing unwarranted variation in the management of common pediatric disorders.[15,18,21] Providers lacking experience with a given disorder may apply management strategies inappropriately. Errors of commission and omission can lead to unnecessary testing and interventions that increase the cost, admission rate, length of stay, and complications of inpatient pediatric care and decrease patient satisfaction.[15,22]

Guidelines are intended to be used flexibly to make health care management decisions, reducing the uncertainties and subsequent variations in care; they are not meant to be rigid principles applied to every child meeting the inclusion criteria for a specific guideline. There should be an understanding that most, but not all, children who satisfy such criteria can be effectively and efficiently managed within the parameters outlined.[2] Guidelines have become an important tool for defining effective care within health care organizations and among practitioners, providing a roadmap for improvement in the quality of care delivered.[3,15,26,27]

ADAPTING NATIONAL GUIDELINES TO THE LOCAL LEVEL

There is evidence that locally developed guidelines affect a higher proportion of patient outcomes than do those developed by national organizations.[28] This may be due to greater awareness and applicability of guidelines when clinicians from local organizations are involved in their development or adaptation. Cincinnati Children's Hospital is one institution that has developed a strategy of adapting national guidelines to local patterns of practice, resources, and health care culture and developing original practice guidelines when nationally recognized organizations have not yet done so.[16,17,29]

In the adaptation process, recommendations in a national guideline are used as an outline for the development of management strategies and answerable clinical questions related to these strategies. These clinical questions are then used to guide literature searches for relevant clinical research evidence; the literature searches go back at least 1 year before the publication date of the national guideline. The evidence retrieved from literature searches is appraised by members of the guideline team for its validity and possible incorporation into the local guideline. This updated evidence is combined with local health services data on the disorder of interest; integrated with the frontline clinical experience of local experts and allied health professionals; and combined with the experiences, values, and preferences of parents and families of children affected by the disorder in developing recommendations.

CHOOSING AN APPROPRIATE CLINICAL AREA FOR GUIDELINE DEVELOPMENT

Choosing an appropriate clinical area for guideline development requires an evaluation of the volume of care, cost of care, and variation in management.[30] Patient populations, target users, and specific goals for guideline-related outcomes should be identified. In particular, patient populations to be included and excluded by the guideline should be clearly delineated.

FORMING A GUIDELINE TEAM

The membership of a guideline team is critical to the quality and applicability of the final product. The leader of the team should be chosen carefully. It is critical that he or she be a clinician experienced in the frontline management of the condition of interest. In addition to having a practical clinical knowledge base, the team leader should have a strong commitment to the pediatric center and the regional area where the guideline will be disseminated and implemented. Further, he or she should be a recognized opinion leader in the community, with strong diplomatic skills.

The team leader is responsible for ensuring that the following are accomplished: (1) developing a list of potential candidates (including patients and parents) for the guideline team; (2) determining the scope of or management steps encompassed by the guideline; (3) compiling a preliminary set of answerable clinical questions, based on the outlined management steps; and (4) performing a literature search of appropriate databases, including MEDLINE and the Cochrane Library (preferably with the assistance of a trained librarian).[31] The team leader's perspective is critical for the successful development, applicability, and eventual implementation of a clinical practice guideline. In the case of topics of interest to frontline general practitioners (e.g., urinary tract infection, community-acquired pneumonia, asthma exacerbation, attention-deficit hyperactivity disorder), it is critical that the team leader maintain a general, population-based approach, free of the dogmatic experiential and referral bias to which a subspecialist may be susceptible.[32] Conversely, when developing a practice guideline specific to a subspecialty (e.g., femur fracture, necrotizing enterocolitis, Fontan procedure for congenital heart disease), it may be most appropriate to have a team leader who is intimately familiar with the management of the disorder (as well as the current literature and research).

Other guideline team members might include interested clinicians (including subspecialists, when appropriate), community practitioners, allied health care professionals (e.g., respiratory therapists, pharmacists, librarians), house staff (where available), and parents of children who are affected by the disorder or have experienced disease-specific care at the local institution. One or more team members may function as "champions" for the guideline, committing themselves to implementation efforts such as educational outreach, marketing, and evaluation of changes in practice, processes, and outcomes after implementation. A guideline methodologist with expertise in clinical epidemiology, statistics, and guideline development (either a clinician or nonclinician, with or without experience related to the guideline-specific disorder), along with one or two administrative staff, can assist the team leader and members. Parents of affected children are essential team members to keep the focus practical and useful.

ASKING CLINICAL QUESTIONS AND SEARCHING THE LITERATURE

Once the team has been formed, answerable clinical questions based on management steps are prepared and reviewed by team members. The PICO—patient, intervention-exposure-test, comparison, outcome—format of question development facilitates the literature search, making it more likely to retrieve relevant clinical research evidence that will impact a guideline recommendation. The revised questions are then forwarded to the team librarian for a final search and compilation into a database. The abstracts of the literature search are reviewed by the guideline methodologist, and poor-quality studies pertaining to treatment, diagnosis, prognosis, etiology, or cost-effectiveness are removed. In the case of Cincinnati Children's Hospital's recently completed guideline on acute exacerbation of asthma in children, an initial database of some 1600 articles was reduced to approximately 400 for mapping to 22 answerable questions outlining management. Only 130 were eventually used to support recommendation statements.[33]

At the initial orientation meeting, complete sets of clinical research articles, grouped by answerable clinical question, are laid out for assignment to one or two team members for critical appraisal and presentation to the larger guideline committee. Not all members of a guideline team will be skilled in critical appraisal or interpretation of the medical literature; however, all team members are expected to contribute to the effort of reviewing the medical literature. The orientation meeting should include a brief review of the evidence-based medicine paradigm, the essentials of critical appraisal of the medical literature, and rules for the functioning of team members, including issues and constraints related to consensus generation for recommendation statements. Also reviewed are the basics of critical appraisal of clinical research articles addressing questions of therapy, diagnosis, prognosis, etiology, harm, systematic reviews, cost-effectiveness, and other types of studies; these are readdressed, as needed, throughout the course of the guideline development process.[34,35] For team members new to the guideline process or unfamiliar with the critical appraisal of relatively new methodologies, such as combining or synthesizing data within a systematic review, the guideline methodologist often meets with them before their team presentation to review the appraisal and methodology of the studies in question.

GRADING THE METHODOLOGIC RIGOR SUPPORTING A RECOMMENDATION

We advocate that recommendation statements be followed by explicit links to the evidence supporting them and some indication (e.g., grade on a scale) of the methodologic rigor of the evidence. In an attempt to enhance reproducibility, many guideline developers and organizations use methods for rating the degree of bias and uncertainty present in the evidence supporting a given recommendation statement. Although there are many versions of such grading scales, we believe that an explicit indication of the methodologic rigor is more objective and essential than an assignment of the "strength" of a recommendation.[36-38] Combining a statement about the quality of the evidence and the strength of the recommendation can create confusion. For example, the American Academy of Pediatrics guideline on the diagnosis and management of acute otitis media (AOM) makes the following recommendation (3A): "Observation without use of antibacterial agents in a child with uncomplicated AOM is an option for selected children based on diagnostic certainty, age, illness severity, and assurance of follow-up."[5] Although the evidence was strong—with at least two double-blind, randomized, controlled trials and one observational study in support—the recommendation was called an "option" (defined as a "course that may be taken when either the quality of the evidence is suspect" or "carefully performed studies have shown little clear advantage to one approach").[39-42] However, many frontline practitioners who are unfamiliar with the recommendation strength scales will likely interpret "option" to mean that they are free to use an observational approach in children that they select at their discretion. In fact, the guideline developers only meant to state that this recommendation was on somewhat shakier ground than other recommendations owing to poor-quality evidence. A better approach might have been to word the recommendation to reflect the developers' uncertainty about this management course. In our opinion, a recommendation using simple, clear language with explicit links to the evidence and a clear indication of its methodologic quality is more likely to be implemented and followed than an unclear statement with both quality and strength grades included.[43]

Evidence alone is never sufficient to draft guideline recommendations or make health care decisions.[25,44] It must be combined with clinical experience, patient biology, and patient and family values and preferences.[25,45,46] After critically appraising the clinical research related to an answerable clinical question, the reviewer, the team leader, or another member of the guideline team develops a draft recommendation statement. The member drafting the statement takes into account his or her clinical experience and combines it with an appraisal of the best available evidence.[25,47] This clinical experience allows the member to determine whether the evidence is valid and applicable. The draft statement is then presented to the group for review and revision before publication and implementation of the final guideline.

DEVELOPING CONSENSUS

The rules for consensus development should be presented, discussed, and agreed on at one of the initial team meetings. There are several commonly used approaches that vary in their scientific rigor and efficiency. The most efficient and perhaps least rigorous method can be termed *informal consensus*, whereby draft statements based on the reviewed evidence are presented in an iterative process of revision and editing before inclusion in the guideline. The advantage of this approach is that it engenders discussion of the nuances of management and the inclusion of alternatives or counterpoints in the wording of draft recommendations. This fosters group buy-in to the final guideline and leverages the various points of view, perspectives, and areas of expertise of team members.

More formal methods for consensus generation are the anonymous vote, nominal group, and Delphi techniques. In anonymous voting, team members might vote on each and every recommendation statement and agree to a majority-rules method. In the nominal group technique, team members meet to suggest, rate, or prioritize a series of questions or recommendations; discuss them; and then rerate and reprioritize them. Alternatively, a committee might use a hybrid approach—informal consensus or nominal group techniques for most statements, and anonymous voting for more controversial statements. Delphi techniques for consensus development, initially piloted in the 1950s by the Department of Defense, involve a series of iterative rankings of statements (or, more commonly, themes) until convergence is achieved.[48-51] Although highly rigorous and reproducible, such methods involve setting up a small infrastructure or using specialized computer software and e-mail or mail-based surveys, greatly adding to the complexity and reducing the efficiency of recommendation development.[52,53]

There is likely to be some variability in how evidence is interpreted and integrated into recommendation statements, regardless of which method of consensus development is used. Therefore, perhaps the most important element is for guideline teams to recognize that all recommendation statements are likely to involve some degree of compromise. Still, the actual wording of a recommendation statement can have a great effect on its utility and likelihood of implementation.[43]

IMPLEMENTING GUIDELINES AND CHANGING PHYSICIAN BEHAVIOR

A great deal has been written about the lack of physician awareness of and adherence to recommendations in clinical practice guidelines,[12,23,54] and several authors have outlined both effective and ineffective strategies for changing physician behavior.[7,55,56] Once a guideline has been finalized (and often beginning before finalization), several support tools should be developed, such as order sets (through computerized order entry systems, when available), patient education materials and links to online resources (including a web-based version of the guideline itself), nursing care pathways, care algorithms, and other documents, to assist health care practitioners, patients, and families in integrating the practice guideline recommendations into frontline management. Barriers to implementation fall into three general domains: physician related (e.g., knowledge, attitudes, behaviors), patient related (e.g., psychological, time, financial), and health system related (e.g., culture, costs, availability of technology).[57] Unfortunately, there are no magic bullets for changing physician behavior and frontline practice to reflect evidence-based guideline recommendations.[55] Dissemination-only strategies, in which recommendations are discussed at conferences or during grand rounds or are mailed out to practitioners, have little effect on physician behavior. In contrast, more complex, multifaceted interventions, such as educational outreach visits, academic detailing, and the use of opinion leaders and champions, sometimes produce a moderate reduction in inappropriate practices and increase in evidence-based processes and practices.[13,56,58,59]

In an overview of interventions, including clinical practice guideline implementation, Grimshaw and colleagues concluded that passive approaches to altering physician behavior (e.g., grand rounds, traditional continuing medical education lectures) are generally ineffective and unlikely to result in behavior change.[58] Most other interventions (e.g., audit and feedback, educational outreach, reminder systems) are effective under some circumstances, especially when information is coupled with performance or outcome measures and social influence or management support. Others have argued that decision aids incorporating best evidence with patient values and preferences result in large and consistent improvements in patients' perception of their care.[45,60] Such aids are a potentially powerful method of partnering with patients and families to implement guideline recommendations.[61] Clearly, there must also be administrative support and resources to implement the infrastructural changes (e.g., computerized order entry systems, guideline development teams) required to shift the culture of a given health care organization toward the support of evidence-based practice. Guidelines should be viewed as stepping-stones to bridge the gap between what best evidence implies for best practice and what actually occurs on the front lines of pediatric care.[23]

The approach at Cincinnati Children's Hospital to the implementation and dissemination of clinical practice guidelines is multifaceted and is based on Rogers' theory of diffusion of innovations and Bandura's theory of human behavior or social cognitive theory (formerly social learning theory).[62,63] Rogers' theoretical models of the diffusion of innovations within an organization and Bandura's theory of the interaction of an individual's behaviors, thoughts, and environment are used to develop a matrix for the generation of multifaceted interventions to foster physician awareness and behavior change consistent with clinical practice guideline recommendations (Table 8-1).

Diffusion theory, originally developed in the agricultural sciences, is derived from a body of research that attempted to identify predictable patterns of program adoption among a variety of population groups and across a range of programs.[64] The diffusion process involves attending to the innovation and the channels used to communicate the innovation, as well as to the characteristics of the systems or environment in which this process takes place (diffusion context). Perceptions of an innovation have a major effect on diffusion. Such perceptions are complex and involve whether there is a perceived benefit related to the innovation; whether it is compatible with the culture, beliefs, and values of the organization; the complexity of the innovation; its trialability (whether an adopter can develop a test of change); and its observability (the ease with which potential adopters can see others try the change first).[64] The five adopter categories identified by Rogers, based on the statistical properties of the diffusion curve (number of standard deviations from the mean time to adoption), are innovators, early adopters, early majority adopters, late majority adopters, and laggards.[63,64] Such categories are the basis for the design and implementation of intervention strategies targeted at particular groups of individuals. The aim of diffusion in evidence-based practice is to maximize the exposure and reach of innovations, strategies, or programs for which there is already established evidence of efficacy and effectiveness. This requires that a guideline move through five recognized stages: development, dissemination, adoption, implementa-

tion, and maintenance (see Table 8-1 for details). Diffusion theory can then act as a framework for concurrent quality improvement efforts.[64]

Social cognitive theory, originally developed by Bandura in the early 1960s and refined during the next several decades, refers to the observation that an individual acquires much of his or her behavior by observing and imitating others within a social context. In the area of clinical practice guidelines, it explains the adoption and use of clinical evidence as a consequence of the interaction of the environment (perceived consequences based on the organizational environment), the person (attitudes or expectations about evidence-based practice), and behavioral experiences within the environment (prior experiences of success, failure, and reinforcement for guideline-specific care).

Cabana and coworkers described the process of behavior change related to clinical practice guidelines within the framework of Bandura's social cognitive theory.[12] According to them, physicians must modify their knowledge of the guideline recommendations, accept them, and finally change their behavior to reflect them. According to social cognitive theory, there exists a dynamic among a person's behavior, a person's thoughts, and the environment in which these occur. Because of these combined, reciprocal influences, physicians and allied health care professionals are both products and producers of their personalities, their behaviors, and their environments. Thus, in the presence of senior management support of evidence-based practice, together with the development of local practice guidelines, individual clinicians on an inpatient service can serve as role models by using evidence-based recommendations and creating a culture of "evidence users."[47] According to Bandura, there are three general factors to consider when changing behavior within an organization: (1) situational or environmental factors (goal-oriented, socially oriented, and task or structural cues) that prompt the use of evidence-based recommendations, (2) personal factors (attitudes, personality characteristics, and other cognitive factors that increase or decrease the likelihood of compliance with guideline recommendations), and (3) consequences or behavioral factors (interpersonal and organizational responses to a person's behavior that increase or decrease the likelihood of the behavior's recurrence). For example, (1) division heads expect their clinicians to be involved in guideline development teams, (2) clinician opinion leaders participate on such teams, and (3) such participation is one benchmark for promotion and tenure. Other examples are listed in the Table 8-1.

There is likely to be some variation in the management of common inpatient pediatric diseases, such as acute asthma or croup, when there is a relative wealth of evidence related to a number of interventions in the form of randomized, controlled trials. A well-developed, disseminated, and implemented clinical practice guideline program should be applicable across a large proportion of children admitted with general pediatric diagnoses. In one study, almost 75% of children admitted to a general inpatient service received evidence-based care for at least one of the interventions addressing the initial diagnosis (the other 25% were admitted for observation).[19] However, there remains much variation in the care provided and in the application of best evidence in pediatric inpatient settings.[12,22,23]

Table 8-1 Applicability of Bandura's and Rogers' Theories to Clinical Practice Guidelines

Bandura's Social Learning Theory Constructs	ROGERS' DIFFUSION OF INNOVATION				
	Guideline Development	*Guideline Dissemination*	*Guideline Adoption*	*Guideline Implementation*	*Guideline Maintenance*
Situational or Environmental Factors Situational cues that prompt the ongoing development of evidence-based practice (e.g., availability of expert models, job and organizational design, imposed standards or goals, culture around evidence use)	Management expectations that divisions will engage in the development of practice guidelines; division involvement in the selection of focus populations; division leaders taking the initiative in developing guidelines and advocating their use; leadership expectations for many to be trained to develop guidelines; provision of effective, efficient models of guideline development	Guidelines available in multiple formats: grand rounds, mailings, educational outreach visits, computerized decision support, opinion leaders; patient guideline education; guidelines built into trainee education	Management expectations for guideline adoption; site care to decide appropriate targets; benchmarking with other sites involved in EBP; public display of various efforts to use evidence; small-group educational visits (ED residents, GIS teams, community practices); reengineering of care process to include EBP, EMR, EMSTAT; guidelines built into COE with "show stoppers"	Reengineering of care process; guidelines built into COE with "show stoppers" (e.g., difficult to discharge, changing process of care from nebulized beta-agonist to MDI in ED; peer review in local networks; patients ask about evidence for treatment given; reminders (manual or computerized); patient-specific audit and feedback; patient-mediated interventions	Audit data are transparent; guidelines built into COE with "show stoppers"; local opinion leaders; individual follow-up; data showing the impact of guideline efforts collected on a regular basis; individual practice data compared with that of peers; reminders (manual or computerized); audit and feedback; patient-mediated interventions; Regular updates on EBP adherence
Personal Factors Factors internal to the target clinician that influence his or her use of evidence (e.g., knowledge, skills, abilities, motives, self-efficacy beliefs, attributional style)	Involvement in successful guideline development teams to change attitudes about EBP; opinion leaders promote the importance of developing EBP; dissemination of tools that make access or use of evidence easier; repeated participation in guideline development teams; local consensus processes	Socialization programs that create culture of evidence users; clinician orientation programs; opinion leaders; individual instruction, training and apprenticeship; interactive educational meetings (GIS, division, community practice, parents); residents report guideline recommendations	Develop separate strategies for early to late adopters; address perceived barriers, fears, or concerns; leadership recognition of importance of evidence; individual-level reassurance and engagement; resident orientation regarding EBP; interactive	Annual EBM workshop; individual instruction; small group support; interactive educational meetings where residents can practice and see how evidence and tools are used; continued training experiences provided to target adopters; seeking of mastery experiences; opportunities	Clinicians see that regular use of evidence results in positive outcomes for staff and patients; peer review in local networks; nonthreatening practice opportunities

Table 8-1   Applicability of Bandura's and Rogers' Theories to Clinical Practice Guidelines—cont'd

Bandura's Social Learning Theory Constructs	ROGERS' DIFFUSION OF INNOVATION				
	Guideline Development	Guideline Dissemination	Guideline Adoption	Guideline Implementation	Guideline Maintenance
		to community practitioners	educational meetings; peer review in local networks; residents observe senior residents or attendings using or quoting guidelines; impact of EBP publicized	provided for training of others	
Consequences and Behavioral Factors Responses to behavior that increase or decrease the likelihood of its occurrence	Provide incentives (individual level, division or group level, business unit level) for guideline development or revision (CME credits, letter for educational portfolio, protected time); faculty and staff encouraged to take leadership roles in further guideline development or revision efforts	Rewards for participation in dissemination efforts (ward or team competition, interdivisional competition); business unit reinforcement (e.g., whose dashboard shows use of EBP?)	Case reports of success (EBP resident clubs); patient-mediated interventions; economic incentives; sanctions; immediate + later reinforcement for EBP (audit and feedback); avoid reinforcing non-EBP behavior or institute disincentives for non-EBP behavior	Establish an evidence use performance grading system; economic incentives; sanctions; educational portfolio, P&T letters; CME credit	Economic incentives; sanctions; regulations, laws, licensing; immediate reinforcement for positive performance in guideline development or revision

CME, continuing medical education; COE, computerized order entry; EBP, evidence-based practice; ED, emergency department; EMR, electronic medical record; EMSTAT, emergency medical information system; GIS, general inpatient service; P&T, promotion and tenure.

DESIGNING AND MEASURING OUTCOMES

When attempting to measure outcomes related to recommendation statements in clinical practice guidelines, an efficient strategy is to focus on those outcomes for which there are (1) satisfactory evidence; (2) little debate as to the appropriate interventions, tests, or management strategies; (3) a high likelihood of an impact on patient well-being or hospital costs; and (4) readily available data to measure changes in the outcome of interest exist. Data collection (e.g., administrative or chart review) and measurement of guideline-related outcomes can be a formidable challenge in the absence of management or institutional support.[65] Nelson and colleagues defined six keys to the measurement of practice improvement efforts[66]:

1. Utility
2. Simplicity
3. Balance
4. Data that tell a story
5. Data that are available to key audiences (clinicians, patients, parents)
6. Transparent measurement goals and processes

In other words, in the early stages of a guideline development program, it may be best to use outcome measures that reflect recommendations with strong supporting evidence (large, high-quality, randomized, controlled trials or well-conducted systematic reviews with clear findings), that are generally accepted by frontline practitioners, and that provide easily measurable outcomes or processes of care that generate little debate as to desirability. Therefore, it is important to have clearly defined goals, measures, and expected tasks for a team involved in a quality improvement effort based on a clinical practice guideline.[51,67] It is best to include all allied health care providers, administrative personnel, and others involved in the daily, routine care of inpatients (from registration to discharge) in the guideline implementation efforts related to collecting data and measuring outcomes. It is more efficient if this quality improvement work is integrated seamlessly into the daily tasks of physicians, nurses, house staff, respiratory therapists, unit or ward administrators, and secretarial staff. Quality improvement should be a team activity that is integrated into the process of pediatric care and based on goals and measures derived from guideline recommendations.[67-69]

CONCLUSION

This chapter's focus is quality improvement through the development of evidence-based clinical practice guidelines. Efforts to define best practices are the jumping-off point for the goal of having inpatient pediatric care reflect the best available evidence and clinical expertise, integrated with family and patient values and preferences. One cannot begin to develop quality improvement without achieving local consensus around best evidence and a health care policy that reflects that consensus. When implementing and disseminating clinical practice guidelines, one must be cognizant of relevant individual and organizational cultural and behavioral factors that may enhance or hinder compliance with recommendations. Finally, when developing quality improvement efforts, evidence-based recommendation statements should be used to define simple, clear processes of care and patient outcomes that are readily obtainable from administrative or other accessible databases. Systems for developing both clinical practice guidelines and associated outcome measures will act to create evidence-based cultures that improve the quality of health care delivered on pediatric inpatient services.

SUGGESTED READING

Eddy DM: Practice policies—what are they? JAMA 1990;263:877-880.

Institute of Medicine: Guidelines for Clinical Practice—From Development to Use. Washington, DC, National Academy Press, 1992.

Institute of Medicine: Applying Evidence to Healthcare Delivery: Crossing the Quality Chasm. Washington, DC, National Academy Press, 2001, pp 148-155.

Leape LL, Berwick DM, Bates DW: What practices will most improve safety? Evidence-based medicine meets patient safety. JAMA 2002;288:501-507.

Wilson M, Hayward R, Tunis SR, et al: Users' guides to the medical literature. VIII. How to use clinical practice guidelines B. What are the recommendations and will they help you in caring for your patients? JAMA 1995;274:1630-1632.

REFERENCES

1. Institute of Medicine: Guidelines for Clinical Practice—From Development to Use. Washington, DC, National Academy Press, 1992.
2. Eddy DM: Practice policies—what are they? JAMA 1990;263:877-880.
3. Institute of Medicine: Applying Evidence to Healthcare Delivery: Crossing the Quality Chasm. Washington, DC, National Academy Press, 2001, pp 148-155.
4. NHLBI Guidelines for the Diagnosis and Management of Asthma. Bethesda, Md, National Institutes of Health, July 1997.
5. American Academy of Pediatrics: Diagnosis and management of acute otitis media. Pediatrics 2004;113:1451-1465.
6. Cincinnati Children's Hospital Medical Center: Evidence Based Clinical Practice Guideline: Bronchiolitis. Division of Health Policy and Clinical Effectiveness. Available at *http://www.cincinnatichildrens.org/NR/rdonlyres/0B7B99D7-DB3E-4186-B2FC-71539E23421E/0/bronchiolitis guideline.pdf.*
7. Grimshaw J, Russell I: Effect of clinical guidelines on medical practice: A systematic review of rigorous evaluations. Lancet 1993;342:1317-1322.
8. AGREE: Appraisal of Guidelines for Research and Evaluation (AGREE) Instrument. London, St. George's Hospital, June 2001.
9. Shiffman RN, Shekelle P, Overhage M, et al: Standardized reporting of clinical practice guidelines: A proposal from the Conference on Guideline Standardization. Ann Intern Med 2003;139:493-498.
10. Shaneyfelt TM, Mayo-Smith MF, Rothwangl J: Are guidelines following guidelines? The methodological quality of clinical practice guidelines in the peer-reviewed medical literature. JAMA 1999;281:1900-1905.
11. Wilson M, Hayward R, Tunis SR, et al: Users' guides to the medical literature. VIII. How to use clinical practice guidelines B. What are the recommendations and will they help you in caring for your patients? JAMA 1995;274:1630-1632.
12. Cabana M, Rand C, Powe N, et al: Why don't physicians follow clinical practice guidelines? A framework for improvement. JAMA 1999;282:1458-1465.
13. Grol R: Successes and failures in the implementation of evidence-based guidelines for clinical practice. Med Care 2001;39(Suppl 2):II46-II54.
14. Welch WP, Miller ME, Welch G, et al: Geographic variation in expenditures for physicians' services in the United States. N Engl J Med 1993;328:621-627.
15. Homer CJ, Szilagyi P, Rodewald L, et al: Does quality of care affect rates of hospitalization for childhood asthma? Pediatrics 1996;98:18-23.
16. Perlstein P, Kotagal U, Bolling C, et al: Evaluation of an evidence-based guideline for bronchiolitis. Pediatrics 1999;104:1334-1341.
17. Perlstein P, Kotagal U, Schoettker P, et al: Sustaining the implementation of an evidence-based guideline for bronchiolitis. Arch Pediatr Adolesc Med 2000;154:1001-1007.
18. Kotagal UR, Robbins JM, Kini NM, et al: Impact of a bronchiolitis guideline—a multisite demonstration project. Chest 2002;121:1789-1797.
19. Moyer VA, Gist AK, Elliott EJ: Is the practice of pediatric inpatient medicine evidence based? J Paediatr Child Health 2002;38:341-342.
20. Ellis J, Mulligan I, Rowe J, Sackett DL: Inpatient general medicine is evidence based: A-team, Nuffield Department of Clinical Medicine. Lancet 1995;346:407-410.
21. Wennberg JE: Unwarranted variations in healthcare delivery: Implications for academic medical centers. BMJ 2002;325:913-914.
22. Willson DF, Horn SD, Hendley O, et al: Effect of practice variation on resource utilization in infants hospitalized for viral lower respiratory illness. Pediatrics 2001;108:851-855.
23. Strand M, Phelan KJ, Donovan EF: Promoting the uptake and use of evidence: An overview of the problem. Clin Perinatol 2003;30:389-402.
24. Sackett D, Rosenberg W, Gray J, et al: Evidence based medicine: What it is and what it isn't. BMJ 1996;312:71.
25. Haynes RB, Devereaux PJ, Guyatt G: Physicians' and patients' choices in evidence based practice—evidence does not make decisions, people do. BMJ 2002;324:1350.
26. Haynes RB: Of studies, syntheses, synopses, and systems: The "4S" evolution of services for finding current best evidence. ACP J Club 2001;134:A11-A13.
27. Mehta RH, Montoye CK, Gallogly M, et al: Improving quality of care for acute myocardial infarction—The guidelines applied in practice (GAP) initiative. JAMA 2002;287:1269-1276.
28. Worrall G, Chaulk P, Freake D: The effects of clinical practice guidelines on patient outcomes in primary care: A systematic review. Can Med Assoc J 1997;156:1705-1712.

29. Evolution in procedures and methods for developing practice guidelines. In Field M, Lohr K (eds): Guidelines for Clinical Practice—From Development to Use. Washington, DC, National Academy Press, 1992, pp 183-187.

30. Fisher ES, Wennberg DE, Stukel TA, et al: The implications of regional variations in Medicare spending. Part 1. The content, quality, and accessibility of care. Ann Intern Med 2003;138:273-287.

31. Hunt DL, Jaeschke R, McKibbon KA, EBM Working Group: Users' guides to the medical literature. XXI. Using electronic health information resources in evidence-based practice. JAMA 2000;283:1875-1879.

32. Newman TB: The power of stories over statistics. BMJ 2003;327:1424-1427.

33. Bacon J, Peltier C, Lierl M, et al: Managing an acute exacerbation of asthma. Available at *http://www.cincinnatichildrens.org/svc/deptdiv/health-policy/ev-based/asthma.htm.* Accessed Nov 2004.

34. Haynes RB, Sackett DL, Gray JAM, et al: Transferring evidence from research into practice. 2. Getting the evidence straight. ACP J Club 1997;126:A-14.

35. User's Guides to the Medical Literature—A Manual for Evidence-Based Clinical Practice. Chicago, AMA Press, 2002.

36. American Academy of Pediatrics: Classifying recommendations for clinical practice guidelines. Pediatrics 2004;114:874-877.

37. Atkins D, Best D, Briss PA, et al: Grading quality of evidence and strength of recommendations. BMJ 2004;328:1490.

38. Lohr K: Rating the strength of scientific evidence: Relevance for quality improvement programs. Int J Qual Health Care 2004;16:9-18.

39. Little P, Gould C, Williamson I, et al: Pragmatic randomised controlled trial of two prescribing strategies for childhood acute otitis media. BMJ 2001;322:336-342.

40. Cates C: An evidence based approach to reducing antibiotic use in children with acute otitis media: Controlled before and after study. BMJ 1999;318:715-716.

41. Damoiseaux RA, van Balen FA, Hoes AW, et al: Primary care based randomized, double blind trial of amoxicillin versus placebo for acute otitis media in children aged under 2 years. BMJ 2000;320:350-354.

42. Siegel RM, Kiely M, Bien JP, et al: Treatment of otitis media with observation and a safety-net antibiotic prescription. Pediatrics 2003;112:527-531.

43. Michie S, Johnston M: Changing clinical behaviour by making guidelines specific. BMJ 2004;328:343-345.

44. Larsen EB: Evidence-based medicine: Is translating evidence into practice a solution to the cost-quality challenges facing medicine? Jt Comm J Qual Improv 1999;25:480-485.

45. O'Connor AM, Mulley AG, Wennberg JE: Standard consultations are not enough to ensure decision quality regarding preference-sensitive options. J Natl Cancer Inst 2003;95:570-571.

46. Hayward R, Wilson M, Tunis SR, et al: Users' guides to the medical literature. VIII. How to use clinical practice guidelines A: Are the recommendations valid? JAMA 1995;274:570-574.

47. Guyatt G, O'Meade M, Jaeschke R, et al: Practitioners of evidence based care—not all clinicians need to appraise evidence from scratch but all need some skills. BMJ 2000;320:954-955.

48. Kaplan A, Skogstad A, Cirshick MA: The Prediction of Social and Technological Events. Los Angeles, Rand Corporation, Apr 1949.

49. Dalkey N: Predicting the Future. Santa Monica, Calif, Rand Corporation, 1968.

50. Dalkey N: An experimental study of group opinion: The Delphi method. Futures I 1969:408-420.

51. Campbell SM, Braspenning J, Hutchinson A, Marshall MN: Improving the quality of health care—research methods used in developing and applying quality indicators in primary care. BMJ 2003;326:816-819.

52. Delfo I—Professional Delphi Scan—an Expert System [computer program]. Finland Futures Research Centre, 2004.

53. Rivara FP, Johansen JM, Thompson DC: Research on injury prevention: Topics for systematic review. Inj Prev 2002;8:161-164.

54. Christakis D, Rivara F: Pediatricians' awareness of and attitudes about four clinical practice guidelines. Pediatrics 1998;101:825-830.

55. Oxman AD, Thomson MA, Davis DA, Haynes RB: No magic bullets: A systematic review of 102 trials of interventions to improve professional practice. Can Med Assoc J 1995;153:1423-1431.

56. Bero L, Grilli R, Grimshaw JM, et al: Closing the gap between research and practice: An overview of systematic reviews of interventions to promote the implementation of research findings. BMJ 1998;317:465-468.

57. Rich MW: From clinical trials to clinical practice—bridging the GAP. JAMA 2002;287:1321-1323.

58. Grimshaw J, Shirran L, Thomas R, et al: Changing provider behavior—an overview of systematic reviews of interventions. Med Care 2001;39:II2-II45.

59. Horbar JD, Carpenter JH, Buzas J, et al: Collaborative quality improvement to promote evidence based surfactant for preterm infants: A cluster randomised trial. BMJ 2004;329:1004.

60. O'Connor AM, Stacey D, Rovner D, et al: Decision aids for people facing health treatment or screening decisions. Cochrane Database Syst Rev 2003;(2):CD001431.

61. Charles C, Whelan T, Gafni A: What do we mean by partnership in making decisions about treatment? BMJ 1999;319:780-782.

62. Bandura A: Social Foundations of Thought and Action—A Social Cognitive Theory. Upper Saddle River, NJ, Prentice Hall, 1986.

63. Rogers EM: Diffusion of Innovations, 3rd ed. New York, Free Press, 1983.

64. Berwick DM: Disseminating innovations in health care. JAMA 2003;289:1969-1975.

65. Mangione-Smith R, Onstad K, Wong L, Roski J: Deciding not to measure performance: The case of acute otitis media. Jt Comm J Qual Saf 2003;29:27-36.

66. Nelson EC, Splaine ME, Batalden PB, Plume SK: Building measurement and data collection into medical practice. Ann Intern Med 1998;128:460-466.

67. Muething S, Schoettker PJ, Gerhardt WE, et al: Decreasing overuse of therapies in the treatment of bronchiolitis by incorporating evidence at the point of care. J Pediatr 2004;144:703-710.

68. Berwick DM: Developing and testing changes in delivery of care. Ann Intern Med 1998;128:651-656.

69. Leape LL, Berwick DM, Bates DW: What practices will most improve safety? Evidence-based medicine meets patient safety. JAMA 2002;288:501-507.

Caring for the Patient

CHAPTER 9

The Approach to the Hospitalized Child and Family

Michael T. Vossmeyer, Grace M. Cheng, Debra Monzack, and Alka Patel

The approach to the hospitalized child and family has changed dramatically over the last decade. Physicians are rarely the sole decision makers when children are hospitalized. Patients and families expect to be actively involved in medical decision making,[1] and this expectation is strongly supported by leaders in health care quality improvement.

In 2001 the Institute of Medicine published a report that outlined six aims of health care delivery systems in the United States.[2] It stated that a health care system should be timely, effective, efficient, patient centered, equitable, and safe, and inpatient care should be focused on achieving these aims.

A hospitalized child requires timely access to services without delays attributable to system design. Clinical care should be evidence based, and the implementation of evidence-based clinical guidelines decreases unnecessary variation in care and improves clinical outcomes (see Chapters 7 and 8). When there are no available guidelines, the original medical literature can be accessed using generally accepted methods of developing clinically answerable questions.[3] Hospital systems should be designed to minimize length of stay while improving clinical outcomes. Equitable care must be available for all hospitalized children without regard to race, national origin, religious or cultural background, gender, or insurance status. Hospital systems must be designed to ensure patient safety and to dramatically decrease preventable sources of error (see Chapter 5). The use of computerized technologies, such as electronic patient records and computerized order entry systems, can increase the reliability of hospital systems.[4]

Hospital cultures need to change from physician centered to patient and family centered and should focus on dimensions of care that patients and families value, including respect for preferences, involvement in decision making, access to care, coordination of care, information and education, physical comfort, emotional support, involvement of family and friends, and continuity in the transition from inpatient to outpatient or home setting.[5]

TRANSITION TO THE INPATIENT SETTING

Hospitalization is a stressful event for both the child and the family. Children and families may experience feelings ranging from fear of the unknown to complete loss of control. These feelings complicate the clinical situation and detract from the development of a healing environment. Physicians and other health care providers should address these stresses directly and provide an environment designed to preserve patient and family control. Whenever possible, the child and family should be prepared for the hospitalization; this allows them to be educated about the proposed care and can help clarify the expectations of the family and the physician. Such preparation also provides an opportunity to initiate discharge planning at the earliest possible time. If the child's primary care physician will not be making rounds in the hospital (as in most hospitalist systems), the family should be told who will provide hospital care and how the physicians will communicate and coordinate care inside and outside the hospital. Physician-to-physician communication should occur near the time of hospitalization to ensure a safe handoff of care. If possible, before the hospitalization, the child and family should be given the opportunity to tour the facility and meet the staff who will be providing care. An active child life service can facilitate much of the prehospitalization activity. When hospitalization occurs urgently or emergently, child life programs can provide support for children and families at the point of contact.

HOSPITAL CARE AND FAMILY-CENTERED ROUNDS

During hospitalization, the process of care can be viewed as the interaction of four separate but interdependent processes: medical decision making, communication, rounds, and discharge planning. All caregivers, as well as the child and family, should participate in each of these processes.

Decision making should be transparent to all involved. The family is often the best source of information about a child, but it is frequently overlooked. Actively taking into account the family's values, culture, race, and socioeconomic background, as well as family members' unique knowledge of the patient, can assist in decision making. All diagnostic and treatment decisions should be made with the full participation of the family. Health care team members must be willing to work constructively with families even when their decisions do not coincide with the advice of the medical team. The use of evidence-based protocols can often facilitate a transparent decision-making process and establish a basis for the discussion of recommended therapies with families. Such protocols decrease the variation among providers, which can confuse patients and families.

Communication that recognizes the family as the driving force in decision making is central to the empowerment process. Simple gestures such as asking patients or families about their preferences regarding rounds allows them to regain a sense of control and involvement. Honest and open communication between medical professionals and families is vital to the success of the hospitalization. Total transparency in all aspects of hospitalization is necessary to maintain optimal lines of communication.

Unless families state otherwise, all critical discussions about medical care should occur in the presence of families. Morning rounds can and should be conducted with the family present. The patient is presented to the medical team in the presence of the family, using language that can be comprehended by the patient and the family. Medical terminology should be minimized or explained in plain language if necessary. Translators should be present if there is a language barrier; it is not advisable to use family members as interpreters.[6] Family-centered rounds allow for a more complete understanding of the patient's medical condition and the development of a treatment plan that is understood and agreed on by all members of the child's health care team. The open communication encouraged by family-centered rounds encourages a dialogue and conveys to family members that they are part of the health care team. Being present during the health care team's discussion gives the family a greater sense of control and dispels some fear of the unknown.

CHILD LIFE SERVICES

Child life services are offered in many inpatient, emergency, and ambulatory settings. The overall objectives of a child life department are to recognize and address developmental issues related to health care experiences and to respond to the fears and concerns of hospitalized children and their families. Child life workers meet these objectives through a variety of activities, including creating opportunities for play and enhanced self-esteem, providing inpatient schoolwork, assessing coping responses, minimizing stress, preparing children and families for health care experiences, facilitating family celebrations, and communicating these goals to the health care team.

Children are encouraged to play in a variety of medical spaces and situations, including intensive care units, clinics, presurgical waiting areas, and emergency departments, during inpatient hospitalization, laboratory testing, and imaging studies. The way a child plays often communicates his or her interpretation of the medical care and illness in a manner that may be inaccessible to other health care providers. Child life specialists can correct misunderstandings that arise during play or relay critical developmental concerns to the family and other specialists on the child's health care team. In addition, play is a method of coping in the foreign environment of the hospital. Therapeutic play can include dramatic play, artistic activity, pet therapy, sensory play (e.g., making dough), games, and attending special events (e.g., musical performances). Medical play provides children with an open-ended opportunity to act, draw, or otherwise use creative media to explore medical equipment, situations, or themes. For example, children at the "Teddy Bear Clinic" bring stuffed toys to different medical stations, giving them casts, intravenous lines, nasogastric tubes, and so forth. These activities familiarize children with their medical surroundings and help them better understand their own medical experiences.

Child life specialists also provide educational resources and environments for family members to help them cope with a child's illness. In-hospital libraries for families, educational video broadcasting in hospitals, and setting aside specific time for siblings in child life rooms can all help alleviate a family's anxiety during a child's illness or hospitalization. Each child life specialist is a member of the comprehensive medical team caring for the patient and can serve as a valuable liaison between the family and child and health care providers.

Hospitalized children and their families frequently misunderstand even the most common medical expressions. For example, "move you to the floor" can be construed as being moved physically to the floor, and "stretcher" can be heard as "stretch her." Child life specialists can help clarify misunderstandings and interpret medical terms for sick children and their families.

TRANSITION FROM THE INPATIENT SETTING

An orderly transition from the inpatient to the outpatient setting is important for continuity of clinical care (see also Chapter 17 on discharge planning). Discharge goals should be established as soon as possible after admission. These goals should be reviewed at least daily and discussed on rounds with the family and nurses. Once established, discharge goals facilitate ongoing care as well as smooth and efficient discharge planning. The use of care coordinators or discharge planners may assist the primary medical team in accessing necessary outpatient services and proactively dealing with insurance issues. Communication with the private physician is also necessary before discharge and sets the stage for the safe handoff of care. Gaining the support and cooperation of the private physician facilitates this transition. Important items to discuss are discharge diagnosis, results of diagnostic testing, outstanding tests that need follow-up, discharge medications, follow-up appointments, and family concerns. This communication should be in addition to a written discharge summary and should optimally occur before the patient's discharge from the hospital.

CONCLUSION

A family-centered approach to the hospitalized child includes evidence-based clinical care and addresses issues of timeliness, access, efficiency, and safety. Care that is systems based and accounts for these aims will produce more satisfactory clinical outcomes. An active child life service can help support hospitalized children and make their care more family and patient centered. Attention must also be paid to the transition from inpatient to outpatient care. Good communication among health care providers supports a safe transition and handoff of care. Involving patients and their families at all levels of the care process can improve satisfaction with the health care delivery system and the quality of care delivered.

REFERENCES

1. Stewart M, Belle Brown J, Weston WW, et al: Patient Centered Medicine: Transforming the Clinical Method. Thousand Oaks, Calif, Sage Publications, 1995.

2. Institute of Medicine: Crossing the Quality Chasm: A New Health Care System for the 21st Century. Washington, DC, National Academy Press, 2001.

3. Moyer V, Williams K, Elliott EJ (eds): Evidence Based Pediatrics and Child Health. London, BMJ Publishing Group, 2000.

4. Upperman JS: The impact of hospitalwide computerized physician order entry on medical errors in a pediatric hospital. J Pediatr Surg 2005;40:57-59.

5. Frampton S, Gilpin L, Charmel P: Putting Patients First: Designing and Practicing Patient-Centered Care. San Francisco, Jossey Bass, 2003.

6. Flores G: Culture and the patient-physician relationship: Achieving cultural competency in health care. J Pediatr 2000;136:14-23.

CHAPTER 10

Hospitalist as Patient Advocate

Susmita Pati

Advocacy has been an integral part of pediatric practice since 1930, when the American Academy of Pediatrics was founded. At that time, 35 pediatricians met in a Detroit hospital library to address the lack of knowledge about children's health care needs, separate and apart from those of adults.[1,2] The idea that children have unique developmental and health needs was novel in the early 20th century. Despite opposition by the Academy of Physicians (which subsequently became the American Medical Association), these pediatricians supported the passage of the Sheppard-Towner Act of 1921, the first federal legislation aimed at benefiting poor mothers and their infants. Since this first act of advocacy, pediatricians have supported a wealth of legislation to promote child health, development, and well-being, including the implementation of vaccination programs, environmental regulations, and safety legislation.

Child advocacy encompasses a wide range of activities conducted in a variety of settings, including clinical, educational, research, and administrative environments. Pediatric hospitalists are uniquely positioned to advocate for the improvement of health care delivery for children in the inpatient setting because they care directly for vulnerable subgroups of hospitalized children and fill leadership roles in children's hospitals. Through administration, medical education, and health care policy development, hospitalists can address the conditions of children's health both locally and nationally.

HOSPITALIST-CLINICIANS AS ADVOCATES FOR INDIVIDUAL PATIENTS

Inpatients stays are challenging for children and their families.[3,4] Hospitalists are adept at managing the medical needs of ill children, providing continuity of care, and developing effective relationships with other health care team members. Ideally, hospitalists' skills as inpatient specialists significantly enhance the quality of health care provided to individual children. Because hospitalists have frequent and regular interaction with nursing staff, social workers, and subspecialists, these groups become familiar with the specific expertise of other team members and their approaches to clinical decision making and management. At the individual level, this familiarity can be used to match the expertise of nurses, social workers, and subspecialists with the specific needs of a given family or patient. From a systems perspective, the continuity of inpatient care available from hospitalists may provide advantages analogous to benefits observed in the outpatient setting.[5]

In their clinical capacity, hospitalists have the ability to improve the efficacy of care for hospitalized children, especially those with chronic illnesses requiring recurrent or prolonged hospitalization. In response to the increasing emphasis on delivering cost-effective and high-quality health care, many hospitals have implemented clinical pathways and protocols that rely on evidence-based guidelines for a variety of common, predictable inpatient illnesses and procedures.[6] Hospitalists can contribute diagnostic, treatment, and procedural expertise to the development of these guidelines, ultimately improving the quality of care delivered to hospitalized children with these conditions. According to recent data, the most common inpatient pediatric diagnoses include respiratory illnesses (e.g., asthma, bronchiolitis), gastrointestinal disorders, and trauma.[7] Although clinical pathways have been widely adopted in the treatment of inpatient respiratory disorders such as asthma and bronchiolitis,[8-12] there is sparse evidence that these pathways have been successful at improving child health outcomes in the long term.[13,14] By contributing to the continuing evaluation of these clinical initiatives, hospitalists advocate for improvements in the quality of health care delivered to children in the inpatient setting.

Hospitalists have additional opportunities to practice clinical advocacy for populations of vulnerable children, including those with chronic conditions and complex social situations (Table 10-1). To improve the outcomes for these children, hospitalists may promote more comprehensive and better-coordinated care for medically complex children, who may depend on a variety of medical technologies (e.g., feeding tubes, ventilators), and those in complex social situations (e.g., those in foster care, adjudicated delinquents). For these children, hospitalists may lead the health care team in advocating for improvements in specific types of care, such as palliative care and transitional care (e.g., to a residential skilled nursing facility or foster care). Just as an office-based pediatrician develops proficiency in ambulatory problems by virtue of experience, a hospitalist acquires clinical fluency with inpatient problems.

HOSPITALIST-RESEARCHERS AS ADVOCATES TO IMPROVE KNOWLEDGE

Stemming from their role as clinicians, pediatric hospitalists are afforded a broad array of opportunities to contribute to the development of evidence-based inpatient clinical practices. Apart from the development of clinical pathways that benefit individual patients directly, research by hospitalists aims to improve the structure and process of inpatient pediatric care to benefit patients more broadly. For example, there are limited data about the effect of hospitalist systems on various dimensions of health care quality because of the challenge of developing measures of quality in pediatrics. Proposed measures have included readmission rates, rates of errors in transfer of care, patient or parent satisfaction, and provider experience. To date, most studies have shown that readmission rates are not affected,[15-18] but the complex interactions that lead to readmission are not well

Table 10-1 Aspects of Clinical Care That May Benefit from Hospitalist Advocacy

Management of complex technologies (e.g., ventilators, feeding tubes)

Management of complex social situations (e.g., foster care entry, intrafamily violence, parental incarceration)

Palliative care

Transitional care (e.g., to a skilled nursing facility)

understood, and the utility of readmission rates as an indicator of quality remains controversial. Results of other studies are self-contained works of advocacy that focus on patient or parent satisfaction. One prospective study of 181 pediatric inpatients with the study hospital's four most common diagnoses—asthma, bronchiolitis, gastroenteritis, and pneumonia—demonstrated the parents were more satisfied with various aspects of care provided by hospitalists as opposed to primary care providers.[18] Another cross-sectional study of pediatric residents and attending physicians performed after the implementation of a system to increase inpatient continuity of care demonstrated uniformly favorable ratings with regard to improved inpatient care, increased efficiency, and better communication with referring physicians.[19] Despite the paucity of data, many pediatric centers continue to adopt pediatric hospitalist systems based on the belief that these systems will ultimately improve inpatient care.[20,21] However, little attention has been given to defining, supporting, or evaluating the role of the hospitalist as an advocate for improving health care quality at multiple levels. Hospitalists are well positioned to further elucidate these areas.

HOSPITALIST-EDUCATORS AS ADVOCATES TO IMPROVE UNDERSTANDING

At the societal level, hospitalists make tremendous contributions to medical education across a variety of disciplines, including nursing, social work, and pharmacy. As in other disciplines, hospitalists' contributions to medical education ensure that emerging health care professionals are adequately trained and that they pursue promising new developments within pediatric inpatient medicine. To date, there have been several studies evaluating the educational experiences of pediatric residents in a hospitalist system. One study of 109 first-year pediatric residents at Children's Hospital in Boston demonstrated that their satisfaction with their educational experience and their self-assessment of general skills and knowledge related to pediatrics improved significantly after the introduction of a hospitalist system in 1998.[22] Compared with traditional attending physicians, hospitalists were rated as more effective role models and teachers and were considered more knowledgeable and accessible.[22] Another study of attending physicians' satisfaction at a rural tertiary care center in West Virginia found that medical student and resident education improved after the inpatient service was restructured using concepts developed by hospitalists.[19] Although long-term outcomes have not

been studied, hospitalists' contributions to medical education are likely to have diffuse effects not only on the immediate experience of trainees but also on their future career development. This is likely to ultimately benefit children by producing health care professionals armed with the knowledge and skills required to evaluate and take advantage of the most promising developments in medical research and technology.

HOSPITALIST-ADMINISTRATORS AS ADVOCATES TO IMPROVE SYSTEMS OF CARE

At the administrative level, the experience of hospitalists can contribute to the development of patient safety procedures, quality assurance protocols, and hospital formularies. As the prevention of inpatient medication errors has become a higher priority,[23] active participation by an interdisciplinary team, including hospitalists, is required to ensure that appropriate and effective measures are implemented and periodically reassessed. With the advent of the rule mandating the testing of pharmaceuticals among children, input from hospitalists is critical to evaluate results and make recommendations for inpatient formularies that meet the unique needs of children.[24,25]

At the community level, hospitalists, like emergency room physicians, are keenly aware of morbidity and mortality rates related to disease trends (e.g., influenza and meningitis epidemics), natural disasters (e.g., earthquakes, floods), preventable injuries, and potential bioterrorist threats (e.g., anthrax). For example, pediatricians in New York City have been collaborating with the Department of Transportation to identify and target street intersections with high rates of motor vehicle–pedestrian accidents for appropriate renovations.[26] To progress beyond our current state of knowledge about injury interventions and other environmental exposures, we will require multidisciplinary input from physicians, epidemiologists, lawyers, and community organizations.[27]

Finally, data gathered by hospitalists can influence national policies to improve health care and stabilize health care financing for children. The passage of the Newborns' and Mothers' Health Protection Act of 1996, mandating a minimum 48-hour stay, was a direct result of advocacy by hospital-based physicians in concert with other health care professionals. Although subsequent research suggests that this mandated minimum stay may not have affected health care utilization,[28] other studies found that this mandate may have reduced neonatal mortality.[29,30] The clinical experience of hospital-based physicians was critical in focusing the evaluation of this legislation on clinical outcomes, such as mortality, rather than on health care utilization or costs. More recently, because the availability and quality of pediatric health care are often dependent on the stability of health care financing for children,[31] efforts have focused on the financing of services such as interpreters for families with limited proficiency in English, child life services, and the specialized procedures required for children (e.g., venipuncture, conscious sedation).[32-37] Consistent with the historical events that led to the formation of the American Academy of Pediatrics, administrative advocacy for children continues to delineate differences between the clinical care of children and that of adults.

Table 10-2 Selected Organizations Focusing on Improving Child Health and Well-Being

Organization	Website
National (United States)	
American Academy of Pediatrics	*www.aap.org*
Children's Defense Fund	*www.childrensdefense.org*
Families USA	*www.familiesusa.org*
Ronald McDonald House Charities	*www.rmhc.com*
International	
CARE	*www.care.org*
Save the Children	*www.savethechildren.org*
UNICEF	*www.unicef.org*

Ultimately, hospitalists have the potential to make important contributions to improved child health at multiple levels in the health care system. As physicians, hospitalists influence children's lives directly by the care they provide. For some, joining larger organizations devoted to improving the health and well-being of children may be another way to give voice to children's health care needs (Table 10-2). By advocating for improvements in the quality of child health care, hospitalists can fulfill their mission to make children's lives better.

REFERENCES

1. American Academy of Pediatrics: AAP Profile Booklet. Elk Grove, Ill, American Academy of Pediatrics, 2004.
2. AAP Fact Sheet. *http://aap.org/visit/facts.htm* (accessed July 13, 2004).
3. Zweig CD: Reducing stress when a child is admitted to the hospital. MCN Am J Matern Child Nurs 1986;11:24-25.
4. Azarnoff P: Preparing well children for possible hospitalization. Pediatr Nurs 1985;11:53-56.
5. Bradford WD, Kaste LM, Nietert PJ: Continuity of medical care, health insurance, and nonmedical advice in the first 3 years of life. Med Care 2004;42:91-98.
6. Morrissey J: The best route: Clinical pathways have become a habit at Children's Hospital in San Diego and the effort is paying off in quantifying quality and cutting costs. Mod Healthcare 2003;33:26-28.
7. Owens PL, Thompson J, Elixhauser A, Ryan K: Care of Children and Adolescents in US Hospitals. AHRQ Publication No. 04-004. Rockville, Md, Agency for Healthcare Research and Quality, 2003.
8. Kelly CS, Andersen CL, Pestian JP, et al: Improved outcomes for hospitalized asthmatic children using a clinical pathway. Ann Allergy Asthma Immunol 2000;84:509-516.
9. Kelly CS, Morrow AL, Shults J, et al: Outcomes evaluation of a comprehensive intervention program for asthmatic children enrolled in Medicaid. Pediatrics 2000;105:1029-1035.
10. Kwan-Gett TS, Lozano P, Mullin K, Marcuse EK: One-year experience with an inpatient asthma clinical pathway. Arch Pediatr Adolesc Med 1997;151:684-689.
11. Johnson KB, Blaisdell CJ, Walker A, Eggleston P: Effectiveness of a clinical pathway for inpatient asthma management. Pediatrics 2000;106:1006-1012.
12. Wilson SD, Dahl BB, Wells RD: An evidence-based clinical pathway for bronchiolitis safely reduces antibiotic overuse. Am J Med Qual 2002;17:195-199.
13. Glauber JH, Farber HJ, Homer CJ: Asthma clinical pathways: Toward what end? Pediatrics 2001;107:590-592.
14. Bergman DA: Evidence-based guidelines and critical pathways for quality improvement. Pediatrics 1999;103(1 Suppl E):225-232.
15. Bellet PS, Whitaker RC: Evaluation of a pediatric hospitalist service: Impact on length of stay and hospital charges. Pediatrics 2000;105:478-484.
16. Landrigan C, Srivastava R, Muret-Wagstaff S, et al: Pediatric hospitalists: What do we know, and where do we go from here? Ambul Pediatr 2001;1:340-345.
17. Seid M, Quinn K, Kurtin PS: Hospital-based and community pediatricians: Comparing outcomes for asthma and bronchiolitis. J Clin Outcomes Manage 1997;4:21-24.
18. Wells RD, Dahl B, Wilson SD: Pediatric hospitalists: Quality care for the underserved? Am J Med Qual 2001;16:174-180.
19. Ogershok PR, Li X, Palmer HC, et al: Restructuring an academic pediatric inpatient service using concepts developed by hospitalists. Clin Pediatr 2001;40:653-660.
20. Srivastava R, Landrigan C, Gidwani P, et al: Pediatric hospitalists in Canada and the United States: A survey of pediatric academic department chairs. Ambul Pediatr 2001;1:338-339.
21. Fernandez A, Grumbach K, Goitein L, et al: Friend or foe? How primary care physicians perceive hospitalists. Arch Intern Med 2000;160:2902-2908.
22. Landrigan CP, Muret-Wagstaff S, Chiang VW, et al: Effect of a pediatric hospitalist system on housestaff education and experience. Arch Pediatr Adolesc Med 2002;156:877-883.
23. Stucky ER: Prevention of medication errors in the pediatric inpatient setting. Pediatrics 2003;112:431-436.
24. Connor JD: A look at the future of pediatric therapeutics: An investigator's perspective of the new pediatric rule. Pediatrics 1999;104:610-613.
25. Keren R, Pati S, Feudtner C: The generation gap: Differences between children and adults pertinent to economic evaluations of health interventions. Pharmacoeconomics 2004;22:71-81.
26. Community Sites: Safety City—Department of Transportation. Anne E. Dyson Community Pediatrics Training Initiative. *http://www.communityped.org/* (accessed July 16, 2004).
27. Winston FK, Schwarz DF, Baker SP: Biomechanical epidemiology: A new approach to injury control research. J Trauma Injury Infect Crit Care 1996;40:820-824.
28. Madden JM, Soumerai SB, Lieu TA, et al: Effects of a law against early postpartum discharge on newborn follow-up, adverse events, and HMO expenditures. N Engl J Med 2002;347:2031-2038.
29. Malkin JD, Garber S, Broder MS, Keeler E: Infant mortality and early postpartum discharge. Obstet Gynecol 2000;96:183-188.
30. Malkin JD, Keeler E, Broder MS, Garber S: Postpartum length of stay and newborn health: A cost-effectiveness analysis. Pediatrics 2003;111:e316-e322.
31. Pati S, Keren R, Alessandrini EA, Schwarz DF: Generational differences in public spending, 1980-2000. Health Aff (Millwood) 2004;23:131-141.
32. Meier P: CMS increases reimbursement for pediatric venipuncture. AAP News 2002;20:5.
33. American Academy of Pediatrics, Committee on Hospital Care: Child life services. Pediatrics 2000;106:1156-1159.
34. AAP Department of Practice and Research: Academy forms team to advise on reimbursement problems. AAP News 2002;21:86.
35. Britton CV: Academy working on issue of how to pay for interpreters. AAP News 2004;24:68.
36. Edwards ES: Appropriate reimbursement among triad of top AAP priorities. AAP News 2003;22:52.
37. Guidelines for monitoring and management of pediatric patients during and after sedation for diagnostic and therapeutic procedures: Addendum. Pediatrics 2002;110:836-838.

CHAPTER 11

Spiritual Care

Chris Feudtner, Mirabai Galashan, Jack Rodgers, and Martha Dimmers

Most Americans regard spirituality as an important part of their lives, and this sense of importance tends to increase during times of illness, injury, or crisis.[1] Patients want their physicians to understand how their spiritual or religious beliefs affect their health and their views about health care. Further, hospitals are now evaluated by the Joint Commission on the Accreditation of Healthcare Organizations regarding how well they provide pastoral care that respects patients' spiritual values and inner spiritual resources.[2]

How should spiritual issues be addressed by pediatric hospitalists? Across the spectrum of illness severity—from healthy newborn care or mild asthma to devastating trauma or end-of-life care—patients and parents are often grappling with spiritual concerns or drawing on sources of spiritual strength and hope. This chapter provides a general overview of some key issues in the domain of spiritual care and some practical guidance on this important but admittedly subtle and sometimes difficult aspect of care.

WHAT IS SPIRITUAL CARE?

Spirituality has many definitions. We embrace the following view:

- Spirituality is intimately related to religion and formal religious affiliation and practices but is a broader concept of one's life view and purpose.
- Spirituality and religion serve a vital role in the lives of humans in terms of mediating the relationship between large, transcendent questions or concerns, such as an intimate God or ultimate Being, on the one hand, and the practical day-to-day realities of life, on the other.

Seen from this perspective, spiritual care aims to facilitate the spiritual dialogue between transcendent and other domains of existence (Fig. 11-1).

Traditionally, spiritual care in hospitals has been the realm of hospital chaplains and spiritual leaders visiting from the community, usually organized by a pastoral care department. Yet spiritually relevant care for children is ultimately delivered by many other people as well. In the classic book *The Spiritual Life of Children*, psychiatrist Robert Coles noted, "we talked with a lot of children whose specific religious customs and beliefs came under discussion; but we also talked with a lot of children whose interest in God, in the supernatural, in the ultimate meaning of life, in the sacred side of things, was not by any means mediated by visits to churches, mosques, or synagogues." Coles also observed that among the children interviewed, "some were the sons and daughters of professed agnostics or atheists; others belonged to 'religious' families but asked spiritual questions that were not at all in keeping with the tenets of their religion."[3]

How can a pediatric hospitalist facilitate this broad-ranging dialogue with a child or the parents in a helpful, competent, and professional manner? A three-step process can be used:

1. Ask patients or parents, "Is there anything I should know about your spiritual or religious beliefs that are important to you and your medical care?"
2. Learn about the spiritual care specialists, allies, and resources available, and make appropriate referrals or consultation requests.
3. Provide some form of follow-up.

Each of these steps is considered in more detail in the following sections.

ADOPT A CURIOUS ATTITUDE AND ASK QUESTIONS

Although most patients would welcome questions about spiritual or religious issues,[4, 5] most physicians do not ask them.[6, 7] There are likely several reasons for this lack of inquiry, but one of the most important is that physicians often do not feel competent in this area and are worried about asking and responding appropriately. We propose that physicians should not be concerned about having sufficient cultural or spiritual competence but rather should focus on approaching these issues with an appropriate degree of cultural or spiritual humility and sensitivity. Typically, patients and parents do not expect physicians to be experts in spiritual matters; most of them simply appreciate a physician who is willing to ask about and be sensitive to their spiritual concerns, acknowledge their importance, and make appropriate referrals or contacts with spiritual care specialists at the hospital.

Although there are several spiritual assessment tools available for health care providers,[8-11] a hospitalist's role is to perform a "spiritual screening," which is brief and less specialized. Its aim is to elicit some basic information while also expressing an appreciation for the potential spiritual dimensions of health, illness, and medical care. For pediatric hospitalists, a simple question might be the best starting point: "Is there anything I should know about your spiritual or religious beliefs that are important to your (or your child's) medical care?" This question can easily be added to the initial history-taking process at the time of admission or can be asked at any subsequent discussion between the patient or parent and the hospitalist. The key is to ask this question with sincerity and sensitivity, and then to use receptive listening with regard to the answer. Once the question has been asked and the invitation to discuss spiritual or religious issues has been extended, the physician must be open and willing to receive what the patient or parent expresses, both verbally and nonverbally. Sometimes, the answer is brief and

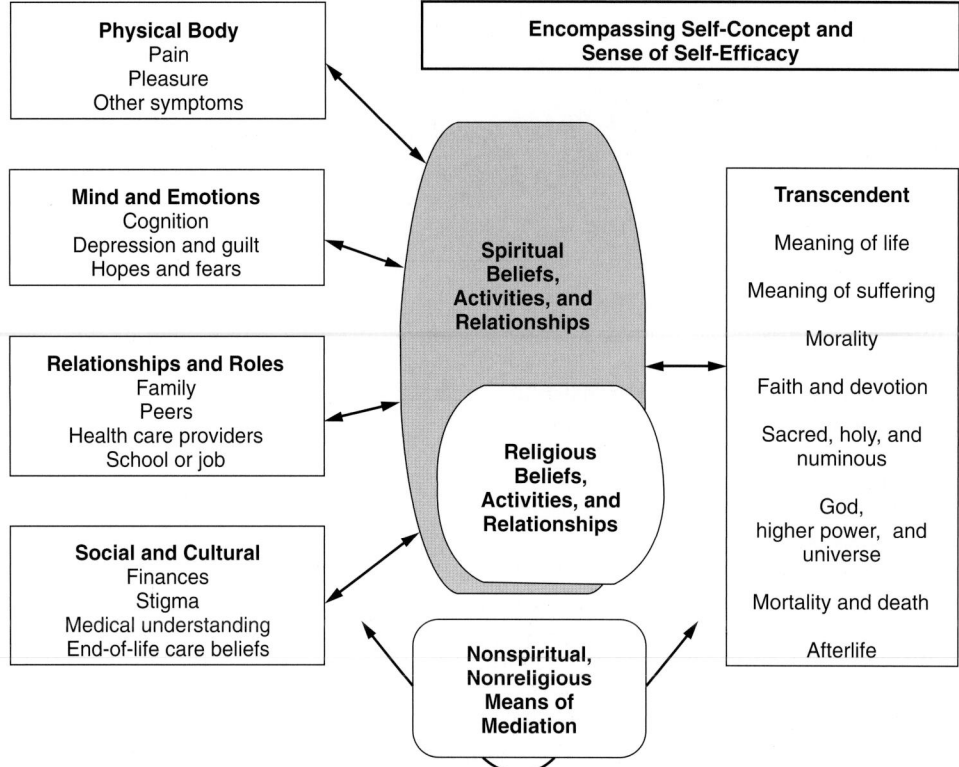

Figure 11-1   The relationship among spiritual, religious, transcendent, and other domains of human lives. (Adapted from Feudtner C, Haney J, Dimmers MA: Spiritual care needs of hospitalized children and their families: A national survey of pastoral care providers' perceptions. Pediatrics 2003;111:e67–e72.)

perfunctory; other times, the response is long and profound. While listening, the physician should be attentive to the following:

- The overall importance of spiritual or religious beliefs or practices to the patient and family. If these matters are a paramount concern, the physician must be cognizant of these issues throughout the hospitalization and draw on all available resources in the hospital and in the patient's home community.
- More specific implications regarding the treatment plan. For instance, if the patient's or family's beliefs preclude the use of certain interventions, or incline them toward a particular set of treatment goals, the physician needs to take these preferences into account when devising therapeutic recommendations.
- Opportunities to connect the patient or parent to spiritual care specialists.

TAKE ADVANTAGE OF SPIRITUAL CARE SPECIALISTS, ALLIES, AND RESOURCES

Pediatric hospitalists are typically surrounded by colleagues who can help provide spiritual care. Chief among these are the professional pastoral care workers or chaplains who are officially part of the hospital. Chaplains can be from any faith or denominational background: Buddhist monks, Christian clergy, Islamic imams, Catholic priests, Jewish rabbis, and numerous others. The chaplain's role is to provide spiritual and emotional support—the spiritual medicine of realistic hope—to patients and their loved ones, as well as to the hospital staff. They provide in-depth spiritual assessments and help patients and their parents use their faith and faith practices to cope with illness. The chaplain is the spiritual care specialist on the multidisciplinary team, as well as a liaison and collaborator with community clergy, outside visitors, and volunteers. Certified chaplains have graduate-level theological education plus one year of clinical pastoral education and are certified through four main organizations: Association of Professional Chaplains, National Association of Catholic Chaplains, National Association of Jewish Chaplains, and Association of Clinical Pastoral Education.

Physicians who want to develop their capacities in the area of spiritual care should first meet with the hospital chaplain. Getting to know each other—perhaps over a cup of coffee or tea—and discussing how the physician might best use the spiritual care specialists at the hospital can greatly facilitate subsequent referrals.

To attend to the spiritual needs of hospitalized children and their families, the physician likely has a legion of allies among child life workers, nurses, and other hospital staff. Often, the most revealing comments offered by children or their parents about matters of faith or the challenges of their illnesses are made not to the physician but to these other members of the health care team. Often, children reveal their views or struggles through their play or drawings, which are witnessed by child life or art therapists. Children may write

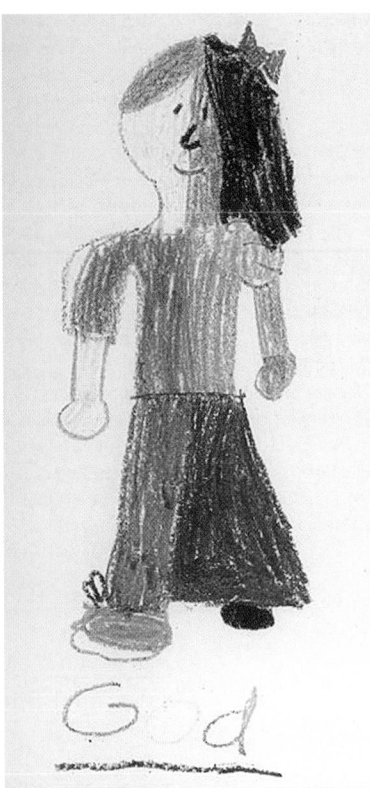

Figure 11-2 A pediatric patient's drawing of God.

prayers or do artwork in a prayer book in the chapel (Fig. 11-2). Adolescents may share their most intimate thoughts and worries to a bedside nurse at 3 AM. Soliciting the input of the entire health care team and incorporating them into the ongoing evaluation and treatment plan can be invaluable.

In addition to regularly scheduled religious denominational or ecumenical services, most hospitals have lovely places devoted to worship, meditation, solitude, or solace. Being able to recommend these places to patients or parents adds to the physician's repertoire. For example, one might ask, "Have you seen the hospital's chapel on the second floor or the butterfly garden outside? They are wonderful places to go when you need some quiet."

FOLLOW UP AND CONTINUE THE DIALOGUE

The delivery of spiritual care should be handled with the same commitment to quality as any other aspect of health care. If a patient has opened the door to a discussion of spiritual matters, the hospitalist should be sure to follow up on the concerns and questions raised, checking in to see how the patient is doing spiritually as well as physically throughout the hospital stay. The physician should make sure that any requests from the patient or parent to meet with a spiritual care specialist have been granted. Concerns at discharge should be conveyed to the primary care provider.

TWO COMMON QUESTIONS

We conclude this chapter with an examination of two questions that often come up in hospital practice.

Should Physicians Pray with Patients and Families?

Views about this issue differ widely, perhaps because no single answer fits all people and all circumstances. Physicians should respond with integrity and compassion when a patient or family requests that they pray. "The physician who is comfortable with doing so may join the patient (and or family) in prayer."[12] This may involve joining verbally in a prayer that is respectful of the patient's beliefs or simply listening as the patient or family prays. This response will likely provide comfort to the patient and engender confidence in the physician. If, however, a physician is not comfortable praying with a patient, does not practice any religious faith, or does not practice one that correlates with the patient's, it is disingenuous to pray with the patient. In this case, the physician should offer to contact the hospital chaplain to pray with the patient. A response such as "I deeply appreciate your inquiry and would like to address your needs the best way I know how" shows both respect and integrity on the part of the physician.

How Should Religion-Related Conflicts Regarding Medical Treatment Be Handled?

Hospital pediatricians are occasionally involved in the care of a child whose family requests that certain forms of medical therapy (e.g., blood products) be withheld because they violate the family's religious or spiritual beliefs or that other forms of therapy (e.g., resuscitation efforts that are highly unlikely to be effective) be delivered in the expectation of a miracle. Regarding the withholding of treatment, the American Academy of Pediatrics' Committee on Bioethics has offered some general guidelines: (1) withholding effective treatments for serious conditions is equivalent to child neglect; (2) in less clear-cut circumstances, parents should control whether their children receive less than highly effective treatments for less than life-threatening conditions; and (3) pediatricians should explore all possible means of conflict resolution before seeking adjudication by the legal system.[13]

Regarding the care of children with severe, life-limiting conditions, guidance about parental demands for potentially inappropriate care has focused largely on the so-called futility of care. Arguments in favor of enforcing rules or policies that limit "futile" care embody a perspective that is both ethically problematic and impractical in clinical practice—namely, that the medical community knows the "truth" and should have the unilateral power to enforce this medical truth. Instead of framing the situation as a conflict regarding the probability of a treatment succeeding, a more effective mind-set is to recognize that families are engaged in an often chaotic and confusing spiritual journey of shifting hope. The role of the healer is to help this hope evolve in realistic directions toward the ultimate best interests of the child. Although there is no simple solution to these situations, involving hospital- and community-based spiritual care specialists and possibly the hospital ethics committee may be extremely helpful. In all cases, open and sustained dialogue, pursued with both tolerance and integrity, is crucial to reaching a satisfactory resolution.[14]

In summary, hospitalists can fill a crucial role in meeting the spiritual as well as physical needs of their patients, but to do so, they must be attuned to their patients' spiritual concerns and willing to listen. Numerous spiritual care resources exist within most hospitals and in the community, and hospitalists should learn to use these as they would any other therapeutic modality.

REFERENCES

1. Gallup G, Jones TK: The Next American Spirituality: Finding God in the Twenty-first Century. Colorado Springs, Colo, Cook Communications, 2000.
2. Joint Commission: Requirements related to the provision of culturally and linguistically appropriate services: Standard RI.2.10. *http://www.jointcommission.org* (accessed April 25, 2006).
3. Coles R: The Spiritual Life of Children. Boston, Houghton Mifflin, 1990.
4. Daaleman TP, Nease DEJ: Patient attitudes regarding physician inquiry into spiritual and religious issues. J Fam Pract 1994;39:564-568.
5. King DE, Bushwick B: Beliefs and attitudes of hospital inpatients about faith healing and prayer. J Fam Pract 1994;39:349-352.
6. Ellis MR, Vinson DC, Ewigman B: Addressing spiritual concerns of patients: Family physicians' attitudes and practices. J Fam Pract 1999;48:105-109.
7. Armbruster CA, Chibnall JT, Legett S: Pediatrician beliefs about spirituality and religion in medicine: Associations with clinical practice. Pediatrics 2003;111:e227-e235.
8. Fitchett G: Assessing Spiritual Needs: A Guide for Caregivers. Minneapolis, Augsburg Fortress, 1993.
9. Maugans TA: The SPIRITual history. Arch Fam Med 1996;5:11-16.
10. Anandarajah G, Hight E: Spirituality and medical practice: Using the HOPE questions as a practical tool for spiritual assessment. Am Fam Physician 2001;63:81-89.
11. Puchalski CM, Larson DB: Developing curricula in spirituality and medicine. Acad Med 1998;73:970-974.
12. Cohen CB, Wheeler SE, Scott DA: Walking a fine line: Physician inquiries into patients' religious and spiritual beliefs. Hastings Cent Rep 2001;31:29-39.
13. Religious objections to medical care. American Academy of Pediatrics Committee on Bioethics. Pediatrics 1997;99:279-281.
14. Feudtner C: Tolerance and integrity. Arch Pediatr Adolesc Med 2005;159:8-9.

CHAPTER 12

Palliative, End-of-Life, and Bereavement Care

Tammy Kang, Sarah Hoehn, Daniel J. Licht, Oscar H. Mayer, Gina Santucci, Jean Marie Carroll, Carolyn M. Long, Malinda Ann Hill, and Chris Feudtner

Children die: as long as this statement is true, hospitals that care for sick or injured children have a cardinal obligation to provide excellent pediatric palliative, end-of-life, and bereavement (P-EOL-B) care.[1] Although far more attention is now given to this area of pediatric medicine than in the past, many health care professionals still find this domain of practice extremely difficult. This chapter addresses the core challenges of providing P-EOL-B care, supplying practical and, to the extent possible, evidence-based answers to these issues.

GOALS OF PALLIATIVE, END-OF-LIFE, AND BEREAVEMENT CARE

Palliative and end-of-life care seeks to minimize distressing or uncomfortable symptoms that patients experience while maximizing the quality of their remaining lives.[2] Collaboration and communication among patients, families, and health care professionals are essential. Bereavement care seeks to mitigate the adverse effects of grieving while honoring the life and memory of the person who died.

IDENTIFYING PATIENTS WHO REQUIRE PALLIATIVE, END-OF-LIFE, OR BEREAVEMENT CARE

Figuring out which patients and their families would benefit from P-EOL-B care, and when, is challenging for two main reasons. First, the prevailing medical model presents palliative care as a mutually exclusive alternative to curative care. This is a false dichotomy: patients can simultaneously receive care that seeks to cure disease or extend life while also receiving complementary care that seeks to minimize bothersome symptoms and maximize the quality of life (Fig. 12-1). Second, among the approximately 55,000 children who die each year in the United States,[3] there are three different trajectories of dying:

1. Children who die suddenly, before any diagnosis (e.g., due to trauma or conditions such as sudden infant death syndrome or occult cardiac arrhythmias). These families warrant bereavement care.
2. Children whose conditions are inevitably fatal. This group can be subdivided into the following groups: (a) Patients who will inevitably die relatively quickly after diagnosis (e.g., nonviable prematurity, inoperable brain tumor). All these patients clearly warrant P-EOL-B care immediately. (b) Patients who will inevitably die, but years to decades after diagnosis (e.g., many neurodegen-

erative disorders). These patients warrant P-EOL-B care, but when to institute such care is debatable. We believe that, along with life-extending care, complementary palliative care and advanced-care planning should be initiated at the time of diagnosis.
3. Children who have conditions that make them extremely frail and vulnerable (e.g., severe spastic quadriplegia with swallowing dysfunction and risk of aspiration pneumonia, cancer that requires debilitating chemotherapy, sepsis that makes the child critically ill). Because of their fragile health, such children have an increased risk of dying on any given day; however, the risk is still low enough so that although death is likely at some point, it is not inevitable in the next year or even the next decade. For these patients, complementary palliative care and advanced-care planning are warranted as early as possible, with a transition toward a more exclusive focus on palliative care if the condition progresses to the point where the benefits of life-extending care are outweighed by the suffering such care imposes.

DISCUSSING PALLIATIVE, END-OF-LIFE, AND BEREAVEMENT CARE

Talking about pediatric P-EOL-B care with families is one of the most demanding and difficult tasks of clinical medicine. Dividing the task into two major components—what the patient and family are up against, and what can and will be done—and having a distinct plan for each aspect of the conversation (which will likely occur over several interactions) can be helpful.

The first component focuses on delivering the bad news itself, which may be a new diagnosis or the latest in a long series of illnesses and deteriorating health.[4] This bad news threatens the goals, plans, and hopes of patients and parents, and the resulting emotional tumult can make even the most seasoned clinician feel overwhelmed and desperate. Preparation is therefore essential: have a precise plan of what information is to be conveyed to whom, allow ample time to hold this meeting, and have the discussion in a private environment with appropriate support persons (e.g., other family members, nursing staff, social workers) present. After briefly reviewing the clinical events, preface your remarks with a warning, such as, "I'm sad to say that the news I have is bad," and then state the new information as simply as possible, such as, "The tests show that your child has cancer." Then stop talking and let the family assimilate this informa-

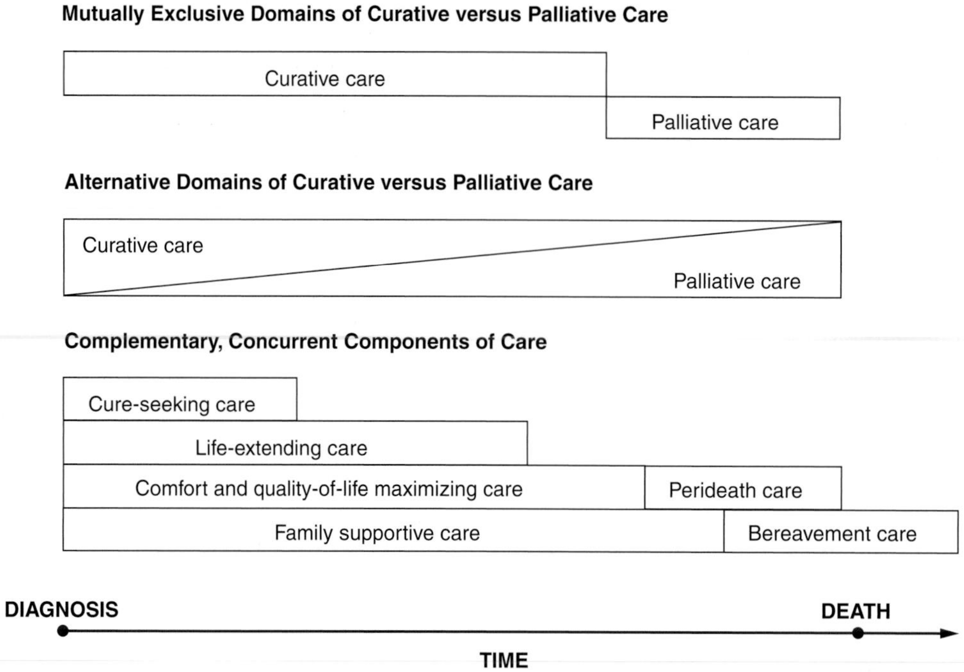

Mutually Exclusive Domains of Curative versus Palliative Care

Curative care

Palliative care

Alternative Domains of Curative versus Palliative Care

Curative care

Palliative care

Complementary, Concurrent Components of Care

Cure-seeking care

Life-extending care

Comfort and quality-of-life maximizing care

Perideath care

Family supportive care

Bereavement care

DIAGNOSIS

DEATH

TIME

Figure 12-1   Palliative care should complement other modes of care.

tion. Your quiet, compassionate presence will be perceived as supportive. Answer questions as they are posed, avoiding the temptation to downplay or sugar-coat the bad news. Given the turmoil that such news often creates in the minds of those who receive it, simply relaying the information and responding to initial questions may be all that can be accomplished at the first meeting. Before ending the meeting, however, propose some specific plans for follow-up conversations or actions. For example, say, "I will be back to check on you and your child in two hours, and I can answer any additional questions that may have occurred to you and start to discuss plans at that point."

The second component of P-EOL-B conversations focuses on possible therapeutic actions and deciding which ones to pursue.[5,6] After the family has had adequate time to absorb the bad news (which, depending on its severity and unexpectedness, can take minutes to hours or days to weeks or even longer), the objective of this conversation is to help formulate new goals, plans, and hopes in light of the constraints imposed by the diagnosis. Instead of focusing on dying and death per se, this conversation focuses on what the therapeutic alliance among patient, family, and care team can strive to accomplish, despite the fact that death is likely to occur in the near future. A useful way to proceed is along the following lines: "Learning that your child has an incurable condition that will shorten her [or his] life has been incredibly upsetting and difficult. Given the problems that the condition creates, I am wondering how we can best care for your child. What are your major hopes for her?" At this juncture, family members often both mourn the loss of hope for a normal life and mention the desire to keep pain or other forms of suffering to a minimum or quality-of-life goals, including social or spiritual concerns. These hopes provide the basic goals of all subsequent palliative and end-of-life care plans, and they are the compass by which the rest of clinical care is oriented.

MINIMIZING UNPLEASANT SYMPTOMS

Children who are dying often suffer with seven main symptoms that are managed most effectively within a holistic framework that includes but extends well beyond pharmacotherapy.[7]

Nausea and Vomiting

Many children experience nausea and vomiting for a variety of reasons, including chemotherapy, other drugs, metabolic disturbances, central nervous system tumors, vestibular or middle ear pathology, gastrointestinal pathology, and anxiety or other conditioned responses. Treatment includes both pharmacologic and nonpharmacologic approaches. Medications commonly used include prochlorperazine, ondansetron, granisetron, scopolamine, metoclopramide, dexamethasone, and benzodiazepines. Unfortunately, scant data support the effectiveness of these drugs in the pediatric palliative care setting. Initial therapy should target the primary cause of the nausea or vomiting (e.g., dexamethasone for vomiting due to raised intracranial pressure from a brain tumor, or a benzodiazepine for nausea caused by anxiety). These medications can then be titrated to a maximal dose, and if that is ineffective, therapeutic control with another agent can be attempted. Often, symptom relief can be achieved only with multiple agents. Some of the most effective nonpharmacologic methods are providing small, frequent meals; giving medications after meals, if possible; and eliminating smells and tastes that exacerbate the symptoms.

Fatigue

Fatigue is one of the most prevalent symptoms in children at the end of life. The definition of fatigue in the palliative care setting varies, but in general, it refers to the subjective feeling of being tired or lacking energy. Fatigue usually stems from several concomitant causes (Table 12-1). Although assessment tools exist for fatigue in children, the diagnosis is based on subjective reports by the patient or parent.[8,9] Treatment begins by addressing any possible underlying causes. Maximizing the patient's rest is important, and this may involve the use of sleep-promoting agents. Increasing wakefulness may also be beneficial; the potent psychostimulant amphetamine has produced consistent improvements in validated measures of fatigue in randomized, controlled trials in adult patients with cancer, human immunodeficiency virus (HIV), chronic fatigue syndrome, and multiple sclerosis. Less potent psychostimulants, such as methylphenidate, dextroamphetamine, or corticosteroids, may also improve fatigue.[10-13]

Pain

Most children experience pain at some point during their illness. Pain is a subjective symptom that is physically and emotionally distressing for both the patient and caregivers. The type of pain may be somatic, visceral, or neuropathic and may be the result of a combination of disease-related, treatment-related, and psychological causes. It is important to make a detailed assessment of pain, including location, duration, and possible causes. It is also important to assess the patient's ability to take oral medications and the family's reaction to the use of pain medications. Many parents are afraid to permit treatment with narcotics, owing to the widespread negative cultural perception of opiates as drugs of abuse, and need reassurance. Any treatment must take into account the developmental level of the child as well as the environment (home, hospital, or health care facility) in which the child lives.

The World Health Organization's treatment ladder is a reliable tool for managing pain (Fig. 12-2); it guides physicians to escalate therapy depending on whether the degree of pain is mild, moderate, or severe and whether the previous level of treatment intensity eliminated the pain. Treatment should begin with mild analgesics such as nonsteroidal anti-inflammatory drugs and acetaminophen and, based on the patient's response, can escalate to narcotics. Two of the essential components of good palliative care are to assess pain frequently and treat it aggressively (see Chapter 197).

Anorexia

Loss of appetite is common and often results from other symptoms, such as nausea, vomiting, constipation, pain, depression, gastritis, and weakness. It is important to treat the underlying causes if possible. As with nausea and vomiting, nonpharmacologic measures may be helpful, including giving small, frequent meals; removing unpleasant odors; and providing a relaxing atmosphere for meals. Pharmacologic therapies include corticosteroids, megestrol acetate, and dronabinol.[14-18] Each of these therapies has adverse effects (e.g., anxiety, dizziness, hypertension, hyperglycemia, adrenal insufficiency, fatigue) that can limit their usage.

Dyspnea

The sensation of breathlessness commonly occurs in conditions with respiratory insufficiency. Patients experiencing dyspnea typically breathe in a shallow, rapid pattern as they struggle with musculoskeletal or pleuritic pain (which restricts the range of chest wall excursion), respiratory muscle weakness (as occurs with myopathies or cachectic states), poorly compliant lung tissue (due to infection, heart failure, and other conditions), or lung lesions that compromise the airway (e.g., bronchiectasis, tumor), fill airspaces (e.g., atelectasis, edema, pneumonia), or occupy space in the chest cavity (e.g., pleural fluid). Dyspnea should first be treated by correcting the underlying cause. The accompanying pain also requires effective treatment. The discomfort or fatigue associated with hypoxemia can be ameliorated by administering supplemental oxygen (recognizing,

Table 12-1 Common Causes of Fatigue in Palliative Care Settings
Depression
Anxiety
Pain
Poor nutrition
Medication side effects
Hypoxia
Infection
Dehydration

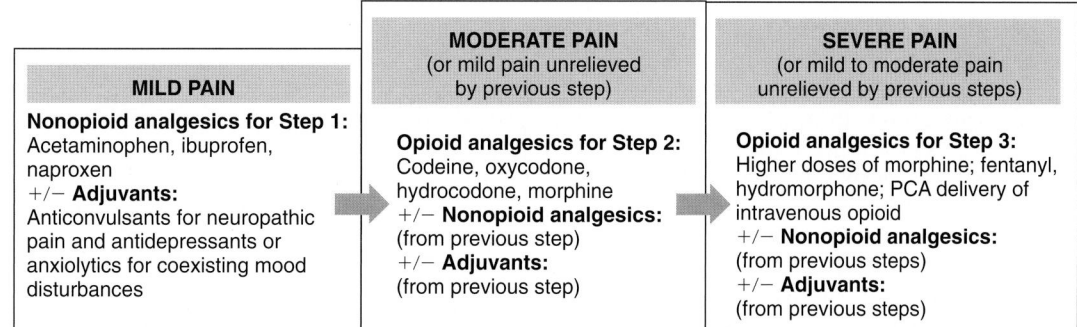

Figure 12-2 Use this "ladder" approach (based on the World Health Organization's approach to cancer pain management) to guide the escalation of pain management for dying children. PCA, patient-controlled analgesia.

however, that for patients with long-standing respiratory insufficiency, supplemental oxygen may suppress the hypoxic drive to breathe and cause respiratory suppression). Fatigued respiratory muscles (which contribute to the sense of dyspnea) can often be supported using noninvasive ventilation through a nasal or oronasal interface (see Chapter 209). With proper fitting of the mask and adjustment of the device, continuous or biphasic airway pressure can be delivered either at home or in a health care institution. Finally, the sensation of dyspnea and the associated anxiety can be abated directly with narcotic agents (e.g., morphine) or with anxiolytics (e.g., benzodiazepines), thereby reducing discomfort and maximizing quality of life.

Constipation

This remarkably common and often neglected complaint of dying children requires a daily assessment of stool output and pain with defecation to determine whether treatment with polyethylene glycol (MiraLax), Colace, or senna is adequate. Treatment failure most often occurs because the starting dose of laxative proves to be too small to produce a soft, painless, daily bowel movement or because the laxative is used only intermittently after constipation recurs. Better results ensue when constipation is assessed every day so that if bowel movements are infrequent or painful, doses can be increased quickly to maximal amounts. Anecdotally, the combination of stool-softening agents (polyethylene glycol and Colace) and a peristalsis-stimulating agent (senna) may work best for patients with difficult-to-manage constipation. Although enemas, suppositories, or GoLYTELY clean-outs may be useful for patients with neurologic bowel dysfunction, such measures should be used sparingly in other patients, whose persistent constipation should be treated with increased maintenance doses of laxatives (see Chapter 94).

Seizures

Convulsions may occur as patients approach the end of life, and they are often particularly distressing to patients and family members. Indeed, many parents who witness their child convulsing express the hope that they never have to see a similar event.[19,20] In the context of end-of-life care, clinical decisions regarding the treatment of seizures are guided by the acuity of presentation, the presence of other organ damage or malfunction, and, most important, the wish to preserve or cloud the patient's consciousness. Benzodiazepines are the mainstay of treating seizures acutely, but they cause substantial sedation and may cause respiratory depression. Newer oral anticonvulsants such as levetiracetam (Keppra) and oxcarbazepine (Trileptal) are options when sedation is undesirable. Both medications are available only in oral formulations, but they achieve good serum concentrations after only two doses, with negligible sedation and good overall tolerance. Valproic acid (Depakote) also causes negligible sedation and is available in both oral and intravenous formulations, but it should not be used in patients younger than 2 years or in those who have bleeding diatheses (valproic acid interferes with platelet function) or liver dysfunction (the metabolism of valproate is dependent on hepatic function and may interfere with the hepatic metabolism of other drugs). For a child in hospice care who experiences a first seizure, a good treatment plan would be the

following: rectal valium (Diastat) (0.5 mg/kg for children younger than 5 years, 0.2 mg/kg for older children and adults) to terminate a seizure in progress, and oxcarbazepine (8 to 10 mg/kg divided twice a day) started as a scheduled medication. The dose of oxcarbazepine can be increased as needed until dose-limiting toxicity is manifested by double vision, vertigo, or ataxia.

MAXIMIZING QUALITY OF LIFE

To support children nearing the end of life, as well as their families, health care professionals need to encourage them to maintain their normal lifestyles to the best of their ability and ensure that their philosophy of life is respected. In any discussion about quality of life, the health care team needs to take into consideration the family's cultural values and traditions.

In conversations with families, it is important to emphasize improving the quality rather than the quantity of one's days. There are many ways to maximize quality of life for dying children. Because time is a paramount consideration, the focus should be on making each day meaningful. Health care providers should encourage the child and family to make memories out of big and small moments and to celebrate milestones—first tooth, first words, birthdays, graduations, religious ceremonies—while the child is still able to participate. Activities such as keeping a journal, making a photo album, videotaping special occasions, making imprints of the child's hands or feet, sharing stories, and keeping locks of hair all help create memories for the whole family.

CHOOSING TO GO HOME

The decision whether to have a child die at home or in the hospital is one of the most difficult that parents face. Not all families are comfortable having a child die at home; the choice depends on many factors, including medical resources, the child's condition, and the family's cultural belief system. Even when families decide to take a child home, they must be reassured that they can always return to the hospital. Going home is often a stressful time, especially for long-term patients, because it represents the first step toward separating from the acute medical facility and team and often symbolizes the beginning of the end-of-life journey. To make the transition as seamless as possible, the health care team needs to have a well-organized plan that is communicated to everyone involved.

The most important consideration in discharge planning is to honor the child's and family's wishes. Ideally, the conversation between the health care team and the family about going home should take place as early as possible so that referrals to hospice or home care services can be made and strategies for improving the quality of life can be implemented. When raising the possibility of involving a hospice agency, one should anticipate several common misperceptions and address them proactively (Table 12-2).

Transitioning a dying patient to home or to a hospice facility is best achieved through a concentrated, multidisciplinary team approach. As an advocate for the child and family, the health care team can help identify appropriate services and providers, as well as clarify the treatment

Table 12-2   Common Misperceptions about Hospice Care

Misconception	Reality
Hospice is about dying and death	Hospice is about living with life-limiting conditions, making the most of one's quality of life
Patients need to be "at death's door," or have less than 6 months to live, to enroll in hospice	Patients with longer life expectancies can enroll in hospice, and physicians should consider hospice enrollment whenever the goals of care are palliative
Enrollment in hospice means that the patient cannot return to the hospital or receive any life-extending care	Hospice patients can reenter the hospital at any time and usually can receive many forms of life-extending care
Hospice enrollment entails stopping all other forms of home nursing care	This is sometimes, but not always, true; direct conversations with the patient's insurance case manager can often result in more flexible arrangements

plan and the patient's needs with third-party payers to ensure maximum utilization of benefits. The health care team can facilitate the discharge planning process by working with its institutional system (e.g., case management, social work) to access all the necessary information and medical orders and to arrange the desired hospice or home care services.

Children and families choose to manage their end-of-life care in a variety of ways. Some continue with home care, others transition to home care with hospice services, and still others choose to end their life's journey in an inpatient hospice or hospital facility. The most important thing to remember is that the journey belongs to the child and the family, and their wishes should be supported.

BEREAVEMENT

Families whose children have died need help to heal and find new ways to live. Each member of the family struggles with intense grief and may experience and express that pain differently.[21]

During the period of grief, the physical and emotional well-being of the bereaved individual may be threatened. Although rigorous evidence is lacking that health risks and psychological problems can be alleviated or avoided if proper support and help are made available,[22] we believe that this absence of evidence should not deter efforts to provide grieving individuals with emotionally supportive interventions to prevent long-term problems.

With advances in diagnostic and therapeutic capabilities, the period between the diagnosis of a terminal illness and the moment of death is becoming longer, and people often have time to consider death and grief before the loved one dies. Known as anticipatory grief, this form of grieving may help families prepare for the loss and lower the degree and

intensity of grief at the time of a child's death. Physicians and nurses who detect that parents or other family members are filled with anticipatory grief and acknowledge this emotion (with simple comments such as "I can see how sad you are") can help them cope.

A comprehensive bereavement program helps families start on the painful journey of grieving. A program should be tailored to meet the unique needs of each family, which includes providing a safe place to sit with sadness, acknowledging the many facets of grief, and helping the family glue the pieces of life back together over time. When parents who have experienced the loss of a child meet together in a grief support group, they often report a sense of peace, healing, and comfort, knowing they are not alone in their grief.

Although the journey is not easy, support, hope, and guidance should be offered to families who must begin the process of healing. Grieving families should be provided with a number of services and encouraged to choose which, if any, suit their particular needs. Bereavement follow-up services may include needs assessments and consultations, crisis intervention and referrals, individual counseling (in person or by telephone), support groups (for parents, siblings, and extended family), follow-up mailings and phone calls, written materials and resources, and memorial services. Little is known, however, about the effectiveness of these interventions in assisting the bereaved.

SPIRITUAL ISSUES

Most Americans have religious or spiritual beliefs of some kind. When people are confronting grave illness or death, these beliefs and associated rituals or practices are often of paramount concern.[23] Accordingly, when caring for a critically ill or dying child, health care professionals should always ask patients or family members whether their religious or spiritual beliefs should be considered in the provision of care, and they should offer to arrange a meeting with the hospital's pastoral care service. For further suggestions, see Chapter 11.

DO-NOT-ATTEMPT-RESUSCITATION ORDERS

Do-not-attempt-resuscitation (DNAR) orders are considered at the end of this chapter because there is so much more involved in pediatric P-EOL-B care (see also Chapter 18 on ethics). Indeed, because DNAR orders require a discussion among the health care team and the patient and family members about values, preferences, and views regarding the quality of life—and about whether the patient's or family's therapeutic goals are best achieved through cardiopulmonary resuscitation or other modes of care—hospitalists who participate in these discussions should thoroughly understand and be capable of providing the other forms of care outlined in this chapter. The conversation, in other words, should be as much about what will be done to promote comfort as about what will not be done. For a more complete discussion of this topic, see Chapter 196. Ultimately, tailoring the DNAR order to fit the personal therapeutic goals set by the patient or family is an expression of the patient- and family-centered philosophy of care that lies at the core of excellent P-EOL-B care.

SUGGESTED READING

American Academy of Pediatrics, Committee on Bioethics and Committee on Hospital Care: Palliative care for children. Pediatrics 2000;106:351-357.

Buckman R, Kason Y: How to Break Bad News: A Guide for Health Care Professionals. Baltimore, Johns Hopkins University Press, 1992.

Carter BS, Levetown M: Palliative Care for Infants, Children, and Adolescents: A Practical Handbook. Baltimore, Johns Hopkins University Press, 2004.

Doyle D: Oxford Textbook of Palliative Medicine, 3rd ed. Oxford, Oxford University Press, 2004.

Field MJ, Behrman RE, Institute of Medicine (US) Committee on Palliative and End-of-Life Care for Children and Their Families: When Children Die: Improving Palliative and End-of-Life Care for Children and Their Families. Washington, DC, National Academy Press, 2003.

REFERENCES

1. Field MJ, Behrman RE, Institute of Medicine (US) Committee on Palliative and End-of-Life Care for Children and Their Families: When Children Die: Improving Palliative and End-of-Life Care for Children and Their Families. Washington, DC, National Academy Press, 2003.

2. Feudtner C: Perspectives on quality at the end of life. Arch Pediatr Adolesc Med 2004;158:415-418.

3. Feudtner C, Hays RM, Haynes G, et al: Deaths attributed to pediatric complex chronic conditions: National trends and implications for supportive care services. Pediatrics 2001;107:E99.

4. Buckman R, Kason Y: How to Break Bad News: A Guide for Health Care Professionals. Baltimore, Johns Hopkins University Press, 1992.

5. Hays RM, Haynes G, Geyer JR, Feudtner C: Communication at the end of life. In Carter BS, Levetown M (eds): Palliative Care for Infants, Children, and Adolescents: A Practical Handbook. Baltimore, Johns Hopkins University Press, 2004, pp 112-140.

6. McConnell Y, Frager G, Levetown M: Decision making in pediatric palliative care. In Carter BS, Levetown M (eds): Palliative Care for Infants, Children, and Adolescents: A Practical Handbook. Baltimore, Johns Hopkins University Press, 2004, pp 69-111.

7. Hain R, Weinstein S, Oleske J, et al: Holistic management of symptoms. In Carter BS, Levetown M (eds): Palliative Care for Infants, Children, and Adolescents: A Practical Handbook. Baltimore, Johns Hopkins University Press, 2004, pp 163-195.

8. Clarke-Steffen L: Cancer-related fatigue in children. J Pediatr Oncol Nurs 2001;18(2 Suppl 1):1-2.

9. Hinds PS, Hockenberry-Eaton M, Gilger E, et al: Comparing patient, parent, and staff descriptions of fatigue in pediatric oncology patients. Cancer Nurs 1999;22:277-288.

10. Breitbart W, Rosenfeld B, Kaim M, Funesti-Esch J: A randomized, double-blind, placebo-controlled trial of psychostimulants for the treatment of fatigue in ambulatory patients with human immunodeficiency virus disease. Arch Intern Med 2001;161:411-420.

11. Sarhill N, Walsh D, Nelson KA, et al: Methylphenidate for fatigue in advanced cancer: A prospective open-label pilot study. Am J Hosp Palliat Care 2001;18:187-192.

12. Wagner GJ, Rabkin JG, Rabkin R: Dextroamphetamine as a treatment for depression and low energy in AIDS patients: A pilot study. J Psychosom Res 1997;42:407-411.

13. Wagner GJ, Rabkin R: Effects of dextroamphetamine on depression and fatigue in men with HIV: A double-blind, placebo-controlled trial. J Clin Psychiatry 2000;61:436-440.

14. McClement SE, Degner LF, Harlos M: Family responses to declining intake and weight loss in a terminally ill relative. Part 1. Fighting back. J Palliat Care 2004;20:93-100.

15. Faull C, Hirsch C: Symptom management in palliative care. Prof Nurse 2000;16:840-843.

16. Sarhill N, Mahmoud F, Walsh D, et al: Evaluation of nutritional status in advanced metastatic cancer. Support Care Cancer 2003;11:652-659.

17. Strasser F, Bruera ED: Update on anorexia and cachexia. Hematol Oncol Clin North Am 2002;16:589-617.

18. Tomiska M, Tomiskova M, Salajka F, et al: Palliative treatment of cancer anorexia with oral suspension of megestrol acetate. Neoplasma 2003;50:227-233.

19. Freeman JM, Vining EPG, Pillas DJ: Seizures and Epilepsy in Childhood: A Guide, 3rd ed. Baltimore, Johns Hopkins University Press, 2002.

20. van Stuijvenberg M, de Vos S, Tjiang GC, et al: Parents' fear regarding fever and febrile seizures. Acta Paediatr 1999;88:618-622.

21. Davies B, Worden JW, Orloff SF, et al: Bereavement. In Carter BS, Levetown M (eds): Palliative Care for Infants, Children, and Adolescents: A Practical Handbook. Baltimore, Johns Hopkins University Press, 2004, pp 196-219.

22. Forte AL, Hill M, Pazder R, Feudtner C: Bereavement care interventions: A systematic review. BMC Palliat Care 2004;3:3.

23. Orloff SF, Quance K, Perszyk S, et al: Psychosocial and spiritual needs of the child and family. In Carter BS, Levetown M (eds): Palliative Care for Infants, Children, and Adolescents: A Practical Handbook. Baltimore, Johns Hopkins University Press, 2004, pp 141-162.

Hospitalist Service Administration

CHAPTER 13

Transitions in Care
Patrick H. Conway and Stephen E. Muething

Transitions in patient care have become common within the health care system and typically involve numerous providers, each of whom is trying to provide optimal care for a patient. To provide the best care possible, tight coordination and standardized processes for the transfer of critical information are essential. Common transfers include those between team members, between teams or units within the hospital, and to or from the outpatient setting. These transfers involve complex communications and therefore pose significant potential risks to patient safety. Few studies in the pediatric inpatient setting have formally evaluated the transition process.

Hospitals need systems to manage transitions, and such systems should be rigorously evaluated. As experts in inpatient care, hospitalists should play a key role in developing and monitoring the processes of patient transitions in an effort to improve the quality of care (Table 13-1). Attention should be paid to several key aspects of successful transitions:

- Decisions to admit, discharge, and transfer care
- Effective communication
- Patient transport
- Safety and error reduction in the transfer of patient care

DECISIONS

No national guidelines exist for general admission and discharge criteria to the inpatient pediatric ward, and the evidence base defining the admission and discharge criteria for common illnesses such as bronchiolitis, pneumonia, and asthma is not robust. There is wide variation in hospitalization rates for common pediatric conditions. Each hospital is organized differently and has different units and specialists available. Additionally, each patient has unique needs and family strengths. Consequently, decisions about hospital admission, discharge, and transfer of care typically fall to the front-line providers directly involved in patient care. Local knowledge and experience of a particular hospital's capabilities may lead to locally accepted criteria for where and when a patient should be admitted.

The decision whether to admit a particular patient usually demands a careful weighing of numerous factors. As the inpatient attending physician, the hospitalist must take into consideration nursing skills, staffing levels, family convenience and proximity, and physician expertise when making decisions about admission or when advising others. Such decisions are typically made at an individual patient level in collaboration with the patient and family, the primary care physician, and possibly the emergency physician caring for the patient in the emergency department. The smooth execution of this task demands excellent communication skills and strong relationships with community and hospital physicians.

Beyond the individual decision-making process, however, hospitalists should seek to establish general admission and discharge criteria for patients at their hospitals, in collaboration with primary care and emergency physicians as well as patient representatives. Such guidelines can help eliminate undesirable variations in policies and improve the quality of care. Models for such guidelines can be drawn to some extent from related fields. The American Academy of Pediatrics (AAP) Committee on Hospital Care and Section on Critical Care have published guidelines on admission and discharge policies for pediatric intensive care units and intermediate-care units.[1,2] These guidelines are meant to be adapted and modified to fit each institution's policies and procedures regarding the nature and scope of the critical illnesses it treats and its interhospital transfer arrangements. The guidelines are delineated by system and include specific physiologic parameters, such as hyperkalemia, and specific conditions, such as spinal cord compression or impending compression.[2]

COMMUNICATION

Good communication is fundamental to a safe and effective transition, whether from one service to another within a hospital or even between providers on the same service. Traditionally, medical education has spent relatively little time teaching sign-out and teamwork skills. Hospitalists should be attuned to the risk of miscommunication and seek to foster (1) an awareness of the importance of communication among hospital personnel during the transition process, (2) good sign-out procedures whenever there is a change of provider or service, and (3) tools to aid in the sign-out process.

Table 13-1 Key Issues in the Transition of Patient Care

Type of Transition	Key Issues	Strategies for Effective Transition
Admission to hospital	Effective communication with ED physicians, PCP, and patient and family regarding workup and plan Knowledge of previous history and treatment	Established, agreed-upon process for communication and transfer between ED and inpatient team Contact PCP to understand history and coordinate treatment plan
Transfer to or from intensive or intermediate-care unit	Decision of when and how to transfer Possible patient decompensation if transfer is not timely	Establish hospital guidelines for conditions requiring intensive care Establish hospital guidelines regarding communication and process of transfer
Transport for test or procedure	Movement of patient has potential to cause patient instability or pain	Preparation and plan for transport of patients within the hospital Plan for appropriately trained staff to accompany patients
Change of covering physician (attending or resident)	Understanding of patient issues and treatment plan Balance of efficient, timely sign-out and provision of all necessary information	Establishment of a sign-out or rounding process that promotes efficient, comprehensive transfer of information Checklist of key items to communicate Systems such as computerized sign-out that facilitate effective communication
Transfer to or from subspecialist team	Substantial overlap between generalist and subspecialist for many inpatient diagnoses (e.g., asthma, seizures) Decisions regarding when subspecialist care is beneficial	Establish hospital policies on when patients with certain diagnoses (e.g., asthma, seizures) should be managed by subspecialty team Subspecialty teams must be available and willing to help manage patients on a general team
Discharge from hospital	Coordination between inpatient team and outpatient PCP Family comfort with discharge plan	Written discharge plan discussed with PCP, including any pending test results, treatment plan, and follow-up appointments Family-centered communication to facilitate family's understanding of discharge plan

ED, emergency department; PCP, primary care physician.

Patients are typically transferred from one location to another because of a change in condition. This is true for patients being admitted to the hospital and for those being transferred to another unit. Treatment plans are often in the process of being revised during such transfers. Timing and accuracy are critical at this juncture, making precise and unambiguous communication essential. Developing a standardized system for communication during transitions is essential and should be a high priority of any hospitalist service.

One key element of transfers (within as well as between institutions; see also Chapter 15 on transport medicine) is the designation of a responsible provider at each stage of the transition. The responsible provider monitors the patient's condition and makes decisions if changes occur. He or she must ensure that all necessary information is transferred to the next provider. In a critical incident analysis of communication failures during patient sign-out, omitted content (e.g., medications, active problems, pending tests) or failure-prone communication processes (e.g., lack of face-to-face discussion) emerged as major categories of failed communication.[3] The system for transfers should designate which information is essential. Many hospitals have begun using communication checklists to standardize the transfer process and ensure that critical information is not lost. The

content of the checklist may vary from site to site but should always contain the following:

- Demographic information
- Allergies and reactions
- Medication doses and frequency
- Diagnoses
- Key history, physical examination, and laboratory findings
- Immediate needs and concerns

Hospitalists should play a key role in developing a safe system that includes appropriate communication. The AAP Committee on Hospital Care published a report summarizing the different roles for hospitalists, subspecialists, and primary care physicians in terms of communication and the coordination of care within and outside the hospital.[4] Often, redesign of existing rounding and sign-out processes is required to ensure safe care.

Communication between the hospitalist and the primary care physician is a key aspect of delivering health care within a child's medical home. This is even more important for children with special health care needs.[5] One survey demonstrated that 60% of primary care pediatricians versus only 30% of hospitalists ($P < .001$) believed that a hospitalist system might impair communication with the primary care physician.[6] However, a recent systematic review demonstrated that in five of five studies, primary care pediatricians rated the quality of care favorably in hospitalist systems, although communication concerns remain.[7] Hospitalists therefore need to focus on communication with primary care physicians, especially at admission and discharge. At the time of discharge, a written summary and recommendations for outpatient care should be provided to families after communication and coordination with the primary care physician[4] (see also Chapter 17 on discharge planning).

PATIENT TRANSPORT

Because patients in transition are usually experiencing a change in their condition and may be deteriorating, the actual movement from one physical location to another within a hospital or between hospitals makes them particularly vulnerable. Hospitalists often play a key role in making transport decisions and performing transport tasks. Proper planning for transport involves three levels of preparedness: routine, clinical change, and emergency. (For a more detailed discussion of transport planning and preparedness, see Chapter 15.)

Routine

During all transports, staff accompanying a patient need to be trained in the use of all applicable equipment and monitors, including intravenous pumps and respiratory equipment. The staff should decide whether treatments should be continued during transport. Because patients may be moved onto a gurney or other transport device, careful attention needs to be paid to airway positioning, intravenous access, and other invasive devices. Sudden deterioration can be secondary to equipment failure during movement. During this vulnerable time, monitoring should be used if there is any significant risk of change in the patient's condition. Adequate staff should accompany the patient.

Clinical Change

Before transport, the responsible provider should have a plan to deal with any anticipated changes; this may include worsening respiratory distress, hemodynamic instability, or increased pain. The plan should also anticipate the possibility of equipment malfunction. Although not all changes can be planned for, preparation allows providers to respond to most problems effectively.

Emergency

Providers transporting a patient need to be skilled in pediatric advanced life support and should be prepared to initiate resuscitation. There should also be a method for alerting the hospital rapid response or code team. If transport involves traveling a distance where phones are unavailable, other means of communication should be established in advance.

SAFETY AND ERROR REDUCTION

The Institute of Medicine report *To Err Is Human* brought patient safety issues to the forefront of efforts to improve the quality of patient care.[8] As suggested earlier, there are many opportunities for errors during the transfer of patient care, and this issue has recently gained renewed attention owing to the Accreditation Council for Graduate Medical Education guidelines and other initiatives seeking to reduce physicians' consecutive work hours. In adults, Petersen and colleagues demonstrated a significant increase in potentially preventable adverse events when a cross-covering physician was providing care.[9] This same research group later demonstrated a reduction in medical errors and a significant decrease in preventable adverse events for cross-covering physicians after the implementation of a computerized sign-out system.[10] Hospitalists play a key role in error reduction and should be leaders in developing systems and creating a culture of safety.

A fundamental step in ensuring the safe transfer of care includes tracking data on the safety of transitions, including arrests, near arrests, medication errors, and other errors. Each hospital should systematically study the causes of errors, develop new processes or adopt proven systems to ensure the safe transition of care, and test their effectiveness.

In summary, transitions in care represent a significant hazard to hospitalized patients, and there is room for considerable improvement. Standardization of communication and transfer procedures is as essential in health care as it is in other high-risk industries. Training of individuals in basic procedures needs to be supplemented by teamwork training, the use of sign-out tools, and practice in managing common problems. Training is particularly effective if scenarios are drawn from previous real-life events. Working with hospital staff and administration to develop systems for safe and effective transitions for patients and their families may be one of the foremost opportunities for hospitalists to improve the quality of hospital care.

REFERENCES

1. Jaimovich DG: Admission and discharge guidelines for the pediatric patient requiring intermediate care. Crit Care Med 2004;32:1215-1218.
2. Guidelines for developing admission and discharge policies for the pediatric intensive care unit. Pediatric Section Task Force on Admission and Discharge Criteria, Society of Critical Care Medicine, in conjunction with the American College of Critical Care Medicine and the Committee on Hospital Care of the American Academy of Pediatrics. Crit Care Med 1999;27:843-845.
3. Arora V, Johnson J, Lovinger D, et al: Communication failures in patient sign-out and suggestions for improvement: A critical incident analysis. Qual Saf Health Care 2005;14:401-407.
4. Percelay JM: Physicians' roles in coordinating care of hospitalized children. Pediatrics 2003;111:707-709.
5. The medical home. Pediatrics 2002;110:184-186.
6. Srivastava R, Norlin C, James BC, et al: Community and hospital-based physicians' attitudes regarding pediatric hospitalist systems. Pediatrics 2005;115:34-38.
7. Landrigan CP, Conway PH, Edwards S, Srivastava R: Pediatric hospitalists: A systematic review of the literature. Pediatrics 2006;117:1736-1744.
8. Kohn LT, Donaldson MS (eds): To Err Is Human: Building a Safer Health System. Washington, DC, National Academy Press, 2000.
9. Petersen LA, Brennan TA, O'Neil AC, et al: Does housestaff discontinuity of care increase the risk for preventable adverse events? Ann Intern Med 1994;121:866-872.
10. Petersen LA, Orav EJ, Teich JM, et al: Using a computerized sign-out program to improve continuity of inpatient care and prevent adverse events. Jt Comm J Qual Improv 1998;24:77-87.

CHAPTER 14

Medical Comanagement and Consultation

Erin R. Stucky and Cynthia L. Kuelbs

Consultation and comanagement are relatively new and evolving roles for the pediatric hospitalist. Typically, hospitalists provide direct care for inpatients, seeking consultation from subspecialty colleagues as needed. Until recently, hospitalists were infrequently called on to serve as consultants themselves or to comanage patients with other physicians in the hospital during an episode of inpatient care. Yet in the broader milieu of patient care, hospitalists practice a certain type of consultation every day. When a primary care provider asks a hospitalist to manage one of his or her inpatients, the hospitalist is in many respects comanaging the patient with the primary care provider. Rather than doing this simultaneously during the hospital stay (as is typically envisioned with comanagement), however, the patient is comanaged by the hospitalist and the primary care provider sequentially. For the patient to receive optimal treatment, it is crucial that the two systems integrate. Viewing this relationship as comanagement rather than care transfer serves as a starting point for the concept of two physicians jointly managing patients, whether horizontally along a timeline or vertically during a single episode of care.

In other countries, hospital-based generalists have long been viewed as consultants to outpatient general practitioners. Studying the United Kingdom's system of pediatrician hospitalists as consultants may aid in defining how hospitalists can serve as consultants in the United States. Specialist registrars in the United Kingdom who were asked to define key attributes of the "ideal hospital doctor" named the following eight areas as essential for consultants: clinical knowledge and skills, clinically related nonclinical skills, self-directed learning and medical education, change management implementation, application of strategic and organizational skills, consultation (history and physical) skills, research, and key personal attributes.[1]

In the United States, hospitalists have recently begun serving as clinical consultants and comanagers during a given hospital admission, working with other providers who serve as the attending physicians of record. Pediatric hospitalists in particular are being called on to provide a pediatrician's view of global issues such as child development, pain management, and home health care, as well as to aid in the diagnosis and management of medically complex children. For hospitalists to provide optimal service to patients and providers in these consultant and comanagement roles, it is essential that definitions, expectations, and goals be clear.

Consultation is defined as "diagnosis and proposed treatment by two or more health care workers at one time"[2] or "a deliberation between physicians on a case or its treatment."[3] *Management,* in contrast, is "to handle or direct with a degree of skill"[3] and "the whole system of care and treatment of a disease or a sick individual."[4] *Comanagement* implies that care is managed by more than one physician. To provide the "whole system of care" that patients deserve, physicians must work synergistically as a team. This chapter reviews consultation and comanagement in the current literature, defines terms and goals, explores existing models, and examines future directions.

EVOLUTION OF HOSPITALISTS AS CONSULTANTS AND COMANAGERS: CURRENT LITERATURE

Little has been written on the specific issue of hospitalist consultation or comanagement. Some work has addressed the use of specialty consultants by hospitalists serving as attending physicians of record for inpatients. Very little work, however, has evaluated the effectiveness of hospitalists serving as consultants or comanagers of care with other hospital providers.

Hospitalists' Use of Subspecialty Consultants

In a study at a community hospital in San Francisco, the number of patients receiving any subspecialty consultation or having more than one consultant was not statistically different whether the primary attending physician of record was a hospitalist or a community physician.[5] Of note, however, the two groups cared for patients with different principal diagnoses. Additionally, the timing of and indications for the consultations requested by the two groups were not specified. Even though the authors concluded that there was no difference in the overall use of consultants by hospitalists and community physicians, they discovered a trend for decreased costs and length of stay over the first year of implementation of the hospitalist model.

Hospitalists as Consultants and Comanagers

The literature regarding the use of hospitalists as consultants is sparse. One retrospective chart review of adult patients for whom hospitalists were consulted by orthopedic surgeons for the care of nonpathologic hip fractures did not demonstrate significant improvements in osteoporosis treatment, as defined by the "addition of a medication for osteoporosis that strengthened treatment."[6] However, these patients had more comorbid illnesses and were significantly older than those receiving no consultation. A separate randomized, controlled trial of adults undergoing elective orthopedic surgery compared standard surgical care with comanagement by a team of hospitalists and orthopedic surgeons.[7] This study demonstrated that comanaged patients were more likely to be discharged without medical postoperative complications, were ready for discharge sooner, and had fewer minor medical complications. Unfortunately, lack of blinding, documentation variation, and age and ethnic characteristics of the patients make generalizability of these findings problematic. However, a similar, more recent study also found lower costs, more efficient care, and shorter lengths of stay when hospitalists were compared with traditional non-hospitalist medical physicians in the comanagement of hip fracture patients.[8] Literature on the effectiveness of pediatric hospitalists as consultants or comanagers has yet to emerge.

PEDIATRIC HOSPITALIST AS CONSULTANT

By definition, a pediatric hospitalist acting as a consultant focuses on a specific question or management issue involving a given patient. Most consultations involve a single interaction. The goal should be to provide either diagnostic and therapeutic treatment options or a single comprehensive pediatric screening examination. Discussion of the findings and options with the requesting physician and communication with the family after that discussion are essential. When a pediatric hospitalist is consulted for a specific question but is interacting with a patient on a daily basis, the service requested is actually comanagement rather than consultation. The factor that distinguishes consultation from comanagement is the lack of expectation for longitudinal care and coordination of all patient care needs. Pediatric hospitalist consultation almost always addresses one or more of the following three questions:

1. Is this child stable for the planned procedure or intervention? This is answered by performing a global screening assessment and plan.
2. Are the evaluation and treatment appropriate? This requires a review of the plan of care.
3. What is the cause of and treatment for this problem? This requires a problem-focused assessment and plan.

Each of these three situations requires a thorough history and physical examination, but with a different emphasis. Even for the problem-focused question, however, the pediatric hospitalist should include relevant issues that are at the heart of general pediatrics and may not be thoroughly considered by consulting services, such as nutrition, pain management, psychosocial factors, and developmental needs.

Any of these three key questions may be asked of a pediatric hospitalist by any physician in the institution; however, certain trends have emerged. In particular, surgeons and specialists treating primarily adults may benefit from consistent, planned pediatric inpatient consultation for their patients.[9] Expectations for facilities and personnel can also be a guide in determining the pediatric hospitalist's level of involvement in acute care settings.[10,11]

Consultation may be requested on a case-by-case basis, or there may be an agreement that all patients in a particular group or setting will have a single initial consultation. Each pediatric hospitalist system must determine the best approach for their patients, community, and facility. Groups for whom routine consultations might be considered include the following:

- Service specific: adult and pediatric surgeons, adult specialists, teaching service, family practitioners
- Acuity or site specific: newborn care (e.g., labor and delivery, nursery, level II neonatal intensive care unit),

pediatric intermediate care, nonpediatric emergency department
- Advice only: remote site, in hospital

Although not as widespread, clinical consultation without chart review or patient examination is performed occasionally by hospitalists for patients both on site and at remote locations. Academically based pediatric hospitalists are often asked diagnostic and treatment plan questions about patients who are not under their care. Although this is often educational and uncompensated, the discussion of a specific patient and options for care is a form of consultation. Remote consultation, usually done by phone, is of value for emergency department physicians as well as local community physicians. Clinical issues can vary from the need for admission to highly complex emergency transport requirements. Pediatric hospitalists involved in coordinating and directing care teams for communitywide emergency transport offer a unique and critical form of consultation (see Chapter 15 for more on this topic).

Regardless of the model used, guidelines should be developed for the hospitalist's role as consultant to ensure that the requesting physician is satisfied, patient care is optimized, redundancies are removed, and communication is streamlined. When establishing guidelines, key issues to consider include defining the question, determining whether consultations are accessed by request only or through service agreements, defining who is responsible for communicating with the primary care physician, and clarifying whether the consultant can write orders without approval of the primary attending physician.

PEDIATRIC HOSPITALIST AS COMANAGER

Comanagement can be defined as a situation in which two or more physicians are involved in the ongoing care of a patient. As stated previously, comanagement routinely occurs between the hospitalist and primary care provider, with each physician filling a specific role. This concept is now moving into the inpatient setting. Just as primary care physicians' office obligations preclude them from being available for inpatient care, surgeons' operating room obligations may preclude them from being available for hospital management and timely discharge planning.[12] In a survey of members of the National Association of Inpatient Physicians (now known as the Society of Hospital Medicine), almost half the respondents were comanaging surgical patients.[13]

Comanagement goals should be clearly laid out for each patient. The hospitalist's role may be to coordinate care, provide general pediatric care, improve discharge planning, or enhance communication with the primary care provider, family, or child. Coordination of care is considered by many to be a significant strength of pediatric hospitalists.[14] The models for comanagement are similar to those described for hospitalist consultation and should be developed to fit individual community and hospital needs.

Again, guidelines must be established if comanagement is to succeed. In particular, care is required when treating physicians are in conflict over clinical management, there are conflicts with the family's wishes, or the requesting physician cannot be on site or is available only by telephone. It is important to define which, if any, physician is the "captain of the ship." Defining lines of authority is crucial, and these should be established upon assuming care. Communication expectations must also be addressed, including who will communicate with the primary care provider, the family, the patient, other consultants, nursing staff, and house staff. Many models can be successful, as long as expectations are clear.

For example, a 3-year-old child with cerebral palsy and a ventriculoperitoneal shunt presents with fever and renal failure. The hospitalist is the primary attending physician, comanaging with the patient's neurologist and neurosurgeon. The decision to consult nephrology or infectious diseases is the hospitalist's decision as the primary attending physician. In comparison, a 6-year-old child with known diabetes is admitted with fever and joint swelling. The patient's endocrinologist manages the diabetes, and the hospitalist manages all other aspects of diagnostic and therapeutic evaluation, including the decision to consult orthopedics, if needed. In this scenario, the specialist manages specialty-related issues, leaving the hospitalist to manage all other aspects of care.

CURRENT DATA

The number of patients for whom pediatric hospitalists provide consultation or comanagement varies significantly by site. Given the varied nature of consultation opportunities, mandated hospitalist programs in some managed care organizations, and differences in night coverage, comparisons of hospitalist models are extremely difficult. Hospitalist surveys have traditionally focused on diagnosis-related groups or bundled admission and consultation data, making extraction and interpretation difficult.[15] Specific billing data from an individual program can, however, supply at least a gross overview and provide opportunities for quality review and growth.

At one tertiary care academic children's hospital with a pediatric emergency department and closed pediatric intensive care unit, hospitalists' consultations on other physicians' patients averaged fewer than 2% of the total charges billed for the 24 months between January 2003 and December 2004.[16] Common reasons for consultation included fever, abdominal pain, seizures, and respiratory concerns. Over this same period, 4892 patients were admitted with hospitalists as the attending physicians of record. Approximately 28% of these patients were comanaged either on admission (20%) or after the first hospital day (8%). Of those comanaged, 17% were general or specialty surgical patients. The low consultation and high comanagement numbers at this site may be related to several factors, including the following: the pediatric emergency department does not require consultation; initial admission to the pediatric hospitalist service occurs frequently, often with a specialist as a comanaging or consulting physician; intensive care patients with a known, focused disease are transferred directly to a specialty service, and others are transferred directly to the pediatric hospitalist service; the postoperative care of cardiothoracic and transplant patients is done by their respective surgical and medical specialty services; and transfer of care rather than consultation occurs for complex patients from primary care providers, when requested. Of the patients comanaged during the period, 18% involved coordination with more than one specialist. These patients often required more coordination of care, social support, or home care. It is unclear whether the time and effort required have a linear relationship with the number of physicians involved. It seems reasonable, however, to draw from studies of management group dynamics, which note more unresolved conflicts and less individual involvement as the group size increases.[17] As the number of physicians involved in care increases, hospitalists will likely have a more difficult time managing or comanaging care.

The myriad settings in which pediatric hospitalists practice require data comparison for groups based on academic affiliation, in-house coverage, and pediatric specialist service availability. Those who are in settings with significant numbers of family practitioners or with emergency departments staffed by general emergency medicine physicians, for example, will likely have many more opportunities for consultations or procedures. As the scope of pediatric hospitalist practice develops, an ability to clarify the details of consultation and comanagement will be important.

OTHER ISSUES

Billing issues arise when the hospitalist serves as a consultant or comanages patients. Knowledge of the initial consultation and follow-up codes can prevent billing confusion and delays. Only one physician per medical group can be the attending physician of record, requiring that other physicians bill as "consultants" (regardless of whether they are serving as consultants or comanagers of care, according to the definitions provided earlier).

Contract, risk management, and Health Insurance Portability and Accountability Act issues should be considered by pediatric hospitalists performing "advice only" consulting. A discussion of these issues is beyond the scope of this chapter, but they are covered to some degree in Chapter 19. Despite these concerns, the role of the pediatric hospitalist as consultant is clearly growing.

Pediatric hospitalists must acquire leadership skills to resolve differences of opinion regarding clinical care, particularly in the arena of comanagement. These skills will also be used at an organizational level to institute consultation and comanagement policies and related changes, improve patient safety, streamline processes, advocate for new technology and services, and control costs.

FUTURE DIRECTIONS

The pediatric hospitalist's role as consultant and as partner in comanagement is growing rapidly. Hospitalist reviews to date have focused primarily on cost and efficiency and on major clinical outcomes, such as mortality.[18] The practice of inpatient and outpatient medicine is changing globally, however. More is expected from outpatient physicians, including the management of complex patients who once would have been managed in inpatient settings. Hospitalist comanagement and coordination of care vertically and horizontally are needed to ensure seamless care. Experiences in the United Kingdom and elsewhere may be useful guides as pediatric hospitalists in the United States move toward defining the scope of practice and postresidency training needs.[19]

Studies are needed to evaluate the variety and sources of consultations and comanagement, as well as the effects on patients, specialist colleagues, resident trainees, hospital staff, and hospital administration. Methods should include surveys of those involved, as well as studies of length of stay, cost, and clinical outcome data by disease type and acuity level. Multicenter data collection will be necessary to validate results in varied hospital settings. The intensity of service needed when multiple services are coordinated by the pediatric hospitalist should be appraised separately. Training for current and future hospitalists should include lessons learned from these studies and from mature systems outside the United States. Groups involved in pediatric hospitalist curriculum development, scope of practice, research, and education include the Society of Hospital Medicine, the Ambulatory Pediatric Association's Special Interest Group on Hospital Medicine, the Pediatric Research in Inpatient Settings network, and the American Academy of Pediatrics Section on Hospital Medicine. These groups are well poised to study and refine current and future expectations for the hospitalist as consultant and comanager as the shape of the specialty becomes more defined and specialty certification is considered.

REFERENCES

1. Khera N, Stroobant J, Primhak RA, et al: Training the ideal hospital doctor: The specialist registrars' perspective. Med Educ 2001;35:957-966.
2. Thomas CL (ed): Taber's Medical Dictionary, 14th ed. Philadelphia, FA Davis, 1981, p 328.
3. Merriam-Webster's Collegiate Dictionary, 10th ed. Springfield, Mass, Merriam-Webster, 1997, p 248.
4. Pease RW Jr (ed): Webster's Medical Desk Dictionary. Springfield, Mass, Merriam-Webster, 1986, p 408.
5. Auerbach AD, Wachter RM, Katz P, et al: Implementation of a voluntary hospitalist service at a community teaching hospital: Improved clinical efficiency and patient outcomes. Ann Intern Med 2002;137:859-865.
6. Jachna CM, Whittle J, Lukert B, et al: Effect of hospitalist consultation on treatment of osteoporosis in hip fracture patients. Osteoporos Int 2003;14:665-671.
7. Huddleston JM, Kirsten HL, Naessens JM, et al: Medical and surgical comanagment after elective hip and knee arthroplasty. Ann Intern Med 2004;141:28-38.
8. Roy A, Heckman MG, Roy V: Associations between the hospitalist model of care and quality-of-care-related outcomes in patients undergoing hip fracture surgery. Mayo Clin Proc 2006;81:28-31.
9. Percelay JM, AAP Committee on Hospital Care: Physicians' roles in coordinating care of hospitalized children. Pediatrics 2003;111:707-709.
10. Jaimovich DG, AAP Committee on Hospital Care and Section on Critical Care: Admission and discharge guidelines for the pediatric patient requiring intermediate care. Pediatrics 2004;113:1430-1433.
11. Rosenberg DI, Moss M, AAP Section on Critical Care and Committee on Hospital Care: Guidelines and levels of care for pediatric intensive care units. Pediatrics 2004;114:1114-1125.
12. Wachter RM, Goldman L: The hospitalist movement 5 years later. JAMA 2002;287:487-494.
13. Lindenauer PK, Pantilat SZ, Katz PP, Wachter RM: Hospitalists and the practice of inpatient medicine: Results of a survey of the National Association of Inpatient Physicians. Ann Intern Med 1999;130:343-349.
14. Gill JM, Daru JA: Community pediatricians collaborate with hospitalists to build a ward service. Pediatr Ann 2003;32:791-796.
15. Bellet PS, Whitaker RC: Evaluation of a pediatric hospitalist service: Impact on length of stay and hospital charges. Pediatrics 2000;105:478-484.
16. Kimmons H, Stucky E: Unpublished data, Pediatrics Hospitalists Division, Children's Specialists of San Diego.
17. Schenke R: American College of Physician Executives, Physician in Management Seminar, "Small group dynamics," Feb 6 1998, Sheraton Grande Torrey Pines, Calif.
18. Wachter RM: Hospitalists in the United States—mission accomplished or work in progress? N Engl J Med 2004;350:1935-1936.
19. Flanders SA, Wachter RM: Hospitalists: The new model of inpatient medical care in the United States. Eur J Int Med 2003;14:65-70.

CHAPTER 15

Transport Medicine

George A. Woodward

Pediatric hospitalists need to be familiar with transport medicine, whether to receive incoming patients or to transfer children from the inpatient stetting to a different level of care. To appropriately manage either subset of patients, one must understand the differences between emergency medical systems and interfacility transport, as well as the variable capabilities of the latter. This chapter reviews issues surrounding patient transport from both the referral and the receiving perspectives. Suggestions for the transport of patients with specific disease processes are beyond the scope of this chapter but can be found elsewhere.[1-16]

It is important to recognize that although transport medicine developed from emergency medical systems and intensive care, emergency, and inpatient medicine, the transport environment presents significant and unique challenges to the provision of optimal care. Nonphysician transport personnel are required to work independently, often without direct physician oversight. The working quarters are small, without the benefits and backup afforded to caretakers in the hospital setting. There are the physical stresses of travel, temperature change, vibration, and noise, as well as the risk of injury and death to the participants, including patients, providers, and crew. Limitations with regard to space, testing, medications, equipment, and additional personnel, along with the mobile environment, may affect the capability of the medical care provider who accompanies a pediatric patient during transport.

Transport medicine offers an opportunity for caretakers from different institutions and backgrounds to function seamlessly as an integrated care team. It also presents potential pitfalls in the management of relatively stable to critically ill patients. It is an environment where care may be less controlled than in the inpatient setting and where capabilities may not be as consistent as an institution may desire. Although a strong critical care transport team can perform almost any intervention or procedure in the transport environment, these locations are always less than ideal when compared with a stable hospital setting with appropriate and often redundant personnel and equipment. Transport vehicles do not have radiographic capability or equipment for surgical interventions other than those needed emergently (e.g., needle thoracotomy, chest tube, central venous access, airway management), and most cannot provide advanced care such as extracorporeal membrane oxygenation or high-frequency ventilation. Certain teams, however, are equipped for these types of transports, and if the patient may require advanced capabilities, it is important to identify those systems before the actual need arises.

HISTORY OF PEDIATRIC TRANSPORT MEDICINE

In the United States, the emergency medical service (EMS) system started in 1973 with the passage of the EMS Act, which authorized the Department of Health, Education, and Welfare to fund 300 regional EMS systems across the country. In 1983 the government funded the Emergency Medical Services for Children legislation, which is administered by the Maternal and Child Health Bureau of the Department of Health and Human Services and the National Highway and Traffic Safety Administration. In 1990 the American Academy of Pediatrics (AAP) designated section status to the specialty of transport medicine, and in 2000 it developed the Pediatric Education for Prehospital Professionals training course to teach such individuals more about children and the intricacies of pediatric transport.[17]

Improved pediatric transport medicine was required after the development of intensive care specialties and practices (e.g., neonatal and intensive care medicine and units), along with the recognition that ill children cared for by trained pediatric transport personnel had improved outcomes.[18,19] Before these advances, pediatric transport medicine was an afterthought in the care continuum. It was often accomplished without appropriate medical personnel or via general EMS teams with little expertise in or specific equipment for children. With recognition of the importance of pediatric transport medicine, especially for the neonatal intensive care, pediatric intensive care, and inpatient pediatric population being referred from nonpediatric caretakers, improved and validated transport standards have been developed. The AAP and several other organizations have developed transport guidelines and standards.[20,21] There is also a transport accreditation body that offers guidelines and an optional (in most areas) accreditation.[22] Other organizations with pediatric transport concerns and expertise include the Air Medical Physicians Association, Air and Surface Transport Nurses Association, Association of Air Medical Services, and National Association of EMS Physicians, as well as specific groups within medicine, nursing, respiratory, and prehospital care societies.[23-26]

PREHOSPITAL AND INTERFACILITY TRANSPORT

Hospitalists often interact with EMS providers on both the receiving and the initiating end of an EMS transport. There are various levels of ambulance personnel and transport capabilities, and understanding these differences is important. Most often, hospitalists interact with ambulance transport teams who have picked patients up from their homes or other nonmedical settings and brought them to the hospital (prehospital transport) or with teams delivering patients between two medical settings (interfacility transport).

An emergency medical technician (EMT) may be the primary provider on a prehospital ambulance transport. EMTs have typically had approximately 40 to 100 hours of medical training, only a small portion of which may be pediatric. They have limited assessment and interventional capabilities, and local statutes govern what procedures EMTs can perform during a transport. For example, most municipalities do not allow EMTs to initiate intravenous (IV) lines or administer IV medications. They are, however, often allowed to provide oxygen, glucose, and occasionally the patient's own medication.

A higher level of EMS transport involves paramedics. Paramedics have approximately 1 year of medical training and usually at least 16 hours and a limited practicum involving pediatrics. On average, children account for only 10% to 15% of prehospital transports, so most paramedics have limited experience with pediatric assessments and procedures. Paramedics have the capability to administer typical pediatric and cardiac advanced life support interventions and medications, although they too are governed by state and local regulations.

EMS transports can also include a higher level of provider, such as a prehospital nurse or physician. These advanced personnel configurations are sometimes used in the prehospital arena and often for interfacility transport.

Interfacility transport can occur from an emergency department or clinic to a hospital or from one hospital to another. Interfacility transport can be used to bring a stable or potentially unstable patient from an initial level of outpatient or inpatient service to a different level of care or even to move a stable patient between institutions for financial or other nonmedical reasons. Interfacility transport is sometimes undertaken by EMS personnel but is more often accomplished by specialized interfacility transport teams. These teams usually consist of two caretakers, often led by a transport nurse. The second member may be a transport nurse, physician, respiratory therapist, or paramedic. The pediatric expertise and level of service that can be provided depend on the configuration of the team and the experience of the team members. A general interfacility transport service is composed of transport personnel who take care of patients of all ages. Although they provide advanced transport care, they may not possess specific pediatric knowledge or expertise.

Pediatric interfacility transport involves personnel with a pediatric or neonatal background and ongoing pediatric training. Pediatric and neonatal transports may be combined or separate entities within a transport service or institution. When choosing a transport service, one should evaluate the capabilities of the transport personnel as well as the types of patients routinely transferred. The transport service and its personnel should have the skills to expertly assess and monitor the types of patients being referred or received and should be able to manage all potential medical contingencies that might occur during the transport process.[27-29]

It is the responsibility of the initiating provider to ensure that the level of competence during the transport process is adequate for the patient's current and expected needs. The initiating provider must also ensure that the mode of transport (i.e., the transport vehicle) matches the requirements of the patient. A transport service should be investigated before it is used to verify that the appropriate expertise will be available during the transport process.

As a general rule, ambulance transport provides direct door-to-door care, with great flexibility in the number and type of personnel involved. The abundance of ground ambulances allows for backup as needed; however, the ground ambulance is limited by issues such as traffic, severe weather, and other uncontrollable factors. The helicopter offers the advantage of speed to the scene or return to the receiving facility, but it often offers less flexibility in terms of administered care during transport, space, and additional personnel. Landing zones must be determined, and this may not be feasible at the site of the patient; if not, additional ground transport must be arranged. Transferring the patient between stretchers and vehicles can be especially hazardous; essential interventions such as endotracheal tubes, venous and arterial lines, and life-sustaining medications can be inadvertently dislodged or interrupted during the transfer process. Minimizing the number of transfers is usually in the patient's best interest. If the time between hospitals needs to be minimized, or if the entire process needs to be accomplished in the shortest time possible, helicopter transport should be considered. Knowledge of transfer times, landing zone locations, and alternative options before the need arises is essential for optimal patient care. In general, ambulance transport takes approximately two to three times as long but is one half to two thirds as expensive as helicopter transport over a similar distance.[30-33]

EXPECTATIONS OF THE TRANSPORT PROCESS

It is helpful to have established guidelines and expectations for the transport process before there is an emergent need for transport. The transport system should provide easy and direct access to the referring population, including both EMS staff initiating prehospital transports and hospitalists or other providers initiating interfacility transports. Receiving providers should be immediately available for a case discussion or transport request and to accept a patient if the institution has capacity, especially if the patient is in need of tertiary care. Transfer agreements between institutions can help elucidate these expectations and relationships before an emergency. One should expect clear, concise, and expert recommendations.

Ideally, the transport system has a communications center staffed by transport communications specialists; this should be the first point of contact for any transport. Although it may seem that contacting a receiving physician or unit directly may be an expedient method to gain patient acceptance and arrange a transfer, it is often not the most efficient way to manage transport referrals. For example, if one were to call an intensive care physician or unit directly, exchange medical information, and ask for acceptance of a patient, the transport service would not be aware of the impending need for transport. If a well-organized transport communications center is contacted, that center can immediately contact the most appropriate receiving physician so that appropriate medical advice and acceptance can be given, as well as arrange the logistics of the transport. This could be as simple as alerting the on-site medical personnel and ambulance or helicopter crew of an incoming transport, or as complicated as triaging or redirecting current patient care responsibilities or vehicles to enable appropriate and timely services to the patients with the most urgent need.

After the transport communications center is contacted, demographics will be requested: the patient's name, age, and birth date; the referring physician's location (facility), name, and contact numbers; and the chief complaint. Emergent referrals should not require insurance information; stable transfers, however, may require this information for precertification of the transport process. This is also required for long-range, fixed-wing airplane transports. There should be a medical command physician or intake caretaker with advanced and appropriate medical knowledge who receives the medical information and can offer medical expertise and advice as required. A succinct discussion should take place that covers the patient's presenting symptoms, relevant past medical history, physical examination findings, laboratory and radiographic assessments, interventions, response to those interventions, and current status. Also included should be full vital signs and other parameters such as ventilator settings, oxygen requirements, and current medications and IV fluids. The receiving physician or intake personnel records this information and offers advice as to the continuation of current therapy or suggests additions or changes to care. Although it is the prerogative and responsibility of the referring physician to accept or decline those suggestions, it is advisable to carefully consider the transport experts' recommendations regarding stabilization and therapy, especially for a critically ill child. The transport service often makes specific recommendations about how the transport should be accomplished. It is important that good relationships be established between transport services and referring and receiving personnel, so that teams can frankly and openly discuss patient care and type of transport. Although the transport system can recommend the best mode of transport from its perspective, it is the legal responsibility of the referring physician to choose the appropriate mode and team to transport each particular patient.

The receiving team should organize the required personnel, diagnostics, and interventions before the patient's arrival and ensure a seamless transition upon presentation to the receiving service.[34] The referring team should anticipate the need for both verbal and written communications regarding the patient's transport, as well as his or her ultimate destination within the receiving hospital. This, of course, must be accomplished in compliance with current Health Insurance Portability and Accountability Act regulations (HIPAA).

EXPECTATIONS OF THE REFERRING TEAM

The referring and receiving teams have many responsibilities during the transport process.[35] The referring team's first priority is to stabilize the patient before transfer. The referring team may prefer to wait for the transport team to provide emergent interventions such as an airway or vascular access, on the assumption that the transport team is more experienced with such procedures and can more efficiently stabilize the patient. This may be true, and if a transport team is immediately available, it may be appropriate to

temporize until its arrival. However, transport arrival times often cannot be guaranteed owing to limited resources, multiple demands, and logistical issues, including personnel and vehicle availability, mechanical breakdown, and traffic delays. Thus, critical interventions should not wait for a transport team to arrive.

The referring physician or team must make the appropriate decision to transfer and choose the appropriate facility. This is especially important when the patient is potentially unstable. It is prudent to consider the majority of patients who are transferred early in their illness to be potentially unstable. The referring team should discuss plans for stabilization and intervention with the transport and receiving teams and initiate those plans. Disagreement about management is not unusual during the transport process, and these issues should be discussed. The referring physicians and nurses are the only ones who actually have their eyes on the patient; the receiving team is gathering information and developing a mental picture of that patient. If suggestions from the receiving team do not seem appropriate, or if the referring team is unable or unwilling to implement those suggestions because of technical, personnel, or equipment limitations, the nature of those limitations should be made clear to the transport team. This may make a difference in the mode of transport, the personnel involved, and possibly even the ultimate destination of the patient.

When the transport team arrives, the referring team should facilitate the transition of the patient to the care of that service. This includes being physically available on team arrival, updating the team regarding the patient's medical care, having all appropriate records copied and all laboratory results and radiographs available, and having a transfer summary completed. Procedures and interventions should be accomplished and verified so that the transport team does not need to spend time managing those aspects of patient care. This is especially important for time-sensitive, critical care transports.

LEGAL ISSUES IN PEDIATRIC INTERFACILITY TRANSPORT

The Emergency Medical Treatment and Labor Act (EMTALA) governs the transfer of patients from one medical facility to another.[36-38] EMTALA guidelines are intended to ensure adequate evaluation and stabilization before and during transfer, not necessarily to prevent transfers. EMTALA dictates that an unstable or potentially unstable patient may not be transferred unless certain criteria are met and consents are obtained. If a patient is stable, EMTALA regulations do not apply, and the patient may be transported for other reasons, including financial. EMTALA sets a bar for transport standards that cannot be lowered or circumvented by local hospital, regional, or state guidelines or legislation. Any law that conflicts with or contradicts EMTALA is considered preempted by EMTALA. When one transfers patients, it is important to understand the "appropriate transfer" concept, which states that the referring hospital has a duty to supply all the stabilizing care that it is able to provide to protect the patient before and during the transport process. It also requires the receiving hospital with capacity to agree to accept the patient and to have the necessary personnel and space to provide appropriate treatment.

As mentioned earlier, the referring physician is required to select an appropriate receiving hospital. If an inappropriate hospital or mode of transport is chosen, the referring physician and institution may be liable under EMTALA.

There are multiple potential risks during the transfer process. These include inappropriate use of resources at the referring hospital, lack of availability of resources at the receiving hospital, failure of timely acceptance of the patient, risks inherent in the chosen method of transport (including limitations in care imposed by the transport process), prolonged duration of the transport, inappropriate medical personnel for the transport, lack of required equipment, and lack of full understanding of the patient's medical diagnosis or prognosis, which may not be clear at the time transport is initiated.

Transport documentation should include the patient's identifying data and condition; risks and benefits of transfer; risks for deterioration; specifics of the receiving hospital, including which hospital, expected location within the institution, and accepting physician; mode of transport; skill level of transport personnel; notation that all pertinent documentation was sent with the patient (if this is not immediately available, it may be sent after the transfer); written consent of the responsible patient or guardian or, if the patient is very unstable and transfer is required for specialized lifesaving therapy, the referring physician; and signatures of the patient (as able), physicians, and witnesses.

The referring team should ensure that consent is obtained for transport. This includes disclosure of the risks and benefits of transport, the mode of transport, the specific team involved, and the receiving location. Discovering that the patient (or family) refuses to be transported, that the chosen hospital is not acceptable, or that they refuse to fly after an air transport team has arrived is not ideal.

One issue that is sometimes not clear during the transport process is who is in charge. It is clear that until the transport team arrives at the referring institution, the referring physician and hospital are entirely responsible and liable for the patient's care, as well as any decisions regarding transport. When the transport team arrives, it is initially acting as a consultant to the referring team, so the referring team should be present and involved in any decision making or interventions. At that time, there is shared responsibility and liability regarding patient care. When the transport team leaves with the patient, it assumes responsibility and a greater level of liability for the patient's care. This process is an opportunity for both teams to work together to ensure optimal patient care. At times, there may be differences of opinion regarding the amount or type of care to be delivered at the bedside. If this happens, it should be discussed away from the bedside, and care should be maintained or initiated to ensure the patient's stability during the transport process.

QUALITY ASSURANCE

Appropriate metrics regarding the quality of transport care may be difficult to identify and measure. Criteria to consider include timeliness of the referral request, team response time, and morbidity or mortality related to the initial care or transport process. Although these may be easy to review in retrospect, they are often difficult to critically assess during the acute phases of transport. Referring and receiving teams should work closely together to identify critical indicators of service and quality of care, including logistics as well as standards of care. These should be benchmarked against local, regional, and national data when these are available. Identification of a less than optimal transport, referring, or receiving experience should be used as an opportunity for cooperative review and education to improve care in the future.

Although it may not be obvious, making the transport process family centered generally improves the quality of care provided. The need for transfer is a stressful situation for a patient and family, and it is important for the patient to have support from his or her family and for parents or guardians to feel involved in the patient's care at the time of transport. It should be noted, however, that although inclusion of the parent or guardian in the transport process is beneficial in the majority of situations, there are times when the parent or guardian should be asked not to accompany the patient. For example, severely distraught, inebriated, or otherwise unstable parents or guardians should not accompany the child. Parents may also need to be excluded if space is not available in the transport vehicle (e.g., in a small helicopter or fixed-wing aircraft).[39,40]

CONCLUSION

Pediatric transport is an integral part of inpatient medicine. Knowledge of the availability and capabilities of local transport teams, as well as the responsibilities involved in optimal and efficient transfer, is beneficial to all involved. Patients are transported to us for care, and we may transport patients to other facilities for escalation of care or rehabilitation, or to home when they are unable to go in the usual fashion. The referring service should critically evaluate transport options before the need arises, and the receiving service must assess the needs and capabilities of the referring community. There is an important role for the hospitalist in this process, because issues identified in the inpatient arena can be easily overlooked by critical care transport services, and vice versa, if clear communication does not occur.

REFERENCES

1. Aoki BY, McCloskey K: Evaluation, Stabilization, and Transport of the Critically Ill Child. St Louis, Mosby Year-Book, 1992.
2. Beyer AJ, Land G, Zaritsky A: Nonphysician transport of intubated pediatric patients: A system evaluation. Crit Care Med 1992;20:961-966.
3. Brink LW, Neuman B, Wynn J: Transport of the critically ill patient with upper airway obstruction. Crit Care Clin 1992;8:633-647.
4. Han YY, Carcillo JA, Dragotta MA, et al: Early reversal of pediatric-neonatal septic shock by community physicians is associated with improved outcome. Pediatrics 2003;112:793-799.
5. Henning R, McNamara V: Difficulties encountered in transport of the critically ill child. Pediatr Emerg Care 1991;7:133-137; comment in Pediatr Emerg Care 1991;7:398.
6. Ishimine P, Zorc JJ, Woodward GA: Sometimes it's not so clear: Altered mental status and transport. Pediatr Emerg Care 2001;17:282-288.
7. Jaimovich DG, Vidyasagar D (eds): Handbook of Pediatric and Neonatal Transport Medicine, 2nd ed. Philadelphia, Hanley & Belfus, 2001.
8. McCloskey KA, Orr RA (eds): Pediatric Transport Medicine. St Louis, Mosby, 1995.
9. Macnab AJ, Wensley DF, Sun C: Cost-benefit of trained transport teams: Estimates for head-injured children. Prehosp Emerg Care 2001;5:1-5.

10. Woodward GA, Wernovsky G, Rhodes LA, et al: Sepsis, septic shock, acute abdomen? The ability of cardiac disease to mimic other illness. Pediatr Emerg Care 1996;12:317-324.

11. Woodward GA, Moore KJ, Needle MN: Oncology and transport: Beware of the presentation and anticipate the clinical course. Pediatr Emerg Care 1996;12:454-459.

12. Woodward GA, King B: "Interfacility" transport from the home or office. Pediatr Emerg Care 1997;13:164-168.

13. Woodward GA, Levy RJ, Weinzimer SA: Diabetes and transport: A potentially bittersweet combination. Pediatr Emerg Care 1998;14:71-76.

14. Woodward GA, Posner JC, Bolte RG, Howell J: Just another asthmatic? The many faces of asthma in pediatric transport. Pediatr Emerg Care 1998;14:237-245.

15. Woodward GA, Chun T, Miles DK: It's not just a seizure: Etiology, management and transport of the seizure patient. Pediatr Emerg Care 1999;15:147-155.

16. Woodward GA: Pediatric head trauma. AirMed 1999;5:6-8.

17. Pediatric Education for Prehospital Professionals. *www.peppsite.com.*

18. Britto J, Nadel S, Maconochie I, et al: Morbidity and severity of illness during interhospital transfer: Impact of a specialized paediatric retrieval team. BMJ 1995;311:836-839.

19. American Academy of Pediatrics, Committee on Pediatric Emergency Medicine, American College of Critical Care Medicine, Society of Critical Care Medicine: Consensus report for regionalization of services for critically ill or injured children. Pediatrics 2000;105:152-155.

20. Guidelines for Air and Ground Transport of Neonatal and Pediatric Patients: Woodward GA, editor-in-chief, Section of Transport Medicine, American Academy of Pediatrics. Elk Grove Village, Ill, 2006.

21. Council of the Society of Critical Care Medicine: Consensus report for regionalization of services for critically ill or injured children. Crit Care Med 2000;28:236-239.

22. Commission on Accreditation of Medical Transport Services. *www.camts.org.*

23. Air Medical Physicians Association. *www.ampa.org.*

24. Air & Surface Transport Nurses Association (ASTNA). *www.astna.org.*

25. Association of Air Medical Services (AAMS). *www.aams.org.*

26. National Association of EMS Physicians (NAEMSP). *www.naemsp.org.*

27. King BR, Foster RL, Woodward GA, McCans K: Procedures performed by pediatric transport nurses: How "advanced" is the practice? Pediatr Emerg Care 2001;17:410-413.

28. King BR, Woodward GA: Procedural training for pediatric and neonatal transport nurses. Part 1. Training methods and airway training. Pediatr Emerg Care 2001;17:461-464.

29. King BR, Woodward GA: Procedural training for pediatric and neonatal transport nurses: Part 2. Procedures, skills assessment, and retention. Pediatr Emerg Care 2002;18:438-441.

30. Arfken CL, Shapiro MJ, Bessey PQ, Littenberg L: Effectiveness of helicopter versus ground ambulance services for interfacility transport. J Trauma Injury Infect Crit Care 1998;45:785-790.

31. Bruhn JD, Williams KA, Aghababian R: True costs of air medical vs ground ambulance systems. Air Med J 1993;August:262-268.

32. Woodward GA, King BR, Garrett AL, Baker MD: Prehospital care and transport medicine. In Fleisher G, Ludwig S, Henretig F (eds): Textbook of Pediatric Emergency Medicine, 5th ed. Philadelphia, Lippincott Williams & Wilkins, 2006, pp 93-134.

33. Woodward GA, Insoft RM, Pearson-Shaver AL, et al: The state of pediatric interfacility transport: Consensus of the Second National Pediatric and Neonatal Interfacility Transport Medicine Leadership Conference. Pediatr Emerg Care 2002;18:38-43.

34. Woodward GA: Responsibilities of the receiving hospital. In McCloskey K, Orr R (eds): Textbook of Pediatric Transport Medicine. St Louis, Mosby-Yearbook, 1995, pp 41-49.

35. Ammon AA, Fath JJ, Brautigan M, et al: Transferring patients to a pediatric trauma center: The transferring hospital's perspective. Pediatr Emerg Care 2000;16:332-334.

36. Frew SA: In Appleton WR (ed): Patient Transfers: How to Comply with the Law, 2nd ed. American College of Emergency Physicians, 1995.

37. Williams A: Outpatient Department EMTALA Handbook 2002. New York, Aspen Publishers, 2001.

38. Woodward GA: Legal issues in pediatric interfacility transport: Ethical and legal issues in pediatric emergency medicine. Clin Pediatr Emerg Med 2003;4:256-264.

39. Woodward GA, Fleegler EW: Should parents accompany pediatric interfacility ground ambulance transports? The parents' perspective. Pediatr Emerg Care 2000;16:383-390.

40. Woodward GA, Fleegler EW: Should parents accompany pediatric interfacility ground ambulance transports? Results of a national survey of pediatric transport team managers. Pediatr Emerg Care 2001;17:22-27.

CHAPTER *16*

Financial Aspects of Pediatric Hospitalist Programs

Sanford M. Melzer

Despite a dramatic increase in the number of pediatric hospitalist programs, there are surprisingly few studies that systematically explore the financial impact of such programs on the child health care delivery system, which includes hospitals, pediatric primary care physicians, and health plans.[1] One of the key economic forces driving the growth of the hospitalist movement has been the pressure to reduce the costs of hospital care. A number of studies in health maintenance organizations, academic medical centers, and children's hospitals comparing hospitalist programs to traditional inpatient care systems have shown a decrease in hospital charges, costs, and length of stay.[2-5] Enhanced availability of hospitalists, a higher level of proficiency in treating inpatient conditions, and judicious use of laboratory and radiology studies have been suggested as possible explanations for the lower costs associated with hospitalist care.

Despite data showing lower costs and shorter lengths of stay, assessment of the economic impact of hospitalist programs on the sponsoring hospital's bottom line is quite complex. The overall result reflects the balance between the costs of hospitalists and the savings or revenue enhancement for the hospital. On the cost side of the economic equation, the financial outcome is greatly influenced by hospitalist program costs and the level of subsidy required. On the revenue side, the shortened length of stay or lower charges attributable to hospitalists may represent a net benefit to the hospital, depending on the proportion of cases paid at a diagnosis-related group (DRG)–based per case rate, at a daily (per diem) rate, or as a percentage of charges. In prospective payment systems such as those used by Medicare and many state Medicaid programs, hospitalists are most likely to have a positive impact on hospital margins through resource reduction and improvement in throughput.[6] The impact of increased throughput is most pronounced when the rapid turnover of patients allows for new patients under per case payment plans to fill available hospital beds.[7] In contrast, in environments where hospital charges are paid on a percentage of charges or per diem basis, the increased efficiency of hospitalists may negatively impact hospital revenue, with the benefits of cost reduction accruing instead to third-party payers.

In some cases, financial results may not be the only criterion used to decide whether to sponsor a hospitalist program. Pediatric hospitalist programs are increasingly being used as a strategy to enhance hospital marketing and increase market share. In competitive health care environments, some hospitals may view pediatric hospitalists as a way to attract more pediatric patients by supporting local pediatricians and surgeons who refer patients to the hospital but choose not to care for their own inpatients. Hospitalists provide a broader scope of pediatric services in the inpatient unit, emergency department, delivery room, and nursery; they may also reduce risks and increase referrals or hospital utilization.[8] In this strategic context, hospitalist programs that effectively drive an increase in pediatric admissions may be considered successful regardless of the increased costs associated with them.

For primary care physicians, declining hospitalization rates, less experience with inpatient care,[9] and increasing pressure to maximize outpatient productivity all contribute to the increased acceptance of hospitalist programs. In a national survey of pediatricians' attitudes toward and experiences with pediatric hospitalists, more than half the respondents who referred patients to hospitalists agreed that attention to inpatients takes too much time away from their office practices, and 78% agreed that using hospitalists makes office practice manageable and predictable.[10] Although there are limited data on the economic impact of hospitalists on pediatricians, a California survey of 524 primary care physicians, including 152 pediatricians, showed that 69% believed that hospitalists had no effect on their income, while 27% reported a decrease and 4% an increase.[11] Another study concluded that adult primary care providers could realize a net gain of $40,000 by replacing hospital care with ambulatory productivity.[12] Clearly, more information is needed on the impact of hospitalists on primary care pediatricians and specialists.

With the increasing demand for pediatric hospitalist services, more community and children's hospitals, physician groups, and managed care organizations are either contemplating or operating pediatric hospitalist programs. The vast majority of these programs, like their counterparts in adult medicine, require some level of institutional support to cover program expenses. Given the potential financial impact that hospitalist programs may have on physician groups, health plans, and hospitals, physician leaders and hospital administrators with responsibility for developing and operating these programs must be familiar with the financial aspects of hospitalist programs. This chapter describes the financial and business principles involved in planning and managing hospitalist programs and provides a framework to evaluate and maximize their financial outcomes.

BUSINESS PLAN FOR A HOSPITALIST PROGRAM

The purpose of a business plan is to project, on a multiyear basis, the overall financial performance (profit or loss) of a hospitalist program. Forward-looking estimates are also called pro forma projections. The key elements included in a business plan that ultimately determines the program's financial performance are projections of clinical activity (demand), revenue associated with the delivery of services, and program expenses associated with the costs of delivering hospitalist services.

Clinical Demand Projections

The business planning process for a hospitalist program begins with an analysis of the present demand for clinical services and a projection of future volume, based on growth scenarios. Demand metrics commonly used in hospitalist planning include number of admissions, number of patient days, and average length of stay. The patient mix may be described using diagnostic categories such as DRGs. The case mix index may be determined using proprietary systems such as the All Payer Related Diagnostic-Related Groups, which provide severity rankings based on number and type of diagnoses, comorbidities, and procedures.

For programs with existing clinical services, it is relatively straightforward to define the present state or volume of inpatient care provided in hospital units and nurseries. Data regarding consultation volume (from the emergency department or inpatient unit) or other outpatient services may be harder to determine because they are typically not tracked as part of the hospital's cost accounting.

Projecting future demand is an imprecise science at best, made complex by the uncertainties of program growth rates, recruitment, and a multitude of external forces, such as competition from other hospitals and changes in the state, federal, or commercial payer environment. Some model growth scenarios are based on projected annual increases in volume from a baseline. In general, program growth estimates should not be overstated; volume growth in excess of 10% a year is unusual for most programs. More sophisticated models take into account evolving practice patterns of community physicians, especially their willingness to refer existing and future patients to hospitalists for care. Other factors that can have an impact on future demand include plans for the acquisition of existing practices, recruitment of new providers, strategic initiatives such as satellite programs, and clinical program development.

When anticipating the volume of a hospitalist program, it is important to define clinical roles and responsibilities and the hospitalists' scope of service, including inpatient care, well-baby or intensive care nursery, emergency department consultations, and other services. It is also important to consider both the total program volume and the proportion of demand that will be served by the hospitalists. For example, in many community hospitals, even after the implementation of a hospitalist program, some proportion of inpatients and newborns will continue to receive care from community physicians and will not be part of the hospitalist revenue stream. For planning purposes, this proportion should be estimated and excluded from the demand model projecting hospitalist revenue.

Clinical Revenue Projections

Cash Collections

Although there are a number of different methods for calculating clinical revenue, they all share the common goal of determining how much cash will be collected for clinical services. The first step in developing the revenue projection is to convert the demand model into an estimate of specific clinical services that will be provided. This is best accomplished using the American Medical Association's current procedural terminology (CPT) codes. Most commonly, these will be evaluation and management (E&M) services, which,

depending on the hospitalists' specific clinical responsibilities, typically include codes for initial and subsequent inpatient care, consultation, observation, and neonatal or intensive care services.

Once the number and frequency of CPT codes are estimated, cash collections can be determined based on a collection rate applied to gross charges, published fee schedules, or the Resource-Based Relative Value System (RBRVS). Using the physician fee schedule and charges per CPT code, it is relatively simple to project the program's gross charges based on the anticipated volume and CPT code mix. Although gross charges are a commonly reported metric for hospitalist programs, the planner still needs to apply a collection rate to determine the actual cash collections. Collection rates reflect the proportion of gross charges that will be collected as cash and generally reflect payer mix and specific payer contracts. Collection rates are typically lowest for Medicaid populations and highest for those insured under commercial contracts. Most hospitals and physician groups will be able to calculate a collection rate based on historical data or, if a program's payer mix is known, by applying the payer-specific collection rate to that portion of charges represented by each payer. Another method of describing cash payments is to calculate contractual allowances, which reflect the proportion of charges not collected. For example, a payer mix that results in a 55% collection rate has a 45% contractual allowance rate. Cash collections can also be calculated using fee schedules in markets where payers (including Medicaid) have established such schedules for specific services and contracted providers.

Regardless of the method used to determine cash collections, allowances should be made during the start-up period for the cash lag that reflects the delay in collecting payments once charges have been reported to the payer. Cash lag may vary by payer, but a period of 90 days is commonly used for purposes of business planning.

The RBRVS, which represents a uniform national benchmark for physician payments, can also be used to project cash collections. This fee schedule, initially developed for reimbursement under the Medicare program but now increasingly used in pediatrics, provides an objective measure of physician work and can be used to describe and compare physician productivity in different clinical settings. The RBRVS is also used to standardize reimbursement by assigning relative value units (RVUs) to each CPT code. The two most commonly used measures are total RVUs, which take into account the physician's work, practice expenses, and professional liability associated with specific CPT codes, and work RVUs, which describe only the physician's work associated with a specific service. For most inpatient services, there are minimal practice expenses, so work RVUs closely approximate total RVUs.

Under the RBRVS, payment is determined by applying a conversion factor, a value that converts total RVUs into reimbursement amounts for physicians. The Medicare conversion factor used nationally is set annually by Congress as part of the budget process. Among other payers using the RVU system, there is wide variation in the conversion factors used to establish payments. This state-by-state variation is particularly striking within the Medicaid program. The conversion factor (dollars paid per RVU) not only provides a method to evaluate and negotiate contracts but also is an effective tool to describe and compare payments in health care environments characterized by different payer mixes and reimbursement rates.

Conversion factors for pediatric hospitalist programs can be expected to vary widely, depending on the local payer environment and the Medicaid mix, which greatly impact the "blended" payment rate per RVU. There are limited national data on which to model conversion factors for pediatric hospitalist programs. Two Seattle studies showed conversion factors of $24.50 and $46 in a children's hospital and a community hospital with a payer mix of 40% and 15% Medicaid, respectively.[13,14] A 2004 survey of productivity and compensation undertaken by the Society for Hospital Medicine, which included 206 pediatric hospitalists, reported mean and median collections per RVU of $55.78 and $54.55, respectively.[15] When RVU production and cash collections are known, a blended conversion factor can be calculated by dividing total cash collected by RVU. This program-specific conversion factor can then be used for planning and applied to projected RVU production by hospitalist physicians.

Pediatric Hospital Physician Productivity

There are limited data describing pediatric hospital physician productivity. A study of faculty physician productivity on a children's hospital inpatient service reported a weekly average of $7014 in gross billings and 109 total RVUs.[13] In its 2004 survey, the Society for Hospital Medicine reported annual median charges of $203,554 per physician and 1990 RVUs among a group of 206 pediatric hospitalists (Table 16-1).

Other Sources of Revenue

Contract or Service Fees

Published and unpublished studies indicate that in most cases, professional fee revenues generated by pediatric hospitalists do not cover physicians' salaries, benefits, and practice expenses.[13-16] These deficits result from a number of factors, including low inpatient volume, the requirement for 24-hour-a-day staffing, poor reimbursement for the time spent managing inpatients (which may include multiple bedside visits and case management), and an unfavorable payer mix. As a result, most pediatric hospitalist groups in both academic and community settings receive financial support for physicians' salaries, benefits, and practice expenses.

One way that hospitals provide support for physicians' expenses is through contract or service fees, which may be defined under the terms of professional service agreements. Professional service agreements may be structured in a variety of ways. In fixed-fee contracts, the hospital pays a fixed sum to the hospitalist group for a prescribed set of services, including on-site clinical care, after-hours call coverage, and other services. The fixed fee is typically intended to cover the difference between projected revenues and practice expenses, with an allowance for some "excess revenue" or profit for the group. These fixed-fee contracts may require the hospitalist group to assume a level of risk. For example, under these arrangements, if revenues do not meet projections, there may be a shortfall in available funds to pay salaries and benefits, requiring the group to either reduce compensation or draw funds from practice reserves. Conversely, with fixed-fee contracts, if the program outperforms the business plan, the hospitalist group is entitled to retain the excess revenue, or profit.

For a hospitalist group seeking to limit its risk, especially in start-up programs with poorly defined volumes, it may be possible to structure variable-fee contracts that ensure the coverage of salaries, benefits, and relevant practice expenses. In this case, the contract fee is prospectively set to cover the difference between actual cash collected from professional fees and a negotiated level of salary and practice expense during a prior period. These types of arrangements require periodic reconciliation and should take into account the lag period between the reporting of gross charges and the collection of actual cash. At a minimum, to avoid operating at a deficit, contract or service fees should cover the difference between available revenues and all relevant practice expenses, plus an amount of net income, or revenue in excess of expenses, as determined by the business plan.

Incentive Payments

Additional fees in the form of incentive payments are sometimes included in hospitalist service agreements. Incentive payments can be used to reward improvement in physician performance. Under these arrangements, an incentive pool is created and distributed according to a predetermined formula and a set of prospectively set targets or goals. For example, hospitals with capacity constraints may wish to reward hospitalists for timely discharge, while those seeking to promote standard practices may reward

Table 16-1 Productivity and Salary of Pediatric Hospital Physicians by Employment Model

Employment Model	No.	Median Charges	Median Collections	Median RVUs	Median Admits and Consults	Median Inpatient Hours	Median Annual Compensation
Hospital or hospital corporation	69	$200,000	$125,000	1,596	450	2,000	$148,000
Hospitalist-only group	10	$350,000	$180,000	NA	149	2,873	$152,500
Multispecialty group	27	$266,610	$205,000	2,856	600	1,938	$167,375
Academic	73	$213,554	$90,043	2,271	502	1,300	$107,500
Other	16	NA	NA	NA	441	2,115	$120,000
All models	206	$236,507	$111,000	1,990	441	1,700	$130,000

NA, not applicable; RVU, relative value unit.
From 2004 Survey on Productivity and Compensation. Philadelphia, Society for Hospital Medicine, 2004.

physicians for the development of or compliance with inpatient care pathways. Patient and referring physician satisfaction may also be used as a criterion for incentive payments.

Regardless of the targets and benchmarks used to determine incentive payments, they should be easily, accurately, and consistently measurable; be prospectively set; and reflect the strategic and operational goals of the sponsoring hospital. Incentive payments should not be tied to referral volume or financial performance. Incentive arrangements should be carefully reviewed by legal counsel experienced in health care law to ensure that they do not place the hospital or providers at risk of noncompliance with federal regulations that prohibit payments for patient referrals.[17]

Teaching, Research, and Administration

For some hospitalist programs, fees for teaching and administrative activities can be an important source of funding to offset the cost of physician salaries and benefits. Although many physicians are expected to participate in resident teaching programs or serve on hospital committees as part of their duties, additional compensation may be provided for functioning as the medical director of inpatient services, supervising training programs, developing or revising policies and procedures, or chairing major hospital committees, such as pharmacy and therapeutics or quality assurance. Fees for these services may be paid on an annual or hourly basis. Physicians engaged in clinical research under federal or other grant programs may also be eligible for funding of a portion of their salaries based on the time devoted to these research activities.

Program Expense Projections
Physician Salaries and Benefits

Physician salaries constitute the largest portion of hospitalist program expenses, and historically, only limited salary benchmark data have been available for pediatric hospitalists. A survey of 36 pediatric hospitalist programs undertaken through the Pediatric Research in Inpatient Settings (PRIS) network found that the median annual salary for pediatric hospital physicians was $120,000 (range, $90,000 to $150,000).[16] The Society for Hospital Medicine published a survey of 160 pediatric hospitalists and reported that the mean and median annual compensation was $128,265 and $130,000, respectively (see Table 16-1).[15] Median compensation was lowest among physicians working in academic centers ($107,500) and highest among physicians working in hospitals or multispecialty groups ($148,00 and $152,500, respectively). Other sources of data for hospitalist salaries include compensation and productivity data published by the Medical Group Management Association (Englewood, Colorado) in its annual *Academic Practice Compensation and Production Survey for Faculty and Management*. Hospitalist salary data for academic physicians may be available through the Association of Administrators in Academic Pediatrics.

Physician Staffing Models and Workload

The Society for Hospital Medicine survey revealed that hospital medicine groups generally work within one of three staffing models: shift based, call based, or mixed.[15] Shift-based models use a schedule of defined hours during which a hospitalist remains in the hospital, even when not providing direct patient care. Call-based models use a schedule of defined hours but allow a hospitalist to leave the hospital when not providing direct patient care; the hospitalist is expected to be available to return to the hospital when direct care is required. Mixed models are a combination of shift- and call-based staffing.

The coverage requirements and daily patient volumes determine total staffing costs. A 7-day-a-week, 24-hour-a-day, in-house or on-call coverage at a single site generally requires three to four full-time-equivalent employees. With in-house residents or other physicians on site, or with low patient volumes, a single physician may be able to cover more than one site, with appropriate contingencies to provide staffing for unanticipated emergencies at both sites. There are few national benchmarks to define pediatric hospital physician workload in terms of hours or patient encounters. The results of the Society for Hospital Medicine survey are shown in Table 16-1.[15]

Other Practice Expenses

All physicians providing inpatient services require malpractice insurance, and these costs should be included in the business plan. Other important practice expenses may include office lease costs, equipment, secretarial support, and an answering service. Billing costs can be quite variable. For those practices using dictation for correspondence and documentation, transcription expenses should be included. Physician professional expenses include state medical license, Drug Enforcement Administration registration, books, journals, and professional society fees. Allowances for continuing medical education should include travel expenses to professional meetings. Depending on the standard within the group, these practice expenses can usually be determined with relative accuracy and budgeted accordingly.

PUTTING IT ALL TOGETHER: THE COMPLETED BUSINESS PLAN

Figure 16-1 shows a sample business plan for a community hospital hospitalist program. For purposes of this illustration, the planning assumptions include benchmarks for physician productivity, charges, collections, salaries, and benefits consistent with those described in the Society for Hospital Medicine survey.[15]

TRACKING HOSPITALIST PROGRAM PERFORMANCE

Tracking hospitalist program performance is a critical component of program management and can be accomplished with regular reporting and review of key performance metrics. At a minimum, performance reports should include the following:

- Program volumes
- Financial results
- Selected quality performance measures
- Physician productivity

Program volumes are a key indicator of performance and should include patient discharges, lengths of stay, total patient days, and discharges by DRG. Financial metrics

Revenue	
Gross charges @ $200,000/FTE	700,000
Contractual allowances @ 45%	(315,000)
Cash collections @ 55%	385,000
Total RVU production (median 2000/FTE)	7,000
Conversion factor	55
Cash collections based on RVUs	385,000
Hospital service fee @ 55,000/FTE	192,500
Inpatient medical administration	15,000
Total revenue	**$ 592,500**

Expense	
Salary	
3.5 FTE @ $130,000/FTE	416,000
Benefits @ $22,000/FTE	77,000
Targeted incentive payment	15,000
Total salary and benefits	**$ 508,000**
Practice expenses	
Billing service fee (9% of cash collections)	34,650
Malpractice expenses @ $6000/FTE	21,000
Answering service ($700/month)	8,400
CME and journals @ $2000/FTE	7,000
Total practice expense	**$ 71,050**
Total physician and practice expense	**$ 572,050**
Excess of revenue over expenses	**$20,450**

Figure 16-1 Sample hospitalist program business plan.

should be examined from both the hospital's and the physician's perspective. Relevant hospital metrics include facility revenue, direct and indirect expenses per case, and profit or loss calculated on a per case and unit basis. These results should always be compared to the projected budget and prior comparable periods. Many institutions also include quality performance measures in their regular reports. These might include patient satisfaction, other quality measures (e.g., medication error rate), and the development of protocols that reflect specific organizational goals. Physician productivity metrics include patient visits and procedure counts; patient care and call hours worked; and charges, cash, and RVUs generated by the physician.

MAXIMIZING HOSPITALIST PROGRAM PERFORMANCE

In community hospitals, where the average daily census of inpatients and consultations does not generate sufficient revenue to cover expenses, some hospitalist physician groups have expanded their scope to include other services, such as newborn care. Maximizing physician efficiency is an important element of hospitalist program performance, especially in settings where the physicians cover multiple sites or provide a high volume of services in the inpatient unit or nursery. Depending on volume, hospitalist groups may find it more efficient to deploy physicians to more than one hospital and thereby minimize coverage costs for multiple institutions. Physicians should also be familiar with methods to improve the efficiency of workflow and throughput, such as "lean processing," an industrial process and quality improvement tool that is now widely used in health care.

In addition to expanding the scope of services, a number of other practice management tools and techniques can be used to maximize the financial performance of hospitalist programs. Charge capture is probably the single most important practice management tool for the hospitalist. Physicians should be formally trained in the appropriate reporting and documentation for the commonly used inpatient CPT codes, including initial and subsequent hospital and observation care and discharge-day management. In addition, physicians should be familiar with the use of add-ons, modifiers, and non–face-to-face codes that allow the provider to report and be paid for additional work beyond the typical time for an inpatient service. These include codes for team conferences, medical report preparation, telephone care, and prolonged services. Accurate coding is critical to ensure compliance with billing regulations for federal programs. Systems should be established to audit provider coding and provide feedback in an accurate and timely manner. There are a number of resources available for physicians that provide background and guidance for CPT coding for inpatient services. The American Academy of Pediatrics' publication *Coding for Pediatrics* is a well-written manual that covers the use of specific codes for inpatient care, along with clinical scenarios and coding and documentation tips.

Program managers should also pay close attention to the revenue cycle. Prompt reporting of services, preferably electronically, on a daily basis rather than batching at the time of discharge can improve cash flow by decreasing the accounts receivable or funds not yet paid. Although revenue enhancement is critical, it is also important to manage program costs. To avoid overpaying for hospitalists, national benchmarks should be used whenever possible to determine salaries, although local market conditions may require higher than normal salaries to meet the staffing needs of a particular program.

CONCLUSION

With the rapid growth in the number of pediatric hospitalist programs, physician managers, hospital administrators, and health care analysts have focused increasing attention on the financial aspects of these programs. Although many studies have shown a reduction in inpatient costs associated with hospitalist models of care, the broader financial effects of hospitalist programs on children's and community hospitals, physicians, and systems of child health care are not yet known. Key elements of business planning for hospitalist programs include projections of demand and clinical revenues and a full accounting of salary, benefit, and practice expenses. Tracking program performance is critical for optimal management and should include regular reporting of metrics describing program volumes, physician productivity, cash collection, and quality indicators. Maximizing the financial performance of pediatric hospitalist programs can be accomplished by paying close attention to physician coding and billing, charge capture, management of the revenue cycle, and hospital physician expenses. The bottom line is that pediatric hospitalist programs represent financial challenges for hospitals, physician groups, and health plans. Even with careful management, many programs do not generate sufficient clinical revenue to cover physician costs and require operational subsidies, generally in the form of institutional support. How this economic reality will influence the long-term success of the hospitalist physician model in pediatrics remains an important and unanswered question.

REFERENCES

1. Landrigan C, Srivastava R, Muret-Wagstaff S, et al: Pediatric hospitalists: What do we know, and where do we go from here? Ambul Pediatr 2001;1:340-345.
2. Ogershok PR, Xiaoming L, Palmer HC, et al: Restructuring an academic pediatric inpatient service using concepts developed by hospitalists. Clin Pediatr 2001;40:653-661.
3. Bellet PS, Whitaker RC: Evaluation of a pediatric hospitalist service: Impact on length of stay and hospital charges. Pediatrics 2000;105:478-484.
4. Landrigan CP, Srivastava R, Muret-Wagstaff S, et al: Impact of a health maintenance organization hospitalist system in academic pediatrics. Pediatrics 2002;105:720-728.
5. Ponitz K, Mortimer J, Berman J: Establishing a pediatric hospitalist program at an academic medical center. Clin Pediatr 2000;39:221-228.
6. Gregory D, Baigelman W, Wilson IB: Hospital economics of the hospitalist. Health Serv Res 2003;38:905-917.
7. Larson E: Twenty first century hospitals: Intensification increases. Health Serv Res 2003;38:919-992.
8. Rogers JC: Pediatric hospitalist programs offer chance to improve quality and cost. Health Care Strategic Manage 2003;21:12-16.
9. Melzer SM, Grossman DG, Rivara FP: Physician experience with inpatient care in Washington State. Pediatrics 1996;97:65-70.
10. Percelay JM, O'Connor KG, Neff JM: Pediatricians' Attitudes toward and Experiences with Pediatric Hospitalists: A National Survey. Oak Grove, Ill, American Academy of Pediatrics, Division of Health Policy Research, 2003.
11. Fernandez A, Grumbach K, Goitein L, et al: Friend or foe? How primary care physicians perceive hospitalists. Arch Intern Med 2000;160:2902-2908.
12. Wachter RM, Goldman L: The hospitalist movement 5 years later. JAMA 2002;297:487-492.
13. Melzer SM, Molteni RA, Marcuse EK, Rivara FP: Characteristics and financial performance of a pediatric faculty inpatient attending service: A resource-based relative value scale analysis. Pediatrics 2001;108:79-84.
14. Tieder J, Migita D, Cowan C, Melzer S: Physician productivity and financial performance in a community hospital–based pediatric hospitalist program. Abstract presented at Pediatric Academic Societies Meeting, 2004.
15. 2004 Survey on Hospitalist Productivity and Compensation. Philadelphia, Society for Hospital Medicine, 2004.
16. Chiang VW, Landrigan CP, Stucky E, Ottoloni M: Financial health of pediatric hospitalist systems: A study from the Pediatric Research in Inpatient Settings (PRIS) network. Abstract presented at Pediatric Academic Societies Meeting, 2004.
17. Kalb PE: Health care fraud and abuse. JAMA 1999;282:1163-1168.

CHAPTER 17

Communication and Discharge Planning

Daniel Rauch and David Zipes

In discussing hospitalist models, it is essential to keep in mind the relationships between hospitalists and the wider pediatric community. Communication is at the forefront of any hospitalist model and can be the Achilles' heel of an otherwise high-quality program. Conversely, excellent communication to and from primary care physicians (PCPs) can help a program thrive and prosper. PCPs who are kept in the loop regarding their patients' hospital course will likely support the hospitalist service. By communicating in an effective and timely manner, one of the major potential downsides (loss of valuable information) of a hospitalist service can be avoided.

Communication can positively or negatively affect a variety of issues, including but not limited to quality of care, cost of care, patient and physician satisfaction, and liability. With excellent communication, the transition from inpatient to outpatient settings (including transitional care units, chronic care facilities, and rehabilitation hospitals) can be smooth, with minimal to no loss of information.

HANDING OFF CARE

The concept of assuming care for other physicians' patients and then returning their care to the PCPs at discharge is an integral component of all hospitalist models. This is generally accomplished via a formal handoff, which is one of the more controversial aspects of hospital medicine. The intentional creation of discontinuity of care permits a physician (hospitalist) to be present in the hospital for an extended period to manage inpatients throughout the day. This omnipresence is one of the biggest advantages of the hospitalist model. As with most things, however, one must accept the good with the bad. As a result of the handoff, the PCP, with whom the patient has fostered a trusting relationship and who knows the patient's medical history best, is not caring for the patient when he or she is most ill. This situation can result in a loss of essential information ("voltage drop") from the outpatient to the inpatient setting and vice versa. Complex and expensive laboratory and radiology data, as well as vital information concerning possible medical allergies, medications, code status, and patient's likes and dislikes, can be lost or poorly or miscommunicated during the transfer. This could result in a variety of negative outcomes—some relatively benign, and others life threatening.

With excellent communication between the PCP and the hospitalist, voltage drop can be minimized. In a study of 400 discharged patients, researchers found that 19% of patients suffered adverse events soon after discharge; about half of these events would have been preventable if communication had been adequate.[1] To date, no standard for communication between the hospitalist and the PCP has been set, and there is significant variation from practice to practice.

Communication may occur in person; via telephone, fax, e-mail, or Internet; or sometimes not at all. A task force formed by the Society of Hospital Medicine and the Society of General Internal Medicine to address continuity-of-care issues found that more than a quarter of PCPs do not receive discharge summaries on their patients. Additionally, the task force discovered that more than half of discharged patients made contact with their PCPs before the PCPs had received any discharge information—many PCPs did not even know that their patients had been admitted to the hospital. Only 17% of those surveyed stated that hospitalists had notified them before their patients were discharged to home.

The growth of information technology and easy access to e-mail, the Internet, faxes, wireless communications, and hand-held devices have created many effective modes of communication. New computer and hand-held device programs to address communications issues have been developing at a rapid pace, and many of them are quite useful. Template-driven discharge summaries can simplify the process and help ensure that essential information is communicated. The technology to create real-time communication exists, although many hospitalist programs have not made the leap because of cost (both financial and time), unwillingness to change, lack of administrative support, inadequate staffing, or a variety of other reasons. The information communicated, such as discharge summaries or laboratory reports, should be filtered appropriately to maximize the efficiency of communication and reduce the time commitment for PCPs. Some information, such as social issues and end-of-life care discussions, does not lend itself well to electronic communication, and in these situations, the value of the telephone or face-to-face communication should not be overlooked.

"Social rounds" by the PCP, either by phone or in person, are an excellent patient satisfaction tool and can help erode the voltage-loss issue and increase the family's confidence in the hospitalist. One effective technique is for the hospitalist to call the PCP while in the patient's room so that the family can hear that everyone is on the same page. Similarly, including the PCP in complicated social and medical discussions, such as end-of-life care, code status, case conferences, and major medical or surgical decisions, can be useful to all involved. One needs to be cognizant that the PCP will be dealing with the aftermath of the hospitalization. By working as a team, the PCP and the hospitalist can maximize the advantages of hospital medicine while minimizing its disadvantages.

DISCHARGE PLANNING

Discharge planning is an integral part of hospitalization and is an area in which hospitalists should have a significant impact. Many of the inherent benefits of a hospitalist service, such as improved quality of care, efficiency, and communication, all culminate in effectively transitioning the patient out of the hospital setting. Discharge planning must begin on admission to the hospital and continue throughout the hospital stay. It should include communication with the PCP and appropriate follow-up services or physicians and must encompass coordination with social services, the payer, and, of course, the family. It must also provide for follow-up with regard to any issues that are still pending at discharge.

As discussed in previous chapters, hospitalists can play a significant role in determining who gets admitted to the inpatient service and in facilitating intrahospital transfers. This involvement may vary from program to program and from patient to patient. Even when the hospitalist plays no role in screening admissions, it is incumbent on the hospitalist to clearly define the goal of an inpatient stay; the discharge criteria should follow from this. Anticipating at the outset the durable medical equipment, medications, and services that will be required at discharge can greatly facilitate timely and efficient discharges, even on the weekends.

Collaboration

Discharge planning, just as inpatient management itself, requires a team approach (Table 17-1). Optimally, the inpatient service has a multidisciplinary approach that includes at least nursing, social services, and a coordinator familiar with local payer structures and other outpatient and community resources, such as home care agencies and alternative care facilities.

Nursing input is vital because nurses interface with patients and families in a different way from physicians; this allows valuable insight into the relative strengths and weaknesses of each patient—information that is critical for appropriate discharge planning. Social workers bring another viewpoint that can shed light on the patient's and family's response to illness and their ability to manage

posthospitalization care. This perspective should help guide the timing of discharge and what postdischarge services will be necessary. The discharge planner begins reviewing charts on admission, looking for medical documentation of discharge goals. This allows the planner to immediately start coordinating with payers on issues such as anticipated length of stay and available outpatient services. For adult patients, experience with nurse discharge planners and comprehensive discharge planning demonstrates reduced costs and lengths of stay.[2,3] Other possible members of a discharge team include therapists, nutritionists, and child life specialists, all of whom may have unique information that impacts discharge planning. Additionally, a postdischarge coordinator can follow up on pending laboratory results and ensure that the family is able to keep or schedule appointments, obtain prescribed medicines, and follow through with other discharge plans. A weekly (or more frequent) meeting of all parties involved in discharge planning to review ongoing cases and the availability of additional consultation is an effective technique used by many hospitalist groups. This type of multidisciplinary approach can identify significant issues that may affect discharge planning and may serve as a source of quality improvement projects. The hospitalist should be involved in developing mechanisms to ensure the timely review of patient charts by related services to identify discharge issues and improve hospital resource utilization.

Most important, patients and families must be partners in the discharge process. Clear goals for admission, as well as discharge criteria and anticipated obstacles, make it easy for the patient and family to follow the course of the hospitalization and prepare for discharge. The hospitalist must be aware of the prevailing Patients' Bill of Rights regarding necessary notification of discharge, as well as the mechanisms for patients to dispute discharge decisions.

Communication with the PCP is essential for appropriate discharge planning,[4] and the American Academy of Pediatrics has established the following guidelines for minimum communication with the PCP: communication on admission, for any significant events, and on discharge.[5] Good relationships and ongoing communication with referring physicians can help define the best means of communication. It is also important to clarify the capacity of outpatient services to handle ongoing medical needs. Because many factors influence the PCP's ability to handle various levels of acuity and necessary follow-up after discharge, these issues must be considered during discharge planning. Likewise, it is important to establish open lines of communication with alternative care facilities so that transfer procedures can be initiated as soon as a potential transfer is anticipated. All communication of patient information must be mindful of Health Insurance Portability and Accountability Act (HIPAA) regulations.[6]

Continuity of Care

Many successful hospitalist practices have the policy of calling PCPs with every discharge—regardless of the time. This avoids middle-of-the-night telephone calls from patients or families to uninformed PCPs. The median time from a patient's discharge to his or her first visit to the PCP is 6 days; knowledge of events in the hospital is often critical to a successful office visit and helps assure the patient

Table 17-1	Discharge Planning Team
Participant	**Role**
Hospitalist	Acts as team leader
Other medical providers with knowledge of current inpatients	Provide medical information
Nursing staff	Provide additional medical information and insight into patient-family dynamics
Social workers	Provide information to patient and family about necessary resources for discharge
Discharge planner	Coordinates discharge needs with outpatient services in context of patient's insurance
Other: therapists (occupational, physical, speech), nutrition, child life	Provide unique patient information that may impact discharge

that his or her care has been adequately coordinated. In addition to a discharge phone call, many practices fax a one-page summary of pertinent information, including dates of admission and discharge, discharge diagnosis, procedures, medicines, change in code status, pertinent laboratory results and pending tests, consultations, disposition, and follow-up appointments. A typed discharge summary can also be generated and sent (generally via fax) for each discharged patient. Although this can be time consuming, the benefits of effective communication are worth the extra effort.

Discharge from the inpatient service is usually not the end of care for a patient. Many patients reach their goals for admission and are successfully discharged with various tests still pending and therapies needed (e.g., antibiotics, respiratory therapy). An important element of discharge communication is conveying information regarding pending tests and studies. This can prevent the repetition of studies that have already been done and ensures that data from the studies are conveyed to the outpatient care providers. The person responsible for following up on pending results can vary from practice to practice, and it is unclear who is medicolegally responsible for following up on tests after discharge. Regardless of the legal implications, the hospitalist should either follow up on pending tests or make sure that the PCP does so.

Many practices have implemented postdischarge follow-up clinics for one to two visits. The PCP must be notified of these visits, and the patient should be "returned" to the PCP as soon as possible. One must be aware of the potential political ramifications of delving into the outpatient arena. Along the same lines, a focused postdischarge phone call from the hospitalist practice can help ferret out problems with prescriptions, follow-up appointments, or the patient's condition.

CONCLUSION

Excellent communication is essential to any successful hospitalist service, and adequate discharge planning is essential to the smooth operation of a hospitalist system. The hallmark of effective discharge planning is that it never unnecessarily extends the inpatient stay. By anticipating patient needs, hospitalists can not only improve the care their patients receive but also maintain efficient throughput and maximize the beds available to the inpatient service and the hospital as a whole. PCPs may be concerned with many aspects of their interaction with a hospitalist service, and effective discharge planning can have an important impact on acceptance.[7,8]

REFERENCES

1. Forster AJ, Murff HJ, Peterson JF, et al: The incidence and severity of adverse events affecting patients after discharge from the hospital. Ann Intern Med 2003;138:161-167.
2. Palmer HC, Armistead NS, Elnicki DM, et al: The effect of a hospitalist service with nurse discharge planner on patient care in an academic teaching hospital. Am J Med 2001;111:627-632.
3. Naylor MD, Brooten DA, Campbell RL, et al: Comprehensive discharge planning for the elderly: A randomized, controlled trial. J Am Geriatr Soc 2004;52:675-684.
4. Goldman L, Patilat SZ, Whitcomb WF: Passing the clinical baton: 6 Principles to guide the hospitalist. Am J Med 2001;111:36S-39S.
5. Percelay JM, Committee on Hospital Care: Physicians' roles in coordinating care of hospitalized children. Pediatrics 2003;111:707-709.
6. American Academy of Pediatrics Security Manual. Oct 2003.
7. Fernandez A, Grumbach K, Goitein L, et al: Friend or foe? How primary care physicians perceive hospitalists. Arch Intern Med 2000;160:2902-2908.
8. Auerbach AD, Aronson MD, Davis RB, Phillips RS: How physicians perceive hospitalist services after implementation: Anticipation vs reality. Arch Intern Med 2003;163:2330-2336.

Ethics, the Law, and Pediatric Clinical Research

CHAPTER 18

Ethical Issues in Pediatric Hospital Practice

K. Sarah Hoehn and Chris Feudtner

The ethical and moral dimensions of health and medicine pervade all aspects of clinical care. Providers of hospital care for children constantly encounter situations in which ethical considerations are vital, ranging from the routine task of obtaining parental permission for medical care to rarer quandaries regarding care that is deemed necessary (yet is refused) or futile (yet is requested). Competence in handling ethically problematic situations can be enhanced by expanding one's perspective on ethical thinking, knowing what institutional resources are available to help resolve ethical problems, and learning how to approach specific common problems.

ETHICAL PERSPECTIVES

Rules and Policies

There are many ways to approach ethical decision making. An important practical starting point is the hospital's rule or policy providing specific instructions regarding the issue at hand. For instance, hospitals typically provide guidance about when the general consent for care granted by a parent at the time of admission is inadequate and specific parental permission to perform certain diagnostic or therapeutic procedures must be obtained and documented. Such rules and policies can often be found in the medical staff bylaws or in national guidelines published by the American Academy of Pediatrics (AAP), American Medical Association, or other organizations. Ethically problematic situations are addressed by asking: What rules and policies (or pertinent state or federal laws) govern our conduct and guide our choices?

Duties, Responsibilities, and Commitments

Similarly, consideration of professionally defined duties and responsibilities can help guide decisions. A growing movement within medicine emphasizes the importance of professional duties, responsibilities, and commitments toward such ends as professional competence, a just distribution of finite resources, the integrity and advancement of scientific knowledge, honesty with patients, patient confidentiality, the maintenance of appropriate relations with patients, improvements in quality of care and access to it, and the maintenance of trust by managing conflicts of interest.[1] Fundamental to nursing codes of ethics are duties such as caring and advocating for patients. To the degree that such commitments reflect professional consensus, they function as informal policies and guide our actions by telling us (less explicitly than policies) how to behave.

Virtues or Personal Traits

An allied approach to ethics focuses on individual character traits such as honesty, compassion, competence, fortitude, temperance, fidelity, integrity, self-effacement, and wise and prudent decision making. Here, however, the emphasis shifts away from what constitutes good behavior (which is the focus of policies or duties) and toward what constitutes a good person who will behave virtuously. When confronting ethically problematic situations, personal traits can be used to evaluate a proposed course of action: If I behave in this manner, will I be acting with honesty, fidelity, and fortitude? If not, why would I pursue this course of action? Can I chart another course with greater integrity and wisdom?

Bioethics Principles

To analyze what would be the "right" course of action, it may also be useful to consider the frequently cited core principles of bioethics. Although these concepts are complex and somewhat abstract, their consideration often yields insight into the fundamental nature of a particular ethical dilemma. Beneficence seeks to maximize the benefits caused by our actions, whereas nonmaleficence seeks to minimize the harm that our actions cause. Many therapeutic decisions involve some trade-off between beneficence and nonmaleficence; simply making a list of the good and bad things that might happen, and how likely they are to happen, can help clarify some dilemmas. Autonomy seeks to enable an individual's values to dictate his or her medical care; this is one example of the broader principle of respect for a person's dignity. Considerations of justice involve how the care of one person fits into the larger system of the care of all persons and can bring up issues of resource allocation and fair procedures to determine who gets what type of care. Understanding how these core principles may be in conflict with one another in specific situations can help elucidate why different individuals may view ethical dilemmas in different ways and may serve as a starting point for discussion and resolution of conflict.

Mediation of Human Social Interactions

A final set of concepts focuses less on ethical theory and more on people's understanding of a situation and their interactive behavior. Poor communication and misunderstandings lie at the heart of many conflicts that are perceived as ethical dilemmas. Patterns of interacting—ranging from hurried attempts to communicate complex information or bad news to vocal or body language expressions of anger or haughtiness—can worsen misunderstanding and intensify noncooperation. If misunderstanding and mistrust are allowed to persist, the lines of the dispute can ossify into entrenched positions (e.g., "I will not permit such-and-such to be done under any circumstances"). Making progress in such cases takes time, patience, and a willingness to share control over the decision-making process. A mediation or negotiation model emphasizes, first and foremost, building mutual understanding and trust; only after these prerequisites have been created can one move on to problem solving.

HOSPITAL RESOURCES

When confronting ethically problematic situations, most pediatric physicians can draw on valuable resources within their hospitals.

Key People

To improve communication, build shared understanding, clarify goals, generate novel solutions, or mediate disputes, physicians may turn to professional translators or cultural mediators, social workers, nurses, pastoral care workers such as chaplains or rabbis, palliative care team members, legal counsel, or other physicians with particular skills in these areas.

Ethics Committees

Institutional ethics committees can develop or review hospital policies, perform clinical ethics consultations, mediate disputes or controversies, and educate health care professionals and patients.[2,3] Seven principles guide the process of ethics consultation (Box 18-1).[2] Overall, the quality of an ethics consultation rests on the committee's preparation, including interviewing key stakeholders, gathering pertinent data, and reviewing pertinent literature,[4] and its ability to provide an open forum for honest and confidential discussion.

Research and Institutional Review Boards

Children are allowed to participate in research only when the institutional review board determines that the risks are minimal or that the pediatric subjects may benefit directly from participation in the research study.[5] As always, fully informed permission or consent is a prerequisite for research conducted on human subjects (yet only a third of published pediatric studies include proper documentation of institutional review board approval and informed permission or consent).[6] (See Chapter 21 for further discussion of children as research subjects.)

Box 18-1 Principles of Ethics Consultations

1. Any patient, parent or guardian, or family member can initiate an ethics consultation.
2. The patient and parent or guardian can refuse to participate in an ethics consultation.
3. The refusal of a patient or parent or guardian to permit an ethics consultation does not hinder the ability of an ethics committee to provide consultation services to physicians, nurses, and other concerned staff.
4. Any physician, nurse, or other health care provider involved in the care of the patient can request an ethics consultation without fear of reprisal.
5. The process of ethics consultation is open to all persons involved in the patient's care but is conducted in a manner that respects patient and family confidentiality.
6. Anonymous requests for ethics consultation are not accepted in the absence of an identified person who is willing to speak to the issue being raised.
7. The primary care pediatrician is invited to participate in the consultation to support existing physician-family relationships.

COMMON PEDIATRIC INPATIENT SITUATIONS

Although rigorous estimates of the prevalence or incidence of ethically significant or problematic incidents in the inpatient setting are lacking, our experience suggests that hospital-based pediatricians will encounter most or all of the following situations.

Obtaining Permission, Assent, or Consent

In pediatric practice, there are three important processes by which parents or patients agree that the patient will receive certain medications, tests, or procedures.[7] Informed permission is used when a pediatric patient lacks the necessary decision-making capacity and legal empowerment to make an autonomous decision, requiring the parent or designated surrogate caregiver to do so. Assent is sought when a child or adolescent has some decision-making capacity but is not yet legally empowered. Informed consent is used when an adolescent or young adult has legal authority to make decisions regarding his or her health care.

The processes of obtaining informed permission and informed consent include four key components: (1) appropriate disclosure of information, (2) adequate personal understanding of the information, (3) emotional capacity to make a decision, and (4) voluntariness or freedom from coercion.[8] The process of seeking assent translates these elements into a developmental framework applicable to pediatric patients (Box 18-2).

Necessary urgent medical care should not be withheld because of a lack of consent.[9] No evaluation of a life-threatening or emergency condition should be delayed because of a perceived problem with consent or payment authorization. A parent's act of leaving his or her child with another custodian or the state represents implied consent when the parent is not immediately available for verbal consent and nonelective medical care is needed. These situations include relief of pain or suffering; suspected serious infectious disease; assessment and treatment of serious injuries and conditions that threaten life, limb, or central nervous system; and potentially other serious conditions.[9]

Determining Decision–Making Capacity and Competence

When can an adolescent consent to medical care? The laws that govern this issue vary by state, so it is prudent to check with your hospital legal counsel. In general, however, persons are judged to be legally competent to consent to care when they are 18 years or older or when they have been emancipated from parental authority by circumstances such as being married, being pregnant or having borne a child, or living on their own. Adolescents seeking care for certain conditions (e.g., reproduction, emergencies, sexually transmitted diseases, drug and alcohol abuse) may also be deemed competent to consent to treatment without parental permission.

Occasionally, pediatric hospitalists may be caring for persons 18 years or older who lack decision-making capacity (e.g., due to mental retardation). In such circumstances, the first step is to determine whether the patient has been determined by the legal system to be incompetent and, if so, who has been specified as the surrogate decision maker through either guardianship or a durable power of attorney. Even more rarely, the decision-making capacity of a younger patient's parent or guardian may be in doubt. In such an event, attending physicians should confer with other members of the health care team and perhaps hospital legal counsel before asking for a legal determination of incompetency and the specification of an authorized surrogate decision maker.

Being Purposefully Deceptive

Although the use of deceptive practices by physicians and health care staff runs counter to the principle of truth-telling and the virtue of forthrightness, such practices still occur—in some cases, perhaps with justification—in the pediatric inpatient setting. Examples include the secretive use of placebos to determine whether a response to therapy is due to physiologic or psychological mechanisms, quasi-investigational feeding trials of a child with growth failure to determine whether the family is noncompliant with nutritional recommendations, and the use of covert surveillance video cameras to investigate potential cases of Munchausen syndrome by proxy. Recourse to these deceptive methods should

be considered only after all other possible nonsecretive means of addressing the situation have been exhausted, and then only if the potential benefits of deception greatly outweigh considerations of truth-telling, trustworthiness, and patient or parent autonomy, and only if the course of action has been evaluated by a sufficiently wide array of hospital staff (e.g., members of the ethics committee) to ensure that the two preceding conditions have been met.

Mediating Disputes Regarding Futile or Essential Care

When parents want an increased level of technologic support for their child and health care providers disagree, the notion of futility is sometimes brought up.[10] The Society for Critical Care Medicine defines futile treatments as those that will not accomplish their intended goal.[11] Attempts have been made to better define futile treatments both quantitatively (e.g., treatment has been useless in the last 100 cases) and qualitatively (e.g., treatment will merely preserve permanent unconsciousness or fail to end total dependence on intensive medical care).[12] Such definitions have been criticized, however, because of the imprecision of medical prognoses and because they are value laden and biased against technology-dependent children.[13] Lacking a consensus definition of futility, many ethicists believe that parents' wishes should be honored[14] and that the treatment team's attention should be focused on improving communication with the family, because poor communication often prompts such disputes.[15,16] Failure to reach consensus after a team's best efforts to improve communication is a good indication for an ethics consultation.

In contrast to futile treatment disputes, parents sometimes refuse care that seems necessary. The AAP believes that all children deserve effective medical treatment that is likely to prevent substantial harm, suffering, or death.[17] In addition, the AAP advocates that all legal interventions should apply equally whenever children are endangered or harmed, with no exemptions based on religious or spiritual beliefs—with the exception of immunizations. The AAP does not support the application of medical neglect laws for failure to vaccinate, although it does endorse universal immunizations. In general, if the benefit of treatment is uncertain, the parents' wishes should be honored; if the treatment is in the child's best interests, all legal means should be used to protect the health and welfare of the child.[17]

Deciding to Withhold or Withdraw Life-Sustaining Treatment

Within the medical ethics community, there is strong consensus that there is no salient ethical difference between withholding (i.e., never starting) and withdrawing (i.e., stopping) treatment. Simply stated, if the initiation or continuation of a potentially life-sustaining therapy adversely affects the likelihood of accomplishing therapeutic goals that the patient values above life (such as quality of life), therapy can be ethically withheld or stopped.

Although most health care professionals are ethically comfortable withholding or withdrawing potentially life-sustaining high-technology therapy, many are uncomfortable with the practice of withholding or withdrawing fluids and nutrition administered through tubes. Ethicists argue that intravenous infusions and tube feedings are no differ-

---

Box 18-3 Four Rules Regarding the Doctrine of Double Effect

1. The intention when instituting treatment (typically, administering a drug) must be solely to relieve the patient's suffering.
2. The treatment must be given in response to a sign or symptom of suffering (not a hypothetical potential for suffering to occur).
3. The potency of the treatment must be commensurate with the degree of suffering (not a massive overdose).
4. The treatment must not be given as a deliberate attempt to cause or hasten death.

---

ent from other forms of therapy that patients have the right to refuse.[18] General consensus on these practices is lacking, however, and many states have ambiguous case law precedents that leave the legally sanctioned course of action unclear.

Distinguishing between Treating Suffering and Performing Euthanasia

Euthanasia is illegal throughout the United States.[19] Yet the proper management of a patient in severe pain or with some other form of intractable suffering sometimes requires doses of medications (especially opiates) that may hasten death and in other clinical circumstances would be considered inappropriate. For example, administration of the drug produces the desired effect, such as reducing suffering, but also produces an undesired but anticipated secondary effect, such as respiratory depression. Physicians committed to minimizing the suffering of dying patients can evaluate the ethical appropriateness of their actions by considering whether they can affirm the four rules of the so-called doctrine of double effect (Box 18-3).

Advocating for Patients and Enhancing Quality of Care

Pediatrics as a profession has long recognized the need to advocate for children. Pediatric hospitalists have ethical obligations to improve how health care is delivered to their patients. Although these obligations are often most compelling on a case-by-case basis, hospitalists involved in the design of hospital practice guidelines or policies should also be mindful of how these practices can be evaluated from an ethical point of view. Enhancing access to care, ensuring that limited resources are allocated fairly, eliminating financial conflicts of interest, and improving the quality of care are all activities that can promote justice, equity, and beneficial outcomes in child health care.

REFERENCES

1. Medical professionalism in the new millennium: A physician charter. Ann Intern Med 2002;136:243-246.
2. American Academy of Pediatrics, Committee on Bioethics: Institutional ethics committees. Pediatrics 2001;107:205-209.
3. Spencer EM: A new role for institutional ethics committees: Organizational ethics. J Clin Ethics 1997;8:372-376.
4. Burns JP: From case to policy: Institutional ethics at a children's hospital. J Clin Ethics 2000;11:175-181.
5. Shah S, Whittle A, Wilfond B, et al: How do institutional review boards apply the federal risk and benefit standards for pediatric research? JAMA 2004;291:476-482.
6. Weil E, Nelson RM, Ross LF: Are research ethics standards satisfied in pediatric journal publications? Pediatrics 2002;110:364-370.
7. American Academy of Pediatrics, Committee on Bioethics: Informed consent, parental permission, and assent in pediatric practice. Pediatrics 1995;95:314-317.
8. Faden R, Beauchamp T: A History and Theory of Informed Consent. New York, Oxford University Press, 1986.
9. American Academy of Pediatrics, Committee on Pediatric Emergency Medicine: Consent for medical services for children and adolescents. Pediatrics 1993;92:290-291.
10. Avery GB: Futility considerations in the neonatal intensive care unit. Semin Perinatol 1998;22:216-222.
11. Consensus statement of the Society of Critical Care Medicine's Ethics Committee regarding futile and other possibly inadvisable treatments. Crit Care Med 1997;25:887-891.
12. Schneiderman LJ, Jecker NS, Jonsen AR: Medical futility: Response to critiques. Ann Intern Med 1996;125:669-674.
13. Truog RD, Brett AS, Frader J: The problem with futility. N Engl J Med 1992;326:1560-1564.
14. Nonbeneficial or futile medical treatment: Conflict resolution guidelines for the San Francisco Bay area. Bay Area Network of Ethics Committees (BANEC) Nonbeneficial Treatment Working Group. West J Med 1999;170:287-290.
15. Fins JJ, Solomon MZ: Communication in intensive care settings: The challenge of futility disputes. Crit Care Med 2001;29(2 Suppl):N10-N15.
16. Cogliano JF: The medical futility controversy: Bioethical implications for the critical care nurse. Crit Care Nurs Q 1999;22:81-88.
17. American Academy of Pediatrics, Committee on Bioethics: Religious objections to medical care. Pediatrics 1997;99:279-281.
18. Casarett D, Kapo J, Caplan A: Appropriate use of artificial nutrition and hydration—fundamental principles and recommendations. N Engl J Med 2005;353:2607-2612.
19. Feudtner C: Control of suffering on the slippery slope of care. Lancet 2005;365:1284-1286.

CHAPTER 19

Medicolegal Issues

Steven M. Selbst and Joel B. Korin

Legal risks are common in the care of hospitalized children. Pediatric hospitalists care for complex patients of all ages with a variety of medical conditions. Many are acutely ill with rapidly changing medical conditions. Hospitalists often find themselves juggling several ill patients simultaneously, and they must make critical decisions rapidly. The risk for error is high, and there is the possibility of a subsequent malpractice suit. In addition, certain hospital processes and situations pose a particular risk for lawsuits, including communication, informed consent, refusal of care, documentation, altering the medical record, use of consultants, treatment of incidental findings, patient confidentiality, restraints, and legal responsibility during discharge. The legal obligations surrounding each of these situations are described in this chapter.

The hospitalist movement is relatively new, and little information has been generated regarding claims against these specialists. Evidence suggests that hospitalists reduce malpractice claims in the inpatient setting by improving quality of care and patient and parent satisfaction.[1,2] In addition to improved quality of care, hospitalists have demonstrated enhanced efficiency.[3,4] They often become team leaders in their hospitals, attempting to optimize quality and continuity while delivering evidence-based care for acutely ill patients.[3] Hospitalists' presence in the hospital enables the discovery and demonstration of best practices in detecting errors.[5,6] Tenner's retrospective study found that the quality of care of critically ill patients improved after hours when more experienced physicians provided care at the bedside; more specifically, patients cared for by pediatric hospitalists (general pediatricians who had completed training) had improved survival rates compared with patients cared for by pediatric residents who were supervised from a distance by intensivists.[7] Thus, the use of hospitalists may lead to safe care, fewer adverse outcomes, and fewer malpractice suits.

Like all physicians, hospitalists may face legal action when pediatric patients in their care have bad outcomes. When a lawsuit is instituted, the plaintiff must show that the physician had a duty to the patient, breached that duty, and did not meet the standard of care. The plaintiff must then show that this breach caused damage or injury to the patient.[8]

COMMUNICATION

Good communication between the hospitalist and the patient and family is essential to prevent lawsuits. Poor communication can lead to angry feelings, omission or distortion of important information, and subsequent injury to the patient. Effective communication with the primary care physician (PCP) and nursing staff is also crucial. One study showed a direct relationship between physicians' enhanced communication skills and fewer malpractice suits.[9] Another study of families that sued physicians (after infants suffered permanent injury or death) found that most were dissatisfied with physician-patient communication. They believed that the physicians would not listen to them (13%), would not talk openly (32%), attempted to mislead them (48%), or did not warn them about long-term neurodevelopmental problems (70%).[10] The patient and family must perceive a caring attitude, openness, professional integrity, and standards of excellence; a sense of trust is also crucial. Patients are not always aware of the physician's competence, but they are keenly aware of his or her manner. They remember how the physician looked, acted, spoke, and listened; whether he or she was neatly dressed; and whether the physician was pleasant or disinterested, serious or cavalier, haughty or condescending, polite or discourteous. Good eye contact and body language are important.[11] No matter how tired, frustrated, or stressed the hospitalist feels, this should not be communicated to the family. Establishing good rapport with the family can sometimes be difficult, but it is essential.

The hospitalist should try to appear unhurried and ready to listen. An adverse outcome—even if inevitable—coupled with the parents' feeling that the physician was rushed or was not sincerely interested in the child may provoke a lawsuit. Thus, when meeting with families, it is advisable to introduce oneself, shake hands, and sit down in the examination room. This gives the parents the message that, at least for the next few minutes, they have your undivided attention, no matter how many other children are in the hospital. Studies have shown that if the physician sits down in the presence of the patient, the perception of the time spent with the patient is doubled.[12,13]

The hospitalist must also establish rapport with the child. Avoid casual teasing, condescension, and talking about the child without attempting to include him or her in the discussion. Be careful not to violate modesty in school-age children. Speak at an age-appropriate level, and remember that even young children understand far more than they say. Try to be flexible, but do not offer choices when none exist.[8]

The hospitalist should keep the family informed about necessary procedures, suspected diagnoses, and the child's overall progress. In addition, the family should understand the makeup of the health care team that is caring for the child. This is especially important at a teaching hospital, where residents, fellows, consulting physicians, and several nurses may participate in patient care. At times, parents might insist on obtaining certain laboratory tests that the medical team believes to be unnecessary. The medical staff must then calmly and skillfully explain why such tests may not be needed. This need not become a point of contention if the parents recognize the physician's sincere interest in the child. One study showed that patient satisfaction with care was related not to whether patients got antibiotics for respiratory infections but rather to their perception of the amount of time the physician spent explaining the illness and their understanding of the treatment.[14] Questions about pain management must be discussed, and the parents must believe that everything possible is being done to relieve their child's pain. Parents should be encouraged to stay with their child for procedures whenever possible. Many parents can nurture the child through a painful procedure if they know what to expect.[8,15]

Care should be taken when discussing the patient's management with other staff members in front of the family. Parents should not witness disagreements over plans for management, such as might occur if one staff member suggests ordering a specific laboratory test and the hospitalist disagrees. Likewise, it is not appropriate to reprimand or correct a nurse or physician-in-training in view of the family. This would undoubtedly create a feeling of uneasiness.

In some cases, communication with a parent is particularly difficult. For example, parental anger can be predicted when they are informed that a report for suspected child abuse is being filed. The physician must remain nonjudgmental in these circumstances. The family should be told that the physician is required by law to file such a report and that the medical staff is not accusing anyone of abuse.[8]

Finally, if a harmful medical error is made, many advise the hospitalist to explain what has happened to the family. It is best to be honest with parents about the mistake. If an error is merely suspected, one should not admit negligence but rather explain that all will be done to investigate the situation and improve results.[16] Lawsuits may be avoided if the physician is honest and forthright. Like in politics, an attempted "cover up" makes the situation worse. In all cases, the hospitalist should follow hospital policies for disclosure of a medical error (see also Chapter 5).

INFORMED DECISION MAKING (INFORMED CONSENT)

Parents have the right to be informed about their child's medical care and to give consent for treatment. Parental rights are limited, however. For instance, adults can refuse treatment—even life-sustaining treatment—for themselves, but not for their children. Parents must act responsibly and in their child's best interests. If they are neglectful or abusive, the courts can relieve them of decision making and, if necessary, custody.[17]

Most states define *informed consent* as providing a description of the procedure or treatment and the risks and alternatives in such a way that a reasonably prudent person would be able to make an informed decision whether to undergo that procedure or treatment. Patients and parents are entitled to know the diagnosis; the nature and purpose of the proposed treatment or procedure; the risks, consequences, and side effects of the proposed procedure; reasonably available alternatives and their risks; and the anticipated prognosis without treatment. The physician must be sure that the patient or parent understands the information given.[18,19]

In a true emergency, informed consent is not needed. When a hospitalist provides care in the emergency department, the legal guardian may not even be present. For an unconscious or severely injured child, no consent for treatment is necessary because it is assumed that a reasonable

parent would want the physician to care for the child immediately. If it is not clear that a true emergency exists, it is generally best to treat the patient and get consent later.[19] A physician is more likely to be sued for failure to treat without consent than for providing reasonable treatment without the guardian's knowledge or approval. However, do not give a blood transfusion to a reasonably stable child or intravenous contrast material for a computed tomography scan if the risks and benefits have not been explained to the parents. It is conceivable that a patient could suffer a reaction to these procedures, and the guardian may sue the physician for failing to inform him or her of the risks involved.[8] No patient or parent should be forced or influenced to make a specific decision; however, no decision by a parent is completely free of outside influences. Most parents need and want the physician's opinion to help them decide what is best for their child.[20] Finally, the physician has an ethical obligation to try to inform a minor child about the proposed treatment, to describe what he or she is likely to experience, and to get his or her assent to care, if possible.[18-20]

Consent forms are widely used at most hospitals and should be written at an appropriate level for most patients or parents (generally, a sixth- to eighth-grade reading level). Parents must be given the opportunity to ask questions after reading the form. Language barriers must be taken into consideration. Parents usually sign a general consent form at the time of presentation to the hospital that allows for a general evaluation and treatment of the child. However, parental signing of such a form does not equate with informed consent. The patient or parent can still claim that the risks and benefits were not adequately explained.[8,18] Patients and parents may not recall what was told to them when they were emotionally stressed. A signed consent form may provide some legal protection for the physician, because it documents that steps were taken to inform the parent about a procedure. However, a signed form is of little value unless a discussion about risks and benefits took place.[18] Clear documentation in the record, noting what was explained to the parent, may be just as valuable as a signed consent form. Remember, informed consent is a process, not a paper. Table 19-1 summarizes procedures for assisting parents with informed decision making.

Table 19-1 Responsibilities for Informed Decision Making (Informed Consent)
Assess the patient's or guardian's decision-making capacity
Provide the patient and guardian with appropriate information 　　Diagnosis 　　Nature of procedure or intervention 　　Purpose of procedure or treatment 　　Risks and benefits of procedure or treatment 　　Alternative treatments and associated risks and benefits 　　Prognosis with and without treatment
Assess the patient's or guardian's comprehension of the discussion
Ensure that the decision is made freely, not coerced
After the discussion, obtain signed consent

REFUSAL OF CARE

Despite all efforts, some patients or parents refuse treatment or leave the hospital against medical advice (AMA). This usually occurs when the patient or parent is angry, afraid, or disoriented or has certain religious beliefs. Emancipated minors and parents generally have the right to refuse treatment for themselves or their child. However, when a patient or family leaves the hospital without a full evaluation and complete treatment, everyone involved may suffer. The child may have persistent or worsening symptoms from a medical problem that has not been addressed. Likewise, the physician usually feels a sense of failure and frustration when advice and recommendations are not heeded. The hospital and physicians may be subjected to a lawsuit if the patient later suffers serious morbidity or dies, even if the family left voluntarily or signed out AMA. Therefore, the goal should always be to keep the child and family from leaving prematurely.[8,21]

Understanding the Patient

Some patients or parents wish to leave the hospital because they are angry about a long wait for medical treatment. Some may fear a prolonged or expensive hospitalization, or they anticipate unnecessary and painful procedures for their child. Others are afraid to learn of a serious diagnosis or are anxious about children left at home. Those who do not speak English may be especially frightened. Still others may fear teaching institutions in particular because they believe that students or residents "practice" on patients.[8] Understandably, families may be less trusting of a hospitalist physician with whom they are not familiar.

Providing Treatment

If a true emergency exists, prompt medical intervention should be provided even over parental objections. It is extremely unlikely that the physician will be successfully sued for intervening and delivering care to a child in an emergency situation.[18,20] In fact, the legal risk is much greater if emergency care is not given.

The hospitalist should first try to learn why the patient or family wishes to leave the hospital. If the patient or parent seems angry, the physician should allow him or her to express concerns without interruption. The hospitalist should remain courteous, concerned, and flexible in the treatment plan. It is never wise to challenge patients to sign out AMA, and they should not be threatened with a call to security officers. Security should be called only if necessary to maintain order.[8]

A social services worker may be extremely helpful in difficult cases. Further, a telephone call to a familiar PCP may allay the parent's fears and convince the family to follow the proposed treatment. If a language barrier is a factor in the misunderstanding, a competent translator should be provided. The physician must be sure the parents understand the risks and benefits of treatment and the risks of refusing treatment. Allow the patient and family to consider options in a low-pressure atmosphere so that they can make a rational decision.

Documenting Events

If a parent still wishes to leave the hospital despite all efforts to reach an agreement, the guardian or emancipated minor should be asked to sign a statement releasing the doctor and the hospital from all liability. Such statements have limited usefulness, however, because parents can later claim that they did not fully understand the risks involved in leaving AMA. However, a signed statement witnessed by one or two staff members may shift some responsibility to the parents in the event of an adverse outcome.[8,20,21]

Exactly what was done for the child and what was told to the parents should be documented in the hospital records. Specifically, if the child was examined, the findings and impression of the limited evaluation should be recorded and what tests or treatment was contemplated. Also, the parents' reason for leaving AMA should be documented, as well as the risks of refusing treatment as they were explained to the parents. Parents should be told (and it should be documented) that they can always return to the hospital for reevaluation if they change their minds or if the child's condition worsens. It may be helpful to volunteer the names of alternative hospitals and doctors and to offer to arrange transportation, if feasible. This shows a sincere interest in the patient and may prevent litigation. Finally, if a parent refuses to officially sign out AMA before leaving the hospital, this should be carefully documented and witnessed in the medical record.[8,20]

In some situations, the patient should not be permitted to leave the hospital under any circumstances. If the guardian is disoriented or intoxicated and cannot understand the risks and benefits of treatment or the consequences of refusing care, the patient should not be allowed to leave. A life-threatening medical problem also mandates immediate medical care. It is always better to win the cooperation of the parents, but if they refuse, the staff is justified in treating the child. The refusal should be reported to the proper authorities as medical neglect, and a court order should be sought while emergency care is being delivered. If it is unclear whether a life-threatening situation is present, err on the side of treatment.[8,20,21]

Similarly, in a case of suspected child abuse in which the perpetrator is unknown, the child should not be released, despite the parents' wishes or protests. In this situation, the security staff should be called to prevent the parents from removing the child from the hospital. The staff must contact the hospital lawyers, administrators, or a judge on emergency call to seek a verbal temporary restraining order. The physician should record the conversation with the judge on the patient's chart, including the specific actions authorized. The procedure to obtain court permission to treat a child may vary in different locales, and the hospitalist should be familiar with local and hospital policies.[8]

Special Cases
HIV Testing

Testing a pediatric patient for human immunodeficiency virus (HIV) is an important issue. HIV testing without a patient's (or guardian's) consent is illegal in almost every state. Occasionally, a staff member may unintentionally injure himself or herself with a needle stick and then request HIV testing of the patient. The specific hospital policy for this event should be followed carefully.

Lumbar Puncture

Lumbar punctures arouse fear and concern among parents. Many parents have misperceptions about the procedure and an unwarranted fear of complications. Parents should be fully informed about the need to do the procedure—for instance, that a lumbar puncture is necessary to determine if a serious disease such as meningitis is present—and that there is no adequate alternative to establish the diagnosis. They should be informed about the most common complications, such as local pain. They should also be told that serious complications, such as apnea in a small infant who is curled for the procedure, are quite rare. There is no need to discuss possible herniation, because this is extremely rare when signs of increased intracranial pressure are absent. If such signs exist, the procedure should be withheld.

If a parent refuses the lumbar puncture, the hospitalist may choose to treat the child for possible meningitis without doing the procedure. Parents should be told of the inherent problems with this alternative plan, and permission for the lumbar puncture can be pursued after treatment is started.[8]

Blood Transfusions and Jehovah's Witnesses

If a parent refuses a blood transfusion because of religious beliefs, legal counsel should be obtained, when time permits. A court order may be necessary. If the child's life or health is in danger, nearly every state allows the physician to override the parents' religious beliefs. Even for an older child or adolescent who holds the same beliefs, it is unlikely that the courts will uphold the minor's right to refuse treatment if doing so means risking death.[22] Still, it is best to avoid court action or coercing a teenager to accept treatment that is unwanted. The hospitalist should try to settle the affair with the patient and family whenever possible. Discuss the use of blood substitutes if time allows and if this is acceptable to the physician. If the patient is in shock and unable to consent, blood can be given as deemed necessary. A transfusion can also be authorized over a teenager's objection if there is a question about the patient's competency or if the state can demonstrate an overriding interest.[18]

DOCUMENTATION—THE MEDICAL RECORD

The importance of careful documentation cannot be overemphasized. Good documentation prevents lawsuits. The patient's chart is almost always the first document reviewed by parents, attorneys, and their consulting physicians. A record that demonstrates a thorough examination and testing may convince the plaintiff's attorney not to proceed further. A record that does not demonstrate conclusively whether an important test or portion of the examination was negative or positive may lead counsel to assume that it was not done. The record can also influence an expert witness hired to advise the attorney whether the case has merit and should be pursued. Because one can never truly predict which patient will have a bad outcome and end up in litigation, each chart should be prepared carefully.[8]

Because of the extended statute of limitations for children, many years may pass before a physician is advised of malpractice litigation. The hospitalist often has little if any recollection of the treatment rendered without referring to

the medical record. This document can prove to be the physician's friend or foe, depending on how well it was prepared at the time of treatment. Many settlements have been offered even when good medical care was rendered but not substantiated in the medical records.[8,23]

The history of the present illness must be described completely but concisely. Even though there may be limited time for recording information, a note that is very brief and barely legible may convey a sense of carelessness and haste to a jury.[23] Any information that seems relevant to the chief complaint must be noted. Also record details about the child's recent diet, level of activity, and medications given at home.

The record for every pediatric patient should include a history of immunizations, allergies to any medications, and underlying medical problems. Also, known exposure to infection may be important in many cases. For an adolescent girl, the last menstrual period should be documented. For an injured child, the medical record should reflect how the injury occurred and whether the history is consistent with the physical examination. If there is a concern about child abuse, this should be described, as well as a decision to file a report with authorities.[8]

A thorough physical examination must be recorded for each child, including a complete, timed set of vital signs. Abnormal vital signs merit repeating. If the blood pressure or pulse is abnormal because the child is crying, this should be stated. Particular emphasis must be given to the child's general appearance, state of hydration, and level of activity or playfulness. Be as descriptive as possible. For instance, "alert, interactive, playing with toys on mother's lap" graphically depicts the general appearance of an infant. Rather than "irritable baby," it is better to note "baby cries when approached but is easily consoled by mother." For a febrile child or a complicated case, the chart should convincingly reflect that the child was well appearing at the time of discharge. In the emergency department, this may require that a second note, or progress note, be included in the chart. Additional paper may be needed for such progress notes; an inability to fit the note on the chart is not an excuse for incomplete documentation. For an injured child, it may be best to use a picture or diagram to describe the trauma in detail.[8,23]

The medical record must reflect a timely process. All entries, including diagnostic or therapeutic orders, must be clearly written and the exact time of the entry noted. Likewise, telephone conversations with consultants should be dated and timed. For example, in the event of delayed surgery, recording the time when a consultant was called and when he or she arrived can prove useful years later when litigation begins. All laboratory test results or reports of procedures performed must be documented.[23]

The medical record must also include the physician's clinical observations of the patient and the diagnostic impression formulated. Documenting one's thought process can be helpful, especially if the case is complicated. For instance, if the physician initially orders laboratory tests and later cancels them, the reasons for this change in the management plan should be justified in the medical records (e.g., "child improved, drinking well, no need for spinal tap").[8,23]

It is important that the hospitalist's final disposition be reasonable and based on the history, physical examination, test results, and impression. For instance, if the final diagnosis is gastroenteritis, the child should be discharged only if the record reflects that he or she is well hydrated.

The medical record should provide meaningful information to another practitioner if additional care is needed at a later time. It should also display a concerned, professional attitude toward the child and family. Although some charts use a checklist system in an effort to save time, pertinent positive and negative findings on the physical examination should always be added. For instance, in the evaluation of the skin of a febrile child, comments such as "no petechiae or purpura" may be quite important. A chart in which the entire examination is merely checked off as "normal" will not convince a jury that a careful examination was performed. The chart should not comment on parts of the examination that were not done. For instance, the rectal examination should not be checked off as normal if no such examination was performed. This will damage the physician's credibility and make a jury doubt that other parts of the examination were truly performed.[8,23]

The medical record will be made public if a lawsuit is filed. Therefore, only comments that one would be proud to read in front of a jury should be included. Illegible records can compromise the quality of care and make the hospitalist appear unprofessional. The record should not contain insensitive terms. A medical term such as "dysmorphic child" serves all parties better than "FLK" (funny looking kid). Avoid derogatory statements or descriptions of the parents as well. If the parents are angry during the evaluation, the note may reflect this; for example, "mother became upset during the exam and her concerns were addressed." No judgmental statements should be added.[8,21,23] If a patient returns to the hospital after a prior admission or emergency department visit, note the earlier treatment but avoid terminology that suggests that the initial care given was incomplete or careless.[21] It is also advisable to avoid self-serving statements in the record that appear defensive. The purpose of the record is primarily to take care of the patient, and it should not look like it was written for legal defense purposes.

The physician's notes should be consistent with the nursing notes and those of any other disciplines. The hospitalist must read and acknowledge the nursing notes. If a physician disagrees with the nursing assessment (e.g., does not believe that a baby is lethargic), this should be emphasized in a noncombative manner in the record. It is important that nurses, physicians, consultants, and other members of the medical staff do not engage in intramural battles on the record.[24] Disagreements should be settled before the patient goes home, and the record should reflect agreement among caretakers whenever possible. Inflammatory remarks should not be written down, and extensive discussions about the frustrations of patient care should be left out of the record.

When a child's care is transferred to another physician, such as at a change of shift, the physician coming on duty can write a brief note to document the patient's condition at that time. Document all procedures in a detailed note, including how the child tolerated the procedure. Include brief descriptions of any conversations with the family and those with the PCP. Use abbreviations sparingly, and use only standard ones accepted by the medical records department of the hospital. Avoid squeezed-in entries or premature conclusions.[21]

Altering the Medical Record

Written errors in a patient's chart should be corrected appropriately. There should be no attempt to cover up mistakes by blacking out words or phrases, which tends to arouse suspicion. Draw a single line drawn through the error, then initial and date it.

Never attempt to "enhance" the medical record after the case is involved in litigation. It is likely that any change made to the record will be discovered and will be seen as a deliberate and dishonest cover-up. In some cases, forensic or handwriting experts may be called to review the records and testify to the alterations. In general, it is easier to defend missing facts or a poor record than an altered one. Credibility is a key factor in any litigation, and an altered record frequently destroys the physician's credibility.[23,25] When there is a need to add clinical information after an untoward event occurs, it is best to do so in a confidential letter to the physician's attorney rather than adding to the chart.

Besides resulting in the loss of a lawsuit, tampering with the record can result in the award of "punitive damages," intended to punish the physician for attempting to mislead the court. Some malpractice policies deny coverage if it is determined that medical records were altered. In some states, altering medical records can be considered a criminal offense in certain circumstances. Finally, any attempt to destroy or "lose" the medical records will seriously hurt the physician's ability to defend against the litigation.[21]

CONSULTANTS

No physician in the hospital works in isolation. There is often a need to consult with the PCP, critical care specialists, surgeons, and other physicians while caring for ill children. The hospitalist should call for help whenever he or she believes that the care required is beyond his or her expertise or when it appears that another opinion will be helpful. Failure to consult appropriately and in a timely manner can result in a lawsuit should there be a poor outcome.[26]

The hospitalist should generally complete a history and physical examination and obtain appropriate laboratory studies to ensure appropriate referral and avoid unnecessary consultation. However, if there is a true emergency, such as a surgical abdomen or testicular torsion, do not delay consultation by waiting for a urinalysis, Doppler studies, or other tests that may postpone definitive care.[27] If the consultant does not arrive in a timely manner, the hospitalist should consider calling the consultant's supervisor, asking other sources for help, or transferring the child to another institution.[26] Document the time the specialist was called, the time he or she arrived, and, if applicable, the time the consultant assumed care of the patient. The hospitalist is also responsible for making sure that the consultant is competent for the case in question. If appropriate consultation is not available, safe transport of the child to another facility should be arranged after discussion with the parents.

If the hospitalist believes that consultation is warranted, he or she should not be dissuaded by the PCP. The opinion of the PCP should be considered advisory only. Further, if the family insists on consultation or a second opinion (e.g., a plastic surgeon to suture a facial laceration), it is wise to comply if the request is reasonable.[28]

Radiology consultation ensures proper reading of a film. The hospitalist may be found liable for misreading a child's radiograph if a radiologist was available. The hospitalist will not be held to the same standard as a radiologist, but rather whatever expertise the jury believes the hospitalist should possess.[8,23]

Communication with the Consultant

Good communication with the consultant is essential. The hospitalist should give appropriate information to the consultant and make certain that the specialist understands the reason for consultation or the question that needs to be addressed. The consultant should discuss his or her findings with the hospitalist, and the two should decide who will relay the information to the parents. Consultants should write complete notes and list clear reasons for their recommendations. For radiology consultations in particular, it is important to have a system in place so that reports of reread radiographs reach the hospitalist, especially any opinion that differs from the hospitalist.

Telephone consultations without direct examination by the consultant pose a risk for both the consultant and the hospitalist. It is always possible that incomplete information will be provided to the consultant, resulting in incorrect advice. In general, the hospitalist should not allow the specialist to dictate care by phone or deem that consultation is unnecessary if the hospitalist is uncomfortable. If only phone advice is sought, the gist of the conversation should be recorded in the patient's chart.[27]

Some hospitals allow the consultant to write orders for the patient, whereas others request that the specialist only give suggestions to the hospitalist. It should be clear to all parties who is placing the orders so that there is no confusion or omission of desired treatment. With most consultations, the hospitalist remains responsible for the patient. If care is to be formally transferred to a consultant who evaluates a child, the time of transfer should be documented.

Disagreements with Consultants

Understandably, there are occasional disagreements about patient management. These should not be taken lightly, because both physicians may be held responsible for a patient's poor outcome. The hospitalist is not legally bound to accept the advice of a consultant. Blind acceptance of the consultant's advice can leave the hospitalist liable if the child suffers.[28] However, it is not advisable to reject the advice of a specialist without careful consideration of the consequences. If there is a poor outcome, the consultant's views as a specialist will be given great weight in court.[26] If there are questions about care, it is best to discuss the case personally with the consultant. If the consultant's recommendations are not followed, the hospitalist should document why suggested studies were not obtained.[26] Disputes about care should not be discussed in front of the patient or family. Instead, it is best to try to resolve these disagreements amicably, away from the patient. If resolution cannot be reached, it may be appropriate to tell the family in a nonjudgmental way about the difference in opinion.[27,28] If the family accepts the opinion of the consultant rather than the hospitalist, this should be noted in the record, and care should be transferred to the consultant. Ideally, actions should be guided by hospital conflict resolution policies. Cordial, honest dialogue is needed to ensure a good outcome.

If the hospitalist evaluates a child in the emergency department and believes that admission to the hospital is warranted, and the consultant disagrees, the specialist must come to the emergency department to evaluate the child. Responsibility for the disposition may still rest with the hospitalist, but there will probably be shared responsibility if both have evaluated the child.

TREATMENT OF INCIDENTAL FINDINGS

Often a child is admitted to the hospital to manage a specific condition and, during the course of treatment, another problem is identified. Whether the hospitalist is responsible for the workup of incidental findings (e.g., hypertension, scoliosis) is unclear.[29,30] It depends somewhat on common practice in the particular area. Hospitalists may be held to the same standard as other pediatricians who discover an unexpected finding during an inpatient stay. It is in everyone's best interest for the hospitalist to clarify who will manage the new incidental finding and whether it needs to be completed in an inpatient or ambulatory setting. If a patient or the family prefers an inpatient workup and it can be expeditiously and safely performed, it is reasonable for a hospitalist to pursue it. Regardless, the patient should be informed of the findings and the need for follow-up.[29] This conversation should be documented.

CONFIDENTIALITY

It is extremely important for the hospitalist to maintain patient confidentiality. Patients have filed many lawsuits because of breach of confidential information. Patient privacy is governed by federal, state, and local laws, and the privacy of patient information has changed extensively with the implementation of the Health Insurance Portability and Accountability Act (HIPAA). Medical notes and patient-identifiable data are confidential and cannot be communicated to any third party without the patient's or parent's written consent. When conversing about a patient, it is important to pay attention to who is nearby and may overhear the conversation. Test results and other confidential information must be securely protected throughout the hospital. Be cautious when using a computer monitor that does not have a privacy screen.[21]

E-mail has become important in the practice of medicine. However, e-mail can result in a breach of privacy if the message is inadvertently sent to the wrong person or left unattended on a computer screen, where it can be viewed by another party.[21] The hospitalist should also understand that e-mail is discoverable in legal proceedings.

Electronic medical records have the capacity to improve quality of care by compiling and centralizing all pertinent information related to the pediatric patient. The electronic medical records system must protect the privacy of patients' health information by restricting access according to local and federal laws and policies.[21]

RESTRAINT OF PATIENTS

Occasionally, a patient must be physically restrained, and hospital staff may use reasonable force to prevent a child from hurting him- or herself or others. Proper monitoring and humane care are required. The hospitalist and hospital staff should adhere to regulations of the Joint Commission on Accreditation of Healthcare Organizations (JCAHO) and state and hospital policies whenever restraints are applied. A patient should not be restrained just for convenience or punishment, because this may cause physical harm and result in litigation.[31] For female patients, always have a female staff member present during the restraint procedure.

Leather restraints are safest for violent patients and should be used instead of bed sheets, intravenous tubing, or other improvised devices that may result in injury to the patient or inadequate immobilization.[31] Locking restraints should not be used because the need for keys is dangerous in the event of a fire or deteriorating medical condition. Avoid restraint if the patient is hypotensive or has respiratory distress, limited chest expansion, or airway obstruction. Avoid restraining the patient in a prone position as this may compromise ventilation and lead to death of the patient.

After restraint, take and document vital signs every 15 minutes, and assess the child's ventilation, circulation, comfort, mobility, need for change in position, defecation, and micturition. To remove a patient from restraints, gather adequate personnel and free only one limb at a time. Debrief the patient while freeing him or her, and observe the patient's behavior to determine whether he or she has regained control.[31]

The hospitalist must always act in the patient's best interests. The medical record should reflect what was done to the patient, why it was done, and that all efforts were made to consider the patient.[31]

DISCHARGE INSTRUCTIONS

At the time of discharge from the hospital or from the emergency department, the hospitalist should review the child's problems and treatment and give directions for ongoing therapy. The physician should write down the diagnosis, give written discharge instructions, and review these carefully with the guardian and the patient if he or she is old enough to understand.[24] Nonspecific instructions to "give fluids" or "return as needed" are not helpful. Abbreviations that may not be familiar to the parents or patient should be avoided. Clear instructions about medication regimens, use of inhalers, and how to taper steroids are needed. The instructions should always include a few examples of worrisome signs to look for at home. Although it is not feasible to list every possible complication, the parents must have a general idea of when to visit the PCP and what warrants an immediate return to the emergency department. If no radiologist is available in the hospital during off-hours, the family should be told that the hospitalist's reading of the radiographs is preliminary and that the films will be reviewed by a radiologist and the family notified of any change in interpretation.[8,24] This strategy may prevent anger or the feeling of poor care if they are called back for additional treatment or referral.

Some authorities recommend that the parents read back the instructions to the physician to indicate that they can comprehend the treatment plan.[24] Logan and colleagues found that most patients discharged from an urban emergency department could not recall and state their diagnoses

or treatment plans completely when interviewed immediately after discharge.[32] Of course, the physician must be sure that the parents understand English, and translators or translation services should be contacted before the patient leaves the hospital whenever there is reason to believe that the family does not understand the instructions.[8]

Computer-generated discharge instructions, commonly used by many hospitals, are advantageous because they are legible and readable if designed at an appropriate reading level. Most can be personalized and edited. Many have the capability to produce the instructions in a foreign language or with large print for the visually impaired. They can be programmed to print disclaimers about final readings of radiographs and electrocardiograms, which many physicians may neglect to do if handwriting is required. Parents who receive written, standardized discharge instructions are more satisfied than those who receive nonuniform instructions from a house officer.[33] An exit interview, during which important information is reviewed with the guardians, also improves their retention of discharge information. Return visits to the emergency department can be avoided with careful discharge instructions, including written material that is geared to the reading level of the patient.[34]

In all cases, the family should be asked to sign that they have received and understand the discharge instructions.[23] A copy must become part of the medical record, because the physician will not remember what was discussed with the family years later. Good discharge instructions may prevent litigation or at least affect negotiations and damages in the event of a lawsuit.[23]

At the time of discharge, it is wise to ask the guardians if they have any questions. Likewise, it is prudent to investigate potential social problems, such as inability to obtain medications, need for transportation home, inability to be seen by the PCP, or other factors that may interfere with the care of the child. This must be done in a caring, nonobtrusive manner.

The hospitalist has an obligation to protect the child if he or she is discharged on medications with potentially serious side effects. For example, if a teenager is discharged on a sedative medication or has an unusual condition that may predispose him or her to seizures or syncope, it may be wise to advise the patient not to drive.[8] Table 19-2 lists responsibilities of the hospitalist at the time of patient discharge from the hospital.

FOLLOW-UP CARE

One particular area of risk involves follow-up care for patients who were treated by the hospitalist. The duty to provide follow-up care is shared by the hospitalist and the PCP.[29,30] The inpatient team is responsible for evaluating whether the outpatient treatment plan is feasible for the child's family and modifying the plan if needed.[29,30] The hospitalist has a duty to provide instructions to patients and parents regarding follow-up care.

Some patients may have trouble getting medications prescribed or could develop new symptoms after discharge. In such cases, the patient needs to know who to call in the interim.[30] If the patient calls the hospitalist about a change in condition, this information should be forwarded to the PCP. Patients should be counseled about the risks of failing

Table 19-2 Hospitalist Responsibilities When Discharging a Pediatric Patient

Give written instructions and review them verbally with the parent or guardian
List medications and treatments clearly
Ensure that the patient or parent understands discharge instructions and the importance of keeping appointments
Have the parent sign a form indicating that he or she received the instructions and understands them
Specify an interim plan if the patient becomes ill before the scheduled appointment with the PCP
Be specific and clear about when to see the PCP and when to return to the emergency department or hospital
Arrange appropriate follow-up care
Communicate with the PCP
Be certain that the discharge summary and important documents reach the PCP
Develop a system to review and forward incoming results and reread radiographs after patient discharge

PCP, primary care provider.

to receive ongoing care, and the hospitalist must also ensure that the PCP has enough information about the hospitalization to provide high-quality care when the patient arrives for follow-up.[29,30]

Despite everyone's best intentions, things can be overlooked during the transition from the hospital to the outpatient setting.[30] Hospitalists may be held liable for failing to inform patients and the PCP of laboratory studies or test results that are received after discharge. Some hospitalists hire physician assistants to provide continuity or to locate charts and test results. At academic medical centers, residents may assist with the review and communication of test results to patients or PCPs.[4,29] Regardless of who is assisting with these important tasks, the hospitalist must ensure that relevant information, including the discharge summary, gets to the PCP. It is not necessary to fax every note from the chart. If the PCP is deluged with too much information, it may be ignored.[30] Timely dictation services are needed to forward complete and legible records.[35] The PCP has a legal obligation to ensure follow-up once the hospitalist has communicated with him or her and an appointment has been scheduled. Be careful of weekends and holidays. For example, telling patients to follow up with the PCP in two days on December 23 would be worthless.

CONCLUSION

Hospitalists have many medicolegal obligations in the care of hospitalized children. The risk of lawsuits can be greatly reduced through an understanding of these risks, good communication and documentation, and attention to the needs and wishes of patients and their families.

REFERENCES

1. Narang AS, Ey J: The emerging role of the pediatric hospitalist. Clin Pediatr 2003;42:295-297.
2. Wachter RM, Goldman L: The hospitalist movement 5 years later. JAMA 2002;287:487-494.
3. Williams MV: The future of hospital medicine: Evolution or revolution? Am J Med 2004;117:446-450.
4. Bellet PS, Wachter RM: The hospitalist movement and its implication for the care of hospitalized children. Pediatrics 1999;103:473-477.
5. Freed DH: Hospitalists: Evolution, evidence, and eventualities. Health Care Manage 2004;23:238-256.
6. Chaudhry SI, Olofinboda KA, Krumhotz HM: Detection of errors by attending physicians on a general medicine service. J Gen Intern Med 2003;18:595-600.
7. Tenner PA, Dibrell H, Taylor RP: Improved survival with hospitalists in a pediatric intensive care unit. Crit Care Med 2003;31:847-852.
8. Selbst SM, Korin JB: Preventing Malpractice Lawsuits in Pediatric Emergency Medicine. Dallas, American College of Emergency Physicians, 1999.
9. Adamson TE, Schann JM, Guillan DS, et al: Physician communication skills and malpractice claims: A complex relationship. West J Med 1989;150:356-360.
10. Hickson GB, Clayton EW, Githens PB, et al: Factors that prompted families to file malpractice claims following perinatal injuries. JAMA 1992;267:1359-1363.
11. Lester GW, Smith SG: Listening and talking to patients: A remedy for malpractice suits? West J Med 1993;158:268-272.
12. Little NE: Image of the emergency physician. In Henry GL, Sullivan DJ (eds): Emergency Medicine Risk Management: A Comprehensive Review, 2nd ed. Dallas, American College of Emergency Physicians, 1997, pp 9-13.
13. Barnett PB: Rapport and the hospitalist. Am J Med 2001;111:31S-35S.
14. Hamm RM: Antibiotics and respiratory infections: Are patients more satisfied when expectations are met? J Fam Pract 1996;43:56.
15. Sachetti A, Guzzetta C, Harris R: Family member presence during resuscitation attempts and invasive procedures: Is there science behind the emotion? Clin Pediatr Emerg Med 2004;4:292-296.
16. Wu AW, Cavanaugh TA, McPhee SL, et al: To tell the truth: Ethical and practical issues in disclosing medical mistakes to patients. J Gen Intern Med 1997;12:770.
17. American Academy of Pediatrics, Committee on Bioethics: Informed consent, parental permission and assent in pediatric practice. Pediatrics 1995;96:314-317.
18. Kassutto Z, Vaught W: Informed decision making and refusal of treatment. Clin Pediatr Emerg Med 2003;4:285-291.
19. American Academy of Pediatrics, Committee on Pediatric Emergency Medicine: Consent for emergency medical services for children and adolescents. Pediatrics 2003;111:703-706.
20. Thewes J, Fitzgerald D, Salmasy DP: Informed consent in emergency medicine: Ethics under fire. Emerg Med Clin North Am 1996;14:245-254.
21. Berger JE, Deitschel CH (eds): Medical Liability for Pediatricians, 6th ed. Elk Grove Village, Ill, American Academy of Pediatrics, 2004.
22. Sheldon M: Ethical issues in the forced transfusion of Jehovah's Witness children. J Emerg Med 1996;14:251-257.
23. Selbst SM, Korin JB: Malpractice and emergency care: Doing right by the patient—and yourself. Contemp Pediatr 2000;17:88-106.
24. SAEM Task Force on Physician-Patient Communication: Physician-patient communication in the emergency department. Part 3. Clinical and educational issues. Ann Emerg Med 1997;4:72-78.
25. Barrah K, Schmid B, Schmid M: Don't doctor your records. West Med J 1996;95:385.
26. Wilde JA, Pedroni AT: The do's and don'ts of consultations. Contemp Pediatr 1991;8:23-28.
27. Holliman CJ: The art of dealing with consultants. J Emerg Med 1993;11:633-640.

28. O' Riordan WD: Consultations. In Henry GL, Sullivan DJ (eds): Emergency Medicine Risk Management: A Comprehensive Review, 2nd ed. Dallas, American College of Emergency Physicians, 1997, pp 329-334.

29. Alpers A: Key legal principles for hospitalists. Am J Med 2001;111:5S-9S.

30. Crane M: When a hospitalist discharges your patients. Med Econ 2000;6:41-54.

31. Dorfman DH: The use of physical and chemical restraints in the pediatric emergency department. Pediatr Emerg Care 2000;16:355-360.

32. Logan PD, Schwab RA, Salomone JA, et al: Patient understanding of emergency department discharge instructions. South Med J 1996;89: 770-773.

33. Issaccman DJ, Purvis K, Gyuro J, et al: Standardized instructions: Do they improve communication of discharge information from the emergency department? Pediatrics 1992;89:1204-1207.

34. Pierce JM, Kellerman AL, Oster C: "Bounces": An analysis of short-term return visits to a public hospital emergency department. Ann Emerg Med 1990;19:752-757.

35. Percelay JM, Committee on Hospital Care, American Academy of Pediatrics: Physician's role in coordinating care of hospitalized children. Pediatrics 2003,111:707-709.

Clinical Research in the Pediatric Inpatient Setting

Sarah C. McBride and Christopher P. Landrigan

There is a national move toward developing pediatric inpatient research that provides a foundation for evidence-based medicine and health policy. Many hospitalists thus find themselves in a position to develop research projects and answer clinical questions in their areas of practice. Unfortunately, pediatric hospitalist medicine currently lacks rigorous studies to guide the management of many conditions for which children are hospitalized, leading to widespread variability in care.[1] There are innumerable gaps in knowledge that hospitalist researchers have an opportunity to address. This chapter outlines key components that aspiring researchers should consider when preparing to study a clinical question. A summary of these components is provided in Box 20-1. These aspects of a research plan form the basis for selecting and refining a high-quality research proposal and, in many cases, for preparing a grant application for a governmental, nonprofit, or commercial entity. (For guidance in applying for federal grants, see *http://www.niaid.nih.gov/ncn/grants/default.htm* and *http://www.ahrq.gov/*.)

GETTING STARTED: TRAINING AND MENTORSHIP

Like clinical medicine, research has its own standards and language that can be daunting to newcomers. Hospitalists undertaking research endeavors for the first time typically need assistance to develop workable proposals and to attract external (or even internal) support for their work. With appropriate guidance and support from senior personnel (who are often collaborators from outside the field of hospital medicine) and some introductory training in research methods, many hospitalists are capable of conducting successful research projects. The importance of mentorship and training should not be overlooked because they greatly increase the chance of success.

Research Training

For clinicians lacking a strong background in research, short courses in research methods (e.g., biostatistics, epidemiology, health services research) are available at many universities affiliated with medical centers. Such courses can help one think critically about how to pursue a research question and refine a general idea into a workable study, especially after an area of interest has been identified. In addition, interaction with senior epidemiologists, biostatisticians, and classmates with similar interests can lead to mentoring and collaborative relationships. For those who are considering research as a primary academic endeavor, such courses can be an initial step toward an advanced research degree.

Mentorship

The development of a working relationship with a senior researcher or researchers is a crucial step for any beginning investigator. Although senior staff members sometimes share this role (a community of mentors), it is best to identify one mentor willing to devote considerable time and resources to a junior investigator's development. Because there are few senior researchers in the field of pediatric hospitalist medicine, given its recent emergence, one should consider working with mentors from outside the field. General pediatric researchers, pediatric subspecialists, internal medicine hospitalists, and nonmedical researchers can all fill this role. Regardless of a mentor's background, both parties should share common, though not necessarily identical, interests. A successful mentoring relationship is one that benefits both parties: the junior researcher has the opportunity to receive frequent feedback and advice from the mentor, and the mentor receives assistance studying a question of interest and the satisfaction of fostering a junior colleague's career. The advice, experience, and training received under the guidance of a mentor can be invaluable.

RESEARCH OBJECTIVE OR HYPOTHESIS

Once appropriate training has been completed and a mentor relationship initiated, the first step in any proposed research project is the development of an answerable, well-formulated question. Although there are many unanswered questions in medicine, a sound research project must be able to identify a focused question that can be addressed in a single study. An appropriate research objective is one that is interesting and relevant, as well as ethical and feasible. Whether a particular question is interesting to a wide medical audience is also relevant.

After an initial question of interest has been identified, it must be refined and specified. For example, an initial question might be: Should all pediatric patients be prescribed inhaled steroids after hospitalization for asthma? To effectively address such a question, both the outcomes of interest and the population of interest need to be specified. A more specific question might be: Do pediatric patients with asthma between the ages of 2 and 18 years who use inhaled steroids after hospitalization have lower readmission rates in the year following initial hospitalization? Or perhaps: How frequently do patients using inhaled steroids suffer side effects, and, on average, does the benefit of inhaled steroids outweigh the risk? Once this question has been formulated, the investigator can construct a testable hypothesis and the specific aims of the project. For example: The specific aim of this study is to determine whether the use of inhaled steroids after hospital discharge decreases readmission rates among pediatric patients aged 2 to 18 years with asthma in the year following initial hospitalization.

In a grant application, an introductory section that describes the overall project goals and then lays out specific aims in detail is crucial. In a proposal, the importance of carefully developing and stating specific aims cannot be overstated. A project that suffers from poorly developed aims may not be feasible, and such studies are unlikely to be funded by experienced grant reviewers.

BACKGROUND AND SIGNIFICANCE

Researching the background of a study is invariably part of developing the initial study questions and hypotheses. As part of a grant proposal, concisely summarizing the existing literature is important to provide the context in which an investigator has developed his or her research questions. This section typically cites prior studies that are relevant to the topic and their findings, any limitations of these studies, and how the current study will address outstanding issues or resolve concerns about past research. While thoroughly reviewing the background literature, one often further refines or modifies the specific aims of the project.

Applications for federal grants and grants from some other agencies also require a "Preliminary Results" subsection as part of the background for a proposal. This section describes the investigator's previous work that is relevant to the proposal at hand. If either the subject or the research method of a senior collaborator's (mentor's) prior research is relevant to one's proposal, that work should be cited here. Citation of this work on a grant application indicates that the requisite experience, skills, and guidance will be available to a junior investigator doing the groundwork for the proposed study.

STUDY DESIGN

There are two main types of study designs: observational and experimental. An observational study monitors events that occur among a study's subjects without any imposed intervention. Cohort studies, in which subjects are followed over time, and cross-sectional studies, in which observations about subjects are made at a single moment in time, are examples of observational studies. Case-control studies are observational studies that compare a group of subjects who possess the condition or disease of interest (cases) with a

group of subjects who do not (controls). Observational studies are also known as descriptive studies and can be used effectively to explore a topic for which there is limited prior research. An example of a question that lends itself to an observational or descriptive study is: Are hospitalized children with asthma being discharged consistently on inhaled steroids?

In contrast, experimental research designs typically apply an intervention to study subjects and describe the effects of the intervention. Randomized, double-blinded, controlled clinical trials are generally considered the gold standard in experimental study design, particularly for evaluating the effectiveness of therapeutic interventions such as medications; however, they are often the most difficult types of studies to design and conduct. As a general rule, observational studies are more feasible and usually precede the justification for conducting a randomized, controlled trial in an area of interest.

New investigators should recognize that studies can be conducted on data that have already been collected. This can be a faster and much less costly way to perform clinical research and, in poorly explored areas (including much of inpatient pediatric medicine), can be fruitful. Secondary data analysis uses previously collected data to answer questions other than those addressed by the initial data collection. Similarly, ancillary studies add newly measured variables to existing data to answer new research questions. Finally, systematic reviews rigorously and systematically summarize the results of multiple prior studies of a single research topic, with the goal of better estimating the effect of their collective findings.

SUBJECTS

Investigators need to determine who the target population will be and how they will be selected or recruited for a study. A primary consideration in selecting study subjects is maximizing the validity of the study so that conclusions drawn from the results can be applied to the real world. The investigator must decide whether to choose subjects who are easily accessible or those who most closely resemble the target population of interest. For example, if the research is targeted toward the general population, subjects selected from a single institution may be less representative than subjects selected from multiple institutions. Conversely, the advantages of conducting a study at a single institution are related to cost and the ease with which the study can be performed.

VARIABLES

No two research subjects are completely identical. Therefore, it is necessary to determine which characteristics or variables will be measured for each subject. Typically, demographic information on subjects is collected, along with other clinical variables relevant to the question being considered. Once variables have been measured, it is often prudent to look for possible associations between them to determine whether they interact to predict the outcome of interest. Variables are either independent (predictor variables) or dependent (outcome variables), based on their suspected relationships. For example, age and gender are independent variables. Respiratory failure and death would be considered dependent variables.

When an experimental study is conducted, its goal is typically to isolate the effect of a single independent variable (e.g., use or nonuse of a particular drug) on the measured outcome variable (e.g., length of hospital stay), while controlling for confounding variables (e.g., age, gender, severity of illness at admission) by either experimental design or statistical analytic techniques. In a randomized, controlled trial, randomization is used to minimize the influence of other independent variables during the interpretation of data (confounding). In cohort studies, statistical methods (e.g., linear or logistic regression modeling) can be used to minimize the effects of known confounders.

STATISTICS

The way data will be analyzed should be decided before conducting the study. This is important for several reasons. First, in devising the research question or objective, it is necessary to know how large a study population will be required to detect an effect. To prove whether a study's hypothesis is true, the investigator must be confident that the sample size—or number of subjects necessary to observe the expected effect or difference in outcome between study groups—is adequate. If so, then the study has the ability (power) to detect this difference between study groups.

Second, determining in advance how data will be classified and analyzed increases the researcher's confidence that an observed result is "true" rather than the result of chance. Performing multiple comparisons on data that were not considered in advance (sometimes referred to as "trolling" the data) can yield results attributable to chance rather than real associations.

Third, laying out a well-formulated statistical plan before conducting a study allows one to carefully consider whether any additional data need to be collected. Finally, a well-formulated statistical plan helps reviewers critically evaluate a proposal and can help convince them of its merit.

ETHICS

Any research involving human subjects requires investigators to respect the participants and make every effort to protect their interests. Specifically, this includes obtaining informed consent from study participants, designing a study that soundly weighs the risks to subjects against the likely benefits of the study, and distributing the benefits and burdens of the research fairly among the study population.

Federal regulations apply to all federally funded projects that involve research on human subjects to ensure that such studies are carried out in an ethical manner (see Chapters 18 and 21 for further details). All research on human subjects must be approved by an institutional review board (IRB). The IRB approves clinical research studies based on whether they meet certain ethical criteria, which include minimizing risks to subjects, ensuring that existing risks are justifiable in the context of the anticipated benefits of the study, selecting participants equitably, obtaining informed consent, and preserving confidentiality. An IRB has the power to exempt certain types of research from review, particularly when a study poses minimal risk to subjects or is limited to secondary analysis of existing data or medical charts only; when obtaining informed consent would make the study impossible to carry out; or, in some cases, when a study is being conducted as a secondary element of a project being carried out primarily for quality improvement purposes. Generally exempt from IRB approval are anonymous surveys, interviews, or studies conducted on existing medical records, data, or specimens using a coded collection method whereby patients' identities cannot be exposed. In contrast, most randomized clinical trials undergo extensive review, and there are criteria for stopping a study if one arm is determined to be significantly more effective or safer. The conditions under which individual IRBs grant exemptions, as well as the safeguards in place for higher-risk protocols, vary considerably, so it is best to check with a local IRB representative before proceeding with a proposed research or quality improvement study, no matter how safe it appears.

TIMELINE

It is helpful for investigators (and usually required by funding agencies) to have a general timeline to map out the expected schedule for the research. Depending on the method of data collection, time requirements differ for each type of study. In general, a timeline gives an estimate in months for study design and organization, data collection, analysis, and manuscript preparation.

CONCLUSION

There is a growing demand in pediatric medicine for research that provides a foundation for evidence-based approaches to care and clinical practice guidelines for common pediatric illnesses.[2] Hospitalists have an opportunity to work as physician-scientists; they have the necessary exposure to these illnesses to develop cogent, unanswered clinical questions that can affect large numbers of pediatric patients. With appropriate training, guidance, and an organized approach, hospitalists are well suited to study important questions in pediatric inpatient care and ultimately improve the quality of hospital care.

SUGGESTED READING

Browner WS: Publishing and Presenting Clinical Research. Baltimore, Lippincott Williams & Wilkins, 1999.

Hulley S, Cummings SR, Browner WS, et al: Designing Clinical Research: An Epidemiologic Approach, 2nd ed. Baltimore, Lippincott Williams & Wilkins, 2001.

REFERENCES

1. Landrigan CP, Stucky E, Chiang VW, Ottolini MC: Variation in inpatient management of common pediatric diseases: A study from the Pediatric Research in Inpatient Settings (PRIS) network. Pediatr Res 2004;55:1792.

2. Evidence-based medicine: A new approach to teaching the practice of medicine. Evidence-Based Medicine Working Group. JAMA 1992;268: 2420.

CHAPTER 21

Institutional Review Boards, Pharmaceutical Trials, and the Protection of Research Subjects

Rupali Gandhi

The Food and Drug Administration (FDA), as well as most federal and nonfederal research granting agencies, requires institutional review board (IRB) approval of all research involving human subjects. The principal purpose of IRBs is to protect the rights of human subjects. IRBs are formed at individual institutions and typically consist of committees of ethicists, clinicians, and nonclinical personnel that develop their own application and approval process to meet the needs of the particular institution, under the guidance of federal oversight bodies.

The Department of Health and Human Services (DHHS) and the FDA have polces designed to ensure the competent functioning of IRBs. The DHHS conducts site visits and audits of IRB records, as well as provides educational activities to assist IRB members in recognizing and considering the ethical issues raised by research involving human subjects. The FDA conducts site inspections and has extensive grounds for disqualifying an IRB if it is not in compliance with regulations.

IRBs are required to approve all research that involves human subjects conducted at their institutions. These may be clinical studies using therapies already in existence, studies involving new drugs, or, in some cases, studies of systemic or nonpharmacologic interventions.

DRUG APPROVAL PROCESS

When a pharmaceutical company wishes to study a new drug for use in humans, there are many steps involved in both the FDA and IRB approval process.[1] First the company must conduct preclinical (i.e., laboratory and animal) studies to determine whether a drug is sufficiently promising for humans. Once these studies are conducted, a drug can be submitted to the FDA as an "investigational new drug." The FDA then decides whether to permit initial research in humans. If approval is granted, the pharmaceutical company must conduct three phases of clinical studies; each phase is also subject to approval by the appropriate local IRBs because human subjects will be involved.

Phase I trials are conducted to assess the safety of an investigational new drug. These studies usually involve healthy subjects or, occasionally, members of a targeted patient population; this phase is designed to determine only the adverse effects of the drug. Phase II trials are conducted to assess the efficacy of the new drug. In these studies, the drug is given to members of the targeted patient population to determine whether it has the desired therapeutic effects. Finally, phase III studies are conducted; these usually involve double-blinded, randomized trials to assess whether the drug can provide a statistically significant benefit over existing therapies or placebos. After at least two adequate phase III studies have been completed, a new drug application can be submitted to the FDA.

When a researcher applies for IRB approval of a study that involves children as subjects, the process is the same, but the evaluation standards are different from those used for adults.

RESEARCH INVOLVING CHILDREN

Children are distinct from other human research subjects because they usually do not have the maturity and knowledge base to make informed decisions and are therefore legally "incompetent." They are also "incapacitated" in the sense that one would not expect a 5-year-old child to comprehend, process, engage in abstract reasoning, or synthesize information in the same way as a 35-year-old person. Children cannot be expected to make fully informed decisions regarding their own participation in clinical trials that may or may not be beneficial to them. To ensure that, to the extent possible, a child truly understands what participation in a research study entails, and to ensure that he or she is not being coerced or improperly informed, special precautions must be used.

Historical Violations of Children's Rights

A historical perspective is helpful to understand why the evaluation standards for children and adults differ. Child research subjects were not always so well protected. Unfortunately, there are countless examples of children being victimized in unethical clinical trials. In one such case from the late 1700s, researchers who were trying to find a smallpox vaccine injected young children, including orphans, with cowpox and then inoculated them with smallpox material to see whether the cowpox would offer protection. Although these vaccination trials posed an obvious danger to the children who were inoculated, it was argued that the possible benefit to children as a group outweighed the risk inflicted on the few children who were the initial subjects. Another infamous example comes from the Willowbrook State School for mentally disabled children, where researchers infected young children with hepatitis virus in order to study the natural course of the disease.[2]

National Commission and Ethical Principles

To ensure that research subjects were better protected, the federal government took a series of steps that ultimately led to the enactment of a law in the 1980s that governs the approval of clinical trials involving children. The Department of Health, Education, and Welfare (DHEW) published the first proposed regulations on the protection of human subjects in

Table 21–1   Federal Regulations for Research Involving Children

Federal Regulation Section	Risk Posed by the Intervention or Procedure	Additional Requirements for Protocol Approval*
45 CFR §46.404	No greater than minimal risk	None
45 CFR §46.405	Greater than minimal risk, with prospect of direct benefit to subject	Risk is justified by anticipated benefit to each subject Anticipated benefit to each subject is at least as favorable as that presented by available alternative approaches
45 CFR §46.406	Greater than minimal risk, with no prospect of direct benefit to subject	Risk represents a minor increase over minimal risk Intervention or procedure involves experiences that are reasonably commensurate with those in the child's actual or expected medical, dental, psychological, social, or educational situation The study is likely to yield generalizable knowledge about the child's disorder or condition that is vital for understanding or ameliorating that disorder or condition
45 CFR §46.407	Research not otherwise approvable	IRB finds that the research presents a reasonable opportunity to further the understanding, prevention, or alleviation of a serious problem affecting the health or welfare of children Approval of the secretary of DHHS after consultation with a panel of experts in pertinent fields, and after opportunity for public review and comment

*All require IRB approval, the child's assent, and permission by a parent or guardian. Under 45 CFR §46.408, the IRB is responsible for soliciting the assent of the child when, in its judgment, the child is capable of providing assent. In determining whether a child is capable of assenting, the IRB must consider the child's age, maturity, and psychological state. Permission from one parent or guardian is acceptable for research covered by 45 CFR §§46.404 and 46.405, but for research covered by §§46.406 and 46.407, both parents must give their permission unless one parent is deceased, unknown, incompetent, or not reasonably available, or unless only one parent has legal responsibility for the care and custody of the child.
CFR, Code of Federal Regulations; DHHS, Department of Health and Human Services; IRB, institutional review board.

1973. In 1974 Congress passed the National Research Act, which created the National Commission for the Protection of Human Subjects of Biomedical and Behavioral Research. The commission's purpose was to develop guidelines for ethical research involving human subjects and to make recommendations to the DHEW for the application of those guidelines.[3] It published a number of reports from 1975 to 1978 on topics such as IRBs, research on fetuses and embryos, and research involving children. During its brief existence, the commission made valuable contributions to the discussions of research ethics and suggested regulating guidelines.

The commission's Belmont Report described three ethical principles that should guide research involving human subjects: respect for persons, beneficence, and justice.[4] Respect for persons requires that individuals be treated as "autonomous agents" and that those with diminished autonomy be protected. Beneficence means that researchers should maximize possible benefits and minimize possible harm to subjects. Justice requires that subjects be chosen fairly and that safety measures be instituted to protect vulnerable populations involved in research. The commission's reports and suggestions were later adapted and added to the Code of Federal Regulations (CFR).

FEDERAL LAW

Research Involving Children

The commission's 1977 report made recommendations that allowed children to be used in research but also protected them from harm. Those recommendations served as the basis for CFR subpart D, which was designed to provide additional protection to children involved in research. Under the law, research involving children is divided into four categories, each of which has different requirements for approval (Table 21-1).

No Greater than Minimal Risk (§404)

The first category of research is that which involves interventions or procedures that pose no greater than minimal risk to research subjects, who may be either healthy children or those with an illness. For this research, the criteria for approval are essentially the same as those for all human subjects, including adults or nonvulnerable populations. The only additional requirements are that the child's assent be obtained (if possible) and that a parent's or guardian's permission be obtained for the child's participation in the study. (Under the law, assent means a child's affirmative agreement to participate in research; failure to object cannot be construed as assent.)

Because the idea of "minimal risk" is subject to multiple interpretations, the regulations attempt to clarify the definition by stating that minimal risk "means that the risks of harm anticipated in the proposed research are not greater, considering probability and magnitude, than those ordinarily encountered in daily life or during the performance of routine physical or psychological examination or tests" (45 CFR §46.102[g]). The idea behind the minimal risk threshold is that it is a socially permissible level of risk to which parents would normally permit their children to be exposed in nonresearch settings. The commission provided some examples of interventions that fall under this category: routine immunizations, modest changes in diet or schedule, physical examination, obtaining blood and urine specimens, and developmental assessments.[3] It is important to remember that for protocols in this category, it does not make any difference whether the intervention has the potential to benefit the subject or whether the child is healthy. As long as the risk posed by the intervention is no more than minimal, there are no additional requirements for review and acceptability.

The National Human Research Protections Advisory Committee (NHRPAC) Children's Workgroup was formed in 2000 and charged with providing advice and recommendations to the Office for Human Research Protections (OHRP). The committee issued a report to clarify the definitions of "minimal risk" and "minor increase over minimal risk" and specifically denied that minimal risk should be a variable standard based on a particular child's circumstance; instead, it defined minimal risk as the level of risk associated with the daily activities of a "normal, healthy, average child."[5] Further, the report states that "indexing the definition of minimal risk to the socially allowable risks to which normal, average children are exposed routinely should take into account the differing risks experienced by children of different ages."

Interventions with a Potential Direct Benefit to the Subject (§405)

The second category includes procedures or interventions that have the potential to benefit the individual subject directly. In these cases, the minimal risk evaluation is not applicable because such studies generally involve children who are *not* average, healthy children in a stable environment, although in unusual circumstances, healthy children may be involved. (For example, the siblings of ill children were allowed to participate in a protocol that involved more than minimal-risk procedures because the healthy siblings were viewed as gaining a direct psychological benefit—that is, the possibility of keeping their ill siblings alive.[6]) When there is the prospect of direct benefit to the individual subject, the research protocol must also show that the risk is justified by the anticipated benefit and that the anticipated benefit is at least as favorable as that presented by available alternatives.

An example of a research protocol that falls into this category is a phase III study of a new chemotherapeutic agent for leukemia. The new drug may pose a significant risk to the subjects, but as long as the anticipated benefits are also high, and as long as the expected benefits are at least as good as the available alternatives, the trial would be approved.

Interventions with No Prospect of Direct Benefit to the Subject (§406)

The third category involves interventions or procedures that provide no direct benefit to the subject. For these types of studies, the intervention must present only a minor increase over minimal risk to the subject, and the study must be likely to yield knowledge that is vital to the understanding or amelioration of the disorder or condition under study. Further, the intervention or procedure must involve experiences that are reasonably commensurate with those inherent to the subject's actual or expected medical, dental, psychological, social, or educational situation. The commensurability requirement exists because children who have had a particular intervention previously are better able to understand what is being asked of them, and their assent to participate in the study will be better informed.[2] There are ongoing questions and disagreements about what constitutes a "minor increase" above minimal risk and what is meant by "disorder or condition" and "reasonably commensurate."

An example of a protocol in this category is one that subjects children with leukemia to an additional bone marrow aspirate to obtain information about the pathogenesis of the disease. It is probable that a child with leukemia has already had a bone marrow aspirate and that another aspirate would be reasonably commensurate with his or her actual experience; thus, this child's assent would be more informed than that of a child who has never experienced a bone marrow aspirate. Further, it is imaginable that such a research study could yield generalizable knowledge about leukemia that is vital to its amelioration, thus fulfilling the requirements of §406. In this hypothetical case, one additional bone marrow aspirate is viewed as only a minor increase over minimal risk, but what if the protocol called for two? Three? Ten? When is the threshold exceeded? Some might argue that it is impossible to set a threshold—that an instinctual "gut feeling" tells reviewers when the limit has been exceeded. However, the "I know it when I see it" standard used by the Supreme Court to recognize pornography may be inappropriate when errors in judgment could expose children to real danger.[7] IRBs would be hard pressed to find a public willing to accept such a subjective interpretation of §406.

The NHRPAC Children's Workgroup report provided some insight when it concluded that "minimal risk" should be an absolute standard but that "minor increase over minimal risk" is a relative standard. The committee acknowledged that the concept of commensurability is crucial to give children and parents a point of reference for making a decision about participation. The report includes lists of specific interventions and how those interventions should be classified (Tables 21-2 and 21-3). Nevertheless, these classifications are not universally accepted, and local IRBs may differ when determining whether a particular research protocol is acceptable. For example, Yale's IRB has approved bone marrow aspirations in children with leukemia, single additional spinal taps in adolescents who have already had at least one for a neurologic disorder, and administration of yohimbine to gain information about the pathogenesis of a neurologic disorder. It rejected a proposal to do left heart catheterization on children at risk for the development of cardiac hemosiderosis.[2]

The §406 requirements have several problems. First, it is very difficult, if not impossible, to generate any control data from healthy children for these types of studies. In the earlier example involving children with leukemia, it would not be permissible to subject a healthy child to a bone marrow aspirate because such a procedure is not reasonably commensurate with the child's actual or expected situation. Second, §406 presupposes a clear distinction between a child with a disease and a child who is healthy; in reality, this is not always so well demarcated.

Table 21-2   Common Procedures and Category of Risk

Procedure*	Minimal Risk	Minor Increase over Minimal Risk	More than Minor Increase over Minimal Risk
Routine history taking	X		
Venipuncture, finger stick, heel stick	X		
Urine collection via bag	X		
Urine collection via catheter		X	
Urine collection via suprapubic tap			X
Chest radiograph	X		
Bone density test	X		
Wrist radiograph for bone age	X		
Lumbar puncture		X	
Collection of saliva	X		
Collection of small sample of hair	X		
Vision testing	X		
Hearing testing	X		
Complete neurologic examination	X		
Oral glucose tolerance test	X		
Skin punch biopsy with topical pain relief		X	
Bone marrow aspirate with topical pain relief		X	
Organ biopsy			X
Standard psychological tests	X		
Classroom observation	X		

*The category of risk is for a single procedure. Multiple or repetitive procedures are likely to affect the level of risk.
From Clarifying Specific Portion of 45 CFR 46 Subpart D that Governs Children's Research. National Human Research Protections Advisory Committee, Children's Workgroup Report. Available at *http://ohrp.osophs.dhhs.gov/nhrpac/documents/nhrpac16.pdf*.

Table 21-3   Interpreting Level of Risk in Common Procedures

Procedure	Determinants of Level of Risk
Indwelling heparin lock catheter	Level of risk may range from minimal to more than a minor increase over minimal, depending on child's age, length of time catheter will be in place, number and volume of samples, and setting of the research
Single subcutaneous or intramuscular injection	Level of risk may range from minimal to more than a minor increase over minimal, depending on the substance injected
Nasogastric tube insertion	Generally minor increase over minimal risk
Small amount of additional tissue obtained at surgery	Generally minor increase over minimal risk, but must take into account any increased operative time, the specific organ or tissue, and likelihood of bleeding and infection
Magnetic resonance imaging	If no sedation, generally minimal risk If procedural sedation, generally minor increase over minimal risk Intubation in the appropriate setting may decrease potential risks for certain children, and its use should be considered on a case-by-case and proposal-by-proposal basis
Psychological test, survey, interview, observation	Generally minimal risk if performed under standardized conditions; level of risk may increase, depending on sensitive nature of questions, possibility of triggering unpleasant memories or emotions, and length of the instrument or observation

From Clarifying Specific Portion of 45 CFR 46 Subpart D that Governs Children's Research. National Human Research Protections Advisory Committee, Children's Workgroup Report. Available at *http://ohrp.osophs.dhhs.gov/nhrpac/documents/nhrpac16.pdf*.

Research Not Otherwise Approvable (§407)

The last category outlined in subpart D involves research that would not be approvable under any of the aforementioned categories. In such cases, if the IRB finds that the research presents a "reasonable opportunity to further understanding, prevention, or alleviation of a serious problem affecting the health or welfare of children," the secretary of the DHHS may consult with a panel of experts, provide an opportunity for public review and comment, and then possibly approve the research. The secretary can deem the protocol acceptable by finding that the research actually does satisfy the conditions of §404, 405, or 406 or by finding that the research (1) presents a reasonable opportunity to further the understanding, prevention, or alleviation of a serious problem affecting the health or welfare of children; (2) will be conducted in accordance with sound ethical principles; and (3) makes adequate provisions for soliciting the assent of children and the permission of their parents or guardians. Although this category has been used infrequently to permit research with children, the OHRP lists nine protocols that were reviewed under §407.[8]

TRANSLATING FEDERAL LAW INTO LOCAL PRACTICE

The definitional ambiguities noted earlier leave considerable power in the hands of IRBs. It is incumbent upon each IRB to carefully review research protocols and determine how to protect pediatric research subjects, with an eye toward their vulnerability and the risks they will be exposed to.

When proposing a research project, hospitalists should be aware of both their own responsibilities to research subjects and the responsibilities of IRBs, and every effort should be made to protect the welfare of children who participate in such studies. When planning any study, whether it involves a prospective test of a new therapeutic agent, a proven agent, a system-level health care intervention, or even a retrospective review of medical records, hospitalist researchers should consult their IRBs. Projects that involve only the retrospective review of medical records or the observation of systemic changes receive expedited review at many centers or may be exempt from review altogether. Researchers would be well advised to discuss all projects with the IRB while they are still in the planning stages, and whenever questions arise about the safety or ethics of a proposed study, consultation with the IRB should be undertaken expeditiously.

CONCLUSION

Children are a vulnerable population and deserve protection from the potential risks posed by research. The federal government has codified many of these protections into law, but because a lot of the language is vague and terms are defined imprecisely, much of the responsibility for their interpretation and application falls to individual IRBs. Even the relatively well-defined term *minimal risk* lends itself to multiple interpretations. Although consensus on the meaning of some of these words is reached eventually, this is not true of all. Hospitalist researchers studying children should carefully consider the risks and benefits of any proposed research protocol and discuss these issues with their IRBs, even if the risk appears to be minimal.

REFERENCES

1. Hutt PB, Merrill RA (eds): Food and Drug Law, Cases and Material, 2nd ed. Westbury, NY, Foundation Press, 1991, pp 513-525.
2. Levine RJ: Ethics and Regulation of Clinical Research, 2nd ed. New Haven, Conn, Yale University Press, 1988.
3. National Commission for the Protection of Human Subjects of Biomedical and Behavioral Research: Research Involving Children: Report and Recommendations. DHEW Publication No. (OS) 77-0004. Washington, DC, 1977.
4. National Commission for the Protection of Human Subjects of Biomedical and Behavioral Research: The Belmont Report: Ethical Principles and Guidelines for the Protection of Human Subjects of Research. DHEW Publication No. (OS) 78-0012, Washington, DC, 1978. Available at *http://www.hhs.gov/ohrp//humansubjects/guidance/belmont.htm*.
5. Clarifying Specific Portion of 45 CFR 46 Subpart D that Governs Children's Research. National Human Research Protections Advisory Committee, Children's Workgroup Report. Available at *http://www.hhs.gov/ohrp/nhrpac/mtg04-01/child-workgroup4-5-01.pdf*.
6. Gordon B, Prentice E, Reitemeier P: The use of normal children as participants in research on therapy. IRB 1996;May-June1;18(3):5-8.
7. Jacobellis v Ohio, 378 US 184, 197 (1964) (6-3 decision).
8. Office for Human Research Protections website: *http://www.hhs.gov/ohrp/*.

Hospitalists' Work: Present and Future

CHAPTER 22

Medical Education

David Rubin and Mary C. Ottolini

The hospitalist movement in internal medicine emerged during the mid-1990s, motivated in large part by issues of cost containment, length of stay, and quality of care. In 1998 Wachter and colleagues' landmark article documented the success of the general medicine hospitalist service in containing costs and decreasing length of stay compared with traditional models of providing inpatient care.[1] The first pediatric hospitalist studies followed a few years later, with evidence of similar success.[2-5] As hospitalists have become more common at pediatric institutions throughout the country, particularly at academic centers, the focus has begun to shift beyond efficient care and patient outcomes to considerations of hospitalists' impact on medical education.[6] Pediatric hospitalists influence medical education at all levels: medical students, who were traditionally trained on teams supervised by academic general pediatricians; pediatric residents; and residency graduates turning to hospital-based general pediatrics as a career.

RESIDENT EDUCATION

Hospitalists in Traditional Attending Roles

Because hospitalists develop expertise in inpatient pediatrics, it has been suggested that they might be able to provide a higher-quality education for residents and medical students. Some limited data have been gathered with regard to this possibility. In 2002, Landrigan and colleagues surveyed the opinions of interns and senior residents on the contribution of pediatric hospitalists to their training, and compared house officers' ratings of their experience and their ratings of attending physicians' teaching skills, in a hospitalist and a traditional system.[7] The authors found that interns generally had a more favorable experience with hospitalists in an attending role, rating them higher than traditional academic general pediatricians as teachers and role models; they also rated their overall educational experience, supervision, and quality of life on the wards higher in the hospitalist system. Senior residents' opinions varied, however. Immediately after the introduction of pediatric hospitalists, senior residents raised concerns about loss of autonomy, increased stress levels, and less availability of bedside teaching, although this concern dissipated over time.

The authors speculated that much of the early negative response by senior residents was attributable to the adjustment to a new system, and that once the system had become common, their concerns lessened.

Other emerging literature examining the introduction of hospitalists at academic teaching centers and community hospitals has similarly found that education in hospitalist systems is rated highly. These studies, though often small and uncontrolled, support the perception that hospitalist attending physicians offer greater advantages to resident education compared with traditional teaching attending physicians. Several studies have shown that residents evaluate the teaching in pediatric hospitalist systems favorably.[8-10] Further, hospitalists are perceived as high-quality teachers of inpatient medicine by their colleagues; a recent survey of physicians with medical staff privileges at a tertiary care pediatric teaching hospital found that 58% of community physicians and 78% of faculty physicians agreed with the statement that hospitalists may be more effective teachers for house staff and medical students.[3]

Although the net results of these studies support the role of hospitalists as educators, concerns remain. Hospitalists tend to be younger and more recently out of training, and some investigators have raised concerns that their emergence in academic centers may pose a threat to resident autonomy.[11] This concern may be greatest for senior pediatric residents, whose supervisory role on a general pediatrics service marks a key point in their training, allowing them to direct patient care and manage the junior residents on their team.

Because limited data exist on the educational impact of pediatric hospitalists on residents, their role should continue to be studied. Such studies are likely to take place on a rapidly changing landscape. As different programs embrace hospitalist teams in their networks, these teams are likely to vary in their composition and their teaching responsibilities. The optimal balance of hospitalists and residents on an inpatient team to promote resident education and high-quality patient care may vary, depending on financial considerations, patient complexity, and rounding style, among other things. The ability to generalize about hospitalists' impact on resident education will be limited by the heterogeneity of these teams as the field evolves.

Effect of Hospitalists in Nonteaching Services

A key limitation of the current literature on hospitalists' impact on medical education is that all prior studies examined traditional medical teams in which the academic teaching attending role was assumed by the hospitalist. However, with the recent emergence of Accreditation Council for Graduate Medical Education (ACGME) work-hour restrictions for residents, teaching hospitals have been forced to consider alternative models of care to relieve residents of coverage that exceeds these restrictions. The result has been an increase in non–resident-covered hospitalist teams, staffed with or without physician extenders, that operate independently from traditional resident services and may have no responsibility for education.[12] These nonresident teams bring their own set of concerns (Table 22-1).

Perhaps the most important concern about independently operating hospitalist teams is that they may siphon patients with core pediatric problems (e.g., asthma) or unusual problems away from resident teams. For example, although there is emerging evidence that hospitalists functioning in pediatric intensive care units without residents resulted in improved quality of care compared with resident-covered services, these teams threatened the proportion of such patients likely to be covered by residents.[13] Similar improvements in length of stay and quality of care have been observed in general inpatients units, but the same concerns remain.[14] For less complex or less severely ill patients, physician extender teams supervised by hospitalists may be able to care for patients with diagnoses such as asthma in a manner that reduces length of stay.[15] Questions arise, however, whether such a division of responsibility may limit resident exposure to the most common conditions in pediatric patients. Conversely, in some settings it may be difficult to recruit hospitalists to care for "pathway" patients with standard evaluation and management issues; such teams may increasingly admit patients with diagnostic and management uncertainties, but this may siphon some of the most unusual patients, with their attendant learning opportunities, away from resident teams.

What is certain is that pediatric hospitalist teams will continue to grow as teaching hospitals look for ways to cut costs, provide higher-quality care, and meet resident work-hour restrictions. Studying the impact of ACGME requirements on hospitalist-resident interaction and educational outcomes will be a critical area for future research. Integrating senior residents into non–resident-covered teams as supervised "attending" physicians can provide a real-world experience for residents considering a career in hospitalist pediatrics.[6] It will also give them an opportunity to integrate the information learned earlier in residency to develop autonomy in their senior year.

MEDICAL STUDENT EDUCATION

The impact of pediatric hospitalists on medical student education, although less studied, may be different from its impact on residents. In particular, there are fewer concerns about autonomy. The data show that with a traditional resident team structure, hospitalists are more likely to be identified as role models and spend time contributing to student education than are traditional teaching attending physicians.[16-19] They are also more likely to practice evidence-based medicine, as recommended by the Institute of Medicine for improving overall quality of care.[20] Bedside teaching as part of the daily structure has been raised as a concern, however, and deserves further study.

For medical students, the benefit of working with hospitalists may be independent of team structure (see Table 22-1). Although cost containment and resident work-hour restrictions may dictate the need for independent hospitalist teams, that arrangement offers unique advantages to medical student education. Nonresident hospitalist teams may be ideal placements for medical students during their core pediatric clerkships. These teams can provide students with direct access to attending physicians, bypassing the junior and senior residents who often act as go-betweens on traditional medical services. For the student, the result is an opportunity for more direct learning and apprenticeship; for

Table 22-1	Pediatric Hospitalist Models and Their Impact on Resident and Student Education	
	Traditional Teaching Service with Hospitalist Attending Physicians	Nonresident Hospitalist Team
Hospitalist	Key responsibility for educating house staff and residents	Limited opportunities for educating house staff unless pursued independently
Senior resident	Increased access to and availability of attending supervision Potential concern for resident autonomy	Potentially increased responsibility and autonomy, with less access to attending supervision Detriment may be decreased experience with general pediatric patients admitted to nonresident service
Junior resident	Improved educational experience Better emphasis on cost containment and evidence-based medicine	Diminished access to attending supervision Detriment may be decreased experience with general pediatric patients admitted to nonresident service
Medical student	Greater access to attending supervision and feedback Greater emphasis on cost containment and evidence-based practice	Opportunity for a more personalized learning experience with direct attending supervision if medical students work on a nonresident service

the pediatric hospitalist, it offers an opportunity to pursue a teaching mission even if one's team is isolated from the pediatric residency program.

CAREER DEVELOPMENT

With an increasing number of pediatric residents choosing careers in hospital pediatrics, there will inevitably be a renewed focus on residency training and the responsibility of preparing trainees for such careers. This focus is already emerging among medicine residency programs. In a survey of medical hospitalists attempting to identify key deficiencies that were not addressed during residency training, deficient areas included hospice and end-of life care, procedures, and experience with sedation techniques.[21]

Beyond the need to cover additional topics in a categorical medical residency program, the debate about career development has centered on whether residency programs should provide a separate residency track for trainees intending to pursue careers in hospital-based medicine. A survey of academic pediatric chairs in the United States and Canada in 2001 found that only one third of respondents saw the need for additional postresidency training for those intending to pursue hospitalist careers.[22] More recently, the Pediatric Research in Inpatient Settings (PRIS) network survey found that the vast majority of pediatric hospitalists believed that further training was needed.[23] Desired training included administrative, clinical, research, and teaching skills not obtained during residency. Fellowship was cited as the most popular means of providing such training, but a substantive minority suggested further training within residency, as an addition to the general curriculum or as a hospital medicine track. Regardless of one's opinion about the need for more hospitalist-directed residency curricula, the PRIS survey clearly illustrates that as more trainees pursue hospitalist careers, key deficiencies in pediatrics training programs are likely to receive even greater attention. In addition, the primary care community already questions whether pediatric training programs have become too hospital focused at the expense of primary care training.

In all likelihood, concerns about balancing diverse training needs will prevent a further subspecialization of most pediatric training programs, but program deficiencies must be carefully studied and addressed. Whether such deficiencies will be addressed through elective rotations (e.g., palliative care or anesthesia) or through the implementation of new required rotations across the curriculum will be up to the individual programs. Further, as hospitalists take on additional roles that differentiate them from other general pediatricians (e.g., sedation, working in intensivist settings), and as the number of hospitalists increases, the issues of board certification and fellowship training are likely to arise. Hospitalist pediatrics may follow the course pursued by pediatric emergency medicine, which split from general pediatrics and received specialty certification in 1992.

RESEARCH

As the pediatric hospitalist role continues to evolve, so does the research mission for this field. Hospitalist research is still in its infancy, with the bulk of articles focusing on the quality of care provided by hospitalist teams. The hospitalist movement in pediatrics was born out of clinical and economic need, so it is not surprising that a research mission has followed more slowly. For those aspiring to academic careers in hospitalist pediatrics, the research opportunities are many, allowing young trainees to emerge as leaders in the field quite quickly. Areas for research include a continued focus on measures of quality and cost-effectiveness (traditional health services research), as well as disease-specific inquiries (clinical epidemiology), improvements in diagnostic accuracy, and clinical trials to identify better treatment strategies.

The evolution of research will inevitably rely on the emergence of fellowship programs that allow candidates for hospitalist careers to pursue masters-level coursework in research. Initially, general pediatric fellowship programs will provide the framework for early trainees to pursue academic careers, but eventually, pediatric hospitalist programs will need to create their own fellowship training programs to compete for federal funding to support research training. A handful of pediatric hospitalist fellowships have already appeared around the country, and more are likely to develop over the next decade.

CONCLUSION

Pediatric hospitalist medicine, which arose out of a need for cost containment and improved quality of care, is only beginning to confront its educational challenges. At all levels—from the medical student to the pediatric resident to the aspiring hospitalist—the emergence of the hospitalist model of care has begun to affect medical education. Residents are likely to see curriculum changes, with a greater focus on the needs of hospitalized patients, and a spirited debate on promoting independent decision making in a system that is becoming increasingly centered on the decisions of hospitalist attending physicians. For the aspiring hospitalist, the growth of this field has provided numerous opportunities in both community and teaching hospitals, but as the field becomes saturated, access to teaching hospitals may become limited to those seeking more formal academic training. Such a shift in the workforce at pediatric teaching hospitals will likely create the need for fellowship training programs specific to hospital-based pediatrics. Whether this will lead to the identification of hospital-based pediatrics as its own boarded specialty remains to be seen.

REFERENCES

1. Wachter R, Katz P, Showstack J, et al: Reorganizing an academic medical service: Impact on cost, quality, patient satisfaction, and education. JAMA 1998;279:1560-1565.
2. Landrigan CP, Srivastava R, Muret-Wagstaff S, et al: Impact of a health maintenance organization hospitalist system in academic pediatrics. Pediatrics 2002;110:720-728.
3. Srivastava R, Norlin C, James BC, et al: Community and hospital-based physicians' attitudes regarding pediatric hospitalist systems. Pediatrics 2005;115:34-38.
4. Wachter R, Goldman L: The hospitalist movement 5 years later. JAMA 2002;287:487-494.
5. Bellet P, Whitaker R: Evaluation of a pediatric hospitalist service: Impact on length of stay and hospital charges. Pediatrics 2000;105:478-484.

6. Kulaga M, Charney P, O'Mahony S, et al: The positive impact of initiation of hospitalist clinician educators. J Gen Intern Med 2004;19:293-301.

7. Landrigan C, Muret-Wagstaff S, Chiang V, et al: Effect of a pediatric hospitalist system on housestaff education and experience. Arch Pediatr Adolesc Med 2002;156:877-883.

8. Ponitz K, Mortimer J, Berman B: Establishing a pediatric hospitalist program at an academic medical center. Clin Pediatr 2000;39:221-227.

9. Ogershok P, Li X, Palmer H, et al: Restructuring an academic pediatric inpatient service using concepts developed by hospitalists. Clin Pediatr 2001;40:653-660.

10. Wilson S: Employing hospitalists to improve residents' inpatient learning. Acad Med 2001;76:556.

11. Kemper A, Freed G: Hospitalists and residency medical education: Measured improvement. Arch Pediatr Adolesc Med 2002;156:858-859.

12. Saint S, Flanders SA: Hospitalists in teaching hospitals: Opportunities but not without danger. J Gen Intern Med 2004;19:392-393.

13. Tenner PA, Dibrell H, Taylor RP: Improved survival with hospitalists in a pediatric intensive care unit. Crit Care Med 2003;31:847-852.

14. Dwight P, MacArthur C, Friedman J, Parkin P: Evaluation of a staff-only hospitalist system in a tertiary care, academic children's hospital. Pediatrics 2004;114:1545-1549.

15. Kessler R, Berlin A: Physician assistants as inpatient caregivers: A new role for mid-level practitioners. Cost Qual 1999;5:32-33.

16. Hauer K, Wachter R: Implications of the hospitalist model for medical students' education. Acad Med 2001;76:324-330.

17. Hauer KE, Wachter RM, McCulloch CE, et al: Effects of hospitalist attending physicians on trainee satisfaction with teaching and with internal medicine rotations. Arch Intern Med 2004;164:1866-1871.

18. Kripalani S, Pope A, Rask K, et al: Hospitalists as teachers. J Gen Intern Med 2004;19:8-15.

19. Hunter A, Desai S, Harrison R, Chan B: Medical student evaluation of the quality of hospitalist and nonhospitalist teaching faculty on inpatient medicine rotations. Acad Med 2004;79:78-82.

20. Institute of Medicine: Crossing the Quality Chasm: A New Health System for the 21st Century. Washington, DC, National Academy Press, 2001.

21. Plauth WH 3rd, Pantilat SZ, Wachter RM, Fenton CL: Hospitalists' perceptions of their residency training needs: Results of a national survey. Am J Med 2001;111:247-254.

22. Srivastava R, Landrigan C, Gidwani P, et al: Pediatric hospitalists in Canada and the United States: A survey of pediatric academic department chairs. Ambul Pediatr 2001;1:338-339.

23. Ottolini M, Landrigan C, Chiang V, Stucky E: PRIS survey: Pediatric hospitalist roles and training needs. Pediatr Res 2004;55:360A.

CHAPTER 23

Pediatric Hospital Medicine Organizations

Jack M. Percelay, Daniel A. Rauch, and David Zipes

Pediatric hospital medicine has benefited from the strong collaborative leadership of three organizations: the American Academy of Pediatrics (AAP), the Ambulatory Pediatric Association (APA), and the Society of Hospital Medicine (SHM) (Table 23-1). The AAP is the umbrella organization for all pediatricians and focuses on the clinical care of children. The APA is the professional organization for academic general pediatricians and focuses on education and research. The SHM focuses on the practice of hospital medicine, with an emphasis on systems of care applicable to both adult and pediatric hospitalists. Together, these organizations contribute synergistically to the care of hospitalized children and the growth of pediatric hospital medicine. This chapter briefly outlines the history and activity of pediatric hospitalists in each organization and highlights their shared accomplishments.

AMERICAN ACADEMY OF PEDIATRICS

The AAP was founded in 1930. Its mission is to "attain optimal physical, mental and social health and well-being for all infants, children, adolescents and young adults."[1] Current membership is approximately 60,000, and many members also serve on AAP committees or sections. Committees consist of 6 to 15 members and are appointed by the board to formulate AAP policy in discrete areas. The Committee on Hospital Care is the one most closely linked to the concerns of hospitalists. Sections are larger groups with open membership based on a shared discipline or interest (e.g., gastroenterology, community pediatrics, practice management, residents). The primary responsibility of sections is to offer educational programs in their particular fields to both section members and at-large AAP members. Additionally, sections routinely review and may author policy statements and technical reports.

The AAP's Section on Hospital Medicine (SOHM) represents pediatric hospitalists. Membership is open to any AAP member with an interest in general inpatient pediatrics and includes primary care pediatricians, intensivists, and emergency medicine physicians, as well as hospitalists. In 1999 the AAP formed the Provisional Section on Hospital Care, with 80 charter members, as the sister section to the Committee on Hospital Care. At that time, the term *hospitalist* was new, and there were fears that hospitalists would "steal" patients, prevent primary care pediatricians from treating inpatients, disrupt continuity of care, and potentially detract from the overall practice of pediatrics. The section's initial efforts concentrated on allaying these fears, highlighting the benefits of hospitalists, promoting best practices, emphasizing close communication with referring physicians, and sponsoring educational programs for both section members and AAP members at large.

Beginning in the early 2000s, the climate within the AAP began to change. Adult hospital medicine programs were growing rapidly at this time, and practicing pediatricians began to see the benefits that their internist colleagues were reaping from adult hospitalist systems; many began to seek the same benefits for their patients and practices. Pediatric hospitalists began advocating for overall improvements in the general pediatric ward and the hospital as a whole. Adult and pediatric peer-reviewed literature demonstrated the effectiveness of hospitalist systems and a high rate of satisfaction with them. Gradually, naysayers became advocates. Quality concerns combined with economic pressures and limited resident availability to further drive program growth.

In 2002, the AAP Provisional Section on Hospital Care achieved full section status, including full-day section programs, rapid membership growth, and active collaboration with the Committee on Hospital Care. In 2004 the section changed its name to the Section on Hospital Medicine to recognize that emerging discipline. By 2006 section membership exceeded 670. Today, the section is clearly the center for hospitalist activity within the AAP, and it regularly reviews and comments on statements and policies relevant to hospitalists and the practice of pediatric hospital medicine.

Concurrent with its rapid membership growth, the SOHM has been active in both research and policy development. In 2002 the section cosponsored a national survey that indicated that approximately 40% of primary care pediatricians in office practice had access to pediatric hospitalists. These pediatricians referred approximately 45% of their general pediatric ward patients to hospitalists. Both patients and referring pediatricians expressed high levels of satisfaction with the care provided by hospitalists.[2] In 2005 the section was the primary author of the AAP policy statement "Guiding Principles for Pediatric Hospitalist Programs," which recommends that referrals to pediatric hospitalist programs be voluntary, programs be designed to meet unique local needs, hospitalists be board certified in pediatrics or have equivalent qualifications, provision for appropriate outpatient follow-up be included in program design, communication be complete and timely among hospitalists and other physicians caring for a child, and outcome measurements be included as part of hospitalist programs.[3]

In keeping with its traditional educational role, the section holds a full-day program at the AAP's annual national conference and exhibition targeted specifically toward hospitalists; it sponsors general educational programs as well. The SOHM produces a semiannual newsletter and hosts the pediatric hospital medicine Listserv. The SOHM webpage archives newsletters, provides links to relevant policies and resources, and maintains an electronic library of volunteer submissions of relevant materials

Table 23-1 Pediatric Hospital Medicine Organizations

Name	Organizational Focus	Website
American Academy of Pediatrics (AAP)	Umbrella organization for all pediatricians Clinical aspects of pediatric hospital medicine Advocacy for children	*www.aap.org*
Ambulatory Pediatric Association (APA)	Academic home for general pediatricians Research and teaching	*www.ambpeds.org*
Society of Hospital Medicine (SHM)	Organizational and systems aspects of hospital medicine practice (adult and pediatric) Advocacy for hospitalists	*www.hospitalmedicine.org*

such as order sets, pathways, coding resources, lectures, and policies.

The section is actively involved in the AAP's evaluation of inpatient management codes and, together with the Committee on Hospital Care, has supported efforts to develop a national database on pediatric hospitalization trends. Within the AAP's educational program AAP Grand Rounds, there is dedicated space for hospital medicine alongside disciplines such as cardiology and infectious disease.

A top priority for the SOHM is to become more involved with the AAP's advocacy efforts for children in general and to ensure that all children have access to high-quality inpatient medical care. The section is also developing subcommittees to focus on specific hospital medicine topics such as palliative care, billing and coding, information technology, community hospitalists, and critical care hospitalists. Chapter liaisons have been established to strengthen interactions with local AAP chapters. Additional projects include developing expanded inpatient coding resources and a hospital medicine performance improvement module that would meet the practice performance requirements of the American Board of Pediatrics for maintenance of certification.

AMBULATORY PEDIATRIC ASSOCIATION

The APA was founded in 1961. According to its mission statement, "the APA fosters the health of children, adolescents and families by promoting generalism in academic pediatrics and academics in general pediatrics."[4] This is accomplished through patient care, teaching, research, and advocacy. Despite its name, the APA is committed to being the academic home for pediatric generalists working in both inpatient and outpatient settings. In fact, the APA mission statement specifically identifies hospital medicine as an academic division that shares a generalist focus. The APA has more than 2000 members. Geographically, the APA is divided into 10 regions, and it has a wide range of standing committees and special-interest groups (SIGs). The APA's SIGs function like AAP sections, with membership open to all members who share the same interest.

In 2001 the APA Hospitalist/Inpatient Medicine SIG was formed, and in 2004 the name was changed to the Hospital Medicine SIG. It emphasizes teaching and research in the inpatient setting and serves as the academic home for pediatric hospitalists. The SIG participates in the annual meeting of the Pediatric Academic Societies, a spring event sponsored by the APA, the American Pediatric Society, the Society for Pediatric Research, and, most recently, the AAP. The meeting includes a hospital medicine plenary session where scientific abstracts are presented. In addition to providing a forum for sharing advances in hospital medicine, these platform and poster sessions have helped advance the field of pediatric hospital medicine as an academic endeavor.

The Hospital Medicine SIG was the driving force behind the APA-sponsored conference "Pediatric Hospitalists in Academic Settings" in San Antonio, Texas, in November 2003. This was the first national meeting specifically focused on the development of pediatric hospital medicine as a field. It helped develop a roadmap for the growth of pediatric hospital medicine as an academic discipline and established a framework for future conferences.[5] In July 2005 the APA served as the primary sponsor of the pediatric hospital medicine meeting in Denver, Colorado, with the AAP and SHM serving as cosponsors.

Other APA SIGs and resources have provided valuable assistance to physicians practicing in the inpatient arena (even before the advent of the term *hospitalist*) and continue to be useful today. These include guidelines for inpatient rotations for pediatric and family practice house staff and guidelines for pediatric clerkships for medical students. The teaching tools, academic career development materials, and research mentoring available through the APA are important resources designed for general academic pediatricians but are of immense value to pediatric hospitalists as well. In addition to its other functions, the APA has served as the reviewing organization for selected pediatric hospital medicine fellowship programs. The APA journal *Ambulatory Pediatrics* welcomes submissions on pediatric hospital medicine topics.

SOCIETY OF HOSPITAL MEDICINE

The SHM was founded in 1997 as the National Association of Inpatient Physicians shortly after Wachter and Goldman coined the term *hospitalist*. The name was changed to the Society of Hospital Medicine in 2003 to recognize hospital medicine as a distinct field. The SHM defines hospitalists as "physicians whose primary professional focus is the general medical care of hospitalized patients."[6]

According to its mission statement, the SHM "is dedicated to promoting the highest quality care for all hospitalized patients. SHM is committed to promoting excellence in the practice of Hospital Medicine through education, advocacy and research."[7] The SHM has outlined six major goals to fulfill this mission: "(1) to promote high quality care for all hospitalized patients, (2) to promote education and research in Hospital Medicine, (3) to promote teamwork to achieve the best possible care for hospitalized patients, (4) to advocate a career path which will attract and retain the highest quality hospitalists, (5) to define the competencies, activities and needs of the hospitalist community, and (6) to support, propose and promote changes to the health care system that lead to higher quality and more efficient care for all hospitalized patients."[7] Thus, compared with the AAP or APA, the SHM advocates more specifically for hospital medicine on a national and local basis and concentrates on the business aspects of practicing hospital medicine.

In 2005 the SHM estimated that there were 15,000 hospitalists in the United States and predicted that there would be 30,000 by 2010.[8] Hospital medicine is growing faster than any other medical specialty in the country. The great majority of hospitalists are internists; pediatricians constitute approximately 8% to 10% of the total.

In 2006 the SHM had more than 6000 members. Although pediatricians account for only 10% of SHM membership, a pediatrician has been on the SHM board since the inception of the organization; in 2005 the bylaws were amended to formalize this arrangement. Within the SHM, the Pediatrics Committee supports, coordinates, and oversees pediatrics-related activities. The SHM does not have a pediatrics SIG or section per se but has been extremely supportive of pediatric hospitalists.

The SHM has enjoyed extraordinary success as a professional organization, in terms of both membership growth and organizational accomplishments. Its initial policy statements confirmed a commitment to voluntary referrals to hospitalists; surveys documented the growth of the field and the satisfaction of providers and payers. Peer-reviewed research by SHM members consistently demonstrated high-quality patient outcomes and cost savings in the 10% to 15% range. As the organization has matured, the SHM has been at the forefront of patient safety and quality initiatives. To this end, the SHM has active relationships with the Joint Commission on Accreditation of Healthcare Organizations, the Institute for Healthcare Improvement, and the American Hospital Association, among other professional organizations. Current SHM projects include web-based resource rooms for common hospital medicine problems such as deep vein thrombosis, catheter-related infection, glycemic control, and heart failure.

In 2006 the SHM published a set of core competencies for (adult) hospitalists covering clinical, procedural, and systems topics.[9] This project, along with the impressive growth in the number of hospitalists, has spurred conversations among the SHM, the American Board of Internal Medicine, and other adult internal medicine organizations about the possibility of designating hospital medicine as a specific area of expertise within internal medicine. This distinction will most likely be effective at recertification rather than at initial board certification and will require documentation of hospital medicine clinical activity in addition to other elements related to the maintenance of certification. The SHM Pediatric Core Curriculum Task Force has been working in parallel with the Adult Core Curriculum Task Force to develop pediatric core competencies. The structure of subspecialty certification developed for hospital medicine within internal medicine will most likely serve as the model for pediatric hospital medicine certification.

The SHM annual meeting is held in the spring and offers specific pediatric clinical content, along with organizational and logistic presentations that require minimal modification to be directly applicable to pediatric hospital medicine practice. These presentations are particularly valuable to leaders of hospital medicine programs (both physicians and administrators) and are available on the SHM website, as are additional practice management resources. The SHM Leadership Academy teaches hospitalists the skills necessary to manage an individual group and to implement change within a hospital system. The SHM's biannual productivity and compensation survey provides comprehensive data for both pediatric and adult hospitalists. According to 2005-2006 survey data for pediatric hospitalists ($n = 261$), the mean annual compensation was $146,000; median annual compensation was $139,000.[10]

The SHM's peer-reviewed publication is the *Journal of Hospital Medicine*. Pediatric submissions are encouraged. The SHM also publishes a monthly newsletter, *The Hospitalist*, which regularly reviews relevant pediatric literature, profiles individual programs, and lists job openings.

COLLABORATIVE EFFORTS

A key factor in the success of the pediatric hospital medicine movement has been cooperation among the three organizations. Respecting the unique strengths of each organization has prevented redundancy and balkanization. In areas where the three organizations' interests overlap, shared structures have been developed to formalize and preserve these collaborative efforts. Foremost among these ventures are the Listserv, the Pediatric Research in Inpatient Settings (PRIS) network, and the annual Pediatric Hospital Medicine meeting.

The Listserv is housed in the AAP, but membership is open to all professionals with a legitimate clinical (i.e., noncommercial) interest in pediatric hospital medicine. This is an active list that addresses clinical, organizational, teaching, and research topics. Job openings are posted weekly. Polite and respectful dialogue on any relevant topic, except actual fee structures, is welcome. All three organizations contribute materially to this service—the AAP by acting as host and making membership open to all, and the APA and SHM by referring members to the AAP Listserv and not creating competing ones.

The PRIS network is another collaborative effort. It is modeled after the AAP Pediatric Research in Office Settings (PROS) network and was founded jointly by all three organizations. The APA houses PRIS administratively for purposes of the receipt and allocation of grant funds and has generously provided staff support. Like the Listserv, PRIS has benefited from the absence of competition among the three organizations.

After the 2005 Pediatric Hospital Medicine meeting in Denver, for which the APA was the lead sponsor, the organizations agreed to rotate primary responsibility for this meeting on an annual basis. This 4-day stand-alone meeting of approximately 250 to 300 pediatric hospitalists is held in the summer, separate from any of the individual organization's larger meetings. Clinical, practice management, educational, research, and policy topics are presented. Future advances in pediatric hospital medicine will likely be presented at this meeting, which will serve as the venue where the community of pediatric hospitalists progresses toward a distinct discipline.

Given the slow pace of change in organized medicine, many of the readers (and the authors) of the first edition of this textbook are likely to see firsthand the initial set of boards or (re-) certifications in pediatric hospital medicine. Prior to this occurring, the AAP, APA and SHM all offer wonderful opportunities to get involved on the ground floor and help shape the field.

CONCLUSION

Pediatric hospital medicine has benefited from the leadership activities provided by the SOHM of the AAP, the APA's Hospital Medicine SIG, and the SHM and its Pediatrics Committee. Broadly speaking, the AAP concentrates on clinical issues related to the care of hospitalized children, the APA focuses on research and educational issues, and the SHM emphasizes logistics and systems issues. These three organizations have worked collaboratively on a number of leading projects, and each one welcomes the participation of readers of this textbook who are interested in promoting the optimal care of hospitalized children, advancing the field of pediatric hospital medicine, and achieving personal career satisfaction. Additional information about these organizations is available through their respective websites (see Table 23-1) and other recent publications.[11]

REFERENCES

1. American Academy of Pediatrics mission statement. Available at *http://www.aap.org/visit/facts.htm.*
2. Percelay J, O'Connor K, Neff J: Pediatricians' attitudes toward and experiences with pediatric hospitalists: A national survey. Available at *http://www.aap.org/research/abstracts/03abstract9.htm.*
3. Section on Hospital Medicine: Guiding principles for pediatric hospitalist programs. Pediatrics 2005;115:1101-1102.
4. Ambulatory Pediatric Association mission statement. Available at *http://www.ambpeds.org/site/about/index.htm.*
5. Lye P, Rauch D, Ottolini M, et al: Pediatric hospitalists: Report of a leadership conference. Pediatrics 2006;117:1122-1130.
6. Society of Hospital Medicine definitions. Available at *http://www.hospitalmedicine.org/Content/NavigationMenu/AboutSHM/DefinitionofaHospitalist/Definition_of_a_Hosp.htm.*
7. Society of Hospital Medicine mission statement. Available at *http://www.hospitalmedicine.org/Content/NavigationMenu/AboutSHM/MissionStatementGoals/Mission_Statement_Go.htm.*
8. Society of Hospital Medicine statistics. Available at *http://www.hospitalmedicine.org/Content/NavigationMenu/Media/GrowthofHospitalMedicineNationwide/Growth_of_Hospital_M.htm.*
9. Pistoria M, Amin A, Dressler D, et al: The core competencies in hospital medicine. J Hosp Med 2006;1 (Suppl 1).
10. Society of Hospital Medicine: 2005-2006 Survey: The authoritative source on the state of the hospital medicine movement. Data presented at Society of Hospital Medicine Annual Meeting, May 4, 2006, Washington, DC. Available as CD-ROM from Society of Hospital Medicine.
11. Rauch D, Percelay J, Zipes D: Introduction to pediatric hospital medicine. Pediatr Clin North Am 2005;52:963-977.

CHAPTER 24

Pediatric Hospital Medicine: Future Directions

Christopher P. Landrigan

Hospital medicine is the fastest growing specialty in the United States, having increased to more than 10,000 practitioners nationwide since its birth in 1996.[1,2] As many as 30,000 hospitalists could be practicing in the United States by 2016 if current workforce projections are accurate.[3] Pediatric hospital medicine has grown in parallel. In 1998, only 2 years after the initial description of the hospitalist model by Wachter and Goldman, 50% of pediatric department chairs reported having pediatric hospitalist systems in their institutions, and another 27% planned to institute them.[4] Current estimates place the number of pediatric hospitalists nationwide at around 1000.[5]

In most institutions, hospitalists were hired initially purely as clinical workers and spent their time almost exclusively in clinical roles. In 2001 half of the department chairs surveyed expected pediatric hospitalists to spend more than 50% of their time engaged in inpatient clinical work.[4] Over the past several years, however, the nature of hospitalist positions has changed as the number and diversity of programs have increased. Hospitalists have increasingly taken on administrative and quality improvement positions within academic and community centers alike. In teaching settings, hospitalists are well positioned to serve as core teachers of medical students and house staff.[6] They have begun to pursue clinical and epidemiologic research germane to the inpatient pediatric population.

Early research on hospitalist systems focused principally on determining whether hospitalists added value in the health care system. The overwhelming majority of studies in both internal medicine and pediatrics found that hospital costs were lower and lengths of stay were shorter in hospitalist compared with traditional systems; referring provider, house staff, and patient and family satisfaction with care was high, but little was known about the quality of care that hospitalists provided[7,8] (see also Chapter 2).

With the growth and development of the field, concerns about quality of care have come to the forefront, and other new questions have been raised. It has become increasingly apparent that the lack of evidence regarding hospitalists' quality of care is largely due to the lack of clarity about what constitutes high-quality pediatric inpatient care in general. With the notable exception of asthma, for which a robust evidence base has been generated, the optimal inpatient management of most common pediatric diseases remains highly variable and poorly understood.[9] Clinical studies of common conditions are urgently needed, and hospitalists are ideally suited to address these questions. Multicenter studies involving hospitalist collaboration across diverse sites may be particularly informative.

Although there is a burgeoning awareness of non–disease-specific quality of care measures (e.g., the Institute of Medicine's push to measure and improve the safety, efficiency, effectiveness, timeliness, equity, and patient centeredness of care; see Chapter 4), implementation is lagging far behind knowledge. Patients have yet to feel the effects of efforts to improve the safety and quality of the health care system.[10] The gap between knowledge and implementation of safety and quality improvement efforts represents a major ongoing opportunity for hospitalists to translate science into real benefits for patients in an unprecedented manner.

With the maturation of the field, concerns about training, credentialing, and fellowships have also arisen. Currently, four pediatric hospitalist fellowships have been launched in the United States and Canada to provide training in research, education, administration, and inpatient clinical medicine. The fellowships established to date are geared primarily toward the academic setting, with the recognition that the long-term success of academic hospitalists will require training beyond that provided in residency. It is likely that the number and size of pediatric hospitalist fellowship programs will increase as the presence of pediatric hospitalists in academic centers grows, but the shape of fellowship training as a whole has yet to be determined. Current issues include the optimal length of fellowship training, development of standard curricula, and whether completion of training toward an advanced degree should be a requirement.

Questions also remain about what clinical training and credentialing, if any, are necessary for hospitalists in academic and community centers. In internal medicine, hospitalists appear to be occupying a clinical niche increasingly distinct from that of their counterparts in primary care practice; consequently, the issue of a hospitalist certification or even subspecialization has been raised.[11] Whether pediatrics will follow suit is unclear.

The long-term funding of pediatric hospitalist programs also remains a concern. Although most programs appear to save money for the health care system as a whole, these savings are generally not credited directly to the hospitalist programs themselves. Most programs seem to be losing money in the current health care market, with salaries and the cost of maintaining hospitalist services generally exceeding revenues collected.[12,13] Determining how to redistribute the savings generated by hospitalists to ensure the fiscal viability of such programs is an important challenge.

Altogether, the health of pediatric hospital medicine is excellent, and its growth and development prodigious. Pediatric hospitalist systems will unquestionably play a major role in the United States and Canada for the foreseeable future, although the mechanisms for organizing and funding these programs are still evolving. The question is no longer whether pediatric hospitalists add value; rather, it is how they can continue to incrementally and measurably improve the quality of hospital care. Although considerable challenges remain, the opportunity for aspiring hospitalists to improve patient care by providing excellent clinical treatment, educating students and house staff, and participating in research and quality improvement activities is extraordinary.

REFERENCES

1. Wachter RM, Goldman L: The emerging role of "hospitalists" in the American health care system. N Engl J Med 1996;335:514-517.
2. Society of Hospital Medicine: Growth of Hospital Medicine Nationwide: 2006. Available at *http://www.hospitalmedicine.org/Content/Navigation Menu/Media/GrowthofHospitalMedicineNationwide/Growth_of_ Hospital_M.htm.*
3. Lurie JD, Miller DP, Lindenauer PK, et al: The potential size of the hospitalist workforce in the United States. Am J Med 1999;106:441-445.
4. Srivastava R, Landrigan C, Gidwani P, et al: Pediatric hospitalists in Canada and the United States: A survey of pediatric academic department chairs. Ambul Pediatr 2001;1:338-339.
5. Lye PS, Rauch DA, Ottolini MC, et al: Pediatric hospitalists: Report of a leadership conference. Pediatrics 2006;117:1122-1130.
6. Landrigan CP, Muret-Wagstaff S, Chiang VW, et al: Effect of a pediatric hospitalist system on housestaff education and experience. Arch Pediatr Adolesc Med 2002;156:877-883.
7. Wachter RM, Goldman L: The hospitalist movement 5 years later. JAMA 2002;287:487-494.
8. Landrigan CP, Conway PH, Edwards S, Srivastava R: Pediatric hospitalists: A systematic review of the literature. Pediatrics 2006;117:1736-1744.
9. Godlee F (ed): Clinical Evidence, 12th ed. London, British Medical Journal Publishing Group, 2004.
10. Altman DE, Clancy C, Blendon RJ: Improving patient safety—five years after the IOM report. N Engl J Med 2004;351:2041-2043.
11. Wellikson L: Come together: Key leaders in internal medicine call for a revision in residency training. Hospitalist 2006;10:5.
12. Melzer SM, Molteni RA, Marcuse EK, Rivara FP: Characteristics and financial performance of a pediatric faculty inpatient attending service: A resource-based relative value scale analysis. Pediatrics 2001;108:79-84.
13. Chiang VW, Landrigan CP, Stucky E, Ottolini MC: Financial health of pediatric hospitalist systems: A study from the Pediatric Research in Inpatient Settings (PRIS) network. Pediatr Res 2004;55:1794.

PART II

Common Presenting Signs and Symptoms

Abdominal Mass

Daniel Rauch

Although the evaluation of an abdominal mass often occurs in an outpatient setting, pediatric hospitalists are often asked to expedite the initial assessment and coordinate the appropriate consultations. The diagnostic possibilities vary considerably, based on the patient's age and associated symptoms. The most urgent considerations are acute surgical conditions and neoplasms. A careful history and physical examination should guide a directed laboratory and imaging evaluation, leading to the diagnosis.

ANATOMY

The abdomen is classically divided in four quadrants. The right upper quadrant contains the liver, gallbladder, and bowel. The liver is often palpated under the costal margin and up to 2 to 3 cm below in infants. The liver may be displaced inferiorly with hyperaeration of the chest cavity. When the liver edge extends to the left of the midline, it is likely enlarged. The left upper quadrant contains the spleen, pancreas, stomach, and bowel. Both the right lower quadrant and the left lower quadrant contain bowel and the female reproductive organs. Aside from the liver, these intraperitoneal structures are not typically palpable. In young infants the bladder may be palpable in the suprapubic area, but this structure becomes intrapelvic in later infancy. Retroperitoneal structures, such as the aorta and kidneys, are not normally palpable. Normal structures may be felt in patients who are very thin and have relaxed abdominal musculature, especially the aorta, which can be appreciated as a pulsatile midline structure, and the tip of the spleen in the left upper quadrant.

There are many structures within the abdomen from which masses can arise (Table 25-1). The gastrointestinal (GI) tract comprises most of the volume of the abdomen. Focal areas of distention can present as a mass, such as in duplication, intussusception, volvulus, and constipation (see Chapter 138). GI duplications are rare and may present with obstruction or bloody diarrhea in addition to a palpable mass. Intussusception uncommonly presents with the classic triad of colicky abdominal pain, vomiting, and currant jelly stool. More typical is some combination of vomiting, lethargy, and abdominal pain, with a right upper quadrant sausage-shaped mass and an empty right lower quadrant (Dance sign) in an infant or toddler. Volvulus also presents with vomiting and pain associated with an acute obstruction. Constipation is the most common cause of a palpable abdominal mass in any of the quadrants; it is usually tubular, mobile, and nontender.

Hepatomegaly is a nonspecific finding that may represent primary liver pathology or myriad secondary processes. Enlargement may be due to an increase in the size or number of cells or structures in the liver, including the hepatocytes (e.g., glycogen storage diseases), biliary tree (cholelithiasis),

and vascular spaces (e.g., congestive heart failure), or to an infiltrative process (e.g., neuroblastoma). A list of possible infectious causes is provided in Table 25-2. Other causes to consider are listed in Table 25-3.

The spleen can enlarge in response to a wide range of insults. Many of the infectious, metabolic, neoplastic, and inflammatory disorders that can cause hepatomegaly can also cause splenomegaly, either in isolation or in combination. Hemolytic disorders can cause chronic splenomegaly or, as in the case of acute splenic sequestration of sickle cell disease, sudden splenic enlargement with profound anemia. Serum sickness and subacute bacterial endocarditis can cause splenomegaly, with deposition of immune complexes in the spleen. Chronic granulomatous disease can cause intrasplenic granuloma formation.

The female reproductive tract resides in the pelvis but can expand into the lower abdomen under certain circumstances. Ovarian cysts or, much less commonly, neoplasms can become large enough to be palpable by direct abdominal examination. An engorged uterus may be palpable in the suprapubic area with congenital vaginal atresia and is seen with hydrometrocolpos. A gravid uterus extends beyond the pelvic brim at approximately 12 weeks' gestation. Ectopic pregnancy within a fallopian tube is usually symptomatic before being palpable but should always be considered in patients with abdominal pain and a positive pregnancy test. An intravaginal-abdominal bimanual examination is appropriate for better palpation of the female reproductive organs.

The bladder, which is a pelvic structure after infancy, can expand into the lower abdomen when enlarged. This may occur with urinary retention.

Retroperitoneal structures such as the kidneys, adrenals, pancreas, and midline paravertebral nodes and vessels can be palpable through the abdomen when there is significant tissue bulk, as may be seen with neoplasms such as Wilms tumor, neuroblastoma, and lymphoma. Cystic kidney disease may present as an abdominal mass. Neonates may have a palpable right kidney, which may be completely normal.

The abdominal wall is a rare source of abdominal masses, taking the form of incarcerated hernias or sarcomas.

ASSOCIATED SYMPTOMS

A painless mass is the classic sign of abdominal malignancy, particularly Wilms tumor and neuroblastoma. However, painless masses may also be completely benign, such as a fecal mass in a constipated child, a horseshoe kidney, or a wandering spleen. Painless masses are usually identified incidentally, often by parents when bathing the child, and sometimes on routine physical examinations. Systemic symptoms such as weight loss, pallor, bruising, or bleeding are suggestive of a malignant process. Masses may

Table 25-1 Possible Diagnoses of Abdominal Masses

Region	Organ or Site	Diagnosis
Epigastrium	Stomach	Distended stomach from pyloric stenosis, duplication
	Pancreas	Pseudocyst
Flank	Kidney	Hydronephrosis, Wilms tumor, dysplastic kidney, ureteral duplication
	Adrenal	Neuroblastoma, ganglioneuroblastoma, ganglioneuroma
	Retroperitoneum	Neuroblastoma, ganglioneuroblastoma, ganglioneuroma, teratoma
Lower abdomen	Ovary	Dermoid, teratoma, ovarian tumor, torsion of ovary
	Kidney	Pelvic kidney
	Urachus	Urachal cyst
	Omentum, mesentery	Omental, mesenteric, peritoneal cysts
Pelvic	Bladder, prostate	Obstructed bladder, rhabdomyosarcoma
	Uterus, vagina	Hydrometrocolpos, hydrocolpos, rhabdomyosarcoma
Right upper quadrant	Biliary tract	Cholecystitis, choledochal cyst
	Liver	Hepatomegaly from congestion, hepatitis, or tumor; mesenchymal hamartoma; hemangioendothelioma; hepatoblastoma; hepatocellular carcinoma; hepatic abscess; hydatid cyst
	Intestine	Intussusception, duplication
Left upper quadrant	Spleen	Splenomegaly from congestion, infectious mononucleosis, leukemic infiltration, or lymphoma; splenic abscess; cyst
Right lower quadrant	Appendix	Appendiceal abscess
	Ileum	Meconium ileus, inflammatory mass (complication of Crohn's disease), intestinal duplication
	Lymphatics	Lymphoma, lymphangioma
Left lower quadrant	Colon	Fecal impaction
	Lymphatics	Lymphoma, lymphangioma

From Zitelli B, Davis H: Atlas of Pediatric Physical Diagnosis, 4th ed. Philadelphia, Elsevier, 2002.

Table 25-2 Infectious Causes of Hepatomegaly

Bacteremia
Infectious hepatitis
Mononucleosis
Syphilis
Leptospirosis
Histoplasmosis
Brucellosis
Toxoplasmosis
Tuberculosis
Ascariasis
Amebiasis
Pyogenic abscess
Visceral larva migrans
Q fever
Gonococcal or chlamydial perihepatitis
AIDS
Neonatal enteroviral infection
Gianottic-Crosti syndrome
Cat-scratch disease (granuloma)

From Green M (ed): The abdomen. In Pediatric Diagnosis: Interpretation of Symptoms and Signs in Children and Adolescents, 6th ed. Philadelphia, Saunders, 1998, pp 97-98.

Table 25-3 Noninfectious Causes of Hepatomegaly

Anemia (sickle cell disease)
Passive vascular congestion (congestive heart failure)
Metabolic disorders (mucopolysaccharidosis)
Cholestatic disorders (biliary atresia)
Neoplastic disease (Hodgkin's disease)
Cysts (congenital hepatic cyst)
Fatty infiltration (idiopathic steatohepatitis)
Trauma (subcapsular hematoma)
Autoimmune (systemic lupus erythematosus)
Hemosiderosis
Poisoning (hypervitaminosis A)

cause or be the result of GI obstruction and can present with vomiting, abdominal pain, and constipation. Masses that are renal in origin can present with symptoms of urinary dysfunction and hematuria. Painful masses require an urgent evaluation for possible surgical issues. Duration of the symptoms is an important consideration. Slowly growing masses are typical of some malignancies, whereas rapidly enlarging masses are more typical of others.

IMAGING

Imaging studies can help localize the mass, determine the origin, or identify the cause. Plain radiographs (flat plates) can identify some abnormalities (e.g., solid tumors with calcifications) but are more useful as part of an obstruction series. The additional views demonstrate the effect of gravity on the intra-abdominal structures and fluids, revealing patterns of bowel obstruction, abscess, or free air.

Ultrasonography is a readily available, nonionizing imaging modality that usually does not require the patient to be sedated. It provides information regarding the consis-

Chapter 25 ABDOMINAL MASS 119

tency of the mass (e.g., solid versus cystic), can readily identify an abscess, and can often identify the organ of origin. Cystic masses are usually from the GI or genitourinary tract and are less likely to be malignant than solid masses are.

Computed tomography and magnetic resonance imaging provide a more complete assessment and greater structural detail. Factors such as need for sedation, radiation exposure, availability, and likely yield are important considerations. In addition, when the diagnosis is likely to be a malignancy and additional body areas will need to be imaged for staging purposes, studies should be coordinated to the extent possible. Further discussion of imaging is provided in Chapter 198.

SUGGESTED READING

Brodeur AE, Brodeur GM: Abdominal masses in children: Neuroblastoma, Wilms tumor, and other considerations. Pediatr Rev 1991;12:196-207.

Golden CB, Feusner JH: Malignant abdominal masses in children: Quick guide to evaluation and diagnosis. Pediatr Clin North Am 2002;49:1369-1392.

Pearl RH, Irish MS, Caty MG, Glick PL: The approach to common abdominal diagnoses in infants and children. Part II. Pediatr Clin North Am 1998;45:1287-1326.

CHAPTER 26

Abdominal Pain

Timothy Gibson

Abdominal pain is one of the most common complaints encountered by pediatric hospitalists. The evaluation can be exceedingly difficult, however, and in many cases, no definitive diagnosis can be made. The most serious disorders causing acute abdominal pain can be rapidly life threatening and are often managed in conjunction with a pediatric surgeon.

BACKGROUND

Abdominal pain can be caused by inflammation of the abdominal organs themselves (or their visceral peritoneum) or by inflammation of the parietal peritoneum lying in proximity to the underlying inflammation. Irritation of the abdominal wall musculature can also lead to pain, and various extra-abdominal processes have been associated with abdominal pain (e.g., diabetic ketoacidosis, porphyria). Pain due to a process in the small intestine is usually felt in the midline around the umbilicus initially; as the inflammation progresses, the parietal peritoneum in the area of inflammation becomes involved, allowing better localization of pain. The classic example is appendicitis, with a dull periumbilical ache early in the course, followed by a progressive shift of pain to the right lower quadrant as the inflammation evolves. Certain elements of the history and physical examination findings may help identify the cause of abdominal pain (Table 26-1).

ASSESSMENT

The differential diagnosis of abdominal pain is extensive (Table 26-2). In addition to the typical history and physical examination, epidemiologic factors are extremely helpful in narrowing the differential diagnosis, including age, gender, season, locale, and the like. The first question to be answered by any physician evaluating a patient with abdominal pain is: Does the patient have an acute or surgical abdomen? A patient with peritonitis requires a timely surgical evaluation. With several conspicuous exceptions, most patients have a gradual progression of pain to the point of peritonitis. On questioning, these patients, if old enough, may report that the bumps in the road on the trip to the emergency department caused pain. These patients prefer to lie motionless and do not want their abdomens palpated. The examiner can check for signs of peritonitis immediately by "inadvertently" bumping the gurney; a wince of pain from the patient is a sign that any movement at all is irritating to the inflamed parietal peritoneum. Bowel sounds may be hypoactive or absent at this late stage, reflecting an ileus. The abdomen may be rigid, caused by stiffening of the abdominal wall musculature to guard the inflamed peritoneum just below from being manipulated. Patients with peritonitis are likely to have rebound tenderness; that is, the pain felt when the

examiner releases the abdomen is greater than that caused by the palpation itself. Patients of any age who fit this classic description of an acute abdomen are highly likely to require surgical intervention and rarely need further evaluation, such as laboratory tests or radiographic studies, except possibly to assess their surgical risk.

Unfortunately for physicians (but fortunately for patients), most cases of abdominal pain are not this clear-cut. For each disease process in the differential diagnosis, there is a wide range of severity. For example, a patient with severe constipation may be in extremis, whereas a patient with early appendicitis may have so little pain (or such a high tolerance for pain) that he or she is sent home without surgical consultation. A full history and physical examination are paramount to determine the cause of the pain. It must be kept in mind that common diagnoses (e.g., viral gastroenteritis, constipation) occur commonly, and it is the examiner's job to triage these patients appropriately, while recognizing the red flags that point to less common entities or those that need more urgent evaluation or intervention.

HISTORY

The timing, location, and progression of the pain should be elicited, as well as its quality and severity. Did the pain begin in the umbilical area and progress to the right lower quadrant, as occurs with appendicitis? Is the pain burning or boring, as in ulcer disease, or sharp and stabbing, as in appendicitis? Does it come in waves, suggesting a blockage of peristalsis in a hollow viscus, such as the small bowel, bile duct, or ureter? Is the pain relieved by meals, as in some peptic ulcer diseases, or is the pain exacerbated by oral intake, as in biliary disease and pancreatitis? Is there vomiting before the pain, as in viral gastroenteritis, or after the pain, as in appendicitis? Is the vomiting bilious, signifying a blockage distal to the sphincter of Oddi? In a verbal child, questions about urinary complaints should be included, such as dysuria, frequency, or discolored urine, suggesting a urinary tract infection, nephrolithiasis, or the nephritis of Henoch-Schönlein purpura. In a younger child, it is important to determine whether the pain is episodic and severe, with intervening periods of lethargy or even apparent wellness, as in intussusception. What is the patient's baseline stooling pattern? Is there a history of constipation? If there is diarrhea, is it bloody, as in inflammatory bowel disease (IBD) or a bacterial infection? Are the stools melanotic, as in a bleeding duodenal ulcer? Are there red flags—weight loss, fatigue, night sweats—for a prolonged systemic disease such as Crohn's disease? Are there extraintestinal manifestations that are suspicious for IBD, such as rash, arthralgias or arthritis, aphthous stomatitis, or eye problems? Is there a family history of gastrointestinal disorders, especially heritable disorders such as IBD? Is the patient on any medications

Table 26-1 Using History and Physical Examination Findings to Diagnose Abdominal Pain

Findings	Possible Diagnosis
History of present illness	
Sudden onset	Ovarian or testicular torsion, intussusception, volvulus, trauma
Bilious emesis	Bowel obstruction
Bloody stools	IBD (older patients), intussusception (younger patients), infectious colitis
Recent weight loss	IBD, malignancy
Travel	Infectious colitis, parasitic infection
Fevers	Infectious colitis, IBD
Rash	Henoch-Schönlein purpura, IBD (erythema nodosum)
Menstrual history	Dysmenorrhea, pregnancy, mittelschmerz
Past medical history	
Pharyngitis	Mesenteric adenitis, EBV-associated splenic distention
Gastroenteritis	Intussusception, postinfectious gastroparesis
Abdominal surgery	Obstruction from adhesions
Family history	
IBD	IBD
Migraines	Abdominal migraines
Social history	
Pets, especially reptiles	Infectious colitis
Sexual history	Pelvic inflammatory disease, pregnancy, ectopic pregnancy
Physical examination	
Clubbing or pallor	IBD
Perianal skin tags	Crohn's disease
Jaundice	Biliary disease
Bluish color of flank or umbilicus	Pancreatic disease, trauma
Hemorrhoids, caput medusae	Chronic liver disease

EBV, Epstein-Barr virus; IBD, inflammatory bowel disease.

that could predispose to abdominal pain, especially nonsteroidial anti-inflammatory drugs (suspected ulcer disease) or recent antibiotics (possible *Clostridium difficile* infection)? Is there anything relevant in the social history, such as recent sexual activity predisposing to a sexually transmitted disease or pelvic inflammatory disease, or difficulties at school or at home causing stress?

PHYSICAL EXAMINATION

The physical examination starts with an evaluation of the vital signs. True abdominal catastrophes with associated abdominal pain (volvulus, perforated duodenal ulcer, splenic rupture following Epstein-Barr virus infection, severe trauma) quickly progress to frank shock, with accompanying changes in hemodynamics and vital signs. Fever is often found with inflammatory and infectious processes. The

degree of fever is not necessarily directly related to the severity of the eventual diagnosis. Fever of 104°F to 105°F is often seen with viral gastroenteritis, whereas the fever of appendicitis starts much lower and spikes to 104°F to 105°F only after perforation.

The importance of the patient's general examination on presentation cannot be overstated. A toxic, shocky child needs emergent evaluation and intervention after ensuring the ABCs (airway, breathing, circulation), whereas a patient with normal vital signs who smiles and jokes while complaining of 10 out of 10 abdominal pain may not warrant admission. Examination of the acute abdomen was addressed earlier, with an emphasis on recognizing the signs of peritonitis. After inspection of the abdomen (for distension, discoloration, visible masses, etc.) bowel sounds should be assessed, because deep palpation can alter their character. Are the bowel sounds present? Are they high pitched, as in a bowel obstruction?

Percussion of the abdomen is invaluable. Are there tympanitic sounds of air, potentially proximal to an obstruction? Is there a fixed area of dullness, signifying organomegaly or a mass (malignant or otherwise, including a firm stool), in the left lower quadrant? Is there a shifting dullness or a fluid wave, suspicious for ascites? Palpation is also important in evaluating for masses and organomegaly and for eliciting pain. One should always begin palpating as far away from the reported location of the patient's pain as possible. Having the child flex the hips and bend the knees is helpful to relax the abdominal musculature. Any child younger than teenaged should be distracted during palpation, and the practitioner's eyes should be fixed on the patient's face, looking for even subtle signs of tenderness. The obturator sign and the psoas sign are suggestive of inflammation in or near those muscles, often secondary to organic abdominal pathology (described in Chapter 143). The Rovsing sign is present when palpation in the left lower quadrant produces pain in the right lower quadrant.

All children should have a full examination in addition to the abdominal examination, with an emphasis on findings that could be causing or contributing to the abdominal pain. Controversy exists over which children need rectal examinations and which females need pelvic examinations. In selected cases, either of these examinations can be immensely informative, and the need for them is dictated by the history.

EVALUATION

As stated earlier, a patient with an obvious surgical abdomen often needs no further evaluation before surgical exploration is undertaken. For other patients, the question is whether to perform radiologic studies and laboratory tests.

Radiology

The simplest and most widely available initial study is a supine plain radiograph of the abdomen (also known as a kidney, ureter, and bladder [KUB] study). Most findings are nonspecific and often just confirm the findings elicited by physical examination. Exceptions include a renal or ureteral calculus or the finding of a fecalith in the right lower quadrant. A fecalith is a small, radiointense mass of hardened stool that obstructs the lumen of the appendix, preventing

Table 26-2   Differential Diagnosis of Abdominal Pain

Gastrointestinal	**Surgical**
Viral gastroenteritis	Appendicitis
Bacterial infectious colitis	Intussusception
Parasitic infection	Malrotation with midgut volvulus
Constipation	Incarcerated inguinal hernia
Colic	Trauma with associated hematoma
Functional abdominal pain	Postsurgical obstruction
Abdominal migraine	Psoas (or other) abscess
Acute cholecystitis, cholelithiasis	**Toxicologic**
Ulcer disease (gastric, peptic)	Heavy metal poisoning
Pancreatitis	Food (toxin-mediated) poisoning
Hepatitis	**Infectious**
Inflammatory bowel disease	Tuberculosis
Gastroesophageal reflux	Zoster
Esophagitis	Mesenteric adenitis
Gastroparesis, ileus	Mononucleosis
Lactose intolerance	Sepsis
Toxic megacolon	**Pulmonary**
Meckel's diverticulum	Lower lobe pneumonia
Hirschsprung disease	Meconium ileus equivalent
Urologic	**Endocrinologic**
Urinary tract infection	Diabetic ketoacidosis
Urolithiasis	**Hematologic**
Testicular torsion	Vaso-occlusive crisis
Gynecologic	Porphyria
Ovarian torsion, cyst	**Oncologic**
Pregnancy, ectopic pregnancy	Tumor (e.g., Wilms)
Pelvic inflammatory disease	**Renal**
Dysmenorrhea	Nephrosis
Endometriosis	Spontaneous bacterial peritonitis
Hematocolpos	Hemolytic uremic syndrome
Ovarian neoplasm	**Cardiovascular**
Rheumatologic	Abdominal aortic aneurysm
Henoch-Schönlein purpura	**Psychiatric**
Familial Mediterranean fever	Somatoform or conversion disorder

the outflow of intestinal bacteria and predisposing the patient to appendicitis. Many surgeons will operate on a patient with an equivocal history based on a radiographic finding of a fecalith. Distended loops of bowel are common and nonspecific, as is scoliosis toward the side of pain. The addition of a second abdominal view in the upright or left lateral decubitus allows for effect of gravity on air and fluid to be examined. Air-fluid levels may be visible within bowel secondary to ileus or obstruction. Free air may be visible on the upright film, but these patients often have peritoneal signs on examination.

Ultrasonography has the advantage of being a real-time study, along with its ability to evaluate blood flow to an organ. This is especially helpful in evaluating female patients in whom ovarian torsion or pelvic inflammatory disease is a consideration. Ultrasonography is frequently used in the evaluation of suspected intussusception to identify a "donut"

(the intussusceptum within the lumen of the intussuscipiens). Air-contrast enema has the advantage of being able to both diagnose and treat intussusception, but because there is a small risk of perforation, this procedure should be performed only in centers staffed by surgeons competent in the care of small children (see Chapter 138).

The radiologic evaluation of patients with suspected appendicitis has changed since the mid-1990s (see Chapter 139). Ultrasonography is useful, and for a female patient with atypical right lower quadrant pain, it may be the preferred study because of the ability to simultaneously evaluate the pelvic organs. Computed tomography, especially when done with effective rectal or oral contrast, has high specificity for appendicitis. The radiologist is able to see signs of inflammation in the right lower quadrant, including free fluid and stranding in the pericecal fat. With effective contrast, an appendix that does not fill is presumed to be obstructed, confirming the diagnosis of appendicitis. The study is quite operator and hospital dependent, however.

Other imaging studies that may be encountered in the evaluation of abdominal pain include barium swallows (effective for the evaluation of malrotation with intermittent volvulus and for IBD) and, rarely, nuclear medicine studies for gastrointestinal bleeding with associated abdominal pain.

Laboratory Studies

As with radiologic studies, the history and physical examination guide the practitioner as far as laboratory studies. The result of all laboratory testing needs to be taken in context and cannot supercede physical findings or discount the importance of serial physical examinations.

In patients with abdominal pain, a complete cell count (CBC) with differential is helpful in the evaluation for inflammation, infection, or anemia. In general, an elevated high white blood cell (WBC) count with a neutrophilic predominance is more suspicious for an acute infectious or inflammatory cause of the patient's pain, including appendicitis. However, a normal WBC count does not rule out appendicitis, and an elevated WBC count does not confirm it. Anemia, if observed, can be very helpful in pointing the practitioner toward a chronic disease like IBD, especially if accompanied by a relative reticulocytopenia. A low mean corpuscular volume (MCV) suggests iron deficiency, perhaps suggestive of chronic blood loss. Sudden, acute blood loss may present with evidence of hemodynamic compromise before there is a fall in the hemoglobin level on an initial CBC.

A basic chemistry panel with serum electrolytes, glucose, creatinine, and blood can help evaluate hydration status, acid-base balance, and electrolyte derangements, especially if vomiting, diarrhea, or inadequate oral intake is part of the clinical picture. These findings are typically less helpful in identifying the etiology of abdominal pain but are often needed for appropriate management.

Evaluation of serum hepatic enzymes and bilirubin levels, often referred to as liver function tests, are useful for patients with right upper quadrant pain or tenderness or with jaundice. These tests usually include alanine aminotransferase (ALT), aspartate aminotransferase (AST), alkaline phosphatase, γ-glutamyl transferase (GGT), and levels of both the conjugated and unconjugated fractions of serum bilirubin (see Chapter 93 for further discussion of these tests). Concern for mononucleosis should prompt testing for Epstein-Barr virus (EBV) with either a heterophil antibody test ("monospot") for children over 4 years of age or EBV serology. Elevations of pancreatic enzymes, amylase, and lipase are quite specific for pancreatitis, and these studies would be warranted in patients with epigastric pain or tenderness or prominent vomiting. They can establish a diagnosis and are often useful in following the course of the illness (see Chapter 100).

The erythrocyte sedimentation rate (ESR) is usually elevated with chronic diseases like IBD, but again they are nonspecific markers for inflammation and therefore can be elevated in many infectious, inflammatory, or malignant conditions. Newer serologic tests for IBD may be helpful in patients with a suggestive clinical picture, but definitive diagnosis still requires endoscopic or imaging studies (see Chapter 98).

Urinalysis can provide information regarding hydration status (specific gravity) as well as indications of genitourinary injury (e.g., red blood cells secondary to ureteral calculus) or infection (e.g., nitrates and white blood cells secondary to pyelonephritis). Note that patients with appendicitis may have sterile pyuria if the inflamed appendix settles on the wall of the bladder. All stools for any child with abdominal pain should be tested for blood, and if there is concern for infectious gastroenteritis or colitis, appropriate samples should be sent to evaluate for the bacteria, toxins, parasites, or viruses of concern. Serologies can be sent for *Helicobacter pylori* if gastritis due to this entity is suspected (see Chapter 95).

TREATMENT

The treatment of abdominal pain obviously depends on what is discovered during the workup. Patients thought to have surgical pathology are given nothing by mouth and often need intravenous fluids for replacement losses or maintenance needs. Particular attention should be paid to pain control, which often requires parenteral opioids. Definitive surgical intervention occurs when the patient is stable enough for anesthesia, or occasionally before this point if the patient is toxic and deteriorating. If bowel perforation is suspected, the patient is started on broad-spectrum antibiotics to cover enteric pathogens, including anaerobes. Patients who are admitted without a definitive diagnosis deserve close monitoring, and the importance of serial examinations cannot be overstated. Recent literature suggests that serial examinations by pediatric surgeons are as effective as radiologic evaluation in patients with suspected early appendicitis. Diligent monitoring of fluid intake and output, along with vital signs, can provide an early clue that a disease process is progressing. If there are stigmata of systemic gastrointestinal disease, consultation with a pediatric gastroenterologist, with an eye toward possible endoscopy, is appropriate. There is a wealth of treatments for constipation, and a child with viral gastroenteritis needs fluid resuscitation and a tincture of time.

As stated earlier, many patients who present with abdominal pain never receive a definitive diagnosis. When a symptomatic patient has been fully evaluated and organic disease has been ruled out, the goal of treatment is to control the patient's symptoms and allow a return to the activities of daily living. A child must be able to tolerate enough by mouth to stay hydrated and prevent weight loss. A schoolage child must be able to attend school on most days. Above all, a patient with pain and a negative workup needs close follow-up, sometimes with a specialist, but always with the primary care physician. It has been reported that patients with depression may present with abdominal pain. In this case, a psychiatrist may need to be involved, both for the evaluation of nonorganic pain and for the teaching of coping strategies.

For patients discharged to home, it should be stressed to parents that the workup is ongoing and will continue in the outpatient setting.

SUGGESTED READING

Ashcraft KW: Consultation with the specialist: Acute abdominal pain. Pediatr Rev 2000;21:363-367.

Boyle JT: Abdominal pain. In Walker WA, Durie P, Hamilton J, et al (eds): Pediatric Gastrointestinal Disease. Hamilton, Ontario, BC Decker, 2000, pp 129-149.

Hrabovsky E: Acute and chronic abdominal pain. In Kliegman R (ed): Practical Strategies in Pediatric Diagnosis and Therapy. Philadelphia, WB Saunders, 1996, pp 258-279.

Kosloske AM, Love CL, Rohrer JE, et al: The diagnosis of appendicitis in children: Outcomes of a strategy based on pediatric surgical evaluation. Pediatrics 2004;113:29-34.

CHAPTER 27

Acidosis

Katherine Ahn Jin

BACKGROUND

Acidosis is defined as an abnormal clinical process that causes a net gain in hydrogen ions (H^+) in the extracellular fluid. Metabolic acidosis occurs when there is an accumulation of H^+ or a loss of bicarbonate ions (HCO_3^-) and is reflected by a decrease in plasma HCO_3^- (<22 mEq/L). Respiratory acidosis occurs when there is an accumulation of carbon dioxide (CO_2) and is reflected by an increase in the arterial partial pressure of carbon dioxide (P_{CO_2} >40 mm Hg).

Clinically, acid-base scenarios can involve a primary acidosis or alkalosis with or without compensation, or a mixed acid-base disorder. The pH reflects the net effect of these processes (Fig. 27-1). The term *acidemia* is defined as an abnormal decrease in blood pH (<7.37).

PATHOPHYSIOLOGY

Maintaining blood pH between 7.37 and 7.43 creates an optimal environment for cellular enzyme activity and membrane integrity. The body has several mechanisms by which it maintains blood pH in that range, despite dietary and endogenous production of acids and bases. It is estimated that the average child generates 1 to 3 mEq/kg of net acid each day.

The body has three main mechanisms to compensate for acid disturbances. The timing of the peak effect of each mechanism varies from seconds to days. The first line of defense consists of the bicarbonate and nonbicarbonate (e.g., hemoglobin, tissue proteins, organophosphate complexes, bone apatite) buffering systems in the plasma and cells. The buffers in the plasma readily accept H^+, providing an immediate defense against life-threatening acidemia. The buffering effect of cells peaks 2 to 4 hours after H^+ has entered the cells.

The second line of defense is the respiratory system. H^+ is combined with HCO_3^- to form carbonic acid (H_2CO_3), which dissociates to water (H_2O) and CO_2. CO_2 freely diffuses across alveolar barriers and is excreted by the lung. The efficacy and potency of this compensatory system are due to the large buffer capacity in this open system and its rapid effect (beginning in 10 to 15 minutes; complete in 12 to 24 hours). The stimulus to hyperventilate likely involves peripheral chemoreceptors that immediately sense a drop in plasma pH; later, the respiratory center senses changes in pH in the cerebrospinal fluid. The utility of this system is, of course, predicated on the ability to ventilate the lungs.

The third line of defense is the renal system. The kidney maintains acid-base homeostasis by the reabsorption of HCO_3^- from the glomerular filtrate and the secretion of H^+ into the urine. Renal acidification rises in a stepwise fashion, and a maximum level is achieved in 3 to 5 days.

Compensatory mechanisms drive the pH *toward* normal, but never to normal or beyond, because the body neither fully compensates nor overcompensates for primary acid-base disorders.

DIFFERENTIAL DIAGNOSIS

The arterial blood gas is important in initially categorizing the primary acid-base disorder (Fig. 27-2). Metabolic acidosis can be categorized as anion gap or non–anion gap acidosis (Table 27-1). The anion gap is approximated by the following formula (all units mEq/L):

$$\text{Anion gap (AG)} = \text{Serum sodium (Na}^+) - (\text{Serum chloride [Cl}^-] + HCO_3^-)$$

The anion gap is normally 12 ± 4 mEq/L. It accounts for unmeasured anions that normally exist in serum, such as anionic proteins (principally albumin), and inorganic and organic anions. Hypoalbuminemia makes the anion gap smaller, potentially masking an anion gap acidosis. In the setting of hypoalbuminemia, the anion gap can be adjusted using the following equation:

$$\text{Adjusted AG (mEq/L)} = \text{Calculated AG (mEq/L)} + 2.5 \times [\text{Normal albumin (g/dL)} - \text{Measured albumin (g/dL)}]$$

In anion gap acidosis, elevation of the anion gap indicates the addition of non-chloride–containing acids in the blood. HCO_3^- neutralizes these acids, leaving the anion to balance the preexisting cationic (Na^+) charge:

$$H^+\text{anion}^- + NaHCO_3 \Longleftrightarrow H_2O + CO_2 + Na^+\text{anion}^-$$

The anions accompanying these acids may not undergo glomerular filtration, they may be filtered but readily reabsorbed, or they cannot be used.

If the anion gap is 20 or greater, a metabolic acidosis is likely to be present, regardless of a concurrent pH or serum HCO_3^- falling in the normal range. An anion gap greater than 20 is more than 4 SD from the mean and is therefore unlikely due to chance. Although a compensatory metabolic acidosis may occur with a primary alkalosis, it would be associated with only a modest increase in the anion gap (not >20). In those with an anion gap greater than 20, a specific cause for the metabolic acidosis will probably be discerned from the usual screening tests.[1]

The osmolal gap can be useful in further identifying toxin-induced anion gap acidosis. Serum osmolality is calculated according to the following equation:

$$\text{Osmolality}_{calc} \text{ (mOsm/kg)} = 2 \times Na^+ \text{ (mEq/L)} + \text{Blood urea nitrogen (mg/dL)}/2.8 + \text{Glucose (mg/dL)}/18$$

The difference between the calculated and measured osmolalities, termed the osmolal gap, is normally 10 to

15 mOsm/kg. If the measured osmolality exceeds the calculated osmolality by more than 15 to 20 mOsm/kg, it indicates an accumulation of osmolytes other than the sodium salts, urea, and glucose used in the formula. A high osmolal gap is commonly associated with the ingestion of ethylene glycol and alcohols.

Non–anion gap acidosis indicates either the loss of HCO_3^- through the kidney or gastrointestinal tract, with the subsequent retention of Cl^-, or the addition of an acid, with the subsequent consumption of HCO_3^-, followed by rapid renal excretion of the accompanying anion and replacement with Cl^-. In both cases, HCO_3^- is effectively replaced by Cl^-, keeping the anion gap within normal limits. Because of this tendency for Cl^- to replace HCO_3^-, non–anion gap acidosis is also known as hyperchloremic metabolic acidosis.

An excess anion gap (calculated AG – normal AG, or calculated AG – 12 mEq/L) might reveal a hidden non–anion gap acidosis. Because 1 mEq of unmeasured acid titrates

with 1 mEq of HCO_3^-, and a 1 mEq/L decrease in HCO_3^- results in a 1 mEq/L contribution to the excess anion gap, the sum of the excess anion gap and measured HCO_3^- should equal a normal HCO_3^- concentration. If the sum is less than 22 mEq/L, this suggests an underlying non–anion gap acidosis. Conversely, if the sum is greater than 26 mEq/L, an underlying metabolic alkalosis should be suspected.[1]

The urinary anion gap can be useful in differentiating between two common causes of non–anion gap acidosis: gastrointestinal losses and renal tubular acidosis (RTA). The urinary anion gap is calculated by obtaining spot measurements of urinary Na^+, potassium (K^+), and Cl^- (all units mEq/L):

$$\text{Urinary anion gap (UAG)} = (Na^+ + K^+)_u - (Cl^-)_u$$

The urinary anion gap is an indirect measure of urinary ammonia (NH_4^+), which is generated in the setting of acidosis. NH_4^+ is assumed to be present if the sum of the major urinary cations ($Na^+ + K^+$) is less than the major anion (Cl^-); because electroneutrality must exist in the urine, some cation must be balancing the apparent surfeit in measured Cl^-. In a metabolic acidosis evolving from chronic diarrhea, the functioning kidneys increase renal NH_4^+ synthesis and excretion, thus providing more urinary buffer. In RTA, the urinary NH_4^+ is low because of the kidney's intrinsic inability to deal with acid loads. Thus, a negative urinary anion gap suggests an extrarenal cause of non–anion gap acidosis, whereas a positive urinary anion gap suggests a renal cause of non–anion gap acidosis.

The urinary anion gap calculation is not useful in the setting of a urinary pH greater than 6.5 because this suggests the presence of bicarbonate in the urine. Urinary bicarbonate is not commonly measured in most laboratories, so if it is present and its concentration is not calculated, the calculated urinary cations may appear to be excessive for the load of chloride alone. In this situation, it is best to calculate the urinary osmolal gap (difference between measured and calculated urinary osmolalities), because urinary NH_4^+ can be estimated as half of the urinary osmolal gap:

$$\text{Urinary } NH_4^+ \text{ (mEq/L)} = 0.5 \times (\text{Measured Uosm} - \text{Calculated Uosm})$$

$$\text{Calculated Uosm (mOsm/kg)} = 2[Na^+_u \text{ (mEq/L)} + K^+_u \text{ (mEq/L)}] + \text{Urea}_u \text{ (mg/dL)}/2.8 + \text{Glucose}_u \text{ (mg/dL)}/18$$

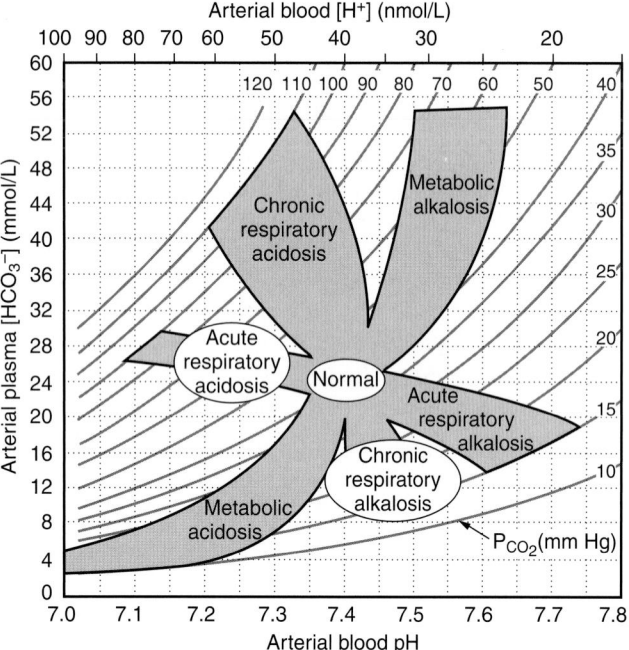

Figure 27-1 Acid-base nomogram showing arterial blood pH, arterial plasma HCO_3^-, and P_{CO_2} values. The central open circle depicts acid-base status in normal people. The shaded areas depict the 95% confidence limits of the normal respiratory and metabolic compensations for primary acid-base disturbances. For values lying outside the shaded areas, a mixed acid-base disorder should be suspected. (From DuBose T Jr: Acid-base disorders. In Brenner BM, Rector FC [eds]: Brenner and Rector's The Kidney, 7th ed. Philadelphia, WB Saunders, 2004, p 938.)

HISTORY AND PHYSICAL EXAMINATION

The history and physical examination should focus on identifying the cause of acidosis as well as any complications related to the severe acidemia (Table 27-2), although the findings are often nonspecific (Tables 27-3 and 27-4). The

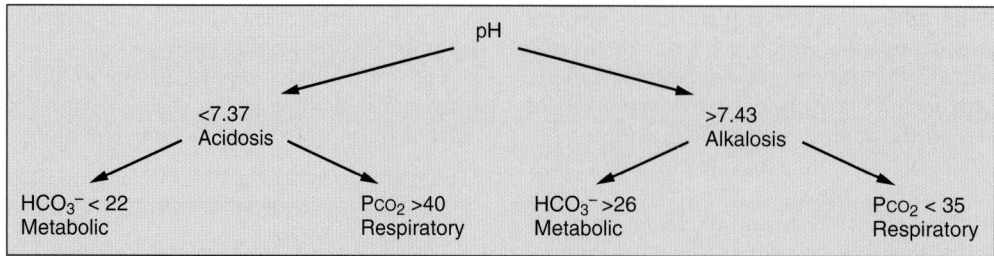

Figure 27-2 Use of arterial blood gas to determine acid-base status.

Table 27-1 Causes of Anion Gap and Non–Anion Gap Metabolic Acidosis

Anion Gap Acidosis
Ketoacidosis
  Diabetic ketoacidosis
  Alcoholic ketoacidosis
  Starvation
Lactic acidosis
  Tissue hypoxia
    Shock
    Dehydration
    Hypoxia
    Carbon monoxide poisoning
  Increased production or decreased clearance of lactate
    Leukemia, lymphoma, large tumors
    Liver or renal failure
Renal failure (especially if GFR <15 mL/min/1.73 m^2; uremia and lactic acidosis)
Toxins or drugs
  High osmolal gap
    Ethylene glycol
    Ethanol
    Methanol
  Normal osmolal gap
    Salicylate
    Paraldehyde
    Toluene inhalation
    Isoniazid
    Iron
    Metformin
Inborn errors of metabolism

Non–Anion Gap Acidosis
Gastrointestinal loss of HCO_3^-
  Diarrhea
  Enteric fistulas (e.g., pancreatic) or enterostomies
  Ureterosigmoidostomy (Cl^-/HCO_3^- exchanger)
  Drugs (e.g., calcium chloride, cholestyramine, magnesium sulfate)
Renal acidosis
  Loss of HCO_3^-
    Proximal RTA (type 2)
    Drugs (e.g., acetazolamide)
  Failure to excrete H^+
    Distal (classic) RTA (type I)
    Drugs (e.g., potassium-sparing diuretics, amphotericin B)
  Decreased ammoniagenesis
    Generalized distal nephron dysfunction (type IV RTA)
    Early and moderate renal insufficiency (GFR 20-50 mL/min/1.73 m^2)
Acid load
  Hyperalimentation
Dilutional
  Rapid saline administration

GFR, glomerular filtration rate; RTA, renal tubular acidosis.

Table 27-2 Major Adverse Consequences of Severe Acidemia

Cardiovascular
  Impairment of cardiac contractility
  Arteriolar dilation, venoconstriction, and centralization of blood volume
  Increased pulmonary vascular resistance
  Reductions in cardiac output, arterial blood pressure, and hepatic and renal blood flow
  Sensitization to reentrant arrhythmias and reduction in threshold of ventricular fibrillation
  Attenuation of cardiovascular responsiveness to catecholamines
Respiratory
  Hyperventilation
  Decreased strength of respiratory muscles and promotion of muscle fatigue
  Dyspnea
Metabolic
  Increased metabolic demands
  Insulin resistance
  Inhibition of anaerobic glycolysis
  Reduction in synthesis of adenosine triphosphate
  Hyperkalemia
  Increased protein degradation
Cerebral
  Inhibition of metabolism and cell volume regulation
  Obtundation and coma

From Adrogue HJ, Madias NE: Management of life-threatening acid-base disorders. N Engl J Med 1998;338:27.

Table 27-3 Elements of a Focused History

Preceding events
  Vomiting, diarrhea
  Fever
  Decreased oral intake
  Changes in urination
  Decreased activity or lethargy
  Changes in respiration
  Rash or edema
  Ingestions or exposures
Past medical history
  Underlying illness (e.g., diabetes, renal disease, metabolic disorder)
  Medications and changes in medications
  Surgical history (e.g., ostomies)
  Developmental and growth history
Family history
  Metabolic disorders
  Renal disease

Table 27-4 Elements of a Directed Physical Examination
Vital signs, including temperature, heart rate, blood pressure, respiratory rate
General
Level of activity (e.g., alert and playful, lethargic, obtunded)
Developmental assessment
Weight and height
Skin
Turgor
Color (pink versus mottled)
Temperature (cool versus warm)
Rash (e.g., petechiae)
Edema (e.g., periorbital, extremity)
Head, eyes, ears, nose, throat
Sunken fontanelle
Pupil size, equality, and reactivity
Sunken eyes
Evidence of tears
Mucous membranes (e.g., moist versus tacky)
Fruity breath
Cardiovascular
Heart rhythm and rate
Extra heart sounds or murmur
Distal pulses
Respiratory
Respiratory rate
Respiratory effort
Rales or evidence of pulmonary edema
Kussmaul breathing
Gastrointestinal
Abdominal tenderness
Ascites
Hepatomegaly

Table 27-5 Initial Laboratory Evaluation for Metabolic Acidosis
Standard
Arterial blood gas
Electrolytes (Na^+, K^+, Cl^-, HCO_3^-)
Blood urea nitrogen, creatinine
Glucose
Urinalysis
Consider urine electrolytes
Based on clinical suspicion
Serum toxicology screen or measurement of specific drug if suspected
Complete blood count
Bacterial cultures
Hepatic enzymes and albumin determinations
Prothrombin time
Screening tests for suspected metabolic disorder (see Table 27-6)
Electrocardiogram

most common cause of metabolic acidosis in children is dehydration.

LABORATORY EVALUATION

Arterial blood gas measurements and electrolytes are the most important initial laboratory tests in making the diagnosis of metabolic acidosis, and a systematic approach can be used to interpret the data (Fig. 27-3). The urgency of obtaining these results depends on whether the patient is showing clinical evidence of severe acidemia or multisystem involvement. As with any critically ill patient, the first priority in management should be stabilizing the ABCs (airway, breathing, and circulation) if necessary. Table 27-5 outlines the initial laboratory evaluation for the workup of a patient with metabolic acidosis.

Arterial blood gas determination is useful in identifying acidosis as well as the degree of acidemia. It can also indicate whether there is appropriate respiratory compensation or if a mixed acid-base disorder exists. Expected respiratory compensation for acute metabolic acidosis can be calculated using the following formulas:

$$PCO_2 \text{ (mm Hg)} = 1.5 \times HCO_3^- \text{ (mEq/L)} + 8 \pm 2$$
$$\downarrow PCO_2 \text{ (mm Hg)} = 1.2 \times \downarrow HCO_3^- \text{ (mEq/L)} \pm 2$$
$$\text{Limit of compensation } PCO_2 = 15 \text{ mm Hg}$$

If the measured PCO_2 is different from the expected PCO_2, it may indicate a mixed acid-base disorder.

A quick way to judge whether the PCO_2 is appropriate is to compare the last two digits of the plasma pH to the PCO_2. In pure metabolic acidosis, they should be equivalent. For example, an arterial pH of 7.25 should result in a PCO_2 of 25.

Electrolytes can be used to calculate the anion gap and the osmolal gap. The pH, specific gravity, and presence of ketones and glucose in the urinalysis might indicate the cause of acidosis. Urine electrolytes can be used to calculate the urinary anion gap or the urinary osmolal gap.

Depending on clinical suspicions about the cause of the acidosis, further studies might be considered. Drug levels can be obtained if there is a history of ingestion or if the examination is suggestive of a toxidrome. The complete blood count may be abnormal in the setting of infection, systemic illness, or malignancy. Elevated liver enzymes and abnormal function test results might indicate hepatic failure. In an infant or toddler with a history of poor growth or development, recurrent vomiting or lethargy, or acidosis or hypoglycemia with illness, a metabolic disorder should be considered, and appropriate screening studies should be performed (Table 27-6). An electrocardiogram should be done if there is evidence of severe acidosis on laboratory evaluation or cardiac involvement on physical examination.

TREATMENT

As in any condition, the first priority in management is stabilizing the ABCs, as necessary.

Management of metabolic acidosis is directed toward treating the underlying cause. In general, treating the causes of anion gap acidosis can regenerate bicarbonate within hours; however, non–anion gap acidosis can take days to resolve and may require exogenous bicarbonate therapy. Insulin, hydration, and electrolyte repletion will correct the acidosis in diabetic ketoacidosis. In addition to treating the underlying condition, lactic acidosis can be resolved by increasing tissue oxygenation using crystalloid, blood products, afterload reduction, inotropic agents (e.g., dopamine,

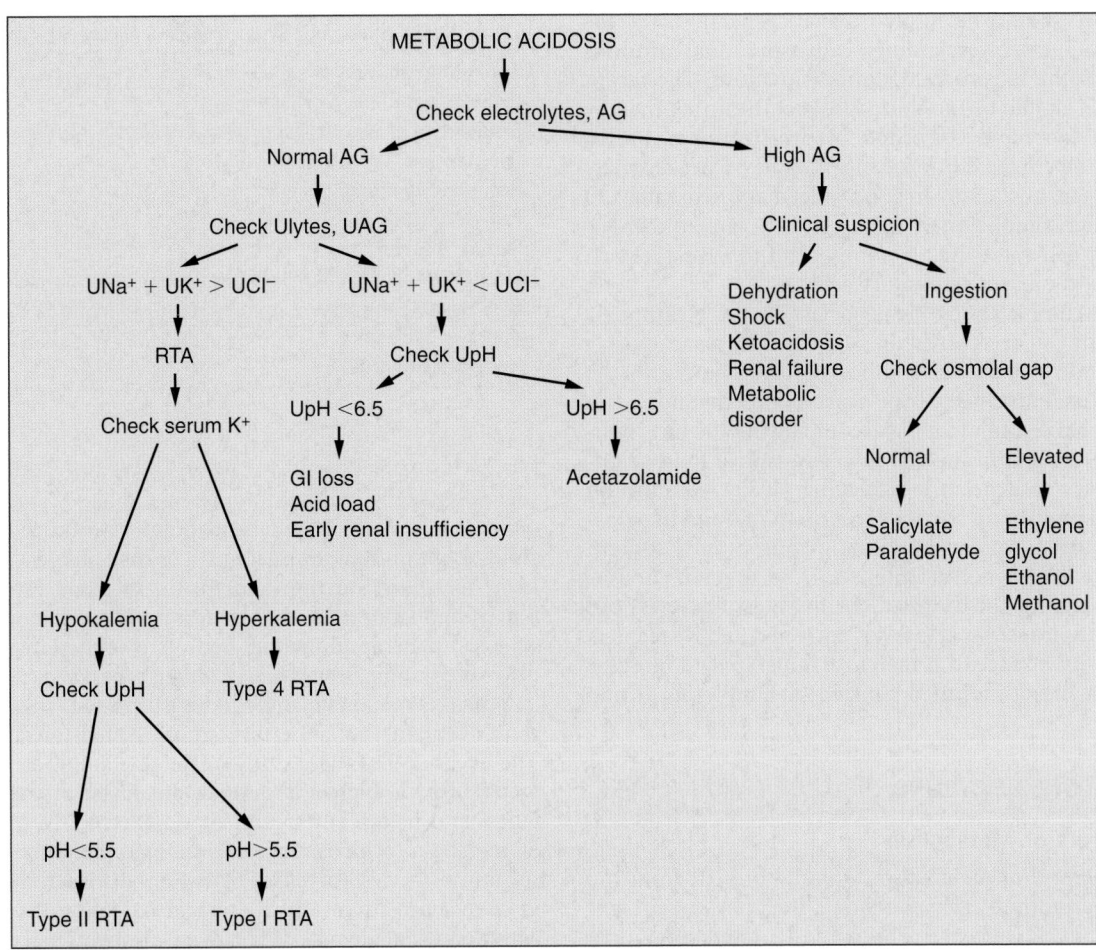

Figure 27-3 Algorithmic approach to a patient with metabolic acidosis. AG, anion gap; GI, gastrointestinal; RTA, renal tubular acidosis; U, urinary.

Table 27-6 Laboratory Studies for Suspected Inborn Error of Metabolism

Blood
 Complete blood count with differential
 Blood gas
 Serum electrolytes
 Glucose
 Ammonia, lactate, and pyruvate
 Amino acid quantification
 Acylcarnitine profile
 Free and total carnitine
Urine
 Urinalysis, including ketones
 Organic acids
 Acylglycines

dobutamine), and oxygen. Renal failure might require dialysis. Ethylene glycol and methanol ingestion can be treated with fomepizole, ethanol, and hemodialysis. Management of salicylate ingestion may include repeated doses of activated charcoal, alkalization of urine to optimize excretion, correction of metabolic derangements such as hypoglycemia and hypokalemia, and hemodialysis for severe ingestion. The guiding principle in treating acidosis secondary to metabolic disorders is to reverse counterregulation and tissue catabolism with appropriate energy substrate. Diarrhea can be managed with fluid and electrolyte repletion. Bicarbonate supplementation and management of calcium and potassium homeostasis are effective in managing RTA, regardless of type.

Sodium bicarbonate infusion is warranted in cases of acute, severe acidemia (pH <7.2 or HCO_3^- <8 mEq/L) to stabilize the myocardium and prevent serious complications (see Table 27-2). If the serum K^+ is less than 3 mEq/L or the ionized calcium (Ca^{2+}) is suspected to be abnormally low, potassium and calcium should be administered along with bicarbonate. Acidemia maintains serum K^+ and ionized Ca^{2+} values at high levels; therefore, correction of acidosis without repletion of potassium and calcium can further decrease these critically low levels.

The goal of bicarbonate therapy is to increase the pH to approximately 7.2 to 7.25 and the serum HCO_3^- to 10 to 12 mEq/L. When administering sodium bicarbonate, one must consider not only the dose but also the rate of correction of acidosis. The dose is dependent on the volume of bicarbonate distribution. In health or mild to moderate acidosis (pH 7.2 to 7.37), this volume is 20% to 50% of body weight in liters. In severe acidosis, this volume is often greater than 50% of body weight in liters; it can even be 100% in severe lactic acidosis. As a first step, the bicarbonate deficit in severe acidosis can be calculated by the following equation:

$$HCO_3^- \text{ deficit (mEq)} = [HCO_{3\ desired}^- \text{ (mEq/L)} -$$
$$HCO_{3\ actual}^- \text{ (mEq/L)}] \times \text{Weight (kg)} \times 0.5 \text{ L/kg}$$

The dose should be infused slowly, generally over the course of minutes or even hours, with more rapid infusions reserved for the most urgent clinical situations. The serum HCO_3^- level should be monitored frequently during therapy to prevent too rapid correction or overtreatment and to determine whether additional bicarbonate is needed. The clinical effects of therapy may be judged approximately 30 minutes after completion of the infusion. Because bicarbonate therapy generates CO_2, it is important to have adequate ventilation to prevent respiratory acidosis.

Certain complications are associated with bicarbonate therapy. One can overcorrect the acidosis and create a poorly tolerated state of alkalosis. Volume overload can occur in the setting of renal insufficiency or heart failure, due in part to the additional sodium loading accompanying the bicarbonate. Rapid correction can lead to cerebrospinal fluid acidosis secondary to a delay in achieving HCO_3^- equilibrium across the blood-brain barrier. Hypernatremia and hyperosmolality can be avoided by diluting concentrated sodium bicarbonate in 25% normal saline or D5W to render an isotonic solution. As noted earlier, serum potassium levels can decline precipitously as acidosis is corrected and K^+ reenters the intracellular space. It is therefore imperative to monitor electrolytes and, if indicated, ionized calcium levels during therapy.

SPECIAL CONSIDERATIONS

Inborn Errors of Metabolism

Inborn errors of metabolism typically present from the neonatal period into early childhood, but they can present later, even in adolescence. The clinical presentation of a metabolic disorder may be nonspecific and is sometimes mistaken for another illness, such as sepsis. Signs and symptoms suggesting a metabolic disorder are listed in Table 27-7.

A child with a metabolic disorder may come to medical attention in several ways. State-mandated newborn screening often detects certain metabolic disorders before babies are even symptomatic. The caveat is that each state tests for a limited number of metabolic disorders, and false-negative results may occur if the test is done too early (e.g., within 24 hours of life) or before the baby is feeding well. A child might also present to the primary pediatrician with a history of

Table 27-7 Signs and Symptoms of a Metabolic Disorder
Severe presentation of simple illness
Lethargy with illness or fasting
Irritability
Poor feeding
Recurrent vomiting
Failure to thrive
Seizure disorder
Loss of developmental milestones or developmental delay
Hypotonia
Apnea or tachypnea
Hepatosplenomegaly

suggestive signs and symptoms (see Table 27-7), and the pediatrician might pursue a laboratory workup. Finally, a child might present to urgent care or the emergency department for the evaluation and treatment of an intercurrent illness, and laboratory abnormalities such as hypoglycemia, acidosis, hyperammonemia, or liver dysfunction might be discovered, indicating a metabolic disorder.

When a metabolic disorder is suspected, the clinician should obtain the laboratory studies listed in Table 27-6. The likelihood of these studies detecting an inborn error of metabolism is higher if samples are taken at the time of illness and before any treatment is delivered. In the setting of metabolic acidosis, hypoketotic hypoglycemia is highly suggestive of a fatty acid oxidation disorder. Hyperammonemia can occur with fatty acid oxidation disorders or with organic acidemias. When lactate levels are elevated, the clinician can calculate the lactate-to-pyruvate ratio. Lactate elevation out of proportion to pyruvate elevation, yielding an increased lactate-to-pyruvate ratio, is most consistent with a mitochondrial disorder. Hypoglycemia in the setting of an elevated lactate level but normal lactate-to-pyruvate ratio suggests a defect in gluconeogenesis, whereas normoglycemia in the setting of an elevated lactate level but normal lactate-to-pyruvate ratio suggests a disorder of pyruvate metabolism (e.g., pyruvate carboxylase deficiency or pyruvate dehydrogenase deficiency) (Fig. 27-4). Other than severe acidosis, the initial laboratory results for organic acidemias are variable; therefore, diagnosis is based on the

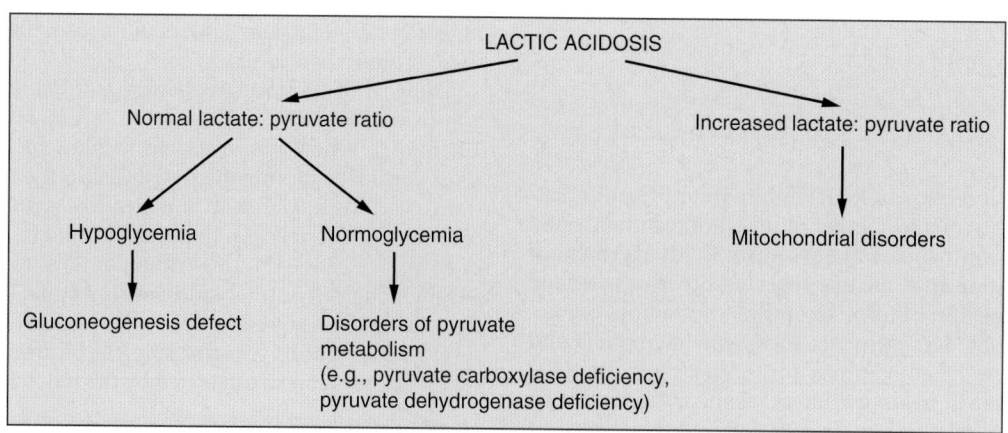

Figure 27-4 Preliminary algorithm for a suspected metabolic disorder in the presence of metabolic acidosis.

characteristic pattern of urine organic acids and urine acylglycines.

Because clinical manifestations occur secondary to toxic metabolites formed during tissue catabolism, the general principle of therapy in cases of a suspected metabolic disorder is to reverse counterregulation and tissue catabolism and to promote an anabolic state. This is done by meeting the body's metabolic needs with energy substrates that can be safely used by the patient. For example, in cases of suspected organic acidemia or a fatty acid oxidation disorder, this can be accomplished by correcting existing hypoglycemia with a bolus of 0.25 to 0.5 g/kg dextrose and then providing basal glucose needs at 10 mg/kg per minute. Practically, this can be accomplished with a 10% dextrose solution at a rate of 1.5 times maintenance or its enteral equivalent. Other methods of lowering counterregulatory hormones include ensuring an adequate circulating volume, controlling vomiting, recognizing and treating any infection or precipitating event, aggressively treating fever, and minimizing pain, stress, and agitation.

Severe presentations of metabolic disorders may require stabilization of the ABCs, correction of severe acidosis, and enhanced excretion or removal of toxic metabolites.

Respiratory Acidosis

Respiratory acidosis is an abnormal clinical process that causes the arterial P_{CO_2} to increase to greater than 40 mm Hg. Increased CO_2 concentration in the blood may be secondary to increased CO_2 production or decreased ventilation. For example, administration of bicarbonate (which the body converts to CO_2) without adequate ventilation can result in respiratory acidosis. Decreased ventilation can result from depressed central respiratory drive, abnormalities in the chest wall or respiratory muscles, or alveolar hypoventilation. Table 27-8 describes some clinical scenarios in which respiratory acidosis can occur. When it does occur, cellular buffering begins within minutes. Renal compensation is optimized in 3 to 5 days.

The history and physical examination should focus on assessing the severity of respiratory symptoms, detecting consequences of acidemia, and identifying the underlying cause. The clinician should elicit any history of trauma, ingestion, or preceding illness, as well as any pertinent past medical history (e.g., severity of asthma exacerbations). The patient's general appearance, mental status, respiratory effort and drive, and cardiovascular examination are particularly relevant. If suspected, one should also look for toxidromes.

The arterial blood gas should be measured. A low pH and high P_{CO_2} indicate respiratory acidosis. For every 10 mm Hg increase in P_{CO_2}, the pH is expected to decrease by 0.08. Expected metabolic compensation for acute respiratory acidosis can be calculated using the following rule: for every 10 mm Hg increase in P_{CO_2}, serum HCO_3^- is expected to increase by 1 mEq/L (limit of compensation HCO_3^- = 38 mEq/L). If the pH or measured HCO_3^- is different from what was expected, a mixed acid-base disorder may be present. The partial pressure of oxygen (P_{O_2}) is useful in assessing oxygenation in the setting of inadequate ventilation. In some situations, it may be useful to calculate the alveolar-arterial P_{O_2} gradient (A-a gradient):

Table 27-8 Clinical Scenarios Causing Respiratory Acidosis

Acute central nervous system depression
  Drug overdose
    Benzodiazepines
    Narcotics
    Barbiturates
  Head trauma
  Cerebrovascular accident
  Central nervous system infection
Acute neuromuscular disease
  Guillain-Barré syndrome
  Spinal cord injury
  Myasthenia gravis
  Toxin mediated (e.g., botulism, tetanus)
Acute pleural or chest wall disease
  Pneumothorax
  Hemothorax
  Flail chest
  Weakness secondary to electrolyte disturbances
    (hypophosphatemia, hypomagnesemia, hypokalemia)
Acute airway disease
  Status asthmaticus
  Upper airway obstruction
Acute parenchymal and vascular disease
  Cardiogenic pulmonary edema
  Acute lung injury
  Multilobar pneumonia
  Massive pulmonary embolism
  Severe pneumonitis

From Epstein SK, Singh N: Respiratory acidosis. Respir Care 2001;46:368.

$$\text{A-a gradient (mm Hg)} = F_{IO_2} \times (P_{atm} - P_{H_2O}) - P_{aCO_2}/RQ - P_{aO_2},$$

where P_{atm} at sea level is 760 mm Hg, P_{H_2O} is 47 mm Hg; F_{IO_2} in room air is 0.21, and RQ is usually 0.8 (see Chapter 38).

Normally, an A-a gradient is less than 15 mm Hg in adults; in children, the upper limit of normal is often estimated as follows: (age/4) + 4. A higher than expected gradient suggests intrinsic lung disease, whereas a lower gradient may point toward hypoventilation from a neurologic or muscular cause. The arterial blood gas results should be considered in the context of the clinical picture. For example, a normal P_{CO_2} in a patient with increased work of breathing and tachypnea may indicate relative hypoventilation and signify impending respiratory fatigue. If available, an end-tidal CO_2 monitor can be helpful in following P_{CO_2} and detecting any significant change.

In addition to arterial blood gas, one should consider a chest radiograph, toxicology screen, electrolytes, lumbar puncture, and head computed tomography, based on clinical suspicion.

Acute respiratory acidosis can be a medical emergency that may require emergent intubation and mechanical ventilation. Otherwise, the underlying disease is treated, and supportive care is provided as necessary. The airway should be assessed and optimized, and oxygen should be administered if the patient is hypoxemic. If the patient is unable to ventilate or oxygenate adequately, or if respiratory acidosis is severe, mechanical ventilation with continuous positive airway pressure, bilevel positive airway pressure (BiPAP), or intubation may be necessary. It is important not to correct acidosis too quickly if prolonged hypercapnia is suspected. Rapid correction can cause cerebrospinal fluid alkalization, which can result in seizures. Medications that suppress respiratory drive, such as narcotics, should be avoided until adequate assistance with ventilation is in place. Electrolytes, particularly phosphate, magnesium, and potassium, should be maintained within normal ranges to optimize respiratory muscle function. Bicarbonate is not typically used to treat respiratory acidosis because it generates more CO_2. However, if there are clinical manifestations of severe acidemia (see Table 27-2) and ventilation is controlled, bicarbonate therapy can be considered.

ACKNOWLEDGMENT

Special thanks to Michael Somers, MD.

SUGGESTED READING

Adrogue HJ, Madias NE: Management of life-threatening acid-base disorders: First of two parts. N Engl J Med 1998;338:26-34.

Burton B: Inborn errors of metabolism in infancy: A guide to diagnosis. Pediatrics 1998;102:e69.

Chan J, Mak R: Acid-base homeostasis. In Avner E, Harmon W, Niaudet P (eds): Pediatric Nephrology, 5th ed. Philadelphia, Lippincott Williams & Wilkins, 2004, pp 189-208.

Cronan K, Norman M: Renal and electrolyte emergencies. In Fleisher G, Ludwig S (eds): Textbook of Pediatric Emergency Medicine, 4th ed. Philadelphia, Lippincott Williams & Wilkins, 2000, pp 828-832.

DuBose T Jr: Acid-base disorders. In Brenner BM, Rector FC (eds): Brenner and Rector's The Kidney, 7th ed. Philadelphia, WB Saunders, 2004, pp 921-996.

Epstein SK, Singh N: Respiratory acidosis. Respir Care 2001;46:366-383.

Gluck S: Acid-base. Lancet 1998;352:474-479.

Haber R: A practical approach to acid-base disorders. West J Med 1991;155:146-151.

Schwaderer A, Schwartz G: Acidosis and alkalosis. Pediatr Rev 2004;25:350-357.

REFERENCE

1. Haber R: A practical approach to acid-base disorders. West J Med 1991;155:146-151.

CHAPTER 28

Altered Mental Status

Daniel J. Lebovitz

From mild confusion to complete unconsciousness, the presentation of a patient with altered mental status is almost as diverse as the possible underlying causes. Although coma is easy to recognize, the more subtle behavioral clues, such as changes in feeding habits, irritability, lethargy, and a child who "just doesn't act right," present more of a challenge. These subtle changes could indicate the beginning of a process that is impairing the normal function of the central nervous system and may lead to deterioration and a life-threatening situation.

The responsibility of the treating physician is to recognize the condition and initiate treatment in an unstable or deteriorating patient and to detect subtle changes in a stable patient by obtaining a focused history and performing a complete physical examination and laboratory evaluation. Subsequently, in a stable patient, the physician needs to select appropriate interventions to prevent further deterioration.

Efficient diagnosis and management require a familiarity with (1) the vocabulary, pathophysiology, and assessment tools used to evaluate altered mental status; (2) the acute common interventions needed in many situations; and (3) an approach to diagnosing the underlying cause for ultimate specific therapeutic intervention.

DEFINITIONS

Consciousness. A state of awareness of oneself and one's environment.[1,2]

Altered Mental Status. Any situation in which the normal state of consciousness is altered or absent.

Alert. Normal state of arousal.

Lethargy. State of minimally reduced wakefulness, with the primary defect being a lack of attention. The patient has difficulty focusing, is intermittently drowsy, and has some faulty memory.

Obtundation. Mild or moderate blunting of alertness, with decreased interest in the environment. Communication is somewhat preserved.

Stupor. State similar to a deep sleep from which the patient is only partially and temporarily arousable with vigorous and repeated stimulation. Communication is minimal or absent.

Coma. State of unarousable unresponsiveness. There are no spontaneous movements, the eyes are closed, and the patient is unable to speak; he or she may have the ability to withdraw from painful stimuli nonspecifically.

PATHOPHYSIOLOGY

Conscious behavior requires both a level of arousal and awareness of the environment. Arousal, a state of alertness or wakefulness, is dependent on the arousal system in the ascending reticular activating system (ARAS), also known as the sleep center. The anatomic location of the ARAS system is thought to be an array of nuclei and tracts extending from the medulla through the tegmentum of the pons and midbrain, continuous caudally with the reticular intermediate gray lamina of the spinal cord and rostrally with the subthalamus, hypothalamus, and thalamus. The specifics of communication to the cortex are unclear, but there appear to be both direct pathways from the reticular formations and indirect pathways through the thalamus-hypothalamus.[1] A simplistic analogy is the "lightbulb-switch" model, where the ARAS is the switch (arousal) and the cerebral hemispheres the lightbulb (awareness). If the ARAS is not working properly, the cerebral hemispheres do not have the opportunity to function properly, representing altered arousability. Conversely, if the ARAS is working properly but both cerebral hemispheres are dysfunctional, this represents altered awareness. Both these systems must be functional to achieve normal consciousness.[3]

INITIAL STABILIZATION

Paramount in the treatment of a patient with altered mental status is remembering that this is a potentially life-threatening emergency. Initial care must focus on minimizing or preventing permanent brain injury from potentially reversible causes while obtaining necessary information from the history and physical examination to determine the underlying cause and thus focus the treatment.

The initial treatment of the patient should occur coincidentally with the initial historical and diagnostic investigation. Subsequent acute management decisions are based on a reevaluation of the patient's clinical response to the initial interventions.

The physical examination includes a rapid overview of the patient, with a focus on derangements of the vital signs and an evaluation of the ABCDs of resuscitation (airway, breathing, circulation, dextrose/disability). Following the initial evaluation and stabilization, a systems-based approach is used for the remainder of the evaluation.

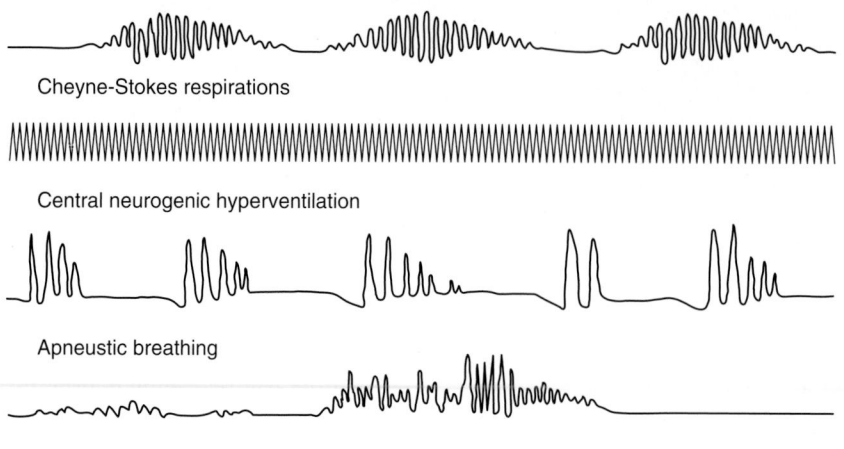

Figure 28-1 Abnormal breathing patterns.

Airway

The patient's ability to maintain a stable, open airway and adequate respiratory drive is assessed. This assessment should differentiate among a clear airway, an airway that is maintainable with positioning, and an airway that is not maintainable. The airway may be compromised by a primary anatomic abnormality or secondarily due to neurologic compromise.

Breathing

The respiratory rate, respiratory effort, and respiratory mechanics are evaluated. Breath sounds should be clearly audible, with good air exchange and chest excursion in all fields. There should be no significant grunting, flaring, or retractions. Increased respiratory drive to hyperventilate, with either a high respiratory rate or deep breathing, is most likely due to hypoxemia, respiratory compensation for metabolic acidosis, or neurogenic hyperventilation, which is seen with increased intracranial pressure or brainstem lesions. Slow, inadequate respirations indicate toxic ingestion or may be a late sign of increased intracranial hypertension (Cushing's triad).[4] The respiratory pattern should also be noted; certain respiratory patterns are identified with specific causes (Fig. 28-1).[3,5]

- Cheyne-Stokes: Hyperpnea in a crescendo-decrescendo pattern followed by apnea is seen in bilateral hemispheric disease, hypertensive encephalopathy, cerebral hypoxia, and metabolic conditions.
- Central neurogenic hyperventilation: Sustained rapid, deep respirations may occur with lesions in the pons.
- Apneustic breathing: End-inspiratory pauses alternating with end-expiratory pauses are seen with damage to the pons.
- Ataxic breathing: A completely irregular pattern may progress to apnea; this is seen with damage to the respiratory centers of the medulla.

Oxygen saturation measured by pulse oximeter should be maintained above 95%. It may be necessary to provide supplemental oxygen via nasal cannula, facemask, or hood to achieve the desired saturation.

Indications for intubation and mechanical ventilation include (1) any compromise during evaluation of the airway or lack of adequate protective airway reflexes, (2) inability to maintain adequate oxygen saturation despite supplemental oxygen, or (3) a Glasgow Coma Scale score of 8 or lower on the initial evaluation or a rapidly declining Glasgow Coma Scale score or deteriorating neurologic condition on serial examinations (Table 28-1).[6]

Intubation, when needed, should be performed using the rapid-sequence technique. If there is a possibility of spinal cord injury, the neck should be placed midline in a cervical spine collar until a spinal cord injury can be ruled out. Gaining access to the airway should take place with the neck stabilized.

Table 28-1	Glasgow Coma Scale	
Activity	Scoring	Pediatric Modification
Eye opening	4 Spontaneous 3 To voice 2 To pain 1 No response	None
Verbal response	5 Oriented and appropriate 4 Disoriented conversation 3 Inappropriate words 2 Incomprehensible sounds 1 No response	5 Coos, babbles 4 Cries irritably 3 Cries to pain 2 Moans to pain 1 None
Motor response	6 Obeys commands 5 Localizes pain 4 Flexion withdrawal 3 Decorticate posturing 2 Decerebrate posturing 1 No response	6 Normal spontaneous, purposeful movement 5 Withdraws to touch 4 Withdraws to pain 3 Abnormal flexion 2 Extensor response 1 None

Table 28-2 Minimally Acceptable Systolic Blood Pressure

Age	Minimum Systolic Blood Pressure* (mm Hg)
0 to 1 mo	60
>1 mo to 1 yr	70
1 to 10 yr	70 + (2 × age in yr)
>10 yr	90

*5th percentile.

Table 28-4 Interpretation of Glasgow Coma Scale Score in the Setting of Head Injury

Score	Interpretation
13-15	Minor head injury
9-12	Moderate head injury
≤8	Severe head injury or coma with significant risk of mortality

After intubation, hyperventilation (carbon dioxide partial pressure <35) should be avoided because it may lead to inadequate cerebral blood flow and oxygen delivery to the brain.[7] With the artificial airway secured, a nasogastric tube for gastric decompression is placed, further decreasing the likelihood of regurgitation or aspiration and providing access to the stomach for lavage or decontamination as indicated.

Circulatory System

Rapid assessment of the patient's hemodynamic status includes evaluation of the heart rate, presence of cardiac murmur, blood pressure, pulse quality in both a central and a peripheral site, skin temperature in the core and periphery, and capillary refill. The heart rate and blood pressure are evaluated in comparison to the normal ranges for the child's age by consulting standard tables. Minimally acceptable systolic blood pressures by age are given in Table 28-2.[8]

Heart rate and blood pressure abnormalities may be indicators of different problems. A high heart rate and low blood pressure may indicate decreased intravascular blood volume from dehydration, sepsis syndrome, cardiogenic dysfunction, or inadequate oxygen delivery. Adequate volume resuscitation should be provided with isotonic fluid boluses (10 to 20 mL/kg) until hemodynamic stability has been achieved. A low heart rate and high blood pressure may indicate increased intracranial pressure (Cushing's triad of hypertension, bradyarrhythmias, and agonal respirations).[4] Other causes of bradycardia may include hypoxemia, hypothermia, and myocardial injury. Tachyarrhythmias may be seen with hypovolemia, fever, or infection. Hypotension is a late finding in septic shock and can be seen with drug ingestion, myocardial injury or disease, and adrenal insufficiency. Hypertension may be a primary abnormality responsible for

Table 28-3 Reed Scale for the Clinical Assessment of Consciousness

Grade	Description
0	Asleep, arousable, answers questions
1	Comatose, withdraws from painful stimuli, intact reflexes
2	Comatose, does not withdraw from painful stimuli, no respiratory or circulatory depression, intact reflexes
3	Comatose, absent reflexes, no circulatory or respiratory depression
4	Comatose, absent reflexes, respiratory or circulatory problems

hypertensive encephalopathy or may be a compensatory response to maintain adequate oxygen delivery in a patient with increased intracranial pressure or a stroke.

Dextrose

Hypoglycemia is a well-known cause of altered mental status. During the initial resuscitation, a bedside serum glucose measurement should be obtained, because prolonged hypoglycemia may lead to irreversible brain injury. If no rapid test is available, empirical treatment with glucose should be initiated. The possibility of transient hyperglycemia from incorrect presumptive treatment is less likely to adversely affect the patient than is a prolonged hypoglycemic state. The treatment of hypoglycemia (blood glucose <60, or <80 with an abnormal neurologic examination) consists of 0.5 to 1 g/kg of intravenous dextrose.

Disability

The need for a more uniform nomenclature to describe the extent of a patient's altered neurologic function has led to the development of a number of different scoring systems. These scoring systems share the advantages of rapid assessment, ease of use, and good interrater reliability. The simplest is the AVPU evaluation tool, which is widely taught in the Pediatric Advanced Life Support courses of the American Heart Association.[8] The tool is named for the key functions it rates: Awake, responsive to Voice, responsive to Pain, or Unresponsive. An alternative is the Reed scale for the clinical assessment of consciousness (Table 28-3).[5]

By far, the most commonly used scoring system is the Glasgow Coma Scale. This evaluation tool yields a score from 3 (worst) to 15 (best) based on a patient's best response to stimuli in three categories: eye opening, verbal response, and motor response. Initially developed in Scotland in 1974 to evaluate adult patients with traumatic brain injury, it has been used to evaluate any circumstance of altered mental status and has been adapted for use in infants and children (see Table 28-1).[9] Table 28-4 provides an interpretation of the Glasgow Coma Scale score in patients with head injury.

The widespread use of these tools has allowed better communication between health care workers and has served as a basis for the study of the treatment of patients with similar neurologic states of altered consciousness.

A general neurologic assessment of disability should include an evaluation of level of consciousness and pupillary size and responsiveness to light. In a patient with altered mental status, a pupillary evaluation is easy to do and provides helpful information. If the pupils are reactive to light, the cause of the altered mental status is likely toxic or metabolic. Miosis, or pupillary constriction, is seen with sympathetic paralysis or parasympathetic excess. With extreme miosis, it may be difficult to see reactivity unless a very bright light is used with a magnifying glass. If reactivity is present, drugs may be responsible—recalled by the mnemonic COPS[10]:

- Cholinergics/clonidine
- Opiates/organophosphates
- Phenothiazines/pilocarpine
- Sedative-hypnotics (benzodiazepines)

Mydriasis is a response to excess sympathetic stimulation or paralysis of the parasympathetic system. Bilaterally dilated but reactive pupils are also indicative of drug intoxication or exposure, and the likely agents can be remembered by the mnemonic AAAS:

- Anticholinergics/atropine
- Antihistamines
- Antidepressants (tricyclic antidepressants)
- Sympathomimetics (cocaine, amphetamines)

When one or both pupils are not reactive to light, this suggests a structural cause leading to increased intracranial pressure and compression of cranial nerve III.[3,7] Immediate institution of neuroprotective therapies for intracranial pressure and computed tomography evaluation of the head should occur, along with a call to an intensivist and neurosurgeon. Anisocoria is also suggestive of a structural abnormality, unless it is associated with exposure to a dilating drug in a single eye. The pupillary response to both light and ocular movements allowing conjugate gaze may provide some indication of where the problem lies, due to the close proximity of these brainstem reflex pathways to the ARAS. Preservation of these reflexes implies an intact ARAS pathway and therefore a likely cerebral hemispheric problem, whereas loss of either of these reflexes implies involvement of the ARAS pathways.[3,9]

Exposure and Environment

Hypothermia is most often seen with ingestions during the colder months of the year and is typically secondary to exposure to the outdoors. Other causes of hypothermia include near drowning, some presentations of severe sepsis (usually in very young patients or late in the course of sepsis), and some drug overdoses, especially sedative-hypnotics. Prolonged exposure to a cool environment in the emergency department or a doctor's office during evaluation places a patient at risk for the development of iatrogenic hypothermia. Hypothermia should be avoided and treated by the use of an overhead heating system, warm blankets, or a similar device. The initial goal should be temperature of approximately 35°C. Severe hypothermia, if left untreated, may lead to cardiac arrhythmias (see Ch. 186).

Hyperthermia is most likely the result of infection, although extreme intracranial hemorrhage, anticholinergic drugs, and heatstroke must be considered, especially with a core temperature of greater than 40°C.[2]

HISTORY

After the patient has been stabilized with the ABCD approach, a focused history and physical examination may provide additional information about the cause of the altered mental status. Direct information from an eyewitness to recent events should be obtained, if possible. Most often, the parent or caretaker is helpful. Questions to be considered are the following:

1. Has this deterioration been a slow progression or an acute, unexpected event? An accurate time sequence may lead to a specific cause. Especially important are the circumstances immediately preceding the altered mental status. Sudden, rapid deterioration to coma in a previously awake, alert patient makes the diagnosis of convulsion, arrhythmia, or intracranial hemorrhage more likely. Slow progression from a normal state to sleepiness, unsteadiness, and then unresponsiveness in a previously healthy child may indicate ingestion of a drug or toxin.
2. Has the deterioration been accompanied by fever or a recent illness? If so, an infectious or postinfectious cause may be implicated.
3. Is there a history of trauma? If there is a vague or no history of trauma yet obvious, unexplained signs of physical injury, shaken baby syndrome or child abuse must be considered and investigated.
4. Is there a recent history of travel? If so, to where? Travel may suggest an indigenous infection not typically considered in the differential diagnosis in the local area.
5. Is there a history of headaches? If so, how long have the headaches been present, and when during the day or night do they occur? Where on the head is the pain focused? What is the duration? Is there an associated aura, such as that which occurs with migraines? Is there a family history of migraines?
6. Are there any underlying acute or chronic illnesses? Does the patient take any chronic medicines? Have there been any recent surgeries? Does the child have access to the medications of others or to poisons?
7. Does the patient have pica, which might suggest lead or other heavy metal poisoning?
8. Is there history of polyuria or polydipsia to suggest diabetes?
9. Is this the first episode like this, or have there been others?

PHYSICAL EXAMINATION

The examination of the head begins with a search for signs of trauma. The presence of a cephalhematoma, lacerations, bulging fontanelle, or bruising may provide keys to the diagnosis of cranial trauma. Blood or clear fluid leaking from the nose, mouth, or ears or trapped behind the tympanic membrane may suggest a basilar skull fracture. Bruises characteristic of abuse should be searched for, especially in a child 2 years old or younger. Retinal examination for hemorrhages is necessary, but the use of eye drops that alter the pupillary response to light should be avoided if an assessment of pupillary reactivity will be performed.

The neck examination includes an evaluation for nuchal rigidity and thyromegaly. The presence of nuchal rigidity in a febrile patient indicates possible meningitis or meningoencephalitis.

If there is a potential for traumatic injury, the neck should be stabilized with a hard collar of the appropriate size until the issue of spinal cord or neck trauma is resolved; evaluation for nuchal rigidity should be temporarily deferred.

Table 28-5 Common Causes of Structural and Medical Alterations of Mental Status

Cause	Examples
Structural*	
Trauma	Concussion, contusion, intracranial hemorrhage (subdural, epidural, intraparenchymal), cerebral edema, shaken baby syndrome, traumatic brain injury
Vascular disease	Arteriovenous malformation, aneurysm, other congenital vascular dysplasias, stroke, embolism, trauma to carotid or vertebral arteries in the neck
Neoplasm	Tumor
Hydrocephalus, focal infection	Empyema, abscess, cerebritis
Medical	Hypoglycemia, electrolyte abnormality, infection (bacterial, viral, rickettsial, acute demyelinating encephalomyelitis), toxin, poison, substance abuse, hypertension, renal failure, child abuse, hypoxemia, metabolic disorder (inborn, acquired), hypoxic-ischemic injury, epilepsy, hemorrhagic shock and encephalopathy, hemolytic uremic syndrome, abdominal pathology (including intussusception), migraine, psychological, vitamin deficiency

*Structural causes that involve the ascending reticular activating system (ARAS) pathway may present with or develop the need for emergent surgical decompression. The anatomic location of the abnormality may assist in determining the need for decompression. Lesions involving a single cerebral hemisphere are unlikely to alter level of consciousness unless there is a coincidental lesion affecting the other hemisphere or the process in one hemisphere results in increased intracranial pressure on the contralateral side of the brain. This is not the case if the lesion involves the brainstem in areas that disrupt the ARAS pathways.[2,3] ADEM, acute disseminated encephalomyelitis.

A skin examination for rashes, bruises, needle tracks, or any abnormal pigmentation should be performed as a clue to trauma, drug use or abuse, systemic infections such as meningococcemia or rickettsial diseases, or an underlying disease associated with intracranial tumors such as neurofibromatosis or tuberous sclerosis.

The patient should be evaluated for abnormal odor from the mouth. This could indicate diabetic ketoacidosis if the odor is sweet and fruity, cyanide poisoning if almond scented, or the ingestion of alcohol or insecticides. Other unusual body odors may suggest inborn errors of metabolism.

Abdominal examination for intra-abdominal pathology, including intussusception, tumor, or hepatomegaly, should be done. Rectal examination, including stool for guaiac, should be done as well.[11]

DIFFERENTIAL DIAGNOSIS

The differential diagnosis for altered mental status in a pediatric patient is extensive. One approach is to first divide the causes into two large categories—structural causes and medical (toxic, infectious, metabolic) causes (Fig. 28-2).

Structural causes are those that lead to altered mental status as a result of compression or dysfunction of the ARAS (including cerebral or brainstem herniation); purely medical causes are more likely to lead to bihemispheric cerebral dysfunction.[3] The most common structural and medical causes of altered mental status are listed in Table 28-5. It is important to recall that in some cases a combination of structural and medical causes may be responsible for the clinical condition. For example, a hypertensive patient may have a hemorrhagic or ischemic stroke. Appropriate laboratory and diagnostic studies to determine the cause of altered mental status are listed in Table 28-6. If there is no concern about an intracranial space-occupying lesion, a diagnostic spinal tap, with measurement of opening and closing pressure, may be performed. If the possibility of an intracranial mass exists,

Table 28-6 Diagnostic Studies in Patients with Altered Mental Status

Glucose, sodium, potassium, chloride, bicarbonate, calcium, phosphorus, urea nitrogen, creatinine, magnesium, serum osmolality, liver function
Serum ammonia (if high, workup for metabolic abnormality)
Complete blood count
Arterial blood gas
If metabolic acidosis is present, serum ketones, lactic acid
Co-oximetry for carbon monoxide poisoning, methemoglobinemia
Directed drug levels (e.g., barbiturates)
Serum toxicology screen
Urinalysis
Urine toxicology screen
Cerebral spinal fluid: cell count, Gram stain, glucose, protein
Electrocardiogram
Computed tomography of head, abdomen
Chest radiograph
Cerebral spine radiographs (if trauma considered)
Stool guaiac
Electroencephalogram

the spinal tap may be deferred until a head computed tomography scan is obtained. Regardless of the diagnostic approach, if there is suspicion of meningitis, the administration of broad-spectrum antibiotics should not be delayed.

Another effective approach to diagnosis is the use of two mnemonics (AEIOU and TIPS) to ascertain the origin of a patient's altered mental status (Table 28-7).

CONCLUSION

A patient presenting with altered mental status presents a diagnostic conundrum to the treating physician. Initial treatment with the ABCDs of resuscitation must occur

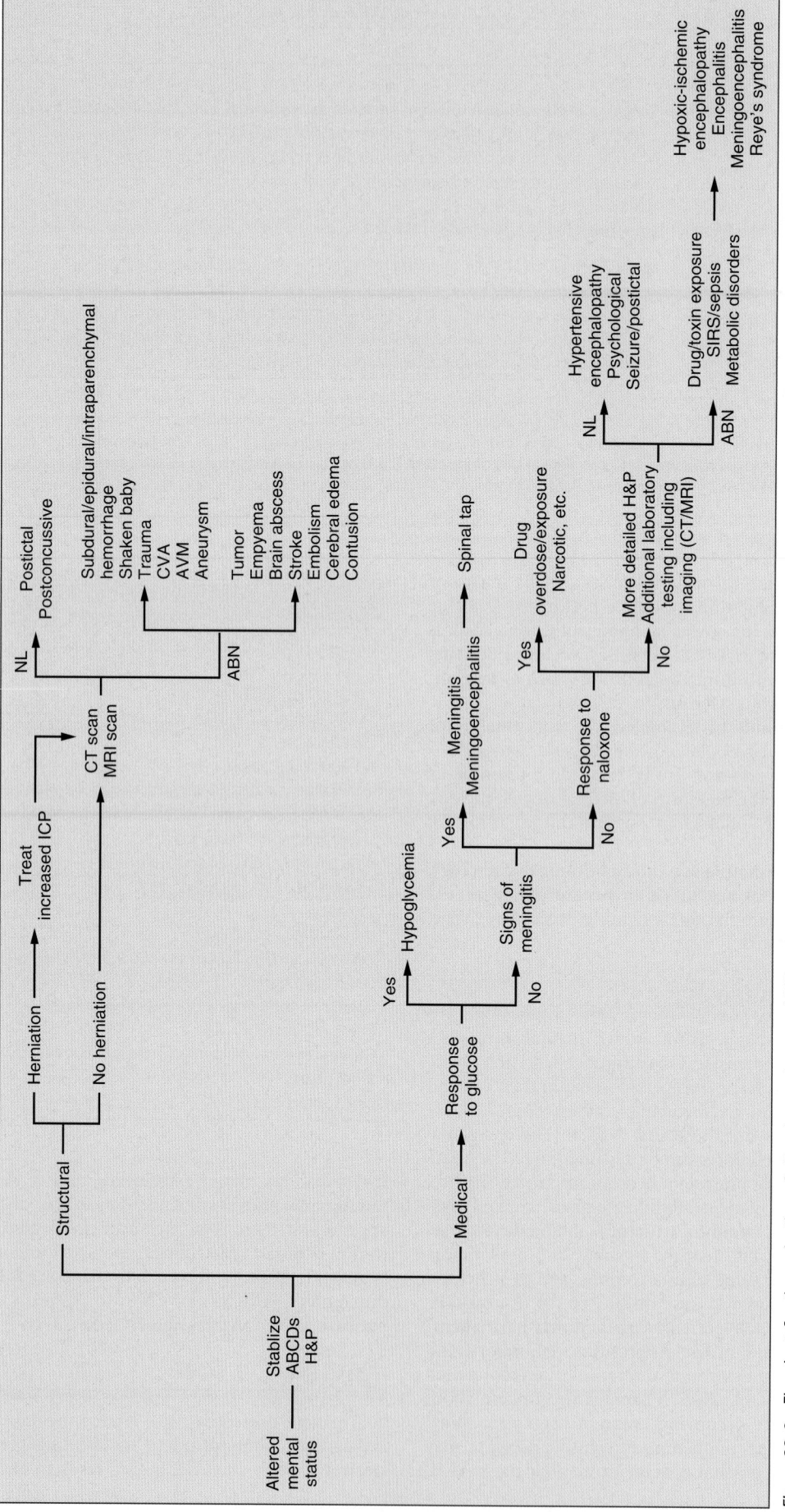

Figure 28–2 Flowchart for the evaluation of altered mental status. ABCDs, airway, breathing, circulation, dextrose/disability; ABN, abnormal; AVM, arteriovenous malformation; CT, computed tomography; CVA, cerebrovascular accident; H&P, history and physical examination; ICP, intracranial pressure; MRI, magnetic resonance imaging; NL, normal; SIRS, systemic inflammatory response syndrome.

Table 28-7	Mnemonics for Causes of Altered Mental Status	
Mnemonic	Initial	Cause
AEIOU	A: alcohol, abuse	Alcohol suppresses the liver's ability to make glucose; therefore, alcohol intoxication increases susceptibility to hypoglycemia
		Abuse includes shaken baby syndrome; altered mental status is due to direct head trauma and diffuse brain injury
	E: epilepsy, electrolyte disorders, encephalopathy, endocrine disorders	Children with epilepsy may have altered mental status during subtle seizures or the postictal state
		Electrolyte disorders involving sodium, calcium, potassium, or magnesium
		Encephalopathy affects the cerebral hemispheres, often resulting in confusion and behavioral changes; it may be due to a number of viruses, Reye syndrome, herpesvirus, cytomegalovirus, and HIV
		Endocrine disorders include hypoglycemia, hyperglycemia, diabetic ketoacidosis, thyroid disorders
	I: insulin, intussusception, intoxication	Insulin shock, due to either insulin overdose or inadequate food intake, can cause hypoglycemia
		Intussusception or other GI processes compromise intestinal blood flow
		Intoxication with drugs, toxins, or heavy metals
	O: overdose, oxygen	Overdose involving sedative-hypnotic agents, particularly when the ingestion involves barbiturates, benzodiazepines, or narcotics; keep in mind that such intoxications may be either accidental or deliberate
		A low blood oxygen level, or hypoxemia, typically causes altered mental status (may be the most common serious cause in children)
	U: uremia (and other metabolic causes)	Usually seen in children with renal failure, uremia arises when abnormal levels of urea nitrogen, a waste product of nitrogen metabolism, accumulate in the blood; urea nitrogen is normally excreted in the urine
		Hemolytic uremic syndrome, with intravascular destruction of erythrocytes, accompanies renal failure and uremia, usually following gastroenteritis or an upper respiratory infection; altered mental status results from the damaging effects of antibodies on small capillaries in the brain
		Other metabolic causes include hepatic problems, adrenal insufficiency, and congenital enzyme defects
TIPS	T: trauma, temperature, tumors, toxicologic syndromes	Head trauma that results in brain injury may cause increased intracranial pressure, hemorrhage, or concussion; any traumatic injury that causes hypoxemia or shock, including that arising from child abuse, may cause altered mental status
		Abnormal body temperature (hypothermia or hyperthermia)
		Tumors or other mass lesions of the brain or brainstem
		Toxicologic syndromes or toxidromes:
		Cholinergic syndrome: SLUDGE—salivation, lacrimation, urination, defecation, GI findings (increased motility), emesis, or DUMBBELS—diarrhea, urination, emesis, lacrimation, salivation
		Anticholinergic syndrome: flushed (red as a beet), febrile (hot as a hare), dry skin (dry as a bone), central nervous system excitation (mad as hatter), mydriasis (blind as a bat), urinary retention (full as a flask)
		Opioid syndrome: miosis, hypotension, hypoventilation, pulmonary edema
	I: infection	Meningitis, encephalitis, sepsis, postinfectious encephalopathy
	P: psychiatric, poisoning	Psychiatric causes exist, but factitious altered mental status is rare in young children; this should be a diagnosis of exclusion
		Unintentional poisoning, intoxication, or ingestion
	S: shock, stroke, space-occupying lesions, subarachnoid hemorrhage, seizures	Shock from any cause
		Stroke is a rare cause; more likely in children with sickle cell anemia or vasculitis
		Space-occupying lesions include brain tumors, hemorrhage, and vascular malformations that leak or bleed
		Subarachnoid hemorrhage from any cause
		Seizures—either nonconvulsive status epilepticus or a postictal state

GI, gastrointestinal; HIV, human immunodeficiency virus.

coincidentally with the history and directed physical examination. This rapid evaluation of the patient, along with directed laboratory and neurologic tests, will determine whether acute neurosurgical consultation is required for catastrophic intracranial processes from a structural cause, or whether focused treatment should be given for a medical cause. Even with close attention to detail, there will be some poor outcomes that result in immediate death, brain death on mechanical ventilators, and varied states of chronic neurologic disability, ranging from mild to severe. The best outcomes result from rapid intervention and determination of a specific cause for more directed treatment.

SUGGESTED READING

Antunes NL: Mental status changes in children with systemic cancer. Pediatr Neurol 2002;27:39-42.

Baxter A: Acute confusional state in the emergency department: Consider a common zebra. Clin Pediatr Emerg Med 2003;4:215-220.

Behrman RE, Busey SL, Kliegman RM: Altered mental status. In Pomeranz AJ, Busey SL, Sabnis S, et al (eds): Pediatric Decision-Making Strategies to Accompany Nelson Textbook of Pediatrics. New York, Elsevier Science Health Science, 2002, pp 216-217.

Byerley JS: Pediatric emergencies in the family practice clinic. Clin Fam Pract 2003;5:445-466.

Fenichel GM: Altered states of consciousness. In Fenichel GM (ed): Clinical Pediatric Neurology: A Signs and Symptoms Approach. Philadelphia, WB Saunders, 2001, pp 47-76.

Glaser N, Barnett P, McCaslin I, et al: Risk factors for cerebral edema in children with diabetic ketoacidosis. N Engl J Med 2001;344:264-269.

Halley MK, Silva PD, Foley J, Rodarte A: Loss of consciousness: When to perform computed tomography. Pediatr Crit Care Med 2004;5:230-233.

Hsia SH, Wu CT, Wang HS, et al: The use of bispectral index to monitor unconscious children. Pediatr Neurol 2004;31:20-23.

Quayle KS, Jaffe DM, Kuppermann N, et al: Diagnostic testing for acute head injury in children: When are head computed tomography and skull radiographs indicated? Pediatrics 1997;99:E11.

REFERENCES

1. Plum F, Posner JB: The Diagnosis of Stupor and Coma, 3rd ed. Philadelphia, FA Davis, 1982.
2. Stubgen J, Caronna JJ: Altered mental status. In Samuels MA (ed): Hospitalist Neurology. Woburn, Mass, Butterworth-Heinemann, 1999, pp 27-43.
3. King D, Avner JR: Altered mental status. Clin Pediatr Emerg Med 2003;4:171-178.
4. Pattisapu JV: Etiology and clinical course of hydrocephalus. Neurosurg Clin N Am 2001;12:651-659.
5. Ellenhorn MJ, Barceloux DG: Medical Toxicology: Diagnosis and Treatment of Human Poisoning. New York, Elsevier, 1988.
6. Teasdale G, Jennett B: Assessment of coma and impaired consciousness: A practical scale. Lancet 1974;2:81-84.
7. Rogers M: Textbook of Pediatric Intensive Care. Philadelphia, Williams & Wilkins, 1996, pp 735-745.
8. Hazinski MF, Zaritsky AL, Nadkarni VM, et al (eds): PALS Provider Manual. Dallas, Tex, American Heart Association, 2002.
9. Taylor DA, Ashwal S: Impairment of consciousness and coma. In Swaiman KF, Ashwal S (eds): Pediatric Neurology: Principles and Practice. St Louis, Mosby, 1999, pp 861-872.
10. Moses S: Ophthalmology. Available at FamilyPracticeNotebook.com.
11. Pumberger W, Dinhobl I, Dremsek P: Altered consciousness and lethargy from compromised intestinal blood flow in children. Am J Emerg Med 2004;22:307-309.

CHAPTER 29

Chest Pain

Chad K. Brands

The hospitalist frequently encounters patients complaining of chest discomfort. Given the myriad causes of chest pain, the hospitalist must begin with a systematic approach to this patient complaint. One relies on a thorough understanding of potential causes and pathophysiology while using the history, physical examination, and laboratory and radiographic information to identify and treat the underlying cause of the discomfort as well as the pain itself.

DIFFERENTIAL DIAGNOSIS

When chest pain is a presenting symptom, the underlying cause must be determined to guide diagnostic studies and appropriate consultation or treatment (Table 29-1).

Cardiovascular

Cardiopulmonary causes of chest pain are at the top of the list of considerations because of their potential to be life threatening. Although infrequently encountered in pediatric or adolescent medicine, chest pain that accompanies the spectrum of myocardial ischemia, injury, and infarction may be described similarly to the classic adult coronary syndromes, such as the "tight" or "squeezing" pain of angina pectoris. This discomfort can be substernal or located over the precordium and may radiate into the arms or upward into the neck and jaw. Physicians continue to appreciate the tremendous variability in the way patients describe symptoms of myocardial ischemia and infarction. Thus, the clinician must be alert to the possibility of myocardial ischemia and seek associated symptoms that typically accompany angina, such as nausea, vomiting, diaphoresis, palpitations, and dizziness. A particularly high degree of suspicion is required in the clinical context of prior cardiac history or surgery, trauma, myocarditis, Kawasaki disease, and illicit drug use. Stimulants such as cocaine may create hypertensive emergencies, with end-organ effects such as cardiac ischemia. Obtaining a confidential history is critical to uncover substance abuse, and the hospitalist should not hesitate to use toxicologic screens when patients present with symptoms and signs of substance use. It should also be noted that hospitalists will increasingly be called on to evaluate young adults with cardiac conditions who are survivors of complex congenital and childhood disease processes such as cancer, heart disease, diabetes, renal failure, and cystic fibrosis.

Pulmonary

The presence of cough with distress in a patient with chest pain points to an airway occlusive process such as epiglottitis, bacterial tracheitis, or a foreign body. If the patient appears toxic or is drooling and sitting forward to splint open the airway, the examiner should simply observe the child, place him or her in a parent's lap for greatest comfort, supply oxygen in a nonthreatening manner, and request urgent consultation with anesthesia and otolaryngology. In an older, nontoxic child, palpation of the neck is important to exclude tenderness and swelling seen in processes such as a parapharyngeal abscess. Stridor is always indicative of an upper airway obstructive process.

The most common cause of chest pain in pediatric medicine is asthma, which is the leading reason for pediatric hospitalization in the United States. However, the hospitalist must remember the dictum that "all that wheezes is not asthma" and considers other diagnoses when evaluating a wheezing patient. Children and even adolescents may have difficulty describing dyspnea and chest discomfort. Episodic coughing and wheezing in response to well-known triggers, such as active or passive cigarette smoke or viral upper respiratory infections, are hallmark clinical findings in asthma. Wheezing has high sensitivity for a diagnosis of asthma, but much less specificity. Signs of air trapping may also manifest as a barrel-chested appearance and prolonged inspiratory-expiratory ratios. The presence of clubbing may be the result of chronic hypoxia and suggests other pulmonary processes, such as bronchiectasis and cystic fibrosis, with potential complications such as pneumothorax.

Central venous catheters are the leading risk factor for deep venous thrombosis (DVT) and subsequent pulmonary embolus (PE). The presence of pain or swelling in an extremity should suggest the possibility of thrombosis and calls for noninvasive investigation of the involved extremity. In the setting of prolonged hospitalization with immobilization, prolonged indwelling catheter use, and the possibility of heparin-associated thrombocytopenia, the hospitalist should have a high degree of suspicion for DVT-PE complex. The symptoms and signs of pulmonary embolism are notoriously nonspecific: chest pain, anxiety, dyspnea, cough, and sinus tachycardia.

Mediastinal

Pneumomediastinum may occur rarely as a spontaneous phenomenon, typically in tall, thin patients; it may also occur in patients with status asthmaticus. If an asthmatic patient experiences distress or deterioration, the clinician should consider these possibilities, in addition to a tension pneumothorax. Pneumopericardium and pneumomediastinum are common in critical care settings in mechanically ventilated patients and in postoperative settings in patients with chest tubes draining pleural or pericardial cavities. Mediastinitis, though distinctly uncommon in pediatrics, can rarely follow esophageal rupture or an infectious process such as histoplasmosis.

Table 29-1   Causes of Chest Pain

Cardiovascular

Myocardial ischemia, injury, infarction spectrum
  Coronary anomalies
  Acute coronary syndromes
  Kawasaki disease
  Stimulant use
Myocardial contusion
Aortic dissection (Marfan syndrome)
Hypertensive emergency
  Illicit substances, including cocaine and stimulants
  Acute or chronic kidney disease
Cardiomyopathies—hypertrophic cardiomyopathy
Congestive heart failure
Arrhythmias
Valvular heart disease
Myocarditis
Pericarditis
Endocarditis
Pancarditis
  Acute rheumatic fever
Pericardial effusion
Cardiac tamponade
Cardiac masses and tumors
Complications of central venous catheters, including thromboses
Substance use—cocaine, inhalants, stimulants

Pulmonary

Diseases of the airways
  Asthma
  Bronchospasm
  Foreign body
Diseases of the parenchyma
  Pneumonia—nosocomial or community acquired
  Pulmonary infarction
  Bronchogenic cyst
  Cystic adenomatoid malformation
  Acute chest syndrome of sickle cell crisis
Diseases of the pleura
  Pneumothorax
  Hemothorax
  Pleural effusion
  Empyema
  Pleuritis of autoimmune diseases (e.g., systemic lupus
    erythematosus)
Diseases of the vasculature
  Pulmonary embolism, air embolism
  Pulmonary hypertension

Mediastinal

Mediastinal air leak
  Barotrauma due to mechanical ventilation
  Pneumopericardium or pneumomediastinum
Masses and malignancies
  Thymoma
  Lymphoma
  Teratoma
Mediastinitis
  Infectious or noninfectious
  Ruptured esophagus

Gastrointestinal

Trauma to organs in the upper abdomen
Esophageal causes
  Foreign body
  Rupture
  Spasm
  Motility disorders, including achalasia
  Esophagitis—infectious or noninfectious
Gastroesophageal reflux disease
Biliary disease, including cholelithiasis and cholecystitis
Pancreatitis
Hepatitis
Subdiagphragmatic processes—inflammation, infection, mass
Referred pain from abdominal processes—splenomegaly,
  malignancy, mass

Musculoskeletal

Costochondritis and chest wall pain
Blunt injury and trauma
Child abuse
Fractures to bones of the chest, including ribs
Pectus deformities
Scoliosis
Myofascial pain syndromes, including fibromyalgia
Precordial catch syndrome
Floating and slipping rib syndromes
Disorders of bone mineralization, including rickets
Pain in and around the breasts

Neuropathic and Psychiatric

Acute anxiety and panic disorders
Mood disorders, including depression and anxiety
Varicella-zoster (pain may precede vesicular eruption)
Postherpetic neuralgia
Chronic pain syndromes
Somatization

Gastrointestinal

During the bedside evaluation of a patient with chest pain, the hospitalist should search for a cause of pain referred from intra-abdominal organs. A patient with gallbladder or biliary disease may report pain in the right shoulder or posterior thorax. A patient with splenomegaly may report pain in the left shoulder. A patient with an abdominal mass may report pain referred to the lower chest wall or even the shoulder region. Stretching of the hepatic capsule or subdiaphragmatic irritation can cause right upper quadrant pain as well as right-sided pain in the lower chest. Esophageal spasm and gastroesophageal reflux commonly cause chest discomfort in children and adolescents.

Musculoskeletal

The chest must be inspected for the presence of visible abnormalities such as bruising and signs of trauma and nonaccidental injury. Palpation is also crucial for the diagnostic assessment of a young patient with chest pain. The examining hand should press on each of the costochondral junctions where the ribs articulate with the sternum. Rib fractures are well described in the child abuse literature, but signs of trauma may not be present. Rib infarction should be suspected in a patient with sickle cell disease who presents with a chest pain crisis. Costochondritis is a common cause of chest pain in young adolescents. Fibromyalgia in adolescents can also present with this type of pain, in addition to pain with light touch in multiple areas, suggestive of a myofascial pain syndrome.

Neuropathic and Psychiatric

Rarely, children or adolescents present with burning pain preceding the eruption of a group of vesicles in a dermatomal distribution that allows a clinical diagnosis of varicella-zoster. The medical literature increasingly points to the presence of underlying depression in adolescents and young adults with chronic pain syndromes. Anxiety is also well known to contribute to intermittent or chronic chest wall pain. Most important, patients who present with acute anxiety or panic symptoms should be evaluated promptly, and the hospitalist must consider medical processes with a pathophysiology that would explain the sudden onset of such symptoms.

EVALUATION

History and Physical Examination

The evaluation of a patient complaining of acute pain is often challenging. The patient may be uncomfortable, anxious, or distressed, and the hospitalist may not have met the patient and family previously. A calm and reassuring presence allows the physician to focus the interview efficiently and thereby quickly obtain the information required to determine potential causes and possible interventions. Table 29-2 provides clues that may help identify the cause of chest pain.

As the evaluation begins, the practitioner seeks to answer the following questions: Is the patient in distress? What is the degree of distress? Is the distress due to cardiorespiratory compromise? Does the patient have a stable airway? If the patient is in pain, what is the anatomic localization of the pain? What are the probable causes of chest pain in this patient at this point in the hospitalization? Is the patient's mental status normal? What processes are suggested by the vital signs and the recent vital sign trends? Are there urgent or emergent diagnostic or therapeutic interventions needed at the bedside?

In urgent or emergent settings, the pace and sequence of the assessment are directed by the acuity of the patient's presentation. Any indication of respiratory distress or hemodynamic instability in a patient with chest pain means that the physician leading the bedside assessment is examining the patient while simultaneously obtaining historical information to answer the preceding questions. For a patient who is unstable, the immediate vital sign assessment focuses on measuring the heart rate, best done by auscultation over the precordium, and counting respirations during the chest examination. Blood pressure and pulse oximetry measurements can be obtained quickly. Additional verbal information can be obtained during the rapid hands-on assessment and thereafter as the physician seeks additional information once it has been determined that the patient is stable.

For a patient reporting sudden-onset or severe chest pain suggestive of cardiopulmonary causes, the physician begins

---

Table 29-2   Clues to the Cause of Chest Pain

Timing
Sudden onset—air embolism, pulmonary embolism, myocardial ischemia or infarction, arrhythmias, air leak during mechanical ventilation, spontaneous pneumothorax
Gradual onset—community-acquired or nosocomial pneumonia and complications such as pleural effusion and empyema

Hospital Setting
Pain on initial presentation
  Toxicologic causes, including inhalants and stimulant use
Pain during the course of hospitalization
  Postoperative complications
  Infection at incisions
  Bleeding
  Barotrauma
  Pneumonia
  DVT-PE complex in native vessels or arising from central catheters
  Myocardial ischemia

Characterization of Pain
Severe—myocardial ischemia or infarction; classically, associated symptoms include nausea, vomiting, radiation of pain to neck, jaw, and arms
Crushing—myocardial ischemia or tamponade
Sharp—pleuritic, pericardial, musculoskeletal, and gastrointestinal causes; arrhythmias
Pleuritic—pericardial or pleural disease

Associated Symptoms and Signs
Abdominal pain—lower lobe pneumonia, pancreatitis, biliary and liver disease
Bruising—nonaccidental trauma of child abuse
Central venous catheters—arrhythmias, pneumothorax, DVT-PE complex
Clubbing—chronic lung disease, such as cystic fibrosis or bronchiectasis
Cough—pneumonia, asthma, pulmonary edema, pleural effusions
Crepitus—subcutaneous air due to air leak secondary to barotrauma
Cyanosis—congenital heart disease, pneumonia, heart failure
Dyspnea—asthma, pulmonary edema, multiple cardiopulmonary causes
Extremity edema—DVT progressing to PE
Gallop—heart failure
Odynophagia—para- or retropharyngeal abscess
Pericardial rub—pericardial effusion, pneumopericardium
Pleural rub—pleural effusion due to inflammation or infection
Stridor—foreign body, occluding infectious process in the airway (e.g., epiglottitis, bacterial tracheitis, croup)
Tall and hypermobile (often with pectus excavatum)—Marfan syndrome
Wheezing—asthma, multiple cardiopulmonary causes

DVT, deep venous thrombosis; PE, pulmonary embolus.

---

the examination by inspecting the chest. Asymmetry, scars, incisions, catheters, chest tubes, and mechanical ventilation equipment settings and data should be noted during the rapid hands-on survey. Auscultation of the heart allows assessment of the apical pulse for rhythm and rate. The examiner's trained ear listens to the first and second heart sounds; he or she then listens separately for sounds in systole and diastole. Cardiac cycles should be assessed at the base and apex of the heart, with specific assessment for pathologic murmurs and sounds that could provide a bedside diagnosis. The respiratory rate and character are assessed as the lung fields are auscultated, moving the stethoscope symmetrically from one side of the chest to the other to ensure the presence of equal breath sounds, in addition to assessing their character and quality in each lobe. During this hands-on evaluation, the physician is searching for clues to life-threatening causes of chest pain, particularly those of cardiopulmonary origin, which include but are not limited to myocardial ischemia, cardiac tamponade, arrhythmia, upper airway obstruction, pneumothorax, pneumomediastinum, and esophageal perforation.

Diagnostic Testing

A bedside 12-lead surface electrocardiogram should be ordered in all patients complaining of chest pain. The clinician must examine the tracing systematically for characterization of rate; rhythm; axis; intervals; P, QRS, and T waves; signs of ischemia, injury, or infarction; voltage; and chamber enlargement. Reference guides provide clinicians with age-specific normative values for pediatric electrocardiogram interpretation. The clinician should keep in mind that although the electrocardiogram may provide useful information, it is notoriously insensitive and nonspecific for the detection of many pathophysiologic processes, including ischemia. Thus, if the patient has a cardiac history or the hospitalist is considering a cardiac cause of the chest pain, timely cardiac consultation is imperative. Blood can be sent for cardiac enzyme levels, and rapid assays exist for the measurement of troponin and myoglobin.

Bedside chest radiographs should be obtained and interpreted for signs of disease in the airway, lungs, pleura, mediastinum, and abdomen. If the patient is stable, a lateral view of the chest obtained in the radiology department can be helpful. Signs of barotrauma and pneumonia should be sought on the chest films of asthmatic patients.

Pulse oximetry is readily available, but below 80%, it does not correlate well with the arterial oxygen concentration as measured by blood gas assessment.

Although the D-dimer enzyme-linked immunosorbent assay (ELISA) assay may be sensitive for DVT-PE complex, it is not specific for this condition. Pulse oximetry may not demonstrate hypoxemia early in the course of the disease process, but arterial blood gas assessment is useful for determining the partial pressure of oxygen and the alveolar-arterial gradient, as well as the patient's acid-base status. Tachypnea and hyperpnea may give rise to an early respiratory alkalosis. A high-resolution spiral computed tomography scan is the test of choice to diagnose pulmonary embolism; it can be obtained quickly and provides additional information about the status of the organs in the chest.

Once cardiopulmonary conditions and other causes of chest pain are excluded, empirical treatment with antacids may be indicated. Esophagoduodenoscopy and pH probe studies are needed to definitively diagnose esophagitis and document reflux, respectively.

SUGGESTED READING

Burns JC, Shike H, Gordon JB, et al: Sequelae of Kawasaki disease in adolescents and young adults. J Am Coll Cardiol 1996;28:1.

Chalumeau M, Le Clainche L, Sayeg N, et al: Spontaneous pneumomediastinum in children. Pediatr Pulmonol 2001;31:1.

Coleman WL: Recurrent chest pain in children. Pediatr Clin North Am 1984;31:5.

Feinstein RA, Daniel WA: Chronic chest pain in children and adolescents. Pediatr Ann 1986;15:10.

Glassman MS, Medow MS, Berezin S, Newman LJ: Spectrum of esophageal disorders in children with chest pain. Dig Dis Sci 1992;37:5.

Rowe BH, Dulberg CS, Peterson RG, et al: Characteristics of children presenting with chest pain to a pediatric emergency department. Can Med Assoc J 1990;143:5.

Selbst SM: Consultation with the specialist: Chest pain in children. Pediatr Rev 1997;18:5.

Selbst SM, Ruddy RM, Clark BJ: Chest pain in children: Follow-up of patients previously reported. Clin Pediatr 1990;29:7.

Selbst SM, Ruddy RM, Clark BJ, et al: Pediatric chest pain: A prospective study. Pediatrics 1988;82:3.

CHAPTER 30

Cyanosis

Diana M. Heinzman

The finding of cyanosis is a concern, and its causes range from insignificant to life threatening. The pediatric hospitalist must be able to accurately and efficiently stabilize, evaluate, and manage a patient who presents with cyanosis.

BACKGROUND

Cyanosis is a bluish discoloration of the skin, mucous membranes, tongue, lips, or nail beds and is due to an increased concentration of reduced hemoglobin (Hb) in the circulation.[1] Clinically evident cyanosis typically occurs at an oxygen saturation of 85% or less.[2] Mild cyanosis may be difficult to detect. Cyanosis is usually easier to detect with natural lighting and is typically more difficult to detect in patients with dark skin pigmentation or with anemia. Long-term complications include clubbing, polycythemia, cerebrovascular accident, brain abscess, platelet abnormalities, lower-than-expected IQ, scoliosis, and hyperuricemia.[1]

Central cyanosis is associated with arterial desaturation and involves the skin, mucous membranes, lips, tongue, and nail beds. Peripheral cyanosis occurs when there is increased oxygen uptake in peripheral tissues; it is not associated with arterial desaturation. Peripheral cyanosis often involves only the extremities.[1] Differential cyanosis, in which the upper extremities are pink and the lower extremities are cyanotic, is associated with conditions such as coarctation of the aorta and interrupted aortic arch when there is right-to-left shunting through a patent ductus arteriosus.[3] In newborns, acrocyanosis, or blueness of exposed extremities, is common and is typically insignificant. Similarly, isolated circumoral cyanosis due to prominent venous plexuses in the skin is insignificant, as long as cardiac output is normal.[1]

PATHOPHYSIOLOGY

Clinically evident cyanosis occurs when the concentration of reduced (or deoxygenated) Hb in the circulation reaches 5 g/dL. Increased levels of reduced Hb occur when there is desaturation of arterial blood (central cyanosis) or when there is increased uptake of oxygen in peripheral tissues (peripheral cyanosis). There is normally 2 g/dL of reduced Hb in the circulation, which means that another 3 g/dL of reduced Hb is needed to produce clinical cyanosis; thus, the total amount of Hb is critical to the development of cyanosis. For this reason, a hypoxic child with anemia may not have enough reduced Hb in the circulation to produce clinical cyanosis; in contrast, in a hypoxic child with polycythemia, a sufficient level of reduced Hb is reached at a higher oxygen saturation level.[3]

Hypoxia results from one or a combination of the following mechanisms:

1. Decreased inspired oxygen content (Fio_2)
2. Decreased respiratory rate or apnea
3. Increased right-to-left shunt
4. Increased ventilation-perfusion mismatch
5. Diffusion abnormality

When the iron in Hb is oxidized to the ferric state (Fe^{3+}), methemoglobin is formed.[4] Methemoglobin is unable to carry oxygen and normally constitutes less than 2% of circulating Hb. With congenital or acquired causes of methemoglobinemia, as well as with certain abnormal Hb variants, such as the Hb M group, elevated levels of methemoglobin cause central cyanosis and give the blood a chocolate brown appearance.[5]

DIFFERENTIAL DIAGNOSIS

Multiple entities can cause cyanosis. Central cyanosis (hypoxia) results from reduced arterial oxygen saturation caused by decreased alveolar ventilation, right-to-left shunting, ventilation-perfusion inequalities, decreased diffusion of the lung, or decreased affinity of Hb for oxygen (Box 30-1). Peripheral cyanosis results from increased oxygen uptake in peripheral tissues (Box 30-2).

INITIAL STABILIZATION

When faced with a patient with cyanosis, the pediatric hospitalist must determine whether immediate intervention is necessary. As always, the ABCs (airway, breathing, and circulation) should be addressed immediately. Supplemental oxygen should be administered. Assisted ventilation or intubation may be necessary if there is cardiorespiratory or neurologic compromise. Intravenous access, continuous pulse oximetry, and continuous cardiac monitoring are indicated. If possible, initial pulse oximetry and arterial blood gas determination should be obtained; however, stabilization should not be delayed to obtain these studies. Patients with cyanosis and a possible obstructed airway should receive emergent therapy to relieve the obstruction. Once the patient is stabilized, a more complete history and physical examination are indicated.

HISTORY AND PHYSICAL EXAMINATION

A careful history and physical examination are essential in the evaluation of cyanosis (Boxes 30-3 and 30-4). The physical examination should concentrate on determining the presence of central cyanosis (cyanosis of the oral mucosa, lips, tongue, and nail beds) and evaluating the cardiac, respiratory, and neurologic systems for involvement that may require urgent intervention.

Box 30-1 Causes of Central Cyanosis

CARDIAC CAUSES

Congenital heart disease with right-to-left shunting or admixture lesions

Congenital heart disease causing obstruction to pulmonary blood flow (e.g., pulmonary atresia with intact ventricular septum)

Congenital heart disease with large left-to-right shunts causing pulmonary vascular congestion (e.g., large ventricular septal defect)

PULMONARY CAUSES

Airway obstruction (congenital or acquired)
Asthma or bronchiolitis
Obstructive (including sleep) apnea
Pneumonia or other infection
Pulmonary hypoplasia
Meconium aspiration (newborn)
Respiratory distress syndrome (newborn)
Transient tachypnea of the newborn
Cystic fibrosis
Pulmonary edema
Intrapulmonary shunting (e.g., pulmonary arteriovenous fistula)
Pulmonary hypertension resulting in right-to-left shunting (e.g., primary pulmonary hypertension, persistent pulmonary hypertension of the newborn)
Pneumothorax
Atelectasis

NEUROLOGIC CAUSES

Intracranial hemorrhage
Maternal sedative administration (newborn) or sedative ingestion
Infection (e.g., meningitis)
Neuromuscular disease
Hypoxic insult
Seizure
Central apnea
Breath holding

GASTROINTESTINAL CAUSES

Diaphragmatic hernia
Gastroesophageal reflux leading to aspiration
Chronic liver disease causing pulmonary arteriovenous fistulas (hepatopulmonary syndrome)[6]

HEMOGLOBIN ABNORMALITIES

Acquired methemoglobinemia (e.g., aniline dye; anesthetics, including topical and oral; nitrates)[7]
Hereditary methemoglobinemia (NADH cytochrome-b_5 reductase deficiency)
Abnormal hemoglobin variants (typically benign cyanosis)[5]

Box 30-2 Causes of Peripheral Cyanosis

Exposure to cold
Acrocyanosis of the newborn
Shock
Sepsis
Hypoglycemia
Acidosis
Breath holding
Raynaud phenomenon[8]
Congestive heart failure
Prominent venous plexuses mimicking cyanosis

---

the blood gas determination while the patient is breathing room air also allows the calculation of an alveolar-arterial (A-a) gradient (see Chapter 38). Hypoxia in the setting of a normal A-a gradient suggests hypoventilation or decreased FIO_2 as the cause, whereas an elevated A-a gradient points to right-to-left shunting, ventilation-perfusion mismatch, or diffusion abnormality as the underlying cause. One may also consider a hyperoxygenation test, which is a repeat arterial PO_2 determination after the patient has been inhaling 100% oxygen via mask or plastic hood for 20 minutes.[9] If there is significant improvement of the arterial PO_2 or if it rises to greater than 150 mm Hg with 100% oxygen, cardiac causes are unlikely.[9] If there is little or no improvement, cyanotic congenital heart disease is suggested.

Methemoglobinemia should be considered when cyanosis is unresponsive to oxygen therapy and there is a normal cardiorespiratory examination. Pulse oximetry is not reliable in the presence of a significant methemoglobin level. A simple bedside procedure to check for the presence of methemoglobin is the filter paper test, whereby a few drops of the patient's blood placed on filter paper turn chocolate brown instead of bright red in the setting of methemoglobinemia. However, to confirm the presence of methemoglobin, one must perform co-oximetry.[7] Many laboratories do not automatically perform co-oximetry on a blood gas sample, so this test must be requested specifically. Further testing, such as red blood cell enzyme activity and DNA analysis, can be performed if congenital methemoglobinemia is suspected.[5] Abnormal Hb variants may be picked up with Hb electrophoresis, which is available on many newborn screens.[4]

Chest radiographs are helpful in evaluating heart size, pulmonary blood flow, and pulmonary parenchymal disease. Laboratory evaluation should include a complete blood count with differential and a glucose level. Other studies to consider include electrolytes, blood urea nitrogen, creatinine, and liver function tests.

Electrocardiography and echocardiography should be performed if a cardiac cause is suggested. If a neurologic cause is suspected, appropriate imaging and drug levels or screens should be performed. If there is an abnormal temperature or other signs of possible sepsis, appropriate cultures should be obtained.

EVALUATION

Once the patient is stabilized, further workup is initiated. The first steps in this evaluation include pulse oximetry and arterial oxygen tension (PO_2) by blood gas determination while the patient is breathing room air, if possible. A low arterial PO_2 confirms the diagnosis of hypoxia. Obtaining

TREATMENT

Treatment is guided by the underlying cause. Supplemental oxygen should be continued. In neonates with suspected cyanotic congenital heart disease, pulmonary blood flow is

Box 30-3 History

<table>
<tr><td>

Description of cyanosis
  Timing of first observation
  Involved body parts
  Severity
  Persistent or episodic
  Exacerbating and alleviating factors
  Timing of episodes (e.g., cyanotic spells of tetralogy of Fallot in the morning)
  Duration
  Worsening, stable, or improving
  Description of typical cyanotic event
Associated symptoms or behaviors
  Effect of crying (e.g., crying may worsen cyanosis with cardiac causes, improve cyanosis with respiratory or neurologic causes)[1]
  Inciting event (e.g., choking with foreign body aspiration)
  Postural changes, such as squatting, with the episodes (e.g., cyanotic spells with tetralogy of Fallot)
  Effect of feedings (e.g., cyanosis after feedings with gastroesophageal reflux)
  Sweating or tachypnea with feeding (e.g., congenital heart disease)
  Occurrence primarily when the child is angry or hurt (e.g., breath holding)
  Recent medications, anesthesia (including topical and oral), or other exposures or ingestions (e.g., methemoglobinemia)
  Syncope (e.g., primary pulmonary hypertension)
Focused review of systems
  Respiratory status
  Recent cold or fever (e.g., infection)

</td><td>

Easy fatigability
Alertness
Difficulty growing or gaining weight
Difficulty or choking during feeding (e.g., aspiration with gastroesophageal reflux)
Developmental milestones
Feeding history
Known heart murmur or cardiac disease
Recurrent respiratory infections or chronic cough
Unusual movements, such as seizures
Birth history (especially important in neonates and infants)
  Gestational age, birth weight, maternal medical history and screening tests, maternal medications or sedatives, delivery complications such as fetal distress or meconium
  Apgar score
  Prenatal ultrasonography and fetal echocardiography results
  Mode of delivery (e.g., scheduled cesarean section with no labor and transient tachypnea of the newborn)
Past medical history
  Known cardiac, pulmonary, or neurologic disease
  Chronic illnesses
  Medications, including over the counter, herbal remedies, teething gel, topical anesthetics
  Prior surgeries or hospitalizations
Other history
  Family history of cyanosis, congenital cardiac disease, pulmonary disease, neuromuscular disease, or early childhood death
  Social history, including potential exposures at home and school

</td></tr>
</table>

often dependent on shunting through a patent ductus arteriosus. In these patients, an intravenous infusion of prostaglandin E_1 should be started, typically at a dose of 0.05 to 0.1 μg/kg per minute, to keep the ductus open while the evaluation progresses.[3] The most serious side effect of prostaglandin E_1 is respiratory depression.[3] Cyanotic congenital heart disease may require cardiac catheterization or prompt corrective surgery.

If airway obstruction is suspected, laryngoscopy or bronchoscopy may be indicated. Other pulmonary therapies are directed at the underlying cause (e.g., bronchodilators for asthma).

In cases of methemoglobinemia, intravenous methylene blue at a typical dose of 1 to 2 mg/kg promptly removes methemoglobin and resolves cyanosis.[10] A repeat dose may be given if needed. If this fails, exchange transfusion and hyperbaric oxygen should be considered.[10] Cyanosis from hereditary methemoglobinemia is treated with daily oral methylene blue, ascorbic acid, or both.[5]

If sepsis is suspected, appropriate intravenous antibiotic therapy should be initiated. Furosemide (Lasix) should be given if congestive heart failure is present. Shock should be aggressively addressed. Electrolyte abnormalities, hypoglycemia, and acidosis should be corrected. Warming or bundling may be effective in peripheral cyanosis secondary to cold exposure.

SPECIAL CONSIDERATIONS

Cyanotic Spells

Cyanotic spells are associated most frequently with tetralogy of Fallot. Typically, uncontrolled crying with rapid, deep breathing is accompanied by deepening of the cyanosis and disappearance of the heart murmur. The patient often squats, which increases the oxygen saturation temporarily. Untreated, these episodes can lead to limpness, convulsions, or death. Treatment is emergent and initially includes calming, morphine, oxygen, and sodium bicarbonate to correct acidosis.[1]

Breath-Holding Spells

Breath-holding spells typically occur when a child is upset or injured. With prolonged crying, the child holds his or her breath in expiration, develops cyanosis and change in postural tone, and may have brief tonic-clonic movements. Most children outgrow this typically benign condition by 6 years of age; however, in extreme cases, permanent pacemakers may be necessary.[11]

Primary Pulmonary Hypertension

Primary pulmonary hypertension is a rare condition in children. Initial complaints are fatigue and slowly progressive exercise intolerance. Cyanosis may be mild, and there

Box 30-4	Physical Examination

Vital signs, including temperature and blood pressures in the right arm and right leg
  Right lower extremity systolic blood pressure 10 mm Hg lower than that in right upper extremity suggests coarctation of the aorta or interrupted aortic arch
General
  Dysmorphic features may indicate syndrome with other congenital anomalies
  Poor growth indicates chronic underlying pathology
  Cyanotic changes with crying or feeding
Skin
  Degree and location of cyanosis; evaluate nail beds
  Jaundice may indicate underlying liver disease
Head, eyes, ears, nose, and throat
  Foreign body or anatomic anomaly causing upper airway obstruction
  Plethoric sclera with CHD
  Icteric sclera with hepatic disease
  Cyanosis of oral mucosa, tongue, and lips with central cyanosis
Neck
  Meningismus suggests meningitis
  Mass causing possible obstruction
Respiratory
  Rales, wheezing, grunting, or flaring suggests pulmonary pathology
  Unequal air entry (e.g., pneumothorax or foreign body aspiration)
  Stridor with upper airway obstruction or laryngeal irritation due to severe gastroesophageal reflux
  Significant retractions and labored breathing indicate pulmonary pathology
  Shallow, irregular respirations or apnea may indicate CNS depression

Tachypnea is common with CHD[2]
Breathing is often minimally affected with CHD unless congestive heart failure, acidosis, or pulmonary edema is present[2]
Cardiovascular
  Hyperactive precordium with CHD
  Arrhythmia may cause congestive heart failure with pulmonary edema and cyanosis
  Murmur is suggestive of CHD, although the absence of murmur does not rule it out (e.g., transposition of the great arteries may have no murmur or only a soft murmur)
  Single, loud S_2 may indicate CHD
  Gallop
  Unequal peripheral pulses or pulse lag suggests coarctation of the aorta or interrupted aortic arch
  Poor peripheral perfusion may indicate sepsis, shock, or low cardiac output
Gastrointestinal
  Hepatosplenomegaly or ascites may indicate congestive heart failure or underlying hepatic disease
Extremities and musculoskeletal
  Clubbing signifies long-standing hypoxemia and cyanosis
  Peripheral edema may indicate heart failure
  Scoliosis is seen with chronic cyanosis and CHD, notably tetralogy of Fallot
  Restrictive chest deformities
Neurologic
  Abnormal head circumference may indicate hypoxic injury or other CNS pathology
  Weakness may suggest neuromuscular disease
  Hypotonia and lethargy may indicate CNS depression
  Inconsolability may indicate meningitis
  Unusual movements or seizures

CHD, congenital heart disease; CNS, central nervous system.

may be associated syncope. On physical examination, there may be a subtle but loud S_2, S_3, or S_4 or a tricuspid regurgitation murmur. Prompt cardiology evaluation is indicated.[12]

SUGGESTED READING

Da Silva SS, Sajan IS, Underwood JP: Congenital methemoglobinemia: A rare cause of cyanosis in the newborn—a case report. Pediatrics 2003;112: e158-e161.

Kelly AM, Coburn JP, McGoon MD, et al: Breath-holding spells associated with significant bradycardia: Successful treatment with permanent pacemaker implantation. Pediatrics 2001;108:698-702.

Park MK: Manifestations of cardiac problems in the newborn. In Pediatric Cardiology for Practitioners. St Louis, Mosby–Year Book, 1996, pp 375-389.

Tingelstad J: Nonrespiratory cyanosis. Pediatr Rev 1999;20:350-352.

REFERENCES

1. Park MK: Pathophysiology of cyanotic congenital heart defects. In Pediatric Cardiology for Practitioners. St Louis, Mosby–Year Book, 1996, pp 114-123.
2. Park MK: Manifestations of cardiac problems in the newborn. In Pediatric Cardiology for Practitioners. St Louis, Mosby–Year Book, 1996, pp 375-377.
3. Tingelstad J: Nonrespiratory cyanosis. Pediatr Rev 1999;20:350-352.
4. Da Silva SS, Sajan IS, Underwood JP: Congenital methemoglobinemia: A rare cause of cyanosis in the newborn—a case report. Pediatrics 2003;112:e158-e161.
5. Honig GR: Hemoglobin disorders. In Nelson WE, et al (eds): Nelson's Textbook of Pediatrics. Philadelphia, WB Saunders, 1996, p 1401.
6. Yuan HC, Wu TC, Huang IF, et al: Hepatopulmonary syndrome in a child. J Chin Med Assoc 2003;66:127-130.
7. Balicer RD, Kitai E: Methemoglobinemia caused by topical teething preparation: A case report. Sci World J 2004;4:517-520.
8. Nigrovic PA, Fuhlbrigge RC, Sundel RP: Raynaud's phenomenon in children: A retrospective review. Pediatrics 2003;111:715-721.
9. Aly H: Respiratory disorders in the newborn. Pediatr Rev 2004;25:201-208.
10. Rumack BH: Chemical and drug poisoning. In Nelson WE, et al (eds): Nelson's Textbook of Pediatrics. Philadelphia, WB Saunders, 1996, p 2014.
11. Kelly AM, Coburn JP, McGoon MD, et al: Breath-holding spells associated with significant bradycardia: Successful treatment with permanent pacemaker implantation. Pediatrics 2001;108:698-702.
12. Gartner JC Jr: Syncope. In Gartner JC Jr, Zitelli BJ (eds): Common and Chronic Symptoms in Pediatrics. St Louis, Mosby–Year Book, 1997, p 165.

CHAPTER 31

Diarrhea

Marin Kiesau

Worldwide, diarrhea causes an estimated 2 million deaths per year in children younger than 5 years. Although the overall morbidity and mortality related to diarrheal illnesses are decreasing, diarrhea continues to be a leading cause of pediatric hospitalization.

BACKGROUND

Diarrhea is simply defined as an increase in stool output. It is typically associated with both increased frequency of bowel movements and liquidity of stool. Normal stool output is approximately 5 g/kg per day for neonates and infants and 50 to 75 g/day for preschool-aged children. Diarrhea typically results in stool losses of more than 10 g/kg per day in children younger than 3 years and more than 200 g/day in children older than 3. Diarrheal illnesses are considered acute if symptoms last less than 14 days and chronic if they last more than 14 days.

PATHOPHYSIOLOGY

In the normally functioning gastrointestinal tract, nutrients are absorbed via active, carrier-mediated transport across the intact mucosal lining. Electrolytes such as sodium, potassium, chloride, and bicarbonate are transported via both active and passive mechanisms, with sodium transport creating the most significant gradient. This sodium gradient is responsible for promoting the passive transport of water across the mucosal lining. Under normal circumstances, there is a balance between the absorptive and secretory functions, which are the opposing unidirectional electrolyte fluxes. This results in a net water absorption, with 90% of this absorption occurring in the small intestine.

Altered pathophysiologic mechanisms resulting in diarrhea can be divided into four categories: osmotic, secretory, inflammatory, and motility disorders. Osmotic diarrhea occurs when solute creates an osmotic load within the lumen of the intestine, resulting in decreased water absorption. Withholding intake of the inciting agent usually results in cessation of the diarrhea. Secretory diarrhea occurs when there is an increase in water and electrolyte secretion in the intestine, leading to excessive water loss. This mechanism is not affected by alterations in enteral intake. Inflammation causes diarrhea by decreasing water absorption and increasing fluid secretion secondary to mucosal damage. This may be associated with mucus, blood, and protein losses in the stool. Lastly, motility disorders can cause either increased or decreased transit time in the intestine, leading to altered water absorption. A decreased transit time (increased motility) results in diarrhea.

DIFFERENTIAL DIAGNOSIS

The list of possible causes of diarrhea is extensive (Table 31-1). Differentiating acute diarrhea from chronic diarrhea can be helpful in narrowing the possibilities. The most common causes of acute diarrhea are infectious. Viral infections (e.g., rotavirus, Norwalk virus, enteric adenovirus, calicivirus) account for most cases of acute diarrhea. Other infectious causes include bacterial pathogens (e.g., *Escherichia coli, Salmonella, Shigella, Campylobacter*) and parasites (e.g., *Giardia*).

Chronic diarrhea involves a much broader list of possible causes. When evaluating chronic diarrhea, the age of the patient is helpful in narrowing the likely diagnosis. A common diagnosis in children younger than 1 year is intractable diarrhea of infancy. This entity is associated with diffuse mucosal injury resulting in persistent diarrhea, malabsorption, and malnutrition beginning before the age of 6 months. It is most commonly related to either cow milk or soy protein intolerance or prolonged postinfectious mucosal injury. Between the ages of 1 and 5 years, postinfectious enteritis, giardiasis, and celiac disease are more common diagnoses. In children older than 5 years, inflammatory bowel disease, constipation with encopresis, and acquired lactose intolerance are frequently diagnosed. It is also important to remember that chronic diarrhea may be a presenting symptom of an immune deficiency.

Treatment of diarrheal illness depends on identification of the underlying cause and institution of appropriate therapy. Because most cases of acute diarrhea are caused by viral infections and are self-limited, the role of the physician is to rule out other causes that may be more serious or require more specific treatment. Pediatric patients with diarrhea are most commonly hospitalized because of dehydration and the need for intravenous fluid.

HISTORY

The frequency, duration, volume, and character of the diarrhea (e.g., smell, color, presence of mucus or blood) should be determined. A sweet odor is sometimes associated with carbohydrate malabsorption, while a rancid odor is encountered with steatorrhea. An understanding of the patient's normal bowel habits is valuable to determine the degree of change from baseline. A careful dietary history can help identify inciting factors that may contribute to an osmotic diarrhea, as well as identify foods or other vectors associated with an increased risk of food- or waterborne pathogens (e.g., *Salmonella, Shigella, E. coli, Giardia*).

Table 31-1 Causes of Diarrhea

Infectious
  Viruses
    Rotavirus
    Norwalk virus
    Enteric adenovirus
    Calcivirus
  Bacteria
    Salmonella
    Shigella
    Campylobacter jejuni
    Escherichia coli
    Clostridium difficile
    Aeromonas hydrophila
    Plesiomonas shigelloides
  Parasites
    Giardiasis
    Amebiasis
    Cryptosporidiosis
Congenital
  Congenital microvillus atrophy
  Autoimmune enteropathy
  Hirschsprung disease
  Congenital chloride-losing diarrhea
  Intractable diarrhea of infancy
  Short-bowel syndrome
Malabsorptive
  Celiac disease
  Cystic fibrosis
  Inflammatory bowel disease
  Monosaccharide deficiencies
  Disaccharide deficiencies
  Postinfectious enteropathy
Motility disorders
  Irritable bowel syndrome
Allergic or intolerance
  Eosinophilic enteropathy
  Cow milk or soy protein intolerance
Systemic
  Hemolytic uremic syndrome
  Hyperthyroidism
  α_1-Antitrypsin deficiency
  Immune deficiency
  Intestinal lymphangiectasia
  Acrodermatitis enteropathica
  Pancreatic insufficiency
  Hormone-secreting tumors
  Adrenal insufficiency
  α-lipoproteinemia
  Protein calorie malnutrition
Miscellaneous
  Toddler's diarrhea
  Constipation with encopresis
  Antibiotic associated

Potential exposures, such as day-care attendance, recent travel, and pets in the home, should be explored. Day-care attendance increases the risk of most infectious diarrheal illness transmitted fecal-orally. *Giardia* and *Salmonella* are the most commonly diagnosed parasitic and bacterial pathogens, respectively, in day-care attendees. One should inquire about exposure to potential zoonotic vectors such as reptiles (e.g., *Salmonella*), as well as travel to areas where endemic parasitic or bacterial infections are common.

Antibiotic-associated diarrhea typically resolves with completion or cessation of the medication. If the symptoms persist, or if blood appears in the stool, colitis secondary to *Clostridium difficile* becomes an important consideration.

Accompanying systemic symptoms are important to illicit. High fever is associated with viral and some bacterial infections. Associated rash or wheezing may accompany allergy-mediated diarrhea. Coincident seizure activity in an otherwise healthy child has been associated with *Shigella* infection.

The growth history and nutritional status are also important when considering the cause of chronic diarrhea. In otherwise well toddler-aged children, one of the most common causes of chronic diarrhea is a disorder of small intestine motility called nonspecific diarrhea of childhood ("toddler's diarrhea"). Postinfectious carbohydrate intolerance causing an osmotic diarrhea should be considered in an otherwise well patient with recent acute gastroenteritis. Both these entities may be related to the ingestion of excessive quantities of fluids with a high sugar content (e.g., juices, soda). Such a limited diet leads to villous atrophy and subsequent malabsorption of these carbohydrates and resultant osmotic diarrhea.

Constipation with encopresis is also seen in healthy children with prolonged "diarrhea," which actually represents leakage of stool through a dilated, impacted colon.

Causes of chronic diarrhea associated with poor growth and nutrition are extensive and varied. Plotting a careful growth curve can assist in making a diagnosis. Patients with cystic fibrosis often have poor growth and nutrition recognizable soon after birth. In contrast, infants with celiac disease exhibit poor growth after 4 to 6 months of age, coincident with the introduction of gluten-containing cereals to the diet.

PHYSICAL EXAMINATION

The physical examination should first focus on the patient's hydration status and hemodynamic stability to determine whether immediate fluid resuscitation is needed. Comparison of the premorbid weight to the weight at presentation is the most reliable method of determining the degree of dehydration, but this is often not feasible. Because chronic diarrhea may represent underlying systemic illness, as well as lead to the loss of calories, protein, and other minerals and vitamins (e.g., zinc, vitamin B_2), the physical examination should also look for evidence of these deficiencies (Table 31-2).

EVALUATION

The laboratory evaluation is individualized, with attention paid to the acute versus chronic nature of the diarrhea and the patient's hydration status and age. In many cases of

Table 31–2   Selected Physical Findings Consistent with Evidence of Malnutrition or Systemic Illness

Area of Examination	Finding	Nutritional Deficiency/Systemic Illness
General	Underweight	↓ Calories
	Edematous	↓ Protein
Hair	Easily pluckable, sparse	↓ Protein, zinc
Skin	Generalized dermatitis	↓ Zinc
	Erythema nodosum	Inflammatory bowel disease
Subcutaneous tissue	Decreased	↓ Calories
Muscles	Decreased mass	↓ Calories, protein
Mouth/tongue	Glossitis, angular stomatitis	↓ Vitamin B_2
Extremities	Digital clubbing	Cystic fibrosis
Anus/rectum	Rectal prolapse	Cystic fibrosis
	Perianal tags, fissures, fistulas	Inflammatory bowel disease

viral gastroenteritis, laboratory evaluation is not performed unless it is necessary to manage dehydration. The search for a specific cause should be undertaken in patients with a high fever, toxic appearance, or grossly bloody stools; in hospitalized patients with nosocomial exposure; in immunocompromised patients; in those with recent antibiotic treatment; and in young infants.

When a definitive diagnosis is necessary, the stool should be examined for any or all of the following, based on the history: occult blood and the presence of white blood cells (suggestive of colonic inflammation), fecal fat (fat malabsorption), bacterial culture, ova and parasites, rotazyme assay, *C. difficile* toxin, *Giardia* antigen assay, and α₁-antitrypsin assay. Different laboratories may have protocols to isolate different pathogens when "routine" bacterial culture is requested. If there is concern about a particular enteric pathogen, this should be communicated to the laboratory so that the specimens can be plated on the appropriate media. If carbohydrate malabsorption is suspected, stool pH (<5.5) and analysis for the presence of reducing substances may be helpful in making a diagnosis.

Depending on the severity of illness, serum laboratory studies may be necessary. Signs of significant dehydration may warrant evaluation of electrolytes and renal function. The hematocrit can identify the presence of anemia associated with acute or chronic hematochezia. If an underlying immune deficiency is suspected, the complete blood count with differential and quantitative immunoglobulin levels may be helpful. The erythrocyte sedimentation rate and C-reactive protein are nonspecific and may be elevated in an infectious or inflammatory process. Total protein, albumin, and prealbumin levels may reflect the extent or chronicity of malnutrition, if present. Vitamin and mineral deficiencies can be identified with further laboratory investigation, if indicated. If celiac disease is suspected, tests for antigliadin, antiendomysial, and tissue transglutaminase antibodies should be performed. A sweat-chloride test should be obtained when cystic fibrosis is a concern.

Imaging or direct visualization studies are rarely helpful in the evaluation of patients with acute diarrheal illness, because most have a viral gastroenteritis. In these patients, plain films typically reveal a nonspecific bowel gas pattern, with or without associated air-fluid levels. Radiographs, computed tomography, or endoscopy may be warranted to evaluate other diagnostic considerations, especially if the symptoms are severe or prolonged.

TREATMENT

Most cases of acute diarrhea are self-limited illnesses that can be managed with oral rehydration therapy and close outpatient follow-up. However, patients who are unable to tolerate adequate enteral hydration, have underlying illnesses that complicate management, or need rapid evaluation for other diagnoses warrant admission.

Initial management consists of fluid resuscitation to achieve hemodynamic stability. Intravenous boluses of an isotonic solution should be administered and repeated until the patient's intravascular volume has been restored. Replacement of any remaining fluid deficits, continued maintenance requirements, and ongoing fluid losses should be handled with infusions of appropriate intravenous solutions (see Chapter 57).

Once a patient is able, oral intake should be initiated as soon as possible, with advancement to solid intake as tolerated.[1] There is no medical reason to delay solid food intake secondary to persistent diarrhea. Although intestinal absorption of nutrients is compromised in the presence of diarrhea, 80% of dietary carbohydrates and 50% of dietary proteins continue to be absorbed.[2] Some studies suggest that early initiation of dietary nutrients may help decrease output or promote the resolution of diarrhea. Avoidance of cow milk protein, although strongly recommended in the past, may not be warranted with acute diarrheal illnesses, because a clinically significant acquired lactase deficiency is uncommon in this setting. In certain cases, additional nutritional support should be considered. For instance, the presence of intractable vomiting may delay the initiation of oral intake. In such cases, placement of a nasogastric or nasojejunal tube may be helpful to avoid prolonged periods of inadequate nutrition. Elemental formulas may be better tolerated in cases of significant malabsorption. Finally, total parenteral nutrition may be necessary in severe cases of malnutrition, especially those associated with an underlying systemic illness.

Pharmacologic treatment is rarely needed for acute diarrhea, although appropriate antibiotic therapy should certainly be given for infectious causes (see Chapter 68). Antidiarrheal agents should be avoided in young children. Although adsorbents (e.g., activated magnesium aluminum silicate and bulk-forming fibers) act to absorb fluid within the intestine, they do not decrease overall fluid losses or the risk of dehydration. Antimotility agents should never be used in the presence of bloody diarrhea or when an infectious cause is suspected; they may prolong the carrier state. Probiotic agents have recently gained increased popularity in the management of diarrhea. *Lactobacillus GG* and *Saccharomyces boulardii* function to alter the intestinal flora in the face of diarrhea, resulting in a modest decrease in stool output. Specifically, *Lactobacillus GG* has been associated with decreased severity of rotavirus infection. Antiemetic therapy may be helpful for patients with associated vomiting.

SUGGESTED READING

Cohen MB: Evaluation and treatment of the child with acute diarrhea. In Rudolph AM, Rudolph CD, Hostetter MK, et al: Rudolph's Pediatrics, 21st ed. Norwalk, Conn, Appleton & Lange, 2002, pp 1363-1366.
Duggan C, Nurko S: "Feeding the gut": The scientific basis for continued enteral nutrition during acute diarrhea. J Pediatr 1997;131:801-808.
Mascarenhas MR, Piccoli DA: Gastroenterology and Nutrition: The Pediatric Clinics of North America. Philadelphia, WB Saunders, 2002.
Silverman A, Roy CC, et al (eds): Pediatric Clinical Gastroenterology. St Louis, Mosby, 1995.

REFERENCES

1. King CK, Glass R, Bresee JS, et al: Managing acute gastroenteritis among children: Oral rehydration, maintenance, and nutritional therapy. MMWR Recomm Rep 2003;52:1-16.
2. Duggan C, Nurko S: "Feeding the gut": The scientific basis for continued enteral nutrition during acute diarrhea. J Pediatr 1997;131:801-808.

CHAPTER 32

Failure to Thrive

Stephen D. Wilson

Failure to thrive (FTT) is among the most challenging diagnostic entities facing pediatric hospitalists. The interaction of psychosocial, behavioral, and physiologic factors can be complex. Because there is no uniformly accepted definition of FTT, the incidence cannot be precisely determined. However, in high-risk populations (e.g., low-birth-weight infants, children living in poverty), estimates run as high as 5% to 10%.[1,2]

FTT represents approximately 1% to 5% of patient referrals to tertiary care pediatric centers. Although the disorder is managed primarily in the outpatient setting, more challenging or severely affected patients, or those whose safety is in question, may require hospitalization. Thus, it is critical for pediatric hospitalists to have a clear approach to this diagnostic challenge.

BACKGROUND

FTT is not a diagnosis but rather a description of undernutrition and deficient growth over time. Owing to the vagary of the term, many specialists have suggested that it be replaced by *growth deficiency, growth failure,* or *undernutrition*. To date, none of these terms has gained widespread acceptance, so they are often used interchangeably with FTT.

Growth failure can occur at any age. However, owing to the vulnerability of infants and toddlers and their complete dependence on caregivers for nutrition, it is most commonly noted in the youngest age groups. Approximately 80% of cases involve infants younger than 6 months; more than 95% of patients are younger than 2 years.[1-3]

Although there is no consensus definition of FTT, it is commonly defined as weight below the 5th percentile or a downward change in growth rate that results in the crossing of two major percentile lines for weight. Additionally, weight for height or height for age below the 10th percentile has been used as an indicator of deficient growth. These rigid criteria, however, greatly oversimplify the complex task of identifying children in whom growth is a problem. As many as 25% of normal infants cross major percentile lines during their first 2 years of life, then maintain growth consistently along the new curve.[4-6] Most of these children show no signs of illness and should not be categorized as failing to thrive. Similarly, there are healthy children who consistently track along a specific growth curve at or below the 5th percentile, usually owing to genetic factors such as diminutive parental height. By definition, such children represent 5% of the normal population and should not be labeled as growth retarded. For these reasons, it preferable to define FTT more generally as inadequate growth over time relative to standardized growth charts, after taking into account genetic background.

In the early stages, undernutrition may be of little obvious consequence to the child. However, more severe or long-standing cases may lead to short stature, reduced muscle mass, impaired brain growth, and behavioral or developmental abnormalities.[6-8] The most severe malnutrition syndromes—marasmus (severe global caloric deficiency) and kwashiorkor (severe protein deficiency)—are rarely seen in the industrialized world but illustrate the dramatic extremes of these effects.

Initially, undernutrition causes an isolated slowing of weight gain. With more long-standing nutritional deficiency, height velocity also slows. Head growth is typically spared until the problem has become severe. Because of this predictable pattern of growth failure, anthropomorphic measurements provide insight into the chronicity of the process.[9]

PATHOPHYSIOLOGY

The cause of FTT is frequently multifactorial. Although the list of possible organic causes is long, psychosocial and behavioral factors play a predominant role in the majority of cases; this is particularly true in patients younger than 2 years. In general, inadequate growth can be caused by any combination of four factors: (1) abnormally low caloric intake, (2) inadequate digestion and absorption of ingested calories, (3) abnormally high metabolic demands, or (4) impaired utilization of calories.

Inadequate caloric intake is most commonly caused by psychosocial or behavioral factors that inhibit appropriate feeding. A chaotic home environment, inadequate bonding between primary caregivers and infant, difficulty with breastfeeding, incorrect preparation of infant formula, parental stress, depression, or substance abuse, and other such factors may inhibit normal feeding. If inadequate feeding continues, the infant or child may lose or fail to develop appropriate hunger-satiety cues, and inadequate intake may become an entrenched behavior.[10]

Anatomic or neurologic abnormalities can also interfere with feeding. Cleft palate or other undetected oropharyngeal anomalies may inhibit an infant's normal suck-swallow mechanism. Brain injury or in utero drug exposure may impair the development of an organized feeding pattern. Delayed gastric emptying may cause early satiety and contribute to gastroesophageal reflux. Gastroesophageal reflux often causes pain immediately after eating and may lead to feeding aversion or habitual early cessation of feeding.[11-13]

Inadequate absorption of ingested calories may stem from inherited or acquired gastrointestinal conditions that result in inadequate growth despite appropriate caloric intake. Malabsorption syndromes typically cause an abnormal stool character, such as smelly, bulky stools suggestive of fat malabsorption, bloody diarrhea with mucus (e.g., milk protein intolerance), or watery stools typical of carbohydrate malabsorption (e.g., persistent diarrhea following a bout of infectious diarrhea).

Increased metabolic demands can stem from innumerable conditions. Major causes include cardiac disease with increased cardiac work, pulmonary disease resulting in chronic increased work of breathing or chronic hypoxemia, chronic inflammation, chronic infection, or malignancy. Impaired utilization of calories can be seen in a variety of metabolic and genetic disorders.

DIFFERENTIAL DIAGNOSIS

Before seeking an underlying cause, it is crucial to ensure that concerns about poor growth are warranted. Inexperienced practitioners may mistake the normal crossing of percentile lines or familial small size for FTT. A multitude of processes can contribute to growth deficiency, many of which are listed in Box 32-1.

INITIAL STABILIZATION

Most patients with FTT, even those who are significantly malnourished, are clinically stable. Signs of critical malnutrition include bradycardia, hypothermia, dehydration, and altered mental status. If any of these signs are present, stabilization of the patient and the acute management of malnutrition or associated dehydration take precedence. Subsequently, nutrition must be reestablished slowly to avoid the complications of refeeding syndrome (see Chapter 99).[14]

If a patient is hospitalized but does not have signs of instability, it is preferable to forgo some common admission procedures, such as placement of an intravenous catheter and continuous monitoring devices. The successful evaluation of FTT inevitably depends on the patient feeling comfortable enough to feed. Minimizing painful or frightening interventions may be crucial to establishing the appropriate environment.

HISTORY AND PHYSICAL EXAMINATION

Because so many cases of FTT are attributable to behavioral and psychosocial factors, obtaining an extremely detailed feeding history is key. This must include details of the child's diet, including volume, frequency, and content of intake; for infants, a careful assessment of the preparation of formula at home is crucial. Other factors include feeding environment (supervision, distractions, feeding position) and feeding behavior (distractibility, food refusal, early satiety). It is also important to ask parents about their perceptions of the child's temperament and about the child's interactions with the rest of the family; if a child is seen as a difficult or troubled member of the family, this may indicate a disordered parent-child bond. A family history regarding growth patterns should also be taken, as well as a detailed social history. Key areas to explore include major stressors in the home, financial difficulties, depression, substance abuse, domestic violence, and a history of prior involvement with a child protective agency. Because these factors are central to understanding feeding difficulties, it is advisable to interview the family more than once and to consider the assistance of a pediatric social worker. Box 32-2 lists important aspects of

Box 32-1   Major Causes of Failure to Thrive
Inadequate intake
Disturbance of parent-child relationship
Neglect
Food aversion, behavioral problems
Incorrectly mixed formula
Improper food choices, inadequate food
Oromotor dyscoordination
Gastroesophageal reflux
Pyloric stenosis
Delayed gastric emptying
Anatomic abnormalities
Central nervous system dysfunction
Malabsorption
Milk protein intolerance
Bacterial overgrowth
Bile acid malabsorption
Hepatobiliary disease
Enzyme deficiencies
Celiac disease
Inflammatory bowel disease
Villous atrophy
Short-bowel syndrome
Acrodermatitis enteropathica
Increased metabolic demands
Congestive heart failure/major heart disease
Chronic hypoxemia
Bronchopulmonary dysplasia
Cystic fibrosis
Restrictive lung disease
Upper airway obstruction
Chronic anemia
Chronic infection (e.g., HIV, tuberculosis)
Chronic renal failure
Chronic inflammatory disease (e.g., inflammatory bowel disease)
Malignancy
Thyroid disease
Spasticity, choreoathetosis
Defective utilization of calories
Inborn errors of metabolism
Chromosomal anomaly
Diabetes mellitus
Renal tubular acidosis

the history for cases of FTT. The remainder of the history is directed toward eliciting symptoms suggestive of an underlying organic disease (Box 32-3).

A directed physical examination (Box 32-4) should begin with carefully measured weight, length, and head circumference. These should be plotted using the 2002 revised growth charts from the Centers for Disease Control, which draw from a more diverse population to determine normal ranges than did previous versions.[15] Wasting should be noted as diminished subcutaneous fat, with attention to the temporal and thenar areas. In addition, the physical examination should be targeted to identify any craniofacial anomalies, signs of chronic cardiac or pulmonary disease, hepatic enlargement, neurodevelopmental abnormalities, or features suggestive of a chromosomal anomaly. Close attention

---

Box 32-2   Focused History

Dietary history
    Details of everything the child eats and drinks
    For infants, check proper formula preparation
    Quantification of caloric intake
    History of excessive juice, soft drinks, or cow's milk
    Vegetarian or other restrictive diet
Feeding history
    When, where, and with whom the child eats
    For infants, feeding or breastfeeding position
    Eye contact while feeding (especially infants)
    Distractions during feeding (e.g., TV, toys, siblings)
    Duration of each feeding
    Hunger at feeding time
    Resistance to eating
Family history
    History of delayed growth in parents or siblings
    Height and weight of both parents
    Family history of major systemic disease
Social history
    Interaction with the family
    Parental description of patient's temperament
    Financial stressors, difficulty buying food
    Identification of all caregivers, especially those who feed the
        patient
    Parental history of depression or other mental illness
    Indicators of substance abuse in the family
    Indicators of domestic violence
    Involvement of a child protective agency with the family

Box 32-3   History Suggestive of Organic Disease

Difficulty initiating suck
Sputtering or choking during feeding
Spitting up, vomiting, or signs of pain after feeding
Early satiety
Abnormal stools (watery, bloody, mucoid, foul smelling)
Indicators of neurodevelopmental delay
History of birth trauma, asphyxia, or postnatal head injury
For infants, diaphoresis or dyspnea when feeding
Chronic shortness of breath, labored breathing, stridor, or
    snoring
Chronic or recurrent fevers
HIV risk factors

Box 32-4   Directed Physical Examination

Vital signs
    Bradycardia, hypothermia (indicative of critical malnutrition)
General
    Height, weight, head circumference, and body mass index
        plotted on growth chart
    Midparental height*
    Subcutaneous fat
    Poor hygiene, dental caries, other signs of possible neglect
    Dysmorphic features
Head, eyes, ears, nose, and throat
    Markedly enlarged tonsils
    Stridor
    Craniofacial anomalies
Chest
    Increased work of breathing
    Chest wall deformities
Cardiovascular
    Signs of increased cardiac work (tachycardia, hyperdynamic
        precordium)
    Pathologic murmur
Abdomen
    Hepatomegaly or jaundice
Extremities
    Clubbing
Skin
    Pallor
    Cyanosis
    Unusual rashes
Neurologic
    Abnormal tone or reflexes
    Developmental delay
    Abnormal affect or social interactions

*Midparental height calculation: boys = (Maternal height + Paternal height + 13 cm)/2; girls = (Maternal height + Paternal height − 13 cm)/2.

should also be paid to any potential signs of abuse or neglect.

EVALUATION

Often, the direct observation of the patient being fed is the most informative evaluation. Typically, multiple feedings must be evaluated, and the environment should be as similar to home as possible.

With infants in particular, careful attention must be paid to the interaction between the infant and the caregiver during feedings. If the parent appears uncomfortable holding or feeding the infant or is quick to relinquish the infant to medical personnel, this suggests psychosocial disruption. An infant with disorganized early feeding behavior or one who becomes easily distracted or fussy during feeding may be demonstrating temperamental or neurodevelopmental characteristics that impair the parents' ability to feed the infant. It is particularly notable if, under these circumstances, the parent stops feeding the baby prematurely.

With toddlers and young children, the initial evaluation also involves close observation of feeding behavior; however, the focus is directed more toward the child. Key elements to evaluate include the patient's overall temperament, his or her ability to focus during mealtimes, food choices, attitudes toward eating and food, and emotional struggles with caregivers regarding food. Specific attention should be paid to consistent food refusal, because this is the hallmark of behavioral FTT in toddlers, also known as infantile anorexia.[16]

As part of the evaluation, consultation with a feeding specialist, typically a pediatric speech or occupational therapist, should be considered. In addition to observing the caregiver's approach to feeding, these professionals may feed the patient themselves and can often identify abnormalities in oromotor coordination or swallowing or certain behaviors that suggest pain with feeding. In addition, during their evaluation sessions, they can experiment with subtle variations in positioning, timing of feeding, nipple types, and feeding environment to determine whether a successful feeding routine can be established.

Even when behavioral or psychosocial issues are identified and feeding disturbances are obviously present, it is often unclear whether these factors are the only explanation for poor growth. Under such circumstances, or when no clear feeding disturbance is identified, the next step is careful daily weight determinations during a period of enforced caloric intake. This may be done with either carefully supervised feedings of a preset caloric content or nasogastric feeding. If appropriate weight gain ensues, the focus can remain on feeding. If appropriate caloric intake does not result in the expected weight gain, a more comprehensive workup should be undertaken to look for organic causes of malabsorption, increased metabolic demand, or impaired utilization. It should be noted that when growth retardation affects length and head circumference along with weight, it is more likely that an organic condition is present.

Laboratory evaluations for organic causes of FTT are often reserved for cases in which feeding disturbances and psychosocial factors do not explain the entire picture. Historical data suggest that without specific evidence of organic disease, laboratory testing is helpful in only about 2% of cases of FTT.[17] When underlying organic disease is suspected, laboratory evaluation should include a complete blood count, serum electrolytes, renal function tests, and stool samples for occult blood, pH, and reducing substances. These tests help rule out anemia, chronic acidosis, renal disease, carbohydrate malabsorption, and milk protein intolerance, all of which may be relatively difficult to diagnose clinically. Many practitioners also include sedimentation rate, thyroid function tests, sweat chloride, and fecal fat quantitation as part of the laboratory evaluation. When indicated by history, pH probe, gastric emptying studies, and echocardiogram may be helpful. Other laboratory tests that may help determine the severity of the malnutrition include serum levels of transaminases, albumin, prealbumin, vitamins, and minerals such as calcium, magnesium, and phosphorus.

TREATMENT

Underlying causes of poor weight gain should be identified and corrected if possible. Organic conditions should be treated, and behavioral and psychosocial problems should be addressed. Frequently, ongoing family counseling and social work support are crucial.

Irrespective of cause, all patients with FTT need caloric supplementation to promote catch-up growth. Caloric requirements vary with the age of the infant, the degree of undernutrition, and the presence or absence of underlying organic disease. Caloric and nutritional goals are best set in consultation with a pediatric nutritionist, but general guidelines are provided in Table 32-1.

Infants should be placed on a feeding schedule with defined volume goals. Many require hypercaloric formula (24 to 30 Calories/ounce) to obtain catch-up growth. In exclusively breastfed infants, hypercaloric supplemental feedings may be provided using expressed breast milk with added human milk fortifier or added powdered formula. For toddlers and children, caloric intake can be increased

Table 32-1 General Guidelines for Caloric Needs in Infancy*

Type of Growth	Caloric Requirements (kcal/kg/day)[†]
Normal	80-120
"Catch up"	140-160

*Consultation with a pediatric nutritionist is recommended for patients with malnutrition.
†Approximate distribution of calories: 10% protein, 50% carbohydrate, 40% fat.

through dietary counseling and the use of high-calorie liquid supplements. Parenteral nutrition may be required for severe malabsorption, usually as a temporizing measure.

Despite dietary modifications of oral intake, it is not uncommon for weight gain to fall short of expectations. Patients who have experienced chronic undernutrition often experience early satiety. In these cases, placement of a nasogastric tube for supplementation is usually effective. It is generally preferable to deliver the nasogastric supplementation at night so as not to interfere with daytime appetite.

For hospitalized patients, the goals before discharge should include identification and treatment of any underlying disease, establishment of a feeding regimen that delivers adequate calories, and parental education about appropriate feeding techniques. Once initial success has been demonstrated, monitoring of long-term weight gain should be undertaken in the outpatient setting.

Long-term success can be improved by involving a multidisciplinary team in the outpatient phase. Frequent follow-up should be arranged with the patient's primary care provider, a nutritionist, and a family counselor.

SPECIAL CONSIDERATIONS

The typical hospital setting contains several challenges to the diagnosis and management of FTT. Hospital rooms are usually noisy and distracting, and busy hospital staff members may consider the needs of these children a lower priority than the needs of those who are acutely ill. Additionally, weight is better followed over weeks rather than days, which makes a primarily hospital-based evaluation problematic. When outpatient management has failed, however, hospitalization may be unavoidable. To facilitate a productive hospital stay, it is preferable for the patient to stay in a private room with his or her primary caregiver. Typical hospital interruptions such as the use of monitors and the taking of nighttime vital signs should be minimized. It may be most practical to limit hospitalization to patient evaluation and initiation of a treatment plan. Weight gain can then be followed during frequent outpatient visits, and contingency plans can be made to rehospitalize the patient if the anticipated weight gain does not occur.

SUGGESTED READING

Berwick DM: Nonorganic failure to thrive. Pediatr Rev 1980;1:265.
Berwick DM, Levey JC, Kleinerman R: Failure to thrive: Diagnostic yield of hospitalization. Arch Dis Child 1982;57:347.

Bithoney WG, Dubowitz H, Harwood E: Failure to thrive/growth deficiency. Pediatr Rev 1992;13:453.

Frank D, Silva M, Needleman R: Failure to thrive: Mystery, myth and method. Contemp Pediatr 1993;10:114.

Gahagan S, Holmes R: A stepwise approach to evaluation of undernutrition and failure to thrive. Pediatr Clin North Am 1998;45:169.

Homer C, Ludwig S: Categorization of etiology of failure to thrive. Am J Dis Child 1981;135:848.

Kessler DB, Dawson P (eds): Failure to Thrive and Pediatric Undernutrition: A Transdisciplinary Approach. Baltimore, Brookes, 1999.

Maggioni A, Lifshitz F: Nutritional management of failure to thrive. Pediatr Clin North Am 1995;42:791.

Rudolph CD, Link DT: Feeding disorders in infants and children. Pediatr Clin North Am 2002;49:97.

Schwartz D: Failure to thrive: An old nemesis in the new millennium. Pediatr Rev 2000;21:257.

REFERENCES

1. Gahagan S, Holmes R: A stepwise approach to evaluation of undernutrition and failure to thrive. Pediatr Clin North Am 1998;45: 169.

2. Sherry B: Epidemiology of inadequate growth. In Kessler DB, Dawson P (eds): Failure to Thrive and Pediatric Undernutrition: A Transdisciplinary Approach. Baltimore, Brookes, 1999, p 19.

3. Bithoney WG, Dubowitz H, Harwood E: Failure to thrive/growth deficiency. Pediatr Rev 1992;13:453.

4. Schwartz D: Failure to thrive: An old nemesis in the new millennium. Pediatr Rev 2000;21:257.

5. Smith DW, Troug W, Rogers JE, et al: Shifting linear growth during infancy: Illustration of genetic factors in growth from fetal life through infancy. J Pediatr 1976;89:225.

6. Corbett SS, Drewett RF, Wright CM: Does a fall down a centile chart matter? The growth and developmental sequelae of mild failure to thrive. Acta Paediatr 1996;85:1278.

7. Mettalinos-Katsaras E, Gorman KS: Effects of undernutrition on growth and development. In Kessler DB, Dawson P (eds): Failure to Thrive and Pediatric Undernutrition: A Transdisciplinary Approach. Baltimore, Brookes, 1999, p 37.

8. Gates RK, Peacock A, Forrest D: Long-term effects of nonorganic failure to thrive. Pediatrics 1985;75:36.

9. Raynor P, Rudolf MC: Anthropomorphic indices of failure to thrive. Arch Dis Child 2000;82:364.

10. Frank DA, Zeisel SH: Failure to thrive. Pediatr Clin North Am 1988; 35:1187.

11. Manikam R, Perman J: Pediatric feeding disorders. J Clin Gastroenterol 2000;30:34.

12. Nelson SP, Chen EH, Syniar GM: Prevalence of symptoms of gastro-esophageal reflux in infancy: A pediatric practice-based survey. Arch Pediatr Adolesc Med 1997;151:569.

13. Fleishe DR: Comprehensive management of infants with gastro-esophageal reflux and failure to thrive. Curr Probl Pediatr 1995;25:247.

14. Solomon SM, Kirby DF: The refeeding syndrome: A review. JPEN J Parenter Enteral Nutr 1990;14:90.

15. Centers for Disease Control growth charts. Available at *www.cdc.gov/growthcharts/*.

16. Chatoor I, Ganiban J, Hirsch R, et al: Maternal characteristics and toddler temperament in infantile anorexia. J Am Acad Child Adolesc Psychiatry 2000;39:743.

17. Sills RH: Failure to thrive: The role of clinical and laboratory evaluation. Am J Dis Child 1978;132:967.

CHAPTER 33

Fever

Rana N. Kronfol

Most children undergo at least one medical evaluation for a febrile illness before their third birthday, and nearly one third of pediatric outpatient visits are for fever. Fever is a controlled increase in body temperature, usually by 1°C to 4°C, that is regulated by the central nervous system and mediated by endocrine, autonomic, and behavioral mechanisms.[1-3] Although fever is a common manifestation of infection, it is a feature of many diseases, both infectious and noninfectious.[3] The classic triad in the differential diagnosis of fever is infectious disease, rheumatic disease, and malignancy.

NORMAL BODY TEMPERATURE AND FEVER PATHOPHYSIOLOGY

There is a diurnal or circadian variation that results in body temperatures that are approximately 0.5°C to 1°C higher in the late afternoon or early evening than in the early morning.[2,3] Body temperature is controlled by the thermoregulatory center in the anterior hypothalamus, where thermosensitive neurons respond to changes in blood temperature and signals from cold and warm receptors in skin and muscle.[2] Thermoregulatory mechanisms include the following:

- Heat production by metabolic activity in the liver and muscles, such as secretion of acute phase reactants, production of glucocorticoids, and decreased secretion of vasopressin.
- Heat dissipation by the skin and lungs via redirection of blood flow to or from cutaneous vascular beds, sweating, tachypnea, and rigors (shivering).
- Behavioral responses, such as thirst or seeking shelter.

Important mediators of fever are endogenous pyrogens, or cytokines, which are small proteins that regulate immune, inflammatory, and hematopoietic processes.[3] The most studied of these are the primary endogenous pyrogens interleukin (IL)-1, IL-6, tumor necrosis factor-α, and interferon-α and -γ. These cytokines are released by leukocytes in response to infectious agents or toxic reactions. Peripheral cytokines, also called acute phase reactants, are released in response to inflammation and use several mechanisms to signal the brain to produce fever. Once the cytokines are released into the bloodstream, they are carried to the hypothalamus, where they stimulate the vascular endothelial cell production of prostaglandin E_2 (PGE_2). Specific E-prostanoid receptors within the hypothalamus then trigger the febrile response after the PGE_2 signal.[4]

The diagnosis of fever is based on the measurement of body or core temperature. Normal diurnal variations in temperature for an individual and normal differences in baseline temperature between individuals may be as much as 1.1°C (2°F). As such, there is no definitive lowest temperature elevation that is considered abnormal. Most clinicians consider any temperature above 38°C (100.4°F) to be a fever, especially in the immediate newborn period. Beyond the first 2 to 3 months of life, a temperature greater than 38.3°C (101°F) is often used as the cutoff for fever, although many consider a temperature of 39°C (102.2°F) or higher the threshold that triggers an evaluation for a serious bacterial illness.

The most accurate method of obtaining body temperature is by a rectal thermometer. Oral, axillary, tympanic, and infrared temperature readings taken at home are less accurate but should be considered when taking a history. A home diary of daily fevers is an extremely valuable tool when evaluating a patient with prolonged fever.

EVALUATION

Fever is a sign of a condition that incites cytokine production. The focus of the evaluation is identifying that inciting condition. Chapter 60 discusses fever in infants and toddlers, and illnesses associated with prolonged fever (i.e., fever of unknown origin) are discussed in Chapter 61. Elevations in body temperature may also occur without an inflammatory trigger, as seen in heat disorders, which are discussed in Chapter 185. Fever in an immunocompromised host is discussed in Chapters 73 and 124.

A thorough history and physical examination usually provide the most important clues in determining the cause of fever. Fever may be a sign of a benign, self-limited condition or may be indicative of a life-threatening illness. As such, the overall appearance of the patient must be assessed. Does the patient appear toxic or well? Are there any associated signs or symptoms? What medications are being used, including antibiotics or folk remedies? Has the patient had contact with any ill individuals with similar symptoms? A travel history and a history of exposure to pets or insects should also be included.

The pattern of the fever itself may provide useful information for diagnosis. A single spike of fever is usually not associated with an infectious disease, although it may be due to manipulation of catheters, drugs, and blood infusions. Table 33-1 lists other common fever patterns and the associated diseases.

When a patient has a fever greater than 41°C, noninfectious conditions should be considered, including central fever resulting from central nervous system dysfunction, drug fever, malignant neuroleptic syndrome, heatstroke, and malignant hyperthermia (see Chapter 185).[2]

Table 33-1 Patterns of Fever

Fever Type	Description
Intermittent	Exaggerated circadian rhythm that includes normal temperatures on most days
Septic	Wide fluctuation in temperatures
Sustained	Persistent fever that does not fluctuate by more than 0.5°C in 24 hr
Remittent	Persistent fever that varies by more than 0.5°C in 24 hr (e.g., tuberculosis, viral fever, many bacterial infections)
Relapsing	Febrile periods separated by intervals of normal temperature (*Borrelia* infection)
Tertian	Fever that occurs on the first and third days (malaria caused by *Plasmodium vivax*)
Quartan	Fever that occurs on the first and fourth days (malaria caused by *Plasmodium malariae*)
Biphasic	Illness with two distinct periods of fever over ≥1 wk (e.g., poliomyelitis)
Periodic	Recurring illnesses with some periodicity (e.g., cyclic neutropenia, familial Mediterranean fever)

The relationship between the patient's pulse rate and fever may also aid diagnosis. Relative tachycardia, in which the pulse rate is elevated out of proportion to temperature, is suggestive of a noninfectious process such as a toxin-mediated illness. Relative bradycardia, when the pulse rate is low despite the temperature elevation, suggests typhoid fever, brucellosis, leptospirosis, Legionnaires' disease, drug fever, or a cardiac conduction defect that may occur with acute rheumatic fever, Lyme disease, viral myocarditis, or infective endocarditis.[2]

Given that an infection anywhere in the body can cause fever, a complete examination with attention to possible signs of infection (pain, erythema, swelling, tenderness) must be done. The skin, in particular, should be examined closely, because a number of rashes with fever may be diagnostic (see Chapter 62).

Postoperative patients may develop fever from a number of causes, including atelectasis, dehydration, wound infection, bacteremia, and deep venous thrombosis. Patients who have had urinary bladder catheters in place are at increased risk for urinary tract infection. Further, any procedure involving the surgical placement of a device such as a catheter, shunt, rod, or other hardware carries a risk of infection (see Chapter 71).

TREATMENT

Antipyresis is controversial among clinicians, scientists, caregivers, and patients. "Fever phobia," or an unrealistic concern based on misperceptions of fever, persists.[3] Many caregivers believe that fever is a disease (rather than a symptom) and that fever itself may have life-threatening or brain-damaging effects. In part, this may be due to the health care system's emphasis on fever when children are being evaluated for illness.

The benefits of fever reduction include patient comfort, improved oral intake, decreased insensible fluid loss, improved ability to assess the patient's demeanor, and potential diminished risk of febrile seizures.[5] Highly febrile children often have a toxic appearance, and it may be useful to evaluate a child with a febrile illness after the fever has been reduced. However, the fever's response to antipyretics is not diagnostic and does not provide information about its cause. Children with serious bacterial infections and children with self-limited, benign viral illnesses defervesce with antipyretic therapy in a similar fashion. There is also some evidence that the same pyrogenic cytokines responsible for fever have potentially detrimental effects.[5]

The concern remains that lowering a fever may impair the body's ability to fight off infection, remove important diagnostic clues regarding the pattern of fever, and interfere with the interpretation of the response to therapy for the inciting condition. For instance, some species of bacteria are killed or have their growth impaired by elevated temperatures.[6] Further data suggest that fever may have a beneficial effect on the outcome of many infections.[7] Recently, fever-induced proteins have been identified that may be protective against oxidative injury.[8]

Antipyresis is most commonly pursued pharmacologically. PGE_2, which is central to the production of fever, is synthesized from arachidonic acid, mediated by the enzyme cyclooxygenase (COX).[4] There are two isoforms of this enzyme, COX-1 and COX-2. COX-1 is expressed throughout the body constitutively and is thought to be important for a variety of "housekeeping" functions to maintain homeostasis. COX-2 is inducible by a number of the pyrogenic cytokines and is thought to be the key provider of PGE_2 during the febrile and inflammatory response.

Aspirin and other nonsteroidal anti-inflammatory drugs (NSAIDs), such as ibuprofen, interfere with prostaglandin production through nonselective COX inhibition and downregulation of the expression of COX enzymes.[4] As a result, they have both antipyretic and anti-inflammatory effects. Newer selective COX-2 inhibitors were created to maintain the antipyretic and anti-inflammatory effects of the nonselective agents but cause fewer unwanted side effects of COX-1 inhibition, such as gastrointestinal bleeding. However, the Food and Drug Administration recently requested that the makers of selective COX-2 inhibitors include a boxed warning on the package insert about the potential gastrointestinal and cardiovascular risks of the drug.[9]

Surprisingly, the exact mechanism of action of acetaminophen, the most commonly used antipyretic in pediatrics, remains unknown. It possesses excellent antipyretic but relatively weak anti-inflammatory effects. It is a weak inhibitor of COX, but its effect may be based on tissue-specific COX inhibitors. Acetaminophen penetrates the blood-brain barrier and causes a fall in central nervous system PGE_2 production.

Despite the controversies and uncertainties, virtually all parents expect their children to be treated for fever. Acetaminophen (15 mg/kg every 4 hours) or ibuprofen (10 mg/kg every 6 hours) is the mainstay of treatment. Tepid sponge baths are not recommended to reduce fever because data have shown that they are no more effective than antipyretics alone and significantly increase patient discomfort scores.[10]

SUGGESTED READING

Aronoff DM, Neilson EG: Antipyretics: Mechanisms of action and clinical use in fever suppression. Am J Med 2001;111:304-315.

Greisman LA, Mackowiak PA: Fever: Beneficial and detrimental effects of antipyretics. Curr Opin Infect Dis 2002;15:241-245.

Lorin MI: Pathophysiology and treatment of fever in infants and children. Up To Date, June 2004.

Powell KR: Fever. In Behrman RE (ed): Nelson Textbook of Pediatrics, 17th ed. Philadelphia, Elsevier, 2004, pp 839-841.

REFERENCES

1. Cotran RS: Acute and chronic inflammation. In Robbins Pathologic Basis of Disease, 6th ed. Philadelphia, WB Saunders, 1999, p 86.
2. Powell KR: Fever. In Behrman RE: Nelson Textbook of Pediatrics, 17th ed. Philadelphia, Elsevier, 2004, p 839.
3. Crocetti M, Moghbeli N, Serwint J: Fever phobia revisited: Have parental misconceptions about fever changed in 20 years? Pediatrics 2001;107: 1241-1246.
4. Aronoff DM, Neilson EG: Antipyretics: Mechanisms of action and clinical use in fever suppression. Am J Med 2001;111:304-315.
5. Greisman LA, Mackowiak PA: Fever: Beneficial and detrimental effects of antipyretics. Curr Opin Infect Dis 2002;15: 241-245.
6. Small PM, Tauber MG, Hackbarth CJ, et al: Influence of body temperature on bacterial growth rates in experimental pneumococcal meningitis in rabbits. Infect Immun 1986;52:484-487.
7. Kluger MJ, Wieslaw K, Conn CA, et al: The adaptive value of fever. In Mackowiak PA (ed): Fever: Basic Mechanisms and Management. 2nd ed. Philadelphia, Lippincott-Raven, 1997, pp 255-266.
8. Singh IS, Calderwood S, Kalvakolanu, et al: Inhibition of tumor necrosis factor-α transcription in macrophages exposed to febrile range temperature: A possible role for heat shock factor-1. J Biol Chem 2000;275: 9841-9848.
9. FDA announces series of changes to the class of marketed non-steroidal anti-inflammatory drugs (NSAIDs). FDA press release, Apr 7, 2005.
10. Sharber J: The efficacy of tepid sponge bathing to reduce fever in young children. Am J Emerg Med 1997;15:188-192.

CHAPTER 34

Gastrointestinal Bleeding

Venus M. Villalva

Gastrointestinal (GI) bleeding is a common complaint in the pediatric population and produces alarm and anxiety in parents and physicians. Most causes of GI bleeding do not result in massive or significant bleeding, and 75% to 85% of acute upper GI bleeding ceases spontaneously.[1,2] However, serious illness can present with GI bleeding, leading to hemodynamic compromise that requires aggressive resuscitation and intervention. The diagnostic possibilities are extensive, and a systematic approach is required, including the following:

1. Assessment of the patient for hemodynamic compromise and initiation of appropriate resuscitation measures
2. Confirmation of the presence of GI bleeding and determination of its level
3. Evaluation, including history and physical examination, appropriate laboratory evaluation, imaging, and endoscopy
4. Theraupeutic intervention based on cause

BACKGROUND

GI hemorrhage refers to blood loss from the GI tract at any level. The clinical presentation and character of the blood loss can help localize the site of the bleeding. *Hematemesis* refers to vomiting of either fresh or altered blood (such as coffee grounds emesis) and implies recent or continuing bleeding proximal to the ligament of Treitz.[3,4] *Hematochezia* refers to bright red blood per rectum or maroon-colored stools and usually originates in the colon. However, upper GI hemorrhage may present with hematochezia in approximately 10% of cases,[3] secondary to increased transit time in young neonates or infants or brisk bleeding. *Melena* refers to dark or black, tarry stools with a characteristic aroma. It is indicative of blood that has been in the GI tract for a long time, allowing the denaturation of hemoglobin by bowel flora. Melenic stools are typically from a hemorrhage originating proximal to the ileocecal valve.[4,5] Blood-streaked stools suggest a bleeding source in the rectum or anal canal. *Occult blood* refers to the presence of blood in the stool that is not visible but is confirmed by chemical testing (i.e., guaiac.)

DIFFERENTIAL DIAGNOSIS

The differential diagnosis of GI hemorrhage is divided into upper and lower GI bleeding. Although the causes are age related, there is considerable overlap between age groups. Patients with complex medical issues have special diagnostic considerations in the evaluation of GI bleeding. The causes of upper and lower GI bleeding are summarized in Tables 34-1 and 34-2, respectively.

Upper Gastrointestinal Bleeding

Some causes of upper GI bleeding are unique to neonates and young infants. Swallowed maternal blood from the birth process or from breastfeeding may cause hematemesis and may be difficult to distinguish from acute bleeding. To differentiate between maternal and fetal blood, an Apt test may be performed, which involves placing a small amount of bloody vomitus on filter paper and then adding 1% sodium hydroxide. An alternative method is to mix one part bloody vomitus or stool with five parts water and centrifuge; then mix the supernatant with 1 mL of 0.1% sodium hydroxide.[2] Adult hemoglobin is reduced to a brown-yellow color, whereas fetal hemoglobin is resistant to reduction and remains pink. This test cannot be applied to denatured blood such as melenic stools or coffee grounds emesis.[3] Necrotizing entercolitis may present with blood-tinged secretions in nasogastric aspirate in neonates and young infants.[6]

Stress gastritis can occur in any age group and may be a complication of an overwhelming or life-threatening illness such as sepsis, shock, severe acidosis, or respiratory failure.[3,7] Gastritis may be induced by many commonly used medications, including nonsteroidal anti-inflammatory drugs and aspirin.[8,9] Gastric or duodenal ulceration may accompany head trauma or increased intracranial pressure (Cushing's ulcer) or significant burns (Curling's ulcer). *Helicobacter pylori* may cause ulceration in children but is more commonly associated with nodular gastritis.[9]

Esophagitis can lead to upper GI bleeding and may manifest with symptoms of dysphagia, regurgitation, cough, arching, or failure to thrive. It may be acid related, infectious, associated with a caustic ingestion, or allergic, as in the case of eosinophilic esophagitis. Children with neuromuscular diseases are more prone to severe gastroesophageal reflux disease that leads to esophagitis.

Esophageal varices can cause sudden, massive hematemesis, which can lead to hemodynamic compromise. Varices are associated with portal hypertension from both intrahepatic and extrahepatic causes. Portal vein thrombosis may be associated with umbilical artery catheterization or omphalitis, but it usually occurs in young, previously healthy children, and the cause is not identified.[10,11] Thrombosis of the hepatic veins (Budd-Chiari syndrome) is usually associated with hypercoagulable states. Portal hypertension is most commonly caused by cirrhosis associated with chronic biliary diseases such as biliary atresia, cystic fibrosis, sclerosing cholangitis, and parenteral nutrition–induced cholestasis. Endoscopic evaluation of patients with known cirrhosis and esophageal varices is important, because the source of bleeding is commonly from gastric and duodenal ulcerations rather than varices.[10] Patients with liver failure may develop GI bleeding from other mechanisms, such as associated coagulopathy.

Table 34-1 Causes of Upper Gastrointestinal Bleeding

Neonates and Young Infants	Older Infants, Children, and Adolescents
Ingested maternal blood	Gastritis
At delivery	Gastroduodenal ulceration
During breastfeeding	Sepsis
	Stress
	Medications
	Ingestion
	Burns
	Increased ICP
	Ischemia
	Acidosis
	*Helicobacter pylori**
Gastritis	Esophagitis
Overwhelming illness	Reflux
Medications	Infectious
Idiopathic	Ingestion
Ischemia	Eosinophilic
Acidosis	Esophageal foreign body
Esophagitis	Gastroesophageal varices
Reflux	Cirrhosis
Infectious	Extrahepatic portal vein
	thrombosis†
	Budd-Chiari syndrome*
Necrotizing enterocolitis	Nasopharyngeal bleeding source
	Epistaxis
	Tonsils
	Tooth extraction
Coagulapathy	Coagulapathy
Congenital malformations	Hemobilia
Duplication cyst	Hepatic injury
	Trauma to intestinal mucosa
	Nasogastric tube
	Gastrostomy tube
	Mallory-Weiss tear
	Prolapse gastropathy
	Vascular anomalies†
	Hemangioma
	Dieulafoy lesion
	Telangiectasia
	Other
	Henoch-Schönlein purpura
	Crohn's disease
	Pulmonary hemorrhage
	Congenital malformations†
	Duplication cyst

*More common in older children and adolescents.
†More common in infants and young children.
ICP, intracranial pressure.

Forceful vomiting or retching may lead to a Mallory-Weiss tear or cause prolapse gastropathy, a phenomenon in which the gastric fundus is prolapsed into the esophagus, resulting in injury to the mucosa. Trauma to the esophageal or gastric mucosa may occur with nasopharyngeal suctioning or from nasogastric or gastrostomy tubes, which can lead to local irritation or laceration.

Lower Gastrointestinal Bleeding

Similar to upper GI bleeding, neonates and young infants have some unique causes of lower GI bleeding. In premature or young infants, necrotizing enterocolitis is a significant cause of morbidity and mortality and is an important diagnosis to exclude when evaluating hematochezia. Necrotizing enterocolitis typically presents with bloody stools, vomiting, abdominal distention, temperature instability, and discoloration or erythema of the abdominal wall.[12] Volvulus is another diagnostic consideration when evaluating lower GI bleeding in neonates and infants. Volvulus leads to ischemic injury of the bowel and can cause active bleeding; it is considered a surgical emergency. Hirschsprung colitis may also cause severe illness in young infants. A more common cause of bloody stools in well-appearing infants is allergic colitis, which is usually due to cow milk protein allergy.[9] Soy protein intolerance is also common in these infants. Breastfed infants can become sensitized to cow milk proteins indirectly when antigens are passed through the breast milk.[3]

Infectious enterocolitis can lead to bloody stools in infants and children. The classic pathogens include *Salmonella, Shigella, Yersinia, Escherichia coli* (enteroinvasive or enterohemorrhagic), *Campylobacter jejuni*, and *Entamoeba histolytica*. Viral pathogens such as rotavirus, Norwalk virus, and adenovirus 40/41 can also cause bloody stools. Antibiotic therapy puts patients at risk for the development of *Clostridium difficile* colitis; this should be considered in any patient who develops bloody stools with a history of recent antibiotic exposure.

Meckel's diverticulum is a remnant of the omphalomesenteric duct that can present with painless rectal bleeding. The rule of twos applies to Meckel's diverticulum: it occurs in approximately 2% of the population, is located within 2 feet of the ileocecal junction, is around 2 inches long and 2 cm in diameter, has two types of ectopic mucosa (gastric and pancreatic), and has a 2:1 male-to-female ratio. In addition, Meckel's presents before 2 years of age in 50% of patients. The bleeding is caused from ectopic gastric mucosa leading to ulceration of the adjacent ileal mucosa.[12,13] Duplications of the bowel may also contain ectopic mucosa and present with bleeding from a similar mechanism. Duplications of the bowel can also act as lead points for intussusception and subsequent ischemic injury.

Painless, intermittent rectal bleeding may be caused by juvenile polyps, which are non-neoplastic inflammatory lesions found in the rectosigmoid region of school-age children.[4,5,9] Bleeding diatheses are another cause of painless rectal bleeding in any age group.

Henoch-Schönlein purpura (HSP) is a systemic vasculitis that affects primarily small vessels of the skin, joints, kidneys, and GI tract. The GI manifestations occur in 50% to 70% of patients and may precede the skin manifestations.[9,12] Bloody stools can result from diffuse mucosal hemorrhage or from intussusception resulting from HSP. Occasionally, HSP may result in massive hemorrhage.

Lymphoid nodular hyperplasia is a benign condition of childhood characterized by multiple mucosal nodules of enlarged lymphoid follicles. This response may be triggered

Table 34-2   Causes of Lower Gastrointestinal Bleeding

Neonates and Infants	Young Children	Older Children and Adolescents
Necrotizing enterocolitis	Anal fissure	Inflamatory bowel disease
Anal fissure	Intussusception	Vasculitis
Allergic colitis	Juvenile polyps (>4 yr)	Henoch-Schönlein purpura
Milk protein	Vascular lesions	Juvenile or inflammatory polyps
Soy protein	Hirschsprung enterocolitis	Colonic or rectal varices
Swallowed maternal blood	Intestinal duplication	Hemorrhoids
Meckel's diverticulum	Infectious enterocolitis	Anal or rectal fissure
Hirschsprung enterocolitis	Inflammatory bowel disease (>4 yr)	Infectious enterocolitis
Infectious enterocolitis	Meckel's diverticulum	Colonic or rectal ulceration
Malrotation or volvulus	Perianal streptococcal cellulitis	Bleeding diathesis
Intestinal duplication	Henoch-Schönlein purpura	Eosinophilic gastroenteropathy
Bleeding diathesis	Hemolytic uremic syndrome	Rectal trauma
	Typhlitis*	Typhlitis*
	Eosinophilic gastroenteropathy	
	Bleeding diathesis	
	Colonic or rectal varices	
	Lymphoid nodular hyperplasia	
	Colonic or rectal ulceration	
	Rectal trauma	

*Immunocompromised patients.

by infection or allergy. Although typically asymptomatic, this condition may present with rectal bleeding. Lymphoid hyperplasia is frequently present in patients with intussusception.[14] Intussusception most frequently occurs in the ileocolic region and presents with colicky abdominal pain and bloody stool in children younger than 2 years.[1]

Inflammatory bowel disease (IBD) is an important diagnostic consideration in older children and adolescents with hematochezia. Ulcerative colitis is a diffuse mucosal inflammation limited to the colon. In contrast, Crohn's disease may occur in any segment of the GI tract. Both may present with bloody mucopurulent diarrhea, abdominal pain, and weight loss, as well as extraintestinal manifestations.[15,16]

Immunocompromised patients may develop GI bleeding from some unique causes. They are at risk for esophagitis secondary to cytomegalovirus and fungus, as well as chemically induced mucositis from chemotherapeutic agents. Typhlitis is an important diagnostic consideration in immunocompromised patients with abdominal pain and lower GI bleeding. Immunocompromised patients with bloody diarrhea should be evaluated for opportunistic infections as well as cytomegaloviral colitis.

HISTORY AND PHYSICAL EXAMINATION

The history and physical examination can be helpful in identifying the cause and location of bleeding in the GI tract. Tables 34-3 and 34-4 outline specific points to be addressed in the history and physical examination, respectively. The first priority is a quick assessment to identify patients in significant distress with hemodynamic compromise or shock who need immediate resuscitation. Vital signs should be monitored closely for evidence of hemodynamic instability. Patients may lose up to 15% of blood volume without evidence of hemodynamic compromise,[3] and the blood

pressure may be maintained until the patient has lost as much as 30% of the blood volume.[6] Once the patient is determined to be stable, a comprehensive history and physical examination should be pursued.

INITIAL STABILIZATION

Patients with GI bleeding who present with evidence of hemodynamic compromise should have the ABCs (airway, breathing, circulation) assessed. Once the airway and respiratory status are stabilized, the volume status should be addressed. Aggressive fluid resuscitation may be necessary, initially with crystalloid. Significant blood loss may require transfusion of blood products (red blood cells or fresh frozen plasma). In the case of any significant GI bleeding episode, a nasogastric tube should be placed and gastric lavage performed to assess for ongoing bleeding. Presence of blood in the nasogastric aspirate can confirm an ongoing upper GI bleed in patients with hematemesis or melena. The absence of blood in the nasogatric aspirate does not exclude upper GI bleeding from the postpyloric region in patients with hematochezia or melena with brisk bleeding. Patients with ongoing, substantial upper GI bleeding should be evaluated with endoscopy as soon as possible. Any patient who has evidence of hemodynamic compromise due to an upper GI bleed should undergo endoscopic evaluation by a gastroenterologist even if the bleeding stops spontaneously.

For lower GI bleeding, it is important to identify patients whose bleeding is associated with an intestinal obstruction such as volvulus, intussusception, or incarcerated hernia, which can lead to ischemic bowel and therefore requires prompt surgical intervention. A gastroenterology consultation should be obtained for lower endoscopy in cases of ongoing or severe bleeding or if a diagnosis cannot be established by other imaging modalities.

Table 34-3   Focused History

Characteristics of Bleeding
Quantity: volume of blood (few drops vs a cup)
Duration: intermittent bleeding, isolated episode, ongoing bleeding
Character: bright red blood, coffee grounds emesis, melena, hematochezia

Abdominal Complaints
Bowel patterns: diarrhea (infectious) or constipation (fissures)
Abdominal pain: indicates inflammation or ischemia of bowel wall
Painless bleeding: indicates Meckel's diverticulum, duplication, vascular malformation, or polyps
Abdominal distention: possible bowel obstruction
Tenesmus or urgency to defecate: consider IBD or infectious colitis

Dietary History
Cow milk or soy formula: consider allergic colitis
Breastfeeding: consider ingested maternal blood
Ingestion of products mistaken for hematemesis: artificial food coloring, gelatin, artificial fruit drinks, certain antibiotics and cough
   syrups
Ingestion of products mistaken for melena: beets, iron supplements, dark chocolate, bismuth, spinach, blueberries, grapes, licorice, and
   others

Review of Systems
General: fever, weight loss or gain, anorexia
Skin: rash, vascular malformations, edema, jaundice, lymphadenopathy
Extremities: arthralgia, arthritis, clubbing
Genitourinary: hematuria
Abdomen: distention, pain, bowel patterns, vomiting
Ears, nose, and throat: pharyngitis, epistaxis

Past Medical History
Previous GI bleeding
Liver disease: indicates possible variceal bleeding or coagulopathy
Previous or recent hospitalization: stress gastritis
Medications or ingestions: NSAIDs, aspirin, steroids, anticoagulants, alcohol, toxins (rat poison)
Umbilical artery catheterization: risk for portal vein thrombosis
Coagulopathy
Recent antibiotic exposure: pseudomembranous colitis
Presence of gastrostomy or nasogastric tube

Family History
IBD, peptic ulcer disease, polyposis, bleeding diatheses

Social History
Immediate contacts with similar symptoms: may indicate infectious cause
Travel, camping, or day care: consider infectious causes

GI, gastrointestinal; IBD, inflammatory bowel disease; NSAID, nonsteroidal anti-inflammatory drug.

DIAGNOSTIC EVALUATION AND INTERVENTION

Laboratory Studies

Laboratory studies are directed at determining both the extent of blood loss and the underlying cause. An initial complete blood count should be followed by serial hemoglobin and hematocrit measurements to assess ongoing bleeding. Thrombocytopenia can be associated with multiple systemic illnesses that cause GI bleeding, such as necrotizing enterocolitis, sepsis, idiopathic thrombocytopenic purpura, and hypersplenism. Eosinophilia may be present in allergic colitis or parasitic infections. Clotting studies should be performed to rule out a bleeding diathesis. Blood typing and crossmatching are necessary if there is any suggestion of profuse or ongoing bleeding or hemodynamic compromise. Routine chemistries, including renal and hepatic function, should be checked. Elevated blood urea nitrogen in the setting of a normal creatinine level may indicate a large amount of intraluminal blood in the small intestine with blood resorption. Azotemia may be present with hemolytic uremic syndrome or HSP. Urinalysis should be performed if renal involvement is suspected. Elevated liver transaminases or bilirubin may indicate hepatic failure or cirrhosis, raising the suspicion for varices. In an ill-appearing neonate with bloody stools, a blood culture should be obtained. Inflammatory markers such as the erythrocyte sedimentation rate

Table 34-4   Directed Physical Examination Findings and Associated Diseases

Vital Signs
Fever: infectious causes or inflammatory diseases (IBD or HSP)
Weight loss: chronic diseases (IBD, cystic fibrosis, liver disease)
Tachypnea: hemodynamic compromise or acidosis
Tachycardia: earliest sign of hemodynamic compromise
Hypotension: present with significant blood volume loss

General
Distressed or toxic-appearing patient: hemodynamic compromise from significant hemorrhage or underlying process causing systemic
   illness (toxic colitis, intussusception, ischemic bowel, necrotizing enterocolitis)
Well-appearing patient: less urgent causes of bleeding
Failure to thrive: malnutrition from chronic diseases (IBD, cystic fibrosis, liver disease)

Head, Eyes, Ears, Nose, and Throat
Nose: evidence of epistaxis
Eyes: scleral icterus (liver disease), iritis (IBD)
Oropharyngeal: mucosal trauma or bleeding from posterior pharynx

Cardiovascular
Evidence of hemodynamic compromise: tachycardia, gallop rhythm, delayed capillary refill, poor perfusion

Abdominal
Abdominal tenderness: nonspecific but indicates inflammation or ischemic injury of the bowel
Abdominal mass: intussusception, intestinal duplication may result in right lower quadrant masses
Evidence of portal hypertension: hepatosplenomegaly, ascites
Rectal examination: stool specimen for Hemoccult testing, palpable polyp
Perineal and anal inspection: skin tags (IBD), fissures, superficial skin breakdown or inflammation (streptococcal cellulitis)

Extremities
Clubbing: chronic diseases (cystic fibrosis, IBD, liver disease)
Arthritis: IBD

Skin
Vascular malformations: syndromes with associated GI vascular malformations (e.g., blue rubber bleb nevus syndrome, Klippel-
   Trénaunay syndrome, Rendu-Osler-Weber syndrome[4,15]
Cutaneous or oral pigmentation: Peutz-Jeghers syndrome
Purpura or petechiae: vasculitis (HSP) or bleeding diathesis
Erythema nodosum: IBD

GI, gastrointestinal; HSP, Henoch-Schönlein purpura; IBD inflammatory bowel disease.

and C-reactive protein may be elevated in inflammatory diseases such as IBD or HSP. Infectious causes may also lead to increased inflammatory markers.

Evaluation of stool to confirm the presence of bleeding is important to rule out other ingested materials that may be mistaken for blood. A stool guaiac test uses a leukodye that has an oxidative reaction in the presence of hemoglobin, producing a blue color. False positives can occur in the presence of certain ingested foods such as rare meat, turnips, tomatoes, horseradish, and cherries. False negatives can occur due to the consumption of vitamin C.[4] The Hemoccult test is accurate on stool but is inactivated by acid; therefore, gastric contents should be tested with the Gastroccult test.[13] Stool studies should include fecal leukocytes, eosinophils, bacterial culture, ova and parasites, viral studies, and screening for *C. difficile* toxin A and B when appropriate.

Endoscopy

Upper GI endoscopy is the preferred procedure for the diagnosis and evaluation of acute, severe upper GI hemorrhage or persistent or recurrent upper GI bleeding.

Endoscopy is sensitive and specific and may allow immediate therapy to be provided. Endoscopic interventions are available for active bleeding ulcers and varices, and tissue specimens can be obtained by biopsy. Endoscopic sclerotherapy and elastic band therapy have been used successfully for esophageal varices in children.[10]

Lower GI bleeding that is persistent or recurrent can also be effectively evaluated by endoscopy; in addition, it may allow for immediate intervention. Flexible sigmoidoscopy is usually sufficient to evaluate for colitis and polyps. Colonoscopy reaching the level of the terminal ileum may be needed to evaluate more proximal lesions. Lower endoscopy is a valuable diagnostic modality to detect vascular lesions.[9] Polyps can frequently be removed with electrocautery through an endoscope.[4]

Imaging

Imaging is an important component in the workup of GI hemorrhage in terms of defining the pathology or pinpointing the bleeding site. Some centers may offer interventional options as well. A barium study can detect abnormalities associated with infectious esophagitis, esophageal varices, or an esophageal foreign body. An upper GI study may demonstrate abnormalities associated with profound reflux, obstructive causes such as malrotation with midgut volvulus, or gastric or duodenal ulcers. Plain abdominal radiographs are helpful in the evaluation of GI bleeding to assess for an obstructive bowel gas pattern, intraperitoneal free air, and pneumatosis coli in necrotizing enterocolitis or typhlitis. However, computed tomography is the preferred imaging modality to confirm the diagnosis of typhlitis in immunocompromised children. A barium enema can reveal mucosal abnormalities associated with IBD and can demonstrate polyps. Extraluminal complications of Crohn's disease, such as adhesions or abscess formation, are better evaluated with computed tomography. An air-contrast enema can be diagnostic and therapeutic for intussusception, with successful reduction in nearly 90% of cases.[1]

Nuclear medicine imaging using a tagged red blood cell scan can be helpful in pinpointing the location of bleeding. In one method, the patient's blood is drawn, labeled with a marker, and then reinjected. The images are evaluated in 5-minute frames for up to 2 hours to localize a bleeding source. Another valuable nuclear medicine technique is the Meckel scan, which is designed to demonstrate the presence of ectopic gastric mucosa within the diverticulum; this occurs in 95% of Meckel's diverticula that are resected for bleeding.[13] Technetium 99m pertechnetate is injected intravenously and concentrates in gastric mucosa. Serial images are then obtained in 5-minute intervals to determine the presence of ectopic mucosa within a Meckel's diverticulum.[1]

In specialized centers, angiography of the celiac or superior mesenteric artery can be performed in cases of brisk bleeding that cannot be diagnosed with other approaches. Arteriography may allow for transcatheter therapy with vasopressin or embolization.[1]

Surgery

Surgical indications include bowel perforation, ischemic bowel from obstructive causes or irreducible intussusception, as well as ongoing or massive bleeding not amenable to control with endoscopy or interventional radiology. In cases of ulcerative colitis refractory to medical management, the disease can be cured with a total colectomy. Complications of Crohn's disease, such as adhesions or fistula formation, may require surgical intervention. There are several surgical treatment options for portal hypertension and esophageal varices, including esophageal transection, portosystemic shunts, and transjugular intrahepatic portosystemic shunts, which are most often used in children with extrahepatic portal vein obstruction. Candidates for these procedures should be determined by consultation with a gastroenterologist and a surgeon.

Pharmacologic Therapy

Gastritis and peptic ulcer disease in children is effectively treated with H_2-antagonists and proton pump inhibitors, as well as bismuth preparations. Early use of acid-suppressive medications in critically ill patients or those on high-dose steroids or anti-inflammatory medications may be prudent. *H. pylori* infection in children is treated similarly to that in adults, with antibiotics, acid suppression, and bismuth preparation.

C. difficile colitis requires antibiotic therapy. However, many bacterial pathogens causing bloody diarrhea do not require antibiotic treatment, and appropriate therapy should be reviewed on a case-by-case basis.

For esophageal varices, intravenous or intra-arterial continuous infusions of vasopressin, somatostatin, or octreotide may be administered.[4,6] These therapies work by reducing splanchnic arterial blood flow, therefore reducing the amount of bleeding from the varices.

There are many pharmacologic therapies available for the management of IBD. Use of these medications should be guided by a gastroenterologist (see Chapter 98).

SUGGESTED READING

Arain Z, Rossi T: Gastrointestinal bleeding in children: An overview of conditions requiring nonoperative management. Semin Pediatr Surg 1999;8: 172-180.
Pearl RH, Irish MS, Caty MG, Glick PL: The approach to common abdominal diagnoses in infants and children. Part II. Pediatr Clin North Am 1998;45: 1287-1326.
Rodgers B: Upper gastrointestinal hemorrhage. Pediatr Rev 1999;20:171-174.
Squires R: Gastrointestinal bleeding. Pediatr Rev 1999;20:95-101.

REFERENCES

1. Racadio JM, Agha AK, Johnson ND, Warner BW: Imaging and radiological interventional techniques for gastrointestinal bleeding in children. Semin Pediatr Surg 1999;8:181-192.
2. Fleisher G, Ludwig S (eds): Pediatric Emergency Medicine, 4th ed. Philadelphia, Lippincott Williams & Wilkins, 2000, pp 275-282.
3. Arain Z, Rossi T: Gastrointestinal bleeding in children: An overview of conditions requiring nonoperative management. Semin Pediatr Surg 1999;8:172-180.
4. Squires R: Gastrointestinal bleeding. Pediatr Rev 1999;20:95-101.
5. Lawrence W, Wright J: Causes of rectal bleeding in children. Pediatr Rev 2001;22:394-395.
6. Rodgers B: Upper gastrointestinal hemorrhage. Pediatr Rev 1999;20: 171-174.
7. Pearl RH, Irish MS, Caty MG, Glick PL: The approach to common abdominal diagnoses in infants and children. Part II. Pediatr Clin North Am 1998;45:1287-1326.
8. Matsubara T, Mason W, Kashani IA, et al: Gastrointestinal hemorrhage complicating aspirin therapy in acute Kawasaki disease. J Pediatr 1996;128:701-703.
9. Fox V: Gastrointestinal bleeding in infancy and childhood. Gastroenterol Clin North Am 2000;29:37-66.
10. Karrer F, Narkewicz M: Esophageal varices: Current management in children. Semin Pediatr Surg 1999;8:193-201.
11. Lykavieris P, Gauthier F, Hadchouel P, et al: Risk of gastrointestinal bleeding during adolescence and early adulthood in children with portal vein obstruction. J Pediatr 2000;136:805-808.
12. Leung A, Wong A: Lower gastrointestinal bleeding in children. Pediatr Emerg Care 2002;18:319-323.
13. Brown R: Gastrointestinal bleeding in infants and children: Meckel's diverticulum and intestinal duplication. Semin Pediatr Surg 1999;8:202-209.
14. DiFiore J: Intussusception. Semin Pediatr Surg 1999;8:214-220.
15. Irish M, Caty M, Azizkhan R: Bleeding in children caused by gastrointestinal vascular lesions. Semin Pediatr Surg 1999;8:210-213.
16. Baldassano R, Piccoli D: Inflammatory bowel disease in pediatric and adolescent patients. Gastroenterol Clin 1999;28:445-458.

CHAPTER 35

Hypertension

Avram Z. Traum and Michael J. G. Somers

Hypertension is a relatively uncommon disorder in pediatrics, but it often suggests the presence of underlying disease. Most adults with hypertension are deemed to have essential, or primary, hypertension and often undergo no diagnostic evaluation; in children, however, primary hypertension is a diagnosis of exclusion. Regardless of its cause, significant elevation of blood pressure can lead to acute organ dysfunction; thus, a child who presents with hypertension often requires treatment while the diagnostic evaluation is performed. In a hospitalized child, there is the additional burden of determining whether hypertension is a primary problem or whether it stems from an ongoing condition or its treatment. The approach to the evaluation and treatment of hypertension is often both more directed and more intensive in a hospitalized child than in an ambulatory setting.

MEASUREMENT OF BLOOD PRESSURE

Blood Pressure Norms

Adult blood pressure standards are based on outcome measures related to chronic end-organ damage. In contrast, blood pressure standards in children are based on statistical population norms stratified by age, gender, and height percentile. The recently published "Fourth Report on the Diagnosis, Evaluation, and Treatment of High Blood Pressure in Children and Adolescents"[1] describes blood pressure ranges similar to previously published standards.[2] Normal blood pressure is defined as that falling below the 90th percentile. Prehypertension (formerly known as high-normal blood pressure) is defined as blood pressure at the 90th percentile or higher but less than the 95th percentile. Hypertension is defined as blood pressure at the 95th percentile or greater, and severe hypertension is that exceeding the 99th percentile.

Auscultation versus Oscillometry

Accurate measurement of blood pressure is essential before management decisions can be made. The accepted statistical blood pressure norms in pediatrics are based on measurement by auscultation. In spite of this, oscillometric (e.g., Dynamap) measurements of blood pressure are widely used because of the ease of obtaining readings, especially in hospitalized children. Oscillometric measurements of blood pressure are typically at least 5 to 10 mm Hg higher than those obtained by auscultation.[3] As a result, any high blood pressure measurements should be confirmed with auscultation.

Cuff Size and Location

Cuff size is another important factor that affects blood pressure measurement. Generally, cuffs that are too small overestimate blood pressure. Conversely, cuffs that are too large may underestimate blood pressure, although not as significantly as the overestimation resulting from small cuffs. The most precise method of measuring cuff size is controversial,[4-6] but the recommendations of the National High Blood Pressure Education Program Working Group on High Blood Pressure in Children and Adolescents should be followed.[1] Those guidelines delineate that the width of the cuff bladder should be at least 40% of the arm circumference measured midway between the olecranon and the acromion. This generally correlates with the bladder length covering 80% to 100% of the arm circumference. Appropriate-sized cuffs should be available from infant up to thigh-sized cuffs. In large or obese adolescents, a thigh cuff may be necessary to cover the arm adequately.

Location of the cuff can also significantly affect the reading. It is important that the measurement is made at the level of the heart. A cuff placed on the upper arm remains at the level of the heart whether the patient is in the upright or supine position. When the cuff is placed on the lower extremity, the patient should be supine for accurate measurement. The measurement will be elevated due to increased hydrostatic pressure if obtained on the lower extremity of a patient in a sitting or upright position.

Auscultation Technique

As noted earlier, auscultation is the ideal way to measure blood pressure. With the child at rest, the diaphragm of the stethoscope is placed over the brachial artery at the antecubital fossa. The right arm is used both for convenience and to allow the diagnosis of coarctation of the aorta; the left subclavian artery usually comes off the aorta after a thoracic coarctation and thus has normal blood pressure. The cuff is inflated to a pressure above which the examiner can no longer auscultate a pulsatile sound, at which point the cuff is deflated slowly. The systolic blood pressure is measured at the onset of the tapping or Korotkoff sounds; the diastolic blood pressure is measured at the disappearance of the Korotkoff sounds. In some children, the Korotkoff sounds may continue until the diastolic blood pressure reaches zero. Although this is unlikely in the presence of significant hypertension, if it occurs, the diastolic blood pressure should be measured at the muffling or fourth Korotkoff sound.

DIAGNOSTIC EVALUATION

Most hospitalized children with identified hypertension have a secondary form; however, as the incidence of obesity rises, so does the incidence of primary hypertension in children.[7] Nonetheless, all children with evidence of sustained or recurrent hypertension should be evaluated for secondary hypertension in an individualized and stepwise fashion,

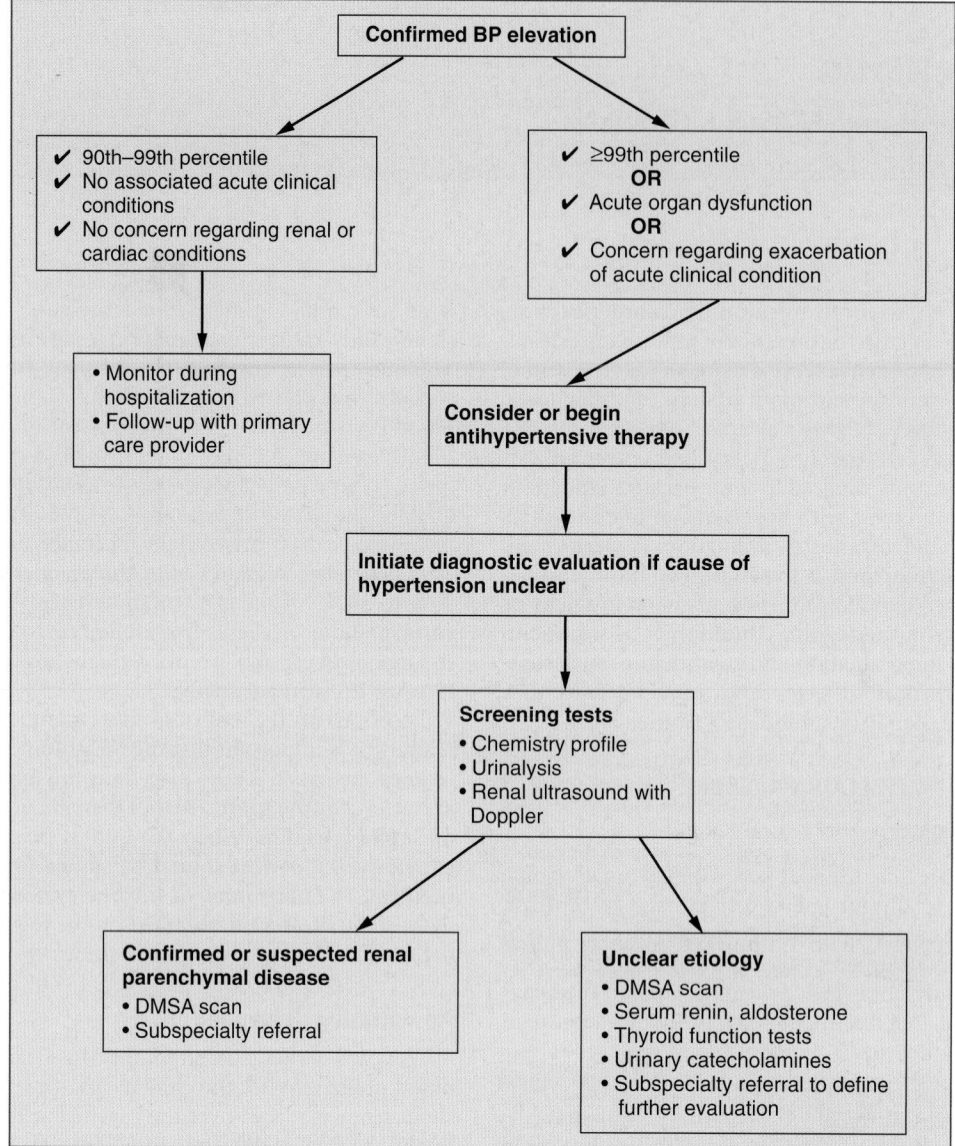

Figure 35-1 Algorithm for the evaluation and management of a hospitalized child with hypertension. BP, blood pressure; DMSA, dimercaptosuccinic acid.

based on the findings of the history, physical examination, and screening tests. Children with more significant elevations of blood pressure, as well as younger children, are more likely to have definable causes of hypertension. The most common cause of secondary hypertension in children is renal parenchymal disease,[8] and the diagnostic evaluation should reflect this. An algorithm for the diagnostic evaluation of hypertension in hospitalized children is provided in Figure 35-1.

HISTORY

The history should focus on disorders or conditions that predispose to hypertension and, in a hospitalized patient, should begin with a history of the present illness leading to the child's admission. For instance, in a postoperative patient who is otherwise healthy, pain or anxiety may play a role in hypertension. In a child hospitalized with severe reactive airway disease, steroid therapy or frequent administration of β-agonists may be problematic. In the absence of an obvious precipitating factor, a careful history is crucial and should begin with the perinatal period. Prematurity itself is a risk factor, as well as interventions in the neonatal period such as placement of umbilical catheters and periods of hypotension leading to hypoperfusion and subsequent renal scarring. Urinary tract infections commonly leave renal parenchymal scars that can lead to hyperreninemic hypertension. These infections may have been undiagnosed, and any history of unexplained recurrent febrile illness should be elicited. Glomerulonephritis presents with edema, hematuria, and hypertension and may be isolated to the kidney or associated with systemic inflammatory disorders such as systemic lupus erythematosus. Relevant findings include joint symptoms, edema, rashes, and recent unexplained fevers. Recent systemic infections may also lead to postinfectious glomerulonephritis and may be associated with gross hematuria.

The family history should focus on relatives with early-onset hypertension and inherited diseases that affect the kidneys, such as the polycystic kidney disease complex, tuberous sclerosis, and neurofibromatosis. A strong family history of cardiovascular disease, such as coronary artery disease, stroke, and hyperlipidemia, suggests a similar risk in a hypertensive child.

Certain medications are known to cause hypertension, including oral contraceptives, corticosteroids, stimulants, decongestants, and the calcineurin inhibitors (cyclosporine, tacrolimus) that are the mainstay of immunosuppression in transplant patients. Recreational drugs with stimulant effects, such as cocaine, nicotine, and ephedra, can also raise blood pressure, as can withdrawal from the effects of central nervous system depressants such as ethanol or narcotic analgesics.

The review of systems should evaluate for symptoms such as headache, chest pain, visual changes, or mental status changes, because these may be related to severe hypertension or end-organ damage. Sweating, palpitations, and flushing are associated with states of catecholamine excess, such as occurs with a pheochromocytoma.

PHYSICAL EXAMINATION

As outlined earlier, accurate measurement of the blood pressure is an essential part of the physical assessment of a child with suspected hypertension. Blood pressure should be measured in all four extremities. The blood pressure in the lower extremities is typically 10 to 20 mm Hg higher than in the right arm. If lower extremity blood pressure is not higher, this suggests a coarctation or other narrowing of the aorta and is often associated with diminished femoral pulses. Height, weight, and body mass index should be measured to assess for poor growth or to document obesity.

The physical examination should look for signs of end-organ damage from hypertension. This involves funduscopy and cardiovascular, pulmonary, and neurologic examinations. Although the finding is uncommon, the abdomen should be auscultated for abdominal bruits, which can be seen in renovascular hypertension.

The physical examination should also seek to uncover evidence of a systemic disease that may explain the elevated blood pressure. Similarly, several genetic syndromes cause elevated blood pressure and have characteristic physical findings. These include neurofibromatosis (café au lait spots, axillary freckling, Lisch nodules), tuberous sclerosis (ash-leaf macules, shagreen patches, adenoma sebaceum, peri- or subungual fibromas, retinal hamartomas), Turner syndrome (short stature, shield chest, upturned mouth, webbed neck), and Williams syndrome (overfriendly personality, cognitive impairment, prominent ears).

LABORATORY AND RADIOLOGIC EVALUATION

A urinalysis should be preformed on a freshly voided urine sample and, if the dipstick is positive for blood or protein, should include microscopy. Screening blood tests include blood urea nitrogen, creatinine, electrolytes, and a complete blood count. This effectively evaluates renal function and screens for states of mineralocorticoid excess that lead to hypokalemia and alkalosis.

Other studies should be based on the history and physical examination findings. For example, tachycardia suggests hyperthyroidism or high-catecholamine states and should trigger blood thyroid function tests and urinary catecholamine quantification. A history of urinary tract infections with unexplained fevers or positive urine cultures should precipitate a dimercaptosuccinic acid (DMSA) scan to determine the presence of cortical scars.

Plasma renin activity and aldosterone levels are helpful only if the results are unequivocally low or high. They are most useful when a diagnosis of mineralocorticoid excess is suspected, because plasma renin activity is typically suppressed. Aldosterone levels may be low or high, depending on the specific cause of the mineralocorticoid excess.

All children with hypertension should undergo renal ultrasonography. An ultrasound study provides information about differential renal size, hydronephrosis, echo texture, and cystic change and is thus a good screening test for many forms of kidney disease. Renal scarring may not be seen on ultrasonography, but a size discrepancy of greater than 1 cm is abnormal and may reflect scarring in the smaller kidney. Doppler studies show changes in flow rates through areas of measurement and, if abnormal, may suggest the presence of renovascular hypertension. A normal Doppler study does not, however, rule out renal artery stenosis, especially stenosis in the smaller segmental arteries that are not well visualized by Doppler.

Echocardiography is necessary in any child suspected of having a structural lesion causing hypertension. In addition, echocardiography may be a sensitive tool to measure cardiac changes such as left ventricular hypertrophy that accompanies sustained hypertension. In some hospitalized patients with hypertension, a careful ophthalmic examination may also provide information about the chronicity of the child's hypertensive state.

TREATMENT

Acute Management

Because hospitalization is an anxiety-producing experience for most children, if the blood pressure is lower than the 99th percentile, it is often best to monitor it with frequent readings to document the trend of measurements. As the child recovers or acclimates to the hospital experience, blood pressure often falls to normal ranges. If blood pressure readings are still consistently between the 90th and 99th percentiles by the time of discharge, it is prudent to arrange follow-up by the child's primary care provider and further evaluation as an outpatient. If there is concern that the blood pressure is directly related to a primary disease process (e.g., glomerulonephritis) or may adversely affect a clinical condition, more immediate measures may be necessary.

In a child with sustained blood pressure exceeding the 99th percentile, diagnostic evaluation and therapy must be carefully considered. The tempo and urgency of the intervention are guided by the individual child's clinical presentation and course.

Children with sustained blood pressure readings more than 30% above the 99th percentile are at particular risk of developing acute sequelae; even if they are asymptomatic, blood pressure control must begin immediately to prevent

Table 35-1   Medications for Pediatric Hypertensive Urgency or Emergency

Drug	Mechanism	Dose	Onset	Duration
Hydralazine	Arteriolar dilator	IV: 0.1–0.4 mg/kg to max dose of 20 mg	5–15 min	3–8 hr
Labetalol	α- and β-adrenergic antagonist	Initial IV bolus: 0.25 mg/kg; repeat q 15 min at increasing doses up to 1 mg/kg until effective or to total dose of 4 mg/kg Maintenance IV drip: 1–3 mg/kg/hr	5 min	2–6 hr
Nitroprusside	Venodilator and arteriolar dilator	IV: start at 0.5 μg/kg/min	1–2 min	3–5 min
Nifedipine	Calcium-channel antagonist	PO: 0.25–0.5 mg/kg	10–20 min	3–6 hr
Nicardipine	Calcium-channel antagonist	IV: 0.5–5 μg/kg/min	10 min	2–6 hr
Esmolol	β-adrenergic antagonist	Loading dose: 500 μg/kg over 2 min Maintenance IV drip: 50–250 μg/kg/min	Seconds	10–20 min
Enalaprilat	ACE inhibitor	IV: 5–10 μg/kg q 8–24 hr	0.5–4 hr	6 hr

ACE, angiotensin-converting enzyme.

progression to a hypertensive urgency (severely elevated blood pressure that is potentially harmful but without evidence of end-organ damage or dysfunction) or emergency (severely elevated blood pressure associated with evidence of secondary end-organ dysfunction, such as hypertensive encephalopathy). Severe hypertension with actual acute end-organ dysfunction or impending end-organ dysfunction should be treated with short-acting intravenous antihypertensive medications. The medications most commonly used in a hypertensive crisis are outlined in Table 35-1. The blood pressure should be lowered by 20% to 30% in the first 2 to 3 hours. Once the blood pressure falls into a range that is not acutely dangerous for the patient, it should be lowered more gradually over the next few days.

Hydralazine is a commonly used vasodilator with a rapid onset that can often be titrated to achieve good blood pressure control. It is generally well tolerated and can be given in a non–intensive care unit setting. Nifedipine is another short-acting agent and has the advantage of oral administration. Its use in adults is rare owing to reports of myocardial infarction.[9] The use of short-acting nifedipine in children is safe, although a higher incidence of adverse events was seen in patients with preexisting central nervous system disease.[10] The sublingual route is somewhat controversial because it requires aspiration of liquid from within the capsule, and its absorption is erratic.

Hypertension refractory to these first-line agents may require continuous infusions to reduce blood pressure. Labetalol and nitroprusside have been used in children with success. Both agents are shorter acting than hydralazine and may be titrated to achieve a target blood pressure. These medications require an intensive care unit setting. Labetalol can be administered via both continuous infusion and scheduled intravenous dosing. It is the only drug that is both an α- and β-adrenergic blocker. Nitroprusside is a vasodilator with a wide dosage range. The drug is photosensitive and must be protected from light. Its use is limited by the toxicity of its metabolites; nitroprusside is converted to cyanide by tissue sulfhydryl groups, and cyanide is converted to thiocyanate in the liver. In patients with liver disease, cyanide levels should be followed. Thiocyanate levels should be monitored in patients on nitroprusside for more than 72 hours and in patients with renal insufficiency. Thiocyanate toxicity manifests primarily as neurotoxicity and includes psychosis, blurred vision, confusion, weakness, tinnitus, and seizures. An early sign of cyanide toxicity includes metabolic acidosis; other signs of toxicity include tachycardia, pink skin, decreased pulse, decreased reflexes, altered consciousness, coma, almond smell on breath, methemoglobinemia, and dilated pupils.

Depending on local experience, continuous infusions of the angiotensin-converting enzyme (ACE) inhibitor enalaprilat, the calcium-channel blocker nicardipine, or the beta-blocker esmolol have also been used in hypertensive children.

Long-Acting Medications

As blood pressure is controlled by intravenous medication, it is important to initiate longer-acting oral antihypertensives to allow weaning off infusions. Table 35-2 reviews the drugs used most often for antihypertensive therapy in pediatrics. The choice of antihypertensive agent should address the presumed underlying pathophysiology of the blood pressure perturbation. For instance, children with fluid overload related to glomerulonephritis should be treated with diuretics and vasodilators. Hyperreninemic hypertension due to renal parenchymal scarring should be treated with ACE inhibitors or angiotensin receptor blockers.

Many of the drugs used to treat hypertension in children have undergone only limited study. The Food and Drug Modernization Act of 1997 created incentives for pharmaceutical companies to obtain pediatric indications; consequently, some of the newer agents have been studied in children.

Calcium-channel blockers are among the most common agents used for pediatric hypertension. These agents are generally well tolerated, and no specific laboratory parameters need to be followed during therapy. At higher doses, they may cause headache and reflex tachycardia. Salt retention

Table 35-2 Long-Acting Antihypertensive Agents in Children

Drug	Initial Dose (mg/kg/day)	Maximal Dose (mg/kg/day)	Dosing Frequency
Calcium channel antagonist			
Nifedipine	0.25	3	XL or SR forms, 2 times/day
Amlodipine	0.1	0.4	1-2 times/day
ACE inhibitor			
Captopril (neonate)	0.03-0.15	2	2-3 times/day
Captopril (child)	1.5	6	2-3 times/day
Enalapril	0.15	Up to 40 mg/day total	1-2 times/day
Diuretic			
Hydrochlorothiazide	1	2-3	1-2 times/day
Furosemide	0.5-1.0	10	1-2 times/day
Adrenergic antagonist			
Atenolol (β)	0.5	2-3	1-2 times/day
Propranolol (β)	1	6-8	2 times/day
Labetalol (α and β)	1	3	2 times/day
Vasodilator			
Hydralazine	0.5	10	3-4 times/day
Minoxidil	0.1-0.2	1	1-2 times/day

ACE, angiotensin-converting enzyme.

may occur with prolonged use, leading to tachyphylaxis, and the addition of a low-dose diuretic augments the antihypertensive effect. Extended-release nifedipine is formulated as a capsule and may be difficult for younger children to swallow. Amlodipine has been studied in children[11-13] and is approved for use in patients older than 6 years.

ACE inhibitors are also used widely in pediatrics, related to both their antihypertensive action and their renoprotective effect in patients with proteinuria and chronic renal insufficiency. Many agents in this class have been studied in children, including a subset that has achieved pediatric indications (enalapril,[14,15] fosinopril, lisinopril, and benazepril). These drugs are especially effective in patients with hyperreninemic hypertension due to renal parenchymal scarring. In patients with suspected renal artery stenosis or in whom the cause of hypertension is unclear, ACE inhibitors should be used with caution because they may precipitate acute renal failure in patients with bilateral renal artery stenosis. ACE inhibitors may cause elevations of serum creatinine and potassium levels, so these biochemical parameters should be followed. They may also lead to anemia, so the complete blood count should be checked periodically. Although cough is reported in adults on ACE inhibitors, this is rarely seen in children unless high doses are used. Finally, this class of drugs is teratogenic, and adolescent females taking these medications should be counseled about contraception or abstinence.

Two angiotensin receptor blockers (irbesartan, losartan) are approved for use in children older than 6 years. These agents have a side effect profile similar to that of ACE inhibitors with respect to biochemical changes and teratogenicity, although the effect on potassium may be less dramatic.

Beta-adrenergic blockers are widely used in adults with primary hypertension because of their ability to decrease mortality after cardiovascular events. These drugs may lead to exercise intolerance owing to the associated decrease in heart rate; they can contribute to depression in some individuals; and they may be problematic in patients with asthma or diabetes.

Diuretic therapy is increasingly recommended as the mainstay of antihypertensive therapy in adult patients. Although diuretics may be necessary in a hospitalized child with volume overload, their use in the ambulatory setting may be complicated by adherence issues.

SUBSPECIALTY REFERRAL

Most hospitalized patients with mild to moderate hypertension requiring admission can be managed effectively without referral. However, certain clinical situations may require specialty input. These include the following:

- Hypertension requiring continuous infusions for blood pressure control (e.g., nitroprusside, labetalol)
- Hypertension requiring multiple medications for control
- Renal insufficiency or other end-organ damage
- Abnormal urine sediment
- Suspicion of renovascular hypertension

CONCLUSION

Hypertension in children is a relatively uncommon phenomenon. When suspected, its presence should be confirmed by multiple readings using auscultation. The evaluation for secondary causes should focus on renal parenchymal disease as well as other causes suspected from the history and physical examination. Sustained or symptomatic hypertension should be treated while the evaluation is ongoing. The choice of medication should be tailored to the suspected cause. Subspecialty referral should be initiated if end-organ damage is discovered, if management becomes complicated, or if an intensive care setting is required. Nonetheless, early diagnosis and management can prevent complications related to this condition.

SUGGESTED READING

Chobanian AV, Bakris GL, Black HR, et al: The seventh report of the Joint National Committee on Prevention, Detection, Evaluation, and Treatment of High Blood Pressure: The JNC 7 report. JAMA 2003;289:2560-2572.

The fourth report on the diagnosis, evaluation, and treatment of high blood pressure in children and adolescents. Pediatrics 2004;114:555-576.

Pappadis SL, Somers MJ: Hypertension in adolescents: A review of diagnosis and management. Curr Opin Pediatr 2003;15:370-378.

REFERENCES

1. The fourth report on the diagnosis, evaluation, and treatment of high blood pressure in children and adolescents. Pediatrics 2004;114:555-576.
2. Chobanian AV, Bakris GL, Black HR, et al: The seventh report of the Joint National Committee on Prevention, Detection, Evaluation, and Treatment of High Blood Pressure: The JNC 7 report. JAMA 2003;289:2560-2572.
3. Park MK, Menard SW, Yuan C: Comparison of auscultatory and oscillometric blood pressures. Arch Pediatr Adolesc Med 2001;155:50-53.
4. Clark JA, Lieh-Lai MW, Sarnaik A, Mattoo TK: Discrepancies between direct and indirect blood pressure measurements using various recommendations for arm cuff selection. Pediatrics 2002;110:920-923.
5. Arafat M, Mattoo TK: Measurement of blood pressure in children: Recommendations and perceptions on cuff selection. Pediatrics 1999;104:e30.
6. Mattoo TK: Arm cuff in the measurement of blood pressure. Am J Hypertens 2002;15:67S-68S.
7. Sorof J, Daniels S: Obesity hypertension in children: A problem of epidemic proportions. Hypertension 2002;40:441-447.
8. Pappadis SL, Somers MJ: Hypertension in adolescents: A review of diagnosis and management. Curr Opin Pediatr 2003;15:370-378.
9. Psaty BM, Heckbert SR, Koepsell TD, et al: The risk of myocardial infarction associated with antihypertensive drug therapies. JAMA 1995;274:620-625.
10. Egger DW, Deming DD, Hamada N, et al: Evaluation of the safety of short-acting nifedipine in children with hypertension. Pediatr Nephrol 2002;17:35-40.
11. Rogan JW, Lyszkiewicz DA, Blowey D, et al: A randomized prospective crossover trial of amlodipine in pediatric hypertension. Pediatr Nephrol 2000;14:1083-1087.
12. Flynn JT, Newburger JW, Daniels SR, et al: A randomized, placebo-controlled trial of amlodipine in children with hypertension. J Pediatr 2004;145:353-359.
13. Tallian KB, Nahata MC, Turman MA, et al: Efficacy of amlodipine in pediatric patients with hypertension. Pediatr Nephrol 1999;13:304-310.
14. Wells TG: Trials of antihypertensive therapies in children. Blood Press Monit 1999;4:189-192.
15. Wells T, Rippley R, Hogg R, et al: The pharmacokinetics of enalapril in children and infants with hypertension. J Clin Pharmacol 2001;41:1064-1074.

CHAPTER 36

Hypoglycemia

Emily Milliken

Normal plasma glucose is maintained by the complex interaction of hormones that regulate the utilization and mobilization of glucose, as well as by the production of glucose from other substrates. The definition of hypoglycemia is controversial and is dependent on the age of the subject. For purposes of this chapter, hypoglycemia is defined as blood glucose less than 50 mg/dL.

CLINICAL FEATURES

The clinical manifestations of hypoglycemia can be divided into two categories: those associated with activation of the autonomic nervous system, and those associated with the effects of decreased cerebral glucose utilization. The autonomic symptoms include diaphoresis, tachycardia, tremulousness, weakness, dizziness, pallor, nausea, and hunger. These symptoms generally occur at blood glucose levels in the 50 to 70 mg/dL range and may serve as a warning to the patient that blood sugar is dropping. The neuroglycopenic symptoms, which typically occur at plasma glucose levels less than 50 mg/dL, include lethargy, irritability, confusion, abnormal behavior, seizure, and coma. Recurrent episodes of hypoglycemia may lead to developmental delays, learning disabilities, and behavioral problems.

EVALUATION

Hypoglycemia can be caused by the body's inability to absorb carbohydrate or convert alternative energy sources into glucose. Other causes include states in which glucose utilization is accelerated or hormone signaling is absent or dysfunctional. Table 36-1 lists the differential diagnosis of hypoglycemia. The first step in narrowing this broad differential diagnosis is obtaining a thorough history and performing a careful physical examination.

History

The history in a hypoglycemic patient can provide important clues to the underlying cause of abnormal glucose homeostasis. First, it is critical to determine whether the hypoglycemia occurs in a fed or a fasting state. If the child develops hypoglycemia just after eating, the specific contents of the preceding meal may point to the cause of the problem. For example, children with galactosemia or defects of organic acid metabolism may develop hypoglycemia shortly after consuming milk products or protein, respectively. In addition, inquiring about food aversions may be helpful, because many children learn to avoid foods that make them sick. Table 36-2 outlines the processes that are primarily responsible for maintaining plasma glucose, based on the time since the last meal. One can therefore gain additional clues to the underlying diagnosis by determining the duration of the fast leading up to the event.

A history of ingestions should also be considered. Hypoglycemia in children can be secondary to the consumption of alcohol, oral hypoglycemic agents, β-adrenergic blockers, or other substances listed in Table 36-1.

The child's past medical history should also be thoroughly explored. If prior episodes of hypoglycemia have occurred, it is important to determine the age of onset. Inborn errors of metabolism generally present in the neonatal period or within the first 1 to 2 years of life, whereas ketotic hypoglycemia, growth hormone deficiency, and cortisol deficiency generally do not present until after 1 year of age. The possibility of past hypoglycemic episodes that were not diagnosed as such should also be considered; a history of unexplained seizures or recurrent respiratory infections (hyperventilation secondary to metabolic acidosis) may actually represent episodes of hypoglycemia. A careful developmental history should also be obtained, because recurrent or prolonged hypoglycemia may manifest as delayed acquisition of milestones.

Finally, the patient's family history may provide clues to a hereditary cause of hypoglycemia. In particular, it is important to inquire about a history of Reye syndrome, sudden infant death syndrome (or unexplained childhood death), and other family members with hypoglycemia.

Physical Examination

In addition to performing a thorough physical examination, clinicians should pay particular attention to physical findings that may be useful in the setting of hypoglycemia. Table 36-3 highlights some of the findings that may suggest a diagnosis.

Laboratory Studies

Blood samples should be obtained before the administration of glucose, if possible. The patient's first voided urine should also be sent for testing. Table 36-4 lists the laboratory tests that should be considered when evaluating a patient with hypoglycemia and the conditions they may help rule in or out.

In a normal host, hypoglycemia induces counterregulatory hormones to stimulate the production of alternative fuels, and a subsequent ketosis occurs. When interpreting the data collected from a hypoglycemic patient, the first step is to determine whether the patient has appropriately devel-

Table 36-1   Differential Diagnosis of Hypoglycemia

Disorders of carbohydrate metabolism
   Glycogen storage diseases
   Galactosemia
   Pyruvate carboxylase deficiency
   Phosphoenolpyruvate carboxykinase deficiency
   Hereditary fructose intolerance
   Liver failure

Disorders of amino acid metabolism
   Maple syrup urine disease
   Methylmalonicacidemia
   Propionicacidemia
   Glutaricaciduria
   Tyrosinemia

Disorders of fat metabolism
   Fatty acid oxidation defects
   Carnitine deficiency

Hormone deficiency
   Growth hormone deficiency
   Adrenocorticotropic hormone deficiency
   Cortisol deficiency
   Panhypopituitarism
   Glucagon deficiency

Ingestions
   Ethanol
   Salicylates
   Quinine
   Oral hypoglycemics
   Insulin
   β-Adrenergic blocking agents
   Ackee fruit

Increased glucose utilization
   Persistent hyperinsulinemic hypoglycemia of infancy
   Beckwith-Wiedemann syndrome
   Sepsis
   Burns
   Hyperthyroidism

Inadequate glucose stores
   Severe malnutrition
   Prematurity

Miscellaneous
   Ketotic hypoglycemia
   Dumping syndrome
   Malaria

Table 36-2   Primary Energy Source Relative to Duration of Fast

Duration of Fast (hr)	Primary Energy Source
0-2	Ingested food
2-6	Glycogen
6-12	Gluconeogenesis
12-24	Fatty acid oxidation

Table 36-3   Physical Findings in Disorders Associated with Hypoglycemia

Finding	Disorder
Short stature	Hypopituitarism, growth hormone deficiency
Failure to thrive	Disorders of carbohydrate, organic acid, or amino acid metabolism
Tachypnea	Inborn errors of metabolism
Midline facial defect	Hypopituitarism, growth hormone deficiency
Nystagmus	Hypopituitarism, growth hormone deficiency
Cryptorchidism, microphallus	Hypopituitarism, growth hormone deficiency
Hyperpigmentation	Adrenal insufficiency
Macrosomia, macroglossia, umbilical hernia	Beckwith-Wiedemann syndrome
Hepatomegaly	Glycogen storage disease, galactosemia, disorders of gluconeogenesis, fructose intolerance

oped ketones. Patients who do not produce ketones in response to hypoglycemia are likely to have either hyperinsulinism (endogenous or exogenous) or a disorder of fatty acid oxidation. Appropriate ketosis, in contrast, suggests signal dysregulation or a disorder of carbohydrate or amino acid metabolism. An algorithm to guide the interpretation of laboratory data is provided in Figure 36-1.

TREATMENT

The initial management of a hypoglycemic patient is to ensure the adequacy of the patient's airway, breathing, and circulation and to raise serum glucose levels by administering a bolus of dextrose at a dose of 0.5 to 1 g/kg. After the initial bolus, patients should be given a dextrose infusion at a rate of 6 to 9 mg/kg per minute. Blood sugar should be monitored frequently (initially every 30 to 60 minutes, then every 2 to 4 hours), with a goal of 80 to 120 mg/dL.

FURTHER EVALUATION

When the evaluation outlined earlier points to a specific disease, confirmatory testing may be possible. For example, fructose tolerance tests can be performed if hereditary fructose intolerance is suspected, or DNA analysis can be done for disorders in which a gene mutation has been identified. In some patients, the cause of hypoglycemia may remain undiagnosed despite obtaining all the aforementioned history, physical examination, and laboratory data. In this setting, additional studies such as glucagon challenge testing or monitored fasting may prove useful. Finally, liver biopsy may be necessary to evaluate for hepatic enzyme deficiencies.

Table 36-4 Blood and Urine Tests Useful in the Evaluation of Hypoglycemia

Test	Associated Diagnosis
Blood tests	
Insulin (plus C peptide)	Hyperinsulinism, exogenous insulin overdose
Cortisol	Cortisol deficiency
Growth hormone	Growth hormone deficiency
Free fatty acids	Fatty acid oxidation defect
β-hydroxybutyrate, acetoacetate	Fatty acid oxidation defect
Amino acids	Organic acidemia
Lactate, pyruvate	Glycogen storage disease, disorders of gluconeogenesis
Carnitine, acylcarnitine	Fatty acid oxidation defect
Electrolytes (with calculated anion gap)	Organic acidemia, maple syrup urine disease, glycogen storage disease, disorders of gluconeogenesis
Ammonia	Organic acidemia
Toxicology screen (alcohol, salicylates)	Ingestions
Venous blood gas	Organic acidemia, maple syrup urine disease, glycogen storage disease, disorders of gluconeogenesis
Urine tests	
Ketones	Hyperinsulinism, fatty acid oxidation defect, fructose intolerance
Glucose, reducing substance	Galactosemia, fructose intolerance
Organic acid	Organic acidemia
Acylglycine	Fatty acid oxidation defect

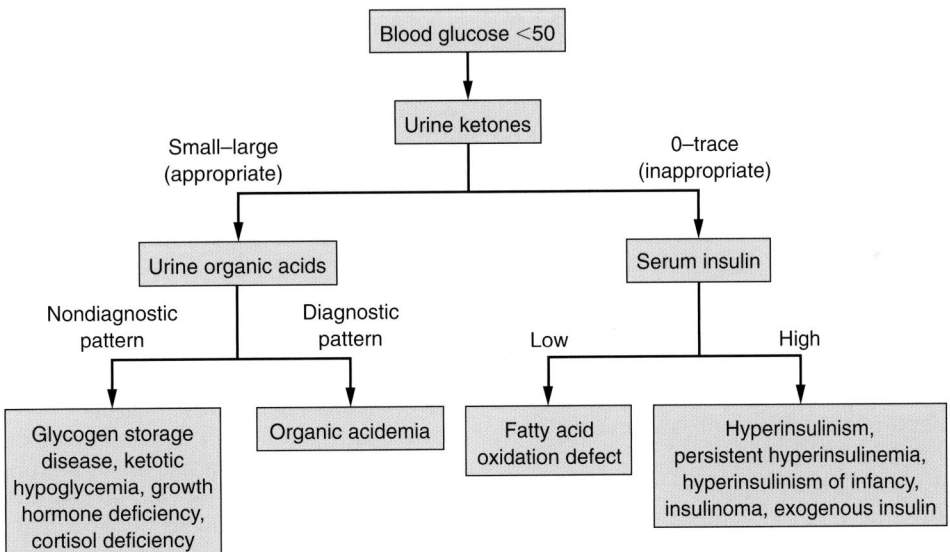

Figure 36-1 Algorithm for the interpretation of laboratory data in the evaluation of hypoglycemia.

SUGGESTED READING

Frier B: Hypoglycaemia—clinical consequences and morbidity. Int J Clin Pract Suppl 2000;112:51-55.

Haymond MW, Sunehag A: Controlling the sugar bowl: Regulation of glucose homeostasis in children. Endocrinol Clin North Am 1999;28:663.

Lteif AN, Schwenk WF: Hypoglycemia in infants and children. Endocrinol Metab Clin North Am 1999;28:619-646.

Ozand PT: Hypoglycemia in association with various organic and amino acid disorders. Semin Perinatol 2000;24:172-193.

Saudubray JM, de Lonlay P, Touati G, et al: Genetic hypoglycaemia in infancy and childhood: Pathophysiology and diagnosis. J Inherit Metab Dis 2000;23:197-214.

Verrotti A, Fusilli P, Pallotta R, et al: Hypoglycemia in childhood: A clinical approach. J Pediatr Endocrinol Metab 1998;11(Suppl 1):147-152.

CHAPTER 37

Shock

Andrew M. Fine

Shock is a clinical condition that occurs when there is inadequate delivery of oxygen and other nutrients to meet the metabolic demands of the tissues. If left untreated, shock results in irreversible cell damage and death. The clinician must be able to recognize shock early, initiate therapy rapidly, and arrange safe transport of the patient to an intensive care facility. These lifesaving tasks require that the clinician have a fundamental knowledge of the causes, presentations, therapies, and complications of shock.

BACKGROUND

Physiologically, shock can be classified as *compensated,* when the patient is able to maintain a normal blood pressure for age, or *decompensated,* when deterioration has led to hypotension. Children can generally maintain a normal blood pressure until advanced stages of shock; therefore, hypotension in a pediatric patient is an ominous sign of impending circulatory collapse. When measuring blood pressure with a sphygmomanometer, it is important to select the smallest cuff that covers two thirds of the upper arm or leg. The minimum systolic blood pressure in children is shown in Table 37-1. In general, compensated shock progresses to decompensated shock if left untreated, which emphasizes the importance of early recognition and intervention.

PATHOPHYSIOLOGY

Shock can also be classified by cause, with the main types being hypovolemic, septic, cardiogenic, and distributive shock. The mechanisms may differ, but inadequate tissue perfusion is the common final pathway.

Hypovolemic Shock

Hypovolemic shock, by far the most common type of shock in children, occurs when a decrease in intravascular volume leads to decreased venous return and, subsequently, decreased preload. Decreased preload results in decreased stroke volume. An increase in heart rate often maintains cardiac output initially, but when this compensatory response is inadequate, cardiac output diminishes. The formula that defines this relationship is as follows:

$$\text{Cardiac output} = \text{Heart rate} \times \text{Stroke volume}$$

Decreased cardiac output results in decreased delivery of oxygen and other substrates to the tissues. The two main categories of hypovolemic shock are hemorrhagic and nonhemorrhagic; examples are provided in Table 37-2.

In the early stage of hypovolemic shock, autoregulatory mechanisms shunt blood flow preferentially to the brain, heart, and adrenal system. Because flow is diverted from less critical organs, patients may present initially with cool or mottled extremities, decreased urine output, and, of note, normal blood pressure. Other signs may include dry mucous membranes, absence of tears, and abnormal skin turgor.

Hemorrhagic shock due to known trauma is typically diagnosed at the initial presentation; however, hemorrhagic shock can present during hospitalization, especially in postoperative patients. Victims of child abuse are also at risk for delayed diagnosis of hemorrhagic shock because the initial history may be incomplete, inaccurate, or misleading, and symptoms may progress over time. Nonhemorrhagic shock may present in patients with ongoing fluid losses (e.g., vomiting, diarrhea, gastric suctioning, burns), especially if there is inadequate replacement.

Septic Shock

Sepsis is a clinical syndrome that results from overwhelming infection and the subsequent development of widespread tissue injury. Shock occurring during sepsis may result from intravascular volume depletion, volume maldistribution, cardiac dysfunction, or metabolic derangements at the cellular level. It is important to consider septic shock early, because a seemingly stable patient with minimal findings of infection can quickly progress to sepsis. In the early (compensated) phase, septic shock may present with decreased vascular resistance, increased cardiac output, tachycardia, warm extremities, and normal urine output. As it progresses to the decompensated phase, patients develop intravascular volume depletion, myocardial depression, cool extremities, central nervous system changes, respiratory distress, and decreased cardiac output.

Although anyone can develop septic shock, risk factors include young age, chronic medical condition, presence of central intravenous (IV) catheters, immunodeficiency, burns, and malnutrition. Septic shock can result from bacterial, viral, or fungal infection. It is important to note that septic shock can occur when cultures or other diagnostic tests do not yield a definitive organism. Shock can also develop from localized bacterial infections that produce toxins; this is referred to as toxic shock (see Chapter 62). This form of shock is most commonly associated with toxin-producing strains of group A streptococci and *Staphylococcus aureus.*

Septic shock is sometimes referred to as "warm shock" because, in the early phase, the patient shows signs of a hyperdynamic state, with warm extremities, bounding pulses, tachycardia, tachypnea, and altered mental status. A patient in septic shock usually has a widened pulse pressure, increased cardiac output, increased mixed venous saturation, and decreased systemic vascular resistance. Laboratory evaluation reveals lactic acidosis. As septic shock progresses, "warm shock" evolves into "cold shock" with a decrease in

Table 37-1	Hypotension Parameters
Age	Minimum Systolic Blood Pressure (mm Hg)
Term neonate (0-28 days)	60
Infant (1-12 mo)	70
Child (1-10 yr)	70 + (2 × age in yr)
Older than 10 yr	90

Table 37-2 Causes of Hypovolemic Shock

Nonhemorrhagic	Hemorrhagic
Vomiting or diarrhea	Trauma
Diabetes insipidus, diabetes mellitus	Gastrointestinal bleeding
Heatstroke	Postsurgical bleeding
Burns	Sequestration crisis
Intestinal obstruction	Splenic rupture
Water deprivation	
Adrenal insufficiency	
Hypothyroidism	

Box 37-1 Causes of Distributive Shock

Anaphylaxis
 Medications
 Foods
 Envenomations or stings
 Blood products
 Latex
Neurologic
 Head injury
 Spinal shock
Septic shock
Drugs

Box 37-2 Causes of Cardiogenic Shock

Cardiomyopathies
 Familial
 Infectious
 Infiltrative
 Idiopathic
Arrhythmias
 Ventricular fibrillation
 Supraventricular tachycardia
 Bradycardia
 Complete heart block
Mechanical defects
 Congenital heart disease
 Coarctation of the aorta
 Cardiac tumor
Obstructive disorders
 Pulmonary embolism
 Tension pneumothorax
 Constrictive pericarditis
 Pericardial tamponade
 Pulmonary hypertension
Ischemia or infarction
 Anomalous coronary artery
 Kawasaki disease

cardiac output. Clinically, the patient may have cyanosis, cool extremities, rapid and thready pulses, and shallow respirations.

Distributive Shock

Distributive shock is caused by a decrease in systemic vascular resistance. Abnormalities in vasomotor tone cause peripheral pooling of blood, which leads to a diminished effective preload, decreased cardiac output, and inadequate tissue perfusion. This process can occur without frank fluid loss. Causes of distributive shock are listed in Box 37-1.

Anaphylactic shock occurs when an exogenous stimulus causes an allergic, systemic, immunoglobulin E–mediated response that triggers the release of histamine and other vasoactive factors from mast cells, with resultant vasodilation (see Chapter 134). Neurogenic shock may occur with spinal cord transection above the first thoracic level, with severe injuries to the brainstem, or with isolated intracranial injuries. An injury to the cervical cord may result in unopposed parasympathetic tone and subsequent vasodilation. Some drugs can cause severe vasodilation, resulting in shock; these drugs include those that cause anaphylaxis and those that cause severe hypotension (e.g., β-antagonists and calcium channel antagonists).

Cardiogenic Shock

Cardiogenic shock occurs when there is decreased cardiac output caused by pump failure. The main causes are listed in Box 37-2. In general, excluding patients with congenital heart disease, cardiogenic shock is much less common in children than in adults because of the relatively low incidence of coronary artery disease and congestive heart failure in the pediatric population. Cardiogenic shock should be strongly considered when there is no history of fluid losses, the physical examination reveals hepatomegaly or rales, the chest radiograph demonstrates cardiomegaly, and there is no clinical improvement despite oxygenation and volume expansion.

Management of cardiogenic shock should focus on correcting arrhythmias if present, improving preload and cardiac contractility, and reducing afterload. The workload of the heart can be minimized by the achievement of normothermia, correction of anemia if present, and sedation, intubation, and mechanical ventilation if necessary.

Although cardiogenic shock is uncommon as the primary cause of shock in children, it may be a late manifestation of other forms of shock.

Box 37-3 Special Considerations in Neonatal Shock

Congenital adrenal hyperplasia
Inborn errors of metabolism
Left-sided cardiac obstructive lesions
   Aortic stenosis
   Hypoplastic left heart syndrome
   Coarctation of the aorta
   Interrupted aortic arch
Blood loss at delivery
Perinatal infection

SPECIAL CONSIDERATIONS

Shock in a neonate may be the result of any of the previously mentioned causes, but the differential diagnosis of neonatal shock should also include those listed in Box 37-3. Likewise, medically complicated patients may be more difficult to diagnose with shock because they may have abnormal vasomotor responses, be unable to mount an adequate immune response, or possess internal hardware that could harbor infection.

PROGRESSION OF SHOCK

In early, or compensated, shock, pediatric patients are able to maintain cardiac output and blood pressure by increasing the heart rate and peripheral vascular resistance. With further compromise of cardiac function, the compensatory tachycardia is insufficient to maintain cardiac output. Decreased perfusion affects many systems, causing metabolic acidosis, oliguria, elevated transaminases from hepatocellular injury, cool extremities, mottling of the skin, and ileus. Tachypnea develops to increase the elimination of carbon dioxide, which helps compensate for the metabolic acidosis.

In the late stages of shock, end-organ failure may manifest as central nervous system depression (ranging from confusion and agitation to coma), anuria, uremia, hyperkalemia, acute respiratory distress syndrome, and coagulopathies.

EVALUATION

Early recognition of shock is important. Box 37-4 identifies patients at increased risk for developing shock. The history (Box 37-5) and physical examination (Box 37-6) should focus on aspects that will help the clinician distinguish among the different causes of shock. Diagnostic tests may help identify the cause of shock, as well as early signs of end-organ dysfunction (Box 37-7).

Box 37-4 Patients at Increased Risk for Shock

Febrile infants
Immunocompromised patients
Neonates
Patients with congenital heart disease
Patients with excessive fluid losses

Box 37-5 Focused History

Initial diagnosis
   Is it consistent with patient's current condition?
Recent exposures
   Trauma
   Infection
   Travel
Recent therapies
   Medications
   Fluids
   Procedures
Past medical history
   Immune status
   Cardiac disease
   Systemic disease
Medications
Allergies
   Medication
   Food
   Latex or other chemicals

Box 37-6 Directed Physical Examination

Vital signs
Skin
   Rash
   Petechiae
   Ecchymosis
   Erythroderma
   Mottling
Head, eyes, ears, nose, and throat
   Evidence of head trauma
   Pupil size and reactivity
   Conjunctival pallor
   Central cyanosis (lips, tongue)
Neck
   Meningismus
   Cervical spine tenderness
Lungs
   Abnormal breathing pattern (e.g., Kussmaul)
   Retractions
   Wheezes or rales (focal or bilateral)
   Diminished breath sounds or dullness to percussion
Heart
   Hyperdynamic
   Murmur
   Rub
   Gallop
Abdomen
   Tenderness, rebound, or guarding
   Distention or ascites
   Mass or organomegaly
Extremities
   Temperature
   Peripheral pulses
   Clubbing
Neurologic
   Mental status
   Focal deficit

INITIAL STABILIZATION

A pediatric patient in shock represents a medical emergency. For this reason, identification of the precise cause of shock may be delayed while resuscitation and stabilization proceed. Attention to the ABCs (airway, breathing, and circulation) remains a basic principle in the initial assessment and management. In general, increasing oxygen delivery to the tissues and decreasing oxygen demand are key. Hypoxemia should be avoided, but if it occurs, it should be corrected with generous oxygen supplementation. If there is suspicion of trauma, cervical spine immobilization should be maintained until the spine can be evaluated. The primary survey of a pediatric patient in shock is directed toward the rapid identification of immediately life-threatening conditions that should be addressed before a more extensive evaluation.

A stable airway should be established and maintained, and supplemental oxygen should be provided to keep arterial oxygen saturation greater than 95%. Evaluating peripheral perfusion and pulses provides a rapid assessment of the circulation. Continuous cardiorespiratory monitoring and frequent blood pressure measurement are important to assess the response to intervention. The standard of two large-bore IV lines may not be feasible, especially in very young pediatric patients in shock, but the goal is to maintain reliable intravascular access through which vigorous resuscitation can proceed. If peripheral IV access is not immediately obtained, intraosseous access should be considered, especially in a child younger than 5 years (see Chapter 203). Unless the patient has myocardial failure, the initial therapy should be 20 mL/kg of isotonic fluid (normal saline or lactated Ringer's) administered intravenously as rapidly as possible. This may be repeated two more times, to a total of 60 mL/kg, with close clinical assessment of vital signs, perfusion, urine output, and mental status for improvement. In the case of hemorrhagic shock, blood products should be used as soon as possible. Until appropriate blood products are available, isotonic IV fluids are used as a temporizing measure to restore intravascular volume.

If the patient remains hypotensive and poorly perfused despite 60 mL/kg of IV fluids, inotropic support should be strongly considered. Dopamine IV infusion is commonly initiated at a rate of 10 μg/kg per minute and then titrated to improve and maintain blood pressure, peripheral perfusion, and urine output. In patients who do not respond to dopamine, IV epinephrine, norepinephrine, or both may be considered. Hydrocortisone should also be considered for patients who show resistance to catecholamines or have adrenal suppression.

A chest radiograph may be helpful to assess the presence of cardiomegaly, fluid overload, pulmonary edema, pneumonia, pleural effusion, or pneumothorax. Central venous pressure is also helpful, if obtainable, so that the degree of volume repletion can be assessed. In a neonate with shock in whom a duct-dependent cardiac lesion is a possible cause, prostaglandin E_1 should be considered to maintain patency of the ductus arteriosus. Preparation should be made for the possibility of intubation, because prostaglandin E_1 may cause apnea. The decision to administer prostaglandin E_1 is usually made in consultation with a neonatologist or pediatric cardiologist.

Antipyretics should be administered, when feasible, to a febrile patient to decrease metabolic demand. Conversely, warming should be instituted in a hypothermic patient (see Chapter 186). Broad-spectrum antibiotics should be given intravenously or intraosseously unless it is known that infection is not the cause of the patient's condition. The choice of antibiotic is driven by the likely pathogens (Table 37-3) and the age of the patient (Table 37-4).

TRANSPORT OF THE PATIENT IN SHOCK

Early initiation of transport can be life and limb saving for patients in shock. The child should be hospitalized in an intensive care unit capable of invasive monitoring and

---

Box 37-7   Diagnostic Tests Considered for Patients in Shock

Complete blood count with differential
Serum chemistries
   Electrolytes
   Blood urea nitrogen
   Creatinine
   Glucose*
   Liver enzymes
   Pancreatic enzymes
   Cardiac enzymes
   Lactic acid
Coagulation studies
   Prothrombin time
   Partial thromboplastin time
   Fibrinogen
   Fibrin split (degradation) products
Arterial blood gas
Type and crossmatch
Cultures
   Blood
   Urine
Toxicology
   Urine
   Serum
Urinalysis
Imaging
   Chest radiograph
   Abdominal radiograph or obstruction series
Electrocardiogram

*Consider a bedside rapid blood glucose test (Dextrostix).

Table 37-3   Pathogens in Septic Shock

Neonate and Young Infant	Infant and Young Child
Group B streptococci	*Neisseria meningitides*
Escherichia coli and other gram-negative bacilli	*Streptococcus pneumoniae*
Enterococci	*Haemophilus influenzae* type B
Herpes simplex virus	Group A streptococci *Staphylococcus aureus* Rickettsieae

Table 37-4 Antimicrobials in Shock

Age	Antimicrobial Agent	Initial IV Dose (mg/kg)
0-4 wk	Ampicillin plus	50-100*
	Gentamicin or	2.5
	Cefotaxime	50
>4 wk	Ceftriaxone	50-100*
	Consider adding vancomycin	10-15*
Immunocompromised	Ceftazidime or	25-75*
	Piperacillin/ tazobactam	100†
	Consider vancomycin	10-15*
Possible rickettsial infection	Add doxycycline	2.2

*Higher dosing recommended for possible meningitis.
†Based on piperacillin component.

airway intervention and with personnel who are experienced in managing critically ill children. If transfer to another institution is necessary, the clinician has the challenging task of weighing the risks and benefits of the different modes of transportation (see Chapter 15). In every case, whether the patient is transferred to another facility or from one unit to another within the same facility, it is essential that the team transporting the patient have the appropriate personnel and equipment to do so safely. In addition, the receiving facility or unit must be ready for the patient's arrival. Communication of the patient's condition and the interventions performed is key, and medical records, imaging studies, and laboratory results should accompany the patient whenever possible.

SUGGESTED READING

Carcillo JA, Fields AI: Clinical practice parameters for hemodynamic support of pediatric and neonatal patients in septic shock. Crit Care Med 2002;30:1365-1378.

Dellinger RP, Carlet JM, Masur H: Surviving Sepsis Campaign guidelines for management of severe sepsis and septic shock. Crit Care Med 2004;32:858-873.

Pediatric Advanced Life Support Provider Manual. Dallas, TX, American Heart Association, 2002.

Saladino RA: Management of septic shock in the pediatric emergency department in 2004. Clin Pediatr Emerg Med 2004;5:20-27.

CHAPTER 38

Hypoxemia

Bryan L. Stone

Hypoxia is a relative or absolute deficiency of oxygen (O_2); anoxia is the complete lack of O_2. Hypoxemia is a subset of hypoxia, referring specifically to low O_2 levels in the blood. There are four broad categories of hypoxia:

1. Hypoxemic hypoxia is due to low blood O_2 levels from pulmonary or environmental causes (e.g., pneumonia, high altitude, chronic lung disease, increased shunt from congenital heart disease).
2. Hypemic hypoxia is due to a decreased blood O_2 carrying capacity (e.g., anemia, carbon monoxide poisoning).
3. Ischemic or stagnant hypoxia is due to decreased tissue O_2 delivery (e.g., shock, arterial occlusive disease).
4. Histotoxic hypoxia is due to mitochondrial cytochrome poisoning (e.g., cyanide, carbon monoxide).[1]

Hypoxia and hypoxemia are common reasons for admission, usually in the context of a primary respiratory illness such as pneumonia or bronchiolitis. An understanding of hypoxia and the evaluation, diagnosis, and monitoring of patients with the condition improves patient care and resource utilization.

BACKGROUND

The process of delivering O_2 to tissues is complex, but knowledge of this process facilitates an understanding of the clinical problems associated with hypoxemia and hypoxia. O_2 moves down the "oxygen cascade" from dry atmospheric air (160 mm Hg at sea level) to the mitochondria in tissues (3 to 20 mm Hg).[1] In contrast, carbon dioxide (CO_2) diffuses readily, dissolves minimally in plasma, is transported primarily by the red blood cells, is a waste product of aerobic metabolism, is eliminated from the body almost uniquely by the lungs, and is a primary driving force for ventilation.

Arterial partial pressure of CO_2 ($PaCO_2$) reflects energy metabolism (production of CO_2) and ventilation. Diet affects the respiratory quotient, which is the ratio of CO_2 to O_2 exchanged across the alveolar membrane. The respiratory quotient on a pure carbohydrate diet is 1.0; on a protein diet, it is 0.81; and on an animal fat diet, it is 0.71. A balanced diet results in a respiratory quotient of about 0.83, the value typically used to calculate alveolar partial pressure of O_2 (PAO_2). CO_2 is also involved in acid-base balance, which has an impact on its rate of elimination.

The fraction of inspired O_2 (FIO_2) constitutes 20.93% of the atmosphere, but the partial pressure of inspired O_2 (PIO_2) is dependent on barometric pressure (P_B) as a function of altitude. Further, O_2 entering the alveolus is "diluted" by CO_2 in the alveolus in relation to the respiratory quotient.

For example, at sea level, the P_B is 760 mm Hg; the partial pressure of O_2 (PO_2) of dry air is 159 mm Hg; and, once humidified at 37°C, the PIO_2 is 149 mm Hg ([760 − 47] × 0.2093). In the alveolus, CO_2 is present in proportion to the respiratory quotient (R), and the final PAO_2 is diminished by the factor $PACO_2$ (FIO_2 − [(1 − FIO_2)/R]). With an alveolar partial pressure of CO_2 ($PACO_2$) of 40 mm Hg and an R of 0.83, the ideal PAO_2 at sea level is 103 mm Hg. In contrast, in Salt Lake City, 1280 m above sea level, the P_B is 647 mm Hg, and the ideal PAO_2 is only 79 mm Hg.

Diffusion of O_2 across the alveolar and pulmonary capillary membranes is less efficient than that of CO_2 and is affected mostly by the diffusion distance, the PAO_2–mixed venous PO_2 gradient, and the transit time of blood through the pulmonary capillary. Arterial O_2 pressure (PaO_2) is also influenced by deoxygenated blood that bypasses the alveolar capillary bed, referred to as the shunt fraction. This results in a "normal" alveolar-arterial (A-a) gradient, or difference between PAO_2 and PaO_2. The anatomic, or fixed, shunt fraction is about 2% of cardiac output and combines with a variable physiologic shunt fraction to create the A-a gradient. Accordingly, the normal PaO_2 of blood would be 95 mm Hg at sea level and 72 mm Hg in Salt Lake City. A PaO_2 of 60 mm Hg is thought to trigger physiologic mechanisms to acclimate to hypoxemia.[2]

Once it crosses the alveolar-pulmonary capillary membranes, a minimal amount of O_2 is dissolved in plasma (0.003 mL per dL of blood for each millimeter of mercury of PaO_2). The majority of the O_2 is transported bound to hemoglobin, reversibly, as oxyhemoglobin. When 100% of the O_2 binding sites are occupied, hemoglobin carries 1.34 mL of O_2 per gram. The O_2 binding relationship with hemoglobin is complex, generating an S-shaped curve of O_2 saturation of hemoglobin binding sites when viewed graphically (Fig. 38-1). Above a PaO_2 of about 50 mm Hg, the curve flattens out so that there is little additional hemoglobin binding despite increases in PaO_2. This hemoglobin saturation-desaturation relationship facilitates both O_2 uptake across the alveolar-pulmonary capillary diffusion gradient and O_2 release in tissues, where O_2 tension levels can be as low as 3 mm Hg at the threshold of anaerobic metabolism.[1] Several substances and conditions can "shift" the oxyhemoglobin saturation curve rightward, toward decreased pulmonary O_2 uptake and improved tissue release, or leftward, leading to improved pulmonary O_2 uptake and inhibited tissue release (see Fig. 38-1). The capacity of blood to carry O_2 is dependent on hemoglobin content and is a combination of dissolved O_2 and that carried by hemoglobin, totaling 20.8 mL O_2 per deciliter of blood at a hemoglobin concentration of 15 g/dL blood.

Because the majority of O_2 carried by the blood is bound to hemoglobin, anemia results in decreased O_2-carrying capacity. Acute euvolemic anemia is probably tolerated to a hemoglobin level of 7 g/dL. Chronic anemia is tolerated below those levels, but the lowest threshold that is incompatible with life is unknown.[3] Cyanosis, which is visible deoxyhemoglobinemia, is not detectable until a concentration of about 4 to 5 g/dL of deoxyhemoglobin is present,[4] or a hemoglobin saturation of about 67% to 73% with hemoglobin levels of 15 mg/dL.

EVALUATION

History

The history related to hypoxemia involves a complete pulmonary systems review, including infectious symptoms; this covers most clinical presentations. A history of possible toxic exposure or inhalation can help diagnose some conditions not easily detected by pulse oximetry (e.g., carbon monoxide poisoning, see Chapter 184). Review of the history with regard to lung disease, cardiovascular disease, medication use, prior thoracic surgery, chest wall deformity or restriction (e.g., scoliosis), allergy, prior or current O_2 baseline use, artificial ventilatory support, and results of prior blood gas testing, pulmonary function tests, or other studies of cardiopulmonary function is also essential.

Physical Examination

The physical examination should include a critical evaluation of the patient's vital signs based on norms for age and altitude (Table 38-1),[5] because tachycardia and tachypnea can be compensations for hypoxia, resulting in a normal pulse oximetry O_2 saturation (SpO_2) reading. This can also help in diagnosing causes of hypoxia not related to hypoxemia. An initial impression of the patient's degree of illness is beneficial, because hypoxia (with or without hypoxemia) may be present if the patient looks ill or uncomfortable. A careful cardiopulmonary examination should include a search for peripheral evidence of hypoperfusion or regional or systemic hypoxia and for chest wall abnormalities. A neurologic evaluation with regard to respiratory drive, strength of the muscles of respiration, and level of consciousness is applicable. If the patient has been placed on O_2, the physical findings may have improved, leaving a false impression of less acute illness. A review of preintervention findings with persons who observed or examined the patient before O_2 was administered can be helpful. It should also be noted that a significant amount of deoxyhemoglobinemia cannot be easily achieved in an anemic patient, so cyanosis is not always a reliable physical finding of hypoxemia with coexistent anemia.

Pulse Oximetry

Pulse oximetry combines the principles of spectrophotometry and optical plethysmography, taking advantage of the differential absorption of light in the red and ultraviolet wavelengths of deoxy- and oxyhemoglobin, and differentiating arterial flow as pulsatile flow. The probe includes two light-emitting diodes, one around 660 nm and the other around 940 nm, and a photodetector placed opposite across a perfused tissue bed. The light transmitted through the

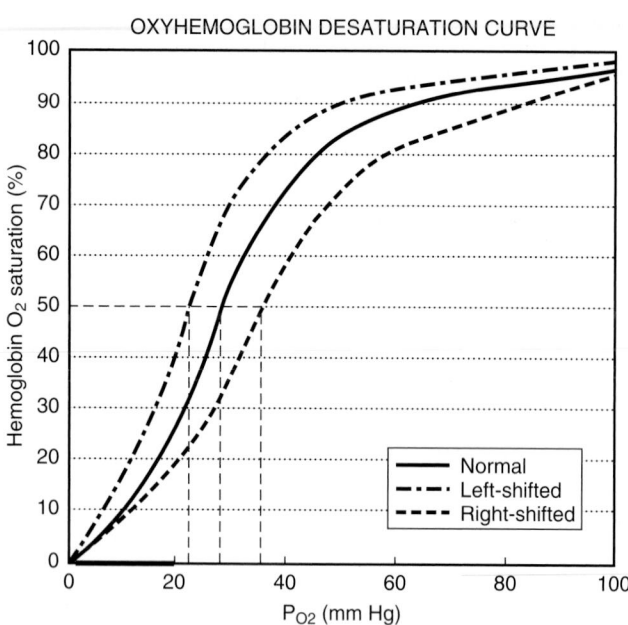

Figure 38-1 Oxyhemoglobin saturation-desaturation curve. The normal curve for adult hemoglobin is depicted, as are examples of left-shifted (poor tissue O_2 unloading) and right-shifted (improved tissue O_2 unloading) curves. The curve is shifted to the left by alkalemia, carboxyhemoglobinemia, hypocarbia, hypothermia, methemoglobinemia, a high fetal hemoglobin content, and low 2,3-diphosphoglycerate (2,3-DPG). The curve is shifted to the right by acidemia, hypercarbia, hyperthermia, sulfhemoglobinemia, and high levels of 2,3-DPG, an end product of red cell metabolism. Note the P_{O_2} at which 50% of the O_2 is unloaded for each curve and the range of tissue P_{O_2} (thick bar from 3 to 20).

Table 38-1	Heart Rate and Respiratory Rate by Age and Altitude, in Awake Subjects at Rest								
	SEA LEVEL		3600-3750 FEET		4100 FEET		PUBLISHED		
Age	HR	RR	HR	RR	HR	RR	HR	RR	Age
0-5 mo			123-155	36-62	140-154	41-51	70-190	24-50	NB
6-11 mo			117-149	31-53	125-136	38-46	80-160	24-38	1-11 mo
12-23 mo			108-138	25-39	120-134	33-41	80-130	22-30	2 yr
24-35 mo			104-140	26-38	105-119	31-36	80-120	20-24	4 yr
36-60 mo			91-123	22-34	103-116	30-35	75-115	20-24	6 yr
2-6 yr	79-93*	18-21*					70-110	18-24	8 yr
7-11 yr	71-81*	17-19*					70-110	16-22	10 yr
12-16 yr	66-71*	17-18*					55-105	14-20	14-18 yr

*Interquartile range.
HR, heart rate (beats/min); NB, newborn; RR, respiratory rate (breaths/min).

Table 38-2 Helpful Formulas and Pearls

DO_2 (mL/min) = CaO_2 (mL/dL) × CO (L/min) × 10 (dL/L)

CO (L/min) = Stroke volume (L/contraction) × Heart rate (contractions/min)

CaO_2 (mL/dL) = [Hb (g/dL) × % saturation × 1.34 mL/g] + PaO_2 × 0.003 (mL/dL)

PIO_2 (mm Hg) = [P_B − P_{H_2O}] × FIO_2

PAO_2 = PIO_2 − [$PACO_2$(FIO_2 − [(1 − FIO_2)/R])], approximated as PAO_2 = PIO_2 − [$PaCO_2$/R]

Normal PaO_2 measured by ABG at sea level $\cong$ 104.2 − 0.27 × age (yr)

A-a gradient = PAO_2 − PaO_2, or [(P_B − 47) × FIO_2] − [($PaCO_2$/0.83)] − PaO_2; A-a gradient = 2.5 + 0.21 × age (yr), or [age + 10]/4

ABG measures pH, PaO_2, $PaCO_2$, Hb, and SaO_2; calculated values are also reported, such as HCO_3

CBG yields reasonably reliable pH, $PaCO_2$, Hb, and SaO_2 values

VBG yields Hb, SaO_2, and, if from the right atrium, mixed venous PO_2

For the desired information, use any of the checked tests:

Parameter	ABG	CBG	VBG	Pulse Oximetry
A-a gradient (must test on a known FIO_2)	X			
Ventilation status	X	X		
Dyshemoglobinemias (SaO_2)	X	X	X	
Oxygenation (PaO_2)	X			
Tissue O_2 consumption (mixed venous PO_2, right atrial sample)			X	
CaO_2	X			
CvO_2 (right atrial sample)			X	
PAO_2 (must know FIO_2)	X	X		
Arterial oxyhemoglobin saturation	X			X*

*Pulse oximetry measures functional Hb O_2 saturation but provides no information about ventilation, O_2-carrying capacity, DO_2, or general tissue oxygenation status. Factors that decrease pulse oximetry accuracy include ambient light, which tends to move the reading toward 85%, with both sensors detecting the same amount of light; probe placement, because both wavelengths of light must traverse an equivalent tissue bed; motion artifact and signal loss; electromagnetic interference (magnetic resonance imaging can cause burns); nail polish (if it absorbs at 660 or 940 nm); hypoperfusion; severe anemia (Hb <5 mg/dL); venous congestion with venous pulsation; and vital dyes (methylene blue, indocyanine green, fluorescein, indigo carmine, and isosulfan blue all lower SpO_2). Skin pigmentation and hyperbilirubinemia do not affect SpO_2. The latest advances in pulse oximetry are addressing artifact due to motion, hypoperfusion, and ambient light. Oximeters advertised to provide fractional oximetry do not actually do so. Readings are simply adjusted for presumed methemoglobin and carboxyhemoglobin levels based on published norms.

A-a, alveolar-arterial; ABG, arterial blood gas; CaO_2, arterial O_2 content; CBG, capillary blood gas; CO, cardiac output; CvO_2, venous O_2 content; DO_2, tissue O_2 delivery; FIO_2, fraction of inspired O_2 (0.21 on room air); Hb, hemoglobin; O_2, oxygen; $PACO_2$, alveolar partial pressure of carbon dioxide; $PaCO_2$, arterial partial pressure of carbon dioxide; PAO_2, alveolar partial pressure of O_2; PaO_2, arterial partial pressure of O_2; P_B, barometric pressure; P_{H_2O}, water pressure (47 mm Hg at 37°C); PIO_2, partial pressure of inspired O_2; PO_2, partial pressure of O_2; R, respiratory quotient (0.83 on a mixed carbohydrate, fat, protein diet); SaO_2, fractional O_2 saturation; SpO_2, pulse oximetry O_2 saturation; VBG, venous blood gas.

tissue bed at each wavelength allows differentiation of oxyhemoglobin and deoxyhemoglobin. Sampling through pulsatile and nonpulsatile flow distinguishes between arterial blood and background absorption by all other tissues, including venous blood. The resulting reading is fed into an algorithm that relates it to empirically obtained hemoglobin saturation values by co-oximetry among normal volunteers in O_2-depleted environments; this is reported as the SpO_2 percentage. It should be noted that each light source must transmit light across an equivalent tissue bed, displayed values are delayed 3 to 6 seconds, artifacts are common, and several factors can affect the accuracy of pulse oximetry (Table 38-2).[1] Nevertheless, compared with pulse oximetry, physical examination findings are often insensitive in diagnosing hypoxemia clnically.[6-9]

The presence or absence of hypoxemia determined by pulse oximetry is a major factor in the decision regarding hospital admission versus outpatient treatment. Pulse oximetry has become known as the "fifth vital sign" owing to its ubiquitous use.[10] The need for supplemental O_2, monitored and titrated by pulse oximetry, is a basis for admission and ongoing hospitalization; resolution of such need is a common criterion for discharge.[11] Pulse oximetry used or interpreted incorrectly, however, can lead to misdiagnosis, inappropriate admission, and delay in discharge. For example, during the 2 decades from the 1980s to the early 2000s, nationwide admissions for bronchiolitis increased 250% largely because of reliance on pulse oximetry, with no apparent change in morbidity and mortality.[11-13]

Important caveats when using pulse oximetry are that SpO_2 is a measure of functional saturation and does not differentiate saturation of dyshemoglobin from saturation of oxyhemoglobin. The hemoglobin saturation curve is not linear, and because of this, SpO_2 is insensitive to large changes in PaO_2 resulting from changes in patient status at the upper, flattened portion of the curve. For instance, PaO_2 would have to fall from 145 to 65 mm Hg before a significant decrease in SpO_2 would occur. Clinically, it would seem that the patient had suddenly worsened, but an appropriately sensitive system would have detected a more gradual decline. Pulse oximetry is also not useful for detecting hyperoxia.[14]

Ventilation status cannot be monitored by pulse oximetry. Hypoventilation leads to a rapid rise in partial pressure of CO_2 (PCO_2), but SpO_2 responses may be delayed for minutes to hours in a well-preoxygenated patient still receiving O_2. Nor does SpO_2 equate with arterial O_2 content (CaO_2), tissue O_2 delivery, or tissue O_2 use. Therefore, one must verify an adequate CaO_2, cardiac output, and tissue O_2 uptake and use if clinical symptoms or suspicion of tissue hypoxia are present despite a normal SpO_2. Pulse oximetry also cannot identify poor O_2-carrying capacity of the blood from causes such as anemia or dyshemoglobinemias (hypemic hypoxia); decreased cardiac output, arterio-occlusive disease, shock, or other causes of stagnant hypoxia; and syndromes that interfere with tissue O_2 use or histotoxic hypoxia. There is also evidence that pulse oximetry may be less accurate clinically than was traditionally assumed.[15,16]

Blood Gas Evaluation

Arterial blood samples that are properly obtained, handled, and analyzed with modern equipment yield information about oxygenation, ventilation, hemoglobin level, hemoglobin fractional saturation (including dyshemoglobinemias), and acid-base status of the patient. When combined with an accurate FIO_2, an A-a gradient and CaO_2 can be calculated. Arterialized capillary blood provides similar information, but fractional saturation (SaO_2), acid-base status, and ventilation data are the most reliable. Venous blood gas analysis is also useful for acid-base information and SaO_2, and mixed venous PO_2 helps determine tissue O_2 consumption and reflects tissue O_2 delivery.[17]

Arterial oximetry, or co-oximetry, is carried out by most modern arterial blood gas analysis equipment. SaO_2 is measured using a cuvette with a defined light path and up to six light sources of differing wavelengths to distinguish oxyhemoglobin, deoxyhemoglobin, carboxyhemoglobin, methemoglobin, and other abnormal hemoglobin saturation levels independently. Table 38-2 provides helpful formulas and other general information.

Other Studies

Other studies to consider in the evaluation of a hypoxic patient are hemoglobin measurement, chest radiograph, surrogate markers of hypoperfusion such as lactate and blood pH, specific toxicology screens, and other studies based on the specific presentation, such as echocardiography, computed tomography, computed tomography-angiography, and arteriography.

MANAGEMENT

Most clinical presentations of hypoxemia are due to ventilation-perfusion mismatch, and patients generally respond to O_2 administration (Table 38-3).[18,19] Patient status and progress can usually be monitored with pulse oximetry. If there is concern about the development of respiratory failure, blood gas determination can help identify the underlying cause of the hypoxia (Table 38-4).

If the response to O_2 is inadequate, intubation for delivery of higher FIO_2 should be considered. The clinician should also consider the possibility of a fixed anatomic shunt, such as an intracardiac shunt due to cyanotic congenital heart disease, which will not respond to any degree of supplemental O_2. Hypoxia that is not due to hypoxemia may not respond as well to O_2 administration and will likely require other interventions based on the underlying cause, such as blood transfusion in severe anemia, hyperbaric O_2 in carbon monoxide poisoning, and pressor agents in shock.

Many clinicians include a room air O_2 saturation goal as one of the discharge criteria. Studies suggest that the use of pulse oximetry criteria may be responsible for significant delays in discharge.[11] Clinicians following other markers of patient improvement often alter the original SpO_2 goal, accepting a lower cutoff as the patient improves otherwise.[11] Data from studies of normal oximetry in healthy children include significant brief, repetitive desaturation events; a drop in saturation of 1% to 2% with sleep or feeding; and an average 1% drop with an upper respiratory infection.[20-36] The limited data available in children living at high altitudes suggest chronic borderline hypoxemia and even more significant intermittent "normal" desaturations.[37-44] There is no known adverse long-term consequence of this condition in otherwise normal children.

SPECIAL CONSIDERATIONS

Special cases of hypoxemia include the dyshemoglobinemias, methemoglobinemia, and carboxyhemoglobinemia. Methemoglobin is hemoglobin with the iron in the ferric state, which is unable to bind O_2 and shifts the oxyhemoglobin dissociation curve to the left in the remaining hemoglobin molecules in the tetramer. Only about 1.5 g/dL methemoglobin in the circulation causes the appearance of cyanosis.[45] A small amount of methemoglobin (1%) is normal, and there are cellular mechanisms to reduce iron back to the ferrous state, although these can be genetically absent (e.g., cytochrome b_5 reductase deficiency). Exogenous agents such as nitrites, phenacetin, sulfonamides, and aniline dyes are known to cause methemoglobinemia. In most cases, discontinuation of the offending agent is adequate treatment. Intravenous methylene blue acts as an electron acceptor in patients who are not glucose-6-phosphate dehydrogenase (G6PD) deficient (pretreatment screening is indicated in populations likely to be G6PD deficient), and ascorbic acid may be useful in G6PD-deficient patients. In severe cases of methemoglobinemia, transfusion and hyperbaric O_2 have been used.[46]

Carboxyhemoglobin is hemoglobin with the iron bound to carbon monoxide (CO). CO binds with an affinity about 240 times stronger than O_2, rendering the molecule unavailable to carry O_2 until the complex dissociates. Carboxyhemoglobin also shifts the oxyhemoglobin dissociation curve leftward. Levels of 2% to 5% are normal, and levels of 5% to 10% are commonly observed in smokers. There are many sources of CO poisoning, including virtually any combustion process without proper venting, smoke inhalation, tobacco smoke exposure, and automobile exhaust. Carboxyhemoglobin is not differentiated from oxyhemoglobin by pulse oximetry. A blood gas sample (arterial, capillary, or venous) to measure SaO_2 is required to determine the carboxyhemoglobin level. Treatment is O_2, which competes with CO and reduces the binding half-life to about 90 minutes. Severe cases may need hyperbaric O_2 treatment (see Chapter 184).[47]

CONCLUSION

Hypoxemia is defined as a low O_2 level in the blood and is one of four major categories of hypoxia. Clinically, hypoxemic hypoxia due to pulmonary infection, chronic lung disease, or both is the most common cause of hypoxia, with

Table 38-3 Oxygen Delivery Systems

O₂ Delivery Device	Flow Rate (L/min)	Theoretical FIO₂ Delivered (%)	Highest FIO₂ (x100)*	Advantages	Disadvantages
Nasal cannula	<1-5	22-40	23.8/25.4/25.2	Ease of use, comfortable, inexpensive, able to eat without removal	Higher flow rates dry out mucous membranes; gastric distention and headache
Simple mask	5-10	35-50	62.7/52.0/42.0	Can deliver higher flow rates than nasal prongs	Must remove to eat and drink and for airway care; insufficient flow rates may cause CO₂ retention
Partial rebreather†	6-15	60-95	NA	Higher FIO₂ with lower flow rates	Same as above; risk of atelectasis and O₂ toxicity with prolonged use
Nonrebreather†	6-15	Approaches 100	98.2/96.1/ 94.2	Same as above	Same as above
Venturi mask‡	4-10	Fixed FIO₂ set by mask design and flow rate	36.4/33.1/ 29.4 (for 40% mask)	More predictable FIO₂ delivered	Same as above; also, high-flow systems are noisy; if backpressure develops on the jet, less room air enters, and FIO₂ can elevate unpredictably
Tracheostomy mask	4-10	Unpredictable unless attached to Venturi circuit	NA	Provides humidity and controlled O₂	FIO₂ should be analyzed for each patient
Oxygen hood/ head box	>10	Approaches 100	NA	High FIO₂ possible	Insufficient flow can lead to CO₂ retention; O₂ gradients develop within the box; patient must be removed for care and feeding; significant temperature effect possible
Oxygen tent	>10	Approximately 50	NA/88/82	Can provide humidification	Same as above; also, combustion hazard; claustrophobia
Reservoir nebulizer‡	Up to 80	Approaches 100	98.2/96.1/ 94.2	Can deliver humidification, and positive pressure	As for masks above; noisy; risk of O₂ toxicity and barotrauma

*Highest reading (at highest theoretical FIO₂) in healthy young adult volunteers measured by intratracheal sensor; the three values represent quiet breathing/normal breathing/hyperventilation.[19] Actual delivered FIO₂ is a function of minute ventilatory volume (MVV) and peak inspiratory flow (PIF). A system that combines a reservoir-flow structure that exceeds the patient's flow volume will deliver 100% FIO₂. Note that as patients hyperventilate, both the MVV and PIF increase, so without changing the O₂ delivery system, the tracheal FIO₂ will drop. In small children, because of the decreased MVV and PIF and the increased reservoir-to-tidal volume ratio (even when the reservoir is only the child's nasal and oral cavities), it is much easier to exceed the limits of safe chronic FIO₂ delivery, increasing the risk of pulmonary edema, atelectasis, and lung injury.

†Mask with reservoir bags attached. A nonrebreather mask-bag set up with sufficient flow to prevent complete collapse of the bag and a tight mask seal will deliver 100% FIO₂.

‡High-flow systems, including continuous positive airway pressure and T-tube.

CO₂, carbon dioxide; FIO₂, fraction of inspired oxygen; NA, not available; O₂, oxygen.

Table 38–4 Differential Diagnosis and Evaluation of Hypoxia

	TYPE OF HYPOXIA				
	Hypoxemic*		Hypemic	Ischemic	Histotoxic
Differential diagnosis	V̇/Q̇ mismatch: pneumonia, bronchiolitis, asthma, pulmonary edema, airway obstruction, RDS, pleural fluid, inhalation lung injury, drowning, inflammatory lung injury, chronic lung disease (BPD, COPD), other	Shunt: congenital heart disease, PE, other	Hypoventilation: CNS depression (central apnea, medication side effect or overdose, CNS injury, intoxication, Ondine's curse); neuromuscular (botulism, tetanus, Guillian-Barré syndrome, myasthenia gravis, muscular dystrophies, polymyositis, spinal cord injury, phrenic nerve injury); extrinsic chest wall pathology (post-thoracotomy, chest wall injury, pleurisy, pneumothorax, pleural fibrosis, abdominal pain); obstructive lung disease (asthma, COPD, BPD); interstitial lung disease, other	Diffusion impairment: interstitial lung disease, other	Anemia, carbon monoxide poisoning (carboxyhemoglobinemia), methemoglobinemia, sulfhemoglobinema, right-shifted oxyhemoglobin desaturation curve (acidosis, hypercarbia, hyperthermia, high 2,3-DPG levels), other	Hypovolemia, shock, sepsis, regional vascular insufficiency (arterial embolization and occlusion), arrhythmia with poor cardiac output, other	Mitochondrial cytochrome poisoning (cyanide), metabolic disease, sepsis, other

Primary defect	Primary lung physiology impairment		Impaired O_2-carrying capacity	Impaired O_2 delivery to tissues	Impaired tissue O_2 use
Evaluation Helpful studies	SpO_2; may need CBG (respiratory failure) or ABG (A-a gradient with shunting); chest radiograph; other tests per diagnosis (e.g., PFTs with lung volumes and diffusion)		SaO_2; Hb level	Vital signs; assessment of perfusion	CaO_2-CvO_2 difference; toxicology
SpO_2 response to O_2	Improved; variable amount	Improved; good	None (O_2 directly treats some)	Variable; may not change	Variable; may not change
CaO_2†	Decreased (SaO_2)	Decreased (SaO_2)	Decreased (drop in usable Hb)	Unchanged	Unchanged
DO_2	Decreased (CaO_2)	Decreased (CaO_2)	Decreased (CaO_2)	Decreased (blood flow)	Unchanged
CaO_2-CvO_2‡	No change	No change	No change	No change	Decreased

*The majority of clinical presentations are of the hypoxemic type, under the $\dot{V}/\dot{Q}$ mismatch subcategory. Several diseases cross categories owing to multiple effects, particularly in the hypoxemic category. Diseases that respond well to oxygen may also present without hypoxemia.

†O_2 administration can overcome the decrease in CaO_2 (and thereby in DO_2) noted in all hypoxemic categories.

‡Arterial-venous O_2 content difference is approximately unchanged due to comparable drops on both sides of the equation, except with histotoxic hypoxia, where mixed venous content increases owing to poor tissue O_2 extraction, decreasing the difference.

A-a, alveolar-arterial; ABG, arterial blood gas; BPD, bronchopulmonary dysplasia; CaO_2, arterial O_2 content; CBG, capillary blood gas; CNS, central nervous system; COPD, chronic obstructive pulmonary disease; CvO_2, venous O_2 content; DO_2, tissue O_2 delivery; Hb, hemoglobin; O_2, oxygen; PE, pulmonary embolism; PFT, pulmonary function test; RDS, respiratory distress syndrome; SaO_2, fractional O_2 saturation; SpO_2, pulse oximetry O_2 saturation; 2,3-DPG, 2,3-diphosphoglycerate; $\dot{V}/\dot{Q}$, ventilation-perfusion.

ventilation-perfusion mismatch the most common pathophysiology. This condition responds to O_2 administration, which is the mainstay of treatment. Pulse oximetry can detect hypoxemia in most circumstances and is adequate for monitoring patient status and titrating therapy, but it has significant limitations that must be understood by the practitioner. Overreliance on and misunderstanding of pulse oximetry may lead to misdiagnosis, inappropriate evaluation, inappropriate treatment, excess hospital admissions, and delay in discharge. Blood gas studies can add significantly to the understanding of a clinical presentation if there is any question. O_2 treatment likewise needs to be understood, particularly the limitations and possible complications of different treatment approaches.

SUGGESTED READING

Silverman M, O'Callaghan CL (eds): Practical Paediatric Respiratory Medicine. London, Arnold Publishing, 2001.

West JB: Pulmonary Pathophysiology: The Essentials. Philadelphia, Lippincott Williams & Wilkins, 2003.

West JB: Respiratory Physiology, 6th ed. Philadelphia, Lippincott Williams & Wilkins, 2000.

REFERENCES

1. Wilson WC, Shapiro B: Perioperative hypoxia: The clinical spectrum and current oxygen monitoring methodology. Anesthesiol Clin North Am 2001;19:769-812.
2. Miller R: Oxygen therapy. In Anesthesia, 5th ed. New York, Churchill Livingstone, 2000, pp 715-718.
3. Miller R: Appendix 1: American Society of Anesthesiologists practice guideline. In Anesthesia, 5th ed. New York, Churchill Livingstone, 2000, pp 2788-2791.
4. Lundsgaard C, Van Slyke DD: Cyanosis. Medicine 1923;2.
5. Bardella IJ: Pediatric advanced life support: A review of the AHA recommendations. Am Fam Physician 1999;60:1743-1750.
6. Wong MW, Tsui HF, Yung SH, et al: Continuous pulse oximeter monitoring for inapparent hypoxemia after long bone fractures. J Trauma 2004;56:356-362.
7. Lodha R, Bhadauria PS, Kuttikat AV, et al: Can clinical symptoms or signs accurately predict hypoxemia in children with acute lower respiratory tract infections? Indian Pediatr 2004;41:129-135.
8. Duke T, Blaschke AJ, Sialis S, Bonkowsky JL: Hypoxaemia in acute respiratory and non-respiratory illnesses in neonates and children in a developing country. Arch Dis Child 2002;86:108-112.
9. Usen S, Webert M: Clinical signs of hypoxaemia in children with acute lower respiratory infection: Indicators of oxygen therapy. Int J Tuberc Lung Dis 2001;5:505-510.
10. Mower WR, Sachs C, Nicklin EL, Baraff LJ: Pulse oximetry as a fifth pediatric vital sign. Pediatrics 1997;99:681-686.
11. Schroeder AR, Marmor AK, Pantell RH, Newman TB: Impact of pulse oximetry and oxygen therapy on length of stay in bronchiolitis hospitalizations. Arch Pediatr Adolesc Med 2004;158:527-530.
12. Mallory MD, Shay DK, Garrett J, Bordley WC: Bronchiolitis management preferences and the influence of pulse oximetry and respiratory rate on the decision to admit. Pediatrics 2003;111:e45-e51.
13. Bergman A: Editorial: Pulse oximetry, good technology misapplied. Arch Pediatr Adolesc Med 2004;158:594-595.
14. Poets CF, Urschitz MS, Bohnhorst B: Pulse oximetry in the neonatal intensive care unit (NICU): Detection of hyperoxemia and false alarm rates. Anesth Analg 2002;94(1 Suppl):S41-S43.
15. Van de Louw A, Cracco C, Cerf C, et al: Accuracy of pulse oximetry in the intensive care unit. Intensive Care Med 2001;27:1606-1613.
16. Gerstmann D, Berg R, Haskell R, et al: Operational evaluation of pulse oximetry in NICU patients with arterial access. J Perinatol 2003;23:378-383.
17. Kirubakaran C, Gnananayagam JE, Sundaravalli EK: Comparison of blood gas values in arterial and venous blood. Indian J Pediatr 2003;70:781-785.
18. Myers T: AARC clinical practice guideline: Selection of an oxygen delivery device for neonatal and pediatric patients—2002 revision and update. Respir Care 2002;47:707-716.
19. Gibson RL, Comer PB, Beckham RW, McGraw CP: Actual tracheal oxygen concentrations with commonly used oxygen equipment. Anesthesiology 1976;44:71-73.
20. Beresford MW, Parry H, Shaw NJ: Twelve-month prospective study of oxygen saturation measurements among term and preterm infants. J Perinatol 2005;25:30-32.
21. Urschitz MS, Wolff J, Von Einem V, et al: Reference values for nocturnal home pulse oximetry during sleep in primary school children. Chest 2003;123:96-101.
22. Thoyre SM, Carlson J: Occurrence of oxygen desaturation events during preterm infant bottle feeding near discharge. Early Hum Dev 2003;72:25-36.
23. Toth B: Oxygen saturation in healthy newborn infants immediately after birth measured by pulse oximetry. Arch Gynecol Obstet 2002;266:105-107.
24. Meyts I, Reempts PV, Boeck KD: Monitoring of haemoglobin oxygen saturation in healthy infants using a new generation pulse oximeter which takes motion artifacts into account. Eur J Pediatr 2002;161:653-655.
25. O'Brien LM, Stebbens VA, Poets CF, et al: Oxygen saturation during the first 24 hours of life. Arch Dis Child Fetal Neonatal Ed 2000;83:F35-F38.
26. Levesque BM, Pollack P, Griffin BE, Nielsen HC: Pulse oximetry: What's normal in the newborn nursery? Pediatr Pulmonol 2000;30:406-412.
27. Horemuzova E, Katz-Salamon M, Milerad J: Breathing patterns, oxygen and carbon dioxide levels in sleeping healthy infants during the first nine months after birth. Acta Paediatr 2000;89:1284-1289.
28. Hunt CE, Corwin MJ, Lister G, et al: Longitudinal assessment of hemoglobin oxygen saturation in healthy infants during the first 6 months of age. Collaborative Home Infant Monitoring Evaluation (CHIME) study group. J Pediatr 1999;135:580-586.
29. Owen G, Canter R: Analysis of pulse oximetry data in normal sleeping children. Clin Otolaryngol 1997;22:13-22.
30. Hunt CE, Hufford DR, Bourguignon C, Oess MA: Home documented monitoring of cardiorespiratory pattern and oxygen saturation in healthy infants. Pediatr Res 1996;39:216-222.
31. Gries RE, Brooks LJ: Normal oxyhemoglobin saturation during sleep: How low does it go? Chest 1996;110:1489-1492.
32. Hammerman C, Kaplan M: Oxygen saturation during and after feeding in healthy term infants. Biol Neonate 1995:67:94-99.
33. Masters IB, Goes AM, Healy L, et al: Age-related changes in oxygen saturation over the first year of life: A longitudinal study. J Paediatr Child Health 1994;30:423-428.
34. Poets CF, Stebbens VA, Samuels MP, Southall DP: Oxygen saturation and breathing patterns in children. Pediatrics 1993;92:686-690.
35. Poets CF, Stebbens VA, Alexander JR, et al: Arterial oxygen saturation in preterm infants at discharge from the hospital and six weeks later. J Pediatr 1992;120:447-454.
36. Stebbens VA, Poets CF, Alexander JR, et al: Oxygen saturation and breathing patterns in infancy. 1. Full term infants in the second month of life. Arch Dis Child 1991;66:569-573.
37. Huicho LP, Pawson IG, León-Velarde F, et al: Oxygen saturation and heart rate in healthy school children and adolescents living at high altitude. Am J Hum Biol 2001;13:761-770.
38. Saleu G, Lupiwa S, Javati A, et al: Arterial oxygen saturation in healthy young infants in the highlands of Papua New Guinea. P N G Med J 1999;42:90-93.
39. Gamponia MJ, Babaali H, Yugar F, Gilman RH: Reference values for pulse oximetry at high altitude. Arch Dis Child 1998;78:461-465.

40. Beebe SA, Heery LB, Magarian S, Culberson J: Pulse oximetry at moderate altitude. Clin Pediatr 1994;33:329-333.
41. Niermeyer S, Shaffer EM, Thilo E, et al: Arterial oxygenation and pulmonary arterial pressure in healthy neonates and infants at high altitude. J Pediatr 1993;123:767-772.
42. Nicholas R, Yaron M, Reeves J: Oxygen saturation in children living at moderate altitude. J Am Board Fam Pract 1993;6:452-456.
43. Lozano JM, Duque OR, Buitrago T, Behaine S: Pulse oximetry reference values at high altitude. Arch Dis Child 1992;67:299-301.
44. Thilo EH, Park-Moore B, Berman ER, Carson BS: Oxygen saturation by pulse oximetry in healthy infants at an altitude of 1610 m (5280 ft): What is normal? Am J Dis Child 1991;145:1137-1140.
45. Jaffe E: Hereditary methemoglobinemias associated with abnormalities in the metabolism of erythrocytes. Am J Med 1962;32:512.
46. Goldstein G, Doull J: Treatment of nitrite-induced methemoglobinemia with hyperbaric oxygen. Proc Soc Exp Biol Med 1971;138:134.
47. Weaver LK, Hoplins RO, Chan KJ, et al: Hyperbaric oxygen for acute carbon monoxide poisoning. N Engl J Med 2002;347:1057-1067.

CHAPTER 39

Irritability and Intractable Crying

Karen E. Schetzina

Irritability and intractable crying may be the presenting complaint for a wide range of medical problems in infants and children, some of which are potentially serious. These symptoms may also begin after hospitalization. Hospitalists must be able to differentiate significant irritability and intractable crying from developmentally appropriate crying. They must also be familiar with the common causes of irritability and intractable crying, which are often identifiable based on a thorough history and physical examination, as well as the more unusual causes and a stepwise approach to evaluation.

BACKGROUND

Irritability is a state of increased sensitivity to stimuli; it may also be described by parents as fussiness, whining, or increased crying. Crying is the primary way that infants and young children express hunger, thirst, fear, fatigue, desire for attention, and discomfort or pain. When caregivers have taken the usual measures to address these common needs, such as feeding and holding the child and changing the diaper, yet the child continues to cry, the child is said to be inconsolable or to have intractable crying.

The quantity as well as the quality of crying behavior should be considered. What qualifies as excessive crying varies based on the age and developmental level of the child, as well as the clinical scenario. Normal infants cry most during the first 3 months of life; during this period, serious illness may present with few or only subtle signs and symptoms, making evaluation in this age group particularly challenging.

Crying should also be evaluated to determine whether it is appropriate for the clinical scenario. For example, a febrile infant with a viral upper respiratory infection is likely to be irritable and may cry more than usual. However, crying with movement of the child's lower extremities should lead to suspicion of an alternative cause, such as meningitis or a septic hip joint. Stranger anxiety—which appears at around 8 to 9 months of age, peaks at 12 to 15 months, and decreases thereafter—may manifest as inconsolable crying during examination; however, an otherwise healthy child should be comforted and calmed in the arms of a caregiver.

A change in the character of a child's cry may also be significant: louder, higher pitch, or more urgent tone or a weak, stridulous, or hoarse cry may suggest the presence of illness.

PATHOPHYSIOLOGY

Irritability may result from pain, discomfort, or fatigue; direct neurologic insult; or altered metabolic or endocrine status. Crying in infants and young children is an involuntary action that serves physiologic and protective purposes. A newborn's first cries enable essential changes in the cardiorespiratory system during the transition to postnatal life. Many studies of normal infants suggest that crying may help maintain homeostasis.[1,2] Crying increases to almost 3 hours per day, on average, by 6 weeks of life and decreases thereafter. During this period of greatest crying, infants cry most during the late afternoon and evening hours, perhaps to release tension accumulated throughout the day from internal and external stimuli. Crying is also a way for infants and children to express their emotional needs.

HISTORY AND PHYSICAL EXAMINATION

It is important to obtain a detailed description of the irritability and crying, as delineated in Box 39-1. When examining the child, it is often helpful to observe respiration, movement, and behavior from across the room at first. This provides useful information and helps eliminate the confounding influences of stranger anxiety. With a frightened toddler, the parents can assist in the physical examination by exposing areas of skin and moving the extremities to check for tenderness while the examiner stands back several feet and observes. Use of distraction techniques can facilitate a complete physical examination. It is essential to examine the child from head to toe, fully exposed (removing clothes, shoes, socks, bracelets, barrettes, and so forth). Growth parameters, including head circumference in infants, should be assessed.

EVALUATION

Because of the extensive differential diagnosis, a stepwise approach is essential. The presence of fever makes an infectious cause more likely; other inflammatory processes and endocrine disorders must also be considered. It is important to remember that serious bacterial infections can be present in the absence of fever, particularly in neonates, and may also coexist with more benign conditions such as viral upper respiratory tract infections. Most common causes of irritability and intractable crying in afebrile patients are apparent after a careful history and physical examination. A period of observation may also be helpful.[3]

Care must be taken not to routinely attribute irritability and crying to otitis media. In older infants with intact tympanic membranes, determining whether otitis media observed on physical examination is the cause of the symptoms can be accomplished by placing anesthetic drops in the affected ear and observing the patient's response. If the irritability does not dramatically improve, another cause should be sought.

Parents may not notice the presence of a hair tourniquet around an appendage such as a digit, penis, or clitoris, which can cause swelling, ischemia, and pain. The band of hair may not be visible if it is buried beneath a fold of edematous

Box 39-1   Elements of the History Relevant to Intractable Crying

Normal or baseline crying behavior
Duration of presenting crying episode
Quality of crying
    Intensity
    Character
    Pitch
Characteristics of crying episodes
    Duration of previous crying episodes
    Time of day
    Circumstances or triggers
Efforts of caregivers to console child
Conditions that make crying better or worse
Associated symptoms
Exposures
Caregivers' ideas regarding causes
Normal and recent feeding patterns
Normal and recent sleep patterns
Growth pattern

tissue. In some cases, the hair may be so tightly wound that it is difficult to release, making it necessary to remove the hair. Applying a hair removal cream, such as Nair, to the affected area for about 10 minutes may dissolve the hair and relieve the constriction.

Ocular abnormalities, including corneal abrasion and acute glaucoma, are difficult to discern by history or physical examination, because tearing and conjunctival injection are difficult to appreciate in the setting of excessive crying. Consider a topical anesthetic, fluorescein stain, ultraviolet light examination of both eyes, and lid eversion to rule out corneal abrasion or foreign body. Tonometry with evidence of increased intraocular pressure indicates acute glaucoma.

There are no standard screening laboratory tests, with the possible exception of urinalysis and culture in females and uncircumcised males younger than 12 months and circumcised males younger than 6 months. Laboratory and radiographic evaluation should be guided by findings from the history and physical examination.

If a child continues to cry inconsolably during a period of observation after the initial examination and no reasonable cause has been identified, admission for further evaluation and observation should be considered, because a serious occult condition may be present. At this point it is essential for the clinician to entertain an extensive differential diagnosis, focusing first on potentially serious or life-threatening conditions.

The presence of tachypnea may suggest metabolic acidosis, respiratory tract infection, or cardiac dysfunction. Foreign body aspiration or other airway obstruction may produce symptoms of respiratory distress such as cyanosis, increased work of breathing, diaphoresis, drooling, stridor, wheezing, or rales.

Evidence of recent trauma ascertained either by history or on physical examination should be investigated further. An assessment of the family environment and social stressors and the observation of interactions among family members are also important to identify possible nonaccidental

trauma, such as shaken baby syndrome (see Ch. 173). Evaluation for the presence of rib bruising or crepitus, a bulging fontanelle, and retinal hemorrhages should be included.

Symptoms of altered sensorium, such as increased somnolence, lethargy, confusion, or agitation, may suggest central nervous system infection or injury, a metabolic disorder, drug ingestion or withdrawal, toxin exposure, or cardiopulmonary failure. It is important to inquire specifically about toxins and medications (prescription, nonprescription, and traditional or homeopathic) that the child may have ingested or been exposed to. Loss of developmental milestones is suggestive of a metabolic or neurodegenerative disorder.

Further investigation of symptoms of gastrointestinal obstruction should be done expeditiously to evaluate for ischemia-inducing gastrointestinal disorders.

Box 39-2 provides a list of causes to consider in the evaluation of prolonged irritability or intractable crying. Box 39-3 provides a list of conditions associated with recurrent irritability or crying episodes.

SPECIAL CONSIDERATIONS

Colic

Clinicians should be familiar with the clinical features of colic—a common cause of excessive and intractable crying in infants—so that they can differentiate it from other conditions. Colic is characterized by episodes of inconsolable crying in an otherwise healthy infant and is a diagnosis of exclusion. The timing of colic parallels the normal peak of infant crying, usually beginning during the third week of life and resolving by 3 or 4 months of age. Colic is commonly defined by the "rule of threes": crying for more than 3 hours per day, on more than 3 days per week, in an infant 3 months of age or younger.[2] The crying episodes tend to occur suddenly during the late afternoon and evening hours and are often described as more intense than the infant's usual crying. The episodes may be associated with facial flushing, abdominal distention, and increased tone.

Colic likely stems from different causes in different infants. Proposed causes include immaturity of the nervous system, impaired intestinal absorption or motility, or a reflection of temperament or parent-child interactions. Parental education, reassurance, and support are important aspects of management, and efforts to soothe the infant and limit air swallowing, improve burping, and minimize stimulation may be helpful. Medications are not recommended for colic; however, a subgroup of infants with a milk protein intolerance may benefit from a change to a hypoallergenic formula.[4] Although not inherently dangerous, colic is extremely stressful for families and may have long-term effects on the parent-child relationship. Therefore, it requires close outpatient follow-up.

New Irritability or Excessive Crying in a Hospitalized Patient

Although the approach to irritability or inconsolability that develops in a hospitalized patient is similar, additional causes must be considered. Dietary, environmental, and sleep-wake schedule changes should be examined. For example, restricting oral intake before procedures could

---

Box 39-2   Causes of Irritability and Intractable Crying

General
  Infection
  Dehydration
  Anemia
  Leukemia
  Kawasaki syndrome
Eyes, ears, nose, and throat
  Corneal abrasion
  Ocular foreign body
  Glaucoma
  Otitis media
  Thrush, herpangina, herpes stomatitis
  Teething
  Nasal, oropharyngeal, or otic foreign body
Cardiovascular and respiratory
  Supraventricular tachycardia
  Myocardial ischemia or infarction
  Congestive heart failure or congenital heart defect
  Respiratory distress or failure
Gastrointestinal
  Incarcerated hernia
  Spontaneous perforation of bile duct
  Appendicitis
  Malrotation, volvulus, intussusception
  Henoch-Schönlein purpura
  Bowel perforation
  Constipation
  Anal fissure
Genitourinary
  Testicular torsion
  Urinary tract obstruction
  Urethritis
  Meatal ulcer
  Sexual abuse
Endocrine and metabolic
  Congenital adrenal hyperplasia
  Hyperthyroidism
  Syndrome of inappropriate antidiuretic hormone

  Hypoglycemia
  Electrolyte abnormalities (sodium, calcium, potassium)
  Hyperammonemia
  Metabolic acidosis
  Pheochromocytoma
  Reye syndrome
Neurologic
  Central nervous system injury, hemorrhage, tumor, shaken baby syndrome
  Meningitis, encephalitis, brain abscess
  Pseudotumor cerebri or hydrocephalus
  Migraine
  Spontaneous epidural hematoma
Drugs and toxins
  Neonatal abstinence or other withdrawal syndromes
  Fetal alcohol syndrome
  Poisoning (e.g., lead, mercury, iron, carbon monoxide)
  Monosodium glutamate reaction
  Drugs (e.g., antihistamines, atropinics, phenothiazines, pseudoephedrine, albuterol, theophylline or other methylxanthines, metoclopramide, promethazine, barbiturates, tricyclic antidepressants, vitamin A, vitamin D, salicylates, amphetamines, cocaine, phencyclidine)
  Vaccine reaction
Skin
  Hair tourniquet
  Insect, arachnid, or arthropod bite or sting
  Burn
  Herpes dermatitis (pain may precede vesicles)
  Paronychia
  Atopic dermatitis, acrodermatitis enteropathica, or other pruritic conditions
Orthopedic
  Fracture
  Acute arthritis (infectious, postinfectious, inflammatory)
  Nursemaid's elbow or joint dislocation
  Diskitis
  Osteomyelitis

Box 39-3   Syndromes and Conditions Associated with Chronic or Recurrent Irritability or Intractable Crying

Anomalous origin of the coronary artery
Congenital heart disease (e.g., "tet" spells of tetralogy of Fallot)
Gastroesophageal reflux, Sandifer syndrome
Colic
Milk protein intolerance
Nutritional deficiencies (e.g., iron, zinc, vitamin C)
Diabetes insipidus
Sickle cell disease
Metabolic and neurodegenerative disorders (e.g., glutaricaciduria type I, acute intermittent porphyria, Pompe disease, pyridoxine deficiency, tryptophan malabsorption, hypoglycinemia, arginemia, tyrosinemia, pyruvate carboxylase deficiency, biotin deficiency, argininosuccinate lyase deficiency, Krabbe disease, lipogranulomatosis)

Genetic syndromes (e.g., Smith-Lemli-Opitz, Williams, de Lange)
Unrecognized deafness
Behavioral problems (e.g., attention-deficit hyperactivity disorder)
Parent-child interactions, problems, or stress
Mental illness (e.g., depression, bipolar disorder)
Rheumatologic disorders (e.g., juvenile rheumatoid arthritis)
Infantile cortical hyperostosis (Caffey disease)

result in crying due to hunger. Patients with prolonged exposure during examinations and monitoring may become too cold, or infants under warmers may become overheated. Intravenous catheter sites should be inspected for any evidence of thrombophlebitis, and the locations of other catheters, tubes, and probes should be examined for skin irritation, excessive traction, and infection. Adverse effects and interactions of medications started in the hospital should also be considered as possible contributors.

ACKNOWLEDGMENTS

I would like to thank Dr. David Price for his review of this chapter.

SUGGESTED READING

Barr RG: Colic and crying syndromes in infants. Pediatrics 1998;102(Suppl E):1282-1286.
Brazelton TB: Crying in infancy. Pediatrics 1962;29:579-588.
Chabali R, Matre WM, Greene MK: Infant with irritability, feeding problems, and progressive developmental abnormalities presenting repeatedly to a pediatric emergency department. Pediatr Emerg Care 1997;13:123-126.
Gatrad AR, Sheikh A: Persistent crying in babies. BMJ 2004;328:330.

Mahle WT: A dangerous case of colic: Anomalous left coronary artery presenting with paroxysms of irritability. Pediatr Emerg Care 1998;14:24-27.
Patel H, Gang BP: Increasing irritability with sudden onset of flaccid weakness. Semin Pediatr Neurol 1996;3:192-197.
Poole SR: The infant with acute, unexplained, excessive crying. Pediatrics 1991;88:450-455.
Reust CA: Diagnostic workup before diagnosing colic. Arch Fam Med 2000;9:282-283.
Valman HB: The first year of life: Crying babies. BMJ 1980;280:1522-1525.
Weinstein M, Bernstein S: Pink ladies: Mercury poisoning in twin girls. CMAJ 2003;168:201.
Wessel MA, Cobb JC, Jackson AB, et al: Paroxysmal fussing in infancy, sometimes called "colic." Pediatrics 1954;14:421-434.
Xanthakos SA, Yazigi NA, Ryckman FC, Arkovitz MS: Spontaneous perforation of the bile duct in infancy: A rare but important cause of irritability and abdominal distention. J Pediatr Gastroenterol Nutr 2003;36:287-291.

REFERENCES

1. Brazelton TB: Crying in infancy. Pediatrics 1962;29:579-588.
2. Wessel MA, Cobb JC, Jackson AB, et al: Paroxysmal fussing in infancy, sometimes called "colic." Pediatrics 1954;14:421-434.
3. Poole SR: The infant with acute, unexplained, excessive crying. Pediatrics 1991;88:450-455.
4. Garrison MM, Christakis DA: A systematic review of treatments for infant colic. Pediatrics 2000;106:184-190.

CHAPTER 40

Limp
Robert Sundel

Musculoskeletal complaints account for a significant number of outpatient visits to the pediatrician—up to 10% of non-well-child appointments in some studies. Only a minority of these visits result in hospitalization, but in many cases, even these admissions could have been avoided if a logical, stepwise approach to evaluation and management had been used. This chapter focuses on the entities to consider in a limping child and the appropriate approaches to take with regard to the history, physical examination, and diagnosis.

PATHOPHYSIOLOGY

The normal gait is the most efficient and stable means for a bipedal creature such as a human being to ambulate. For this gait to be altered, strong countervailing forces must be applied. These forces may be anatomic (e.g., broken bone, unstable skeleton) or sensory (loss of proprioception or balance) in nature. Pain is the most common cause of a disrupted gait in children.

Different types of pathology result in predictable alterations in a child's gait. Although formal gait analysis is not necessary, recognizing specific abnormalities can facilitate the localization and identification of specific conditions. For example, a psoas abscess is often difficult to diagnose because of the poor localization of pathology within the pelvis; pain may be perceived as occurring anywhere from above the knee to the diaphragm. Trying to walk with a psoas abscess, however, results in a characteristically altered gait owing to the pain associated with use of the psoas muscle. Use of the psoas muscle is avoided during all aspects of the stance and swing phases to minimize discomfort. This causes leaning to the involved side and using the bones of the pelvis and upper leg to substitute for the usual contraction of the psoas muscle. Further, the contralateral hemipelvis dips to keep the psoas muscle level and thus avoid pain. The result is the Trendelenburg gait, which can be caused only by a pathologic condition involving the proximal femur or muscles of the pelvis (Fig. 40-1). Similar relationships for other sites of pathology are listed in Table 40-1.

DIFFERENTIAL DIAGNOSIS

When a child presents with a complaint referable to the lower extremities, the list of possible causes is long and varied. In the absence of an obvious explanation, such as known trauma, it is helpful to start the evaluation by categorizing the type of pain or discomfort according to the nature of its onset (acute versus chronic), the number of joints involved, and whether extra-articular signs or symptoms are present. It is also important to remember that most normally active children have some history of trauma during the preceding 24 hours; however, unless the trauma is sig-

nificant (e.g., football injury, automobile accident, bicycle fall), it is more likely to have unmasked a preexisting pathologic condition than to have caused damage to the child's resilient tissues. For example, 10% to 20% of osteogenic sarcomas present after trauma, but in all cases, the accident is only a signpost for the problem.

HISTORY

The key elements of the medical history that help identify the cause of pain include the timing of the pain; the nature of the pain with regard to alleviating and exacerbating factors, particularly response to activity (Table 40-2); and the character of the pain, such as dull, sharp, radiating, or burning. In young or nonverbal children who are unable to articulate the specifics of their symptoms, the observations of parents and other caregivers substitute for the patient's description.

Inflammatory Pain

The most characteristic feature of discomfort related to inflammatory processes is the classic morning stiffness of arthritis. Difficulty is also reported after naps or other periods of inactivity, such as long car rides or sitting in school. The stiffness is caused by the gelling of joint fluid as a result of decreased hyaluronic acid production by inflamed synovial tissue. This, in turn, leads to reduced lubrication, which can be reversed by warming of the joint, which returns the synovial fluid to the liquid state, permitting efficient lubrication. Thus, children with arthritis typically feel better after a warm bath or after several minutes of activity. These children may suffer joint stiffness in the morning but may be quite comfortable exercising strenuously later in the day. Cold, damp weather or swimming in cool water also tends to affect children with arthritis adversely, whereas warm weather generally relieves symptoms. Nighttime awakening is unusual with arthritis. Any atypical symptoms—especially nighttime pain or discomfort with activity—should raise the suspicion of an alternative diagnosis, even in the setting of otherwise typical joint inflammation.

Mechanical Pain

The timing of mechanical pain is essentially the mirror image of inflammatory pain. Children typically feel well in the morning, but the more active they become, the more discomfort they have. Like inflammation, however, mechanical pain generally does not awaken children from sleep. Rest and ice tend to alleviate mechanical symptoms, as opposed to the activity and heat that typically relieve arthritis pain. The precise type of overuse syndrome or injury causing a child's symptoms can generally be determined from a careful history (e.g., Osgood-Schlatter syndrome in an adolescent male athlete, iliotibial band syndrome in an adolescent female runner) and physical examination.

Bone Pain

Pain originating in the osseous compartment tends to be constant and does not change significantly with activity. Bone pain raises concern for infection, trauma, and malignancy. This type of pain may awaken a child at night, particularly when it is related to leukemia or a tumor. Consequently, when a history of nighttime awakening is elicited, special consideration must be given to oncologic causes. Cytopenias are typically seen with leukemia, although a normal complete blood count does not exclude the possibility. Other tumors, such as sarcoma or metastatic neuroblastoma, are far less common, but they must be considered

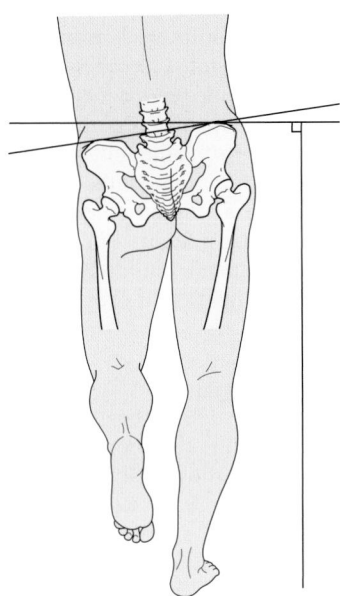

Figure 40-1 Trendelenburg gait, with pathology of the right proximal femur or adjacent muscles causing characteristic dipping of the contralateral hemipelvis.

in children with more nighttime pain than morning stiffness.

Neuropathic Pain

Nerve pain tends to be worst at bedtime, when the usual distractions of daily activities disappear. In children old enough to describe the sensation, neuropathic pain typically has a burning or shooting character. It is also commonly associated with allodynia, a severe hypersensitivity of overlying normal soft tissues. Although joints may be involved, neuropathic pain generally encompasses extra-articular areas as well and can follow a dermatomal distribution. Activity does not have a significant effect on neuropathic pain. When nerve pathology due to severe trauma, tumor, or vasculitis cannot be identified, pain syndromes such as fibromyalgia or reflex sympathetic dystrophy should be considered in children with such pain.

Pattern of Joint Involvement

In addition to categorizing the type of pain a child is experiencing, it is critical to determine how many joints are affected. The potential causes of a monoarticular process differ significantly from those of polyarticular conditions (Table 40-3), so careful examination of all the joints is mandatory, even when it is believed that only a single joint is involved. It is also important to determine the type of onset (sudden or gradual), duration of symptoms, and any associated systemic features, such as fever or rash.

Monoarthritis

The potential causes of a monoarticular process can be narrowed down by considering the onset and duration of symptoms.

Acute Onset

When pain and swelling of a single joint start acutely, traumatic injury must always be considered. Documentation of an antecedent trauma is helpful, but this may be difficult to elicit in young children who are unable to verbalize the specifics of the history. In patients with an underlying bleed-

Table 40-1	Characteristic Alterations in Gait Based on Location of Pathology		
Location	Effect on Gait	Example	Result
Hip	Decreased or eliminated swing phase	Septic arthritis Inguinal tendinitis	Refusal to bear weight Circumduction or dragging of involved side
Knee	Decreased extension > flexion	Lyme disease	Stiff-kneed gait
Ankle	Decreased dorsiflexion	Juvenile rheumatoid arthritis	Ginger gait, like walking on coals

Table 40-2	Characteristics of Musculoskeletal Pain			
Pain Type	Morning	Afternoon	Nighttime	Activity
Inflammatory (e.g., arthritis)	+++	+	−	Improves
Mechanical (e.g., overuse syndromes)	+/−	++	+/−	Worsens
Bone (e.g., tumors)	++	++	++	No change
Neuropathic (e.g., neuropathy)	+	++	+++	No change

Table 40–3 Common Causes of Arthritis
Monoarticular
Acute onset
Septic arthritis
Reactive arthritis
Trauma
Hemophilia
Lyme disease
Chronic
Juvenile rheumatoid arthritis
Lyme disease
Tuberculosis (rare without pulmonary disease)
Tumor (pigmented villonodular synovitis most common, but rare)
Polyarticular
Juvenile rheumatoid arthritis
Spondyloarthropathies
Systemic autoimmune diseases
Systemic lupus erythematosus
Vasculitis
Arthritis associated with inflammatory bowel disease
Viral arthritis
Reactive arthritis
Serum sickness
Rheumatic fever (migratory arthritis)
Malignancies
Periodic fever syndromes

ing disorder, such as hemophilia, routine daily activities may cause hemarthrosis. Once this possibility is excluded, bacterial infection must be considered. A history of fever associated with a red, swollen, painful, or hot joint necessitates arthrocentesis for cell count and culture. Treatment of septic arthritis must not be postponed (in contrast, for most types of inflammatory arthritis, a delay in the diagnosis by days or weeks has few long-term implications). Postinfectious or "reactive" arthritis may involve one or many joints, but it characteristically causes less inflammation than that seen with acute infection. Thus, postinfectious arthritis usually does not cause erythema overlying the joint, and although it may be uncomfortable, excruciating pain is uncommon. Reactive arthritis generally responds well to nonsteroidal anti-inflammatory agents and is typically transient. Lyme disease may also be difficult to distinguish clinically from septic arthritis, although it generally causes more indolent symptoms.

Subacute Onset

The diagnostic considerations in cases of an isolated, chronically swollen joint differ from those related to an acute arthritis. Bacterial infection is far less likely, but lower-grade infections, especially Lyme disease in endemic areas, must be excluded. Chronic monoarthritis also may be caused by *Mycobacterium tuberculosis*, particularly in immunocompromised children. This category also includes chronic forms of juvenile arthritis, especially pauciarticular juvenile idiopathic (rheumatoid) arthritis, psoriatic arthritis, and juvenile spondyloarthritides. Rarer inflammatory arthropathies, such as arthritis due to sarcoidosis, may also cause

monoarthritis. Tumors of the cartilage and synovium, though extremely rare, are also more likely to present in an indolent manner. The most common of these, pigmented villonodular synovitis, typically causes a chronically painful and swollen knee. A nontraumatic arthrocentesis that yields bloody fluid increases the likelihood of an articular tumor.

Polyarthritis

When several joints are involved, rheumatologic conditions rise to the top of the differential diagnosis. Most common among these is polyarticular juvenile idiopathic (rheumatoid) arthritis (JIA, previously known as JRA), although other autoimmune diseases, such as systemic lupus erythematosus and vasculitis, typically involve multiple joints as well. Infection is progressively less common as more joints are involved, with the exception of gonococcal arthritis in sexually active or abused children and salmonella arthritis in immunocompromised patients. Arthritis associated with systemic conditions, such as inflammatory bowel disease or cystic fibrosis, must also be considered. Usually, extra-articular involvement (e.g., a new murmur in rheumatic fever, hives in serum sickness) offers a clue to these conditions. The pattern of joint involvement may also be suggestive: rheumatic fever, vasculitis, and serum sickness characteristically cause a migratory polyarthritis, whereas most other conditions cause additive or fixed involvement of multiple joints. In general, children with polyarticular arthritis are likely to benefit from consultation with a pediatric rheumatologist.

PHYSICAL EXAMINATION

Signs of inflammation are the hallmark of arthritis. Warmth and swelling are most characteristic; overlying erythema is more characteristic of septic arthritis. The child may report discomfort that is more commonly described as stiffness rather than pain. In fact, at least 20% of children with juvenile arthritis never complain of pain, and a recent study from Oklahoma found that only 13 of 226 children referred to a rheumatology clinic with joint pain actually had arthritis.[1]

The knee may exhibit a ballotable effusion, meaning that applying pressure directly to the patella forces it downward, displacing synovial fluid and causing it to bounce against the femur. The characteristic springiness is not noted when fluid does not intervene between the patella and femur, as in healthy children. The joint may also be swollen from synovial proliferation, which has a boggier consistency than the free fluid of a joint effusion.

Careful examination of an inflamed joint may allow an estimation of the duration of the arthritis. Synovitis is characterized by increased blood flow, typically more pronounced in the portion of the joint compartment subjected to the maximal force. In the knee, this is the medial aspect, where hyperemia leads to increased delivery of nutrients and accelerated growth. This may manifest initially as prominence of the medial femoral condyle, and later as genu valgus. Ultimately, the leg with the inflamed knee grows more rapidly, and a leg length discrepancy develops. The lower leg may bow to compensate for the greater length of the upper leg. At the same time, the knee loses extension and develops a flexion contracture, with resultant atrophy of the vastus medialis and wasting of the quadriceps muscle. In contrast, significant inflammation in the hip often damages the growth plate and leads to foreshortening of the involved leg. Because minimal longitudinal growth occurs at the distal tibia, ankle arthritis causes little if any discrepancy in leg length.

EVALUATION

Laboratory Studies

Laboratory studies may be helpful in excluding infectious and malignant causes of a swollen joint, but they cannot confirm a diagnosis of arthritis; a child may have JIA despite uniformly normal laboratory studies. Even when laboratory studies support a diagnosis of JIA, they are nonspecific and must be interpreted in the context of the patient's clinical presentation. Ultimately, a diagnosis of JIA rests on the history and physical examination.

The laboratory studies that are most characteristic of arthritis are those that reflect systemic inflammation: elevated erythrocyte sedimentation rate, C-reactive protein, and platelet count. In general, the elevation of acute-phase reactants is proportional to the number of joints involved. In a case of monoarticular arthritis, therefore, normal laboratory studies are the rule. Leukocytosis may be present in JIA, particularly in children with systemic-onset JIA; a mild to moderate anemia may also be seen in the setting of chronic inflammation.

The serum antinuclear antibody (ANA) level is usually measured when a child is being evaluated for possible arthritis. This is rarely diagnostic, although an ANA at a titer of 1:1024 or higher is strongly suggestive of an autoimmune condition. At lower titers, a positive ANA result is nonspecific, occurring in conditions from arthritis and lupus to viral illnesses. Thus, up to 2% of children have a positive ANA (typically low titer) result at any time, and most are healthy. A positive ANA assay in a child with known arthritis is a marker for an increased risk of developing anterior uveitis.

One of the most overused tests in children with swollen joints is the rheumatoid factor (RF), an autoantibody directed against the Fc portion of the immunoglobulin G molecule. Unlike in adult rheumatoid arthritis, in which 80% of cases are associated with a positive RF result, this test is rarely positive in children. Only 2% of more than 400 children seen at a rheumatology clinic in Philadelphia had a positive RF result, and many of these were considered to be false positives.[2] The only setting in which RF is helpful in children is in the case of polyarticular JIA; those with a positive RF are more likely to have a severe, erosive course, warranting more aggressive management. Even in such cases, however, the test is nonspecific, and children with infections and other conditions associated with circulating immune complexes may have a positive RF result.

Radiographic Studies

Imaging studies are essential for evaluating children with musculoskeletal pathology. They may be particularly helpful in confirming a clinical impression of arthritis by excluding other causes of joint pathology and by showing the characteristic changes caused by disease progression.

Plain films are usually the first imaging modality used to evaluate a child with joint complaints. They are generally normal during the initial stages of arthritis, or there may be nonspecific findings such as soft tissue swelling, joint effusion, periarticular osteopenia, or periosteal new bone formation.[3] Radiographs may help rule out fractures or foreign bodies. It is important to remember, however, that bony demineralization or callus formation takes 7 to 10 days to become visible on radiographs.

In longer-standing arthritis, more severe changes are evident on plain radiographs. Joint space narrowing reflects cartilage destruction, and it may be accompanied by other signs of inflammatory damage, including bony erosions and subchondral cysts. Such changes may be evident after several weeks in the case of untreated articular infection or after months to years in inflammatory conditions. Epiphyseal maturation also tends to be accelerated in JIA, leading to asymmetric growth. Thus, bilateral films to compare structures on the uninvolved side may be particularly helpful. Later signs of inadequately controlled arthritis, including bony ankylosis, subluxation, epiphyseal fracture, and avascular necrosis, are rare today with the more effective medications available to treat children with arthritis.

Plain radiographs provide limited information on the soft tissues of joints, restricting their utility in the evaluation of synovitis or abscess. Accordingly, other imaging modalities may be preferable, particularly for detecting and assessing early disease. Magnetic resonance imaging (MRI) is able to demonstrate soft tissue masses, cartilage thinning, meniscal changes, joint effusions, and popliteal cysts. The sensitivity of MRI increases significantly when performed with gadolinium enhancement. Following its intravenous administration, gadolinium accumulates quickly in tissues with increased vascularity, including inflamed synovium.[4] The utility of MRI is limited primarily by its cost and by the need to sedate young children to prevent movement artifact.

Ultrasonography is another imaging modality that may be used to assess arthritic joints. In the hands of experienced operators, ultrasonography may be useful for detecting joint effusions, popliteal cysts, lymph nodes, and, to some degree, changes in articular cartilage. Although MRI is more sensitive than ultrasonography for most purposes, the latter is less expensive, and ultrasound images can be acquired rapidly, avoiding the need for sedation or anesthesia in children who cannot remain still.[5]

TREATMENT

Treatment of a limping child depends on the cause. If a child is unable to ambulate and initial outpatient or emergency department screening does not confirm a diagnosis, admission is generally appropriate. In general, the goal of therapy is to exclude acutely dangerous conditions, prevent irreversible sequelae, and restore full functioning. This is particularly important in a growing child, in whom inflammation may result in permanent derangements in joint development and function.[6] Conversely, a growing child is also far better able to heal damage to cartilage and bone if the pathologic process is completely suppressed, increasing the incentive for adequate disease control. In the case of inflammatory arthropathies, the argument for aggressive and rapid control of joint inflammation is bolstered by evidence that the longer an autoimmune condition persists, the more resistant to therapy it becomes.[7]

Treatments for extremity abnormalities can be divided into those that relieve symptoms but do not prevent joint damage, and specific therapies that alter the biology of the process. Although symptomatic relief may or may not be necessary, depending on a child's level of discomfort, disease control is essential for preventing chronic joint changes due to ongoing inflammation.[8]

Nonsteroidal Anti-inflammatory Drugs

First-line agents for the symptomatic relief of musculoskeletal pain are nonsteroidal anti-inflammatory drugs (NSAIDs). Although dozens of medications in this category are available, only a handful have been approved by the Food and Drug Administration for use in children. Aspirin is the prototype NSAID, although it has fallen out of favor in pediatrics owing to concern about Reye syndrome and because of its very short serum half-life. Ibuprofen is available over the counter as a suspension, so it is often prescribed for children. Anti-inflammatory doses are 10 mg/kg three or four times daily, with the caveat that the medication must be given every 6 hours to achieve maximal anti-inflammatory effect. Naproxen (Aleve) may be more convenient because its long half-life allows twice-daily dosing (10 mg/kg every 12 hours). Although all NSAIDs have potential gastrointestinal, hepatic, and renal toxicities, naproxen has an additional predilection for causing pseudoporphyria, especially in fair-skinned children. Up to 12% of children develop this potentially scarring photosensitive eruption, so patients must be diligent about using sunscreen if they must take naproxen for extended periods. Parenteral NSAIDs such as ketorolac offer no advantage over their oral counterparts. In rare cases (e.g., reactive arthritis), a parenteral anti-inflammatory agent may be essential for treatment when oral administration is not possible. Generally, however, parenteral narcotics and oral NSAIDs offer a cheaper, safer alternative.

Adjunct Therapies

The major goal of therapy in children with chronic musculoskeletal complaints is to maintain as normal a life as possible. Reassurance that most children recover with minimal residual problems can provide emotional support. Simple measures, such as warm baths and the use of electric blankets at night, can help control morning stiffness. For children with minimal joint involvement, regular daily activities, including participation in physical education classes, should be encouraged, although high-impact activities should be avoided. In the presence of muscle wasting, weakness, or restricted range of motion in any joint, an active physical therapy program is indicated.

Arthritis of the knee causes pain as a result of stretching of the joint capsule by synovial fluid. A position of about 30 degrees flexion provides maximal volume and therefore minimal capsular stretching, so children with knee synovitis prefer moderate flexion; full flexion or extension is most painful. The vastus medialis muscle provides the final 5 degrees of extension, and this is the first to atrophy when splinting of the knee due to effusion leads to a joint contracture. Aquatic therapy in a heated pool is particularly helpful early in the course, because this allows effective therapy with no impact on the inflamed joint. Patients are transitioned to land therapy as the knee improves.

Nighttime splinting and serial casting are sometimes used in severe flexion contractures to maximize extension. In the setting of significant leg length discrepancies, children may require shoe lifts. Rarely, surgical correction of flexion deformities or leg length discrepancies may be necessary, although these conditions generally resolve spontaneously, provided sufficient potential for growth remains at the time the synovitis is controlled.

Advanced Therapies

Children with JIA or other chronic inflammatory diseases generally require treatment with so-called disease-modifying antirheumatic drugs. In general, this class of medications is quite effective in the treatment of childhood inflammatory joint diseases, altering the arthritis without causing significant immunosuppression.[9] Although they differ chemically, one feature that such agents have in common is that their clinical benefits manifest slowly, over weeks to months. As aggressive treatment of juvenile arthritis becomes the standard of practice, it is increasingly important that hospital-based physicians be familiar with these medications and their potential side effects (Table 40-4).

Disease-modifying agents used for the treatment of chronic arthritis, including sulfasalazine, hydroxychloroquine, and methotrexate, are often used in inflammatory bowel disease and inflammatory lung conditions as well. Practitioners choose an agent based on the child's age, the severity of the inflammation, and the speed with which control must be achieved. Sulfasalazine is used most often in children with inflammatory bowel disease or spondyloarthropathy, but it also has a role in mild cases of JIA. It is typically administered at a dosage of 40 to 70 mg/kg per day, divided into two or three doses. Sulfasalazine is a sulfa drug, and its most severe side effects are typical of this class of medication. Headache and gastrointestinal upset—especially with preparations that are not enterically coated—are most common. Rarer but more troubling side effects are bone marrow suppression, agranulocytosis, photosensitive eruptions, and hypersensitivity reactions, including Stevens-Johnson syndrome (see Chapter 161). Sulfasalazine is contraindicated in children with a known intolerance of sulfa drugs and in children younger than 2 years, in whom neurotoxicity may occur.

Hydroxychloroquine is an antimalarial agent with mild immunomodulatory effects. Such agents must be administered judiciously because of their ability to cause irreversible ocular toxicity at doses greater than 7 mg/kg per day. Even at lower doses, children may develop rashes, gastric upset, or reversible visual disturbances secondary to altered accommodation. Finally, children with glucose-6-phosphate deficiency who receive hydroxychloroquine may develop hemolytic anemia, especially during intercurrent infections.

Methotrexate is the most commonly used second-line agent in JIA, and it is the first drug shown to prevent erosive changes. Doses of 0.5 to 1 mg/kg are usually employed in arthritis and inflammatory bowel disease. This is several orders of magnitude lower than chemotherapeutic doses, so most of the toxicity associated with this agent in patients with cancer is not seen in children with JIA. Live viral vac-

Table 40-4 Adverse Effects of Medications Used to Treat Juvenile Rheumatoid Arthritis

Drug Class	Side Effects
Nonsteroidal anti-inflammatory drugs Ibuprofen, naproxen, indomethacin, tolmetin sodium	Gastric irritation, hepatotoxicity, nephrotoxicity, headache, rash
Disease-modifying antirheumatic drugs Methotrexate	Nausea, oral ulcers, hepatotoxicity, cytopenias, pulmonary hypersensitivity (rare), infection
Sulfasalazine (Azulfidine)	Gastrointestinal upset, aplastic anemia, photosensitive eruptions, Stevens-Johnson syndrome
Hydroxychloroquine (Plaquenil)	Gastrointestinal upset, retinal toxicity
Biologic agents Etanercept (Enbrel)	Injection site reactions, infections (mild to severe; mycobacteria a particular concern)

cines are nonetheless generally avoided in children receiving methotrexate, but reported cases of opportunistic or unusually severe infections are rare.

Despite its favorable therapeutic profile, methotrexate is an antimetabolite with the potential to cause oral ulcers, nausea, and abdominal pain. These adverse effects can be minimized by supplementation with folic acid. Children must be monitored regularly for evidence of hepatic toxicity; persistent elevation of hepatic transaminases identifies those at risk for hepatic fibrosis or cirrhosis. Methotrexate may also cause lymphopenia, especially with prolonged use, or even pancytopenia due to bone marrow suppression. Ten percent of children receiving methotrexate for arthritis may develop mild hypogammaglobulinemia, but this usually is not clinically significant. Concurrent use of other dihydrofolate reductase inhibitors, such as trimethoprim-sulfamethoxazole, potentiates these risks and should be avoided.

Rarely, methotrexate is associated with the development of pulmonary hypersensitivity. This most commonly occurs during the first 6 to 12 months of use and may be marked by dyspnea, cough, fever, and fluffy infiltrates on chest radiographs. Although such symptoms can be conclusively distinguished from viral pneumonitis only by lung biopsy, suspicion of this complication necessitates the discontinuation of methotrexate and the addition of systemic corticosteroids. Failure to stop the drug, or a rechallenge with methotrexate, may cause fatal respiratory failure.

Other agents are used rarely in the United States, although an occasional patient receiving intramuscular or oral gold or D-penicillamine may present for evaluation. The major side effects from gold compounds are rash, bone marrow suppression with cytopenias, and proteinuria. Penicillamine may cause rash, bone marrow suppression, nephrotoxicity, myasthenia gravis, and Goodpasture syndrome. In view of their low benefit-to-risk ratios and prolonged duration of action, these agents should be discontinued whenever toxicity is suspected. If subsequent investigations identify another explanation for the apparent drug reaction, the drug can be restarted after a hiatus of days or weeks, with little effect on arthritis control.

Biologic Response Modifiers

The newest agents in the anti-inflammatory armamentarium are the biologic response modifiers, medications that specifically target inflammatory cytokines, cellular receptors, and adhesion molecules. Etanercept, which blocks tumor necrosis factor (TNF), was the first biologic agent approved for use in children. The route of administration is subcutaneous injection, generally at a dose of 0.4 to 0.8 mg/week, given once a week or in two divided doses, depending on the size of the child. The most common side effects of etanercept are generally mild, including injection site reactions, upper respiratory tract infections, and abdominal complaints. Nonetheless, this and other biologic agents are immunosuppressive, necessitating caution in children who develop signs of a possible infection. Although most patients note only an increased frequency of mild upper respiratory tract illnesses, treatment with TNF inhibitors also increases one's susceptibility to potentially serious mycobacterial, bacterial, and herpes infections. Patients should therefore be screened with purified protein derivative before initiating anti-TNF therapies, and doses should be withheld during febrile illnesses. Additionally, as with methotrexate, live viral vaccines are generally avoided while children are receiving biologic agents.

The long-term effects of altering the immune response with these new anti-TNF medications are not known. In adults, the appearance of new autoantibodies, including ANA and anti–double-stranded DNA, and rare cases of central nervous system disorders, including multiple sclerosis, have been reported. A causal relationship between these complications and etanercept or infliximab has not been proved, but these reports should be taken into account if a child on etanercept develops new neurologic or rheumatologic complaints.

Corticosteroids must be administered judiciously owing to the significant toxicity associated with their use. Systemic steroids are typically reserved for children with severe cardiac or pulmonary symptoms, during brief flares of severe arthritis, or while waiting for slower-acting agents to take effect. Topical steroids are also effective for localized manifestations of JIA. Intra-articular steroids may be used in patients with pauciarthritis or in children with polyarticular disease in whom selected joints require particularly aggressive management. Ocular steroids are the linchpin of therapy for iridocyclitis. Among the long list of potential side effects of systemic corticosteroids, their mood-altering effects in the acute setting have the greatest impact on the clinical management of JIA. It is important to remember that these agents also increase susceptibility to herpesviruses (especially disseminated varicella) and intracellular pathogens such as mycobacteria and *Listeria*. Although steroids have little effect on susceptibility to other bacterial pathogens, their anti-inflammatory effects tend to mask clinical signs of infection, accentuating the need for vigilance on the part of clinicians.

CONCLUSION

Musculoskeletal complaints are common in children, but for the most part, they can be managed in an outpatient setting. Even children with chronic conditions such as JIA—one of the most prevalent chronic diseases of childhood, affecting an estimated 100,000 children in the United States[10]—rarely require hospitalization. Whatever the cause of joint pain, the major goal of therapy is to help the child and his or her family maintain as normal a life as possible. Most children with arthritis are referred first to orthopedists, who must be able to recognize inflammatory joint disease that is best treated medically rather than surgically. Expeditious and accurate diagnosis allows the condition to be treated before chronic damage occurs. Whether this involves appropriate antibiotics for Lyme arthritis, disease-modifying agents for JIA, or novel biologic response modifiers for recalcitrant joint inflammation, few if any children need to suffer chronic consequences. Emotional support, including the fact that most children recover with minimal residual problems, adds reassurance to this prescription.

SUGGESTED READING

Gerber MA, Zemel LS, Shapiro ED: Lyme arthritis in children: Clinical epidemiology and long-term outcomes. Pediatrics 1998;102:905-908.

Hashkes PJ, Laxer RM: Medical treatment of juvenile idiopathic arthritis. JAMA 2005;294:1671-1684.

Lovell DJ, Giannini EH, Reiff A, et al: Etanercept in children with polyarticular juvenile rheumatoid arthritis. Pediatric Rheumatology Collaborative Study Group. N Engl J Med 2000;342:763-769.

Murray KJ: Advanced therapy for juvenile arthritis. Best Pract Res Clin Rheumatol 2002;16:361-378.

Willis AA, Widmann RF, Flynn JM, et al: Lyme arthritis presenting as acute septic arthritis in children. J Pediatr Orthop 2003;23:114-118.

REFERENCES

1. McGhee JL, Burks FN, Sheckels JL, Jarvis JN: Identifying children with chronic arthritis based on chief complaints: Absence of predictive value for musculoskeletal pain as an indicator of rheumatic disease in children. Pediatrics 2002;110:354-359.

2. Eichenfield AH, Athreya BH, Doughty RA, Cebul RD: Utility of rheumatoid factor in the diagnosis of juvenile rheumatoid arthritis. Pediatrics 1986;78:480-484.

3. Cassidy J, Martel W: Juvenile rheumatoid arthritis: Clinicoradiologic correlations. Arthritis Rheum 1977;20:207-211.

4. Gylys-Morin VM, Graham TB, Blebea JS, et al: Knee in early juvenile rheumatoid arthritis: MR imaging findings. Radiology 2001;220:696-706.

5. El-Miedany YM, Housny IH, Mansour HM, et al: Ultrasound versus MRI in the evaluation of juvenile idiopathic arthritis of the knee. Joint Bone Spine 2001;68:222-230.

6. Ilowite NT: Current treatment of juvenile rheumatoid arthritis. Pediatrics 2002;109:109-115.

7. Turvey SE, Sundel RP: Autoimmune diseases. In Leung DYM, Sampson HA, Geha RS, Szefler SJ (eds): Pediatric Allergy: Principles and Practice. St Louis, Mosby, 2003, pp 159-169.

8. Oen K: Long-term outcomes and predictors of outcomes for patients with juvenile idiopathic arthritis. Best Pract Res Clin Rheumatol 2002;16:347-360.

9. Fleischmann R: Safety and efficacy of disease-modifying antirheumatic agents in rheumatoid arthritis and juvenile rheumatoid arthritis. Expert Opin Drug Safety 2003;2:347-365.

10. Gare BA: Juvenile arthritis: Who gets it, where and when? A review of current data on incidence and prevalence. Clin Exp Rheumatol 1999;17:367-374.

CHAPTER 41

Lymphadenitis
Catherine Cross

BACKGROUND

Lymphadenitis, a localized infection of lymph glands, is a common reason for hospital admission in pediatric patients. The cells in lymph glands typically proliferate in the setting of infection; a focal lymph node infection can proceed to cellulitis of the overlying skin and organization of a focal abscess in the soft tissue, with subsequent spread.[1] Because lymphatic drainage is regional, the involved nodes often reflect a distal primary infection or a systemic illness affecting multiple groups of lymph nodes. It is important to distinguish lymphadenitis from nonlymphatic processes and from lymphadenopathy—swollen, reactive nodes—secondary to other diseases.

HISTORY AND PHYSICAL EXAMINATION

A detailed history and physical examination can be invaluable in determining the likely causes of localized swelling in a pediatric patient (Tables 41-1 and 41-2). The history can help determine systemic involvement, the risk of serious underlying diagnoses, causes of the presenting process other than lymph node infection, and possible infectious exposure. In describing the swelling itself, it is useful to define the chronology of the illness and the location and progression of the process. The pertinent health history includes any major illnesses, dysmorphologies, or diagnosed syndromes; previous dental and surgical procedures; prior swellings; and recent infections, including upper respiratory infections.

The physical examination includes evaluation of the region of the lymphadenitis, as well as a general examination of other lymph nodes and organ systems. The extent of local erythema along with possible tracks or defined margins should be delineated.[1] To follow the progression of the process during subsequent evaluations, it can be useful to outline the borders of the indurated or erythematous area with a nontoxic marking pen.

DIFFERENTIAL DIAGNOSIS

In determining possible causes of suspected lymphadenitis, the location of the lesion plays an important role, as do other components of the history and physical examination. Lymphadenitis can affect any regional lymph nodes, including pre- and postauricular, submandibular, submental, anterior and posterior cervical, supraclavicular, axillary, epitrochlear, inguinal, femoral, and popliteal. Head and neck, axillary, and inguinal nodes are the most common sites of infection in children. The differential diagnosis for involved lesions includes bacterial, mycobacterial, fungal, and viral processes, as well as noninfectious causes (Table 41-3).

The organisms most commonly responsible for lymphadenitis are the gram-positive *Staphylococcus aureus* and group A β-hemolytic *Streptococcus* species.[1] Other *Staphylococcus* and *Streptococcus* species (particularly group B streptococci in neonates) are implicated less frequently, but because they are common skin and nasopharyngeal flora, they should be considered in the differential diagnosis of lymphadenitis resulting from breaks in the skin secondary to lacerations, insect bites, eczema, or other forms of dermatitis.[2] A dental source can result in infections from gram-negative organisms such as *Bacteroides* and *Prevotella*[2] or anaerobic bacteria such as *Actinomyces*.[1]

Mycobacteria can also cause lymphadenitis, particularly in the cervical lymph node chains. *Mycobacterium tuberculosis* can cause focal lymphadenitis or generalized lymphadenopathy, but atypical mycobacteria are usually the culprit organisms in focal soft tissue infections.[1] The most common mycobacteria species implicated in lymphadenitis is *Mycobacterium avium* complex.[2]

Close attention should be paid to possible cutaneous sources of drainage to and infection of a regional lymph node. Lymphadenitis can result from progression of local inoculation and trauma, such as with gram-negative *Bartonella henselae*, resulting in cat-scratch disease; gram-negative *Pasteurella multocida* after a cat or dog bite; local fungal infection such as tinea capitis; unusual skin infections such as sporotrichosis from the fungus *Sporothrix schenckii*, after gardening exposure; cellulitis caused by gram-negative anaerobic *Vibrio* species, after abrasions in seawater; genital chancroid infection caused by sexually transmitted gram-negative *Haemophilus ducreyi*; filariasis after mosquito exposure to nematodes of the *Wuchereria bancrofti* or *Brugia* species in developing countries; or other rare organisms causing soft tissue infections in patients with compromised immune function, such as *Burkholderia cepacia* in patients with chronic granulomatous disease.[1,2]

With a worrisome clinical presentation in the setting of possible arthropod or zoonotic exposure to rare organisms, the differential diagnosis should be widened to include tularemia, anthrax, and bubonic plague.[2] Although these diseases are uncommon in developed countries, they can present with a focal lesion that becomes a regional lymphadenitis before progressing to systemic disease. With these illnesses, timely recognition and aggressive antibiotic treatment may save a patient from significant morbidity and possible mortality.

It is important to distinguish infectious lymphadenitis from lymphadenopathy. Generalized lymphadenopathy can be found with a multitude of systemic infections, including

Table 41-1 **History**

Area of swelling
 Location, prior swellings in that location
 Chronology, progression, local symptoms
 Recent injuries, infections, or breaks in skin distal to
  involved site

Review of systems
 Fever course
 Malaise
 Bruising or bleeding
 Weight loss

Exposures
 Geography—residence and travel
 Sick contacts
 Family members or caretakers with chronic cough
 Contact with prison or homeless populations
 Insect bites
 Exposure to pets, farm animals, or wild animals, or to their
  meat or carcasses

Past medical history
 Recent infections, including upper respiratory infections
 History of prior infections
 Past dental or surgical procedures
 Major illnesses, dysmorphologies, diagnosed syndromes

Table 41-2 **Physical Examination**

Vital signs with temperature

Thorough head and neck examination, including scalp

Cardiac examination

Pulmonary examination

Abdominal examination, including assessment for
 hepatomegaly, splenomegaly, masses

Dermatologic examination, with particular focus on distal sites
 in area of lymphatic drainage

Description of involved site
 Location
 Erythema
 Warmth
 Tenderness
 Swelling
 Size
 Heterogeneity, focal nodules
 Fluctuance
 Skin openings, discharge
 Mobility or matted quality
 Margins

General lymph node examination, including the following
  regions:
 Posterior and anterior cervical
 Supraclavicular
 Axillary
 Inguinal

Neurologic and other examinations as indicated

those secondary to Epstein-Barr virus (EBV), cytomegalovirus, varicella, adenovirus, Coxsackievirus, herpes simplex virus, human herpesvirus 6, and human immunodeficiency virus (HIV).[1] Reactive lymph nodes may be tender, and in the setting of a viral infection, they may induce surrounding inflammation, which can present similarly to bacterial infection of nodes.

Noninfectious causes of lymphadenopathy, or focal swelling that mimics it, may be rheumatologic, immunologic, inflammatory, or oncologic in nature. Kawasaki disease is a vasculitis that often presents with focal lymph node swelling and tenderness in the setting of fever; a careful history and physical examination should rule out conjunctivitis with limbic sparing, rash, and oral mucosal findings, other signs of Kawasaki disease that typically distinguish it from lymphadenitis (see Ch. 102). A variety of immune deficiencies and inflammatory processes, such as sarcoidosis,[3] can also present with lymphadenopathy. Oncologic causes of lymph node swelling include lymphoma, lymphoproliferative disorders, and metastatic lymph nodes from primary tumors situated elsewhere. Focal oncologic processes such as soft tissue neoplasms may also mimic lymph node swelling.

The location of the process plays an important role in determining whether congenital malformations and anatomic abnormalities are possible causes. In the head and neck region, midline thyroglossal duct cysts, lateral branchial cleft cysts, and dermoid cysts in a variety of locations may present with swelling, with or without superinfection; parotid or submental salivary gland dysfunction or infection may also be present. In the inguinal area, hydroceles and undescended testes or testicular torsion should be added to the differential diagnosis in males, whereas in females an entrapped ovary may present in the setting of a hernia. In either sex, entrapped intestine or omentum may be present in a hernia.[4]

EVALUATION

Laboratory testing is indicated if there is suspicion of a disease other than localized *Staphylococcus* or *Streptococcus* infection, thereby affecting treatment decisions. Bacteremia can occur in pediatric patients—particularly young patients with high fevers—with significant focal bacterial lymph node infections,[1] so obtaining blood cultures can help identify a bacterial organism as well as its sensitivities. A complete blood count with leukocyte differential may be helpful to determine leukocytosis and indicate possible infectious mononucleosis or oncologic processes. Infectious mononucleosis is caused by EBV and commonly presents with atypical lymphocytosis, lymphadenopathy, and fever, as well as exudative pharyngitis and hepatosplenomegaly.[2] Initial testing for EBV may include heterophil antibody testing—most sensitive in patients older than 4 years—as well as EBV serum titers for immunoglobulins M and G; it is important to keep in mind that these tests are most sensitive after 2 to 3 weeks of illness.[2] Cytomegalovirus infections can present similarly to EBV infections, so serum cytomegalovirus titers may be helpful. Depending on the differential diagnosis for a given patient, serologies for *Bartonella henselae* and *Francisella tularensis* (the gram-negative bacterium that causes tularemia) may also be indicated. HIV testing should be

Table 41-3 Differential Diagnosis

Lymphadenitis Due to the Following Organisms	Other Causes of Focal Swelling that Can Mimic Lymphadenitis

Common skin and nasopharyngeal flora
  Staphylococcus aureus
  Streptococcus species, particularly group A
Bacteria from a dental source
  Bacteroides, Prevotella, other gram-negative dental organisms
  Actinomyces and other anaerobes
Mycobacteria
  Atypical mycobacteria, particularly *Mycobacterium avium* complex
  Mycobacterium tuberculosis
Less common organisms that can infect lymph nodes after local infection
  Bartonella henselae (cat-scratch disease)
  Trichophyton or *Microsporum* species (resulting in tinea capitis)
  Sporothrix schenckii (after gardening)
  Vibrio species and other water-based organisms
  Haemophilus ducreyi (after genital chancroid)
  Filariasis due to *Wuchereria bancrofti* or *Brugia* species
Special organisms in immunocompromised patients
  Burkholderia cepacia
After exposure in relevant geographic regions
  Francisella tularensis (tularemia)
  Bacillus anthracis (anthrax)
  Yersinia pestis (bubonic plague)
	Lymphadenopathy
	  Viral infections
	    Epstein-Barr virus
	    Cytomegalovirus
	    Varicella-zoster virus
	    Adenovirus
	    Coxsackievirus
	    Herpes simplex virus
	    Human herpesvirus 6 (roseola)
	    Human immunodeficiency virus
	  Tuberculosis
	  Rheumatologic causes
	    Kawasaki disease
	  Immune deficiencies
	  Inflammatory processes
	    Sarcoidosis
	  Oncologic processes
	    Lymphoma
	    Lymphoproliferative disorders
	    Metastatic lymph nodes from other primary tumors
	Primary neoplastic processes
	  Soft tissue neoplasms
	Anatomic malformations
	  Head and neck area
	    Thyroglossal duct cyst (midline)
	    Branchial cleft cyst (lateral)
	    Dermoid cyst
	    Salivary gland processes
	  Inguinal region
	    Hernia with or without entrapped intestine or omentum
	    Ovary entrapped in hernia (females)
	    Hydrocele, undescended testis, testicular torsion (males)

performed if there is any history of HIV exposure or if the clinical history leads to suspicion of an underlying immune deficiency. In the setting of recurrent infections, an immunology consultation may be helpful in recommending further testing.[1]

If there is a history of travel to developing countries or other possible exposure to tuberculosis (TB), a Mantoux tuberculin purified protein derivative (PPD) test should be done. A negative PPD test should not be considered definitive in the setting of high clinical suspicion for TB, however, because 10% of immunocompetent children with culture-documented TB may have a negative PPD; this number is higher in immunocompromised patients and in those with disseminated TB.[2] Atypical mycobacterial disease can sometimes cause a positive PPD.[2] In the setting of a positive PPD test or supraclavicular adenopathy on examination, a chest radiograph can screen for pulmonary TB or other diseases, particularly oncologic processes in the chest, whose lymphatics may drain to a sentinel supraclavicular node.

To visualize the presenting lesion itself—particularly if it is rapidly progressive, fluctuant, or close to vital structures—ultrasonography often provides distinct images of a superficial process without exposing the patient to radiation. If there is concern for a deeper or more widespread process, a computed tomography scan may be more helpful.

If the infection has a loculated component or an organized abscess, drainage may be therapeutic as well as diagnostic. Fine-needle aspiration, under ultrasound guidance if necessary, is a useful method of obtaining a fluid sample for bacterial, mycobacterial, and fungal stains and cultures. It is important to note that many lymphadenitis organisms, especially mycobacteria, are fastidious and may not grow in culture.[2] Incision for drainage can lead to a chronically draining sinus tract, particularly in the setting of a mycobacterial infection; in these cases, excisional biopsy is the preferred approach. If there is little concern about rare or resistant organisms and if a good response to antibiotic treatment alone is expected in a given patient, treatment is often initiated without obtaining microbiologic studies from the site of infection.

TREATMENT

After the initial assessment, which often occurs in a primary care setting, an important issue is whether a patient requires hospitalization. Possible criteria for hospital admission include toxic appearance, rapid progression of infection, airway involvement of a neck process, inability to tolerate enteral antibiotics or lack of clinical improvement on a prior trial of outpatient antibiotics, comorbid conditions, suspicion of an underlying secondary diagnosis, and possible bacteremia, particularly in a febrile infant or young child.

If a case of likely bacterial lymphadenitis warrants hospital admission, intravenous (IV) antibiotics are usually the initial treatment. Antibiotic choice should be directed by the likely bacteria, mycobacteria, or fungi responsible for the process, as well as by patient allergies and recent antibiotic exposures.

For lymphadenitis due to *S. aureus* or *Streptococcus* species, a β-lactamase–resistant β-lactam antibiotic such as oxacillin or nafcillin is indicated; a combination of the β-lactam ampicillin and the β-lactamase inhibitor sulbactam sodium is also an option.[2] With the rise in hospital- and community-acquired methicillin-resistant *S. aureus* (MRSA), the past medical history of the patient and community resistance rates should be taken into account. Clindamycin may be another good option for empirical treatment of these common pathogens. However, susceptibility to MRSA varies widely by region and empirical therapy should be guided by local patterns of antibiotic resistance. If there is suspected or documented MRSA, IV vancomycin should be administered; for serious infections, it should be combined with a β-lactamase–resistant β-lactam antibiotic.[2]

For lymphadenitis due to other bacterial, mycobacterial, or fungal causes, medication choices should be based on the likely organisms involved and their susceptibility profiles in the geographic region. The treatment course can be adjusted based on culture results and tested susceptibilities when those are available.

Lack of clinical improvement typically dictates further therapeutic interventions or changes. An initial consideration is whether an unusual organism may be responsible for the process or whether the organism involved may demonstrate a degree of antibiotic resistance. In these cases, identifying the organism via stained and cultured tissue samples can be invaluable; consultation with an infectious disease specialist is also helpful. The possibility of immunocompromise in a patient who is not responding to conventional therapy should be reconsidered. The lymphadenitis lesion can be imaged or reimaged if it is not regressing. One possible reason for failed treatment response is low antibiotic penetrance into an organized, circumscribed abscess; penetrance into a walled-off loculation may be low despite relatively high vascular flow to inflamed surrounding tissues.

For an identified abscess, drainage is often the most appropriate course of treatment. This can be performed via needle aspiration rather than open incision and drainage to reduce the risk of chronic drainage and scar formation.[1] Excision is indicated for lesions with chronic drainage (as can occur with *M. tuberculosis* lymphadenitis) and for atypical mycobacteria, which are often multidrug resistant.[1] For lymphadenitis caused by *M. avium* complex, excision is

indicated, and antituberculosis medications are ineffective.[2] Depending on the site in question, consultation with a general surgeon or otorhinolaryngologist is recommended.

Discharge criteria for pediatric patients admitted with lymphadenitis include demonstration of significant clinical improvement, nontoxic appearance, ability to receive enteral antibiotics for the remainder of the required course, and family support for treatment and follow-up. Worrisome signs and symptoms should be reviewed with the patient and family, and criteria for when to seek immediate medical attention should be discussed; medication instructions and follow-up plans should also be given. The choice of discharge antibiotics for likely or identified bacterial processes depends largely on the organisms involved and the IV antibiotics used during the hospital stay. Common conversions to oral (PO) medications for pediatric lymphadenitis patients include IV oxacillin to PO dicloxacillin, IV ampicillin–sulbactam sodium to PO amoxicillin-clavulanate, IV to PO clindamycin, and IV cefazolin to PO cephalexin. These PO medications can also be given through a gastric tube, if necessary.

When planning for discharge, communication with the primary care physician should include details about pending laboratory studies, such as final results of blood cultures; planned antibiotic course; any concerns about the patient's underlying immune status or other secondary diagnoses; information regarding specialty clinic follow-up for issues such as directly observed therapy for TB, and the recommended time interval for clinical follow-up with the primary care physician.

SUGGESTED READING

Camitta BM: The lymphatic system. In Behrman RE, Kliegman RM, Jenson HB (eds): Nelson Textbook of Pediatrics, 17th ed. Philadelphia, WB Saunders, 2004, pp 1677-1678.

Davis HW, Michaels MG: Infectious disease. In Zitelli BJ, Davis HW (eds): Atlas of Pediatric Physical Diagnosis, 4th ed. Philadelphia, Mosby, 2002, pp 396-454.

Liu JH, Myer CM: Evaluation of head and neck masses. In Rudolph CD, Rudolph AM, Hostetter MK, et al (eds): Rudolph's Pediatrics, 21st ed. New York, McGraw-Hill, 2003, pp 1279-1281.

Pickering LK (ed): Red Book: 2003 Report of the Committee on Infectious Diseases, 26th ed. Elk Grove Village, III, American Academy of Pediatrics, 2003, pp 189-692.

REFERENCES

1. Davis HW, Michaels MG: Infectious disease. In Zitelli BJ, Davis HW (eds): Atlas of Pediatric Physical Diagnosis, 4th ed. Philadelphia, Mosby, 2002, pp 396-454.

2. Pickering LK (ed): Red Book: 2003 Report of the Committee on Infectious Diseases, 26th ed. Elk Grove Village, III, American Academy of Pediatrics, 2003, pp 189-692.

3. Liu JH, Myer CM: Evaluation of head and neck masses. In Rudolph CD, Rudolph AM, Hostetter MK, et al (eds): Rudolph's Pediatrics, 21st ed. New York, McGraw-Hill, 2003, pp 1279-1281.

4. Fink DL, Serwint JR: The knotty problem in an infant girl's groin. Contemp Pediatr 2005;22:24.

CHAPTER 42

Oral Lesions

Suzanne Swanson

Oral lesions can result from a broad spectrum of both local and systemic pathophysiologic processes, as well as from direct injury. Oral lesions may be the primary concern in children requiring hospital admission, or these lesions may be important clues to an underlying condition (Table 42-1). Dental anomalies, especially delayed eruption, are often associated with genetic syndromes such as those listed in Table 42-2. This chapter focuses on acute infectious, inflammatory, and traumatic lesions of the mouth and teeth that may warrant hospitalization.

INFECTIOUS ORAL LESIONS

Most pediatric patients admitted with infectious oral lesions are hospitalized due to their inability to tolerate oral intake because of the associated pain and often present with dehydration. Typically, these lesions are self-limited, and treatment is mainly supportive. Discharge criteria are usually satisfied once the patient is able to tolerate oral intake, with or without medication for pain control.

Viral causes of oral infections are listed in Table 42-3.[1] Two of the more common viral causes—herpes simplex virus (HSV) and enterovirus—are discussed here, along with candidiasis, which is caused by a fungus.

Herpes Simplex Virus

Primary HSV gingivostomatitis results from direct contact with infected oral secretions or lesions (Fig. 42-1). Approximately two thirds of these infections are caused by HSV type 1, and the balance are caused by type 2. The incubation period varies from 2 days to 2 weeks. Characteristic oral lesions occur (see Table 42-3), along with tender anterior cervical and submental lymphadenitis, fever, malaise, drooling, and anorexia. No specific treatment is currently recommended for immunocompetent patients other than antipyretics, analgesics, hydration, and perhaps mouth rinses (e.g., chlorhexidine) to provide relief and reduce the risk of secondary infection. Oral or intravenous acyclovir may help shorten the duration of symptoms if it is initiated within the first 48 to 72 hours.[1]

With recurrent HSV episodes, small clusters of ulcers without halos form on the hard palate, lips (herpes labialis), or attached gingival surfaces. Healing should be expected within 7 to 14 days. Systemic symptoms are uncommon, but localized lymphadenitis is often seen. No treatment is needed unless the child has frequent recurrences.

Enterovirus

Enteroviruses, including coxsackie- and echoviruses, can cause oral ulcers in the context of either hand-foot-and-mouth disease or herpangina. Hand-foot-and-mouth disease is most commonly associated with coxsackievirus A16 and is characterized by shallow, yellow ulcers with red halos found on mucosal surfaces, including the mouth and genital areas. Cutaneous involvement occurs in two thirds of cases of hand-foot-and-mouth disease and is characterized by the formation of tender vesicles on the palms, the soles, and occasionally the buttocks. Herpangina has similar oral lesions, but they usually occur more posteriorly in the mouth, commonly involving the tonsillar pillars and the soft palate. Treatment for both hand-foot-and-mouth disease and herpangina is mainly supportive, but oral analgesics and anesthetic mouth rinses may provide some relief. Cold drinks and foods may also help keep the child hydrated.

Although the distribution of the lesions may be helpful in making the diagnosis, the initial presentation may be difficult to differentiate from herpetic lesions. Children with primary herpetic gingivostomatitis tend to have more severe mouth pain, a higher fever, gingival bleeding, and an ill appearance.[2]

Candida

Oral candidiasis, also known as thrush, is seen in young infants, immunosuppressed individuals, children on antibiotic therapy or using inhaled corticosteroids, and those with underlying systemic conditions. By far the most common cause is *Candida albicans*. Candidiasis appears as a white, cheesy, adherent plaque on the buccal mucosa, tongue, or palate or at the commissures of the lips (cheilitis). This plaque cannot be "wiped off," but if it is removed, the underlying tissue is raw and red. Treatment involves topical or systemic oral antifungal agents.[3]

ODONTOGENIC INFECTIONS

Dental Caries

Dental caries rarely require hospital admission (Figs. 42-2 and 42-3). Patients may present, however, with associated dental infections, or caries may be the predisposing condition for more serious infections of the head and neck. Significant dental decay noted incidentally during a hospitalization presents an opportunity for appropriate outpatient referral.

Gingivitis

The gingiva is the pink-colored keratinized mucosa that surrounds the teeth. Pericoronitis is a local infection of the gingiva surrounding an erupting tooth. In acute necrotizing ulcerative gingivitis (also known as trench mouth or Vincent angina), the interdental gingival papillae become ulcerated and friable, and pseudomembrane formation may occur.

Table 42-1 Conditions with Oral Manifestations

Condition	Oral Signs or Symptoms
Cyclic neutropenia	Oral ulcers, early loss of primary teeth
Leukocyte adhesion deficiency disorder	Severe gingival inflammation around primary teeth, increased tooth mobility, early tooth loss
Submucosal cleft palate	May present with bifid or notched uvula
Systemic lupus erythematosus	Oral or nasal mucocutaneous ulcerations
Kawasaki syndrome	Dry, fissured lips and "strawberry tongue"
Stevens-Johnson syndrome	Fragile mucosal bullae, shallow oral ulcers with a gray or white membrane
Peutz-Jeghers syndrome	Melanotic spots on lips and buccal mucosa
Osler-Weber-Rendu disease	Telangiectasia of oral mucosa
Porphyria	Possibly reddish brown discoloration of teeth
Acute myelogenous leukemia	Subtypes can present with gingival hyperplasia, oral ulcers
Primary HIV infection	Oral ulcers, pharyngitis, cervical lymphadenopathy

HIV, human immunodeficiency virus.

Table 42-2 Syndromes Associated with Delayed Tooth Eruption

Albright hereditary osteodystrophy
Apert syndrome
Cornelia de Lange syndrome
Hunter syndrome
Incontinentia pigmenti
Miller-Dieker syndrome
Osteogenesis imperfecta type I
Progeria syndrome

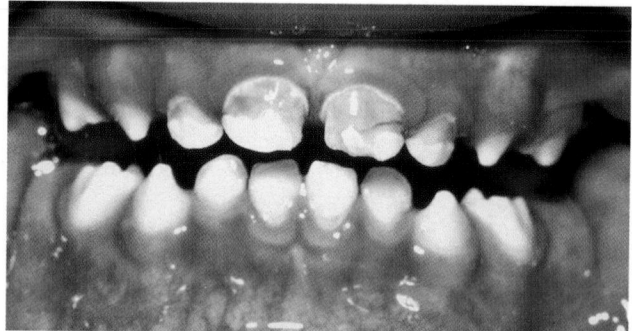

Figure 42-2 Moderate early childhood caries characterized by brownish discoloration of teeth with defects in tooth surfaces.

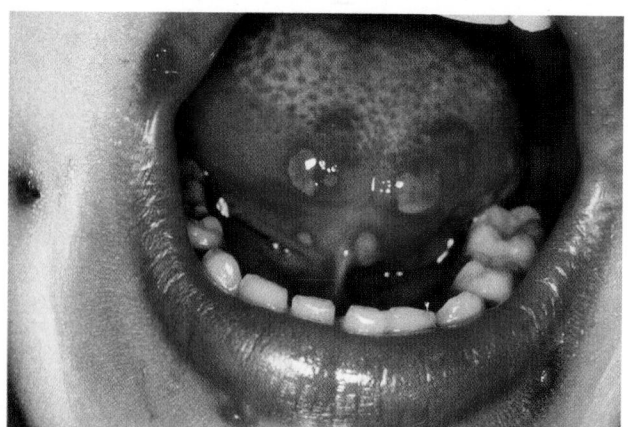

Figure 42-1 Primary herpetic gingivostomatitis with ulcers and vesicles seen on the anterior tongue, lips, and perioral area.

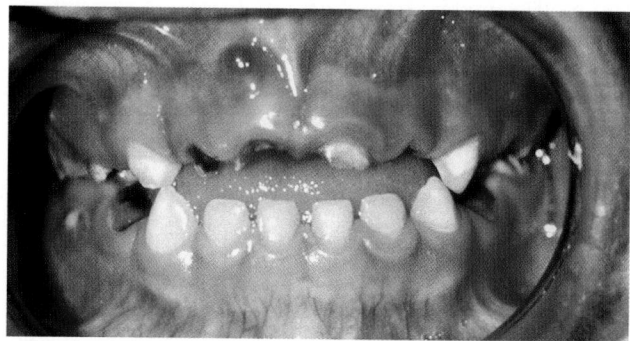

Figure 42-3 Severe early childhood caries characterized by discoloration and destruction of teeth.

Table 42-3 Viral Oral Mucosal Infections

Cause	Lesion	Site and Distribution
HSV		
Primary (herpes stomatitis)	Inflamed gingiva and mucosa, followed by vesicles that promptly rupture to reveal characteristic irregular, painful, superficial ulcers	Anterior: gingival, labial, lingual, and buccal mucosa; floor of mouth; extension to perioral skin involvement and "drop" lesions Posterior: hard palate and tonsils
Recurrent	Single or small clusters of vesicles	Mucocutaneous junction of lips
Varicella-zoster HHV-6	Shallow, nonpainful ulcers Erythematous papules	Palate Soft palate and base of uvula
Rubeola (measles)	Mottled erythema in prodromal phase; grayish white granular lesions on pronounced erythematous mucosa (Koplik spots) on about day 10	Prodromal findings: palate Koplik spots: initially, buccal mucosa adjacent to lower molars; subsequently extends throughout oral mucosa
Enteroviruses Several coxsackie- and echoviruses Coxsackievirus A16 (hand-foot-and-mouth disease)	Tiny yellowish papules or ulcers on erythematous base	Lingual and buccal surfaces; soft palate

HHV-6, human herpesvirus 6; HSV, herpes simplex virus.
Adapted from Long SS, Pickering LK, Prober CG (eds): Principles and Practice of Pediatric Infectious Diseases. New York, Churchill Livingstone, 1997, p 183.

Patients are typically adolescents who present with pain, bleeding gums, bad breath, and occasionally fever. These infections are often polymicrobial and can include anaerobes, spirochetes, and fusobacteria. Treatment consists of antibiotic therapy, such as penicillin with or without metronidazole, first-generation cephalosporins, macrolides, or clindamycin. Oral rinses with dilute hydrogen peroxide or chlorhexidine are often offered. Occasionally, local débridement may be necessary.

Periapical Abscess

Oral bacteria that enter erosions in the dental enamel (caries) can track through the dentin to the pulp. This pulpitis can result in a periapical abscess or penetration into the bone causing an acute alveolar abscess. Patients present with pain, especially with percussion of the affected tooth, and overlying facial swelling. Depending on the location, extension of these infections can cause myriad complications (Fig. 42-4; Box 42-1), including acutely life-threatening entities (discussed in Chapter 65).

APHTHOUS ULCERS

Aphthous ulcers are common in teenagers and young adults and are not of infectious origin. The lesions are larger than herpetic ulcers, but there is no preceding vesicle formation. Most commonly found on movable tissue, the lesion consists of a white crater with an erythematous halo. Aphthous ulcers may be triggered by stress, sunlight, or hormonal changes, but they can also occur with systemic disorders such as iron, folate, or vitamin B_{12} deficiency;

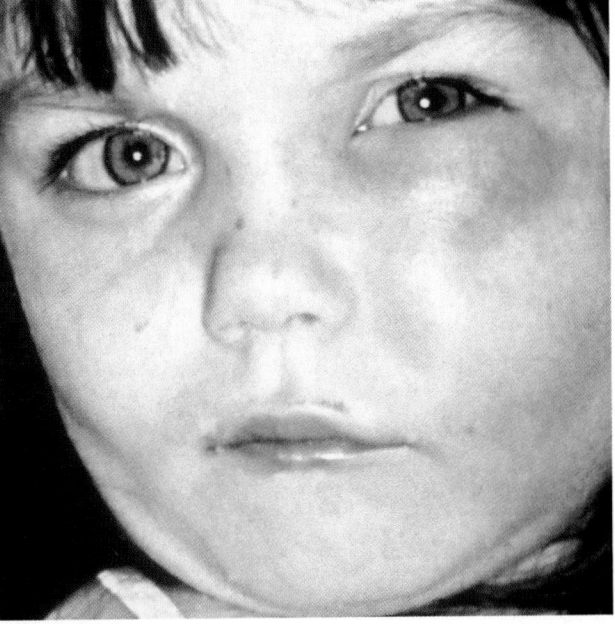

Figure 42-4 Facial cellulitis from untreated left maxillary dental abscess demonstrating swelling of the left face and periorbital area and patches of diffuse erythema.

Crohn's disease; celiac disease; Behçet syndrome; Sweet syndrome; human immunodeficiency virus infection; neutropenia; and other immunodeficiencies. The lesions may coalesce into larger lesions. They are often painful but resolve in 7 to 10 days without scarring.

| Box 42-1 | Complications of Periapical Dental Infections |

Maxillary sinusitis
Intraoral or cutaneous fistula
Osteomyelitis
Palatal cellulitis or abscess
Buccal or facial cellulitis
Sublingual or submandibular cellulitis (Ludwig angina)
Suppurative jugular thrombophlebitis (Lemierre syndrome)

ORAL TRAUMA

Traumatic mucosal injuries are the most common type of oral injury in infants and young children and may be caused by burns, either chemical (e.g., alkali) or thermal (e.g., hot drinks); by sucking on a pacifier or finger; by sharp objects inserted into the mouth, resulting in abrasions or lacerations; or by blunt trauma (accidental or nonaccidental).

Thermal or chemical burns may result in areas of mucosal erythema or sloughing, and adherent white material appears as healing proceeds. The distribution may include the palate, the lips, or the peripheral areas of the tongue. These lesions may be painful but generally heal within 2 weeks.[3] Ulcers from sucking are usually found on the hard palate.

The head, face, and neck are the most common sites affected by physical abuse and may be the only manifestation on physical examination. Orofacial injuries suggestive of child abuse include lacerations of the oral frenulae, swollen lips with underlying ecchymoses, and tooth fractures without an adequate history. Radiographs may reveal multiple healed fractures of the teeth and jaw. Unexplained oral bleeding in an infant warrants investigation. Neglect may be suspected in a child with severe, untreated dental caries and oral infection, but this can be difficult to differentiate from parental ignorance of proper dental hygiene. Sexual abuse may present with oral findings, such as bruising of the hard and soft palates, tears of the lingual frenulum, or oral lesions associated with a sexually transmitted disease.[3]

ACKNOWLEDGMENTS

Special thanks to Dr. Charles Klass and Dr. Arthur J. Nowak for their assistance in editing this chapter.

SUGGESTED READING

Nowak AJ: A Health Professional's Guide to Pediatric Oral Health Management. National Maternal and Child Oral Health Resource Center, 2004. Available at *http://www.mchoralhealth.org/PediatricOH/index.htm.*

REFERENCES

1. Long SS, Pickering LK, Prober CG (eds): Principles and Practice of Pediatric Infectious Diseases. New York, Churchill Livingstone, 1997, p 183.
2. Lotstein SK: Photoclinic: Hand-foot-and-mouth disease. Consult Pediatr 2004;3:246-247.
3. Nowak AJ: A Health Professional's Guide to Pediatric Oral Health Management. National Maternal and Child Oral Health Resource Center, 2004. Available at *http://www.mchoralhealth.org/PediatricOH/index.htm.*

CHAPTER 43

Neck Pain

Nicole R. Frei

Neck pain is a nonspecific presenting symptom in children, and patients are more likely to be seen in the emergency department or outpatient settings than in the hospital. Because neck pain is a symptom with a number of possible causes, the primary responsibility of the evaluating physician is to recognize those conditions that require urgent management, especially those for which surgery may be required.

BACKGROUND

Although neck pain is a common presenting symptom, it is rarely a discharge diagnosis. Estimates of the incidence of neck pain necessitating admission to an inpatient service do not exist, but data from a regional children's hospital with 40,000 emergency department visits per year suggest that less than 10% of patients seen in the emergency department with a complaint of neck pain are admitted to the hospital. Among those not requiring hospitalization, the most common discharge diagnosis is neck strain or neck spasm. Children with neck pain who are admitted to the hospital generally have serious infections requiring intravenous antibiotics, a condition requiring emergent management by a specialist, or both (see Chapter 65).

DIFFERENTIAL DIAGNOSIS

When neck pain is a presenting symptom, the underlying cause must be determined to guide diagnostic studies and appropriate consultation or treatment (Table 43-1).

Infectious Causes

Primary Lymphadenitis

The most common cause of neck pain requiring admission to an inpatient service is infection, and the most common infection is cervical lymphadenitis. This infection can often be treated on an outpatient basis with oral antibiotics, but progression of infection despite such treatment is a common reason for admission to the hospital. Often these infections resolve with intravenous antibiotics alone, but they may require surgical drainage if an abscess forms. Children typically present with a unilateral enlarged, tender lymph node or nodes with overlying erythema; most have fever. The most common causative bacteria are *Staphylococcus aureus* and group A β-hemolytic streptococcus (GABHS). Cervical lymphadenitis can also be caused by viruses, mycobacteria, and other atypical organisms. This infection can present at any age. The diagnosis is often made based on the clinical presentation, but a computed tomography (CT) scan may be indicated to identify other causes of a neck mass or abscess formation. Ultrasonography or biopsy can be useful in certain situations if the diagnosis is in question or if the patient is not responding to treatment

as expected. Successful treatment depends on an accurate assessment of the underlying cause.

Meningitis

The classic clinical presentation of meningitis is fever, nuchal rigidity, irritability, and vomiting in a toxic-appearing patient. The most common causes are viral or bacterial. The most common bacterial causes in this era are *Streptococcus pneumoniae* and *Neisseria meningitidis*. Viral causes vary from season to season. Diagnosis is made by evaluation of cerebral spinal fluid (CSF) from a lumbar puncture; CSF pleocytosis is required for diagnosis. Bacterial culture and viral studies can provide a definitive diagnosis. Appropriate treatment includes supportive care and antimicrobial treatment as dictated by the causative organism.

Cervical Osteomyelitis

The most common location for osteomyelitis is the long bones, but up to 20% of reported cases involve other bones. The clinical presentation of osteomyelitis of the cervical spine includes focal tenderness, limited range of motion, and fever. This infection occurs most often in children older than 8 years. The most common organism identified is *S. aureus*. Evidence of infection is supported by magnetic resonance imaging (MRI) or bone scan. Cultures of the blood or bone obtained by biopsy are useful in choosing antibiotics, but in their absence, treatment should be a prolonged course of intravenous antibiotics covering *Staphylococcus* and GABHS (see Chapter 70). Surgical débridement is indicated if the patient does not demonstrate clinical improvement after appropriate treatment.

Suppurative Thyroiditis

This uncommon disease typically occurs after an upper respiratory infection and presents with the acute onset of fever, chills, and a tender, enlarged thyroid gland. Infection can be caused by *S. aureus*, GABHS, and oral flora. Diagnosis is made by needle aspiration or biopsy with culture. Thyroid function tests are rarely abnormal. Many cases are associated with a persistent thyroglossal duct or a piriform sinus anomaly. A barium swallow is recommended to identify persistent embryonic communication with the alimentary tract. Initial treatment is empirical intravenous antibiotics to cover *S. aureus*, *S. pneumoniae*, and oral flora. Treatment can be narrowed based on culture results.

Deep Neck Infection

Retropharyngeal or peritonsillar phlegmon or abscess occurs most commonly in preschool children. Most patients with deep neck infections appear ill and usually have drool-

Table 43–1   Differential Diagnosis of Neck Pain

Diagnostic Category	Diagnosis
Infectious	
Complications of oropharyngeal infection	Retropharyngeal or peritonsillar abscess
	Dental abscess
	Submandibular space infection (Ludwig's angina)
	Jugular septic thrombophlebitis (Lemierre disease)
Other infections	Cervical adenitis
	Meningitis
	Cervical osteomyelitis
	Suppurative thyroiditis
	Infected branchial cleft cyst
	Infected thyroglossal duct cyst
	Infected cystic hygroma
Traumatic	Vertebral fracture
	Spinal epidural hematoma
	Esophageal injury
	Laryngotracheal injury
Orthopedic	Osteoid osteoma
	Cervical spine stenosis
	Acute cervical disk calcification
	Atlantoaxial instability
	Atlantoaxial rotatory subluxation
Neurologic	Chiari I malformation
	Syrinx
Musculoskeletal	Strain
Vascular	Vertebral artery dissection
	Stroke
Oncologic	Posterior fossa tumor
	Spinal canal tumor
	Neck soft tissue tumor
Rheumatologic	Juvenile rheumatoid arthritis
	Spondyloarthropathies
Other	Pneumomediastinum

ing, limited neck movement, and a muffled voice; they prefer sitting in an upright position. *Staphylococcus* and GABHS are the most common pathogens, although the infection is often polymicrobial. The most useful imaging study is a CT scan with contrast to define the area involved and to determine whether there is abscess formation. Lateral neck radiographs show less detail but are abnormal about 90% of the time in the presence of a retropharyngeal process. Treatment involves broad empirical coverage with intravenous antibiotics. If there is no response to medical therapy within 24 to 72 hours, incision and drainage may be necessary.

Submandibular Space Infection (Ludwig's Angina)

Ludwig's angina is a cellulitis of the connective tissue, fascia, and muscles of the submandibular space. It is usually a complication of an odontogenic infection. It occurs most

often in older children and adolescents. The clinical presentation includes a toxic-looking patient with a swollen and tender neck, fever, dysphagia, foul breath, and drooling. The tongue is typically elevated, and the patient has trismus. This is a rapidly progressive illness and represents a true airway emergency. Nearly all children require emergent intubation or tracheotomy. Treatment involves controlling the airway and administering broad-spectrum intravenous antibiotics.

Jugular Septic Thrombophlebitis (Lemierre Disease)

Patients with Lemierre disease present with systemic findings following tonsillopharyngitis, dental infection, mastoiditis, or sinusitis. The typical presentation is associated with a dental infection and foul-smelling breath. About half of patients with jugular septic thrombophlebitis have unilateral neck pain and swelling; somewhat fewer have trismus. Most have signs of metastatic infectious disease, including pulmonary infiltrates, hepatosplenomegaly, increased liver enzymes, or disseminated intravascular coagulation. Infection is thought to spread into the lateral pharyngeal space, which contains the internal jugular vein. The most common organism identified is *Fusobacterium necrophorum*, although this infection is usually polymicrobial with aerobic and anaerobic organisms. The diagnosis is suggested if *F. necrophorum* grows from a blood culture, and it can be confirmed by contrast CT scan of the neck. Treatment is a 4- to 6-week course of broad-spectrum antibiotics to cover aerobic and anaerobic bacteria and supportive care. Anticoagulation is recommended only if there is evidence of continued propagation of the thrombus.

Dental Abscess

Dental abscess is typically caused by mouth flora in the setting of dental caries. It can occur at any age and typically presents with face or neck swelling, pain, and fever. A fluctuant area near the affected tooth or gum is sometimes palpable. The acute treatment is intravenous or oral antibiotics to cover aerobic and anaerobic organisms, followed by definitive dental treatment.

Traumatic Causes

Discussion of traumatic causes of neck pain is beyond the scope of this chapter. Most significant trauma in children is managed by a designated trauma team. Less obvious forms of trauma, such as an unwitnessed fall from a bed or a hyperextension injury from gymnastics, are important considerations when a child presents with neck pain that does not appear to have an infectious cause. In nonverbal children, it is important to consider nonaccidental trauma as a possible cause of neck pain.

Orthopedic Causes

Upper Cervical Spine Instability

Atlantoaxial instability is typically caused by congenital abnormalities of the odontoid process or ligamentous hyperlaxity. It can also be caused by inflammatory conditions such as juvenile idiopathic (rheumatoid) arthritis. The age range for symptoms due to instability varies, as does the severity of symptoms; patients with cervical spine instability may be totally asymptomatic, or they may have severe neck pain with limitation of movement and neurologic deficits. The diagnosis is made using plain films of the cervical spine with open-mouth anteroposterior and lateral in neutral, flexion, and extension views. Three-dimensional CT reconstruction can also be used to diagnose instability. Treatment is surgical fusion; however, the decision to treat should be individualized, because many children with radiographic evidence of instability do not exhibit symptoms. As many as 15% of children with Down syndrome have cervical spine instability, but most experts agree that operative fusion should be performed only on those who are symptomatic. The one absolute indication for surgical fusion is the presence of neurologic symptoms, which may include difficulty walking, abnormal gait, neck pain, decreased mobility, sensory deficits, hyperreflexia, clonus, or other motor abnormalities.

Atlantoaxial Rotatory Subluxation (Grisel Syndrome)

Grisel syndrome is rare and presents with painful torticollis, most commonly after otolaryngologic procedures or upper respiratory infections. The cause is thought to be hyperemia of the tissues, leading to laxity of the atlantoaxial joint. The diagnosis is made by CT scan with three-dimensional reconstruction. Treatment consists of a cervical collar and anti-inflammatory medications until symptoms resolve. If reduction does not occur, cervical traction may be necessary. Rarely, a patient may require surgical fusion to maintain reduction.

Osteoid Osteoma

Osteoid osteomas are benign bone tumors characterized clinically by localized pain over the affected region. They most commonly occur in the lower extremities but may occur in the spine as well, in which case a painful secondary scoliosis may be evident. The cause of these lesions is unclear. They most commonly occur in older children and adolescents, with a 2:1 male predominance. The diagnosis can be made by plain films; a bone scan or CT provides more detail if the radiographs fail to show the typical appearance. Most osteoid osteomas are self-limited and gradually calcify and blend into surrounding bone. Depending on the location and degree of symptoms, treatment with nonsteroidal anti-inflammatory drugs may be sufficient. If not, surgical excision of the nidus is extremely effective.

Cervical Stenosis

In children, cervical stenosis is most often associated with achondroplasia. All children with this condition have abnormal growth of the pedicles with associated spinal stenosis. One third of patients with achondroplasia have symptomatic stenosis by age 15 years. Patients present with pain in the lower back and legs that is exacerbated by activity. MRI is diagnostic and can identify the extent of the stenosis. The treatment is surgical decompression.

Acute Cervical Disk Calcification

Disk calcification is thought to be due to a nonspecific inflammatory process. The average age at diagnosis is 7 years, with a 2:1 male predisposition. The child usually presents with fever and a painful, stiff neck. Examination reveals tenderness over the affected disk, most commonly in the cervical area. Radiographs show calcification of the intervertebral disk space 1 to 3 weeks after the onset of symptoms.

Treatment is symptomatic, with a cervical collar and anti-inflammatory medication. Most cases resolve within 2 to 3 weeks.

Neurologic Causes
Chiari I Malformation

Type I Chiari malformation is defined as descent of the cerebellar tonsils more than 5 mm below the foramen magnum. The cause is unknown. Classically, it presents with occipital headache or posterior neck pain lasting seconds to minutes, which is worsened by Valsalva maneuvers. The symptoms vary with the age of presentation. A review by Greenlee and coworkers showed that children younger than 3 years often present with oropharyngeal dysfunction, and older children present with more classic symptoms.[1] Although associated neurologic deficits are common, many patients with this malformation are asymptomatic. Up to 50% of individuals with type I Chiari malformation have an associated syrinx, or a collection of fluid caused by obstruction of CSF flow. The incidence of Chiari malformation has dramatically increased with the advent of MRI scanning, the diagnostic test of choice. Treatment, when indicated, is surgical decompression. Surgical treatment usually results in a decrease in size or resolution of an associated syrinx.

Vascular Causes
Spontaneous Arterial Dissection

Dissection of the cervical and intracranial portions of the carotid and vertebrobasilar arteries may occur spontaneously or in association with trauma or other underlying risk factors. Classically, patients present with head and neck pain in association with ataxia, vomiting, or other focal neurologic signs. Dissection is a known cause of stroke in children. In one study of vertebral artery dissection in children, half of those who had cervical radiographs had associated cervical anomalies.[2] Other possible causes of dissection include trauma and vasculopathy; in some cases, the cause is unknown. Dissection can occur at any age. A review of 68 cases by Hasan and colleagues showed a 6.6:1 male predominance and a median age of 9 years.[2] The diagnosis is made most accurately by angiography; in the future, magnetic resonance angiography may become the study of choice. Limited data are available regarding the most effective medical treatment of dissection in children and young adults. Most physicians consider antiplatelet or anticoagulation therapy, or both, even though there are no prospective studies evaluating the safety and efficacy of such treatments. Interventional neuroradiology may offer a new approach in difficult cases.

Oncologic Causes

Tumors causing neck pain can occur in a variety of locations, and the signs and symptoms vary with location. In general, pain is a prominent symptom. Patients often have associated neurologic deficits involving the cranial nerves or motor function. Sensory deficits are uncommon. Up to 25% of patients with neck or spinal tumors present with secondary scoliosis. Diagnosis is usually made by CT scan or MRI of the neck or spine. Treatment is dependent on the cause of the tumor.

Rheumatologic Causes
Arthritis and Spondyloarthropathy

The clinical picture of neck pain due to arthritis or other inflammatory conditions is typically an insidious onset of swelling in multiple joints in addition to the neck. The affected joints have limited motion and are warm, tender, and swollen. The cause of most inflammatory joint diseases is unknown. Polyarticular juvenile idiopathic (rheumatoid) arthritis has a biphasic incidence; onset is typically between 1 and 3 years or 8 and 10 years. There is a female predominance in the older group. With the spondyloarthropathies, involvement of the cervical spine increases with age and disease duration. The diagnosis is made by history and physical examination findings. Laboratory tests such as sedimentation rate, HLA typing, or specific antibodies may help support those findings (see Chapter 105).

Other Causes
Pneumomediastinum

Children with pneumomediastinum present with subcutaneous emphysema, throat or neck pain, and a crunching sound with systole (Hamman sign). The possible causes include trauma, with esophageal or tracheal disruption, and parenchymal lung disease, such as asthma or cystic fibrosis; it may also occur spontaneously or idiopathically. The age at presentation is variable, based on the underlying cause. In one review of the medical causes of pneumomediastinum, there was a 2:1 male predominance.[3] The diagnosis can be made by physical examination and by chest radiography. Treatment is usually supportive if there is a medical cause. If there is a history of trauma, surgical exploration may be indicated.

HISTORY AND PHYSICAL EXAMINATION

A thorough history and physical examination are warranted in all children presenting with neck pain. A few pieces of information from the history can quickly guide the examiner. Specifically, the presence or absence of fever and related complaints such as a sore throat, ear pain, headache, or vomiting might point one toward an infectious or inflammatory cause. Important information in the history of present illness includes the temporal onset of pain (acute, subacute, or chronic), whether it is progressive or static, location of pain, radiation of pain, and presence of associated neurologic symptoms, including bowel or bladder dysfunction, gait disturbance, or mental status change. Often a history of trauma is obvious or known, but eliciting a history of more subtle trauma is important. Family history can be helpful in some cases if the cause is rheumatologic or vascular. Because of the known associations among some conditions or syndromes, it is important to obtain a thorough past medical and surgical history, including medication use, genetic syndromes, bleeding disorders, and immunodeficiency.

The physical examination is extremely useful and can often point to a category of disease, if not a specific cause. It is important to note the general appearance of the patient, including his or her position of comfort. A thorough head, eyes, ears, nose, and throat examination should be performed, taking note of the oral structures, including the teeth and gums; nasal cavity; soft tissues of the lateral neck; ears; thyroid gland; and cervical vertebrae. It is important to look for any signs of respiratory distress, drooling, dental caries or oral abscess, enlarged or asymmetric tonsils, pharyngeal exudate, and facial or neck swelling. Special attention to the neck includes inspection for torticollis, head tilt, and skin lesions. Palpation is used to assess for masses, lymph nodes, fluctuance, and tenderness. In addition, one should note any decrease in neck mobility. Finally a complete neurologic examination is important to rule out nerve palsy, motor weakness, sensory deficit, and gait abnormality.

EVALUATION AND TREATMENT

The diagnostic evaluation of neck pain is guided by findings from the history and physical examination. It is critical to determine the adequacy of the airway in children who look toxic or are in acute distress. A lumbar puncture should be performed if meningitis is suspected. Other laboratory studies that can aid in the diagnosis include a rapid strep antigen test or culture of any purulent material obtained. If acute infection is suspected, markers of inflammation, including a complete blood count, erythrocyte sedimentation rate, and C-reactive protein, are useful. Radiologic studies are often helpful in the diagnosis of neck pain. Depending on the history and physical examination findings, a cervical spine series can identify any fracture, dislocation, or instability. A CT scan with contrast is useful for evaluating the soft tissue structures of the neck and can suggest a diagnosis of deep cellulitis or abscess. Following trauma, in addition to identifying fractures or dislocations and evaluating for soft tissue injury, a CT scan can identify injury to the trachea or esophagus. MRI is indicated if cervical osteomyelitis is suspected and for the evaluation of certain tumors. Magnetic resonance angiography may be necessary if vasculitis, penetrating trauma, or dissection of a vessel is suspected. Appropriate treatment of neck pain can be initiated once its cause has been determined.

SUGGESTED READING

Atlantoaxial instability in Down syndrome: Subject review. American Academy of Pediatrics Committee on Sports Medicine and Fitness. Pediatrics 1995;96:151-154.

Bliss SJ, Flanders SA, Saint S: Clinical problem-solving: A pain in the neck. N Engl J Med 2004;350:1037-1042.

Craig FW, Schunk JE: Retropharyngeal abscess in children: Clinical presentation, utility of imaging, and current management. Pediatrics 2003;111:1394-1398.

Greenlee JD, Donovan KA, Hasan DM, Menezes AH: Chiari I malformation in the very young child: The spectrum of presentations and experience in 31 children under age 6 years. Pediatrics 2002;110:1212-1219.

Nicklaus PJ, Kelley PE: Management of deep neck infection. Pediatr Clin North Am 1996;43:1277-1296.

Peters TR, Edwards KM: Cervical lymphadenopathy and adenitis. Pediatr Rev 2000;21:399-405.

Silverboard G, Tart R: Cerebrovascular arterial dissection in children and young adults. Semin Pediatr Neurol 2000;7:289-300.

Subach BR, McLaughlin MR, Albright AL, Pollack IF: Current management of pediatric atlantoaxial rotatory subluxation. Spine 1998;23:2174-2179.

Yassari R, Frim D: Evaluation and management of the Chiari malformation type 1 for the primary care pediatrician. Pediatr Clin North Am 2004;51:477-490.

REFERENCES

1. Greenlee JD, Donovan KA, Hasan DM, Menezes AH: Chiari I malformation in the very young child: The spectrum of presentations and experience in 31 children under age 6 years. Pediatrics 2002;110:1212-1219.

2. Hasan I, Wapnick S, Tenner MS, Couldwell WT: Vertebral artery dissection in children: A comprehensive review. Pediatr Neurosurg 2002;37:168-177.

3. Damore DT, Dayan PS: Medical causes of pneumomediastinum in children. Clin Pediatr (Phila) 2001;40:87-91.

CHAPTER 44

Petechiae and Purpura

Susan H. Frangiskakis

Petechial and purpuric rashes can cause even seasoned clinicians to become very concerned because they can signify dangerous disease such as meningococcemia, as well as more benign disorders such as viral infections. It is important for the pediatric hospitalist to have an approach to the evaluation and management of patients with petechiae or purpura. A more complete discussion of the individual disease entities associated with petechiae and purpura is provided in Chapter 150.

BACKGROUND

Petechiae and *purpura* are hemorrhages in skin or mucous membranes that are less than 2 mm in diameter or greater than 2 mm in diameter, respectively. These lesions do not blanch under diascopy. *Ecchymoses* are subcutaneous hemorrhages that are greater than 1 cm. *Purpura fulminans* is a progressive condition in which cutaneous infarctions occur and result in extensive skin necrosis.

PATHOPHYSIOLOGY

Petechiae and purpura can occur from a variety of pathophysiologic mechanisms that interfere with the complex process of hemostasis. Platelets, von Willebrand factor, and the coagulation cascade are essential for hemostasis. Thrombocytopenia, abnormal platelet function, von Willebrand factor defects, and clotting factor deficits can result in petechiae and purpura. Disruption of normal vascular integrity, such as occurs with endothelial injury as a result of infection or inflammation, can cause petechiae and purpura. Mechanical causes, such as trauma or increased intravascular pressure from coughing or vomiting, can cause petechiae and purpura by this mechanism as well. Intrinsically abnormal vascular components, such as collagen defects in connective tissue disorders, can result in these lesions. Ecchymoses are most often caused by trauma. Purpura fulminans typically occurs in the setting of bacterial sepsis and disseminated intravascular coagulopathy (DIC).

DIFFERENTIAL DIAGNOSIS

Because a number of different pathophysiologic mechanisms can cause petechiae or purpura, the differential diagnosis is extensive (Table 44-1). The clinical manifestations of bleeding disorders vary according to the underlying defect. Thrombocytopenia and abnormal platelet function typically result in petechiae, ecchymoses, and persistent bleeding from superficial cuts and mucosal membranes. Infection and vasculitis can cause petechiae or purpura, which can be palpable. Clotting factor deficits and other coagulation disorders typically cause hemarthroses, soft tissue bleeding, and prolonged bleeding, but they can also cause petechiae or

purpura. Von Willebrand disease is usually manifested as mucosal membrane bleeding, postsurgical bleeding, and menorrhagia, but it can result in petechiae. Disorders of vascular fragility can give rise to ecchymoses, as well as petechiae and purpura.

HISTORY AND PHYSICAL EXAMINATION

Some key information from the history and physical examination can help determine the most likely cause of the petechiae or purpura and help direct the appropriate steps in evaluation of the patient. See Table 44-2 for focused history questions and Table 44-3 for directed physical examination items.

The anatomic location of the skin lesions is suggestive but not definitive of certain disease processes. In general, petechiae solely above the nipple line suggest a benign cause such as vomiting or coughing. These Valsalve-like maneuvers cause spikes in intravascular pressure in the venous system of the head and neck. Lesions primarily on the buttocks and lower extremities are suggestive of Henoch-Schönlein purpura. Lesions in a stocking-glove or generalized distribution are more concerning for bacterial disease, although viruses can also give rise to this pattern, for instance, papular-pruritic glove-and-stocking syndrome caused by parvovirus B19.

EVALUATION

Children presenting with petechiae and purpura often warrant a complete blood count (CBC), including a platelet count and white blood cell (WBC) differential, peripheral blood smear, partial thromboplastin time (PTT), and prothrombin time (PT) performed to direct the remainder of the evaluation.

Children who present with fever and petechiae or purpura warrant immediate attention because this can be a medical emergency (see Chapter 62). Approximately 0.5% to 11% of children presenting with fever and petechiae or purpura have a serious bacterial infection. In addition to the initial screening laboratory tests mentioned, a blood culture and cerebrospinal fluid (CSF) studies, including cell counts, glucose, protein, Gram stain, and culture, should be obtained. If infection by group A β-hemolytic streptococcus is suspected, a rapid streptococcal test or culture of the oropharynx, or both, are indicated. Testing for viruses, such as adenovirus and influenza, may be performed, depending on the level of clinical suspicion. Other studies such as enteroviral polymerase chain reaction assay on CSF or Rocky Mountain spotted fever antibody titers may also be helpful in some settings. If DIC is suspected, fibrinogen, fibrin degradation product, and D-dimer studies of blood should be obtained.

Table 44-1   Causes of Petechiae and Purpura

General Mechanism	Categories	Examples
Disrupted vascular integrity	Infection	Bacterial (meningococcemia, pneumococcal or *Haemophilus influenzae* sepsis, group A streptococcal infections)
		Viral (adenovirus, enteroviruses, influenza A virus, Epstein-Barr virus, parvovirus B19)
		Rickettsial (Rocky Mountain spotted fever)
	Vasculitis	Henoch-Schönlein purpura, Kawasaki disease, systemic lupus erythematosus
	Mechanical	Trauma (accidental, nonaccidental, or birth related), coughing, vomiting
	Abnormal vascular components	Collagen vascular disorders (Ehlers-Danlos syndrome), vitamin C deficiency (scurvy)
Thrombocytopenia	Decreased platelet production	Leukemia, aplastic anemia, medications (sulfonamides, carbamazepine, valproic acid), vitamin B_{12} or folate deficiency
	Increased platelet destruction	Idiopathic thrombocytopenic purpura, hemolytic uremic syndrome, thrombotic thrombocytopenic purpura
	Splenic sequestration	Hypersplenism, consumptive hemangioma (Kasabach-Merritt syndrome)
Platelet dysfunction	Hereditary	Bernard-Soulier syndrome, Glanzmann thrombasthenia, storage pool disease
	Acquired	Medications (aspirin, nonsteroidal anti-inflammatory drugs), uremia
Coagulation defects	Hereditary	Factor deficiencies, factors VIII and IX most commonly (hemophilia A and B); von Willebrand disease; fibrinogen disorders
	Acquired	Liver disease, vitamin K deficiency, medications (heparin, warfarin), disseminated intravascular coagulopathy, clotting factor inhibitors

Note: Some causes may result in petechiae or purpura by more than one mechanism.

Table 44-2   Focused History

Characteristic	Questions
Onset and duration of lesions	Acute? Rapidly progressing? Recurrent or chronic?
Location of the lesions	Only above the nipple line? Only on the buttocks and lower extremities? In a stocking-glove distribution? Generalized? Involving the mucous membranes?
Predisposing factors	Coughing? Vomiting? Recent trauma? Recent illness such as an upper respiratory infection? Bloody diarrhea? Medications?
Systemic signs or symptoms	Fever? Irritability? Lethargy?
Review of systems	Headache? Stiff neck? Bleeding from other sites such as epistaxis or per rectum? Darkened urine? Joint pain or swelling? Abdominal pain? Bone pain? Myalgias?
Past medical history	Immunization status? History of prolonged bleeding?
Birth history for neonates	Was the mother ill? Did the mother have any medical conditions such as preeclampsia or lupus? Was the mother taking any medications?
Family history	Bleeding disorders? Siblings with conditions such as neonatal thrombocytopenia?

Children with an ill appearance, hypotension, decreased perfusion, or mental status changes, including irritability or lethargy, are more likely to have a serious bacterial infection. Laboratory evidence supporting a potential serious bacterial cause includes an abnormal peripheral WBC count, elevated C-reactive protein, abnormal PT, and abnormal CSF studies.

If the child does not have a fever or does not appear acutely ill and infection is not likely, the evaluation should be directed by the type of bleeding and clinical scenario. See Table 44-4 for suggested studies to work up various causes.

Some conditions such as viral infections, idiopathic thrombocytopenic purpura, and Henoch-Schönlein purpura are more common causes of petechiae and purpura in children. If the child is otherwise well and recently had a viral infection, idiopathic thrombocytopenic purpura would be likely. The child would be expected to have a decreased platelet count with a normal WBC count and hemoglobin. If this patient has an abnormal WBC count or is anemic, in addition to having thrombocytopenia, evaluation of a peripheral blood smear and assessment by a hematologist for condi-

Table 44-3 Directed Physical Examination

System	Physical Examination Findings
Vital signs	Febrile? Hypotensive?
General	Well or toxic appearing? Irritable? Lethargic?
HEENT	Bulging fontanelle? Pupils equal and reactive? Photophobia? Palatal petechiae? Erythematous oropharynx? Tonsillar exudates?
Neck	Nuchal rigidity? Kernig or Brudzinski signs?
Cardiovascular	New murmur? Capillary refill and extremity perfusion?
Abdomen	Hepatomegaly or splenomegaly? Tenderness?
Musculoskeletal	Joint swelling? Joint pain on movement?
Neurologic	Mental status? Focal findings?
Skin	Location of the lesions (e.g., at the site of the blood pressure cuff? Above the nipple line only? On the buttocks and lower extremities primarily? In a stocking-glove distribution or generalized?) Characteristics of the lesions (e.g., are the lesions palpable?). Quantity of lesions present?

HEENT, head, ears, eyes, nose, and throat.

Table 44-4 Evaluation of Petechiae and Purpura

Condition Suspected	Recommended Studies
Acute lymphocystic leukemia	CBC with platelet count and WBC differential, peripheral blood smear, PT, and PTT
Infection	Blood culture, CSF studies, CRP; consider a rapid streptococcal antigen test or oropharyngeal culture, respiratory viral cultures, specific viral antibody titers, RMSF antibody titers
Vasculitis	ESR, CRP, ANA, anti–double-stranded DNA antibody, complement levels (C3, C4, CH50); consider other specific autoantibody titers
Mechanical	Imaging studies for trauma, including head CT scan and skeletal survey for suspected nonaccidental trauma
Abnormal vascular components	Skin biopsy for Ehlers-Danlos syndrome or other collagen vascular disorders, ascorbic acid level
Thrombocytopenia	Consider bone marrow biopsy; urinalysis, BUN, creatinine
Platelet dysfunction	Bleeding time, platelet aggregation studies, clot retraction assay, BUN, creatinine
Coagulation defect	Specific clotting factor assays, thrombin time, fibrinogen level; bleeding time, factor VIII activity, von Willebrand factor antigen level, and ristocetin cofactor activity for von Willebrand disease; liver function tests, correction of PT and PTT after administration of vitamin K, mixing studies to detect factor inhibitors

ANA, antinuclear antibody; BUN, blood urea nitrogen; CBC, complete blood count; CH50, 50% hemolyzing dose of complement; CRP, C-reactive protein; CSF, cerebrospinal fluid; CT, computed tomography; ESR, erythrocyte sedimentation rate; PT, prothrombin time; PTT, partial thromboplastin time; RMSF, Rocky Mountain spotted fever; WBC, white blood cell.

tions such as leukemia are indicated. If the child has abdominal pain, arthritis, and hematuria, Henoch-Schönlein purpura should be considered, provided that the CBC, peripheral smear, PT, and PTT are normal (see Chapter 103).

TREATMENT

Treatment of petechiae and purpura is based on the underlying cause. Aggressive management with the administration of antibiotics and supportive care is warranted in cases concerning possible serious infectious disease (see Chapter 62). For example, meningococcemia can progress

very rapidly because of the release of a potent endotoxin, with the development of shock, purpura fulminans, and respiratory failure, and the patient can potentially die within hours of presenting. It is imperative that the administration of antibiotics not be delayed if there is difficulty obtaining the screening tests or cultures. Admission to a pediatric intensive care unit in cases of suspected bacterial sepsis is warranted for supportive care and frequent monitoring of vital signs, mental status, and the development of shock, respiratory failure, or DIC.

Hemorrhage from other sites needs to be evaluated in these patients. In some circumstances patients may require transfusions with red blood cells, platelets, fresh frozen plasma, or cryoprecipitate (see Chapters 119, 120, and 121).

SPECIAL CONSIDERATIONS

Neonatal Petechiae or Purpura

Petechiae and purpura in a neonate can be due to a number of unique causes in addition to those listed earlier, including birth trauma, TORCH (toxoplasmosis, other infection, rubella, cytomegalovirus, herpes simplex virus), other infections such as syphilis or human immunodeficiency virus infection, neonatal alloimmune thrombocytopenic purpura, congenital thrombocytopenic syndromes such as thrombocytopenia–absent radius syndrome, and congenital abnormalities of platelet function. It is critical to determine whether the neonate is well or ill in order to direct the investigation. If the neonate is ill, sepsis

and DIC must be strongly considered and addressed appropriately. If the neonate is well, one can proceed with the basic screening laboratory tests as stated earlier. Depending on these results, further investigation under the guidance of a hematologist or neonatologist may be helpful.

SUGGESTED READING

Brogan PA, Raffles A: The management of fever and petechiae: Making sense of rash decisions. Arch Dis Child 2000;83:506-507.
Mandl KD, Stack AM, Fleisher GR: Incidence of bacteremia in infants and children with fever and petechiae. J Pediatr 1997;131:398-404.
Nielsen HE, Anderson EA, Anderson J, et al: Diagnostic assessment of haemorrhagic rash and fever. Arch Dis Child 2001;85:160-165.
Wells LC, Smith JC, Weston VC, et al: How likely is meningococcal disease in a child with a non-blanching rash: A prospective cohort study. Arch Dis Child 2001;84(suppl 1):A10-A68.

CHAPTER 45

Respiratory Distress

Juliann Lipps Kim

Respiratory distress is one of the most common reasons for a child to present to the emergency department or a practitioner's office. Respiratory distress can result from disorders in the respiratory system or in organ systems that control or influence respiration. Young children have an increased risk for respiratory distress because of their anatomy and physiology. Nearly 20% of all emergency department visits for children younger than 2 years are for respiratory disease.[1] The causes of respiratory distress are vast, and practitioners caring for children should have a systematic approach to its diagnosis and management. Cardiopulmonary arrest in children is largely due to respiratory failure (in adults, cardiac causes are most common). Rapid evaluation and management of severe pediatric respiratory disease may be necessary to prevent respiratory failure.

PATHOPHYSIOLOGY

Understanding respiratory physiology can aid the practitioner in diagnosing the cause of respiratory symptoms. The main goals of respiration are oxygen uptake and elimination of carbon dioxide. Secondary goals include acid-base buffering, hormonal regulation, and host defense. To achieve the goals of respiration, three main functional components of the respiratory system are used: (1) mechanical structures (including chest wall, respiratory muscles, and pulmonary circulation), (2) membrane gas exchanger (interface between airspace and pulmonary circulation), and (3) regulatory system (network of chemical and mechanical sensors throughout the circulatory and respiratory systems). All three components are tightly integrated, and dysfunction of one can lead to respiratory distress or failure.

Respiratory function is tightly controlled by a complex network of central and peripheral chemoreceptors and mechanoreceptors responding to information from the body about the status of the respiratory system. This network modulates the neural output to the respiratory muscles, affecting the timing and force of respiratory effort. Central chemoreceptors in the ventral reticular nuclei of the medulla are sensitive to changes in pH and partial pressure of carbon dioxide (PCO_2) of cerebrospinal fluid. The intrinsic brainstem function of the dorsal and ventral respiratory centers of the medulla controls inspiration and expiration, respectively. The apneustic center in the pons increases the depth and duration of inspiration, whereas the pneumotaxic center decreases depth and duration. The cerebellum, hypothalamus, motor cerebral cortex, and limbic system also play a role in mediating respiration. Carotid and aortic bodies are peripheral chemoreceptors sensitive to the partial pressure of oxygen (PO_2), PCO_2, and pH in arterial blood. Mechanoreceptors (stretch, juxtacapillary, and irritant reflex) distributed along the airways, lung parenchyma, and chest wall respond to lung volume, changes in pulmonary microvasculature, chest wall muscle activity, and environmental irritants.

Information from central and peripheral receptors is integrated in the brainstem, and efferent impulses are transmitted to alter respiratory function and maintain homeostasis. Even slight alterations in arterial pH, PO_2, or PCO_2 stimulate the respiratory centers to modify the respiratory pattern. Increased arterial PCO_2 and decreased arterial PO_2 lead to an increase in respiratory drive and increased neural output to respiratory muscles. The resulting increase in ventilation can be achieved by increases in tidal volume or respiratory rate, because the product of these two factors determines the minute ventilation. Respiratory insufficiency or the more severe entity, respiratory failure, occurs when regulatory systems or the effector organs (lungs, respiratory muscles) are impaired or overwhelmed. This results in diminished oxygenation (decreased arterial PO_2), retention of carbon dioxide (increased arterial PCO_2), and acidosis (decreased arterial pH).

Disruption of the mechanics of the lung or chest wall results in the majority of respiratory disease in children.[2] Obstructive or restrictive disease leads to increased work of breathing and increased energy demands on the respiratory muscles to meet the body's needs. This increased work manifests itself clinically as respiratory distress, evidenced by increased work of breathing. When demand exceeds capability, the result is respiratory insufficiency, which can progress to respiratory failure. In respiratory muscle dysfunction, neural output is sent to the respiratory muscles, but they are unable to respond adequately to increase respiratory effort. The physical signs of respiratory failure in this setting are more subtle, and the signs of increased work of breathing may not be present. When the difficulty involves the control of breathing, there is an inadequate neural response to hypoxemia or hypercarbia. Arterial hypoxemia or hypercarbia without an increase in respiratory effort should lead one to suspect an anomaly in the neural control of breathing caused by central nervous system injury, drug-induced inhibition, or dysfunction of spinal motor neurons or nerve fibers innervating the respiratory muscles.

DIFFERENTIAL DIAGNOSIS

Respiratory difficulties may result from abnormalities within the respiratory system or from the dysfunction of organ systems influencing the respiratory system. Within the respiratory system, problems can arise from upper airway obstruction, lower airway obstruction, changes in gas diffusion from the alveolus to the capillary, abnormal pulmonary blood flow, or alterations in nerves and muscles that control breathing. Disease in other organ systems can compromise respiratory function directly or may induce compensatory respiratory mechanisms (Tables 45-1 and 45-2).

Table 45-1 Differential Diagnosis of Respiratory Distress

Respiratory System	Other Organ Systems
Upper airway (nasopharynx, oropharynx, larynx, trachea, bronchi) Anatomic: craniofacial abnormalities, choanal atresia, tonsillar hypertrophy, macroglossia, midface hypoplasia, micrognathia, laryngomalacia, tracheomalacia, hemangioma, webs, cysts, laryngotracheal cleft, papilloma, subglottic stenosis, vocal cord paralysis, tracheal stenosis, fistula, bronchomalacia, bronchogenic cyst Infectious: nasal congestion, peritonsillar abscess, tonsillitis, croup, epiglottitis, retropharyngeal abscess, tracheitis, bronchitis Environmental or traumatic: chemical or thermal burn, aspiration of foreign body Mass, including malignancy Inflammatory: angioneurotic edema, anaphylaxis	**Central nervous system** Structural abnormality: agenesis, hydrocephalus, mass, arteriovenous malformation Infectious: meningitis, encephalitis, abscess, poliomyelitis Dysfunction or immaturity: apnea, hypoventilation, hyperventilation Inherited degenerative disease: spinal muscular atrophy Intoxication or toxins: alcohol, barbiturates, benzodiazepines, opiates, tetanus Seizure Trauma: hemorrhage, birth asphyxia, spinal cord injury, anoxic encephalopathy Other: transverse myelitis, acute paralysis, myopathy
Lower airway (bronchioles, acini, interstitium) Inflammatory: asthma, allergy, angioneurotic edema, meconium aspiration, near drowning, gastroesophageal reflux, aspiration Infectious: bronchiolitis, pneumonia (bacterial, viral, atypical bacterial, *Chlamydia*, *Pertussis*, fungal, *Pneumocystis*), abscess Congenital malformation: congenital emphysema; cystic adenomatoid malformation; sequestration; pulmonary agenesis, aplasia, or hypoplasia; pulmonary cyst Environmental or traumatic: thermal or chemical burn, smoke, carbon monoxide, hydrocarbon, drug-induced pulmonary fibrosis, bronchopulmonary traumatic disruption, pulmonary contusion Other: bronchiectasis, interstitial lung disease, bronchopulmonary dysplasia, cystic fibrosis, pulmonary edema, hemorrhage, embolism, atelectasis, mass	**Peripheral nervous system** Phrenic nerve injury Environmental or toxins: tick paralysis, heavy metal poisoning, organophosphates, botulism, snakebite Metabolic: inborn errors of metabolism, carnitine deficiency, porphyria Inflammatory: dermatomyositis, polymyositis Other: Guillain-Barré syndrome, multiple sclerosis, myasthenia gravis, muscular or myotonic dystrophy, muscle fatigue
Chest wall and intrathoracic Pneumothorax, tension pneumothorax Pneumomediastinum Pleural effusion Empyema Chylothorax Hemothorax Diaphragmatic hernia Cyst, mass Spinal deformity (kyphoscoliosis) Pectus excavatum or carinatum Rib fracture, flail chest	**Cardiovascular** Structural: congenital heart disease, pericardial effusion, pericardial tamponade, aortic dissection or rupture, mass, coronary artery dilation or aneurysm, pneumopericardium, great vessel anomalies Other: arrhythmia, myocarditis, myocardial ischemia or infarction, congestive heart failure
	Gastrointestinal Appendicitis Necrotizing enterocolitis Mass (including hepatomegaly, splenomegaly) Ascites Obstruction Perforation, laceration Hematoma Contusion Esophageal foreign body
	Metabolic and endocrine Acidosis: fever, hypothermia, dehydration, sepsis, shock, inborn errors of metabolism, liver disease, renal disease, diabetic ketoacidosis, salicylates

Table 45-2 Common Causes of Respiratory Distress

Neonate	Infant or Child
Transient tachypnea of the newborn	Bronchiolitis
Sepsis	Pneumonia
Respiratory distress syndrome	Asthma
Pneumonia	Croup
Nasal obstruction or airway anomalies	Foreign body
Congenital heart disease	aspiration
	Fever
	Sepsis
	Metabolic
	derangements
	Allergy

INITIAL STABILIZATION

The first priority in evaluating a child with respiratory distress is to assess the airway, breathing, and circulation (ABCs). Rapid assessment and intervention can prevent the progression from respiratory compromise to respiratory failure. To assess the airway, determine whether it is patent, stable, and maintainable. If not, such an airway must be established (e.g., repositioning, instrumentation). Once these three criteria are met, the breathing process is evaluated by determining the respiratory rate, oxygen saturation, adequacy of breath sounds, and quality of respiratory effort (e.g., labored, use of accessory muscles). Determination of arterial blood gas levels may be needed if there is evidence of respiratory insufficiency or failure. If spontaneous ventilation is inadequate, assisted breathing with positive pressure, initially via a bag-mask device, is indicated. Assessment of the patient's circulation and mental status are other key aspects of the initial evaluation. Based on this rapid assessment, the clinician obtains information about the severity of the patient's condition and how rapidly interventions must be performed.

Providing supplemental oxygen is an important first step for a child presenting in distress, especially with hypoxemia demonstrated by oximetry. Oxygen can be delivered by multiple devices, and the choice depends on the child's clinical status and oxygen needs (see Chapter 38). Some of these devices can agitate a child further, worsening respiratory compromise. Allow the child to remain with the parent as much as possible, and use the least noxious form of oxygen delivery necessary. In a small number of children, airway adjuncts such as a nasopharyngeal airway, oropharyngeal airway, or assisted ventilation are needed. An oropharyngeal airway holds the tongue forward to prevent airway obstruction, so it will not be tolerated in a conscious or semiconscious patient with an intact gag reflex, and it may induce vomiting. A nasopharyngeal airway can be used in a conscious or unconscious patient but should be avoided in those with facial trauma. Continuous positive airway pressure may assist inspiratory efforts as well as provide positive end-expiratory pressure (PEEP). PEEP provides resistance to expiration, which may help expand atelectatic portions of the lung and thereby reduce ventilation-perfusion mismatch. Bilevel positive airway pressure provides inspiratory and expiratory

pressure via a firmly fitting facemask, which may be uncomfortable and not well tolerated in infants or young children (see Chapter 209).

Careful reevaluation after every intervention is critical to the care of a child with respiratory compromise. This confirms proper application of the intervention and monitors the patient's response.

HISTORY AND PHYSICAL EXAMINATION

Therapeutic interventions in an ill child should not be delayed to perform a detailed history. A focused history includes an assessment of respiratory and systemic symptoms (Box 45-1). For children with special needs or chronic respiratory problems, ask about the child's baseline respiratory status and how this episode is different.

Certain features of the physical examination are particularly important in determining the severity of respiratory distress and localizing the primary cause (Box 45-2). Vital signs help determine cardiopulmonary status but may be influenced by various factors. Fever increases the respiratory rate by approximately three breaths per minute for each degree Celsius above normal. Tachycardia commonly occurs as a response to the increased sympathetic tone in a child with respiratory distress; sympathetic tone is also increased with fever. Bradycardia is a late and ominous sign of severe hypoxia. Pulsus paradoxus (>10 mm Hg decrease in blood pressure during inspiration) can occur with severe pulmonary disease. Cyanosis is not evident until more than 5 g of hemoglobin are desaturated, which correlates with an oxygen saturation of less than 70% to 75%. Central cyanosis is evidenced by blue, gray, or dark purple discoloration of mucous membranes, most reliably assessed at the lips and tongue. Perioral cyanosis is not indicative of central cyanosis and likely represents local venous congestion. It is often seen with Valsalva-like maneuvers (e.g., crying) in fair-skinned infants. Acrocyanosis is often present in healthy newborns; in older children, it may be more suggestive of cardiovascular status (e.g., peripheral vasoconstriction secondary to hypotension). Pulse oximetry is a useful, noninvasive means of assessing hypoxia, but it has some limitations. It can be unreliable with low blood pressure, movement, or arterial PO_2 less than 50 mm Hg; if hemoglobin is bound to molecules other than oxygen (e.g., carbon monoxide); or if significant methemoglobinemia is present.

Restlessness or anxiety is associated with early hypoxia ("air hunger"), but the mental status can progress to somnolence and lethargy with hypercarbia and severe hypoxemia. The position of comfort can provide information about the location of dysfunction. Children with upper airway obstruction often sit upright with the neck extended to open the airway. Infants with laryngomalacia have more pronounced stridor in the supine position compared with the prone position. Inspiratory and expiratory noises can help localize the underlying process and may suggest cause. Stridor is a predominantly inspiratory monophasic noise indicating an extrathoracic airway obstruction. Upper airway obstruction can lead to acute deterioration and severe morbidity and mortality. Expiratory wheezing or stridor usually reflects intrathoracic obstruction; however, biphasic stridor may suggest a fixed lesion at any point along the airway. Grunting represents a child's attempt to increase the

Box 45-1   Components of a Focused History
Onset, duration, chronicity, character of symptoms
Alleviating and provoking factors
Treatment to date
Activity level
Respiratory symptoms
Cold symptoms
Cough (wet, dry, time of day)
Trouble breathing (rapid breathing, retractions, abdominal muscle use, "seesaw" respirations, positional distress)
Color change (pale, cyanotic)
Altered pattern of breathing (periodic, shallow or deep, bradypnea, apnea)
Inability to clear upper respiratory tract because of weakness or poor gag
Systemic symptoms
Fever
Poor feeding, fluid intake
Urine output
Weight loss or failure to gain weight
Emesis or diarrhea
Past medical history
Special health care needs or preexisting medical conditions (complex heart disease, chronic infections, prematurity)
Respiratory disease (asthma, cystic fibrosis)
Medications (respiratory treatments, oral medications, herbal supplements)
Allergies (medications, foods, environment)
Immunization status
Last oral intake (in case airway management becomes necessary)

Box 45-2   Directed Physical Examination
General
Level of consciousness (alertness, responsiveness)
Preferred position of child
Failure to thrive
Signs of prematurity
Respiratory
Airway
Nasal flaring
Inspiratory noises: seal-like barking, sonorous (nasal or pharyngeal), harsh (tracheal), high pitched (intrathoracic)
Symmetry of palate and tonsils
Prominence of posterior pharynx
Drooling
Inspection
Depth and quality of respirations
Retractions (subcostal, supraclavicular, intercostal)
Accessory muscle use
Symmetry of chest wall movement
Shape of chest (scoliosis, pectus excavatum or carinatum)
Auscultation
Air entry
Inspiration-to-expiration ratio
Rales or crackles
Wheezing (inspiratory or expiratory)
Symmetry of breath sounds
Presence of pleural rub
Cardiac
Murmur
Rhythm
Heart sounds
Thrill, rub, gallop
Quality of pulses
Capillary refill time
Color
Abdomen
Hepatomegaly
Splenomegaly
Mass
Ascites
Extremities
Clubbing
Deformities
Neurologic
Focal deficit
Cranial nerves
Muscle tone and strength
Evidence of increased intracranial pressure

PEEP and raise the functional residual capacity by closing the glottis during expiration.

Auscultation along the entire airway, including the nose, mouth, neck, and chest, may provide localizing information. The presence of rales, wheezing, or asymmetrical breath sounds and the duration of inspiration versus expiration are particularly noteworthy. The ratio of inspiration to expiration (I/E) is normally 1:1. Extrathoracic obstruction tends to prolong the inspiratory phase (e.g., I/E ratio of 3:1), whereas lower airway obstructive pathology, such as asthma or bronchiolitis, produces a prolonged expiratory phase (e.g., I/E ratio of 1:3).

Respiratory distress may be caused by nonrespiratory pathology or may have an impact on other organ systems. Detailed cardiac, abdominal, musculoskeletal, skin, and neurologic examinations should be performed.

EVALUATION

Further workup may be indicated to evaluate the severity of illness or its cause and should be guided by the clinical assessment. In children with chronic disease, compare laboratory studies and radiographs to previous studies, if available.

Pulse oximetry can detect hypoxemia but does not provide direct information about the adequacy of ventilation. Exhaled carbon dioxide levels can be measured with noninvasive devices, but this determination is used most often in the setting of endotracheal intubation. Arterial blood gas analysis can assess oxygenation (arterial PO_2) and ventilation (arterial PCO_2) and detect metabolic derangements of pH, bicarbonate, and base excess. Venous blood samples can provide some information about ventilation but are less useful for assessing oxygenation. The utility of obtaining other laboratory studies depends on the clinical setting and the diagnostic considerations.

Radiographs may be an important adjunct in the evaluation of a child with respiratory disease. Chest radiographs (anteroposterior and lateral views) are performed upright and on full inspiration whenever possible. Quality images can assist in the identification of airspace disease, hyperinflation, effusion, mass, foreign body, chest wall deformity or trauma, or cardiac abnormality. If an effusion is suspected, decubitus films may be helpful to determine whether the fluid shifts with gravity ("layers out"). Inspiratory and forced expiratory or bilateral decubitus chest films are useful to evaluate for the presence of a foreign body or other localized lower airway obstruction. An obstructing lesion can cause air trapping distal to the site. On an expiratory film, the unobstructed lung tissue decreases in volume and appears more dense, whereas the obstructed region is relatively hyperlucent. With decubitus films, the dependent (inferiorly positioned) lung should decrease in volume and appear denser, except for an obstructed region that remains inflated due to air trapping. When the patient's position is switched, the affected lung is superior and appears fully aerated, making the obstructed portion difficult to appreciate. If the obstruction is long standing, the obstructed portion may become atelectatic or fluid filled and appear as a persistent density in the various views.

Lateral and anteroposterior radiographs of the neck are useful for the evaluation of upper airway obstruction, allowing the visualization of retropharyngeal, supraglottic, and subglottic spaces. These films may be useful to diagnose retropharyngeal abscess, epiglottitis, foreign body aspiration, or tracheitis. Ill children with suspected upper airway obstruction should not be sent to the radiology department unattended or should have films deferred until they are stabilized.

Other imaging modalities to consider are computed tomography (CT), magnetic resonance imaging (MRI), airway fluoroscopy, and barium swallow studies. CT evaluates cervical and thoracic structures in greater detail and may help identify areas of intrinsic or extrinsic compression. Mediastinal, pleural, and pulmonary parenchymal abnormalities are well identified with CT. MRI is particularly helpful to delineate hilar and vascular anatomy. Airway fluoroscopy provides dynamic pictures of the respiratory system, including the airways and diaphragm. Barium swallow studies are helpful in the evaluation of patients with recurrent pneumonia, persistent cough, stridor, or wheezing. The anatomy of the gastrointestinal tract from the mouth to the stomach is revealed, and compression along the esophagus may suggest a lesion that is compressing the airway as well. Contrast material is mixed with substances of different consistencies and textures, ranging from thin liquids to thick liquids to solids. Barium swallow studies evaluate swallowing mechanics and the presence of vascular rings, tracheoesophageal fistulas, and gastroesophageal reflux.

TREATMENT

Acute interventions should not be delayed in a child with respiratory distress, regardless of the underlying cause. Restoration of oxygenation and ventilation is the main priority. Airway patency should be established and maintained, followed by a rapid assessment of breathing and circulation. Oxygen delivery should be initiated using the least noxious form possible that provides an adequate fraction of inspired oxygen (FIO_2), and the child should be placed on cardiopulmonary monitors, including pulse oximetry. Airway adjuncts may be necessary to maintain patency. If these are unsuccessful, or if oxygenation and ventilation are inadequate, endotracheal intubation may be indicated. Breathing treatments (albuterol, racemic epinephrine, ipratropium bromide) may be useful in certain clinical situations, including asthma, bronchiolitis, or croup. Further therapies are determined by the underlying cause of respiratory distress.

SUGGESTED READING

Barren JM, Zorc JJ: Contemporary approach to the emergency department management of pediatric asthma. Emerg Med Clin North Am 2002;20:1.

Haddad GG, Palazzo RM: Diagnostic approach to respiratory disease. In Behrman RE, Kliegman RM, Jenson HB (eds): Nelson Textbook of Pediatrics. Philadelphia, WB Saunders, 2004, pp 1363-1370.

Infosino A: Pediatric upper airway and congenital anomalies. Anesthesiol Clin North Am 2003;20:4.

Perez Fontan JJ, Haddad GG: Respiratory pathophysiology. In Behrman RE, Kliegman RM, Jenson HB (eds): Nelson Textbook of Pediatrics. Philadelphia, WB Saunders, 2004, pp 1376-1379.

Ruddy RM: Evaluation of respiratory emergencies in infants and children. Clin Pediatr Emerg Med 2002;3:156-162.

Stevenson MD, Gonzalez del Rey JA: Upper airway obstruction: Infectious cases. Clin Pediatr Emerg Med 2002;3:163-172.

REFERENCES

1. Weiner DL: Respiratory distress. In Fleisher GR, Ludwig S (eds): Textbook of Pediatric Emergency Medicine. Philadelphia, Lippincott Williams & Wilkins, 2000, pp 553-564.

2. Perez Fontan JJ, Haddad GG: Respiratory pathophysiology. In Behrman RE, Kliegman RM, Jenson HB (eds): Nelson Textbook of Pediatrics. Philadelphia, WB Saunders, 2004, pp 1376-1379..

CHAPTER 46

Syncope

Sarah C. McBride

Syncope is defined as an abrupt and transient loss of consciousness. Patients experience an altered level of cognitive ability followed by a brief period of unconsciousness that resolves spontaneously to a baseline level of function. The causes of syncope are heterogeneous among pediatric patients, but the autonomic nervous system is commonly involved. Less frequently, syncope is due to neurologic or cardiac causes. Despite its common occurrence during childhood, syncope can cause significant anxiety among patients, families, school personnel, and physicians. It is important for the pediatric hospitalist to develop a practical approach to the evaluation of syncope, with the goal of identifying the rare individual at risk for serious underlying pathology.

BACKGROUND

Syncope, also known as fainting, blackout spells, or falling out, occurs when inadequate cerebral perfusion results in a transient loss of consciousness and postural tone. Presyncope describes an event that does not include full loss of consciousness. Girls more commonly present for the evaluation of syncope than do boys, with a peak incidence between 15 and 19 years of age.[1] Most causes of syncope in pediatric patients are isolated and benign in nature. In fact, the risk of sudden death among patients with prior syncopal events is equivalent to the risk of sudden death in the general population.[1]

Syncope can be classified into three major categories: cardiac, autonomic (neurocardiogenic or vasovagal), and metabolic. Regardless of the cause, syncope is the end result of inadequate cerebral perfusion. This may be due to ineffective systemic blood flow (autonomic, cardiogenic) or compromised capacity to provide oxygen or glucose (metabolic).

CARDIAC SYNCOPE

Syncope may occur when there is obstruction to cardiac outflow, myocardial dysfunction, or a cardiac arrhythmia (Table 46-1). Patients who have a prior history of surgery for congenital cardiac lesions are often at increased risk for acquired and residual structural lesions, myocardial dysfunction, and supraventricular or ventricular arrhythmias. Therefore, a cardiologist should evaluate any patient with a prior cardiac history who presents with syncope.

Cardiac syncope caused by an obstruction to blood flow usually occurs in association with exertion or exercise. It is often related to a fixed or dynamic obstruction due to a structural lesion or an obstruction resulting from pulmonary vascular disease. Myocardial dysfunction commonly results in syncope due to an associated cardiac arrhythmia. However, when the dysfunction leads to poor stroke volume, cardiac output is inadequate to meet increased demands

(e.g., exertion), and syncope can result. Although mitral valve prolapse is generally asymptomatic in the pediatric population, it is worth mentioning because of its prevalence. It is now believed that when syncope occurs in patients with mitral valve prolapse, the causes are multifactorial and may involve either autonomic dysfunction or arrhythmia, depending on the nature and severity of mitral valve dysfunction.[2]

The diagnosis of myocardial dysfunction can usually be achieved by clinical examination, electrocardiogram (ECG), and echocardiography. Cardiac arrhythmias causing syncope are unusual in patients with structurally normal hearts. Supraventricular arrhythmias generally cause palpitations rather than syncope. However, atrioventricular nodal bypass tracts, which occur in Wolff-Parkinson-White syndrome, may cause rapid conduction of atrial flutter or fibrillation to the ventricles, resulting in syncope or sudden death. Ventricular arrhythmias occur more frequently in postoperative patients with congenital heart disease but may also be seen in patients with structurally normal hearts. Long QT syndrome predisposes patients to ventricular arrhythmias by its characteristic prolongation of the QT interval corrected for heart rate (QTc), which places patients at risk for a polymorphic ventricular tachycardia known as torsades de pointes. Tachycardia begins with a characteristic short-long-short sequence caused by premature ventricular depolarization, followed by a long pause. The escape complex that forms in response to this pause is associated with a prolonged repolarization, which causes premature ventricular depolarization that can initiate tachycardia. If prolonged, torsades de pointes can lead to cardiac arrest or death as it degenerates into ventricular fibrillation. In some patients, an ECG demonstrating borderline Q-Tc prolongation may be consistent with the upper range of normal. However, many ECG findings become more exaggerated with an increased heart rate as the Q-Tc fails to shorten appropriately with the R-R interval. Brief and self-resolving periods of rhythm disturbances causing syncope may be precipitated by exercise or a startling experience. Other reported ECG manifestations of long QT syndrome include bradycardia, atrioventricular block, and abnormal T-wave morphologies. Congenital causes of long QT syndrome include Jervell and Lange-Nielsen syndrome and Romano-Ward syndrome. Acquired causes include electrolyte disturbances (e.g., hypokalemia, hypocalcemia, hypomagnesemia), increased intracranial pressure, and medications (e.g., tricyclic antidepressants, phenothiazines, antiarrhythmics).

AUTONOMIC SYNCOPE

Also known as neurocardiogenic, vasovagal, or vasodepressor syncope, autonomic syncope is responsible for the majority of childhood syncopal episodes. A common

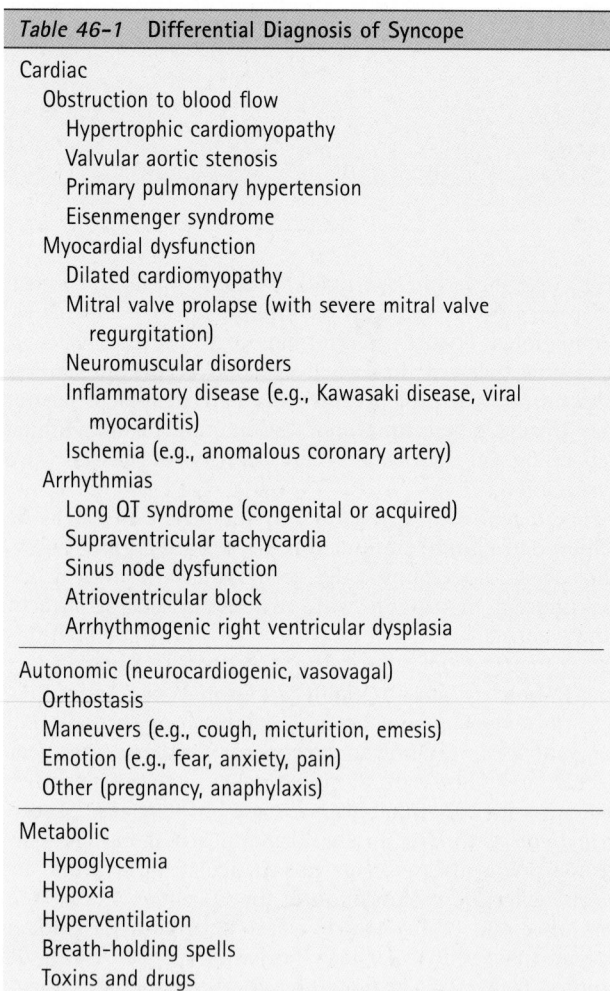

Table 46-1 Differential Diagnosis of Syncope

Cardiac
  Obstruction to blood flow
    Hypertrophic cardiomyopathy
    Valvular aortic stenosis
    Primary pulmonary hypertension
    Eisenmenger syndrome
  Myocardial dysfunction
    Dilated cardiomyopathy
    Mitral valve prolapse (with severe mitral valve
      regurgitation)
    Neuromuscular disorders
    Inflammatory disease (e.g., Kawasaki disease, viral
      myocarditis)
    Ischemia (e.g., anomalous coronary artery)
  Arrhythmias
    Long QT syndrome (congenital or acquired)
    Supraventricular tachycardia
    Sinus node dysfunction
    Atrioventricular block
    Arrhythmogenic right ventricular dysplasia

Autonomic (neurocardiogenic, vasovagal)
  Orthostasis
  Maneuvers (e.g., cough, micturition, emesis)
  Emotion (e.g., fear, anxiety, pain)
  Other (pregnancy, anaphylaxis)

Metabolic
  Hypoglycemia
  Hypoxia
  Hyperventilation
  Breath-holding spells
  Toxins and drugs

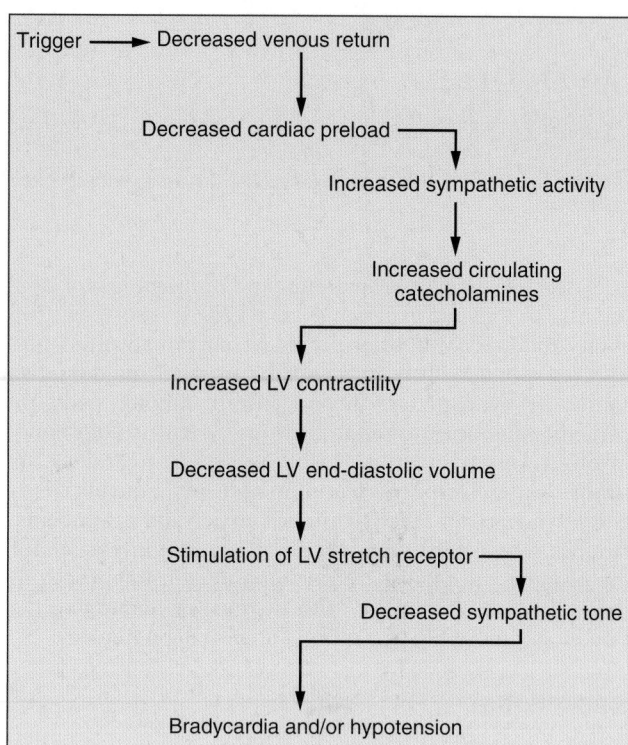

Figure 46-1 Autonomic syncope cascade. LV, left ventricular.

progression of symptoms begins with a prodrome lasting seconds to minutes, followed by a brief period of unconsciousness, after which the patient arouses to a previous level of alertness. The premonitory symptoms may include lightheadedness, dizziness, nausea, pallor, shortness of breath, diaphoresis, and visual changes.

The mechanism of autonomic syncope is likely a cascade of events. Many triggers are known to precipitate autonomic syncope, although their exact mechanisms of action are not clearly understood. Physical stressors such as anemia, dehydration, hunger, illness, and physical exhaustion can predispose patients to syncopal episodes. Orthostatic hypotensive syncope occurs during an excessive or prolonged decrease in blood pressure upon assuming an upright position. When an individual assumes an upright posture or is exposed to a sudden physical or emotional stress, a sequence of events that culminates in syncope is triggered (Fig. 46-1). In this scheme, the hypotensive cardioinhibitory response, which is mediated by the left ventricular stretch receptors, causes a paradoxical withdrawal of sympathetic activity in response to myocardial stretch. This normal response to stretch receptor stimulation, as occurs in hypertension or hypervolemia, results in hypotension. Meanwhile, enhanced parasympathetic activity leads to bradycardia. Therefore, before syncope itself occurs, patients exhibit variable degrees of

both bradycardia and hypotension. It is unknown why this abnormal progression of events occurs.

METABOLIC SYNCOPE

Metabolic derangements that can lead to syncope include hypoglycemia, hypoxia, and hyperventilation. In general, these conditions produce more persistent symptoms that require intervention and are usually unaffected by position or activity. Presentations may include a depressed level or loss of consciousness or seizure activity. Diaphoresis, tremor, and altered mental status may precede hypoglycemic syncope. Hypoxia may initially present with agitation, but increasing somnolence ensues as the hypoxemic state continues. Hyperventilation may lead to loss of consciousness if cerebral vasoconstriction occurs due to resultant hypocapnia. Drugs and toxin exposure can cause syncope in addition to altering consciousness, and some can induce cardiac arrhythmias, which may also present as syncope.

Breath-holding spells are common among young children. They typically start with crying, followed by apnea (often at end-expiration), then cyanosis or pallor, and ultimately a brief syncopal event with limpness. A prompt return to a normal level of consciousness occurs following the event. Hypoxia and hypocapnia are thought to be significant factors that lead to the loss of consciousness.

CONDITIONS THAT MIMIC SYNCOPE

Table 46-2 lists a number of conditions that can mimic syncope. For example, a seizure may mimic a syncopal episode, but a seizure generally lasts longer than several seconds and may include a preceding aura, abnormal move-

Table 46-2	Conditions That Mimic Syncope
Neurologic	
Seizure	
Migraine	
Cerebrovascular accident	
Psychogenic	
Hysteria	
Malingering	
Munchausen syndrome	
Munchausen syndrome by proxy	

ments, and a postictal period. Atypical migraines can present with syncope-like spells and may include a preceding aura or severe headache.

Spells caused by hysteria can mimic true syncope and occur mostly in adolescent patients. A detailed history of the event usually supports this diagnosis and may include a preceding period of stress or hyperventilation while in the presence of others. Patients who have a full recollection of the event are less likely to have suffered a full loss of consciousness. Although uncommon, malingering, Munchausen syndrome, or Munchausen syndrome by proxy may present with a history of a syncope-like episode. Features that support these diagnoses include the patient's or parent's strong desire for extensive or invasive evaluation or therapy.

EVALUATION

The patient history and physical examination can provide valuable clues to the diagnosis and may curtail or circumvent the need for further diagnostic evaluation.

Recent circumstances and those immediately preceding the event should be thoroughly explored. Because patients are often unable to provide details of an episode, witnesses to the event are important. Past medical history, especially with regard to previous syncopal episodes, cardiac or neurologic conditions, and medications, should always be obtained. Specific inquiries into the family history should include sudden death, syncope, sudden infant death syndrome, congenital heart disease, seizures, and congenital deafness (associated with Jervell and Lange-Nielsen syndrome).

Although the findings are often normal, a thorough physical examination should be performed. Blood pressure measurements and evaluation of distal pulses in both the supine and upright positions and from both upper extremities and a lower extremity should be obtained. Cardiac examination may reveal a gallop, murmur, or click, which raises the concern for a primary cardiac cause.

An ECG should be performed as part of all initial evaluations for syncope, with special attention paid to the Q-Tc interval and T-wave morphology for evidence of long QT syndrome. In addition, voltage criteria for ventricular hypertrophy suggestive of an obstructive lesion, the preexcitation of Wolff-Parkinson-White syndrome, and ectopy and conduction disturbances should be ruled out during ECG interpretation. In a patient with a normal ECG but a history suspicious for a cardiac arrhythmia, a 24-hour ambulatory Holter monitor may aid in the diagnosis if the episodes are frequent. In a patient whose episodes are isolated or less frequent, an event monitor that can be turned on to record during symptomatic events may be more appropriate. In general, a more extensive cardiovascular evaluation is indicated if syncope occurs with exertion and in cases in which there is chest pain preceding the loss of consciousness, seizure activity, recurrent syncope, or an abnormal cardiac examination.

Laboratory testing is easily performed and, if indicated, should include a blood glucose level and complete blood count. If a toxic ingestion is suspected, a serum and urine toxicology screen should be obtained. Because hypoxia due to carbon monoxide poisoning can lead to syncope, co-oximetry with a carboxyhemoglobin level should be considered when indicated by the circumstances. A pregnancy test is indicated in teenaged girls with syncope.

An electroencephalogram or imaging of the central nervous system is often part of an evaluation when epilepsy or other neurologic causes are being considered.

TREATMENT

Standard resuscitative interventions should be instituted for acute syncopal events. Therapeutic intervention to prevent or treat recurrent syncope depends on the pathogenic cause and the frequency and severity of the episodes.

The treatment of cardiogenic syncope is generally overseen by a cardiologist and is based on a careful and thorough diagnostic evaluation to determine the underlying abnormality. Suppression of symptomatic supraventricular arrhythmias is often managed with medication, but treatment varies based on the inciting or propagating feature of the disorder. Patients with long QT syndrome may benefit from β-adrenergic antagonists to prevent exercise-induced ventricular arrhythmia, but pacemakers or implanted cardiac defibrillators are necessary in some cases. Surgical intervention may be needed for structural abnormalities, and intensive care interventions are required for those with progressive or unstable conditions.

Autonomic syncope is considered a benign illness, and in most cases, prophylaxis against presyncope or near syncope is sufficient intervention. Educating patients and families generally results in earlier awareness of symptoms and the ability to abort episodes by assuming a recumbent posture. Additional measures for prophylaxis include the avoidance of dehydration, a salt-enriched diet, and, in some cases, the use of mineralocorticoids to induce salt and water retention. When simple prevention strategies fail, treatment with β-adrenergic receptor blockade is often used to decrease stimulation of the cardiac mechanoreceptors. Disopyramide, an anticholinergic, negative inotropic, and vasoconstrictive agent, is effective in some patients. Finally, direct α-adrenergic receptor stimulation and stimulation of peripheral norepinephrine release can be tried. It is important to remember that no pharmacologic agent has been consistently efficacious in clinical trials.[3] Atrioventricular pacing has been used in patients with frequent episodes of symptomatic bradycardia, but this is reserved for refractory cases when pharmacologic agents are unsuccessful.

The treatment of metabolic syncope focuses on the underlying process, both in the acute resuscitation phase and in the prevention stage. Identification of a causative entity often allows patients and families to prevent future syncopal events or to manage such events safely if they occur.

SUGGESTED READING

Mark AL: The Benzold-Jarisch reflex revisited: Clinical implications of inhibitory reflexes originating in the heart. J Am Coll Cardiol 1983;1:90-102.

Sapin SO: Autonomic syncope in pediatrics: A practice-oriented approach to classification, pathophysiology, diagnosis, and management. Clin Pediatr 2004;43:17-23.

Scott W: Syncope and the assessment of the autonomic nervous system. In Allen HD, Gutgesell HP, Clark EB, Driscoll DJ (eds): Moss and Adam's Heart Disease in Infants, Children, and Adolescents, 6th ed. Philadelphia, Lippincott Williams & Wilkins, 2001, pp 443-451.

Tanel RE, Walsh EP: Syncope in the pediatric patient. Cardiol Clin 1997;15:277-294.

REFERENCES

1. Driscoll DJ, Jacobsen SJ, Porter CJ, Wollan PC: Syncope in children and adolescents. J Am Coll Cardiol 1997;29:1039-1045.

2. Boudoulas H, Wooley CF: The floppy mitral valve, mitral valve prolapse, and mitral valvular regurgitation. In Allen HD, Gutgesell HP, Clark EB, Driscoll DJ (eds): Moss and Adam's Heart Disease in Infants, Children, and Adolescents, 6th ed. Philadelphia, Lippincott Williams & Wilkins, 2001, p 964.

3. Calkins H: Pharmacologic approaches to therapy for vasovagal syncope. Am J Cardiol 1999;84:20Q-25Q.

CHAPTER 47

Vomiting

Amber M. Hoffman

Vomiting is a common symptom in childhood and is a common complaint or diagnosis for pediatric patients admitted to the hospital. It can lead to dehydration, hypokalemia, hypochloremia, metabolic alkalosis, aspiration pneumonia, esophagitis, Mallory-Weiss tears, gastritis and hematemesis, and weight loss. Most commonly, vomiting is caused by a self-limited infectious gastroenteritis, but it can be a presenting sign of illness in nearly every organ system.

PATHOPHYSIOLOGY

Vomiting occurs when the contents of the stomach (and occasionally the small intestine) are forcefully expelled out of the mouth. This simple description belies the fact that vomiting is an extremely complex process that is mediated both locally and centrally.

The vomiting centers of the brain lie in the reticular formation of the medulla. Here they receive signals from a number of sources that trigger vomiting:

- Chemoreceptor zone in the brainstem, which lies under the floor of the fourth ventricle. These receptors detect chemical abnormalities in the body (e.g., uremia, ketoacidosis, emetic drugs) and trigger the vomiting centers.
- Afferent signals from the gastrointestinal (GI) tract. These signals come from the vagus and other sympathetic nerves due to gastrointestinal distention or mucosal irritation.
- Afferent signals from outside the GI tract. These signals come from other organs located in the thorax and abdomen. This explains why a disease outside of the GI tract (e.g., urinary tract infection) often presents with vomiting.
- Afferent signals from extramedullary centers in the brain. There are a number of other triggers caused by signals from other parts of the brain. Examples include vomiting due to cerebral trauma (e.g., concussion, increased intracranial pressure), vestibular disturbance (e.g., motion sickness), or other stimuli (e.g., fear, anxiety, noxious odors).

DIFFERENTIAL DIAGNOSIS

It is important for the hospitalist to remember that vomiting is rarely a diagnosis; it is far more often a symptom of another process. Owing to the numerous signals that can trigger vomiting, illness in virtually every organ system can cause vomiting. The occurrence of these diseases also varies considerably by age (Tables 47-1 to 47-3).

Gastrointestinal Causes

Vomiting is often associated with the GI tract, and the causes of vomiting in this organ system are numerous. They can be divided into obstructive and nonobstructive causes.

Among the obstructive forms, many present early in life with nonbilious emesis if the obstruction is proximal to the ampulla of Vater, and bilious emesis when it is distal. Esophageal atresia causes nonbilious emesis with feeding. In this condition, a nasogastric tube cannot pass to the abdomen, and a gasless abdomen is seen on the abdominal radiograph unless there is also a tracheoesophageal fistula that can deliver air into the stomach by a connection distal to the atretic portion of the esophagus. Duodenal atresia has the classic "double bubble" appearance on radiographs, showing air in the stomach and air that has passed by the pylorus and remains trapped in the duodenum. This can cause either bilious or nonbilious emesis, depending on the level of atresia. Between the age of 2 weeks and 2 months, pyloric stenosis results in projectile nonbilious emesis that can eventually lead to hypochloremic metabolic alkalosis. On abdominal examination, one can occasionally palpate an "olive" in the epigastric region, which is the hypertrophied pylorus. Ultrasonography can confirm the diagnosis.

Obstructive intestinal disorders beyond the ampulla of Vater often present with bilious emesis. Malrotation with midgut volvulus is a surgical emergency that can occur at any age but generally presents in infancy. Any infant with bilious emesis should be suspected of having intestinal malrotation. It can be evaluated with a barium swallow followed at least to the ligament of Treitz. Ileal and jejunal atresia, stenosis, or duplication may also cause emesis that can become bilious. Echogenic loops of bowel on prenatal ultrasonography can be an indication of intestinal atresia.

Meconium plugs can cause vomiting that improves once the obstruction has passed. They sometimes pass on their own or may require surgical excision. Meconium plugs have a much higher incidence in children with cystic fibrosis. Colonic atresia or stenosis, imperforate anus, microcolon, or Hirschsprung disease should also be considered in cases of colonic obstruction.

Intussusception can have a variety of presentations, including vomiting. Paroxysms of severe abdominal pain, vomiting, and lethargy often occur. Occasionally a sausage-shaped mass can be palpated in the right lower quadrant, which is the ileum invaginating though the ileocecal valve into the colon. "Currant jelly" stools present late in the course as the lining of the intestine becomes ischemic and necrotic.

Complications from torsion of Meckel's diverticulum around its fibrous attachment to the abdominal wall, incarcerated hernias, and adhesions from prior abdominal surgeries can all cause obstruction and vomiting. Foreign bodies can obstruct the pylorus or esophagus in toddlers who often swallow nonfood items such as coins; nonmetal items are sometimes radiopaque. It is helpful for parents to bring along any items they think the child might have swallowed

Table 47-1 Common Causes of Vomiting in Newborns and Infants

Benign
　Overfeeding
　Aerophagia
　Innocent spitting
　Excessive handling
　Parental anxiety

Neurologic
　Hydrocephalus
　Subdural bleeding
　Cerebral edema
　Kernicterus

Genitourinary
　Obstructive uropathy
　Pyelonephritis

Pulmonary
　Bronchiolitis
　Pertussis
　Reactive airway disease
　Pneumonia

Metabolic or endocrine
　Urea acid cycle defects
　Aminoacidopathies
　Organic acidopathies
　Hypercalcemia
　Glycogen storage disease
　Fatty acid oxidation defects—MCAD deficiency
　Galactosemia
　Congenital adrenal hyperplasia

Gastrointestinal
　Gastroesophageal reflux
　Milk protein intolerance
　Allergy
　Eosinophilic enteritis
　Lactobezoar
　Gastritis
　Intestinal atresia or stenosis
　Intestinal duplication
　Hiatal or diaphragmatic hernia
　Pyloric stenosis
　Malrotation
　Vovulus
　Meconium plug or ileus
　Annular pancreas
　Hirschsprung disease
　Hepatitis
　Pancreatitis, necrotizing enterocolitis, imperforate anus, microcolon

Other infections
　Meningitis (viral or bacterial)
　Gastroenteritis (viral or bacterial)

Other
　Medications
　Munchausen syndrome by proxy

MCAD, medium-chain acyl-CoA dehydrogenase.

Table 47-2 Common Causes of Vomiting in Infants and Toddlers

Neurologic
　Hydrocephalus
　Subdural bleeding
　Cerebral edema
　Kernicterus
　Benign paroxysmal vertigo
　Migraine
　Cyclic vomiting
　Tumor or mass

Genitourinary
　Obstructive uropathy
　Pyelonephritis
　Renal failure
　Ovarian or testicular torsion

Pulmonary
　Bronchiolitis
　Pertussis
　Reactive airway disease or asthma
　Pneumonia

Metabolic or endocrine
　Urea acid cycle defects
　Aminoacidopathies
　Hypercalcemia
　Glycogen storage disease
　Congenital adrenal hyperplasia
　Fatty acid oxidation defects—MCAD deficiency

Gastrointestinal
　Gastroesophageal reflux
　Milk protein intolerance
　Lactose intolerance
　Allergy
　Eosinophilic enteritis
　Celiac disease
　Bezoar
　Foreign body
　Gastritis
　Intestinal stenosis or adhesions
　Intestinal duplication
　Hiatal hernia
　Malrotation
　Volvulus
　Annular pancreas
　Hepatitis
　Pancreatitis
　Intussusception
　Incarcerated hernia
　Meckel's diverticulum

Other infections
　Meningitis (viral or bacterial)
　Gastroenteritis (viral or bacterial)
　Appendicitis
　Otitis
　Sinusitis
　Postviral gastroparesis

Other
　Medications
　Poisoning
　Munchausen syndrome by proxy
　Psychogenic

Table 47-3 Common Causes of Vomiting in Children and Adolescents

Neurologic	**Gastric or duodenal ulcer**
Subdural bleeding	Intestinal stenosis or adhesions
Cerebral edema	Hiatal hernia
Benign paroxysmal vertigo	Malrotation
Migraine	Volvulus
Cyclic vomiting	Annular pancreas
Tumor or mass	Hepatitis
Concussion	Pancreatitis
	Cholecystitis, cholelithiasis
Genitourinary	Intussusception
Obstructive uropathy	Incarcerated hernia
Pyelonephritis	Meckel's diverticulum
Renal failure	
Ovarian or testicular torsion	**Other infections**
Pregnancy	Meningitis (viral or bacterial)
	Gastroenteritis (viral or bacterial)
Pulmonary	Appendicitis
Pertussis	Otitis
Reactive airway disease or asthma	Sinusitis
Pneumonia	*Helicobacter pylori*
	Postviral gastroparesis
Metabolic or endocrine	
Inborn errors of metabolism	**Rheumatologic or immunologic**
Diabetic ketoacidosis	Crohn's disease
Addison's disease	Scleroderma
	Chronic granulomatous disease
Gastrointestinal	
Gastroesophageal relux	**Other**
Lactose intolerance	Medications
Allergy	Poisoning
Eosinophilic enteritis	Munchausen syndrome by proxy
Celiac disease	Psychogenic
Bezoar	Anorexia
Foreign body	Bulimia
Gastritis	

so that they can be radiographed alongside the child to determine whether they are radiopaque. Bezoars are more common in toddlers or older children with developmental delays who eat hair, carpet, or other unusual items that build up over time. Lactobezoars can occur in young infants.

Achalasia, cricopharyngeal incoordination, hiatal and diaphragmatic hernias, duodenal webs, duodenal hematomas, intestinal strictures, and vascular rings or slings can also cause emesis. An aberrant subclavian artery can compress the esophagus as well as the upper airway. If a child has stridor or monophonic midline wheezing, this type of compression should be considered. Superior mesenteric artery syndrome can occur in children who have lost weight, have prominent lordosis, or are bed ridden for a period of time. The duodenum is thought to become compressed between the aorta and the artery, and food cannot pass this obstruction easily.

Vomiting in infants and young children can also have a variety of nonobstructive GI causes. Many infants have effortless emesis or regurgitation after feeding or handling that does not cause discomfort or other signs of systemic problems. Rumination can occur in young or older children.

Improper mixing of formula, generally rendering it too concentrated, can cause emesis. Overfeeding is a notorious cause of vomiting in infancy. Aerophagia from crying, gulping formula or breast milk, inadequate burping, excessive handling after feeding, and parental nervousness or stress are also nonorganic causes of vomiting in young children and infants.

More aggressive investigations or interventions should be undertaken when the emesis is persistent or forceful or leads to other complications. Gastroesophageal reflux alone can lead to hematemesis, apnea, aspiration pneumonia, failure to thrive, wheezing, coughing, and Sandifer syndrome. A history of spitting up after feeding, back arching, crying with feeding, or increased symptoms when supine should increase one's suspicion for gastroesophageal reflux. Necrotizing enterocolitis should be suspected in a newborn or premature baby with vomiting followed by abdominal distention or a toxic appearance. The classic radiographic findings are pneumatosis intestinalis and, after perforation, hepatic portal venous gas. Necrotizing enterocolitis can be managed with antibiotics early in the course when there is just feeding intolerance, distention, and mild pneumatosis intestinalis; if it is not identified quickly, however, it may progress and require surgical intervention when perforation occurs.

Another GI cause of emesis is related to allergy or intolerance. Milk protein intolerance or enteropathy can cause severe vomiting, diarrhea, bloody stools, and failure to thrive. It responds to elemental formulas. Lactose intolerance can run in families and may be the source of vomiting in a child. Isolated food allergies can cause both vomiting and abdominal pain, as well as rash, urticaria, respiratory distress, swelling, and anaphylaxis. Eosinophilic enteritis can present with emesis, reflux, and abdominal pain. It may be isolated to the esophagus, stomach, or intestine or involve multiple regions. It is often associated with food and environmental allergies. Identification of allergens by serum testing, skin-prick testing, and delayed hypersensitivity patch testing is important to allow removal of the allergen. Current treatments include elemental formulas, topical steroids such as fluticasone (which is swallowed rather than inhaled), and systemic steroids.

Celiac disease classically presents as vomiting, weight loss, behavior problems, diarrhea, and failure to thrive in children 9 months to toddler age. It can also present later in life with less classic symptoms. It is caused by gluten sensitivity that leads to villus atrophy and subsequent malabsorption. Once gluten is completely removed from the diet, the vomiting stops and the symptoms improve as the villi have time to recover.

Cholecystitis, cholelithiasis, and choledocholithiasis can present with colicky, right upper quadrant pain after meals. These conditions occur more commonly in children with rapid red blood cell turnover, such as occurs in sickle cell disease or hereditary spherocytosis. They can also be seen in children subjected to prolonged total parenteral nutrition or may be secondary to medications.

Pancreatitis in children is often viral in origin, but it can also be secondary to structural abnormalities. An annular pancreas or pancreas divisum can cause pancreatitis due to intrinsic ductal abnormalities or, in the case of annular pancreas, due to obstruction of the duodenum by wrapping around it. Stress, drugs, and trauma are also common causes of pancreatitis in children. Children with cystic fibrosis as well as those who carry the *CFTR* gene mutation are at higher risk for pancreatitis. In fact, several genes have been implicated in hereditary forms of pancreatitis.

Hepatitis from viruses, toxins, drugs, or metabolic causes such as Reye syndrome may cause emesis. Gastritis and gastric or duodenal ulcers can be stress induced, secondary to allergy or medicine, or caused by *Helicobactor pylori*.

Nongastrointestinal Causes

Numerous medications can cause vomiting either by direct gastric irritation or the stimulation of nausea. Chronic nonsteroidal anti-inflammatory drugs can cause a severe gastritis that leads to ulceration and hematemesis. Common antibiotics, particularly amoxicillin–clavulanic acid and erythromycin, can cause both vomiting and diarrhea as unwanted side effects. Chemotherapeutic agents and radiation are notorious for causing nausea and vomiting. Some children develop vomiting before receiving these therapies as a behavioral response secondary to prior negative experiences.

There are several neurologic causes of vomiting. Migraine headaches can affect even young children, who may be unable to identify the location of pain, aura, or scotoma. Caregivers note only the vomiting. Motion sickness can cause significant nausea and vomiting and often exists in families with a history of migraines. Cyclic vomiting presents primarily with vomiting and abdominal pain, but children may also report headache or vertigo. Cyclic vomiting sometimes responds to cyproheptadine, antiemetics, or intravenous fluids until the episode has passed. Familial dysautonomia is an autosomal recessive autonomic neuropathy that can result in vomiting crises, along with excessive sweating, rashes, ataxia, seizures, and irritability.

Increased intracranial pressure may initially present with nausea and headache. If the intracranial pressure is from an expanding mass such as a tumor, hydrocephalus, or vascular malformation, intractable vomiting can develop. Accompanying features may include headache and visual changes. A headache that awakens a child from sleep, is constant, or worsens with Valsalva maneuvers is worrisome. Blurry vision, diplopia, and visual field cuts are also suggestive of increased intracranial pressure. Idiopathic intracranial hypertension can stimulate nausea and vomiting as well as cause headache. It has a higher incidence in obese females and in teenagers on acne medications such as isotretinoin, tetracycline, or minocycline. Subdural hematomas from accidental or nonaccidental trauma, as well as cerebral edema from trauma or infection such as meningitis, may present with vomiting before other neurologic signs are seen. Vomiting can also occur during or after a seizure or following a concussion.

Otitis media and benign paroxysmal positional vertigo (BPPV) are two otologic causes of vomiting. Otitis media can disturb the vestibular system, and the vomiting improves with treatment of the infection. In older patients, BPPV can be diagnosed by using the Dix-Hallpike maneuver to elicit vertical-torsional nystagmus characteristic of BPPV. The symptoms often respond to physical maneuvers to reposition loosened particles from the utricular macula that float in the long arm of the posterior semicircular canal and stimulate the sensation of vertigo. In young children with BPPV, cyproheptadine and other antihistamines are sometimes helpful. Sinusitis can also stimulate vomiting secondary to persistent postnasal drip. Posterior oropharyngeal bleeding from epistaxis or bleeding after a tonsillectomy and adenoidectomy can lead to hematemesis.

Infectious causes of vomiting are numerous, with the majority being viruses. Norovirus, rotavirus, enterovirus, and adenovirus often cause self-limited episodes of emesis. Bacterial causes include but are not limited to *Staphylococcus aureus* (toxin mediated), *Bacillus cereus, Shigella, Salmonella, Escherichia coli, Yersinia enterocolitica,* and *Campylobacter jejuni*. Group A streptococcal pharyngitis often causes vomiting in children. Appendicitis presents with nausea, vomiting, anorexia, fever, and periumbilical pain that migrates to the right lower quadrant. Children with peritonitis from a perforation or those with severe inflammation often demonstrate rebound, guarding, or a Rovsing sign on examination. Appendicitis in young children can be difficult to diagnose because they may have no signs of anorexia and appear to have only diffuse abdominal pain. Viral or bacterial meningitis also stimulates nausea and vomiting. A postviral gastroparesis can delay gastric emptying and cause vomiting and decreased appetite that can last for months. Parasitic infections, such as ascariasis, can also cause obstructions leading to vomiting.

The respiratory system is occasionally responsible for emesis. Children with pertussis can have such violent paroxysms of coughing that they have post-tussive emesis. The respiratory signs of lower lobe pneumonia in children can be overshadowed by such severe abdominal pain and emesis that children sometimes undergo evaluations for appendicitis that reveal pneumonia on the higher cuts of an abdominal computed tomography scan. Bronchiolitis or excessive crying can cause aerophagia, which can stimulate emesis.

Cardiovascular causes of vomiting are generally related to arrhythmia or heart failure. Supraventricular tachycardia in a young infant can cause irritability and feeding intolerance. A child with heart failure secondary to a ventricular septal defect or other congenital or acquired cardiac abnormality can also have emesis or feeding intolerance. Vomiting can also be a sign of heart transplant rejection.

The genitourinary system can cause vomiting in several ways. Pyelonephritis, nephrolithiasis, ureteropelvic junction obstruction, and renal insufficiency can all present at various ages with emesis. Torsion of the ovary or testis causes severe pain along with emesis in some cases. Nausea from pregnancy is a cause of vomiting not to be overlooked in teenaged girls.

The endocrine system can be implicated in vomiting in several ways. Children with diabetic ketoacidosis begin to have intractable vomiting as they become more ketotic and acidotic, leading to further dehydration and worsening of their condition. Vomiting is a prominent feature of salt-wasting congenital adrenal hyperplasia, which should be suspected in a female infant with any sign of virilization. Male infants with this form of congenital adrenal hyperplasia usually have normal genitals, and their condition may be mistaken for gastroesophageal reflux or pyloric stenosis. Addison's disease can present with vomiting during a crisis.

Metabolic and mitochondrial diseases should also be considered in a young child or infant with persistent vomiting. Hypercalcemia, hypokalemia, hypoglycemia, and hyperammonemia can all cause emesis. Urea acid cycle defects such as ornithine transcarbamylase deficiency generally present in newborns with emesis, lethargy, coma, and death if not recognized and treated aggressively. Even those with partial defects may have more exaggerated vomiting illnesses in childhood. Aminoacidopathies such as tyrosinemia can present with vomiting in children aged 2 weeks to 1 year. Organic acidopathies such as maple syrup urine disease, isovalericacidemia, mevalonicacidemia, propionicacidemia, and methylmalonicacidemia present with vomiting in infancy. Lactic acidosis, fatty acid oxidation defects, particularly medium-chain acyl-CoA dehydrogenase deficiency, glycogen storage disease, and galactosemia have vomiting as a primary presenting feature as well. Porphyria can present with periods of vomiting, change in mental status, or rash, depending on the subtype. Mitochondrial diseases are often associated with intestinal dysmotility or pseudo-obstruction. These children often have a long history of gastroesophageal reflux, feeding intolerance, abdominal pain, constipation or diarrhea, and failure to thrive. Leigh disease, also known as subacute necrotizing encephalomyelopathy, usually presents in infancy with feeding or swallowing difficulties, failure to thrive, and vomiting.

Psychological causes of vomiting include anorexia nervosa, bulimia, hyperventilation, and severe anxiety. Accidental and nonaccidental poisoning with toxins such as lead, household cleaners, or medications such as acetaminophen, aspirin, or digitalis can stimulate emesis.

Munchausen syndrome by proxy should be suspected in cases of recurrent emesis that occurs only when a certain caregiver is present or when there are discrepancies in the case. Vomiting can be induced with drugs such as ipecac. Some medications and toxins can be found by urine, stool, or serum toxicology screens. Video surveillance is the easiest way to capture the perpetrator; however, this can be difficult to do for legal reasons, and many hospitals are not equipped for covert video surveillance. Apparent hematemesis can also be secondary to Munchausen syndrome by proxy. A transfusion with tagged red blood cells and a nuclear scan right after an episode of hematemesis can prove that the blood is not from the child.

Drug and alcohol abuse in children and teenagers can lead to emesis. Alcohol can cause emesis due to overdose as well as withdrawal. Withdrawal symptoms can begin anywhere from hours to a week after the cessation of alcohol ingestion. Patients can have tremor, anxiety, depression, nausea, vomiting, diaphoresis, tachycardia, hallucinations, seizures, and delirium tremens in severe cases. Abused opioids such as heroin, codeine, and hydromorphone can cause vomiting within hours of ingestion or during the withdrawal period, which can last for weeks. Other associated signs of withdrawal include tachycardia, irritability, pupillary dilation, diarrhea, and rhinorrhea.

Some recreational drugs can cause emesis during acute intoxication. Gamma hydroxybutyrate (GHB)—also known as Liquid Ecstasy, Liquid X, Georgia Home Boy, Grievous Bodily Harm, and Easy Lay—is a date-rape drug that causes sedation, amnesia, euphoria, and hallucinations. The more toxic effects include nausea, vomiting, loss of peripheral vision, respiratory depression, and coma. Ketamine can be ingested orally or nasally, smoked, or injected. It has dissociative effects and causes nystagmus, hallucinations, and vomiting.

HISTORY AND PHYSICAL EXAMINATION

A thorough history and physical examination are warranted in all children presenting with vomiting. A few pieces of information from the history can quickly guide the examiner: How old is the patient? What is the nature of the emesis? Bilious or nonbilious? Bloody or nonbloody? Is the vomiting associated with eating? Are there associated GI complaints, such as diarrhea? Are there associated systemic signs, such as fever or failure to thrive? A complete review of systems can help find associations that either rule in or rule out serious disease. Timing of the emesis, progression of symptoms, and exposures are important historical factors to investigate.

The physical examination is directed first at an overall assessment of the patient: Does the patient appear well, ill, or toxic? Is the patient febrile or afebrile? Are there signs of cardiovascular instability? What is the patient's hydration status? Careful examination of the abdomen is also required.

Does the patient try to avoid unnecessary movement, suggesting peritonitis? Are there signs of nonfocal tenderness or abdominal distention, suggesting obstruction? A complete physical examination must be performed to assess for nongastrointestinal causes of vomiting.

EVALUATION AND TREATMENT

Given the extensive differential diagnosis of vomiting, there is no such thing as a routine workup. Laboratory and radiographic studies should be ordered only after a complete history and physical examination are completed, to at least guide the evaluation process. For example, bilious emesis in a neonate necessitates an emergent evaluation for malrotation. In contrast, an older child with dehydration due to vomiting and diarrhea from an apparent viral gastroenteritis may need no evaluation beyond the history and physical examination.

Treatment also varies significantly, based on the cause. Oral rehydration can be used in those with less pathologic causes of vomiting and in those who can tolerate it. Isotonic intravenous fluids should be given during fluid resuscitation in children with life-threatening disease or in those who cannot tolerate oral rehydration. Correctly diagnosing the vomiting disorder is the key to determining additional treatment beyond rehydration.

SUGGESTED READING

Behrman RE, Kliegman RM, Jenson HB (eds): Nelson's Textbook of Pediatrics, 16th ed. Philadelphia, WB Saunders, 2000, pp 347-348, 354-362, 377-378, 406, 413, 1846.

Green M (ed): Pediatric Diagnosis. Interpretation of Symptoms and Signs in Children and Adolescents, 6th ed. Philadelphia, WB Saunders, 1998, pp 212-223.

Koesters SC, Rogers PD, Rajasingham CR: MDMA ("ecstasy") and other "club drugs": The new epidemic. Pediatr Clin North Am 2002;49:415-433.

McRae AL, Brady KT, Sonne SC: Alcohol and substance abuse. Med Clin North Am 2001;85:799-801.

Morinville V, Perrault J: Genetic disorders of the pancreas. Gastroenterol Clin North Am 2003;32:763-787.

Tunnessen W Jr (ed): Signs and Symptoms in Pediatrics, 3rd ed. Philadelphia, Lippincott Williams & Wilkins, 1999, pp 491-507.

Zitelli BJ: Persistent vomiting. In Gartner JC Jr, Zitelli BJ (eds): Common and Chronic Symptoms in Pediatrics. St Louis, Mosby, 1997, pp 275-289.

PART III

Systems Approach

Neonatology

CHAPTER 48

Delivery Room Medicine

Marissa de Ungria and Jennifer Daru

The transition from fetal to newborn physiology is a complicated process. For a normal transition to occur, a well-orchestrated sequence of physiologic changes must transpire. Difficulties encountered may be due to prenatal events, events that occur as a result of the delivery process itself, or events caused by influences that occur in the immediate postnatal period. Conditions that may be tolerated in utero may be ill suited to extrauterine life. The rapidity with which the changeover occurs makes prompt assessment and intervention important.

PHYSIOLOGY

Fetal physiology relies on the placenta as the organ of gas exchange, nutrition, metabolism, and excretion. In the fetoplacental circulation, most of the oxygenated blood flows from the placenta through the umbilical vein and is shunted away from the high-resistance pulmonary circuit of the lungs, via the foramen ovale and the ductus arteriosus, into the low-resistance systemic circuit. Fetal blood is relatively hypoxemic, with an arterial PaO_2 of 20 to 30 mm Hg and oxyhemoglobin saturation of 75% to 85%. However, compensatory mechanisms are in place that allow adequate tissue oxygenation and growth of the fetus to occur. Fetal oxygen consumption is decreased and the red cell mass is increased in comparison to that of a newly born infant. In addition, fetal hemoglobin has increased affinity for oxygen.

The adaptation from intrauterine life to extrauterine life starts during the process of labor. Labor not only increases oxygen consumption in the transitioning fetus but also causes brief periods of asphyxia during contractions as umbilical venous blood flow is briefly interrupted. The fetus tolerates this interruption in blood flow because fetal tissue beds have greater resistance to acidosis than adult tissue beds do. The fetus responds to bradycardia with the "diving reflex" whereby blood preferentially flows to the brain, heart, and adrenal glands. Finally, the fetus is capable of switching to anaerobic sugar production, provided that liver glycogen stores are adequate.

During labor and delivery, catecholamine levels surge and increase lung fluid resorption, release of surfactant, and stimulation of gluconeogenesis. This surge also helps direct blood flow to vital organs such as the heart and brain. With clamping of the umbilical cord, the low-resistance placental circuit is removed from the newborn's circulation. Systemic blood pressure increases, and transition to the postnatal circulation begins.

As a newly born infant takes the first few breaths, negative intrathoracic pressure is generated, which helps the lungs expand and become filled with air. Alveolar oxygenation increases as air replaces the fetal lung fluid. The negative intrathoracic pressure, however, is countered by lung compliance, lung fluid viscosity, and surface tension forces. Because these factors need to be overcome to establish adequate alveolar expansion, the infant must take deep enough breaths to create the large transpulmonary pressure initially required after birth. Surfactant, a phospholipid-protein complex that is produced by type II pneumocytes and is deposited along the alveolar surfaces, also helps counteract alveolar surface tension and promote alveolar stability. As a result of the increasing effect of surfactant, less transpulmonary pressure is needed for subsequent breaths, and functional residual capacity (FRC) is soon established. Pulmonary blood flow increases as the lungs expand, and pulmonary vascular resistance declines under the influence of oxygen-mediated relaxation of the pulmonary arterioles. This increase in pulmonary blood flow in turn allows the patent foramen ovale and the patent ductus arteriosus to functionally close, thereby allowing further blood flow to the lungs. The postnatal circulation is now that of a low-resistance pulmonary circuit and high-resistance systemic circuit, and the lungs assume the responsibility of gas exchange and oxygenation.[1]

Amazingly, the majority of newly born infants make the transition from fetal to postnatal circulation without significant difficulty. However, it is estimated that 5% to 10% of newborn infants need some degree of resuscitation in the delivery room.[2] One percent of newborn infants require intensive delivery room resuscitation to survive. Birth asphyxia accounts for approximately 19% of the 5 million neonatal deaths per year.[3] Delays in establishing effective cardiorespiratory function could increase the risk for hypoxic-ischemic cerebral injury, pulmonary hypertension, and systemic organ dysfunction. Some of these injuries may be preventable with prompt and appropriate resuscitation. However, some of these outcomes are related to events or exposures that precede the birth process, such as prenatal injuries, abnormal development, and insults to the intrauterine environment, among many others.

Multiple maternal, placental, mechanical, and fetal problems may occur at any point in the process of pregnancy, labor, or delivery and can jeopardize a smooth fetus-to-newborn transition. The fetoplacental circulation can be compromised for a variety of reasons. All of these circumstances may cause deceleration of the fetal heart rate and in turn can result in hypoxia and ischemia. In the case of maternal hypotension, the maternal side of the placenta is inadequately perfused. In placental abruption, gas exchange between the fetus and mother is impaired. Blood flow from the placenta or through the umbilical cord (or both) may be compromised, such as with cord compression. A fetus with intrauterine growth restriction may be intolerant of even brief and intermittent interruptions of umbilical blood flow during contractions.

Insufficient respiratory effort as a result of respiratory distress syndrome, maternal narcotic administration, or anesthesia will hamper lung expansion and replacement of fetal lung fluid with air. Abnormal ion transport within the lung interstitium can also lead to retained fetal lung fluid.[4,5] Foreign material such as meconium or blood may obstruct the neonate's airway and prevent adequate lung inflation. The end result of any of these situations is inadequate alveolar oxygenation, which in turn sets the stage for the development of persistent pulmonary hypertension of the newborn (PPHN). In this condition, which is also known as persistent fetal circulation, the pulmonary arterioles remain constricted, thereby preventing adequate blood flow to the lungs and resulting in hypoxia and acidosis. Hypoxia and acidosis mediate sustained constriction of the pulmonary arterioles, and a vicious cycle ensues as progressively deoxygenated blood circulates. Transitional physiology does not occur normally, and unoxygenated blood is shunted away from the high-pressure lung circuit. Systemic organ dysfunction and, more importantly, long-term neurologic compromise may result. Other causes of PPHN include problems that cause systemic hypotension, such as excessive blood loss or hypoxia-induced cardiac dysfunction.

Asphyxia is defined as failure of gas exchange leading to a combination of hypoxemia, hypercapnia, and metabolic acidemia. If adequate ventilation and pulmonary perfusion are not rapidly established, a progressive cycle of worsening hypoxemia, hypercapnia, and metabolic acidemia ensues. Initially, blood flow to the brain and heart is preserved, whereas blood flow to the intestines, kidneys, muscles, and skin is sacrificed. However, maintenance of blood flow, even to vital organs, cannot be sustained endlessly. Ultimately, ongoing ischemia, hypoxia, and acidosis result in myocardial dysfunction and impaired cardiac output. Inadequate blood flow, perfusion, and tissue oxygenation result in brain injury, multiorgan injury, and even death.

CLINICAL PRESENTATION

Clinical signs and symptoms of disrupted fetal-to-neonatal transition include cyanosis, bradycardia, hypotension, decreased peripheral perfusion, depressed respiratory drive, and poor muscle tone. Apgar scoring is an assessment tool used in the first minutes of life. It helps guide initial resuscitation needs, but early scores are not reliable predictors of long-term outcome. Table 48-4 provides the scoring system. The newborn is assessed at 1, 5, and 10 minutes, and if the infant remains unstable, an assessment may be performed at 20 minutes. A score of 0 to 3 indicates the need for immediate or ongoing resuscitation. A commonly used mnemonic for this tool is APGAR:

A = appearance (color)
P = pulse (heart rate)
G = grimace (reflex irritability)
A = activity (muscle tone)
R = respirations (respiratory effort)

Asphyxia is a medical condition manifested by

1. Profound umbilical arterial metabolic or mixed acidemia with a pH lower than 7
2. An Apgar score of 0 to 3 beyond 5 minutes of life
3. Neonatal sequelae such as seizures, hypotonia, or coma
4. Multiple organ dysfunction

Gestational Age Assessment

Assessing the gestational age of an infant at delivery is a crucial element of both a full-term and premature newborn's physical examination. Infants may mature and grow at different rates, so an assessment of gestational age by physical examination should be done after birth, regardless of a mother's last menstrual period or ultrasound examination. In 1991 the "New Ballard Score" was published to include an assessment of the gestational age of infants ranging from mature to extremely premature. This assessment tool (Fig. 48-1) requires the examiner to perform a detailed neuromuscular and physical evaluation.

The Ballard Score may be calculated by first tallying a score for the neuromuscular section of the examination:

1. Posture: Examine the supine infant's tone at rest. To elicit, gently stimulate the extremities of the supine infant and see what position the infant returns to. This "preferred position" should be scored according to the diagram.
2. Square window: Extend the infant's fingers and gently press the palm of the hand toward the forearm. The resulting distance between the palm and the forearm is then scored.
3. Arm recoil: Support the elbow of a supine infant and gently flex and then extend the arm. Let go of the arm and record the angle to which it recoils.
4. Popliteal angle: The supine, undiapered infant's leg is pressed up toward the abdomen. Once the infant is comfortable, gently extend the lower part of the leg by grasping the foot while supporting the upper part of the leg. When resistance to extension is felt, score the angle between the upper and lower part of the leg.
5. Scarf sign: The supine infant's head is placed midline, and then the hand is moved across the chest. Gentle pressure is put on the elbow to extend the arm further across the chest. When resistance is felt, the score is based on elbow position relative to the body.
6. Heel to ear: The supine undiapered infant's leg is supported laterally against the body with the hip in a flexed position. The lower part of the leg is extended until resistance is felt at the pelvic girdle. The position of the heel relative to the ear is recorded.

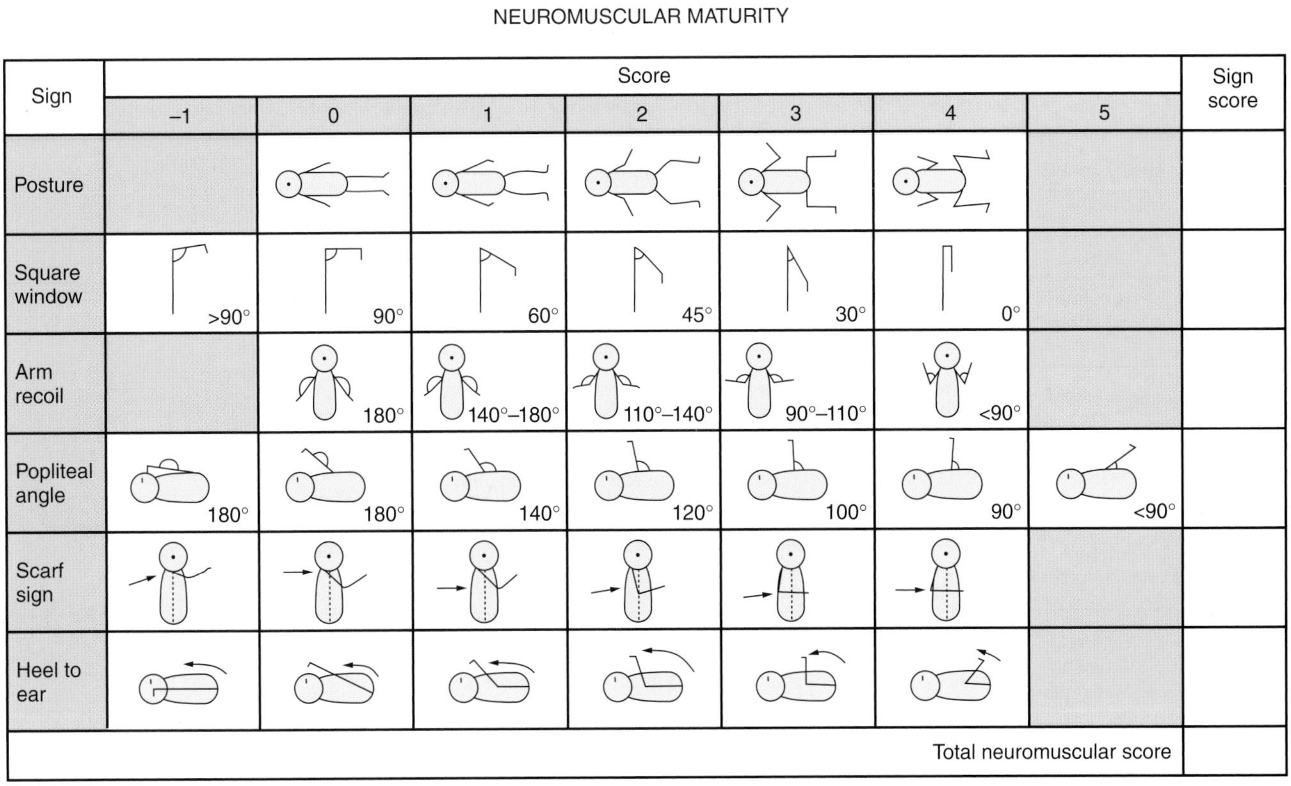

NEUROMUSCULAR MATURITY

Sign	Score							Sign score
	−1	0	1	2	3	4	5	
Posture								
Square window	>90°	90°	60°	45°	30°	0°		
Arm recoil		180°	140°–180°	110°–140°	90°–110°	<90°		
Popliteal angle	180°	180°	140°	120°	100°	90°	<90°	
Scarf sign								
Heel to ear								
						Total neuromuscular score		

A

Figure 48-1 New Ballard Score sheet. Use this score sheet to assess the gestational maturity of your baby. At the end of the examination the total score determines the gestational maturity in weeks. (From Ballard JL, Khoury JC, Wedig K, et al: New Ballard Score, expanded to include extremely premature infants. J Pediatr 1991;119:417–423.)

The second portion of the Ballard examination is performed through simple observation by scoring skin maturity, the fine hair or lanugo of the infant, and the infant's plantar surface, breast, eye/ear, and genital maturity. A score is then tallied for the physical maturity section of the Ballard instrument.

The two sections are then added together and the total placed on a chart corresponding to the gestational age of the infant. It is crucial that the examiner does not add the two halves of the examination and consider this score the gestational age of the infant.

The final score should be used to plot the infant for length, head circumference, and weight and will help determine whether an infant is appropriate, large, or small for gestational age and thus indicate whether treatment or tests are required. In addition, premature infants may require different therapies based on the Ballard examination (such as prophylaxis for respiratory syncytial virus).

TREATMENT

Optimizing Delivery Room Resuscitation

Anticipation, adequate preparation, accurate evaluation, and prompt initiation of support are critical for successful neonatal resuscitation. High-risk infants should be identified early. Many of the conditions that place newly born infants at risk for disrupted transition are listed in Table 48-1. Communication between physicians delivering infants and the resuscitation team is essential. If a high-risk delivery is antic-

ipated, a prenatal consultation by the pediatric team should be performed if time permits. Resuscitation equipment should be readily available for each and every birth, and personnel attending deliveries should be familiar with the organization of the equipment so that resuscitation can be promptly initiated and support provided. Equipment should be checked at regular intervals and immediately before any delivery. Expiration dates of medications should be monitored periodically. Table 48-2 provides a list of supplies and equipment necessary for most neonatal resuscitations.

Well-trained personnel must be immediately available in any setting in which an infant might be delivered. Every birth should be attended by at least one person whose primary responsibility is the newly born infant and who is therefore able to initiate resuscitation if needed. Such personnel will vary according to local circumstances. If a high-risk delivery is anticipated in which significant resuscitative intervention may be necessary, additional skilled personnel should be present. Such is the case in a 32-week twin gestation delivery, for which separate personnel are required for each infant. The resuscitation team should be easily and rapidly activated. Not only should each member of the team understand the physiologic mechanisms of adaptation, but they must also maintain their resuscitative skills and familiarize themselves with any new guidelines as outlined by the American Academy of Pediatrics and the American Heart Association. In institutions in which resuscitations are uncommon, periodic mock codes may be helpful. It is imperative that the resuscitation team know conditions that place the infant at

PHYSICAL MATURITY

Sign	Score							Sign score
	-1	0	1	2	3	4	5	
Skin	Sticky, friable, transparent	Gelatinous, red, translucent	Smooth pink, visible veins	Superficial peeling and/or rash, few veins	Cracking, pale areas, rare veins	Parchment, deep cracking, no vessels	Leathery, cracked, wrinkled	
Lanugo	None	Sparse	Abundant	Thinning	Bald areas	Mostly bald		
Plantar surface	Heel-toe 40–50 mm: -1 <40 mm: -2	>50 mm No crease	Faint red marks	Anterior transverse crease only	Creases ant. 2/3	Creases over entire sole		
Breast	Imperceptible	Barely perceptible	Flat areola No bud	Stippled areola 1–2 mm bud	Raised areola 3–4 mm bud	Full areola 5–10 mm bud		
Eye/ear	Lids fused loosely: -1 tightly: -2	Lids open Pinna flat Stays folded	Sl. curved pinna; soft; slow recoil	Well-curved pinna; soft but ready recoil	Formed and firm instant recoil	Thick cartilage Ear stiff		
Genitals (male)	Scrotum flat, smooth	Scrotum empty, faint rugae	Testes in upper canal, rare rugae	Testes descending, few rugae	Testes down, good rugae	Testes pendulous, deep rugae		
Genitals (female)	Clitoris prominent and labia flat	Prominent clitoris and small labia minora	Prominent clitoris and enlarging minora	Majora and minora equally prominent	Majora large, minora small	Majora cover clitoris and minora		
						Total physical maturity score		

B

MATURITY RATING

Total score (neuromuscular + physical)	Weeks
-10	20
-5	22
0	24
5	26
10	28
15	30
20	32
25	34
30	36
35	38
40	40
45	42
50	44

C

Figure 48-1, cont'd

risk. Significant maternal medical history, gestational age, prenatal complications, medications, illicit drug use, and prenatal laboratory values should be recorded. Risk factors for sepsis, including group B streptococcus carrier status, length of rupture of membranes, maternal fever, evidence of chorioamnionitis, and use of intrapartum antibiotics, should be assessed. Specific indicators of fetal condition such as heart rate monitoring, lung maturity, and antenatal ultrasound findings should be communicated.

Initial Steps of Delivery Room Resuscitation

The initial focus at delivery should be on preventing cold stress in the infant and minimizing heat loss. Cold stress not only increases oxygen consumption but can also induce peripheral vasoconstriction, which if persists, will lead to acidosis.[6] To mitigate convective heat loss, the delivery room should be free of any draft. The radiant warmer should be preheated and blankets should be prewarmed. A hat should be available because the surface area of a newborn head is larger than the body and therefore a potentially significant source of heat loss. To prevent evaporative heat loss, the infant should be dried rapidly and the wet linens removed immediately. Of note, hyperthermia should be avoided as well, given the association with perinatal respiratory depression, in addition to increased oxygen consumption.[7,8]

The next step focuses on clearing and opening the airway. The infant's head should be placed in a neutral or "sniffing" position (Fig. 48-2). This position allows alignment of the

Table 48-1 Conditions Associated with Risk to Newborns

Antepartum Risk Factors
Maternal diabetes
Pregnancy-induced hypertension
Chronic hypertension
Chronic maternal illness
   Cardiovascular
   Thyroid
   Neurologic
   Pulmonary
   Renal
Anemia or isoimmunization
Previous fetal or neonatal death
Bleeding in second or third trimester
Maternal infection
Polyhydramnios or oligohydramnios
Premature rupture of membranes
Postterm gestation
Multiple gestation
Size-date discrepancy
Drug therapy, e.g., lithium carbonate or magnesium
Adrenergic-blocking drugs
Maternal substance abuse
Fetal malformation
Diminished fetal activity
No prenatal care
Age ≤16 or ≥35 years

Intrapartum Risk Factors
Emergency cesarean section
Forceps- or vacuum-assisted delivery
Breech or other abnormal presentation
Premature labor
Precipitous labor
Chorioamnionitis
Prolonged rupture of membranes (>18 hours before delivery)
Prolonged labor (>24 hours)
Prolonged second stage of labor (>2 hours)
Fetal bradycardia
Nonreassuring fetal heart rate patterns
Use of general anesthesia
Uterine tetany
Narcotics administered to the mother within 4 hours of
   delivery
Meconium-stained amniotic fluid
Prolapsed cord
Abruptio placentae
Placenta previa

Modified from American Heart Association/American Academy of
Pediatrics: Textbook of Neonatal Resuscitation. Elk Grove Village, Ill,
American Academy of Pediatrics, 2006.

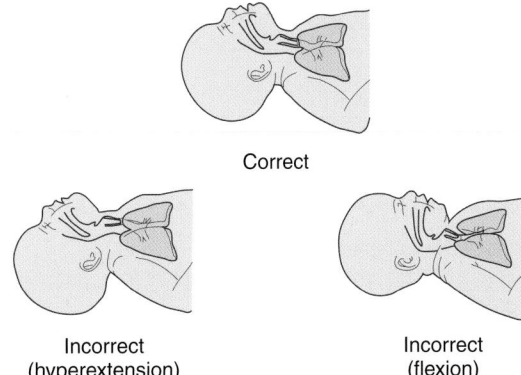

Correct

Incorrect (hyperextension)   Incorrect (flexion)

Figure 48-2 Correct and incorrect head positions for resuscitation.
(From American Heart Association/American Academy of Pediatrics:
Textbook of Neonatal Resuscitation. Elk Grove Village, Ill,, American
Academy of Pediatrics, 2006.)

posterior pharynx, larynx, and trachea such that the airway is maximally patent. The newborn head is larger than the body, so the neck has a tendency to either be flexed (underextended) or be hyperextended. In either of these positions, flow through the airway will be obstructed. A blanket roll beneath the shoulders may be helpful in attaining the neutral or "sniffing" position. Next, either a bulb syringe or a suction catheter should be used to clear the airway of any potential obstructions. The mouth should be suctioned first because suctioning the nose and nasopharynx may cause gagging and aspiration of oral secretions. Vigorous suctioning of the posterior pharynx should be avoided because laryngeal spasm and a vagal response may result.[9] Subsequent apnea or bradycardia, or both, may delay the onset of spontaneous breathing.

Respirations may be encouraged by providing tactile stimulation to the infant by gentle rubbing of the back or flicking of the heels. If an infant remains cyanotic, oxygen should be provided at a flow rate of 5 L/min via face mask and a flow-inflating bag, oxygen mask, or oxygen tubing encircled by a cupped hand. Initially, the oxygen source should be held as close to the infant's face as possible and then slowly withdrawn as the infant responds.

These initial steps of neonatal resuscitation should take less than 30 seconds, at which point the infant's respirations, heart rate, and color should be evaluated. If there is no improvement or if the infant's response is inadequate, the subsequent steps of active resuscitation should be performed (Fig. 48-3). The infant's response to resuscitation, including heart rate, respirations, and color, should be reassessed after every intervention.

Positive-Pressure Ventilation and Endotracheal Intubation

Four percent of newly born infants require bag-mask ventilation with supplemental oxygen. In fact, if there is any evidence of perinatal depression, vigorous resuscitation should be initiated early to counteract any hypoxemia or acidemia that may be present. Clinical signs of perinatal depression include an insufficient respiratory pattern manifested by gasping or apnea (or both), persistent heart rate lower than 60 beats per minute (bpm), or persistent central cyanosis despite providing 100% oxygen. In this scenario, bag-mask ventilation provides adequate ventilation, and immediate intubation is not necessary. In contrast, rapid intubation is indicated for an infant with a known congenital diaphragmatic hernia or, more commonly, for a depressed infant with meconium-stained amniotic fluid whose airway needs to be cleared.

Two types of bags, each with advantages and disadvantages, are available for resuscitation. A self-inflating bag (Ambu) may be easier to use, especially by less experienced

---

Table 48-2 Neonatal Resuscitation Supplies and Equipment

Suction Equipment
Bulb syringe
Mechanical suction and tubing
Suction catheters: 5F or 6F, 8F, and 10F or 12F
8F feeding tube and 20-mL syringe
Meconium aspiration device

Bag-and-Mask Equipment
Neonatal resuscitation bag with a pressure-release valve or pressure manometer (the bag must be capable of delivering 90% to 100% oxygen)
Face masks, newborn and premature sizes (masks with a cushioned rim preferred)
Oxygen with flowmeter (flow rate up to 10 L/min) and tubing (including portable oxygen cylinders)

Intubation Equipment
Laryngoscope with straight blades, No. 0 (preterm) and No. 1 (term)
Extra bulbs and batteries for the laryngoscope
Tracheal tubes: 2.5-, 3.0-, 3.5-, and 4.0-mm inner diameter
Stylet (optional)
Scissors
Tape or securing device for the tracheal tube
Alcohol sponges
CO_2 detector (optional)
Laryngeal mask airway (optional, requires additional training and expertise)

Medications
Epinephrine 1:10,000 (0.1 mg/mL)—3- or 10-mL ampules
Isotonic crystalloid (normal saline or lactated Ringer's solution) for volume expansion—100 or 250 mL
Sodium bicarbonate 4.2% (5 mEq/10 mL)—10-mL ampules
Naloxone hydrochloride, 0.4 mg/mL (1-mL ampules) or 1.0 mg/mL (2-mL ampules)
Normal saline, 30 mL
Dextrose 10%, 250 mL
Normal saline ampule (also known as "fish" or "bullet") (optional)
Feeding tube, 5F (optional)
Umbilical vessel catheterization supplies
Sterile gloves
Scalpel or scissors
Povidone-iodine solution
Umbilical tape
Umbilical catheters: 3.5F, 5F
Three-way stopcocks
Syringes: 1, 3, 5, 10, 20, and 50 mL
Needles: 25, 21, and 18 gauge or puncture device for needleless system

Miscellaneous
Gloves and appropriate personal protection for universal precautions
Radiant warmer or other heat source
Firm, padded resuscitation surface
Clock (timer optional)
Warmed linens
Stethoscope
Tape: $^1/_2$ or $^3/_4$ inch
Cardiac monitor and electrodes and/or pulse oximeter with probe (optional for delivery room)
Oropharyngeal airways

Modified from American Heart Association/American Academy of Pediatrics: Textbook of Neonatal Resuscitation. Elk Grove Village, Ill, American Academy of Pediatrics, 2006.

resuscitators. However, the valve assembly allows free flow of oxygen only when the bag is compressed or squeezed and therefore cannot deliver blow-by oxygen. Significant mixing with room air occurs, thereby limiting maximal oxygen delivery to only 40%, unless an oxygen reservoir is attached. The flow-inflating or "anesthesia" bag requires continual flow for inflation. More experienced resuscitators are necessary for several reasons. First, it is more prone to mechanical failure, which may occur at several points along the system. Gas must flow into the gas inlet, gas must flow out through the flow control valve, the mask must be securely attached to the bag, and the mask must make a tight seal with

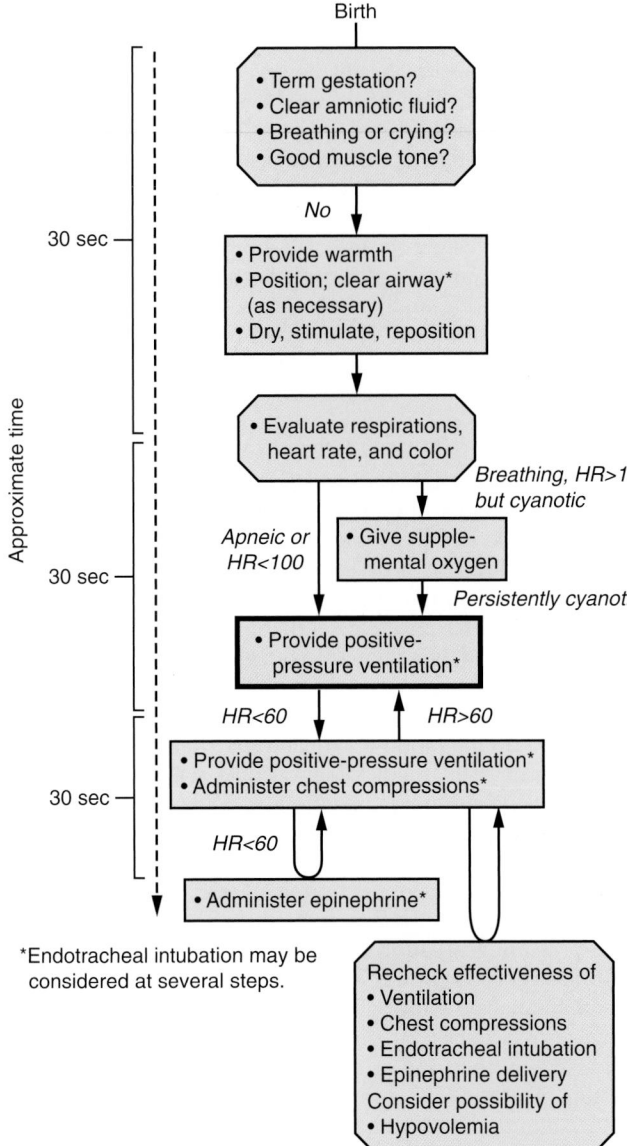

Birth

- Term gestation?
- Clear amniotic fluid?
- Breathing or crying?
- Good muscle tone?

No

- Provide warmth
- Position; clear airway*
  (as necessary)
- Dry, stimulate, reposition

- Evaluate respirations,
  heart rate, and color

*Breathing, HR>100
but cyanotic*

*Apneic or
HR<100*
- Give supple-
  mental oxygen

Persistently cyanotic

- Provide positive-
  pressure ventilation*

HR<60   *HR>60*

- Provide positive-pressure ventilation*
- Administer chest compressions*

HR<60

- Administer epinephrine*

*Endotracheal intubation may be considered at several steps.

Recheck effectiveness of
- Ventilation
- Chest compressions
- Endotracheal intubation
- Epinephrine delivery
Consider possibility of
- Hypovolemia

Approximate time — 30 sec, 30 sec, 30 sec

Figure 48-3 Algorithm for resuscitation of a newly born infant. HR, heart rate. (From American Heart Association/American Academy of Pediatrics: Textbook of Neonatal Resuscitation. Elk Grove Village, Ill, American Academy of Pediatrics, 2006.)

with air-filled cushions help maintain a tight seal without inflicting facial or ocular injury. Supporting the chin while holding it to the mask helps preserve a tight seal. It also serves to elevate the angle of the jaw, which brings the tongue forward and opens the airway.

Care should be taken to prevent overdistention and hyperventilation during resuscitation. Overdistention from bag-mask ventilation using high airway pressure—and therefore applying large tidal volumes—may impair venous return to the heart and may also lead to air leak syndromes. Of specific concern, overdistention may exacerbate intracranial hemorrhage because of transmission of transthoracic pressure to the pressure-passive cerebral circulation. Hyperventilation with resultant hypocapnia decreases both cerebral and myocardial perfusion. Positive-pressure ventilation should be performed at a rate of 30 to 60 breaths per minute (bpm). Often, this is the only resuscitative maneuver required. Efficacy is judged by chest movement or chest rise, audible symmetrical breath sounds, and improvement in heart rate and color. If the infant's response is inadequate, endotracheal intubation is required. This procedure is detailed in Chapter 208. Table 48-3 details correct tube sizes and insertion depth based on infant gastational age and weight.

In the delivery room, assessment of endotracheal tube (ETT) position after intubation in the setting of resuscitation is particularly challenging. Clinical assessments can have shortcomings. In extremely preterm infants it is often difficult to distinguish sounds in the lungs from those occurring over the stomach. If an infant has received positive-pressure ventilation before intubation, the stomach may already be inflated. Condensation has been observed within an ETT misplaced in the esophagus.

A CO_2 detector will assist in determining that an ETT is in the trachea. When attached to the end of an ETT placed in the airway, a CO_2 detector will change color as the level of CO_2 rises during exhalation after breaths are given (i.e., from purple to yellow and back again). Falsely positive color changes of a CO_2 detector are very unlikely.[12] However, a CO_2 detector may not change color if adequate circulation has not been established despite proper ETT placement, such as in the case of a patient in cardiopulmonary arrest. Moreover, a CO_2 detector will not indicate whether an ETT is in the correct position along the trachea. Given these caveats, it is recommended that a CO_2 detector be used during initial intubation to verify ETT placement in the trachea but that ultimately, a chest radiograph be taken to confirm appropriate position of the ETT.

Chest Compressions or External Cardiac Massage

Bradycardia, decreased perfusion, and decreased blood pressure will ensue after only a few minutes of hypoxia. Heart rate is assessed either by feeling pulsations at the base of the umbilical cord or by auscultating over the precordium with a stethoscope. Chest compressions or external cardiac massage is indicated if the heart rate is absent or remains less than 60 bpm after 30 seconds of effective ventilation. Two techniques may be used to administer external cardiac massage, either the two-finger method or the two thumb–encircling method. Both techniques are demonstrated in Figure 48-4. Although either method is acceptable, the two thumb–encircling method is preferred because it results in better peak systolic and coronary perfusion pressure.[13] However, one must be careful to avoid limiting chest

the infant's face. Additionally, higher pressure can be delivered with a flow-inflating versus a self-inflating bag. If the delivered pressure exceeds what is needed, air leak syndromes such as pneumomediastinum, pneumothorax, or pneumopericardium may result.[10] Hence it is crucial to observe the pressure applied via a manometer and make adjustments as lung compliance changes with fetal-newborn transition. The first breath must be large enough to ensure alveolar expansion such that FRC is established.[11] This sometimes requires initial breaths with a pressure of 25 to 40 mm Hg. Once FRC is established, less pressure is likely to be necessary. The greatest advantage, therefore, of a flow-inflating bag is that a greater range of peak inspiratory pressure is possible. A tight seal between the infant's face and the mask is essential to provide adequate ventilation. Using the appropriate equipment is a key component. The mask should cover the nose and mouth but be clear of the eyes. Masks

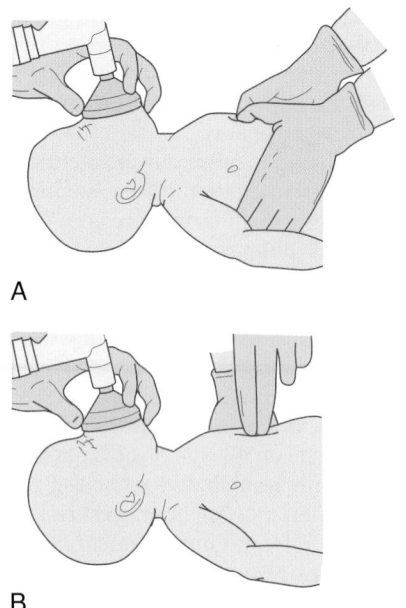

A

B

Figure 48-4 Two techniques for providing chest compressions: thumb (A) and two finger (B). (From American Heart Association/American Academy of Pediatrics: Textbook of Neonatal Resuscitation. Elk Grove Village, Ill, American Academy of Pediatrics, 2006.)

expansion during ventilation with this method. Chest compressions are performed on the lower third of the sternum immediately above the xiphoid process to a depth of one third the anteroposterior diameter of the chest. The goal is to generate a palpable pulse. Chest compressions are performed in coordination with ventilations at a 3:1 ratio such that 90 compressions and 30 ventilations occur in 1 minute. The infant should be reassessed 30 seconds after initiation of chest compressions.

Vascular Access

If the infant's response to the aforementioned resuscitative measures continues to be poor, the next intervention is the administration of medications. Epinephrine is the only resuscitative medication that can be administered intratracheally. Therefore, vascular access should be attained. Peripheral intravenous access can be difficult and time consuming, especially if hypoxia or acidosis is present. Emergency vascular access can be achieved via the umbilical vein. See Chapter 205 for a description of this procedure. If the umbilical vein cannot be cannulated and peripheral access is unsuccessful, intraosseous access can be used as an alternative route for medications or volume expansion.[14] This procedure is described in Chapter 203.

Medications

Bradycardia is most often the result of hypoventilation or hypoxia. Thus, adequate ventilation with supplemental oxygen is the most important step in correcting bradycardia. Drugs are rarely, but sometimes necessary in resuscitation of a newly born infant. Epinephrine is indicated when the heart rate remains lower than 60 bpm after 30 seconds of effective ventilation and external cardiac massage. The α-vasoconstrictive properties and the positive cardiac chronotropic effects of epinephrine aid in improving spontaneous cir-

culation. A 1:10,000 solution is administered in a dose of 0.1 to 0.3 mL/kg. As noted previously, epinephrine may be administered intratracheally; however, the intravenous route is preferred.[15-17] The dose can be repeated every 3 to 5 minutes as needed.

Correction of metabolic acidosis may increase pulmonary blood flow and enhance the effect of epinephrine. However, to be effective, adequate ventilation and circulation need to be established before the use of sodium bicarbonate.[18] Blood pH will not improve significantly in the absence of adequate ventilation. Additionally, respiratory acidosis, which may develop as bicarbonate is converted to carbon dioxide, can augment the preexisting metabolic acidosis. Sodium bicarbonate, at a dose of 1 to 2 mEq/kg, should always be diluted 1:1 with sterile water or saline and given slowly over at least a 2-minute period. Rapid infusions may be associated with intracranial hemorrhage,[19] which is especially of concern in premature infants. Sodium bicarbonate administration may also unmask any hypovolemia that had previously been inapparent because of peripheral vasoconstriction.

Not unlike sodium bicarbonate, naloxone should be considered only after effective ventilation and circulation have been established. It is a narcotic antagonist that may be effective against the narcotics used for labor analgesia. However, significant respiratory depression because of peripartum narcotic administration is rare and may in fact be related to other peripartum medications against which naloxone is ineffective. For example, magnesium sulfate, often used for preeclampsia, may cause respiratory depression in an infant that will not be reversed by naloxone. The only indication for naloxone is severe respiratory depression that persists despite a normal heart rate and color after delivery of positive-pressure ventilation in the setting of maternal narcotic administration within 4 hours of delivery. Naloxone may precipitate acute withdrawal, including severe seizures and long-term sequelae, if given to the infant of an opioid-addicted mother and is therefore contraindicated in this setting. Naloxone has a rapid onset of action, acting within 1 to 2 minutes, but has a fairly short duration of action. In fact, the duration of narcotics used for labor analgesia is greater than that of naloxone, and repeated doses of naloxone may thus be needed. The dosage of naloxone is 0.1 mg/kg, and it can be administered intratracheally, subcutaneously, intramuscularly, or intravenously.

Volume expansion should be considered in situations in which hypovolemia progresses to hypovolemic shock. Clinical manifestations of shock include weak pulses, poor capillary filling, and low blood pressure. Hypovolemia occurs as a result of inadequate supply or increased loss of blood. Significant hemorrhage may be due to placenta previa or placental abruption, fetomaternal bleeding, internal hemorrhage, or twin-twin transfusion syndrome in the donor twin. In the scenarios of cord accidents, a tight nuchal cord, or umbilical cord compression by the after-coming head in a breech delivery, umbilical venous blood flow may be impeded while umbilical arterial blood flow is uninterrupted. In these situations, circulating blood volume in the infant may be decreased by as much as 20%. Options for volume resuscitation include normal saline or lactated Ringer's solution, which are readily available, 5% albumin, or type O-negative packed red blood cells. Whatever solution is used, it should be administered slowly and in aliquots

Table 48-3   Suggested Tracheal Tube Size and Depth of Insertion According to Weight and Gestational Age

Weight (g)	Gestational Age (wk)	Tube Size (mm, ID)	Depth of Insertion from the Upper Lip (cm)
<1000	<28	2.5	6.5-7
1000-2000	28-34	3.0	7-8
2000-3000	34-38	3.5	8-9
>3000	>38	3.5-4.0	>9

ID, inner diameter.
Modified from American Heart Association/American Academy of Pediatrics: Textbook of Neonatal Resuscitation. Elk Grove Village, Ill, American Academy of Pediatrics, 2006.

of 10 mL/kg. Cardiac function may be compromised during shock and may be exacerbated by an acutely expanded preload volume. In addition, some vascular beds, in particular, the vasculature of the brain, will be maximally dilated in response to hypotension, so intracranial hemorrhage is a possible consequence of rapid volume expansion, especially in preterm infants. As with any intervention, reassessment, including blood pressure, perfusion, and oxygenation, is essential before additional doses.

SPECIAL CIRCUMSTANCES

Meconium-Stained Amniotic Fluid

Meconium-stained amniotic fluid (MSAF) occurs in 10% to 15% of all pregnancies and is caused by a reaction to fetal hypoxemia, acidemia, stress, or any combination of these precipitants. If the stress is significant in utero, the meconium may be aspirated into the airways before birth. MSAF is rare before 34 weeks' gestation and occurs more commonly in postterm gestations. At least 2% of infants with MSAF will manifest some degree of aspiration; the clinical spectrum ranges from mild tachypnea after birth to severe pneumonitis and pulmonary hypertension.[20,21] Pulmonary disease is more likely if MSAF occurs before the second stage of labor, if the meconium is thick with particulate material, or if meconium is present below the vocal cords. In the past, attempts at preventing meconium aspiration syndrome (MAS) in infants have included amniotic infusion of the uterus before birth and suctioning of the infant on delivery of the head. Unfortunately, recent studies have shown that amniotic infusion does not prevent moderate or severe MAS.[22] Furthermore, routine suctioning of the infant's oropharynx on delivery of the head but before delivery of the shoulders is no longer recommended.[23,24] However, obstetricians have been able to reduce the incidence of MAS by decreasing the number of postterm deliveries (>41 weeks).[25]

Endotracheal intubation to prevent MAS is indicated only in certain scenarios. On delivery of an infant with MSAF, if the infant is vigorous, especially if the infant is crying, tracheal suctioning is not necessary because it does not reduce the incidence of MAS or improve outcome.[26,27] In fact, attempting to suction an infant in this situation may not only be difficult but may also result in esophageal or tracheal injury, or both. These infants require routine resuscitation and suctioning only. If the infant is nonvigorous or depressed, intubation and tracheal suctioning should be performed before any stimulation or positive-pressure ventila-

tion.[28] The ETT should be large enough to remove thick copious meconium yet fit easily into the infant's trachea (Table 48-3). A meconium aspirator should be placed directly onto the end of the ETT and connected to suction at 80 to 100 cm H_2O pressure. The entire apparatus, including the ETT, should then be withdrawn slowly. It is prudent to have a few endotracheal tubes available and ready because repeat intubation and tracheal suctioning with a clean ETT may be necessary. Suctioning should be performed until the return is clear or other resuscitation priorities take precedence (e.g., sustained infant heart rate <80 bpm). Once the infant has been resuscitated, the stomach should be suctioned as well to avoid the potential aspiration of swallowed meconium. If respiratory distress develops after delivery with MSAF, there should be a high index of suspicion for the development of pneumothorax given the ball valve–like properties that can occur with meconium plugs. Pneumothorax can be identified clinically from asymmetry of chest movements or breath sounds, or both. If a tension pneumothorax develops, venous return and cardiac output are compromised and cardiac arrest may occur. Transillumination may be helpful, particularly in preterm infants. When a light is placed next to the newborn's chest on the side of the pneumothorax, it will light up the air pocket of the pneumothorax more brightly than when it is placed against the side with normal lung tissue. A chest radiograph is diagnostic, but diagnostic thoracentesis should be considered in life-threatening cases, even before a radiograph is available (see Chapters 147, and 210).

Multiple Gestations

Separate teams of skilled personnel are required for each infant of a multiple gestation. Multiple gestations are associated with an increased incidence of preterm labor and delivery, as well as an increased risk for intrauterine growth retardation in at least one fetus. Postnatally, there is a risk of higher sensitivity to asphyxia, hypoglycemia, or polycythemia in each infant. Monozygotic twins are especially at high risk not only because of the potential for twin-twin transfusion syndrome, possibly with hydrops in either twin, but also because of the increased incidence of congenital anomalies.

Extremely Premature Infants (<1000 g)

These infants should be delivered in a perinatal center with skilled personnel in obstetrics, anesthesia, and neonatology. Because this is not always possible, each hospital with labor and delivery capabilities should be part of a perinatal network or center such that the infant, once stabilized, can be transferred to a high-level center. Whenever possible, a conference should take place with the parents before delivery. The incidence of perinatal depression is markedly increased in this population because of physiologic immaturity and lability.

The potential for significant heat and insensible water loss exists in this population of infants. They have decreased amounts of subcutaneous tissue and fat, their skin is immature and prone to epidermal heat and water loss, and they have a high surface area–to–body mass ratio. Therefore, although difficult, it is imperative to dry these infants thoroughly and provide warmth. In addition to the preheated radiant warmer, linens, and hat previously mentioned, a warming mattress may be helpful, as well as the use of warm, humidified air and oxygen. Polyethylene wrap may decrease not only convective heat loss but also evaporative heat and water loss through the very thin, translucent skin of these infants.

These small infants have weaker muscles of respiration and are therefore less likely to either establish or maintain FRC. The resultant inadequate ventilation may be compounded by decreased lung compliance as a result of surfactant deficiency. Hence intubation and administration of large tidal volumes by applying high peak pressure may be necessary until exogenous surfactant is administered. These interventions may further complicate the course of these infants. They are at increased risk for the development of air leak syndromes not only because the surfactant-deficient lungs are stiff and noncompliant but also because of changes in lung compliance after surfactant replacement. Overventilation may impair cardiac output as a result of compromised venous return and may reduce cerebral blood flow because of the resultant hypocapnia.

Alteration of cerebral blood flow may heighten an already high risk for intracranial hemorrhage in this vulnerable population of infants. Any acute and dramatic changes in intracranial pressure, vascular volume, oxygen tension, osmolarity, or cerebral circulation pressure may promote or exacerbate the development of an intracranial hemorrhage.[29] The pressure generated with positive-pressure ventilation, especially with large tidal volumes, and with chest compressions can be transmitted to the pressure-passive cerebral circulation. Rapid changes in cardiac output, as may occur with rapid volume expansion or with the hypertension associated with epinephrine, can play a part as well. Sodium bicarbonate, a hyperosmolar solution, can alter the osmotic gradient of the circulation, especially if given rapidly.

For infants at the threshold of viability, it is especially important to provide antenatal counseling, as well as maintain an ongoing dialogue with the family. Assessment of gestational age both antenatally, by ultrasound, and postnatally, by a gestational age examination such as the Ballard Score (see earlier), is accurate only to within 1 to 2 weeks. Therefore, if there is any question of gestational age, it is reasonable to provide aggressive resuscitative support, which allows ongoing assessment of the infant. The infant's response to therapy is an important factor in assessment, and if response to resuscitation is poor or if severe complications develop, withdrawal of support may be offered.

Hydrops Fetalis

This condition occurs in 1 in 1500 to 4000 deliveries and is usually detected by prenatal ultrasound. Excessive fluid accumulation in utero leads to generalized skin thickening, ascites, pleural effusion, pericardial effusion, cystic hygroma, a thick placenta, or any combination of these findings. At birth, infants are very ill and require extended resuscitation. The potential causes are vast; major causes include hematologic, cardiac, vascular malformation, infection, genetic, metabolic, endocrine, and pulmonary. If the condition is detected before birth, it is helpful to establish the presence and size of pleural effusions or peritoneal fluid (or both) immediately before delivery by prenatal ultrasound. These fluid collections may hinder ventilation and may need to be evacuated. If so, additional skilled personnel will be needed to perform the thoracentesis or paracentesis, or both. If the pleural effusions have been long-standing, pulmonary hypoplasia may be an issue. In this situation, high inflating pressure and positive end-expiratory pressure are required to overcome noncompliant lungs, and pulmonary hypertension is common. As previously described with noncompliant lungs, the development of pneumothorax is a potential complication. Frequently, death occurs in utero or shortly after birth.

ADMISSION CRITERIA AND CONSULTATION

Transfer from the delivery room to a neonatal intensive care unit or consultation with a neonatologist (or both) is recommended in the following circumstances:

- Existence of or suspicion of a significant fetal anomaly, including Down syndrome, ambiguous genitalia, or cardiac or gastrointestinal malformation
- Respiratory distress/tachypnea
- Infants requiring respiratory or cardiac support
- Prolonged resuscitation or delivery or infants requiring cardiac compressions

Of note, many infants with minor concerns can remain in a mother's room to facilitate parent-infant bonding. Infants with simple anomalies such as extra digits, hypospadias, or a cleft lip or palate do not require admission to the neonatal intensive care unit.

OUTCOMES

Indicators of a poor outcome in terms of both survival and subsequent neurodevelopment include Apgar scores of less than 3 at 5 and 10 minutes (Table 48-4), cord or newborn blood pH less than 7.0 in the first 2 hours of life, absence of a heartbeat at 5 minutes of life, and seizures in the first 24 hours of life.[29] The occurrence of seizures within the first 12 hours of life is particularly ominous. Resuscitation should rarely be continued longer than 15 to 20 minutes in an infant with an initial Apgar score of 0 who does not respond rapidly to resuscitation. In these infants, the incidence of death or severe, irreversible neurologic damage is very high.[30-32]

Table 48-4 Apgar Scoring

Sign	SCORE		
	0	*1*	*2*
Heart rate	Absent	Slow (<100 bpm)	>100 bpm
Respirations	Absent	Slow, irregular	Good, crying
Muscle tone	Limp	Some flexion	Active motion
Reflex irritability (catheter in nares, tactile stimulation)	No response	Grimace	Cough, sneeze, cry
Color	Blue or pale	Pink body, blue extremities	Completely pink

bpm, beats per minute.
Modified from American Heart Association/American Academy of Pediatrics: Textbook of Neonatal Resuscitation. Elk Grove Village, Ill, American Academy of Pediatrics, 2006.

IN A NUTSHELL

- The transition from fetal to newborn physiology is complicated and requires the support of at least one neonatal resuscitation provider at delivery.
- Multiple problems can occur at any point during pregnancy, labor, and delivery for which the delivery room should remain prepared.
- The Apgar score is used to assess an infant during the first few minutes of life, but it should not take precedence over neonatal resuscitation.
- Neonatal resuscitation steps include maintaining an infant's temperature while clearing the airway and stimulating the infant.
- Nonvigorous meconium-stained infants will need to be intubated and suctioned before initiating other resuscitative steps.
- A CO_2 detector should be used to ensure that an ETT has been placed in the trachea, but it will not work in the case of cardiopulmonary arrest.
- Resuscitation medicines work best when given intravenously.

ON THE HORIZON

- New neonatal resuscitation program guidelines will change recommendations on epinephrine dosing during neonatal resuscitation to up to 0.3 to 1 mL/kg when given through the ETT. Laryngeal mask airways will also be part of the equipment recommended for assisting ventilation when bag-and-mask ventilation or endotracheal intubation has failed. These guidelines will also include recommendations for resuscitation of infants less than 32 weeks with blended rather than 100% oxygen.

SUGGESTED READING

Ballard JL, Khoury JC, Wedig K, et al: New Ballard Score, expanded to include extremely premature infants. J Pediatr 1991;119:417-423.

Care of the neonate: Delivery room care. In Guidelines for Perinatal Care, 5th ed. Elk Grove Village, Ill, American Academy of Pediatrics and American College of Obstetrician and Gynecologists, 2002, pp 187-198.

Fowlie PW, Booth P, Skeoch CH: Moving the preterm infant. BMJ 2004;329:904-906.

Fowlie PW, McGuire W: Immediate care of the preterm infant. BMJ 2004;329:845-848.

Hamilton P: ABC of labour care: Care of the newborn in the delivery room. BMJ 1999;318:1403-1406.

http://www.ballardscore.com/index.htm, accessed on 5/14/2006.

International Guidelines for Neonatal Resuscitation: An excerpt from the Guidelines 2000 for Cardiopulmonary Resuscitation and Emergency Cardiovascular Care: International Consensus on Science. Pediatrics 2000;106:e29.

Kattwinkel J (ed): Textbook of Neonatal Resuscitation, 4th ed. Elk Grove Village, Ill, American Academy of Pediatrics and American Heart Association, 2000.

Wolkoff LI, Davis JM: Delivery room resuscitation of the newborn. Clin Perinatol 1999;26:641-658.

REFERENCES

1. Nelson NM: Respiration and circulation before birth. In Smith CA, Nelson NM (eds): The Physiology of the Newborn Infant. Springfield, Ill, Charles C Thomas, 1976, pp 15-117.
2. Saugstad OD: Practical aspects of resuscitating asphyxiated newborn infants. Eur J Pediatr 1998;157(Suppl 1):S11-S15.
3. World Health Organization: World Health Report. Geneva, Switzerland, WHO, 1997, p 21.
4. O'Brodovich H: Epithelial ion transport in fetal and perinatal lung. Am J Physiol 1991;261:C555-C564.
5. Bland RD, Carlton DP, Scheerer RG, et al: Lung fluid balance in lambs before and after premature birth. J Clin Invest 1989;84:568-576.
6. Gandy GM, Adamson SK Jr, Cunningham N, et al: Thermal environment and acid-base homeostasis in human infants during the first few hours of life. J Clin Invest 1964;43:751-758.
7. Perlman JM: Maternal fever and neonatal depression: Preliminary observations. Clin Pediatr (Phila) 1999;38:287-291.
8. Lieberman E, Lang J, Richardson DK, et al: Intrapartum maternal fever and neonatal outcome. Pediatrics 2000;105:8-13.
9. Cordero L Jr, Hon EH: Neonatal bradycardia following nasopharyngeal stimulation. J Pediatr 1971;78:441-447.
10. Vyas H, Milner AD, Hopkin IE, Boon AW: Physiologic responses to prolonged and slow-rise inflation in the resuscitation of the asphyxiated newborn infant. J Pediatr 1981;99:635-639.
11. Vyas H, Field D, Milner AD, Hopkin IE: Determinants of the first inspiratory volume and functional residual capacity at birth. Pediatr Pulmonol 1986;2:189-193.
12. Aziz HF, Martin JB, Moore JJ: The pediatric disposable end-tidal carbon dioxide detector role in endotracheal intubation in newborns. J Perinatol 1999;19:110-113.
13. Todres ID, Rogers MC: Methods of external cardiac massage in the newborn infant. J Pediatr 1975;86:781-782.

14. Ellemunter H, Simma B, Trawoger R, Maurer H: Intraosseous lines in preterm and full term neonates. Arch Dis Child Fetal Neonatal Ed 1999;80:F74-F75.

15. Berg RA, Otto CW, Kern KB, et al: A randomized, blinded trial of high-dose epinephrine versus standard-dose epinephrine in a swine model or pediatric asphyxial cardiac arrest. Crit Care Med 1996;24:1695-1700.

16. Burchfield DJ, Preziosi MP, Lucas VW, Fan J: Effects of graded doses of epinephrine during asphyxia-induced bradycardia in newborn lambs. Resuscitation 1993;25:235-244.

17. Pasternak JF, Groothuis DR, Fischer JM, Fischer DP: Regional cerebral blood flow in the beagle puppy model of neonatal intraventricular hemorrhage: Studies during systemic hypertension. Neurology 1983;33:559-566.

18. Hein HA: The use of sodium bicarbonate in neonatal resuscitation: Help or harm? Pediatrics 1993;91:496-497.

19. Papile LA, Burstein J, Burstein R, et al: Relationship of intravenous sodium bicarbonate infusions and cerebral intraventricular hemorrhage. J Pediatr 1978;93:834-836.

20. Wiswell TE, Fuloria M: Resuscitation of the meconium-stained infant and prevention of meconium aspiration syndrome. J Perinatol 1999;19:234-241.

21. Wiswell TE, Tuggle JM, Turner BS: Meconium aspiration syndrome: Have we made a difference? Pediatrics 1990;85:715-721.

22. Fraser WD, Hofmeyr J, Lede R, et al: Amnioinfusion for the prevention of meconium aspiration infusion. N Engl J Med 2005;353:909-917.

23. Vain NE, Szyld EG, Prudent LM, et al: Oropharyngeal and nasopharyngeal suctioning of meconium-stained neonates before delivery of their shoulders: Multicentre, randomised controlled trial. Lancet 2004;364:597-602.

24. Carson BS, Losey RW, Bowes WA Jr, Simmons MA: Combined obstetric and pediatric approach to prevent meconium aspiration syndrome. Am J Obstet Gynecol 1976;126:712-715.

25. Yoder BA, Kirsch EA, Barth WH, Gordon MC: Changing obstetric practices with decreasing incidence of meconium aspiration syndrome. Obstet Gynecol 2002;99:731-739.

26. Wiswell TE, Gannon CM, Jacob J, et al: Delivery room management of the apparently vigorous meconium-stained neonate: Results of the multicenter collaborative trial. Pediatrics 2000;105:1-7.

27. Halliday HL: Endotracheal intubation at birth for preventing morbidity and mortality in vigorous, meconium-stained infants born at term. Cochrane Database Syst Rev 2001;1:CD000500.

28. Greenough A: Meconium aspiration syndrome—prevention and treatment. Early Hum Dev 1995;41:183-192.

29. Hambleton G, Wigglesworth JS: Origin of intraventricular hemorrhage in the preterm infant. Arch Dis Child 1976;51:651-659.

30. Casalaz DM, Marlow N, Speidel BD: Outcome of resuscitation following unexpected apparent stillbirth. Arch Dis Child Fetal Neonatal Ed 1998;78:F112-F115.

31. Jain L, Ferre C, Vidyasagar D, et al: Cardiopulmonary resuscitation of apparently stillborn infants: Survival and long-term outcome. J Pediatr 1991;118:778-782.

32. Yeo CL, Tudehope DI: Outcome of resuscitated apparently stillborn infants: A ten year review. J Pediatr Child Health 1994;30:129-133.

CHAPTER 49

The Well Newborn

Katarzyna Madejczyk

The majority of full-term newborns have an uneventful postnatal course. Once the newborn makes the transition from the intrauterine world to the outside environment, nursery management centers on routine infant care and anticipatory parental guidance. However, certain disease states may not manifest in the immediate newborn period, and their early detection may prevent long-term morbidity or even death. Therefore, proper parental education not only makes the mother's and father's transition into parenthood easier but also prevents potential adverse outcomes for the infant.

EVALUATION

Assessment of the newborn begins with review of the maternal history, the pregnancy, and the delivery (Table 49-1).

A physician must perform a thorough head-to-toe examination of the newborn infant within 24 hours of birth and daily while the infant is in the hospital. Every examination should start with a review of the vital signs; the range of normal values for newborns is provided in Table 49-2. The initial examination should also include measurements of birth weight, length, and head circumference. These are plotted on standard growth curves to determine whether they are proportional and appropriate for the gestational age.

The infant should be completely undressed and observed for any signs of distress, dysmorphology, asymmetry, or abnormal color. Pertinent findings of the newborn examination are summarized in Table 49-3. Abnormalities, including vital signs outside the normal range, often require further investigation or follow-up.

DEVELOPMENTAL DYSPLASIA OF THE HIP

Developmental dysplasia of the hip (DDH) is defined as an abnormal relationship of the femoral head and acetabulum. It includes frank dislocation (luxation), partial dislocation (subluxation), femoral head instability, and any malformation of the acetabulum. Screening for DDH should start in the nursery and continue at each scheduled well-child visit until age 18 months. By that age, normal children should be walking well, and any hip abnormality will manifest as an abnormal gait. The earlier the diagnosis is made, the sooner proper treatment can be instituted to prevent long-term morbidity. The true incidence of DDH is unknown, but it is estimated that 1 in 100 newborns has hip instability and 1 to 1.5 per 1000 has dislocation. The left hip is involved three times more often than the right hip. Factors that increase the risk for DDH include female gender, breech position, positive family history, and oligohydramnios.[1]

Physical Examination

The hip examination should be carried out in a systematic manner while the infant is quiet and relaxed. Although no physical examination signs are pathognomonic for a dislocated hip, findings that should raise the examiner's suspicion include asymmetry of thigh or gluteal folds, apparent limb length discrepancy, and restricted mobility of the hip, especially abduction. The Barlow, Ortolani, and Galeazzi tests are physical maneuvers that suggest hip dislocation and should prompt the physician to undertake further action. These maneuvers are detailed in Table 49-4. It is not unusual for hip "clicks" to be elicited during the initial newborn examination; these usually represent ligamentous laxity that tends to resolve by 2 weeks of age.

Management

If a "clunk" is obtained during the examination, the infant should be referred to an orthopedic surgeon. There is no need to confirm the dislocation by radiographic studies; the physical examination should guide treatment. The infant will likely be placed in a Pavlik harness and followed with ultrasound studies and physical examinations by the orthopedic specialist. Double and triple diapering of infants to stabilize the hip is not recommended. A click present in the nursery should be reevaluated at 2 weeks of age. If the finding persists or there are other suspicious findings (e.g., unequal gluteal folds) but no evidence of true hip dislocation, the physician may refer the patient to an orthopedist or perform ultrasonography of the hips at 3 to 4 weeks of age.

If the examination is normal at 2 weeks of age, routine periodic examinations should be continued. Certain risk factors may prompt the physician to pursue further evaluation, even when the examination is normal. Boys with a positive family history of DDH have a newborn risk of 9.4 in 1000 and may be followed clinically; girls with a positive family history have a newborn risk of 44 in 1000 and may benefit from an ultrasound study at 6 weeks of age or radiographs of the hips at 4 months. Breech-born boys, with an estimated newborn risk of 26 in 1000, can be followed clinically but might benefit from radiographic evaluation; breech-born girls, with a newborn risk of 120 in 1000, should undergo either hip ultrasonography at 6 weeks or hip radiography at 4 months of age.[1]

When imaging pediatric hips, one must remember that because the femoral head is mostly cartilaginous in the first weeks of life, plain radiographs are not useful. Ultrasonography is a reliable method of evaluating hips in the first 4 months of life. After age 4 months, the femoral head should be well ossified, and plain radiographs can be obtained. Between 4 and 6 months of age, either method is acceptable.

Table 49-5 summarizes the evaluation and management of DDH.

Table 49-1   Perinatal History Assessment

Maternal	Fetus	Labor
Illnesses (current or past)	CVS or amniocentesis	Gestational age at delivery
Medications	Prenatal ultrasonography	Progression of labor (e.g., duration of rupture of membranes, maternal fever)
Drug, alcohol, or tobacco use	In utero interventions (e.g., surgery, infusions, selective reductions)	Delivery (induced, spontaneous, vaginal, forceps or vacuum assisted, cesarean, presentation)
Prenatal care		Medications (analgesia, antibiotics)
Prenatal testing (CVS, amniocentesis, hepatitis B, HIV, RPR, other STDs, PPD, GBS, blood type)		Fetal distress, presence of meconium, evidence of chorioamnionitis
Complication of this pregnancy (e.g., premature labor, bleeding)		Resuscitation
Complications of previous pregnancies		Apgar scores
Disorders in other children or family members		Complications

CVS, chorionic villus sampling; GBS, group B streptococci; HIV, human immunodeficiency virus; PPD, purified protein derivative (for tuberculosis); RPR, rapid plasma reagin (for syphilis); STD, sexually transmitted disease.

Table 49-2   Vital Signs in Full-term Newborns

Vital Sign	Normal Range
Temperature	Rectal: >36.5°C and <38°C*
Heart rate	90-150 beats/min
Respiratory rate[†]	30-60 breaths/min

*Corresponds to >97.7°F and <100.4°F.
[†]The respiratory rate should be obtained by counting breaths for 60 seconds, because newborns often exhibit periodic breathing.

NURSERY MANAGEMENT AND ANTICIPATORY GUIDANCE FOR WELL NEWBORNS

After delivery, all infants should receive prophylaxis against hemorrhagic disease of the newborn with the intramuscular administration of 1 mg of vitamin K_1 (phytonadione) and against ophthalmia neonatorum with one application of a topical antimicrobial agent to the eyes. Accepted antimicrobials are 1% silver nitrate solution, 0.5% erythromycin ointment, 1% tetracycline ointment, and 2.5% povidone-iodine solution. Although topical agents work well against many of the typical organisms, including *Neisseria gonorrhoeae*, their effectiveness against *Chlamydia trachomatis* has not been established.

Blood typing is not mandatory in all newborns. Routine blood typing is currently recommended in infants of Rh-negative mothers and in those whose mothers have an unknown blood type. All nurseries must have protocols for assessing newborns for jaundice. The routine checking of hemoglobin, glucose, and blood pressure in well-appearing infants with no risk factors is not indicated.[2] Some clinicians recommend a single postductal pulse oximetry check on all newborns before discharge (or at 24 to 48 hours of life) as a

method of detecting certain forms of congenital heart disease in asymptomatic infants.

Further management of the well newborn centers on parental guidance and support. Social service consultation may be indicated in cases of poor prenatal care, drug use during pregnancy, teen pregnancy, maternal mental illness, or lack of family support or resources.

Feeding and Elimination

All mothers should be asked about their desire to breast-feed and should be offered lactation support. Each newborn record must be reviewed daily for feeding and elimination patterns.

Breastfeeding

The newborn infant does not feed much in the first 24 hours of life. If the mother wishes to breastfeed, the infant should be put to the breast as soon as possible after birth. In the first 24 to 72 hours, the breast produces a few milliliters of colostrum, which is generally enough to sustain the newborn. The mother should be encouraged to breastfeed on demand, but no less frequently than every 3 hours, from 5 to 15 minutes on each breast.[3,4]

Some mothers and babies may have a difficult time establishing proper breastfeeding habits, which may result in dehydration of the infant. Lactation support and counseling by a trained professional can often remedy the situation. Although bottle feeding should generally be avoided in the first 2 weeks of life to establish a good milk supply and breastfeeding patterns, supplementation may be medically necessary.

When supplementation is indicated, the mother should breastfeed every 2 hours, 15 minutes on each breast, and then offer formula. Putting the infant to the breast stimulates milk production, and formula supplementation prevents dehydration. Putting the infant to the breast before offering

Site or System	Pertinent Findings
Table 49-3	Newborn Examination
General	Vital signs, anthropomorphic measurements Evidence of distress Symmetry of movements Dysmorphic or asymmetric features Jaundice
Head	Skull shape, irregularities Swelling or discoloration of scalp Appearance of fontanelle
Eyes	Shape, size, spontaneous opening Red reflex Subconjuctival hemorrhage or discharge
Ears	Shape and position Patency of external canals Preauricular pits or tags
Nose	Shape Patency of nares
Mouth	Natal teeth, alveolar cysts Cleft lip, palate, or uvula Short lingular frenulum ("tongue-tie")
Neck	Range of motion (e.g., torticollis) Masses, sinuses, pits
Chest	Shape, symmetry of motion Breast tissue, supernumerary nipples Clavicular fracture
Lungs	Symmetry of air entry, retractions Adventitial sounds
Cardiovascular	Heart rate, rhythm, sounds, murmurs, point of maximum impulse Pulses, capillary refill
Abdomen	Distention Presence of bowel sounds Organomegaly, masses Hernia Umbilical stump
Genitourinary	Female genitalia: size of clitoris and labia, presence of vaginal opening and hymenal tissue, discharge Males: presence of both testes, presence of epi- or hypospadias, hydrocele, inguinal hernia
Extremities	Symmetry and range of motion Hips: symmetry of thigh and gluteal folds, symmetry of abduction, Barlow and Ortolani maneuvers*, acrocyanosis, extranumerary digits, clubfeet
Neurologic	Tone Reflexes: Moro, suck, palmar, plantar, deep tendon
Back	Asymmetry Midline lesions (tufts, pits, masses) Position and patency of anus
Skin	Birthmarks Rashes Abrasions, lacerations, contusions

*See Table 49-4.

Table 49-4	Newborn Examination of the Hips	
Maneuver	Procedure	Abnormal Findings Suggestive of DDH
Barlow	Infant is placed in supine position Examiner holds infant's hip and knee in flexion, with lower leg in examiner's first web space Examiner places index and middle fingers over infant's greater trochanter Examiner places thumb on infant's inner thigh over lesser trochanter Examiner adducts the hip while pressing the femur posteriorly	A "clunk" with this maneuver represents dislocation of the femoral head from the acetabulum
Ortolani	Infant is placed in supine position Examiner holds infant's hip and knee in flexion, with lower leg in examiner's first web space Examiner places index and middle fingers over infant's greater trochanter Examiner places thumb on infant's inner thigh over lesser trochanter Examiner abducts the hip and lifts femur anteriorly	A "clunk" with this maneuver represents reduction of the femoral head into the acetabulum
Galeazzi	Infant is placed in supine position Adducted femurs are aligned, with hips and knees flexed and dorsum of feet on firm surface	Uneven knee height if unilateral dislocation is present; discrepancy may not be evident with bilateral DDH

DDH, developmental dysplasia of the hip.

Table 49-5	Approach to Developmental Dysplasia of the Hip	
DDH Examination	Risk Factors	Recommended Action
Positive	NA	Refer to orthopedist
Equivocal at birth	NA	Repeat at 2 wk
Equivocal at 2 wk	NA	Refer to orthopedist or perform ultrasonography at 3–4 wk, determine risk factors
Negative	Girl with breech delivery	Recommend ultrasonography at 6 wk or radiographs at 4 mo
Negative	Boy with breech delivery	Reevaluate at well-child visits and consider ultrasonography at 6 wk or radiographs at 4 mo
Negative	Girl with family history of DDH	Reevaluate at well-child visits and consider ultrasonography at 6 wk or radiographs at 4 mo
Negative	Boy with family history of DDH	Reevaluate at well-child visits
Negative	No risk factors	Reevaluate at well-child visits

DDH, developmental dysplasia of the hip; NA, not applicable.

formula usually prevents any problems with subsequent breastfeeding. Once breastfeeding is well established, offering a bottle for one or two feedings is usually not a problem. Cup feeding of formula is an alternative to bottle feeding when the mother wishes to avoid artificial nipples. Although cup feeding is safe when done properly, mothers should be counseled regarding the potential for aspiration.

In the United States, contraindications to breastfeeding include maternal human immunodeficiency virus (HIV) infection, active tuberculosis infection, human T-lymphotropic virus type I and II infection, herpes simplex virus lesions on the breast, and certain drugs, including drugs of abuse, cytotoxic drugs, and radioactive compounds. Medications taken by the breastfeeding mother should be reviewed to ensure that their transfer via breast milk will not adversely affect the infant. A complete list of drugs compatible with breastfeeding is available from the American Academy of Pediatrics. Maternal use of methadone is no longer a contraindication to breastfeeding.[3,4]

Formula Feeding

Formula-fed infants usually take between $1/4$ and 1 ounce (approximately 50 to 30 mL) per feeding in the first 24 hours of life. This amount increases in subsequent days. At discharge, most infants take 2 to 3 ounces (60 to 90 mL) of formula every 3 to 4 hours.

Formula-fed infants can be started on any of the standard formulas. Although there are differences among the various brand-name formulas, they all meet nutritional standards and provide adequate calories and nutrients to full-term infants. Premature infants have special needs and may require special formulas. All infants should be fed iron-fortified formula. Although low-iron formulas are available, there is no medical reason to use such formulas, which provide inadequate amounts of this essential element.

Soy formulas may be fed to infants whose parents want a formula that is free of animal products. However, soy formulas should not be fed to premature infants because of the poor bone mineralization associated with their use. Soy and hydrolysate formulas may be used in infants with cow's milk protein intolerance; however, signs and symptoms of allergy usually do not become evident until after the newborn is discharged home. Therefore, unless there is a strong family history of milk-protein intolerance, standard formula should be offered to all infants in the nursery. If a switch to a soy formula is planned, the physician must keep in mind that there is a 10% to 30% cross-reactivity between cow-milk and soy proteins. Because true primary lactase deficiency is extremely rare in infancy, there is no reason to offer lactose-free formulas in the nursery.

Urine

Many infants urinate in the delivery room, and most void within hours of birth. A normal infant should urinate within 24 hours of birth, and if no urine output is recorded within that time frame, the cause should be investigated. Well infants have multiple wet diapers in 24 hours but should void at least once every 6 hours. An infant with decreased urine output may be dehydrated; this is more common in infants who are having difficulty breastfeeding and thus taking in an inadequate amount of fluid. Other considerations are anatomic or functional abnormalities that prevent normal urination.

Stool

Most full-term infants pass meconium in the first 24 hours of life. A delay in the passage of meconium may be a variant of normal or may signal a problem, such as meconium plugging, Hirschsprung disease, or dehydration. When addressing a lack of stool production, it should be noted whether there was meconium staining of the amniotic fluid. An infant who has not produced a stool in 48 hours should undergo investigation for an underlying pathology.

Healthy infants have frequent stools—on average, at least four per day in the first 2 to 4 weeks of life. Breastfed infants tend to have more frequent bowel movements and often stool after every feeding. The first stools are meconium (thick, sticky, dark green or black with a "tarry" appearance). These transition to yellow, seedy stools in the first 48 hours of life.

Weight

Normal infants typically lose weight in the first few days of life as they diurese the excess fluid not needed for extrauterine life. Weight should be monitored daily in the nursery because a weight loss of more than 7% may indicate a potential problem, usually inadequate intake. Loss of more than 10% of birth weight for an appropriate for gestational age infant should be considered a significant problem that requires exploration and rectification before discharge and close follow-up afterward. Parents should be reassured that infants usually regain their birth weight in the first 10 to 14 days of life.

Cord Care

The umbilical stump usually falls off in the first 2 weeks of life. Depending on the institution, the umbilical stump may be treated with triple dye or alcohol. Some hospitals now advocate dry cord care, whereby the stump is cleansed with soap and water and allowed to dry.[5] Whatever method is used, caretakers must be instructed in how to keep the stump clean and dry. Old blood and discharge accumulated between the skin and the base of the stump may serve as a nidus for infection. Omphalitis is uncommon and usually presents with erythema and induration around the umbilical stump and foul-smelling discharge, with or without fever. It usually occurs after the newborn has left the hospital. Parents should be taught to recognize signs of omphalitis and instructed to bring the infant to medical attention immediately if these signs develop.

Parental Bonding

During the hospital encounter, one must assess not only the health of the newborn but also the bonding that should be taking place between the newborn and the mother. Postpartum "blues" or depression is very common and may manifest in the hospital with a mother who is emotionally labile or withdrawn. A mother may leave her newborn in the nursery while she is resting, but a mother who does not feed or visit her baby may be having difficulty bonding. Breastfeeding is often a challenge, especially for first-time mothers. Feelings of inadequacy may ensue in the first few days and interfere with bonding. Reassurance, professional guidance, and family support should be instituted in the hospital and continued after discharge. Awareness of cultural differences is also important. In some cultures it is expected that the infant will spend most of its time in the nursery or in the care of others while the mother recuperates.

Circumcision

Whether to circumcise a newborn male is a personal choice, and many parents base their decision on religious or cultural factors. Various studies have shown some potential medical benefits, but there is no consensus in the medical community. The American Academy of Pediatrics issued a statement in 1999 that "existing scientific evidence demonstrates potential medical benefits of newborn male circumcision; however, these data are not sufficient to recommend routine neonatal circumcision."[6] Potential medical benefits include decreased risk of urinary tract infection in the first year of life, decreased risk of penile cancer, and possibly decreased risk of syphilis and HIV susceptibility when sexually active. The risks of circumcision are minor but include bleeding, infection, poor cosmetic result, surgical trauma, meatal stenosis, skin bridges, and inclusion cysts. Infants undergoing circumcision experience pain, as demonstrated by increased heart rate, blood pressure, and cortisol levels and changes in oxygen saturation. They may also exhibit a stronger pain response to later immunizations. Therefore, all infants undergoing circumcision should receive proper analgesia. Options to reduce pain include topical anesthetic application, dorsal penile nerve block, and subcutaneous ring block, along with sucrose on a pacifier and proper positioning during the procedure. Potential but rare complications of analgesia include methemoglobinemia and hematoma. Infants with penile anomalies, such as hypo- or epispadias, should not be circumcised in the newborn period because the foreskin may be needed during subsequent repair.

Care of the Circumcised Penis

Immediately after circumcision, there is swelling and oozing of the glans and subcorona. Depending on te method of circumcision, gauze with lubricant may be applied to the area to prevent adherence to the diaper and repeated trauma to the healing tissue. This should be continued until the area is well healed, usually by the fifth day. The area can be cleansed with water as needed.

Care of the Uncircumcised Penis

The uncircumcised penis requires little care, but parents need to be warned against retracting the foreskin. Many parents are under the impression that the foreskin is always retractile. However, separation of the skin and glans usually takes several years to develop. In most cases, the foreskin can be retracted by age 4 to 5 years, but in some boys this may not happen until adolescence. Forceful retraction of the foreskin is painful and can lead to scarring and permanent adhesion. Until the foreskin separates on its own, only cleansing the external tissue with warm water and later with mild soap is recommended. If the foreskin is retracted down, parents should be advised to pull it back over the glans to prevent paraphimosis.

Care of the Female Genitalia

White, mucus-like vaginal discharge, secondary to maternal hormone exposure, is normal and common in newborn female infants. As it resolves, blood streaking from the vagina may be noted due to maternal hormone withdrawal. Hymenal tissue is often hypertrophied and may protrude from the vaginal opening. It regresses as the effects of maternal hormones on the genitalia resolve. Gentle cleaning with water-soaked gauze or a cotton ball between the labia is all that is necessary to keep the area clean.

Hepatitis B Vaccine

Hepatitis B infection is a worldwide problem, with up to 300 million carriers. It causes acute as well as chronic hepatitis and cirrhosis and is responsible for up to 80% of hepatocellular carcinomas. Although there is an age-specific decline in immunogenicity, the hepatitis B vaccine series is very effective and provides adequate immunity in 90% of adults and more than 95% of children. Routinely, the hepatitis B vaccine is initiated in the nursery.[7]

Perinatal transmission of hepatitis B is very efficient. If the mother is positive for both hepatitis B surface antigen (HBsAg) and hepatitis B e antigen, 70% to 90% of exposed infants will become infected if no postexposure prophylaxis is provided. If the mother is positive only for HBsAg, up to 20% of infants will be infected. Among these congenitally infected infants, up to 90% will become chronic carriers; of these, up to 25% will die of secondary liver failure.[7,8]

Decisions to provide postexposure prophylaxis to infants are based on the mother's HBsAg status. If the mother is HBsAg positive, the infant should receive both hepatitis B immune globulin (HBIG) and the first dose of the hepatitis B vaccine administered as soon as possible within the first 12 hours of life. If HBIG is not available, the vaccine alone should be administered. The vaccine alone is 70% to 95% effective, and the combination of hepatitis B vaccine and HBIG is 85% to 95% effective in preventing infection in the infant.

If the mother's hepatitis B status is unknown, full-term infants with birth weight over 2000 g should receive the hepatitis B vaccine as soon as possible within the first 12 hours of life and the mother should be tested to determine her status. If the test comes back positive, HBIG should be administered as soon as possible. If the results of the HBsAg test are unavailable when the infant reaches 7 days of age, some experts recommend that the infant receive HBIG. Infants should complete the vaccine series based on the maternal hepatitis B status and current recommendations by the American Academy of Pediatrics *Red Book*. Infants of mothers with positive or unknown HBsAg results should be tested at 9 to 18 months of age for evidence of hepatitis B infection.[7,8]

Hearing Screening

All newborns should undergo a hearing screen before discharge from the hospital.[9,10] Between 1 and 3 per 1000 well newborns have some form of hearing loss. Until universal hearing screening was implemented, most of these children were not identified until 14 to 30 months of age. Studies have shown that if intervention is instituted by 6 months of age, the child's language development will be equal to that of normal peers.

There are two accepted and commonly used methods for screening hearing in newborns: the otoacoustic emissions (OAE) test and the auditory brainstem response (ABR) test. The OAE test measures sound waves generated by outer hair cells in the cochlea in response to clicks emitted and recorded by microphones in the outer ear canal. It detects sensory or inner ear hearing loss but not neural hearing loss. It is easy and quick to perform but may produce false failures if there is debris or fluid in the ear canal or effusion in the middle ear. The ABR test measures the activity of the cochlea, auditory nerve, and auditory brainstem pathways. Three electrodes placed on the infant's scalp measure waves generated in response to clicks emitted in the ear canal. It is not affected by conditions of the middle or external ear but requires a quiet infant and environment.

It is recommended that an infant who fails the initial hearing test have a second test before discharge. An infant who fails the second test should be referred for outpatient screening at 1 month of age. A referral for full audiologic evaluation is warranted for infants who fail this series of tests, and this referral should take place before the infant reaches 3 months of age.

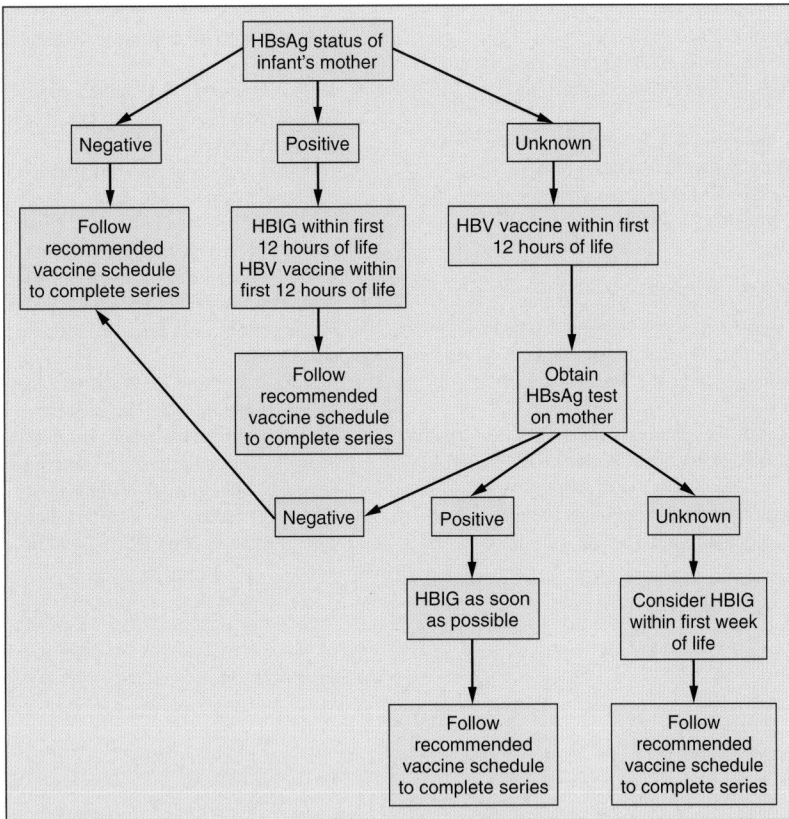

Figure 49-1 Recommendations for the prevention of perinatal transmission of hepatitis B virus in term infants with birth weight over 2000 g. HBV, hepatitis B virus; HBIG, hepatitis B immune globulin; HBsAg, hepatitis B surface antigen.

Metabolic Screening

Newborn screening for certain metabolic and genetic disorders began in the 1960s when Robert Guthrie devised a test that screened for phenylketonuria (PKU). He also developed a simple and inexpensive way of collecting blood samples from the heel of newborns on filter paper. Since then, screening for other disorders has become possible. The goal of newborn screening is to detect certain disorders early and provide treatment to prevent their clinical manifestations and subsequent morbidity and mortality. Today, all 50 states test for PKU and hypothyroidism; however, because there is no federal law regulating newborn screening programs, there is state-to-state variation in the testing for other disorders. Many states test for medium-chain acyl-CoA dehydrogenase deficiency, congenital adrenal hyperplasia, biotinidase deficiency, cystic fibrosis, maple syrup disease, galactosemia, homocystinuria, and sickle cell anemia. Clinicians must be familiar with the tests performed in the states where they practice and counsel parents appropriately about these conditions. It is important to ensure that the specimen is collected at least 24 hours after birth, because many of the disorders are based on abnormal protein metabolism. Some state laboratories may require specimen collection 24 hours after initiation of feedings. With the development of tandem mass spectrometry and DNA-based testing, it is now possible to screen for a number of other metabolic, genetic, and infectious diseases. Clinicians should be aware of the facilities that offer these expanded screenings so that they can provide that information to parents.

Discharge and Follow-up

The nursery clinician is responsible not only for providing guidance to parents regarding the care of their infants but also for ensuring that they have the necessary resources and support. All newborns should have a designated physician for follow-up care. Infants discharged within 24 hours of life (early discharge) need to be seen by a health care professional within 48 hours of discharge. Infants with feeding issues, significant weight loss, temperature instability, significant jaundice, or social issues are not candidates for early discharge. The 2004 American Academy of Pediatrics policy statement outlines the criteria for newborn discharge before 48 hours of life.

At discharge, parents should be specifically counseled with regard to temperature measurement, how to recognize jaundice, the need for a car seat when transporting the infant in a vehicle, positioning the child on the back for sleep, and when to call the physician. Parents should be provided with a telephone number where they can reach a medical professional if questions arise.

SUGGESTED READING

American Academy of Pediatrics: Circumcision policy statement. Pediatrics 1999;103:686-693.

American Academy of Pediatrics: Clinical practice guideline: Early detection of developmental dysplasia of the hip. Pediatrics 2000;105:896-904.

American Academy of Pediatrics: Hospital stay for healthy term newborns. Pediatrics 2004;113:1434-1436.

American Academy of Pediatrics: Newborn and infant hearing loss: Detection and intervention. Pediatrics 1999;103:527-530.

American Academy of Pediatrics: Red Book—2006 Report of the Committee on Infectious Diseases, 27th ed. Elk Grove Village, Illinois, 2006, pp 335-355.

American Academy of Pediatrics: Routine evaluation of blood pressure, hematocrit, and glucose in newborns. Pediatrics 1993;92:474-476.

American Academy of Pediatrics: The transfer of drugs and other chemicals into human milk. Pediatrics 2001;108:776-789.

REFERENCES

1. American Academy of Pediatrics: Clinical practice guideline: Early detection of developmental dysplasia of the hip. Pediatrics 2000;105:896-904.
2. American Academy of Pediatrics: Routine evaluation of blood pressure, hematocrit, and glucose in newborns. Pediatrics 1993;92:474-476.
3. American Academy of Pediatrics: The transfer of drugs and other chemicals into human milk. Pediatrics 2001;108:776-789.
4. American Academy of Pediatrics: Red Book—2006 Report of the Committee on Infectious Diseases, 27th ed. Elk Grove Village, Illinois, 2006, pp 123-127.
5. Janssen P, Selwood B, Dobson S, et al: To dye or not to dye: A randomized, clinical trial of a triple dye/alcohol regime versus dry cord care. Pediatrics 2003;111:15-20.
6. American Academy of Pediatrics: Circumcision policy statement. Pediatrics 1999;103:686-693.
7. Centers for Disease Control and Prevention: Epidemiology and Prevention of Vaccine-Preventable Diseases: The Pink Book, 9th ed. Washington, DC, Public Health Foundation, 2006, pp 191-212.
8. American Academy of Pediatrics: Red Book—2006 Report of the Committee on Infectious Diseases, 27th ed. Elk Grove Village, Illinois, 2006, pp 335-355.
9. American Academy of Pediatrics: Newborn and infant hearing loss: Detection and intervention. Pediatrics 1999;103:527-530.
10. Joint Committee on Infant Hearing: Year 2000 position statement: Principles and guidelines for early hearing detection and intervention programs. Pediatrics 2000;106:798-817.
11. American Academy of Pediatrics: Hospital stay for healthy term newborns. Pediatrics 2004;113:1434-1436.

CHAPTER 50

Birth Injury

Mark D. Hormann

Birth injuries are an uncommon complication of vaginal and cesarean delivery. Injuries range from those that are minor and require no further diagnostic evaluation or treatment to those that are life threatening or associated with long-term morbidity. Risk factors for injury include macrosomia, precipitous or prolonged delivery, breech presentation, cephalopelvic disproportion, shoulder dystocia, and the use of forceps or vacuum to assist extraction.

FRACTURES

Fractures as complications of the delivery process most commonly occur in the clavicle, humerus, and femur. Skull fractures are also reported, usually in association with forceps delivery. Long bone fractures generally require evaluation by an orthopedic specialist, whereas skull fractures are usually simple linear fractures that do not require intervention. Infants rarely have more than one fracture; for those with multiple fractures, diagnoses such as osteogenesis imperfecta should be considered.

Clavicular Fractures

Clavicle fractures occur as a complication of the delivery process in approximately 0.5%[1] to 1.7%[2] of all live births. Historically, clavicle fractures were thought to be a result of obstetric mismanagement. Recent studies, however, have shown that little can be done to prevent this complication. Clavicle fractures are most commonly reported with vaginal deliveries, but they are also reported with cesarean sections. Risk factors proposed by various studies include fetal macrosomia, instrumented delivery, and a prolonged second stage of labor, but predictive models based on these factors have a high false-positive rate and have not been clinically useful.

Clinical Presentation

Clavicular fractures are sometimes overlooked, particularly in the case of a nondisplaced fracture. Acutely, the examiner may feel crepitus, and irritability may be noted with pressure over the bone. In displaced fractures, a bony ledge may be palpated. The infant may have decreased movement of the ipsilateral arm with an asymmetric Moro response. This pseudoparalysis is typically related to pain but may also be the result of associated nerve damage. Frequently, the fracture is first diagnosed as normal healing occurs and the callus forms, which may be noted as early as the second week of life.

Diagnosis

The diagnosis of neonatal clavicle fracture may be made clinically either at the time of delivery or in the first month of life. A single anteroposterior radiograph of the chest is sufficient to confirm the fracture if the diagnosis is in question.

Treatment

Clavicular fractures usually heal without sequelae or deformity. Management is conservative and involves keeping the infant off the affected side; immobilization of the arm may help decrease pain. Healing should occur within 2 weeks, and callus formation may be seen radiographically in several weeks. Parents may complain of a bony irregularity as the clavicle heals, but it will become less prominent as the child grows.

Long Bone Fractures

The humerus is occasionally fractured during the delivery process, typically with a difficult vertex delivery of the shoulder or a breech delivery. The fracture may result from direct pressure or traction. A greenstick fracture is most common, but displaced fractures may also occur. Clinically, there may be swelling and pain; in the case of a displaced fracture an obvious deformity will be noted. The infant may refuse to move the affected arm, thereby resulting in an asymmetric Moro reflex and pseudoparalysis; however, nerve involvement may occur as well. Plain films will confirm the diagnosis of fracture. Treatment is generally limited to immobilization for 2 to 4 weeks in the adducted position, and the prognosis is excellent.

Breech deliveries may also result in a femur fracture; most are complete fractures that result in obvious deformity. Plain films are usually sufficient to confirm the diagnosis. Treatment is 3 to 4 weeks of traction and suspension of both lower extremities. The prognosis is excellent.

In a Nutshell

- Clavicle fractures are the most common fracture seen in the newborn.
- Although unlikely, evaluation for an associated brachial plexus injury should be considered.
- Clavicle fractures generally heal rapidly without specific treatment and without sequelae.
- Humerus and femur fractures occur infrequently and have an excellent prognosis for full healing.
- Multiple fractures in a newborn should suggest other musculoskeletal abnormalities such as osteogenesis imperfecta.

PERIPHERAL NERVE INJURIES

Nerve damage is an infrequent, but important complication of the birthing process. Injury results from traction on the neck and thus on the brachial plexus during delivery. Severity can range from mild stretching of the nerve to nerve root avulsion. Brachial plexus injury is documented in 0.038

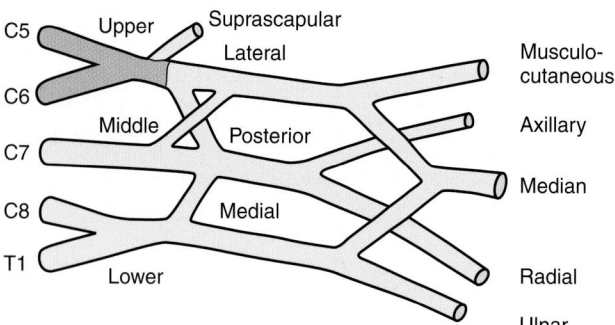

Figure 50-1   Schematic of the brachial nerve plexus. (From Piatt JH: Birth injuries of the brachial plexus. Pediatr Clin North Am 2004;51:421–440.

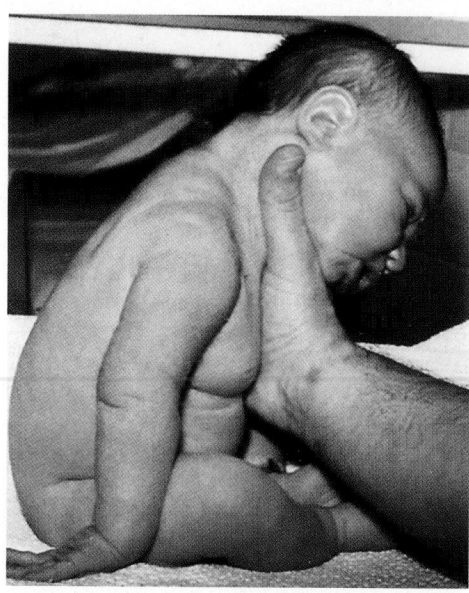

Figure 50-2   Waiter's tip position of Erb palsy. (From Brozanski BS, Bogen DL: Neonatology. In Zitelli BJ, Davis HW [eds]: Atlas of Pediatric Physical Diagnosis. Philadelphia, CV Mosby, 2002.)

to 0.2% of all live births.[3,4] Incidence rates rise with birth weight; in one study of infants weighing more than 4500 g and born vaginally, the incidence of brachial plexus injury was 3.6%.[5] Risk factors include macrosomia, shoulder dystocia, breech presentation, and instrumented delivery. However, because many cases of brachial plexus injury occur without these risk factors, an effective predictive model has not been established.

Clinical Presentation

Injury to the fifth and sixth cervical (C5 and C6) nerve roots is the most common nerve injury (Fig. 50-1) and results in partial paralysis of the upper extremity, known as Erb-Duchenne paralysis. Affected infants have unilateral arm weakness and an asymmetric Moro response. The hypotonic extremity is adducted, internally rotated, and pronated at the forearm. Additional involvement of the seventh cervical (C7) root results in paralysis of the wrist and finger extensors, which causes unopposed flexion of the hand. Together, this is described as the "waiter's tip" position (Fig. 50-2).

Klumpke paralysis is very rare and involves isolated injury to the seventh and eighth cervical (C8) and first thoracic (T1) nerve roots. These infants have normal shoulder and elbow position but a weak or paralyzed hand. If the sympathetic fibers of T1 are also affected, miosis, ptosis, anhidrosis, and enophthalmos (Horner syndrome) are additional findings.

Infants may also have injury to the third and fourth cervical nerve roots (C3 and C4), which results in unilateral diaphragmatic paralysis from phrenic nerve involvement. These infants may present with respiratory distress, hypoxia, asymmetric chest wall movement, and diminished breath sounds on the affected side.

Total plexus injury (C5-T1) accounts for approximately 20% of all plexus injuries and results in a flaccid upper extremity. Involvement of C4 with or without C3 may accompany this severe form of plexus injury.

Diagnosis

The diagnosis of nerve root injury is usually made clinically and based on the finding of an upper extremity with abnormal tone and movement. Plain radiography can rule out an associated fracture of the clavicle or humerus. Electromyography and nerve conduction studies may help clarify the injury in anticipation of surgical repair, but they are rarely necessary otherwise. These studies are typically performed several weeks after birth. When required, magnetic resonance imaging (MRI) can define the anatomy and extent of injury.

The diagnosis of diaphragmatic paralysis is made by demonstrating an elevated hemidiaphragm on the same side as the affected arm on an inspiratory radiograph. Real-time visualization with ultrasound or fluoroscopy will reveal paradoxical movement.

The differential diagnosis includes a clavicular or humeral fracture that may cause the infant pain and result in a pseudoparalysis that is not associated with nerve root damage. Pseudoparalysis of Parrot involving the upper extremity caused by a painful osteochondritis secondary to congenital syphilis can also mimic a brachial plexus injury. However, in this condition multiple long bones are generally involved and other features of congenital syphilis are often present.

Treatment and Outcome

There is some debate about how many infants have complete resolution of their injury without surgical intervention. Recent reports vary in their findings of full recovery from 66%[6] to 92%[7] of affected infants, with the rest displaying varying degrees of residual weakness. Infants with upper arm paralysis do better than those with lower arm involvement. Other features associated with a less favorable outcome include diaphragmatic paralysis and Horner syndrome. Early signs of recovery, which may be noted by 2 weeks of age, clearly favor complete resolution. Some prospective studies suggest that if significant weakness is still present at 4 to 6 months, there is a good chance of permanent weakness.[6]

Initial management is rapid initiation of physical therapy. Therapy needs to include range-of-motion, stretching, and strengthening exercises. The therapist also needs to educate

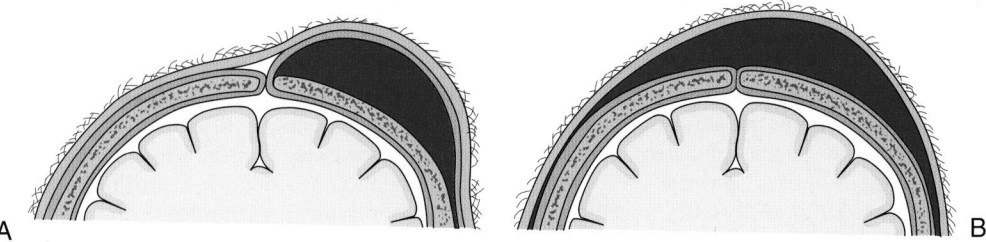

Figure 50-3 Drawing of cephalohematoma (A) versus subgaleal hemorrhage (B). (From Vacca A: Handbook of Vacuum Extraction in Obstetric Practice, 1999, p 71).

the parents of the infant in appropriate exercises at home. These exercises decrease the risk for contractures. Additionally, early involvement of an occupational therapist and a brachial plexus surgeon may be helpful.

Nerve reconstruction is an emerging technique that has shown promise in improving function in certain patients. The best timing for the procedure is not yet clear, but several studies suggest that early repair may have a better long-term outcome. If the infant has no detectable muscle strength of the biceps by 3 months, surgical evaluation is indicated.

In a Nutshell

- Brachial plexus injury may occur with shoulder dystocia, but it also occurs in otherwise normal deliveries.
- Erb-Duchenne paralysis, involving C5, C6, and C7, results in an upper extremity that is internally rotated with flexion at the wrist ("waiter's tip" position).
- Klumpke paralysis is very rare and may be associated with Horner syndrome.
- Although most patients improve with physical therapy and time, nerve reconstruction may be indicated for those with significant deficits at 3 to 6 months of age.

EXTRACRANIAL HEMORRHAGE

Injuries to the scalp, subcutaneous tissue, and skull usually result in swelling that is apparent at birth or shortly thereafter. These extracranial injuries may occur from soft tissue swelling or hemorrhage and often resolve without treatment. However, the clinician needs to be able to accurately recognize these entities and be aware of the complications that may occur with each.

Clinical Presentation

Caput Succedaneum

Pressure applied to the scalp by the uterus, cervix, or pelvis during vaginal delivery results in a localized swelling outside the cranial aponeurosis known as caput succedaneum. It appears as a circular boggy area of edema with indistinct borders that typically crosses cranial suture lines. There may be overlying ecchymosis. Vacuum extraction can cause a more pronounced caput as the presenting region of the scalp receives negative pressure in addition to the positive pressure from below. A chignon is a vacuum-induced caput succedaneum.

Cephalohematoma

It is estimated that up to 2.5%[8] of infants present with a subperiosteal hemorrhage known as a cephalohematoma. It represents hemorrhage between the cranial periosteum and the bony skull and presents as a fluid-filled mass that does not cross suture lines (Fig. 50-3A). Cephalohematoma is often not present at the time of delivery but develops over the first few hours of life. Most commonly it appears in the parietal bone, but more than one cranial bone may be involved. Risk factors for cephalohematoma include a primiparous mother, forceps- or vacuum-assisted delivery, and prolonged labor. In one study, 90% of infants with cephalohematoma had an occiput anterior presentation. In the same study, 7% of cephalohematomas were associated with an underlying skull fracture, with all these injuries being related to the use of forceps.[8]

Subgaleal Hemorrhage

Bleeding that occurs beneath the aponeurosis of the scalp but outside the cranial periosteum is termed a subgaleal or subaponeurotic hemorrhage (Fig. 50-3B). Similar to a cephalohematoma, a subgaleal hemorrhage is fluctuant because of the fluid collection that is present, but it extends over suture lines. Unlike a cephalohematoma, the bleeding into the subgaleal space is not restricted by the boundaries of the sutures. Extensive bleeding may occur and the infant may present with signs of hypovolemic shock.

Diagnosis

The diagnosis is based on the feel and location of the scalp swelling. Ultrasonography is helpful when the clinical examination is not definitive. Because fractures are only occasionally associated with cephalohematoma and the majority of these fractures are benign linear skull fractures, routine skull radiographs are not generally necessary.

Other entities to consider are subarachnoid cyst, meningocele, or leptomeningeal cyst.

Treatment

Caput succedaneum resolves spontaneously over a period of several days; no management is needed other than parental reassurance. Cranial molding and prominent bony ridges as a result of overriding sutures may become more apparent as the soft tissue swelling improves. Parents can be reassured that these bony changes will improve over the next few weeks.

Cephalohematoma takes weeks to months to resolve. As resorption proceeds, the additional red cell destruction may cause or contribute to indirect hyperbilirubinemia. As the hematoma resolves, a firm calcified ring may form around the hematoma and cause the illusion of a depressed skull fracture. In fact, cephalohematomas are uncommonly associated with skull fractures, and they are almost always linear skull fractures that require no specific management.

Subgaleal hemorrhage requires prompt recognition because it is a much more serious entity with mortality estimated at up to 20%. Rapid bleeding can occur and may lead to hypovolemic shock. Serial hemoglobin and bilirubin levels, as well as coagulation studies, are indicated. Volume replacement or red cell transfusion may be needed. Surgical management is rarely indicated because the source of bleeding is typically not identifiable.

Aspiration of these fluid collections is discouraged because the procedure is rarely therapeutic or diagnostic. Imaging studies can determine the anatomic level of the bleeding and do not have the attendant risk of introducing infection.

Infection of the fluid collection can occur, especially when there is an overlying laceration or puncture secondary to forceps, scalp probes, or aspiration attempts. The area becomes erythematous and warm, and fever often develops. When infection is present, aspiration for Gram stain and bacterial culture and sensitivity studies is warranted while empirical antibiotic therapy is initiated. Coverage of skin flora and newborn pathogens is recommended.

In a Nutshell

- Caput succedaneum is edema that resolves in a few days; it crosses the midline.
- Cephalohematoma is a subperiosteal collection of blood that does not cross suture lines. It takes several weeks to months to resolve.
- Subgaleal hemorrhage presents as a fluctuant mass that crosses suture lines. Blood loss can be extensive and lead to hypovolemic shock.

INTRACRANIAL HEMORRHAGE

With advances in obstetric practices, hemorrhage within the bony skull is an increasingly uncommon occurrence in full-term infants. Risk factors are similar to those for other birth injuries, including macrosomia and precipitous or instrument-assisted deliveries. Intraventricular hemorrhage is a significant consideration in premature infants, but not in full-term infants.

Subdural Hemorrhage

Although often associated with vacuum-assisted deliveries, subdural hemorrhage is now known to occur in spontaneous vaginal deliveries, as well as in utero before delivery.

The clinical manifestations range from asymptomatic infants with no long-term sequelae to serious neurologic injury. The location of the hemorrhage can alter the presentation, but the most common locations are tentorial and intrahemispheric. Apnea or cyanotic episodes are the most common initial symptoms, although seizure, focal neurologic deficits, lethargy, or other global nonspecific findings may be the presenting early symptoms. Commonly, infants become symptomatic on the first day of life, but sometimes the findings are not apparent until several days after birth.

Computed tomography (CT) of the head is the diagnostic tool of choice; MRI may be needed to clearly visualize bleeding in the posterior fossa. Because of the risk for an underlying coagulopathy, a prothrombin time and partial thromboplastin time should be obtained. Surgical intervention is usually reserved for infants with evidence of brainstem compression.

Epidural Hemorrhage

Bleeding into the epidural space is the least common form of intracranial hemorrhage. The cause is injury to the middle meningeal artery, which is almost uniformly associated with an overlying fracture of the temporal bone and cephalohematoma. Focal or generalized neurologic symptoms are present shortly after birth, and evidence of raised intracranial pressure may be demonstrated by a bulging fontanelle. CT of the head is diagnostic and may also show the associated skull fracture. Surgical drainage is necessary for most newborns.

Subarachnoid Hemorrhage

In older children and adults, subarachnoid hemorrhage is most often due to aneurysms or arteriovenous malformations. By contrast, subarachnoid hemorrhage in newborns is due to rupture of small bridging veins of the subarachnoid space and is more common with vacuum- or forceps-assisted deliveries than with vaginal deliveries.

The typical presentation in newborns with subarachnoid bleeding is seizure activity that starts on the second day of life, with normal neurologic findings between seizures. CT of the head confirms the diagnosis.

The prognosis is very good, with complete resolution of the hemorrhage and no neurologic sequelae. Most infants do not require intervention unless the hemorrhage is very extensive. Children with asphyxia or underlying cortical injury are at risk for permanent deficits. Posthemorrhagic hydrocephalus may develop in the first few weeks of life and can be detected by routine monitoring of head circumference.

In a Nutshell

- Intracranial hemorrhages are uncommon and may be asymptomatic or life-threatening events.
- CT of the head is the imaging study of choice to diagnose or assess the severity of the bleeding.
- Coagulation studies are indicated as part of the workup for children or infants with an intracranial hemorrhage.
- Surgical intervention is often needed for the management of epidural hemorrhage, but infrequently for subdural or subarachnoid bleeding.

PNEUMOTHORAX

Spontaneous pneumothorax in a term newborn has a reported incidence of 1% to 2%, although many are asymptomatic.[9] It is thought to be the result of the intrathoracic pressure created by the infant during the first few attempts at respiration. Pneumothorax may also be seen in infants with meconium aspiration or pneumonia and in those with a history of receiving positive-pressure ventilation at delivery.

Clinical Presentation

Most spontaneous pneumothoraces in newborns are not clinically apparent. However, if the volume of air in the pleural space is large or under pressure (tension pneumothorax), the infant will display signs of respiratory distress, including grunting, flaring, and retracting, with decreased breath sounds on the involved side. A tension pneumothorax may cause a shift in location of the point of maximal impulse of the heart, deviation of the trachea, or a distended hemithorax.

Diagnosis

If the diagnosis of pneumothorax is suspected and the infant is not clinically stable, intervention should not be delayed to obtain a chest radiograph. Initially, needle thoracostomy may be performed until a definitive chest tube can be inserted (see Treatment). An audible release of air under pressure along with an associated improvement in the patient's clinical status confirms the diagnosis.

If the diagnosis is in question and the infant is clinically stable, a chest radiograph is appropriate to confirm the presence and severity of the pneumothorax. Pneumothorax appears as a dark (radiolucent) area in the chest, without overlying lung markings (Fig. 50-4). A radiograph of an infant with tension pneumothorax also displays a shift of the mediastinum and airway away from the affected side.

Treatment

A small pneumothorax generally resolves spontaneously in a few days and may be monitored clinically or radiographically. Large pneumothoraces and those under pressure

require evacuation of the air and continued drainage with a chest tube and negative pressure. When the air leak has stopped, the tube may be clamped. Without further evidence of reaccumulation, the chest tube may be removed (see Chapter 147).

In a Nutshell

- Small pneumothoraces are common in term infants, are not usually significant, and resolve spontaneously.
- In an infant with cardiopulmonary instability in whom a pneumothorax is suspected, immediate intervention is indicated, such as needle thoracostomy.

On the Horizon

- With advances in obstetric practice, the incidence of certain birth injuries has been reduced. Risk factors for birth injuries continue to be defined, and prevention strategies are being explored.
- Surgical techniques for the repair of brachial plexus injuries are being refined and continue to offer improved outcomes for infants with severe and persistent impairment.

SUGGESTED READING

Beall MH, Ross MG: Clavicle fracture in labor: Risk factors and associated morbidities. J Perinatol 2001;21:513-515.

Dodds SD, Wolfe SW: Perinatal brachial plexus palsy. Curr Opin Pediatr 2000;12:40-47.

Steele RW, Metz JR, Bass JW, DuBois JJ: Pneumothorax and pneumomediastinum in the newborn. Radiology 1971;98:629-632.

Tasunaga S, Rivera R: Cephalohematoma in the newborn. Clin Pediatr (Phila) 1974;13:256-260.

REFERENCES

1. Beall MH, Ross MG: Clavicle fracture in labor: Risk factors and associated morbidities. J Perinatol 2001;21:513-515.
2. Kaplan B, Rabinerson D, Avrech OM, et al: Fracture of the clavicle in the newborn following normal labor and delivery. Int J Gynecol Obstet 1998;63:15-20.
3. Dodds SD, Wolfe SW: Perinatal brachial plexus palsy. Curr Opin Pediatr 2000;12:40-47.
4. Greenwald AG, Schute PC, Shiveley JL: Brachial plexus birth palsy: A 10-year report on the incidence and prognosis. J Pediatr Orthop 1984;4:689-692.
5. Raio L, Ghezzi F, Di Naro E, et al: Perinatal outcome of fetuses with a birth weight greater than 4500 g: An analysis of 3356 cases. Eur J Obstet Gynecol Reprod Biol 2003;109:160-165.
6. Noetzel MJ, Park TS, Robinson S, Kaufman B: Prospective study of recovery following neonatal brachial plexus injury. J Child Neurol 2001;16:488-492.
7. Michelow BJ, Clarke HM, Curtis CG, et al: The natural history of obstetrical brachial plexus palsy. Plast Reconstr Surg 1994;93:675-680; discussion 681.
8. Tasunaga S, Rivera R: Cephalohematoma in the newborn. Clin Pediatr (Phila) 1974;13:256-260.
9. Steele RW, Metz JR, Bass JW, DuBois JJ: Pneumothorax and pneumomediastinum in the newborn. Radiology 1971;98:629-632.

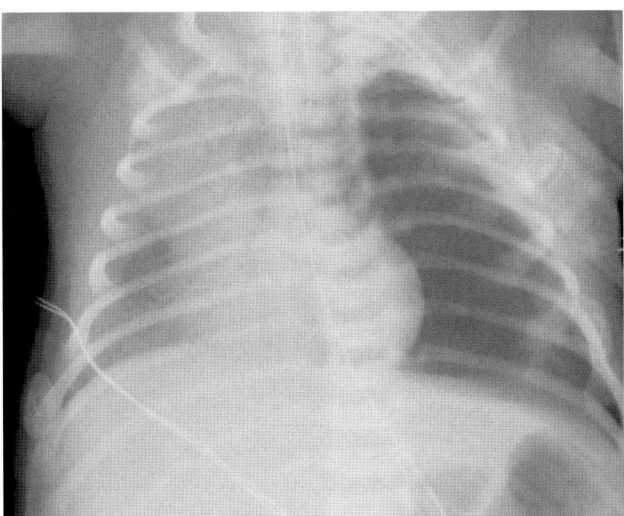

Figure 50-4 Radiograph of a newborn with a large left-sided pneumothorax displacing the mediastinal structures to the right. The mass effect from the pneumothorax is also causing compressive atelectasis in the right upper lung field.

CHAPTER 51

Congenital Anomalies

Mary Beth Madonna and Bill Chiu

Congenital anomalies range from small, barely detectable variations to significant dysmorphologies. They may be caused by recognized genetic mutations (e.g., trisomy 21), toxin-driven syndromes (e.g., fetal alcohol syndrome), deformities due to mechanical in utero effects (e.g., amniotic constriction band syndrome, leading to amputation), or myriad entities of unknown cause. Anomalies frequently occur in a pattern, and the identification of one anomaly raises the possibility that other anomalies may be present, warranting further evaluation.

When approaching a family whose child has either a prenatally diagnosed abnormality or an anticipated birth defect, it is important to be sensitive to the parents' perception of the abnormality, encourage infant-parent bonding, and diplomatically explore possible contributory influences (e.g., drug use, work exposure, consanguinity, family history). This chapter addresses the identification, initial management, and appropriate referral for common congenital anomalies.

ABDOMINAL WALL DEFECTS

Gastroschisis and omphalocele are the most common abdominal wall defects in neonates. In the United States, the combined incidence is estimated to be 1 in 2000 live births. These defects are commonly detected during prenatal ultrasound examinations, which allows delivery at a facility that offers the complete range of expertise needed.

Pathophysiology

During normal fetal development, the gut protrudes from the umbilical ring and then retracts into the abdominal cavity by the 11th week of gestation. When the series of events needed to complete this process fail to occur, abdominal wall defects result. Gastroschisis is not commonly associated with other congenital anomalies, with the exception of intestinal atresia in up to 15% to 25% of cases and cryptorchidism in up to 30%.

An omphalocele results from failed growth and fusion of the lateral folds early in gestation. This creates a central defect of the umbilical ring and allows the bowel to remain herniated. Up to 80% patients with omphalocele have associated anomalies, which are usually midline. These include cardiac defects, colonic atresia, imperforate anus, sacral and vertebral anomalies, and genitourinary malformations. Syndromes associated with omphalocele include pentalogy of Cantrell (sternal cleft; pericardial, cardiac, and diaphragmatic defects), Beckwith-Wiedemann syndrome (macroglossia, macrosomia, and hypoglycemia), and trisomy 13, 18, and 21.

Clinical Presentation and Diagnosis

Patients with gastroschisis commonly present with a defect to the right of the umbilicus and herniation of the abdominal contents through the umbilical ring. The bowel frequently appears thickened, with a fibrous peel, owing to prolonged intrauterine exposure to amniotic fluid. The bowel is not contained within a sac. Complications include intestinal malrotation, volvulus, stenosis, or atresia.

An omphalocele presents as a central defect in the abdominal wall, commonly inferior to the umbilical ring. The opening is generally greater than 4 cm, and a membranous sac covers the contents, unless it ruptured before delivery. The liver and intestines herniate through the opening in 10% of these patients, resulting in a giant omphalocele.

Management

The initial management of an infant with either gastroschisis or omphalocele is the same. The abdominal contents are wrapped in moistened sterile saline gauze. Intravenous fluids at 1.5 times the maintenance rate are started. Parenteral antibiotics that cover bowel flora are given (e.g., ampicillin + gentamicin + metronidazole or ampicillin-sulbactam + gentamicin). A thorough physical examination should be performed to detect any associated anomalies or clinical deterioration. Eventually, radiographic studies ("babygram"), echocardiogram, renal ultrasound, and chromosomal analysis should be obtained.

After initial stabilization, the newborn requires prompt transfer to a neonatal intensive care unit (NICU), with a pediatric surgeon available for further evaluation, management, and treatment.

CONGENITAL DIAPHRAGMATIC HERNIA

Congenital diaphragmatic hernia (CDH) represents one of the most challenging conditions in neonates. As the understanding of this condition evolves, initial stabilization of the patient has taken precedence over immediate surgical repair.

The incidence of CDH is between 1 in 2000 and 1 in 5000 live births, and the majority are on the left side. In utero compression of the developing lung by the bowel may result in pulmonary hypoplasia.

Clinical Presentation

Immediately after birth or within the first 48 hours, neonates with CDH present with respiratory distress, which can include tachypnea, grunting respirations, chest retractions, cyanosis, and pallor. Physical examination reveals a scaphoid abdomen and bowel sounds within the chest. Heart sounds are heard on the right, and breath sounds are decreased bilaterally. Persistent fetal circulation may be demonstrated by the difference in pre- and postductal oxygen saturation measurements.

Differential Diagnosis

Many neonatal conditions can present with respiratory distress (see Chapter 52). Other unusual conditions include pulmonary sequestration, bronchogenic cyst, cystic adenomatoid malformation, pleural effusion, pulmonary consolidation, cystic teratoma, and neurogenic tumor.

Diagnosis and Evaluation

CDH is frequently diagnosed by fetal ultrasonography after 25 weeks' gestation. At birth, a whole-body radiograph (babygram) demonstrates an intestinal air-fluid level within the chest, mediastinal shift, and intrathoracic gastric bubble. A nasogastric tube frequently coils in the chest cavity. Echocardiography and renal ultrasonography are performed to assess for any associated anomalies.

Management

Initial stabilization and delayed surgical intervention constitute the principal strategy. Treatment of respiratory distress includes endotracheal intubation and positive-pressure ventilation. A nasogastric tube is inserted to decompress the stomach, optimizing the respiratory status. Efforts should be directed toward maintaining euvolemia and avoiding acidosis or hypoxemia. After the patient has been stabilized, transfer to a NICU with pediatric surgery availability is required.

VACTERL ANOMALIES

VACTERL association is an acronym to describe a spectrum of Vertebral, Anorectal, Cardiac, Tracheoesophageal, Renal, and Radial Limb malformations. Other malformations include inguinal hernia, small intestinal malformation, choanal atresia, and cleft lip or palate.[3]

Clinical Presentation

Vertebral anomalies include malformation of the vertebrae, myelodysplasia (myelomeningocele, meningocele, lipomeningocele), or even central nervous system disorders. Flaccid paralysis or anesthesia beyond the spinal lesion may be evident.

The most common anorectal malformation is imperforate anus. No anal opening is visible, and no meconium is passed. Other findings may include the presence of a perineal fistula or anal pit.

Cardiac defects can include tetralogy of Fallot, atrial septal defect, ventricular septal defect, truncus arteriosus, patent ductus arteriosus, and coarctation of the aorta.

Tracheoesophageal malformations can include tracheoesophageal fistula and esophageal atresia. Polyhydramnios, resulting from the inability to swallow amniotic fluid, may be noted prenatally if renal agenesis does not exist. After birth, patients present with excessive salivation from pooling of secretions in the posterior pharynx and esophageal pouch. Feeding leads to regurgitation, choking, and cyanosis. Inspired air enters the gastrointestinal tract, causing abdominal distention. Inability to pass a nasogastric tube is another important finding.

Renal anomalies can include agenesis, horseshoe kidney, hypoplastic kidney, or ureteric duplication. Some patients present with early renal failure, requiring kidney transplantation.

Limb deformities include absent radius, absent or displaced thumb, polydactyly, or syndactyly.

Diagnosis and Evaluation

Appropriate imaging is used to evaluate vertebral malformation (spine radiography), limb defects (radiography), cardiac defects (echocardiography), and renal anomalies (renal ultrasonography). Anorectal anomalies are first evaluated by physical examination; a cross-table lateral radiograph can assist in locating the rectal terminus. Tracheoesophageal malformations are revealed on radiographs of the chest and abdomen, which can demonstrate coiling of a nasogastric tube in the esophageal pouch and the presence of bowel gas in the stomach and small intestine.

Management

Most vertebral anomalies are evaluated and managed according to the severity of the defect. Patients presenting with myelomeningoceles require special handling (see the section on spina bifida) and prompt referral to a NICU that can provide multidisciplinary services.

Patients with anorectal malformations, especially imperforate anus, should have nothing by mouth and should be placed on peripheral intravenous fluids. A pediatric surgeon should be consulted for further evaluation and management.

A cardiologist should be involved in the echocardiographic evaluation of cardiac defects, along with a cardiac surgeon, if needed.

Patients with tracheoesophageal fistula and esophageal atresia should be placed on aspiration precautions, with suction to control pooled secretions. Conventional endotracheal intubation should be avoided. Pediatric surgical consultation and transfer to a NICU are required.

Specialists in urology and nephrology are involved in the management of renal anomalies. Patients with limb deformities are referred to orthopedic surgeons.

SACRAL DIMPLES

A sacral dimple or pit, also known as a pilonidal dimple, is a small indentation in the crease between the base of the coccyx and the buttocks. The presence of a sacral dimple may signify the presence of spinal or vertebral anomalies. Approximately 80% of such anomalies have skin lesions overlying the sacral area, but the overwhelming majority are benign.

Sacral dimples may or may not have a clearly visible base. In some cases, hair, skin tags, or nevi may be growing out of the lesion.

Any suspicious lesion should be evaluated by spinal sonography. If the baby is more than 2 to 3 months old, magnetic resonance imaging of the spinal cord is the best study.

If spinal or vertebral anomalies are found, referral to a neurologist or neurosurgeon is warranted.

AMBIGUOUS GENITALIA

Many enzyme or receptor defects and chromosomal abnormalities produce a wide range of abnormalities of the gonads and external genitalia that may be evident in a newborn. The development of genitalia in utero is influenced by many factors. Male sexual differentiation occurs when müllerian inhibiting substance and testosterone are produced by the fetal testis and the Y chromosome is present. If these substances are absent, female development ensues. Testosterone stimulates the development of the internal male (wolffian) structures, and müllerian inhibiting substance inhibits development of the internal female structures.

The most common intersex anomaly in the United States and Europe is congenital adrenal hyperplasia (CAH), also known as female pseudohermaphroditism when it occurs in girls. CAH may be due to different enzyme deficiencies in the steroidogenesis pathway, but 90% of cases are due to a deficiency of the 21-hydroxylase enzyme. The defect in the cortisol pathway leads to increased production of corticotropin and adrenocorticotropic hormone, which results in overproduction of the steroids proximal to the defect—namely, the androgenic steroids and melanocyte-stimulating hormone. Approximately 75% of these patients are salt losers.

CAH may present with virilized genitalia in girls, but boys have normal-appearing genitalia at birth. For this reason, girls are more likely to be identified immediately. Undetected salt-wasting CAH presents in the first few weeks of life with nonspecific symptoms, including poor feeding, lack of weight gain, vomiting, and lethargy. As adrenal crisis progresses, the infant becomes severely dehydrated and can present in extremis.

Initial Management

A patient presenting with ambiguous genitalia at birth faces complex problems that are best treated at a specialized center as soon as the condition is recognized. Rapid gender assignment minimizes emotional trauma to the family but must be done only after the diagnostic workup is complete.

A complete history should be performed, including a pedigree, drug use in the mother, and assessment of maternal virilization. The physical examination should assess the size of the phallus and the symmetry of the gonads. Because mineralocorticoids may be deficient or overabundant, chemistries and serum sugar should be rapidly assessed, and vital signs should be closely monitored. To identify the hormonal abnormalities, serum levels of cortisone, testosterone, dihydrotestosterone, luteinizing hormone, follicle-stimulating hormone, serum 17-hydroxyprogesterone, and dehydroepiandrosterone should be obtained. The latter two are elevated in 21-hydroxylase–deficient CAH. A rapid evaluation of chromosomes should also be performed. More elaborate testing can be done at a specialized center to look for a specific genetic defect.

Patients with salt-wasting CAH develop adrenal crisis with severe dehydration and electrolyte abnormalities. Initial stabilization involves volume expansion with intravenous normal (0.9%) saline. This fluid resuscitation also corrects the hyponatremia and hyperkalemia caused by the mineralocorticoid deficiency. Hypoglycemia is common and should be treated with intravenous dextrose. If possible, baseline laboratory studies should be obtained before steroid replacement, but steroid administration should not be delayed. Intravenous hydrocortisone (50 mg/m^2) is given as a bolus, followed by an infusion to deliver 50 mg/m^2 over the first 24 hours; this should provide sufficient glucocorticoid and mineralocorticoid activity.

CLEFT LIP AND PALATE

One in every 700 infants has cleft lip or palate, or both. Cleft lip and palate are associated with other anomalies in up to 63% of cases, most often as part of a well-recognized syndrome. Failure of the facial prominences to fuse leads to cleft lip; failure of the palatal shelves to fuse leads to cleft palate.

Diagnosis

Patients who have cleft lip are easily identified at birth, which should prompt the examiner to check for an associated abnormality of the palate. Visualization can also identify isolated cleft palate; however, because palatal defects may exist despite a normal appearance, palpation of the anterior and posterior palate is required to detect submucosal abnormalities. In addition, an assessment of hearing is important because there may be associated auditory abnormalities.

Management

Feeding is a major concern in the postnatal period. A physician should evaluate the infant's cough and gag reflex before attempting the various methods available for oral feeding. Although some infants may be able to breastfeed, many infants with cleft lip and palate cannot generate enough suction to draw milk from the breast or from a standard bottle. A special nipple with an enlarged slitlike aperture and a squeezable bottle (Haberman bottle) are often effective. A speech therapist should be involved early to assist in assessing and implementing safe and effective feeding regimens. The patient should be referred to a center that can provide the multidisciplinary services required by these children and their families.

In the past, cleft lip repair was delayed until the child weighed more than 10 pounds and was 10 weeks old, to lower the risk of anesthesia. Today, with advances in anesthesia, the repair is performed earlier, usually around 6 weeks.

SPINA BIFIDA

A neural tube defect (NTD) is any defect in the morphogenesis of the neural tube, ranging from anencephaly to spina bifida occulta. The cause of NTDs is unknown, but some mulitfactorial genetic and environmental factors have been implicated, including deficiencies in folic acid and zinc.

Diagnosis

Prenatal diagnosis of NTDs allows improved obstetric care or the option of pregnancy termination. Chorionic villus sampling can be done at 8 weeks and is a reliable method of diagnosis. Maternal serum α-fetoprotein is a good mass screening tool and can identify pregnancies that require further evaluation. Amniocentesis is performed in suspicious cases after 16 weeks, and the amniotic fluid is tested for α-fetoprotein and acetylcholinesterase levels, which are markers for NTDs. Prenatal ultrasonography is also a useful screening tool.

Classification, Management, and Outcome

Spina bifida occulta refers to a form of spinal dysraphism that is not accompanied by extrusion of the contents of the vertebral column. If there is no external evidence, this condition is rarely diagnosed in the newborn period. Occasionally, this lesion produces a neurologic deficit over time due to cord tethering; this may manifest as urinary problems or motor or sensory deficits such as muscle weakness, pelvic tilt, or trophic ulceration. Radiographs of the spine show the anomalies. Spinal ultrasonography is useful in the newborn period, and magnetic resonance imaging may be required later. Surgical correction may be necessary.

A meningocele, which is a form of spina bifida cystica, is an epithelium-lined sac filled with cerebrospinal fluid that does not contain neural elements. It communicates with the spinal subarachnoid space. The meningocele is covered with skin and protrudes through an incomplete posterior arch. The site of predilection is the lumbar region. A cranial meningocele is most commonly found at the occiput; it is usually not associated with neurologic deficit or hydrocephalus. Early operative intervention is recommended to prevent infection and restore continuity. The prognosis for normal development is good.

A myelomeningocele is a vertebral defect producing a cystic lesion with attenuated meninges and skin that may contain neural tissue. The lumbar region is most commonly involved (80%), because this is the last region of the neural tube to close. The defect can also occur in the cervical, thoracic, or sacral region, however, or there may be multiple defects. There is often marked kyphosis or scoliosis and almost always some degree of paralysis, sensory loss, and bladder and bowel abnormalities. The paralysis is usually flaccid but can occasionally be spastic. The sensory loss is determined by pinprick, and the level of anesthesia is an indicator of the myotomic defect and a predictor of the handicap. Approximately 85% to 95% of patients develop hydrocephalus, although only 15% present with it at birth. Clubfoot is the most common associated skeletal anomaly.

Encephaloceles are cystic lesions that contain cerebrospinal fluid and brain tissue and are most commonly located in the occipital region. Children with this defect are at increased risk for hydrocephalus and often have significant neurologic deficits.

The initial management of meningoceles, myelomeningoceles, and encephaloceles involves protection of the protruding lesion. The sac is wrapped in a nonstick dressing, and the patient is placed in a prone or side-lying position. Empirical antibiotic therapy is considered, especially if there is evidence of a cerebrospinal fluid leak. These children should be transferred to a center that can provide multidisciplinary coordinated care involving neurosurgery, urology, orthopedics, physical therapy, and social work. The timing of surgical repair is controversial; it is based on many factors and varies among institutions.

IN A NUTSHELL

- Abdominal wall defects are often detected prenatally.
- Gastroschisis is generally to the right of the umbilical ring, lacks a membranous sac, and is not commonly associated with other anomalies.
- Omphalocele is centrally located inferior to the umbilicus, is generally covered by a sac, and is usually associated with other major congenital malformations.
- CDH is usually detected prenatally by ultrasonography. Postnatally, patients present with respiratory distress; a chest radiograph demonstrates a stomach bubble in the lung field.
- At birth, patients with CDH require rapid intubation, followed by prompt transfer to a NICU.
- VACTERL association involves vertebral, anorectal, cardiac, tracheoesophageal, renal, and limb abnormalities. Any newborn with both esophageal and renal abnormalities should be evaluated for VACTERL association.
- Superficial sacral abnormalities may indicate the presence of underlying spinal malformations.
- Ambiguous genitalia occurs due to a range of abnormalities. Gender assignment should be timely, but not rushed, and should take multiple concerns into consideration.
- CAH often presents with ambiguous genitalia in girls but may present with adrenal crisis in the first few weeks of life.
- The palate of every infant should be assessed visually and manually for defects. Patients with cleft lip and palate need early feeding assistance.
- Spina bifida ranges from subclinical (spina bifida occulta) to neurologically devastating neural tube defects.
- Patients with meningocele, myelomeningocele, or encephalocele are best managed by centers that can provide specialized multidisciplinary services.

ON THE HORIZON

- The prediction, detection, and management of congenital abnormalities continue to evolve as genetic mutations are identified, prenatal ultrasound and other diagnostic techniques improve, and both fetal and post-delivery surgical techniques advance.
- In utero repair of CDH, treatment of tracheal occlusion, and lung transplantation have been attempted either in humans or in experimental models. Selected centers have used novel techniques to provide early intervention, but the results are still under investigation.
- Studies of VACTERL association are ongoing to better delineate associated abnormalities.
- In utero repair of cleft lip and palate is being explored to reduce the typical scar formation.
- Folic acid supplementation in bread may help reduce the incidence of spina bifida.

SUGGESTED READING

Bohn D: Congenital diaphragmatic hernia. Am J Respir Crit Care Med 2002;166:911-915.

Donahoe PK, Schnitzer JJ: Ambiguous genitalia in the newborn. In O'Neill JA, Rowe MI, Gorsfeld JL, et al (eds): Pediatric Surgery. St Louis, Mosby, 1998, pp 1797-1818.

Dykes EH: Prenatal diagnosis and management of abdominal wall defects. Semin Pediatr Surg 1996;5:90-94.

Geissler GH: Abdominal wall defects. In Arensman RM, Bambini DA, Almond PS (eds): Pediatric Surgery. Georgetown, Tex, Landes Bioscience, 2000, pp 361-365.

Gibson PJ, Britton J, Hall DM, et al: Lumbosacral skin markers and identification of occult spinal dysraphism in neonates. Acta Paediatr 1995;84:208-209.

Witt PD: Cleft lip and palate. In Oldlam KT, Columbani PM, Foglia RP (eds): Surgery of Infants and Children: Scientific Principles and Practice. Philadelphia, Lippincott-Raven, 1997, pp 815-824.

REFERENCES

1. Townsend CM Jr: Sabiston Textbook of Surgery, 17th ed. Philadelphia, Elsevier, 2004, p 2116.
2. Weber T, Au-Fliegner M, Downard C, Fishman S: Abdominal wall defects. Curr Opin Pediatr 2002;14:491-497.
3. Weaver DD: The VATER association: Analysis of 46 patients. Am J Dis Child 1986;140:225-229.

Respiratory Distress and Transient Tachypnea of the Newborn

Nicola Klein

Respiratory distress occurs frequently in newborns and can be a presenting symptom of both benign and life-threatening diseases. A detailed discussion of the complex series of cardiovascular and pulmonary modifications that help the neonate make the transition to extrauterine life can be found in Chapter 48. Failure of any of these adaptations to perinatal life can manifest as neonatal respiratory distress. Clinical features of a newborn in respiratory distress include tachypnea of more than 60 breaths per minute; cyanosis; expiratory grunting; intercostal, subcostal, or supraclavicular retractions; and nasal flaring. Although the causes of respiratory distress are numerous, this chapter focuses on a relatively common cause of respiratory distress known as transient tachypnea of the newborn (TTN) and the identification of a more serious condition, persistent pulmonary hypertension of the newborn (PPHN).

PATHOPHYSIOLOGY

TTN is a benign, self-limited disorder that occurs during the transition from uterine to extrauterine life and results from the delayed clearance of excess lung fluid. TTN was first described in 1966 when it was observed that a subset of newborns exhibited respiratory distress, consisting primarily of tachypnea, at or shortly after birth. Although the tachypnea persisted for several days, it subsequently resolved completely without sequelae.[1]

Inadequate or delayed clearance of fetal lung fluid results in TTN, whereas surfactant deficiency results in respiratory distress syndrome. These categorizations are not absolute, however; some have suggested that TTN is associated with a relative surfactant dysfunction,[2] but other studies found no association between TTN and surfactant mutation.[3]

Delivery via elective cesarean section increases the risk for TTN. Although the physiologic mechanisms are not understood, this risk is significantly decreased if the mother undergoes a trial of labor.[4-6] Additional risk factors for TTN include male sex and macrosomia.[7] Although the mechanism is obscure, being born to an asthmatic mother appears to be a risk factor for TTN.[8] Infants born to women with gestational diabetes also appear to be at increased risk. This observation may be related to a corresponding increase in the rate of cesarean sections among these mothers.[9]

PPHN commonly occurs in full-term and near-term infants (>34 weeks) and has an estimated incidence of 0.2% of live births.[10] After birth, PPHN occurs when there is an insufficient or delayed decrease in pulmonary vascular resistance, which results in right-to-left shunting of blood through the ductus arteriosus or foramen ovale and severe hypoxemia. PPHN typically arises in the setting of a structurally normal heart, either with or without associated pulmonary disease. Perinatal risk factors that increase pulmonary vasoconstriction include hypoxia, acidosis, alveolar atelectasis, sepsis, direct lung injury, hypoglycemia, and cold stress.[11,12] The most common causes are meconium aspiration syndrome (50%), idiopathic PPHN (20%), sepsis (20%), and respiratory distress syndrome (5%).[11]

Despite the array of conditions associated with PPHN, one common feature is an underlying abnormality of the pulmonary vasculature. This abnormality can be broadly categorized into three groups.[10,11] In the first group, the vasculature is abnormally constricted due to parenchymal lung disease. This group is the most common and includes meconium aspiration syndrome, sepsis, and respiratory distress. The second group is associated with structurally abnormal pulmonary vasculature and includes idiopathic PPHN. The pulmonary vasculature of these infants shows significant thickening and does not appropriately vasodilate in response to birth stimuli (particularly nitric oxide and endothelin signaling pathways). The vasculature of the third group is hypoplastic, usually due to congenital diaphragmatic hernia or, much less commonly, a rare malformation of lung development known as alveolar-capillary dysplasia.[10]

CLINICAL PRESENTATION

TTN presents within the first few hours of life with respiratory rates greater than 60 breaths per minute. Infants typically have shallow respirations, which may be accompanied by mild cyanosis. Increased work of breathing, including subcostal retractions, expiratory grunting, and nasal flaring, may also be present. Auscultation of the chest reveals clear breath sounds without rales, rhonchi, or crackles. Most infants do not require high levels of exogenous oxygen to ensure adequate oxygenation. Although symptoms usually resolve within the first 24 hours, TTN can persist for as long as 72 hours.

Early signs of PPHN may overlap with those of TTN, but there are distinguishing features. As unoxygenated blood is shunted away from the high-pressure circuit of the lungs through the patent ductus arteriosus in PPHN, the blood that reaches postductal areas of the systemic circulation is mixed, or lower in saturation, than the blood that circulates to the preductal regions. Pulse oximeters placed on both a preductal (right upper) and a postductal (left upper, right or left lower) extremity yield discrepancies. If the preductal oxygen saturation exceeds the postductal oxygen saturation by more than one or two percentage points, a diagnosis of PPHN must be considered. These infants may deteriorate

Table 52-1   Causes of Respiratory Distress in the Newborn

Structural and anatomic
  Diaphragmatic hernia
  Choanal atresia
  Tracheomalacia
  Laryngomalacia
  Tracheoesophageal fistula
  Vocal cord paralysis
  Excessive nasal secretions

Pulmonary
  Transient tachypnea of the newborn
  Respiratory distress syndrome
  Meconium aspiration syndrome
  Persistant pulmonary hypertension of the newborn
  Pulmonary hypoplasia
  Pneumothorax
  Neonatal pneumonia
  Pulmonary cysts

Infectious
  Neonatal pneumonia
  Sepsis

Systemic
  Metabolic acidosis
  Hypothermia
  Encephalopathy

Cardiac
  Congenital heart disease

rapidly, with systemic hypotension and severe respiratory distress, if their pulmonary arterioles cannot be dilated.

DIFFERENTIAL DIAGNOSIS

As mentioned earlier, the differential diagnosis for a newborn in respiratory distress is extensive (Table 52-1). Infants with TTN generally do not require high levels of oxygen (>60%) or respiratory support such as mechanical ventilation. PPHN is one of the more serious conditions that presents with respiratory distress, but others must also be considered. A newborn exhibiting prolonged, significant respiratory distress or requiring a high level of respiratory support may be suffering from neonatal sepsis, pneumonia, pneumothorax, respiratory distress syndrome, or cardiac disease.

Significant cardiac malformations causing respiratory distress can be differentiated from TTN and other causes of respiratory distress. The initial evaluation should include auscultation for the existence of a pathologic murmur. In infants with significant cyanotic cardiac lesions, blood is shunted away from the lungs through the lesion. Therefore, when these infants are given exogenous oxygen, their oxygen saturation or arterial oxygen tension improves only minimally (or not at all). Measurements of upper and lower extremity blood pressures may reveal a difference between the two, suggestive of coarctation of the aorta. In the presence of critical lung disease or a more subtle cardiac lesion,

echocardiography may be necessary to detect or confirm a diagnosis.

DIAGNOSIS AND EVALUATION

TTN is a clinical diagnosis. PPHN is also suggested by the clinical presentation, but further diagnostic testing is usually performed to confirm the diagnosis or assess the severity.

The initial evaluation may include a complete blood count and a chest radiograph. If there are clinical features (e.g., temperature instability, lethargy) or risk factors (e.g., maternal fever, chorioamnionitis, incomplete treatment of maternal group B streptococcal colonization) for infection, appropriate cultures should also be obtained (see Chapter 53). In addition, measurement of C-reactive protein levels may be helpful, although these results may be unreliable when obtained shortly after birth if there has been insufficient time for an inflammatory response to occur.[13] In TTN, an arterial blood gas evaluation reveals a mild respiratory acidosis due to mild hypoxemia and hypercapnia; the complete blood count and C-reactive protein are typically normal. On chest radiographs, classic findings of TTN include prominent central markings suggestive of vascular engorgement, moderate cardiomegaly, increased lung volume, and increased anteroposterior chest diameter.[1] A study conducted of more than 2800 babies reported in 2003 found a subset of infants whose clinical appearance indicated TTN but whose chest films were clear. This suggests that TTN can occur despite normal chest findings.[14] Unless the infant's clinical symptoms suggest more serious disease, other studies are usually not necessary.

In PPHN, chest radiographs typically reveal a normal or slightly enlarged heart with normal or reduced blood flow. The arterial blood gas evaluation reflects a low oxygen tension for the inspired oxygen content; carbon dioxide levels may be normal if there is no parenchymal lung disease. The presence of a gradient between pre- and postductal oxygen saturation may also be helpful in the diagnosis (see earlier). However, to diagnose PPHN definitively, an echocardiogram must be obtained to exclude structural heart lesions as the cause of the severe hypoxemia. In PPHN, the echocardiogram reveals normal structural anatomy with evidence of pulmonary hypertension.

MANAGEMENT

Management of TTN is supportive. Although an infant exhibiting mild tachypnea can usually be observed for a few hours in the newborn nursery, significant tachypnea (>60 to 80 breaths per minute) prevents oral feeding and necessitates transfer to a higher level of care for initiation of intravenous fluids and monitoring. In selected situations, an orogastric or nasogastric tube can be placed for assistance with feeding, but only after determining that the infant is unlikely to require ventilatory support. Because of concerns about gastroesophageal reflux and aspiration, infants with respiratory rates greater than 90 to 100 breaths per minute should not receive oral or gastric feedings. However, placement of an orogastric or nasogastric tube for stomach decompression may be helpful to maximize lung volume expansion. Supplemental oxygen may be needed, and nasal continuous positive airway pressure may be required for infants exhibiting persistent and significant work of breathing. Although some have proposed that furosemide may be useful in the treatment of TTN, studies have not confirmed that it has any role.[15]

Whenever there is concern about PPHN, the infant should be placed on 100% oxygen and transferred to a neonatal intensive care unit. While awaiting transfer, any metabolic abnormalities should be corrected, including metabolic acidosis (although the use of alkalizing agents is controversial), hypoglycemia, hypothermia, hypovolemia, anemia, and hypocalcemia.[10]

CRITERIA FOR TRANSFER TO A NEONATAL INTENSIVE CARE UNIT

- Suspected or proven PPHN
- Respiratory distress requiring supplemental oxygen
- Significant tachypnea (>60 to 80 breaths per minute) that requires frequent reassessment or precludes oral feeding
- Prolonged tachypnea (>4 to 6 hours)
- Respiratory distress that may require the administration of continuous positive airway pressure or other ventilatory support
- Suspected or proven infection
- Suspected or proven cardiac disease
- Respiratory distress for which there is an unclear diagnosis

DISCHARGE CRITERIA

Transient Tachypnea of the Newborn

- Resolved respiratory distress
- No exogenous oxygen requirement for at least 24 hours
- Able to feed adequately by mouth
- Reliable outpatient follow-up

Persistent Pulmonary Hypertension of the Newborn

- Management and discharge criteria determined by the neonatologist

IN A NUTSHELL

- TTN is a common cause of neonatal respiratory distress that usually presents in the first few hours of life with tachypnea, mild cyanosis, and mildly increased work of breathing.
- TTN is a clinical diagnosis but may require diagnostic tests to exclude other causes of respiratory distress, based on a history of risk factors and typical findings on chest radiographs.
- TTN has a benign and self-limited course, and treatment is supportive.
- PPHN usually occurs in term or near-term infants and presents with severe cyanosis and tachypnea. The findings on chest radiographs depend on the presence of associated lung disease. For any infant suspected of having PPHN, an echocardiogram is required to

- exclude structural heart defects as the cause of hypoxemia.
- PPHN is a life-threatening condition that requires management in an intensive care setting.

ON THE HORIZON

- A recent report describes the use of the stable microbubble test to identify a subset of infants who initially present with the characteristic symptoms of TTN but subsequently develop more severe and progressive respiratory distress. Such patients may benefit from surfactant therapy.[2]

SUGGESTED READING

Agrawal V, David RJ, Harris VJ: Classification of acute respiratory disorders of all newborns in a tertiary care center. J Natl Med Assoc 2003;95:585-595.

Farrow KN, Fliman P, Steinhorn RH: The diseases treated with ECMO: Focus on PPHN. Semin Perinatol 2005;29:8-14.

Hook B, Kiwi R, Amini SB, et al: Neonatal morbidity after elective repeat cesarean section and trial of labor. Pediatrics 1997;100:348-353.

Levine EM, Ghai V, Barton JJ, Strom CM: Mode of delivery and risk of respiratory diseases in newborns. Obstet Gynecol 2001;97:439-442.

REFERENCES

1. Avery ME, Gatewood OB, Brumley G: Transient tachypnea of newborn. Am J Dis Child 1966;111:380-385.
2. Fiori H, Henn R, Baldisserotto M, et al: Evaluation of surfactant function at birth determined by the stable microbubble test in term and near term infants with respiratory distress. Eur J Pediatr 2004;163:443-448.
3. Tutdibi E, Hospes B, Landmann E, et al: Transient tachypnea of the newborn (TTN): A role for polymorphisms of surfactant protein B (SP-B) encoding gene? Klin Padiatr 2003;215:248-252.
4. Morrison JJ, Rennie JM, Milton PJ: Neonatal respiratory morbidity and mode of delivery at term: Influence of timing of elective caesarean section. Br J Obstet Gynaecol 1995;102:101-106.
5. Hook B, Kiwi R, Amini SB, et al: Neonatal morbidity after elective repeat cesarean section and trial of labor. Pediatrics 1997;100:348-353.
6. Levine EM, Ghai V, Barton JJ, Strom CM: Mode of delivery and risk of respiratory diseases in newborns. Obstet Gynecol 2001;97:439-442.
7. Rawlings J, Smith FR: Transient tachypnea of the newborn: An analysis of neonatal and obstetric risk factors. Am J Dis Child 1984;138:869-871.
8. Schatz M, Zeiger RS, Hoffman CP, et al: Increased transient tachypnea of the newborn in infants of asthmatic mothers. Am J Dis Child 1991;145:156-158.
9. Persson B, Hanson U: Neonatal morbidities in gestational diabetes mellitus. Diabetes Care 1998;21(Suppl 2):B79-B84.
10. Farrow KN, Fliman P, Steinhorn RH: The diseases treated with ECMO: Focus on PPHN. Semin Perinatol 2005;29:8-14.
11. Konduri GG: New approaches for persistent pulmonary hypertension of newborn. Clin Perinatol 2004;31:591-611.
12. Dakshinamurti S: Pathophysiologic mechanisms of persistent pulmonary hypertension of the newborn. Pediatr Pulmonol 2005;39:492-503.
13. Polin R: The "ins and outs" of neonatal sepsis. J Pediatr 2003;143:3-4.
14. Agrawal V, David RJ, Harris VJ: Classification of acute respiratory disorders of all newborns in a tertiary care center. J Natl Med Assoc 2003;95:585-595.
15. Lewis V, Whitelaw A: Furosemide for transient tachypnea of the newborn. Cochrane Database Syst Rev 2002;1.

CHAPTER 53

Congenital and Perinatal Infections

Eric Frehm and Mary Catherine Harris

Congenital and perinatal infections are a major cause of ill health in children. Although many infections of the fetus and neonate can be treated effectively, others may result in lengthy hospitalization, prolonged suffering, lifelong disability, and even death. The list of responsible pathogens includes bacteria, viruses, fungi, and protozoa. The modes of transmission are similarly varied, including transplacental spread, intrauterine contamination, and exposure at the time of delivery and beyond. Expert care of the newborn requires a thorough understanding of the presentation, diagnosis, and treatment of these diverse infectious conditions.

CONGENITAL INFECTIONS

Congenital infections are a significant source of pediatric morbidity and occasional neonatal mortality. Their long-term sequelae can include feeding problems, sensorineural impairment, seizures, and mental retardation. Congenital infections typically result from primary maternal infection during pregnancy, although some cases result from the reactivation of previous disease. Unfortunately, the TORCH acronym (toxoplasmosis, other agents, rubella, cytomegalovirus, herpes simplex) no longer encompasses the full spectrum of true congenital infections. Although cytomegalovirus (CMV) and toxoplasmosis remain important clinical entities, congenital rubella has become a rarity in the United States, and herpes simplex virus (HSV) is more typically a perinatally or postnatally acquired infection. The "other" category unjustly lumps together *Treponema pallidum*, varicella-zoster, parvovirus B19, human immunodeficiency virus (HIV), and many other important pathogens.

Clinical Presentation

Many congenital infections remain asymptomatic in the newborn period. When clinical signs are readily apparent (e.g., growth retardation, intracranial calcification), the constellation of findings is rarely specific enough to be pathognomonic for one particular disease.

CMV, from the Herpesviridae family of viruses, is the most common congenital viral infection in the United States, affecting as many as 1% of newborns.[1] Although congenital infection is much more likely to occur with primary maternal disease than with recurrent maternal infection, intrauterine CMV transmission is possible in women with preconceptual immunity. Virus can also be passed during delivery or postnatally (e.g., through breast milk), but these infections are usually mild. The clinical presentation of congenital CMV may include intrauterine growth retardation, hepatosplenomegaly, petechiae or purpura, and jaundice. Central nervous system (CNS) involvement can include microcephaly, intracranial calcification, retinitis, and hearing loss. Pneumonitis and viral sepsis are also possible.

The great majority of infants with congenital CMV, however, are asymptomatic in the newborn period.

Toxoplasma gondii is a protozoan parasite transmittable through contact with cat feces or the consumption of contaminated foods, such as meat containing infective tissue cysts or unwashed produce from contaminated soil. Congenital infection with *Toxoplasma* is usually subclinical, but it can present with hepatosplenomegaly, lymphadenopathy, maculopapular rash (see Chapter 164), jaundice, anemia, and thrombocytopenia. Early CNS manifestations may include chorioretinitis, microcephaly or hydrocephalus, and intracranial calcifications. Congenital toxoplasmosis can be severe enough to result in stillbirth or neonatal death.[2]

Rubella virus remains a serious threat to infant health worldwide, but vaccination has made it an infrequent cause of congenital infection in the United States. Manifestations may include intrauterine growth retardation; cataracts, retinopathy, and other eye disorders; cardiac structural defects (e.g., pulmonary artery stenosis, patent ductus arteriosus) and myocarditis; hepatosplenomegaly; thrombocytopenia; purpuric rash; and neurologic effects such as hearing loss, meningoencephalitis, and mental retardation.[3]

Congenital syphilis, caused by the spirochete *Treponema pallidum*, can result in stillbirth, preterm delivery, and a wide range of early clinical signs, including hepatosplenomegaly, jaundice, lymphadenopathy, osteochondritis, periostitis, "snuffles" (syphilitic rhinitis), and mucocutaneous findings such as maculopapular erythema, bullae, desquamation, and even condylomas (see Chapter 164).[4]

Other pathogens that may warrant diagnostic consideration in the evaluation of congenital infection include parvovirus B19, varicella, HIV, enteroviruses, HSV, and lymphocytic choriomeningitis virus.

Differential Diagnosis

The clinical presentation of congenital infection often overlaps with that of noninfectious diseases, such as genetic conditions (e.g., pseudo-TORCH syndrome), metabolic disorders, or antenatal teratogen or drug exposure. Conversely, congenital infection often tops the list of differential diagnoses for a multitude of fetal and neonatal conditions, such as intrauterine growth retardation, hydrocephalus, conjugated hyperbilirubinemia, hepatosplenomegaly, and assorted cytopenias.

Diagnosis and Evaluation

The diagnosis of congenital CMV is best made by isolating shed virus from urine or saliva before 3 weeks of age. After that time, the shedding could represent infection acquired perinatally or postnatally. Tissue culture and shell vial assay are common techniques for isolating CMV. Detection of CMV DNA by polymerase chain reaction (PCR) and characteristic histopathologic changes (e.g., in the placenta) can also suggest or support the diagnosis. Serologic testing is possible but is less precise.

Recommendations of the American Academy of Pediatrics for the evaluation of infants with suspected congenital syphilis include a complete physical examination, quantitative nontreponemal serologic testing of the infant's serum (e.g., VDRL, RPR), lumbar puncture for routine cerebrospinal fluid (CSF) testing and VDRL, complete blood count, radiographs of the long bones, and a focused pathologic examination of the placenta (if possible). Laboratory abnormalities in infants with syphilis include hemolytic anemia, thrombocytopenia, and signs of liver dysfunction.

Congenital rubella can be diagnosed by demonstration of virus or, more typically, by serologic or PCR-based laboratory methods. Likewise, toxoplasmosis can be diagnosed by isolation of the parasite from the placenta, blood, or CSF; PCR methods; or serologic assays.

Course of Illness

Although congenital infections can present as acute neonatal illnesses, these conditions are often clinically silent in the newborn period. More commonly, manifestations occur later in childhood as learning disability, growth disturbance, mental retardation, and sensorineural impairment. Infants diagnosed with congenital CMV, for example, require close surveillance of growth and development, including serial audiologic examinations, as well as ophthalmologic and rehabilitative follow-up, as indicated.

The classic (but infrequently observed) triad of congenital toxoplasmosis includes chorioretinitis, hydrocephalus, and intracranial calcification, highlighting that pathogen's predilection for the brain and eyes. Almost all newborns with congenital toxoplasmosis infection go on to develop ocular sequelae at some point in childhood; seizures and developmental disabilities are also common.

Although congenital syphilis can cause hydrops fetalis, stillbirth, and preterm delivery, it is often clinically inapparent in the nursery. Untreated congenital syphilis can progress to involve the reticuloendothelial system, skin, skeleton, bone marrow, CNS, and eyes.

Treatment

Treatment of the sickest infants with congenital CMV, such as those with pneumonia or sepsis syndrome, may require ventilator, vasopressor, and transfusion support. Short-term ganciclovir is indicated to reduce viral replication in these acutely ill infants and those with active retinitis. Whether ganciclovir improves long-term neurodevelopmental outcomes is not known. When its use is considered, consultation with an infectious disease specialist is warranted.

Parenteral penicillin remains the standard treatment for congenital syphilis. Factors to consider in determining the course of treatment include the timing, effectiveness, and adequacy of maternal therapy. Infants treated for congenital syphilis require regular follow-up with serial antibody titers; retreatment with penicillin is sometimes required.

The specific treatment of infants with congenital toxoplasmosis consists of a prolonged course of pyrimethamine

and sulfadiazine with folinic acid supplementation. Prednisone is indicated for severe chorioretinitis or CSF protein elevation of 1000 mg/dL or higher.

There is no specific antiviral treatment for congenital rubella.

Prevention

Congenital CMV infection is best avoided by preventing primary infection during pregnancy. Transmission occurs through direct contact with infected body fluids, usually from asymptomatic infants, children, and adults. Good hygiene (e.g., hand washing) may reduce the risk of infection. No vaccine for CMV is currently available, but research is ongoing.

Widespread immunization is responsible for the enormous reduction in congenital rubella infection. Pregnant women identified as rubella nonimmune should be immunized in the immediate postpartum period to protect future pregnancies, but because rubella is a live-virus vaccine, immunization is contraindicated during pregnancy and in the 3 months before conception.

Congenital syphilis is best prevented by routine, prenatal serologic screening of the mother; cord blood or infant samples alone are susceptible to false-negative results. Newborns at high risk for congenital syphilis must be identified; at-risk infants include those born to women whose syphilis infection was treated incompletely, ineffectively, without penicillin, or within 1 month of delivery.

Preventing maternal toxoplasmosis is the best way of preventing congenital infection. Pregnant women should be counseled about the importance of proper food handling and the need to avoid exposure to cat feces.

PERINATAL INFECTIONS

An acutely ill and potentially infected neonate presents the hospital-based clinician with multiple diagnostic and therapeutic challenges. The ability to rule in or rule out a perinatally acquired infection requires an understanding of disease characteristics and thoughtful interpretation of historical information, physical examination findings, and laboratory data. Acute infections have a relatively low incidence in term neonates but account for a significant proportion of neonatal morbidity and mortality. Although some definitions of neonatal sepsis are limited to bacterial infections, this section addresses nonbacterial pathogens as well. Table 53-1 lists the common pathogens implicated in neonatal sepsis.

Clinical Presentation

Signs of emerging neonatal sepsis include vital sign derangements such as hyper- or hypothermia, tachycardia, and tachypnea. Other respiratory signs (e.g., apnea, grunting, flaring, cyanosis) are common, as are lethargy, irritability, abdominal distention, and poor feeding.[5] Although focal examination findings are uncommon in neonatal sepsis, the skin deserves careful examination; in particular, vesicles or oral lesions should raise the possibility of perinatally transmitted HSV. When neonatal sepsis becomes fulminant, cardiorespiratory compromise, hematologic abnormalities, hepatic and renal failure, adrenal insufficiency, CNS impair-

Table 53-1   Common Pathogens Associated with Neonatal Sepsis

Group B streptococcus *(Streptococcus agalactiae)*
Escherichia coli and other gram-negative bacilli
Listeria monocytogenes
Staphylococcus aureus
Group A streptococcus *(Streptococcus pyogenes)*
Streptococcus viridans
Enterococcus species
Herpes simplex virus 1 and 2
Enteroviruses
Fungi (especially *Candida* species)

ment, and even death may result. Sepsis-like viral syndromes, such as those caused by HSV or enteroviruses, require a high index of suspicion. They may present as "culture-negative sepsis" that is clinically indistinguishable from bacterial disease. Presentations of perinatal HSV infections include skin-eye-mouth disease, localized CNS infection, and disseminated disease; true congenital HSV infection is rare. Disseminated HSV disease often appears in the first 7 to 10 days of life, whereas herpes CNS infection typically presents in the second or third week.

In a newborn's first few hours of life, tachypnea, hypoglycemia, or low temperature may be present as part of the normal transition to extrauterine life. When such findings are both mild and transient and the perinatal history is reassuring, affected infants may merit only close monitoring. If symptoms worsen or fail to resolve promptly, careful evaluation for infection and other pathophysiology is required. Fever may be the earliest sign of serious bacterial or viral disease in a neonate and is always a red flag. Various noninfectious causes of neonatal fever—environmental overwarming, excessive bundling, intrapartum epidural analgesia, breastfeeding dehydration—may be considered when determining the appropriate sepsis evaluation and treatment course.

Differential Diagnosis

The differential diagnosis for an acutely ill neonate is broad. Infectious conditions (e.g., sepsis, meningitis, pneumonia) are typically considered first. Bacteria and viruses are the usual pathogens, although fungi (e.g., *Candida* species) and other organisms (e.g., parasites) are occasional culprits. Critical congenital heart disease is another essential consideration; many duct-dependent anatomic lesions and tachyarrhythmias manifest early in life with initial presentations ranging from mild (e.g., asymptomatic hypoxemia or murmur) to severe (e.g., profound cardiovascular collapse). Hypovolemia resulting from acute perinatal blood loss may present with signs of shock (e.g., tachycardia, pallor, hypotension). Likewise, a wide spectrum of multiorgan dysfunction can present in an asphyxiated neonate. Common causes of abnormal breathing in infants include transient

tachypnea of the newborn and primary pulmonary disorders such as pneumothorax, pulmonary hypertension, aspiration, and respiratory distress syndrome. Other noninfectious causes of sepsis-like symptoms include congenital anatomic lesions (e.g., congenital diaphragmatic hernia, choanal atresia), the effects of maternal medication or withdrawal from illicit drugs, polycythemia, and an array of endocrine and metabolic abnormalities.

Among the common bacterial causes of neonatal sepsis, group B streptococcal infection is most important because of its high prevalence and substantial preventability.[6] *Escherichia coli* and, to a lesser extent, other gram-negative bacilli are also significant causes of neonatal sepsis and meningitis. Other noteworthy gram-positive pathogens include *Staphylococcus aureus*, non–group B streptococci (including *Streptococcus viridans*, group A streptococcus), and *Enterococcus* species. *Listeria monocytogenes*, a gram-positive bacillus, is a less common but well-established cause of neonatal sepsis, meningitis, and pneumonia, as well as amnionitis, pregnancy loss, and prematurity. Herpes simplex viruses 1 and 2 and enteroviruses are commonly implicated in nonbacterial neonatal sepsis.

Diagnosis and Evaluation

History taking for an infant with suspected sepsis should focus on risk factors: prolonged rupture of membranes (>18 hours), evidence of maternal chorioamnionitis, group B streptococcus (GBS) colonization, and preterm delivery. A maternal history of sexually transmitted disease (e.g., HSV, chlamydia) or other infection during pregnancy (e.g., urinary tract infection), or the previous delivery of a GBS-infected infant, can also offer clues to a diagnosis.

Microbiologic and viral diagnostic techniques include cultures, PCR tests, and many others. It must be recognized that the neonatal blood culture, despite its obvious centrality to the sepsis evaluation, has a low sensitivity that is decreased even further by maternal antibiotic pretreatment. Recovery rates for bacterial pathogens improve somewhat with larger blood samples; a full 1 mL should be obtained whenever possible. Gram stain and culture of the CSF are also essential components of the sepsis evaluation. Urine cultures have little diagnostic utility in the first 72 hours of life but should be obtained thereafter. Tracheal cultures may be useful in infants requiring intubation.

Among the techniques available for identifying suspected viral pathogens are viral cultures (e.g., for enteroviruses or HSV), which can be obtained from the nasopharynx, stool or rectum, blood, CSF, urine, skin lesions, or conjunctiva (for HSV). HSV in particular is a robust virus that grows well in culture. Tzanck smear analysis of skin lesion scrapings has been largely supplanted by more sophisticated immunofluorescence and enzyme immunoassay techniques. Virus-specific PCR methods for urine, CSF, and blood are becoming available and offer superior viral detection.

Beyond the pathogen-identifying diagnostics, no single test (or combination of tests) is optimal for establishing the diagnosis of neonatal sepsis. The complete blood count is a time-honored component of the evaluation, but its interpretation is made difficult by broad, fluctuating normal ranges and by factors that can influence the results (e.g., maternal hypertension, site of blood collection). Abnor-

Table 53-2 Complete Blood Count Abnormalities Suggestive of Neonatal Sepsis

Component	Value
White blood cell count	<5000/mm^3
Absolute neutrophil count	<1750/mm^3
I/T ratio*	≥0.2
Platelet count	<100,000/mm^3

*Ratio of immature neutrophils to total neutrophils.

Table 53-3 Medications for Treating Neonatal* Sepsis

Medication	Dose (per kg)	Interval (hr)
Acyclovir	20 mg	8
Ampicillin	50-100 mg	12
Cefotaxime	50 mg	12
Gentamicin	2.5 mg	12
Penicillin G	50000-150,000 units	8-12
Vancomycin	10-15 mg	12

*Term infants younger than 7 days.

malities widely considered suspicious for neonatal sepsis include thrombocytopenia, leukopenia, neutropenia, and an increased proportion of immature neutrophil forms (Table 53-2). A ratio of immature neutrophils to total neutrophils that is 0.2 or greater has been reported to be 90% to 100% sensitive, with a negative predictive value approaching 99% to 100%.[7] Recent data suggest, however, that these indices may be less useful than previously believed. Another measurement noteworthy for its negative predictive value is the acute-phase reactant C-reactive protein.[8] Well-appearing babies with normal serial C-reactive protein levels (<1 mg/dL) are highly unlikely to have sepsis; antibiotics can often be discontinued after 48 hours if their examination and hospital course remain reassuring.

Neonatal meningitis can exist even when blood cultures remain sterile. Because the presentation of meningitis can be nonspecific and clinically indistinguishable from that of sepsis alone, lumbar puncture should be performed in any infant with presumed sepsis, possible meningeal signs (e.g., apnea, lethargy, irritability), or culture-positive bacteremia. CSF should be sent for bacterial culture, Gram stain, cell count, and measurements of protein and glucose. If HSV, enterovirus, or syphilis is suspected, pathogen-specific CSF testing should also be performed. Lumbar puncture should be postponed in the face of cardiorespiratory instability or thrombocytopenia.

Other tests to consider in a potentially septic neonate include liver function tests, which often reveal hepatitis in viral disease; placental pathology, when signs of chorioamnionitis are present at delivery; and neuroimaging and ophthalmic evaluation if HSV disease is strongly suspected. A chest radiograph should be obtained whenever respiratory signs are present. Group B streptococcal pneumonia, for example, can be radiographically identical to respiratory distress syndrome.

Course of Illness

Neonatal sepsis can vary widely in its presentation, from asymptomatic bacteremia (e.g., in a screened, at-risk newborn) to fulminant, life-threatening disease. Case-fatality rates for neonatal group B streptococcal infection, for example, are 4% to 8%. The majority of neonatal group B streptococcal disease occurs as early-onset (0 to 6 days) sepsis or pneumonia; meningitis and other focal infections (e.g., osteomyelitis, septic arthritis, adenitis) become more common with late-onset (7 to 30 days) disease.

Localized CNS and disseminated HSV disease have mortality rates of 5% and 30%, respectively, and both presenta-tions can leave survivors with serious neurologic sequelae.[9] The prognosis is more favorable for infants with skin-eye-mouth disease alone. Perinatal enteroviral disease is often relatively mild, but severe meningoencephalitis, multiorgan system failure, and death are possible.

Treatment

Physicians should not hesitate to embark on a sepsis evaluation in an at-risk or symptomatic neonate. Though relatively infrequent in term babies, neonatal sepsis is a potentially lethal, progressive condition that can present with subtle, inconsistent signs. Neonatal sepsis attacks distinctly vulnerable hosts. It is best treated as early as possible, and therapy is generally well tolerated. Once the decision is made to evaluate and treat, a careful review of the infant's clinical course and laboratory data helps bring the picture into sharper focus.

Prompt initiation of empirical antibiotic therapy is essential (Table 53-3). Ampicillin plus an aminoglycoside (e.g., gentamicin) provides excellent coverage for the likeliest pathogens, namely GBS and *E. coli*, as well as less common agents, such as *Listeria* and enterococci. Measurement of serum aminoglycoside peak and trough levels is necessary if treatment extends beyond 48 hours. When the evaluation suggests meningitis, a third-generation cephalosporin (e.g., cefotaxime) is frequently used in place of the aminoglycoside. When GBS is the established pathogen, penicillin G may be substituted for ampicillin. Once a microbiologic and clinical response to penicillin is confirmed, neonatal group B streptococcal sepsis can be treated with penicillin G monotherapy for 10 days; uncomplicated meningitis warrants 14 days of therapy. The treatment of gram-negative sepsis and meningitis should be tailored to the individual antimicrobial susceptibilities of the offending pathogen. The treatment for known or suspected neonatal HSV infection is intravenous acyclovir for 14 days for skin-eye-mouth disease and 21 days for disseminated or CNS disease. Patients should be monitored for neutropenia, which may necessitate dosing adjustments or granulocyte colony-stimulating factor administration. No specific antienteroviral therapy is currently available.

Supportive measures in the treatment of neonatal sepsis include assisted oxygenation and ventilation; cardiovascular support; management of fluid, electrolyte, and acid-base balance; and treatment of coagulation and CNS disturbances (e.g., seizures).

Prevention

Prevention strategies have substantially reduced the burden of invasive group B streptococcal disease in neonates.[10] The 2002 Centers for Disease Control and Prevention (CDC) guidelines recommend that all pregnant women be screened for vaginal and rectal colonization between 35 and 37 weeks' gestation. Any woman with a positive screen, a history of group B streptococcal bacteriuria during the pregnancy, or previous delivery of an infant with group B streptococcal disease should be considered colonized with GBS. These women require antibiotic chemoprophylaxis at the time of labor onset or membrane rupture; a planned cesarean delivery obviates the need for antibiotics if labor has not begun and the membranes have not ruptured. Women with an unknown GBS status and prolonged membrane rupture, intrapartum temperature of 38° C or higher, or preterm (<37 weeks) delivery also warrant antibiotic chemoprophylaxis for GBS. Adequate prophylaxis is defined as at least 4 hours of intrapartum exposure to penicillin, ampicillin, or cefazolin.

The CDC also provides recommendations for the management of a term newborn whose mother received intrapartum antibiotics (Fig. 53-1).[10] Uncertainty persists as to how to best manage a term newborn whose mother did not receive antibiotics despite an indication to do so. Common practice varies from full or limited septic evaluation to observation only.

Current practices for reducing neonatal HSV disease include cesarean section—before the onset of labor, if possible—for women with clinically apparent genital lesions. Even if performed within 4 to 6 hours after membrane rupture, cesarean section may decrease the risk of HSV disease.[11] These infants should have screening cultures from the nasopharynx, mouth, urine, and stool or rectum at 24 to 48 hours, at which time positive viral cultures are more likely to reflect true infection rather than surface contamination. These babies should be kept in contact isolation and closely observed, with thorough parental education at the time of discharge. Infants delivered vaginally are at much greater risk of vertical transmission of HSV, especially when mothers are experiencing primary infections. For vaginally delivered HSV-exposed neonates, the American Academy of Pediatrics also recommends HSV surveillance cultures at 24 to 48 hours. Expert opinion varies on whether asymptomatic, HSV-exposed neonates should receive empirical treatment while viral cultures are pending.

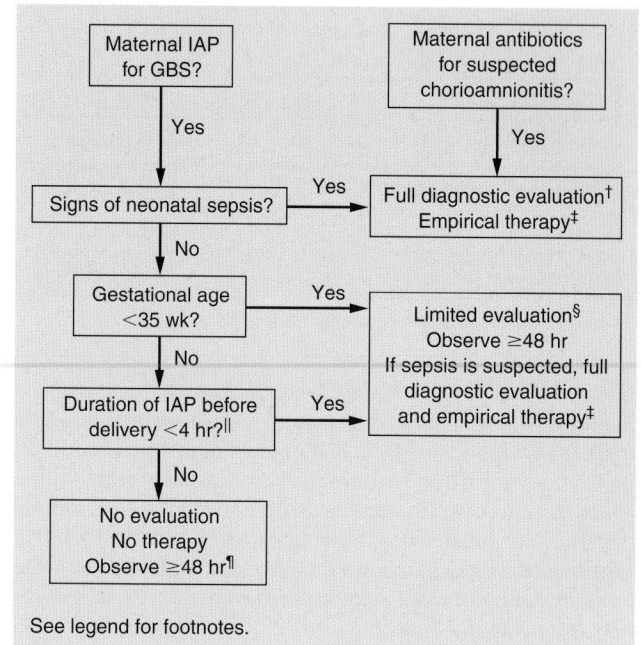

Figure 53-1   Sample algorithm for the management of a newborn whose mother received intrapartum antimicrobial prophylaxis (IAP) for the prevention of early-onset group B streptococcal disease (GBS)* or suspected chorioamnionitis. This algorithm is not the only acceptable course of management; variations that incorporate individual circumstances or institutional preferences may be appropriate.
*If no maternal intrapartum prophylaxis for GBS was administered despite an indication being present, data are insufficient to recommend a single management strategy.
†Includes complete blood cell count (CBC) and differential, blood culture, and chest radiograph if respiratory abnormalities are present. When signs of sepsis are present, a lumbar puncture, if feasible, should be performed.
‡Duration of therapy varies, depending on the results of blood culture, cerebrospinal fluid findings (if obtained), and the infant's clinical course. If laboratory results and clinical course do not indicate bacterial infection, duration may be as short as 48 hours.
§CBC with differential and blood culture.
||Applies only to penicillin, ampicillin, or cefazolin and assumes recommended dosing regimens.
¶A healthy-appearing infant who was ≥38 weeks' gestation at delivery and whose mother received ≥4 hours of IAP before delivery may be discharged home after 24 hours if other discharge criteria have been met and if a person capable of complying with instructions for home observation will be present. If any one of these conditions is not met, the infant should be observed in the hospital for at least 48 hours and until discharge criteria are achieved.
From Schrag S, Gorwitz R, Fultz-Butts K, Schuchat A: Prevention of perinatal group B streptococcal disease: Revised guidelines from CDC. MMWR Recomm Rep 2002;51[RR-11]:1-22.

IN A NUTSHELL

- Congenital infections, though often asymptomatic in the neonatal period, are associated with significant long-term morbidity and mortality.
- Perinatal sepsis is an infrequent but potentially fatal affliction in term newborns.
- Although early therapy may improve outcome, the morbidity and mortality from both congenital infections and perinatal sepsis remain substantial.

ON THE HORIZON

- Increased reliance on PCR techniques for the diagnosis of bacterial and viral pathogens.
- Development of immunoprophylactic strategies for the prevention of group B streptococcal disease.
- Evaluation of CMV vaccines.
- Concerns about the development of antibiotic resistance as a result of the widespread use of intrapartum chemoprophylaxis for GBS.

SUGGESTED READING

Gerdes JS: Diagnosis and management of bacterial infections in the neonate. Pediatr Clin North Am 2004;51:939-959.
Polin RA, Parravicini E, Regan JA, Taeusch HW: Bacterial sepsis and meningitis. In Taeusch HW, Ballard RA, Gleason CA (eds): Avery's Diseases of the Newborn, 8th ed. Philadelphia, Elsevier, 2005, pp 551-577.
Schrag S, Gorwitz R, Fultz-Butts K, Schuchat A: Prevention of perinatal group B streptococcal disease: Revised guidelines from CDC. MMWR Recomm Rep 2002;51(RR-11):1-22.

REFERENCES

1. Pan ES, Cole FS, Weintrub PS: Viral infections of the fetus and newborn. In Taeusch HW, Ballard RA, Gleason CA (eds): Avery's Diseases of the Newborn, 8th ed. Philadelphia, Elsevier, 2005, pp 495-529.
2. Montoya JG, Liesenfeld O: Toxoplasmosis. Lancet 2004;363:1965-1976.
3. American Academy of Pediatrics: Rubella. In Red Book 2003: Report of the Committee on Infectious Diseases, 26th ed. Elk Grove Village, Ill, American Academy of Pediatrics, 2003, pp 536-541.
4. Sanchez PJ, Ahmed A: Toxoplasmosis, syphilis, malaria, and tuberculosis. In Gershon AA, Hotez PJ, Katz SL (eds): Krugman's Infectious Diseases of Children, 11th ed. St. Louis, Mosby, 2004, pp 530-550.
5. Edwards M, Baker CJ: Sepsis in the newborn. In Gershon AA, Hotez PJ, Katz SL (eds): Krugman's Infectious Diseases of Children, 11th ed. St. Louis, Mosby, 2004, pp 545-561.
6. Harris MC, Polin RA: Diagnosis of neonatal sepsis. In Spitzer AR (ed): Intensive Care of the Fetus and Neonate, 3rd ed. Philadelphia, Hanley & Belfus, 2005, pp 1115-1124.
7. Gerdes JS: Diagnosis and management of bacterial infections in the neonate. Pediatr Clin North Am 2004;51:939-959.
8. Polin RA, Parravicini E, Regan JA, Taeusch HW: Bacterial sepsis and meningitis. In Taeusch HW, Ballard RA, Gleason CA (eds): Avery's Diseases of the Newborn, 8th ed. Philadelphia, Elsevier, 2005, pp 551-577.
9. Whitley R: Neonatal herpes simplex virus infection. Curr Opin Infect Dis 2004;17:243-246.
10. Schrag S, Gorwitz R, Fultz-Butts K, Schuchat A: Prevention of perinatal group B streptococcal disease: Revised guidelines from CDC. MMWR Recomm Rep 2002;51(RR-11):1-22.
11. American Academy of Pediatrics: Herpes simplex. In Red Book 2003: Report of the Committee on Infectious Diseases, 26th ed. Elk Grove Village, Ill, American Academy of Pediatrics, 2003, pp 344-353.

CHAPTER 54

Hypoglycemia and Infants of Diabetic Mothers

Laura J. Mirkinson

Glucose is the preferred oxidative energy source for the central nervous system. At birth, the sudden loss of a continuous maternal glucose supply requires a neonatal response that maintains adequate serum glucose levels throughout the early feeding and fasting periods. Adaptive changes in hormonal regulation at birth conspire to maintain the newborn's plasma glucose concentration, reserve glucose for the central nervous system, and avoid hypoglycemia. Finally, counterregulatory hormones, including glucagon, growth hormone, cortisol, and epinephrine, act together to increase blood glucose via glycogenolysis, gluconeogenesis, ketogenesis, and inhibition of peripheral glucose uptake and insulin release. The failure of one or several parts of this process can result in hypoglycemia. Additional metabolic challenges such as immaturity, low glycogen reserves, and thermal stress increase the risk of neonatal hypoglycemia.

HYPOGLYCEMIA

Clinical Presentation

In healthy adults, a decrease in blood glucose concentration inhibits the production of insulin and stimulates the production of glucagon. This prevents the blood glucose from dropping to less than 60 mg/dL, thus avoiding the development of typical symptoms of hypoglycemia such as diaphoresis, headache, and dizziness. In neonates there is a weaker clinical correlation between blood glucose concentrations and symptoms of hypoglycemia. The newborn's plasma glucose level drops quickly after delivery to about 60% to 80% of maternal glucose levels, or approximately 50 mg/dL by 2 hours of age. Although some newborns may display nonspecific signs and symptoms of hypoglycemia (Table 54-1), others may appear completely asymptomatic despite low blood and cerebral glucose levels. For this reason, many newborn nursery protocols are designed to anticipate neonatal hypoglycemia and suggest evaluation at glucose levels of 25 to 50 mg/dL. This reflects the uncertainty about where the lower limit of normal is for newborns, as well as the limitations of a single cutoff value. In general, to avoid the systemic effects and potential neurologic sequelae of hypoglycemia, a conservative threshold for defining hypoglycemia is useful. An "operational threshold" has been suggested that takes into consideration the unstable relationship between plasma glucose levels and clinical signs of hypoglycemia. The operational threshold has been defined as "that concentration of plasma or whole blood glucose at which clinicians should consider intervention."[1]

Infants at higher risk for hypoglycemia are those with diminished hepatic glucose production, increased metabolic need versus substrate availability, or increased insulin production (Table 54-2). The American Academy of Pediatrics recommends selective screening for high-risk infants but does not currently support universal screening, except in nurseries where a large number of infants meet high-risk criteria.[2] Thus, normal full-term infants who are delivered without complications after a normal pregnancy do not require glucose monitoring. Regardless of risk factors, any infant with clinical signs consistent with hypoglycemia requires evaluation (see Table 54-1).

Differential Diagnosis

The presence of hypoglycemia is most often the result of a healthy newborn's inability to quickly and adequately respond to the dramatic loss of maternal sources of glucose. However, hypoglycemia may also be a signal of other stresses, including sepsis, inborn errors of metabolism, hyperinsulinism, polycythemia, and congenital hypopituitarism (see Table 54-2). Symptoms of hypoglycemia are nonspecific and overlap with abnormalities of nearly every organ system (e.g., seizure disorder) and with other systemic conditions (e.g., narcotic abstinence syndrome). In addition, hypoglycemia may be one feature of a syndrome or multifaceted disorder (e.g., Beckwith-Wiedemann syndrome).

Diagnosis and Treatment

In healthy neonates, blood glucose levels fall in the first 1 to 2 hours after birth, stabilize at a minimum of about 40 mg/dL, and then rise to 50 to 80 mg/dL by 3 hours of life. Hypoglycemia in newborns generally appears at around 2 to 6 hours of life. Glucose monitoring should begin within 30 to 60 minutes after birth in infants at risk for hypoglycemia. A threshold for intervention of 40 mg/dL (2.2 mmol/L) and a post-treatment goal of greater than 45 mg/dL (2.5 mmol/L) are suggested for healthy newborns. Glucose reagent strips may be used as a screening method to evaluate blood glucose, but laboratory confirmation of plasma glucose levels is necessary.

Because of the potential risk to the central nervous system, neonatal hypoglycemia is treated aggressively with the early institution of oral feedings. Infants with low serum glucose levels of 26 to 40 mg/dL are effectively treated with 30 to 60 mL of standard infant formula or breast milk by oral or gavage feeding. This increases blood glucose concentrations by about 30 mg/dL.[3] Infants with glucose levels less than 20 to 25 mg/dL (1.1 to 1.4 mmol/L) should be treated with intravenous glucose. An intravenous bolus of 2 to 4 mL/kg of 10% dextrose (D10W) is followed by a maintenance infusion of 6 to 8 mg/kg per minute of D10W (equivalent to 85 to 115 mL/kg per day).[3,4] Infants who do not respond to an initial bolus followed by maintenance infusions may require an increase in the volume of fluid or the concentration of glucose. Infants who require greater than 100 mL/kg per day of D10W to maintain adequate serum

Table 54-1 Symptoms of Hypoglycemia in Neonates
Irritability
Abnormal or high-pitched cry
Tremors
Jitteriness
Lethargy
Hypotonia
Poor suck reflex, poor feeding
Apnea
Tachypnea
Cyanosis
Seizures
Hypothermia
Vasomotor instability
Temperature instability
Cardiac arrest

glucose levels can be treated with D12.5W via a peripheral intravenous line. Concentrations greater than this, such as D15W or D20W, require central venous access. Once a neonate's glucose has stabilized, glucose infusions can be decreased by approximately 2 mL/hour while providing oral feedings. Glucose levels should be assessed before each oral feeding while the intravenous infusion is being decreased (Table 54-3). Infants who require more than 100 mL/kg per day or concentrations greater than D12.5W, or who are unable to be weaned off intravenous fluids within 48 hours, should be considered at risk for neonatal hyperinsulinemia.

INFANTS OF DIABETIC MOTHERS

Hypoglycemia

A unique metabolic consequence of pregnancy is a blunting of the effects of insulin in the mother. The normal clearance of glucose is delayed, which helps maintain a consistent level of maternal glucose for the fetus. Pregestational maternal diabetes potentiates these anti-insulin effects and causes an additional increase in glucose in the fetal environment. Excessive glucose in the fetal environment (fetal hyperglycemia) induces fetal pancreatic islet hypertrophy and beta cell hyperplasia. This results in an elevation in fetal and, later,

Table 54-2 Infants at Risk for Hypoglycemia*

Risk Due to Diminished Hepatic Glucose Production	Risk Due to Increased Glucose Utilization (Increased Metabolic Demand)	Risk Due to Excessive Transient Pancreatic Insulin Production (Hyperinsulinism)	Risk Due to Excessive and Persistent Pancreatic Insulin Production (Hyperinsulinism)	Other
SGA infant IUGR	Perinatal stress Hypoxia	Infant of diabetic mother	Congenital hyperinsulinism	Endocrine Adrenal insufficiency (CAH) Congenital hypopituitarism Hypothyroidism
Prematurity	Thermal stress	LGA infant	Beckwith-Wiedemann syndrome	Delayed feeding
IUGR and infant of diabetic mother	Polycythemia-hyperviscosity	Severe Rh incompatibility (erythroblastosis fetalis)	Pancreatic islet cell adenoma	Iatrogenic
Post-term gestation	Congenital heart disease	Iatrogenic (maternal drugs)†	Adenomatosis	
Infants of multiple gestations	CNS abnormalities	High umbilical artery catheter		
Inborn errors of metabolism Glycogen storage disease Galactosemia Tyrosinemia Hereditary fructose intolerance α_1-Antitrypsin deficiency	Sepsis	Exchange transfusion		

*Infants with hypoglycemia due to a lack of available glucose generally have ketones in the urine; infants with hypoglycemia due to excess insulin do not.
†Chlorpropamide, diazoxide, diuretics, salicyclates, alcohol, terbutaline, ritodrine.
CAH, congenital adrenal hyperplasia; CNS, central nervous system; IUGR, intrauterine growth retardation; LGA, large for gestational age; SGA, small for gestational age.

Table 54-3   Assessment and Treatment of Healthy Infants at Risk for Hypoglycemia or Those with Symptoms Consistent with Hypoglycemia

Assess blood glucose (BG) concentration by rapid method and laboratory confirmation for screening BG <45 mg/dL at 30-60 min after delivery

↓

BG 20-25 mg/dL	BG 26-40 mg/dL	BG >40-45 mg/dL and Symptomatic	BG >40-45 mg/dL and Asymptomatic
2 mL/kg IV D10W, followed by 6-8 mg/kg/min D10W ↓ Continuous monitoring with frequent glucose assessment in a setting allowing close observation	30-60 mL standard infant formula, or IV bolus 2 mg/kg D10W if unable to tolerate oral feeds ↓ Recheck BG in 30-60 min If BG >45 mg/dL, recheck within 1 hr If BG continues >45 mg/dL, institute oral feeds every 2-3 hr Recheck BG before the next 2 consecutive feeds If within normal range for 3 feedings, may discontinue BG checks	30-60 mL standard infant formula ↓ Recheck BG in 30-60 min If BG >45 mg/dL, recheck within 1 hr If BG continues >45 mg/dL, institute oral feeds every 2-3 hr Recheck BG before the next 2 consecutive feeds If within normal range for 3 feedings, may discontinue BG checks	Routine care ↓ Recheck BG before the next 2 consecutive feeds If within normal range for 3 feedings, may discontinue BG checks

Table 54-4   Laboratory Abnormalities in Infants of Diabetic Mothers

Abnormality	Proposed Cause
Hyperinsulinemia	Maternal hyperglycemia
Hypoglycemia	Hyperinsulinemia
Hypomagnesemia	? Maternal magnesium losses
Hypocalcemia	? Magnesium deficiency (functional hypoparathyroidism)
Polycythemia and hyperviscosity	Decreased fetal arterial O_2 content, increased erythropoiesis
Hyperbilirubinemia	Increased bilirubin production, impaired hepatic function, polycythemia

neonatal plasma insulin concentrations. The normal shift in energy metabolism that allows the infant to use fat and amino acids may be hampered by hyperinsulinemia. Of interest, infants with hypoglycemia due to a lack of available glucose generally have ketones in the urine, whereas infants with hypoglycemia due to excess insulin do not.

Up to 50% of infants of diabetic mothers (IDMs) experience hypoglycemia in the first hours of life. Other metabolic abnormalities seen in IDMs include hypocalcemia, hypomagnesemia, polycythemia, and hyperbilirubinemia (Table 54-4).

Macrosomia

Insulin acts as an anabolic growth hormone. In the presence of elevated fetal insulin levels, an increased growth of insulin-sensitive tissues occurs. Macrosomia, noted in up to 40% of diabetic pregnancies, is characterized by birth weight above the 90th percentile, increased body fat, visceral organ hypertrophy, and increased skeletal growth. Owing to their large size, IDMs are more likely to be delivered by cesarean section and to experience complications of delivery, such as shoulder dystocia and brachial and facial nerve palsies (see Chapter 50). In fact, the fetus of a diabetic mother that appears to be following a normal intrauterine growth curve may actually be comparatively small and may be at risk for the complications noted in other small-for-gestational-age infants. Although macrosomia is the most common growth abnormality of IDMs, intrauterine growth restriction (IUGR) can occur in the presence of advanced vascular disease and hypertension in the mother. IUGR can lead to significantly reduced hepatic glycogen stores, making IDMs particularly vulnerable and dependent on exogenous glucose supplies. Macrosomic IDMs have adequate glycogen and lipid stores but cannot use them efficiently owing to the antagonistic effects of high insulin levels on glycogenolysis, gluconeogenesis, ketogenesis, and lipolysis.

Congenital Malformations

In addition to macrosomia and hypoglycemia, there is an estimated 5% to 10% incidence of major congenital malformations in infants born to women with pregestational diabetes. The degree of risk is related to the timing and intensity of the teratogenic effects of hyperglycemia and to the level of glycemic control during the first trimester. Although strict glycemic control during pregnancy, especially during the period of organogenesis, is thought to be optimal, it does not appear to lower the rate of congenital malformations (or the incidence of macrosomia) to that seen among the normal population. Diabetic embryopathy is a major cause of perinatal mortality in diabetic pregnancies. A 10-fold

Table 54-5 Congenital Malformations in Infants of Diabetic Mothers

System Affected	Defect
Neural tube	Caudal regression syndromes Holoprosencephaly
Gastrointestinal	Duodenal atresia Microcolon Anorectal atresia
Vertebral	Lumbosacral agenesis
Cardiac	Hypertrophic cardiomyopathy Ventricular septal defect Atrial septal defect Transposition of the great arteries Coarctation of the aorta
Skeletal	Femoral hypoplasia
Renal	Hydronephrosis Renal agenesis
Craniofacial	Oculoauriculovertebral abnormalities Hemifacial microsomia

Table 54-6 Laboratory Evaluation for Infants with Suspected Hyperinsulinism*

Blood	Urine
Glucose	pH
Electrolytes	Ketones
Free fatty acids	Reducing substances
Lactate	Organic acids
Pyruvate	Amino acids
Amino acids	
Ammonia	
Insulin	
C-peptide	
Cortisol	
Growth hormone	

*Sampling is done at the time of hypoglycemia.[3]

Table 54-7 Criteria Suggestive of Hyperinsulinism in Infancy[7]

Persistent glucose requirement >6-8 mg/kg/min to maintain blood glucose >45 mg/dL (2.5 mmol/L)

Laboratory blood glucose concentration <40 mg/dL (2.2 mmol/L)

Detectable insulin at the point of hypoglycemia

Elevated C-peptide concentration at the point of hypoglycemia

Inappropriately low free fatty acid and ketone body concentrations at the time of hypoglycemia

No ketones in urine

Elevation in plasma glucose concentration after glucagon injection when hypoglycemic

increase in risk has been described, compared with the general population.[4]

The association between congenital malformations and gestational diabetes and type 2 non–insulin-dependent diabetes mellitus is more controversial, but it is likely that in women with gestational diabetes who have greater glucose intolerance and poor first trimester glycemic control, the rate of congenital malformations is similar to that in women with pregestational diabetes. Transient hypertrophic cardiomyopathy is an example of the visceromegaly seen in IDMs. Most infants are asymptomatic, and the septal and wall hypertrophy spontaneously resolves over several months. Congenital malformations associated with maternal diabetes are listed in Table 54-5.

Large-for-Gestational-Age Infants

Maternal diabetes is the most common cause of large-for-gestational-age (LGA) infants; however, post-term pregnancies (>42 weeks' gestational age), excessive maternal weight gain, multigravidity, and familial genetic factors (large parental size) can contribute to the incidence of LGA newborns. Fetal hyperinsulinism and excessive intrauterine growth is the fetal response to an abundance of glucose in the intrauterine environment. Hypoglycemia has been estimated to occur in 16% of term LGA infants within the first 24 hours of life.[5] Hypoglycemia in LGA infants is generally transient and usually responds well to oral feedings (see Table 54-3 for treatment recommendations).

HYPERINSULINISM OF INFANCY

Hyperinsulinism of infancy presents with persistent and recurrent hypoglycemia. It is a heterogeneous disorder with several different pathophysiologies resulting in excessive insulin secretion from the pancreatic beta cells. It has been described as "hyperinsulinemic, hypofattyacidemic, hypoketonemic, hypoglycemia."[6] Long-term neurologic morbidity is a serious concern owing to the repeated episodes of severe and often unpredictable hypoglycemia. Infants with hyperinsulinism can require glucose infusions of more than 20 mg/kg per minute. Infants with persistent hypoglycemia and suspected hyperinsulinism require a diagnostic laboratory evaluation that includes analysis of hormones and metabolites associated with hyperinsulinism (Table 54-6). Diagnostic criteria suggestive of hyperinsulinism are noted in Table 54-7.[7] Medical therapy includes diazoxide and chlorothiazide. Other medical therapies, such as calcium channel antagonists, have also been used in the treatment of hyperinsulinism. Refractory cases sometimes require surgical intervention in the form of partial pancreatectomy.[8]

CONSULTATION

Infants with persistent hypoglycemia despite oral or gavage feedings with breast milk, infant formula, or glucose water should receive evaluation and treatment in a setting where close observation and parenteral therapy are available. Significant and persistent hypoglycemia despite parenteral therapy suggests the need for subspecialty evaluation by a neonatologist or pediatric endocrinologist.

ADMISSION OR TRANSFER CRITERIA

Admission or transfer to a neonatal intensive care unit is appropriate in the following circumstances:

- Persistent hypoglycemia despite adequate oral or gavage feeding
- Inability to tolerate an oral or gavage glucose load
- Presence of nonspecific signs of hypoglycemia (see Table 54-1) despite normalized serum glucose

DISCHARGE CRITERIA

- Clinically asymptomatic infant with the ability to take breast milk or infant formula by mouth at age-appropriate intervals
- Stable glucose level greater than 50 mg/dL

IN A NUTSHELL

- Infants may present with typical signs and symptoms of hypoglycemia or be completely asymptomatic.
- Screening glucose monitoring is recommended for newborns with risk factors for hypoglycemia and for symptomatic newborns.
- Infants of diabetic mothers are at risk for hypoglycemia as well as other abnormalities, such as macrosomia, electrolyte abnormalities, organomegaly, and congenital anomalies.
- Initial management depends on the degree of hypoglycemia and the infant's ability to maintain safe blood glucose levels (>45 mg/dL).
- Persistent hypoglycemia requires consideration of hyperinsulinemia.

ON THE HORIZON

- Identification of new causes of hypoglycemia, including glucose transporter disorders, respiratory chain disorders, mitochondrial fatty oxidation disorders, and congenital disorders of glycosylation.
- Isolation of specific genetic abnormalities responsible for congenital hyperinsulinism and Beckwith-Wiedemann syndrome.
- Completion of long-term follow-up studies of the neurologic outcomes of infants with congenital hyperinsulinism.

SUGGESTED READING

Cornblath M, Hawdon JM, Williams AF, et al: Controversies regarding definition of neonatal hypoglycemia: Suggested operational thresholds. Pediatrics 2000;105:1141-1145.

Cowett RM, Loughead JL: Neonatal glucose metabolism: Differential diagnoses, evaluation and treatment of hypoglycemia. Neonatal Netw 2002;21:9-19.

Perlman D, Southgate WM, Purohit DM: Neonatal hypoglycemia. J S C Med Assoc 2002;98:99-104.

REFERENCES

1. Cornblath M, Hawdon JM, Williams AF, et al: Controversies regarding definition of neonatal hypoglycemia: Suggested operational thresholds. Pediatrics 2000;105:1141-1145.
2. American Academy of Pediatrics Committee on Fetus and Newborn: Routine evaluation of blood pressure, hematocrit and glucose in newborns. Pediatrics 1993;92:474-476.
3. Perlman D, Southgate WM, Purohit DM: Neonatal hypoglycemia. J S C Med Assoc 2002;98:99-104.
4. Casson IF, Clarke CA, Howard CV, et al: Outcomes of pregnancy in insulin dependent diabetic women: Results of a five year population cohort study. BMJ 1997;315:275-278.
5. Schaefer-Graf UM, Ross R, Buhrer C, et al: Rate and risk factors of hypoglycemia in large-for-gestational-age newborn infants of nondiabetic mothers. Am J Obstet Gynecol 2002;187:913-917.
6. Hussain K, Aynsley-Green A: Hyperinsulinism in infancy: Understanding the pathophysiology. Int J Biochem Cell Biol 2003;35:1312-1317.
7. Hussain K, Aynsley-Green A: Management of hyperinsulinism in infancy and childhood. Ann Med 2000;32:544-551.
8. Meissner T, Wendel U, Burgard P, et al: Long term follow-up of 114 patients with congenital hyperinsulinism. Eur J Endocrinol 2003;149:43-51.

CHAPTER 55

Neonatal Hyperbilirubinemia

Ron Keren

Sixty percent of term infants have clinically apparent jaundice associated with transient elevations of serum bilirubin.[1] Only 5% to 15% develop bilirubin levels greater than 12.9 mg/dL, and even fewer have higher bilirubin levels.[2,3] Nonetheless, each year approximately 1% of all term infants born in the United States are hospitalized in the first 2 weeks of life for the treatment of hyperbilirubinemia. This accounts for more than half of all readmissions in the first month of life and considerable health care expenditures.[4,5] Health care providers monitor newborn jaundice and bilirubin levels and provide treatment to prevent the development of kernicterus (bilirubin encephalopathy), a neurologically devastating condition caused by neurotoxic levels of bilirubin in the basal ganglia and brainstem nuclei. Although it is rare, since the mid-1990s there has been an increase in reports of kernicterus in term and near-term infants.[6-8] In an effort to prevent the occurrence of severe hyperbilirubinemia and kernicterus, in 2004 the American Academy of Pediatrics (AAP) published an updated clinical practice guideline on the management of newborn jaundice.[9] The guideline emphasizes the importance of predischarge risk assessment, risk-specific follow-up after discharge, and new hour-specific bilirubin thresholds for initiating phototherapy and exchange transfusion.

PATHOPHYSIOLOGY

Bilirubin is a breakdown product of heme, which is contained primarily in hemoglobin but also in myoglobin and cytochromes. Microsomal heme oxygenase catabolizes heme to biliverdin, which is then reduced to bilirubin by biliverdin reductase. The resulting unconjugated biliruibin is a nonpolar, lipid-soluble molecule that is transported to the liver in plasma bound to albumin. In the endoplasmic reticulum of the hepatocytes, bilirubin uridine diphosphate glucuronosyl transferase (UDPGT) conjugates bilirubin with glucuronic acid. Conjugated bilirubin is a polar, water-soluble molecule that is excreted from the hepatocyte to the bile canaliculi, through the biliary tree, and into the duodenum. In the colon, bacterial β-glucuronidase converts conjugated bilirubin to urobilinogen. A small amount of urobilinogen is absorbed and returned to the liver (enterohepatic circulation) or excreted by the kidneys. The rest is converted to stercobilin and excreted in the feces.

Hyperbilirubinemia is classified as either conjugated or unconjugated (also known as direct or indirect, referring to the van den Bergh reaction used to measure bilirubin). Unconjugated hyperbilirubinemia is caused by increased production, decreased hepatic uptake or metabolism, or increased enterohepatic circulation of bilirubin. Newborn infants are particularly susceptible to unconjugated hyperbilirubinemia because, compared with adults, they have more red cells with a higher turnover and a shorter life span, and a limited ability to conjugate bilirubin. Newborn bilirubin levels typically peak on days 3 to 5 of life at about 5 to 6 mg/dL and then decrease over the next few weeks to adult levels. Exaggerated physiologic jaundice occurs at values above this threshold (7 to 17 mg/dL). Bilirubin levels higher than 17 mg/dL are not generally considered physiologic, and a cause of pathologic jaundice should be sought (see the section on differential diagnosis).[10]

Conjugated hyperbilirubinemia can occur with hepatocellular or cholestatic disease that causes a decreased secretion of bilirubin into the canaliculi or decreased drainage through the biliary tree.

Unconjugated bilirubin that exceeds the binding threshold of albumin (maximum of 8.2 mg bilirubin per gram of albumin) enters the brain and deposits primarily in neurons in the basal ganglia, hippocampus, cerebellum, and brainstem nuclei for oculomotor function and hearing. Bilirubin's neurotoxicity is mediated through a variety of mechanisms, including impaired mitochondrial function, DNA and protein synthesis, and synaptic transmission. Factors that increase bilirubin neurotoxicity include the concentration of bilirubin and the duration of exposure to it, albumin levels, and conditions that increase blood-brain barrier permeability (e.g., infection, acidosis, hyperoxia, sepsis, prematurity, hyperosmolarity).[11]

CLINICAL PRESENTATION

Jaundice, the yellow discoloration of the skin and sclerae, may be present at birth or appear any time in the first month of life. It generally starts on the face and spreads down the body in a cephalocaudal progression. Dermal pressure can be applied to reveal the anatomic progression of jaundice but cannot be used to reliably estimate serum bilirubin levels. Unconjugated bilirubin in the skin appears bright yellow or orange, whereas conjugated bilirubin appears more greenish or muddy yellow. Jaundice may be difficult to detect in darker-skinned infants. Infants who are jaundiced secondary to insufficient milk intake may be dehydrated, appear lethargic, and have significant weight loss (>10% of birth weight), dry mucous membranes, poor capillary refill, sunken eyes and fontanelle, and poor skin turgor.

Signs of acute bilirubin encephalopathy usually appear 2 to 5 days after birth but may occur any time during the neonatal period. In the early phase, infants display lethargy, hypotonia, and poor ability to suck. In the intermediate phase, infants have stupor, irritability, and hypertonia (retrocollis-opisthotonos) alternating with drowsiness and hypotonia. They may also develop a fever and high-pitched cry. Infants who reach the late phase may have increased retrocollis-opisthotonos, cessation of feeding, bicycling movements, inconsolable irritability and crying, seizures, fever, and coma. Many of these infants die, and the survivors are likely

Table 55-1   Differential Diagnosis of Pathologic Jaundice

Finding	Diagnosis
Unconjugated hyperbilirubinemia	
Increased production	Isoimmune hemolysis (ABO, Rh, other)
	Cephalohematoma
	Ecchymoses
	Sepsis
	Polycythemia
	Congenital hemolytic anemias (spherocytosis, elliptocytosis, pyknocytosis)
	Erythrocyte enzyme defects (G6PD, pyruvate kinase, hexokinase)
	Medicines (vitamin K, maternal oxytocin)
Decreased uptake, storage, or metabolism	Crigler-Najjar syndrome (I or II)
	Gilbert syndrome
	Lucey-Driscoll syndrome
	Hypothyroidism or hypopituitarism
	Sepsis
	Hepatitis
	Congestive heart failure
	Hypoxia
	Acidosis
Increased enterohepatic circulation	Breastfeeding jaundice
	Breast milk jaundice
	Intestinal obstruction (ileal atresia, Hirschsprung disease, cystic fibrosis)
Conjugated hyperbilirubinemia	Sepsis
	Extrahepatic biliary atresia
	Intrahepatic cholestasis
	Metabolic disorders
	Congenital viral infections

G6PD, glucose-6-phosphate dehydrogenase.

to have severe kernicteric sequelae, even after intensive treatment. The rate of progression of clinical signs depends on the rate of bilirubin rise, duration of hyperbilirubinemia, host susceptibility, and presence of comorbidities.[11]

Infants who survive acute bilirubin encephalopathy may have kernicteric sequelae such as extrapyramidal movement disorders (dystonia and athetosis), gaze abnormalities (especially upward gaze), auditory disturbances (especially sensorineural hearing loss with central processing disorders or auditory neuropathy), and enamel dysplasia of the deciduous teeth. Cognitive deficits are unusual. Earlier reports of mental retardation in children with kernicterus probably reflected an inability to accurately assess intelligence in children with hearing, communication, and coordination problems.

DIFFERENTIAL DIAGNOSIS

Many authors distinguish between physiologic and pathologic jaundice. The distinction has more to do with the timing, rate of rise, and extent of hyperbilirubinemia than its cause, because some of the same processes that cause physiologic jaundice (e.g., large red blood cell mass, decreased capacity for bilirubin conjugation, increased enterohepatic circulation) can also cause pathologic jaundice. Jaundice that appears in the first 24 hours of life and bilirubin levels that exceed 17 mg/dL or rise more than 5 mg/dL per day should be considered pathologic, and a specific cause should be sought. Direct bilirubin fractions

greater than 10% of the total bilirubin should also be considered abnormal.

The differential diagnosis for pathologic jaundice is extensive (Table 55-1). Processes that lead to increased bilirubin production include isoimmune hemolysis (due to ABO, Rh, or other minor blood group incompatibility), extravascular hemolysis (cephalohematoma and skin bruising), polycythemia, and glucose-6-phosphate dehydrogenase (G6PD) deficiency. Genetic and metabolic disorders resulting in decreased uptake, storage, or metabolism of bilirubin include Crigler-Najjar syndrome (I or II), Gilbert syndrome, Lucey-Driscoll syndrome, hypothyroidism, and hypopituitarism. These rare disorders should be considered when bilirubin levels are greater than 10 mg/dL beyond the first week of life. Processes that result in increased enterohepatic circulation, such as breastfeeding and intestinal obstruction, may also cause pathologic jaundice. Breastfeeding is one of the strongest risk factors for significant hyperbilirubinemia. Infants who are breastfed have higher average peak bilirubin levels than do formula-fed infants. The hyperbilirubinemia observed with breastfeeding is likely multifactorial in origin. Decreased milk intake before maternal milk production is established results in dehydration, which hemoconcentrates bilirubin. Poor milk intake results in fewer bowel movements, which in turn increases the enterohepatic circulation of bilirubin.

Breastfeeding jaundice, which occurs in the first week of life, should be distinguished from breast milk jaundice,

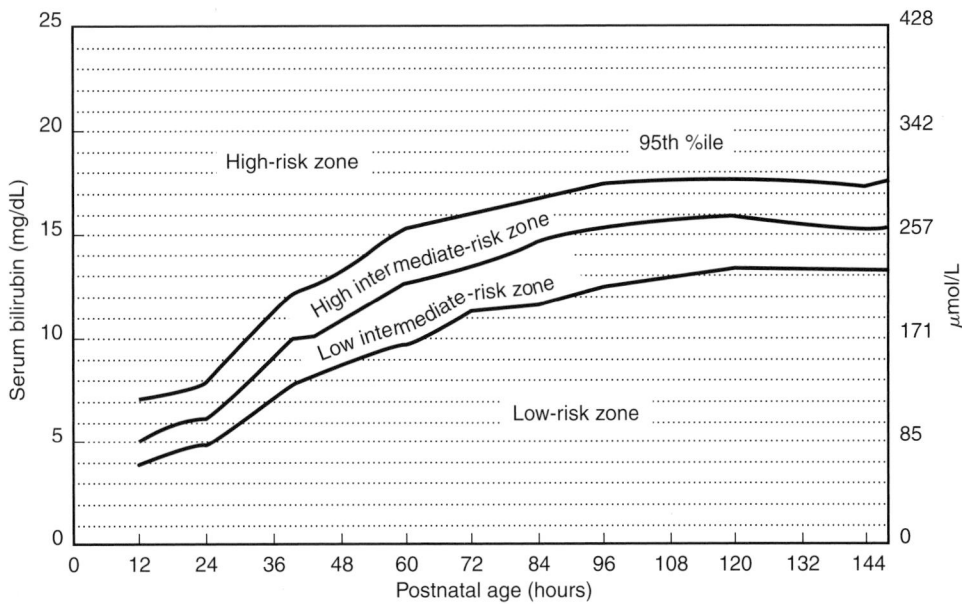

Figure 55-1 Hour-specific bilirubin nomogram for predischarge risk assessment. (From Bhutani VK, Johnson L, Sivieri EM: Predictive ability of a predischarge hour-specific serum bilirubin for subsequent significant hyperbilirubinemia in healthy term and near-term newborns. Pediatrics 1999;103:6-14.)

which refers to the jaundice that persists beyond the first week of life in approximately 2% of breastfed infants. With breast milk jaundice, bilirubin levels can rise as high as 10 to 30 mg/dL in the second to third week and then decrease, but jaundice may persist for up to 10 weeks. Discontinuation of breastfeeding and substitution of formula for 1 to 2 days results in a rapid and sustained decline in serum bilirubin, but this is generally not recommended unless bilirubin levels approach treatment thresholds. The cause of breast milk jaundice is not known with certainty, although β-glucuronidase (resulting in deconjugation of bilirubin and increased enterohepatic circulation) and other factors in breast milk that might interfere with bilirubin conjugation (e.g., pregnanediol and free fatty acids) have been implicated as potential causes.

Congenital causes of conjugated hyperbilirubinemia include extrahepatic biliary atresia, intrahepatic cholestasis, metabolic disorders, and congenital viral infections.

EVALUATION

The 2004 AAP clinical practice guidelines provide detailed recommendations for the evaluation and treatment of hyperbilirubinemia.[9] Evaluation begins in the prenatal period, with maternal blood testing for ABO and Rh (D) blood types and isoimmune antibodies, and continues through the first few days and weeks of the infant's life. If the mother has not had prenatal blood grouping or is Rh-negative, the infant's cord blood should be tested for blood type and Rh (D). Routine testing of infant cord blood for blood type and direct (Coombs) antibody when the maternal blood is group O, Rh-positive, is no longer recommended, as long as appropriate surveillance and follow-up for hyperbilirubinemia are performed.

During an infant's postbirth hospitalization, a jaundice assessment should be performed no less than every 8 to 12

hours, preferably in natural light near a window. Any infant who is jaundiced in the first 24 hours after birth should have a transcutaneous bilirubin (TcB) or total serum bilirubin (TSB) measurement, or both. Infants who appear excessively jaundiced for their age in hours should also have TcB or TSB measured. Bilirubin levels must be interpreted with respect to the age of the infant in hours, not days. The hour-specific bilirubin nomogram in Figure 55-1 can be used to evaluate an infant's bilirubin level on an age-adjusted percentile basis.[12]

Before discharge, all infants (but especially those discharged before 72 hours) should be evaluated for the risk of developing severe hyperbilirubinemia. The AAP recommends two methods for risk assessment: measurement of TcB or TSB (plotted on an hour-specific bilirubin nomogram) and clinical risk factor assessment. Predischarge bilirubin measurement can be performed at the time of the newborn screen or earlier, if clinically indicated. Infants whose predischarge bilirubin level is in the low-risk zone (see Fig. 55-1) are at very low risk of developing severe hyperbilirubinemia (defined as postdischarge bilirubin >95th percentile), whereas those with predischarge bilirubin in the high-risk zone are at significantly increased risk (>40%) of developing severe hyperbilirubinemia. Clinical risk factor assessment using the factors listed in Box 55-1 can also be performed to determine the nature and timing of follow-up. The risk of severe hyperbilirubinemia is directly proportional to the number of clinical risk factors present; therefore, those with more risk factors should be seen earlier and more often, and those with no risk factors can be followed up at longer intervals.

Infants whose TSB levels are rising rapidly (crossing percentiles) or who require phototherapy should have fractionated (conjugated and unconjugated) bilirubin levels checked, as well as blood type, Coombs test, complete blood count and smear, reticulocyte count, and G6PD levels (if available), to evaluate for hemolysis and congenital red blood cell membrane defects. Infants with elevated direct bilirubin levels should have urinalysis and urine culture to rule out urinary tract infection. Infants who are jaundiced beyond 2 weeks of age should have total and direct bilirubin levels measured and should undergo evaluation for the cause of cholestasis if the direct bilirubin level is elevated. The results of the newborn screen can be used to evaluate for congenital hypothyroidism and galactosemia as causes of jaundice.

FOLLOW-UP AND TREATMENT

Infants discharged before 24 hours, between 24 and 47.9 hours, and between 48 and 72 hours should be seen by age 72 hours, 96 hours, and 120 hours, respectively. Earlier or more frequent follow-up may be needed for infants who have elevated hour-specific bilirubin values or clinical risk factors for hyperbilirubinemia. If an infant's predischarge bilirubin level remains in, or is crossing percentile tracks into, the high-risk zone and appropriate follow-up cannot be assured, a clinician may opt to delay discharge until the

bilirubin trajectory is elucidated and a decision can be made about the need for phototherapy or discharge home.

Hour-specific bilirubin thresholds for initiating phototherapy and exchange transfusion have been recommended by the AAP (Figs. 55-2 and 55-3, respectively). Clinicians should use the TSB, not the indirect (or unconjugated) fraction, in applying these treatment guidelines. Treatment thresholds are dependent on the infant's gestational age, appearance (well versus ill), and other clinical risk factors, all of which modify the infant's susceptibility to bilirubin neurotoxicity.

Phototherapy achieves reduction of hyperbilirubinemia by two mechanisms: (1) reversible photoisomerization of the nonpolar native unconjugated 4Z, 15Z-bilirubin into the polar configurational isomer 4Z, 15E-bilirubin, which is excreted in the bile without need for conjugation; and (2) irreversible conversion of native unconjugated bilirubin into the structural isomer lumirubin, which is excreted by the kidneys. Phototherapy must contain light in the blue range (420 to 470 nm) and be of sufficient intensity to efficiently reduce hyperbilirubinemia. The AAP recommends that hospitals use intensive phototherapy light of at least $30\,\mu W/cm^2/nm$ measured by a radiometer at the infant's skin directly below the center of the unit. Intensive phototherapy can be expected to decrease the initial bilirubin level by 30% to 40% in the first 24 hours, with the most significant drop in the first 4 to 6 hours. For infants who are discharged after birth and then readmitted, phototherapy should be continued until the TSB is less than 13 to 14 mg/dL. Though uncommon, rebound hyperbilirubinemia requiring another course of phototherapy can occur, particularly in infants with hemolytic disease or those in whom phototherapy was initiated early and discontinued before 3 to 4 days of life. Discharge from the hospital need not be delayed because of the potential for rebound bilirubin; however, these infants should have a follow-up bilirubin measurement within 24 hours after discontinuation of phototherapy.

Exchange transfusion is the last therapeutic resort if the TSB level does not decrease despite intensive phototherapy or if an infant presents with signs of acute bilirubin encephalopathy. When the TSB level exceeds the recommended threshold for exchange transfusion, intensive phototherapy should be administered, the TSB measurement should be repeated every 2 to 3 hours, preparations for exchange transfusion should be made, and exchange transfusion should be performed if the TSB remains above the recommended threshold after 6 hours of intensive phototherapy. The bilirubin-to-albumin ratio can also be used, together with TSB level, as an additional risk factor in determining the need for exchange transfusion (Table 55-2). For infants with isoimmune hemolytic disease whose TSB is rising despite intensive phototherapy or whose TSB is within 2 to 3 mg/dL of the exchange level, intravenous gamma globulin (0.5 to 1 g/kg over 2 hours) should be administered, because it has been shown to reduce the need for exchange transfusion in these infants.

ADMISSION CRITERIA

Jaundiced infants who require intensive phototherapy, exchange transfusion, or management of dehydration should be admitted to the hospital. Infants with profound

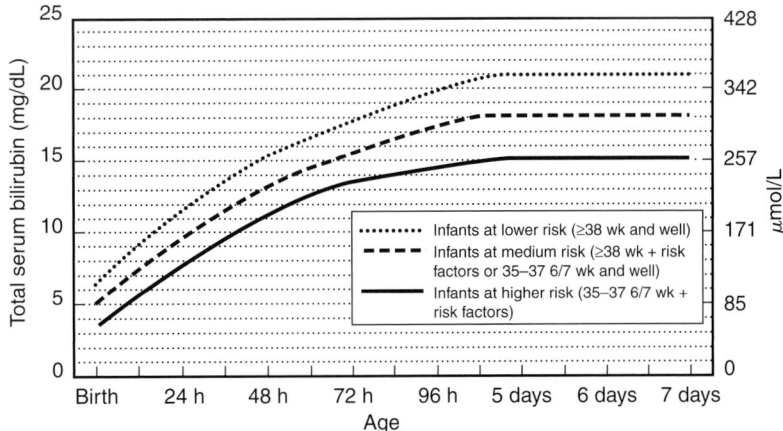

• Use total bilirubin. Do not subtract direct-reacting or conjugated bilirubin.

• Risk factors = isoimmune hemolytic disease, G6PD deficiency, asphyxia, significant lethargy, temperature instability, sepsis, acidosis, or albumin <3.0 g/dL (if measured).

• For well infants 35–37 6/7 wk, can adjust TSB levels for intervention around the medium risk line. It is an option to intervene at lower TSB levels for infants closer to 35 wk and at higher TSB levels for those closer to 37 6/7 wk.

• It is an option to provide conventional phototherapy in hospital or at home at TSB levels 2–3 mg/dL (35–50 mmol/L) below those shown, but home phototherapy should not be used in any infant with risk factors.

Figure 55-2 Guidelines for phototherapy in hospitalized infants of 35 or more weeks' gestation. G6PD, glucose-6-phosphate dehydrogenase; TSB, total serum bilirubin. (From American Academy of Pediatrics Subcommittee on Hyperbilirubinemia: Management of hyperbilirubinemia in the newborn infant 35 or more weeks of gestation. Pediatrics 2004;114:297–316.)

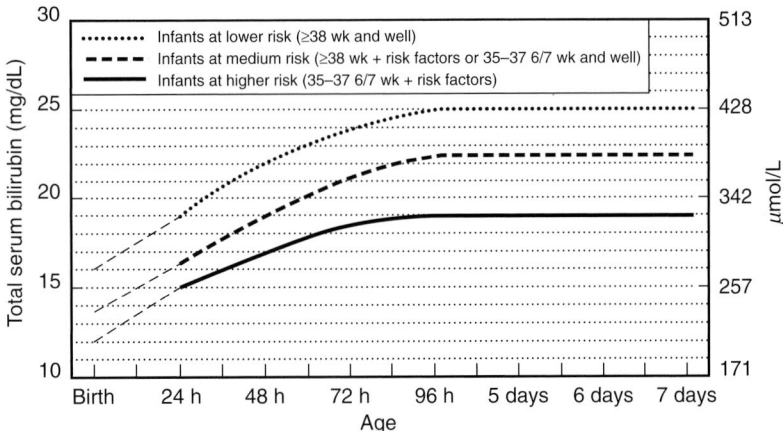

• The dashed lines for the first 24 hours indicate uncertainty due to a wide range of clinical circumstances and a range of responses to phototherapy.

• Immediate exchange transfusion is recommended if infant shows signs of acute bilirubin encephalopathy (hypertonia, arching, retrocollis, opisthotonos, fever, high-pitched cry) or if TSB is ≥5 mg/dL (85 μmol/L) above these lines.

• Risk factors—isoimmune hemolytic disease, G6PD deficiency, asphyxia, significant lethargy, temperature instability, sepsis, acidosis.

• Measure serum albumin and calculate B/A ratio.

• Use total bilirubin. Do not subtract direct-reacting or conjugated bilirubin.

• If infant is well and 35–37 6/7 wk (median risk), can individualize TSB levels for exchange based on actual gestational age.

Figure 55-3 Guidelines for exchange transfusion in infants 35 or more weeks' gestation. B/A, bilirubin-albumin; G6PD, glucose-6-phosphate dehydrogenase; TSB, total serum bilirubin. (From American Academy of Pediatrics Subcommittee on Hyperbilirubinemia: Management of hyperbilirubinemia in the newborn infant 35 or more weeks of gestation. Pediatrics 2004;114:297-316.)

Table 55-2 Bilirubin–Albumin Ratio as an Additional Risk Factor When Considering Exchange Transfusion

Risk Category	Total Serum Bilirubin (mg/dL)-to-Albumin (g/dL) Ratio
Infants ≥38⁰/₇ wk	8.0
Infants 35⁰/₇ to 36⁶/₇ wk and well or ≥38⁰/₇ wk if higher risk or with isoimmune hemolytic disease or G6PD deficiency	7.2
Infants 35⁰/₇ to 37⁶/₇ wk if higher risk or with isoimmune hemolytic disease or G6PD deficiency	6.8

G6PD, glucose-6-phosphate dehydrogenase.
From American Academy of Pediatrics Subcommittee on Hyperbilirubinemia: Management of hyperbilirubinemia in the newborn infant 35 or more weeks of gestation. Pediatrics 2004;114:297-316.

dehydration or with bilirubin levels approaching or exceeding exchange transfusion thresholds should be admitted to a neonatal intensive care facility, if available. Infants with mild to moderate dehydration and bilirubin levels requiring phototherapy alone can be monitored and treated in a pediatric inpatient ward or newborn nursery setting.

DISCHARGE CRITERIA

Infants who are discharged and then readmitted should receive phototherapy until the TSB is less than 13 to 14 mg/dL. For infants treated during the initial birth hospitalization, the TSB thresholds for discontinuing phototherapy are less clear, but reducing the TSB level below the 40th percentile can be used as a treatment goal. Before discharge, infants must be well hydrated and feeding well, with frequent wet diapers and stools. For breastfed infants, particularly those whose jaundice can be attributed to lactation or breastfeeding problems, both the parents and the health care providers must be confident that the infant will have an adequate milk supply through either lactation interventions (e.g., pumping) or supplemental feedings.

PREVENTION

Primary prevention of severe hyperbilirubinemia, acute bilirubin encephalopathy, and kernicterus is dependent on a systems-based approach to ensure newborn infant safety. As recommended by the AAP, this approach includes the following:

- The establishment of standing protocols for nurses' assessment of jaundice, including measurement of TcB and TSB levels, without requiring a physician's order (similar to the protocols in place for measuring serum glucose levels)
- Routine, frequent, and multilevel (physician, nurse, lactation consultant) support and advice for breastfeeding mothers to increase the probability of successful breastfeeding
- Checklists or reminders to prompt providers to consider risk factors and age at discharge, and laboratory test results that guide appropriate follow-up
- Educational materials for parents concerning the identification of jaundice

IN A NUTSHELL

- Pathologic jaundice is caused by increased production, impaired metabolism, or increased enterohepatic circulation of bilirubin.
- Early identification of infants at risk of severe hyperbilirubinemia, early follow-up for high-risk infants, and prompt phototherapy for those who exceed treatment thresholds can prevent the neurologic sequelae of extreme hyperbilirubinemia.
- The 2004 AAP clinical practice guidelines for the management of hyperbilirubinemia provide specific recommendations for evaluation and treatment.

ON THE HORIZON

- Transcutaneous bilirubin meters that use multiwavelength spectral reflectance analysis are now available for point-of-care estimation of bilirubin levels.[13] Use of these devices should be reserved for bilirubin screening before discharge, when bilirubin levels are likely to be lower, because they are less reliable at higher levels.
- Synthetic metalloporphyrins are being developed that inhibit bilirubin production. Tin-mesoporphyrin is effective in both premature and full-term infants with severe hyperbilirubinemia, but it has not yet been approved by the Food and Drug Administration.[14]

SUGGESTED READING

American Academy of Pediatrics Subcommittee on Hyperbilirubinemia: Management of hyperbilirubinemia in the newborn infant 35 or more weeks of gestation. Pediatrics 2004;114:297-316.

Bhutani VK, Johnson L, Sivieri EM: Predictive ability of a predischarge hour-specific serum bilirubin for subsequent significant hyperbilirubinemia in healthy term and near-term newborns. Pediatrics 1999;103:6-14.

Dennery PA, Seidman DS, Stevenson DK: Neonatal hyperbilirubinemia. N Engl J Med 2001;344:581-590.

Kappas A: A method for interdicting the development of severe jaundice in newborns by inhibiting the production of bilirubin [see comment]. Pediatrics 2004;113:119-123.

Maisels MJ, Gifford K: Normal serum bilirubin levels in the newborn and the effect of breast-feeding. Pediatrics 1986;78:837-843.

Moyer VA, Ahn C, Sneed S: Accuracy of clinical judgment in neonatal jaundice. Arch Pediatr Adolesc Med 2000;154:391-394.

Newman TB, Xiong B, Gonzales VM, Escobar GJ: Prediction and prevention of extreme neonatal hyperbilirubinemia in a mature health maintenance organization. Arch Pediatr Adolesc Med 2000;154:1140-1147.

REFERENCES

1. Rudolph CD, Rudolph AM, Hoffman JIE: Rudolph's Pediatrics, 20th ed. Norwalk, CT, Appleton & Lange, 1996.
2. Hardy JB, Drage JS, Jackson EC: The First Year of Life, the Collaborative Perinatal Project of the National Institutes of Neurological and Communicative Disorders and Stroke. Baltimore, The Johns Hopkins University Press, 1979.
3. Maisels MJ, Gifford K: Normal serum bilirubin levels in the newborn and the effect of breast-feeding. Pediatrics 1986;78:837-843.
4. Liu LL, Clemens CJ, Shay DK, et al: The safety of newborn early discharge. The Washington State experience. JAMA 1997;278:293-298.
5. Maisels MJ, Kring E: Length of stay, jaundice, and hospital readmission. Pediatrics 1998;101:995-998.
6. Johnson LH, Bhutani VK, Brown AK: System-based approach to management of neonatal jaundice and prevention of kernicterus. J Pediatr 2002;140:396-403.
7. Maisels MJ, Newman TB: Kernicterus in otherwise healthy, breast-fed term newborns. Pediatrics 1995;96:730-733.
8. Kernicterus in full-term infants—United States, 1994-1998. MMWR 2001;50(23):491-494.
9. Management of hyperbilirubinemia in the newborn infant 35 or more weeks of gestation. Pediatrics 2004;114:297-316.
10. Dennery PA, Seidman DS, Stevenson DK: Neonatal hyperbilirubinemia. N Engl J Med 2001;344:581-590.
11. Volpe JJ: Neurology of the Newborn, 4th ed. Philadelphia, WB Saunders, 2001.
12. Bhutani VK, Johnson L, Sivieri EM: Predictive ability of a predischarge hour-specific serum bilirubin for subsequent significant hyperbilirubinemia in healthy term and near-term newborns. Pediatrics 1999;103:6-14.
13. Bhutani VK, Gourley GR, Adler S, et al: Noninvasive measurement of total serum bilirubin in a multiracial predischarge newborn population to assess the risk of severe hyperbilirubinemia. Pediatrics 2000;106:E17.
14. Kappas A: A method for interdicting the development of severe jaundice in newborns by inhibiting the production of bilirubin [see comment]. Pediatrics 2004;113:119-123.

CHAPTER 56

Neonatal Abstinence Syndrome

William McNett

Infants born to mothers who habitually use opiates or their derivatives (heroin, methadone, morphine, meperidine, or codeine) have physical manifestations of opiate withdrawal. This phenomenon was observed by Hippocrates in the 5th century BC and has been described in medical literature since the 19th century. Heroin, a chemically processed form of naturally occurring morphine, was developed in the 1870s. By the 1950s, heroin had become readily available in North America and Europe, which led to its widespread use as a drug of abuse. It became apparent in the following decades that significant mortality and morbidity were associated with infants born to heroin-addicted mothers, including prematurity, low birth weight, seizures, and poor weight gain. As a disease process, neonatal abstinence syndrome (NAS) was not identified until the 1970s, when a systematic approach for diagnosis, monitoring, and treatment was developed.[1,2]

Approximately 3% of women of childbearing years use illicit drugs or abuse prescription medications, including marijuana, cocaine, hallucinogens, heroin, sedatives, and stimulants.[3] In addition, alcohol abuse during pregnancy is one of the leading causes of preventable birth defects. Infants born to mothers who abuse drugs suffer adverse effects at birth, including drug intoxication and drug withdrawal. NAS focuses on opiate withdrawal, but similar symptoms often occur in infants who have been exposed in utero to other drugs of abuse.

CLINICAL PRESENTATION

Nearly all infants exposed to opiates in utero on a continuing basis have some symptoms of NAS. Of these exposed infants, 60% to 80% have moderate to severe symptoms, as defined by an NAS scoring system (Table 56-1), and require medical intervention.[4] Infants born to mothers who use opiates usually present with symptoms within the first 72 to 96 hours of life. Withdrawal symptoms can be classified into three areas: central nervous system (CNS), autonomic nervous system, and gastrointestinal (GI) symptoms (Table 56-2). Skin excoriation on the buttocks (due to excessive stooling) and the elbows and knees (due to friction burns secondary to tremors) is also well described.

The severity and timing of the onset of symptoms vary, based on the type of opiate involved, the amount used, and the interval between last exposure to the drug and delivery. Infants exposed to codeine generally have mild manifestations of withdrawal and commonly need only supportive care. Those exposed to heroin or methadone have much more pronounced symptoms. Although the symptoms of heroin exposure develop more quickly after birth and are less severe than those seen with methadone exposure, pregnant women using heroin are encouraged to enter a methadone maintenance program to avoid complications associated with ongoing heroin use. Women who become pregnant while addicted to opiates are also advised to avoid acute withdrawal during pregnancy owing to the risk of spontaneous abortion, intrauterine growth restriction, prematurity, and antepartum hemorrhage.

A delayed onset of NAS symptoms is associated with maternal polydrug use. Opiate use combined with sedative use during pregnancy may mask infant withdrawal symptoms for up to 2 weeks. Another factor known to cause delayed or protracted infant withdrawal is prolonged maternal use of high-dose methadone.[4] Complete withdrawal for these infants can take 2 weeks to 4 months.

DIFFERENTIAL DIAGNOSIS

In infants younger than 2 weeks who present with symptoms consistent with NAS, other considerations are sepsis, electrolyte abnormalities (glucose, magnesium, calcium), neonatal hyperthyroidism, CNS hemorrhage, GI obstruction, colic, or congenital infections such as toxoplasmosis and cytomegalovirus (CMV).

DIAGNOSIS AND EVALUATION

In the case of known in utero exposure to opiates or other illicit drugs, no laboratory studies are warranted except a urine toxicology screen on both mother and infant. This may detect polydrug use that might not have been revealed in the maternal history. In addition, child protective services frequently require a positive urine toxicology screen to investigate a case. Other laboratory studies can be directed by clinical impression and other birth history as necessary.

If an infant presents with symptoms consistent with NAS and there is no reported history of maternal drug use, maternal drug use is still a possibility, but other conditions should also be considered. Each institution should develop objective criteria to screen for illicit drug use in pregnant women at the time of delivery (Table 56-3). If maternal drug abuse is verified, it is important to test the mother for sexually transmitted diseases, such as human immunodeficiency virus (HIV), hepatitis B, hepatitis C, syphilis, gonorrhea, and chlamydia, because of the higher incidence of these infections in women who use illicit drugs. Because maternal information is frequently unreliable, an infant urine toxicology screen is useful. Of note, if the mother abstained from drug use just before delivery, both she and her infant may have negative urine toxicology screens in the peripartum period. Nonetheless, previous habitual drug use puts the infant at risk for NAS. In the case of a negative urine toxicology screen on the infant, meconium analysis (if available) for illicit drugs may be useful to identify maternal drug use

Table 56-1 Classification of Neonatal Abstinence Syndrome Based on Finnegan Scoring System

	Mild	Moderate	Severe
Score	<8	8-16	>16
Treatment	Supportive care	Supportive care NOS	Supportive care NOS Adjunctive therapy
	Social services	Social Services	Social services
Outcome	Discharge after 72-96 hr Close outpatient monitoring	Hospitalization for 1-3 wk	Hospitalization for >3wk Comorbidities (e.g., GERD, nosocomial infection)

GERD, gastroesophageal reflux disease, NOS, neonatal opiate solution.

Table 56-2 Symptoms of Neonatal Abstinence Syndrome

Central nervous system
  Irritability
  Jitteriness
  Tremors
  Excessive crying
  High-pitched cry
  Hyperreflexia
  Sleep disturbance
  Seizures

Autonomic nervous system
  Hyperthermia
  Excessive sweating
  Mottling
  Tachypnea
  Nasal congestion
  Sneezing
  Hiccupping
  Yawning

Gastrointestinal system
  Hyperphagia
  Excessive sucking
  Suck-swallow incoordination
  Vomiting
  Diarrhea
  Poor weight gain

Table 56-3 Criteria for Checking Maternal and Infant Toxicologies

Inadequate prenatal care (e.g., missed appointments, late initiation of care, absence of care)

Unexplained prematurity (<35 weeks' gestation)

Unexplained late fetal loss

Unexplained intrauterine growth restriction

Abruptio placentae without maternal hypertension

Precipitous labor or delivery

Maternal history of drug abuse

that occurred after 20 weeks' gestation. Unfortunately, meconium screening is costly, takes time to process, and may not have a direct impact on immediate management.

To explore the diagnostic possibilities in an infant with a negative maternal history and negative toxicology studies, the following laboratory tests should be performed: complete blood count with differential of the white cell count, C-reactive protein level, basic metabolic panel, serum calcium, and serum magnesium. Evaluation for toxoplasmosis and CMV includes urine culture for CMV, *Toxoplasma* serology, brain imaging, and ophthalmology consultation to evaluate for retinal abnormalities.

To assess the severity of NAS and determine the need for medical intervention, it is important to use a tool that is objective, is reproducible, and has low interobserver variability. Multiple assessments performed over time are more informative than a single assessment performed at one point in time. There are currently four NAS scoring systems that can help determine the severity of withdrawal and guide the weaning process:

1. Neonatal abstinence scoring system by Finnegan[5]
2. Neonatal drug withdrawal scoring system by Lipsitz[2]
3. Neonatal narcotic withdrawal index by Green and Suffet[6]
4. Neonatal withdrawal inventory by Zahorodny and colleagues[7]

Each scoring system includes recommendations for starting treatment and guidelines for weaning or increasing medication. Finnegan's system was developed in the 1970s and is the most comprehensive and widely used tool for infants with NAS (Table 56-4). It is designed to be used for bedside assessment every 3 to 4 hours when feedings occur. The neonatal withdrawal inventory is as effective as and less time-consuming than the neonatal abstinence scoring system, but not as comprehensive.

MANAGEMENT

Nonpharmacologic

Initial intervention for NAS starts with supportive care, which may suffice for mild withdrawal symptoms. This includes keeping the infant tightly swaddled in a dimly lit, quiet environment, with minimal interruptions between feedings. Parents can be taught how to minimize external disturbances and help with the infant's care by allowing them to do as many feedings as possible and reinforcing basic parenting skills in the nursery.

Table 56-4 Finnegan Scoring Criteria

Neonatal Abstinence Score

Evaluator should place a number next to each sign or symptom observed at various time intervals, then add scores for total score.																			
Date:				Daily Weight:															
System	**Signs and Symptoms**	**Score**	**AM**							**PM**								**Comments**	
Central Nervous System Disturbances	Excessive High Pitched (other) Cry Continuous High Pitched (other) Cry	2 3																	
	Sleeps < 1 hour after feeding Sleeps < 2 hours after feeding Sleeps < 3 hours after feeding	3 2 1																	
	Hyperactive Moro reflex Markedly Hyperactive Moro reflex	2 3																	
	Mild Tremors Disturbed Moderate-Severe Tremors Disturbed	1 2																	
	Mild Tremors Undisturbed Moderate-Severe Tremors Undisturbed	3 4																	
	Increased Muscle Tone	2																	
	Excoriation (specific areas)	1																	
	Myoclonic jerks	3																	
	Generalized Convulsions	5																	
Metabolic/Vasomotor/Respiratory Disturbances	Sweating	1																	
	Fever < 101 (99–100.8F./37.2–38.2C.) Fever > 101 (38.4C. and higher)	1 2																	
	Frequent Yawning (>3–4 times/interval)	1																	
	Mottling	1																	
	Nasal Stuffiness	1																	
	Sneezing (>3–4 times/interval)	1																	
	Nasal Flaring	2																	
	Respiratory rate >60/min. Respiratory rate >60/min. with Retractions	1 2																	
Gastrointestinal Disturbances	Excessive Sucking	1																	
	Poor Feeding	2																	
	Regurgitation Projectile Vomiting	2 3																	
	Loose Stools Watery Stools	2 3																	
Total Score																			
Initials of Scorer																			

Initials	Signature		Initials	Signature

From Finnegan LP, Kaltenbach K: The assessment and management of neonatal abstinence syndrome. In Hockelmann R, Nelson N: Primary Pediatric Care, 3rd ed. St. Louis, Mosby, 1992, pp 1367-1378.

Social services should be involved as soon as an infant with NAS is identified or when infant drug exposure is confirmed without NAS symptoms. Social services can assess parenting behavior and the safety of the home environment and help mothers get into a recovery program if this has not already occurred. Infants with NAS are at high risk for developmental and behavioral problems, and arrangements for early intervention and follow-up are indicated for all infants with in utero drug exposure. If a drug-using mother is not in a recovery program before delivery or is not compliant in her program, child protective services should be informed at the time of delivery or when the infant is diagnosed

Table 56-5 Goals of Therapy for Neonatal Abstinence Syndrome
Reduce central and autonomic nervous system symptoms
Induce regular feeding cycles
Induce regular sleep cycles
Establish adequate weight gain (>15 g/day)
Provide parental preparation and education

with NAS. The child protective services agency determines whether the infant can go home with the mother at the time of discharge or whether foster placement is necessary.

The weight of infants with withdrawal must be carefully monitored during and after the initial hospital stay. To achieve good nutrition, either breast milk or formula can be used. For mothers in a recovery program and drug-free, breastfeeding is still recommended unless there are other contraindications, such as HIV infection.[4] Methadone does cross into breast milk, but it is considered safe for breast-feeding infants. Adjunctive nutritional therapy includes using a hypercaloric formula (22 to 27 kcal/oz) for infants showing poor weight gain and hypoallergenic formula for infants with continued watery stools. Vomiting, irritability, and poor feeding may continue even after good control of other NAS symptoms, and evaluation and treatment for gastroesophageal reflux may be warranted. A feeding evaluation should be considered if there is evidence of disorganized swallowing.

Pharmacologic

Although the mortality rate is low among infants with NAS, pharmacologic intervention is recommended in moderately to severely affected infants to achieve symptomatic relief and adequate weight gain. The goals of treating NAS are listed in Table 56-5. Historically, opiates, phenobarbital, and benzodiazepines have been used as single agents to treat NAS. The Cochrane Neonatal Group, in its most recent reviews, concluded that opiates are preferred for an infant whose mother used only opiates during the pregnancy; opiates will improve the CNS, GI, and autonomic nervous system symptoms.[8] Benzodiazepines are not recommended as a single agent for the treatment of NAS.[9]

Neonatal opiate solution (NOS) is an aqueous solution containing 0.4 mg/mL of morphine sulfate; it has replaced paregoric as a treatment for NAS. Paregoric contains additives, including camphor and benzoic acid, that are associated with adverse effects. The starting dosage for NOS is 0.2 to 0.5 mg/kg per day orally, divided into six to eight doses, depending on the frequency of feedings. This initial dosage is continued for 48 to 72 hours to stabilize the infant. The four screening tools mentioned earlier can be used to help guide the weaning process. If the infant responds with improved feeding, sleeping, and comfort and reduced GI symptoms (NAS score consistently <8), the NOS dosage can be decreased by 10% every 24 to 48 hours, as long as the symptoms remain under control. If the initial dosage does not significantly improve the infant's symptoms, it can be increased by 10% until treatment goals are met. Maximum dosing of 1 to 2 mg/kg per day has been used, but adding phenobarbital as an adjunctive therapy should be considered with NOS doses higher than 1 mg/kg per day.

Phenobarbital as a single agent is an alternative treatment for NAS. Unfortunately, it does not ameliorate GI symptoms such as emesis and diarrhea, which may be clinically significant. In addition, it may not control withdrawal-induced seizures as well as opiates do, and there are concerns about the long-term adverse affects of phenobarbital on the newborn brain.[9] If phenobarbital is used, a loading dose of 15 to 20 mg/kg intramuscularly or orally is recommended, followed by 4 to 6 mg/kg per day divided for twice-a-day dosing. Phenobarbital can be weaned by 10% after successful stabilization, much like NOS, or increased by 10% until adequate control is achieved. For an infant who is having a difficult withdrawal or whose mother used sedatives in addition to opiates during pregnancy, a combination of NOS and phenobarbital may be beneficial. Other medications such as clonidine and chlorpromazine are currently being studied, but no data support their use as adjunctive therapy with NOS for withdrawal.

Methadone as a therapy for NAS has not been adequately studied in newborns, although it is used at many centers at dosages of 0.05 to 0.1 mg/kg orally every 6 hours, increasing the dosage by 0.05 mg/kg until symptoms are controlled, and then weaning as with NOS.

COURSE OF ILLNESS

Mild NAS symptoms may persist until age 4 months, even after successful medical management.[3] Sleep may continue to be disorganized, and hyperreflexia may continue, but tremor and jitteriness usually resolve earlier. GI disturbances such as loose stools, emesis, and colic also tend to resolve later in the withdrawal process. An increased incidence of sudden infant death syndrome has been reported in this population. In addition, there is a higher incidence of child abuse, possibly associated with maternal isolation, poor parenting preparation and skills, increased infant irritability, and the stresses of ongoing maternal drug use or recovery.[3]

Long-term effects of opioid withdrawal are not clearly defined. There is some evidence that in utero exposure to opiates leads to learning behaviors that may interfere with school performance, such as attention-deficit hyperactivity disorder, cognitive deficits, and poorly developed organizational and adaptive skills. There is also evidence that these behaviors may be more dependent on the home and social environment and not directly related to in utero drug exposure.[10]

ADMISSION CRITERIA

- Infants born to mothers with known opiate or other illicit drug use. These infants should remain hospitalized for a minimum of 72 to 96 hours to observe for symptoms of moderate to severe NAS and to allow proper social services intervention to ensure the safety of the home before discharge.
- Infants without known in utero drug exposure but exhibiting symptoms consistent with NAS. These infants

should be observed for at least 48 hours, and appropriate studies should be performed.

- Infants with known in utero drug exposure who have been discharged from the nursery after the initial observation period and then develop symptoms of significant NAS or have dehydration, persistent emesis, failure to thrive, CNS disorganization, or seizures.

DISCHARGE CRITERIA

- Infant is no longer receiving opiate medication for at least 48 hours without reemergence of moderate or severe symptoms.
- Infant achieves adequate oral intake and consistent weight gain.
- Social services personnel have contacted the local child protective agency, and an appropriate primary caregiver and safe home environment for the infant have been assured.
- Close medical and social follow-up is ensured.
- Elucidation of neonatal withdrawal associated with maternal use of selective serotonin reuptake inhibitors during pregnancy.[11]

PREVENTION

Prevention of NAS and in utero drug exposure is a complicated medical and socioeconomic problem. Solutions include improved drug prevention in high-risk areas and for high-risk groups and increased access to and promotion of health care during pregnancy.

IN A NUTSHELL

- Consider NAS or neonatal intoxication in infants who have neurologic, GI, or autonomic symptoms, even without a maternal history of drug use.
- Use an assessment and scoring system that support staff have been trained to administer with consistency and low interobserver variability.
- Involve social services early, and report the patient to the appropriate child welfare agencies.
- Provide NOS for moderate to severe withdrawal symptoms.
- Provide aggressive nutritional support, if needed, including feeding evaluation, nutritional supplementation, or alternative feeding methods.
- Refer the patient to early intervention services before discharge from the hospital.

ON THE HORIZON

- Home therapy after initial inpatient stabilization to promote maternal involvement and decrease hospital costs.

- Increased understanding of the utility of other medications for the treatment of NAS, such as selective serotonin reuptake inhibitors.
- Improved recognition of infants with disorders related to in utero alcohol and drug exposure.
- Use of shorter-acting pharmacologic agents (e.g., buprenorphine) during pregnancy to control maternal addiction and possibly alter the severity and duration of NAS.

SUGGESTED READING

AAP Committee on Drugs: Neonatal drug withdrawal. Pediatrics 1998; 101:1079-1088.
Kandall SR: Treatment strategies for drug-exposed neonates. Clin Perinatol 1000;26:231-243.
Martinez A, Partridge JC, Taeusch HW: Perinatal substance abuse. In Taeusch HW, Ballard RA, Gleason CA (eds): Avery's Diseases of the Newborn. Philadelphia, Elsevier Saunders, 2004, pp 106-126.
Osborn DA, Cole MJ, Jeffery HE: Opiate treatment for opiate withdrawal in newborn infants. Cochrane Database Syst Rev 2004;3.
Osborn DA, Jeffry HE, Cole MJ: Sedatives for opiate withdrawal in newborn infants. Cochrane Database Syst Rev 2004;3.

REFERENCES

1. Finnegan LP, Kron RE, Connaughton JF, Emich JP: Assessment and treatment of abstinence in the infant of the drug-dependent mother. Int J Clin Pharmacol 1975;12:19-32.
2. Lipsitz P: A proposed narcotic withdrawal score for use with newborn infants. Clin Pediatr 1975;14:592-594.
3. Ostrea E, Posecion J, Villanueva M: The infant of the drug-dependent mother. In Avery G, Fletcher MA, MacDonald M (eds): Neonatology, Pathophysiology and Management of the Newborn. Philadelphia, Lippincott Williams & Wilkins, 1999, pp 1407-1445.
4. Kandall SR: Treatment strategies for drug-exposed neonates. Clin Perinatol 1999;26:231-243.
5. Finnegan LP: Neonatal abstinence syndrome. In Nelson NM (ed): Current Therapy in Neonatal-Perinatal Medicine, 2nd ed. Philadelphia, BC Decker, 1990, pp 314-320.
6. Green M, Suffet F: The neonatal narcotic withdrawal index: A device for the improvement of care in the abstinence syndrome. Am J Drug Alcohol Abuse 1981;8:203-213.
7. Zahorodny W, Rom C, Whitney W, et al: The neonatal withdrawal inventory: A simplified score of newborn withdrawal. J Dev Behav Pediatr 1998;19:89-93.
8. Osborn DA, Cole MJ, Jeffery HE: Opiate treatment for opiate withdrawal in newborn infants. Cochrane Database Syst Rev 2004;3.
9. Osborn DA, Jeffry HE, Cole MJ: Sedatives for opiate withdrawal in newborn infants. Cochrane Database Syst Rev 2004;3.
10. Martinez A, Partridge JC, Taeusch HW: Perinatal substance abuse. In Taeusch HW, Ballard RA, Gleason CA (eds): Avery's Diseases of the Newborn. Philadelphia, Elsevier Saunders, 2004, pp 106-126.
11. Sanz EJ, Detas-Cuevas C, Kiuro A, et al: Selective serotonin reuptake inhibitors in pregnant women and neonatal withdrawal syndrome: A database analysis. Lancet 2005;365:482-487.

Fluids and Electrolytes

CHAPTER 57

Dehydration

Philip R. Spandorfer

Dehydration occurs when there is fluid loss in excess of intake. Although fluid losses can occur from several different sources, gastrointestinal losses are the most common. Dehydration is one of the most frequent reasons for hospitalization in children. Furthermore, rotavirus, which is the most commonly identified cause of viral gastroenteritis, is a ubiquitous problem in children worldwide. In fact, it has been shown that almost all children are exposed to rotavirus by age 5 years.

Dehydration can be classified as mild, moderate, or severe. Mild dehydration represents a less than 5% loss of body weight; moderate, 5% to 10%; and severe, greater than 10%. Isonatremic dehydration occurs when the serum sodium level is between 130 and 150 mEq/L. This type of dehydration, which is the most common, is the focus of this chapter.

PATHOPHYSIOLOGY

Dehydration is a general state in which there is a total-body fluid deficit. Under normal physiologic conditions, water constitutes 70% of lean body mass. In infants, the proportion is approximately 75%. Two thirds of the fluid is intracellular, and one third is extracellular. Of the extracellular fluid, 75% is interstitial and 25% is intravascular. Fluid that is lost from the body often has an electrolyte composition similar to that of plasma. Most of the fluid deficit during the early stages of dehydration is from the extracellular space, but over time, the fluid losses equilibrate, and fluid leaves the intracellular space. During the recovery phase, fluid administered to the patient is located in the extracellular space and needs time to equilibrate with the intracellular space.

DIFFERENTIAL DIAGNOSIS

Dehydration is not a disease but rather a symptom or consequence of another process. It can be thought of as a common final pathway. The clinician must search for the cause of dehydration, which can be due to decreased intake, increased losses, or a combination of the two (Table 57-1). Among the myriad causes of dehydration, a few stand out. The most common cause that brings patients to medical attention is acute gastroenteritis. Decreased intake secondary to stomatitis or pharyngitis is also fairly common.

EVALUATION

Initial Stabilization

Careful attention to the ABCs (airway, breathing, circulation) is required for appropriate stabilization in any emergent situation. However, with dehydration, derangements are most common. In particular, it is important to identify signs of shock, which include poor peripheral perfusion, obtundation, severe tachycardia, and blood pressure changes—either narrowed pulse pressure or frank hypotension. Any dehydrated patient in shock should receive large amounts of isotonic fluid administered via large-bore intravenous lines in 20 mL/kg boluses. Constant reassessment of the patient's vital signs, urine output, and physical findings can assist in determining the appropriate duration of therapy. Even in initially stable-appearing patients, paying careful attention to early indicators of shock can avoid a precipitous deterioration in their condition. A substantial percentage of moderately and severely dehydrated patients is also hypoglycemic, making it important to consider checking the bedside glucose level in dehydrated patients.

History and Physical Examination

Because almost all treatment depends on the degree of dehydration, it is important to be as accurate as possible in this respect. In the setting of acute illness (<5 days of symptoms), acute weight loss is the best indicator of the fluid deficit; each kilogram of weight loss indicates a deficit of 1 L. Unfortunately, a recent "well" weight is rarely known in children being treated for dehydration; thus, an estimate of the deficit must be made on the basis of the clinical evaluation (discussed later in this section).

The history is perhaps most helpful in determining the cause of dehydration, particularly the symptoms present, their duration, and what therapies have been implemented (Table 57-2). Of specific interest are the presence, quality, and quantity of both vomiting and diarrhea. Determining whether there has been a reduction in urine output is

Table 57-1   Causes of Dehydration
Increased Losses
Gastroenteritis* (viral or bacterial)
Vomiting
Pyloric stenosis
Pyelonephritis
Increased intracranial pressure
Abdominal obstruction
Appendicitis
Pancreatitis
Hepatitis
Diarrhea
Carbohydrate or other malabsorption
Milk protein allergy
Inflammatory bowel disease
Cystic fibrosis
Increased insensible losses (fever, tachypnea)
Burns
Diabetes insipidus
Diabetic ketoacidosis
Cystic fibrosis
Decreased Intake
Gingivostomatitis*
Pharyngitis*
Febrile episode*
Altered mental status
Physical restriction
Dependence on caregiver

*The most common causes.

Table 57-2   Focused History
Description of the illness
How many days has the child been sick?
Does the child have vomiting, and if so, how many times per day?
Does the child have diarrhea, and if so, how many times per day?
Did the abdominal pain start before the vomiting?
What has the urine output been?
Who else has been ill?
Does the child have fever?
Description of treatment administered
What has been tried at home?
How is the infant formula made?
What other health care providers have been involved?
Past medical history
Does the child have any cardiac, renal, or metabolic disorders?
If yes, is the child on fluid restriction?
Any other relevant past medical or surgical history
Other history
Does the family use well water?
Was there any recent travel?
Was there any recent antibiotic use?

Table 57-3   Dehydration Scoring System
Decreased skin elasticity
Capillary refill >2 seconds (measured at the volar aspect of the fingertip)*
Ill appearance (tired, somnolent, "washed out")*
Absent tears*
Abnormal respirations
Dry mucous membranes*
Sunken eyes
Abnormal radial pulse
Tachycardia (heart rate >150 beats/min)
Decreased urine output (parental report)

*Subset of items included in a 4-point scoring system.

helpful; although decreased urination has a low positive predictive value for dehydration, a history of normal urine output is reassuring.

It is medically accurate to reserve the diagnosis of gastroenteritis for those patients who have diarrhea with or without vomiting. Numerous diseases can be confused with gastroenteritis if the cause of the emesis is not elucidated. Common diseases occasionally misdiagnosed as gastroenteritis include urinary tract infection, pyelonephritis, lower lobe pneumonia, and appendicitis.

Because dehydration is such a ubiquitous problem in ill children, an overall assessment of hydration status should be part of the routine physical assessment of all patients. The dehydration scoring system presented in Table 57-3 offers an evidence-based approach to determining the degree of dehydration.[1] With this system, the patient is assessed on 10 individual features, receiving 1 point for each feature present. A score of 0 indicates no dehydration. A score of 1 or 2 indicates mild dehydration, or less than 5% loss of total body weight. A score of 3 to 6 indicates moderate dehydration, or 5% to 10% body weight loss. A score of 7 to 10 indicates severe dehydration. A 4-point scoring system based on overall ill appearance, decreased tear production, dry mucous membranes, and delayed capillary refill time appears to have the same diagnostic accuracy as the full 10-point system. Using this limited subset, a score of 0 indicates no dehydration, 1 indicates mild dehydration, and 2 or higher indicates moderate to severe dehydration. Children with hyponatremia have a greater relative loss of extracellular fluid and may manifest more marked clinical findings for a given degree of dehydration; conversely, hypernatremia leads to relative preservation of the extracellular fluid compartment and the consequent amelioration of clinical signs.

Ancillary Studies

The majority of children with uncomplicated dehydration do not require laboratory testing. A decreased serum bicarbonate concentration is often associated with dehydration; however, this usually reflects the ketoacidosis that accompanies not eating. The measurement of serum bicarbonate may

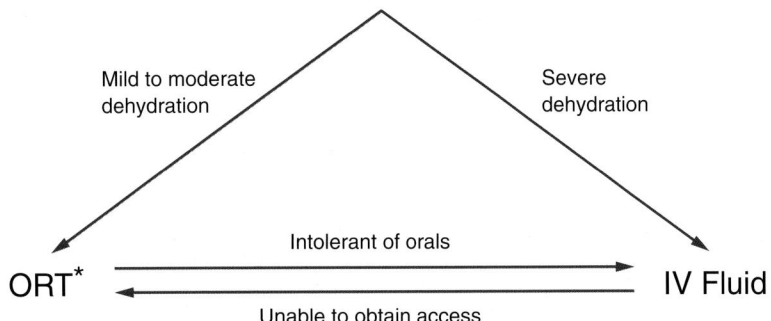

Assessment
Determine degree of dehydration
Determine etiology of dehydration

Mild to moderate dehydration

Severe dehydration

Intolerant of orals

ORT* ⟵⟶ IV Fluid

Unable to obtain access

* If intolerant of orals, a nasogastric tube may be used to administer appropriate electrolyte solutions.

ORT medical personnel directions:
- ORT works via the sodium glucose cotransport mechanism.
- Utilizing the correct electrolyte solution is critical for its success.
- Choose appropriate solution:
  - Maintenance electrolyte solution (e.g., Pedialyte) as first line
  - May use ½-strength sports beverage (e.g., Gatorade) with saltine crackers in older patients.
- Caution: Do not add juice to the Pedialyte as it alters the sodium-to-glucose concentration, which is important for fluid absorption across the GI tract.
- Calculate total volume to be administered over 4-hr rehydration phase.
  - Mild dehydration: 50 mL/kg
  - Moderate dehydration: 100 mL/kg
  - Severe dehydration: 150 mL/kg
- Calculate 5-min aliquot volume
  - (Total volume) ÷ 4 ÷ 12, i.e., 4-hr rehydration period and 12 five-min blocks in an hour
- Administer the aliquot over the 5-min period.
- Increase volume as tolerated.

ORT family directions:
- ORT is a specific treatment technique for dehydrated patients.
- A small amount of liquid is administered every few minutes with a syringe—although the child may want more, the stomach needs a chance to digest the liquid before the next syringe feed.
- If the child has been vomiting, he or she may continue to vomit.
- Please try to collect the vomit in a bucket so we can measure it.
- If it is only a small amount of vomit, we will continue.
- If it is a large amount of vomit, we may need to stop and place on IV.
- You should watch the clock and every 5 min give the syringe.
- It may be hard at first, but with a few feeds it gets much easier and the child begins to take the feeds.
- If your child refuses the feeds, then we may need to place an IV as well.
- This is a treatment that you are able to do at home to continue treating this illness as well as any future cases of dehydration that may occur.

Figure 57-1   Algorithm for the treatment of dehydration. GI, gastrointestinal; IV, intravenous line; ORT, oral rehydration therapy.

be a useful adjunct if the diagnosis is unclear, but by itself, it does not determine the need for hospitalization.[2] Measurement of serum electrolytes is indicated for children with severe dehydration or those with risk factors for hypo- or hypernatremia (see Chapter 58). Blood glucose should be measured when intravenous therapy is chosen over oral treatment, because glucose-containing fluids are not routinely used in initial parenteral therapy unless there is documented hypoglycemia.

TREATMENT

Oral Rehydration Therapy

Oral rehydration therapy (ORT) is recommended by the American Academy of Pediatrics and the World Health Organization (WHO) as the treatment of choice for mildly

and moderately dehydrated patients.[3,4] Contraindications to ORT include shock or suspected acute abdomen. Vomiting itself is not a contraindication to a trial of ORT. Because ORT can be instituted rapidly, and treatment failure is typically apparent early on, it is reasonable to start with ORT and, if it is unsuccessful, progress to intravenous fluids (Fig. 57-1). However, if ORT has already been attempted without success, initial parenteral therapy may be appropriate.

ORT uses the sodium-glucose cotransport mechanism to passively absorb water across the intestinal mucosa. Hence, the oral rehydration solution (ORS) should have the correct sodium-to-glucose ratio,[5] which is optimally 1:1. Rehydralyte and the WHO ORS packets are examples of appropriate solutions for the rehydration phase of treatment. The WHO ORS has a 1:1 ratio, whereas Rehydralyte has a 1:2 ratio. Maintenance solutions, such as Pedialyte, are acceptable alternatives for mildly and moderately dehydrated patients.

The ratio of sodium to glucose in Pedialyte is 1 : 3. The proper procedure for administering ORT is shown in Figure 57-1. The aim is to replace fluid losses over 4 to 6 hours. When vomiting is a prominent part of the clinical picture, administration of small, frequent aliquots is necessary. Ongoing assessment, including serial weight measurement, is necessary to evaluate the progress of treatment. ORT failure is defined as progression of signs of dehydration, failure to replace the deficit over 8 hours, or the presence of intractable vomiting.

Once patients are better able to tolerate oral intake, the normal diet can be reintroduced. If the gastroenteritis is severe, the brush border of the small bowel may be injured, causing a temporary secondary lactase deficiency. Lactose-free milk may be recommended for 48 hours to 1 week, depending on the severity of diarrhea, but lactose restriction is not necessary in most children.

Despite the recommendations and evidence that ORT is as effective as intravenous fluids for mild and moderate dehydration, in North America ORT is used in less than 30% of the cases for which it is indicated.[6]

Intravenous Fluid Therapy

Intravenous fluid therapy is needed when ORT fails or is contraindicated. The usual approach is to administer 20 mL/kg aliquots of isotonic fluid (e.g., normal saline) over 20 to 60 minutes, with frequent reexamination to determine the need for additional bolus administration. After bolus therapy has been administered, intravenous fluids can be administered at a rate calculated to replace the entire deficit over a 24- to 48-hour period (see Chapter 58). Alternatively, for children with isonatremic dehydration, it is reasonable to provide this additional fluid in the form of 5% dextrose with $\frac{1}{4}$ to $\frac{1}{2}$ normal saline at a rate of 1.5 to 2 times maintenance to account for ongoing losses until intravenous therapy is no longer needed. Intravenous fluids may be discontinued when clinical signs are improving and the patient is able to take sufficient oral fluids to meet maintenance needs and ongoing losses.

Antiemetics

The routine use of antiemetics is discouraged in pediatric patients owing to the side effects of the commonly used drugs. However, ondansetron, which selectively blocks serotonin 5-HT$_3$ receptors, has an acceptable side effect profile. Approximately 80% of these receptors are located in the emetic center in the brain. Ondansetron can be administered either orally or intravenously, but it should be instituted early in the rehydration phase in patients with persistent vomiting. Several recent studies showed that ondansetron reduces emesis in patients with viral gastroenteritis.[7,8] Although a majority of patients stop vomiting with routine rehydration measures alone, these studies found that 20% more patients stop vomiting after ondansetron administration. Patients who are more ill may derive an additional benefit. The high cost of the medication has been cited as a downside.

ADMISSION CRITERIA

- Inability to tolerate ORT due to persistent vomiting, high stool output, or inability to cooperate, requiring ongoing intravenous fluid therapy.

- Signs or symptoms of severe dehydration (>10% loss of body weight).
- Significant electrolyte abnormalities (see Chapter 58).

DISCHARGE CRITERIA

- Ability to maintain hydration status orally.
- Correction of abnormal electrolyte status.

IN A NUTSHELL

- Dehydration is one of the most common reasons for hospitalization in children.
- ORT is the treatment of choice for mildly and moderately dehydrated patients.
- Intravenous fluid therapy is needed when ORT fails or is contraindicated.
- Ondansetron appears to reduce emesis in patients with viral gastroenteritis.

ON THE HORIZON

- A growing literature suggests that isotonic fluid administration may help prevent many cases of iatrogenic hyponatremia.[9-11] These studies are based in part on the recognition of nonosmotic stimulation of antidiuretic hormone secretion, especially in hospitalized children. In the future, hypotonic replacement fluids may be reserved only for those patients with ongoing free water losses or hypernatremia (i.e., existing free water deficit).
- There is growing evidence that rapid intravenous fluid replacement—the concept of administering intravenous boluses as indicated and then allowing the child to continue oral hydration either in the medical setting or at home—is both safe and effective, allowing more than two thirds of patients to be discharged from the emergency department or observation unit.[12,13]

SUGGESTED READING

Centers for Disease Control and Prevention: Managing acute gastroenteritis among children: Oral rehydration, maintenance, and nutritional therapy. MMWR 2003;52:1-16.

Gorelick MH, Shaw KN, Murphy KO: Validity and reliability of clinical signs in the diagnosis of dehydration in children. Pediatrics 1997;99:e6.

Spandorfer PR, Alessandrini EA, Joffe M, et al: Oral vs intravenous rehydration of moderately dehydrated children: A randomized controlled trial. Pediatrics 2005;115:295-301.

Steiner MJ, DeWalt DA, Byerley JS: Is this child dehydrated? JAMA 2004;291:2746-2754.

The Treatment of Diarrhoea: A Manual for Physicians and Other Senior Health Workers, 3rd ed. WHO/CDD/SER/80.2. Geneva, World Health Organization, Division of Diarrhoeal and Acute Respiratory Disease Control.

REFERENCES

1. Gorelick MH, Shaw KN, Murphy KO: Validity and reliability of clinical signs in the diagnosis of dehydration in children. Pediatrics 1997;99: e6.

2. Wathen JE, MacKenzie T, Bothner JP: Usefulness of the serum electrolyte panel in the management of pediatric dehydration treated with intravenously administered fluids. Pediatrics 2004;114:1227-1234.

3. American Academy of Pediatrics, Provisional Committee on Quality Improvement, Subcommittee on Acute Gastroenteritis: Practice parameter: The management of acute gastroenteritis in young children. Pediatrics 1996;97:424.

4. The Treatment of Diarrhoea: A Manual for Physicians and Other Senior Health Workers, 3rd ed. WHO/CDD/SER/80.2. Geneva, World Health Organization, Division of Diarrhoeal and Acute Respiratory Disease Control.

5. Centers for Disease Control and Prevention: Managing acute gastroenteritis among children: Oral rehydration, maintenance, and nutritional therapy. MMWR 2003;52:1-16.

6. Conners GP, Barker WH, Mushlin AI, Goepp JG: Oral versus intravenous: Rehydration preferences of pediatric emergency medicine fellowship directors. Pediatr Emerg Care 2000;16:335-338.

7. Freedman SB, Adler M, Seshadri R, Powell EC: Oral ondansetron for gastroenteritis in a pediatric emergency department. N Engl J Med 2006; 354:1698-1705.

8. Reeves JJ, Shannon MW, Fleisher GR: Ondansetron decreases vomiting associated with acute gastroenteritis: A randomized, controlled trial. Pediatrics 2002;109:e62.

9. Hoorn EJ, Geary D, Robb M, et al: Acute hyponatremia related to intravenous fluid administration in hospitalized children: An observational study. Pediatrics 2004;113:1279-1284.

10. Neville KA, Verge CF, O'Meara MW, Walker JL: High antidiuretic hormone levels and hyponatremia in children with gastroenteritis. Pediatrics 2005;116:1401-1407.

11. Moritz ML, Ayus JC: Prevention of hospital-acquired hyponatremia: A case for using isotonic saline. Pediatrics 2003;111:227-230.

12. Reid SR, Bonadio WA: Outpatient rapid intravenous rehydration to correct dehydration and resolve vomiting in children with acute gastroenteritis. Ann Emerg Med 1996;28:318-332.

13. Phin SJ, McCaskill ME, Browne GJ, Lam LT: Clinical pathway using rapid rehydration for children with gastroenteritis. J Paediatr Child Health 2003;39:343-348.

CHAPTER 58

Fluid and Electrolyte Therapy

Mary Ottolini

An understanding of pediatric fluid therapy is one of the most important advances in pediatric medicine and a cornerstone of current inpatient practice for children with a wide range of acute and chronic conditions.

Before beginning to calculate deficit fluid replacement and manage electrolyte disturbances, it is important to understand the pathophysiology behind water homeostasis and maintenance fluid calculations. Body water and sodium retention are regulated by the hormones antidiuretic hormone (ADH) and aldosterone in response to renin-angiotensin production. Renin and ADH are secreted in reaction to output from sensors detecting changes in circulating blood volume and serum osmolality. These volume receptors are located in the left atrium, carotids, and the aortic arch, and the osmolar receptors are located in the hypothalamus, as well as elsewhere in the body. There are also nonosmotic triggers of ADH secretion, such as pain, stress, vomiting, and a number of pulmonary processes, that in particular affect hospitalized patients. Because sodium is the predominant extracellular cation, its regulation is essential to maintaining water homeostasis. Disturbances in ADH, aldosterone, and sodium will therefore have significant effects on water and electrolyte homeostasis.[1]

MAINTENANCE FLUIDS

Infants kept without oral intake (NPO) for diagnostic studies frequently need maintenance intravenous fluids if they are not allowed to drink for more than 4 to 6 hours. Two methods commonly used to calculate maintenance requirements of fluid are the Holliday-Segar formula and use of the patient's body surface area (BSA). Both formulas assume that the patient is healthy and do not take ongoing losses or additional sources of metabolic stress, such as fever, into account. Furthermore, the Holliday-Segar formula bases fluid requirements on calorie expenditure in healthy children by calculating basal metabolic rates and total energy requirements during normal activity.

The Holliday-Segar method uses the caloric expenditure of the "average patient" to determine fluid needs. By adding up normal insensible water loss from the skin and lungs as a result of metabolic activity and losses in urine and the gastrointestinal tract and then subtracting net gain from water oxidation, essentially 1 mL of water is needed for each kilocalorie of energy expended. Because the metabolic rate is inversely proportional to weight (Fig. 58-1), younger infants and children have higher metabolic rates and therefore require more fluids per unit of body weight than adolescents and adults do.

The Holliday-Segar formula can be simplified and used to calculate fluids on a daily or hourly basis (Table 58-1).

Note that the hourly calculation is often referred to as the "4-2-1" rule.[2-7]

The Holliday-Segar formula refers only to water requirements and does not take into consideration electrolyte losses and needs. In healthy children, most electrolyte loss is through urine. An average of 3 mEq of Na^+ and 2 mEq of K^+ is lost for every 100 kcal of energy expended or 100 mL of maintenance fluid required per 24 hours. Alternatively, one can estimate electrolyte requirements by BSA:

$$BSA\ (m^2) = Height\ (cm) \times Weight\ (kg)/3600$$

Using the BSA method, the electrolyte requirements are as follows:

$Na^+ = 30$ to $50\ mEq/m^2/day$
$K^+ = 30$ to $40\ mEq/m^2/day$
$Cl^- = 30\ mEq/m^2/day$

Example: Maintenance Fluids

An 8-month-old needs to be NPO after midnight for his hernia repair tomorrow. What maintenance fluid would you order for him? He weighs 23 lb (10 kg).

Calculation

	Water	Sodium
Maintenance	1000 mL/day	30 mEq

We use the Holliday-Segar formula, which states that 100 mL of fluid is needed per day for the first 10 kg of body weight. Therefore he would need a total of 1000 mL/day (100 mL/kg/day × 10 kg). A total of 3 mEq of Na^+ is needed for every 100 mL of fluid, so he would need 30 mEq Na^+ (3 mEq/100 mL × 1000 mL). If this quantity of Na^+ were provided as NaCl in the 1000 mL of water, it would be 30 mEq/L. Since the concentration of Na^+ in normal saline (NS) is 154 mEq/L, $\frac{1}{4}$ NS should be used for this infant (30 mEq/L is close to 38.5 mEq/L in $\frac{1}{4}$ NS). Because 2 mEq of K^+ is needed per every 100 mL, 20 mEq of KCl is added per liter. To determine the hourly rate, we divide the total volume needed each day, 1000 mL, by 24.

Answer

Order: 5% dextrose (D5)/$\frac{1}{4}$NS + 20 mEq KCl/L to run at 42 mL/hr.

It should be noted that much has been published regarding use of the Holliday-Segar formula for calculating maintenance fluids. Several authors have suggested that administration of isotonic fluid may help prevent many cases of iatrogenic hyponatremia. This is based in part on the recognition of nonosmotic stimulation of ADH secretion, especially in hospitalized ill children. Many centers are now reserving the use of hypotonic solutions such as

D5/^{1}/$_{4}$NS for children in the first several months of life and have changed to using D5/^{1}/$_{2}$NS as routine maintenance fluid.[8,9]

Ongoing Losses

In addition to maintenance needs of water and electrolytes, ongoing losses are also important to take into account during hospitalization. Losses may result from conditions in which one is continuing to lose fluid (e.g., ongoing diarrhea) or from conditions associated with increased insensible losses (e.g., fever, which results in a 12% increase in maintenance fluid requirements for every 1° C increase over 38° C) or injury to the skin (e.g., burns). Ongoing gastrointestinal losses are another common problem (e.g., continuing diarrhea). Table 58-2 gives the typical electrolyte content of various body fluids to help estimate salt and water losses from various gastrointestinal sites.[10,11]

Dehydration

In treating patients with dehydration, it is important to determine both the quantity (mild, moderate, or severe) and quality (hypo-osmolar, iso-osmolar, or hyperosmolar) of the fluid deficit.

In calculating fluid deficits it is useful to calculate the water component separately from the sodium component and combine them to determine the final fluid concentra-

Table 58-1 Fluid Requirements Based on the Holliday-Segar Formula

Patient Weight	24-Hour Calculation	Hourly Calculation
3-10 kg	100 mL/kg	4 mL/kg
>10 but <20 kg	1000 mL + 50 mL/kg*	40 mL + 2 mL/kg
>20 kg	1500 mL + 20 mL/kg†	60 mL + 1 mL/kg

*This additional amount for the weight >10 kg only.
†This additional amount for the weight >20 kg only.

Table 58-2 Electrolyte Content of Various Fluids

Site	Na$^+$ (mEq/L)	K$^+$ (mEq/L)	Cl$^-$ (mEq/L)	HCO$_3^-$ (mEq/L)
Gastric	20-80	5-30	100-140	0
Small intestine	100-140	5-25	90-135	0
Ileostomy	45-135	3-15	20-115	110
Diarrhea	50-100	5-80	10-110	15-50

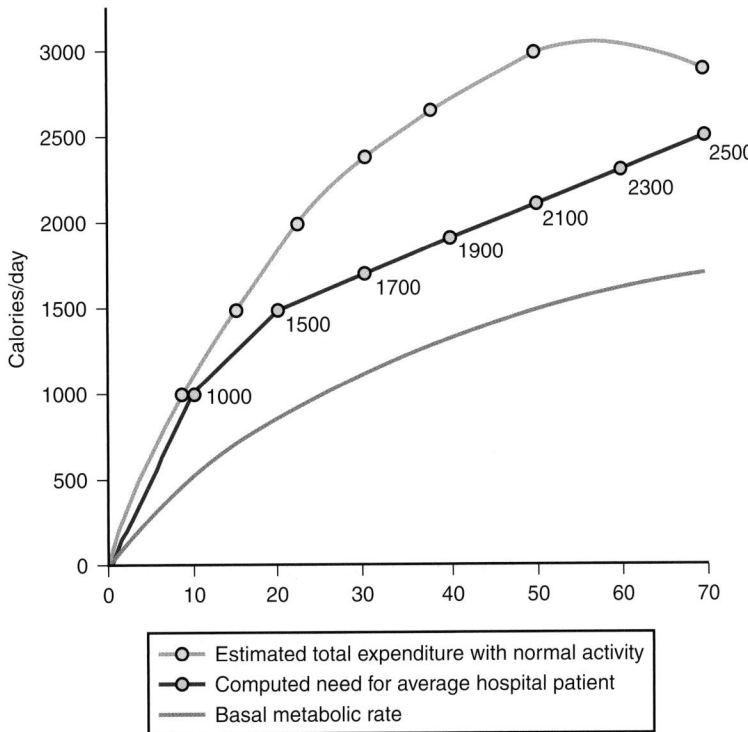

Figure 58-1   Comparison of energy expenditure and basal and ideal state. (From Holliday MA, Segar WE: The maintenance need for water in parenteral fluid therapy. Pediatrics 1957;19:823-832.)

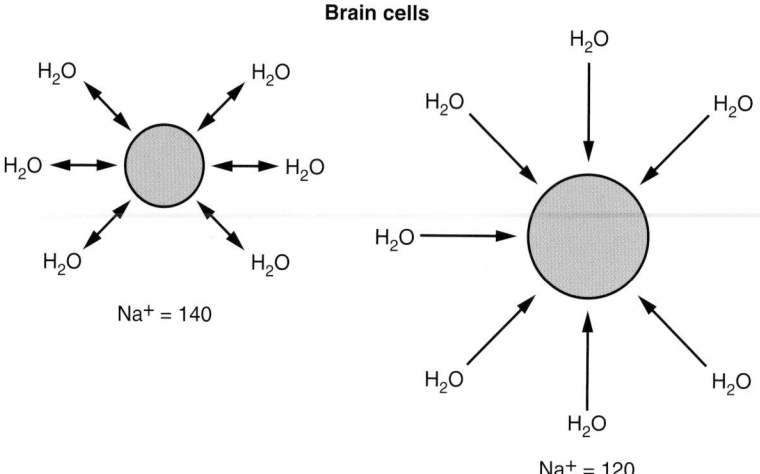

Tonicity:
Measure of the "effective osmols"
(impermeable) in a particular weight of
solvent

Brain cells

$Na^+ = 140$

$Na^+ = 120$

H_2O moves across cell membrane
from "low" tonicity to "high" tonicity

Figure 58-2   Changes in osmolarity can result in cerebral edema.

tion. To determine the rate of fluid administration after the initial bolus, the maintenance and deficit fluid volumes are combined and given at a fixed rate over the first 24 to 48 hours.[12]

Example: Isonatremic Dehydration

See Table 58-3.

OSMOLAR DISTURBANCES

Osmolality is a measure of all solute particles per weight of solvent and can be estimated according to the following formula:

$$2(Na^+) + (Blood\ urea\ nitrogen/2.8) + (Glucose/18)$$

Normal osmolality is 280 to 295 mOsm/kg. Generally, patients who are hypernatremic (Na^+ >150 mEq/L) will be hyperosmolar. Conversely, hyponatremic (Na^+ <130 mEq/L) patients will be hypo-osmolar. Water will shift from a low-osmolar space to a higher-osmolar space. This is important because rapid shifts in osmolality caused by correcting sodium disturbances too quickly (>0.5 mEq/hr) can cause fluid shifts within the brain that lead to brain injury (Fig. 58-2).

Hyponatremia

Clinical Presentation

Brain edema caused by fluid shifts with hypo-osmolarity is manifested as nausea, vomiting, muscular weakness, headaches, lethargy, ataxia, and psychosis in patients with moderate hyponatremia. Severe hyponatremia leads to increased intracranial pressure with seizures, coma, tentorial herniation, respiratory depression, and death. Certain disease states and pathogens, including pyloric stenosis and gastrointestinal pathogens such as rotavirus and cholera, are more likely to produce hyponatremic dehydration. Too rapid a correction of hyponatremic dehydration (>0.5 to 1 mEq/L/hr) may lead to central pontine myelinolysis characterized by a persistent "locked in" neurologic state.

Hyponatremia is usually caused by sodium loss in excess of free water loss. It is important to note that the serum sodium concentration does not accurately reflect total body sodium; rather, hyponatremia reflects a relative excess of free water. Although the cause of the hyponatremia is often obvious, it can be more of a diagnostic dilemma than is the case with hypernatremia. To determine the cause and treatment of hyponatremia, three factors are most important: the patient's volume status and urine sodium and osmolality.

Before beginning therapy it is important to determine whether "true" or hypo-osmotic hyponatremia is present. "Pseudohyponatremia" exists when serum is either isotonic, as in severe hyperlipidemia or hyperproteinemia, or hypertonic, as in hyperglycemia. In isotonic pseudohyponatremia caused by hyperlipidemia or hyperproteinemia, the volume of lipid or protein displaces plasma water so that a smaller volume of sodium-containing plasma is measured. In the past, chemistry laboratories used indirect potentiometry, in which the total volume of the specimen is used in calculating the sodium concentration, not just the aqueous sodium-containing portion. Now, virtually all laboratories measure sodium with ion-selective electrodes, and as a result, this error no longer occurs. In hypertonic or "dilutional" hyponatremia, hyperglycemia causes intracellular fluid to shift into the vascular space such that a decrease in serum Na^+ of 1.6 mEq/L occurs for every 100-mg/dL elevation in serum glucose (e.g., a serum glucose concentration of 800 results in a sodium concentration of 124; 800 − 100 = 700, 1.6 × 7 = 11, 135 − 11 = 124).[13]

Table 58-3 **Example: Isonatremic Dehydration**

A 7-year-old boy is admitted with a 2-day history of vomiting and diarrhea. He is estimated to be 7% dehydrated and vomited all attempts at oral rehydration in the emergency department. He was given a 20 mL/kg bolus of IV normal saline prior to transfer to the inpatient unit. His weight is 23 kg and his serum sodium level is 139 mEq/L.

	Water		Sodium	
	Calculation	Result	Calculation	Result
Maintenance 1st 10 kg = 100 mL/kg 2nd 10 kg = 50 mL/kg >20 kg = 20 mL/kg	10 kg × 100 mL/kg = 1000 mL 10 kg × 50 mL/kg = 500 mL 3 kg × 20 mL/kg = 30 mL	1560 mL	1560 mL × 3 mEq/100 mL	47 mEq
Total Fluid Deficit = weight × % dehydration × 1000 mL/kg or = (normal wt − dehydrated wt) × 1000 mL/kg	23 kg × 0.07 × 1000 mL/kg	1610 mL	—	—
ECF Na⁺ Deficit = 0.6 × total fluid deficit × 140 mEq/L	—	—	1.61 L × 0.6 × 140 mEq/L	135 mEq
Correction for Sodium Derangement No sodium derangement	—	—	—	—
Total Requirements	—	3170 mL	—	182 mEq
Previous Replacement	23 kg × 20 mL/kg	−460 mL	0.46 L × 154 mEq/L	−71 mEq
Balance of Requirements	3170 mL − 460 mL	2710 mL	182 mEq − 71 mEq	111 mEq
Concentration of Saline Solution	111 mEq ÷ 2.71 L	41 mEq/L		

Note: numbers that are highlighted in blue are specific for the patient data provided in the example.

Maintenance:
This boy's maintenance water needs for the first 24 hours are 100 mL/kg for his first 10 kg of body weight (1000 mL) plus 50 mL/kg for the second 10 kg of body weight (500 mL) plus 20 mL/kg for the last 3 kg of body weight, which yields a total of 1560 mL. Only a current weight is available for this child but provides a sufficiently close approximation of his normal body weight to be used in these calculations. His daily maintenance sodium needs are 3 mEq for each 100 mL of water, or 47 mEq.

Total Fluid Deficit:
This child's weight loss is used to approximate his total fluid loss. Since he is estimated to be 7% dehydrated, the weight loss can be calculated by multiplying his body weight by the estimated percent of dehydration (23 kg × 0.07). Since each kilogram of weight loss is equivalent to 1000 mL, the total fluid loss would be 1610 mL.

ECF Sodium Deficit:
The sodium content of this total fluid deficit is based on the proportion of the fluid that is made up by the extracellular fluid (ECF), which is 60% of the total. The sodium concentration is normally 140 mEq/L; therefore the sodium content in the total fluid deficit is found by multiplying this concentration by the volume of ECF deficit (1.61 L × 0.6), which yields 135 mEq.

Correction for Sodium Derangement:
Since this child is isonatremic, no additional water or sodium deficits beyond that already approximated above are expected.

Total Requirements:
The total water requirements are equal to the sum of the maintenance (1560 mL) and volume of the total fluid deficit (1610 mL), which is 3170 mL. The total sodium requirements are the maintenance sodium needs (47 mEq) plus the amount of sodium in the ECF deficit volume (135 mEq), which is 182 mEq.

Previous Replacement/Balance of Requirements:
This boy received a bolus of 20 mL/kg of normal saline, which provided some portion of his total water and sodium needs. The total volume of water in this saline bolus is equal to the total volume (23 kg × 20 mL/kg = 460 mL = 0.46 L). Since the concentration of normal saline solution is 154 mEq/L, the amount of sodium in that volume is 71 mEq (= 0.46 L × 154 mEq/L). These amounts of water and sodium are subtracted from the total requirements, which leaves the balances of 2710 mL of water and 111 mEq of sodium.

Concentration of Saline Solution:
An appropriate concentration of intravenous saline would be 111 mEq of sodium in 2710 mL (2.71 L) of water, or 41 mEq/L. Since normal saline is 154 mEq/L, this would be proportional to approximately ¼ normal saline solution (41 mEq/L ÷ 154 mEq/L = 0.27 ≈ ¼).

The potassium needs are estimated by multiplying the daily maintenance potassium needs (2 mEq/100 mL) by the maintenance daily fluid requirements (1560 mL), which would be 31 mEq. This amount should be added to the balance of fluids that he will receive in the first day (2710 mL, or 2.71 L), which is equivalent to 11 mEq/L (31 mEq ÷ 2.71 L). A standard or "stock" solution that contains 10 or 20 mEq/L KCl can be used. Potassium should not be added routinely to an intravenous solution if renal failure is suspected.

To provide some caloric support and to deliver a more isotonic fluid through the vein, the saline is provided in a 5% dextrose solution. The hourly rate at which the fluids should be delivered is calculated by dividing the balance of the fluids needed in the first day (2710 mL) by 24 hours, or 113 mL/hour for the first 24 hours.

Answer: D5/¼ NS + 20 mEq/L KCl at 113 mL/hour (or D5/¼ NS + 10 mEq/L KCl at 113 mL/hour).

CLASSIFICATION, DIAGNOSIS AND TREATMENT

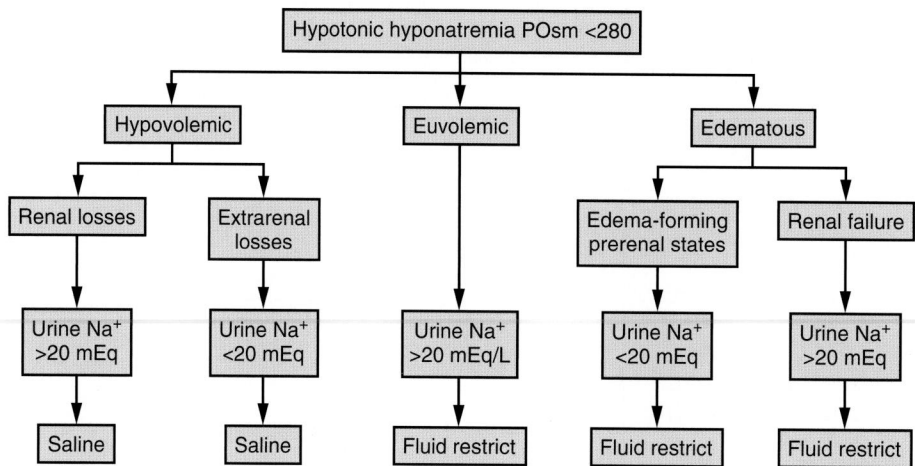

Figure 58-3   Diagnostic algorithm for hyponatremia. (From Berl T, Anderson RJ, McDonald KM, et al: Clinical disorders of water metabolism. Kidney Int 1976;10:117.)

True hyponatremia (Na^+ <130 mEq/L) occurs when serum is hypotonic. True hyponatremia may be associated with changes in total body water and categorized as hypovolemic, euvolemic, or edematous. A treatment algorithm for hyponatremia is presented in Figure 58-3.

Hyponatremic hypovolemia or dehydration occurs when there is a decrease in total body water, as well as sodium. Urine osmolality is greater than 100 mOsm/kg. If urine Na^+ is less than 20 mEq/L, hyponatremia is due to extrarenal losses such as vomiting and diarrhea. If urine Na^+ is greater than 20 mEq/L, renal losses are occurring as a result of diuretics, mineralocorticoid deficiency, salt-losing nephropathy, bicarbonaturia, ketonuria, or osmotic diuresis.

Treatment

In hyponatremic dehydration, aside from the sodium and water deficit that would be expected with isonatremic dehydration, an additional amount of sodium must be given to correct the sodium deficit. The following formula is used to calculate the additional sodium deficit that occurs:

$$0.6 \times Wt \times (Desired\ Na^+ - Current\ Na^+)$$

The "desired" sodium should be 12 to 14 mEq/L above the current sodium level so that a rapid shift in fluid does not ensue. Electrolytes should be monitored closely until serum sodium is in the 130-mEq/L range.

Example: Hypovolemic Hyponatremia

A 6-month-old girl presents with a 4-day history of vomiting and diarrhea. Her parents have been giving her apple juice for fluid replacement. Her weight is 8 kg, and she weighed 9 kg at her well-child visit 5 days ago.

Physical Examination

The girl's temperature is 36.7° C with a heart rate of 145, respiratory rate of 40, blood pressure of 78/44, and weight of 8.0 kg. She is difficult to arouse and has sunken eyes and dry, tacky mucous membranes. Her serum sodium is 122 mEq/L. The patient received 20 mL/kg of NS. What fluid order would you write? See Table 58-4 for an example calculation.

Hyponatremia with Edema

Edema exists when renal mechanisms inappropriately conserve excessive sodium and water. Urine osmolality is greater than 100 mOsm/kg. This may be due to acute or chronic renal failure with urine Na^+ greater than 20 mEq/L or due to decreased effective circulating blood volume because of decreased cardiac output (congestive heart failure) or decreased oncotic pressure (cirrhosis or nephrotic syndrome). In addition to treating the underlying disorder, hyponatremia is treated by sodium and fluid restriction and use of a loop diuretic and potentially an angiotensin-converting enzyme inhibitor.[14]

Hyponatremia with Euvolemia

Hyponatremia associated with euvolemia is most commonly seen in the syndrome of inappropriate antidiuretic hormone (SIADH) secretion, which may be due to glucocorticoid deficiency, hypothyroidism, stress (especially pain in the postoperative period), drugs (including selective serotonin reuptake inhibitors, antineoplastic agents, and anticonvulsants), or positive-pressure ventilation. Urine osmolality is greater than 100 mOsm/kg and urine Na^+ is greater than 20 mEq/L. Euvolemic hyponatremia with urine osmolality less than 100 mOsm/kg is due to water intoxication. Treatment should be focused on the underlying disease. Fluid restriction and administration of NS and a loop diuretic may be indicated.[15]

Emergency Treatment of Hyponatremia

Patients with significant hyponatremia can present with generalized seizure activity. If a patient's seizure activity is due to hyponatremia, raising Na^+ by 5 mEq/L or increasing the serum sodium level above 125 mEq/L will typically stop the seizure activity. Note that this rate of rapid correction of

Table 58-4 Example: Hypovolemic Hyponatremia

	Water		Sodium	
	Calculation	Result	Calculation	Result
Maintenance 1st 10 kg = 100 mL/kg 2nd 10 kg = 50 mL/kg >20 kg = 20 mL/kg	9 kg × 100 mL/kg	900 mL	900 mL × 3 mEq/100 mL	27 mEq
Total Fluid Deficit = weight × % dehydration × 1000 mL/kg or = (normal wt − dehydrated wt) × 1000 mL/kg	(9 kg − 8 kg) × 1000 mL/kg	1000 mL	—	—
ECF Na⁺ Deficit = 0.6 × total fluid deficit × 140 mEq/L	—	—	1 L × 0.6 × 140 mEq/L	84 mEq
Correction for Sodium Derangement Sodium Deficit: = (desired Na⁺ − current Na⁺) × wt × 0.6	—	—	(134 − 122) × 9 kg × 0.6	65 mEq
Total Requirements	—	1900 mL	—	176 mEq
Previous Replacement	9 kg × 20 mL/kg	−180 mL	0.18 L × 154 mEq/L	−28 mEq
Balance of Requirements	1900 mL − 180 mL	1720 mL	183 mEq − 28 mEq	148 mEq
Concentration of Saline Solution	148 mEq ÷ 1.72 L	86 mEq/L		

Note: numbers that are highlighted in blue are specific for the patient data provided in the example.

Maintenance:
This child's maintenance water needs for the first 24 hours are 100 mL/kg for each of her 9 kg of body weight, or 900 mL. Her maintenance sodium needs for this time period are 3 mEq for each 100 mL of water, or 27 mEq.

Total Fluid Deficit:
Her total fluid deficit is calculated by the difference between her pre-illness weight (9 kg) and her weight at the time she presented with dehydration (8 kg), which is 1 kg. This indicates that she is 11% dehydrated, i.e., 1 kg is 11% of her pre-illness weight (9 kg). If a pre-illness weight were not available, estimates of degree of dehydration would be made based on physical findings (see Chapter 57). Since each 1000 mL weighs 1 kg, her total fluid deficit is 1000 mL.

ECF Sodium Deficit:
The sodium content of this total fluid deficit is based on the proportion made up by her extracellular fluid (ECF) compartment, which is 60% of the total fluid deficit. The sodium concentration in the ECF is normally 140 mEq/L; therefore this little girl's estimated sodium deficit is the product of her ECF deficit (expressed in liters) and the normal sodium concentration, or 84 mEq.

Correction for Sodium Derangement:
However, this child is hyponatremic; therefore she has an additional sodium deficit, beyond that already approximated above. The additional sodium deficit is estimated by the difference between her current serum sodium level and her desired serum sodium level for her whole body ECF compartment. The whole body ECF volume is 60% of the total body weight. Rather than target a complete correction of her serum sodium level, a desired sodium level 12 mEq/L higher than her current level, or 134 mEq/L, is used. Therefore, the sodium deficit is calculated by multiplying her ECF volume (body weight × 0.6) by the difference between her desired and current serum sodium level. For this example the sodium deficit would be 65 mEq.

Total Requirements:
The maintenance water (900 mL) and total fluid deficit (1000 mL) are added to determine the total water requirements for the first 24 hours (1900 mL). The total sodium requirements are the sum of the maintenance sodium needs (27 mEq), the amount of sodium in the ECF deficit (84 mEq), and the additional sodium deficit due to her hyponatremia (65 mEq), which is 176 mEq.

Previous Replacement/Balance of Requirements:
However, her initial resuscitation included 20 mL/kg of normal saline. This provided her with 180 mL of water and 28 mEq of sodium, which are subtracted from the total needs. This leaves the balances of water and sodium needed in the first 24 hours of 1720 mL and 148 mEq, respectively.

Concentration of Saline Solution:
If a saline solution containing the proportions of salt and water from the balance of requirements were prepared, it would yield a saline concentration of 79 mEq/L. Since normal saline is 154 mEq/L, this would be approximately equivalent to a ½ normal saline solution.

The potassium needs are approximated by multiplying the daily maintenance potassium needs (2 mEq/100 mL each day) by the maintenance fluid requirements (900 mL), which yields 18 mEq/day. This amount should be added to the balance of fluids that she will receive in the first 24 hours (1720 mL, or 1.72 L), which is equivalent to 10 mEq/L (18 mEq ÷ 1.72 L = 10 mEq/L). Potassium should not be added routinely to intravenous solutions if renal failure is suspected.

To provide some caloric support and to deliver a more isotonic fluid through the vein, the saline is provided in a 5% dextrose solution. The total volume should be delivered over 24 hours, so one would divide 1720 mL by 24 hours to provide a rate of 72 mL/hour.

Answer: D5/½ NS + 10 mEq/L KCl to run at 72 mL/hour.

For patients with hyponatremia secondary to excessive renal sodium loss, the underlying disorder should be corrected if possible. Mineralocorticoid supplementation should be given for deficient states such as congenital adrenal hyperplasia. Long-term oral sodium supplementation is often needed if the underlying defects cannot be completely corrected.

sodium is reserved only for patients presenting with seizure activity.[16] Usually, giving 1 mL/kg of hypertonic (3%) saline will raise serum Na^+ by approximately 1 mEq/L. Generally, 2 to 6 mL/kg of 3% saline administered IV over an hour is used to treat seizure due to hyponatremia.

Hypernatremia

Clinical Presentation

Patients with hypernatremia present with hyperpnea, muscle weakness, restlessness, a high-pitched cry, lethargy, coma, and convulsions. Hypernatremia equates with hyperosmolality and leads to cellular dehydration, and with resultant areas of ischemia secondary to blood vessel sludging or bleeding from tension on bridging vessels. Diabetes insipidus can also result in hyperosmolar dehydration if the patient is unable to drink enough to compensate for deficient levels of ADH. Breastfeeding failure, especially in older first-time mothers, has been associated with hypernatremic dehydration in the newborn. Severe hypernatremic dehydration is sometimes also associated with hyperglycemia and hypocalcemia. Too rapid a correction of hypernatremic dehydration may result in cerebral edema and brainstem herniation.

The goal in treatment is to avoid cerebral edema by decreasing serum sodium slowly, by 1 mEq/L/hr with acute hypernatremia or by 0.5 mEq/L/hr with chronic hypernatremia. Figure 58-4 presents a treatment algorithm for hypernatremia.[17-21]

Hypernatremia secondary to sodium and water loss results in hypertonic dehydration. In hypernatremic dehydration the skin may feel "doughy." In addition, in contrast to patients with hyponatremic dehydration, patients with hypernatremic dehydration have less prominent signs and symptoms of dehydration because circulating blood volume is preserved. Renal losses from osmotic diuresis, as in diabetes mellitus (mannitol, glucose, or urea), result in urine Na^+ less than 20 mEq/L. Extrarenal losses caused by vomiting and diarrhea, excessive sweating, or breastfeeding failure result in urine Na^+ less than 20 mEq/L.

Treatment

In hypernatremic dehydration, there is a loss of water and sodium as with isonatremic dehydration but there are additional free water losses. Maintenance and deficit needs are calculated as for isonatremic dehydration. The additional free water deficit is determined next, and is calculated as

$$(Current~Na^+ - Desired~Na^+) \times 4~mL/kg \times Patient~weight$$

In this formula, the desired sodium is generally 145 mEq/L to prevent overly rapid correction. The patient weight in the formula should be expressed in kilograms.

Generally, half the free water deficit, along with all of the maintenance and solute deficit, is administered in the first 24 hours.

When treating hypernatremic dehydration, one must take care not to correct the sodium by hydrating too quickly. Treat shock with 0.9% saline (20 mL/kg) administered over a 30-minute period, but do not give a bolus unless necessary. Although the formula for calculating the free water deficit is a good general staring point, the rate of decrease in serum sodium is not as predictable as the rate of rise is for hyponatremic dehydration. No formula can replace frequent reassessment of the patent's sodium level and mental status. It is important to check electrolytes frequently to be sure that the sodium level does not drop too quickly, that is, a rate of decrease no greater than 0.5 mEq/L per hour.

HYPERNATREMIA: DIAGNOSTIC AND THERAPEUTIC APPROACH

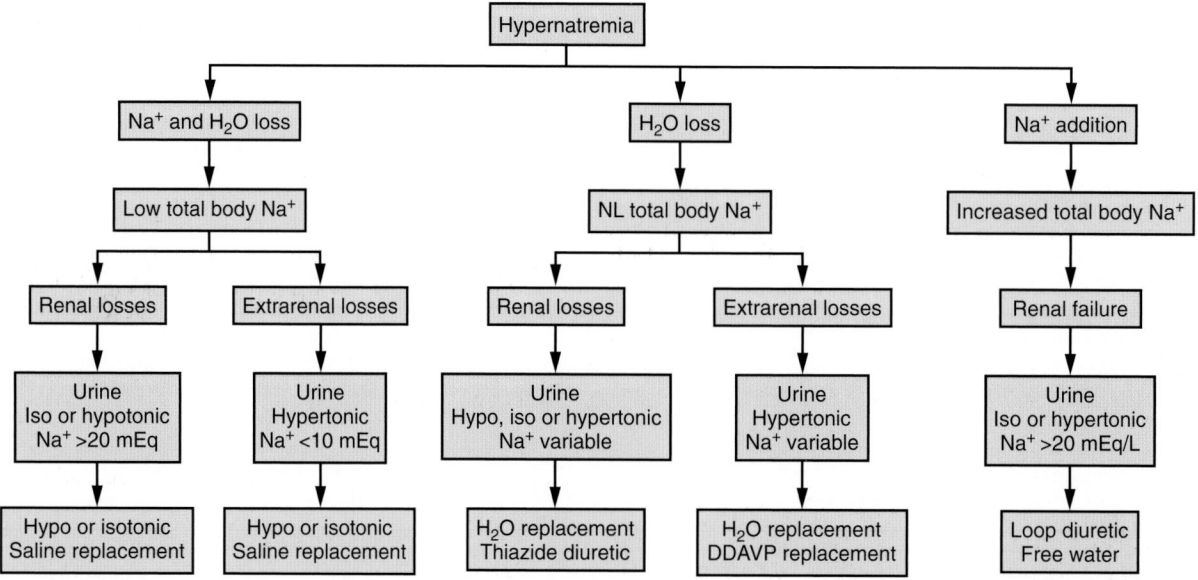

Figure 58–4 Diagnostic algorithm for hypernatremia. (From Berl T, Anderson RJ, McDonald KM, et al: Clinical disorders of water metabolism. Kidney Int 1976;10:117.)

The duration of correction is based on serum Na^+:

150 to 170 mEq/L: correct over a 48-hour period.
Greater than 170 mEq/L: correct over a 72-hour period.
Greater than 200 mEq/L: consider dialysis.

Patients with a serum sodium concentration higher than 170 should be managed in an intensive care unit (ICU) setting for close monitoring of electrolytes and cardiovascular and neurologic status.

Example: Hypernatremic Dehydration

A 5-month-old infant presents with vomiting and diarrhea. He weighed 7 kg at his last checkup 1 week ago. His current weight is 6.2 kg. The infant has a sunken fontanelle, decreased urine output, no tears, and dry lips, but his capillary refill time is well maintained and his skin feels "doughy." His serum Na^+ concentration is 155 mEq/L. What would your initial fluid order be? See Table 58-5.

Diabetes Insipidus

Hypernatremia secondary to water loss with normal total body sodium is due to inadequate secretion of ADH by the posterior pituitary gland (central diabetes insipidus) or inappropriate response by the renal collecting tubule to reabsorb water (nephrogenic diabetes insipidus). Central diabetes insipidus occurs more commonly and is often due to injury or destruction of the hypothalamus or posterior pituitary from meningitis or tumor (craniopharyngioma, histiocytosis X) and less commonly due to autosomal dominant or recessive defects in ADH synthesis and release. Nephrogenic diabetes insipidus may be due to an autosomal or sex-linked recessive defect in the membrane receptor protein. It may also be acquired as a result of an illness or insult that damages the renal medulla, such as from medication, obstructive uropathy, or electrolyte disturbances, including hypokalemia and hypercalcemia. Infants with nephrogenic diabetes insipidus may be febrile in association with hypernatremic dehydration.

The diagnosis is made by finding an inappropriately low urine osmolality (specific gravity <1.005, urine osmolarity of 50 to 200) with a low serum ADH level in the face of increased serum osmolality after a period of water deprivation.

Primary treatment is to administer free water. Inadequate endogenous ADH may be treated by replacement with desmopressin (DDAVP), a synthetic analogue. DDAVP is given as a nasal spray (3 months to 12 years of age, 5 to 30 μg/24 hr divided daily or twice daily with a maximum of 40 μg in 24 hours), orally (begin with 0.05 mg per dose daily or twice daily and titrate to achieve control of excessive thirst and urination), or intravenously/subcutaneously (children ≥ 12 years and adults, 2 to 4 μg/24 hr divided twice daily) as replacement therapy for central diabetes insipidus. Patients with nephrogenic diabetes insipidus may benefit from the addition of a thiazide diuretic. Hydrochlorothiazide dosing for neonates and infants younger than 6 months is 2 to 4 mg/kg/day in 2 divided doses (maximum daily dosage: 37.5 mg) and for older infants and children dosing is 2 mg/kg/day in 2 divided doses (maximum daily dosage: 200 mg).[22-26]

Hypernatremia with edema means that there is increased total body sodium and an increase in total body water. Urine Na^+ is greater than 20 mEq/L. The cause is usually iatrogenic and due to excessive administration of hypertonic dialysis fluid, $NaHCO_3$ or NaCl, or saline for therapeutic abortion. Primary hyperaldosteronism and Cushing syndrome are rare causes of edema and hypernatremia in childhood. Treatment is a loop diuretic along with administration of free water.

Potassium

Ninety-five percent of total body potassium is intracellular, mostly in muscle cells in a concentration of 150 mEq/L. Most (90%) potassium is excreted in urine under normal conditions. Renal excretion of potassium is very efficient, but unlike sodium, conservation is not efficient and occurs only in states of extreme deprivation. Aldosterone plays a critical role in potassium secretion in the distal tubule in exchange for sodium or hydrogen ions, or both. Delivery of sodium to the distal tubule for reabsorption is necessary for normal potassium excretion.

Most conditions resulting in dehydration cause depletion of total body potassium and sodium. Because potassium is an intracellular cation, serum potassium represents only 2% of total body potassium. Good general rules regarding potassium therapy are never to institute K^+ repletion until the patient has established urine output and not to exceed 4 mEq/kg/day of K^+ repletion. The potassium requirement for maintenance fluid in a patient with normal body potassium is approximately 2 mEq/100 kcal or per 100 mL of fluid. In practice, giving a patient 10 to 20 mEq/L of fluid provides adequate maintenance potassium.

Hyperkalemia
Clinical Presentation

True hyperkalemia is defined as serum K^+ greater than 5.5 mEq/L. Moderate to severe hyperkalemia (K^+ >6.1 to 6.9 mEq/L) is potentially life threatening because high serum potassium disrupts the normal electrical conduction system. Within the muscular system hyperkalemia causes skeletal muscle weakness and fatigue, whereas smooth muscle inhibition can cause respiratory depression. Most seriously, disruption of the cardiac conduction system, manifested as electrocardiographic changes such as prolongation of the PR interval, widening of the QRS complex, and peaked T waves, can lead to cardiac arrhythmias and ultimately to cardiac arrest.

Differential Diagnosis of Hyperkalemia

"Pseudohyperkalemia" is very common and usually due to inappropriate specimen collection, such as squeezing a digit too strenuously when obtaining a finger-stick blood draw, which causes the blood collected to be hemolyzed and release of potassium from red blood cells.

Severe leukocytosis greater than 70,000/cm³ or thrombocytosis greater than 1,000,000/cm³ can also result in pseudohyperkalemia.

True Hyperkalemia

True hyperkalemia most commonly results from a decrease in potassium excretion in the kidney or redistribution of potassium from the intracellular to the extracellular space (Table 58-6). A decrease in renal potassium excretion can occur in either acute or chronic renal failure, as a result

Table 58–5   Example: Hypernatremic Dehydration

	Water		Sodium	
	Calculation	Result	Calculation	Result
Maintenance 1st 10 kg = 100 mL/kg 2nd 10 kg = 50 mL/kg >20 kg = 20 mL/kg	7 kg × 100 mL/kg	700 mL	700 mL × 3 mEq/100 mL	21 mEq
Total Fluid Deficit = weight × % dehydration × 1000 mL/kg or = (normal wt − dehydrated wt) × 1000 mL/kg	(7 kg − 6.2 kg) × 1000 mL/kg	800 mL	—	—
ECF Na⁺ Deficit = total fluid deficit × 0.6 × 140 mEq/L		—	0.8 L × 0.6 × 140 mEq/L	67 mEq
Correction for Sodium Derangement $\frac{1}{2}$ free water deficit = (current Na⁺ − desired Na⁺) × wt × 4 mL/kg ÷ 2	(155 − 145) × 7 kg × 4 mL/kg ÷ 2	140 mL	—	—
Total Requirements		1640 mL		88 mEq
Previous Replacement		0		0
Balance of Requirements		1640 mL		88 mEq
Concentration of Saline Solution	88 mEq ÷ 1640 L	54 mEq/L		

Note: numbers that are highlighted in blue are specific for the patient data provided in the example.

Maintenance:
For this 7-kg boy, his maintenance water needs are 10 mL/kg for each of his 7 kg of body weight, or 700 mL each day. His maintenance sodium needs for this time period are 3 mEq for each 100 mL of water, or 27 mEq/day.

Total Fluid Deficit:
The difference between his pre-illness weight (7.0 kg) and his weight at the time of presentation (6.2 kg) indicates the total fluid deficit, which is 0.8 kg, or equivalent to 800 mL.

ECF Sodium Deficit:
Despite the fact that this child is hypernatremic, he still has a sodium deficit due to fluid losses from the ECF, which makes up 60% of the total fluid deficit. The sodium content of this total fluid deficit is calculated by multiplying the ECF proportion of the total fluid deficit (0.6 × 800 mL) by the sodium concentration of the ECF (approximately 140 mEq/L), which yields 67 mEq/L.

Correction for Sodium Derangement:
However, this boy's hypernatremia is caused by an additional loss of free water, which needs to be replaced. The amount of free water is calculated based on the difference between the current serum sodium level and the desired serum sodium (155 − 145), which is multiplied by a factor of 4 mL/kg and the patient's weight. Since corrections of hypernatremia should proceed more slowly, only half of the estimated free water deficit is replaced in the first 24 hours, which yields a result of 140 mL.

Total Requirements:
The water and sodium requirements are totaled, which indicated that this patient should receive 1640 mL of water and 88 mEq of sodium in the first 24 hours.

Previous Replacement/Balance of Requirements:
In this example, the patient did not receive a normal saline bolus or any other replacement therapy, so the balance of water and sodium requirements are the same as for the total requirements.

Concentration of Saline Solution:
If the sodium requirements were mixed in the amount of water required, it would yield a saline solution containing 54 mEq/L, which is equivalent to $\frac{1}{3}$ normal saline solution. To avoid the risk of correcting the serum sodium level too quickly, i.e., more than 0.5 mEq/L per hour, most clinicians would select a stock solution of $\frac{1}{2}$ normal saline for this patient.

As previously calculated, the potassium needs are estimated by multiplying the daily maintenance potassium needs (2 mEq/100 mL each day) by the maintenance fluid requirements (700 mL), which yields 14 mEq/day. This amount should be added to the total fluids that this boy will receive in the first 24 hours (1640 mL), which is equivalent to 9 mEq/L (14 mEq ÷ 1640 mL = 8.5 mEq/L). A standard solution that contains 10 mEq/L of KCl can be used. Potassium should not be added routinely to intravenous solutions if renal failure is suspected.

To provide some caloric support and to deliver a more isotonic fluid through the vein, the saline solution is provided with 5% dextrose solution. The total volume should be delivered over 24 hours, so one would divide 1640 mL by 24 hours to provide a rate of 68 mL/hour.

Answer: D5/$\frac{1}{2}$ NS + 10 mEq/L KCl to run at 68 mL/hour.

Subsequent Therapy: The entire deficit of ECF, along with half of the additional free water deficit, is replaced during the first 24 hours. The remaining free water deficit is then replaced over the next 24 hours. For this period, the maintenance needs remain the same: 700 mL of water, 21 mEq of sodium, and 14 mEq of potassium per day. Adding the 140 mL of free water yields a total of 840 mL of water with 21 mEq of sodium, or 25 mEq/L, which is equivalent to $\frac{1}{6}$ normal saline with 17 mEq/L of potassium. A stock solution of D5$\frac{1}{4}$ normal saline with 10 or 20 mEq/L of KCl may be used at a rate of 35 mL/hr (840 mL ÷ 24 hours).

Table 58-6 Causes of Hyperkalemia

Decrease in K^+ Excretion
Acute or chronic kidney disease
Aldosterone deficiency: Addison's disease or congenital adrenal
    hyperplasia
Drugs
    Potassium-sparing agents
    Angiotensin-converting enzyme inhibitors
    Nonsteroidal anti-inflammatory drugs
    Miscellaneous (trimethoprim-sulfamethoxazole, heparin,
        pentamidine, alpha- and beta-blockers)

Increase in K^+ Load: Cellular Destruction
Ingestion of a K^+-rich diet
Tumor lysis syndrome
Rhabdomyolysis
Trauma
Intravascular hemolysis
Transfusion of stored red blood cells
Catabolic states

Redistribution of K^+
Metabolic acidosis
Infusion of hypertonic solution
Hyperkalemic periodic paralysis
Nonselective beta-blockers

Tubular Unresponsiveness to Aldosterone
Sickle cell anemia
Systemic lupus erythematosus
Amyloidosis
Renal transplantation

of tubular dysfunction, or because of impairment of aldosterone production by the adrenal gland, as in some forms of congenital adrenal hyperplasia (21-hydroxylase deficiency). Drugs that decrease glomerular filtration rates (such as angiotensin-converting enzyme inhibitors and nonsteroidal anti-inflammatory agents) or inhibit the action of aldosterone (potassium-sparing diuretics) can increase serum and total body potassium. Shifts in potassium from the intracellular to the extracellular space, as in metabolic acidosis or with nonselective beta-blockers, can lead to an increase in serum potassium, although total body potassium is normal. Extreme and rapid cellular destruction can overwhelm the kidney's ability to excrete the increased potassium load. This can occur as a result of tumor lysis, intravascular hemolysis such as with a transfusion reaction, rhabdomyolysis or tissue destruction secondary to a crush injury or burn, and extreme catabolic states. Tubular unresponsiveness to aldosterone is unusual but may occur as an isolated defect or in association with systemic lupus erythematosus, sickle cell disease, amyloidosis, and renal transplantation.

Treatment of Hyperkalemia

If the patient has none of the aforementioned causes of hyperkalemia and the serum potassium level is reported as high, it is often prudent to recheck the potassium from a venous, easy-flowing blood draw and minimize the use of a tourniquet to avoid pseudohyperkalemia from a hemolyzed blood specimen. In metabolic acidosis from bicarbonate losses in diarrhea or from diabetic ketoacidosis, buffering occurs at the cellular level as potassium shifts from the intracellular to the extracellular space while hydrogen ion shifts to the intracellular space. Correction of the acidosis will usually correct the hyperkalemia.

If true hyperkalemia exists, check an electrocardiogram for prolongation of the PR or QRS intervals and for peaked T waves. If any of these changes exist, urgent action must be taken to lower the potassium level before a life-threatening arrhythmia develops. The patient should be placed on a cardiorespiratory monitor and transferred to an ICU setting. Immediately discontinue any potassium intake.

To block the effects of hyperkalemia on the cardiac conduction system, the following infusion is administered:

- 10% calcium gluconate, 0.5 to 1 mL/kg intravenously (50 to 100 mg/kg per dose) peripherally, or 27% calcium chloride, 0.2 mL/kg (20 mg/kg per dose) through a central venous line, not to exceed 100 mg/min.

Potassium can be shifted from the extracellular to the intracellular space by

- Infusing $NaHCO_3$, 1 to 2 mEq/kg per dose intravenously; this works best in the presence of metabolic acidosis.
- Infusing dextrose, 0.5 to 1 g/kg (e.g., 2 to 4 mL/kg of 25% dextrose) with 0.1 U/kg of insulin.

Potassium can be removed from the body by

- Sodium polystyrene sulfonate (Kayexalate) with sorbitol (1 g/kg per dose) orally or per rectum.
- Diuresis if the patient has normal renal function by a combination of an NS bolus, 10 to 20 mL/kg per dose, and furosemide, 0.5 to 1 mg/kg per dose intravenously.
- Hemodialysis or peritoneal dialysis, which can also be used in patients with renal failure or severe poisoning.[27-29]

Hypokalemia

Hypokalemia is defined as a serum potassium concentration less than 3.5 mEq/L. Moderate to severe hypokalemia exists when serum K^+ is less than 2.5 to 3.0 mEq/L.

Clinical Presentation

The most common clinical signs and symptoms are caused by disordered electrical conduction in cardiac, skeletal, and smooth muscle that results in electrocardiographic changes such as the presence of U waves and arrhythmias, generalized muscle weakness, paralytic ileus, and impaired respiration. In addition, hypokalemia impairs the ability of the kidneys to reabsorb hydrogen ion, thereby promoting metabolic alkalosis and renal medullary dysfunction with an inability to dilute or concentrate the urine.

Causes of Hypokalemia

Causes of hypokalemia can be divided into increased potassium losses or shift of potassium into the intracellular space. Stool losses occur as a result of diarrhea or laxative abuse. Increases in renal potassium excretion can be seen with metabolic alkalosis, metabolic acidosis, or administration of drugs such as diuretics and high doses of penicillin. If the cause of the hypokalemia is not clear, a urine potassium level higher than 10 indicates excess urine loss. In the face of

Table 58-7   Causes of Hypokalemia

Increase in Renal K⁺ Excretion
Metabolic alkalosis
   Chloride responsive
      Volume contraction
   Chloride unresponsive
      Primary hyperaldosteronism
      Hypertension
         Liddle syndrome
         11β-Hydroxysteroid dehydrogenase deficiency
      No hypertension
         Bartter syndrome
         Gitelman syndrome
Metabolic acidosis
   Type I and II renal tubular acidosis
Drugs
   Diuretics
   Fluorinated steroids
   Penicillins

Transcellular K⁺ Shift
β-Adrenergic agonists
Insulin administration
Theophylline and caffeine
Verapamil and chloroquine ingestion
Hyperthyroidism
Familial hypokalemic paralysis

Excessive K⁺ Loss in Stool
Laxative abuse
Diarrheal illness

Miscellaneous
Mg^{2+} depletion

hypokalemia, a potassium bolus may be given intravenously during close cardiac monitoring (dose of 0.25 to 0.5 mEq/kg with a maximum dose of 40 mEq over a 2-hour period; the concentration should not exceed 0.1 mEq/mL in a peripheral line and 0.2 mEq/mL in a central line). In the non-ICU setting, KCl infusion should not exceed 0.25 mEq/kg/hour. Enteral replacement (oral or via nasogastric tube) can supplement repletion efforts or, in less severe setting, can be used instead. For hypokalemia in the face of metabolic acidosis, potassium may be given as phosphate or acetate, whereas with metabolic alkalosis it is given as KCl.[1,2,5-7]

CONSULTATION

Given the myriad of disease states that can lead to electrolyte disturbances, the hospitalist may consult any number of specialists, including renal, endocrine, and critical care colleagues, to assist in the management of these patients, especially if the electrolyte derangements are severe.

ADMISSION CRITERIA

- Any patient with a significant fluid or electrolyte disturbance should be admitted, especially if the cause of the abnormality is unclear.

DISCHARGE CRITERIA

- Correction of abnormal electrolyte status
- Presence of a treatment plan to maintain normal electrolyte status

IN A NUTSHELL

- An understanding of pediatric fluid and electrolyte therapy is one of the most important aspects of pediatric hospital medicine. In general, the approach to patients with various electrolyte disturbances is based on the underlying physiology of how the body handles water and the specific electrolyte itself. The further from normal at the time of presentation, the greater the care and need for monitoring during the correction process.

ON THE HORIZON

- As stated earlier, there is a growing literature suggesting that administration of isotonic fluid may help prevent many cases of iatrogenic hyponatremia and that many centers are reducing their use of hypotonic intravenous fluids.
- Recently, the Food and Drug Administration approved the first human recombinant hyaluronidase, which degrades hyaluronic acid into smaller tetrasaccharide blocks, thus opening up the interstitial space and allowing coinjected fluid or drugs, or both, to be more readily absorbed into the bloodstream. This may allow subcutaneous delivery of drugs and fluids and be a potential solution for patients with poor venous access.

volume contraction, as seen in chloride-responsive metabolic alkalosis, urine Cl⁻ is less than 25 mEq/L and the renin-angiotensin system is activated by the low circulating blood volume, which leads to increased aldosterone secretion to retain sodium and chloride and results in continued potassium excretion by the kidney. Chloride-unresponsive metabolic alkalosis (urine Cl⁻ >40 mEq/L) can occur with primary mineralocorticoid excess, either associated with hypertension (Liddle syndrome or 11β-hydroxysteroid dehydrogenase deficiency) or with renal tubular dysfunction and normal blood pressure as in Bartter or Gitelman syndrome. Renal tubular acidosis can also be associated with hypokalemia inasmuch as potassium is excreted with unabsorbed bicarbonate or instead of hydrogen ion in the distal tubule. Potassium is wasted with furosemide or thiazide diuretics.

Potassium can also shift into the intracellular space in association with diseases such as hyperthyroidism and familial hypokalemic paralysis, as well as a variety of drugs such as β-adrenergic agonists, insulin, theophylline, caffeine, verapamil, and chloroquine (Table 58-7).

Treatment of hypokalemia is potassium repletion. Up to 40 mEq of KCl/L intravenously can be safely given on the floor. If infusions of 40 to 80 mEq/L are needed, patients should be monitored in an ICU setting and a central line should be used for administration. For symptomatic/severe

SUGGESTED READING

Hoorn EJ, Geary D, Robb M, et al: Acute hyponatremia related to intravenous fluid administration in hospitalized children: An observational study. Pediatrics 2004;113:1279-1284.

Moritz ML, Ayus JC: Prevention of hospital-acquired hyponatremia: A case for using isotonic saline. Pediatrics 2003;111:227-230.

Roberts KB: Fluid and electrolytes: Parenteral fluid therapy. Pediatr Rev 2001;22:380-387.

Rose BD, Post TW: Clinical Physiology of Acid-Base and Electrolyte Disorders, 5th ed. New York, McGraw-Hill, 2001.

REFERENCES

1. Rose BD, Post TW: Clinical Physiology of Acid-Base and Electrolyte Disorders, 5th ed. New York, McGraw-Hill, 2001.
2. Finberg L, Kravath RE, Hellerstein S: Water and Electrolytes in Pediatrics, 2nd ed. Philadelphia, WB Saunders, 1993.
3. Holliday M: The evolution of therapy for dehydration: Should deficit therapy still be taught? Pediatrics 1996;98:171-177.
4. Winters RW: Principles of Pediatric Fluid Therapy. Chicago, Abbott Laboratories, 1982.
5. Feld LG, Kaskel FJ, Schoeneman MJ: The approach to fluid and electrolyte therapy in pediatrics. Adv Pediatr 1988;35:497-536.
6. Chesney RW, Batisky DL: Fluid and electrolyte therapy in infants and children. In Arieff AI, DeFronzo RA (eds): Fluid and Base Disorders, 2nd ed. New York, Churchill Livingstone, 1995, pp 877-904.
7. Roberts KB: Fluid and electrolytes: Parenteral fluid therapy. Pediatr Rev 2001;22:380-387.
8. Moritz ML, Ayus JC: Prevention of hospital-acquired hyponatremia: A case for using isotonic saline. Pediatrics 2003;111:227-230.
9. Hoorn EJ, Geary D, Robb M, et al: Acute hyponatremia related to intravenous fluid administration in hospitalized children: An observational study. Pediatrics 2004;113:1279-1284.
10. Welt LG: Clinical Disorders of Hydration and Acid-Base Equilibrium. Boston, Little, Brown, 1955.
11. Finberg L: Dehydration in infancy and childhood. Pediatr Rev 2002;23:277-282.
12. Steiner MJ, DeWalt DA, Byerley JS: Is this child dehydrated? JAMA 2004;291:2746-2754.
13. Moritz ML, Ayus JC: Disorders of water metabolism in children: Hyponatremia and hypernatremia. Pediatr Rev 2002;23:371-380.
14. Rose BD: Hypoosmolal states—hyponatremia. In Clinical Physiology of Acid-Base and Electrolyte Disorders, 4th ed. New York, McGraw-Hill, 1994, pp 651-694.
15. Keating JP, Schears GJ, Dodge PR: Oral water intoxication in infants: An American epidemic. Am J Dis Child 1997;145:985-990.
16. Sarnaik AP, Meert K, Hackbarth R, Fleischmann L: Management of hyponatremic seizures in children with hypertonic saline: A safe and effective strategy. Crit Care Med 1994;19:758-762.
17. Finberg L: Hypernatremic (hypertonic) dehydration in infants. N Engl J Med 1973;289:196-198.
18. Cooper WO, Atherton HD, Kahana M, et al: Increased incidence of severe breastfeeding malnutrition and hypernatremia in a metropolitan area. Pediatrics 1995;96:957-960.
19. Moritz ML, Ayus JC: The changing pattern of hypernatremia in hospitalized children. Pediatrics 1999;104:435-439.
20. Morris-Jones PH, Houston IB: Prognosis of the neurological complication of acute hypernatremia. Lancet 1967;2:1385-1389.
21. Rose BD: Hyperosmolal states—hypernatremia. In Clinical Physiology of Acid-Base and Electrolyte Disorders, 4th ed. New York, McGraw-Hill, 1994, pp 695-736.
22. Saborio P, Tipton GA, Chan JCM: Diabetes insipidus. Pediatr Rev 2000;21:122-129.
23. Alon U, Chan JCM: Hydrochlorothiazide-amiloride in the treatment of nephrogenic diabetes insipidus. Am J Nephrol 1985;5:9-13.
24. Leung AKC, Robson WLM, Halperin ML: Polyuria in childhood. Clin Pediatr (Phila) 1991;11:634-640.
25. Mulders SM, Bichet DG, Rijss JPL, et al: An aquaporin-2 water channel mutant which causes autosomal dominant nephrogenic diabetes insipidus is retained in the Golgi complex. J Clin Invest 1998;102:57-66.
26. Yamamoto T, Sasaki S: Aquaporins in the kidney: Emerging new aspects. Kidney Int 1998;54:1041-1051.
27. Fuhrman BP, Zimmerman JJ: Pediatric Critical Care, 2nd ed. St Louis, Mosby-Year Book, 1998, p 713.
28. Allon M, Dunlay R, Copney C: Nebulized albuterol for acute hyperkalemia in patients on hemodialysis. Ann Intern Med 1998;110:426-429.
29. Montoliu J, Lens XM, Rovert L: Potassium-lowering effect of albuterol of hyperkalemia in renal failure. Arch Intern Med 1985;147:713-717.

Infectious Diseases

CHAPTER 59

Empirical Treatment of Bacterial Infections

Talene A. Metjian and Samir S. Shah

A common challenge for clinicians caring for hospitalized patients is the initiation of antibiotic therapy. Many factors influence the choice of whether to start antibiotics, when to start, and which agent or agents to employ. Often the decision to initiate antibiotics, and to select appropriate antibiotic agents, happens before confirmation of the presence of a treatable infection and before its precise location, severity, and specific infectious cause are identified. Some of the factors to consider include the likelihood of a treatable infection actually being present, the risks of an untreated infection, the odds of predicting the correct pathogen involved, the chances of resolution without antibiotic therapy, and the need to identify the organism definitively. Other antibiotic-related factors include the toxicity of empirical treatment and the pharmacodynamic parameters of the antibiotic.

This chapter provides guidance for antibiotic selection according to common pediatric bacterial infections and bacteria targeted for treatment. The antibiotic susceptibilities of organisms vary by region, by hospital, and, in some cases, by units within a hospital. For proper treatment and appropriate use, the clinician must remain cognizant of these ever-changing antibiotic-susceptibility profiles by reviewing the current literature and antibiograms (local and hospital). If culture and sensitivity results become available, the medical professional should modify antibiotic coverage to the narrowest spectrum that effectively treats the pathogen of concern and adequately targets the site of infection.

Table 59–1 Empirical Treatment for Common Childhood Infections*

	ANTIBIOTIC	
Bacterial Infection	*First Choices*	*Others*
Adenitis	Clindamycin	Ampicillin-sulbactam or cephalexin, or oxacillin if low MRSA prevalence
Arthritis, septic		
Neonate	Clindamycin + gentamicin	Clindamycin + cefotaxime or vancomycin + cefotaxime
School age	Clindamycin	Vancomcyin
Adolescent	Clindamycin	Vancomycin (add ceftriaxone if gonococcus suspected)
Brain abscess	Vancomycin + metronidazole + either cefotaxime or ceftriaxone	Vancomycin + carbapenem
Cellulitis	Clindamycin	Cephalexin if low MRSA prevalence
Deep soft tissue abscess	Clindamycin	Trimethoprim-sulfamethoxazole
Facial/orbital cellulitis	Ampicillin-sulbactam	Cefotaxime or ceftriaxone (consider clindamycin or vancomycin if signs of external trauma)
Epiglottitis	Cefotaxime or ceftriaxone	Ampicillin-sulbactam
Intra-abdominal abscess	Ampicillin + gentamicin + metronidazole or cefoxitin	Ampicillin-sulbactam or ciprofloxacin[†] + metronidazole or pipercillin-tazobactam or ticarcillin-clavulanate or carbapenem

Continued

Table 59–1 Empirical Treatment for Common Childhood Infections*—cont'd

Bacterial Infection	ANTIBIOTIC	
	First Choices	*Others*[†]
Meningitis	Vancomycin + either cefotaxime or ceftriaxone	Vancomycin + levofloxacin[†] or vancomycin + carbapenem if cephalosporin allergy
Osteomyelitis, acute		
Neonate	Clindamycin + gentamicin	Vancomycin + gentamicin (may use cefotaxime instead of gentamicin)
Older child	Clindamycin	Vancomycin or linezolid
Osteomyelitis, puncture wound	Ticarcillin-clavulanic acid + gentamicin	Ceftazidime + gentamicin or ciprofloxacin[†] + gentamicin
Otitis media, acute	Amoxicillin[†]	Amoxicillin-clavulanate or ceftriaxone
Pelvic inflammatory disease	Doxycycline (PO or IV)[§] + cefoxitin	Clindamycin + gentamicin
Pharyngitis (group A streptococcus)	Penicillin V (PO), benzathine penicillin G (IM) (can combine with procaine penicillin 3:1 ratio)	Amoxicillin or cephalexin or clindamycin or azithromycin
Pneumonia		
Neonate	Ampicillin + gentamicin	Ampicillin + cefotaxime or consider azithromycin
Older child (mild/moderate)	Ampicillin or amoxicillin	Clindamycin or cefotaxime or ceftriaxone
Older child (severe)	Cefotaxime or ceftriaxone	Vancomycin (consider adding azithromcyin or levofloxacin)
Complicated (empyema or necrotizing)	Clindamycin + cefotaxime	Vancomycin + cefotaxime
Retropharyngeal/peritonsillar abscess	Ampicillin-sulbactam	Clindamycin + either cefotaxime or ceftriaxone, or cefoxitin or oxacillin + metronidazole
Sepsis (immunocompetent)	Vancomycin + either ceftriaxone or cefotaxime	Vancomycin + one of the following: ceftazidime, cefepime, ciprofloxacin,[†] or carbapenem
Sepsis (immunocompromised)	Vancomycin + one of the following: ceftazidime, cefepime, ciprofloxacin,[†] or carbapenem	Linezolid + one of the following: ceftazidime, cefepime, ciprofloxacin,[†] or carbapenem
Sinusitis (acute)	Amoxicillin[†]	Clindamycin or amoxicillin-clavulanic acid or levofloxacin[†]
Urinary tract infection		
Outpatient	Trimethoprim-sulfamethoxazole or cefixime or ceftibuten	Amoxicillin or cefprozil or cephalexin
Inpatient	Ampicillin + gentamicin	Cefotaxime or ceftriaxone or ciprofloxacin[†]

*Definitive therapy should be based on the availability of additional information, including culture results.

[†]Ciprofloxacin is approved for complicated urinary tract infections and pyelonephritis in children. Levofloxacin is approved only for patients >18 years of age; used off-label in children <18 years of age if no other alternatives are available.

[†]If no antibiotics were administered in the prior month, use regular-dose or high-dose amoxicillin (80 to 90 mg/kg divided every 12 hours). If antibiotics were given previously, use high-dose amoxicillin or amoxicillin-clavulanic acid (80 to 90 mg/kg amoxicillin component divided every 12 hours); if clavulanic acid component exceeds 10 mg/kg/day, use a preparation with a higher ratio of amoxicillin-to-clavulanic acid (e.g., 14:1 or higher ratio of amoxicillin-to-clavulanic acid).

[§]Avoid doxycycline use in children ≤8 years of age.

MRSA, methicillin-resistant *Staphylococcus aureus*.

Table 59-2 Empirical Treatment of Bacterial Infections by Common Organisms*

Organisms	First Choice	Others
Acinetobacter spp.	Cefepime ± aminoglycoside or carbapenem ± aminoglycoside	Trimethoprim-sulfamethoxazole or ciprofloxacin
Bacteroides fragilis group	Metronidazole	Clindamycin or ampicillin-sulbactam or cefoxitin
Bordetella pertussis	Erythromycin or azithromycin	Trimethoprim-sulfamethoxazole or clarithromycin
Burkholderia cepacia	Meropenem + infectious diseases consultation	Trimethoprim-sulfamethoxazole or ceftazidime or doxycycline or chloramphenicol
Campylobacter jejuni	Erythromycin or azithromycin	Ciprofloxacin or doxycycline[†]
Chlamydia trachomatis	Erythromycin	Azithromycin or doxycycline[†]
Citrobacter spp.	Cefepime ± aminoglycoside or carbapenem ± aminoglycoside	Trimethoprim-sulfamethoxazole or ciprofloxacin
Clostridium difficile	Metronidazole (PO)	Vancomycin (PO) or metronidazole (IV)
Enterobacter spp.	Cefepime ± aminoglycoside or carbapenem ± aminoglycoside	Trimethoprim-sulfamethoxazole or ciprofloxacin
Enterococcus faecalis	Ampicillin + gentamicin	Vancomycin or linezolid or quinupristin-dalfopristin
Enterococcus faecium	Vancomycin + gentamicin	Linezolid or quinupristin-dalfopristin
Escherichia coli	Cefotaxime or ceftriaxone	Aztreonam or carbapenem or trimethoprim-sulfamethoxazole or ciprofloxacin
Fusobacterium spp.	Penicillin	Clindamycin or metronidazole or ampicillin-sulbactam
Haemophilus influenzae	Cefotaxime or ceftriaxone	Amoxicillin-clavulanate
Klebsiella spp.	Cefotaxime or ceftriaxone	Trimethoprim-sulfamethoxazole or aztreonam
Listeria monocytogenes	Ampicillin ± gentamicin	Trimethoprim-sulfamethoxazole
Moraxella catarrhalis	Cefuroxime or amoxicillin-clavulanate	Ampicillin-sulbactam or trimethoprim-sulfamethoxazole
Mycoplasma pneumoniae	Azithromycin	Doxycycline[†] or erythromycin, clarithromycin, levofloxacin[†]
Neisseria gonorrhoeae	Ceftriaxone or cefotaxime	Ofloxacin[†] or ciprofloxacin (see pelvic inflammatory disease chapter); infectious diseases consultation if recent travel outside the United States
Neisseria meningitidis	Penicillin G	Cefotaxime or ceftriaxone
Pasteurella multocida	Penicillin or ampicillin or amoxicillin	Doxycycline[†] or 2nd- or 3rd-generation cephalosporins or amoxicillin-clavulanic acid
Proteus mirabilis	Ampicillin + gentamicin	Cefuroxime or trimethoprim-sulfamethoxazole
Providencia and *Morganella* spp.	Cefotaxime ± gentamicin	Ciprofloxacin or aztreonum
Pseudomonas aeruginosa	Ceftazidime + aminoglycoside or piperacillin + aminoglycoside	Ticarcillin-clavulanic acid + aminoglycoside or ciprofloxacin[†] + aminoglycoside or cefepime + aminoglycoside
Prevotella spp.	Clindamycin	Metronidazole or ampicillin-sulbactam or cefoxitin
Salmonella (systemic)	Cefotaxime or ceftriaxone	Trimethoprim-sulfamethoxazole or ampicillin or ciprofloxacin

Continued

Table 59-2   Empirical Treatment of Bacterial Infections by Common Organisms*—cont'd

Organisms	First Choice	Others
Serratia spp.	Cefepime ± aminoglycoside or carbapenem ± aminoglycoside	Trimethoprim-sulfamethoxazole or ciprofloxacin
Shigella, intestinal	Cefotaxime or ceftriaxone	Azithromycin or ampicillin or trimethoprim-sulfamethoxazole or ciprofloxacin
Staphylococcus aureus		
MSSA	Oxacillin	Cefazolin or nafcillin
MRSA, community acquired§	Clindamycin	Vancomycin or trimethoprim-sulfamethoxazole
MRSA, hospital acquired or serious infection	Vancomycin	Linezolid or quinupristin-dalfopristin
Staphylococcus epidermidis (and other coagulase-negative staphylococci in context of an indwelling device)	Vancomycin	Linezolid or may use oxacillin if isolate is susceptible
Streptococcus pneumoniae		
Meningitis or critically ill	Cefotaxime + vancomycin	Levofloxacin[†] + vancomycin or carbapenem + vancomycin
Pneumonia	Ampicillin or cefotaxime or ceftriaxone	Levofloxacin[†]
Streptococcus pyogenes (group A streptococcus)	Penicillin	Erythromycin[¶] or cefazolin or clindamycin
Streptococcus agalactiae (group B streptococcus)	Penicillin ± gentamicin	Cefotaxime or ceftriaxone or vancomycin[¶]
Treponema pallidum	Penicillin	Erythromycin[¶] or tetracycline[†] or ceftriaxone
Yersinia enterocolitica (invasive)	Trimethoprim-sulfamethoxazole	Cefotaxime or ciprofloxacin

*Empirical treatment should be guided by local and hospital sensitivity patterns. After sensitivities are known, use the effective antibiotic with the narrowest spectrum.
[†]Patient age, 8 years or older.
[‡]Levofloxacin is approved for patients >18 years of age; used off-label in children <18 years of age if no other alternatives are available.
[§]Clindamycin can be used if the test for inducible resistance ("D-test") is negative; otherwise, use vancomycin.
[¶]Penicillin-allergic patient.

SUGGESTED READING

American Academy of Pediatrics, Subcommittee on Management of Acute Otitis Media: Clinical Practice Guideline: Diagnosis and Management of Acute Otitis Media. Pediatrics 2004;113:1451-1465.

American Academy of Pediatrics, Subcommittee on Management of Sinusitis and Committee on Quality Improvement: Clinical Practice Guideline: Management of Sinusitis. Pediatrics 2001;108:798-808.

American Academy of Pediatrics, Subcommittee on Urinary Tract Infections and Committee on Quality Improvement: Practice Parameter: The Diagnosis, Treatment, and Evaluation of the Initial Urinary Tract Infection in Febrile Infants and Young Children. Pediatrics 1999;103:843-852.

Bisson G, Fishman NO, Patel JB, et al: Extended-spectrum β-lactamase-producing *Escherichia coli* and *Klebsiella* species: Risk factors for colonization and impact of antimicrobial formulary interventions on colonization prevalence. Infect Control Hosp Epidemiol 2002;254-260.

Bliziotis IA, Samonis G, Vardakas KZ, et al: Effect of aminoglycoside and β-lactam combination therapy versus β-lactam monotherapy on the emergence of antimicrobial resistance: A meta-analysis of randomized, controlled trials. Clin Infect Dis 2005;41:149-158.

British Thoracic Society Standards of Care Committee: BTS Guidelines for the management of community acquired pneumonia in childhood. Thorax 2002;57(Suppl 1):i1-124.

Cherry JD, Shapiro NL, Deville JG: Sinusitis. In Feigin RD, Cherry JD, Demmler GJ, Kaplan SL (eds): Textbook of Pediatric Infectious Diseases, 5th ed. Philadelphia, Saunders, 2004, pp 201-212.

Cosgrove SE: The relationship between antimicrobial resistance and patient outcomes: Mortality, length of hospital stay, and health care costs. Clin Infect Dis 2006;42(Suppl 2):S82-S89.

Cosgrove SE, Carroll KC, Perl TM: *Staphylococcus aureus* with reduced susceptibility to vancomycin. Clin Infect Dis 2004;39:539-545.

Craig FW, Schunk JE: Retropharyngeal abscess in children: Clinical presentation, utility of imaging, and current management. Pediatrics 2003;111:1394-1398.

Hilf M, Yu VL, Sharp J, et al: Antibiotic therapy for *Pseudomonas aeruginosa* bacteremia: Outcome correlations in a prospective study of 200 patients. Am J Med 1989;87:540-546.

Ibia EO, Imoisili M, Pikis A: Group A beta-hemolytic streptococcal osteomyelitis in children. Pediatrics 2003;112:e22-e26.

Kaplan SL: Osteomyelitis in children. Infect Dis Clin North Am 2005;19:787-797.

Klein JO: Bacterial pneumonias. In Feigin RD, Cherry JD, Demmler GJ, Kaplan SL (eds): Textbook of Pediatric Infectious Disease, 5th ed. Philadelphia, Saunders, 2004, pp 299-310.

Korick JA, Bryan CS, Farber B, et al: Prospective observational study of *Klebsiella* bacteremia in 230 patients: Outcome for antibiotic combinations versus monotherapy. Antimicrob Agent Chemother 1992;36:2639-2644.

Lautenbach E, Patel JB, Bilker WB, et al: Extended-spectrum β-lactamase-producing *Escherichia coli* and *Klebsiella pneumoniae*: Risk factors for infection and impact on outcomes. Clin Infect Dis 2001;32:1162-1171.

Leibovici L, Paul M, Poznanski O, et al: Monotherapy versus β-lactam-aminoglycoside combination treatment for gram-negative bacteremia: A prospective, observational study. Antimicrob Agent Chemother 1997; 41:1127-1133.

Martinez-Aguilar G, Avalos-Mishaan A, Hulten K: Community-acquired, methicillin-resistant and methicillin-susceptible *Staphylococcus aureus* musculoskeletal infections in children. Pediatr Infect Dis J 2004;23:701-706.

Mermel LA, Farr BM, Sherertz RJ, et al: Guidelines for the management of intravascular catheter-related infections. Clin Infect Dis 2001;32:1249-1272.

Moellering RC Jr, Eliopoulos GM: Principles of anti-infective therapy. In Mandell GL, Douglas RG Jr, Bennett JE (eds): Principles and Practice of Infectious Diseases, 6th ed. New York, John Wiley & Sons, 2005, pp 242-253.

Muder RR: *Providencia Species*: Antimicrobial Therapy and Vaccines. New York, Apple Trees Productions, 2002, pp 545-548.

Rubenstein E, Lode H, Grassi C, et al: Ceftazidime monotherapy vs. ceftriaxone/tobramycin for serious hospital-acquired gram-negative infections. Clin Infect Dis 1995;20:1217-1228.

Nageswaran S, Woods CR, Benjamin DK Jr, et al: Orbital cellulitis in children. Pediatr Infect Dis J 2006;25:695-699.

Shlaes DM, Gerding DN, John JF, et al: Society for Healthcare Epidemiology of America and Infectious Diseases Society of America Joint Committee on the Prevention of Antimicrobial Resistance: Guidelines for the Prevention of Antimicrobial Resistance in Hospitals. Clin Infect Dis 1997;25:584-599.

Tiwari T, Murphy TV, Moran J: Recommended Antimicrobial Agents for the Treatment and Postexposure Prophylaxis of Pertussis: 2005 CDC Guidelines. MMWR 2005;54(RR-14):1-16.

Tunkel AR, Hartman BJ, Kaplan SL: Practice guidelines for the management of bacterial meningitis. Clin Infect Dis 2004;39:1267-1284.

Wald ER: Cystitis and pyelonephritis. In Feigin RD, Cherry JD, Demmler GJ, Kaplan SL (eds): Textbook of Pediatric Infectious Diseases, 5th ed. Philadelphia Saunders, 2004, pp 541-555.

Yogev R, Bar-Meir M: Management of brain abscesses in children. Pediatr Infect Dis J 2004;23:157-159.

CHAPTER 60

Fever

Samir S. Shah and Elizabeth R. Alpern

Fever, a pyrogen-mediated increase in body temperature, may have a multitude of disparate causes, including infection, inflammation, or malignancy. Therefore, the most important goal when confronted with a febrile patient is to determine the underlying cause. Owing to a differential risk of disease, the cutoff point of abnormal temperature is determined by the age of the child and the presence of any underlying immunodeficiencies. Although there is some ovelap, in this chapter the discussion of fever is divided into two age groups: (1) neonates and young infants and (2) older infants and toddlers.

FEVER IN NEONATES AND YOUNG INFANTS

Fever frequently prompts the medical evaluation of neonates (younger than 28 days) and young infants (aged 29 to 90 days). In this age group, fever is generally defined as a temperature greater than 38.0°C (100.5°F). Up to 15% of neonates and young infants with fever have a serious bacterial infection (SBI). The risk appears to be lower in certain subgroups, such as those with normal laboratory studies or with bronchiolitis.

The most common SBIs in febrile infants are urinary tract infection (UTI; 5% to 10%), bacteremia (1% to 2%), and meningitis (0.5% to 1%). Bacterial pneumonia, gastroenteritis, septic arthritis, osteomyelitis, cellulitis, omphalitis, and mastitis also occur. Infecting organisms vary by the site of infection (Table 60-1). UTIs caused by *Staphylococcus aureus* and *Citrobacter* species are often associated with urinary tract abnormalities and extrarenal sites of infection. Early-onset (age younger than 1 week) group B streptococcal infections are typically associated with bacteremia, pneumonia, and meningitis; late-onset (older than 1 week) infections include septic arthritis, osteomyelitis, cellulitis, and adenitis. *Streptococcus pneumoniae* is responsible for 5% of cases of meningitis in neonates and a slightly greater proportion in infants 1 to 3 months of age.[1] Brain abscesses are more likely in cases of meningitis caused by *Citrobacter koseri*, *Enterobacter sakazakii*, *Bacteroides fragilis*, and *Serratia marcescens*. Bacteremia complicates *Salmonella* gastroenteritis in 5% to 10% of cases.[2] In contrast to older children, young infants with *Salmonella* bacteremia rarely have other immunocompromising conditions. Omphalitis, an infection of the umbilical stump, affects 0.2% to 0.7% of newborn infants; it occurs most often among hospitalized preterm infants undergoing umbilical catheterization. Gram-negative organisms have emerged as an important cause of omphalitis since the introduction of antistaphylococcal cord care (e.g., triple dye). Predominant pathogens causing omphalitis now include *S. aureus*, group A β-hemolytic streptococci, *Escherichia coli*, *Klebsiella pneumoniae*, and *Proteus mirabilis*; anaerobes are involved in one third of cases. *S. aureus* causes most cases of neonatal mastitis.[3]

Case reports occasionally implicate group A β-hemolytic streptococci, group B streptococci (GBS), and enteric gram-negative rods.

Herpes simplex virus (HSV) infection should also be considered in acutely ill infants younger than 1 month of age. Most HSV infections (75%) in neonates are caused by HSV type 2; the remainder are caused by HSV type 1. Fetal scalp electrode use increases the risk of neonatal HSV infection. The higher infection rate after primary maternal genital HSV infection (compared with recurrent infection) may be related to the higher viral load, the longer duration of viral excretion, and the absence of transplacentally acquired protective antibodies in infants born to mothers with primary HSV infection.[4] Although the onset is typically between 11 and 17 days, 9% of infants develop symptoms within the first 24 hours of life. Most infants with skin, eye, and mouth involvement or disseminated disease present between 10 and 14 days of life. In contrast, most infants with isolated central nervous system involvement present on day 18 to 21 of life.[5]

Clinical Presentation

Symptoms and signs of illness vary considerably. Up to two thirds of infants younger than 2 months appear well and have a normal physical examination at the initial evaluation, despite the presence of SBI. Signs of sepsis or other systemic disease are often nonspecific and include disturbances of thermoregulation, such as fever (temperature >38°C) or hypothermia (temperature <36°C); poor feeding; and evidence of organ dysfunction. Potential cardiovascular disturbances include tachycardia (pulse >180 beats per minute), bradycardia (pulse <95 beats per minute), hypotension (systolic blood pressure <60 mm Hg in full-term infants), weak or bounding femoral pulses, mottled skin, and delayed capillary refill (>2 to 3 seconds). Respiratory abnormalities include apnea, tachypnea (respirations >60 per minute), grunting, nasal flaring, intercostal or subcostal retractions, and hypoxemia. Signs of gastrointestinal tract disturbances include a rigid or distended abdomen, absent bowel sounds, diarrhea, or bloody stools. Cutaneous findings such as jaundice, petechiae, and cyanosis may be present. Neurologic abnormalities can occur with any serious infection and include irritability, lethargy, hypotonia, and hypertonia.

Signs of a specific disease process may also be detected. Infants with meningitis may have a tense or bulging fontanelle, and up to one third may develop seizures. The presence of vesicles warrants consideration of HSV infection; vesicles are detected in two thirds of children with either central nervous system or disseminated HSV infection.[5] Erythema, edema, induration, and tenderness of the breast tissue herald mastitis. Although most cases of mastitis are mild, the infection can progress rapidly. Involvement may extend beyond the breast tissue to involve the

Table 60-1 Bacterial Pathogens Causing Urinary Tract Infection, Gastroenteritis, and Bacteremia and Meningitis in Infants Younger than 90 Days

Frequency	Urinary Tract Infection	Gastroenteritis	Bacteremia and Meningitis
Common	*Escherichia coli* *Klebsiella* species	*Salmonella* species	Group B streptococci *Escherichia coli** *Klebsiella* species* *Listeria monocytogenes**
Less common	Group B streptococci *Enterococcus* species *Pseudomonas aeruginosa* *Staphylococcus aureus* *Citrobacter* species	*Campylobacter jejuni* *Yersinia enterocolitica* *Shigella* species	*Streptococcus pneumoniae* *Neisseria meningitidis* *Salmonella* species Group A β-hemolytic streptococci Other gram-negative bacilli†

*Less common in infants older than 1 month.
†Includes *Serratia marcescens, Citrobacter* species, *Enterobacter* species.

subcutaneous tissue around the shoulder and the abdomen. Periumbilical erythema, ecchymosis, edema, induration, or crepitus suggests omphalitis. Extremity abnormalities may be more noticeable to the parents. Local signs of septic arthritis or osteomyelitis include swelling, erythema, warmth, exquisite tenderness, and diminished range of motion of the affected joint or extremity. These infants often demonstrate an unwillingness to move the extremity, a finding known as pseudoparalysis.

Differential Diagnosis

The management of febrile infants younger than 90 days poses a challenge because of the relatively high prevalence of SBI and the inability to easily distinguish those with serious bacterial disease or HSV from those with uncomplicated, common viral illnesses caused by respiratory syncytial virus (RSV), parainfluenza viruses, influenza viruses, adenovirus, human metapneumovirus, and enteroviruses.

Evaluation

The diagnostic evaluation of young febrile infants is controversial. Because this group is at higher risk for SBI than are older infants and children, management traditionally involved a complete evaluation, including complete blood counts, chemistries, and cultures of urine, blood, and cerebrospinal fluid (CSF); hospitalization; and empirical antibiotic administration for all infants younger than 60 to 90 days. Because this strategy leads to the unnecessary hospitalization of many infants without SBI, several studies focused on the development of clinical screening tools to identify selected groups who are at low risk for SBI and can be safely managed in the outpatient setting. The Boston,[6] Philadelphia,[7,8] and Rochester[9,10] protocols are commonly used screening strategies (Table 60-2), but they apply only to infants with stable home situations (including a telephone to receive culture results) and who do not appear ill.

The Boston and Philadelphia protocols exclude febrile infants younger than 1 month of age from consideration for outpatient management. In studies that applied the Philadelphia or Boston protocol to neonates, 3% to 5% of infants younger than 1 month who were identified as low risk had

SBI.[11,12] The investigators advocated that these protocols not be applied to neonates and concluded that all infants with fever in the first month of life require hospitalization for empirical antibiotic therapy. In contrast, the Rochester criteria do not take a different approach to febrile infants in the first month of life; however, this protocol has a lower sensitivity for detecting SBI than either the Boston or the Philadelphia protocol.

In summary, no clear consensus exists regarding the optimal approach to febrile infants younger than 90 days. In deciding on a course of evaluation, clinicians must determine the degree of diagnostic uncertainty they are willing to tolerate when attempting to exclude SBI. Institutional or regional practice variations and personal preferences regarding test minimization and risk minimization may influence individual practice patterns. We discuss the components of evaluation included in the various protocols in the following sections.

Complete Blood Count

The total peripheral white blood cell (WBC) count, in combination with other laboratory parameters (see Table 60-2), can contribute to the identification of infants with SBI. Although less than half of practitioners surveyed are compliant with published guidelines for the management of febrile infants younger than 90 days, 96% of practitioners surveyed routinely obtain peripheral WBC counts.[13] Unfortunately, the complete blood count alone is an inaccurate screen for SBI in infants younger than 90 days. Using WBC cutoffs of less than 5000/mm^3 or greater than 15,000/mm^3 fails to identify at least 33% of infants with bacteremia and 40% of infants with meningitis.[14,15]

Urinalysis

Several rapid screening tests are available to identify UTI. The traditional urinalysis (UA) involves a combination of urine dipstick (uncentrifuged urine) detection of leukocyte esterase and nitrites plus microscopic (centrifuged urine) detection of WBCs per high-power field and bacteria per high-power field. The enhanced UA uses a combination of hemocytometry to provide a WBC count per cubic millime-

Table 60-2 Comparison of Protocols to Identify Febrile Infants with a Low Risk of Serious Bacterial Infection*

Variable	Boston[†]	Philadelphia[†]	Rochester
Age (days)	28-89	29-56	0-60
Temperature (°C)	≥38.0	≥38.0	≥38.0
History and physical examination	Normal	Normal	Normal
Peripheral WBC count (per mm³)	<20,000	<15,000	5000-15,000
Differential count	N/A	Band-neutrophil ratio <0.2	Absolute band count <1500/mm³
Urinalysis	No leukocyte esterase	<10 WBCs/hpf No bacteria on Gram stain	<10 WBCs/hpf No bacteria on Gram stain
CSF WBC count (per mm³)	<10	<8	N/A[†]
CSF Gram stain	Negative	Negative	N/A[†]
Chest radiograph	No discrete infiltrate[§]	No discrete infiltrate	No discrete infiltrate[§]
Stool	N/A	If diarrhea: few or no WBCs on smear	If diarrhea: ≤5 WBC/hpf
Treatment option for low-risk infants	Discharge after one dose of parenteral ceftriaxone; 24 hr follow-up	Discharge without antibiotics; 24 hr follow-up	Discharge without antibiotics; 24 hr follow-up
Risk of SBI if low risk (%)	5.4	0	1.1
Negative predictive value for SBI (%)	94.6	99-100	88-99[¶]

*Infants not meeting the low-risk criteria require hospitalization for empirical antibiotic therapy.
[†]In the Boston and Philadelphia protocols, infants younger than the age criterion should receive a complete evaluation and require hospitalization for empirical antibiotic therapy.
[†]Infants not meeting the low-risk criteria also require lumbar puncture.
[§]Chest radiograph is unnecessary in the absence of signs of respiratory illness such as cough, tachypnea, abnormal findings on auscultation, or hypoxia.
[¶]This range of values includes extrapolation of data to account for infants excluded from the study owing to incomplete evaluation.
CSF, cerebrospinal fluid; hpf, high-power field; N/A, not applicable to screening protocol; SBI, serious bacterial infection; WBC, white blood cell.

ter and Gram stain for bacteria on uncentrifuged urine specimens; it has a higher negative predictive value and sensitivity compared with the traditional UA. An abnormal enhanced UA (>10 WBCs/mm³ or positive Gram stain) has a sensitivity of 94% to 96% and a specificity of 84% to 99%.[16,17] The Boston, Philadelphia, and Rochester protocols have not yet been studied using the enhanced UA; however, inclusion of the enhanced UA in these protocols would likely improve the detection of SBI in young febrile infants but might also result in more infants falsely classified as high risk. The positive predictive value of the enhanced UA (10% to 17%) is substantially lower than that of urine dipstick tests (38% to 54%).[16]

Chest Radiograph

Chest radiographs are no longer considered a routine part of most protocols. Several studies specifically evaluated the need for routine chest radiographs in febrile infants, but they are of limited value because they included any radiographic abnormality (e.g., peribronchial thickening) rather than the more clinically meaningful but more difficult to define finding of pneumonia.[18-20] A reasonable approach is to limit the use of chest radiographs to infants with abnormal respiratory signs (e.g., cough, tachypnea, hypoxia, abnormal lung auscultation).

Blood Culture

Several important variables affect the volume of blood necessary for culture. The magnitude of bacteremia affects blood culture yield, especially when small blood volumes are used. Although it is often difficult to obtain adequate blood samples in pediatric patients, the volume of blood in a single blood culture bottle matters more than the total number of blood cultures obtained.[21,22] A single culture containing 1 to 2 mL of blood is sufficient for the detection of most clinically important bacteremias; a 0.5-mL blood sample, though not ideal, permits the detection of some clinically important bacteremias.[23]

Lumbar Puncture

CSF should routinely be sent for Gram stain and culture, glucose, protein, and cell count. An additional tube is occasionally collected and held in the microbiology or chemistry laboratory in case other studies are required. Interpretation of CSF values varies by age (Table 60-3).[24-27] Bacteria are evident on CSF Gram stain in up to 75% of infants with bacterial meningitis; premature infants with bacterial meningitis are less likely to have organisms detected by Gram stain. Because of the relatively low concentration of organisms, infants with *Listeria monocytogenes* meningitis rarely have bacteria detectable by Gram stain.

Table 60-3 Guidelines for the Interpretation of Cerebrospinal Fluid Studies in Neonates and Young Infants*

Age	Cell Count (per mm³)	Protein (mg/dL)	Glucose (mg/dL)†
Preterm newborn	<25	65-150	>40
Term newborn	<22	20-170	>40
<4 wk	<15	20-170	>40
4-8 wk	<10	35-85	>40

*Data pooled from references 24-27. Infants with central nervous system infection may have cerebrospinal fluid values in the normal range; therefore, these values should be interpreted in the context of the infant's clinical status.

†Cerebrospinal fluid glucose values are typically >40 mg/dL, or one half to two thirds of serum values.

Detection of bacterial antigens in the CSF by latex particle agglutination (*S. pneumoniae, Neisseria meningitidis, Haemophilus influenzae*) or counterimmunoelectrophoresis (*E. coli*) has been described. Moderate sensitivity (70% to 80%), changing antibiotic susceptibility patterns, and the availability of broad-spectrum antimicrobial therapy limit the current usefulness of these tests. Polymerase chain reaction (PCR) assays for *S. pneumoniae* and *N. meningitidis* result in fewer false-negative results than do bacterial antigen detection tests, but additional research is required.

Contamination of CSF with blood during a traumatic lumbar puncture confounds the accurate interpretation of results. If the ratio of WBCs to red blood cells (RBCs) in the peripheral blood remains constant when peripheral blood is introduced into the subarachnoid space during lumbar puncture, comparing the ratio of observed to predicted CSF WBCs may raise or lower the suspicion for bacterial meningitis. A predicted CSF WBC count can be calculated using the following formula:

Predicted CSF WBCs
= CSF RBCs × (Blood WBCs/Blood RBCs)

A retrospective study determined that an observed-predicted CSF WBC ratio less than 0.01 had a sensitivity of 100% (95% confidence interval, 74% to 100%) in predicting the *absence* of bacterial meningitis.[28] Some experts dispute the assumption of a fixed ratio of WBCs in the CSF and peripheral blood. In the Boston and Philadelphia screening protocols, infants with difficult to interpret (e.g., grossly bloody) lumbar punctures are *not* considered low risk; these infants are hospitalized and receive empirical antibiotic therapy. In certain situations, a repeat lumbar puncture 12 to 24 hours later may clarify the ambiguity of the initial results.

Additional Studies

When HSV is a concern, CSF should be sent for PCR testing. This technique has a sensitivity and specificity of 96% and 99%, respectively.[29] In infants with skin, eye, or mucous membrane HSV disease, and in many with either central nervous system or disseminated disease, HSV can often be isolated from conjunctival, throat, and rectal swabs by culture or PCR. HSV from these cutaneous sites can usually be detected by culture within 48 hours. Although a negative culture result cannot completely exclude HSV infection, most infants with HSV infection have positive culture results from cutaneous sites.[5] False-negative PCR results are rare but may occur when CSF specimens are obtained very early in the course of HSV illness. In such cases, repeat testing 2 to 3 days later confirms the diagnosis. PCR testing of CSF remains reliable for up to 7 days after the initiation of acyclovir; 50% of specimens remain PCR-positive 8 to 14 days after the initiation of acyclovir.[30] Infants with disseminated HSV may also have laboratory evidence of hepatitis, coagulopathy, and thrombocytopenia.

Other Considerations

The prevalence of SBI may be lower among some febrile infants with a bronchiolitis syndrome. In a prospective, multicenter study, RSV-positive infants younger than 60 days were less likely to have an SBI than were RSV-negative infants (7% versus 12.5%).[31] However, the subanalysis found some differences by age. Infants 28 days or younger had an overall SBI rate of 13.3%, *regardless of RSV status*. In contrast, RSV-positive infants 29 to 60 days of age had a lower risk of SBI than did RSV-negative infants (5.5% versus 11.7%; relative risk, 0.5). The SBIs in RSV-positive infants aged 29 to 60 days were due solely to UTI; no RSV-positive patient in this age group had bacteremia or meningitis.

In summary, among infants 28 days and younger, the risk of SBI is substantial and is not altered by the presence of RSV. In these children, we continue to perform a complete evaluation, including urine, blood, and CSF studies. RSV-positive infants 29 to 60 days of age have a clinically important rate of UTI, and because we cannot exclude SBI in any febrile infant in this age group without a complete evaluation, blood and urine cultures are routinely performed in hospitalized infants. In well-appearing infants, the lumbar puncture is occasionally deferred unless changes in the patient's condition warrant additional evaluation. In infants 29 to 60 days of age who will be discharged home from the emergency department, a complete evaluation, including lumbar puncture, may be appropriate. In determining the extent of laboratory evaluation, clinicians should consider these data in combination with other factors, including the family's reliability to assess the infant's clinical deterioration, access to a telephone, proximity to medical care, and likelihood of follow-up evaluation within 24 hours after emergency department discharge or availability of 24-hour physician support for hospitalized patients.

Office-Based Strategies

The protocols summarized in Table 60-2 were developed for use in the emergency department setting. A large proportion of office-based physicians do not routinely follow any of these strategies.[32] In an office-based study of 3066 febrile infants younger than 3 months, the overall rate of SBI was similar to the rates found in studies conducted in the emergency department: UTI (5.4%), bacteremia (2.4%), and meningitis (0.5%).[33] Most cases of bacteremia or meningitis occurred during the first month of life, when 4.1% of infants were affected; in contrast, 1.9% and 0.7% of cases occurred during the second and third months of life, respectively. Practitioners in this study followed current guidelines in

42% of cases; however, they correctly treated 61 of 63 cases of bacteremia or bacterial meningitis with empirical antibiotics during the initial visit. These findings suggest that if close follow-up care is attainable in an office-based setting (most infants in the study had more than one office visit and multiple telephone contacts), the management of selected cases by an experienced clinician may be more important than strict adherence to published recommendations. This strategy can reduce costs and complications associated with routine evaluation and hospitalization. This study, however, illustrated limitations that warrant consideration. Two infants with life-threatening infections did not receive antibiotics initially; both these infants would have been treated initially if they had been evaluated by at least one of the commonly used screening protocols. Given the relatively high prevalence of UTI and the wide availability of screening UA tests, practitioners should strongly consider routine UA in all young febrile infants.

Admission Criteria

In each of the protocols outlined (see Table 60-2), all infants not meeting low-risk criteria require hospitalization and empirical antibiotic therapy. Any ill-appearing infant, regardless of laboratory test results, also requires hospitalization and empirical antibiotic therapy.

Treatment

Infants hospitalized for suspected SBI should receive broad-spectrum antimicrobial therapy. During the first month of life, either ampicillin plus an aminoglycoside (e.g., gentamicin) or ampicillin plus a third-generation cephalosporin (e.g., cefotaxime) is recommended. Between 30 and 90 days of life, cefotaxime alone is usually sufficient. A systematic review determined that the prevalence of infections caused by either *L. monocytogenes* or enterococci (organisms for which cephalosporins are not effective) was 0.7% among febrile infants younger than 30 days but only 0.2% among infants 31 to 60 days of age. In this review, no case of *Listeria* infection was seen in infants older than 1 month.[34] The combination of vancomycin and cefotaxime should be considered for infants with CSF parameters suggestive of bacterial meningitis or those with gram-positive cocci identified on CSF Gram stain until cultures have excluded drug-resistant *S. pneumoniae*. Infants with gram-negative meningitis should receive an empirical aminoglycoside plus either ceftazidime or imipenem.

Duration of therapy is discussed in detail in Chapter 63 on central nervous system infections, Chapter 69 on UTIs, and Chapter 67 on lower respiratory tract infections. In general, infants with bacteremia or UTI should receive at least 2 weeks of therapy. Meningitis should be treated for approximately 2 weeks after bacteriologic cure. For meningitis caused by GBS, *L. monocytogenes*, or *S. pneumoniae*, 2 weeks of total therapy is usually sufficient. Delayed sterilization is common for infants with gram-negative meningitis; therefore, they should receive a minimum of 3 weeks of therapy. Infants with complicated disease (e.g., brain abscess) may require a longer duration of therapy. Repeat lumbar puncture after 48 to 72 hours of therapy is routinely recommended for meningitis due to drug-resistant *S. pneumoniae* or gram-negative organisms.

Infants with suspected HSV infection should receive high-dose acyclovir (60 mg/kg per day).[35] Infants with skin, eye, or mucous membrane disease receive 14 days of intravenous therapy. Infants with disseminated or central nervous system disease require at least 21 days of therapy. Many experts suggest repeating the lumbar puncture upon completion of the 21-day acyclovir course and extending the duration of acyclovir therapy if the CSF PCR remains positive for HSV. In such situations, consultation with a pediatric infectious disease specialist is recommended.

Discharge Criteria
Emergency Department Discharge

The Boston protocol includes administering ceftriaxone to all low-risk infants before discharge. Infants subsequently identified to have positive culture results return for continuation of parenteral antibiotic therapy.

The Philadelphia protocol requires hospitalization and empirical antibiotic therapy for all febrile infants younger than 28 days of age, but it allows low-risk febrile infants 29 to 56 days of age to be managed in the outpatient setting without antibiotics. Approximately 40% of presenting febrile infants are classified as low risk by the Philadelphia protocol.

The Rochester protocol permits discharge of approximately 45% of febrile infants younger than 60 days without antibiotics; however, 1% to 12% of these infants may have an SBI.

Hospital Discharge

Historically, infants were discharged if the concern for SBI no longer existed, the infant was clinically stable, and culture results had been negative for at least 48 hours. Earlier hospital discharge may be possible for some infants, because most pathogens grow from culture within 24 hours. A pathogen was detected in culture after 24 hours in 1.1% of 3166 febrile 28- to 90-day-old infants; however, all 8 infants with meningitis had growth from CSF cultures less than 24 hours after specimen collection.[36] Additional data on time to pathogen detection are presented later in this chapter. The patient's diagnosis (e.g., UTI, bacteremia, meningitis) and clinical response ultimately determine the duration of hospitalization.

Prevention
Group B Streptococcal Infection

Maternal intrapartum chemoprophylaxis with at least two doses of penicillin or ampicillin reduces the vertical transmission of GBS from colonized mothers to their neonates. Women allergic to penicillin can receive clindamycin, erythromycin, or, in the absence of immediate-type hypersensitivity, a first-generation cephalosporin. Approximately 20% of pregnant women require intrapartum chemoprophylaxis, based on current protocols. These strategies have dramatically decreased the incidence of early-onset group B streptococcal disease. However, because intrapartum penicillin administration does not reliably eradicate GBS from the colonized infant, its impact on late-onset disease is less significant. Some studies raised the concern that intrapartum ampicillin use led to an increase in neonatal infections with ampicillin-resistant pathogens[37,38] and gram-negative bacteremia.[39]

Recurrent group B streptococcal disease occasionally occurs. Most GBS isolates in recurrent infections are genotypically identical to isolates from the initial infection. The likely mechanism involves recurrent infection due to persistent colonization with the original strain. In patients with recurrent infection, the penicillin susceptibility of the isolate should be determined by minimum inhibitory concentration (MIC) testing. Additional evaluation of the infant may include testing for human immunodeficiency virus (HIV) and analysis of B-lymphocyte function. Consultation with pediatric infectious disease or immunology specialists is warranted. Oral rifampin therapy (20 mg/kg per day during the last 4 days of parenteral therapy) may be used in an attempt to eradicate mucosal GBS colonization. This regimen successfully eradicates mucosal colonization in 50% of cases.[40,41]

Herpes Simplex Virus Infection

Cesarean section within 4 hours of membrane rupture in a mother with active genital herpes at the time of delivery can prevent many neonatal HSV infections. However, three fourths of mothers of infants with neonatal HSV infection are asymptomatic or have unrecognized infection, and neonatal infection can occur in an infant delivered by cesarean section in the presence of intact membranes. Symptomatic infants and those with findings that suggest a high likelihood of HSV infection (e.g., vesicles) should receive intravenous acyclovir while awaiting study results. For asymptomatic infants born to mothers with active genital HSV lesions, HSV cultures should be obtained at 24 to 48 hours of life from the conjunctiva, mouth, or nasopharynx and from the rectum or stool. Asymptomatic infants do not require any antiviral therapy while awaiting HSV culture results, although many experts suggest empirical acyclovir in those delivered vaginally.

In a Nutshell

- Up to 15% of febrile infants younger than 90 days have an SBI.
- Screening protocols can identify infants younger than 90 days who are at low risk for SBI. These infants may be candidates for outpatient management.
- RSV-infected infants aged 29 days and older have a lower risk of bacteremia and meningitis than do infants who are not infected with RSV; however, the risk of UTI in this population remains significant. In contrast, infants 28 days and younger have a high risk of SBI regardless of their RSV status.
- Intrapartum prophylaxis for GBS dramatically decreases the rate of early-onset group B streptococcal disease in neonates but is less effective in the prevention of late-onset disease.

On the Horizon

- PCR-based tests to rapidly identify bacterial causes of meningitis and bloodstream infection.
- Further clarification of the role of viral pathogen testing on the management of young febrile infants.
- Inclusion of enhanced UA in the protocols that identify young infants at low risk for SBI.

FEVER IN OLDER INFANTS AND TODDLERS

Although there is some overlap with the previously discussed age group, fever in older infants and toddlers (2 to 24 months) is generally defined as body temperature greater than 38.5°C (101.3°F). These young children have waning maternal antibodies and increasing exposure to contagious illnesses and may experience multiple febrile illnesses each year. Differentiating serious illness from benign viral syndromes is the most important aspect of care of these febrile children. Several clinical entities are of particular importance in this population. Healthy, well-appearing young children with fever but without an identifiable focal bacterial infection may have an occult infection, including bacteremia, UTI, and pneumonia. Occult UTI and pneumonia are discussed in detail in Chapters 69 and 67, respectively. Occult bacteremia is discussed in the following sections.

Clinical Presentation

Occult bacteremia is defined as the presence of bacteria in the blood of a well-appearing febrile child (temperature >39°C [102.2°F]) between the ages of 2 and 24 (or 36) months.[42] By definition, these children have an intact immune system and lack an identifiable focal bacterial infection (e.g., abscess, cellulitis, pneumonia) or pathognomonic viral entity (e.g., herpes stomatitis, varicella).

Historically, occult bacteremia has overwhelmingly been due to *S. pneumoniae* and *H. influenzae* type B (HIB).[43-45] Other causative organisms include *Salmonella* species, nontypeable *H. influenzae*, group A β-hemolytic streptococci, *Enterococcus* species, and *N. meningitidis*. Recently, the overall risk of occult bacteremia among febrile infants and toddlers has been significantly reduced by administration of the HIB and heptavalent pneumococcal conjugate (PCV7) vaccines.[1,46-51] Before the licensure of the HIB vaccine in 1987, the prevalence of occult bacteremia among febrile young children was between 3% and 11%.[43-45,52,53] However, after widespread use of the HIB vaccine, the reported overall rate of occult bacteremia in immunized children is less than 2%.[54,55] With the release of PCV7 in 2000, there has been nearly a 70% decrease in the rate of invasive pneumoccocal disease[56]; in addition, the overall prevalence of occult bacteremia declined to less than 1%.[57]

The risk of occult bacteremia is determined by the age of the child, his or her immunization status, and clinical parameters such as height of fever. Occult bacteremia is a concern because of its possible progression to deep-seated focal infection, such as osteomyelitis or meningitis, or to sepsis syndrome. The risk of invasive disease due to occult bacteremia depends on the infecting organism. When HIB was a prominent causative organism, the risk of invasive disease with known occult HIB bacteremia was between 25% and 44%.[45,58] However, occult pneumococcal bacteremia is associated with a significantly smaller risk (0.6%) of invasive disease.[45] Because HIB is no longer a major concern in immunized populations, the risk of progression to meningitis or death is substantially reduced. Currently, the overall risk of meningitis or death in children with occult bacteremia is approximately 1.8%.[54]

Differential Diagnosis

The differential diagnosis of fever in a young child is extremely broad. It is important to differentiate children at risk for occult bacteremia from those at risk for nonoccult bacteremia. Children with identifiable signs and symptoms of invasive disease, those with focal bacterial infections, and those ill enough to warrant lumbar puncture and hospital admission are certainly at risk for bacteremia, but they fail to meet the definition of children at risk for occult bacteremia.

Viral syndromes, otitis media, bronchiolitis, and unidentified pneumonia or UTI are common entities that have presentations similar to that of occult bacteremia. Some of these entities may be complicated by the presence of occult bacteremia, and some may even predispose patients to develop bacteremia, further complicating the evaluation and management of these febrile children.

Diagnosis

The diagnosis of occult bacteremia is dependent on a complete history and physical examination. Immunization status is an important component of the history to determine the risk of occult bacteremia by specific organisms; those who have not been immunized for HIB or *S. pneumoniae* are at increased risk. The risk of occult bacteremia also increases with increasing body temperature. The risk in children with fevers higher than 40°C is approximately twice the risk in those with fevers lower than 40°C.[59] However, many children with occult bacteremia do not have fevers greater than 40°C, and the vast majority of children with fevers that high do not have occult bacteremia. The response to antipyretics does not reflect the risk for occult bacteremia. Children with identifiable otitis media have the same overall risk for occult bacteremia as do those without this discernible infection.[54,58] Children presenting with simple (also known as "typical") febrile seizures and no evidence of focal infection also have a similar prevalence of occult bacteremia.[60,61] In contrast, children in this age group diagnosed clinically with bronchiolitis, croup, or stomatitis have a decreased risk for occult bacteremia associated with the febrile illness.[31,62,63]

Many screening laboratory studies have been evaluated as markers for occult bacteremia. However, because of the low overall prevalence of occult bacteremia in the population, these studies are limited in their positive predictive value. The complete blood count is the most widely studied diagnostic test.[43,53,55,57,59,64] In one study, a WBC count greater than 15,000/mm³ was associated with a positive predictive value of 5%[55]; another study found that an absolute neutrophil count greater than 10,000/mm³ yielded a positive predictive value of 8%.[59] Therefore, although the risk of occult bacteremia increases with an increasing WBC count or absolute neutrophil count, the vast majority of patients with a leukocytosis or increased neutrophil count do not have occult bacteremia.

C-reactive protein (CRP) has been studied as a marker for SBI and occult bacteremia.[65,66] Although the risk of SBI increases with an increasing CRP level, its utility in detecting occult bacteremia is modest.[65] Using a CRP value of 4.4 mg/dL or greater, the positive predictive value is only 30% (i.e., only 30% of patients with a CRP level ≥4.4 mg/dL have occult bacteremia). However, the negative predictive value is 94% (i.e., 94% of patients with a CRP level <4.4 mg/dL do not have occult bacteremia).[66]

Blood culture remains the gold standard for diagnosing occult bacteremia. The most important limitation of a blood culture is the delay in identifying positive cultures. If a continuously monitored carbon dioxide production pediatric system is used, 94% of pathogenic cultures will be identified as positive within 18 hours.[54] The prevalence of occult bacteremia has decreased, and the prevalence of contaminated cultures now approximates the prevalence of true pathogens.

Treatment

The evaluation and treatment of patients at risk for occult bacteremia are controversial. Owing to the difficulty of diagnosing occult bacteremia without waiting for test results, expectant antibiotic use has been advocated by some to decrease the risk of adverse outcomes such as meningitis or sepsis. In the pre-HIB vaccine era, amoxicillin, amoxicillin–clavulanic acid, and ceftriaxone were studied as expectant treatment and were determined to have no statistically significant effect on serious adverse outcomes.[44,53] In another study, ceftriaxone was noted to decrease the risk of "definite" focal infections but was not effective in decreasing the risk of acquiring a "definite or probable" focal infection.[45] In this study, *H. influenzae* and *Salmonella* species were the only causes of subsequent meningitis in patients with occult bacteremia.[45,67] Because occult bacteremia has changed owing to the availability of immunizations and the changing epidemiology of causative organisms, many advocate treating only patients with documented bacteremia, rather than treating all patients at higher risk. This has been supported in several meta-analyses and comparison studies.[68-70]

If gram-positive cocci are identified, empiric therapy for *S. pneumoniae*, the most likely pathogen, with amoxicillin, ampicillin, or ceftriaxone is reasonable. The well-appearing patient in whom fever has resolved may be managed in the outpatient setting. If the patient appears ill, empiric coverage should be broadened to provide coverage against methicillin-resistant *S. aureus* with vancomycin. If gram-negative rods are identified, *Salmonella* and *H. influenzae* are most likely. The patient requires hospitalization and empiric therapy may include a third-generation cephalosporin with or without an aminoglycoside. Ill-appearing patients should receive either a carbapenem or a beta-lactam/beta-lactamase inhibitor combination.

Admission Criteria

If a child evaluated for occult bacteremia has a positive blood culture within 18 to 24 hours, there is a high probability that the positive culture indicates a true pathogen. Currently, *S. pneumoniae* causes most episodes of occult bacteremia and has a very high spontaneous resolution rate. However, the bacteremia still creates a risk of hematogenously seeded infection. A patient with a positive blood culture result but resolution of fever and lack of signs or symptoms of focal infection upon reevaluation can be safely assessed with a repeat blood culture and followed as an outpatient.[71] However, persistently febrile or ill-appearing patients with positive blood cultures require a full evaluation to assess for new focal infections, including meningitis. If no antibiotics have been prescribed previously, the physical examination may reliably indicate the presence or absence of focal infection. Complete blood count, blood culture, UA and urine culture, chest radiograph, and lumbar puncture should be considered in an ill-appearing febrile child with bacteremia. Hospital admission and treatment with a broad-spectrum antibiotic, such as ceftriaxone, are indicated. Vancomycin is added in cases of suspected meningitis.

Discharge Criteria

When children with positive initial blood cultures warrant admission (i.e., their clinical appearance or laboratory studies are not reassuring), the repeat culture is followed closely for the first 24 hours. Several studies using continuously monitored carbon dioxide blood culture systems have documented that the great majority of pathogens from immunocompetent hosts are detected within 24 hours.[54,72,73] Therefore, well-appearing immunocompetent patients may be safely discharged home if their repeat blood cultures remain negative for at least 24 hours. Total length of treatment is determined by the presence or absence of any particular focal infection that may have developed and should be tailored to the identified infection.

Prevention

The HIB and conjugate pneumococcal vaccines are the most effective means of preventing occult bacteremia. The conjugate pneumococcal vaccine is immunogenic for 7 of the 90 *S. pneumoniae* serotypes. Although early data are promising, there is theoretical concern about serotype shift due to nonvaccine organisms.

In a Nutshell

- Occult bacteremia is the presence of pathogenic bacteria in the blood of a well-appearing febrile child aged 2 to 24 (or 36) months who lacks a focal bacterial infection.
- Occult bacteremia has the potential to progress to focal infection (including meningitis) or sepsis.
- The overall prevalence of occult bacteremia in at-risk children is less than 2%.
- Widespread HIB vaccination had dramatically decreased the prevalence of occult bacteremia, and use of the heptavalent pneumococcal conjugate vaccine may lead to an even further decrease.
- *S. pneumoniae* is the most common causative organism and has a very high spontaneous resolution rate. The overall risk of meningitis or death in children with occult bacteremia is approximately 1.8%.
- Expectant antibiotic treatment of patients with possible occult bacteremia has not been shown to definitively prevent subsequent focal or systemic infection.
- Patients with positive blood culture results should be carefully evaluated for focal infections and admitted to the hospital if they appear ill or are persistently febrile.

On the Horizon

- Procalcitonin and urine antigen assays are being evaluated as improved rapid diagnostic studies to evaluate patients at risk for occult bacteremia.[74,75]
- Further study of the changes in the epidemiology of occult bacteremia due to the pneumococcal vaccine is warranted, with particular attention to decreased prevalence, possible seroreplacement, and cross-immunogenicity between vaccine serotypes and closely related nonvaccine serotypes.

SUGGESTED READING

Alpern ER, Alessandrini EA, Bell LM, et al: Occult bacteremia from a pediatric emergency department: Current prevalence, time to detection, and outcome. Pediatrics 2000;106:505-511.

Bachur R, Harper MB: Reevaluation of outpatients with *Streptococcus pneumoniae* bacteremia. Pediatrics 2000;105:502-509.

Baker MD, Bell LM, Avner JR: Outpatient management without antibiotics of fever in selected infants. N Engl J Med 1993;329:1437-1441.

Bulloch B, Craig WR, Klassen TP: The use of antibiotics to prevent serious sequelae in children at risk for occult bacteremia: A meta-analysis. Acad Emerg Med 1997;4:679-683.

Lee GM, Harper MB: Risk of bacteremia for febrile young children in the post–*Haemophilus influenzae* type B era. Arch Pediatr Adolesc Med 1998;152:624-628.

Levine DA, Platt SL, Dayan PS, et al: Risk of serious bacterial infection in young febrile infants with respiratory syncytial virus infections. Pediatrics 2004;113:1728-1734.

Pantell RH, Newman TB, Bernzweig J, et al: Management and outcomes of care of fever in early infancy. JAMA 2004;291:1203-1212.

Schuchat A, Robinson K, Wenger J, et al: Bacterial meningitis in the United States in 1995. N Engl J Med 1997;337:970-976.

REFERENCES

1. Schuchat A, Robinson K, Wenger JD, et al: Bacterial meningitis in the United States in 1995. N Engl J Med 1997;337:970-976.
2. Torrey S, Fleisher G, Jaffe D: Incidence of *Salmonella* bacteremia in infants with *Salmonella* gastroenteritis. J Pediatr 1986;108:718-721.
3. Walsh M, McIntosh K: Neonatal mastitis. Clin Pediatr 1986;25:395-399.
4. Brown ZA, Benedetti J, Ashley R, et al: Neonatal herpes simplex virus infection in relation to asymptomatic maternal infection at the time of labor. N Engl J Med 1991;324:1247-1252.
5. Kimberlin DW, Lin CY, Jacobs RF, et al: Natural history of neonatal herpes simplex virus infections in the acyclovir era. Pediatrics 2001;108:223-229.
6. Baskin MN, O'Rourke EJ, Fleisher GR: Outpatient treatment of febrile infants 28 to 89 days of age with intramuscular administration of ceftriaxone. J Pediatr 1992;120:22-27.
7. Baker MD, Bell LM, Avner JR: Outpatient management without antibiotics of fever in selected infants. N Engl J Med 1993;329:1437-1441.
8. Baker MD, Bell LM, Avner JR: The efficacy of routine outpatient management without antibiotics of fever in selected infants. Pediatrics 1999;103:627-631.
9. Dagan R, Powell KR, Hall CB, Menegus MA: Identification of infants unlikely to have serious bacterial infection although hospitalized for suspected sepsis. J Pediatr 1985;107:855-860.
10. Jaskiewicz KA, McCarthy CA, Richardson AC, et al: Febrile infants at low risk for serious bacterial infection—an appraisal of the Rochester criteria and implications for management. Pediatrics 1994;94:390-396.

11. Baker MD, Avner JR, Bell LM: Failure of infant observation scales in detecting serious illness in febrile, 4- to 8-week-old infants. Pediatrics 1990;85:1040-1043.

12. Kadish HA, Loveridge B, Tobey J, et al: Applying outpatient protocols in febrile infants 1-28 days of age: Can the threshold be lowered? Clin Pediatr 2000;39:81-88.

13. Belfer RA, Gittelman MA, Muniz AE: Management of febrile infants and children by pediatric emergency medicine and emergency medicine: Comparison with practice guidelines. Pediatr Emerg Care 2001;17:83-87.

14. Bonsu BK, Harper MB: Utility of the peripheral blood white blood cell count for identifying sick young infants who need lumbar puncture. Ann Emerg Med 2003;41:206-214.

15. Bonsu BK, Harper MB: Identifying febrile young infants with bacteremia: Is the peripheral white blood cell count an accurate screen? Ann Emerg Med 2003;42:216-225.

16. Shaw KN, McGowan KL, Gorelick MH, Schwartz JS: Screening for urinary tract infection in infants in the emergency department: Which test is best? Pediatrics 1998;101:e1. Available at http://www.pediatrics.org/cgi/content/full/101/6/e1.

17. Herr SM, Wald ER, Pitetti RD, Choi SS: Enhanced urinalysis improves identification of febrile infants ages 60 days and younger at low risk of serious bacterial illness. Pediatrics 2001;108:866-871.

18. Crain EF, Bulas D, Bijur PE, Goldman HS: Is a chest radiograph necessary in the evaluation of every febrile infant less than 8 weeks of age? Pediatrics 1991;88:821-824.

19. Heulitt MG, Ablow RC, Santos CC, et al: Febrile infants less than 3 months old: Value of chest radiography. Radiology 1988;167:135-137.

20. Bramson RT, Meyer TL, Silbiger ML, et al: The futility of the chest radiograph in the febrile infant without respiratory symptoms. Pediatrics 1993;92:524-526.

21. Mermel LA, Maki DG: Detection of bacteremia in adults: Consequences of culturing an inadequate volume of blood. Ann Intern Med 1993;119:270-272.

22. Isaacman DJ, Karasic RB, Reynolds EA, Kost SI: Effect of number of blood cultures and volume of blood on detection of bacteremia in children. J Pediatr 1996;128:190-195.

23. Schelonka RL, Chai MK, Yoder BA, et al: Volume of blood required to detect common neonatal pathogens. J Pediatr 1996;129:275-278.

24. Bonadio WA, Stanco L, Bruce R, et al: Reference values of normal cerebrospinal fluid composition in infants ages 0 to 8 weeks. Pediatr Infect Dis J 1992;11:589-591.

25. Bonadio WA: The cerebrospinal fluid: Physiologic aspects and alterations associated with bacterial meningitis. Pediatr Infect Dis J 1992;11:423-432.

26. Sarff LD, Platt LH, McCracken GH: Cerebrospinal fluid evaluation in neonates: Comparison of high-risk infants with and without meningitis. J Pediatr 1976;88:473-477.

27. Portnoy JM, Olson LC: Normal cerebrospinal fluid values in children: Another look. Pediatrics 1985;75:484-487.

28. Mazor SS, McNulty JE, Roosevelt GE: Interpretation of traumatic lumbar punctures: Who can go home? Pediatrics 2003;111:525-528.

29. Tebas P, Nease RF, Storch GA: Use of the polymerase chain reaction in the diagnosis of herpes simplex encephalitis: A decision analysis mode. Am J Med 1998;105:287-295.

30. Lakeman FD, Whitley RJ: Diagnosis of herpes simplex virus encephalitis: Application of polymerase chain reaction to cerebrospinal fluid from brain-biopsied patients and correlation with disease. J Infect Dis 1995;171:857-863.

31. Levine DA, Platt SL, Dayan PS, et al: Risk of serious bacterial infection in young febrile infants with respiratory syncytial virus infections. Pediatrics 2004;113:1728-1734.

32. Young PC: The management of febrile infants by primary-care pediatricians in Utah: Comparison with published practice guidelines. Pediatrics 1995;95:623-627.

33. Pantell RH, Newman TB, Bernzweig J, et al: Management and outcomes of care of fever in early infancy. JAMA 2004;291:1203-1212.

34. Brown JC, Burns JL, Cummings P: Ampicillin use in infant fever: A systematic review. Arch Pediatr Adolesc Med 2002;156:27-32.

35. Kimberlin DW, Lin CY, Jacobs RF, et al: Safety and efficacy of high-dose intravenous acyclovir in the management of neonatal herpes simplex virus infections. Pediatrics 2001;108:230-238.

36. Kaplan RL, Harper MB, Baskin MN, et al: Time to detection of positive cultures in 28- to 90-day-old infants. Pediatrics 2000;106:e74. Available at http://www.pediatrics.org/cgi/content/full/106/6/e74.

37. Joseph TA, Pyati SP, Jacobs N: Neonatal early-onset Escherichia coli disease: The effect of intrapartum ampicillin. Arch Pediatr Adolesc Med 1998;152:35-40.

38. Mercer BM, Carr TL, Beazley DD, et al: Antibiotic use in pregnancy and drug-resistant infant sepsis. Am J Obstet Gynecol 1999;181:816-821.

39. Shah SS, Ehrenkranz RA, Gallagher PG: Increasing incidence of gram-negative rod bacteremia in a newborn intensive care unit. Pediatr Infect Dis J 1999;18:591-595.

40. Fernandez M, Rench MA, Albanyan EA, et al: Failure of rifampin to eradicate group B streptococcal colonization in infants. Pediatr Infect Dis J 2001;20:371-376.

41. Atkins JT, Heresi GP, Coque TM, Baker CJ: Recurrent group B streptococcal disease in infants: Who should receive rifampin? J Pediatr 1998;132:537-539.

42. American College of Emergency Physicians Clinical Policies Committee, American College of Emergency Physicians Clinical Policies Subcommittee on Pediatric Fever: Clinical policy for children younger than three years presenting to the emergency department with fever. Ann Emerg Med 2003;42:530-545.

43. McGowan J, Bratton L, Klein J, Finland M: Bacteremia in febrile children seen in a "walk-in" pediatric clinic. N Engl J Med 1973;288:1309-1312.

44. Jaffe D, Tanz R, Davis T, et al: Antibiotic administration to treat possible occult bacteremia in febrile children. N Engl J Med 1987;317:1175-1180.

45. Fleisher GR, Rosenberg N, Vinci R, et al: Intramuscular versus oral antibiotic therapy for the prevention of meningitis and other bacterial sequelae in young, febrile children at risk for occult bacteremia. J Pediatr 1994;124:504-512.

46. Centers for Disease Control and Prevention: Progress toward elimination of Haemophilus influenzae type B disease among infants and children—United States, 1987-1995. MMWR Morb Mortal Wkly Rep 1996;45:901-906.

47. Black S, Shinefield H, Fireman B, et al: Efficacy, safety and immunogenicity of heptavalent pneumococcal conjugate vaccine in children. Northern California Kaiser Permanente Vaccine Study Center Group. Pediatr Infect Dis J 2000;19:187-195.

48. Black S, Shinefield H, Baxter R, et al: Postlicensure surveillance for pneumococcal invasive disease after use of heptavalent pneumococcal conjugate vaccine in Northern California Kaiser Permanente. Pediatr Infect Dis J 2004;23:485-489.

49. Kaplan SL, Mason EO Jr, Wald ER, et al: Decrease of invasive pneumococcal infections in children among 8 children's hospitals in the United States after the introduction of the 7-valent pneumococcal conjugate vaccine. Pediatrics 2004;113:443-449.

50. Lin PL, Michaels MG, Janosky J, et al: Incidence of invasive pneumococcal disease in children 3 to 36 months of age at a tertiary care pediatric center 2 years after licensure of the pneumococcal conjugate vaccine. Pediatrics 2003;111:896-899.

51. Poehling KA, Lafleur BJ, Szilagyi PG, et al: Population-based impact of pneumococcal conjugate vaccine in young children. Pediatrics 2004;114:755-761.

52. Teele DW, Pelton SI, Grant MJ, et al: Bacteremia in febrile children under 2 years of age: Results of cultures of blood of 600 consecutive febrile children seen in a "walk-in" clinic. J Pediatr 1975;87:227-230.

53. Bass J, Steele R, Wittler R, et al: Antimicrobial treatment of occult bacteremia: A multicenter cooperative study. Pediatr Infect Dis J 1993;12:466-473.

54. Alpern ER, Alessandrini EA, Bell LM, et al: Occult bacteremia from a pediatric emergency department: Current prevalence, time to detection, and outcome. Pediatrics 2000;106:505-511.

55. Lee GM, Harper MB: Risk of bacteremia for febrile young children in the post–*Haemophilus influenzae* type B era. Arch Pediatr Adolesc Med 1998;152:624-628.

56. Whitney CG, Farley MM, Hadler J, et al: Decline in invasive pneumococcal disease after the introduction of protein-polysaccharide conjugate vaccine. N Engl J Med 2003;348:1737-1746.

57. Stoll ML, Rubin LG: Incidence of occult bacteremia among highly febrile young children in the era of the pneumococcal conjugate vaccine. Arch Pediatr Adolesc Med 2004;158:671-675.

58. Schutzman S, Petrycki S, Fleisher G: Bacteremia with otitis media. Pediatrics 1991;87:48-53.

59. Kuppermann N, Fleisher GR, Jaffe DM:. Predictors of occult pneumococcal bacteremia in young febrile children. Ann Emerg Med 1998; 31:679-687.

60. Shah SS, Alpern ER, Zwerling L, et al: Low risk of bacteremia in children with febrile seizures. Arch Pediatr Adolesc Med 2002;156:469-472.

61. Trainor JL, Hampers LC, Krug SE, Listernick R: Children with first-time simple febrile seizures are at low risk of serious bacterial illness. Acad Emerg Med 2001;8:781-787.

62. Kuppermann N, Bank DE, Walton EA, et al: Risks for bacteremia and urinary tract infections in young febrile children with bronchiolitis. Arch Pediatr Adolesc Med 1997;15:1207-1214.

63. Greenes DS, Harper MB: Low risk of bacteremia in febrile children with recognizable viral syndromes. Pediatr Infect Dis J 1999;18:258-261.

64. Jaffe D, Fleisher G: Temperature and total white blood cell count as indicators of bacteremia. Pediatrics 1991;87:670-674.

65. Pulliam PN, Attia MW, Cronan KM: C-reactive protein in febrile children 1 to 36 months of age with clinically undetectable serious bacterial infection. Pediatrics 2001;108:1275-1279.

66. Isaacman DJ, Burke BL: Utility of the serum C-reactive protein for detection of occult bacterial infection in children. Arch Pediatr Adolesc Med 2002;156:905-909.

67. Long SS: Antibiotic therapy in febrile children: "Best-laid schemes." J Pediatr 1994;124:585-588.

68. Rothrock SG, Harper MB, Green SM, et al: Do oral antibiotics prevent meningitis and serious bacterial infections in children with *Streptococcus pneumoniae* occult bacteremia? A meta-analysis. Pediatrics 1997;99:438-444.

69. Bulloch B, Craig WR, Klassen TP: The use of antibiotics to prevent serious sequelae in children at risk for occult bacteremia: A meta-analysis. Acad Emerg Med 1997;4:679-683.

70. Bandyopadhyay S, Bergholte J, Blackwell CD: Risk of serious bacterial infection in children with fever without a source in the post–*Haemophilus influenzae* era when antibiotics are reserved for culture-proven bacteremia. Arch Pediatr Adolesc Med 2002;156:512-517.

71. Bachur R, Harper MB: Reevaluation of outpatients with *Streptococcus pneumoniae* bacteremia. Pediatrics 2000;105:502-509.

72. McGowan KL, Foster JA, Coffin SE: Outpatient pediatric blood cultures: Time to positivity. Pediatrics 2000;106:251-255.

73. Neuman MI, Harper MB: Time to positivity of blood cultures for children with *Streptococcus pneumoniae* bacteremia. Clin Infect Dis 2001;33: 1324-1328.

74. Neuman MI, Harper MB: Evaluation of a rapid urine antigen assay for the detection of invasive pneumococcal disease in children. Pediatrics 2003;112:1279-1282.

75. Galetto-Lacour A, Zamora SA, Gervaix A: Bedside procalcitonin and C-reactive protein tests in children with fever without localizing signs of infection seen in a referral center. Pediatrics 2003;112:1054-1060.

CHAPTER 61

Prolonged Fever and Fever of Unknown Origin

Samir S. Shah and Elizabeth R. Alpern

In 1961, Petersdorf and Beeson proposed their now classic criteria for fever of unknown origin (FUO): (1) an illness of at least 3 weeks' duration, (2) measured temperatures greater than 38.3°C on several occasions, and (3) no diagnosis after 1 week of hospitalization.[1] For adult patients, Durack and Street modified the third criterion of this definition to account for potential outpatient evaluation by substituting "3 outpatient visits or at least 3 days in the hospital" for "1 week of hospitalization."[2] Studies focusing on pediatric patients have occasionally used a fever duration of 2 rather than 3 weeks. Patients presenting with 2 to 3 weeks of fever but not meeting all the criteria for FUO are often referred to as having prolonged fever. Differentiating prolonged fever from FUO can be impractical, because the diagnostic criteria for FUO do not specify the type or extent of evaluation required. Final diagnoses are determined in a number of ways (e.g., natural history, biopsy, imaging, serologic studies), and no single patient either receives or requires every diagnostic test. This chapter discusses the evaluation of a child with prolonged fever in whom the cause of fever is not readily apparent.

CLINICAL PRESENTATION

For purposes of this chapter, FUO means (1) fever of prolonged duration (>2 weeks), (2) documented temperature higher than 38.3°C (101°F) on multiple occasions, and (3) uncertain cause. Up to 50% of patients referred for evaluation of FUO have multiple, unrelated, self-limited infections, parental misinterpretation of normal temperature variation, or complete absence of fever at the time of referral.[3-5] Therefore, the initial history should include the method used to determine temperature (e.g., "felt warm" versus actual measurement), the duration of thermometer insertion, location of insertion (tympanic membrane, oral, axillary, rectal), time of day, and confirmation by more than one person. Studies examining parents' ability to subjectively determine the presence of fever found a sensitivity of 74% to 84% and a specificity of 76% to 91% for tactile examination.[6-9] Some studies of tactile examination reveal more accurate results for higher temperatures (>38.9°C) than for lower ones. The location of measurement also affects the accuracy of the reading. The oral temperature can be 0.3°C to 0.7°C lower than a simultaneous rectal measurement.[10] Oral measurements are more easily influenced by other factors such as oral liquid intake and respiratory rate. Tandberg and Sklar reported that the difference between rectal and oral measurements increased from 0.5°C to almost 1°C in patients with tachypnea.[11] Axillary and tympanic measurements are at least 0.5°C lower than simultaneous oral measurements.[12] To compensate for such discrepancies, parents are sometimes instructed to add 0.5°C or 1°C to oral or axillary measurements to approximate the "real" temperature. Such corrections are often inaccurate, however, because the amount of underestimation varies from person to person and with the body temperature (differences are exacerbated at higher body temperatures); these corrections may further cloud the evaluation of a febrile child. The timing of measurement is also important because children's body temperature exhibits a daily variation; the normal temperature may be as high as 37.4°C (99.3°F) orally or 38.0°C (100.4°F) rectally in children older than 2 months and peaks in the early evening.[3]

DIFFERENTIAL DIAGNOSIS

New and more sensitive laboratory assays (e.g., polymerase chain reaction) and radiologic scanning procedures (e.g., magnetic resonance imaging) permit the earlier detection of many conditions. As a result, the differential diagnosis of FUO has evolved. In the 1960s and 1970s only 10% to 25% of children presenting with FUO had fever resolution without determination of a cause.[4,5,13-17] In more recent studies, the fever resolved in up to two thirds of children without a specific discharge diagnosis. Infection remains the most common cause of FUO; rheumatologic diseases and malignancy are much less common (Table 61-1). A comprehensive list of causes is provided (Table 61-2).[3,18] In most cases of FUO, the cause of the fever is a common pediatric infection with an uncommonly long time course. In a series by Jacobs and Schutze, Epstein-Barr viral infections (15%), osteomyelitis 10%), cat-scratch disease (5%), and urinary tract infection (4%) were the most frequent causes of FUO.[17] Some infections caused by typical pathogens may be partially treated, blunting other manifestations of the disease. The causes of recurrent fevers differ from those of prolonged fever and FUO (Table 61-3).[19,20] Recurrent fevers are not discussed in detail in this chapter.

DIAGNOSIS

A thorough history and physical examination are paramount in safely managing a child with FUO. In studies by Pizzo and colleagues,[4] McClung,[14] and Lohr and Hendley,[15] a careful history and physical examination yielded the ultimate diagnosis in more than two thirds of patients, usually after repeated encounters. The pattern and duration of fever, response to antipyretic therapy, and presence of nonspecific complaints (e.g., anorexia, fatigue, weight loss) did not accurately predict the patient's diagnosis.[4]

A number of specific questions can contribute to making the diagnosis. The physician should attempt to clarify exposure to animals, travel history, pica, antecedent illnesses, family history, and medication use. Animal exposure includes not only pets within the home but also contact with animals owned by friends and acquaintances or encountered at school. Household contacts may have occupational

Table 61-1 Diagnoses in Pediatric Case Series of Prolonged Fever or Fever of Unknown Origin Including at Least 50 Patients*

	Brewis (1965)[13]	McClung (1972)[14]	Pizzo et al (1975)[4]	Feigin & Shearer (1976)[5]	Lohr & Hendley (1977)[15]	Steele et al (1991)[16]	Jacobs & Schutze (1998)[17]	Total
No. of patients	165	99	100	146	54	109	146	819
No established diagnosis	44 (27)	32 (32)	12 (12)	24 (16)	10 (19)	73 (67)	62 (42)	257 (31)
Infection	91 (55)	29 (29)	52 (52)	88 (60)	18 (33)	24 (22)	64 (44)	366 (45)
Rheumatologic	9 (5)	11 (11)	20 (20)	10 (7)	11 (20)	7 (6)	11 (8)	79 (10)
Malignancy	3 (2)	8 (8)	6 (6)	2 (1)	7 (13)	2 (2)	4 (3)	32 (4)
Other[†]	18 (11)	19 (19)	10 (10)	22 (15)	8 (15)	3 (3)	5 (3)	85 (10)

*Values listed are numbers of cases, with percentages in parentheses. Percentage values may not total 100 owing to rounding.
[†]Includes drug fever, central nervous system fever, heavy metal poisoning, factitious fever, inflammatory bowel disease, and other conditions.

Table 61-2 Causes of Prolonged Fever and Fever of Unknown Origin in Previously Healthy Children

Infection
Common infections
  Respiratory infection
    Otitis media, mastoiditis
    Sinusitis
    Cervical adenitis
    Peritonsillar or retropharyngeal abscess
    Pneumonia
  Systemic viral syndrome
  Urinary tract infection
  Central nervous system infection
    Meningitis, meningoencephalitis
    Intracranial abscess
  Bone or joint infection
    Osteomyelitis
    Septic arthritis
    Paravertebral abscess
  Enteric infection (e.g., *Salmonella, Shigella*)
  Cat-scratch disease
Less common infections
  Tuberculosis
  Infectious mononucleosis (Epstein-Barr virus, cytomegalovirus)
  Tick-borne diseases (e.g., Lyme disease, Rocky Mountain spotted fever, ehrlichiosis)
  Malaria
  Periodontal infection
  Endocarditis or endovascular infection
  Human immunodeficiency virus (HIV) infection
  Acute rheumatic fever
Uncommon infections
  Other zoonoses (brucellosis, leptospirosis, Q fever, tularemia)
  Intra-abdominal abscess
  Toxoplasmosis
  Syphilis
  Parvovirus B19 infection
  Rubella
  Endemic mycoses (e.g., histoplasmosis, blastomycosis, coccidioidomycosis)
  Psittacosis
  Chronic meningococcemia

Collagen Vascular Disease
Juvenile rheumatoid arthritis
Systemic lupus erythematosus
Dermatomyositis
Scleroderma
Sarcoidosis
Vasculitis (Wegener granulomatosis, polyarteritis nodosa, Behçet syndrome)

Malignancy*
Leukemia
Lymphoma

Drug Fever*
Penicillins
Cephalosporins
Sulfonamides
Phenytoin
Methylphenidate
Acetaminophen

Factitious Fever
Pseudofever
Munchausen syndrome
Munchausen syndrome by proxy

Other Considerations
Central fever
Kawasaki syndrome
Inflammatory bowel disease
Hemophagocytic syndrome

*Only common causes listed.

Table 61-3 Causes of Recurrent Fever

Regular Intervals
Cyclic neutropenia
Epstein-Barr virus infection*
Familial Mediterranean fever
Hyperimmunoglobulinemia D syndrome
Periodic fever with aphthous stomatitis, pharyngitis, and
   adenitis (PFAPA) syndrome
Relapsing fever (*Borrelia* species other than *burgdorferi*)*

Less Predictable Intervals
Behçet disease
Brucellosis
Central nervous system abnormalities (e.g., hypothalamic
   dysfunction)
Chronic meningococcemia
Familial dysautonomia (Riley-Day syndrome)
Inflammatory bowel disease
Lymphoma
Muckle-Wells syndrome
Nontuberculous mycobacteria
Parvovirus B19
Relapsing malaria *(Plasmodium vivax, Plasmodium ovale)*
Serial viral infections
Systemic-onset juvenile rheumatoid arthritis
Tuberculosis
Tumor necrosis factor receptor–associated periodic fever
   syndrome (TRAPS)
Yersinia enterocolitica

*May also occur at less predictable intervals.

exposure to farm animals or rodents. The animal exposure history should also include questions regarding the consumption of unpasteurized dairy products and raw or undercooked meats, as well as participation in recreational activities such as hunting. Travel-related questions should elicit details about foreign travel, appropriate pretravel immunizations, antimalarial prophylaxis, and measures taken to avoid contaminated food and water (*Salmonella typhi, Shigella* species, and others). The physician should also inquire about artifacts from distant regions, which may harbor disease-causing organisms. Travel to or past residence in certain areas within the United States may also clarify the cause of fever. For example, the endemic mycoses are related to travel to the Southeast (blastomycosis), Southwest (coccidioidomycosis), and Midwest (histoplasmosis). A family history of hemoglobinopathy, immune deficiency, and autoimmune disease can guide the evaluation. The patient's ethnicity may also suggest a cause, because some diseases are more prevalent among certain ethnic groups—for example, familial Mediterranean fever (Armenian, Arab, Turkish, Sephardic Jew), hyperimmunoglobulinemia D syndrome (Dutch, French), and tumor necrosis factor receptor–associated periodic fever syndrome (TRAPS) (Irish, Scottish).

Medications are often associated with fever. Drug fever, defined as a febrile response to a drug in the absence of cutaneous manifestations, may be difficult to recognize because the presentation is often subtle. The mechanisms of drug fever remain poorly understood. Five main pathophysiologic mechanisms are used to classify drug fever: (1) altered thermoregulatory mechanism (e.g., cimetidine, anticholinergic agents), (2) drug administration-related fever (e.g., amphotericin B, vancomycin, streptomycin), (3) fevers relating to the pharmacologic action of a drug (e.g., Jarisch-Herxheimer reaction in the treatment of spirochete-induced illness), (4) idiosyncratic reaction, and (5) hypersensitivity reaction.[21] Drug fevers may occur any time after the initiation of therapy, but they frequently appear after 1 to 2 weeks of therapy. The patient usually appears remarkably well despite the presence of fever; however, rigors and other symptoms of systemic toxicity do not preclude a medication-related fever. Drug fever should be considered in a person receiving a potentially sensitizing medication with an otherwise unexplained fever. Medications implicated in drug fevers are extensive and include β-lactam antibiotics, pain medications (acetaminophen, ibuprofen, aspirin), antireflux agents (metoclopramide, cimetidine), corticosteroids, methylphenidate, anticonvulsants, and sulfa-containing medications, including some stool softeners. Discontinuation of the offending agent results in resolution of the fever within 72 hours. Failure to recognize drug fever can lead to prolonged hospitalization, unnecessary diagnostic testing, and continuation or readministration of the sensitizing medication.

EVALUATION

The approach to a child with FUO involves (1) documenting the fever, (2) completing a thorough history and physical examination, (3) creating a broad differential diagnosis, (4) performing the initial laboratory evaluation (accounting for relevant findings on the history and physical examination) and tailoring it to the severity of the patient's illness, and (5) basing the subsequent evaluation on results of the initial laboratory studies and a repeated history and physical examination (Table 61-4). Early in the diagnostic process, the child's caretaker should be urged to keep a fever diary or calendar documenting the temperature and time of measurement. Such documentation can clarify the presence or absence of a true fever, as well as determine whether the fever is prolonged or recurrent; this latter distinction has implications for the differential diagnosis (see Table 61-3). Pizzo and colleagues emphasized the importance of carefully reviewing laboratory data. Failure to correctly use existing data occurred in the evaluation of 50% of their cases; this was the most important reason for failure to make the diagnosis before hospitalization.[4]

A "shotgun" approach to the evaluation of FUO is seldom useful. Such an approach often creates misleading false-positive results and additional unnecessary testing. Steele and coworkers evaluated the benefit of radiologic scanning procedures in children with FUO.[16] Children with fever higher than 38.0°C, a fever duration of longer than 3 weeks, and a normal initial physical examination were included in the study. A specific diagnosis was determined in 36 of 109 children (33%). Abnormal results were detected in 8 of 43 (19%) abdominal ultrasound procedures, 5 of 11 (45%) indium scans, 1 of 4 (25%) gallium scans, 2 of 13 (15%) upper gastrointestinal barium studies with small bowel follow-through, 2 of 15 (13%) bone scans, and 1 of 16 (6%) bone marrow examinations. However, the abnormalities identified by these studies suggested a specific

Table 61-4 Studies to Consider in the Initial and Subsequent Diagnostic Evaluations* of Children with Prolonged Fever or Fever of Unknown Origin

Specimen	Initial Investigation	Subsequent Investigation
Blood	Blood culture Complete blood count Peripheral blood smear C-reactive protein Erythrocyte sedimentation rate Hepatic function panel Human immunodeficiency virus (HIV) antibodies Initial infectious disease serologic studies[†] Antinuclear antibody	Repeat blood culture (×3) Second-line infectious disease serologic studies[†]
Urine	Urinalysis Urine culture	Repeat urinalysis Repeat urine culture
Stool	Hemoccult testing Culture (bacterial and viral) Ova and parasite examination (×3)[§]	*Clostridium difficile* toxins A and B
Radiologic	Chest radiograph	Sinus CT Upper GI barium study with small bowel follow-through Abdominal CT or ultrasonography MRI of pelvis, spine, or specific extremities Bone or gallium scan Echocardiogram
Other	Tuberculin skin test Nasal aspirate for rapid viral antigen detection[¶] Throat swab for rapid streptococcal antigen testing and culture	Ophthalmic examination Lumbar puncture Bone marrow biopsy Evaluation for primary immune deficiency

*Findings on the history and physical examination should direct the initial evaluation. Findings on the history, physical examination, and initial laboratory evaluation should direct the subsequent evaluation. A patient usually does not require all the tests listed.

[†]If relevant exposures can be documented, consider serologic testing for hepatitis A, B, and C; tularemia; brucellosis; leptospirosis; Rocky Mountain spotted fever; ehrlichiosis; Q fever; dengue fever; or leptospirosis.

[‡]Potential serologic studies include Epstein-Barr virus, cytomegalovirus, *Bartonella henselae* (cat-scratch disease), *Borrelia burgdorferi* (Lyme disease), antistreptolysin-O and anti-DNase B (group A β-hemolytic streptococci).

[§]Antigen testing is available for some organisms, including *Giardia lamblia*, *Cryptosporidium parvum*, and *Entamoeba histolytica*.

[¶]Viral antigens detectable by immunofluorescence include respiratory syncytial virus, influenza viruses A and B, parainfluenza viruses types 1 to 3, and adenovirus. A polymerase chain reaction–based assay provides a highly sensitive method of detecting adenovirus from nasopharyngeal aspirates, sputum, and conjunctival swabs.

CT, computed tomography; GI, gastrointestinal; MRI, magnetic resonance imaging.

diagnosis in only 7 children; in many of the other cases, the significance of the abnormalities evident on imaging was not known.[16]

Routine echocardiography is also a low-yield procedure in the evaluation of a child with FUO. In one study examining the role of echocardiography in the diagnosis of endocarditis, persistent fever was the most common reason for performing an echocardiogram.[22] Endocarditis was associated with at least two positive blood culture results, congestive heart failure, a new or changing heart murmur, and hematuria; no patient had fever as the sole manifestation of endocarditis. The Duke criteria may facilitate the evaluation for endocarditis (see Chapter 84).[23]

Other tests listed in Table 61-4 are performed even less often. Uveitis, detected by ophthalmic examination, suggests Behçet disease, Kawasaki syndrome, tuberculosis, syphilis, sarcoidosis, inflammatory bowel disease, or juvenile rheumatoid arthritis (polyarticular or pauciarticular, but not systemic). Bone marrow biopsy can detect some malignan-

cies and some infections. Certain organisms that cause FUO readily grow in culture of bone marrow specimens: *Salmonella* species, mycobacteria, *Brucella*, and *Histoplasma capsulatum*. Lumbar puncture occasionally diagnoses the cause of FUO in patients with chronic headache or other signs of central nervous system infection. Organisms and the appropriate tests to detect them include the following:

- Enterovirus: serum, urine, and cerebrospinal fluid (CSF) polymerase chain reaction (PCR)
- Herpes simplex virus: CSF PCR
- *Cryptococcus neoformans*: serum and CSF cryptococcal antigen and CSF culture and India ink stain
- *Mycobacterium tuberculosis*: CSF acid-fast smear and culture
- West Nile virus: serum antibodies and CSF PCR
- *Borrelia burgdorferi*: serum and CSF antibodies
- *Mycoplasma pneumoniae*: nasopharyngeal, throat, and CSF PCR

ADMISSION CRITERIA

Ill-appearing children require hospitalization. There are no firm criteria for the hospitalization of well-appearing patients with FUO. Generally, all the initial investigations (see Table 61-4) can be performed in the outpatient setting. Hospitalization should be considered for children requiring extensive subspecialist consultation or invasive procedures (e.g., lumbar puncture).

TREATMENT

Treatment depends on the diagnosis. The utility of empirical therapy, such as antibiotics, antituberculosis agents, or corticosteroids, has not been studied in FUO. In children who appear well, empirical therapy may further cloud the diagnosis.

DISCHARGE CRITERIA

The diagnosis determines the appropriate time for discharge. For patients in whom a diagnosis cannot be ascertained, outpatient follow-up is appropriate. Talano and Katz described the long-term outcome in children with FUO in whom no diagnosis was established after inpatient evaluation.[24] Among the 19 patients studied, 16 had resolution of fever without recurrence, 2 were diagnosed with juvenile rheumatoid arthritis, and 1 patient had recurrent intussusception. Follow-up information was available for 63 of 73 patients studied by Steele and colleagues for whom no diagnosis could be established.[16] Most of these children recovered uneventfully; 9 of them had continuation or recurrence of fever for brief periods, with ultimate resolution and no specific diagnosis (one patient's fevers resolved after 3 years). Nine additional patients were initially diagnosed with juvenile rheumatoid arthritis; on follow-up, 5 had resolution of fever without further recurrence, and 4 had evidence of infectious processes, including Lyme disease, psittacosis, toxoplasmosis, and cat-scratch disease.

IN A NUTSHELL

- Fifty percent of cases referred for evaluation of FUO have multiple, unrelated, self-limited infections; parental misinterpretation of normal temperature variations; or absence of fever at the time of evaluation.
- Most cases of FUO resolve without determination of a specific cause, but infections are the most common identifiable cause of FUO.
- The evaluation of FUO should include confirmation of fever, a thorough history and physical examination, and a targeted laboratory evaluation guided by the patient's signs and symptoms.

ON THE HORIZON

- PCR-based assays for additional bacteria and viruses.

SUGGESTED READING

Jacobs RF, Schutze GE: *Bartonella henselae* as a cause of prolonged fever and fever of unknown origin in children. Clin Infect Dis 1998;26:80-84.

Li JS, Sexton DJ, Mick N, et al: Proposed modifications to the Duke criteria for the diagnosis of infective endocarditis. Clin Infect Dis 2000;30:633-638.

Steele RW, Jones SM, Lowe BA, Glasier CM: Usefulness of scanning procedures for diagnosis of fever of unknown origin in children. J Pediatr 1991;119:526-530.

REFERENCES

1. Petersdorf RB, Beeson PB: Fever of unexplained origin: Report on 100 cases. Medicine 1961;40:1-30.
2. Durack DT, Street AC: Fever of unknown origin—reexamined and redefined. In Remington JS, Swartz MN (eds): Current Clinical Topics in Infectious Diseases. Boston, Blackwell Science, 1991, pp 35-51.
3. Calello DP, Shah SS: The child with fever of unknown origin. Pediatr Case Rev 2002;2:226-239.
4. Pizzo PA, Lovejoy FH Jr, Smith DH: Prolonged fever in children: Review of 100 cases. Pediatrics 1975;55:468-473.
5. Feigin RD, Shearer WT: Fever of unknown origin in children. Curr Probl Pediatr 1976;6:2-65.
6. Banco L, Veltri D: Ability of mothers to subjectively assess the presence of fever in their children. Am J Dis Child 1984;138:976-978.
7. Alves JG, Correia J: Ability of mothers to assess the presence of fever in their children without using a thermometer. Trop Doct 2002;32:145-146.
8. Hooker EA, Smith SW, Miles T, King L: Subjective assessment of fever by parents: Comparison with measurement by noncontact tympanic thermometer and calibrated rectal glass mercury thermometer. Ann Emerg Med 1996;28:313-317.
9. Graneto JW, Soglin DF: Maternal screening of childhood fever by palpation. Pediatr Emerg Care 1996;12:183-184.
10. Gartner JC Jr: Fever of unknown origin. Adv Pediatr Infect Dis 1992;7:1-24.
11. Tandberg D, Sklar D: Effect of tachypnea on the estimation of body temperature by an oral thermometer. N Engl J Med 1983;308:945-946.
12. Falzon A, Grech V, Caruana B, et al: How reliable is axillary temperature measurement? Acta Paediatr 2003;92:309-313.
13. Brewis EG: Undiagnosed fever. BMJ 1965;9:107-109.
14. McClung HJ: Prolonged fever of unknown origin in children. Am J Dis Child 1972;124:544-550.
15. Lohr JA, Hendley JO: Prolonged fever of unknown origin: A record of experiences with 54 childhood patients. Clin Pediatr 1977;16:768-773.
16. Steele RW, Jones SM, Lowe BA, Glasier CM: Usefulness of scanning procedures for diagnosis of fever of unknown origin in children. J Pediatr 1991;119:526-530.
17. Jacobs RF, Schutze GE: *Bartonella henselae* as a cause of prolonged fever and fever of unknown origin in children. Clin Infect Dis 1998;26:80-84.
18. Shah SS: Fever. In Shah SS, Ludwig S (eds): Pediatric Complaints and Diagnostic Dilemmas: A Case-Based Approach. Philadelphia, Lippincott Williams & Wilkins, 2004, pp 291-317.
19. John CC, Gilsdorf JR: Recurrent fever in children. Pediatr Infect Dis J 2002;21:1071-1080.
20. Drenth JPH, Van Der Meer JWM: Hereditary periodic fever. N Engl J Med 2001;345:1748-1757.
21. Johnson DH, Cunha BA: Drug fever. Infect Dis Clin North Am 1996;10:85-91.
22. Aly AM, Simpson PM, Humes RA: The role of transthoracic echocardiography in the diagnosis of infective endocarditis in children. Arch Pediatr Adolesc Med 1999;153:950-954.
23. Li JS, Sexton DJ, Mick N, et al: Proposed modifications to the Duke criteria for the diagnosis of infective endocarditis. Clin Infect Dis 2000;30:633-638.
24. Talano JM, Katz BZ: Long-term follow-up of children with fever of unknown origin. Clin Pediatr 2000;39:715-717.

CHAPTER 62

Fever and Rash

E. Douglas Thompson and Keith D. Herzog

Fever is one of the most common presenting complaints in the acute care setting, and rash is frequently an associated sign. The disorders that present with these two features range from benign and self-limited to rapidly progressive and life threatening. When evaluating a patient with fever and rash, the entire clinical picture must be considered to narrow down the broad range of possible illnesses.

Skin lesions can be characterized by their morphology, color, distribution, and pattern. Based on this characterization, rash associated with fever can be broken down into six major categories:

1. Morbilliform
2. Vesiculobullous
3. Erythema multiforme
4. Scarlatiniform
5. Erythroderma
6. Petechia or purpura

The character of the rash, combined with other signs and symptoms, frequently suggests a specific cause of a febrile illness.

Morbilliform rash is described as a generalized erythematous to pink maculopapular rash that demonstrates blanching with pressure. Measles and rubella are the classic infections falling into this category; however, widespread vaccination makes these causes unlikely. Features of the classic viral exanthems, including measles and rubella, are outlined in Table 62-1. Studies evaluating immunized pediatric patients with morbilliform rash identified specific causes in 37% to 48% of cases.[1,2] Parvovirus, human herpesvirus 6, enteroviruses, and adenovirus were implicated, in descending order of frequency. Group A streptococcus was isolated from throat cultures in about 15% of patients in one study, although streptococcal infections are typically associated with a scarlatiniform rash. The remaining patients presumably had other unspecified self-limited viral infections, although drug eruption and Kawasaki disease should be considered in the differential diagnosis. Fever, rhinorrhea, and cough were the most frequent symptoms associated with these illnesses.

The causes of vesiculobullous rash and fever are better defined. A generalized pattern of vesicles on an erythematous base ("dewdrops on a rose petal") in various stages of eruption is characteristic of varicella (chickenpox). A dermatomal distribution suggests herpes zoster, particularly in patients with a history of previous varicella infection or vaccination. Vesicular lesions distributed on the palms and soles associated with mouth ulcers suggest hand-foot-and-mouth disease secondary to enterovirus infection, most commonly caused by coxsackievirus A16. Herpes simplex virus (HSV) causes localized vesicular lesions such as gingivostomatitis,

herpes labialis and other genital infections, herpetic whitlow, and keratoconjunctivitis, typically with periocular skin involvement. A vesicular eruption in the neonatal period, with or without fever, raises the suspicion for neonatal HSV infection (see Chapter 53). Bullae associated with erythema multiforme and mucosal involvement are characteristic of Stevens-Johnson syndrome. Staphylococcal scalded skin syndrome (see Chapter 157) and toxic epidermal necrolysis (see Chapter 161) result in bullae with significant skin peeling. See Chapter 151 for a more complete discussion of disorders associated with vesicular and bullous lesions.

Target lesions are the hallmark of erythema multiforme, appearing as fixed, symmetrical, round lesions with concentric rings and central duskiness. The distribution is typically acral. Erythema multiforme major and minor are differentiated by the presence or absence of mucosal involvement (Fig. 62-1). The diagnosis of erythema multiforme major requires the involvement of two or more mucous membrane surfaces, and the lesions may develop bullae (Fig. 62-2). Many experts believe that erythema multiforme major and Stevens-Johnson syndrome are synonymous. Others differentiate the two, with the presence of bullae and a more truncal distribution defining Stevens-Johnson syndrome. In both entities, the histopathology of early lesions is similar, demonstrating perivascular mononuclear cell infiltrates.[3] Although a host of infectious diseases can be associated with erythema multiforme, HSV is associated with more than 50% of cases of the minor type, whereas *Mycoplasma pneumoniae* is the agent most commonly implicated in patients with Stevens-Johnson syndrome.[3] Kawasaki disease may also present with erythema multiforme. Erythema multiforme is discussed in Chapter 160.

Petechiae are small red or purple lesions that do not blanch with pressure. Purpura are larger, nonblanching, brown or purple lesions that can be palpable or nonpalpable. Fever associated with these lesions may represent life-threatening conditions such as meningococcal and rickettsial infections. Scarlatina is a diffuse, fine papular rash with a "sandpaper" texture. A characteristic of this rash is exaggeration in the antecubital, axillary, and inguinal folds known as Pastia lines (Fig. 62-3). Erythroderma is a diffuse erythema of the skin that is similar in appearance to sunburn (Fig. 62-4). A distinguishing feature is extensive involvement of the skin that does not follow the pattern of sun exposure seen with sunburn. Scarlatina and erythroderma raise the possibility of bacterial toxin production and toxic shock syndrome.

The remainder of this chapter focuses on specific infectious diseases, including further discussion of the differential diagnoses of febrile illnesses associated with these dermatologic manifestations.

Table 62-1   Key Features of Classic Childhood Exanthems

Disease	Cause	Rash	Clinical Findings	Complications
Measles	Measles virus	Morbilliform rash, spreads from head to feet	Koplik spots, fever, cough, coryza, conjunctivitis	Bronchopneumonia, encephalitis, otitis media, myocarditis, encephalomyelitis, subacute sclerosing panencephalitis
Rubella (German measles)	Rubella virus	Discrete papular rash, spreads from head to feet	Enanthema, rhinorrhea, tender adenopathy (postauricular, posterior cervical, postoccipital), low-grade fever	Congenital rubella syndrome, arthritis, neuritis, encephalitis
Chickenpox	Varicella virus	Generalized, vesicular; "dewdrop on a rose petal"	Fever, malaise, myalgias, pruritus	Bacterial skin infection, pneumonia, hepatitis, encephalitis, cerebellar ataxia, other postinfectious neurologic syndromes, Reye syndrome
Erythema infectiosum (fifth disease)	Parvovirus B19	Erythematous, lacy, reticular rash on trunk and extremities; "slapped cheek" appearance	Mild symptoms: headache, coryza, myalgia, arthralgia	Aplastic crisis in patients with chronic hemolysis, chronic anemia in those with immunodeficiency, arthritis
Exanthema subitum (roseola)	Human herpesvirus 6	Centrally located, pink macular rash; onset as fever dissipates	No symptoms common; mild rhinorrhea occasionally	Febrile seizures
Scarlet fever	*Streptococcus pyogenes*	Tiny, papular "sandpaper" rash; predilection for skin folds	Exudative pharyngitis, "strawberry" tongue, late desquamation	Postinfectious sequelae (rheumatic fever, glomerulonephritis)

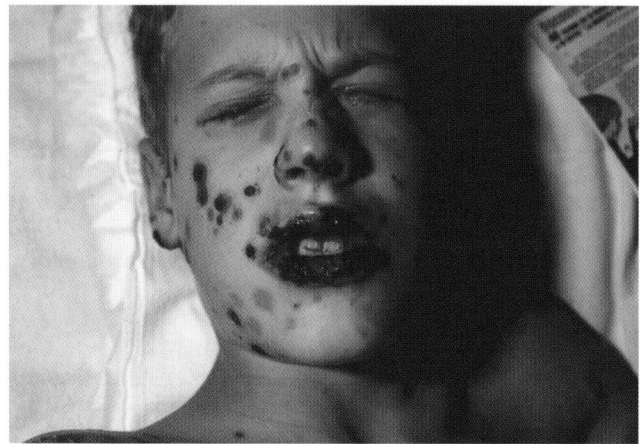

Figure 62-1   Stevens-Johnson syndrome with hemorrhagic crusting of the oral mucosa.

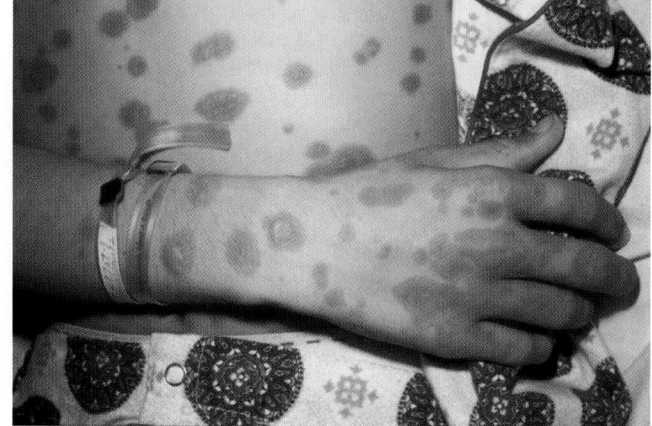

Figure 62-2   Erythema multiforme rash in an 8-year-old boy demonstrating discrete target lesions on the trunk and extremity, with confluence distally. Central bullae are seen in the lesion of the dorsal wrist.

MENINGOCOCCAL INFECTIONS

Meningococcal infections are caused by the gram-negative diplococcus *Neisseria meningitidis*. The peak incidence of these infections is during the first year of life, after passive maternal antibody protection begins to wane; 40% of cases occur in children younger than 5 years. A smaller peak occurs during adolescence and young adulthood, with military recruits and college freshmen living in dormitories considered at higher risk. Asplenia, complement deficiencies, immunoglobulin deficiencies, and infection with human immunodeficiency virus (HIV) are risk factors for the development of meningococcal infections.

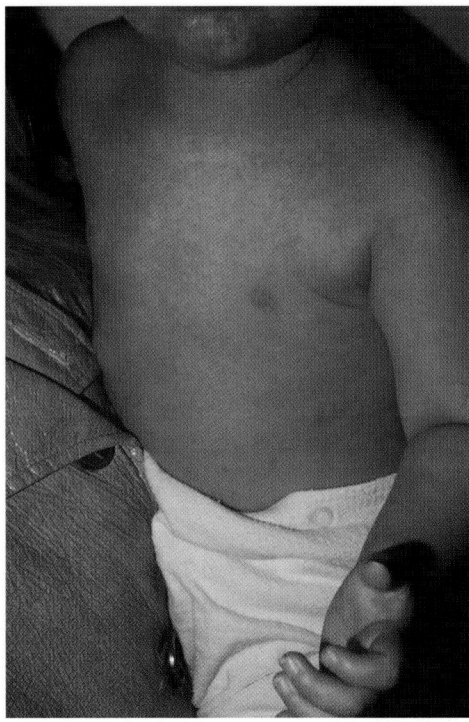

Figure 62-3 Scarlatina in an 18-month-old child with group A streptococcal pharyngitis.

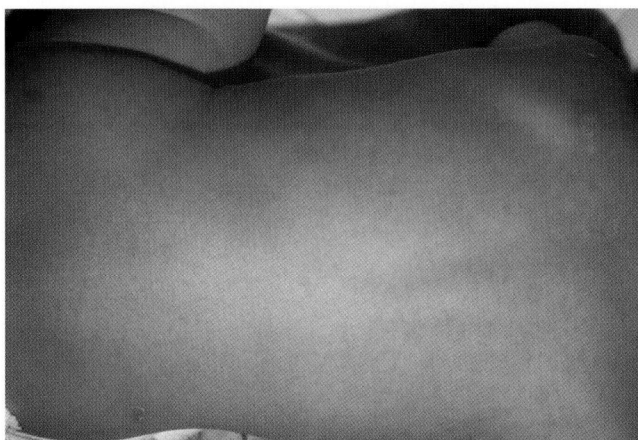

Figure 62-4 Erythroderma.

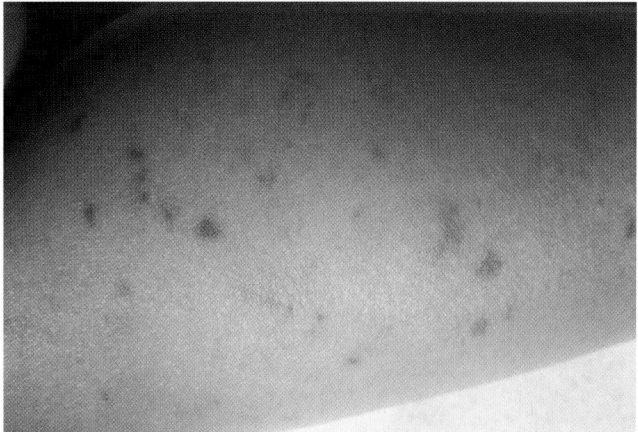

Figure 62-5 Maculopapular rash early in the course of meningococcemia.

Humans are the only reservoir for *N. meningitidis,* and the bacteria reside in the nasopharynx. In nonendemic areas, 5% to 10% of individuals are asymptomatic carriers. Transmission is person to person through respiratory droplets or direct contact with secretions through activities such as kissing or the sharing of drinking glasses. Disease develops when a pathogenic strain of *N. meningitidis* translocates across the mucosal barrier, with subsequent bacteremia. Exposure to cigarette smoke and concurrent upper respiratory infection are risk factors for this process. Once the bacteria enter the bloodstream, the release of lipopolysaccharides and other bacterial factors results in the release of cytokines and tumor necrosis factor, activation of the complement system, and subsequent development of the systemic inflammatory response. This response, in conjunction with a bacteria-induced procoagulant state, results in the clinical features seen in meningococcemia. Purpura develops as a result of vasculitis and thrombosis in the blood vessels of the skin. Meningococcal meningitis is secondary to bacterial seeding of the meninges subsequent to bacteremia.

Clinical Presentation

The classic presentation of meningococcemia is the acute onset of fever in association with petechiae or purpura. Headache, myalgia, nausea, and vomiting may be present. Altered mental status, photophobia, and neck stiffness suggest meningitis. Tachycardia, hypotension, and poor perfusion are evidence of septic shock. Early in the course of disease, the rash can appear to be a nonspecific, erythematous, maculopapular rash that blanches (Fig. 62-5), followed by rapid progression to petechiae (Fig. 62-6). Rash is absent in up to 20% of cases.

Differential Diagnosis

Studies of patients presenting to the emergency department with fever and petechiae show that the incidence of invasive bacterial infections ranges from 2% to 8%, and the incidence of meningococcal infections ranges from 0.5% to 7%.[4-7] In studies of pediatric patients hospitalized for fever and petechiae, the incidence of meningococcal infections is 10% to 15%.[8,9] Invasive infections other than *N. meningitidis* causing fever and petechiae include *Staphylococcal aureus,*

N. meningitidis is classified into serotypes based on the immunologic response to polysaccharides in the capsule. Further subclassification is based on outer membrane proteins and genetic sequencing of the bacteria. Historically, serotypes B and C accounted for the majority of meningococcal infections in the United States and the rest of the industrialized world. In the United States, however, there has been a recent increase in the number of cases attributable to serotype Y; as a result, serotypes B, C, and Y each account for approximately 30% of the total cases. Less common strains, such as W-135, account for the remainder of cases in the United States. Serotype A is responsible for meningococcal epidemics, particularly in sub-Saharan Africa, or the so-called meningitis belt.

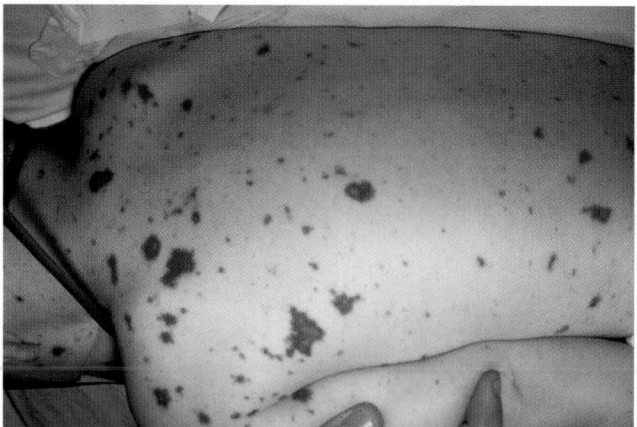

Figure 62-6 Purpuric rash in a 3-year-old with meningococcemia.

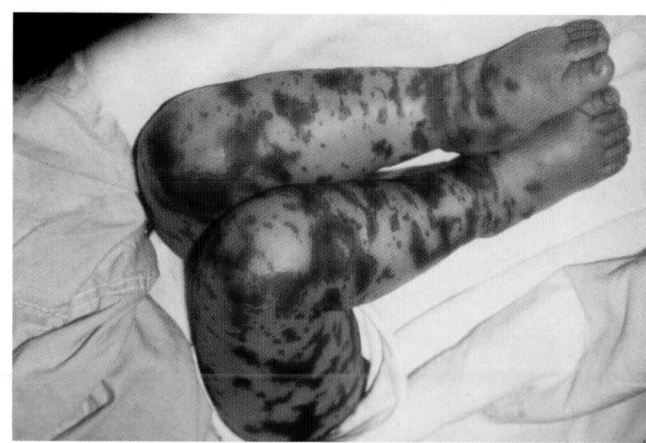

Figure 62-7 Purpura fulminans in an 11-month-old with meningococcemia.

Table 62-2   Noninvasive Causes of Fever and Petechiae
Infectious
Group A streptococcal pharyngitis
Enterovirus infections
Rotavirus gastroenteritis
Respiratory syncytial virus
Mycoplasma pneumoniae
Adenovirus
Epstein-Barr virus
Mechanical
Vomiting
Cough
Blood pressure cuff
Tourniquet
Other
Henoch-Schönlein purpura
Kawasaki disease
Idiopathic thrombocytopenic purpura
Leukemia
Drug rash
Febrile seizures
Immunization reaction (measles-mumps-rubella vaccine)

group A streptococci, *Streptococcus pneumoniae*, *Escherichia coli*, *Rickettsia rickettsii*, and *Ehrlichia chaffeensis*. *Haemophilus influenzae* type B should be considered in an unimmunized population. Noninvasive causes of fever and petechiae are listed in Table 62-2. The mechanism of petechiae secondary to infections such as respiratory syncytial virus and rotavirus are likely mechanical.

Diagnosis and Evaluation

Laboratory abnormalities often include an elevated white blood cell (WBC) count, anemia, acidosis, electrolyte abnormalities, and uremia. Thrombocytopenia, prolonged prothrombin time and partial thromboplastin time, elevated fibrin degradation products, and depressed fibrinogen levels are characteristic of the disseminated intravascular coagulopathy of bacterial sepsis. In patients with meningitis,

cerebrospinal fluid analysis may show an elevated WBC count with high protein and depressed glucose levels, and gram-negative diplococci may be seen on Gram stain.

A number of studies have evaluated clinical and laboratory features in an attempt to exclude meningococcal infection at presentation.[4-9] Petechiae limited to the distribution of the superior vena cava (superior to the nipple line), particularly if associated with coughing or vomiting, make meningococcal infection unlikely. Worrisome findings include ill appearance, evidence of shock, the presence of purpura, WBC count less than 5000 cells/dL or greater than 15,000 cells/dL, and C-reactive protein level greater than 5 mg/L. One study found a 100% negative predictive value for invasive bacterial infections using the criteria of well appearance, no evidence of shock, and normal values for WBC count and C-reactive protein.[4]

Positive culture results of blood or spinal fluid confirm the diagnosis. Gram stain and culture of skin lesions are helpful, particularly when antibiotics are given before the collection of samples. Frequently these cultures are sterile, however, and the diagnosis is made on clinical grounds. Antigen testing is unreliable.

Course of Illness

Rapid progression to multiorgan failure can occur; complications include shock, acute respiratory distress syndrome, seizures, increased intracranial pressure, electrolyte abnormalities, renal failure, adrenal hemorrhage, anemia, thrombocytopenia, coagulopathy, pancreatitis, myocardial dysfunction, and compartment syndrome. Purpura fulminans (Fig. 62-7), with necrosis of the skin and extremities (Fig. 62-8), can develop (see Chapter 150).

Mortality is approximately 20% for meningococcemia and 5% for meningococcal meningitis. The difference in mortality rates is explained by the belief that patients who survive the initial bacteremia long enough to develop meningitis have a less pathogenic strain of meningococcus. Among survivors, neurologic impairment occurs in 5%; sensorineural deafness is the most common deficit. Extremity or skin necrosis requiring amputation or skin grafting occurs in 2% to 5% of survivors. Chronic renal failure and myocardial dysfunction are rare.

Admission Criteria

All patients in whom meningococcal infection is suspected should be admitted to the hospital for prompt intravenous antibiotic therapy and monitoring of clinical status. Those with evidence of cardiovascular instability or multiorgan failure should be admitted to a pediatric critical care unit.

Treatment

The most important components of therapy include antimicrobial therapy in association with supportive care. A third-generation cephalosporin, such as ceftriaxone or cefotaxime, is standard for meningococcal infections. In the past, penicillin was used, but intermediate resistance to penicillin through altered penicillin-binding proteins may exist, and rare reports of clinical failure make the use of penicillin less reliable. Frequently, pneumococcal sepsis or meningitis is being considered in the differential diagnosis of patients presenting with signs and symptoms of meningococcal infection, and vancomycin is added to cover the possibility of resistant pneumococcus. Vancomycin can be discontinued if meningococcal infection is confirmed. Chloramphenicol can also be useful, although resistance exists. A 7-day course of antibiotics is effective therapy for both meningococcemia and meningococcal meningitis.

Supportive care is based on the principles outlined elsewhere in this book. Of note, the need for pharmacologic vasoconstrictors (pressors) should be weighed carefully against the risk of extremity necrosis. Fasciotomy, amputation, and skin grafts are sometimes required.

Discharge Criteria

Patients are discharged from the hospital after completion of an appropriate course of antibiotics, provided that any complications are stable and amenable to outpatient management.

Prevention

Chemoprophylaxis is recommended for household members, day-care contacts, and individuals with direct contact with the patient's secretions within 7 days of the onset of disease. Chemoprophylaxis of other contacts is recommended only during outbreaks or clusters of cases. Rifampin, ceftriaxone, and ciprofloxacin are efficacious (Table 62-3).

Polysaccharide vaccines against serotypes A, C, Y, and W-135 have an efficacy of approximately 85% in children older than 2 years but poor immunogenicity in younger children.[10] Vaccines for serogroup B are currently unavailable. In the United States, where serogroup B accounts for one third of cases and young children are at highest risk, benefits from vaccination are small, and routine vaccination during early childhood is not recommended. Young children at higher risk of meningococcal infection because of anatomic or functional asplenia, terminal complement deficiencies, or properdin deficiency should be vaccinated. Routine immunization of 11- to 12-year-olds with meningococcal

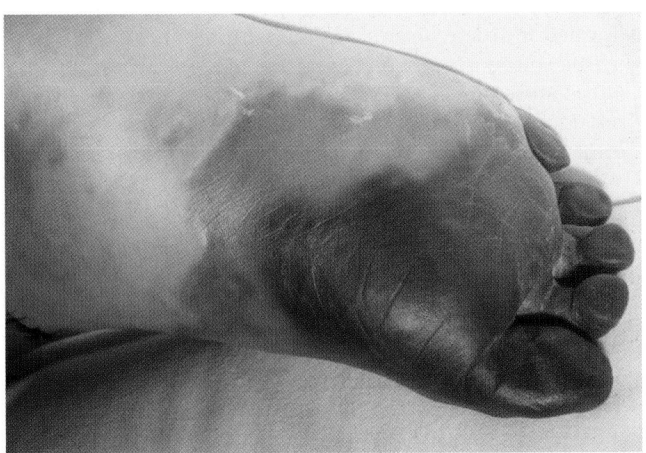

Figure 62-8 Necrosis and early gangrene in the toes and distal foot of a 14-month-old with meningococcemia.

Table 62-3 Chemoprophylaxis for *Neisseria meningitidis*				
Drug/Patient's Age	Dose	Duration	Efficacy (%)	Cautions
Rifampin			72–90	May interfere with efficacy of oral contraceptives and some seizure prevention and anticoagulant medications; may stain soft contact lenses
≤1 mo	5 mg/kg PO q12 h	2 days		
>1 mo	10 mg/kg PO q12h (max 600 mg)	2 days		
Ceftriaxone			97	To decrease pain at injection site, dilute with 1% lidocaine
≤15 yr	125 mg IM	1 dose		
>15 yr	250 mg IM	1 dose		
Ciprofloxacin			90–95	Not licensed for people younger than 18 yr
≥18 yr	500 mg PO	1 dose		

Adapted from Red Book, 26th ed. American Academy of Pediatrics, Elk Grove Village, Ill, 2003.

conjugate vaccine against serotypes A, C, Y, and W-135 (MCV4) is recommended. Catch-up immunization is recommended for previously unvaccinated adolescents entering high school, 15-year-olds, students entering college who plan to live in dormitories, and other high-risk individuals.

TOXIC SHOCK SYNDROME

Toxic shock syndrome (TSS) is a life-threatening condition characterized by rash, fever, multiorgan failure, and shock. *Staphylococcus aureus* and *Streptococcus pyogenes* are the causative agents, and each organism results in a distinct clinical syndrome.

Menstruation-related staphylococcal TSS was first described in the 1970s, and an association with tampon use was noted in the 1980s. Subsequently, cases of TSS both with and without a link to menstruation have been reported. The clinical features of staphylococcal TSS result from the toxin produced by a strain of *S. aureus*. Toxic shock syndrome toxin-1 (TSST-1) accounts for nearly all cases of menstruation-related TSS. TSST-1 production is enhanced by the neutral pH and high protein levels associated with menstruation. Tampon insertion contributes by elevating oxygen levels in a normally anaerobic environment. Elevation of intravaginal carbon dioxide levels with prolonged tampon insertion also contributes, especially with high-absorbency, rayon tampons. Unlike some of the other staphylococcal toxins, TSST-1 can easily cross the mucosal barrier, enter the bloodstream, and cause systemic manifestations. Menstruation-related TSS has declined secondary to public awareness of this entity and removal of high-absorbency rayon-containing tampons from the market. Menstruation-related TSS typically occurs within 2 to 3 days of the onset of menses. Nonmenstruation-related TSS is caused by TSST-1 and staphylococcal enterotoxin serotypes B and C; it occurs in association with surgery, influenza infections, skin lesions and infections, foreign bodies, burns, and sometimes with no obvious focus of infection (e.g., sinusitis).

Streptococcal TSS became known in the 1990s with a resurgence of invasive group A streptococcal infections. Its association with soft tissue infections such as pyomyositis and necrotizing fasciitis brought public recognition as the "flesh-eating bacteria." Preceding skin lesions or infections, particularly varicella in the prevaccination era, are risk factors.

Although bacteremia is common in streptococcal TSS, toxin production plays an important causative role in the clinical manifestations. Streptococcal pyogenic exotoxin serotypes A and C are most commonly associated with severe disease. In addition, M typing appears to play an important role in evasion of the host immune response, with M types 1 and 3 being most common. These toxins can stimulate massive T-cell proliferation. Traditional antigens require recognition at multiple sites on the antigen-presenting cell, whereas these toxins require recognition at only one β-chain variable region. More than 20% of all T cells can be stimulated by these toxins, compared with less than 1% of T cells stimulated by traditional antigens. This ability has led these toxins to be called "superantigens."[11] Massive cytokine release results, which can lead to capillary leak, hypotension, shock, multiorgan failure, and death.

Clinical Presentation

Staphylococcal TSS begins with a 2- to 3-day prodromal phase characterized by malaise, myalgia, fever, and chills.[12,13] Mental status changes, including lightheadedness, lethargy, and confusion, frequently bring the patient to medical attention. Diarrhea is common. Tachycardia and hypotension are usually evident at presentation. Generalized or patchy erythroderma is observed in many patients.

Streptococcal TSS has two major presentations. Some patients present with the acute onset of severe pain and fever. The pain is usually in an extremity, is out of proportion to the physical findings, and results from an underlying soft tissue infection such as necrotizing fasciitis (see Chapter 70).[12,13] Alternatively, patients present with an influenza-like syndrome characterized by fever, chills, myalgias, headache, nausea, vomiting, and diarrhea. Mental status changes ranging from confusion to coma occur in more than 50% of cases. Sore throat is unusual. The heart rate should be assessed carefully, because tachycardia out of proportion to the degree of fever may be the only evidence of impending cardiovascular collapse. Many patients are hypotensive on presentation, but commonly, blood pressure is initially normal and deteriorates rapidly within 4 hours. Erythroderma is seen in a minority of patients. Careful examination of the musculoskeletal system is important, because signs of soft tissue infection may not be obvious. When signs are present, they can range from local swelling to violaceous bullae suggestive of tissue necrosis. Diffuse edema from capillary leak may be evident in either form of TSS.

Differential Diagnosis

The differential diagnosis of fever and shock is broad. Presence of the typical rash should make TSS a strong consideration, but its absence should not exclude the possibility. In addition to TSS, gram-negative sepsis should be considered. Heatstroke presents with hyperthermia and renal dysfunction and may have erythroderma. Meningococcal infections and Rocky Mountain spotted fever present with fever and shock, but the rash, when present, is petechial in nature. Pyomyositis and necrotizing fasciitis can occur without the shock or organ dysfunction associated with TSS. Kawasaki disease may present with fever, mucous membrane involvement, and scarlatina or erythroderma, but shock occurs in only a small percentage of patients. Kawasaki disease also has a younger age distribution than does TSS. Purulent conjunctivitis and the absence of shock differentiate viral infections, such as adenovirus and measles, from TSS. Normal heart rate and blood pressure in association with a scarlatiniform rash and exudative pharyngitis support the diagnosis of uncomplicated scarlet fever.

Diagnosis and Evaluation

The diagnosis of TSS is based on the clinical criteria outlined in Table 62-4. WBC counts are elevated in staphylococcal TSS, with an elevation of immature neutrophils. In streptococcal TSS, WBC counts are frequently normal to mildly elevated, with immature neutrophils accounting for as much as 50% to 60% of the total. Thrombocytopenia with an abnormal coagulation panel suggests the consumptive coagulopathy known to complicate these illnesses. Isolated

Table 62-4 Clinical Criteria for Toxic Shock Syndrome

Streptococcal Toxic Shock Syndrome
Hypotension
Clinical or laboratory evidence of multisystem organ
   involvement (≥2 of the following)
   Renal impairment
   Coagulopathy
   Liver abnormalities
   Acute respiratory distress syndrome
   Extensive tissue necrosis
   Erythematous rash
Definite case: above criteria plus isolation of group A
   β-hemolytic streptococcus from sterile site
Probable case: above criteria plus isolation of group A
   β-hemolytic streptococcus from nonsterile site

Staphylococcal Toxic Shock Syndrome
Major criteria (3 of 3):
   Acute fever ≥38.8°C
   Hypotension
   Characteristic rash
Minor criteria (3 of 7):
   Mucous membrane involvement (conjunctival, oropharyngeal
      erythema)
   Gastrointestinal abnormalities (vomiting, diarrhea)
   Muscle abnormalities (myalgia, elevated creatine
      phosphokinase)
   Central nervous system abnormalities (coma, obtundation)
   Hepatic abnormalities
   Renal abnormalities (pyuria, uremia)
   Thrombocytopenia
Exclusionary criteria
   Another explanation
   Positive blood culture for an organism other than
      Staphylococcus aureus

thrombocytopenia is common with staphylococcal disease. Elevated blood urea nitrogen and serum creatinine are often evident at presentation and can occur before the onset of hypotension in streptococcal TSS. Elevated serum transaminases, bilirubin, and prothrombin time are evidence of liver involvement. Direct hyperbilirubinemia out of proportion to other abnormalities in liver enzymes suggests hydrops of the gallbladder. Hypoalbuminemia can be secondary to capillary leak and liver dysfunction. Hypocalcemia can be significant. Creatine phosphokinase levels are elevated in both types of TSS and correlate with the degree of myositis in streptococcal TSS. Blood cultures are positive in 60% of those with streptococcal TSS but in only a minority of those with staphylococcal disease. *S. aureus* can be isolated from cultures of the anterior nares, rectum, and vagina, and throat culture can identify *S. pyogenes*. Cultures of wounds are helpful in isolating either organism.

Course of Illness

Staphylococcal TSS can progress to shock and multiorgan failure. Aggressive supportive care has decreased mortality to less than 5%.

The outcome of streptococcal TSS is worse. Despite appropriate treatment, shock and renal dysfunction are nearly universal and often progress over 48 to 72 hours. More than 50% of patients develop acute respiratory distress syndrome, with the majority requiring some degree of respiratory support. Mortality ranges from 30% to 70%. Those with deep soft tissue infections fare the worst. Renal dysfunction often persists for 4 to 6 weeks in survivors.

Admission Criteria

All patients with suspected TSS should be hospitalized for intravenous antibiotics and careful monitoring; rapid clinical deterioration is common, and further cardiovascular support may be necessary. Any indication of cardiovascular instability or acute respiratory distress syndrome warrants transfer to a critical care setting.

Treatment

Treatment for TSS involves appropriate intravenous antibiotics in combination with aggressive supportive care. Traditionally, use of a semisynthetic penicillin such as nafcillin provided good bactericidal coverage against *S. aureus* and *S. pyogenes*. In geographic areas demonstrating a significant presence of community-acquired methicillin-resistant *S. aureus*, vancomycin should be used instead. Adequate coverage for gram-negative organisms should be added when these organisms are being considered in the differential diagnosis. A third-generation cephalosporin such as ceftriaxone is appropriate. Many experts advocate the use of clindamycin in addition to the previously mentioned antibiotics. Animal models of streptococcal TSS demonstrate improved survival in clindamycin-treated mice versus those treated with penicillin. The decreased efficacy of penicillin is explained by the high inoculum of *S. pyogenes* in these infections, resulting in a static growth phase and decreased demonstration of penicillin-binding proteins. In addition, clindamycin inhibits bacterial protein synthesis and thus decreases the production of toxin and antiphagocytic M proteins. Last, clindamycin may modulate the host immune response by inhibiting tumor necrosis factor production by monocytes.[13] The antibiotic regimen can be narrowed when a causative agent is identified and antibiotic sensitivities are available for guidance. The benefits of clindamycin as an adjunct agent probably do not continue once the patient is stable and soft tissue collections have been adequately drained. A total course of 10 to 14 days of antibiotics is commonly prescribed. Transition to oral antibiotics at the time of discharge to complete this course is appropriate.

Supportive care for shock and multiorgan failure should be aggressive and is outlined in other sections of this book.

Aggressive surgical débridement of deep soft tissue infections improves outcomes and is required in about 50% of patients with streptococcal TSS.

Discharge Criteria

Patients can be discharged to home when:

- They are afebrile.
- They have negative blood culture results.
- They are cardiovascularly stable.

- Complications are stable and manageable on an outpatient basis.

Prevention

Judicious use of tampons is an important measure to prevent staphylococcal TSS. Recommendations include using tampons of minimal absorbency, avoiding prolonged insertion of tampons (<4 to 8 hours), and alternating tampon and pad use. Patients with staphylococcal TSS who survive are at higher risk of recurrence and should be instructed not to use tampons. There are no preventive measures for streptococcal TSS. Vaccinations are not available for either entity.

DISEASES CAUSED BY RICKETTSIA, EHRLICHIA, AND ANAPLASMA

A dramatic petechial rash is frequently cited as the hallmark of Rocky Mountain spotted fever (RMSF), a potentially severe disease. However, the rash in RMSF, as with other rickettsial diseases and similar zoonoses, is a late clinical phenomenon. A delay in diagnosis is common, and few of these diseases are diagnosed at the first presentation of the illness. In addition, the empirical antimicrobial agents frequently prescribed for suspected systemic bacterial infections (e.g., β-lactams) are ineffective against these organisms. Because morbidity and mortality are significant, clinicians must consider proper empirical therapy for these diseases based on epidemiologic, clinical, and laboratory features.

Rocky Mountain Spotted Fever

Rickettsia rickettsii is a gram-negative coccobacillus that is an obligate intracellular pathogen; it cannot be cultured on routine microbiologic media. Ticks are the vector by which *R. rickettsii* is transmitted. *Dermacentor variabilis* (American dog tick) and *Dermacentor andersonii* (Rocky Mountain wood tick) are the vectors in the eastern and western United States, respectively. The primary targets are the endothelial cells of small blood vessels of all major tissues and organs. This accounts for the protean manifestations of RMSF, including the rash, and the significant morbidity and mortality of the illness.

The incidence of RMSF is approximately 3.5 cases per million population. Although RMSF has been described in most of the continental United States, 80% of cases occur in the southeastern and south-central states, with highly endemic areas in Oklahoma, North Carolina, and Virginia. Up to 50% of patients are children, with an age-specific peak in the 5- to 9-year-old age group. There is a 1.5:1 male-to-female predominance. As would be expected with a tick-borne illness, the majority of cases occur in rural areas, and there is usually a history suggesting significant tick exposure; however, up to 30% to 40% of patients do not recall a tick bite. Ninety percent of infections occur between April and September (50% in May and June), correlating with outdoor recreation and tick activity.

Clinical Presentation

The classic triad of fever, rash, and history of a tick bite is found in the minority of patients when they first present for medical care. Most of the initial symptoms are nonspecific.

After an incubation of 3 to 12 days, patients often present with high fever (as high as 41°C) accompanied by severe myalgias and headache, which is usually frontal in location. Abdominal pain may be prominent and, in some cases, severe enough to suggest an acute surgical abdomen. Findings on physical examination may include splenomegaly, conjunctivitis, and periorbital edema. Central nervous system findings may include neck stiffness, mental status changes, and focal neurologic deficits that may present a confusing clinical picture. The characteristic centripetally spreading rash, if it occurs, appears on about the fourth day of illness. Diagnosis of RMSF should *not* await the appearance of a rash, because data suggest that a delay in initiating therapy of more than 5 days is associated with increased mortality.[14] In fact, the rash may be entirely absent in 10% of cases.[15] When it does appear, the rash frequently begins as macular or maculopapular lesions on the wrists and ankles and spreads to the palms and soles and centrally to the trunk. Because RMSF is a vasculitic illness, it is not surprising that the lesions often become petechial and occasionally purpuric; gangrene may occur.

Differential Diagnosis

The differential diagnosis includes bacterial sepsis, especially meningococcemia. The clinical picture of ehrlichiosis, especially the monocytic form, may be quite similar (see later). Enteroviral infections may be associated with a petechial rash, headache, and myalgias, but clinical manifestations are usually not as severe as with RMSF.

Diagnosis and Evaluation

The peripheral WBC count is often normal, especially early in the illness. Later determinations may show either an increase or a decrease in the WBC count, making this test useless for diagnosis. Thrombocytopenia, with values below 100,000/mm^3, is relatively common. This may be secondary to the vasculitis and endothelial expression of platelet-binding substances produced by *R. rickettsii*. A helpful diagnostic clue is that thrombocytopenia may be found in the absence of evidence of a consumptive coagulopathy. Hyponatremia is also common and is likely a result of disrupted vascular integrity and capillary leakage. Cerebrospinal fluid analysis reveals a mild pleocytosis (polymorphonuclear or mononuclear) in approximately one third of cases; protein may be elevated in an equal proportion, but this is seen less frequently in children than in adults. Serum transaminase, blood urea nitrogen, and serum creatinine levels are frequently elevated and represent end-organ injury from vasculitis. Evidence of renal insufficiency may signal a poor prognosis.[16]

Unfortunately, there are no generally available tests for rapid diagnosis during the acute illness. Serologic evaluation by the indirect fluorescent antibody test can establish a diagnosis 10 to 14 days after the onset of illness with 90% sensitivity and is available at most state health departments and some commercial laboratories. The use of paired acute and convalescent sera demonstrating a fourfold rise in titers against *R. rickettsii* is also diagnostic. *R. rickettsii* may be identified in biopsy specimens by direct immunofluorescent microscopy or immunoperoxidase staining, but this is not widely available.

Course of Illness

Vasculitis and intravascular volume depletion secondary to vascular leak lead to multiorgan involvement. Renal complications include prerenal failure, acute tubular necrosis, and intrinsic renal failure. Hypotension is common, and cardiovascular collapse and myocarditis may occur in severe disease. Neurologic complications include headache, seizures, coma, cerebral edema, and intracranial hemorrhage. Pulmonary edema and hemorrhage and respiratory failure are rare. Mortality can be 10% or higher, although mortality is lower in children than in adults older than 40 years.[14]

Admission Criteria

Abnormal vital signs (other than fever) and evidence of end-organ damage (e.g., mental status changes, renal dysfunction) are clear indications for hospital admission. Oral outpatient therapy may be used for patients with normal vital signs, absence of end-organ damage, tolerance of oral therapy, and assurance of excellent follow-up.

Treatment

As noted earlier, the antibiotics used for typical bacterial agents (e.g., β-lactams) have no activity against *R. rickettsii*. The drug of choice, even in children, is doxycycline. Intravenous therapy with doxycycline should be initiated at 2 to 4 mg/kg every 12 hours, with a maximum dose of 100 mg. The consequences of RMSF far outweigh the small risk of dental staining from the use of tetracyclines (usually associated with repeated and prolonged courses). Uncontrolled data suggest that chloramphenicol is an inferior agent; its only place may be in the treatment of pregnant women. There is a suggestion that some drugs, specifically sulfonamides, may actually worsen the disease.

Discharge Criteria

Therapy should continue for at least 2 days after defervescence, with a minimum course of 5 days. Seven to 10 days of therapy is not uncommon. Although therapy for hospitalized patients is often completed intravenously, rapid improvement may allow completion of therapy with oral doxycycline.

Prevention

Avoidance of ticks should be attempted in tick-endemic areas. This can be accomplished by avoiding bushy areas, wearing long sleeves and pants, and using insect repellents that contain DEET. Careful inspection of the body for ticks during the summer months may also decrease the risk of exposure. Prophylactic antibiotics after a tick bite are not recommended. No vaccine is available.

Other Rickettsial Infections

Historically, a number of other rickettsial diseases have been responsible for significant morbidity and mortality worldwide, but these are rare in the United States. Murine typhus (caused by *Rickettsia typhi*) occurs in pockets in Texas (80%), California, and Hawaii.[17] Rickettsialpox has been described in a number of U.S. cities. Unlike RMSF, these rickettsial diseases are often associated with crowding and urban settings. Lice, fleas, and mites transmit most of these diseases. Although symptoms vary somewhat by pathogen, fever, chills, headaches, and myalgias are common. Rashes frequently occur but are often late findings. As with RMSF, treatment is doxycycline 2 to 4 mg/kg (maximum dose 100 mg) twice daily.

Ehrlichioses

Other zoonoses whose epidemiologic, clinical, and laboratory features mimic RMSF may actually be more common. They are represented predominantly by the ehrlichioses. Like RMSF, the ehrlichioses represent a diagnostic challenge, but fortunately, therapy is much the same as for RMSF.

Ehrlichia chaffeensis and *Anaplasma* (formerly *Ehrlichia phagocytophila*) belong to the family Rickettsiaceae, but the nomenclature of the species is in flux, so phylogenetic name changes can be anticipated. As with *R. rickettsii*, the agents of ehrlichiosis are obligate intracellular bacteria with tick vectors and mammalian hosts. Target cells are mononuclear phagocytic cells for *E. chaffeensis* and neutrophils for *A. phagocytophila*. The clinical syndromes, human monocytic ehrlichiosis (HME) and human granulocytic ehrlichiosis (HGE), correlate with these target cells.

Although HME has been reported in most of the continental United States, the highest incidence is in the southeastern, south-central, and mid-Atlantic states, as well as California. Missouri, Oklahoma, North Carolina, and Arkansas are states with a high incidence of this disease. The vectors are *Amblyomma americanum* (Lone Star tick) and *Dermacentor variabilis* (American dog tick). Deer are the natural reservoir. The geographic distribution of HME significantly overlaps that of RMSF, but the incidence of the former may be severalfold higher than that of the latter.[18] HME occurs in rural and suburban areas, with the highest incidence in the summer months. In contrast to RMSF, only 10% of reported HME cases occur in children, and there is a much more pronounced male predominance. The tick probably needs to be attached 24 to 48 hours before transmission, and incubation is typically 7 to 10 days (but can be as long as 3 weeks).

The distribution of HGE is predominantly in the northeastern, mid-Atlantic, and upper midwestern (Minnesota and Wisconsin) United States, as well as northern California. The vector is *Ixodes scapularis* (*Ixodes pacificus* in California), with deer and white-footed mice serving as reservoirs. The zoonotic cycle is similar to that of *Borrelia burgdorferi*, the agent of Lyme disease. Coinfection with *B. burgdorferi* can occur, but it is unclear how often this occurs. Although there have been fewer than 1000 reported cases of HGE, seroprevalence studies suggest that infection is often unrecognized. The incidence is highest in the summer months and in rural and suburban areas, with a male predominance. The bite may be unrecognized because of the small size of the tick. Incubation averages 8 days, but it can be 3 weeks or more.

Clinical Presentation

The disease ranges from subclinical or asymptomatic cases to severe, life-threatening, and fatal illnesses. Initial symptoms are nonspecific and include fever, chills, severe headache, myalgias, arthralgias, abdominal pain, and weight loss. Central nervous system symptoms can include ataxia, vertigo, and delirium. Lymphadenopathy, which is uncommon with RMSF, may be noted. Organomegaly may result from granulomatous infiltration. Most of the information about the clinical spectrum of human ehrlichioses is derived from the adult literature because of the scarcity of data in the pediatric population. A rash eventually appears in 40% of adults but is present in only 25% by the end of the first week of illness. Rash is more common in children, occurring in two thirds of cases. The rash involves the trunk and extremities and may be macular, maculopapular, or petechial.

Differential Diagnosis

The differential diagnosis of ehrlichiosis is similar to that of RMSF. Most of the entities discussed in the previous sections of this chapter are given greater consideration than ehrlichiosis in patients with fever and rash; however, in patients with tick exposure in endemic areas and suspicious laboratory findings, ehrlichiosis should be considered.

Diagnosis and Evaluation

Laboratory features of HME and HGE are nonspecific but may provide helpful clues to the diagnosis. Abnormalities, particularly hematologic, are more common in children. Leukopenia, with WBC counts in the range of 1 to 4000, may be present early in the course of the illness, along with lymphopenia or neutropenia. During the second week of illness these counts may be elevated; therefore, the timing of laboratory studies relative to the duration of the illness should be considered when interpreting these values. Leukopenia is probably due to peripheral destruction, margination, and sequestration of WBCs rather than bone marrow suppression. Decreased platelet counts (in the range of 50 to 100,000/mm^3) are seen in 80% of patients; anemia is present in 33% of children. A coagulation profile may be normal or abnormal. Moderate serum transaminase elevations (two to eight times normal) are present in 90%, and 67% demonstrate mild to moderate hyponatremia. Cerebrospinal fluid may be normal or show a lymphocytic pleocytosis.[18] In adults, increased protein levels in the cerebrospinal fluid have been observed.

Serologic evaluation (immunoglobulin G and immunoglobulin M) for *E. chaffeensis* (HME) is available by indirect immunofluorescence. Single titers of 1:64 or 1:128 are considered evidence of probable infection, and titers greater than or equal to 1:256 are diagnostic. Alternatively, a fourfold increase in titers or seroconversion in samples 2 to 4 weeks apart is considered diagnostic.

As with HME and RMSF, the serologic diagnosis of HGE is usually retrospective. Titers are not positive during the first week of illness. Indirect immunofluorescent serology is available, with a titer greater than 1:80 considered positive. Acute and convalescent titers demonstrating seroconversion or a fourfold increase confirm the diagnosis.

Tools for the rapid diagnosis of these infections are being investigated.

Course of Illness

Complications of HME include coagulopathy, hypotension, acute respiratory distress syndrome, and renal failure. An interesting observation in adults is the evolution of a poorly understood immune dysfunction, with the emergence of opportunistic infections (fungal and viral) in a small percentage of patients.[19] Mortality can result from gastrointestinal or pulmonary hemorrhage, with case fatality rates of approximately 2%.

Complications of HGE can include acute respiratory distress syndrome and neuropathy. The illness tends to be less severe than HME, with less frequent central nervous system involvement, organomegaly, and mortality.

Admission Criteria

Many cases of ehrlichiosis are unrecognized, but most patients who present to a hospital setting are admitted owing to diagnostic confusion or severe symptoms. In general, admission should be prompted by central nervous system dysfunction, cardiovascular dysfunction, hematologic abnormalities, or electrolyte abnormalities.

Treatment

The initial treatment is frequently empirical, given the difficulty of obtaining timely confirmation of the diagnosis. Therapy should not await serologic confirmation. As with RMSF, doxycycline is the drug of choice in a dose of 2 to 4 mg/kg (maximum 100 mg) every 12 hours. Therapy for 10 to 14 days has been recommended, although few controlled data are available. Chloramphenicol is not recommended. Response to therapy should be seen within 48 hours. It should be restated that coinfection with *B. burgdorferi* and *A. phagocytophila* has been reported in a number of cases, and empirical therapy for Lyme disease with β-lactams (e.g., the treatment of young children with amoxicillin) is not adequate for HGE.

Discharge Criteria

Patients should be hospitalized until central nervous system or cardiovascular instability resolves and there is improvement in hematologic and electrolyte abnormalities.

Prevention

Prevention is similar to that for RMSF.

CONSULTATION

- Critical care for patients who demonstrate cardiovascular instability, respiratory insufficiency or acute respiratory distress syndrome, or other features of sepsis.
- Infectious disease consultation, if necessary, for assistance with initial evaluation, empirical therapy, or management.
- Plastic, general, or orthopedic surgery for débridement of deep soft tissue infections or gangrene, amputation of necrotic segments of extremities, or grafting of large areas of skin loss.
- Nephrology for management of renal insufficiency or failure.
- Physical and occupational therapy for reconditioning, prevention of contractures, and other rehabilitative needs, especially if there is extensive skin involvement or limb loss.

IN A NUTSHELL

- The combination of fever and rash is a common clinical scenario, but careful characterization of the rash in conjunction with a consideration of other clinical features can provide clues to the cause of the illness.
- The characteristic rash may be absent in all the severe infections discussed.
- Although the presence of fever and petechiae usually raises concern for meningococcemia, other severe infections should be considered. Noninvasive infections account for the majority of these illnesses.
- In patients with fever and erythroderma or scarlatina, TSS should be considered in the differential diagnosis.
- TSS may present without obvious signs of shock, and tachycardia out of proportion to the fever may be an early sign of cardiovascular instability.
- Epidemiology, including a history of tick exposure, is key when considering the diagnoses of RMSF and ehrlichiosis.
- Thrombocytopenia and hyponatremia may be helpful clues to the diagnosis of RMSF and ehrlichiosis.
- Early and aggressive therapy improves the outcomes for meningococcemia, TSS, and rickettsial diseases. Therapy should be initiated at the first suspicion of these entities rather than waiting for confirmation.
- Antibiotics commonly used for the empirical treatment of serious bacterial infections are ineffective against RMSF and ehrlichiosis. Doxycycline is the drug of choice.

ON THE HORIZON

- Use of immunomodulators is being investigated for acute therapy for meningococcal infection. Bactericidal permeability increasing protein has the ability to bind and neutralize endotoxin and kill gram-negative bacteria. Monoclonal antibody against endotoxin (HA-1A) is also being studied. Both these agents, in addition to the use of activated protein C to correct coagulation disorders, have shown promise but require further study.
- The use of intravenous immune globulin (IVIG) has anecdotal success in treating streptococcal TSS. Potential mechanisms of this benefit include neutralization of bacterial toxins, increased bacterial phagocytosis related to anti-M protein antibodies, and nonspecific inhibition of tumor necrosis factor production. Randomized studies are unlikely to be performed, and the use of IVIG should be considered in patients with prolonged, intractable shock.
- The organisms responsible for RMSF, HME, and HGE demonstrate in vitro sensitivity to some quinolones, but clinical data in children are unavailable.

REFERENCES

1. Ramsay M, Reacher M, O'Flynn C, et al: Causes of morbilliform rash in a highly immunised English population. Arch Dis Child 2002;87:202-206.
2. Davidkin I, Valle M, Peltola H, et al: Etiology of measles- and rubella-like illnesses in measles, mumps, and rubella-vaccinated children. J Infect Dis 1998;178:1567-1570.
3. Leaute-Labreze C, Lamireau T, Chawki D, et al: Diagnosis, classification, and management of erythema multiforme and Stevens-Johnson syndrome. Arch Dis Child 2000;83:347-352.
4. Brogan PA, Raffles A: The management of fever and petechiae: Making sense of rash decisions. Arch Dis Child 2000;83:506-507.
5. Baker RC, Seguin JH, Leslie N, et al: Fever and petechiae in children. Pediatrics 1989;84(6):1051-1055.
6. Mandl KD, Stack AM, Fleisher GR: Incidence of bacteremia in infants and children with fever and petechiae. J Pediatr 1997;131:398-404.
7. Wells LC, Smith JC, Weston VC, et al: The child with a non-blanching rash: How likely is meningococcal disease? Arch Dis Child 2001;85:218-222.
8. Nguyen QV, Nguyen EA, Weiner LB: Incidence of bacterial disease in children with fever and petechiae. Pediatrics 1984;74:77-80.
9. Nielsen HE, Anderson EA, Anderson J, et al: Diagnostic assessment of haemorrhagic rash and fever. Arch Dis Child 2001;85:160-165.
10. Peter G: Update on meningococcal vaccine. Pediatr Infect Dis J 2001;20:311-312.
11. McCormick JK, Yarwood JM, Schlievert PM: Toxic shock syndrome and bacterial superantigens: An update. Annu Rev Microbiol 2001;55:77-104.
12. Stevens DL: Streptococcal toxic-shock syndrome: Spectrum of disease, pathogenesis, and new concepts in treatment. Emerging Infectious Diseases 1995;1:69-78.
13. Stevens DL: The toxic shock syndromes. Infect Dis Clin North Am 1996;10:727-746.
14. Sexton DJ, Kaye KS: Rocky Mountain spotted fever. Med Clin North Am 2002;86:351-360.
15. Drage LA: Life-threatening rashes: Dermatologic signs of four infectious diseases. Mayo Clin Proc 1999;74:68-72.
16. Colon PJ, Procop GW, Fowler V, et al: Predictors of prognosis and risk of acute renal failure in patients with Rocky Mountain spotted fever. Am J Med 1996;101:621-626.
17. Godbole A: Pediatric puzzler. Contemp Pediatr 2004;21:24-26.
18. Jacobs RF, Schutze GE: Ehrlichioses in children. J Pediatr 1997;131:184-192.
19. Olano JP, Walker DH: Human ehrlichioses. Med Clin North Am 2002;86:375-379.
20. Committee on Infectious Diseases, American Academy of Pediatrics, Pickering LK (ed): Red Book: 2003 Report of the Committee on Infectious Diseases, 26th ed. Elk Grove Village, Ill, American Academy of Pediatrics, 2003, p 434.

CHAPTER 63

Central Nervous System Infections

Angela C. Mix and José R. Romero

Infections of the central nervous system (CNS) in children continue to pose a diagnostic and therapeutic challenge to clinicians. Because of the plethora of bacterial, viral, fungal, and protozoan agents capable of infecting the CNS, it is not possible to discuss them all within the context of this chapter. As such, this chapter focuses on agents most likely to be encountered by hospitalists in the course of their activities.

Simply defined, meningitis is an inflammation of the membranes (i.e., arachnoid, dura, and pia mater) surrounding the brain and spinal cord. Encephalitis involves an inflammatory process of the cerebrum. Although it is common to discuss each as separate entities, in many cases, particularly with viral infections of the CNS, they occur together as meningoencephalitis.

EPIDEMIOLOGY

Bacterial Meningitis

Over the last 2 decades the number of cases of bacterial meningitis in the United States has declined from 10,000 to 20,000 cases per year to approximately 6000 cases annually.[1,2] Approximately 50% of cases occur in children younger than 18 years.[3] In large part as a result of the development of conjugate vaccines against *Haemophilus influenzae* type b (Hib) and *Streptococcus pneumoniae*, the overall incidence of bacterial meningitis has continued to decline in the United States. Before the introduction of conjugate vaccines for the prevention of childhood infections caused by Hib, this agent was the principal cause of bacterial meningitis in the United States, as well as invasive bacterial infections.[3] Inclusion of Hib conjugate vaccines in the routine immunization schedule of children has resulted in the virtual disappearance of invasive Hib disease in children younger than 5 years[4] and a fall in the incidence of Hib meningitis from 2.9 to 0.2 cases per 100,000 population. Coincident with this decline has been a shift in the median age of all patients with meningitis from 15 months to 25 years.[3]

As a result of the licensure of a heptavalent (serotypes 4, 6B, 9V, 14, 18C, 19F, 23) pneumococcal conjugate vaccine in 2000, a significant decrease in reported cases of *S. pneumoniae* invasive disease is being observed.[5] A report noted a decline of 59% in the rate of pneumococcal meningitis after the introduction of pneumococcal conjugate vaccine.[6]

The possible causes of bacterial meningitis are numerous (Table 63-1) and depend on such factors as age, immunization status, and underlying clinical condition (e.g., inherited or acquired immunodeficiency states, ventriculoperitoneal shunts, cochlear implants, cerebrospinal fluid [CSF] leaks). Immunocompromised hosts deserve special consideration when meningitis is suspected. Opportunistic infections caused by *Cryptococcus neoformans*, *Toxoplasma*, tuberculosis, and fungi (e.g., *Aspergillus* species) must be considered.

Despite a significant reduction in the incidence of early-onset *Streptococcus agalactiae* (group B streptococcus) disease in the neonatal period through the use of intrapartum prophylactic antibiotics, group B streptococcus continues to contribute to the burden of disease in this age group.[7] Group B streptococcus, primarily subtype III strains, remains a significant cause of late-onset disease in the form of meningitis in neonates.[8] Coliform bacteria, in particular, K1 antigen–possessing *Escherichia coli*, constitute the second largest group of causes of neonatal meningitis. Other gram-negative enteric bacilli such as *Klebsiella*, *Enterobacter*, and *Salmonella* may also cause sporadic cases of meningitis. *Listeria monocytogenes* occurs only rarely and may be associated with zoonotic outbreaks.[9,10] Other unusual yet notable causes of neonatal meningitis include *Enterobacter sakazakii*[11-13] and *Citrobacter koseri*.[14]

Worldwide and in the areas of the United States with poor vaccination coverage, *S. pneumoniae*, *Neisseria meningitidis*, and Hib are the most common pathogens in infants and young children.[8] As mentioned, the routine use of conjugated Hib vaccines has resulted in virtual disappearance of this organism as a pathogen of children in most of the United States. These vaccines, however, have not had an impact on sporadic cases of nontypable *H. influenzae*–related meningitis or those caused by strains of *H. influenzae* other than type b.

Before the advent of conjugated pneumococcal vaccines, children younger than 2 years were overwhelmingly the group at highest risk for bacterial meningitis from this organism. Use of the hepatavalent conjugated pneumococcal vaccine has dramatically reduced the incidence of invasive disease, including meningitis, in this age group.[6] Recently, an association between the use of cochlear implants and pneumococcal meningitis has been established.[15,16] The rate of pneumococcal meningitis in children in whom cochlear implants with positioners were used was 214 cases per 100,000 person-years 24 to 47 months after surgery.[16]

The age distribution of cases of meningococcal meningitis and disease in the United States is biphasic, with infants younger than 1 year exhibiting the highest incidence of the disease. A second, smaller and broader peak is observed in children and adolescents aged 11 to 19 years.[17] More than half of cases in infants younger than 1 year are due to serogroup B, whereas in individuals older than 11 years, three quarters are the due to serogroups C, Y, or W-135. These latter three serogroups are included in a recently licensed tetravalent (serogroups A, C, Y, W-135) conjugated meningococcal vaccine approved for use in older children and adolescents.[17] It is expected that this vaccine will have an impact on the incidence of meningococcal meningitis in adolescents once it is widely embraced.

Table 63-1 Common Bacterial Pathogens Causing Meningitis by Age and Recommended Empirical Antimicrobial Therapy

Age or Condition	Common Pathogens	Empirical Antimicrobial Therapy
<1 month		
Early onset	*Streptococcus agalactiae, Escherichia coli, Listeria monocytogenes*	Ampicillin plus an aminoglycoside or ampicillin plus cefotaxime
Late onset	*Streptococcus agalactiae, Escherichia coli, Listeria monocytogenes,* coagulase-negative staphylococci, *Staphylococcus aureus, Klebsiella* species, *Enterobacter* species	Nafcillin or vancomycin plus cefotaxime or ceftazidime or cefepime with or without an aminoglycoside
1-3 months	*Streptococcus agalactiae, Escherichia coli, Listeria monocytogenes, Streptococcus pneumoniae, Haemophilus influenzae, Neisseria meningitidis*	Cefotaxime or ceftriaxone plus ampicillin
4-23 months	*Streptococcus pneumoniae, Haemophilus influenzae, Neisseria meningitidis*	Cefotaxime or ceftriaxone plus vancomycin
2-18 years	*Streptococcus pneumoniae, Neisseria meningitidis*	Cefotaxime or ceftriaxone plus vancomycin

Data from Saez-Llorens X, McCracken GH Jr: Bacterial meningitis in children. Lancet 2003;361:2139; and Tunkel AR, Hartman BJ, Kaplan SL, et al: Practice guidelines for the management of bacterial meningitis. Clin Infect Dis 2004;39:1267.

Brain Abscess

Brain abscess is a relatively rare CNS infection. However, nearly 25% of all brain abscesses occur in individuals younger than 15 years, with a peak incidence at 4 to 7 years of age.[18] In up to 30% of all cases, no predisposing factor can be identified.[19] The most common source of infection of the brain comes from the middle ear, paranasal sinuses, or teeth. Children with congenital cardiac defects associated with right-to-left shunts are also at risk for the development of brain abscess.

The location of the brain abscess is related to the underlying condition of its genesis. Additionally, the location and predisposing condition may suggest the possible bacterial cause of the abscess. Dental and sinus infections may result in frontal lobe abscesses. Mastoiditis or chronic ear infections result in abscesses located in the temporal lobe or cerebellum. Abscesses from hematogenous spread secondary to endocarditis may occur throughout the parenchyma of the brain. Finally, abscesses arising from penetrating head trauma or that are postoperative in nature tend to be located adjacent to the site of the cranial breech.

The most commonly involved microorganisms in the etiology of brain abscess in children are aerobic and anaerobic streptococci (60% to 70%), gram-negative anaerobic bacilli (20% to 40%), Enterobacteriaceae (20% to 30%), *Staphylococcus aureus* (10% to 15%), and fungi (1% to 5%).[20] In approximately a third of cases, the brain abscess is polymicrobial in origin and includes both aerobic and anaerobic organisms. In as many as 30% of cases no organism is found.

Herpesviridae Encephalitis

In the United States, the herpes simplex viruses (HSVs) are the most common cause of sporadic, fatal encephalitis.[21,22] These viruses are distributed worldwide, with no seasonal variation in the incidence of infection. Acquisition occurs solely by human-to-human transmission.

Non-neonatal HSV encephalitis is estimated to occur in approximately 1 in 250,000 to 500,000 individuals per year.[23]

Virtually all cases are the result of HSV type 1. In approximately 50% of cases of non-neonatal HSV encephalitis, the CNS infection appears to occur coincident with the primary infection. In the remainder, it is the result of reactivation of previous infection.[24,25]

The estimated incidence of neonatal herpes is approximately 1 in 3200 deliveries, which results in approximately 1500 cases of neonatal HSV infection annually.[22] Approximately 75% of cases of neonatal HSV infection are the result of HSV type 2. A third of all neonates with HSV infection are categorized as having CNS disease (see Chapter 53).[26]

In healthy children, the nonsimplex members of the Herpesviridae family (varicella-zoster virus, human herpesvirus 6, cytomegalovirus, and Epstein-Barr virus) infrequently cause meningitis and encephalitis.[27] Varicella-zoster virus and human herpesvirus 6 have been shown to be rare causes of meningoencephalitis and encephalitis in immunocompetent children.[27] Neurologic complications[27,28] occur in less than 1% of healthy children infected with varicella-zoster virus. Cerebellar ataxia is the most common (1 in 4000) neurologic complication after primary varicella-zoster virus infection. Varicella-zoster virus encephalitis is a serious complication with an incidence of 1 to 2 per 10,000 cases of varicella in healthy persons and is seen more frequently in infants and adults.[27,28]

Enteroviral Meningitis and Encephalitis

The genus Enterovirus is composed of the polioviruses, echoviruses, group A and six group B coxsackieviruses, and numbered enteroviruses. Humans are the only natural hosts for enteroviruses. The principal mode of human-to-human transmission is fecal-oral. Respiratory transmission and self-inoculation are important routes of transmission for some enteroviruses. Vertical transmission may also occur. Enterovirus infections occur predominantly during the summer and early fall. With the eradication of wild-type poliovirus transmission from the Americas, the predominant CNS syndromes associated with enterovirus infection are now meningitis and encephalitis.

The enteroviruses are the preeminent cause of viral meningitis in the United States.[29] Conservative estimates of the annual number of cases of enterovirus meningitis range from 30,000 to 50,000. The highest incidence of disease occurs in infants younger than 1 year and children 5 to 10 years of age.[29] The echoviruses and group B coxsackieviruses are the principal enteroviruses associated with meningitis. Enteroviruses are reported to be responsible for 10% to 20% of identifiable cases of viral encephalitis.[30] The group A coxsackieviruses are the predominant enterovirus subgroup associated with encephalitis.

Arboviral Encephalitis

The arboviruses represent a heterogeneous group of viruses from distinct viral families linked by a common mode of transmission to humans: the bite of an insect or arthropod.[31] Arboviral infections occur during the summer months and coincide with periods of increased activity of their insect and arthropod vectors. The primary arboviral encephalitides in the United States are La Crosse encephalitis, West Nile virus encephalitis, and St. Louis encephalitis. Other, less common forms include eastern and western equine encephalitis and Powassan encephalitis.

The majority of human arboviral infections result in subclinical disease or febrile syndromes that do not involve the CNS. When the CNS is involved, meningitis, encephalitis, or meningoencephalitides commonly result.[32]

La Crosse Encephalitis

The cause of La Crosse encephalitis is an RNA virus of the same name. Most cases occur from July to early October. Cases of La Crosse encephalitis are predominantly reported from the northern Midwestern states and West Virginia. In areas endemic for La Crosse virus, the annual incidence of the disease is approximately 10 to 30 cases per 100,000 in individuals younger than 15 years.[33] Only 0.3% to 4% of La Crosse virus infections result in symptomatic disease.[34] Nearly all cases of La Crosse encephalitis occur in individuals 14 years or younger.[33-36] Males account for the majority of cases.[33,36-38]

West Nile Neuroinvasive Syndromes

West Nile virus, the etiologic agent of West Nile fever and West Nile neuroinvasive syndromes, is a virus found worldwide that made its American debut in 1999.[39] Currently, West Nile virus has superseded all autochthonous North American arboviruses as the single most important cause of arboviral CNS disease in the United States.

St. Louis Encephalitis

St. Louis encephalitis virus is widely distributed in the United States. Until the introduction of West Nile virus to North America in 1999, St. Louis encephalitis virus was the single major cause of epidemic encephalitis in the United States.[40,41]

CLINICAL PRESENTATION

Bacterial Meningitis

The clinical presentation of bacterial meningitis is varied and influenced greatly by the age of the patient. A history of antecedent upper respiratory tract infection may be reported

in up to 75% of children with meningitis.[42,43] The presence of fever is noted in more than 85% of patients; however, fever is rarely the sole complaint, the exception being neonates and very young infants, whose presentation may consist of only fever without an identifiable focus of infection. As such, these infants present a particular diagnostic challenge to the clinician because they often exhibit only nonspecific signs such as irritability, somnolence, and low-grade fever.[8,44]

CNS findings such as headache, photophobia, and neck or back pain are more common in older children and adolescents. In infants, a full fontanelle may be present. Seizures are noted in 20% to 30% of children before or within 3 days after the diagnosis and tend to be more frequently associated with meningitis secondary to *S. pneumoniae* and *H. influenzae*.[44] The seizures may be partial, generalized with focal predominance, or partial with secondary generalization.[45]

Findings on physical examination include alterations in level of consciousness that can range from irritability, to somnolence and lethargy, to coma. Up to 10% of patients at any age are comatose at the time of admission.[44,46] Findings of nuchal rigidity or presence of the Brudzinski and Kernig signs are indicators of meningeal irritation. However, their absence does not exclude the diagnosis of meningitis.

Skin findings such as petechiae and purpura are commonly associated with meningococcal meningitis, but they can be seen in association with *S. pneumoniae* and *H. influenzae* infections as well. It is important to keep in mind that the development of petechiae or purpura may be preceded by a maculopapular rash (see Chapter 62).

Focal neurologic abnormalities serve as indicators of compromised cerebral blood flow or increased intracranial pressure (ICP). Cranial nerve palsies, nystagmus, aphasia, hemiparesis, ataxia, hearing loss, and visual field defects may be present. Papilledema is a relatively late finding and not commonly associated with the acute phase of bacterial meningitis.[44]

Patients may present with evidence of hemodynamic instability or shock. Approximately 15% of children with pneumococcal meningitis present in shock.[47,48]

Brain Abscess

Factors influencing the clinical presentation of brain abscesses in children are the size and location of the abscess, as well as the age and immune status of the child. As is the case with bacterial meningitis, the presentation of brain abscess in infants and children can be nonspecific. The classic triad of fever, headache, and focal neurologic deficits occurs in less than 30% of all cases. In children who are able to report headache, it is the most common symptom. Fever may be seen in half to three quarters of cases. Vomiting, seizures, and focal neurologic deficits occur in a third to half of all cases. Focal neurologic signs reflect the location of the abscess. Lethargy, stupor, and coma are seen late in the course of the illness. Papilledema is seen in less than a quarter of cases.

Herpesviridae Encephalitis

Regardless of age, HSV infection of the brain results in necrotizing encephalitis. The virus demonstrates a particular predilection for the temporal lobes. In older patients, the signs and symptoms of HSV encephalitis are the result of the area or areas of the brain affected.[49,50] Symptoms include fever, altered consciousness, bizarre behavior, disorientation, and localized neurologic findings. In infants, clinical findings include seizures, which may be focal or generalized, irritability, lethargy, tremors, poor feeding, temperature instability, and a bulging fontanelle.

In cerebellar ataxia caused by varicella, the onset of ataxia is generally coincident with appearance of the exanthem. However, the ataxia may begin several days before onset of the rash to up to 2 weeks after its appearance. Other symptoms include vomiting, nystagmus, headache, and nuchal rigidity. In contrast, the onset, which may be sudden or gradual, of varicella-zoster virus encephalitis occurs approximately 1 week after appearance of the rash and consists of headache, altered sensorium, and vomiting.[28] Seizures occur in approximately a third to half of cases. Additional neurologic findings include abnormal plantar reflexes, hyporeflexia or hyperreflexia, hypotonia or hypertonia, hemiparesis, and sensory changes.

Enteroviral Meningitis and Encephalitis

Enteroviral meningitis has an abrupt onset associated with fever. The fever may be biphasic: initially associated with nonspecific constitutional symptoms and then subsiding and returning at the onset of neurologic symptoms. Infants exhibit nonspecific symptoms such as poor feeding, vomiting, exanthems, and respiratory tract findings. In older children and adolescents, symptoms may include anorexia, vomiting, headache, exanthems, myalgia, upper and lower respiratory tract symptoms, and abdominal pain.[31] In young infants, neurologic findings are minimal or absent and may consist of irritability, lethargy, a bulging fontanelle, and nuchal rigidity. In 10% of infants, acute CNS complication (seizures, increased ICP, and depressed mental state) may occur.[30] Headache is almost invariably present in older children and adolescents. Nuchal rigidity is mild and more frequently present in older toddlers, children, and adolescents. Photophobia is also a common finding in older patients.

In addition to the nonspecific symptoms described for meningitis, children with enteroviral encephalitis have mental status changes that range from lethargy and mild disorientation to frank coma. Focal neurologic findings similar to those in HSV encephalitis may occur.[30] Infection with some strains of enterovirus 71 may result in severe brainstem encephalitis in children.[51]

Arboviral Encephalitides
La Crosse Encephalitis

The incubation period for La Crosse encephalitis ranges from 5 to 15 days.[34] Typically, the onset of illness is characterized by a prodrome lasting 2 to 3 days that consists of fever, headache, malaise, and gastrointestinal symptoms.[33,35-38,52,53] Lethargy or an altered sensorium follow, and up to a third of children progress to coma. Seizures have been reported in 46% to 62% of children and may be generalized, focal, partial, partial complex, or status. Some patients have a sudden onset of fever and headache, followed 12 to 24 hours later by abrupt, prolonged, and difficult-to-control seizures.[36] Signs of meningeal irritation are reported in up to 60%, and focal neurologic findings occur in 16% to 25%.

Clinical deterioration during the first 4 days of admission to the hospital is not uncommon.[33] Nearly 60% of hospitalized children require admission to the intensive care unit and a quarter require mechanical ventilation.

West Nile Neuroinvasive Syndromes

The majority of human West Nile virus infections are subclinical. West Nile fever develops in approximately 20% of those infected.[54-57] Neuroinvasive forms of infection, which include encephalitis, meningitis, meningoencephalitis, and acute flaccid paralysis, develop in less than 1% of infected individuals (1 in 140 to 320).[56,57] The overwhelming majority of reported cases of neuroinvasive disease have been in adults.[56,58] The single most significant risk factor for the development of neuroinvasive disease and an adverse outcome is increasing age.

In 2002, 4156 cases of West Nile virus disease were reported, with clinical and demographic information available for 4146.[58] Only 150 (3.6%) cases occurred in individuals younger than 19 years. Of these, 27% were classified as West Nile fever, 70% had neuroinvasive disease (38% meningitis, 28% encephalitis, 34% unspecified), and 2.7% were classified as unknown illness. Thirty-seven percent of children were younger than 10 years.

The incubation period of West Nile virus infection is usually 2 to 6 days but can range from 2 to 14 days.[54,59] The symptoms of neuroinvasive West Nile virus infection, primarily described in adults, include fever, headache, altered mental status, weakness, neck stiffness, seizures, gastrointestinal symptoms, and rash.[56,60,61] Patients with the acute flaccid paralysis syndrome exhibit asymmetric weakness, hypotonia, and absent or diminished deep tendon reflexes, without pain or sensory loss in the affected limb or limbs.[61-63]

Limited reports of the clinical presentations of West Nile virus–associated encephalitis, meningoencephalitis, acute flaccid paralysis, and meningitis in children do exist,[58,64-69] but overall, the presentations are similar to those seen in adults.

St. Louis Encephalitis

The clinical presentation of St. Louis encephalitis virus infection is age dependent and varies from subclinical infection to fatal encephalitis.[31,70,71] The overwhelming majority of St. Louis encephalitis virus infections in humans are asymptomatic. The ratio of clinical to subclinical infection varies from 1:800 in children younger than 10 years to 1:85 in adults.[71]

Three neurologic syndromes associated with St. Louis encephalitis virus infection have been reported: encephalitis, aseptic meningitis, and febrile headache alone.[31] In infants, children, and adolescents, encephalitis, aseptic meningitis, and febrile headache occur in 56%, 38%, and 6% of cases, respectively.

The incubation period of St. Louis encephalitis ranges from 4 to 21 days.[31,72] The onset of neurologic illness may be heralded by nonspecific symptoms of malaise, fever, headache, somnolence, myalgias, abdominal and back pain, and occasionally, conjunctivitis, photophobia, and upper respiratory tract symptoms.[73] Fever is nearly universal. Headache is present in most children capable of reporting it. Nausea and vomiting occur in approximately three quarters of children.[74,75] Abnormal neurologic signs and symptoms include seizures, altered sensorium, including coma, evidence of meningeal irritation, seizures, and cranial nerve palsies.[74-77]

DIAGNOSIS AND EVALUATION

Evaluation of any patient with suspected meningitis or encephalitis requires CSF examination. Although routine neuroimaging of all patients before the performance of lumbar puncture is not required,[78,79] it should be performed in the settings of papilledema, altered mental status, focal neurologic findings, or suspicion of an intracranial mass lesion. Regardless of the decision to perform or delay the lumbar puncture, antibiotic therapy should not be delayed. If a decision is made to delay lumbar puncture, blood should be obtained for culture before the administration of antibiotics.

Ideally, collection of CSF should be performed before the administration of antibiotics because sterilization of CSF can occur rapidly after their administration. Indeed, one report found that sterilization of meningococci from the CSF occurred within 2 hours of the administration of parenteral antibiotics. In the case of pneumococci, sterilization of CSF began by 4 hours into parenteral therapy.[80]

Cytochemical evaluation of CSF should include a cell count and differential, as well as protein and glucose concentrations. CSF opening and closing pressure should be measured whenever possible. An attempt to identify the causal organism should be made by performing a Gram stain, culture, and in selected cases, nucleic acid amplification assays on CSF (i.e., polymerase chain reaction [PCR] and reverse transcription PCR [RT-PCR]).

Pyogenic meningitides generally result in CSF with a white blood cell (WBC) count consisting predominantly of polymorphonuclear cells ($>1000/mm^3$), elevated protein concentration, and depressed glucose concentration relative to that of serum. Rarely, all CSF parameters may be normal despite identification of a pathogen in CSF. In tuberculous meningitis, the CSF protein concentration may be so high that a pellicle forms at the air-fluid interface. In addition, the glucose concentration may be depressed to the point of being undetectable.

Two situations can be vexing in the interpretation of CSF findings: administration of antibiotics before lumbar puncture and a traumatic lumbar puncture. Although the yield of positive CSF cultures may fall to below 50% in patients previously treated with antibiotics,[8] the CSF parameters can still be indicative of infection. The leukocyte count can continue to increase and glucose and protein concentrations in the CSF can remain abnormal for several days.[81] Interpretation of the CSF cell count may be significantly confounded by blood introduced during a traumatic lumbar puncture. Although multiple published reports have attempted to define parameters for interpretation of the WBC count in this scenario, none has been demonstrated to be uniformly useful.[82-88] In 2006 in a retrospective study of 2900 CSF specimens contaminated by blood, it was concluded that adjusted WBC counts offer no advantage over uncorrected counts for predicting bacterial meningitis.[89] It is therefore best to exercise caution in interpreting the CSF findings from traumatic lumbar punctures.

All CSF specimens should be examined by Gram stain because it is positive in up to 80% to 90% of untreated cases of bacterial meningitis.[90,91] However, the decision to initiate antimicrobial therapy should not be based solely on the Gram stain.

Isolates recovered from broth cultures alone and not on agar plate cultures are infrequently true pathogens.[92,93] An exception may be the case of organisms recovered from CSF sampled from a ventriculoperitoneal shunt suspected of being infected. In these cases, organisms such as *Propionibacterium acnes* may be true pathogens and not contaminants.[94]

If CSF indices or the clinical or epidemiologic picture suggests viral, fungal, or tuberculous disease, specific stains and cultures should be requested. Detection of cryptococcal antigen in CSF provides rapid identification of this pathogen in immunocompromised hosts. If available, detection of the *Mycobacterium tuberculosis* genome by PCR may aid in the diagnosis of this infection.

In general, routine neuroimaging studies are not indicated in children with bacterial meningitis, with the exception of newborns. Magnetic resonance imaging (MRI) or computed tomography (CT) of the brain should be considered in the following circumstances: prolonged obtundation, intractable seizures or those that start 72 hours after treatment, focal neurologic findings, and suspicion of subdural empyema or hydrocephalus.[95] Additional diagnostic evaluations for children suspected of having meningitis include blood culture, urinalysis, and urine culture. Other baseline studies include a complete blood count, platelet count, and serum electrolyte concentrations.

Because of the risk for brainstem herniation and the low yield of diagnostic information, lumbar puncture is generally contraindicated in patients suspected of having a brain abscess. For this neuroinfectious process, neuroimaging remains the diagnostic study of choice for establishing the diagnosis (Fig. 63-1). MRI is superior to CT for the diagnosis of brain abscess. The former is more sensitive in detecting early cerebritis and edema formation. If CT is to be used, contrast studies must be included. When used serially, MRI and CT performed at weekly or biweekly intervals is useful in evaluating the response to therapy.

Herpesviridae Encephalitis

The CSF findings in HSV encephalitis are nonspecific and, in up to 10% of children, are normal on initial examination.[23] The average CSF lymphocytic pleocytosis is 100 cells/mm^3 with a protein concentration of 100 mg/dL. These values tend to increase as the disease progresses.

Neuroimaging with MRI or CT reveals changes in the temporal lobes, although MRI has been shown to be more sensitive in detecting early brain changes.[96] Electroencephalographic examination may reveal focal changes arising from the temporal lobe that consist of spike and slow-wave activity and periodic lateralized epileptiform discharges,[97-99] which are usually unilateral initially but spread to the contralateral side as the infection advances.

HSV can be isolated from CSF by culture in only 40% of patients with neonatal HSV encephalitis and 2% of older children and adults with HSV encephalitis.[104,105] Consequently, detection of HSV DNA in CSF by PCR has become

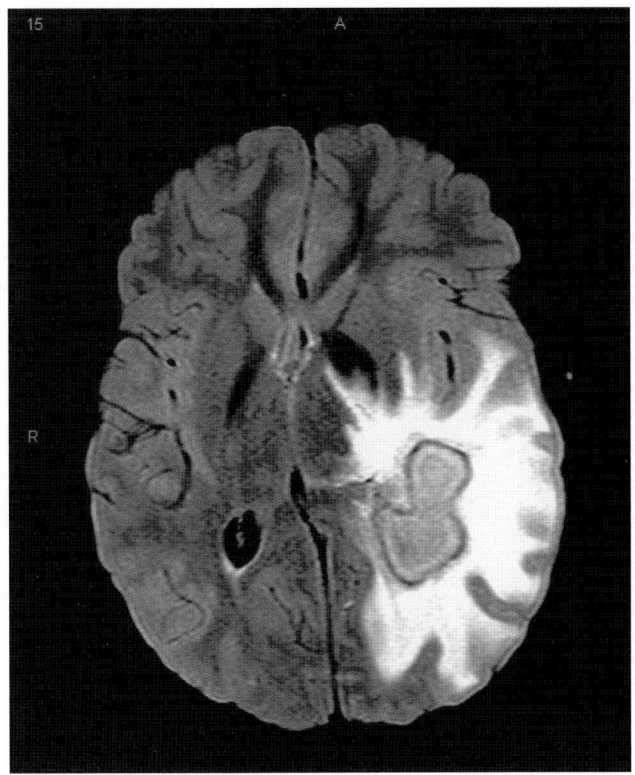

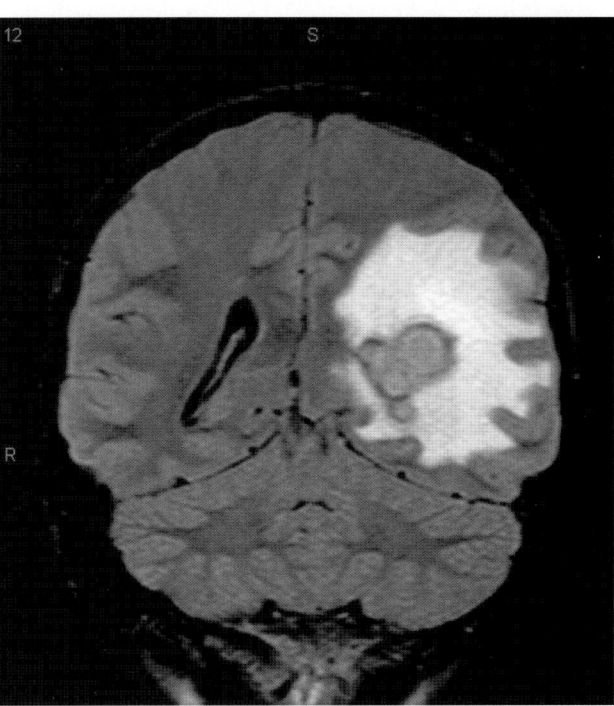

A   B

Figure 63-1 Brain magnetic resonance imaging in a 12-year-old girl demonstrates a multiloculated abscess in the left temporoparietal region. Thick rim enhancement (appears dark on these T2 images) is seen on both the axial (A) and coronal (B) views. Large amounts of vasogenic edema (appears bright white) is seen extending into the left cerebral hemisphere.

the diagnostic method of choice for establishing the diagnosis.[23,101] Data from the Collaborative Antiviral Study Group found the sensitivity and specificity of PCR to be 94% and 98%, respectively, when compared with brain biopsy–confirmed cases.[102]

In the majority of patients with varicella cerebellar ataxia, examination of CSF fails to reveal abnormalities. A mild (<100 cells/mm^3) lymphocytic pleocytosis with a mild elevation in CSF protein concentration is present in 20% to 30% of cases.[28] CSF abnormalities in varicella encephalitis are common and similar to those described for cerebellar ataxia. In addition, an elevated opening pressure is common.

The diagnosis of cerebellar ataxia is established clinically by the concurrent appearance of the rash of varicella in association with ataxia. Cerebellar or brainstem lesions may rarely be demonstrated by MRI.[103] To further substantiate the diagnosis, varicella-zoster virus can be detected in CSF by PCR.[103] In varicella encephalitis, electroencephalography reveals a diffuse encephalopathy consisting of slow-wave activity. Neuroimaging may show cerebral edema or findings of demyelination.[28]

Regardless of age, HSV encephalitis is a devastating infection. Without treatment, non-neonatal HSV encephalitis carries a 70% mortality rate, and only 2.5% of survivors recover complete neurologic function. Despite the advent of effective antiviral therapy, the mortality rate remains significant at 19%, and 62% of survivors are left with considerable neurologic sequelae.[104] As is the case with non-neonatal

HSV encephalitis, although mortality from neonatal HSV encephalitis has been significantly reduced (4%), 69% of survivors are left with major neurologic sequelae.[22,100]

Even without treatment, complete recovery from cerebellar ataxia is almost universally the rule. Although patients who survive varicella encephalitis usually do so without sequelae, there is a 5% to 10% mortality rate associated with this syndrome.

Enteroviral Meningitis and Encephalitis

In cases of enteroviral meningitis, CSF WBC counts may vary from no cells to several thousand but tend to be less than 1000 cells/mm^3. Typically, there is a predominance of mononuclear cells, but if lumbar puncture is performed early in the course of illness, CSF may have a predominance of polymorphonuclear leukocytes. Mild elevations of CSF protein in association with normal glucose concentrations are the general rule.

The CSF findings in enteroviral encephalitis may be minimal with only a few WBCs and a mildly elevated protein concentration. Focal changes may be found on electroencephalography.[30,51] Diffuse or focal brain lesions may occur in cases of encephalitis.

Although commonly used for the diagnosis of enteroviral infections, cell culture suffers from a lack of sensitivity (65% to 75%).[105] An additional limitation is the time required for identification of enteroviruses from CSF, which is reported to range from a mean of 4 to 8 days. The most sensitive, specific, and rapid method currently available for detection of enteroviruses is the use of RT-PCR for detection of the viral RNA genome.[101,105,106] The sensitivity and specificity of RT-PCR range from 86% to 100% and 92% to 100%, respectively. The time needed for identification of enteroviruses in clinical samples is reduced to hours with RT-PCR. The reduction in detection time is clinically meaningful in the management of patients with meningitis by shortening hospitalization and the use of antibiotics and reducing the need for ancillary diagnostic tests.[106,107]

Arbovirus Encephalitis

Typically, CSF analysis in cases of arboviral encephalitis reveals a mild lymphocytic pleocytosis. CSF glucose is normal and protein is mildly increased. However, early in the disease a predominance of polymorphonuclear cells may be present.

Electroencephalographic abnormalities are seen in the majority of cases of La Crosse, West Nile, and St. Louis encephalitis.[31,33,35-37,53,74,108-110] In acute flaccid paralysis, electromyography and nerve conduction studies document evidence of denervation.[61,63,68]

MRI is more sensitive than CT in identifying CNS abnormalities for these encephalitides.[34,56,57,60,111,112] In a child with acute flaccid paralysis, MRI of the spine documented edema of the anterior horns of the cervical spinal cord.[68,113]

The diagnosis of La Crosse encephalitis is established through serologic methods seeking the presence of virus-specific IgM in CSF or serum. More than 90% will have IgM virus-specific antibodies by the fifth day of illness.[114] Serum IgM antibodies may persist for longer than 6 months. Similarly, the diagnosis of West Nile and St. Louis encephalitis virus infections is established by serologic assays.[31] Virus-specific IgM antibody is present in the CSF or serum, or both, of 40% of infected individuals by the fourth day after the onset of illness and in virtually all individuals by day 10 of illness.[31] The finding of West Nile or St. Louis encephalitis virus–specific IgM in CSF is diagnostic of acute infection. However, the same may not be said to be true of finding West Nile virus IgM antibodies in serum. Virus-specific IgM has been shown to persist in serum for up to a year and a half after primary infection.[31,115,116] When only serum is used for diagnosis, a second serum sample should be obtained at least 2 weeks later to document a fourfold increase in specific antibody titer[58] because cross-reactions between St. Louis encephalitis virus, West Nile virus, and Powassan virus can occur.[31]

TREATMENT

Bacterial Meningitis

Recommendations for the management of bacterial meningitis have been published by the Infectious Diseases Society of America.[117] Selection of empirical antibiotic therapy for bacterial meningitis should be based on the most likely pathogen for the child's age group (Table 63-1), known resistance patterns, and the ability of the antibiotic to achieve adequate concentrations in CSF.[2,20,78,118] Once the specific pathogen has been identified and the results of antimicrobial susceptibility testing are known, specific antimicrobial therapy may be selected (Table 63-2).

Table 63-2   Dosages of Intravenous Antibiotics

Antibiotic	Age (Days)	Total Daily Dosage	Divided Dosing Interval
Amikacin	0-7	15-20 mg/kg	Every 12 hours
	8-28	30 mg/kg	Every 8 hours
	>28	20-30 mg/kg	Every 8 hours
Ampicillin	0-7	150 mg/kg	Every 8 hours
	8-28	200 mg/kg	Every 6 hours
	>28	200-300 mg/kg	Every 6 hours
Cefepime	0-7	—	—
	8-28	—	—
	>28	150 mg/kg	Every 8 hours
Cefotaxime	0-7	100-150 mg/kg	Every 8-12 hours
	8-28	150-200 mg/kg	Every 6-8 hours
	>28	225-300 mg/kg	Every 6-8 hours
Ceftazidime	0-7	100-150 mg/kg	Every 8-12 hours
	8-28	150 mg/kg	Every 8 hours
	>28	150 mg/kg	Every 8 hours
Ceftriaxone	0-7	—	—
	8-28	—	—
	>28	80-100 mg/kg	Every 12-24 hours
Gentamicin	0-7	5 mg/kg	Every 12 hours
	8-28	7.5 mg/kg	Every 8 hours
	>28	7.5 mg/kg	Every 8 hours
Meropenem	0-7	—	—
	8-28	—	—
	>28	120 mg/kg	Every 8 hours
Nafcillin	0-7	75 mg/kg	Every 8-12 hours
	8-28	100-150 mg/kg	Every 6-8 hours
	>28	200 mg/kg	Every 6 hours
Oxacillin	0-7	75 mg/kg	Every 8-12 hours
	8-28	150-200 mg/kg	Every 6-8 hours
	>28	200 mg/kg	Every 6 hours
Penicillin G	0-7	150,000 U/kg	Every 8-12 hours
	8-28	200,000 U/kg	Every 6-8 hours
	>28	300,000 U/kg	Every 4-6 hours
Rifampin	0-7	—	—
	8-28	10-20 mg/kg	Every 12 hours
	>28	10-20 mg/kg	Every 12-24 hours
Tobramycin	0-7	5 mg/kg	Every 12 hours
	8-28	7.5 mg/kg	Every 8 hours
	>28	7.5 mg/kg	Every 8 hours
Vancomycin	0-7	20-30 mg/kg	Every 8-12 hours
	8-28	30-45 mg/kg	Every 6-8 hours
	>28	60 mg/kg	Every 6 hours

From Tunkel AR, Hartman BJ, Kaplan SL, et al: Practice guidelines for the management of bacterial meningitis. Clin Infect Dis 2004;39:1267.

Traditionally, for empirical treatment of early-onset neonatal meningitis, ampicillin in combination with an aminoglycoside, usually gentamicin, is recommended. An alternative may be ampicillin in combination with a third-generation cephalosporin (e.g., cefotaxime). In the case of late-onset neonatal meningitis, expansion of the antimicrobial spectrum to provide therapy against staphylococci and other gram-negative organisms may be desirable. In such cases, an antistaphylococcal antibiotic (e.g., nafcillin or vancomycin) in combination with cefotaxime or ceftazidime, with or without an aminoglycoside, provides a broad range of coverage. Because of significant rates of penicillin resistance among pneumococcal isolates in the United States, empirical therapy for meningitis in infants older than 1 month, children, and adolescents should include a third-generation cephalosporin (e.g., ceftriaxone or cefotaxime) along with vancomycin.[2,8,78,117] Some authorities recommend that because of the potential overlap between pathogens in the neonatal period and those found in young infants, coverage with ampicillin and cefotaxime or ceftriaxone be provided for infants 1 to 3 months of age.[8]

Based on numerous published reports, evidence exists for the use of dexamethasone as an adjunct in therapy for Hib meningitis in infants and children. Similar evidence for the strong support of its use in cases of pneumococcal meningitis and in neonates is lacking.[117,119,120] Ideally, dexamethasone should be administered 10 to 20 minutes before the first dose of antibiotic or in no case later than coincident with the first dose. Dexamethasone should not be administered to children who have already initiated antibiotic therapy. The recommended dose of dexamethasone is 0.15 mg/kg every 6 hours for 2 to 4 days.

Although recommendations for the duration of therapy exist, it is important to note that they are based on tradition rather than on controlled clinical trials.[2,8,78,117] As such, they serve only as guides. Decisions regarding the length of treatment must be individualized by taking into account such factors as age, organism and susceptibility, clinical response, and complications. It is generally accepted that 4 to 7 days of therapy is sufficient for the treatment of meningococcal meningitis, whereas 7 to 10 days is adequate for Hib. Ten to 14 days suffices for the treatment of uncomplicated cases of pneumococcal meningitis. In the case of S. agalactiae, if the infant responds rapidly, a 14-day course may be sufficient. Alternatively, up to 21 days may be required. Treatment of gram-negative aerobic bacilli generally requires 21 days. Finally, for L. monocytogenes, treatment for 14 to 21 days or longer is recommended.[2,8,117]

In certain circumstances it may be appropriate or necessary to repeat the lumbar puncture for reexamination of CSF during the course of therapy. In general, if appropriate antibiotics are selected, it is to be expected that CSF will become sterile within 24 to 36 hours after the initiation of therapy.[121] Repeat lumbar puncture is indicated 24 to 48 hours after starting treatment if the infection is caused by a gram-negative bacillus or a penicillin-resistant strain of S. pneumoniae or if the patient is failing to respond appropriately to treatment.[117] Additionally, some experts suggest that all neonates with meningitis undergo repeat CSF examination.[2]

Fluid management in a child with meningitis is an integral and important part of the treatment of this disease and prevention of complications. Maintenance of adequate vascular volume is essential for sustaining adequate cerebral perfusion and managing increased ICP. Even though it had traditionally been taught that fluid restriction should be a component of the management of meningitis, several studies have demonstrated that liberal use of fluids can be beneficial.[122-125] Because most patients are fluid depleted at the time of presentation, fluids should not be restricted in the initial phases of management. Fluid restriction in this setting could compromise cerebral blood flow as a result of decreased blood pressure. In some cases, maintenance of normal blood pressure may necessitate the use of pressors. All patients require close monitoring of volume status, fluid input and loss, weight, serum electrolytes, osmolality, and urine specific gravity.

Measures designed to reduce increased ICP and preserve cerebral perfusion, as well as oxygenation, include administration of supplemental oxygen, control of fever, elevation of the head of the bed, short-term hyperventilation, use of mannitol, and avoidance of frequent suctioning. Seizures should be prevented or controlled. Audiologic screening is indicated for children with meningitis.

Brain Abscess

Management of brain abscess in children requires a multidisciplinary approach. Medical treatment alone may be successful in neurologically intact children whose illness is less than 2 weeks old, who have no signs of increased ICP, and whose abscess is smaller than 3 cm in diameter. If a medical approach is selected, patients should be monitored closely with neuroimaging once a week.

For most brain abscesses, surgical drainage, in combination with antimicrobial therapy, remains the treatment of choice. Currently, MRI- or CT-guided stereotactic aspiration is the procedure of choice for drainage. Material obtained at the time of aspiration should be sent for Gram stain and culture of anaerobic and aerobic bacteria, fungi, and mycobacteria.

In patients with suspected brain abscess, antimicrobial therapy should be initiated immediately. For the empirical treatment of brain abscesses that arise as a result of sinusitis, mastoiditis, otitis, or heart disease associated with left-to-right shunts, a combination of a third-generation cephalosporin (e.g., ceftriaxone, cefotaxime, or ceftazidime) plus metronidazole is generally recommended. Brain abscess associated with penetrating head trauma, endocarditis, or ventriculoperitoneal shunts warrant a third-generation cephalosporin in combination with vancomycin and, possibly, metronidazole. For brain abscesses that arise as a result of S. pneumoniae meningitis, a third-generation cephalosporin plus vancomycin should be used.

The duration of antimicrobial therapy should be individualized. In general, intravenous therapy is continued for 4 to 8 weeks. Some authorities recommend an additional 2 to 3 months of oral antibiotics. Response to therapy should be monitored with neuroimaging techniques. Even with therapy, mortality from brain abscesses remains relatively high. A third of survivors are left with neurologic sequelae. Poor prognostic indicators include age younger than 1 year, rapid neurologic impairment, multiple foci, and coma at the time of diagnosis.

Herpesviridae Encephalitis

Acyclovir is the treatment of choice for HSV encephalitis[104] and should be initiated immediately when signs and symptoms consistent with the diagnosis are identified. In children and adolescents, acyclovir is administered at a dosage of 10 mg/kg every 8 hours (30 mg/kg/day) for a period of 14 to 21 days.[23] For the treatment of neonates, it is administered at a dosage of 20 mg/kg every 8 hours (60 mg/kg/day) for a similar length of time.

Although no conclusive evidence exists that acyclovir therapy alters the course of cerebellar ataxia, its use has been recommended by some experts.[28] The use of intravenous acyclovir is also recommended for the treatment of patients with varicella encephalitis, even though no controlled clinic trials have been conducted.[28]

Enteroviral Infections of the Central Nervous System

Management of enteroviral infections is supportive and includes symptomatic relief and maintenance of hydration. Children with severe encephalitis may require cardiorespiratory support in an intensive care setting. Control of the seizures that can accompany encephalitis may require antiepileptic drugs.

Arbovirus Encephalitis

Management of arboviral encephalitides is primarily supportive. Because of the risk of progressive worsening of neurologic status in 5% to 15% of La Crosse encephalitis cases, close observation with frequent neurologic monitoring is

a key component in management. Deterioration of the patient's Glasgow coma scale score should warrant transfer to an intensive care setting. Attention to airway patency is critical, particularly in cases of West Nile and La Crosse encephalitis. In the former, severe muscle weakness or paralysis may require the use of mechanical ventilation.

In severe cases of encephalitis, monitoring of ICP may be warranted. Close attention to fluid and electrolyte status is important because the development of hyponatremia and the syndrome of inappropriate antidiuretic hormone secretion has been documented. Seizures should be treated with anticonvulsants.

PREVENTION

Primary prevention of bacterial meningitis caused by Hib, *N. meningitidis*, and *S. pneumoniae* is based on the timely administration of conjugated polysaccharide vaccines. Chemoprophylaxis for the prevention of secondary cases of meningitis is indicated for close contacts of cases of meningitis caused by Hib and meningococcus (Tables 63-3 and 63-4). For close contacts of cases of pneumococcal meningitis, chemoprophylaxis is not indicated.

Table 63-3 Chemoprophylaxis Guidelines for Contacts of Index Cases of *Haemophilus influenzae* Type b Meningitis

Chemoprophylaxis Recommended	Antibiotic and Dosage

All close household contacts as follows:
  Household with at least 1 contact younger than 4 years of age who is not immunized or incompletely immunized
  Household with a child younger than 12 months if the child has not received the primary series
  Household with an immunocompromised child, regardless of Hib vaccine status
For nursery school and child care centers, regardless of age, when 2 or more cases of Hib invasive disease have occurred within 60 days
For the index case treated with a regimen other than cefotaxime or ceftriaxone if <2 years old or if a member of a household with a susceptible contact
	Rifampin, 20 mg/kg/day (maximum dose, 600 mg/day) administered once daily for 4 days
	For infants <1 month of age, the dose should be lowered to 10 mg/kg/day

Modified from the American Academy of Pediatrics: *Haemophilus influenzae* infections. In Pickering LK (ed): Red Book: 2003 Report of the Committee on Infectious Diseases, 26th ed. Elk Grove Village, IL, American Academy of Pediatrics, 2003, pp 295-297.

Table 63-4 Chemoprophylaxis Guidelines for Contacts of Index Cases of Meningococcal Meningitis

Chemoprophylaxis Recommended	Antibiotic and Dosage
A household contact, in particular, young children Child care or nursery school contacts during the 7 days before the onset of illness Direct exposure to the index patient's secretions through kissing, sharing of toothbrushes or eating utensils, or close social contact during the 7 days before the onset of illness Mouth-to-mouth resuscitation or unprotected contact during endotracheal intubation during the 7 days before the onset of illness Frequently slept or ate in same dwelling as the index patient during the 7 days before the onset of illness	Rifampin* ≤1 month of age, 5 mg/kg orally every 12 hours for 2 days >1 month of age, 10 mg/kg orally every 12 hours for 2 days (maximum dose, 600 mg orally every 12 hours) Ceftriaxone ≤15 years of age, 125 mg intramuscularly, single dose >15 years of age, 250 mg intramuscularly, single dose Ciprofloxacin* ≥18 years of age, 500 mg orally, single dose

*Not recommended for use in pregnant women.
Modified from the American Academy of Pediatrics: Meningococcal infections. In Pickering LK (ed): Red Book: 2003 Report of the Committee on Infectious Diseases, 26th ed. Elk Grove Village, IL, American Academy of Pediatrics, 2003, pp 433-434.

Prevention of arboviral encephalitides requires a combination of public health and personal protective measures. The former include control of mosquito breeding habitats, judicious use of mosquito larvicides, and active surveillance of arboviral-infected mosquitoes. Individuals should use insect repellents, protective clothing, and insecticides. Screening of windows and the use of mosquito bed nets may also be warranted.

SUGGESTED READING

Bonsu BK, Harper MB: Corrections for leukocytes and percent of neutrophils do not match observations in blood-contaminated cerebrospinal fluid and have no value over uncorrected cells for diagnosis. Pediatr Infect Dis J 2006;25:8-11.

Kimberlin DW, Lin CY, Jacobs RF, et al, for the National Institute of Allergy and Infectious Diseases Collaborative Antiviral Study Group: Natural history of neonatal herpes simplex virus infections in the acyclovir era. Pediatrics 2001;108:223-238.

Rotbart HA: Viral meningitis. Semin Neurol 2000;20:277-292.

Saez-Llorens X, McCracken GH Jr: Bacterial meningitis in children. Lancet 2003;361:2139-2148.

Yogev R, Bar-Meir M: Management of brain abscesses in children. Pediatr Infect Dis J 2004;23:157-159.

REFERENCES

1. Wenger JD, Hightower AW, Facklam RR, et al: Bacterial meningitis in the United States, 1986: Report of a multistate surveillance study. The Bacterial Meningitis Study Group. J Infect Dis 1990;162:1316-1323.
2. Chavez-Bueno S, McCracken GH Jr: Bacterial meningitis in children. Pediatr Clin North Am 2005;52:795-810.
3. Schuchat A, Robinson K, Wegner JD, et al: Bacterial meningitis in the United States in 1995. Active Surveillance Team. N Engl J Med 1997;337:970-976.
4. Centers for Disease Control and Prevention (CDC): Progress toward elimination of *Haemophilus influenzae* type b invasive disease among infants and children—United States, 1998-2000. MMWR Morb Mortal Wkly Rep 2002;51(11):234-237.
5. Advisory Committee on Immunization Practices: Preventing pneumococcal disease among infants and young children: Recommendations of the Advisory Committee on Immunization Practices (ACIP). MMWR Recomm Rep 2000;49(RR-9):1-35.
6. Whitney CG, Farley MM, Hadler J, et al: Decline in invasive pneumococcal disease after the introduction of protein-conjugate polysaccharide conjugate vaccine. N Engl J Med 2003;348:1737-1746.
7. Schraq S, Gorwitz R, Faltz-Butts K, Schuchat A: Prevention of perinatal group B streptococcal disease: Revised guidelines from CDC. MMWR Recomm Rep 2002;51(RR-11):1-22.
8. Saez-Llorens X, McCracken GH Jr: Bacterial meningitis in children. Lancet 2003;361:2139-2148.
9. Kessler SL, Dajani AS: *Listeria* meningitis in infants and children. Pediatr Infect Dis 1990;9:61-63.
10. Linnan MJ, Mascola L, Lou XD, et al: Epidemic listeriosis associated with Mexican-style cheese. N Engl J Med 1988;319:823-828.
11. Willis J, Robinson JE: *Enterobacter sakazakii* meningitis in neonates. Pediatr Infect Dis J 1988;7:196-199.
12. Lai KK: *Enterobacter sakazakii* infections among neonates, infants, children, and adults. Case reports and a review of the literature. Medicine (Baltimore) 2001;80:113-122.
13. Stoll BJ, Hansen N, Fanaroff AA, Lemons JA: *Enterobacter sakazakii* is a rare cause of neonatal septicemia or meningitis in VLBW infants. J Pediatr 2004;144:821-823.
14. Doran TI: The role of *Citrobacter* in clinical disease of children: Review. Clin Infect Dis 1999;28:384-394.
15. Reefhuis J, Honein MA, Whitney CG, et al: Risk of bacterial meningitis in children with cochlear implants. N Engl J Med 2003;349:435-445.
16. Biernath KR, Reefhuis J, Whitney CG, et al: Bacterial meningitis among children with cochlear implants beyond 24 months after implantation. Pediatrics 2006;117:284-289.
17. Bilukha OO, Rosenstein N; National Center for Infectious Diseases, Centers for Disease Control and Prevention (CDC): Prevention and control of meningococcal disease: Recommendations of the Advisory Committee on Immunization Practices (ACIP). MMWR Recomm Rep 2005;54(RR-7):1-21.
18. Yogev R, Bar-Meir M: Management of brain abscesses in children. Pediatr Infect Dis J 2004;23:157-159.
19. Yogev R: Suppurative intracranial complications of upper respiratory tract infections. Pediatr Infect Dis J 1987;6:324-327.
20. Saez-Llorens X, McCracken GH Jr: Antimicrobial and anti-inflammatory treatment of bacterial meningitis. Infect Dis Clin North Am 1999;13: 619-636.
21. Olson LC, Buescher EL, Artenstein MS, et al: Herpesvirus infections of the human central nervous system. N Engl J Med 1967;277:1271-1277.
22. Kimberlin DW: Neonatal herpes simplex infection. Clin Microbiol Rev 2004;17:1-13.
23. Whitley RJ, Kimberlin DW: Herpes simplex encephalitis: Children and adolescents. Semin Pediatr Infect Dis 2005;16:17-23.
24. Whitley R, Lakeman AD, Nahmias A: DNA restriction-enzyme analysis of herpes simplex virus isolates obtained from patients with encephalitis. N Engl J Med 1982;307:1060-1062.
25. Nahmias AJ, Whitley RJ, Visintine AN, et al: Herpes simplex virus encephalitis: Laboratory evaluations and their diagnostic significance. J Infect Dis 1982;145:829-836.
26. Whitley RJ, Corey L, Arvin A, et al: Changing presentation of herpes simplex virus infection in neonates. J Infect Dis 1988;158:109-116.
27. Kleinschmidt-DeMasters BK, Gilden DH: The expanding spectrum of herpesvirus infections of the nervous system. Brain Pathol 2001;11:440-451.
28. Gnann JW Jr: Varicella-zoster virus: Atypical presentations and unusual complications. J Infect Dis 2002;186(Suppl 1):S91-S98.
29. Rotbart HA: Viral meningitis. Semin Neurol 2000;20:277-292.
30. Modlin JF, Dagan R, Berlin LE, et al: Focal encephalitis with enterovirus infections. Pediatrics 1991;88:841-845.
31. Tsai TF, Chandler LJ: Arboviruses. In Murray PR, Baron EJ, Jorgensen JH, et al (eds): Manual of Clinical Microbiology, 8th ed. Washington, DC, American Society for Microbiology Press, 2003, pp 1553-1569.
32. Brinker KR, Monath TP: The acute disease. In Monath TP (ed): St. Louis Encephalitis. Washington, DC, American Public Health Association, 1980, pp 503-534.
33. McJunkin JE, de los Reyes EC, Irazuzta JE, et al: La Crosse encephalitis in children. N Engl J Med 2001;344:801-807.
34. McJunkin JE, Khan RR, Tsai TF: California-La Crosse encephalitis. Infect Dis Clin North Am 1998;12:83-93.
35. Cramblett HG, Stegmiller H, Spencer C: California encephalitis virus infections in children. Clinical and laboratory studies. JAMA 1966;198: 108-112.
36. Balfour HH Jr, Siem RA, Bauer H, Quie PG: California arbovirus (La Crosse) infections. I. Clinical and laboratory findings in 66 children with meningoencephalitis. Pediatrics 1973;52:680-691.
37. Chun RW, Thompson WH, Grabow JD, Matthews CG: California arbovirus encephalitis in children. Neurology 1968;18:369-375.
38. Erwin PC, Jones TF, Gerhardt RR, et al: La Crosse encephalitis in eastern Tennessee: Clinical, environmental, and entomologic characteristics from a blinded cohort study. Am J Epidemiol 2002;155:1060-1065.
39. Asnis DS, Conetta R, Teixeira AA, et al: The West Nile virus outbreak of 1999 in New York: The Flushing Hospital experience. Clin Infect Dis 2000;30:413-418.
40. Centers for Disease Control and Prevention (CDC): Summary of notifiable diseases—United States, 2001. MMWR Morb Mortal Wkly Rep 2003;50(53):i-xxiv, 1-108.
41. Groseclose SL, Brathwaite WS, Hall PS, et al: Summary of notifiable diseases—United States, 2002. MMWR Morb Mortal Wkly Rep 2004; 51(53):1-84.

42. Kaplan SL, Taber LH, Frank AL, et al: Nasopharyngeal viral isolates in children with *Haemophilus influenzae* type b meningitis. J Pediatr 1981;99:591-593.

43. Kilpi T, Anttila M, Kallis MJT, Peltola H: Severity of childhood bacterial meningitis and duration of illness before diagnosis. Lancet 1991;338:406-409.

44. Kaplan SL: Clinical presentations, diagnosis, and prognostic factors of bacterial meningitis. Infect Dis Clin North Am 1999;13:579-594.

45. Pomeroy SL, Homes SJ, Dodge PR, Feigin RD: Seizures and other neurologic sequelae of bacterial meningitis in children. N Engl J Med 1990;323:1651-1657.

46. Feigin RD, McCracken GH Jr, Klein JO: Diagnosis and management of meningitis. Pediatr Infect Dis J 1992;11:785-814.

47. Arditi M, Mason EO Jr, Bradley JS, et al: Three-year multicenter surveillance of pneumococcal meningitis in children: Clinical characteristics and outcome related to penicillin susceptibility and dexamethasone use. Pediatrics 1998;102:1087-1097.

48. Kornelisse RF, Westerbeek CML, Spoor AB, et al: Pneumococcal meningitis in children: Prognostic indicators and outcome. Clin Infect Dis 1995;21:1390-1397.

49. Whitley RJ, Soong SJ, Dolin R, et al: Adenine arabinoside therapy of biopsy-proved herpes simplex encephalitis. N Engl J Med 1977;297:289-294.

50. Whitley RJ, Soong SJ, Hirsch MS, et al: Herpes simplex encephalitis: Vidarabine therapy and diagnostic problems. N Engl J Med 1981;304:313-318.

51. Huang CC, Liu CC, Chang YC, et al: Neurologic complications in children with enterovirus 71 infection. N Engl J Med 1999;341:936-942.

52. Balkhy HH, Schreiber JR: Severe La Crosse encephalitis with significant neurologic sequelae. Pediatr Infect Dis J 2000;19:77-80.

53. Hilty MD, Haynes RE, Azimi PH, Cramblett HG: California encephalitis in children. Am J Dis Child 1972;124:530-533.

54. Campbell GL, Marfin AA, Lanciotti RR, Gubler DJ: West Nile virus. Lancet Infect Dis 2002;2:519-529.

55. Watson JT, Pertel PE, Jones RC, et al: Clinical characteristics and functional outcomes of West Nile fever. Ann Intern Med 2004;141:360-365.

56. Nash D, Mostashari F, Fine A, et al, for the West Nile Outbreak Response Working Group: The outbreak of West Nile virus infection in the New York City area in 1999. N Engl J Med 2001;344:1807-1814.

57. Petersen LR, Marfin AA: West Nile virus: A primer for the clinician. Ann Intern Med 2002;137:173-179.

58. Hayes EB, O'Leary DR: West Nile virus infection: A pediatric perspective. Pediatrics 2004;113:1375-1381.

59. Komar N: West Nile virus: Epidemiology and ecology in North America. Adv Virus Res 2003;61:185-234.

60. Weiss D, Carr D, Kellachan J, et al, for the West Nile Virus Outbreak Response Working Group: Clinical findings of West Nile virus infection in hospitalized patients, New York and New Jersey, 2000. Emerg Infect Dis 2001;7:654-658.

61. Centers for Disease Control and Prevention (CDC): Acute flaccid paralysis syndrome associated with West Nile virus infection—Mississippi and Louisiana, July-August 2002. MMWR Morb Mortal Wkly Rep 2002;51(37):825-828.

62. Chowers MY, Lang R, Nassar F, et al: Clinical characteristics of the West Nile fever outbreak, Israel, 2000. Emerg Infect Dis 2001;7:675-678.

63. Sejvar JJ, Leis AA, Stokic DS, et al: Acute flaccid paralysis and West Nile virus infection. Emerg Infect Dis 2003;9:788-793.

64. Yim R, Posfay-Barbe KM, Holt D, et al: Spectrum of clinical manifestations of West Nile virus infection in children. Pediatrics 2004;4:1673-1675.

65. George S, Gourie-Devi M, Rao JA, et al: Isolation of West Nile virus from the brains of children who had died of encephalitis. Bull World Health Organ 1984;62:879-882.

66. Vidwan G, Bryant KK, Puri V, et al: West Nile virus encephalitis in a child with left-side weakness. Clin Infect Dis 2003;37:e91-e94.

67. Weinstein M: Atypical West Nile virus infection in a child. Pediatr Infect Dis J 2003;22:842-844.

68. Heresi GP, Mancias P, Mazur LJ, et al: Poliomyelitis-like syndrome in a child with West Nile virus infection. Pediatr Infect Dis J 2004;23:788-789.

69. Horga MA, Fine A: West Nile virus. Pediatr Infect Dis J 2001;20:801-802.

70. Report on the St. Louis Outbreak of Encephalitis, Public Health Bulletin 214. Washington, DC, U.S. Government Printing Office, 1935.

71. Monath TP, Tsai T: Flaviviruses. 2002. In Richman DD, Whitley RJ, Hayden FG (eds): Clinical Virology, 2nd ed. Washington DC, American Society for Microbiology, 2002, pp 1097-1151.

72. Leake JP, Musson EK, Chope HD: Epidemiology of epidemic encephalitis, St. Louis type. JAMA 1934;103:728-731.

73. Muckenfuss RS: Clinical observations and laboratory investigations of the 1933 epidemic of encephalitis in St. Louis. Bull N Y Acad Med 1934;10:444-453.

74. Barret FF, Yow MD, Phillips CA: St. Louis encephalitis in children during the 1964 epidemic. JAMA 1965;193:381-385.

75. Blattner RJ, Heys FM: The occurrence of St. Louis encephalitis in children in the St. Louis area during nonepidemic years, 1939-44. JAMA 1945;129:854-857.

76. Quick DT, Thompson JM, Bond JO: The 1962 epidemic of St. Louis encephalitis in Florida. IV. Clinical features of cases occurring in the Tampa Bay area. Am J Epidemiol 1965;681:415-427.

77. Beckman JW: Neurologic aspects of the epidemic of encephalitis in St. Louis. Arch Neurol Psychiatry 1935;33:732.

78. El Bashir H, Laundy M, Booy R: Diagnosis and treatment of bacterial meningitis. Arch Dis Child 2003;88:615-620.

79. Mellor DH: The place of computed tomography and lumbar puncture in suspected bacterial meningitis. Arch Dis Child 1992;67:1417-1419.

80. Kanegaye JT, Soliemanzadeh P, Bradley JS: Lumbar puncture in pediatric bacterial meningitis: Defining the time interval for recovery of cerebrospinal fluid pathogens after parental antibiotic pretreatment. Pediatrics 2001;108:1169-1174.

81. Converse GM, Gwaltney JM Jr, Strassburg DA, Hendley JD: Alteration of cerebrospinal fluid findings by partial treatment of bacterial meningitis. J Pediatr 1973;83:220-225.

82. Osborne JP, Pizer B: Effect on the white blood cell count of contaminating cerebrospinal fluid with blood. Arch Dis Child 1981;56:400-401.

83. Novak RW: Lack of validity of standard corrections for white blood cell counts of blood-contaminated cerebrospinal fluid in infants. Am J Clin Pathol 1984;82:95-97.

84. Rubenstein JS, Yogev R: What represents pleocytosis in blood contaminated ("traumatic tap") cerebrospinal fluid in children? J Pediatr 1985;107:249-251.

85. Mehl AL: Interpretation of traumatic lumbar puncture. Predictive value in the presence of meningitis. Clin Pediatr (Phila) 1986;25:575-577.

86. Mayefsky JH, Roghmann KJ: Determination of leukocytosis in traumatic spinal tap specimens. Am J Med 1987;82:1175-1181.

87. Bonadio WA, Smith DS, Goddard S, et al: Distinguishing cerebrospinal fluid abnormalities in children with bacterial meningitis and traumatic lumbar puncture. J Infect Dis 1990;162:251-254.

88. Mazor SS, McNulty JE, Roosevelt GE: Interpretation of traumatic lumbar punctures: Who can go home? Pediatrics 2003;111:525-528.

89. Bonsu BK, Harper MB: Corrections for leukocytes and percent of neutrophils do not match observations in blood-contaminated cerebrospinal fluid and have no value over uncorrected cells for diagnosis. Pediatr Infect Dis J 2006;25:8-11.

90. Saez-Llorens X, McCracken G: Acute bacterial meningitis. In Long SS (ed): Principles and Practice of Pediatric Infectious Diseases, 2nd ed. Philadelphia, Churchill Livingstone, 2003, pp 264-271.

91. Feldman WE: Concentrations of bacteria in cerebrospinal fluid of patients with bacterial meningitis J Pediatr 1976;88:549-552.

92. Meredith FT, Phillips HK, Reller LB: Clinical utility of broth cultures of cerebrospinal fluid from patients at risk for shunt infections. J Clin Microbiol 1997;35:3109-3111.

93. Stugis CD, Peterson LR, Warren JR: Cerebrospinal fluid broth culture isolates: Their significance for antibiotic treatment. Am J Clin Pathol 1997;108:217-221.

94. Thompson TP, Albright AL: *Propionibacterium acnes* infections of cerebrospinal fluid shunts. Childs Nerv Syst 1998;14:378-380.

95. Wubbel L, McCracken GH Jr: Management of bacterial meningitis: 1998. Pediatr Rev 1998;19:78-84.

96. Schlesinger Y, Buller RS, Brunstrom JE, et al: Expanded spectrum of herpes simplex encephalitis in childhood. J Pediatr 1995;126:234-241.

97. Smith JB, Westmoreland BF, Reagan TJ, Sandok BA: A distinctive clinical EEG profile in herpes simplex encephalitis. Mayo Clin Proc 1975;50:469-474.

98. Chien LT, Boehm RM, Robinson H, et al: Characteristic early electroencephalographic changes in herpes simplex encephalitis. Arch Neurol 1977;34:361-364.

99. Upton A, Grumpert J: Electroencephalography in diagnosis of herpes-simplex encephalitis. Lancet 1970;1:650-652.

100. Kimberlin DW, Lin CY, Jacobs RF, et al: Safety and efficacy of high-dose intravenous acyclovir in the management of neonatal herpes simplex virus infections. Pediatrics 2001;108:230-238.

101. Romero JR, Kimberlin DW: Molecular diagnosis of viral infections of the central nervous system. Clin Lab Med 2003;23:843-865.

102. Lakeman FD, Whitley RJ: Diagnosis of herpes simplex encephalitis: Application of polymerase chain reaction to cerebrospinal fluid from brain biopsied patients and correlation with disease. National Institute of Allergy and Infectious Diseases Collaborative Antiviral Study Group. J Infect Dis 1995;172:857-863.

103. Kleinschmidt-DeMasters BK, Gilden DH: Varicella-zoster virus infections of the nervous system: Clinical and pathologic correlates. Arch Pathol Lab Med 2001;125:770-780.

104. Whitley RJ, Alford CA Jr, Hirsch MS, et al: Vidarabine versus acyclovir therapy in herpes simplex encephalitis. N Engl J Med 1986;314:144-149.

105. Romero JR, Rotbart HA: Enteroviruses. In Murray PR, Baron EJ, Pfaller MA, et al (eds): Manual of Clinical Microbiology, 8th ed. Washington DC, American Society for Microbiology, 2003, pp 1427-1438.

106. Romero JR: Reverse-transcription polymerase chain reaction detection of the enteroviruses: Overview and clinical utility in pediatric enteroviral infections. Arch Pathol Lab Med 1999;123:1161-1169.

107. Ramers C, Billman G, Hartin M, et al: Impact of a diagnostic cerebrospinal fluid enterovirus polymerase chain reaction test on patient management. JAMA 2000;283:2680-2685.

108. Southern PM Jr, Smith JW, Luby JP, et al: Clinical and laboratory features of epidemic St. Louis encephalitis. Ann Intern Med 1969;71:681-689.

109. Brinker KR, Paulson G, Monath TP, et al: St Louis encephalitis in Ohio, September 1975: Clinical and EEG studies in 16 cases. Arch Intern Med 1979;139:561-566.

110. Wasay M, Diaz-Arrastia R, Suss RA, et al: St Louis encephalitis: A review of 11 cases in a 1995 Dallas, Texas epidemic. Arch Neurol 2000;57:114-118.

111. Bosanko CM, Gilroy J, Wang AM, et al: West Nile virus encephalitis involving the substantia nigra: Neuroimaging and pathologic findings with literature review. Arch Neurol 2003;60:1448-1452.

112. Solomon T: Flavivirus encephalitis. N Engl J Med 2004;351;370-378.

113. Cerna F, Mehrad B, Luby JP, et al: St. Louis encephalitis and the substantia nigra: MR imaging evaluation. AJNR Am J Neuroradiol 1999;20:1281-1283.

114. McJunkin JE, Khan R, de los Reyes EC, et al: Treatment of severe La Crosse encephalitis with intravenous ribavirin following diagnosis by brain biopsy. Pediatrics 1997;99:261-267.

115. Roehrig JT, Nash D, Maldin B, et al: Persistence of virus-reactive serum immunoglobulin M antibody in confirmed West Nile virus encephalitis cases. Emerg Infect Dis 2003;9:376-379.

116. Kuno G: Serodiagnosis of flaviviral infections and vaccinations in humans. Adv Virus Res 2003;61:3-65.

117. Tunkel AR, Hartman BJ, Kaplan SL, et al: Practice guidelines for the management of bacterial meningitis. Clin Infect Dis 2004;39:1267-1284.

118. Sinner SW, Tunkel AR: Antimicrobial agents in the treatment of bacterial meningitis. Infect Dis Clin North Am 2004;18:581-602.

119. McIntyre PB, Berkey CS, King SM, et al: Dexamethasone as adjunctive therapy in bacterial meningitis: A meta-analysis of randomized clinical trials since 1988. JAMA 1997;278:925-931.

120. American Academy of Pediatrics: Pneumococcal infections. In Pickering LK (ed): Red Book: 2003 Report of the Committee on Infectious Diseases, 26th ed. Elk Grove Village, IL, American Academy of Pediatrics, 2003, pp 490-500.

121. Bonadio WA: The cerebrospinal fluid: Physiologic aspects and alterations associated with bacterial meningitis. Pediatr Infect Dis J 1992;11:423-431.

122. Moller K, Larsen FS, Bie P, Skinhoj P: The syndrome of inappropriate secretion of antidiuretic hormone and fluid restriction in meningitis—how strong is the evidence? Scand J Infect Dis 2001;33:13-26.

123. Powell KR, Sugarman LI, Eskanazi AE, et al: Normalization of plasma arginine vasopressin concentrations when children with meningitis are given maintenance plus replacement fluid therapy. J Pediatr 1990;117:515-522.

124. Singhi SC, Singhi PD, Srinivas B, et al: Fluid restriction does not improve the outcome of acute meningitis. Pediatr Infect Dis J 1995;14:495-503.

125. Duke T, Mokela D, Frank D, et al: Management of meningitis in children with oral fluid restriction intravenous fluid at maintenance volumes: A randomised trial. Ann Trop Paediatr 2002;22:145-157.

CHAPTER 64

Complications of Acute Otitis Media and Sinusitis

Megan H. Bair-Merritt and Samir S. Shah

Uncomplicated acute otitis media (AOM) and sinusitis are generally managed in the outpatient setting with excellent outcomes. Occasionally, complications from these infections arise, and a subset of these complications requires immediate intervention and hospitalization (Table 64-1).

AOM is one of the most common childhood illnesses. By 1 year of age, two thirds of all children will have had at least one ear infection, and 17% of children will have had more than three episodes of AOM. The prevalence of AOM is higher in children younger than 3 years because of narrower and more horizontal positioning of the eustachian tubes. In addition, these children have a relatively immature immune system in comparison to older children, thus making them more susceptible to infection.[1]

AOM is defined as inflammation of the mucoperiosteal lining of the middle ear.[1] An upper respiratory tract infection (URI) precedes most episodes of AOM and causes edema and obstruction of the eustachian tube, which then impedes drainage of middle ear fluid (Fig. 64-1).[2] If pathogenic bacteria are present in the middle ear fluid, suppurative infection may follow.

Sinusitis develops in 5% to 10% of episodes of URI, and because children average from six to eight URIs each year, sinusitis becomes a very common entity. URIs facilitate the development of sinusitis by causing mucosal edema with subsequent obstruction of the ostia and by impairing ciliary clearance of bacteria. Whereas adults possess well-developed bilateral frontal, ethmoid, sphenoid, and maxillary sinuses (Fig. 64-2), the presence of these sinuses in children varies with age. The maxillary and ethmoid sinuses begin to develop during the third month of gestation and are therefore present at the time of birth.[3] In contrast, the frontal and sphenoid sinuses do not pneumatize until a child is approximately 5 or 6 years of age and are not completely developed until late adolescence.[3] Features useful for the clinical diagnosis of various categories of sinusitis are detailed in Table 64-2.

Children with AOM and sinusitis are predisposed to infectious and inflammatory complications because of their close proximity to orbital and parameningeal structures. The separation between these structures and the middle ear or sinuses may be breached by various means. There is direct communication between the middle ear and the mastoid airspace. Thin bony walls separate the sinuses from intraorbital areas, which may be eroded with infection. Penetrating veins may allow spread of infection from infected sinuses or mastoid spaces to the intracranial region.

Mastoiditis, meningitis, intracranial abscess, orbital and periorbital cellulitis, and lateral sinus thrombosis are serious complications of AOM or sinusitis (or both) that routinely require hospitalization. In the postantibiotic era, these complications occur in only 0.04% to 0.15% of children with AOM.[4] Although serious infectious complications are rare, the associated mortality is between 10% and 31%.[5]

MASTOIDITIS

The mastoid is the inferior posterior portion of the temporal bone and consists of air cells separated by bony septa. Although present at birth, the air cells are not fully pneumatized until 2 to 3 years of age.[1] The mastoid air cells are adjacent to the middle ear, and the two are connected via a narrow opening called the aditus ad antrum. The middle ear and the mastoid share a continuous mucoperiosteum, so the mastoid air cells often become inflamed with middle ear infection.[1] In cases of acute mastoiditis, the aditus ad antrum becomes obstructed and the inflammation within the mastoid air cells progresses to suppuration and necrosis.[1,6]

Acute mastoiditis, defined as the presence of symptoms for less than a month, may be classified into several stages: mastoiditis with periosteitis, mastoiditis with osteitis, and subperiosteal abscess.[7,8] In mastoiditis with periosteitis, the inflammation extends from the mastoid to the periosteum via the venous system, but the infection is limited to the periosteum.[7,9,10] Untreated mastoiditis with periosteitis may progress to mastoiditis with osteitis, also known as acute coalescent mastoiditis. It occurs secondary to swelling of the periosteum and results in obstruction of drainage of purulent material, followed by activation of osteoclastic activity.[10] Destruction of the bony septa separating the air cells and subsequent suppuration are the result of this sequence of events. A subperiosteal abscess may further complicate this picture if the infection extends to and penetrates the external cortex of the mastoid.[7,9]

Clinical Presentation

The age-related incidence of mastoiditis mirrors that of otitis media.[11] Some controversy exists regarding whether infants, whose mastoids are not fully formed, can truly have classic mastoiditis. However, inflammation and suppuration of the mastoid or antrum, or both, have been observed in this age group.[10]

Children with mastoiditis generally present with fever, ear pain, and postauricular erythema, edema, and tenderness several days to weeks after an episode of treated or untreated AOM.[2,11] The tympanic membrane appears abnormal in approximately 90% of cases. Rarely, it may appear normal if the mastoiditis is secondary to obstruction of the aditus ad

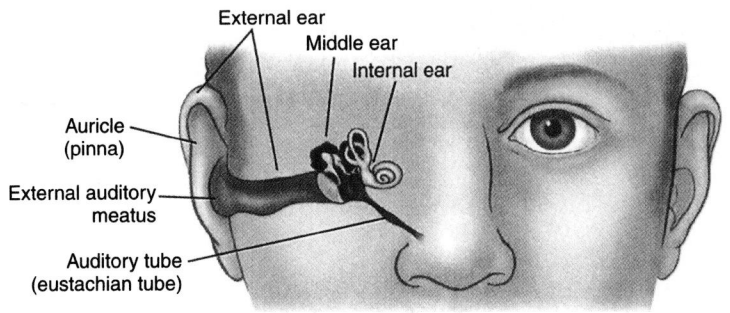

Figure 64-1 Anatomy of the inner ear and mastoid. (From Dorland's Illustrated Medical Dictionary, 30th ed. Philadelphia, WB Saunders, 2003, p 583.)

Table 64-1 Complications of Acute Otitis Media and Sinusitis	
AOM	Hearing loss
	Cholesteatoma
	Tympanosclerosis
	Mastoiditis
	Labyrinthitis
	Meningitis
	Facial nerve palsy
	Intracranial abscess
Sinusitis	Periorbital cellulitis
	Orbital cellulitis
	Meningitis, subdural/epidural abscess
	Intraparenchymal abscess
	Pott puffy tumor

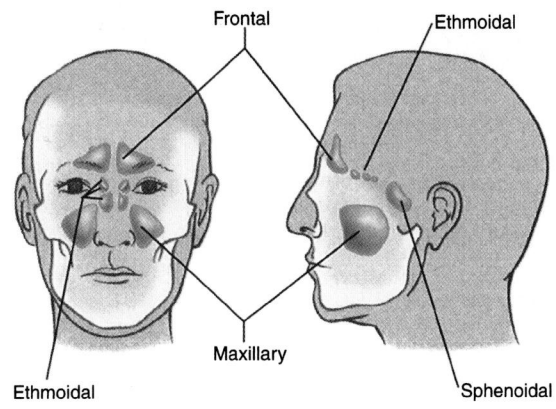

■ Sinus paranasales (paranasal sinuses).

Figure 64-2 Anatomy of the sinuses. (From Dorland's Illustrated Medical Dictionary, 30th ed. Philadelphia, WB Saunders, 2003, p 1707.)

Table 64-2 Sinusitis: Clinically Based Diagnoses	
Entity	Clinical Findings
Acute bacterial sinusitis	Persistent: Nasal discharge or postnasal discharge with daytime cough (with or without nighttime cough) Temperature ≥39° C and purulent nasal discharge for ≥3-4 consecutive days in an ill-appearing child Complete resolution of symptoms within 30 days
Subacute bacterial sinusitis	Symptoms lasting 30-90 days
Recurrent acute bacterial sinusitis	Repeated episodes lasting <30 days each, with symptom-free intervals >10 days
Chronic sinusitis	Persistent symptoms, including cough, rhinorrhea, or nasal obstruction, lasting >90 days
Acute bacterial sinusitis superimposed on chronic sinusitis	Persistent residual upper respiratory tract symptoms with development of an episode of acute bacterial sinusitis that resolves and subsequent continuation of the previous residual symptoms

From American Academy of Pediatrics: Clinical practice guideline: Management of sinusitis. Pediatrics 2001;108:798-808.

antrum from granulation tissue.[11] The examiner should look for the presence of a cholesteatoma because it is frequently associated with subperiosteal abscesses in older children.[8] If a subperiosteal abscess is present, the area posterior to the ear may be fluctuant and tender. In children younger than 1 year, the fluctuance is typically superior and posterior to the ear and displaces the pinna downward and outward.[2] In children older than 1 year, the fluctuance is most commonly posterior and inferior to the ear and displaces the pinna upward and outward.

Differential Diagnosis

The differential diagnosis of mastoiditis includes lymphadenopathy, parotitis, lateral sinus thrombosis, mastoid tumors, and branchial cleft cysts.

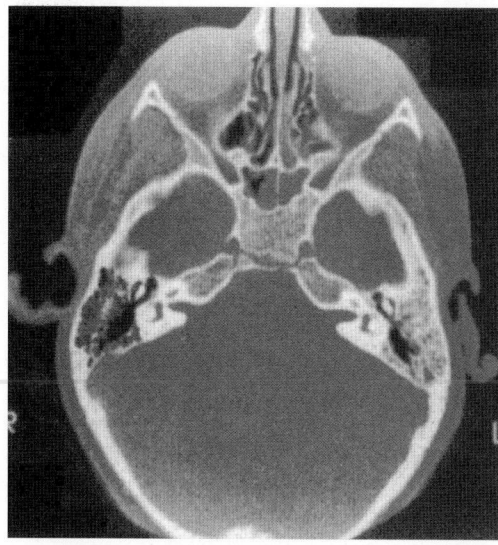

Figure 64-3 Computed tomographic scan of mastoiditis without periosteitis/osteitis. Opacification of the mastoid air cells is present on the left (*arrow*). (From Bluestone CD, Klein JO: Intratemporal complications and sequelae of otitis media. In Bluestone CD, Stool DE, Cuneyt M, et al [eds]: Pediatric Otolaryngology, vol 1, 4th ed. Philadelphia, WB Saunders, 2003, p 716.)

Diagnosis and Evaluation

Computed tomography (CT) of the mastoid/temporal bone with contrast enhancement is the study of choice for diagnosis. On CT, children with early mastoiditis will demonstrate clouding or opacification of the mastoid air cells, indicative of mastoiditis (Fig. 64-3). Destruction of the bony septa and empyema formation indicate mastoiditis with osteitis.[1,8,11] Subperiosteal abscess is also readily visualized by CT.

An elevated C-reactive protein (CRP), erythrocyte sedimentation rate (ESR), and white blood cell count, with a predominance of neutrophils or band forms, may be observed with mastoiditis; however, these tests are neither sensitive nor specific. A blood culture should be considered.[11] Middle ear fluid samples collected after tympanocentesis or placement of a myringotomy tube should be sent for aerobic and anaerobic culture. Culture of fluid in the canal is less reliable than culture of the middle ear or the mastoid because of possible contamination with ear canal flora.

Course of Illness

Although most cases of mastoiditis are isolated, a small percentage may be complicated by one of the following: intracranial extension of infection (meningitis, epidural abscess, subdural abscess, intraparenchymal abscess), lateral sinus thrombosis, Bezold abscess (see later), or facial nerve palsy.[1] The possibility of extension of the mastoiditis necessitates frequent assessment of the patient's neurologic status and neck examination.

Intracranial complications occur either by hematogenous (venous) spread or by bony erosion leading to direct extension. Children with these complications frequently present with headache, fevers, and vomiting and may or may not demonstrate neurologic impairment. If intracranial complications are suspected, CT with contrast or magnetic reso-

nance imaging (MRI) of the brain should be performed immediately, and neurosurgical consultation should be sought.[1]

Lateral sinus thrombosis occurs as a result of the proximity of the mastoid to the sigmoid sinus. If inflammation and infection extend from the mastoid to the adventitia of this venous sinus, a thrombus forms.[1,12] The thrombus may obstruct the sinus lumen or may embolize. Children with lateral sinus thrombosis present with spiking fevers (often called "picket fence" fevers), neck pain, headache, emesis, neurologic signs and symptoms, or any combination of these findings.[1,5,12] They may also demonstrate evidence of distant septic thromboemboli such as pneumonia.

Lateral sinus thrombosis may lead to otitic hydrocephalus with increased intracranial pressure as a result of decreased absorption of cerebrospinal fluid secondary to venous sinus obstruction. Children with otitic hydrocephalus may present with headache, papilledema, and ipsilateral abducens nerve palsy.[5,12]

A Bezold abscess occurs if the infection progresses inferiorly and extends into the deep tissues of the neck. It results in a collection beneath the sternocleidomastoid with swelling and tenderness.[1]

The facial nerve courses through the middle ear, thus making it susceptible to inflammation if bony dehiscence with otitis media is present. Facial nerve palsy is usually unilateral, and paresis of the lower part of the face, as well as the forehead, would be seen, as expected with this peripheral neuritis. CT can identify the bony erosions and is important to rule out cholesteatoma or other middle ear tumor.[5] The facial nerve palsy generally improves as the infection is treated, usually with intravenous antibiotics and surgical drainage with placement of myringotomy tubes.[5]

If the infection extends into the petrous portion of the temporal bone (petrositis), Gradenigo syndrome, a triad of pain behind the eye, ear discharge, and abducens nerve palsy, may develop.[1]

Treatment

Input from otolaryngology should be sought in the management of children with mastoiditis. Neurosurgical involvement should be considered if the potential for intracranial complications exists. Antibiotic coverage should include the most common pathogens with cognizance of local resistance patterns. The microbiology of mastoiditis and AOM differs to some degree. As in AOM, *Streptococcus pneumoniae* is the most common pathogen. However, whereas *Moraxella catarrhalis* and nontypable *Haemophilus influenzae* are the second and third most common organisms responsible for AOM, *Staphylococcus aureus* and *Streptococcus pyogenes* are the next most common bacteria found in mastoiditis.[1] Anaerobes, *S. pyogenes, Pseudomonas aeruginosa* (usually with chronic mastoiditis), and *Proteus* species, in addition to *M. catarrhalis* and nontypable *H. influenzae*, also have been implicated.

Empirical antibiotic regimens typically include a third-generation cephalosporin with either an antistaphylococcal penicillin or clindamycin. Ampicillin-sulbactam would provide similar coverage. Vancomycin should be considered in place of oxacillin or clindamycin in severe cases; vancomycin and clindamycin are appropriate instead of an antistaphylococcal penicillin in areas with a high prevalence of community-acquired methicillin-resistant *S. aureus* (MRSA). Typical antibiotic courses range from 4 to 6 weeks, and some experts suggest that therapy may be switched from intravenous antibiotics to oral antibiotics if a good clinical response has been established.[2] In addition to antibiotic therapy, an otolaryngologist should perform tympanocentesis for culture and place myringotomy tubes.

Indications for mastoidectomy include (1) concern for osteitis, (2) subperiosteal abscess, (3) poor response to medical therapy, or (4) complications.[1,2,12] Treatment of petrositis involves intravenous antibiotics, placement of myringotomy tubes, and surgical drainage of the petrous portion of the temporal bone.[5] Surgical decompression of the facial nerve is considered in some cases of facial nerve palsy associated with AOM/mastoiditis.[5,11] Surgical drainage may also be indicated for a Bezold abscess that does not respond to antibiotic therapy.

Concern for lateral sinus thrombosis warrants MRI with angiography/venography (MRA/MRV).[5,12] Additionally, if deemed safe after head imaging, lumbar puncture with measurement of opening pressure may be both diagnostic and therapeutic for otitic hydrocephalus. Repeat lumbar puncture may be necessary to manage the increased intracranial pressure associated with otitic hydrocephalus. Acetazolamide may be helpful by reducing production of cerebrospinal fluid. Surgical removal of the thrombus by otolaryngology or neurosurgery is a treatment option. The role of anticoagulation is controversial, and therefore guidance from hematology and neurology is recommended.

All children with mastoiditis should have an audiogram performed after completion of therapy.[1]

Admission Criteria

Children with suspected mastoiditis, with or without evidence of further complications, should be hospitalized for intravenous antibiotics, definitive diagnosis, and potential surgical management.

Discharge Criteria

- Afebrile for 48 hours with an improving overall clinical picture
- Ability to tolerate oral/enteral nutrition and antibiotics
- Reliable follow-up with a generalist and otolaryngologist
- No evidence of further complications (normal, improving, or stable neurologic findings)
- Completion of intravenous antibiotic therapy or the ability to complete this treatment at home

Prevention

When considering prevention of mastoiditis, one must consider whether antibiotic treatment of AOM prevents the development of complications. Up to 80% of children with untreated AOM will have resolution of symptoms within 7 to 14 days. Because of the frequency of spontaneous resolution, practitioners in some countries, such as the Netherlands, rarely treat AOM with antibiotics. In a systematic review of the literature, updated in 2003, the Cochrane Library analyzed eight randomized controlled trials investigating patient-related outcomes for treated versus untreated AOM. This review concluded that 15 children with AOM must be treated with antibiotics to improve the clinical outcome (pain at 2 days) of 1 of these children.[6] The authors noted that the prevalence of complications, such as mastoiditis, was low in both treated and untreated children, thereby limiting their ability to make definitive claims about the relationship between treatment and complications, especially in areas with a high prevalence of complications. In their 2004 clinical guidelines, the American Academy of Pediatrics considered this review, along with others indicating that withholding antibiotics initially and watchful waiting did not increase the risk for mastoiditis, and concluded that physicians may withhold antibiotic treatment in children older than 2 years with a definite diagnosis of AOM but without severe illness or in children between 6 months and 2 years of age without systemic illness and without a certain diagnosis of AOM.[13] This age-stratified recommendation was based on evidence indicating higher risk for severe illness and poor outcomes in children younger than 2 years with definite AOM.[13]

In a Nutshell

- Clinical presentation: Fever, posterior auricular pain and swelling, and displacement of the pinna, usually after an episode of AOM.
- Complications: Progression to meningitis with or without intracranial abscess, lateral sinus thrombosis, Bezold abscess, or facial nerve palsy.
- Diagnosis: Clinical diagnosis with a contrast-enhanced CT scan of the mastoid/temporal bone for confirmation and for evaluation of severity or extension.
- Treatment: Intravenous antibiotics, drainage of middle ear fluid, and placement of myringotomy tubes. Further surgical intervention may be necessary if there is progression to osteitis or complications.

On the Horizon

- As resistant strains of *S. pneumoniae* and *S. aureus* increase in prevalence, new antibiotic regimens will be recommended.
- The role of *S. pneumoniae* in AOM will be revisited as the seven-valent pneumococcal vaccine becomes widely instituted.
- Look for continuing research regarding the benefits and risks of anticoagulation for lateral sinus thrombosis.

PERIORBITAL CELLULITIS

Periorbital cellulitis involves inflammation anterior to the orbital septum (Fig. 64-4) and is also referred to as preseptal cellulitis. The orbital septum, which extends from the periosteum of the inferior and superior orbital rims to the tarsal plates of the eyelids, provides a protective barrier for the deeper orbital structures,[1,14,15] as well as structural support for the lids. Periorbital cellulitis may result from inoculation of bacteria into the skin surrounding the eye, such as from abrasions, lacerations, or insect bites or stings. Occasionally, it may develop secondary to hematogenous

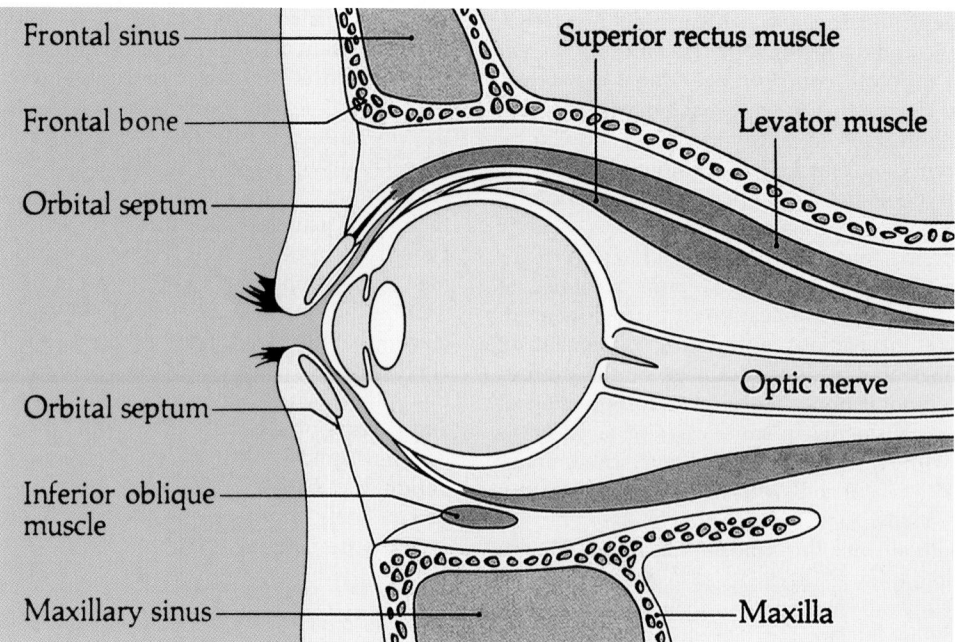

Figure 64-4   Anatomy of the eye. (From Yellon RF, McBride TP, Davis HW: Otolaryngology. In Zitelli BJ, Davis HW [eds]: Atlas of Pediatric Physical Diagnosis, 4th ed. Philadelphia, CV Mosby, 2003.)

spread of bacteria.[1] Conjunctivitis may cause inflammation of the periorbital skin, which may allow cellulitis to develop. Additionally, periorbital swelling may accompany underlying sinusitis but is thought to be sympathetic inflammation caused by poor venous drainage. Uncommonly, sinus infection may extend to the periorbital tissue and result in true periorbital cellulitis.[1,15,16]

Clinical Presentation

Periorbital cellulitis occurs most commonly in children younger than 5 years.[14,15] Hallmarks of the clinical presentation include unilateral eyelid erythema, edema, and tenderness (Fig. 64-5).[1,7] The skin may display evidence of recent trauma or a break in the skin. The contralateral eye may appear mildly edematous secondary to associated compression of the superior and inferior ophthalmic veins. Proptosis, chemosis, pain with extraocular movements, limitation of extraocular movements, and diminished visual acuity are not consistent with a periorbital process and suggest orbital involvement.[17] Constitutional features such as fever or a toxic appearance are uncommon. Tearing may occur, but purulent drainage and pronounced conjunctival injection are not usual unless concomitant conjunctivitis is present.

Differentiating preseptal swelling from proptosis by physical examination is challenging because protrusion of the lid is present with both. Furthermore, retracting the lid is often difficult because of soft tissue swelling, tenderness, and poor cooperation from young children, which makes evaluation of the appearance and function of the globe especially problematic.

Differential Diagnosis

The clinician must distinguish between periorbital cellulitis and orbital cellulitis. Other diagnoses to consider include allergic reaction, chemical irritation, trauma (espe-

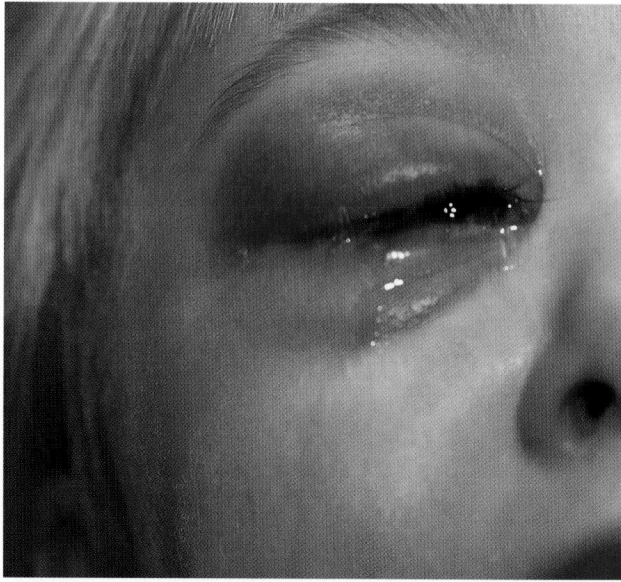

Figure 64-5   Child with periorbital cellulitis.

cially nasal and zygomatic fractures), stye or chalazion, dacryocystitis, and conjunctivitis.

Diagnosis and Evaluation

Visual acuity should always be assessed, with glasses worn by patients who require them. Contrast CT of the brain and orbits should be performed if orbital involvement is a consideration. CT will delineate the extent of the infection and provide information about the presence or absence of an orbital or subperiosteal abscess. Blood cultures should be considered for children younger than 2 years.[1] Leukocytosis and an elevated ESR and CRP are common but, as with mastoiditis, are neither sensitive nor specific. Culture of the eye discharge is rarely diagnostic.

Course of Illness

The majority of cases of periorbital cellulitis resolve without complication after antibiotic therapy.

Treatment

The most common organisms responsible for periorbital cellulitis secondary to trauma are *S. aureus* and *S. pyogenes*,[14] but anaerobic bacteria are also seen. When associated with sinusitis, the practitioner should base treatment on common sinusitis pathogens. Before widespread immunization against Hib, this organism was a common, virulent cause of hematogenously seeded bacteremic periorbital cellulitis. Today, *S. pneumoniae* is most often implicated in periorbital infection by this route.[1,14] Of note, adenovirus is a causative agent that can mimic bacterial infection. With adenoviral conjunctivitis, the eye and surrounding tissues are edematous, the conjunctiva is hyperemic, and copious mucopurulent discharge is present.[15] The periorbital inflammation may allow invasion of bacteria and progression to secondary periorbital cellulitis.

The choice of antibiotic should be guided by the most frequent pathogens. Amoxicillin-clavulanate is an appropriate oral antibiotic. Because of the increasing prevalence of community-acquired MRSA in many areas, clindamycin (to which many of these MRSA strains are susceptible) is an appropriate alternative. If a patient is treated as an outpatient for periorbital cellulitis, close monitoring by a pediatrician is recommended, and the patient should be advised to return to the hospital in the event of any photophobia, decreased vision, pain with eye movement, or diplopia.

Children who are hospitalized should be administered intravenous antibiotics. Ampicillin-sulbactam is an appropriate choice. Clindamycin should be considered if there is concern for MRSA. Antibiotic therapy (intravenous plus oral) should be continued for a total of 7 to 10 days.

Admission Criteria

Most patients with periorbital cellulitis are managed successfully with oral antibiotic therapy in the outpatient setting. Hospitalization and intravenous antibiotics should be considered in the following situations:

- Younger than 1 year
- Incomplete vaccination against *H. influenzae* type b (HIB)
- Toxic appearance
- Inability to tolerate oral/enteral feedings or antibiotics
- Failure of outpatient management
- Concern for orbital involvement

Discharge Criteria

- Afebrile for 24 hours with improving clinical findings
- Ability to tolerate oral/enteral feeding and antibiotics
- Reliable outpatient follow-up

Prevention

Hematogenously seeded periorbital cellulitis secondary to HIB has been nearly eradicated in immunized children. Because minor trauma, insect bites, and conjunctivitis are the most common preceding events that lead to periorbital cellulitis, a prevention strategy would be difficult.

In a Nutshell

- Clinical presentation: Soft tissue swelling and erythema around the eye without proptosis, visual changes, or pain on extraocular movement.
- Diagnosis: Diagnosed clinically, but CT of the orbits and brain should be performed if concern for orbital cellulitis exists.
- Treatment: Usually outpatient with oral antibiotics to cover *S. aureus* and *S. pyogenes*, the most common organisms. Hospitalization may be required for severe cases or for definitive diagnosis.

On the Horizon

- Data regarding the effect of the seven-valent pneumococcal vaccine on prevention of periorbital cellulitis

---

ORBITAL CELLULITIS

With orbital cellulitis, the infection is deep to the orbital septum and involves the bony orbit or the intraorbital structures (see Fig. 64-4). Most commonly, orbital cellulitis results from extension of sinusitis (usually ethmoid), but it can also occur secondary to direct inoculation from penetrating trauma to the intraorbital or postseptal areas or, rarely, from hematogenous spread.[1] Multiple factors facilitate direct extension of sinusitis into the orbits. First, the orbit is surrounded by and in close proximity to the paranasal sinuses. Second, the bony walls that separate the paranasal sinuses from the orbit are thin, thereby providing a permeable barrier. For example, the lamina papyracea is a paper-thin bone that separates the ethmoid sinus from the medial aspect of the intraorbital structures. Extension of infection from this sinus is the most common route by which orbital cellulitis develops. Finally, the veins that drain the sinuses (the orbital veins) are valveless, which allows both anterograde and retrograde spread of infections.[17] With progression, orbital cellulitis may lead to a subperiosteal or orbital abscess.[14]

Clinical Presentation

In contrast to periorbital cellulitis, orbital cellulitis occurs most commonly in older children. Similar to children with periorbital cellulitis, those with orbital cellulitis present with edema and erythema around the eye. However, children with orbital cellulitis may also have painful, limited extraocular movement and proptosis,[1,6,14] as well as conjunctival injection with chemosis. Fever is a common presenting sign, and children with orbital cellulitis are often more ill appearing than those with periorbital cellulitis. Pupillary function and visual acuity should be carefully assessed because optic dysfunction is a worrisome and vision-threatening complication.[1,14]

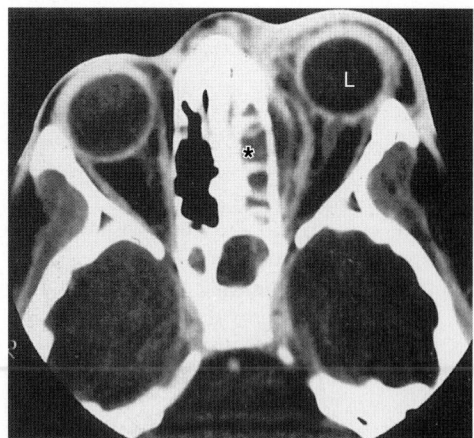

Figure 64-6 Computed tomographic scan of orbital cellulitis demonstrating proptosis of the left eye (*L*) and temporal displacement of the medial rectus muscle (*arrow*), and partial opacification of the ethmoid sinus (*asterisk*). (From Yellon RF, McBride TP, Davis HW: Otolaryngology. In Zitelli BJ, Davis HW [eds]: Atlas of Pediatric Physical Diagnosis, 4th ed. Philadelphia, CV Mosby, 2003, p 849.)

Differential Diagnosis

The differential diagnosis of orbital cellulitis is similar to that for periorbital cellulitis. Orbital pseudotumor and intraocular masses/tumors, including retinoblastoma, lymphoma, and rhabdomyosarcoma, must also be considered.

Diagnosis and Evaluation

A contrast-enhanced CT scan of the brain and the orbits should be performed if there is concern for orbital cellulitis (Fig. 64-6). Such imaging can delineate the extent of the infection and determine whether a subperiosteal or orbital abscess is present.[1,15] Concurrent bacteremia has been reported in up to a third of cases in children younger than 4 years; therefore, a blood culture should be obtained.[17]

Course of Illness

Although most cases of orbital cellulitis resolve with proper therapy, serious sequelae are possible, including loss of vision and central nervous system (CNS) infection. Visual loss is most frequently due to traction on the optic nerve with progressive proptosis or compression of the optic nerve from adjacent abscess or foraminal impingement. The resultant nerve injury is not always reversible.[17]

Treatment

Ideally, children with orbital cellulitis should be managed with input from ophthalmology and otolaryngology. The physical examination should be monitored closely because progression of the infectious process is usually heralded by clinical deterioration. If a child does not demonstrate improvement with intravenous antibiotics in 24 to 48 hours, repeat imaging is warranted to check for the development of an abscess.[1]

Because orbital cellulitis is most frequently a complication of sinusitis, the organisms associated with these diseases are similar and include *S. pneumoniae*, nontypable *H. influenzae*, *M. catarrhalis*, and anaerobes. Additionally, orbital cellulitis may be caused by *S. aureus* and *S. pyogenes*.[1]

Ampicillin-sulbactam is a reasonable choice for empirical intravenous therapy, with a high dose of the ampicillin component used to cover most of the resistant *S. pneumoniae*. Clindamycin plus a third-generation cephalosporin is another reasonable empirical choice. The total duration of antibiotic therapy is 14 to 21 days.

The need for prompt surgical drainage of a subperiosteal abscess is controversial. Medical management may be appropriate for a small subperiosteal abscess that does not impair vision or cause excessive pain.[16,18,19] A large subperiosteal abscess or an abscess that results in impaired vision requires prompt surgical drainage.[1,14,19] If the surgeons elect to not drain a subperiosteal abscess immediately, the patient's clinical status should be frequently assessed for any changes. If there is worsening or no clinical improvement, surgical drainage is important for resolution.

Admission Criteria

Children with suspected or confirmed orbital cellulitis should be admitted for intravenous antibiotics, subspecialty consultation, definitive diagnosis, and possible surgical drainage.

Discharge Criteria

- Improving physical examination findings/resolving symptoms
- Afebrile for 24 to 48 hours
- Ability to tolerate oral/enteral feeding and antibiotics
- Appropriate outpatient follow-up with a generalist, an ophthalmologist, and if appropriate, an otolaryngologist.

Prevention

Because orbital cellulitis is most commonly a sequela of sinusitis, prevention focuses on treatment of paranasal sinusitis. Timely and accurate recognition, as well as appropriate treatment of sinusitis, is important. However, in view of the impressive frequency of childhood sinusitis, the high rate of spontaneous resolution, the small proportion that progress to complications, and the conflicting data available in the literature, diagnosis and treatment remain a challenge for primary care clinicians.

In a Nutshell

- Clinical presentation: Swelling and redness around the eye, which may be accompanied by fever, proptosis, change in vision, or limited or painful extraocular movements
- Diagnosis: Clinical suspicion followed by confirmation with contrast-enhanced CT of the orbits and brain
- Treatment: Hospitalization for intravenous antibiotics, consultation with ophthalmology and otolaryngology, and possible surgical drainage

On the Horizon

- Ongoing studies evaluating management of sinusitis and its effect on prevention of orbital cellulitis
- Controlled trials investigating the benefits of surgical versus medical management

INTRACRANIAL COMPLICATIONS

Perhaps the most serious complication of sinusitis involves extension of infection into the intracranial space and progression to meningitis, epidural abscess, subdural abscess, or intraparenchymal abscess. Although these complications are rare, the morbidity and mortality are significant, with as many as 12% of children with an intracranial abscess dying and a third having continuing neurologic sequelae.[20,21]

Most commonly, intracranial complications result either from direct extension from the sinuses or from hematogenous spread via thrombophlebitis of the valveless diploic veins that connect the sinuses to the dura.[22] Frontal sinusitis is more likely than maxillary, ethmoid, or sphenoid sinusitis to lead to intracranial complications, possibly because the dura around the frontal sinus is less adherent than in other areas and thus creates a potential space for abscess formation.[22]

Frontal sinusitis resulting in osteomyelitis of the frontal bone may lead to intracranial extension, but extension anteriorly is also seen. When the infection progresses in this direction, a subperiosteal abscess known as a Pott puffy tumor develops. Intracranial extension may coexist with this condition, and evaluation for intracranial involvement is recommended.

Sagittal venous sinus thrombosis is a rare complication of sinusitis in children. Most cases are caused by thrombophlebitis of the valveless diploic veins that drain from the sinuses into the superior sagittal venous sinus.

Clinical Presentation

Intracranial complications of sinusitis are most common in adolescent boys. The increased rate of intracranial infection in adolescents is due to the peak growth of their frontal sinus, with resultant increased vascularity.[22] It is unclear why boys are affected more often than girls.[21]

The most common presenting signs and symptoms of the suppurative intracranial complications of sinusitis include headache, vomiting, and fever.[21,23] Neurologic symptoms are present in only a third to half of patients at presentation. Case series have differing views about the frequency of upper respiratory tract symptoms at the time of presentation, with reports varying from approximately 20% to 50% of patients.[21,24]

A Pott puffy tumor presents as a painful, tender, erythematous, and often fluctuant mass adjacent to the glabella. The patient complains of headache, fever, and concomitant or recent symptoms of sinusitis. Clinical signs of coexisting intracranial involvement may be present.

Differential Diagnosis

The differential diagnosis includes other CNS infections, CNS tumor, intracranial hemorrhage, and toxin ingestion.

Treatment

Further discussion of intracranial infections is provided in Chapter 63.

SUGGESTED READING

American Academy of Pediatrics: Clinical practice guideline: Management of sinusitis. Pediatrics 2001;108:798-808.

Myer CM: The diagnosis and management of mastoiditis in children. Pediatr Ann 1991;20:622-626.

Ong YK, Tan HK: Suppurative intracranial complications of sinusitis in children. Int J Pediatr Otorhinolaryngol 2002;66:49.

REFERENCES

1. Feigen R, Cherry J, Demmler G, Kaplan L (eds): Textbook of Pediatric Infectious Diseases. Philadelphia, WB Saunders, 2004.
2. Garfunkel L, Kaczorowski J, Christy C (eds): Mosby's Pediatric Clinical Advisor: Instant Diagnosis and Treatment. St Louis, CV Mosby, 2002.
3. Newton DA: Sinusitis in children and adolescents. Prim Care 1996;23:701-717.
4. Lalwani AK, Grudfast KM (eds): Pediatric Otology and Neurotology. New York, Lippincott-Raven, 1998.
5. Wetmore RF: Complications of otitis media. Pediatr Ann 2000;29:637-646.
6. Glasziou PP, Del Mar CB, Sanders SL, Hayem M: Antibiotics for acute otitis media in children. Cochrane Database Syst Rev 2004;2:CD000219.
7. Behrman R, Kliegman R, Nelson W, Vaughan V: Nelson Textbook of Pediatrics, 14th ed. Philadelphia, WB Saunders, 1992.
8. Fliss DM, Leiberman A, Dagan R: Acute and chronic mastoiditis in children. Adv Pediatr Infect Dis 1997;13:165-185.
9. Haddad J: Treatment of acute otitis media and its complications. Otolaryngol Clin North Am 1994;27:431-441.
10. Wang NE, Burg JM: Mastoiditis: A case-based review. Pediatr Emerg Care 1998;14:290-292.
11. Nadol JB, Eavey RD: Acute and chronic mastoiditis: Clinical presentation, diagnosis and management. Curr Clin Top Infect Dis 1995;15:204-229.
12. Garcia RDJ, Baker AS, Cunninghma MJ, Weber AL: Lateral sinus thrombosis associated with otitis media and mastoiditis in children. Pediatr Infect Dis J 1995;4:617-623.
13. American Academy of Pediatrics and American Academy of Family Physicians: Clinical practice guideline: Diagnosis and management of acute otitis media. Pediatrics 2004;113:1451-1465.
14. Powell KR: Orbital and periorbital cellulitis. Pediatr Rev 1995;16:163-167.
15. Malinow I, Powell KR: Periorbital cellulitis. Pediatr Ann 1993;22:241-246.
16. Givner LB: Periorbital versus orbital cellulitis. Pediatr Infect Dis J 2002;21:1157-1158.
17. Jain A, Rubin PA: Orbital cellulitis in children. Int Ophthalmol Clin 2001;41:71-86.
18. Starkey CR, Steele RW: Medical management of orbital cellulitis. Pediatr Infect Dis J 2001;20:1002-1005.
19. Sobol SE, Marchand J, Tewfik TL, et al: Orbital complications of sinusitis in children. J Otolaryngol 2002;31:131-136.
20. Goldberg AN, Oroszlan G, Anderson TD: Complications of frontal sinusitis and their management. Otolaryngol Clin North Am 2001;34:211-225.
21. Ong YK, Tan HK: Suppurative intracranial complications of sinusitis in children. Int J Pediatr Otorhinolaryngol 2002;66:49.
22. Lerner DN, Choi SS, Zalzai GH, Johnson DL: Intracranial complications of sinusitis in childhood. Ann Otorhinolaryngol 1995;104:288-293.
23. Bairo-Merritt MH, Shah SS, Zaoutis LG, et al: Suppurative intracranial complications of sinusitis in previously healthy children. Pediatr Infect Dis J 2005;24:384-386.
24. Giannoni C, Sulek M, Friedman EM: Intracranial complications of sinusitis: A pediatric review. Am J Rhinol 1998;12:173-178.

CHAPTER 65

Neck and Oral Cavity Infections

Jeffrey L. Sperring

In the 1970s, admission for tonsillectomy was the most common reason for pediatric hospitalization, and it accounted for nearly 20% of all pediatric hospital admissions. Although these rates have decreased significantly over the past few decades, infections of the neck and oral cavity continue to be a significant cause of childhood morbidity and an indication for admission to the hospital. These infections are even more worrisome given their proximity to vital structures, including the upper airway and major blood vessels of the neck. Careful recognition and prompt treatment are essential to prevent significant or even life-threatening complications.

STOMATITIS

Stomatitis is defined as inflammation of the mucous membranes of the oral cavity and can be caused by multiple infectious as well as noninfectious causes. The location of lesions and associated symptoms can often guide correct identification and management. Most cases of stomatitis are benign, self-limited illnesses, but some cases, particularly in special patient populations, cause significant morbidity and require inpatient care.

Clinical Presentation

The three most common infectious causes of stomatitis in children are recurrent aphthous ulcers, herpangina, and herpes gingivostomatitis. These conditions are usually distinguishable by appearance alone.

Recurrent aphthous ulcers, more commonly known as canker sores, are the most common cause of stomatitis. They occur primarily in older children and adolescents. No clear cause has been identified for aphthous stomatitis, although it is thought to be secondary to an infectious agent. Recurrences have also been linked to trauma, periods of emotional stress, and multiple nutritional and vitamin deficiencies. Aphthous ulcers are typically solitary or associated with only a few other lesions and are most commonly found on the inner lip. There is often a pattern of recurrence, and the lesions, although painful, are not generally associated with fever or other symptoms.

Herpangina is associated most commonly with group A coxsackieviruses and is seen most frequently in children 1 to 4 years of age. It presents acutely with fever and eruption of distinct ulcerations of the oropharynx. There is a clear seasonal predominance, with more cases occurring in the summer and early fall. Herpangina lesions occur near the tonsillar pillars and soft palate while sparing the anterior portion of the oral cavity. These lesions are temporally related to the onset of fever, typically start as small vesicles, and progress to ulceration (Fig. 65-1). They have sharp borders and usually cluster in groups of no more than 5 to 10 lesions.

Herpetic gingivostomatitis is the most frequent clinical manifestation of primary herpes simplex virus (HSV) infection. It is classically associated with HSV type 1 and occurs most commonly from infancy to early school age. It is distinguished from other causes of stomatitis by its characteristic lesions. HSV gingivostomatitis is unique in its predominance in the anterior aspect of the mouth and involvement of the gingiva and lips (Fig. 65-2). Perioral involvement may occur as a result of local extension. Autoinoculation can be seen as herpetic whitlow in children who suck their fingers. "Drop" lesions can occur in the path of saliva from drooling children. The ulcerations are identified by their ragged borders, which frequently coalesce as they progress. The lesions are generally preceded by a prodrome of high fever, malaise, and other constitutional symptoms. Feeding aversion is common.

Differential Diagnosis

Stomatitis and oral cavity lesions have been associated with multiple viruses, including HSV, varicella, human immunodeficiency virus (HIV), and the entire family of enteroviruses (specifically, coxsackieviruses and echoviruses.) Hand-foot-and-mouth disease, caused by coxsackieviruses, produces ulcerations of the oral mucosa in association with a vesicular rash on the palms, soles, and sometimes the buttocks. Candidal infections of the mouth (thrush) typically produce white plaques over the mucous membranes and are more likely to be seen in newborns or immunocompromised children. Any break in the mucosal lining can result in ulceration, whether from direct trauma or from chemical irritation as a result of medications or toxins. Because patients receiving chemotherapy are at risk for life-threatening mucositis, immediate recognition and supportive care are essential. Inflammatory or rheumatologic conditions such as Crohn's disease, Reiter syndrome, and Behçet syndrome may present with oral ulcerations in association with systemic signs and symptoms. Hemorrhagic lesions with discoloration of the mucous membranes should suggest Stevens-Johnson syndrome, another life-threatening illness that requires prompt recognition and management (see Chapter 161).

Diagnosis

Diagnosis and management of stomatitis do not usually require laboratory testing. Testing is necessary only in cases in which the cause of the lesions is unclear or the presence of a specific virus might alter therapy. HSV can be readily isolated by culture of the mucous membranes within 48

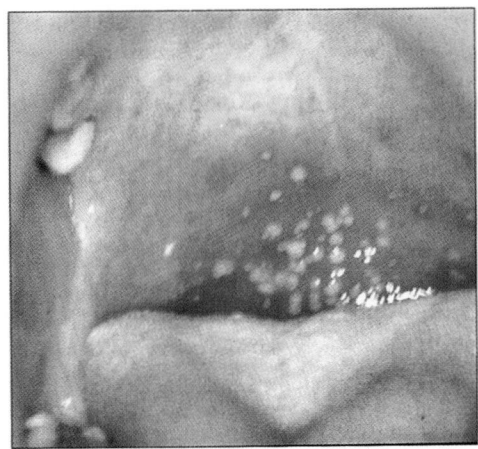

Figure 65-1 Gingivostomatitis caused by coxsackievirus. (From Read RC: Orocervical and esophageal infection. In Cohen J, Powderly W [eds]: Infectious Diseases, 2nd ed. Philadelphia, CV Mosby, 2004, p 463.)

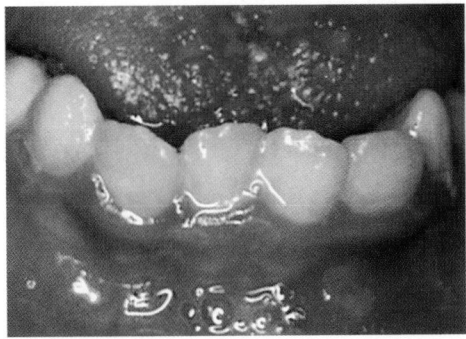

Figure 65-2 Gingivostomatitis caused by herpes simplex virus. (From Nazif MM, Martin BS, McKibben DH et al: Oral disorders. In Zitelli BJ, Davis HW [eds]: Atlas of Pediatric Physical Diagnosis, 4th ed. Philadelphia, CV Mosby, 2002, p 706.)

hours. Direct fluorescent antibody testing of vesicle scrapings can provide diagnostic confirmation within several hours; this method is highly specific but much less sensitive than culture. Detection of HSV by polymerase chain reaction (PCR) is both highly specific and sensitive and is increasingly becoming available. Enteroviruses, including coxsackieviruses, can be detected by PCR on specimens from the throat, respiratory secretions, blood, and urine. Enteroviruses can also be isolated from culture of multiple sites, including respiratory secretions and stool; characteristic cytopathic changes in cell culture are generally detected 2 to 5 days after inoculation. The opportunity to recover the virus is optimized by sampling multiple sites. Given the high sensitivity of PCR-based assays, culture is not routinely used to detect enteroviruses. Determination of serum electrolytes should be considered in children with moderate or severe dehydration. A blood culture and complete blood count should be obtained in ill-appearing patients and those with suspected secondary bacterial infection.

Treatment

Treatment of stomatitis is usually empirical and focused on pain management and hydration. Oral acetaminophen or ibuprofen is typically helpful for analgesia. An equal-parts mixture of Maalox, 2% viscous lidocaine, and diphenhy-

dramine ("magic mouthwash") can be applied topically in older children, but lidocaine should be avoided in younger patients because of concern about systemic absorption. Kenalog in Orabase (triamcinolone) is a compounded mixture of steroid in a dental paste that has been effective in the treatment of aphthous ulcers. Oral acyclovir may have a role in treatment of HSV gingivostomatitis, but it must be given within the first 48 hours after the onset of lesions to be most effective.

Admission Criteria

- Inability to maintain adequate hydration
- Inadequate pain control with oral medications
- Evidence of secondary bacterial infection
- Stomatitis in an immunocompromised patient or a child undergoing chemotherapy
- Concern for more serious or progressive conditions (e.g., Stevens-Johnson syndrome)

Prevention

It is important to educate patients and their families that many forms of stomatitis can be contagious and careful hand washing along with reduced contact with oral secretions should be encouraged to minimize spread. Hospitalized patients with suspected infectious stomatitis should be placed in contact isolation.

PHARYNGITIS

Acute care visits for sore throat are among the most common encountered by health care providers for children. Viruses cause the majority of cases of pharyngitis in children, and it is most often treated with supportive care alone. Bacterial pharyngitis is not uncommon, however, and as many as 30% of all cases of pharyngitis may be due to group A β-hemolytic streptococcus (GABHS). Clinical diagnosis of streptococcal pharyngitis is made more difficult by frequent absence of a classic presentation of symptoms. Most pediatric patients with acute GABHS pharyngitis present with some combination of fever, tender anterior lymph nodes, and pharyngeal erythema in the absence of concurrent viral upper respiratory tract symptoms (cough, congestion, and rhinorrhea). Exudative tonsillitis is another nonspecific finding that may be seen. Not all of these symptoms may be present, however, and less typical symptoms of headache or abdominal pain may predominate. Diagnosis based on symptoms and examination findings has typically lacked the necessary specificity, which has led to an increased role for laboratory testing. Identification of streptococcal pharyngitis by either throat culture or optical immunoassay testing should prompt treatment with an appropriate antibiotic regimen to lessen the incidence of complications, including rheumatic fever. Care should be taken by clinicians to distinguish a positive test in patients with acute infection versus those who are chronically colonized with group A streptococcus. Some studies have shown colonization rates as high as 10% to 15% in children, and these patients may have positive culture on antigen testing even in the absence of acute symptoms. Table 65-1 summarizes several acceptable treatment regimens for acute GABHS pharyngitis, but penicillin remains the cornerstone of treatment. Erythromycin may be

Table 65-1 Antimicrobial Treatment Regimens for Group A Streptococcal Pharyngitis

Drug*	Dosage	Duration
Penicillin V	Children: 250 mg PO bid-tid Adolescents: 500 mg PO bid-tid	10 days
Penicillin G	<27 kg: 600,000 units IM >27 kg: 1,200,000 units IM	1 dose
Amoxicillin	25-50 mg/kg/day PO divided bid-tid	10 days
Erythromycin estolate	30-50 mg/kg/day PO divided tid-qid	10 days
Erythromycin ethylsuccinate	40 mg/kg/day PO divided tid-qid	10 days
Azithromycin	12 mg/kg/day PO once daily	5 days

*A 10-day course of a narrow-spectrum (first-generation) cephalosporin is an acceptable alternative. The additional cost of many cephalosporins and their wider range of antibacterial activity compared with penicillin preclude recommending them for routine use in children with GABHS pharyngitis.

used for penicillin-allergic patients, although the increasing use of macrolide antibiotics, including azithromycin, has raised concern for the development of erythromycin resistance. One regional study showed erythromycin resistance rates for group A streptococci to be as high as 48%, although results have varied by location.[1]

Rarely, more serious deep tissue neck infections can occur in children, either from direct extension of pharyngitis/tonsillitis or from another primary process. Differentiating these infections from uncomplicated pharyngitis can sometimes be subtle, but differentiation is imperative to reduce potential airway compromise and other complications. Peritonsillar and retropharyngeal abscesses are discussed later in further detail.

PERITONSILLAR ABSCESS

A peritonsillar abscess, or "quinsy," is a collection of purulence in the peritonsillar fossa, between the tonsillar capsule and the superior constrictor muscle. It typically results from direct extension of local pharyngitis or tonsillitis. Peritonsillar abscess is more common in adolescents and older children, whereas retropharyngeal and parapharyngeal abscesses are more commonly seen in young children. The most common bacteria isolated are GABHS, but other organisms, including other streptococci, oral cavity anaerobes, and *Staphylococcus aureus*, have been identified.

Clinical Presentation

Most children with a peritonsillar abscess have a preceding pharyngitis with sore throat, fever, and malaise. This diagnosis should be suspected when more significant symptoms are present, including dysphagia, drooling, voice changes (the "hot potato voice"), and trismus.

On physical examination both tonsils may be enlarged, but the affected tonsil is typically more prominent. The mass effect from the abscess will commonly push the tonsil forward and medially and deviate the uvula away from the affected side. There is typically erythema, but tonsillar exudates may or may not be present. These examination findings may be difficult to visualize in a patient with significant trismus. Anterior cervical lymph node enlargement is frequently palpated and can be more prominent on the affected side. Laboratory evaluation often reveals an elevated white blood cell count with a predominance of neutrophils. The diagnosis of peritonsillar abscess is almost exclusively made by the history and physical examination; radiographic studies are not necessary unless there is concern for a deeper abscess or other mass effect.

Differential Diagnosis

Peritonsillar cellulitis, an extension of bacterial pharyngitis to the peritonsillar space with resultant erythema and inflammation but no discrete abscess formation, has similar symptoms, but on examination the uvula remains in the midline. *Epiglottitis* is now a rare entity since implementation of *Haemophilus influenzae* type b vaccination, but it can also present with fever, drooling, and airway compromise. *Retropharyngeal/parapharyngeal abscesses* are additional considerations and are discussed later in this chapter.

Treatment

The standard treatment of a peritonsillar abscess consists of decompression of the abscess and parenteral antibiotics. Patients with peritonsillar abscess should be evaluated by an otolaryngologist for surgical intervention. Several procedural approaches to treatment of peritonsillar abscess have been used, including needle aspiration (repeated if needed), traditional incision and drainage, and immediate tonsillectomy with drainage of the abscess ("quinsy tonsillectomy"). Evidence-based reviews of the literature have not demonstrated a clear advantage of one procedure over another, and treatment is typically guided by otolaryngology preference.[2] Immediate aspiration of the abscess may be required in an emergency setting if there is obvious airway compromise. Intravenous penicillin is an acceptable antibiotic regimen after surgical management, but broader-spectrum antibiotics, including nafcillin, clindamycin, or ampicillin-sulbactam, should be considered if the patient is not responding to therapy or another organism such as *S. aureus* or anaerobes are suspected. Fluid aspirated from the abscess can often be used to identify the infecting organism or organisms, which aids in targeted antibiotic therapy. The use of steroids has been controversial, and no clear role for them in the treatment of peritonsillar abscess has been established. Appropriate treatment after early recognition typically results in a very prompt response. Recurrences have been reported, however, and should be suspected with any return of symptoms.

If the diagnosis of peritonsillar cellulitis is suspected and the patient does not have evidence of airway compromise, a trial of parenteral antibiotics for 24 to 48 hours without surgical treatment may be effective. Any worsening of symptoms or lack of response to antibiotic therapy should prompt reevaluation for surgical treatment.

Consultation

Consultation with otolaryngology is appropriate, especially when surgical intervention is a consideration.

Admission Criteria

Patients with peritonsillar abscess typically are admitted for observation after surgical management and for parenteral antibiotics. Intravenous fluids are generally required, but most patients can be discharged home within 24 to 48 hours on a regimen of oral antibiotics once clinical improvement has occurred. There is growing evidence that a subset of patients with uncomplicated presentations can be managed effectively as outpatients after needle aspiration.

RETROPHARYNGEAL/PARAPHARYNGEAL ABSCESS

The retropharyngeal space is a potential midline space located between the posterior wall of the esophagus and the anterior cervical fascia. This space contains a pair of lymph node chains that drain the nasopharynx, adenoids, and paranasal sinuses. Suppurative infection of these nodes can fill this cavity and result in a *retropharyngeal abscess*. A similar infection may also form in the lateral deep neck tissues and result in a *parapharyngeal abscess*. These abscesses most commonly result from direct extension of pharyngitis/tonsillitis. Other causes may include medial expansion of cervical adenitis, penetrating trauma to the posterior pharynx (seen most commonly when children fall with a foreign object in their mouth), and anterior spread of cervical vertebral osteomyelitis. Retropharyngeal and parapharyngeal infections are uncommon and usually present in preschool children; the mean age in one study was 4 years. The retropharyngeal lymph node chains begin to recede around this age, with a resultant decreased incidence of these deep neck infections in older children. The most common organisms isolated from these abscesses are identical to those found in peritonsillar abscesses and include *Streptococcus* species (usually GABHS), anaerobes, and *S. aureus*.

Clinical Presentation

Children with a retropharyngeal or parapharyngeal abscess can present at various levels of toxicity and airway involvement, depending on the stage of their illness. Early in the course, such abscesses may be indistinguishable from uncomplicated pharyngitis. As the abscess develops, inflammation and a mass effect pushing anteriorly may cause more noticeable symptoms, including stridor, trismus, drooling, and torticollis. Pain with neck extension is found in up to 40% of children with retropharyngeal abscess.[3] Neck stiffness may progress to frank nuchal rigidity and can easily be mistaken for meningismus. Stridor has traditionally been thought to be a common finding, but it may be a late presentation; absence of stridor should not rule out consideration of a retropharyngeal/parapharyngeal abscess. In one study, only 5% of children in whom a retropharyngeal abscess was diagnosed presented with stridor, whereas 38% had neck pain or stiffness.[3]

Physical examination is often difficult because of the patient's age and level of toxicity. Visualization of the posterior pharynx is often impeded by neck pain and drooling. Unlike a peritonsillar abscess with its obvious changes in the oropharynx, examination of a child with a retropharyngeal or parapharyngeal abscess may reveal only a slight asymmetry or fullness of the posterior pharyngeal wall. There may be no obvious findings on visual inspection. Palpation of the neck frequently elicits tender anterior cervical lymph nodes or, in the case of a parapharyngeal abscess, a frank neck mass.

A retropharyngeal or parapharyngeal abscess can spread to local vital structures. Although rare, these complications are acutely life threatening and should be considered in hospitalized children with worrisome findings. A retropharyngeal abscess may track inferiorly into the mediastinum and cause an acute suppurative mediastinitis or track through the prevertebral "danger space" as far as the psoas muscle.

Parapharyngeal extension to the carotid artery may progress from arteritis to aneurysm formation with rupture. Extension into the jugular vein may cause thrombophlebitis of the jugular vein. When caused by *Fusobacterium necrophorum*, this entity is referred to as Lemierre syndrome, although other anaerobic organisms have been identified. More common in previously healthy adolescents, the clinical presentation often includes a toxic appearance, high fever, dysphagia, trismus, torticollis, and tenderness along the anterior sternocleidomastoid muscle. Bacteremia, septic emboli to the lungs, cavernous venous thrombosis, and septic shock are all associated with this serious infection.

Diagnosis

Laboratory abnormalities are usually nonspecific. A complete blood count may show an elevated white blood cell count with neutrophil predominance. Electrolytes may be consistent with dehydration. There are rare reports of associated bacteremia, and a blood culture may yield the pathogen and should be considered in a toxic-appearing child.

Historically, radiographic evaluation of a suspected retropharyngeal abscess began with a lateral neck radiograph. Widening of the retropharyngeal soft tissue was considered indicative of an abscess. In general, the width of the soft tissue between the posterior esophagus and anterior vertebral body should be no more than half the width of the adjacent vertebral body (Fig. 65-3). Proper technique is essential; the patient's neck should be extended and the film taken during inspiration to obtain the most accurate measurement, which can obviously be difficult in a young, ill-appearing child. Although this approach may continue to be used today, neck computed tomography (CT) has become more widely used and offers the clinician two distinct advantages: (1) better localization of the abscess for the consideration of drainage, especially if located in the lateral or parapharyngeal spaces, and (2) better differentiation between a true abscess and a "phlegmon" (defined as a soft tissue suppurative inflammation without a distinct or drainable fluid collection), which may be suitable for medical treatment alone without the need for surgical intervention.

Treatment

The initial priority in the management of a child with a retropharyngeal or parapharyngeal abscess is maintenance of a patent airway. In cases in which the airway is compromised, immediate endotracheal intubation may be necessary. In such cases, emergency consultation with the surgical team should be initiated. More commonly, however, children will present for care before the airway has been clinically compromised. The recent literature has documented a clear trend away from early surgical intervention for patients with

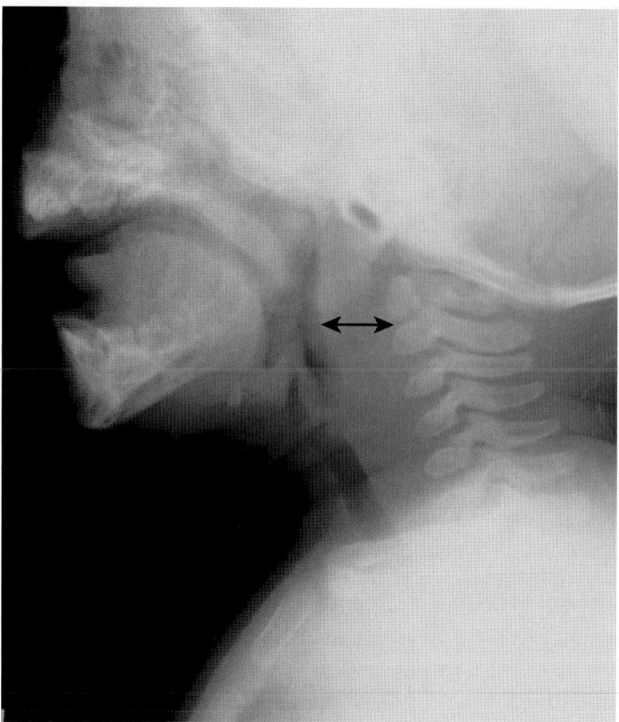

Figure 65-3 Lateral neck radiograph demonstrating a widened prevertebral space in a patient with a retropharyngeal abscess.

retropharyngeal or parapharyngeal abscesses when the fluid collection is limited and the patient does not appear to be in any apparent distress. This trend is even clearer when evaluation of the area by CT shows only evidence of cellulitis or phlegmon rather than a true abscess. These patients should be admitted for 24 to 48 hours of parenteral antibiotics in close consultation with an otolaryngologist. Antibiotics should be targeted to provide adequate coverage of gram-positive and anaerobic organisms. Intravenous clindamycin and ampicillin-sulbactam are appropriate initial choices for therapy. The antibiotic spectrum can be narrowed if surgical drainage is needed and adequate Gram stain, cultures, and sensitivity studies are performed.

If the child shows clinical improvement in response to intravenous antibiotics, surgical intervention is not needed and the child can be transitioned to oral antibiotics and discharged home to complete a 10- to 14-day course. Recommendations for oral antibiotic therapy may include amoxicillin-clavulanate or clindamycin, although clindamycin requires more frequent dosing and the oral liquid preparation is distinctly distasteful. Recent reviews and case series reports have quoted success rates ranging from 18% to almost 60% with an antibiotics-only strategy.[4,5]

If there is clinical worsening or inadequate response, reconsultation with otolaryngology should be obtained in anticipation of surgical drainage. Needle aspiration and decompression at this point may serve as an intermediate step for both treatment and collection of fluid for culture and identification of organisms. If the child fails to respond to this step or significant worsening has occurred, the classic open incision plus drainage of the area is necessary. Retropharyngeal abscesses are usually approached from an intraoral incision, whereas parapharyngeal or larger abscesses may require an external anterior neck approach.

Immediate surgical consultation should be obtained for any hospitalized child who is suspected of having one of the life-threatening complications resulting from extension of the condition, and transfer to an intensive care facility may be warranted.

Consultation

Consultation with otolaryngology should be considered for all patients with a retropharyngeal or parapharyngeal abscess. Ongoing assessment, as well as determination of the need for or the timing of surgical intervention, is best accomplished in collaboration with these colleagues.

Admission Criteria

All children suspected of having a retropharyngeal or parapharyngeal abscess should be admitted for intravenous antibiotics and careful observation with or without surgical intervention.

Discharge Criteria

- Obvious clinical improvement with reduction of symptoms and resolution of any airway compromise
- Ability to tolerate antibiotics and adequate fluids orally
- Careful outpatient follow-up with appropriate discharge instructions to seek care for any worsening symptoms

CERVICAL LYMPHADENITIS

Enlargement of the cervical lymph nodes is one of the more challenging diagnostic dilemmas to pediatricians, with causes ranging from a benign inflammatory response to malignancy. The anterior and posterior cervical lymph node chains along with the submandibular lymph nodes represent the major drainage routes for most of the head and neck. They are most commonly inflamed and enlarged as a secondary reaction to an upper respiratory infection and may be routinely found on neck examination in an otherwise well child.

Infections of these nodes, or *cervical lymphadenitis*, make up a large portion of the differential diagnosis for cervical node enlargement (Table 65-2). The key to accurate diagnosis lies in a thorough history with attention to environmental exposure and associated symptoms.

Epidemiology

Viral infections are the most common cause of cervical lymph node inflammation, particularly Epstein-Barr virus (EBV) and cytomegalovirus (CMV). Other more common upper respiratory tract viruses, including adenovirus, parainfluenza viruses, and respiratory syncytial virus, have also been identified. These viruses are usually transmitted by respiratory droplet or direct contact and are therefore more common in younger children, particularly in day-care and school settings. HIV infection may also present with tender inflammation of the cervical lymph nodes and should be considered in the differential diagnosis, particularly with other supporting evidence of an immunocompromised state.

Table 65-2 Infectious Causes of Cervical Lymphadenitis

Viral	Bacterial	Fungal	Parasitic
Epstein-Barr virus	*Staphylococcus aureus*	*Aspergillus fumigatus*	*Toxoplasma gondii*
Herpes simplex virus	*Streptococcus pyogenes**	*Candida*	
Cytomegalovirus	Anaerobes	Coccidioidomycosis	
Adenovirus	*Bartonella henselae*	*Cryptococcus neoformans*	
Enterovirus	*Brucella* spp. *Francisella tularensis*	*Histoplasma capsulatum* *Nocardia* spp.	
Human herpesvirus 6	Atypical *Mycobacterium*		
Varicella	*Mycobacterium tuberculosis*		
Human immunodeficiency virus	*Nocardia asteroides* *Salmonella typhi* *Yersinia pestis*		

*Also known as group A β-hemolytic streptococcus.

Table 65-3 Common Exposures Associated with Pathogens for Cervical Lymphadenitis

Exposure	Organism
Cats, kittens	*Bartonella henselae*
Cat excrement and undercooked meat	*Toxoplasma gondii*
Ticks or other biting insects, wild rabbits or other infected animals	*Francisella tularensis*
Food or water contaminated with human feces	*Salmonella typhi*
Unpasteurized milk or milk products, especially soft cheese	*Brucella* spp.
Oriental rat fleas from dead rats	*Yersinia pestis*
Soil, house dust, sand, swimming pools	*Nocardia* spp.
Ubiquitous (soil, water, food, animals)	Nontuberculous *Mycobacterium*
Exposure to infected contagious individuals, visiting an endemic area (e.g., Mexico, Philippines, India, South Korea, Haiti) or high-risk facility (e.g., prison, homeless shelter)	*Mycobacterium tuberculosis*
Residence in the Ohio or Mississippi River valleys, with high-risk exposure in caves and barns	*Histoplasma capsulatum*

The bacterial agents that most commonly cause cervical lymphadenitis are similar to those associated with other head and neck infections and include GABHS, *S. aureus*, and various oral anaerobes. Cervical lymph adenitis with these organisms is generally a result of direct extension of a local infection such as pharyngitis or dental infection.

Atypical bacteria play a major role in the differential diagnosis of cervical lymphadenitis, with the diagnosis often being aided by important environmental factors. Key exposures and the corresponding organisms are presented in Table 65-3.

Clinical Presentation

Cervical lymphadenitis usually presents with tenderness, erythema, or enlargement of one or more cervical lymph nodes (or any combination of these findings). The presentation varies with the infecting agent. Classification is generally based on the duration of symptoms (acute versus chronic) and distribution of the nodes (unilateral versus bilateral).

Most cases of cervical lymphadenitis present as acute infections. Young children and infants presenting acutely with solitary or unilateral node inflammation and swelling are more likely to have a bacterial cause. GABHS and *S. aureus* are most commonly isolated in culture, with *S. aureus* being more likely in infants and younger toddlers. Although rare, group B streptococcus has been a reported pathogen in early infancy.[6] Anaerobes are more likely if the adenitis is associated with a dental infection. Patients do not generally have systemic or prodromal symptoms. The infection may be a primary process or a complication/extension from another infection, particularly pharyngitis/tonsillitis, dental abscess, or facial impetigo. The nodes are more likely to be found in the upper cervical chain or submandibular region and can vary in size from 1.5 to 6 to 8 cm. Larger nodes may demonstrate fluctuance on palpation.

Viral infections and pharyngitis are more likely to cause bilateral lymphadenopathy than lymphadenitis. Lymphadenopathy is defined as a simple reactive enlargement of the lymph nodes in response to regional infection or inflammation. The nodes are usually mildly or moderately tender and lack the overlying erythema or skin changes that are more common with lymphadenitis. Suppuration with fluctuance is very uncommon and usually represents bacterial superinfection, such as pyogenic lymph adenitis. Patients with lymphadenopathy caused by a viral illness often have fever and may have other associated symptoms (e.g., rash, sore throat, liver and spleen enlargement, fatigue) that aid in diagnosis of the primary infection. These infections most commonly present in the preschool to adolescent age range. Infectious mononucleosis has a predilection for the posterior cervical nodes, but it may present with generalized lymphadenopathy. Other common viruses associated with acute bilateral lymphadenopathy include CMV, HSV, human herpesvirus 6, adenovirus, enteroviruses, and parvovirus B19.

Cervical node enlargement with tenderness lasting more than 2 weeks is classified as subacute or chronic lymphadenitis. Presentations vary, depending on the cause, with cat-scratch disease and mycobacterial and fungal infections being the most common. Patients with cat-scratch disease can be of any age. There is a clear history of exposure to cats or kittens in approximately 90% of cases, and it may occur with or without a history of scratches or bites from a cat. A papule or pustule forms at the site of inoculation in more than 50% of cases. Lymphadenitis usually presents 1 to several weeks after the initial inoculation as firm nodes 1 to 6 cm in size. Affected nodes are proximal to the area of inoculation, most commonly in the axillary and cervical regions. Associated symptoms of fever, malaise, and headache may be present, but they have often resolved by the time that the nodes appear.

Chronic lymphadenitis from mycobacteria may be caused by either nontuberculous mycobacteria or *Mycobacterium tuberculosis*. Infection with nontuberculous mycobacteria is more likely to be unilateral and affect younger children (<6 years). The nodes are commonly nontender, gradually progress over a period of 1 to 4 weeks from erythema to violaceous discoloration, and if not resected, may spontaneously drain and create a fistulous tract. When compared with patients with tuberculosis, these patients are unlikely to have a positive purified protein derivative (PPD) reaction; if reactive, the PPD is typically less than 10 mm in induration. Patients with tuberculosis tend to be older and have the classically associated risk factors. The adenitis is more likely to be bilateral and associated with systemic symptoms and generalized lymphadenopathy, and the patient would demonstrate a positive PPD reaction.

Differential Diagnosis

In addition to the infectious causes already described, the differential diagnosis of a cervical neck mass or swelling includes several noninfectious conditions. Malignancies such as leukemias, lymphomas, or rhabdomyosarcoma can present as node enlargement in the neck. These nodes are most often painless, firm, and fixed to adjacent tissue. They classically present in the posterior cervical and supraclavicular region, whereas the more common infectious causes

present in the anterior and superior aspects. Congenital lesions can frequently be misinterpreted as cervical lymphadenitis, particularly when they are secondarily infected. Such lesions include thyroglossal duct cysts (midline), branchial cleft cysts (anterior along the sternocleidomastoid muscle), and cystic hygromas (posterior above the clavicles). Other causes include Kawasaki disease (see Chapter 102), Castleman disease (giant lymph node hyperplasia), Kikuchi-Fujimoto disease (histiocytic necrotizing lymphadenitis), and Rosai-Dorfman disease (sinus histiocytosis with lymphadenopathy).

Diagnosis

The initial evaluation of cervical lymphadenitis should be guided by the history (duration of enlargement, associated symptoms, and environmental exposure) and physical examination (location of the nodes, tenderness, and other systemic findings). Describing the involvement as unilateral versus bilateral and acute versus subacute/chronic will help limit the probable causes and therefore focus the diagnostic evaluation.

A solitary node with erythema and tenderness of an acute nature may not require further evaluation because a bacterial cause, specifically GABHS, would be most likely. A positive GABHS antigen test or throat culture may be confirmatory, although care must again be taken to differentiate a positive test in a patient with acute infection versus one who may be chronically colonized. Needle aspiration of any fluctuant node may be helpful in identifying the causative organism; the aspirate should be sent for Gram stain and acid-fast bacillus stain, in addition to bacterial (aerobic and anaerobic), fungal, and mycobacterial culture.

In cases in which the diagnosis is not as obvious, an initial workup should include a complete blood count with differential, pharyngeal swab for GABHS, placement of a PPD tuberculin test, and serologic evaluation for *Bartonella henselae*. Serology for viruses, including EBV and CMV, and other organisms (i.e., toxoplasmosis, histoplasmosis, coccidioidomycosis) may be considered if suggested by the history or physical findings. Further testing may be deferred until a trial of antimicrobial therapy is unsuccessful or there is further advancement of disease. Excisional biopsy is reserved for persistent symptoms, when nontuberculous mycobacterial infection is suspected, or when the nodes are nontender and fixed to adjacent tissue, suggestive of malignancy.

Occasionally, CT of the neck may be helpful in diagnosis but is more often used to detect suppurative lymph nodes, assess the extent of infection, and guide surgical management.

Treatment

Treatment of patients with cervical lymphadenitis should be directed at the most likely organisms based on the patient's age and clinical presentation. Most children who are nontoxic and well hydrated can be managed with oral antibiotics in the outpatient setting. Recommended antibiotic regimens have been diverse, with most focusing on providing adequate coverage for GABHS and *S. aureus* with cephalexin or dicloxacillin. Oral amoxicillin/clavulanic acid and clindamycin also provide appropriate gram-positive coverage and additionally provide anaerobic coverage for patients with suspected primary dental causes. It is important to note the recent increase in prevalence of community-associated methicillin-resistant *S. aureus* (CA-MRSA) as a cause of skin and soft tissue infections. These isolates are often (but not always) susceptible to clindamycin. Trimethoprim-sulfamethoxazole also provides activity against many CA-MRSA isolates; however, it does not have sufficient activity against GABHS. Other options to treat MRSA infections (e.g., linezolid, vancomycin, quinupristin-dalfopristin) should be discussed in consultation with an infectious disease specialist.

Patients younger than 6 months, those who appear toxic or dehydrated, and those who have failed an outpatient trial of oral therapy warrant admission to the hospital and treatment with intravenous antibiotics. Nafcillin, oxacillin, ampicillin-sulbactam, and clindamycin are acceptable intravenous antibiotics for children who require hospitalization. In regions where CA-MRSA accounts for greater than 10% to 15% of *S. aureus* isolates, empirical therapy with β-lactams is not recommended. In this setting, clindamycin or, in severely ill patients, vancomycin is an appropriate option. Clinical improvement should generally be expected within 48 hours of initiation of therapy, and treatment should last for 10 to 14 days. Conversion from an intravenous to an oral regimen is appropriate at the time of discharge.

Consultation with an infectious disease specialist is recommended when other infectious causes are suspected or the patient does not respond to the initial choice of therapy. Such consultation can help guide the management of more difficult cases because treatment recommendations change frequently and are often based on local resistance patterns.

Treatment of cat-scratch disease has been controversial inasmuch as this illness is typically self-limited. Bass and colleagues performed a randomized placebo-controlled study for the treatment of typical cat-scratch lymphadenitis. In this study, a 5-day course of azithromycin was more effective in reducing the size of the lymph node at 1 month, but there was no difference in time to complete resolution between the two groups.[7] Additional published studies, however, have failed to consistently document a role for antimicrobial therapy for this infection.

Consultation

- Infectious disease: Management guidance for atypical cases or patients not responding to initial therapy
- Surgery: Possible excisional biopsy of affected nodes in difficult diagnostic cases
- Pediatric oncology: Evaluation of patients whose nodes are nonacute, nontender, fixed, or located in worrisome areas (supraclavicular)

Admission Criteria

- Patient younger than 6 months
- Toxic appearance or dehydration
- Failed a trial of oral antibiotics as an outpatient

IN A NUTSHELL

- Attention to the location and appearance of oral lesions is the key to diagnosing the correct cause of stomatitis.
- The most common bacterial causes of head and neck infections are group A streptococci, *S. aureus*, and oral anaerobes.
- Neck CT has replaced lateral neck radiographs as the study of choice for any suspected retropharyngeal/parapharyngeal abscess or cellulitis.
- Classification of cervical lymphadenitis as acute versus chronic and unilateral versus bilateral will help limit the differential diagnosis significantly and make the evaluation more straightforward.

ON THE HORIZON

- Infections of the neck and oral cavity should continue to be a diagnostic challenge for clinicians taking care of hospitalized patients for years to come. The recent emergence of CA-MRSA may demand a change in our standard empirical therapy and culture evaluation for soft tissue infections of the neck. There are continued concerns about the further development of antibiotic resistance, even among common bacteria. A practical diagnostic approach to acute streptococcal pharyngitis remains elusive, but with future generations of antigen detection testing there is hope that adequate sensitivity can be achieved to allow timely diagnosis and treatment. A better understanding of the "carrier state" of patients who are chronically colonized with GABHS and improved irradiation therapies should be developed with future study. In the end, however, proper diagnosis and treatment of these conditions will continue to be dependent on an astute clinician who is able to recognize the key details in the clinical presentation and physical examination.

SUGGESTED READING

Craig FW, Schunk JE: Retropharyngeal abscess in children: Clinical presentation, utility of imaging, and current management. Pediatrics 2003;111: 1394-1398.

Herzon FS, Nicklaus P: Pediatric peritonsillar abscess: Management guidelines. Curr Probl Pediatr 1996;26:270-278.

Johnson RF, Stewart MG, Wright CC: An evidence-based review of the treatment of peritonsillar abscess. Otolaryngol Head Neck Surg 2003;128:332-343.

Lalakea M, Messner AH: Retropharyngeal abscess management in children: Current practices. Otolaryngol Head Neck Surg 1999;121:398-405.

Nicklaus PJ, Kelley PE: Management of deep neck infection. Pediatr Clin North Am 1996;43:1277-1297.

Peters TR, Edwards KM: Cervical lymphadenopathy and adenitis. Pediatr Rev 2000;21:399-405.

REFERENCES

1. Martin JM, Green M, Barbadora KA, Wald ER: Erythromycin-resistant group A streptococci in schoolchildren in Pittsburgh. N Engl J Med 2002;346:1200-1206.

2. Johnson RF, Stewart MG, Wright CC: An evidence-based review of the treatment of peritonsillar abscess. Otolaryngol Head Neck Surg 2003;128:332-343.

3. Craig FW, Schunk JE: Retropharyngeal abscess in children: Clinical presentation, utility of imaging, and current management. Pediatrics 2003;111:1394-1398.

4. Lee SS, Schwartz RH, Bahadori RS: Retropharyngeal abscess: Epiglottitis of the new millennium. J Pediatr 2001;138:435-437.

5. Lalakea M, Messner AH: Retropharyngeal abscess management in children: Current practices. Otolaryngol Head Neck Surg 1999;121:398-405.

6. Barton LL, Ramsey RA, Raval DS: Neonatal group B streptococcal cellulitis-adenitis. Pediatr Dermatol 1993;10:58-60.

7. Bass JW, Freitas BC, Freitas AD, et al: Prospective randomized double blind placebo-controlled evaluation of azithromycin for treatment of cat-scratch disease. Pediatr Infect Dis J 1998;17:447-452.

CHAPTER 66

Middle Respiratory Tract Infections and Bronchiolitis

Samir S. Shah, Patricia M. Hopkins, and Jason G. Newland

A large portion of a pediatric hospitalist's time is spent caring for infants and children with bronchiolitis and with infections of the middle respiratory tract. Bronchiolitis and laryngotracheobronchitis (croup) are common and lead to significant morbidity. Epiglottitis, although rare since introduction of the *Haemophilus influenzae* type b (Hib) vaccine, warrants inclusion because of its life-threatening nature.

BRONCHIOLITIS

Bronchiolitis, a common communicable respiratory illness, is accompanied by signs and symptoms of both upper and lower respiratory tract infection. Most episodes occur in otherwise healthy children younger than 2 years. Children younger than 3 months are at high risk for severe disease. Other groups at risk for serious illness secondary to bronchiolitis include young infants less than 32 weeks' gestation with and without chronic lung disease, children with cyanotic congenital heart disease, and those with severe immune deficiency such as hematopoietic stem cell transplantation, solid organ transplantation, and cellular immune deficiencies (e.g., 22q11.2 chromosome deletions).

Respiratory syncytial virus (RSV), a single-stranded RNA paramyxovirus, accounts for 50% to 70% of cases of bronchiolitis. Less common causes of bronchiolitis include parainfluenza virus types 1, 2, and 3, influenza viruses A and B, and adenovirus. More recently, human metapneumovirus (hMPV) has been recognized as a cause of bronchiolitis. hMPV has been detected in 20% to 25% of children with bronchiolitis and negative direct fluorescent antibody testing of nasal aspirates for RSV, parainfluenza types 1 to 3, influenza A and B, and adenovirus.[1,2] Rare causes of bronchiolitis include *Mycoplasma pneumoniae* and enteroviruses.

Overall, bronchiolitis is most prevalent between October and May, although sporadic cases occur throughout the year. Epidemic RSV bronchiolitis displays remarkable seasonality with a peak occurrence between December and April and virtually no occurrence between June and October. Peak activity of hMPV occurs in March and April, just as RSV activity begins to wane. The seasonal prevalence of specific pathogens is shown in Figure 66-1. In the United States, 1% to 3% of affected infants require hospital care; most hospital admissions for bronchiolitis occur between December and March.

Although the clinical manifestations of bronchiolitis and asthma overlap to some extent, the pathogenesis of the two conditions differs, a fact that has important therapeutic implications. In bronchiolitis, progressive infection of the respiratory mucosa induces desquamation of ciliated respiratory epithelial cells and lymphocytic infiltration of peribronchial epithelial cells. These changes lead to small-airway obstruction as intraluminal cellular debris accumulates and mucosal edema worsens. The concomitant increase in mucus production and, in some children, enhanced airway smooth muscle reactivity compound the small-airway obstruction that characterizes bronchiolitis. The relatively small caliber of their distal airways predisposes young infants to more severe obstructive symptoms.

Clinical Presentation

Symptoms appear 5 to 7 days after exposure, although the incubation period is often shorter for parainfluenza (2 to 4 days) and influenza (1 to 7 days) viruses. The initial symptoms include nasal congestion, rhinorrhea, and cough. Poor feeding, posttussive emesis, and irritability may accompany these symptoms. Fever develops in a half to three fourths of patients. These findings persist for several days, and then lower respiratory tract involvement develops precipitously. Dyspnea and audible wheezing are common. In younger infants, especially those younger than 2 months, apnea may develop as the initial manifestation of bronchiolitis.

At the time of evaluation, tachypnea, tachycardia, and mild to moderate hypoxemia are often present. The infant frequently appears barrel-chested because of air trapping. The breathing may be labored with flaring of the alae nasi, grunting, abdominal breathing, and suprasternal, intercostal, subcostal, and supraclavicular retractions. On auscultation, harsh rhonchi, expiratory wheezing, and rales are heard diffusely throughout the chest. The respiratory noise can be loud enough to obscure the heart sounds. As the illness progresses, wheezing is often heard without the aid of a stethoscope. In children with severe lower airway obstruction, wheezing may not be readily appreciated because of poor aeration. Marked prolongation of the expiratory phase of breathing also occurs with more severe lower airway obstruction, although it is not common in a tachypneic young infant.

Other findings in children with bronchiolitis include conjunctivitis, otitis media (5% to 20% of cases), and pharyngitis. The liver and spleen are frequently palpable because of air trapping and flattening of the diaphragm. Signs of dehydration may be noted in children with cough or respiratory distress sufficient to substantially decrease fluid intake; additionally, if posttussive vomiting is present, the dehydration may worsen.

In older children and adults, infections caused by RSV and hMPV usually cause symptoms of upper respiratory tract involvement such as rhinorrhea, cough, coryza, and pharyngitis. Any of the agents that cause bronchiolitis in younger children can exacerbate asthma or other chronic lung diseases in older children and adults.

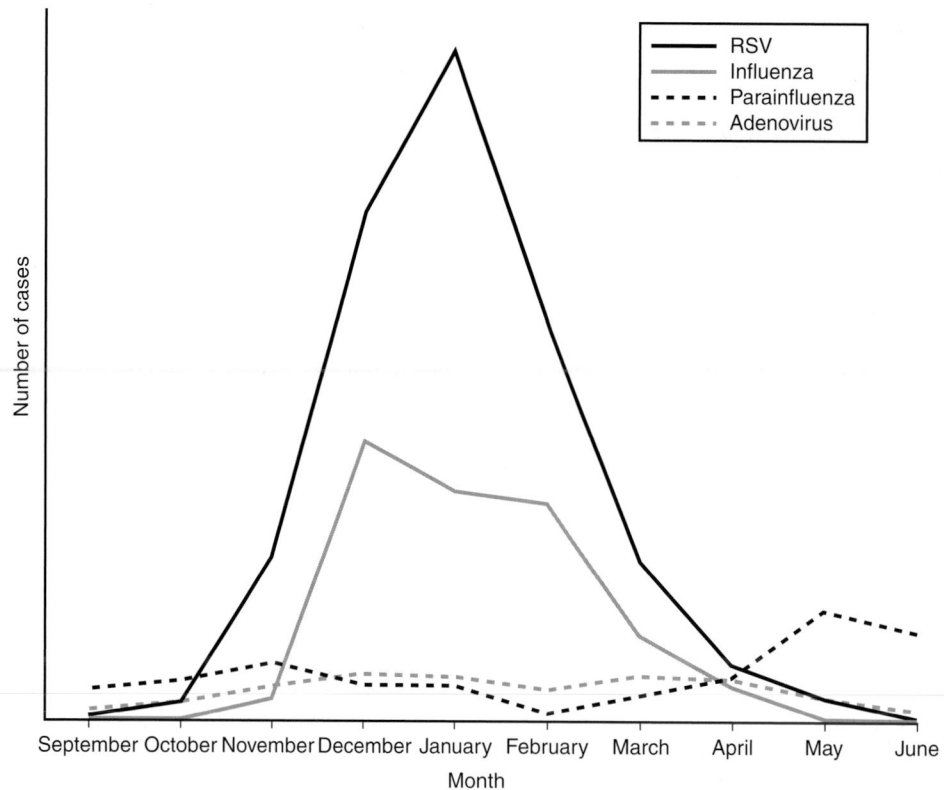

Figure 66-1 The seasonal prevalence of bronchiolitis caused by specific pathogens. The number of cases represents the mean number of cases per year from 2000 to 2004. RSV, respiratory syncytial virus. (Published with permission from Dr. Richard L. Hodinka, Clinical Virology Laboratory, The Children's Hospital of Philadelphia.)

Differential Diagnosis

In young infants early in the course of illness, the cough is occasionally staccato in nature, which makes it difficult to differentiate clinically from infection with *Bordetella pertussis* or *Chlamydia trachomatis*. Asthma, as well as other conditions that cause wheezing (see Chapter 75), must also be considered in the differential diagnosis.[3]

Diagnosis

The diagnosis of bronchiolitis can generally be made by the history and physical examination findings alone. No tests are routinely required.

In the hospital setting, an etiologic diagnosis may facilitate the implementation of strategies to limit nosocomial transmission of respiratory viruses (e.g., type of precautions, patient cohorting). However, institution of these interventions can often be based on the clinical diagnosis (e.g., bronchiolitis) rather than the specific infectious agent.

Rapid viral antigen diagnostic tests are becoming more widely available and have supplanted viral culture of nasal aspirates as the initial diagnostic test for most clinical situations. Types of antigen detection tests include direct and indirect fluorescent antibody tests and "point-of-care" tests. Fluorescent antibody techniques are available to identify RSV, influenza viruses A and B, parainfluenza virus types 1 to 3, and adenoviruses. In the fluorescent antibody tests, binding of viral antigen to an antibody-fluorescein complex can be visualized with the aid of a fluorescence microscope. Virology laboratories can complete these tests in 2 to 4 hours. The sensitivity and specificity of these tests range from 80% to 90% and 92% to 99%, respectively. The exception is adenovirus detection, for which the sensitivity is 40% to 60% by fluorescent antibody techniques.

More rapid tests, known as "point-of-care" tests or solid-phase immunoassays, are currently available for influenza viruses A and B and for RSV. In these rapid tests, binding of viral antigen to an antibody is indicated by a color change on the test cartridge. This reaction is visible without the aid of a microscope. With appropriate facilities and trained personnel, these tests can be completed in an emergency department or office setting in less than 30 minutes. The sensitivity and specificity of these tests vary by manufacturer. Typically, the sensitivity is 75% to 82% and the specificity is 92% to 98%. During the influenza or RSV season, some laboratories initially perform these tests and reserve fluorescent antibody testing for specimens negative by "point-of-care" tests.

Genome detection by polymerase chain reaction (PCR) can be used to detect adenovirus, hMPV, *M. pneumoniae, B. pertussis*, and enteroviruses in nasal aspirates. Adenovirus and enteroviruses can also often be detected in urine and blood samples of infected patients by PCR. The sensitivity and specificity of PCR in detecting adenovirus from respiratory secretions are 99% and 95% to 98%, respectively. Sending specimens from multiple sites (e.g., nasal aspirate, conjunctival swab, urine, and blood) for testing will increase the yield of the test.

Limited evidence does not support the routine use of chest radiography for infants with clinically suspected bronchiolitis. However, chest radiographs should be obtained in children with severe illness or hypoxia and when concern for bacterial pneumonia or other complications (e.g., pneumothorax) exists.[4] Radiographic findings in bronchiolitis include hyperinflation with flattening of the diaphragm, peribronchial thickening, and patchy infiltrates. The infiltrates are usually due to atelectasis; they occur as a consequence of airway narrowing and mucous plugging. Unfortunately, radiographic differentiation of atelectasis, pneumonitis, and bacterial pneumonia is sometimes difficult. Concomitant bacterial pneumonia should be suspected in infants with stable (as opposed to migratory) radiographic infiltrates, persistent fever (longer than 2 to 3 days), and lack of clinical improvement with supportive care only. The presence of a pleural effusion also suggests bacterial superinfection.

Infants with poor oral intake may require evaluation for electrolyte abnormalities. Arterial blood gas studies may be useful when there is concern for or evidence of respiratory failure.

The issue of whether children with bronchiolitis merit additional testing to exclude serious bacterial infection (SBI) remains controversial.[5] The risk for SBI differs by age group. Infants and children older than 2 months who are evaluated during the bronchiolitis season and have fever, clear symptoms and signs of bronchiolitis, and no evidence of lobar pneumonia do not routinely require additional testing; the risk for concomitant SBI is low. However, high fever in boys younger than 6 months and in young girls raises suspicion for urinary tract infection. A screening urinalysis and urine culture should be considered in these children.[6] Clinicians should consider further evaluation, including cultures of blood, urine, and possibly cerebrospinal fluid, in any child with an ill appearance or an atypical clinical course.

Febrile children younger than 2 months with bronchiolitis may be at lower risk for SBI than those without bronchiolitis. However, the risk is not zero. The rate of urinary tract infection, in particular, remains appreciable. Most current studies assessing the risk for SBI in children with bronchiolitis contain important methodologic flaws that limit their generalizability. Levine and colleagues conducted the first prospective multicenter trial in which the risk for SBI was compared in young febrile infants who tested positive for RSV and those who tested negative for RSV. Rates of SBI in the RSV-positive ($n = 269$) versus the RSV-negative ($n = 979$) group were as follows: urinary tract infection, 5.4% (95% confidence interval [CI], 3.0% to 8.8%) versus 10.1% (95% CI, 8.3% to 12.2%); bacteremia, 1.1% (95% CI, 0.2% to 3.2%) versus 2.3% (95% CI, 1.4% to 3.4%); and meningitis, 0% (95% CI, 0% to 1.2%) versus 0.9% (95% CI, 0.4% to 1.7%).[6] Evaluation of children younger than 2 months with bronchiolitis is addressed in more detail elsewhere in this book (see Chapter 63).

Course of Illness

Generally, bronchiolitis is a self-limited disease. Apnea associated with bronchiolitis usually resolves within 48 to 72 hours, although some infants may need longer periods of hospitalization and monitoring. The typical acute bronchiolitis illness lasts 3 to 7 days. Infants hospitalized relatively early in their illness may demonstrate clinical worsening for several days before improving. Improvement is gradual and heralded by decreases in the respiratory rate, retractions, and duration of the expiratory phase. Wheezing generally per-

sists for more than a week after hospital discharge. Oxygen saturation as measured percutaneously by pulse oximeter may hover between 92% and 96% for several weeks. Other symptoms, including cough and noisy breathing, take longer to resolve. Among 181 children with bronchiolitis studied by Swingler and associates, these symptoms were present 3 and 4 weeks after the onset of illness in 18% and 9% of children, respectively.[7]

Mortality is less than 0.1% overall but approaches 5% in those with high-risk conditions, including young age (<2 months), chronic lung disease, cyanotic heart disease, and immune deficiency.

Pulse oximetry is often used as a surveillance tool for respiratory failure, but it does not detect hypoventilation. Hypoventilation leading to significant hypercapnia results in only modest decreases in oxygen saturation. Recalling the hemoglobin-oxygen dissociation curve, oxygen saturation does not diminish significantly until the partial pressure of oxygen (PO_2) falls to the range of 60 mm Hg (i.e., the steep part of the curve) (Fig. 66-2). In addition, small amounts of supplemental oxygen will restore PO_2, thereby normalizing oxygen saturation, which would allow unrecognized inadequate ventilation to progress without further derangements in pulse oximeter readings. Respiratory acidosis ensues with increasing hypercapnia. Bedside evaluation of an infant with respiratory failure would reveal somnolence and tachypnea with shallow respirations, which can progress to bradypnea or apnea. Expected derangements in arterial blood gas results would progress from hypocapnia associated with tachypnea and hyperventilation to the normal-range partial pressure of carbon dioxide (PCO_2). This "normal" PCO_2 would be inappropriate in the setting of hyperventilation and should be considered a harbinger of respiratory insufficiency. Progression to respiratory failure would be confirmed by worsening hypercapnia and respiratory acidosis (i.e., falling blood pH on an arterial blood gas specimen).

Treatment

The primary care physician manages most infants and children with bronchiolitis in the outpatient setting. Certain high-risk children and children with severe symptoms require closer monitoring and often hospitalization.

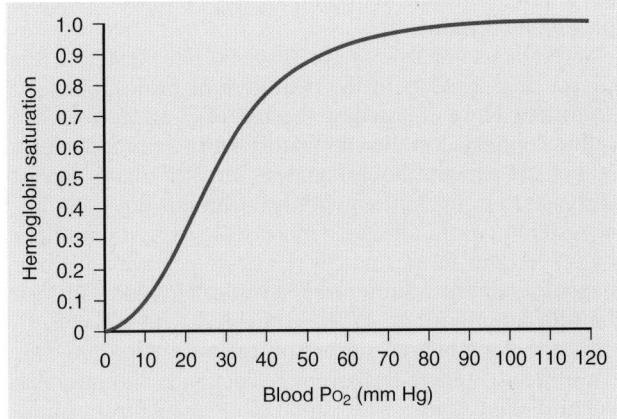

Figure 66-2 Hemoglobin-oxygen dissociation curve. (From Tecklenburg F, McKee TW: Pediatric resuscitation and fluid management. In Haddad LM, Shannon MW, Winchester JF [eds]: Clinical Management of Poisoning and Drug Overdose. Philadelphia, WB Saunders, 1998, p 33.)

The mainstay of treatment in infants and children with bronchiolitis is supportive. Infants and children admitted with bronchiolitis and hypoxia require supplemental oxygen. The appropriate lower limits for oxygen saturation in children with bronchiolitis are not known, but various guidelines suggest values ranging from 90% to 94%. However, no guideline specifies the acceptable duration of desaturation below these values. Furthermore, normal transient desaturation and measurement error because of poor pulse pressure and motion artifact occur frequently. Considerable uncertainty remains over when to begin, increase, or discontinue supplemental oxygen therapy. As a consequence, abnormalities in pulse oximetry readings alone often unnecessarily prolong hospitalization in children with bronchiolitis as a result of the perceived requirement for supplemental oxygen. Schroeder and coworkers propose the following strategies to limit overreliance on pulse oximetry:

1. Discontinue the use of pulse oximetry or transition to intermittent pulse oximetry during the convalescent stage of illness.
2. Initiate or increase supplemental oxygen therapy only in children with increasing respiratory distress or when other maneuvers such as stimulation, suctioning, or repositioning fail to improve oxygenation.
3. Establish a hospital-wide consensus on an acceptable level and duration of desaturation.
4. Increase physician involvement in decisions to initiate and increase oxygen therapy; such decisions are often made independently by nurses or respiratory therapists.[8]

Other potential interventions include heliox therapy, nasal continuous positive airway pressure, and endotracheal intubation with mechanical ventilation. Administration of heliox (70% helium, 30% oxygen) through a non-rebreather (reservoir) face mask may improve respiratory effort by preserving laminar airflow at higher flow rates.[9] Mechanical ventilation should be considered for infants with signs of respiratory failure, shock, or persistent apnea.

Maintaining hydration with intravenous fluids may be necessary, but nasogastric feeding is an alternative. Infusing nasogastric feeding slowly tends to minimize gastric distention and vomiting. Daily weights, as well as careful documentation of intake and output, are helpful in assessing and tracking fluid status.

Several meta-analyses have systematically reviewed the efficacy of β-agonists in the treatment of bronchiolitis.[10,11] Flores and Horwitz assessed the use of β-agonists in five studies conducted in the ambulatory setting that included a total of 251 patients. Pooled analysis revealed that β-agonist administration to children with bronchiolitis did not affect the respiratory rate. Observed increases in oxygen saturation (by 1.2%) and heart rate (by 15 beats per minute) after β-agonist administration were statistically significant but clinically unimportant. When compared with placebo, β-agonist therapy had no impact on the hospitalization rate. In a subsequent meta-analysis by Kellner and colleagues that included eight studies with a total of 394 patients, hospitalization was required in 18% of patients treated with β-agonists versus 26% of untreated patients (odds ratio, 0.7; 95% CI, 0.4 to 1.5); this difference was not statistically significant.[12]

Among hospitalized patients in the eight studies reviewed by Kellner and coworkers, the duration of hospitalization was 0.12 day shorter (95% CI, 0.3 day longer to 0.5 day shorter) in the group treated with β-agonists than in those not treated.[12] A total of 13 trials consisting of 956 patients were included in the subsequent systematic review by King and associates.[11] Most of the studies used nebulized albuterol versus nebulized saline, unspecified placebo, or no treatment, whereas four studies also did comparisons with nebulized ipratropium bromide. Nine of the 13 trials showed no difference in various clinical measures (e.g., oxygen saturation, respiratory rate) between children treated with and without β-agonist therapy, 3 trials demonstrated short-term improvement in various clinical measures, and 1 trial demonstrated a worsening of these parameters. Seven of the 13 trials examined a primary outcome measure related to the need for or length of hospitalization; none reported significant differences between the groups. In summary, although some trials of β-agonist therapy demonstrated mild improvement in some clinical features of bronchiolitis, there was no significant decrease in either the rate or duration of hospitalization.

In addition to the bronchodilating effects of β-agonists, nebulized racemic epinephrine adds α-agonist properties that are thought to reduce airway edema and mucus production by inducing vasoconstriction of the bronchial vasculature. Meta-analyses of clinical trials of epinephrine for bronchiolitis in the outpatient and inpatient setting suggest modest improvements in short-term outcomes (clinical scores, oxygen saturation), but no effect on hospitalization rates or length of stay.[13,14]

Although the benefit of administering bronchodilators has not been established, they are often used in clinical practice. Bronchodilators should be considered in patients with severe respiratory distress, hypoxia, or impending respiratory failure. If no significant improvement occurs within 60 minutes of administration, they should be discontinued.

The role of corticosteroids in the treatment of bronchiolitis is controversial as well. Studies have typically used 3- to 5-day courses of either dexamethasone (0.6 mg/kg to a maximum of 15 mg orally once daily) or prednisolone (1 to 2 mg/kg/day to a maximum of 60 mg orally divided twice daily). A meta-analysis of six placebo-controlled studies (347 total patients) of corticosteroid therapy demonstrated a small but statistically significant reduction in the length of hospital stay; the mean duration of hospitalization was 0.43 day (95% CI, 0.05 to 0.81) shorter in the corticosteroid group than in the placebo group.[15] When the studies that included patients with a history of wheezing were omitted from the analysis, this difference was no longer significant,[15] a finding that supports the notion that certain subgroups with bronchiolitis may benefit from corticosteroid treatment. In a study of mechanically ventilated patients with bronchiolitis, the authors found that the mean length of stay was 6 days (95% CI, 1.8 to 10.2) shorter for the corticosteroid group than for the placebo group.[16]

Overall, the risks and benefits of corticosteroid administration must be weighed. Because bronchiolitis is generally self-limited and corticosteroid use prolongs viral shedding in RSV bronchiolitis, many clinicians do not favor their routine use in the treatment of children with bronchiolitis. However, subgroups that may benefit from corticosteroid administration include those with recurrent wheezing in the context of a strong family history of atopy and asthma (provided that evaluation for other causes of recurrent wheezing has been undertaken) and those with severe illness or respiratory failure.

Ribavirin, a synthetic purine nucleoside analogue, exerts its effect by lethally mutating the viral RNA genome. Ribavirin exhibits activity against many RNA viruses, including paramyxoviruses and adenoviruses. In bronchiolitis, the drug is administered by aerosolized delivery via face masks, oxygen tents, or oxygen hoods. Five studies (167 patients) examined the effect of ribavirin on clinically pertinent outcomes such as duration of hospitalization, illness, and mechanical ventilation in patients with RSV bronchiolitis. Four of these studies found no differences between ribavirin and placebo. The trial by Smith and colleagues found a shorter duration of mechanical ventilation and hospitalization in the ribavirin-treated group; however, the control group received nebulized sterile water, a known precipitant of bronchospasm, thus making the true benefit of ribavirin in this study unclear.[17] When administered orally or intravenously, ribavirin causes dose-related reversible anemia. Low doses cause extravascular hemolysis, whereas higher doses induce bone marrow suppression. Aerosolized administration results in conjunctival irritation and possibly transient worsening of pulmonary function. Although hematologic effects are not usually encountered with aerosol delivery, the potential toxicity to exposed health care workers prompted the development of stringent administration protocols. The limited data do not suggest a significant benefit of ribavirin therapy. The revised American Academy of Pediatrics position states that ribavirin "may be considered" in infants at high risk for serious RSV disease.[18]

Consultation

- Pediatric critical care for an infant or child with respiratory distress requiring intensive monitoring and mechanical ventilation
- Pediatric infectious diseases for a child with concern over an alternative infectious process or for a child at risk for severe disease in whom ribavirin is being considered
- Pediatric pulmonology for an infant or child with severe or persistent symptoms requiring further evaluation or follow-up

Admission Criteria

Hospitalization may be considered for the following reasons:

- Respiratory distress or respiratory difficulties requiring close monitoring, especially in young infants early in the course of their illness
- Hypoxia
- Evidence of respiratory insufficiency by clinical evaluation or arterial blood gas findings of hypercapnia or respiratory acidosis
- Severe symptoms interfering with feeding, dehydration, or both
- Apnea
- Infant with risk factors for severe disease
- Unstable social situation or lack of outpatient support and follow-up, or both

Criteria for Discharge

- Resolution of respiratory distress with stable or improving respiratory status that is well tolerated
- Resolution of hypoxia
- Resolution of apnea
- Ability to maintain adequate hydration
- Ability of a caregiver to provide adequate support at home
- Appropriate outpatient follow-up

Prevention

The goals of prevention are to minimize nosocomial transmission of the viruses that cause bronchiolitis and reduce the risk for RSV infection in high-risk infants by providing immunoprophylaxis.

Infection Control Measures

RSV is the leading cause of nosocomial respiratory illness. Several factors contribute to the frequency of nosocomial RSV infection:

- RSV can be spread by large-particle droplets or by contaminated secretions carried on infected patients, health care workers, and fomites.
- Transmission to 45% of contacts may occur in the absence of infection control measures.
- Repeat infections may be acquired by both adults and children because RSV infection does not induce long-term immunity.

Control measures that have been shown to reduce rates of nosocomial infection and save money include[19]

- Recognizing patients with respiratory symptoms early
- Confirming RSV infection by laboratory testing
- Establishing cohorts of patients and nursing staff
- Instituting gown-and-glove barrier precautions
- Monitoring and education of staff

Immunoprophylaxis

Two options for immunoprophylaxis to prevent RSV infection are available: RSV immunoglobulin intravenous (RSV-IGIV; RespiGam) and palivizumab (Synagis) (Table 66-1).[18,20] These products provide passive immunity for infants at high risk for a poor outcome if infected with RSV.

Developed in the early 1990s, RSV-IGIV consists of polyclonal hyperimmune globulin prepared from donors with high serum titers of RSV-neutralizing antibody. Monthly administration (750 mg/kg intravenously) during the RSV season decreases the incidence of infection and the need for hospitalization in high-risk children. Furthermore, children contracting RSV suffer a milder spectrum of illness and require a shorter duration of hospitalization than do those not receiving RSV-IGIV. The PREVENT study included 510 preterm infants younger than 24 months.[21] Monthly RSV-IGIV decreased the frequency and severity of RSV-associated illness by 41% to 60%. Hospitalization rates for RSV were also lower in the RSV-IGIV group than in the placebo group: 8.9% versus 17.4%, respectively, for infants with chronic lung disease; 6.5% versus 8.1%, respectively, for infants without chronic lung disease. Potential adverse reactions

Table 66-1   Indications for Prophylaxis against Respiratory Syncytial Virus

Children <2 years of age with chronic lung disease who have required therapy (e.g., supplemental oxygen, diuretics, corticosteroids, bronchodilators) less than 6 months before the start of the RSV season

Premature infants less than 32 weeks' gestational age*
   Infants 28 weeks' gestation or less if younger than 12 months at the start of the RSV season
   Infants 29-32 weeks' gestational age if younger than 6 months at the start of the RSV season
   Infants 32-35 weeks' gestational age if younger than 6 months at the start of the RSV season *and* 2 or more risk factors
      Child care attendance
      School-aged siblings
      Exposure to environmental air pollutants
      Congenital anomaly of the airways
      Severe neuromuscular disease

Children younger than 2 years with hemodynamically significant cyanotic or acyanotic congenital heart disease (use palivizumab for this population)†

Consider prophylaxis for children with severe immune deficiency (e.g., severe combined immune deficiency, severe acquired immunodeficiency syndrome)

*Once a child qualifies for initiation of prophylaxis at the start of the RSV season, administration should continue throughout the season and not stop when an infant reaches either 6 or 12 months of age.
†Infants with lesions adequately corrected by surgery do not require prophylaxis unless they continue to need medication for congestive heart failure.
Summarized from AAP Policy Statement: Revised indications for the use of palivizumab and respiratory syncytial virus immune globulin intravenous for the prevention of respiratory syncytial virus infections. Pediatrics 2003;112:1442-1446.

attributable to RSV-IGIV include fever and mild decreases in oxygen saturation during infusion. Disadvantages of RSV-IGIV include

- Requirement for intravenous access followed by a prolonged infusion time (4 to 6 hours)
- Interference with the immune response to some live vaccines (live virus vaccines, specifically measles, mumps, and rubella [MMR] and varicella, must be delayed for 9 months after the last RSV-IGIV infusion)
- Occasional problems with volume overload
- Theoretical risk for contamination of the infusate with infectious agents
- Contraindicated in patients with cyanotic congenital heart disease

Palivizumab, developed in the late 1990s as an alternative to RSV-IGIV, is a genetically engineered humanized murine monoclonal antibody to RSV. It is given at monthly intervals (15 mg/kg intramuscularly) during the RSV season. Several randomized, multicenter placebo-controlled trials have demonstrated the safety and efficacy of palivizumab in children. The IMpact-RSV trial enrolled 1502 patients.[22] Prophylaxis decreased RSV-related hospitalization rates from 10.6% to 4.8% in the placebo versus palivizumab recipients, respectively ($P < .01$). This study also demonstrated decreases in the duration of hospitalization, requirement for supplemental oxygen, and need for intensive care unit admission in the palivizumab versus the placebo group. Among 1287 infants with hemodynamically significant congenital heart disease, palivizumab recipients had lower hospitalization rates than placebo recipients did (5.3% versus 9.7%; $P = .003$). No serious adverse events were attributed to palivizumab. Advantages of palivizumab include its safety in children with cyanotic congenital heart disease, ease of intramuscular versus intravenous administration, and low complication rate. Moreover, immunizations do not need to be

delayed after palivizumab administration. Palivizumab is the current preferred mode of passive immunization.

Both RSV-IVIG and palivizumab are expensive and use a significant amount of health care resources. Therefore, their use is restricted to groups that would most benefit from passive immunization (see Table 66-1). If an infant or child receiving immunoprophylaxis experiences a breakthrough RSV infection, prophylaxis should continue through the RSV season. This recommendation is based on the observation that high-risk infants may be hospitalized more than once in the same season with RSV lower respiratory tract disease and the fact that more than one RSV strain often cocirculates in a community. The families of all high-risk infants should receive counseling regarding smoking cessation and influenza vaccination for all family members, including infants older than 6 months.

In a Nutshell

- Clinical presentation: viral infection of the middle and lower respiratory tract presenting as cough, wheezing, or crackles and varying degrees of respiratory distress most often caused by RSV.
- Hospitalized patients require supportive care, usually for inadequate oral intake, respiratory distress, or hypoxemia.
- Bronchodilators are used often but have not been proved to be effective.
- Steroids may be of benefit to children with a personal or family history of asthma or atopy.
- Prophylaxis is indicated during the RSV season for children at high risk for significant morbidity or mortality.

On the Horizon

- Development of an RSV vaccine that would provide active immunity, in contrast to the passive immunity provided by palivizumab or RSV-IGIV
- Advances toward understanding the role of RSV infection in recurrent wheezing
- Clearer understanding of the role of corticosteroids and bronchodilators in the management of RSV bronchiolitis

CROUP

Croup, or laryngotracheitis, is a common acute respiratory tract infection in children. Children between the ages of 6 months and 6 years are most commonly affected, and highest incidence of disease occurs during a child's second year of life.[23] Each year up to 6 cases per 100 children are evaluated in primary care offices and emergency departments. The seasonal predilection of croup is the fall and early winter, but cases occur throughout the year.

Parainfluenza viruses type 1 to 3, members of the Paramyxoviridae family, account for almost three quarters of all cases of croup. Type 1 is most commonly isolated, followed by type 3 and then type 2. Other viral causes of croup include RSV, influenza A and B, adenovirus, and the newly recognized hMPV. Rare causes of croup include *M. pneumoniae* and, in unimmunized children, measles and diphtheria.

Croup results from an infection of the upper and middle respiratory tract and is manifested as inflammation and edema of the larynx, trachea, and bronchi. The inflammation and edema lead to narrowing of the airway and increased resistance to airflow. In young children this becomes problematic because of the funnel-like anatomy of their airway. The increased resistance causes the classic "croupy" or barky cough and inspiratory stridor. In severe cases, respiratory distress or respiratory failure can occur.

Clinical Presentation

Croup is an illness characterized by a barklike cough, hoarseness, inspiratory stridor, and potentially, respiratory distress. Commonly, a child initially experiences nasal congestion and cough. After 12 to 48 hours the cough progressively worsens and becomes barky in nature, and hoarseness and intermittent inspiratory stridor arise. For reasons that are unclear, the cough and stridor are more severe during the night. Mild pharyngeal erythema, coryza, and fever are common. The symptoms of croup often progress along a spectrum classically divided into mild, moderate, and severe based on the level of respiratory distress. In mild croup, physical examination reveals a comfortable patient who is mildly tachypneic with a hoarse voice. Stridor is generally absent or observed only when the child is agitated. In moderate croup, the child appears uncomfortable, is tachypneic, and has a pronounced cough. Inspiratory stridor is present at rest and suprasternal and intercostal retractions may be present. Children with severe croup have significant respiratory distress with tachypnea, nasal flaring, and retractions and may appear agitated or lethargic. Stridor occurs at rest and, with increasing airway narrowing, may be present with inspiration and expiration. Tachycardia and, in some cases, pulsus paradoxus are observed.

Differential Diagnosis

The differential diagnosis for croup should focus on the potential causes of stridor. Stridor is defined as a medium-pitched respiratory sound, usually with inspiration, that represents resistance to airflow through the airway. The level of resistance determines the timing of the stridor. During inspiration, negative pressure is transmitted to the intraluminal space of the extrathoracic airway and leads to narrowing of the upper airway and partial obstruction, and thus inspiratory stridor is produced. Within the chest cavity, the downward excursion of the diaphragm with inspiration produces negative pressure in the pleural space, thereby allowing expansion of the intrathoracic airways. This increased airway diameter would reduce or relieve partial obstruction of these airways.

Conversely, on expiration, positive pressure is created within the extrathoracic (upper) airway and expands its luminal diameter. With expiration, there is a relative positive pressure in the intrapleural space in comparison to the intraluminal space of the intrathoracic airways. This would lead to narrowing of these airways, worsening of any partial obstruction, and therefore causing expiratory stridor.

Biphasic stridor represents a fixed obstruction that is unaltered by changes in intraluminal diameter or a combination of upper and lower airway involvement. The differential diagnosis for stridor is presented in Table 66-2.

Diagnosis and Evaluation

Croup is a clinical diagnosis that can safely be made by pediatricians without the use of diagnostic tests. Performing diagnostic tests has the potential to agitate the patient and further worsen the respiratory distress. In hospitalized patients, some believe that knowing the cause aids in infection control practices to prevent nosocomial spread of respiratory viruses. See the section Bronchiolitis for discussion of isolation and information on specific diagnostic methods.

In most instances, radiographic studies are not necessary. However, anteroposterior and lateral neck radiographs may confirm typical changes in the contour of the airway seen in croup. These films are particularly useful if there is concern for an airway foreign body. In the anteroposterior view the "steeple sign," the classic finding in croup, reveals narrowing of the subglottic air column. Widening of the hypopharynx is observed in the lateral view. This finding is not present in all children with croup and can be found in some healthy children, depending on the phase of inspiration[24] and positioning of the child when the radiographs are obtained.

In the outpatient setting, routine laboratory testing in children with croup is not needed. However, patients sufficiently ill to warrant hospitalization may require additional laboratory evaluation. Pulse oximetry is a useful tool for detecting oxygen desaturation. In patients with severe respiratory distress, arterial blood gas analysis would be helpful in evaluation of the potential respiratory insufficiency or failure (see discussion in the Bronchiolitis section). Electrolytes may be appropriate in patients with significant dehydration. Concurrent bacterial infections in the setting of croup are rare. However, patients with high spiking fevers

Table 66-2 Differential Diagnosis of Stridor

Quality of stridor	Inspiratory	Biphasic	Expiratory
Location of pathology	Supraglottic	Glottic	Subglottic
Condition	Croup Epiglottitis Peritonsillar abscess Retropharyngeal abscess Foreign body Laryngomalacia Hemangioma Supraglottic web	Croup Bacterial tracheitis Foreign body Laryngomalacia Laryngeal web Vascular ring Hemangioma Vocal cord paralysis	Bacterial tracheitis Foreign body Tracheomalacia Hemangioma Subglottic stenosis Pulmonary sling

Table 66-3 Treatment of Croup

Severity of Symptoms	Management
Mild	Anticipatory guidance Ensure appropriate follow-up and access to medical services Consider dexamethasone, 0.16 mg/kg orally × 1 dose
Moderate	Dexamethasone, 0.16-0.6 mg/kg orally × 1 dose; consider IM or IV if unable to take PO Racemic epinephrine, 0.25-0.75 mL of a 2.25% solution with 2.5 mL normal saline via nebulizer Consider hospital admission if repeated doses of racemic epinephrine are needed or if patient has 1 or more criteria for admission
Severe	Secure the airway if necessary Racemic epinephrine, 0.25-0.75 mL of a 2.25% solution with 2.5 mL normal saline via nebulizer Dexamethasone, 0.6 mg/kg IV or IM Consider heliox (70%-80% helium) via face mask Close observation for possible respiratory decompensation Admit to the hospital; consider admission to the intensive care unit

who continue to worsen despite proper treatment should be evaluated for a secondary bacterial infection. Studies to consider include chest radiography, as well as blood and urine cultures and a complete blood count.

Children with uncomplicated croup do not require routine direct visualization of the airway by laryngoscopy. This test should be considered in children with noisy breathing or a hoarse cry between croup illnesses, frequent or progressively worsening episodes of croup, a severe episode requiring intubation, and a history of intubation in the neonatal period. Children with an episode of choking or gagging at the onset of the illness should be evaluated for foreign body aspiration.

Course of Illness

Croup is a self-limited disease. Symptoms typically worsen during the first 2 to 3 days of the illness and then remit over the next 3 to 7 days. A decrease in oral intake can occur as a result of a sore throat or respiratory distress. Hospitalization occurs in less than 2% of children with croup. Of those hospitalized, less than 1.5% require endotracheal intubation. Long-term sequelae and death are rare. Bacterial tracheitis is a potentially severe complication of croup. There are also sporadic reports of tracheitis caused by *Candida* species after prolonged corticosteroid administration for recurrent stridor.

Treatment

The majority of children with a clear diagnosis of croup can safely be managed as outpatients. Outpatient management includes supportive care and often corticosteroids. Parents must be aware of the signs and symptoms of respiratory distress, and access to medical care should be ensured.

Therapy for croup is aimed at supportive care and reducing airway inflammation and edema if necessary. Table 66-3 outlines management for a child with croup.

Supportive care is an important aspect in the management of croup. Adequate hydration should be ensured; consider administering intravenous isotonic saline. Although hypoxemia is rare, oxygen should be administered in cases associated with low oxygen saturation.

Heliox can be used to prevent or delay endotracheal intubation in children with severe respiratory distress. Heliox increases laminar flow through the narrowed airway. Administration of heliox occurs through a non-rebreather face mask with a helium-to-oxygen ratio of 80:20 or 70:30. If the hypoxia is severe, this modality may provide insufficient supplemental oxygen support.

If respiratory failure or complete airway obstruction is imminent, the airway should be secured by tracheal intubation or tracheostomy. In children who require intubation, the endotracheal tube should be 0.5 to 1 mm smaller than the predicted size for age. Extubation is recommended when a positive pressure of 25 cm H_2O causes a significant air leak.

Corticosteroids act on the anti-inflammatory pathway and lead to a decrease in inflammation and edema of the laryngeal mucosa. Multiple clinical trials and meta-analyses have demonstrated their utility in reducing the duration and severity of symptoms, return office visits, hospitalization rates, length of stay in the emergency department and ward, and need for intubation and reintubation.[25-34] Recent studies have concluded that oral dexamethasone is the optimal treatment modality because of its ease of administration, low cost, and widespread availability.[27,35,36] Investigations of the smallest effective dose of corticosteroids have been conducted. Geelhoed and Macdonald demonstrated that a dose of 0.15 mg/kg was as effective as 0.3 and 0.6 mg/kg of dexamethasone in the treatment of mild to moderate croup.[37] Adverse events from the use of corticosteroids for croup have been rare. Corticosteroids should not be administered to patients with tuberculosis unless they are receiving appropriate antituberculosis treatment or to patients with varicella.

A study from 1971 reported croup-associated tracheotomy rates of 2.9% to 13% and mortality rates of 0.09% to 2.7%. In this study the authors concluded that the use of racemic epinephrine over the preceding 10-year period prevented all deaths and tracheotomies in 351 hospitalized patients with viral croup.[38] Additional studies have confirmed these results.

Aerosolized racemic epinephrine improves symptoms by its α-adrenergic properties. It is composed of an equal mixture of the *d*- and *l*-isomer of epinephrine. The *l*-isomer binds the α-receptors on the precapillary arterioles and causes fluid resorption and a decrease in laryngeal edema. The dose of racemic epinephrine is 0.25 to 0.75 mL of a 2.25% solution. Racemic epinephrine was initially used because it was thought to be associated with less tachycardia and hypertension. It has been shown that *l*-epinephrine is as effective and the cardiovascular effects are similar to those of racemic epinephrine.

Aerosolized racemic epinephrine has an onset of action of 10 minutes and lasts approximately 2 hours. Some children return to their pretreatment state once the effect of the medication dissipates. This return of symptoms has historically been referred to as the "rebound phenomenon." Initially, it was believed that all children receiving racemic epinephrine required hospitalization. Ledwith and coworkers performed a study to evaluate the safety of sending children treated with racemic epinephrine home.[39] In patients with severe respiratory distress after 20 minutes of mist therapy, they administered 0.5 mL of 2.25% racemic epinephrine and 0.6 mg/kg of oral dexamethasone. After 3 hours if a child had a sustained response without return of symptoms, the child was discharged home. Of the patients discharged, none had a return of their respiratory distress. Two additional studies have found similar results. Therefore, children receiving racemic epinephrine in the emergency department require (1) corticosteroids, (2) clinical monitoring for 3 to 4 hours, (3) demonstration of lack of stridor at rest, and (4) a normal level of consciousness before discharge.

The initial therapies thought to be beneficial to croup patients were steam and cool night air. These two treatments are still recommended for patients at home with evidence of mild croup. A "croup tent" was developed for the hospital administration of cool mist into a closed crib containing the child. Moist air theoretically soothes the inflamed mucosa and moistens secretions to facilitate their clearance. However, such therapy has not been shown to be of benefit. One study observed that airway resistance did not decrease after the administration of nebulized air. However, only eight patients were evaluated for 30 minutes. Bourchier and colleagues randomized 16 patients to receive room air or humidified air.[40] After 12 hours of observation, clinical symptoms were unchanged. A recent randomized, blinded controlled study of humidified air and mist therapy failed to demonstrate benefit for patients presenting to the emergency department with moderate croup.[41] Nebulized saline may precipitate bronchospasm in children with underlying airway hyperreactivity and is not recommended.

Problems do exist with the use of mist tents in the hospital setting. First, mist therapy can worsen bronchospasm in children with wheezing. Second, it separates children from their parents, which may cause anxiety and potentially worsen a child's respiratory status. Finally, the cumbersome tent precludes frequent reevaluation, an important aspect of croup management. Therefore, the use of mist tents in the hospital is no longer recommended.

Consultation

- Critical care: Children with respiratory distress requiring intensive monitoring and the possibility of endotracheal intubation or tracheostomy
- Ear, nose, and throat or pulmonology (or both): Children with unusual or persistent symptoms for which laryngoscopy or bronchoscopy may be warranted
- Infectious diseases: Children with suspected alternative infectious processes (e.g., epiglottitis, bacterial tracheitis)

Admission Criteria

Hospitalization may be considered for any of the following reasons:

- Persistent moderate to severe symptoms despite outpatient therapy (corticosteroids and aerosolized epinephrine)
- Respiratory distress
- Hypoxemia
- Young infant, for example, one younger than 4 to 6 months
- Dehydration or inability to tolerate feeding
- Unstable social situation or inability to ensure follow-up, or both
- Uncertain diagnosis in which further evaluation and treatment are necessary

Discharge Criteria

- Resolution of respiratory distress
- Resolution of hypoxemia
- Tolerating sufficient fluids
- Ability of caregivers to provide appropriate support at home and to understand the signs of a worsening clinical condition
- Establishment of appropriate outpatient follow-up

Prevention

Prudent hand washing is the mainstay of prevention for exposed individuals. Adherence to the immunization guidelines will prevent the rare cases caused by measles and diphtheria.

In a Nutshell

- Clinical presentation: A short nonspecific upper airway illness followed by a barking cough, hoarse voice, and stridor.
- Diagnosis: Clinically diagnosed. Neck radiographs, viral testing, and laryngoscopy are reserved for patients with atypical presentations or severe symptoms.
- Treatment: Often managed on an outpatient basis. Corticosteroids are beneficial in mild, moderate, and severe cases. Aerosolized epinephrine can improve airway edema acutely.

On the Horizon

- The optimal dosing and route of administration of steroids will be further delineated. The role of adjunctive supportive therapies will be further investigated.

EPIGLOTTITIS

Acute epiglottitis, an illness characterized by fever, dysphagia, and dysphonia, rapidly progresses to upper airway obstruction secondary to edema of the epiglottis and aryepiglottic folds. In the past it was predominantly a disease of otherwise healthy children. More recent reports emphasize the development of epiglottitis in immunocompromised patients. After the 1988 introduction of the conjugate Hib vaccine and the 1991 recommendation to routinely immunize all infants starting at 2 months of age, invasive Hib disease, including epiglottitis, declined by more than 99%.[42,43] Affected children are now also older than in the pre-Hib vaccine licensure period; the typical age presently ranges from 5 to 12 years rather than 3 to 6 years.[42,44] In the prevaccination era, Hib accounted for up to 90% of cases.[45] Currently, Hib is responsible for approximately 25% of cases of epiglottitis; other bacteria, viruses, and noninfectious agents now cause most cases.[46] Responsible organisms include group A β-hemolytic streptococcus; *Staphylococcus aureus*; nontypable and type a *H. influenzae*; group B, C, and G streptococci; viridans group streptococci; *Streptococcus pneumoniae*; and *Candida* species. Among immunosuppressed patients *S. pneumoniae* and *Candida* species have been reported more commonly than other organisms. Bacterial superinfection causing epiglottitis may follow viral respiratory infections, particularly herpes simplex virus, varicella-zoster virus, Epstein-Barr virus, and parainfluenza viruses. Noninfectious causes include thermal injuries, trauma, and posttransplant lymphoproliferative disorder.

Clinical Presentation

A child with acute bacterial epiglottitis initially has a fever and dysphagia.[47] Antecedent cough and upper respiratory tract infection are uncommon. The illness evolves rapidly over a 12- to 24-hour period with the development of drooling, dysphonia (usually a muffled or "thick-sounding" voice), and progressive irritability, restlessness, and anxiety.[43]

Hoarseness of the voice is uncommon. On physical examination the child appears extremely toxic. The child may sit in the tripod position (sitting up and leaning forward with the neck hyperextended and the mouth open) to maximize airway diameter. Often there is drooling. In contrast to croup, stridor in epiglottitis is rarely severe. However, its presence indicates impending complete airway obstruction. Hypoxia, hypercapnia, and acidosis worsen with the progressive deterioration in air exchange.

Differential Diagnosis

The differential diagnosis for epiglottitis is that of edema and inflammation of the upper airway. An aspirated foreign body can present with a sudden onset of respiratory distress and may be accompanied by drooling. It should be considered in a child with a history of a choking episode that precedes the development of respiratory distress. Laryngotracheobronchitis, or croup, can present with stridor and respiratory distress and should be considered, especially if the child has the associated barky cough and hoarse voice. Bacterial tracheitis can present with respiratory distress in a toxic-appearing child and should be considered in a child with a more slowly evolving course. Peritonsillar abscess and retropharyngeal abscess should be considered. Angioneurotic edema that involves the epiglottis resembles epiglottitis; however, fever is noticeably absent. Isolated uvulitis can cause dysphonia. Although usually viral in origin, cases of bacterial uvulitis with concomitant epiglottitis have been described.

Diagnosis and Treatment

Management of epiglottitis involves securing the airway and then administering appropriate antibiotics.[48] Most epiglottitis-related deaths occur en route to the hospital or within the first few hours of evaluation. Epiglottitis represents an airway emergency; delays of even a few hours may prove fatal. In cases in which suspicion of epiglottitis is high, radiographic confirmation of the diagnosis causes unnecessary delay and should not be considered until airway patency has been established.

Care should be taken to keep the child calm and comfortable. Anxiety-provoking maneuvers such as phlebotomy, intraoral examination, or removal of the child from the comfort of a caregiver's arms should be avoided. Agitation of the child can lead to obstruction of the airway and decompensation. For this reason most institutions have "epiglottitis protocols" delineating the management of children with suspected epiglottitis. A clinician with experience in pediatric airway management should perform a diagnostic evaluation by direct laryngoscopy with endotracheal intubation, and tracheostomy equipment should be available at bedside. This evaluation should take place in the operating suite whenever possible, but the emergency department and pediatric critical care unit are other good options. Direct visualization of the epiglottis provides the definitive diagnosis. The epiglottis and aryepiglottic folds appear inflamed, often described as a "cherry red" epiglottis. An abscess on the lingual surface of the epiglottis may obscure some landmarks.

A child with epiglottitis requires endotracheal intubation, with nasotracheal placement preferred. Age-appropriate endotracheal tubes as well as several smaller tubes should be readily available. Supplies should also be available to perform a tracheostomy if required. In a true emergency, experienced personnel can insert a 13- or 15-gauge needle through the cricothyroid membrane. This needle thoracostomy can provide temporary means of oxygenation while more definitive methods to secure the airway are being established. Culture specimens from the surface of the epiglottis and from blood should be obtained after establishment of an artificial airway. Cultures are particularly important given the diversity of organisms causing epiglottitis.

Once the airway has been secured, the child should be examined for secondary sites of infection, which are present more than half the time and include otitis media, pneumonia, meningitis, and cellulitis.

Culture of blood or epiglottitis may identify the causative organism. Blood cultures were positive in approximately 75% of patients in the pre-Hib vaccine era. Limited data suggest that the yield of positive blood cultures in the post-Hib era ranges from 40% to 60%.[42,49] A complete blood count may reveal leukocytosis with a predominance of neutrophils and band forms. Additional diagnostic evaluation is unnecessary except for studies pertaining to evaluation of respiratory status and to assessment of end-organ damage (e.g., liver, kidneys, brain) as required.

In patients with a high likelihood of epiglottitis, radiography should be deferred until after endotracheal intubation. In stable patients in whom clinical suspicion is low, a lateral radiograph of the neck should be obtained and examined to determine whether it suggests epiglottitis or other pathology. Positioning for radiographs should not compromise the patient's comfort, so flexion of the neck to a neutral position or supine positioning may need to be avoided. On a lateral soft tissue radiograph, the epiglottis appears rounded and thickened (thumb sign) with loss of the vallecular airspace (Fig. 66-3). The aryepiglottic folds may be thickened and the hypopharynx distended. Anteroposterior views of the neck reveal a normal-caliber subglottic space. A clinician skilled

in airway management should accompany the child if radiographic studies are performed, and whenever possible, obtaining portable (bedside) films is preferred.

Ceftriaxone, cefotaxime, and ampicillin-sulbactam are reasonable options for empirical therapy in a child with suspected epiglottitis. Alternative choices in patients with hypersensitivity reactions to β-lactam antibiotics include carbapenem-class (e.g., imipenem, meropenem) and fluoroquinolone-class (e.g., levofloxacin) antibiotics. Therapy should be continued for 7 to 10 days. The therapeutic agent should be altered according to the results of culture and antimicrobial susceptibility testing.

Course of Illness

Epiglottitis is a life-threatening illness. Mortality in various studies has ranged from less than 1% to 30%. Early and aggressive airway management increases survival. Complications include postobstructive pulmonary edema after insertion of the endotracheal tube to relieve laryngeal obstruction and metastatic foci of infection. In the Hib era, epiglottitis was often associated with pneumonia, cervical adenitis, and otitis media and rarely with meningitis, septic arthritis, and cellulitis. Other complications occur as a consequence of initial hypoxia or subsequent mechanical ventilation.

Consultation

- Pediatric critical care: Airway and ventilator management and treatment of hemodynamic complications.
- Pediatric anesthesiology, otolaryngology: Assistance with airway management. Emergency tracheostomy, if needed, may require the assistance of general surgeons.
- Pediatric infectious disease: Antibiotic selection.

Admission Criteria

- All children with suspected epiglottitis require hospitalization for diagnostic evaluation. Those with proven epiglottitis require hospitalization in an intensive care setting for intravenous antibiotics, endotracheal intubation, and monitoring.
- Evaluation and treatment should follow the institutional "epiglottitis protocol," with the person most skilled in pediatric airway management securing the airway.

Discharge Criteria

- No airway compromise is present.
- Completed antibiotic therapy or appropriate oral antibiotics are available.
- Parents/caregivers understand the disease course, treatment, and follow-up.

Prevention

The mainstay of prevention of epiglottitis secondary to Hib is adherence to the immunization guidelines. Secondary disease may occur in contacts of patients with Hib disease. Although the rate of secondary illness after cases of Hib-related epiglottitis is less than that after other invasive Hib infections, prophylaxis of contacts is still recommended as follows: Rifampin prophylaxis (20 mg/kg/day once daily, maximum of 600 mg/dose), when prescribed, should

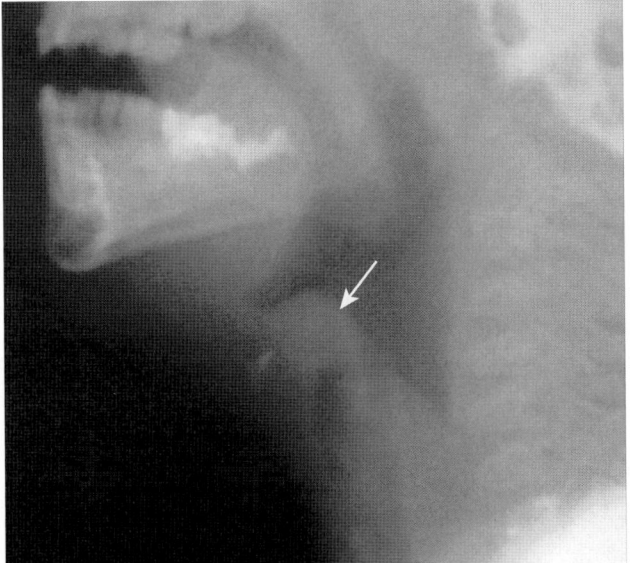

Figure 66-3 Lateral neck radiograph demonstrating epiglottis with the "thumb sign."

continue for 4 days. In households with one or more infants younger than 12 months, the index case and all household contacts should receive rifampin prophylaxis. The same applies in households with children younger than 4 years who are incompletely vaccinated and in families with a fully vaccinated but immunocompromised child. For school or child care contacts, chemoprophylaxis is not indicated unless there is more than one case of invasive Hib disease. Local public health officials, as well as hospital infection control personnel, can assist in identification of individuals requiring prophylaxis.

In a Nutshell

- Epiglottitis is an airway emergency characterized by fever, dysphagia, and dyspnea. The child is often drooling and sitting in the tripod position with a toxic appearance.
- A child with suspected epiglottitis should be cared for by the person most skilled in pediatric airway management and intubated in a controlled setting. Laryngoscopy will support the diagnosis by revealing a "cherry red" swollen epiglottis.
- In fully vaccinated patients, a diversity of organisms may cause epiglottitis.
- Treatment involves securing the airway and systemic antibiotics.

SUGGESTED READING

American Academy of Pediatrics, Committee on Infectious Diseases, and Committee on Fetus and Newborn: Revised indications for the use of palivizumab and respiratory syncytial virus immune globulin intravenous for the prevention of respiratory syncytial virus infections. Pediatrics 2003;112:1442-1446.

Bordley WC, Viswanathan M, King VJ, et al: Diagnosis and testing in bronchiolitis: A systematic review. Arch Pediatr Adolesc Med 2004;158:119-126.

Flores G, Horwitz RI: Efficacy of β_2-agonists in bronchiolitis: A reappraisal and meta-analysis. Pediatrics 1997;100:233-239.

Garrison MM, Christakis DA, Harvey E, et al: Systemic corticosteroids in infant bronchiolitis: A meta-analysis. Pediatrics 2000;105(4):E44.

Hartling L, Wiebe N, Russell K, et al: A meta-analysis of randomized controlled trials evaluating the efficacy of epinephrine for the treatment of acute viral bronchiolitis. Arch Pediatr Adolesc Med 2003;157:957-964.

Kaditis AG, Wald ER: Viral croup: Current diagnosis and treatment. Pediatr Infect Dis J 1998;17:827-834.

Klassen TP: Croup: A current perspective. Pediatr Clin North Am 1999;46:1167-1178.

Kellner JD, Ohlsson A, Gadomski AM, Wang EE: Bronchodilators for bronchiolitis. Cochrane Database Syst Rev 2000;2:CD001266.

King VJ, Viswanathan M, Bordley WC, et al: Pharmacologic treatment of bronchiolitis in infants and children: A systematic review. Arch Pediatr Adolesc Med 2004;158:127-137.

Levine DA, Platt SL, Dayan PS, et al: Risk of serious bacterial infection in young febrile infants with respiratory syncytial virus infections. Pediatrics 2004;113:1728-1734.

McEwan J, Firidharan W, Clarke RW, Shears P: Paediatric acute epiglottitis: Not a disappearing entity. Int J Pediatr Otorhinolaryngol 2003;67:317-321.

Mull CC, Scarfone RJ, Ferri LR, et al: A randomized trial of nebulized epinephrine vs albuterol in the emergency department treatment of bronchiolitis. Arch Pediatr Adolesc Med 2004;158:113-118.

Russell K, Wiebe N, Saenz A, et al: Glucocorticoids for croup. Cochrane Database Syst Rev 2004;1:CD001955.

Schroeder AR, Marmor AK, Pantell RH, Newman TB: Impact of pulse oximetry and oxygen therapy on length of stay in bronchiolitis hospitalizations. Arch Pediatr Adolesc Med 2004;158:527-530.

Shah RK, Roberson DW, Jones DT: Epiglottitis in the *Hemophilus influenzae* type b vaccine era: Changing trends. Laryngoscope 2004;114:557-560.

Stroud RH, Friedman NR: An update on inflammatory disorders of the pediatric airway: Epiglottitis, croup, and tracheitis. Am J Otolaryngol 2001;22:268-275.

REFERENCES

1. Esper F, Boucher D, Weibel C, et al: Human metapneumovirus infection in the United States: Clinical manifestations associated with a newly emerging respiratory infection in children. Pediatrics 2003;111:1407-1410.
2. Williams JV, Harris PA, Tolletson SJ, et al: Human metapneumovirus and lower respiratory tract disease in otherwise healthy infants and children. N Engl J Med 2004;350:443-450.
3. Shah SS: Wheezing. In Shah SS, Ludwig S (eds): Pediatrics Complaints and Diagnostic Dilemmas: A Case-Based Approach. Philadelphia, Lippincott Williams & Wilkins, 2004, pp 1-32.
4. Shaw KN, Bell LM, Sherman NH: Outpatient assessment of infants with bronchiolitis. Am J Dis Child 1991;145:151-155.
5. Bordley WC, Viswanathan M, King VJ, et al: Diagnosis and testing in bronchiolitis: A systematic review. Arch Pediatr Adolesc Med 2004;158:119-126.
6. Levine DA, Platt SL, Dayan PS, et al: Risk of serious bacterial infection in young febrile infants with respiratory syncytial virus infections. Pediatrics 2004;113:1728-1734.
7. Swingler GH, Hussey GD, Zwarenstein M: Duration of illness in ambulatory children diagnosed with bronchiolitis. Arch Pediatr Adolesc Med 2000;154:997-1000.
8. Schroeder AR, Marmor AK, Pantell RH, Newman TB: Impact of pulse oximetry and oxygen therapy on length of stay in bronchiolitis hospitalizations. Arch Pediatr Adolesc Med 2004;158:527-530.
9. Martinon-Torres F, Rodriguez-Nunez A, Martinon-Sanchez JM: Heliox therapy in infants with acute bronchiolitis. Pediatrics 2002;109:68-73.
10. Flores G, Horwitz RI: Efficacy of β_2-agonists in bronchiolitis: A reappraisal and meta-analysis. Pediatrics 1997;100:233-239.
11. King VJ, Viswanathan M, Bordley WC, et al: Pharmacologic treatment of bronchiolitis in infants and children: A systematic review. Arch Pediatr Adolesc Med 2004;158:127-137.
12. Kellner JD, Ohlsson A, Gadomski AM, Wang EE: Bronchodilators for bronchiolitis. Cochrane Database Syst Rev 2000;2:CD001266.
13. Hartling L, Wiebe N, Russell K, et al: A meta-analysis of randomized controlled trials evaluating the efficacy of epinephrine for the treatment of acute viral bronchiolitis. Arch Pediatr Adolesc Med 2003;157:957-964.
14. Mull CC, Scarfone RJ, Ferri LR, et al: A randomized trial of nebulized epinephrine vs albuterol in the emergency department treatment of bronchiolitis. Arch Pediatr Adolesc Med 2004;158:113-118.
15. Garrison MM, Christakis DA, Harvey E, et al: Systemic corticosteroids in infant bronchiolitis: A meta-analysis. Pediatrics 2000;105(4):E44.
16. van Woensel JB, van Aalderen WM, de Weerd W, et al: Dexamethasone for treatment of patients mechanically ventilated for lower respiratory tract infection caused by respiratory syncytial virus. Thorax 2003;58:383-387.
17. Smith DW, Frankel LR, Mathers LH, et al: A controlled trial of aerosolized ribavirin in infants receiving mechanical ventilation for severe respiratory syncytial virus infection. N Engl J Med 1991;325:24-29.
18. Revised indications for the use of palivizumab and respiratory syncytial virus immune globulin intravenous for the prevention of respiratory syncytial virus infections. Pediatrics 2003;112:1442-1446.
19. Macartney KK, Gorelick MH, Manning ML, et al: Nosocomial respiratory syncytial virus infections: The cost-effectiveness and cost-benefit of infection control. Pediatrics 2000;106:520-526.

20. Feltes TF, Cabalka AK, Meissner HC, et al: Palivizumab prophylaxis reduces hospitalization due to respiratory syncytial virus in young children with hemodynamically significant congenital heart disease. J Pediatr 2003;143:532-540.

21. Reduction of respiratory syncytial virus hospitalization among premature infants and infants with bronchopulmonary dysplasia using respiratory syncytial virus immune globulin prophylaxis. The PREVENT Study Group. Pediatrics 1997;99:93-99.

22. Palivizumab, a humanized respiratory syncytial virus monoclonal antibody, reduces hospitalization from respiratory syncytial virus infection in high-risk infants. Pediatrics 1998;102:531-537.

23. Kaditis AG, Wald ER: Viral croup: Current diagnosis and treatment. Pediatr Infect Dis J 1998;17:827-834.

24. Mills JL, Spackman TJ, Borns P, et al: The usefulness of lateral neck roentgenograms in laryngotracheobronchitis. Am J Dis Child 1979;133:1140-1142.

25. Kairys SW, Olmstead EM, O'Connor GT: Steroid treatment of laryngotracheitis: A meta-analysis of the evidence from randomized trials. Pediatrics 1989;83:683-693.

26. Tibballs J, Shann FA, Landau LI: Placebo-controlled trial of prednisolone in children intubated for croup. Lancet 1992;340:745-748.

27. Bjornson CL, Klassen TP, Williamson J, et al: A randomized trial of a single dose of oral dexamethasone for mild croup. N Engl J Med 2004;351:1306-1313.

28. Klassen TP, Craig WR, Moher D, et al: Nebulized budesonide and oral dexamethasone for treatment of croup: A randomized controlled trial. JAMA 1998;279:1629-1632.

29. Klassen TP, Feldman TP, Watters LK, et al: Nebulized budesonide for children with mild-to-moderate croup. N Engl J Med 1994;331:285-289.

30. Klassen TP, Watters LK, Feldman ME, et al: The efficacy of nebulized budesonide in dexamethasone-treated outpatients with croup. Pediatrics 1996;97:463-466.

31. Johnson DW, Jacobson S, Edney PC, et al: A comparison of nebulized budesonide, intramuscular dexamethasone, and placebo for moderately severe croup. N Engl J Med 1998;339:498-503.

32. Geelhoed GC, Macdonald WB: Oral and inhaled steroids in croup: A randomized, placebo-controlled trial. Pediatr Pulmonol 1995;20:355-361.

33. Geelhoed GC, Turner J, Macdonald WB: Efficacy of a small single dose of oral dexamethasone for outpatient croup: A double blind placebo controlled clinical trial. BMJ 1996;313:140-142.

34. Rittichier KK, Ledwith CA: Outpatient treatment of moderate croup with dexamethasone: Intramuscular versus oral dosing. Pediatrics 2000;106:1344-1348.

35. Super DM, Cartelli NA, Brooks LJ, et al: A prospective randomized double-blind study to evaluate the effect of dexamethasone in acute laryngotracheitis. J Pediatr 1989;115:323-329.

36. Kuusela AL, Vesikari T: A randomized double-blind, placebo-controlled trial of dexamethasone and racemic epinephrine in the treatment of croup. Acta Paediatr Scand 1988;77:99-104.

37. Geelhoed GC, Macdonald WB: Oral dexamethasone in the treatment of croup: 0.15 mg/kg versus 0.3 mg/kg versus 0.6 mg/kg. Pediatr Pulmonol 1995;20:362-368.

38. Adair JC, Ring WH, Jordan WS, Elwyn RA: Ten-year experience with IPPB in the treatment of acute laryngotracheobronchitis. Anesth Analg 1971;50:649-655.

39. Ledwith CA, Shea LM, Mauro RD: Safety and efficacy of nebulized racemic epinephrine in conjunction with oral dexamethasone and mist in the outpatient treatment of croup. Ann Emerg Med 1995;25:331-337.

40. Bourchier D, Dawson KP, Fergusson DM: Humidification in viral croup: A controlled trial. Aust Paediatr J 1984;20:289-291.

41. Scolnik D, Coates AL, Stephens D, et al: Controlled delivery of high vs. slow humidity vs mist therapy for croup in emergency departments. JAMA 2006;295:1274-1280.

42. Gorelick MH, Baker MD: Epiglottitis in children, 1979 through 1992. Effects of *Haemophilus influenzae* type b immunization. Arch Pediatr Adolesc Med 1994;148:47-50.

43. Gonzalez Valdepena H, Wald ER, Rose E, et al: Epiglottitis and *Haemophilus influenzae* immunization: The Pittsburgh experience—a five-year review. Pediatrics 1995;96:424-427.

44. Shah RK, Roberson DW, Jones DT: Epiglottitis in the *Hemophilus influenzae* type B vaccine era: Changing trends. Laryngoscope 2004;114:557-560.

45. Glode MP, Halsey NA, Murray M, et al: Epiglottitis in adults: Association with *Haemophilus influenzae* type b colonization and disease in children. Pediatr Infect Dis 1984;3:548-551.

46. Senior BA, Radkowski D, MacArthus C, et al: Changing patterns in pediatric supraglottitis: A multi-institutional review, 1980 to 1992. Laryngoscope 1994;104:1314-1322.

47. Stroud RH, Friedman NR: An update on inflammatory disorders of the pediatric airway: Epiglottitis, croup, and tracheitis. Am J Otolaryngol 2001;22:268-275.

48. Crysdale WS, Sendi K: Evolution in the management of acute epiglottitis: A 10-year experience with 242 children. Int Anesthesiol Clin 1988;26:32-38.

49. McEwan J, Giridharan W, Clarke RW, Shears P: Paediatric acute epiglottitis: Not a disappearing entity. Int J Pediatr Otorhinolaryngol 2003;67:317-321.

CHAPTER 67

Lower Respiratory Tract Infections

Michael Weinstein and Lucinda P. Leung

PNEUMONIA

Approximately 80% of all episodes of pneumonia occur in children younger than 8 years, with the highest incidence in children between 2 and 4 years of age.[1] Pneumonia accounts for up to 20% of all pediatric hospital admissions.[2] Although most deaths due to pneumonia occur in the developing world, where it is the leading cause of mortality among children, pneumonia was responsible for 800 childhood deaths in the United States in 1996.[3] Despite the frequency with which pneumonia is encountered in hospitalized children, its management remains a source of controversy. The reasons for this controversy include a lack of practical, sensitive, and specific diagnostic tests for determining the causative agents of pneumonia (the cause is identified in less than half of cases) and a shortage of clinical studies comparing antibiotic regimens and adjunctive therapies in a methodologically rigorous manner.

Differential Diagnosis

Because standard diagnostic testing is often unrevealing, management is guided by epidemiologic studies. The most helpful predictor of the responsible pathogen is the child's age (Table 67-1). In young infants, *Chlamydia trachomatis* and respiratory viruses, including respiratory syncytial virus, influenza, parainfluenza, adenovirus, and metapneumovirus, predominate. *C. trachomatis* typically causes an afebrile pneumonitis syndrome characterized by diffuse pulmonary infiltrates and air trapping, with radiographic findings more severe than the clinical presentation. Severely ill infants who present with high fever, toxicity, or large effusions or lung abscess are much more likely to have a bacterial infection caused by *Streptococcus pneumoniae* (most common), *Streptococcus pyogenes* (group A streptococcus), *Staphylococcus aureus,* or *Haemophilus influenzae.*

In preschool children, the incidence of viral pneumonia declines, and bacterial pathogens, particularly *S. pneumoniae,* predominate. Although these generalities hold true across most epidemiologic studies, exceptions must be considered. For example, *Mycoplasma pneumoniae* is an important pathogen in older preschool-age children. In school-age children and adolescents, *M. pneumoniae, Chlamydophila pneumoniae,* and *S. pneumoniae* are the most common causes, and disease due to respiratory viruses is much less frequent.[4]

Clinical Presentation

Fever, cough, tachypnea, respiratory distress, and the finding of decreased breath sounds and crackles on auscultation are the hallmarks of pneumonia. Auscultatory findings may be normal and unreliable in young infants. Fever and abdominal pain suggestive of an acute abdomen are not uncommon, particularly in the presence of lobar consolidation adjacent to the diaphragm or a parapneumonic effusion. For practical purposes, pneumonia can be defined as the presence of fever or acute respiratory symptoms accompanied by a new parenchymal infiltrate on a chest radiograph. A clinical diagnosis of pneumonia can be made reliably with careful observation and a physical examination, and the clinical assessment guides the decision whether to perform chest radiography. Since tachypnea is nearly always present, lack of this sign can help eliminate the diagnosis of pneumonia. When counted over two 30-second intervals in a quiet child, tachypnea is defined as greater than 60 breaths per minute in infants younger than 2 months, greater than 50 breaths per minute in children 2 to 12 months old, and greater than 40 breaths per minute in children older than 12 months.[5] Because tachypnea is also observed in other conditions (e.g., metabolic acidosis), chest retractions, other signs of increased work of breathing, and auscultatory findings are more specific physical signs. The absence of tachypnea, increased work of breathing, abnormal auscultatory findings, and hypoxemia estimated by pulse oximetry reliably excludes the presence of pneumonia and the need for radiologic evaluation.[5]

Diagnosis

A pathogen is identified in 40% to 60% of cases, depending on the diagnostic tests used and the population studied.[6] The lack of practical, noninvasive, specific diagnostic tests means that treatment is usually empirical, guided by epidemiologic studies. The inclusion of discordant patient populations (e.g., hospitalized versus ambulatory) hampers the interpretation of these studies. Further, isolation of a pathogen from nasopharyngeal secretions (e.g., respiratory syncytial virus by antigen detection) does not exclude bacterial coinfection. Although serologic tests have been widely used in population-based epidemiologic studies, the need for convalescent titers makes this an impractical tool in individual cases. Distinguishing between viral and bacterial pathogens based on clinical, radiographic, and indirect laboratory signs is unreliable. The presence of features such as coryza, conjunctivitis, myalgia, and ill contacts, typically thought to be an indicator of viral pathogens, is actually not helpful in distinguishing between bacterial and viral causes.[7] Similarly, laboratory tests such as complete blood count, erythrocyte sedimentation rate, and C-reactive protein, though abnormal in children with pneumonia, lack specificity.

Few radiographic features are useful in distinguishing between viral and bacterial pathogens. Pneumonia secondary to viral causes typically has an interstitial pattern on chest radiographs, but lobar consolidation, typical of bacterial pathogens, may also be seen, particularly with respiratory syncytial virus infection. *M. pneumoniae* infection

Table 67-1   Common Causes of Pneumonia by Age

Age	Pathogen
1–3 mo	*Chlamydia trachomatis* Respiratory syncytial virus Parainfluenza virus Metapneumovirus *Streptococcus pneumoniae* *Bordetella pertussis* *Staphylococcus aureus*
3 mo–5 yr	Respiratory syncytial virus Parainfluenza virus Metapneumovirus Influenza Adenovirus *Streptococcus pneumoniae* *Haemophilus influenzae*, nontypable* *Mycoplasma pneumoniae* *Streptococcus pyogenes* *Mycobacterium tuberculosis*
5–15 yr	*Mycoplasma pneumoniae* *Chlamydophila pneumoniae* *Streptococcus pneumoniae* *Mycobacterium tuberculosis*

*Rarely seen in immunocompetent children in developed nations.

characteristically produces diffuse interstitial infiltrates out of proportion to the clinical findings, but it occasionally causes lobar consolidation, pleural effusion (usually small and bilateral, if present), and atelectasis. The most helpful radiographic finding is a significant parapneumonic effusion, which is almost always due to bacterial pathogens. Similarly, the finding of a round infiltrate ("round pneumonia") is suggestive of pneumococcal pneumonia. Blood cultures are seldom positive in cases of pneumonia. In one study, the rate of bacteremia in children with pneumonia who required hospitalization was approximately 7%.[8] In contrast, bacteremia was detected in only 9 of 580 children (1.6%; 95% confidence interval, 0.7 to 2.9) aged 2 to 24 months with pneumonia who were treated as outpatients.[9] Both these studies were conducted before introduction of the pneumococcal conjugate vaccine.

The epidemiology of childhood pneumonia continues to change as new diagnostic tests identify previously unknown pathogens (e.g., human metapneumovirus)[10] and vaccination alters the incidence of other infections. *H. influenzae* type B, previously a common cause of childhood pneumonia, has been virtually eradicated, and there is evidence that the pneumococcal conjugate vaccine may reduce the incidence of pneumonia by up to 20% in the first 2 years of life.[11]

Treatment

In infants and children diagnosed with pneumonia, indications for hospitalization include young age (younger than 3 months), immunocompromised status, significant pleural effusion or respiratory distress, signs of toxicity, dehydration, inability to tolerate oral antibiotics, lack of response to prior oral antibiotic therapy, and caregivers' inability to provide adequate care. Children with hypoxia

necessitating supplemental oxygen at presentation require initial hospitalization.

In practice, the most useful diagnostic tests in identifying a pathogen are blood culture, despite its low yield, and viral antigen detection by immunofluorescence on a nasal or nasopharyngeal swab. Bacterial cultures of nasopharyngeal or throat swabs are not indicated because they do not accurately reflect lower respiratory tract flora. Serology for *S. pneumoniae* and *M. pneumoniae* may play a role but does not provide results rapidly enough to be practically useful. *S. pneumoniae* urinary antigen detection tests demonstrate high sensitivity and specificity for diagnosing pneumococcal pneumonia in adults; however, this test is not useful in children because a positive result is strongly associated with nasopharyngeal *S. pneumoniae* colonization.[12,13] Detection of the *M. pneumoniae* genome in nasopharyngeal secretions by polymerase chain reaction is highly sensitive but not widely available. Thoracentesis performed for a significant parapneumonic effusion can be helpful for diagnostic purposes if the child has not already received prolonged antibiotic therapy (see the later discussion of complicated pneumonia). Tuberculin skin testing and testing of gastric aspirates or induced sputum for mycobacterial culture, acid-fast staining, and nucleic acid amplification should be done if tuberculosis is suspected.

Antibiotic therapy is usually empirical (Table 67-2), reflecting the most likely pathogen based on the child's age (see Table 67-1), clinical presentation, and local resistance patterns. *S. pneumoniae* is the most frequent cause of bacterial pneumonia in children requiring hospitalization, but it has become increasingly resistant to β-lactam antibiotics. With pneumococci, penicillin resistance is mediated by an alteration in penicillin-binding proteins; therefore, the minimum inhibitory concentrations of all β-lactams increase with those of penicillin. Despite the increase in pneumococcal resistance, β-lactam agents, including penicillin G and ampicillin, are still effective for the treatment of penicillin-nonsusceptible pneumococcal pneumonia, and good outcomes can be achieved with high doses of these agents. Along with penicillin and ampicilln, ceftriaxone and cefotaxime are considered the parenteral drugs of choice for pneumococcal pneumonia. Penicillin resistance in pneumococci does not involve β-lactamse production; therefore, use of a β-lactam–β-lactamase inhibitor combination (e.g., ampicillin-sulbactam) does not provide a therapeutic advantage against penicillin-resistant *S. pneumoniae*. Vancomycin is the only effective agent in vitro against highly penicillin-resistant strains, but there is little role for this drug in the treatment of community-acquired pneumonia. When broader-spectrum coverage is desired (e.g., against *S. aureus*), combination coverage with a β-lactam that provides antistaphylococcal activity (e.g., oxacillin, ampicillin-sulbactam) or clindamycin should be used. The addition of a macrolide (erythromycin, azithromycin, clarithromycin) can be considered in children older than 5 years and in cases of suspected atypical pneumonia. Telithromycin, a ketolide class antibiotic, was approved in 2004 by the U.S. Food and Drug Administration (FDA) for patients 18 years of age or older. This agent has high activity against respiratory tract pathogens, including penicillin-resistant pneumococci, and in trials it proved to be at least as effective and safe as clarithromycin and azithromycin.[14,15] However, recent concerns

Table 67-2 Empirical Antibiotics for Pneumonia by Age		
Age	Parenteral Therapy	Oral Therapy
1-3 mo	Penicillin G, ampicillin, or ceftriaxone or cefotaxime, ± erythromycin 40 mg/kg/day	Not recommended
3 mo-5 yr	Penicillin G, ampicillin, or ceftriaxone or cefotaxime, ± macrolide (erythromycin, azithromycin)	Amoxicillin (high dose)* Alternative: cefuroxime
5-15 yr	Penicillin G, ampicillin, or ceftriaxone or cefotaxime, ± macrolide (erythromycin, azithromycin)	Clarithromycin, azithromycin or erythromycin Alternative: amoxicillin (high dose) or cefuroxime or levofloxacin

*High-dose amoxicillin (80-100 mg/kg/d) is used to treat strains of pneumococcus that have some degree of penicillin resistance.

about telithromycin-related hepatotoxicity should prompt pediatricians to consider this medication only if other options are not available. Amoxicillin has the lowest minimum inhibitory concentration against penicillin-resistant strains of *S. pneumoniae* compared with other oral β-lactams and is the oral drug of choice for the treatment of suspected pneumococcal pneumonia. High-dose ampicillin (200 mg/kg per day) is effective in children with pneumonia caused by even resistant pneumococcal strains.[16] Although cefuroxime has been used effectively for the treatment of pneumococcal disease, bacteriologic failure and subsequent increased mortality have been reported in adults.[17] Step-down to oral therapy is appropriate once a clinical response has been observed and the child can tolerate oral antibiotics.

Chest physiotherapy generally does not have a role in the treatment of uncomplicated community-acquired pneumonia. It may be effective in a child with neurologic or swallowing dysfunction and aspiration pneumonia, helping to mobilize and clear secretions. Follow-up chest radiographs to document resolution are unnecessary in a child with uncomplicated pneumonia who does not have persistent symptoms or signs.[18] Repeat radiographs should be reserved for children with complicated pneumonia (e.g., empyema, loculated effusions, pneumatoceles, air leak).

SPECIAL CONSIDERATIONS

Aspiration Pneumonia

Aspiration pneumonia is a frequent reason for hospital admission and an important cause of morbidity and mortality in neurologically impaired children. Although feeding tubes are now widely used in children with neurologic dysfunction and have led to improved nutritional status and prolonged survival, aspiration pneumonia remains a significant problem and challenge. Aspiration pneumonia and pneumonitis are discussed in Chapter 76.

Tuberculosis

One third of the world's population is infected with *Mycobacterium tuberculosis*, and between 2 million and 3 million people die from the disease each year.[19] The 1990s saw a resurgence of tuberculosis (TB) and increasing drug resistance in North America. In children, the TB risk is greatest in those from endemic areas or those having contact with caregivers or visitors from endemic areas, including Asia, Africa, the Caribbean, Latin America, and the Middle East. Aboriginal and disadvantaged populations are also at greater risk.

Pulmonary TB is the most common clinical presentation of the disease in children. Nearly 50% of children with active pulmonary TB are asymptomatic and come to attention when a chest radiograph is performed for other indications. Symptomatic children may present with cough, fever, weight loss, or failure to thrive. Night sweats are uncommon in young children. Extrapulmonary disease, most commonly lymphadenitis, bone and joint infections, and meningitis, can present concurrently. The most common radiographic finding is mediastinal lymphadenopathy; other findings include signs of airway obstruction such as consolidation or atelectasis, miliary disease, and pleural effusions. Cavitary disease, usually seen with reactivation of latent TB, is generally not encountered in young children.

Diagnosis is made by isolation of *M. tuberculosis* by acid-fast bacilli staining, culture, or nucleic acid amplification from early-morning gastric aspirates or induced sputum, usually done on 3 consecutive days. However, cultures generally take 2 to 3 weeks to grow, and gastric aspirates are diagnostic in less than 50% of children with pulmonary TB. Therefore, the combination of a positive tuberculin skin test, signs and symptoms consistent with TB disease, and consistent findings on chest radiographs is adequate to identify a case of TB. The tuberculin skin test is interpreted as positive with induration of 5 mm or more in children suspected of having contact with an individual with contagious TB disease, suspected of having TB disease, or with immunosuppression, including human immunodeficiency virus (HIV). Induration of 10 mm or more is considered positive in children younger than 4 years, those with chronic medical conditions (e.g., diabetes), or children with increased exposure to TB (e.g., child or caregiver from a high-prevalence region). Induration of 15 mm or more is considered positive in all individuals.[20]

Treatment of pan-susceptible pulmonary TB usually consists of isoniazid, rifampin, and pyrazinamide for 2 months, followed by isoniazid and rifampin alone for an additional 4 months. If resistant TB is suspected or proved, four-drug therapy with isoniazid, rifampin, pyrazinamide, and ethambutol is usually recommended for at least 6 months.

COMPLICATED PNEUMONIA

Parapneumonic effusions are frequently present in children with community-acquired pneumonia. Most of these effusions are small and resolve with successful treatment of the underlying pneumonia. However, some effusions are large or composed of fibrinous loculations, leading to a complex, persistent collection that can cause significant morbidity and requires intervention. Complicated pneumonia can thus be defined as a pneumonic process accompanied by such an effusion, lung abscess, or pneumatocele; complicated parapneumonic effusions are the focus here. There is evidence that the incidence of complicated parapneumonic effusions has been increasing in recent years in both Europe and North America. This is a puzzling development, especially in light of the introduction of the conjugate pneumococcal vaccine, which in some studies has been associated with a reduction in the incidence of pneumococcal lower respiratory tract infection—probably the most common cause of complicated pneumonia in children.[21]

Pathophysiology

Parapneumonic effusions develop in three characteristic stages defined by the length of time and the type of constituent cells and inflammatory response evident in the pleural fluid. The first stage consists of an acute exudative phase characterized by free-flowing fluid composed of acute inflammatory cells in the pleural fluid as a consequence of the adjacent pneumonic process. This stage is relatively brief (<24 to 48 hours), and there may be no further progression if the effusion is small and the underlying pneumonia is treated expeditiously. The second stage is termed the fibrinopurulent phase (lasting 2 to 14 days); it develops after 24 to 48 hours and is characterized by the presence of fibrin, which leads to the formation of strands and pockets of inflammatory fluid that can organize and develop into a chronic collection that does not easily resolve. If parapneumonic effusions are not dealt with in the first and second stages, a third organizing stage can ensue, characterized by the formation of collagen in the pleural space and an inelastic pleural peel that develops around the lung, preventing proper expansion. Stage 3 parapneumonic effusions may require decortication to allow proper lung expansion.

It is important to note, however, that this traditional three-stage concept is based primarily on findings in adults with parapneumonic effusions and that in children, this clinical entity has a distinctly different natural history. Further, much of the early literature dealing with parapneumonic effusions dealt specifically with tuberculous infections; this scenario is not easily generalizable to previously healthy children with parapneumonic effusions secondary to community-acquired pneumonia. Thus, it is more practical to think of parapneumonic effusions as existing on a continuum, with free-flowing exudative fluid on one end and multiple loculations or frank pus (empyema) on the other.

Significant parapneumonic effusions are generally a consequence of bacterial pneumonia. Although *S. aureus* was thought to play a significant role in the past, the primary culprit is now *S. pneumoniae,* with an increasing incidence of group A β-hemolytic streptococcal infections appearing as well. As is the case with community-acquired pneumonia in general, studies of parapneumonic effusions in children are limited by the infrequent identification of a causative organism. This is partly attributable to the fact that diagnostic thoracentesis is seldom performed in children and to the fact that children are often treated with antibiotics before a significant parapneumonic effusion develops or is recognized.

Clinical Presentation

The presence of a significant parapneumonic effusion is heralded by a combination of signs and symptoms, including persistent fever despite empirical antibiotic therapy for community-acquired pneumonia; respiratory distress; pleuritic chest, shoulder, or abdominal pain; tracheal deviation; scoliosis; and auscultatory findings such as reduced air entry, bronchial breath sounds and egophony above the area of effusion, dullness to percussion, and reduced tactile fremitus in the area of dullness. These auscultatory findings are less reliable in young children.

Diagnosis

Features to be assessed on plain radiographs include opacification of the pleural space with an underlying parenchymal consolidation, blunting of the costophrenic angle, mediastinal shift, and other features of complicated pneumonia, including air leak, pneumatocele, and lung abscess. A lateral decubitus film can provide further evidence of pleural effusion if doubt exists and can help determine whether the fluid is free-flowing. A width of 10 mm on a decubitus film is considered significant; although this is based on adult literature, it is a practical benchmark for determining whether an effusion needs further investigation and treatment.

Ultrasonography can also provide helpful diagnostic information, including a more accurate estimation of the size of the pleural fluid collection and the composition of the effusion. In addition, the presence of stranding and loculations can be determined. In adults, the presence of multiple fluid loculations is predictive of effusions that will not resolve with antibiotic therapy alone and will likely require further intervention.[22] Similar prognostic value has been shown in children, but it is not as widely established or accepted. Ultrasonography can be performed without sedation, is not associated with radiation risks, and provides a helpful adjunctive diagnostic modality in children who might require intervention for a parapneumonic effusion. Computed tomography can further delineate the lung parenchyma; this might be useful if a large pneumatocele or abscess develops. In the case of pleural effusion, however, computed tomography does not provide additional relevant information, and it often requires sedation and involves significant radiation exposure.

The size of the parapneumonic effusion can help guide management (Fig. 67-1). Small effusions (<10 mm on decubitus films) are likely to resolve without intervention with resolution of the underlying pneumonia. Moderate effusions (>10 mm but less than half the hemithorax) may also resolve with conservative management, but diagnostic thoracentesis should be strongly considered before beginning antibiotic therapy. Large effusions (more than half the hemithorax) are much more likely to require therapeutic as well as diagnostic intervention.[22] Thoracentesis can provide helpful diagnostic information in addition to identifying an organism by

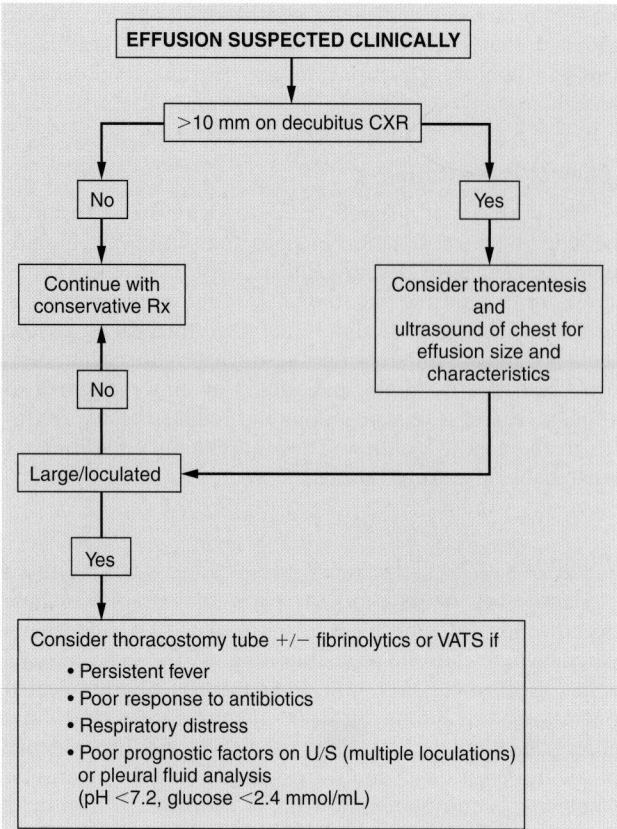

Figure 67-1 Algorithm for the management of parapneumonic effusion. CXR, chest x-ray; Rx, treatment; U/S, ultrasonography; VATS, video–assisted thoracoscopic surgery.

culture. Pleural pH less than 7.20 and a glucose level less than 2.4 mmol/L have been associated with complicated effusions that are likely to require intervention (Table 67-3).[22] Once again, these criteria have been established in adults; it is unclear whether they have similar diagnostic utility in children.

Treatment

Antibiotic Therapy

Various studies of the epidemiology of parapneumonic effusions have identified the importance of *S. pneumoniae*, group A streptococci, and, to a lesser extent, *S. aureus* as the most important causative agents. Cefuroxime provides good empirical coverage against these pathogens; others advocate more extended combination therapy consisting of cefotaxime and either an antistaphylococcal penicillin (e.g., cloxacillin, oxacillin, nafcillin) or clindamycin. Treatment can be narrowed if an organism is identified through blood or pleural fluid culture. In areas with a high prevalence of methicillin-resistant *S. aureus*, empirical therapy should include either clindamycin or vancomycin. Data on the optimal duration of treatment are lacking. Once the fever resolves, children with a relatively straightforward course can receive oral antibiotic therapy for an additional 7 to 10 days. In children with more complicated courses, an additional 7 to 14 days of intravenous antibiotic therapy should be considered after the resolution of fever. The typical duration of therapy is 21 days.

Adjunctive Therapy

A major clinical decision is whether further therapy should be undertaken for a significant parapneumonic effu-

---

Table 67-3   Pleural Fluid Studies in Complicated Pneumonia

Study	Comments
Routine	
Cell count and differential	Usually >10,000 U/mL in parapneumonic effusion
	PMN predominance in bacterial PPE
	Lymphocytes and mononuclear cells predominate in TB, lymphoma, chylothorax
Glucose	Low glucose (<40 mg/dL) more likely to require intervention
pH	Low pH (<7.20) more likely to require intervention
LDH	If high (>1000 U/mL) or pleural fluid-plasma ratio >0.6, more likely to be exudative effusion and require intervention
Gram stain	If positive, more likely to require intervention
Acid fast stain	May be positive with *Myocbacterium tuberculosis* or *Nocardia*
Cultures*	Insensitive in setting of prior antibiotic therapy
Additional studies to consider	
Mycoplasma PCR	Also obtain PCR of nasal aspirate
Viral antigen immunofluorescence	Also obtain immunofluorescence of nasal aspirate; consider PCR testing for adenovirus
Viral culture	May be positive with negative immunofluorescence
Total protein	Indicative of exudates if >3 g/dL and pleural-serum ratio >0.5
Amylase	If concern for pancreatic disease or esophageal rupture
Cholesterol	If >60 mg/dL and pleural fluid-cholesterol ratio >0.3, indicative of exudate
Cytology	To exclude malignancy
Chylomicrons, triglycerides	Along with cholesterol if chylothorax suspected

*Aerobic and anaerobic; consider mycobacterial and fungal.
LDH, lactate dehydrogenase; PCR, polymerase chain reaction; PMN, polymorphonuclear neutrophils; PPE, parapneumonic effusion; TB, tuberculosis.

sion, and what that therapy should be. Severe respiratory distress with or without a mediastinal shift in the setting of a large effusion is a clear indication for drainage, but this scenario is uncommon. The most common factors taken into consideration include persistent fever after initial parenteral antibiotic therapy has begun, significant chest pain, large-sized effusions, and inadequate improvement with conservative therapy alone. The results of ultrasound studies and pleural fluid analysis may be predictive of effusions that are destined to fail antibiotic therapy and warrant early intervention. The available options include prolonged antibiotic therapy alone, serial therapeutic thoracentesis, thoracostomy tube drainage, thoracostomy tube insertion with intrapleural fibrinolytic therapy, video-assisted thoracoscopic surgery (VATS), and open surgical intervention. In adults, a clinical practice guideline has advocated fibrinolytic therapy, VATS, or open surgery in the management of high-risk parapneumonic effusions, as defined by radiographic and pleural fluid criteria.[22] However, adult studies and guidelines are not easily applicable to children. Parapneumonic effusions are associated with significant mortality in adults—an outcome that is very uncommon in children—and adults frequently have comorbid conditions. Disease in adults is thus more severe and justifies a more aggressive treatment approach. In children, outcomes such as length of hospital stay, need for second procedures, time to recovery, school absenteeism, effect on pulmonary function and radiographic tests, and cost are more important measures of efficacy.

Few studies have been performed in children comparing the various treatment options. One randomized study compared intrapleural fibrinolytic therapy with saline placebo in children who had undergone thoracostomy tube insertion for drainage of a parapneumonic effusion.[23] The rationale for using intrapleural fibrinolytics is that they break down the fibrin loculations in the effusion, leading to increased drainage and subsequent resolution of the effusion. The study found a significant reduction in hospital stay in the group treated with intrapleural urokinase. It also found that the use of small-caliber, flexible catheters, which can be inserted by interventional radiologists, was associated with less discomfort. Urokinase has been unavailable in recent years, however, owing to its derivation from human urine. Similarly, streptokinase has been used as an intrapleural fibrinolytic, but because of the relatively high incidence of adverse reactions, such as fever and chest wall pain, physicians are reluctant to use it. A recent nonrandomized study found intrapleural recombinant tissue plasminogen activator to be an effective and safe fibrinolytic therapy in children who did not respond well to thoracostomy tube drainage alone.[24] Studies in both adults and children have shown intrapleural fibrinolysis to be a safe therapy, with infrequent local or systemic bleeding owing to its minimal systemic absorption. Most studies describe using either one dose or multiple (up to six) doses of fibrinolytics instilled into the pleural cavity through a thoracostomy tube and left in place for 1 to 12 hours before resuming drainage. The dose of tissue plasminogen activator used in published studies has ranged from 2 mg (the standard dose for treatment of blocked venous catheters) to 4 mg diluted in 20 to 50 mL of saline.

Recent authors have advocated early surgical management, including VATS, as the preferred treatment for parapneumonic effusions. They cite nonrandomized studies describing reduced hospital stays in children treated with primary surgical intervention compared with those treated initially with fibrinolytics or thoracostomy drainage alone.[25] VATS involves the insertion of instruments and cameras through small keyhole incisions, disrupting the fibrinous loculations and effecting drainage and lung reexpansion. Thoracostomy tubes are left in place after the procedure. Disadvantages of VATS include the requirement for general anesthesia (thoracostomy tube insertion can be achieved with sedation or local anesthesia), the need for multiple incisions, and the learning curve for surgeons to achieve proficiency in the procedure.

A meta-analysis was performed of studies comparing primary nonoperative therapy (e.g., thoracentesis, thoracostomy tube drainage) with primary operative therapy (e.g., thoracotomy, VATS).[26] The primary outcome assessed was therapeutic failure—defined as failure of a primary intervention, necessitating subsequent operative intervention. Among the eight studies included in this analysis, patients undergoing primary operative intervention had a lower risk of therapeutic failure (relative risk, 0.09; 95% confidence interval, 0.04 to 0.23) compared with those receiving nonoperative therapy. However, the meta-analysis was limited by the fact that all the included studies were retrospective and nonrandomized and that none had been adjusted for potentially important confounding variables such as age, organism, or use of fibrinolytic therapy. Further, contrasting the available treatment options by comparing outcomes is difficult. Studies included different patient populations, and management strategies varied dramatically by center. For example, some studies addressing parapneumonic effusions included only children who had failed prolonged conservative therapy with thoracostomy tube drainage and antibiotics alone. Others studied children treated with various therapies early in the course of the disease, when a benefit was more likely to be observed. These confounding variables are highlighted by the fact that some series reported a need for open surgical procedures in nearly 20% of patients, while others reported no need for surgical intervention. These limitations underscore the need for large prospective, controlled trials to determine which children with complicated parapneumonic effusions benefit from further treatment and which option is the preferred therapy. To obtain adequately powered studies, it is likely that multicenter trials will be necessary.

Course of Illness

Once the child has improved clinically, a step-down to oral antibiotics is appropriate. Children who respond rapidly to treatment are often treated for 10 to 14 days, or for a week after defervescence. Those with a more protracted illness and slow radiographic resolution may be treated empirically for several more weeks. Follow-up chest radiographs are indicated for children with complicated pneumonia to ensure resolution. Radiographic resolution generally takes weeks to months, and pleural thickening months after the illness is not uncommon. Few studies have addressed long-term outcomes; however, in the small number of children who have undergone pulmonary function testing, few abnormalities were found.[27]

Admission Criteria

In infants and children with a diagnosis of pneumonia, factors to consider when decision regarding hospitalization is made include
- Young age (<3 months)
- Immunocompromised status
- Significant pleural effusion
Indications for admission would include
- Respiratory distress
- Hypoxemia
- Signs of toxicity
- Lack of response to prior oral antibiotic therapy
- Inability to maintain hydration status and tolerate oral antibiotics
- Inability of caregivers to manage patients at home

Consultation

- Consultation with general surgery or cardiothoracic surgery can assist with diagnostic evaluation and management, including diagnostic/therapeutic thoracentesis, chest tube, or definitive surgery (decortication or VATS).
- Consultation with infectious diseases can provide guidance regarding empiric antibiotic therapy, especially since the organisms are not commonly isolated.

Discharge Criteria

- Resolution of toxicity, respiratory distress, and hypoxemia
- Removal of chest tubes and confirmation that follow-up chest radiographs show no recurrence of significant effusion or pneumothorax
- Ability to maintain hydration and to tolerate oral medications, including antibiotics and pain medication if needed
- Adequate follow-up with primary care physician or, if needed, subspecialist

On the Horizon

- Pneumonia will clearly be an important condition encountered in the hospitalized child. Many of the upcoming developments are likely to relate to the increasing array of practical diagnostic tests that are available to the clinician to better identify causal pathogens and to allow anti-infective therapy to be appropriately tailored. Nucleic acid amplification techniques are likely to become more widely used and standardized. The effect of the conjugate pneumococcal vaccine on the incidence of pneumococcal pneumonia and lower respiratory tract infections in general in children will be further elucidated, and the epidemiology may be further altered by future vaccinations. Concerns regarding increased antibiotic resistance as well the potential increase in tuberculosis and emerging infections are just several potential sources of concern.
- The incidence of complicated pneumonias has been increasing. Despite this recognition, there is a lack of adequate studies relating to the epidemiology, natural history, diagnosis, and treatment of this condition. Future studies will need to address these issues so that more rational and informed management decisions can be made. Collaboration among centers will be required for adequately powered studies to be achieved.

In a Nutshell

- Fever, cough, tachpnea, and focal findings on auscultation or chest radiography are characteristic of pneumonia.
- Pathogens that cause pneumonia are not commonly isolated; therefore, antibiotic coverage is usually empirically based on the most likely pathogen. Factors such as the patient's age, clinical presentation, and local antibiotic resistance patterns are guiding factors.
- Parapneuomonic effusions generally progress from a free-flowing to fibropurulent fluid in the first few days. A third organizing stage with development of an inelastic pleural peel can ensue over the following days to weeks.
- The size and nature of pleural effusions as well as the patient's condition can help guide medical and interventional management of complicated pneumonia.

SUGGESTED READING

Colice GL, Curtis A, Deslauriers J, et al: Medical and surgical treatment of parapneumonic effusions: An evidence-based guideline. Chest 2000;18:1158-1171.
Hilliard TN, Henderson AJ, Langton Hewer SC: Management of parapneumonic effusion and empyema. Arch Dis Child 2003;88:915-917.
Lichenstein R, Suggs AH, Campbell J: Pediatric pneumonia. Emerg Med Clin North Am 2003;21(2):451-473.

PERTUSSIS

Pertussis is an acute infectious disease caused by the bacterium *Bordetella pertussis*. Outbreaks of pertussis were described as early as the 15th century, but the causative bacterium was not isolated until 1906. Pertussis is also called whooping cough, which is descriptive of the high-pitched inspiratory noise ("whoop") made by infected children.

Pertussis was one of the most common childhood diseases in the 20th century and a major cause of childhood mortality in the United States. There were more than 200,000 cases of pertussis reported annually before pertussis vaccine became available in the 1940s. With the advent of widespread vaccination in the United States, the incidence has decreased more than 80% compared with the prevaccine era. Pertussis remains a major health problem among children in developing countries, however, with an estimated 285,000 deaths resulting from the disease worldwide in 2001. In the United States, adolescents and adults have accounted for more than half of reported pertussis cases in recent years. There are periods of increased disease that occur in 3- to 5-year cycles.

Pathophysiology

Pertussis is primarily a toxin-mediated disease, and *B. pertussis* is only infectious in humans. *B. pertussis* is a gram-negative nonmotile coccobacillus that is acquired by contact with aerosolized droplets from infected patients, and infection is limited to the ciliated epithelium of the respiratory tract. The bacteria attach to the respiratory cilia and produce toxins that paralyze the cilia, cause inflammation of the respiratory tract, and impair clearance of pulmonary secretions.

A variety of pertussis components and their contribution to disease have been studied. The antigenic and biologically active components currently thought to be responsible for the clinical features of pertussis disease include pertussis toxin, filamentous hemagglutinin, agglutinogens, adenylate cyclase, pertactin, and tracheal cytotoxin. The pertussis toxin is the major virulence protein and is expressed only by *B. pertussis*. It aids attachment of the bacteria to respiratory epithelium and has multiple systemic effects, including enhancement of insulin secretion, inhibition of leukocyte phagocytic function, and induction of lymphocytosis by inhibition of migration from the bloodstream. Filamentous hemagglutinin, pertactin, and agglutinogens play a role in the attachment to respiratory epithelium. Adenylate cyclase contributes to impairing the phagocytic function of lymphocytes, and tracheal toxin has a role in ciliary stasis. An immune response to one or more of these components produces immunity to subsequent clinical illness, although that immunity is not permanent.

Clinical Presentation

B. pertussis disease presents with a wide clinical spectrum, and several clinical case definitions for pertussis exist. Pertussis is defined by the World Health Organization as a case diagnosed as pertussis by a physician in a person with a cough lasting at least 2 weeks with at least one of the following symptoms: paroxysms of coughing, inspiratory whooping, and post-tussive vomiting without other apparent cause. The incubation period is commonly 7 to 10 days, with a range of 4 to 21 days. The clinical course of the illness is typically divided into three stages: catarrhal, paroxysmal, and convalescent.

The first stage, the catarrhal stage, is characterized by nonspecific symptoms such as rhinorrhea, sneezing, low-grade fever, and a mild cough. Caregivers often do not seek medical attention for these common symptoms, especially in infants and young children. These nondistinctive symptoms rarely prompt investigation even if such patients are brought to medical attention. Over the subsequent 1 to 2 weeks the cough gradually becomes more severe and the second stage, the paroxysmal stage, begins. Fever is usually minimal through the course of illness.

During the paroxysmal stage of classic pertussis disease the patient has bursts of numerous, rapid coughs, and at the end of the paroxysm, a long inspiratory effort is usually accompanied by a characteristic high-pitched crowing or whoop as air is inspired across an inflamed partially closed glottis. Patients younger than 6 months of age may not have the strength to have a whoop, but they will have paroxysms of coughing and may also have choking, gasping, or apnea. Thick, clear mucus may be discharged with the coughing spells. Children and young infants often appear ill and distressed during the attack. A range of color changes may be seen, including cyanosis or pallor, and some children may develop a plethoric appearance to the face during coughing spells. Post-tussive emesis and exhaustion commonly follow the event. The patient's appearance is usually normal after recovery from the coughing paroxysm. During the first 1 or 2 weeks of the paroxysmal stage, the coughing spells typically increase in frequency, then remain at the same level for 2 to 3 weeks, and then will gradually decrease. Paroxysms may occur more frequently at night. The paroxysmal stage usually lasts 1 to 6 weeks but may persist for up to 10 weeks before entering the third stage.

In the third stage, the convalescent stage, the cough becomes less paroxysmal and gradually disappears over several weeks. Paroxysms often recur, especially with subsequent respiratory infections, for many months after the onset of pertussis. This is not due to reactivation or reinfection with *B. pertussis*.

Adolescents, adults, and those partially protected by vaccination may still become infected with *B. pertussis* but will often have milder disease and usually do not demonstrate three distinct stages of disease. They may be asymptomatic or may present with illness ranging from a mild cough to classic pertussis, with persistent cough lasting more than 7 days. Inspiratory whoop is uncommon in this population.

Differential Diagnosis

Prolonged cough may be seen with adenovirus, parainfluenza, influenza, respiratory syncytial virus (RSV), or *Mycoplasma pneumoniae* infection and may be difficult to distinguish from pertussis. Co-infection with more than one respiratory pathogen is not uncommon. Adenovirus may present with sore throat and conjunctivitis not typical of pertussis. Mycoplasma may also present with fever, headache, and lung examination findings, such as rales, with patchy infiltrates on chest radiograph that are not common with pertussis. Pneumonia due to *Chlamydia trachomatis* or *pneumoniae* classically presents with a staccato cough, which implies a breath with each cough. Tachypnea, rales, and wheezes are often present. Patients with RSV infection often have prominent rhinorrhea with bronchiolitis symptoms that accompany or closely follow the nasal symptoms. *Bordetella parapertussis* causes a similar although milder disease and is seen predominantly in Europe. Infection with *Bordetella bronchiseptica* is more commonly an animal infection although there are case reports of human infection.

Foreign body aspiration, gastroesophageal reflux, aspiration pneumonia, and asthma/reactive airways disease are noninfectious processes that may also present with intractable or prolonged cough (see Chapter 45).

Diagnosis

The gold standard for diagnosis of pertussis is isolation of *B. pertussis* by culture. The fastidious nature of this organism results in the need for careful collection and culture methods. Isolation of *B. pertussis* using direct plating is most successful during the catarrhal stage. Specimens should be obtained from the posterior nasopharynx, not from the throat. Cotton swabs should not be used because they will inhibit the growth of *B. pertussis*. Samples should be obtained using Dacron or calcium alginate swabs or by aspiration and should be plated directly onto the selective media. A holding broth or transport medium should be used if plating is not performed immediately. The cultures are grown for 10 to 14 days. Success in isolating the organism declines if the patient has had prior antibiotic therapy effective against *B. pertussis*, if specimen collection is delayed beyond the first 2 weeks of illness, or if the patient has been vaccinated.

Polymerase chain reaction (PCR) testing of nasopharyngeal swabs or aspirates is an increasingly available rapid, sensitive, and specific method of diagnosing pertussis. However, there are currently no FDA-licensed PCR tests available. Many recommend the use of PCR in addition to culture, not as a replacement for culture, because bacterial isolates may be required for evaluation of antimicrobial resistance or for molecular typing. Dacron swab or nasal wash is the recommended method of collection; calcium alginate swabs inhibit PCR and therefore should not be used for PCR testing.[28]

Direct fluorescent antibody (DFA) testing of nasopharyngeal specimens may be useful as a screening test for pertussis. However, DFA testing of nasopharyngeal secretions has been shown in some studies to have low sensitivity and variable specificity.

An elevated IgG titer to pertussis toxin is suggestive of recent infection in an individual who has not received immunization within 2 years. However, there are currently no commercially available serologic tests that are approved by the FDA and diagnostic levels have not been established.[28]

Leukocytosis due to lymphocytosis occurs in the late catarrhal and paroxysmal stages in unimmunized patients who may present with classic disease. Lymphocyte counts above the mean are seen in more than 75% of unimmunized patients with pertussis but only one third of pertussis patients demonstrate a significant lymphocytosis (values above the upper limit of the 95% confidence interval of the age-specific mean).[29] The lymphocytes seen in pertussis are not atypical cells. Patients with mild or modified cases of pertussis and adolescents may not present with lymphocytosis.

Complications

Complications of pertussis may include pneumonia, middle ear infection, anorexia, dehydration, failure to thrive, seizures, rectal prolapse, encephalopathy, pulmonary hypertension, apneic episodes, and death. Eighty percent of deaths from pertussis occur in children under age 1 year.[30-32] The case fatality rate in 1990-1999 was 1% in infants 0 to 2 months of age and 0.5% in infants 2 to 11 months of age.[33] The most common complication, as well as the cause of most pertussis-related deaths, is secondary bacterial pneumonia. Neurologic complications such as seizures and encephalopathy may occur as a result of hypoxia from coughing, or possibly from toxin. Neurologic complications of pertussis are more common among infants. Complications resulting from pressure effects of severe paroxysms include pneumothorax, epistaxis, hernias, and rectal prolapse. Adolescents and adults may also develop complications of pertussis such as difficulty sleeping, urinary incontinence, and pneumonia.

Treatment/Management

The single most effective control measure is maintaining the highest possible level of immunization in the community. Anyone who comes into close contact with a person who has pertussis should receive antibiotics to prevent spread of the disease. People who have or may have pertussis should stay away from young children and infants until properly treated. Treatment during the catarrhal stage may lead to resolution of the infection or may alleviate symptoms. Treatment during the paroxysmal or convalescent phases will have limited effect on established paroxysms, emesis, or apnea but is recommended in order to limit the spread of disease to others. Prophylaxis is recommended for household contacts.

Macrolide agents are the first-line treatment choices. According to Centers for Disease Control and Prevention (CDC) guidelines published in 2005, for patients greater than 1 month of age, azithromycin, clarithromycin, or erythromycin is preferred for treatment. For infants less than 1 month of age, azithromycin is the drug of choice, and clarithromycin and erythromycin are not recommended. In these neonates, trimethoprim-sulfamethoxazole (TMP-SMZ) is the recommended alternative agent.[28,34] These recommendations from the CDC are provided despite the fact that the FDA has not licensed any macrolide for use in infants less than 6 months of age. Specific dosing recommendations are provided in Table 67-4.

Postexposure prophylaxis is recommended for household contacts and those in close contact with an infectious patient. Dosing is the same as for treatment (see Table 67-4).

Admission Criteria

Indications for admission include severe paroxysms of cough, cyanosis or apnea with or without cough, extreme fatigue or apnea after cough, obstruction after cough (from mucous plugs), inability to feed, and seizures. Children may also need to be hospitalized for pneumonia, the most common complication of pertussis. Infants younger than 6 months commonly require hospitalization for management of apnea, hypoxia, and feeding difficulties. Intensive care may be required for infants with severe respiratory failure, pulmonary hypertension, or severe apnea and hypoxia requiring ventilator support.

Supportive care is the mainstay of management. Environmental stimulation should be limited, a detailed cough record should be maintained, and oral intake with daily weights should be recorded. Electronic monitoring for heart rate, respiratory rate, and oxygen saturation is also indicated. Patients should be placed on standard and droplet precautions for the first 5 days on effective treatment or for 21 days after the onset of symptoms if untreated.

Discharge Criteria

- Infant can tolerate adequate oral or enteral fluids and nutrition to maintain hydration and gain weight.
- Infant does not become hypoxic or bradycradic with coughing episodes.
- Caretakers are reliable and comfortable with infant's condition.
- Reliable outpatient follow-up has been established.

Table 67-4   Recommended Antimicrobial Treatment and Postexposure Prophylaxis for Pertussis, by Age Group

Age Group	PRIMARY AGENTS			ALTERNATE AGENT*
	Azithromycin	*Erythromycin*	*Clarithromycin*	*TMP-SMZ*
<1 month	Recommended agent; 10 mg/kg per day in a single dose for 5 days (only limited safety data available)	Not preferred; erythromycin is associated with infantile hypertrophic pyloric stenosis; use if azithromycin is unavailable; 40-50 mg/kg per day in 4 divided doses for 14 days	Not recommended (safety data unavailable)	Contraindicated for infants aged <2 months (risk for kernicterus)
1-5 months	10 mg/kg per day in a single dose for 5 days	40-50 mg/kg per day in 4 divided doses for 14 days	15 mg/kg per day in 2 divided doses for 7 days	Contraindicated at age <2 months; for infants aged ≥2 months, TMP 8 mg/kg per day, SMZ 40 mg/kg per day in 2 divided doses for 14 days
Infants (aged ≥6 months) and children	10 mg/kg in a single dose on day 1 then 5 mg/kg per day (maximum: 500 mg) on days 2-5	40-50 mg/kg per day (maximum: 2 g per day) in 4 divided doses for 14 days	15 mg/kg per day in 2 divided doses (maximum: 1 g per day) for 7 days	TMP 8 mg/kg per day, SMZ 40 mg/kg per day in 2 divided doses for 14 days
Adults	500 mg in a single dose on day 1 then 250 mg per day on days 2-5	2 g per day in 4 divided doses for 14 days	1 g per day in 2 divided doses for 7 days	TMP 320 mg per day, SMZ 1600 mg per day in 2 divided doses for 14 days

*Trimethoprim sulfamethoxazole (TMP-SMZ) can be used as an alternative agent to macrolides in patients aged ≥2 months who are allergic to macrolides, who cannot tolerate macrolides, or who are infected with a rare macrolide-resistant strain of *Bordetella pertussis*.
From Centers for Disease Control and Prevention: Recommended antimicrobial agents for the treatment and postexposure prophylaxis of pertussis: 2005 CDC guidelines. MMWR 2005;54(No. RR-14):1-16.

Consultation

The need for cardiorespiratory support warrants involvement with intensivists. Subspecialty consultation is usually prompted by the development of specific complications (e.g., if seizures or encephalopathy develop, input from pediatric neurologists may be appropriate).

Prevention

The incidence of pertussis has markedly decreased worldwide with the advent of effective vaccinations. Major epidemics have been mostly eliminated. Current vaccination strategies fail to control the circulation of *B. pertussis* in part because they do not capture the adolescent and adult reservoirs and in part because there is inadequate adherence to immunization guidelines worldwide. The vaccination effort has shifted pertussis epidemiology and now we see a reported increase in the incidence of pertussis among adolescents and adults, who function as a reservoir of pertussis for neonates and infants.

Studies suggest that vaccine-induced cellular and humoral immunity lasts 3 to 5 years. Booster vaccination induces another 7 to 8 years of immunity. Natural infection with *B. pertussis* seems to confer a similar length of immunity as vaccination with whole cell pertussis (5 to 8 years).

Children who have recovered from documented pertussis do not need additional doses of pertussis vaccine. Satisfactory documentation includes recovery of *B. pertussis* on culture or typical symptoms and clinical course when these are epidemiologically linked to a culture-confirmed case. If confirmation of pertussis infection is lacking, vaccination should be completed.

In 2005, the FDA licensed two new Tdap (tetanus toxoid, reduced diphtheria toxoid, and acellular pertussis) vaccines for adolescents and adults.

On the Horizon

- Pertussis has persisted in the adult and adolescent reservoir. The emergence of new pertussis variants from the strains that form the basis for the pertussis vaccines (whole cell and acellular) raises concerns for future vaccine effectiveness. There is no current laboratory or epidemiologic evidence to indicate a relationship between the genetic variations among the isolates and the effectiveness of current immunization practices, vaccine types, or the increasing incidence of pertussis. Recently licensed (2005) vaccines targeting adolescents (10 to 18 years of age) and people 11 to 64

years of age should offer immune boosting to our reservoir and should also reduce the incidence of disease in infants and young children. Vaccines that target the reservoir of pertussis infection can help achieve herd immunity and possible eradication.
- Resistance of *B. pertussis* to macrolide agents has been reported rarely. Monitoring of the resistance pattern is ongoing.

In a Nutshell

- Pertussis should be suspected in infants and children with paroxysmal cough or severe cough for more than 5 to 7 days. Infants who develop apnea, cyanosis, or gagging with cough should be evaluated for pertussis.
- Culture is the gold standard when pertussis is suspected, but polymerase chain reaction testing is becoming a more widely available test that provides more rapid results.
- Confirmed cases of pertussis should be reported.
- Macrolide antibiotics are the first choice for treatment and postexposure prophylaxis of pertussis. All close contacts should receive prophylaxis.
- Management is primarily supportive care.
- Immunization is essential for control and goals of future eradication of this disease. Adolescents and adults are currently the reservoir for this disease and should also be evaluated for delayed or inadequate immunization to pertussis.

Suggested Reading

American Academy of Pediatrics: Pertussis. In Pickering LK (ed): Red Book: 2006 Report of the Committee on Infectious Diseases, 27th ed. Elk Grove Village, IL: American Academy of Pediatrics, 2006, pp 498-520.

Centers for Disease Control and Prevention: Recommended antimicrobial agents for the treatment and postexposure prophylaxis of pertussis. 2005 CDC Guidelines. MMWR 2005;54(No. RR-14):1-16.

Tan T: Summary: Epidemiology of pertussis. Pediatr Infect Dis J 2005;24(5 Suppl):S35-38.

References

1. Low DE, Kellner JD, Allen U, et al: Community-acquired pneumonia in children: A multidisciplinary consensus review. Can J Infect Dis 2003; 14(Suppl B):3B-11B.
2. Lichenstein R, Suggs AH, Campbell J: Pediatric pneumonia. Emerg Med Clin North Am 2003;21:451-473.
3. Dowell SF, Kupronis BA, Zell ER: Mortality from pneumonia in children in the United States, 1939 through 1996. N Engl J Med 2000;342:1399-1407.
4. Wubbel L, Muniz L, Ahmed A, et al: Etiology and treatment of community-acquired pneumonia in ambulatory children. Pediatr Infect Dis J 1999;18:98-104.
5. Margolis P, Gadomski A: Does this infant have pneumonia. JAMA 1998;279:308-313.
6. Jadavji T, Law B, Lebel MH, et al: A practical guide for the diagnosis and treatment of pediatric pneumonia. Can Med Assoc J 1997;156:S703-S711.
7. Turner RB, Lande AE, Chase P, et al: Pneumonia in pediatric outpatients: Cause and clinical manifestations. J Pediatr 1987;111:194-200.
8. Byington CL, Spencer LY, Johnson TA, et al: An epidemiological investigation of a sustained high rate of pediatric parapneumonic empyema R risk factors and microbiological associations. Clin Infect Dis 2002;34:434-440.
9. Shah SS, Alpern ER, Zwerling L, et al: Risk of bacteremia in young children with pneumonia treated as outpatients. Arch Pediatr Adolesc Med 2003;157:389-392.
10. Williams JV, Harris PA, Tollefson SJ, et al: Human metapneumovirus and lower respiratory tract disease in otherwise healthy infants and children. N Engl J Med 2004;350:443-450.
11. Black SB, Shinefield HR, Ling S, et al: Effectiveness of heptavalent pneumococcal conjugate vaccine in children younger than five years of age for prevention of pneumonia. Pediatr Infect Dis J 2002;21:810-815.
12. Dowell SF, Garman RL, Liu G, et al: Evaluation of Binax Now, an assay for detection of pneumococcal antigen in urine samples, performed among pediatric patients. Clin Infect Dis 2001;32:824-825.
13. Dominguez J, Blanco S, Rodrigo C, et al: Usefulness of urinary antigen detection by an immunochromatographic test for diagnosis of pneumococcal pneumonia in children. J Clin Microbiol 2003;41:2161-2163.
14. Stratton CW, Brown SD: Comparative in vitro activity of telithromycin and beta-lactam antimicrobials against community-acquired bacterial respiratory tract pathogens in the United States: Findings from the PROTEKT US study, 2000-2001. Clin Ther 2004;26:522-530.
15. Tellier G, Niederman MS, Nusrat R, et al: Clinical and bacteriological efficacy and safety of 5 and 7 day regimen of clarithromycin twice daily in patients with mild to moderate community-acquired pneumonia. J Antimicrob Ther 2004;54:515-523.
16. Pallares R, Linares J, Vadillo M, et al: Resistance to penicillin and cephalosporin and mortality from severe pneumococcal pneumonia from Barcelona, Spain. N Engl J Med 1995;333:474-480.
17. Yu VL, Chiou CC, Feldman C, et al: An international prospective study of pneumococcal bacteremia: Correlation with in vitro resistance, antibiotics administered, and clinical outcome. Clin Infect Dis 2003;37:230-237.
18. Gibson NA, Hollman AS, Paton JY: Value of radiological follow up of childhood pneumonia. BMJ 1993;307:1117.
19. Smith KC: Tuberculosis in children. Curr Probl Pediatr 2001;1:5-30.
20. American Academy of Pediatrics: Tuberculosis. In Pickering LK (ed): Red Book: 2003 Report of the Committee on Infectious Diseases, 26th ed. Elk Grove Village, Ill, American Academy of Pediatrics, 2003, p 643.
21. Byington CL, Spencer LY, Johnson TA, et al: An epidemiological investigation of a sustained high rate of pediatric parapneumonic empyema: Risk factors and microbiological associations. Clin Infect Dis 2002;34:434-440.
22. Colice GL, Curtis A, Deslauriers J, et al: Medical and surgical treatment of parapneumonic effusions: An evidence-based guideline. Chest 2000;18:1158-1171.
23. Thomson AH, Hull J, Kumar MR, et al: Randomized trial of intrapleural urokinase in the treatment of childhood empyema. Thorax 2002;57:343-347.
24. Weinstein M, Restrepo R, Chait PG, et al: Effectiveness and safety of tissue plasminogen activator in the management of complicated parapneumonic effusions. Pediatrics 2004;113:e182-e185.
25. Hilliard TN, Henderson AJ, Langton Hewer SC: Management of parapneumonic effusion and empyema. Arch Dis Child 2003;88:915-917.
26. Avansino JR, Goldman B, Sawin RS, Flum DR: Primary operative versus nonoperative therapy for pediatric empyema: A meta-analysis. Pediatrics 2005;115:1652-1659.
27. Redding GJ, Walund L, Walund D, et al: Lung function in children following empyema. Am J Dis Child 1990;144:1337-1342.
28. American Academy of Pediatrics: Pertussis. In Pickering LK, Baker CJ, Long SS, McMillan JA (eds): Red Book: 2006 Report of the Committee on Infectious Diseases, 27th ed. Elk Grove Village, IL: American Academy of Pediatrics, 2006, pp 498-520.
29. Heininger U, Klich K, Stehr K, Cherry JD: Clinical findings in *Bordetella pertussis* infections: Results of a prospective multicenter surveillance study. Pediatrics 1997;100:10.

30. Crowcroft NS, Andrews N, Rooney C, et al: Deaths from pertussis are underestimated in England. Arch Dis Child 2002;86:336-338.
31. Van Buynder PG, Owen D, Vurdien JE, et al: *Bordetella pertussis* surveillance in England and Wales: 1995-1997. Epidemiol Infect 1999;123:403.
32. Crowcroft NS, Pebody RG: Recent developments in pertussis. Lancet 2006;367;1926-1936.
33. Vitek CR, Pascual FB, Baughman A-I, Murphy TV: Increase in deaths from pertussis among young infants in the United States in the 1990s. Pediatr Infect Dis J 2003;22:628-634.
34. Centers for Disease Control and Prevention: Recommended antimicrobial agents for the treatment and postexposure prophylaxis of pertussis: 2005 CDC guidelines. MMWR 2005;54(No. RR-14):1-16.

CHAPTER 68

Gastrointestinal Diseases

Miriam Laufer and George Siberry

ACUTE GASTROENTERITIS

Acute gastroenteritis is a common infection, with an estimated two to three episodes per year occurring in preschool children. Only a small percentage of children with gastroenteritis require hospitalization, but in the United States, more than 4 million children receive medical care for this illness annually, with more than 200,000 hospitalizations and approximately 300 deaths each year. Worldwide, infectious diarrhea is a leading cause of mortality because of the high burden of disease in developing countries. Causes of infectious diarrhea include bacteria, viruses, and parasites, as well as preformed toxins produced by bacteria.

The term *gastroenteritis* is used as a collective term for intraluminal infections of the gastrointestinal tract involving any regions from the stomach through the colon. Other terms are used to emphasize the predominant areas of involvement, such as *enteritis* (small intestine), *enterocolitis* (small and large intestines), and *colitis* (large intestine).

Viral pathogens are the leading cause of diarrhea, with rotavirus being the most frequent etiologic agent in children who require hospitalization. Most children are infected by school age. Other important viruses that can cause diarrhea include caliciviruses (such as Norwalk virus), enteric adenoviruses, and astroviruses.

The bacteria that most commonly cause inflammatory enteritis in the United States are *Salmonella* and *Campylobacter* species. However, among children younger than 1 year, *Salmonella* infection is more frequent.

Clinical Presentation

Viral Gastroenteritis

With rotavirus gastroenteritis, symptoms usually begin 2 to 4 days after exposure and the diarrhea is loose or watery, with a frequency of up to 10 to 20 times per day. Vomiting is common, particularly in children who require hospitalization, and the vomiting precedes the diarrheal symptoms in approximately half the cases. The presence of fever is variable. Recovery with complete resolution of symptoms generally occurs within 7 days. Mucus or gross blood in the stool, high fevers, and ill appearance suggest a nonviral cause. Rotavirus has a distinct seasonal pattern in temperate climates, with a predictable migration pattern that crosses the United States from west to east starting in the fall. Rotavirus typically begins with fever and vomiting, followed by frequent watery diarrhea.

Other viral agents produce similar symptoms, but they tend to be less severe and of shorter duration. Caliciviruses (including noroviruses and sapoviruses) do not have a seasonal pattern but occur commonly in outbreaks and may be associated with contaminated shellfish or water sources. The pattern of a short incubation period, very short duration of illness, and clustering of cases in relatively closed settings makes it similar in presentation to outbreaks caused by preformed bacterial toxin. However, unlike illness caused by preformed toxins, caliciviruses cause secondary infections, which confirm the contagious nature of the outbreak. Enteric adenoviral infections are seen throughout the year, but some increase is noted in the summer. The diarrheal symptoms are somewhat more prolonged (7 to 10 days), and person-to-person transmission of this pathogen requires close contact. Astroviruses cause a short course of illness usually without significant vomiting, and the diarrheal symptoms generally resolve within 5 days. Winter is the peak season for this pathogen. Enteric adenovirus infections may mimic rotavirus disease, but they occur year-round.

Bacterial Gastroenteritis

The signs and symptoms of bacterial gastroenteritides overlap considerably with those of other causes. In general, bacterial infections cause significant colitis that results in diarrhea with gross blood and mucus, constitutional symptoms such as fever and myalgia, abdominal pain and tenderness, and tenesmus. This bacterial inflammatory diarrhea is often referred to as *dysentery*. Extraintestinal manifestations that may accompany or follow the bacterial diarrheal illness are listed in Table 68-1.

Salmonella can cause enterocolitis, a prolonged illness known as enteric fever, and an asymptomatic carrier state. The enterocolitis is usually caused by non-*typhi* strains and presents with fever and a watery secretory diarrhea, although a more inflammatory stool with blood and mucus can be seen. Bacteremia may complicate the illness, which is most common in children younger than 1 year. Immunocompromised hosts or those with inflammatory bowel disease are also at increased risk. Hematogenous seeding of focal infections, such as meningitis or osteomyelitis, can result from the bacteremia even if spontaneous clearance of the bloodstream occurs. Important vectors for infection include reptiles (e.g., turtles, iguanas, and snakes) and contaminated food such as eggs, milk products, and sprouts.

Salmonella typhi and *paratyphi* can cause enteric or typhoid fever. This progressive illness begins with remitting fever that becomes sustained with increasing constitutional symptoms through the first week. During the second week, hepatosplenomegaly and rose spots (blanching macular or maculopapular rash on the trunk) are seen, and progressive deterioration in mental status ensues. Intestinal hemorrhage and microperforations may develop in the third to fourth week. In uncomplicated untreated cases, resolution of symptoms usually begins within 4 to 6 weeks. Abnormal consciousness and shock are associated with the highest case fatality rate.

Enterocolitis from *Shigella* ranges from a mild illness with watery stools and a paucity of systemic symptoms to a more severe colitis with typical bacterial dysentery symptoms. Some species (*Shigella dysenteriae* type 1) can produce a Shiga toxin that causes endothelial damage and hemolytic uremic syndrome (HUS).

Campylobacter is a major cause of bacterial enterocolitis worldwide and in the United States. Fever, chills, and crampy abdominal pain with bloody mucoid diarrhea are typical, and frank rectal bleeding may occur with mucosal invasion by this pathogen. This clinical picture may be difficult to distinguish from the presentation or recurrent episode of inflammatory bowel disease. This illness is predominantly contracted through food-borne sources, especially poultry and eggs.

In contrast, *Yersinia* is an uncommon infection in the United States but much more common in Europe and Canada. In young children, the illness is usually a self-limited gastroenteritis with stools that range from watery to more inflammatory. Older children present with prominent abdominal pain and tenderness secondary to mesenteric adenitis, which may be confused with acute appendicitis.

Escherichia coli can cause a variety of diarrheal illnesses and is generally grouped by the class of the infecting organism (Table 68-2). The Shiga-producing organism *E. coli* O157:H7 is an important cause of HUS in the United States and is the leading cause of acquired renal failure in children. Transmis-sion from undercooked ground beef and raw milk is a recognized cause of outbreaks and fresh meat and occasionally raw vegetables may be contaminated with this pathogen. The enterotoxigenic classes are the major causative agents of travelers' diarrhea.

Food-borne and waterborne infectious enteritis can be caused by bacteria, preformed bacterial toxins, viruses, or parasites. When evaluating a possible food-borne pathogen, three key points should be considered: the clinical syndrome, the incubation period, and the epidemiology. A food-borne exposure should be considered when two or more people consume the same food and a similar acute illness develops at the same time. The clinical syndromes, including timing and predominant symptoms, point to specific pathogens (Table 68-3). The bacterial pathogens and general exposure are listed in Table 68-4. Some food-borne diseases present as fulminant, aggressive infections in special hosts. Listeriosis generally affects pregnant women, infants, and immuno-compromised hosts. *Vibrio vulnificus*, associated with the consumption of raw oysters, usually affects individuals with underlying liver disease.

Parasitic Gastroenteritis

Protozoa are the most common parasites that cause diar-rhea in the United States. Gastrointestinal illnesses caused by protozoa more commonly present with chronic diarrhea (i.e., lasting more than 2 to 4 weeks). The stools are usually watery, but some exceptions can occur.

Infection by *Entamoeba histolytica* causes a range of ill-nesses, including intestinal amebiasis, amebic dysentery, hepatic amebiasis, and an asymptomatic carrier state. Intesti-nal amebiasis produces increasing intestinal colic and loose stools, but a paucity of constitutional symptoms. Amebic dysentery causes a bloody or mucoid diarrhea, which may be profuse and lead to dehydration or electrolyte imbalances. Hepatic amebiasis is limited to abscess formation in the liver, which may occur with or without intestinal disease.

Giardia lamblia is the leading cause of waterborne disease in the United States and is also seen in day-care centers, where diaper hygiene is difficult to maintain. This flagellate attaches to the mucosa of the proximal part of the small intestine and causes a prolonged diarrheal illness character-ized by episodes of explosive, foul-smelling, watery diarrhea with nausea, abdominal cramps, and bloating. Malabsorp-tion of fats and fat-soluble vitamins can occur if the parasite load is high.

Table 68-1   Extraintestinal Manifestations of Enteric Infections

Reactive arthritis	*Salmonella, Shigella, Yersinia, Campylobacter, Clostridium difficile*
Reiter syndrome	*Shigella*
Guillain-Barré syndrome	*Campylobacter*
Glomerulonephritis	*Shigella, Campylobacter, Yersinia*
Erythema nodosum	*Yersinia, Campylobacter, Salmonella*
Hemolytic anemia	*Campylobacter, Yersinia*
Hemolytic uremic syndrome	*Escherichia coli, Shigella dysenteriae* 1
Seizure or encephalopathy	*Shigella*

Table 68-2   Pathogenic *Escherichia coli* Associated with Acute Infectious Diarrhea

Class of *E. coli*	Abbreviation	Usual Presentation of Disease
Enterohemorrhagic	EHEC	Bloody diarrhea, water- and food-borne outbreaks, associated with hemorrhagic colitis and hemolytic uremic syndrome
Enterotoxigenic	ETEC	Watery diarrhea in children living in and travelers visiting developing countries
Enteroinvasive	EIEC	Dysentery in adults and watery diarrhea, occasionally food-borne outbreaks
Enteropathogenic	EPEC	Acute and chronic diarrhea in infants in nurseries, diarrhea in children <1 year of age in developing countries
Enteroaggregative	EAEC	Acute and chronic watery diarrhea in children worldwide

From Feigin RD, Cherry JD (eds): Textbook of Pediatric Infectious Diseases, 5th ed. Philadelphia, WB Saunders, 2004, p 616.

Table 68-3   Clinical Characteristics of Food–Borne or Water–Borne Outbreaks of Diarrhea

| Usual Incubation Period | CLINICAL ILLNESS | | | Causative Agent | Epidemiologic and Laboratory Diagnosis |
	Fever	*Diarrhea*	*Vomiting*		
5 min–6 hr	Rare	Occasional	Common	Chemical or toxin	Demonstration of toxin or chemical from food or epidemiologic incrimination of food
1–6 hr	Rare	Occasional	Profuse	*Staphylococcus aureus* enterotoxin *Bacillus cereus* emetic toxin	Detection of toxin in food, isolation of organism in food ($>10^5$/g) or in vomitus or stool
8–16 hr	Rare	Typical	Occasional	*Clostridium perfringens* enterotoxin *B. cereus* enterotoxin	Isolation of organisms or toxin from food ($>10^5$/g) or stools of ill persons, epidemiologic incrimination of food
16–96 hr	Common	Typical	Occasional	*Shigella* *Salmonella* *Vibrio parahaemolyticus* Enteroinvasive *Escherichia coli* *Yersinia enterocolitica*	Isolation of organisms from food or stools of ill persons
12–72 hr	Clinical syndrome of botulism			*Clostridium botulinum*	Isolation of organism or toxin from food (10^5/g) or stool, demonstration of toxin in serum or food
16–96 hr	Occasional	Typical	Occasional	*E. coli* enterotoxin *V. parahaemolyticus* enterotoxin *Vibrio cholerae* enterotoxin *Y. enterocolitica* enterotoxin *Listeria monocytogenes*	Isolation of organism from food and stools of ill persons, identification of toxin, epidemiologic incrimination of food
1–15 days	Common	Typical	Common	Rotavirus Enteric adenovirus Astrovirus	Antigen detection by enzyme immunoassay in stool (not available for astrovirus)
1–7 days	Uncommon	Typical	Frequent	*E. coli* O157:H7 and other Shiga toxin–producing *E. coli*	Isolation of organism from food or stool or identification of toxin in stools of ill persons, epidemiologic incrimination of food
1–11 days	Occasional	Common	Occasional	*Cryptosporidium parvum* *Cyclospora cayetanensis*	Request special stool examination; may need to examine water or food
2–5 days	Occasional	Typical	Occasional	*Campylobacter jejuni*	Isolation of organisms from food or stools of ill persons, epidemiologic incrimination of food
2 days–weeks	Common	Typical	Frequent	*Bacillus anthracis*	Isolation of organism from blood or contaminated meat
2 days–8 wk	Common	Common	Common	*Trichinella spiralis*	Serology, muscle biopsy
7–21 days	Common	Common	Rare	*Brucella abortus*, *melitensis*, and *suis*	Blood culture and positive serology
1–4 wk	Rare	Common	Rare	*Giardia lamblia*	Stool for ova and parasite examination, enzyme assay

Table 68-4 Pathogenic Bacteria and Associated Exposure

Agent	Exposure
Aeromonas hydrophila	Water, food, or animal
Bacillus cereus	Food
Campylobacter jejuni	Animal or food, especially poultry
Clostridium difficile	Antimicrobial agents
Clostridium perfringens	Food
Listeria monocytogenes	Food
Plesiomonas shigelloides	Water, fish, or animal
Salmonella species	Meat and dairy products, reptile contact, contaminated food, human carrier
Shigella species	Infected person, contaminated food or object
Staphylococcus aureus	Food
Vibrio cholerae 01, 0139	Food or water
Vibrio parahaemolyticus, vulnificus	Seafood
Yersinia enterocolitica	Food or animal

From Feigin RD, Cherry JD (eds): Textbook of Pediatric Infectious Diseases, 5th ed. Philadelphia, WB Saunders, 2004, page 616.

Table 68-5 Syndromic Approach to Food-Borne Illness

Nausea, vomiting, diarrhea within 16 hours	*Staphylococcus aureus* *Bacillus cereus* *Clostridium perfringens*
Watery diarrhea and cramps within 16-72 hours	Viral agents (e.g., Norwalk) *Escherichia coli* *Vibrio* spp. Rarely other bacteria
Fever, diarrhea, and cramps within 16-72 hours	*Salmonella* *Shigella* *Campylobacter jejuni* *Yersinia* *E. coli*
Abdominal cramps and bloody diarrhea without fever within 3-5 days	*E. coli* 0157:H7 and other Shiga toxin–producing *E. coli*
Paresthesias and neurologic disorders within 0-6 hours	Histamine fish poisoning Ciguatera Paralytic and neurotoxic shellfish poisoning Monosodium glutamate reaction *Clostridium botulinum* (descending paralysis) *C. jejuni* (Guillain-Barré syndrome)

Children in the first 2 years of life are at particularly high risk for infection with *Cryptosporidium*. It is a recognized cause of travelers' diarrhea but is also known to spread through day-care centers through person-to-person spread and in waterborne outbreaks due to the organism's ability to withstand chlorine. It typically presents as an acute or chronic diarrhea with frequent watery stools that may be accompanied by vomiting or low-grade fever.

Outbreaks of diarrhea secondary to *Cyclospora* have followed the ingestion of contaminated water or fresh fruit in developed countries, but travelers to developing countries may also acquire it. Most cases are seen in the spring and summer months. The nonspecific clinical picture includes acute watery diarrhea or a more prolonged course with episodic exacerbations.

Differential Diagnosis

The physician should also consider noninfectious systemic diseases that frequently present with gastrointestinal complaints. Such disease processes include autoimmune diseases (inflammatory bowel disease, Henoch-Schönlein purpura, systemic lupus erythematosus, malabsorption syndromes (congenital disaccharidase deficiency, cystic fibrosis, celiac disease), and endocrine disorders. Some neoplasms present with diarrhea. Infections outside the gastrointestinal tract, such as urinary tract infections and pneumonia, may be associated with acute diarrhea. In addition, significant abdominal pain should raise suspicion of other infectious processes in the abdomen such as appendicitis and pelvic inflammatory disease. Prominent vomiting and abdominal pain make pancreatitis, appendicitis, and cholecystitis diagnostic considerations. Bacterial causes of chronic diarrhea include those already discussed, as well as *Aeromonas*, *Plesiomonas*, and *Mycobacterium tuberculosis*. Table 68-5 reviews the various presentations associated with food-borne infections.

Diagnosis and Evaluation

In the initial evaluation of a patient with acute gastroenteritis, the physician must evaluate and attend to the patient's hydration status. Once the patient has been stabilized, the history and physical examination should focus on detecting signs and symptoms of inflammatory enteritis that may be caused by bacteria or parasites that require specific therapy. Report of fever, tenesmus, or blood, mucus, or pus in stool raises concern for bacterial or parasitic enteritis, although inflammatory bowel disease may share some of these features. A careful history of medication use is important to determine whether the diarrhea is associated with antimicrobial agents. Specific exposures to food, animals, and water are associated with particular enteric pathogens (Table 68-6). Extraintestinal manifestations of gastrointestinal infections might provide information about the etiology of the infection (see Table 68-1).

Most cases of acute diarrhea do not require laboratory testing, so the physician caring for a hospitalized child with diarrhea must determine the extent of the diagnostic evaluation. Identification of a causative agent that might require specific therapy or cohorting of patients to limit the spread of infection may necessitate laboratory investigation.

Table 68-6   Exposures Associated with Specific Pathogens That Cause Diarrhea

Travel to developing countries	*Escherichia coli*, *Shigella*, *Salmonella*, *Campylobacter*, *Entamoeba*
Brackish water	*Vibrio parahaemolyticus*
Institutional exposure or day care	*Shigella*, *Cryptosporidium*, *Giardia*, hepatitis A virus
Unpasteurized milk	*Salmonella*, *Campylobacter*, *Yersinia*, *Listeria*, *Mycobacterium bovis*
Antibiotic therapy	*Clostridium difficile*
Swimming in fresh water	*E. coli*, *Leptospira*, *Cryptosporidium*, *Giardia*
Consumption of raw or undercooked meat	*E. coli*, *Salmonella*, *Campylobacter*, *Yersinia* (chitterlings)
Hemochromatosis	*Yersinia*, *Listeria*, *Vibrio vulnificus*
Underlying immunocompromising condition	Cytomegalovirus, rotavirus, adenovirus, *Salmonella*, *Listeria*, mycobacteria, parasites
Raw oysters and undercooked seafood	*Plesiomonas*, *Vibrio* spp.
Private well	*Aeromonas*, *Giardia*, *Yersinia*
Home canned food	*Clostridium botulinum*

Stool can be examined for mucus, blood, and leukocytes. White blood cells in stool can be assessed through direct microscopic examination, which requires skill on the part of the examiner, or by using commercially available kits to detect lactoferrin in stool. Lactoferrin is a product of neutrophils and is sensitive for detection of these white blood cells in stool. Because lactoferrin is also secreted in breast milk, breastfeeding may cause a false-positive result. Both tests are best performed on fresh stool specimens. The finding of more than five leukocytes per high-power field or a positive lactoferrin assay suggests invasive or toxin-producing bacterial infection, although some patients with colitis will have negative tests. Stool cultures should be performed in patients who have an illness in which a bacterial infection is suspected because of the clinical presentation or stool examination or as part of investigation of an outbreak. If the stool specimen cannot be inoculated immediately in the laboratory, it should be collected in special transport medium that prevents dehydration and bacterial overgrowth. Standard stool culture processing in microbiology laboratories can recover *Shigella* and *Salmonella* species, and most laboratories routinely use special media to isolate *Campylobacter* and *Yersinia*. All bloody stools should also be inoculated into special media for detection of *E. coli* O157:H7 or directly tested for the presence of Shiga-like toxin (or both). Some enteric pathogens are difficult to cultivate in the laboratory. If infections with *Vibrio*, *Aeromonas*, *Plesiomonas*, and *Yersinia* species (varies by laboratory) are suspected, the laboratory should be specifically notified. Because acquisition of a bacterial enteric pathogen in the hospital is very unlikely, stool cultures from patients in whom diarrhea develops more than 3 days after admission are not generally indicated except for patients who are immunocompromised or to investigate a hospital outbreak.

For children older than 1 year who have recently received antibiotics, evaluation for *Clostridium difficile* infection may be appropriate. The cytotoxin assay detects toxin B, the primary cytotoxin, but testing for toxin A is also available at some laboratories. Samples from several occasions should be sent to increase the sensitivity of the test. Direct culture

of the organism is helpful for epidemiologic purposes, but 2 to 5 days is required to obtain results. Testing for *C. difficile* toxin in children younger than 1 year is discouraged because the organism and its toxins are commonly detected in asymptomatic infants.

Rapid tests are available to detect rotavirus and enteric adenoviruses but are not available to test for astroviruses or noroviruses.

Evaluation for intestinal parasites that cause diarrhea focuses on protozoa and is usually indicated in patients who have a travel history, contact with untreated water, or prolonged symptoms. Direct microscopic examination of stool can often reveal parasites, eggs, and cysts. Analyzing three specimens from separate days optimizes the sesitivity of the test. Commercially available enzyme immunoassays and immunofluorescence tests are available for common parasites that are difficult to detect on direct examination, such as *Giardia*, *Cryptosporidium*, and *Entamoeba*.

A complete blood count and blood culture should be obtained if there is concern for systemic bacterial infection. In cases of suspected HUS, a complete blood count with review of the peripheral smear, as well as serum electrolytes and renal function tests, should be performed.

If diarrhea persists with no cause identified, endoscopic evaluation may be indicated. Biopsy specimens help in diagnosing inflammatory bowel disease or identifying infecting agents that may mimic it. A purified protein derivative (PPD) skin test should be performed if no cause is initially identified or the patient is at risk for tuberculosis. Most children with abdominal or intestinal tuberculosis have a positive PPD test, but peritoneal or intestinal biopsy is generally required to confirm the diagnosis. A sweat test is warranted if cystic fibrosis is suspected.

Course of Illness

Viral gastroenteritis illnesses are usually self-limited and resolve after several days. Supportive care with either oral/enteral or intravenous hydration prevents the most common complications related to dehydration, electrolyte abnormalities, or acid-base derangements. Rarely, intussusception may be triggered by lymphoid hyperplasia associated with viral gastroenteritis. Prolonged limitation of the diet may lead to prolonged diarrheal symptoms. Reestablishing a normal diet generally restores villous anatomy and function with resolution of the loose stools.

Many enteric bacterial infections resolve spontaneously, but invasion of the gut wall, bacteremia, perforation, or metastatic spread of infection can complicate the illness. Toxin production can produce systemic illnesses such as HUS or botulism. Extraintestinal manifestations may accompany the gastrointestinal symptoms or develop after the symptoms have resolved.

The time from onset of diarrhea due to *E. coli* O157:H7 to development of HUS is 5 to 13 days. Thrombocytopenia may develop early in the course of the disease and may stabilize and resolve spontaneously or may progress to HUS.

Protozoan infections also tend to be prolonged but self-limited illnesses. However, they may lead to weight loss, malnutrition, or vitamin deficiencies. Infection with *Entamoeba* can cause severe ulcerating colitis, colonic dilation, and perforation. The parasite may spread systemically, most commonly causing liver abscesses. It is critical to exclude *Entamoeba* infection and tuberculosis before initiating corticosteroids for presumed ulcerative colitis.

Treatment

Oral rehydration therapy is the mainstay of management of children with mild to moderate dehydration. Intravenous fluids are appropriate for children who are severely dehydrated, are moderately dehydrated with persistent vomiting, or have an underlying condition that can be exacerbated by dehydration. As soon as the hydration status has normalized and oral/enteral fluids are tolerated, attempts at refeeding should be instituted. Early refeeding with complex carbohydrates, lean meats, fruits, and vegetables, as well as milk products and infant formula, is recommended. Normalized diet has been shown to decrease the duration of diarrhea when compared with oral or intravenous hydration alone.

The American Academy of Pediatrics suggests that antimotility agents should be avoided in children with acute gastroenteritis.

Children with diarrhea should be placed on contact isolation to avoid spread to hospital personnel and other patients. Special care should be taken with children who require diaper changing.

Antibiotic treatment of bacterial gastroenteritides varies by the organism, the clinical syndrome, and the host (Table 68-7). The rationale for treating many enteric infections is to decrease the duration of symptoms if treatment is initiated

Table 68-7 Therapy for Bacterial Enteric Pathogens		
Pathogen Recovered from Stool Culture	Indication for Therapy	Antibiotic Selection (Until Susceptibility of Organism Is Available)
Shigella spp.	Treatment indicated if the patient has severe symptoms or to prevent spread	Ampicillin* TMP-SMZ* Cefixime Fluoroquinolone Ceftriaxone Azithromycin
Salmonella	Children <3 mo Bacteremia Chronic gastrointestinal disease Immunocompromised state *Salmonella typhi* (typhoid fever) Extraintestinal disease Sickle cell disease Comment: may lead to prolonged excretion	Amoxicillin* TMP-SMZ* Fluoroquinolone Ceftriaxone Azithromycin
Campylobacter spp.	Symptomatic If bacteremia suspected	Erythromycin Azithromycin Doxycycline If bacteremic, aminoglycoside or imipenem until susceptibilities are known
Escherichia coli spp. without Shiga toxin production	Treat to shorten duration of symptoms if not Shiga toxin producing	Ampicillin* TMP-SMZ* Fluoroquinolone
Escherichia coli with Shiga toxin production	Avoid administration of antimicrobials	
Aeromonas	Role of treatment unclear May be of benefit for chronic diarrhea Immunocompromised hosts	TMP-SMZ Fluoroquinolone

*Indicates high rates of resistance reported. Consider other options if possible until the susceptibility pattern is known.
TMP-SMZ, trimethoprim-sulfamethoxazole.

early in the course of the illness. In cases of shigellosis, treatment may limit spread of the infection. If results of the stool culture become available after resolution of the patient's symptoms, antimicrobial therapy may be unwarranted.

Antimicrobial treatment of Shiga toxin–producing *E. coli* O157:H7 infection is not recommended because some studies suggest that children treated with antibiotics are at higher risk for the development of HUS. If the renal function is normal, patients should receive intravenous hydration as volume expansion may mitigate renal damage during HUS. As soon as renal dysfunction occurs, fluids should be restricted.

Antimicrobial therapy for parasitic infections is listed in Table 68-8.

CONSULTATION

- Gastroenterology to evaluate persistent diarrhea, significant gastrointestinal bleeding, or suspected inflammatory bowel disease
- Nephrology for HUS
- Surgery for evaluation of acute abdomen
- Intensive care for suspected botulism

Admission Criteria

- Severe dehydration or moderate dehydration with vomiting
- Suspected bacteremia, sepsis, or metastatic bacterial infection
- Suspected HUS
- Suspected intra-abdominal complication (e.g., intussusception, perforation)

Discharge Criteria

- Able to maintain adequate oral/enteral hydration.
- If a bacterial infection is identified and the patient requires therapy, the patient can be discharged if treatment is complete, if an appropriate oral antibiotic is available, or if intravenous therapy can be administered at home.

Special Considerations
Antibiotic–Associated Diarrhea

Diarrhea frequently complicates antibiotic therapy, and if severe, it may lead to discontinuation of the medication. Most cases are mild with no definitive cause and resolve with discontinuation of the antibiotic.

C. difficile is found in approximately 20% of cases of antibiotic-associated diarrhea. *C. difficile* diarrhea has been reported with many antibiotics; however, β-lactams and clindamycin are the most frequently implicated. It causes a broad spectrum of disease from asymptomatic colonization, to mild diarrhea, to life-threatening enterocolitis. *C. difficile* colitis is a systemic illness, and pseudomembranous colitis is a more severe form of the disease. Among adults, fulminant colitis occurs in 3% of patients with *C. difficile* infection. In cases of fulminant colitis, endoscopy is not recommended because of the fragility of the colon. Exploratory laparotomy may be required for diagnosis and management.

The most important intervention for *C. difficile* infection is removal of the offending antibiotic, if possible. Some authors suggest that switching to an antibiotic that causes *C. difficile* diarrhea less frequently may be helpful. Antibiotic therapy directed against *C. difficile* should be instituted if the symptoms are severe or persistent. Oral vancomycin and metronidazole for 7 to 14 days are first-line agents. Because both drugs displayed equivalent efficacy in a prospective randomized trial, metronidazole is preferred because of lower cost and the potential for growth of vancomycin-resistant enterococci as a result of vancomycin therapy. Intravenous metronidazole can be used to treat patients who cannot tolerate oral therapy. Intravenous vancomycin does not penetrate the intestinal lumen and is not effective. Fifteen percent

Table 68-8 Treatment of Intestinal Parasites		
	First–Line Therapy	Alternative
Giardia lamblia	Metronidazole for 5-7 days Nitazoxanide for 3 days Tinidazole once	Furazolidone Albendazole
Strongyloides stercoralis	Ivermectin for 2 days	Albendazole Thiabendazole
Cryptosporidium	Nitazoxanide for 3 days	Paromomycin
Cyclospora	TMP-SMX for 7-10 days	
Amebiasis	Metronidazole for 5-10 days Tinidazole for 3 days (mild to moderate) or 5 days (severe, or extraintestinal)	Iodoquinol or paromomycin to prevent relapse
Isospora	TMP-SMX for 7-10 days	Ciprofloxacin
Trichuris trichiura	Mebendazole for 3 days	Albendazole Ivermectin
Blastocystis hominis	Metronidazole for 10 days	Iodoquinol TMP-SMX

TMP-SMX, trimethoprim-sulfamethoxazole.

to 20% of patients treated for *C. difficile* diarrhea have a relapse. The first relapse should be treated with another course of antibiotics. For recurrent disease, tapering of metronidazole or vancomycin doses over a 4- to 6-week period has been proposed, as well as the addition of cholestyramine or bacitracin. In the absence of ongoing symptoms, a test of cure is not necessary.

The role of probiotics in the management of diarrhea has not been clearly established. Lactobacillus may help to control antibiotic-associated diarrhea in children.

Newborn infants become colonized with *C. difficile* at birth, without any evidence of disease. Between 25% and 65% of healthy infants younger than 1 year are colonized with toxin-producing *C. difficile*. Therefore, isolation of the organism or identification of the toxin from children younger than 1 year and possibly those younger than 2 years may represent nonpathologic bowel flora.

Traveler's Diarrhea

Empirical antibiotics are generally recommended to treat traveler's diarrhea when the traveler is still abroad. The probable causes are enterotoxigenic *E. coli*, *Salmonella*, *Shigella*, and *Campylobacter*. Children younger than 2 years are at higher risk for traveler's diarrhea, as well as more severe disease. For treatment of children, trimethoprim-sulfamethoxazole has been the drug of choice. However, this medication has become much less effective because of increasing rates of drug resistance worldwide. In older children and adults, a fluoroquinolone is recommended. For young children, in whom fluoroquinolones are generally avoided, azithromycin may be considered, although its effectiveness against traveler's diarrhea has not been studied. If the patient has returned home with diarrhea, a microbiologic evaluation can be obtained before initiating antibiotic therapy. Prolonged diarrhea should prompt further investigation into possible parasitic infections. The Centers for Disease Control and Prevention currently does not recommend prophylactic antibiotics for travelers.

Prevention

A rotavirus vaccine was licensed in 2006. It is an oral vaccine, composed of 5 reassortant viruses from human and bovine rotavirus strains. The vaccine is administered during infancy at 2, 4, and 6 months. For travelers, two forms of typhoid fever vaccine are available: a polysaccharide vaccine delivered intramuscularly that can be administered to children older than 2 years and an oral, live attenuated vaccine that can be administered to children over 6 years of age. An effective cholera vaccine is not yet available in the United States.

Transmission of enteric infections via the fecal-oral route can be interrupted by vigilant hand hygiene, especially in centers that provide care for children in diapers. Attention to food preparation and adequate cooking of meat can prevent many food-borne infections. Maintenance of a clean water supply is a most important intervention to prevent bacterial and parasitic infections worldwide.

IN A NUTSHELL

- Clinical presentation: Viral gastroenteritis generally presents with vomiting and diarrhea without blood or mucus, whereas bacterial infections may present with bloody or mucoid stools.
- Diagnosis: Pursue a bacterial or parasitic diagnosis if blood or mucus is present in stool or if there is high fever, a history of travel, or prolonged illness.
- Treatment: Rehydration is the most important intervention. Antimicrobial therapy should be initiated after identification of an infectious organism.
- Antibiotic-associated diarrhea: Antibiotics should be discontinued if possible.

ON THE HORIZON

- New vaccines against important enteric bacterial and viral infections.
- Increasing bacterial resistance worldwide, including high rates of fluoroquinolone resistance in South and Southeast Asia.

HEPATITIS

Hepatitis is a final common pathway of hepatocyte injury by both infectious and noninfectious causes. Infectious causes of hepatitis include hepatotropic and systemic viral infections, as well as bacterial, parasitic, and fungal pathogens. The identified infecting agents that cause primary hepatitis include hepatitis A virus (HAV); hepatitis B virus (HBV); hepatitis C virus (HCV); hepatitis D virus (HDV); hepatitis E virus (HEV), which was previously referred to as non-A, non-B hepatitis; and hepatitis G virus (HGV). Other pathogens can cause hepatitis, but usually as part of a more generalized illness that does not primarily target the liver (Table 68-9).

HAV is spread via the fecal-oral route, and identification of a case requires epidemiologic investigation to provide appropriate postexposure prophylaxis and vaccination. HBV and HCV are transmitted through blood or body fluids. Both percutaneous and nonpercutaneous transmission of HBV is highly efficient, which should be kept in mind when evaluating sexual contacts, occupational exposure, human bites, and perinatal exposure. In contrast, nonpercutaneous transmission of HCV, such as sexual contact and perinatal transmission, is low, estimated at 1.5% and 5%, respectively. The virus is transmitted primarily through contact with infected blood. The seroprevalence is high among intravenous drug users. Screening of the blood supply for HCV was instituted in 1991; therefore, older children and adolescents who had blood or blood product transfusions before 1991 may have been exposed to HCV. HDV is transmitted through blood products, sexual contact, and tattooing or drug use with contaminated needles. It can cause infection only in patients with active HBV infection. HEV infection is acquired by the fecal-oral route, and epidemics have occurred from contaminated water sources. It is rare in the United States and most developed countries but is endemic in South Asia and North Africa. HGV is a

Table 68-9   Infections That Can Cause Hepatitis as Part of a Generalized Illness

Epstein-Barr virus
Cytomegalovirus
Varicella-zoster virus
Herpes simplex virus
Yellow fever
Measles
Mumps
Rubeola
Rubella
Enterovirus
Adenovirus
Human immunodeficiency virus
Syphilis
Toxoplasmosis

Modified from Zaoutis LB: Infectious hepatitis. In Zaoutis TE, Klein JD (eds): Pediatric Infectious Disease Secrets. Philadelphia, Hanley & Belfus, 2003.

recently identified virus that is transmitted percutaneously through blood products, hemodialysis, and transplants and vertically from mother to child.

Clinical Presentation and Course of Illness

The clinical presentation of hepatitis is often nonspecific, and because the symptoms can be insidious, identifying the onset of the disease can be challenging. In addition to jaundice, scleral icterus, right upper quadrant tenderness, and hepatomegaly, constitutional symptoms of poor oral intake, lethargy, fever, arthralgia, rash, or pruritus may be reported. Physical examination may reveal ascites, arthritis, or manifestations of more systemic illness in which liver involvement is not the primary process.

Hepatitis A

Infection with HAV causes an acute illness with two phases. The prodromic phase consists of fever and diarrhea and usually lasts 1 to 7 days. The icteric phase follows with poor appetite, nausea, fatigue, jaundice, and dark urine and lasts 2 to 10 weeks. Children younger than 2 years are generally asymptomatic, but by 5 years of age, most infections with HAV cause symptomatic illness. Fulminant hepatitis is rare, but patients coinfected with HCV are at risk for more severe infection. Prolonged cholestasis lasting more than 12 weeks and relapsing hepatitis can occur. Chronic HAV infection does not occur.

Hepatitis B

HBV infection produces a wide range of illness, including asymptomatic infection, a self-limited moderate illness with features typical of clinical hepatitis, a fulminant lethal hepatitis, and chronic disease. Usually, symptomatic illness begins with the prodromal phase and a gradual onset of malaise and nausea, which may be accompanied by extrahepatic complaints of arthralgia or rash. The icteric phase follows and may last for weeks, after which the convalescent phase occurs and can last many weeks to months.

Although neonates who are infected during the perinatal period are at highest risk for the development of chronic infection with HBV, their infection is generally clinically silent in infancy. Chronic infection occurs in approximately 90% of infants with perinatal infection, whereas the risk for young children who become infected is 25% to 50% and that for older children is 6% to 10%.

Patients with chronic HBV infection may have normal physical examination findings and normal liver function test results or only subtle signs of liver disease unless fulminant hepatic failure develops. Patients with chronic HBV infection are at risk for cirrhosis, hepatic failure, and hepatocellular carcinoma (HCC). Patients with chronic infection, especially those with cirrhosis or a family history of HCC, should be monitored for the development of HCC.

Hepatitis C

Most children are asymptomatic and have normal or nearly normal liver function test values. However, the virus is rarely cleared. The natural progression of hepatitis C is very slow. Over decades, mild, stable hepatic inflammation, severe progression to cirrhosis or fibrosis without cirrhosis, and infrequently, HCC may develop. Severe liver disease may develop in a small percentage of children during childhood.

Hepatitis D, E, and G

HDV can cause coinfection or superinfection with underlying HBV infection. The features of these conditions are those of the underlying HBV infection but may be more severe because of HDV.

HEV infection causes a clinical picture similar to that of HAV, but it is associated with significant mortality in pregnant women.

HGV infection is usually asymptomatic, and despite a high viral load, the liver damage remains mild.

Differential Diagnosis

A wide range of infectious and noninfectious processes can lead to hepatic inflammation and damage. Infections that cause systemic illness including hepatitis are listed in Table 68-9. Noninfectious causes of hepatitis that should be considered include cystic fibrosis, metabolic disorders, Wilson disease, α_1-antitrypsin deficiency, and autoimmune hepatitis. Toxins, including medications such as acetaminophen, accidental ingestions, and complementary and alternative medicine, can cause hepatic injury. In newborns, hepatic injury is frequently due to congenital anatomic abnormalities such as biliary atresia and choledochal cysts.

Diagnosis and Evaluation

To explore the possible cause of liver injury, the physician should ask about the progression of symptoms; potential exposure to toxins, medications, or infected individuals; associated medical problems or symptoms; and travel and family history. Patients should be specifically questioned

Table 68-10 Recommended Evaluation of Patients with Hepatitis

Laboratory Test	Utility of Test
Bilirubin—total and direct	Nearly equal proportions in viral hepatitis If direct <20%, suggests hemolysis or Gilbert syndrome
Alanine transaminase (ALT) and aspartate transaminase	Indicators of hepatocyte damage ALT is more specific to the liver 10- to 100-fold elevations in acute viral hepatitis Chronic viral or metabolic disease usually <300 IU/mL
Alkaline phosphatase	Found in liver, bone predominantly Levels may be much higher in growing children than in adults
γ-Glutamyl transpeptidase	>300 IU/mL in cases of biliary atresia and α_1-antitrypsin deficiency
Albumin	Reduced levels indicate long-standing liver dysfunction or malnutrition
Prothrombin	Factors I, II, V, VII, and X are synthesized in the liver Acute assessment of liver dysfunction May predict a more complicated course
Ammonia	Evaluation of hepatic encephalopathy

Table 68-11 Serologic Diagnosis of Hepatitis B

HBsAg	Anti-HBc	Anti-HBs	IgM anti-HBc	Interpretation
–	–	–		Susceptible to infection
–	+	+		Immune because of natural infection
–	–	+		Immune because of vaccination
+/–	+	–	+	Acutely infected (HBsAg may be below the level of detection)
+	+	–	–	Chronic infection

HBc, hepatitis B core antigen; HBsAg, hepatitis B surface antigen.

about a history of blood transfusion and, in older children and adolescents, sexual activity and the use of intravenous drugs. The physical examination should focus on physical findings associated with liver disease and also signs of extra-hepatic disease.

The initial laboratory evaluation should focus on identifying the extent of liver injury (Table 68-10). Elevation of transaminases reflects the amount of hepatocyte injury. In general, alanine and aspartate transaminase levels greater than 10,000 IU/mL are found in patients with toxin- or ischemia-mediated hepatocyte injury, whereas levels of 1000 to 3000 IU/mL are more typical of acute viral hepatitis. Lower degrees of elevation are seen in chronic viral infection and metabolic disorders. Elevated bilirubin should be further fractionated into direct and indirect bilirubin and, in conjunction with alkaline phosphatase and γ-glutamyltransferase, used to assess hepatic excretory function. Serum albumin and the prothrombin time are a measure of the liver's synthetic function.

Once the diagnosis of hepatitis has been made, the cause should be identified, if possible. The initial evaluation for infectious causes should include studies for HAV, HBV, and HCV. The test for diagnosis of hepatitis A is detection of IgM antibody to HAV.

To evaluate for acute or chronic hepatitis B, studies should be sent for hepatitis B surface antigen (HBsAg), as well as antibodies against hepatitis B core antigen (anti-HBc) and surface antigen (anti-HBs), as detailed in Table 68-11. Persistent hepatitis B e antigen (HBeAg) detection in serum indicates a high risk for progression to chronic infection. Patients who have detectable HBeAg, without antibody formation, are at highest risk for transmission. When HBsAg clears, the infection is considered resolved, although it may reactivate with immunosuppression. The diagnosis of chronic HBV infection is made when HBsAg is present for more than 6 months.

The screening test for hepatitis C is detection of immunoglobulin (IgG) antibody to HCV; however, antibodies may not develop for 6 weeks. If there is a suspicion of acute infection, HCV RNA detection is required. Once it has been present for 3 months, the virus is unlikely to be cleared. The diagnosis of chronic disease is established by the presence of HCV RNA with elevated alanine transaminase, positive serology for 6 months, or positive HCV RNA with liver biopsy–proven chronic hepatitis.

Because HDV infection occurs solely with acute or chronic hepatitis B, testing for antibody against HDV is considered only if HBsAg is present. The virus is found most often in southern Italy, eastern Europe, South America, Africa, and the Middle East. HEV infection, which is the cause of endemic non-A non-B hepatitis, is exceedingly rare in developed countries but should be considered if there is a history of recent travel to the Indian subcontinent, Asia, Africa, or Mexico. Antibody testing or assay for HEV RNA is performed only at reference laboratories. If a systemic viral infection is clinically suspected or the initial hepatitis serology is negative, evaluation for other infectious agents should be considered (see Table 68-9).

In infants and young children with jaundice, imaging of the liver is important because anatomic abnormalities are a leading cause of hepatitis. Ultrasound of the liver is often the first imaging study obtained. It can demonstrate its size, uniformity of composition, and blood flow and can identify most anatomic abnormalities. Although sedation may be required in younger children, computed tomography or magnetic resonance imaging may more accurately detect small tumors or abscesses.

In some cases, liver biopsy may be necessary to determine the cause of the hepatitis, assess the extent of liver injury, and determine the need for therapy.

Treatment

Most cases of infectious hepatitis are managed successfully on an outpatient basis with supportive care and serial office visits to monitor the course of the illness. Acute hepatitis with inadequate oral/enteral intake may require intravenous hydration. Cases of hepatic failure with impaired synthetic function require in-patient management. Coagulopathies with or without active bleeding may necessitate replacement of clotting factors or parenteral administration of vitamin K, or both.

Ascites may develop in patients with severe or chronic liver involvement. Dietary salt restriction and diuretics are often helpful. Spontaneous bacterial peritonitis is a known complication and is discussed in detail in the later section on peritonitis.

If mental status changes occur, consider the complication of hyperammonemia due to liver failure. Deterioration of renal function as evidenced by oliguria, azotemia, acidosis, or hyperkalemia indicates hepatorenal failure. These conditions are usually managed in intensive care units. Progressive, irreversible liver failure with or without renal involvement warrants prompt referral for possible liver transplantation.

Treatment options for hepatitis B include interferon, which cannot be used in patients with severe cirrhosis, and lamivudine. Patients with HCV infection can be treated with standard or long-acting (pegylated) interferons combined with oral ribavirin.

Consultation

- Gastroenterology if liver biopsy may be needed and for further evaluation and treatment recommendations for patients with hepatitis C; hepatitis B with persistently elevated transaminases, increased α-fetoprotein concentration, or abnormal ultrasound findings; active gastrointestinal bleeding; and hepatitis that does not resolve
- Rheumatology for evaluation of autoimmune hepatitis
- Hematology for management of coagulopathy

- Infectious diseases for guidance regarding diagnosis, therapy, isolation, and prophylaxis
- Intensive care for evidence of acute hepatic failure with or without renal insufficiency/failure and severe gastrointestinal bleeding

Admission Criteria

- Inadequate oral/enteral intake
- Worsening liver function (coagulopathy, encephalopathy)
- Renal dysfunction
- Severe ascites or pleural effusion
- Need for further evaluation, including liver biopsy

Discharge Criteria

- Stable liver function
- Control of coagulopathy, active bleeding, and encephalopathy
- Appropriate primary care and subspecialty follow-up

Prevention

HAV vaccine is safe and highly immunogenic. It is currently approved by the Food and Drug Administration for children 1 year of age and older. The two-dose series is recommended for children greater than or equal to 1 year of age, individuals traveling to endemic countries, children living in U.S. communities with high rates of hepatitis A, and patients with chronic liver disease and clotting factor disorders.

After identification of an index case of HAV infection, pooled human immune globulin should be administered to all unimmunized household members, sexual contacts, and child care contacts. The immune globulin should be given within 2 weeks of exposure and may be administered at the same time as the HAV vaccine.

HBV vaccine is recommended for all infants, for children and adolescents who were not vaccinated in infancy, and for individuals at risk for occupational exposure. The vaccine elicits a protective immune response in more than 95% of infants and 90% of adults. Patients who are seronegative despite vaccination should be revaccinated. Pooled hepatitis B immune globulin (HBIG) is available for exposure of nonimmune individuals. Patients with chronic hepatitis B should be vaccinated against HAV if they are not immune.

Full-term and preterm infants born to mothers with HBV infection should receive the initial dose of HBV vaccine within 12 hours of birth. HBIG should be administered at the same time, but at a different site. If the mother's hepatitis B status is unknown, the infant should receive the vaccine within the first 12 hours. If the mother is found to be HBV-positive, HBIG should be administered as soon as possible, but within the first 7 days of life.

Children with chronic HBV infection should undergo periodic screening for disease progression and development of HCC. Screening should include serum transaminase levels, α-fetoprotein concentration, and abdominal ultrasound.

Patients with HCV infection should be vaccinated against HAV and HBV. The rate of vertical transmission of HCV from mother to child is increased from 5% to 12% if the mother is positive for human immunodeficiency virus (HIV). There is no clear evidence that cesarean section prevents mother-to-child transmission of HCV. At this time the risk for transmission of HCV through breast milk is considered negligible. Anti-HCV antibodies can cross the placenta, so exposed infants should not undergo antibody testing until 12 months of age.

IN A NUTSHELL

- Clinical presentation: Clinical findings include jaundice and hepatomegaly but can otherwise be nonspecific. Infections with hepatotropic viruses are often asymptomatic in children.
- Diagnosis: Laboratory tests to assess the extent of hepatocyte damage, excretory function, synthetic function, and cause.
- Treatment: Supportive care is usually sufficient for uncomplicated cases. Complications often warrant subspecialty input and transfer to an intensive care unit. Hepatic failure may necessitate liver transplantation.
- Prophylaxis: Both primary prophylaxis and postexposure prophylaxis are important, and recommendations vary according to the specific infecting agent.

ON THE HORIZON

- Genotyping of HBV and HCV to aid in prognosis and the choice of therapy
- Further information about hepatitis and HIV coinfection

PERITONITIS

Peritonitis refers to inflammation of any aspect of the peritoneum. Infectious peritonitis can be considered as a primary or secondary disease. Bacterial infection of the peritoneum that arises from the bloodstream or lymphatics is termed primary, or spontaneous, peritonitis. It is much more frequently found in patients with ascites secondary to nephrotic syndrome or cirrhosis. Secondary peritonitis develops from contamination of the peritoneal cavity by contents of the gastrointestinal tract or by indwelling devices such as peritoneal dialysis catheters or ventriculoperitoneal shunts.

Clinical Presentation

Children with peritonitis are ill appearing and febrile. They complain of abdominal pain and distention and often have vomiting as a result of ileus. The abdomen is usually distended, and with severe disease, the overlying skin may appear shiny and erythematous. On auscultation, bowel sounds are absent or decreased. The abdomen may be rigid, or rebound tenderness or tenderness with percussion may be elicited.

Diagnosis and Evaluation

An obstruction series may reveal an air-fluid level indicative of bowel obstruction, free air found with perforation, or a ground-glass appearance suggesting the presence of intraperitoneal fluid. Ultrasound may demonstrate intra-

peritoneal fluid, as well as bowel wall inflammation, masses, and organomegaly. The most sensitive study is computed tomography with contrast enhancement to delineate the extent of the disease and identify causes of secondary peritonitis such as a ruptured viscus or abscess.

Because ascites may be present in many conditions and may be a baseline finding in some patients being evaluated for peritonitis, direct examination of the fluid is essential. More than 50 white blood cells/mm^3 is abnormal; however, the white blood cell count in peritoneal fluid in patients with peritonitis generally reaches 5000 to 10,000 cells/mm^3. Cultures for bacteria, fungi, and mycobacteria should be obtained, and specific stains for these organisms should be performed on fresh specimens. Multiple organisms or the presence of anaerobes should raise concern for secondary peritonitis. If tuberculous peritonitis is suspected, skin testing, direct visualization of the abdomen, and peritoneal biopsy aid in the diagnosis.

Children with a catheter in place for peritoneal dialysis are at high risk for the development of peritonitis, with the potential loss of peritoneal membrane transport capacity. Peritonitis is generally suspected when fever with abdominal pain and tenderness develops. The effluent appears cloudy and demonstrates an elevated leukocyte count (>100 cells/mm^3) with greater than 50% polymorphonuclear leukocytes. When infection is suspected, peritoneal fluid should be obtained for analysis and culture as described earlier.

Blood cultures are frequently positive in children with primary peritonitis but generally negative in children with secondary peritonitis.

Differential Diagnosis

When children initially have a peritoneal catheter placed for dialysis, an eosinophilic peritonitis often develops but is usually self-limited. A mild to moderate elevation in the peritoneal leukocyte concentration has been attributed to chemical peritonitis in these patients as well.

Intra-abdominal infections such as hepatitis, cholecystitis, or early appendicitis may cause fever and inflammation of the visceral peritoneum without frank infection of the peritoneal space. Symptoms tend to be more localized, but rebound tenderness may be present. Girls or young women with pelvic infections or ovarian torsion may present similarly.

Bowel obstruction or severe ileus may also produce abdominal distention and tenderness. Fever is usually absent, and significant ascites is not common (unless the ileus is occurring secondary to infected intraperitoneal fluid).

Children with a ventriculoperitoneal shunt generally have a low level of peritoneal inflammation with some abnormal fluid collection in the abdomen. When the fluid becomes infected, clinical signs of peritonitis or central nervous system infection generally develop.

Treatment

In children with a previously normal peritoneum and also those with ascites but without indwelling catheters, *Streptococcus pneumoniae* is the most common cause of primary bacterial peritonitis. Empirical therapy with parenteral third-generation cephalosporins should be administered to treat possible penicillin-resistant *S. pneumoniae* until culture and susceptibility results are known. Children with ascites are also at risk for peritonitis with gram-negative organisms, even in the absence of intestinal pathology. If the patient does not clinically improve after 1 to 2 days, repeat paracentesis should be performed. In children without any complicating factors, systemic antibiotics alone are sufficient to treat primary peritonitis, without drainage of the infected fluid. Treatment for 14 days is usually adequate. In patients with nephrotic syndrome or cirrhosis, data are insufficient to determine whether drainage of the infected fluid improves outcomes. Management of any underlying disease is often needed to achieve a clinical cure.

In children who have peritoneal dialysis catheters in place, gram-positive cocci from the skin are the most common organisms that cause peritonitis. Gram-negative rods, including *Pseudomonas*, can also cause peritonitis in this population. Because of the risk for loss of functional membrane, antimicrobial therapy should be started promptly. If the patient is not systemically ill and the catheter is still in place, adequate levels of antimicrobial agents to treat peritonitis can be achieved by intraperitoneal administration. Because peritonitis associated with a peritoneal catheter is considered a localized infection, guidelines from the International Society for Peritoneal Dialysis recommend empirical intraperitoneal antibiotic treatment with cefazolin and ceftazidime. In addition, these guidelines suggest that vancomycin replace the first-generation cephalosporin if the patient is younger than 2 years or has severe symptoms. Aminoglycosides can also be administered into the peritoneum but are often avoided to preserve any remaining kidney function.

The duration of intraperitoneal treatment of peritonitis in children with peritoneal catheters in place is usually 2 weeks for coagulase-negative staphylococci and 3 weeks for *Staphylococcus aureus* and gram-negative infection. Fungi have been associated with peritonitis in this population, although it has not been well studied. Amphotericin B (intravenously) or fluconazole (orally or intravenously) is recommended for the treatment of *Candida* peritonitis. If a peritoneal catheter is present, removal of the catheter to help clear the fungus is recommended. If no organism is identified but evaluation of peritoneal fluid supports the diagnosis of peritonitis, the initial empirical therapy should be continued.

Patients who fail to improve may require a change in antibiotic therapy or catheter removal. Experts generally recommend that once removed, the catheter can be replaced after 2 to 3 weeks, although there have been some reports of success with simultaneous removal of the infected catheter and replacement with a new catheter.

Consultation

- Nephrology for patients maintained on peritoneal dialysis to ascertain that the membrane is functioning properly and for management of intraperitoneal antibiotic therapy
- Surgery for patients with possible secondary peritonitis or if removal of the peritoneal catheter may be necessary

Admission Criteria

- Children with suspected bacterial or fungal peritonitis require inpatient evaluation.

Discharge Criteria

- Defervescence and overall clinical improvement
- Ability to complete the antibiotic regimen after discharge
- Stability or improvement of any underlying medical condition
- Appropriate follow-up with primary care or subspecialists, or both

IN A NUTSHELL

- Clinical presentation: Fever, abdominal pain, and tenderness, especially in children with ascites, or indwelling peritoneal catheters or ventriculoperitoneal shunts
- Diagnosis: Paracentesis, except when the peritonitis is secondary to gastrointestinal perforation
- Treatment: Intravenous or intraperitoneal antibiotics or laparotomy if a ruptured viscus is suspected or confirmed

SUGGESTED READING

Craig AS, Schaffner W: Prevention of hepatitis A with the hepatitis A vaccine. N Engl J Med 2004;350:476-481.

Demmler GJ: Hepatitis. In Feigin RD, Cherry JD (eds): Textbook of Pediatric Infectious Diseases, 5th ed. Philadelphia, WB Saunders, 2004.

Fine KD, Schiller LR: AGA technical review on the evaluation and management of chronic diarrhea. Gastroenterology 1999;116:1464-1486.

King CK, Glass R, Bresse JS, Duggan C: Managing acute gastroenteritis among children: Oral rehydration, maintenance, and nutritional therapy. MMWR Recomm Rep 2003;52(RR-16):1-16.

Oldfield EC, Wallace MR: The role of antibiotics in the treatment of infectious diarrhea. Gastroenterol Clin North Am 2001;30:817-836.

Pickering LK, Cleary TG: Approach to patients with gastrointestinal tract infections and food poisoning. In Feigin RD, Cherry JD (eds): Textbook of Pediatric Infectious Diseases, 5th ed. Philadelphia, WB Saunders, 2004.

Schaefer F: Management of peritonitis in children receiving chronic peritoneal dialysis. Paediatr Drugs 2003;5:315-325.

Wilcox MH: Treatment of *Clostridium difficile* infection. J Antimicrob Chemother 1998;41(Suppl C):41-46.

Wong CS, Jelacic S, Habeeb RL, et al: The risk of the hemolytic-uremic syndrome after antibiotic treatment of *Escherichia coli* O157:H7 infections. N Engl J Med 2000;342:1930-1936.

www.cdc.gov/foodnet for information on food-borne illnesses.

www.cdc.gov/narms for information about antibiotic resistance among enteric bacteria.

http://www.cdc.gov/ncidod/diseases/hepatitis/ for information about hepatitis in the United States.

www.peritonitis.org: Website of the International Pediatric Peritonitis Registry.

http://www.who.int/csr/disease/hepatitis/en and *http://www.who.int/health_topics/hepatitis/en* for an international perspective.

Yuen MF, Lai CL: Natural history of chronic hepatitis B virus infection. J Gastroenterol Hepatol 2000;15(Suppl):E20-E24.

CHAPTER 69

Urinary Tract Infections in Childhood

Nader Shaikh and Alejandro Hoberman

Urinary tract infections (UTIs) are a common and important clinical problem in childhood and may lead to systemic illness and renal injury in the short term; with repeated infections, renal scarring, hypertension, and end-stage renal dysfunction may develop.

The overall prevalence of UTI is estimated at 5% in febrile infants but varies widely by race and gender.[1,2] The highest prevalence rates of childhood UTI occur in uncircumcised male infants under 3 months of age (prevalence ~20%), and among females (prevalence ~8%). Uncircumcised older male children have the lowest prevalence of UTI (~1%).

PATHOGENESIS

Most UTIs beyond the newborn period represent an ascending infection. Colonization of the periurethral area by uropathogenic enteric organisms is the first step. The most common bacterial species is *Escherichia coli*, which accounts for about 80% of UTIs in children. Other bacteria include both gram-negative species *(Klebsiella, Proteus, Enterobacter,* and *Citrobacter)* and gram-positive species *(Staphylococcus saprophyticus, Enterococcus,* and rarely, *Staphylococcus aureus).* The presence of pathogens on the periurethral mucosa is not sufficient to cause UTIs.[3] Attachment of bacteria to uroepithelial cells is an active process mediated by specific bacterial adhesins and specific receptor sites on the epithelial cells. This process allows bacteria to ascend into the kidney, even in children without vesicoureteral reflux (VUR). In the kidney, the bacterial inoculum can produce an infection with an intense inflammatory response that may ultimately lead to renal scarring.

Many host factors influence the predisposition that children may have to UTI, including familial predisposition, genitourinary anatomy and function, instrumentation, and sexual activity, as well as periurethral flora. The determination of risk factors in a child presenting with UTI is important in preventing further recurrences.

First-degree relatives of children with UTIs are more likely to have UTIs,[4] and adherence of bacteria may, at least in part, be genetically determined.

Uncircumcised febrile male infants have a four- to tenfold higher prevalence of UTIs than circumcised males do.[5] Although uncircumcised males are at increased risk for the development of a UTI, it is important to point out that UTIs do not develop in most uncircumcised boys.[6] It is estimated that 195 circumcisions would be needed to prevent one hospital admission for UTI in the first year of life.[5]

Dysfunctional elimination syndrome (DES) refers to a functional disorder of unknown etiology characterized by the features delineated in Table 69-1. DES, also known as voiding dysfunction, usually appears in healthy school-aged children and may persist for months to years. Although DES is a relatively common condition in the pediatric population, with a prevalence estimated at 15%,[7] it is often underdiagnosed and undertreated by primary care physicians.[8] Approximately 40% of toilet-trained children with their first UTI[9-11] and 80% of children with recurrent UTI[12] report symptoms of DES. In a study of 141 girls older than 3 years with recurrent (more than three) UTIs, 108 had DES.[12] This syndrome is also a risk factor for VUR persistence[13-15] and renal scarring.[10,15]

VUR is the most frequently occurring urologic abnormality in children, with an overall prevalence of 1% and a prevalence of 40% in young children with febrile UTIs. A strong genetic predisposition for VUR exists and has been identified in up to 40% of siblings of children with VUR. The incidence of VUR is markedly lower in the African American population. VUR is graded according to the international classification from grade 1 to grade 5 (Fig. 69-1). In children presenting with their first UTI to a primary care physician, 95% of cases of VUR have been found to be grades 1 to 3.[16] Most VUR improves or resolves as the child ages, with resolution occurring more frequently in children with low-grade and unilateral disease.[17,18] The likelihood of resolution of VUR, 5 years after detection, as derived from a large meta-analysis, is summarized in Figure 69-2.[19]

It has been widely believed that VUR is the major risk factor for pyelonephritis and renal scarring in young children. The role of VUR in initiating pyelonephritis and scarring, however, has been poorly documented in the literature, and there is evidence that its importance in the pathophysiology of pyelonephritis and renal scarring may have been overstated.[20] Current evidence implies that VUR is neither necessary nor sufficient to cause renal scarring and that exclusive focus on VUR, without a search for other modifiable risk factors (such as DES), may be inadequate.

Children with obstructive abnormalities, whether anatomic (e.g., posterior urethral valves, ureteropelvic junction obstruction, constipation), neurologic (e.g., myelomeningocele with neurogenic bladder), or functional (e.g., DES), are at increased risk for the development of UTIs. Stagnant urine is an excellent culture medium for most uropathogens. However, obstructive anatomic abnormalities in children presenting with their first UTI are infrequent (1% to 4%) in nonsyndromic children.[16,21-23] Obstruction should be suspected when other family members have had urologic abnormalities, when dysmorphic features are detected on physical examination, or when symptoms do not respond to appropriate therapy.

There is indirect evidence that alteration of the normal periurethral flora in females (*Lactobacillus* and *Corynebacterium* spp.) promotes attachment of pathogenic bacteria.

Table 69-1	Dysfunctional Elimination Syndrome
Clinical Triad	**Symptoms**
Abnormal elimination pattern	Frequent voiding (>10 times/day) Infrequent voiding (≤3 times/day) Urgency (often runs to the bathroom) Infrequent hard painful stools (ask the child, not the parent)
Incontinence	Bladder (ask about damp underwear) Bowel (ask about streaks of stool in underwear)
Withholding maneuvers	Pee dance Kneeling with the perineum on the heel (Vincent's curtsey)

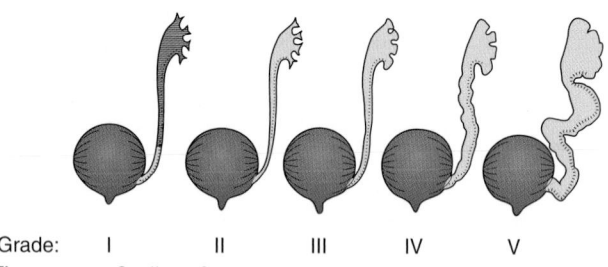

Grade: I II III IV V

Figure 69-1 Grading of vesicoureteral reflux.

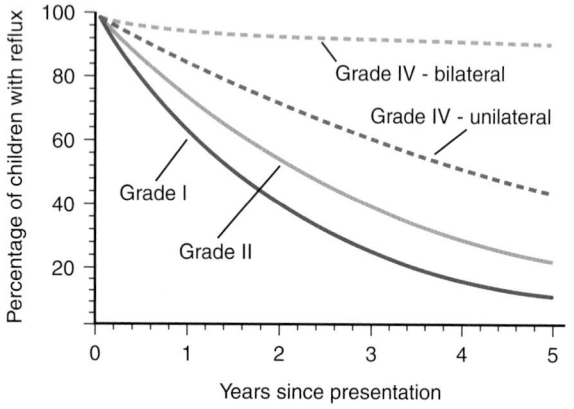

Figure 69-2 Persistence of vesicoureteral reflux in young children.

Sexual activity is also associated with UTI in women. In a prospective study of young sexually active women, recent intercourse was independently associated with the development of UTIs.[24] The use of spermicidal condoms and spermicidal jelly with diaphragms has been independently associated with *E. coli* bacteriuria, thus suggesting that these agents predispose to UTI by altering the vaginal flora.[24]

The risk for UTI increases with increasing duration of catheterization. In a 7-year retrospective study, nosocomial UTIs were found to be the fifth most common infection in hospitalized children. However, only 50% of children with nosocomial UTIs were catheterized, and nosocomial UTIs occurred with a disproportionately high rate in newborns.[25]

CLINICAL PRESENTATION

In general, the younger the child, the less specific the presenting signs and symptoms of UTI. Many infants with UTI are described as "well appearing."

Several prospective studies have shown that infants and young children can present with fever as the sole manifestation of UTI.[1,2] Furthermore, the presence of another potential source for fever (upper respiratory tract infection, acute otitis media, acute gastroenteritis, etc.) does not rule out the possibility of UTI. In one study, the prevalence of UTI in infants and young girls with fever was 6% if no other potential source of fever was identified, but the prevalence was 3% even if another potential source of fever was identified.[2] This finding highlights the importance of considering urine cultures in all febrile infants without a definite source for fever. Parental reporting of foul-smelling urine[26] or the presence of gastrointestinal symptoms (vomiting, diarrhea, and poor feeding[1,2]) does not correlate with the presence of UTIs. Other less common symptoms of UTI in infants include conjugated hyperbilirubinemia and failure to thrive.

Symptoms of UTI in older children may include fever, urinary symptoms (dysuria, urgency, frequency, incontinence, macroscopic hematuria), and abdominal pain.[27,28] Suprapubic tenderness and costovertebral angle tenderness may be present on examination. Occasionally, older children may present with failure to thrive, nephropathy, or hypertension secondary to unrecognized UTIs earlier in childhood.[29]

DIFFERENTIAL DIAGNOSIS

The differential diagnosis of a well-appearing infant or young child with "fever without a definite source" is extensive but most commonly includes UTI, occult bacteremia, and viral infections. In children vaccinated against *Haemophilus influenzae* and *Streptococcus pneumoniae*, the odds of UTI are much higher than the odds of occult bacteremia. The differential diagnosis of an older child presenting with urinary symptoms and bacteriuria includes nonspecific vulvovaginitis, an abdominal process such as appendicitis, urinary calculi, urethritis secondary to sexually transmitted disease, and a vaginal foreign body. Patients with group A streptococcal infection, appendicitis, and Kawasaki disease may present with fever, abdominal pain, and pyuria.

DIAGNOSIS AND EVALUATION

Particular elements of the history of the acute illness should include the height and duration of fever and the presence of urinary symptoms, hematuria, vomiting, nonurinary symptoms (rash, rhinorrhea, cough, etc.), genitourinary instrumentation, sexual activity, and method of contraception. The past history should include any history of chronic constipation, chronic urinary symptoms (incontinence, lack of proper stream, frequency, urgency, withholding maneuvers), previous UTIs, VUR, and previous undiagnosed febrile illnesses. Relevant family history would include frequent UTIs, VUR, and other genitourinary abnormalities in close relatives.

Key elements of the physical examination include blood pressure and temperature, assessment of suprapubic and costovertebral tenderness, and if febrile, a search for signs of other sources of fever. The external genitalia should be examined for signs of vulvovaginitis, vaginal foreign body, sexually transmitted diseases, and anatomic abnormalities.

Given that the signs and symptoms of UTI in children are nonspecific, diagnosis of UTI requires laboratory confirmation. A clean-catch specimen and a catheterized specimen are the preferred methods of urine collection in a toilet-trained and a diapered child, respectively. Suprapubic aspiration may also be used to collect a specimen in young children. The use of a sterile bag is not generally recommended because up to 85% of positive cultures from bag urine specimens will represent false-positive results[30]; therefore, results are useful only if negative. The high false-positive rate of bag specimens can lead to unnecessary and even harmful interventions.[31] Specimens should be examined soon after collection inasmuch as delay of even a few hours increases both false-positive and false-negative rates substantially.[30]

The accuracy of the various diagnostic tests for UTI has been the subject of two meta-analyses.[32,33] The sensitivity, specificity, and likelihood ratios of bedside tests available to diagnose UTIs in children are summarized in Table 69-2.

Dipstick tests are convenient and inexpensive and require little training for proper use, but they may miss some children with UTI (88% sensitivity at best).[33] Furthermore, a positive leukocyte esterase test does not always confirm the diagnosis of UTI.

Microscopic examination requires more equipment and training than dipstick tests do. Traditionally, a centrifuged sample of unstained urine is examined for the presence of bacteria and white cells. The accuracy of microscopic analysis is improved by using (1) an uncentrifuged specimen,[32] (2) a Gram-stained specimen,[33] and (3) a hemocytometer (results reported as white blood cells/mm³).[34] Examination of urine with these three techniques has been termed "enhanced urinalysis."[34] In young children, in whom prompt diagnosis and treatment are paramount, enhanced urinalysis offers the best combination of sensitivity and specificity. A child with neither pyuria nor bacteriuria on enhanced urinalysis is very unlikely to have a UTI, whereas a child with both pyuria and bacteriuria is very likely to have a UTI.

UTI is best defined as significant bacteriuria on urine culture in a patient with abnormal urinalysis findings (leukocyturia or bacteriuria). Determination of "significant" bacteriuria by culture depends on the method of collection. Guidelines are provided in Table 69-3.

A high white blood cell count or elevated C-reactive protein does not reliably differentiate between children with cystitis and pyelonephritis. Accordingly, these tests are not necessary in the initial evaluation of children with suspected UTIs. Determination of serum creatinine is appropriate in a child with multiple UTIs and suspected renal involvement. Although 4% to 9%[35,36] of infants with UTI are bacteremic and although fever in bacteremic infants with UTI may persist on average 1 day longer than in nonbacteremic children,[37] the organisms isolated from blood and urine are identical, as is the prognosis. For this reason, routine performance of a blood culture in children older than 2 months with a UTI is not necessary because it does not alter management in the vast majority of children. Children younger than 1 month with high fever and abnormal urinalysis results should undergo lumbar puncture as part of the initial evaluation inasmuch as some neonates (≈1%) with UTI may also have bacterial meningitis.[38]

COURSE OF ILLNESS

In two large studies, details of the hospital course were documented. Mean time to defervescence was approximately 24 hours.[39] Approximately 90% of children were afebrile by 48 hours, and only 5% of children remained febrile for longer than 72 hours.[40] None of the follow-up urine cultures, including cultures from children with fever that lasted longer than 48 hours, were positive. No renal abscesses were found. Since the incidence of renal abscess formation is very low,

Table 69-2 Diagnostic Indicators of Urinary Tract Infection					
	Sensitivity	Specificity	Positive Likelihood Ratio	1/Negative Likelihood Ratio	Reference
Dipstick					
Leukocyte esterase (LE)	84%	78%	4	5	33
Nitrite	50%	98%	25	2	33
Nitrite or LE	88%	93%	13	8	33
Nitrite and LE	72%	96%	18	3	33
Microscopy					
Uncentrifuged					
Pyuria (<10/mm³) (all ages)	77%	89%	7	4	33
Pyuria (<10/mm³) (>2 yr)	90%	95%	18	10	33, 34
Bacteriuria (by Gram stain)	93%	95%	19	14	33
Overall (P and B)*	85%	99.9%	85	7	33
Overall (P or B)	95%	89%	9	17	33
Centrifuged					
Pyuria (<5/hpf)	67%	79%	3	2	33
Bacteriuria	81%	83%	5	5	30
Overall (P and B)	66%	99%	7	2	34

*Represents enhanced urinalysis.
B, bacteriuria; hpf, high-power field; P, pyuria.

Table 69-3   Guidelines for Determining Urinary Tract Infection from Quantitative Urine Cultures

| Method of Collection | COLONY-FORMING UNITS PER MILLILITER | | |
	Definite*	Indeterminant†	Contaminant
Suprapubic	Any growth		Growth of nonpathogens Mixed culture‡
Catheterization	>50,000	10,000–50,000, single pathogen	Growth of nonpathogens Mixed culture‡ <10,000
Clean catch	>100,000	50,000–100,000, single pathogen	Growth of nonpathogens Mixed culture‡ <10,000

*If accompanied by abnormal urinalysis findings (leukocyturia or bacteriuria).
†Need to obtain a repeat specimen.
‡Mixed culture = uropathogen + nonpathogen *or* two uropathogens.

Table 69-4   Imaging Studies in Children

Diagnostic Study	Purpose/Indications	Comments
Renal ultrasound	To determine the presence of anatomic abnormalities or complications of UTI such as renal abscess	Currently not recommended with a 1st UTI if normal prenatal ultrasound results (beyond 30 weeks' gestation)*

Voiding cystourethrogram
  Radiographic
  Nuclear
	To determine the presence of VUR or urinary outflow obstruction	Currently recommended with/after a 1st UTI to determine the presence of VUR

Renal scintigraphy (DMSA scan)	To determine the presence of pyelonephritis or extent of renal scarring	Not routinely performed; may be useful in the diagnosis and management of certain children
Intravenous pyelogram	To determine the ability of the kidneys to filter and excrete radiopaque material and to delineate the anatomy of the urinary system	Rarely used in children Adequate hydration and good renal function must be ensured before conducting this study

*See text regarding clarification of this recommendation.
DMSA, 99mTc-labeled dimercaptosuccinic acid; UTI, urinary tract infection; VUR, vesicoureteral reflux.

children who are clinically improving do not routinely need a repeat urine culture or a renal ultrasound despite persistent fever. A renal ultrasound is indicated in children who are clinically deteriorating.

TREATMENT

Treatment of children with presumed UTI depends on a number of factors, including age, degree of toxicity, presence of vomiting, duration of fever, underlying disorders, availability of outpatient follow-up, and antimicrobial resistance patterns in the community.

The probable organisms and local resistance patterns should guide the practitioner in the choice of initial antimicrobial agent. Gram staining of urine, if readily available, provides additional guidance for this choice. Given that *E. coli* is the most common pathogen causing UTI and that many *E. coli* strains are resistant to amoxicillin or ampicillin (≈50%),[38,41] these agents cannot be recommended routinely

for the empirical treatment of a young child with UTI. First-generation cephalosporins,[38] amoxicillin-clavulanate or ampicillin-sulbactam,[40] and trimethoprim-sulfamethoxazole[38,42] should be used with caution because increasing rates of resistance to these antibiotics have been reported in some communities. Alternatives include second- and third-generation cephalosporins and gentamicin, although they would not be good choices if enterococcus is a probable pathogen. Quinolones are effective and resistance is rare, but safety of these antimicrobials in children is still under study, so quinolones are not appropriate choices for first-line therapy at this time. The ultimate choice of antimicrobial therapy should be based on the resistance pattern of the organism or organisms cultured from the patient's urine.

Currently, routine imaging is recommended for children less than 3 years of age with their first febrile UTI, and boys with an afebrile UTI. Evidence supporting the utility of routine imaging studies in children, however, is limited. The various imaging studies available provide different diagnostic information, as depicted in Table 69-4.

Renal ultrasonography is a noninvasive test that does not expose the patient to ionizing radiation. It can demonstrate the size and shape of the kidneys and the presence of duplication and dilation of the ureters, gross anatomic abnormalities, or renal abscess. However, routine ultrasonography in the setting of a first UTI is being reconsidered. In a prospective study of 306 children younger than 2 years with their first UTI in whom ultrasound and voiding cystourethrography (VCUG) were performed, the results of renal ultrasound did not identify obstruction nor alter patient management in any instance.[16] In addition, most children with obstructive uropathy are now identified through prenatal ultrasonography. Furthermore, renal ultrasound is not reliable in detecting renal scarring or VUR.[16] Therefore, routine performance of renal ultrasonography after the diagnosis of a first UTI in children with normal prenatal ultrasonographic findings (beyond 30 weeks' gestation) is not recommended.

VCUG is an excellent test to establish the presence and degree of VUR. Two types of VCUG are available: fluoroscopic (radiographic) contrast VCUG and radionuclide (nuclear) VCUG. The procedures involve catheterization to fill the bladder with either a radiopaque or radioactive liquid and then imaging to detect VUR during voiding. Radiographic VCUG allows precise determination of the grade of VUR, whereas nuclear VCUG can only grossly categorize the degree of VUR. Either study can identify outflow obstruction. The amount of radiation exposure used to be less with nuclear VCUG, but this largely depends on the technique and equipment used. Although medical management of children with VUR and UTI includes ongoing antibiotic prophylaxis, it is not clearly established that this provides long-term benefit (reduced renal scarring and reduced risk for hypertension, renal dysfunction, or renal failure later in life). Therefore, the utility of routine VCUG in the evaluation of children with UTI has recently been questioned.[16] Until a large randomized placebo-controlled treatment trial of antimicrobial prophylaxis for VUR is conducted, the current recommendation is for children younger than 3 years with a febrile UTI to have VCUG performed.

The timing of VCUG is often questioned regarding the reliability of the results and need for a test of cure before performing the study. In two of the studies, rates of VUR and the severity of VUR were compared in patients who had VCUG performed "early" (<7 days) or "late" (>7 days) from the time of hospitalization for UTI. Neither the incidence nor the severity of VUR varied according to the timing of the test. A key finding in one of these studies was that 100% of children in the "early" group had VCUG performed, whereas in the late group, the "no show" rate was 50%, even though the tests were scheduled for the patient before discharge.[35,43-45] For these reasons, there is an increasing push to perform VCUG before discharge.

Renal scintigraphy with technetium 99m–labeled dimercaptosuccinic acid (DMSA) is used to detect acute pyelonephritis and renal scarring. DMSA is injected intravenously, and uptake by the renal tubules is measured 2 to 4 hours later. An area of decreased uptake represents an area of pyelonephritis or scarring. Scans may be used in the acute setting to determine the degree and site of involvement. Most initial areas of decreased uptake on DMSA resolve on follow-up.[46] DMSA scanning may also be used to determine the presence and extent of scarring on follow-up. DMSA scans have been shown to be several times more sensitive in the detection of renal scarring than intravenous pyelography. Although some experts recommend prophylactic antimicrobial therapy when a DMSA scan shows a pattern consistent with acute pyelonephritis, the benefits of this strategy have not been evaluated. Because the majority of young febrile children with UTI, in whom imaging is recommended, have pyelonephritis, one strategy is for the clinician to assume that all have pyelonephritis and act accordingly. In most cases, the additional information provided by scintigraphy does not lead to a change in the management or follow-up of patients with pyelonephritis, and its routine use may not be justified. Its use may be warranted in the acute setting if urinalysis and culture results are equivocal. Similarly, the use of follow-up scintigraphy to establish the presence of scarring is not routinely necessary.

ADMISSION CRITERIA

Traditionally, young children with pyelonephritis were managed as inpatients. In a double-blind randomized controlled trial of 306 children 1 to 24 months of age with a febrile UTI, rates of symptom resolution, reinfection, and renal scarring were no different in children receiving an oral third-generation cephalosporin or intravenous therapy.[35] This study would indicate that most infants older than 2 months with pyelonephritis may be managed safely as outpatients with close follow-up.

The following children should be hospitalized:

- Those with vomiting who cannot tolerate oral medications or cannot maintain adequate hydration
- Those who have significant underlying medical disorders that may complicate management of the underlying illness or the UTI
- Those with inadequate outpatient support or follow-up
- Those who have responded inadequately to outpatient therapy

DISCHARGE CRITERIA

Children who are clinically improving and who are tolerating oral feeding may be discharged from the hospital on a regimen of oral antibiotics. Follow-up studies (e.g., VCUG) may be completed before discharge or scheduled on an outpatient basis.

POSTDISCHARGE CONSIDERATIONS

Children with Recurrent Urinary Tract Symptoms

Approximately 8% to 30% of children with UTI experience one or more symptomatic reinfections,[35,45,47] usually within the first 6 months after the initial UTI, and require prompt reevaluation. Prompt recognition and treatment of UTIs may be the most important factor in the prevention of renal scarring. Routine surveillance of asymptomatic children with monthly urine studies has not been shown to be associated with a better prognosis and is therefore not recommended. Children with recurrent febrile UTIs may be candidates for low-dose long-term antimicrobial therapy, although there is no evidence demonstrating the efficacy of this approach. When these children present with fever without a clear focus of infection, evaluation for possible UTI is strongly recommended.

Children with Vesicoureteral Reflux

The goal of treating VUR is to prevent progressive renal damage. The majority of young children with VUR will have low-grade VUR (grades 1 to 3), which will often resolve spontaneously as the child ages. Children with grades 4 and 5 VUR and older children are less likely to experience spontaneous resolution. Children with VUR have traditionally been treated either medically, with low-dose long-term antimicrobials, or surgically. Surgical treatment involves reimplantation of the ureter or ureters into the bladder and creation of a longer mucosal tunnel. Several large prospective studies[18,48] have demonstrated that the incidence of renal scarring in children with persistent grade 3 and 4 VUR is equivalent in medically and surgically treated children. Therefore, it has been recommended[19] that young children with mild to moderate VUR receive treatment with low-dose long-term antimicrobials until resolution of VUR. Antimicrobial agents most appropriate for prophylaxis include trimethoprim-sulfamethoxazole and nitrofurantoin in half the usual therapeutic doses given once daily.[49]

The routine use of long-term antimicrobial therapy in children with mild or moderate VUR has recently been questioned. A significant proportion of children receiving antimicrobial prophylaxis continue to have breakthrough febrile UTIs (30%)[18,48] and scarring (6% to 32% by intravenous pyelography). Furthermore, approximately 10% of children treated with long-term antimicrobials experienced adverse reactions, mostly gastrointestinal and dermatologic, and most adverse events occurred in the first 6 months of therapy.[49,50] No experimental trial to date has satisfactorily compared long-term antimicrobial prophylaxis with placebo in children with VUR. Perhaps prompt treatment of intercurrent episodes of UTI and treatment of underlying dysfunctional elimination, if present, will prove to be as effective as antimicrobial prophylaxis in the care of children with UTI and VUR. Until more research occurs in this area, we recommend antimicrobial prophylaxis for children with VUR until repeat VCUG demonstrates resolution of VUR.

Older children with persistent severe VUR (grades 4 or 5) and those with lesser degrees of VUR but with progressive scarring while receiving prophylaxis may benefit from ureteral reimplantation. The efficacy of endoscopic therapy, a newer, less invasive modality, is currently under investigation. This procedure involves the use of an endoscope introduced via the urethra to implant dextranomer/hyaluronic acid (Deflux) underneath the refluxing ureter.

Determination of children at risk for renal damage from childhood UTI remains difficult. Renal scarring is currently the best indicator of renal damage in children. The long-term significance of scarring identified by DMSA remains to be determined. Modifiable risk factors for renal scarring include pyelonephritis, VUR, and DES. Close attention to these three factors in children with a history of UTI may help prevent further renal compromise.

IN A NUTSHELL

- UTI is the most frequent serious bacterial infection in childhood.
- UTI should be suspected in young children presenting with fever.
- Collection of urine with a bag should be discouraged.
- Enhanced urinalysis is the most accurate bedside test for UTI.
- Dysfunctional elimination is an underrecognized risk factor for UTI.

ON THE HORIZON

- Efficacy and safety of endoscopic subureteral injection in the treatment of VUR.
- Multicenter VUR study to determine the utility of antibiotic prophylaxis.

SUGGESTED READING

Hoberman A, Chao HP, Keller DM, et al: Prevalence of urinary tract infection in febrile infants. J Pediatr 1993;123:17-23.

Hoberman A, Charron M, Hickey RW, et al: Imaging studies after a first febrile urinary tract infection in young children. N Engl J Med 2003;348:195-202.

Hoberman A, Wald ER, Penchansky L, et al: Enhanced urinalysis as a screening test for urinary tract infection. Pediatrics 1993;91:1196-1199.

Koff SA, Wagner TT, Jayanthi VR: The relationship among dysfunctional elimination syndromes, primary vesicoureteral reflux and urinary tract infections in children. J Urol 1998;160:1019-1922.

Shaikh N, Hoberman A, Wise B, et al: Dysfunctional elimination syndrome: Is it related to urinary tract infection or vesicoureteral reflux diagnosed early in life? Pediatrics 2003;112:1134-1137.

Shaw KN, Gorelick M, McGowan KL, et al: Prevalence of urinary tract infection in febrile young children in the emergency department. Pediatrics 1998;102:e16.

REFERENCES

1. Hoberman A, Chao HP, Keller DM, et al: Prevalence of urinary tract infection in febrile infants. J Pediatr 1993;123:17-23.

2. Shaw KN, Gorelick M, McGowan KL, et al: Prevalence of urinary tract infection in febrile young children in the emergency department. Pediatrics 1998;102:e16.

3. Schlager TA, Whittam TS, Hendley JO, et al: Comparison of expression of virulence factors by *Escherichia coli* causing cystitis and *E. coli* colonizing the periurethra of healthy girls. J Infect Dis 1995;172:772-777.

4. Marild S, Wettergren B, Hellstrom M, et al: Bacterial virulence and inflammatory response in infants with febrile urinary tract infection or screening bacteriuria. J Pediatr 1988;112:348-354.

5. To T, Agha M, Dick PT, Feldman W: Cohort study on circumcision of newborn boys and subsequent risk of urinary-tract infection. Lancet 1998;352:1813-1816.

6. Circumcision policy statement. American Academy of Pediatrics. Task Force on Circumcision. Pediatrics 1999;103:686-693.

7. Hellstrom A, Hanson E, Hansson S, et al: Association between urinary symptoms at 7 years old and previous urinary tract infection. Arch Dis Child 1991;66:232-234.

8. Shaikh N, Hoberman A, Wise B, et al: Dysfunctional elimination syndrome: Is it related to urinary tract infection or vesicoureteral reflux diagnosed early in life? Pediatrics 2003;112:1134-1137.

9. Snodgrass W: Relationship of voiding dysfunction to urinary tract infection and vesicoureteral reflux in children. Urology 1991;38:341-344.

10. Naseer SR, Steinhardt GF: New renal scars in children with urinary tract infections, vesicoureteral reflux and voiding dysfunction: A prospective evaluation. J Urol 1997;158:566-568.

11. Wan J, Kaplinsky R, Greenfield S: Toilet habits of children evaluated for urinary tract infection. J Urol 1995;154:797-799.

12. Mazzola BL, von Vigier RO, Marchand S, et al: Behavioral and functional abnormalities linked with recurrent urinary tract infections in girls. J Nephrol 2003;16:133-138.

13. van Gool JD, Hjalmas K, Tamminen-Mobius T, Olbing H: Historical clues to the complex of dysfunctional voiding, urinary tract infection and vesicoureteral reflux. The International Reflux Study in Children. J Urol 1992;148:1699-1702.

14. Koff SA, Wagner TT, Jayanthi VR: The relationship among dysfunctional elimination syndromes, primary vesicoureteral reflux and urinary tract infections in children. J Urol 1998;160:1019-1022.

15. Seruca H: Vesicoureteral reflux and voiding dysfunction: A prospective study. J Urol 1989;142:494-498; discussion 501.

16. Hoberman A, Charron M, Hickey RW, et al: Imaging studies after a first febrile urinary tract infection in young children. N Engl J Med 2003;348:195-202.

17. Arant BS Jr: Medical management of mild and moderate vesicoureteral reflux: Followup studies of infants and young children. A preliminary report of the Southwest Pediatric Nephrology Study Group. J Urol 1992;148:1683-1687.

18. Tamminen-Mobius T, Brunier E, Ebel KD, et al: Cessation of vesicoureteral reflux for 5 years in infants and children allocated to medical treatment. The International Reflux Study in Children. J Urol 1992;148:1662-1666.

19. Elder JS, Peters CA, Arant BS Jr, et al: Pediatric Vesicoureteral Reflux Guidelines Panel summary report on the management of primary vesicoureteral reflux in children. J Urol 1997;157:1846-1851.

20. Garin EH, Campos A, Homsy Y: Primary vesicoureteral reflux: Review of current concepts. Pediatr Nephrol 1998;12:249-256.

21. Alon US, Ganapathy S: Should renal ultrasonography be done routinely in children with first urinary tract infection? Clin Pediatr (Phila) 1999;38:21-25.

22. Dick PT, Feldman W: Routine diagnostic imaging for childhood urinary tract infections: A systematic overview. J Pediatr 1996;128:15-22.

23. Wennerstrom M, Hansson S, Jodal U, et al: Renal function 16 to 26 years after the first urinary tract infection in childhood. Arch Pediatr Adolesc Med 2000;154:339-345.

24. Hooton TM, Scholes D, Stapleton AE, et al: A prospective study of asymptomatic bacteriuria in sexually active young women. N Engl J Med 2000;343:992-997.

25. Tambyah PA, Maki DG: Catheter-associated urinary tract infection is rarely symptomatic: A prospective study of 1,497 catheterized patients. Arch Intern Med 2000;160:678-682.

26. Struthers S, Scanlon J, Parker K, et al: Parental reporting of smelly urine and urinary tract infection. Arch Dis Child 2003;88:250-252.

27. Pylkkanen J, Vilska J, Koskimies O: Diagnostic value of symptoms and clean-voided urine specimen in childhood urinary tract infection. Acta Paediatr Scand 1979;68:341-344.

28. Craig JC, Irwig LM, Knight JF, et al: Symptomatic urinary tract infection in preschool Australian children. J Paediatr Child Health 1998;34:154-159.

29. Smellie JM, Poulton A, Prescod NP: Retrospective study of children with renal scarring associated with reflux and urinary infection. BMJ 1994;308:1193-1196.

30. Downs SM: Technical report: Urinary tract infections in febrile infants and young children. The Urinary Tract Subcommittee of the American Academy of Pediatrics Committee on Quality Improvement. Pediatrics 1999;103:e54.

31. Al-Orifi F, McGillivray D, Tange S, Kramer MS: Urine culture from bag specimens in young children: Are the risks too high? J Pediatr 2000;137:221-226.

32. Huicho L, Campos-Sanchez M, Alamo C: Metaanalysis of urine screening tests for determining the risk of urinary tract infection in children. Pediatr Infect Dis J 2002;21:1-11, 88.

33. Gorelick MH, Shaw KN: Screening tests for urinary tract infection in children: A meta-analysis. Pediatrics 1999;104:e54.

34. Hoberman A, Wald ER, Penchansky L, et al: Enhanced urinalysis as a screening test for urinary tract infection. Pediatrics 1993;91:1196-1199.

35. Allen UD, MacDonald N, Fuite L, et al: Risk factors for resistance to "first-line" antimicrobials among urinary tract isolates of *Escherichia coli* in children. Can Med Assoc J 1999;160:1436-1440.

36. Honkinen O, Jahnukainen T, Mertsola J, et al: Bacteremic urinary tract infection in children. Pediatr Infect Dis J 2000;19:630-634.

37. Bachur R, Caputo GL: Bacteremia and meningitis among infants with urinary tract infections. Pediatr Emerg Care 1995;11:280-284.

38. Goldraich NP, Manfroi A: Febrile urinary tract infection: *Escherichia coli* susceptibility to oral antimicrobials. Pediatr Nephrol 2002;17:173-176.

39. Hoberman A, Wald ER, Hickey RW, et al: Oral versus initial intravenous therapy for urinary tract infections in young febrile children. Pediatrics 1999;104:79-86.

40. Bachur R, Harper MB: Reliability of the urinalysis for predicting urinary tract infections in young febrile children. Arch Pediatr Adolesc Med 2001;155:60-65.

41. McLoughlin TG Jr, Joseph MM: Antibiotic resistance patterns of uropathogens in pediatric emergency department patients. Acad Emerg Med 2003;10:347-351.

42. Ladhani S, Gransden W: Increasing antibiotic resistance among urinary tract isolates. Arch Dis Child 2003;88:444-445.

43. Mahant S, To T, Friedman J: Timing of voiding cystourethrogram in the investigation of urinary tract infections in children. J Pediatr 2001;139:568-571.

44. Winberg J, Andersen HJ, Bergstrom T, et al: Epidemiology of symptomatic urinary tract infection in childhood. Acta Paediatr Scand Suppl 1974;252:1-20.

45. Ditchfield MR, Summerville D, Grimwood K, et al: Time course of transient cortical scintigraphic defects associated with acute pyelonephritis. Pediatr Radiol 2002;32:849-852.

46. Bachur R: Nonresponders: Prolonged fever among infants with urinary tract infections. Pediatrics 2000;105(5):E59.

47. Panaretto K, Craig J, Knight J, et al: Risk factors for recurrent urinary tract infection in preschool children. J Paediatr Child Health 1999;35:454-459.

48. Weiss R, Duckett J, Spitzer A: Results of a randomized clinical trial of medical versus surgical management of infants and children with grades III and IV primary vesicoureteral reflux (United States). The International Reflux Study in Children. J Urol 1992;148:1667-1673.

49. Williams GJ, Lee A, Craig JC: Long-term antibiotics for preventing recurrent urinary tract infection in children. Cochrane Database Syst Rev 2001;4:CD001534.

50. Uhari M, Nuutinen M, Turtinen J: Adverse reactions in children during long-term antimicrobial therapy. Pediatr Infect Dis J 1996;15:404-408.

CHAPTER 70

Bone, Joint, and Soft Tissue Infections

Gary Frank and Stephen C. Eppes

Most soft tissue infections can be managed successfully in the outpatient setting. However, soft tissue infections with signs of systemic illness or infections involving bones or joints often require hospitalization for timely and definitive diagnosis, subspecialty consultation, or prompt initiation of optimal therapy.

NECROTIZING FASCIITIS

Necrotizing fasciitis (also known as hospital gangrene or hemolytic streptococcal gangrene) is a rapidly progressive, deep-seated infection of the subcutaneous soft tissues that can involve any part of the body. Infection spreads in the plane between the subcutaneous tissue and the superficial muscle fascia, resulting in the progressive destruction of fascia and fat. It often follows a fulminant course and has a high mortality rate. These characteristics led the British tabloids to label necrotizing fasciitis the disease of "flesh-eating bacteria." In fact, necrotizing fasciitis was first described by Hippocrates in the 5th century BC when he wrote, "flesh, sinews and bones fell away in large quantities. The flux which formed was not like pus but a different sort of putrefaction with a copious and varied flux. . . . There were many deaths."[1]

Although there have been more than 500 cases of necrotizing fasciitis reported in North America,[2] it is an uncommon disease whose true incidence is not known. An increased frequency is reported in diabetics, intravenous drug users, alcoholics, immunosuppressed patients, and patients with peripheral vascular disease, but necrotizing fasciitis also occurs in young, previously healthy patients, including children. Mortality rates as high as 50% have been reported, but they tend to be much lower in children.[3]

Although group A β-hemolytic streptococcus (GABHS) is the most common organism identified in children with necrotizing fasciitis, the disease is often polymicrobial, involving gram-negative bacilli, enterococci, streptococci, *Staphylococcus aureus,* and anaerobes such as *Bacteroides, Peptostreptococcus,* and *Clostridium* species (Table 70-1).

Necrotizing fasciitis has been reported in a number of cases as a complication of varicella infection.[4] Other predisposing factors include trauma, surgery, burns, and eczema. In neonates, necrotizing fasciitis may complicate omphalitis or circumcision.

The multiple names and causes of necrotizing fasciitis are a common source of confusion. Necrotizing fasciitis type 1 is a mixed infection of anaerobes, gram-negative aerobic bacilli, and enterococci; it is often seen postoperatively or in patients with diabetes mellitus or peripheral vascular disease. Necrotizing fasciitis type 2 is an infection with GABHS that may occur postoperatively or as a result of penetrating trauma, varicella infection, burns, or minor cuts; it is characterized by rapidly extending necrosis as well as systemic toxicity, which can rapidly lead to multiorgan failure and shock. Necrotizing fasciitis type 3 is caused by marine *Vibrio* species that enter through skin lesions exposed to seawater or marine animals.

A number of other related syndromes have been described. Fournier gangrene (named after French dermatologist Jean Alfred Fournier) is necrotizing fasciitis of the scrotum. Gas gangrene is the result of clostridial infection (*Clostridium perfringens, Clostridium histolyticum, Clostridium septicum*) that is often secondary to trauma or crush injury. It is a myonecrotic disease that quickly leads to systemic toxicity and shock. Meleney synergistic gangrene is a slowly progressive infection of the dermis and occasionally the fascia that is characterized by a chronic enlarging ulcer due to infection with *S. aureus* and microaerophilic streptococci.

An association between the use of nonsteroidal anti-inflammatory drugs (NSAIDs) and necrotizing fasciitis has been reported.[5] However, given the frequency of NSAID use worldwide, most authors believe that patients with necrotizing fasciitis used NSAIDs for their analgesic and anti-inflammatory properties and that a true cause-and-effect relationship is unlikely.

Clinical Presentation

In children, necrotizing fasciitis often presents 1 to 4 days after trauma. Other common associated factors are contamination of a surgical wound, omphalitis, and varicella infection. Less common associated factors include insect bite, perirectal abscess, incarcerated hernia, and subcutaneous insulin injection. Necrotizing fasciitis may also occur with a preceding streptococcal pharyngitis or without any previous evidence of trauma or infection.

Patients with necrotizing fasciitis present initially with soft tissue swelling and pain near the infected area. When associated with varicella, the findings typically begin 3 to 4 days after the onset of the exanthem. Infants and toddlers may be extremely fussy or irritable. Toddlers and young children may present with a limp or refusal to bear weight if a lower extremity or the lower trunk is involved. Initially, pain with manipulation of an affected extremity or tenderness with palpation of the affected area tends to be out of proportion to the cutaneous signs of infection.

Induration and edema are generally apparent within the first 24 hours, followed rapidly by blistering and bleb formation. Extension of the infection along fascial planes leads to necrosis of the superficial muscle fascia and the deeper layers of the dermis. Destruction and thrombosis of the small blood vessels in the area lead to necrosis of the surrounding tissues. The skin takes on a dusky appearance, and a thick, foul-smelling fluid is noted if drainage occurs. Destruction of nerves may lead to anesthesia of the overly-

Table 70-1	Bacteria Associated with Necrotizing Fasciitis
Category	Organism
Gram-positive aerobes	Group A β-hemolytic streptococci
	Staphylococcus aureus
	Other *Staphylococcus* and
	Streptococcus species
	Enterococci
Gram-negative aerobes	*Escherichia coli*
	Pseudomonas aeruginosa
	Enterobacter cloacae
	Klebsiella species
	Proteus species
	Serratia species
	Acinetobacter calcoaceticus
	Citrobacter freundii
	Pasteurella multocida
Anaerobes	*Bacteroides* species
	Clostridium species
	Vibrio species
	Peptostreptococcus species

Adapted from Green RJ, Dafoe DC, Raffin TA: Necrotizing fasciitis. Chest 1996;110:219-229.

ing skin. High fevers are common. Severe systemic toxicities include renal and hepatic failure, acute respiratory distress syndrome, and decreased myocardial contractility.

Diagnosis and Evaluation

White blood cell counts may be normal or elevated, but there is often a pronounced bandemia. Thrombocytopenia and evidence of a coagulopathy may also be apparent. Hypocalcemia may occur due to necrosis and saponification of subcutaneous fat. Anaerobic and aerobic blood cultures should be obtained, although they are frequently negative. Other initial laboratory studies to consider include serum electrolytes, arterial blood gas, and urinalysis.

Plain radiographs may show gas or soft tissue edema but are otherwise nonspecific. Although computed tomography (CT) may be useful in defining the extent of soft tissue involvement, magnetic resonance imaging (MRI) is the preferred modality. However, imaging studies should not delay surgical intervention.

Surgeons may note the ability to easily pass an instrument along a fascial plane. Aerobic and anaerobic cultures should be obtained. Frozen section biopsies can be extremely helpful in making a timely diagnosis.

Treatment

Emergent wide surgical débridement is critical and may need to be repeated in 24 to 48 hours. Delays in surgery are associated with increased mortality, and antibiotic therapy in the absence of surgical débridement is ineffective.

Gram stain of surgical or aspirated material from the infected site may be helpful in guiding the selection of antibiotics. In patients with suspected GABHS infection, the antibiotic regimen should include penicillin (150,000 U/kg per day, divided every 4 to 6 hours) and clindamycin

(40 mg/kg per day, divided every 6 hours). Clindamycin is added for the Eagle effect, which can be explained as follows: Group A streptococcus initially proliferates rapidly until a steady state of growth is reached. β-Lactam antibiotics are less effective during the steady-state phase, because they inhibit cell wall synthesis of actively replicating organisms. Clindamycin, however, is not affected by the decreased growth rate, and it also reduces toxin synthesis at the ribosomal level. In patients with polymicrobial infections, consider a β-lactam–β-lactamase inhibitor combination such as ampicillin-sulbactam or piperacillin-tazobactam.

Supportive therapy includes careful fluid management, pain control, and, if present, management of multisystem organ failure, usually in an intensive care setting. Patients with group A streptococcal necrotizing fasciitis are at risk for toxic shock syndrome, and many experts recommend intravenous immunoglobulin in this situation. The role of hyperbaric oxygen therapy is controversial. Patients who survive may require amputation, skin grafting, or reconstructive surgery.

Discharge Criteria

- No evidence of systemic toxicity, such as fever or hypotension.
- No evidence of active local infection.
- Surgical wounds should be healing well.
- Ability to complete antibiotic therapy as an outpatient.

In A Nutshell

- Presentation: rapidly progressive infection of the subcutaneous tissues, which often follows a fulminant course and has a high mortality rate.
- Diagnosis: generally clinical; radiologic studies may be helpful but should not delay surgical intervention.
- Treatment: aggressive surgical débridement, appropriate intravenous antibiotics, and supportive therapy for multisystem organ failure.

OSTEOMYELITIS

Osteomyelitis is an infection of the bone and bone marrow that is generally bacterial in origin. The most common form in childhood is acute hematogenous osteomyelitis (AHO), which affects children younger than 5 years in about 50% of cases.[6,7] The incidence of AHO is approximately 60 in 100,000 children,[8] and boys are about twice as likely to be affected as girls.[6,7] The majority of cases occur in long bones, with the femur and tibia accounting for almost half of all cases. Most cases are limited to a single site.

S. aureus is the most commonly identified organism, accounting for 60% to 89% of cases of AHO,[9,10] with GABHS next in frequency. In the past, *Haemophilus influenzae* accounted for 5% to 7% of cases,[6,9,10] but the advent of effective immunization has decreased this incidence dramatically. *Streptococcus pneumoniae* is another relatively common organism in patients with AHO. *Kingella kingae* is a common cause of osteomyelitis in the Middle East and is being recognized increasingly in the United States. Osteomyelitis due to *K. kingae* tends to occur in young children following an upper respiratory tract infection or stomatitis. Group B streptococcus and enteric gram-negative organisms such as *Escherichia coli* may be identified in neonates with osteomyelitis but are rare in older children. *Salmonella* species are commonly identified in patients with sickle cell disease, and *Pseudomonas aeruginosa* is often identified in cases of osteochondritis following puncture wounds of the feet. Mycobacteria and fungi are rare causes of osteomyelitis. *Bartonella henselae* is an atypical cause of osteomyelitis in patients with cat-scratch disease.

Several routes of infection are hypothesized in the pathogenesis of osteomyelitis. In children, most cases result from hematogenous spread after a transient episode of bacteremia. About one third of patients report a history of blunt trauma,[9] which increases the likelihood of seeding an infection during an episode of bacteremia. Direct inoculation of bacteria into bone may occur during surgery or as a result of penetrating trauma.

Osteomyelitis most commonly begins in the metaphysis of long bones, which are highly vascular structures. Certain bacteria such as *S. aureus* adhere to bone by expressing receptors (adhesins) for a component of the bone matrix. Growing colonies of bacteria surround themselves with a protective glycocalyx, shielding them from circulating white blood cells. As infection advances, cortical bone is destroyed, and infection and inflammation may extend into the subperiosteal space.

The periosteum in young infants is thin and is not tightly adherent to the underlying bone. As a result, the periosteum is more likely to perforate, spreading infection into the surrounding tissues. In young infants, blood vessels extend into the epiphyses, which increases the likelihood of growth plate damage as well as septic arthritis. The hips and shoulders are common sites of epiphyseal infection.

Clinical Presentation

Patients often present after experiencing symptoms for days to weeks, most commonly complaining of fever and pain at the affected site. Infants and toddlers may present with irritability, refusal to bear weight on or use an extremity, or limp. Erythema, warmth, and swelling of the affected site may be noted. Young patients may present with a fever of unknown origin.

Differential Diagnosis

The differential diagnosis for osteomyelitis includes cellulitis, septic arthritis, toxic synovitis, thrombophlebitis, trauma, fracture, rheumatologic disease such as juvenile rheumatoid arthritis, pain crisis in sickle cell disease, Ewing sarcoma, osteosarcoma, and leukemia.

Diagnosis and Evaluation

A complete blood count is likely to reveal a leukocytosis with a left shift, as well as reactive thrombocytosis. Inflammatory markers such as the erythrocyte sedimentation rate (ESR) and C-reactive protein are usually elevated and can be used to follow response to therapy. Needle aspiration is likely to yield an organism in approximately 70% of cases,[9,11] whereas blood cultures are positive in 36% to 55% of cases.[7,11] Open procedures involving metaphyseal drilling may enhance the yield and can also be therapeutic.

The value of various imaging techniques is summarized in Table 70-2. For plain radiographs (Fig. 70-1), the yield depends on the duration of active disease. In the first 3 days, these films may reveal soft tissue swelling; by days 3 to 7, swelling of the surrounding muscle leads to obliteration of the normally translucent fat planes. Osteolytic lesions are generally not apparent until days 10 to 21, at which point there has been greater than 50% loss of bone density.[12]

Nuclear scintigraphy is helpful in young patients who are unable to verbalize the location of their pain, when multiple sites are suspected, and in differentiating osteomyelitis from cellulitis (see Fig. 70-1). Technetium 99m methylene diphosphonate has increased uptake in areas of osteoblastic activity, and the three-phase bone scan is the study of choice. Gallium 67 citrate may be used in conjunction with technetium but is not specific for infection. Tagged leukocyte scans (e.g., indium 111 or technetium 99m) can be used but require special technical skills and may yield false-positive results.

CT allows a cross-sectional assessment and can reveal areas of cortical bone destruction, periosteal reaction,

Table 70-2 Advantages and Disadvantages of Imaging Modalities for the Diagnosis of Osteomyelitis		
Modality	Advantages	Disadvantages
Plain radiographs	Inexpensive Quick Easy	Insensitive in early disease
Computed tomography	Improved sensitivity Relatively quick	Radiation exposure May require sedation
Magnetic resonance imaging	Very sensitive, even in early disease May reveal pus collections or extension into adjacent joint or soft tissue	Long study Often requires sedation Expensive
Three-phase nuclear bone scan (technetium 99m methylene diphosphonate)	Very sensitive Identifies multifocal disease May reveal unsuspected sites in preverbal children	Long study Often requires sedation Expensive Radiation exposure

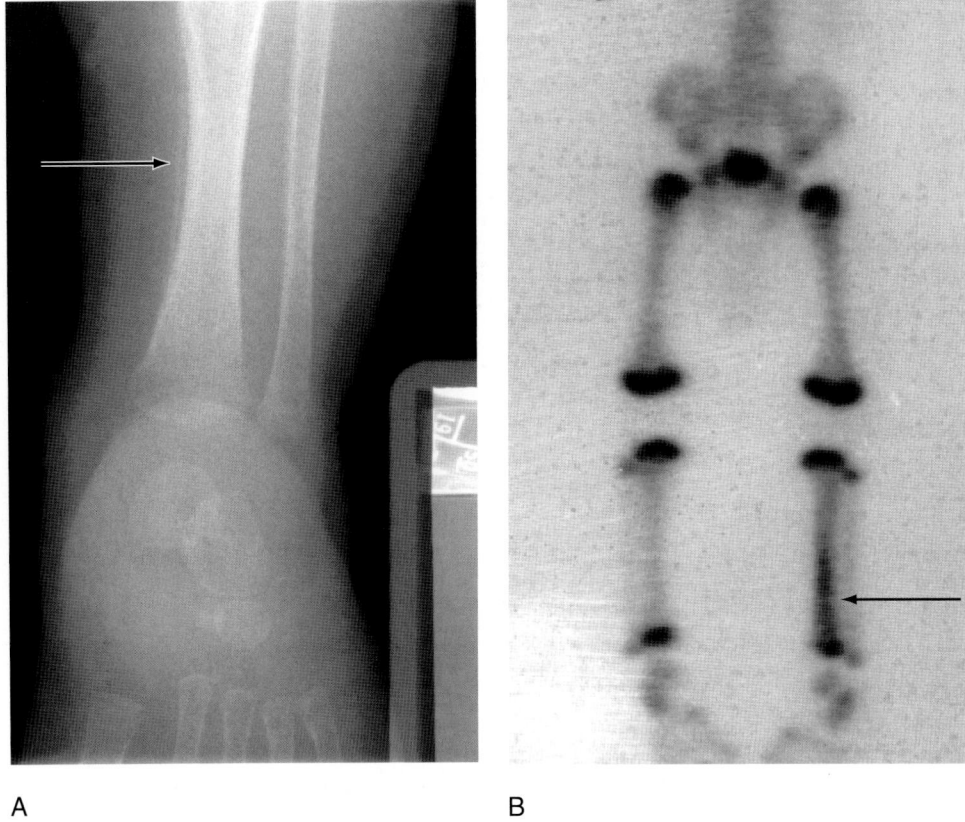

A   B

Figure 70-1 A, Anteroposterior radiograph of the leg in a 6-month-old infant reveals periosteal new bone formation along the tibial diaphysis (*arrow*). B, Anterior bone scan of the same patient reveals increased uptake along the distal tibial diaphysis extending into the metaphysis (*arrow*). These images are consistent with osteomyelitis. (Courtesy of Lisa States, MD, Al duPont Hospital for Children.)

sequestration, and soft tissue abscesses. Images should be obtained with and without enhancement.

With a reported sensitivity as high as 97%,[13] MRI is becoming the modality of choice in patients with a high suspicion for osteomyelitis. Edema and exudate of the medullary space may be noted in early osteomyelitis (Fig. 70-2). Coronal or sagittal images are especially useful for planning surgical procedures and assessing the growth plates and epiphyses. Gadolinium enhancement is recommended.

Treatment

Upon admission, an orthopedist should be consulted, especially if imaging reveals subperiosteal or soft tissue abscesses, sequestra, intramedullary purulence, or involvement of the growth plate. The surgeon's role includes performing the diagnostic procedure, decompression and drainage (when necessary), and long-tem follow-up in complicated cases. Empirical therapy should cover *S. aureus* and GABHS. Traditionally, a semisynthetic penicillinase-resistant penicillin was recommended (e.g., nafcillin or oxacillin 150 to 200 mg/kg per day, divided in four doses). However, a number of recent reports indicate a sharp increase in the number of cases of community-acquired methicillin-resistant *S. aureus* (MRSA) infections. In communities with a high incidence of MRSA, vancomycin should be considered for empirical therapy of osteomyelitis until sensitivities are available. Alternatively, clindamycin may be effective against MRSA, but inducible resistance

(which can be detected by the microbiology laboratory) may reduce its effectiveness.

Neonates with osteomyelitis often have a history of a preceding infection, and about half have involvement of multiple sites. Empirical therapy should cover group B streptococci and enteric gram-negative rods in addition to the pathogens common in older infants and children. A third-generation cephalosporin may be used for empirical therapy, and coverage can be narrowed once culture results and sensitivities are available.

In patients with presumed *Pseudomonas* infection (e.g., puncture wound osteochondritis in the foot), consider an extended-spectrum β-lactam (e.g., ceftazidime, cefepime, piperacillin-tazobactam) plus an aminoglycoside for at least the first 2 weeks. In infants and children up to 5 years old, consider a second- or third-generation cephalosporin (e.g., cefuroxime, cefotaxime, ceftriaxone) for coverage against *S. aureus*, streptococci, and *K. kingae*.

Once an organism has been identified, coverage can be narrowed. The minimum recommended length of treatment is 3 weeks, but most authors recommend treatment for 4 to 6 weeks.[9,14] If long-term intravenous antibiotics will be administered, placement of a peripherally inserted central catheter should be considered. Studies support switching to an oral antibiotic if there is a high likelihood of compliance, an organism has been identified, clinical improvement is noted, the patient is afebrile, and inflammatory markers begin to normalize.

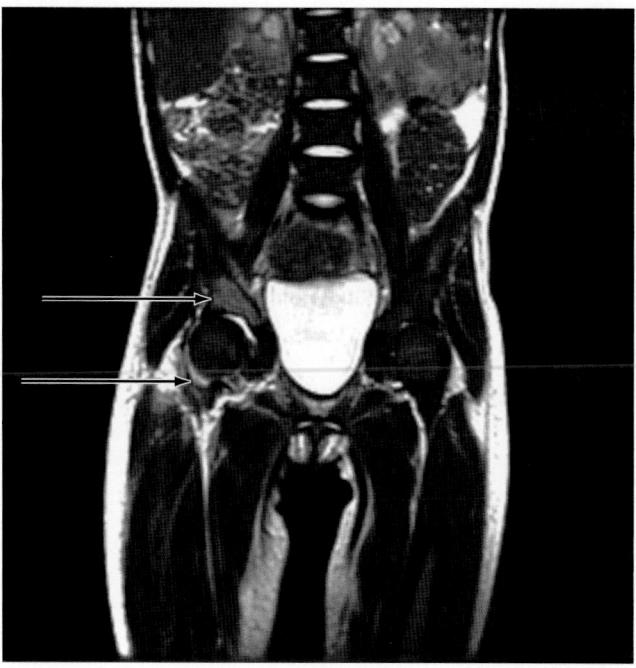

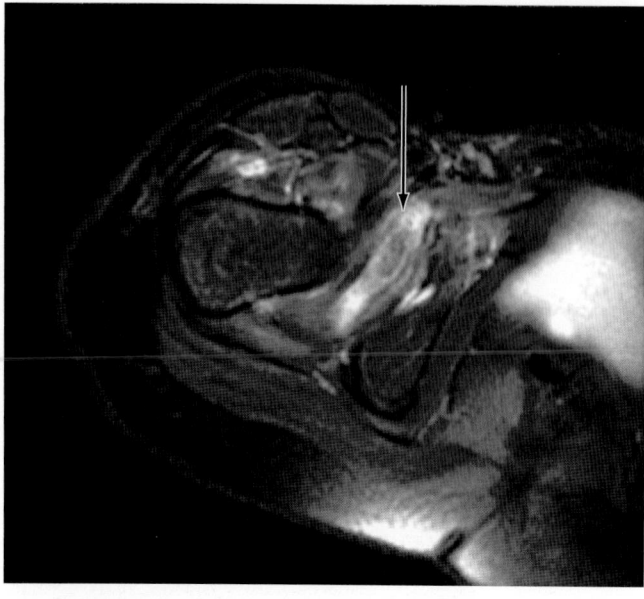

B

A

Figure 70-2 A, T2-weighted coronal MRI scan in a 4-year-old girl demonstrates increased signal in the right ischium due to marrow edema, consistent with osteomyelitis *(upper arrow)*. Also noted is increased signal in the joint space, consistent with a small joint effusion *(lower arrow)*. B, T2-weighted axial image in the same patient reveals increased signal in the deep muscles of the pelvis, consistent with myositis. (Courtesy of Lisa States, MD, Al duPont Hospital for Children.)

When switching to oral antibiotics, two to three times the normal recommended doses are often used. Some authors recommend obtaining serum bactericidal titers to establish an adequate dose.[11] The patient's blood is drawn 1 to 2 hours after administration of the antibiotic, and studies are performed to establish the highest dilution of serum that kills 99.9% of inoculated bacteria after 18 hours of culture. Dilutions of at least 1:8 are desirable.

Special Circumstances
Chronic Osteomyelitis

Two percent to 5% of patients with AHO develop a chronic, suppurative course with intermittent acute exacerbations.[9,14] This occurs more commonly in boys and may develop after an open fracture. Treatment consists of long-term antibiotics (up to 6 to 12 months) and may include surgical débridement, local administration of antibiotics, and reconstructive surgery.

Chronic Recurrent Multifocal Osteomyelitis

Chronic recurrent multifocal osteomyelitis (CRMO) is characterized by recurrent episodes of bony inflammation, pain, and fever with periodic exacerbations and remissions. Cultures are negative, and antibiotics do not alter the course of the disease. CRMO is more common in girls, and the median age of onset is 10 years. CRMO is associated with Sweet syndrome, psoriasis, and pustulosis palmaris et plantaris. Plain radiographs may demonstrate multiple areas of osteolysis and sclerosis, especially in the long bones and clavicles. Treatment generally involves glucocorticoids and

NSAIDs. Other reported therapies include immune modulators, antimetabolites, calcium modulators, colchicine, and hyperbaric oxygen.

Brodie Abscess

A Brodie abscess is a subacute form of osteomyelitis that results in a collection of necrotic bone and pus in a fibrous capsule. It occurs most commonly in the long bones of adolescents. The defect may be seen on plain radiographs, and the ESR is usually elevated. Management involves surgical drainage followed by antibiotic therapy.

Osteomyelitis in Patients with Sickle Hemoglobinopathies

Osteomyelitis may be difficult to differentiate from vaso-occlusive crises in patients with sickle cell disease, because both syndromes can present with fever, bone pain, and tenderness. Spiking fevers above 39°C, chills, toxic appearance, and leukocytosis are indicative of osteomyelitis in this population. Infection can be difficult to differentiate from infarction on imaging studies, and needle aspiration or biopsy of the affected site may be required. In addition to *S. aureus*, *Salmonella* species are common causative agents, and empirical therapy should be chosen accordingly. Prolonged parenteral therapy (at least 6 to 8 weeks) is often required.

Pelvic Osteomyelitis

Osteomyelitis of the pelvis should be considered in children presenting with fever and gait abnormalities. Pain is often localized to the hip, groin, or buttocks, or it may be poorly localized. Patients may also present with abdominal pain mimicking appendicitis. Point tenderness may be elicited over the affected bone, and rocking of the pelvis is often painful. As with other forms of osteomyelitis, *S. aureus* is the most commonly identified organism. Surgical drainage is often required, and antibiotics are continued for at least 4 weeks.

Pseudomonas Osteochondritis

Pseudomonas aeruginosa infection of the bones and cartilage in the feet complicates up to 2% of puncture wounds.[15] *P. aeruginosa* can be found in the linings of sneakers, although infection may occur after puncture wounds through other types of shoes or even bare feet. Management generally involves surgery to remove necrotic cartilage and to obtain a specimen for culture. Traditionally, an intravenous antibiotic with coverage for *Pseudomonas* as well as the more common pathogens (e.g., cefepime, ceftazidime, piperacillin-tazobactam) was used for 7 to 14 days. However, adult studies indicate that oral ciprofloxacin for 7 to 14 days is usually adequate.[15] Anecdotally, the use of prophylactic ciprofloxacin in patients with puncture wounds may prevent the development of osteochondritis.

Spinal Osteomyelitis

Osteomyelitis of the spine may take the form of diskitis or vertebral osteomyelitis. Diskitis is an inflammatory process, usually of a lumbar disk, and is most common in children younger than 5 years. Diskitis generally results from a low-grade bacterial infection, although some authors believe that it can be noninfectious (e.g., following trauma to the spine). Patients may present with a limp, backache, or refusal to walk. Fever is generally absent or low grade. Plain radiographs may demonstrate narrowing of the disk space. Antibiotic therapy should cover *S. aureus* and GABHS and may be given orally for the entire course or intravenously for 5 to 7 days followed by oral administration for another 7 to 14 days.

Vertebral osteomyelitis occurs in 1% to 3% of cases of osteomyelitis and is more common in boys.[16] It may result from hematologic seeding of the vertebrae or through extension of a local infection such as diskitis. *S. aureus* is the most common organism, but others, including *B. henselae* (cat-scratch disease), have been reported. In some areas of the world, tuberculosis of the spine (Pott disease) is not uncommon. Patients may manifest neurologic deficits or loss of normal spinal curvature, and surgery may be required urgently if there is evidence of spinal cord compression. Diagnosis is often based on MRI of the spine. Antibiotics should be administered for at least 4 weeks.

Discharge Criteria

- Afebrile for at least 24 to 48 hours and general clinical improvement.
- Improvement in inflammatory markers such as ESR and C-reactive protein.
- Ability to complete intravenous or oral antibiotic therapy as an outpatient.

In A Nutshell

- Presentation: often presents after days to weeks of symptoms with fever and pain.
- Diagnosis: MRI and triple-phase bone scans are most sensitive for early osteomyelitis.
- Treatment: at least 4 weeks of total antibiotics; some authors advocate switching to oral antibiotics once an organism is identified, sensitivities are available, and clinical improvement is noted.

PYOMYOSITIS

Pyomyositis (also known as tropical myositis and bacterial myositis) is a bacterial infection of skeletal muscle that often results in localized abscess formation. Pyomyositis was well described at the turn of the 20th century as the British and French expanded their colonial empires into tropical parts of Africa and Asia. Although relatively uncommon in more temperate areas such as North America, pyomyositis accounts for up to 4% of surgical admissions in some tropical areas.[17] In North America, the highest incidence of pyomyositis is in the southernmost regions.

Pyomyositis is thought to occur when a transient bacteremia seeds a site of local muscle trauma or strain. Often, patients are able to recall a history of minor trauma or vigorous exercise. In general, the trauma is nonpenetrating, and there is no obvious portal of entry for the infecting organism.

S. aureus is the most commonly identified organism, accounting for more than 90% of cases of pyomyositis in tropical areas and approximately 70% of cases in more temperate regions.[18,19] GABHS, nonhemolytic streptococcal species, and certain gram-negative rods (e.g., *E. coli, Salmonella enteritidis*) also account for a significant number of cases (Box 70-1). Clostridial infections can lead to a fulminant form of myonecrosis that is often fatal. Additionally, a number of nonbacterial organisms are associated with infectious myositis syndromes, such as transient acute myositis and chronic inflammatory myositis (Table 70-3).

Although pyomyositis can occur in all age groups, including neonates and the elderly, it is reported most commonly in children and young adults. There is a 2:1 to 3:1 male predominance,[18,20] although the incidence seems to be increasing in females as more women participate in com-

---

Box 70-1 Bacterial Causes of Pyomyositis

Staphylococcus aureus
Group A β-hemolytic streptococci
Other *Staphylococcus* and *Streptococcus* species
Esherichia coli
Salmonella enteritidis
Clostridium species
Serratia species
Klebsiella species
Yersinia species
Pasteurella species
Mycobacterium tuberculosis

Table 70–3 Nonbacterial Causes of Infectious Myositis	
Category	Organism
Viral	Enteroviruses
	Influenza viruses
	Parainfluenza viruses
	Herpesviruses
	Human immunodeficiency virus
Fungal	*Candida albicans*
Parasitic	*Trichinella spiralis*
	Toxoplasma gondii
	Taenia solium

petitive sports. Although pyomyositis occurs most frequently in young, healthy individuals, there is an increased incidence in patients with chronic diseases such as diabetes mellitus, autoimmune diseases, and immunodeficiency syndromes.

Clinical Presentation

Pyomyositis occurs in three stages. The invasive stage is characterized by low-grade fever, general malaise, and dull, cramping pain. The overlying skin often appears normal; however, a firm or "woody" texture may be appreciated on deep palpation. The insidious nature of the invasive stage of pyomyositis results in many missed diagnoses, especially in temperate climates, where pyomyositis is rarer.

Abscess formation occurs during the suppurative stage, and patients tend to have more focal complaints. Often there is increased tenderness with overlying erythema and swelling. Most patients present during this stage of the disease.

During the late stage of pyomyositis, patients develop high fevers, exhibit more local signs of infection, and complain of severe pain. Patients in the late stage of pyomyositis can develop systemic manifestations, including metastatic abscesses, arthritis, renal failure, septic shock, or toxic shock. If urgent management is not initiated at this late stage, mortality rates of 10% have been reported.[18,21]

Pyomyositis most commonly affects the quadriceps, gluteal, and iliopsoas muscles. Other affected areas include the paraspinous, psoas, shoulder girdle, extremities (e.g., gastrocnemius), and chest wall. Patients with psoas muscle involvement may present with limp, hip pain, or back pain. Multiple sites are involved in 11% to 43% of patients.[18,20]

More rapidly necrotizing infections of muscle have also been described. GABHS infections often occur in patients with a primary varicella infection and can cause a rapidly progressive, necrotizing form of pyomyositis (see also "Necrotizing Fasciitis"). Within hours of presentation, patients can develop hypotension, oliguria, lethargy, and toxic shock; a scarlatiniform rash may be present.

Clostridial myonecrosis (gas gangrene) generally occurs 2 to 3 days after wound contamination with *C. perfringens* and is characterized by myonecrosis, gas production, and sepsis. Patients may present initially with localized pain and pallor, and subcutaneous emphysema and crepitus may be appreciated. Symptoms can progress rapidly, with the appearance of

hemorrhagic bullae and the development of cutaneous necrosis, acidosis, coagulopathy, and shock.

Differential Diagnosis

The broad differential diagnosis of pyomyositis includes other infectious processes such as septic arthritis, cellulitis, acute appendicitis, and osteomyelitis. Inflammatory processes that may mimic pyomyositis include thrombophlebitis, polymyositis, bursitis, and other rheumatic diseases. Pyomyositis may also be confused with muscle strain, viral myositis (e.g., influenza, enterovirus), deep venous thrombosis, hematoma, contusion, or sarcoma.

Diagnosis and Evaluation

Plain radiographs may demonstrate soft tissue swelling or osteomyelitis but are of little help in defining the extent of muscle involvement. Ultrasonography is a quick and inexpensive study that can detect muscle abscesses and is often used in the diagnosis of pyomyositis. Alternatively, CT provides good delineation of muscle structure and may demonstrate a fluid collection. MRI with gadolinium is the most sensitive study for detecting early inflammatory changes. MRI can also define the extent of muscle involvement and may help identify those patients with early disease who do not require surgical intervention (see Fig. 70-2).

Laboratory tests tend to be less specific in diagnosing pyomyositis. A complete blood count generally demonstrates a leukocytosis with a left shift. Eosinophilia is more common in patients from the tropics. The ESR is often elevated, but muscle enzymes, such as creatine kinase and aldolase, are generally normal. Blood cultures are positive in approximately 30% of patients,[21] but fluid aspirated from the site of infection is more likely to yield an organism.

Treatment

Surgical incision and drainage are generally required, although certain patients who present with muscle inflammation before abscess formation can be managed with antibiotic therapy alone. CT- or ultrasound-guided percutaneous drainage is another alternative to surgical management in some patients.

Because *S. aureus* accounts for the majority of infections, a semisynthetic penicillinase-resistant penicillin such as nafcillin or oxacillin (150 mg/kg per day, divided every 6 hours) is the traditional choice for empirical therapy. Clindamycin (40 mg/kg per day, divided every 8 hours) is an alternative in patients with penicillin allergies. However, owing to the increasing frequency of community-acquired MRSA, vancomycin should be considered until sensitivities are available. Intravenous antibiotics should be continued until clinical improvement is evident. Based on sensitivities, appropriate oral antibiotics should be continued for another 2 to 3 weeks. If an organism is not identified, an oral antibiotic that provides similar coverage to the intravenous antibiotic that led to clinical improvement should be used.

Necrotizing GABHS infections require immediate surgical exploration and débridement and possible fasciotomy. Therapy should include clindamycin for the Eagle effect (discussed earlier), because most cases of pyomyositis are diagnosed after the organisms have reached a steady-state growth phase.

The prognosis for patients with pyomyositis is generally good, and most recover without sequelae. However, osteomyelitis, muscle scarring, residual weakness, and functional impairment are possible outcomes.

Discharge Criteria

- Afebrile for at least 24 to 48 hours.
- General clinical improvement.
- Ability to complete the appropriate course of antibiotic therapy as an outpatient.

In a Nutshell

- Presentation: characterized by three stages—invasive, suppurative, and late.
- Diagnosis: ultrasonography is a quick and inexpensive tool for diagnosing pyomyositis, although CT and MRI also have a role if better delineation is needed.
- Treatment: incision and drainage are often required, although some patients who present before abscess formation can be managed with antibiotics alone.

SEPTIC ARTHRITIS

Septic arthritis refers to bacterial invasion of the joint space by viable bacteria. The synovium is a highly vascular layer of connective tissue that lacks a limiting basement membrane, which allows bacteria to enter the joint space more readily. Septic arthritis may occur as a result of hematogenous seeding of the synovium during a transient episode of bacteremia, contiguous spread of an adjacent infection such as osteomyelitis, or direct inoculation during surgery or as a result of penetrating trauma.

In response to bacterial endotoxin, cytokines such as tumor necrosis factor and interleukin-1 are released, which in turn stimulate the release of proteolytic enzymes and increase leukocyte migration. This combination of factors leads to destruction of the synovium and cartilage matrix. When the hip is involved, increased pressure within the joint can interrupt blood flow, leading to avascular necrosis of the femoral head. Although septic arthritis is rarely fatal since the introduction of antibiotics, destruction of the joint space leads to long-term sequelae in a significant percentage of patients. Prompt recognition and aggressive management are therefore critical.

Septic arthritis is commonly a disease of childhood, with approximately half of all cases occurring in patients younger than 20 years.[22] The peak incidence is in children younger than 3 years, and boys are affected approximately twice as often as girls.[22,23]

S. aureus is the most common organism identified in patients with septic arthritis. Other frequently identified organisms include GABHS and *S. pneumoniae*. Now an unusual cause of septic arthritis, *H. influenzae* type B was commonly identified before the introduction of an effective vaccine. *K. kingae* may be identified in toddlers with a preceding history of an upper respiratory tract infection. In addition to *S. aureus*, neonates are also at risk for group B streptococci and gram-negative enteric bacilli. Neonates and sexually active adolescents are at risk for infection by *Neisseria gonorrhoeae*. In addition to the usual organisms, patients with sickle cell disease are at risk for bone and joint infections caused by *Salmonella* species. *Neisseria meningitidis* is a rare cause of septic arthritis, but a reactive arthritis is not uncommon following bacteremia or meningitis secondary to this organism.

Clinical Presentation

Septic arthritis usually presents with systemic symptoms such as fever, malaise, and poor appetite. Local findings at the infected joint include edema, erythema, and tenderness, and patients tend to keep the affected joint in a position that maximizes intracapsular volume and therefore comfort. Knees are held moderately flexed, and hips are kept flexed, abducted, and externally rotated. Refusal to move an affected joint is referred to as pseudoparalysis, and even passive movement may be extremely painful.

Approximately 75% to 80% of cases involve joints of the lower extremities, with the knees and hips most commonly affected.[23,24] Other commonly affected joints include the ankles, wrists, elbows, and shoulders. Small, distal joints are less likely to be involved.

Differential Diagnosis

Multiple entities can be confused with septic arthritis, including trauma, transient synovitis, reactive arthritis, Lyme disease, juvenile rheumatoid arthritis, acute rheumatic fever, osteomyelitis, tumor, slipped capital femoral epiphysis, and Legg-Calvé-Perthes disease. In particular, transient synovitis (also known as toxic synovitis) often mimics septic arthritis. Transient synovitis is presumed to be a postviral phenomenon, often affecting the hip in boys between the ages of 3 and 10 years. The arthritis that occurs with Lyme disease is also a great imitator of septic arthritis and must be considered in endemic areas. In addition, multiple bacteria, including *N. meningitidis*, *Streptococcus* species, *Salmonella* species, and *Mycoplasma pneumoniae*, are associated with postinfectious reactive arthritides that may be difficult to differentiate from septic arthritis. In cases of suspected septic arthritis, concomitant osteomyelitis of an adjacent bone should also be suspected.

Diagnosis and Evaluation

In general, the white blood cell count, C-reactive protein, and ESR are elevated in patients with septic arthritis, but some patients present with normal inflammatory markers. Blood cultures are positive in about one third of cases,[25] and they occasionally yield the pathogen even when culture of the synovial fluid is negative.

The cornerstone of diagnosis is the evaluation of aspirated joint fluid. Synovial fluid should be aspirated into a heparinized syringe. If *K. kingae* is a concern, synovial fluid should be inoculated directly into a blood culture bottle to increase the chance of recovering this organism. The fluid should be sent for Gram stain, aerobic and anaerobic culture, and cell count with differential. Typical findings of aspirated synovial fluid are presented in Table 70-4.

Plain radiographs may demonstrate a widened joint space in a patient with a septic hip, but they are most useful for

Table 70-4   Typical Synovial Fluid Findings

Finding	Septic Arthritis	Transient Synovitis	Normal Joint
Color	Serosanguineous	Yellow	Yellow
Clarity	Turbid	Generally clear, but depends on number of white blood cells	Clear
White blood cells	>50,000-100,000/mm^3	5000-15,000/mm^3	<200/mm^3
% Neutrophils	>75	<25	<25
Culture	Positive in 70%-80%	Negative	Negative
Glucose	<40 mg/dL	Equal to serum	Equal to serum

eliminating other conditions such as fractures, Legg-Calvé-Perthes disease, and slipped capital femoral epiphysis. Ultrasonography is useful for identifying and quantifying a joint effusion, especially in deeper joints such as the hips, and it may be used to guide needle aspiration of these joints. Bone scan and MRI are often performed and may play a critical role in diagnosing concomitant osteomyelitis. However, these imaging studies should not delay aspiration of the joint or prompt surgical and antibiotic management when septic arthritis is suspected.

Treatment

Antibiotic therapy should be initiated immediately after blood and synovial fluid cultures have been obtained. The Gram stain can help guide the initial antibiotic choice; however, antibiotic therapy should not be delayed if these specimens cannot be obtained promptly. If gram-positive cocci are seen, empirical therapy with a semisynthetic penicillinase-resistant penicillin such as oxacillin (150 mg/kg per day, divided in four doses) is the traditional choice, but vancomycin should be considered in areas with high rates of community-acquired MRSA. If gram-negative organisms are found, or if no organisms are identified, a third-generation cephalosporin such as cefotaxime or ceftriaxone will cover most gram-positive organisms, as well as *K. kingae*, *Salmonella* species, and *H. influenzae*. In sexually active adolescents, ceftriaxone or cefotaxime may be used to cover *N. gonorrhoeae*. Neonates are often treated with oxacillin or nafcillin plus cefotaxime or gentamicin, although cefotaxime alone covers the most likely causative agents. Coverage can be narrowed once identification of the organism and susceptibilities are available.

Most authors agree that septic arthritis of the hip is a medical emergency requiring immediate surgical drainage. Infants with septic arthritis of the shoulder are also treated with emergent surgical drainage. When other joints are affected, some authors advocate repeated daily aspiration, which proved to be superior to surgical drainage in an adult study.[26] However, if there is a large amount of fibrin or debris, the infection is loculated, or there is a lack of improvement within 3 days, surgical drainage is recommended. Physical therapy may be beneficial as adjunctive management in some cases, especially when the child is reluctant to use the joint.

In uncomplicated cases, the total duration of therapy should be at least 3 weeks, with at least 1 week of antibiotics given intravenously. If the patient is clinically improved after 1 week and inflammatory markers are normalizing, the remaining 2 weeks of antibiotics may be given orally. Despite appropriate management, approximately 40% of patients with hip involvement and 10% of patients with knee involvement suffer significant sequelae such as growth plate damage and loss of joint function.[25,26,28] Close follow-up in all patients and physical therapy in selected patients are therefore essential.

Discharge Criteria

- Clinical improvement with resolution of fever and improved range of motion of the affected joint, along with decreased edema, erythema, and tenderness.
- At least 1 week of intravenous antibiotics, and provision for completion of oral treatment at home.
- Reliable outpatient follow-up with orthopedics and potentially with physical therapy.

In a Nutshell

- Presentation: systemic symptoms such as fever and malaise may accompany a tender, erythematous, swollen joint.
- Diagnosis: aspiration and analysis of synovial fluid is the cornerstone.
- Treatment: in addition to intravenous antibiotics, emergent surgical drainage or repeated daily aspiration is essential to prevent long-term sequelae.

SUGGESTED READING

Bickels J, Ben-Sira L, Kessler A, et al: Primary pyomyositis. J Bone Joint Surg Am 2002;84:2277-2286.

Bisno AL, Stevens DL: Current concepts: Streptococcal infections of skin and soft tissues. N Engl J Med 1996;334:240-245.

Darville T, Jacobs RF: Management of acute hematogenous osteomyelitis in children. Pediatr Infect Dis J 2004;23:255-257.

Green RJ, Dafoe DC, Raffin TA: Necrotizing fasciitis. Chest 1996;110:219-229.

Gubbay AJ, Isaacs D: Pyomyositis in children. Pediatr Infect Dis J 2000; 19:1009-1013.

Lew DP, Waldvogel FA: Current concepts: Osteomyelitis. N Engl J Med 1997;336:999-1007.

Matan AJ, Smith JT: Pediatric septic arthritis. Orthopedics 1997;20:630-635.

Rose CD, Eppes SC: Infection-related arthritis. Rheum Dis Clin North Am 1997;23:677-695.

Shetty A, Gedalia A: Septic arthritis in children. Rheum Dis Clin North Am 1998;24:287-304.

Spiegel DA, Meyer JS, Dormans JP, et al: Pyomyositis in children and adolescents: Report of 12 cases and review of the literature. J Pediatr Orthop 1999;19:143-150.

Stevens DL: The flesh-eating bacterium: What's next? J Infect Dis 1999;179(Suppl 2):S366-S374.

Vazquez M: Osteomyelitis in children. Curr Opin Pediatr 2002;14:112-115.

REFERENCES

1. Descamps V, Aitken J, Lee MG: Hippocrates on necrotising fasciitis. Lancet 1994;344:55.

2. CDC editorial: Invasive group A streptococcal infections—United Kingdom, 1994. JAMA 1994;272:16.

3. Francis KR, LaMaute HR, Davis JM, Pizzi WF: Implications of risk factors in necrotizing fasciitis. Am Surg 1993;59:304-308.

4. Brogan TV, Nizet V, Waldhausen JH, et al: Group A streptococcal necrotizing fasciitis complicating primary varicella: A series of fourteen patients. Pediatr Infect Dis J 1996;15:556-557.

5. Aronoff DM, Bloch KC: Assessing the relationship between the use of nonsteroidal antiinflammatory drugs and necrotizing fasciitis caused by group A streptococcus. Medicine 2003;82:225-235.

6. LaMont RL, Anderson PA, Dajani AS, Thirumoorthi MC: Acute hematogenous osteomyelitis in children. J Pediatr Orthop 1987;7:579-583.

7. Nelson JD: Acute osteomyelitis in children. Infect Dis Clin North Am 1990;4:513-522.

8. Gillespie WJ: Epidemiology in bone and joint infection. Infect Dis Clin North Am 1990;4:361-375.

9. Dich VQ, Nelson JD, Haltalin KC: Osteomyelitis in infants and children. Am J Dis Child 1975;129:1273-1275.

10. Unkila-Kallio L, Kallio M, Eskola J, Peltola H: Serum C-reactive protein, erythrocyte sedimentation rate, and white blood cell count in acute hematogenous osteomyelitis of children. Pediatrics 1993;92:800-804.

11. Vaughan PA, Newman NM, Rosman MA: Acute hematogenous osteomyelitis in children. J Pediatr Orthop 1987;7:652-655.

12. Darville T, Jacobs R: Management of acute hematogenous osteomyelitis in children. Pediatr Infect Dis J 2004;23:255-257.

13. Mazur JM, Ross G, Cummings J, et al: Usefulness of magnetic resonance imaging for the diagnosis of acute musculoskeletal infections in children. J Pediatr Orthop 1995;15:144-147.

14. Vasquez M: Osteomyelitis in children. Curr Opin Pediatr 2002;14:112-115.

15. Raz R, Miron D: Oral ciprofloxacin for treatment of infection following nail puncture wounds of the foot. Clin Infect Dis 1995;21:194-195.

16. Fernandez M, Carrol C, Baker C: Discitis and vertebral osteomyelitis in children: An 18-year review. Pediatrics 2000;105:1299-1304.

17. Horn CV, Master S: Pyomyositis tropicans in Uganda. East Afr Med J 1968;45:463-471.

18. Chiedozi LC: Pyomyositis: Review of 205 cases in 112 patients. Am J Surg 1979;137:255-259.

19. Christin L, Sarosi GA: Pyomyositis in North America: Case reports and review. Clin Infect Dis 1992;15:668-677.

20. Chacha PB: Muscle abscesses in children. Clin Orthop 1970;70:174-180.

21. Brown JD, Wheeler B: Pyomyositis: Report of 18 cases in Hawaii. Arch Intern Med 1984;144:1749-1751.

22. Baitch A: Recent observations of acute suppurative arthritis. Clin Orthop 1962;22:153-165.

23. Chartier Y, Martin WJ, Kelly PJ: Bacterial arthritis: Experiences in the treatment of 77 patients. Ann Intern Med 1939;50:1462-1473.

24. Heberling JA: A review of two hundred and one cases of suppurative arthritis. J Bone Joint Surg 1941;23:917-921.

25. Morrey BF, Bianco AJ, Rhodes KH: Septic arthritis in children. Orthop Clin North Am 1975;6:923-934.

26. Goldenberg DL, Brandt KD, Cohen AS, Cathcart ES: Treatment of septic arthritis: Comparison of needle aspiration and surgery as initial modes of joint drainage. Arthritis Rheum 1975;18:83-90.

27. Samilson RL, Bersani FA, Watkins MB: Acute suppurative arthritis in infants and children: The importance of early diagnosis and surgical drainage. Pediatrics 1958;21:798-803.

28. Betz RR, Cooperman DR, Wopperer JM, et al: Late sequelae of septic arthritis of the hip in infancy and childhood. J Pediatr Orthop 1990;10:365-372.

CHAPTER 71

Device-Related Infections

Samir S. Shah, Michael J. Smith, and Theoklis E. Zaoutis

Medical devices such as central venous catheters and ventricular shunts are commonly used in children. Catheter-related bloodstream infections are frequent complications of the use of long-term vascular access devices, with more than 200,000 cases occurring each year in the United States.[1] A catheter-related bloodstream infection is defined as bacteremia or fungemia in a patient with an intravascular catheter that is the presumed source of infection. Local infections at insertion sites are another important catheter-associated complication. Insertion of a ventriculoperitoneal (VP) shunt is one of the most commonly performed operations in children.[2] These devices greatly increase the risk of infection by disrupting host defenses and providing a portal of entry for organisms to migrate from the skin and mucous membranes to sterile body sites. These devices also supply a site that is relatively sequestered from immune system surveillance, allowing bacteria to flourish unperturbed. Further, indwelling devices such as catheters can become seeded with bacteria as a result of bacteremia arising at a distant site. This chapter discusses the infectious complications of central venous catheters and ventricular shunts.

In the past, catheter-related infections were primarily the purview of the intensivists, oncologists, gastroenterologists, or other clinicians caring for patients with indwelling catheters. The use of central venous catheters is increasing in both inpatient and outpatient settings. Previously healthy children with isolated infectious processes that require extended intravenous antibiotic therapy (e.g., osteomyelitis, Lyme meningitis) often have these intravascular lines placed. Hospitalists are increasingly called on to assess patients for possible infectious complications in emergency departments, in medical pediatric inpatient units, or through consultations requested by surgical or medical subspecialists. In many institutions, general pediatric hospitalist practice includes the coverage of neonatal and pediatric intensive care units (NICUs and PICUs), where central catheters are commonly used. Knowledge and expertise in assessing and managing catheter-associated infections are becoming increasingly important in many settings.

The medical literature available to guide clinicians comes predominantly from adult studies, studies performed in PICU or NICU settings, or data collected from pediatric oncology patients. The generalizability of such information has yet to be determined, but until studies are performed in broader populations of pediatric patients, data from these more specialized populations must serve as the basis for our understanding of catheter-related infections.

CENTRAL VENOUS CATHETER–RELATED INFECTIONS

Background

Bloodstream infections are the most common infections acquired by hospitalized children, accounting for 21% to 34% of all nosocomial infections in PICU patients.[3-5] Most of these bloodstream infections occur as a consequence of intravascular catheterization.[3] The attributable cost of these infections in PICU patients is approximately $39,000 per episode,[6] and it is an increasingly common problem.

Infection rates are affected by many factors, including the patient's location, comorbid illnesses,[7] and catheter type (Table 71-1) Nontunneled catheters appear to have the highest rate of infection, and totally implanted venous access devices have the lowest rate of infection.[8]

Clinical Presentation

A catheter-related infection may be local or systemic. In local infection, examination of the exit site may reveal erythema, induration, tenderness, fluctuance, and purulent or foul-smelling discharge. Although the infection may appear to be limited to the superficial structures (i.e., skin), it may also extend to deeper soft tissue structures such as fat, fascia, or muscle (Table 71-2).[1] Soft tissue infections are discussed in Chapter 70.

In a patient with a bloodstream infection in the context of a central venous catheter, any of the following circumstances may be occurring (Fig. 71-1):

- The bloodstream infection may be due to an infection at a site distant from the catheter, with the catheter remaining uninfected. It is extremely rare for the catheter to become infected by bacteremia.
- The infusate may be contaminated with microorganisms.
- Microorganisms from the skin can migrate along the percutaneous tract to infect the external (extraluminal) surface of the catheter.
- Contamination of the catheter hub can lead to intraluminal colonization and infection.

These various processes may affect the clinical presentation, although it is often similar.

In catheter-related bloodstream infection, fever is the most common presenting finding, occurring in 62% of children diagnosed with such an infection after emergency department evaluation.[9] However, most children with fever in the context of a central venous catheter do not have

Table 71-1 Commonly Used Central Venous Catheters

Catheter Type	Description
Peripherally inserted central catheter	Inserted via a peripheral vein (usually basilic, cephalic, or brachial) into the superior vena cava
Nontunneled CVC	Inserted directly into a central vein (usually subclavian, internal jugular, or femoral) through a skin incision
Tunneled CVC	Inserted through a subcutaneous tunnel on the chest wall before entering the superior vena cava (e.g., Broviac, Hickman, Groshong, Quinton catheters); a Dacron cuff located at the tunnel exit site contributes to long-term catheter stability by stimulating tissue growth around the tunneled portion of the catheter
Totally implanted venous access device ("port")	Subcutaneous port or reservoir with self-sealing septum accessed by a needle through intact skin; the catheter tip is located in the subclavian or internal jugular vein

CVC, central venous catheter.

Table 71-2 Types of Catheter-Related Infections

Infection Type	Clinical Findings
Exit site	Erythema or induration within 2 cm of catheter exit site
Tunnel	Tenderness, erythema, or induration along subcutaneous tract of tunneled catheter and more than 2 cm from catheter exit site
Pocket	Purulent fluid in subcutaneous pocket of totally implanted venous access device; may be accompanied by overlying tenderness, erythema, induration, visible drainage, and skin necrosis
Infusate-related bloodstream	Growth of the same organism from infusate and bloodstream
Catheter-associated bloodstream	Positive simultaneous blood cultures from central venous catheter and peripheral vein yielding the same organism in the presence of at least one of the following: Simultaneous quantitative blood cultures in which the number of CFUs isolated from blood drawn through the central catheter is at least fivefold greater than the number isolated from blood drawn peripherally Positive semiquantitative (≥15 CFUs/catheter segment) or quantitative (≥100 CFUs/catheter segment) catheter tip cultures Simultaneous blood cultures in which the central blood culture grows ≥2 hr earlier than the peripheral blood culture

CFU, colony-forming unit.

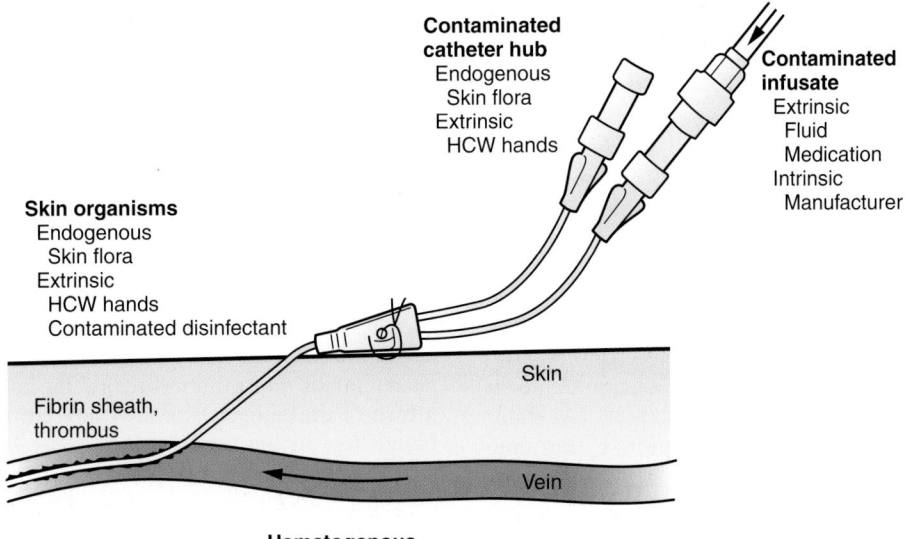

Figure 71-1 Potential sources of infection with a central venous catheter. HCW, health care worker. (From Crnich C: The promise of novel technology for the prevention of intravascular device-related bloodstream infection. I. Pathogenesis and short-term devices. Clin Infect Dis 2002;34:1232-1242.)

catheter-related bloodstream infections. Among cancer patients with fever and indwelling catheters, only 10% and 24% of all episodes of fever were associated with bacteremia in neutropenic and non-neutropenic patients, respectively.[10] A positive blood culture may be the initial presenting feature, especially in the setting of an inpatient consultation or referral from an outpatient location.

A sudden onset of symptoms or recurrent symptoms, such as fever or hypotension, that correlates with the timing of the infusion are important clues. These suggest the introduction of contaminated fluid through the catheter, whether from the hub, the infusion fluid, or the intraluminal catheter space.

Complications of bacteremia may be the presenting symptoms, including sepsis and disseminated infection with emboli in the retinas, skin, bones, heart, and visceral organs (lungs, liver, spleen, kidneys). Organ system dysfunction is another complication that can occur from immune complex deposition (e.g., nephritis).

Differential Diagnosis

As previously mentioned, fever in the setting of an indwelling catheter is usually not caused by a catheter-related bloodstream infection. Therefore, the broad differential diagnosis of fever must be explored, taking into consideration the special circumstances of these patients. Most patients with indwelling catheters have preexisting conditions such as immunocompromised states, previously diagnosed primary infections, or multiorgan system disease.

A coexisting distant infection may present with fever and positive blood culture and should be included in the differential diagnosis. These include dental abscess, distant intravascular septic thrombus, pyelonephritis, and pneumonia, among many others. Possible translocation of bacteria from the intestinal mucosa, especially in patients with abnormalities of this organ system (e.g., necrotizing enterocolitis, short-intestine syndrome), is another factor to consider. When the catheter is placed for treatment of a bacterial or fungal infection, treatment failure with recurrence of the primary infection is an important possibility.

Catheter malfunction can also be a manifestation of catheter-related infection. Thrombi and fibrin deposits on catheters impair blood flow through the catheter and serve as a nidus for microbial colonization and subsequent infection.[11]

Intravenous preparations contaminated with infectious agents are an important consideration in the differential diagnosis, especially in the appropriate clinical setting.

Diagnosis

Local Infections

Local infections attributable to the central venous catheter include exit, tunnel, and pocket infections, and the physical examination can establish the diagnosis (see Table 71-2) or guide the need for further evaluation. Ultrasonography may be useful to demonstrate a fluid collection in the subcutaneous tissue.

Catheter-Related Bloodstream Infections

Identifying the catheter as the source of a bloodstream infection is not always straightforward. In adult patients, only 15% to 20% of central catheters removed in the context of a bloodstream infection are ultimately implicated as the source of infection. Several methods have been proposed to improve the diagnosis of catheter-related bloodstream infections, including quantitative cultures of blood obtained through the catheter and a peripheral vein, quantitative and semiquantitative cultures of a catheter segment, and differential time to blood culture positivity (see Table 71-2).[1]

Diagnosis of a catheter-related bloodstream infection can be made by comparing quantitative differences in colony counts of a pathogen isolated from a blood culture obtained through the catheter and colony counts from a simultaneously obtained peripheral blood culture. A catheter-related bloodstream infection is diagnosed when there is an incremental increase in the quantity of bacteria obtained through the catheter compared with that obtained from peripheral venipuncture (see Table 71-2). Owing to the cost and the limited availability of quantitative blood cultures, this technique is not widely used.

Differential time to positivity of blood cultures—defined as the difference in time necessary for the blood cultures taken by peripheral venipuncture and through the catheter to become positive using a continuous monitoring blood culture system—is the simplest of the three methods and does not require either specialized laboratory culture techniques or catheter removal. This method is accurate only if the peripheral and central cultures are of equal volume because, as discussed later, the volume of blood in the bottle influences the time to positivity. A differential time to positivity of 2 hours or longer has a sensitivity of 93% and a specificity of 75% for catheters in place for greater than 30 days and a sensitivity of 81% and a specificity of 92% for catheters in place for less than 30 days.[12] Several smaller studies demonstrated similar results.[13-15]

Until recently, the most widely accepted methods of diagnosing a catheter-related bloodstream infection involved either quantitative or semiquantitative culture of the catheter tip, which requires removal of the catheter. Quantitative culture of a catheter segment requires slicing the catheter and either flushing the segment with broth or vortexing it in broth, followed by culture of the broth on agar plates.[16] Semiquantitative culture methods, also known as roll-plate methods, involve rolling a sliced segment of the removed catheter across the surface of an agar plate; colony-forming units are counted after overnight incubation.[17]

Timing of Blood Culture

Few studies have evaluated the optimal timing of blood cultures. In clinical conditions with continuous bacteremia, such as endocarditis or septic thrombophlebitis, this issue is less relevant. In catheter-related bloodstream infections, the bacteremia is intermittent because the bacteria reside in the lumen of the catheter and are not continuously exposed to blood flow in the intravascular space. Traditional wisdom suggests that bacteremia precedes the onset of fever and chills by 1 hour or more, implying that blood cultures obtained at the time of fever onset may not reliably detect intermittent bacteremia. Interestingly, there are no data regarding the yield of positive blood cultures and the timing of collection in relation to the onset of fever to support this supposition. However, drawing multiple culture sets within a 24-hour period appears to accurately detect intermittent bacteremia,[15] even if all the specimens are obtained at the same time.[18] In critically ill patients who are hemodynamically unstable, two blood culture sets should be drawn promptly before the initiation of empirical antibiotic treatment. In less urgent cases, blood can be drawn at least twice within a 24-hour period. In patients who are already receiving antibiotics, obtaining samples close to the time of antibiotic trough levels (i.e., just before next dose) theoretically improves blood culture yield.[19] However, this issue has not been studied and may not be clinically practical.

Volume of Blood for Culture

Several important variables, including the magnitude of bacteremia and the sensitivity of the blood culture detection system, affect the volume of blood necessary for culture. The magnitude of bacteremia affects blood culture yield, especially when small blood volumes are used. The likelihood of growth is lower and the median time to detection is later when small volumes (<0.5 mL) are used, particularly at ultralow concentrations of bacteria.[20] The volume of blood in the blood culture bottle is more important than the total number of blood cultures obtained. One study found that the pathogen recovery rate at 24 hours was 72% for a large-volume (6-mL) single culture, compared with a 47% combined yield of two smaller (2-mL) samples inoculated into separate culture bottles.[21] Similar results were found in studies in adult patients; standard adult-volume cultures (mean, 8.7 mL) had a 92% detection rate, whereas low-volume cultures (mean, 2.7 mL) had a detection rate of only 69%.[22] It is estimated that the yield of adult blood cultures increases approximately 3% per milliliter of blood cultured.

Although it is often difficult to obtain peripheral blood specimens in pediatric patients, too much blood can influence the culture yield, just as too little blood can. Diluting the blood into the blood culture broth enhances the recovery of pathogens, perhaps by diluting antimicrobial agents (if the patient is receiving antibiotic therapy) and blood components such as phagocytes, antibodies, and complement factors that are known to have bactericidal activity.[23] Too much blood in the bottle may result in insufficient dilution of these factors. Too little blood also affects the likelihood of bacterial growth in culture, because blood contains factors that enhance the growth of some bacteria (e.g., *Haemophilus influenzae*). In such cases, too little blood volume leads to dilution of these factors by the blood culture bottle's nutrient broth. The ideal blood-broth ratio depends on the blood culture system used, but a ratio between 1:5 and 1:10 is generally considered optimal.[24] For example, the PediBacT system, used at many institutions, contains 20 mL of broth. Therefore, a 2-mL inoculum of blood provides a blood-broth ratio of 1:10, and a 4-mL inoculum provides a ratio of 1:5. Because many systems supplement the broth with other materials that may help compensate for cultures inoculated with suboptimal blood-broth ratios, slightly smaller blood volumes may be acceptable. A single culture containing 1 to 2 mL of blood is considered sufficient for the detection of most clinically important bacteremias, and a 0.5-mL blood sample, though not ideal, permits the detection of some clinically important bacteremias.

Primary Bloodstream Infection versus Contaminated Culture

Distinguishing between true bloodstream infections and contaminated cultures poses a challenge when skin flora (e.g., coagulase-negative staphylococci, *Bacillus* species, micrococci) are isolated from blood culture. If multiple cultures are obtained before antibiotic administration, the situation is less ambiguous, because when multiple cultures yield the same pathogen, the likelihood of repeated contaminated specimens is diminished. Surveillance definitions proposed by the American Academy of Pediatrics and the Centers for Disease Control and Prevention provide a highly sensitive method for detecting primary bloodstream infections; however, from a clinical perspective, these definitions may overestimate the incidence of bloodstream infection.[8]

Causes

Surveillance for nosocomial bloodstream infection is usually performed in high-risk patient areas such as PICUs, NICUs, and oncololgy units. As a result, the majority of data on the causes of nosocomial bloodstream infection are derived from patients in these units. We would expect the spectrum of organisms causing nosocomial catheter-related bloodstream infections in children hospitalized in non-ICU settings to be similar, but there is limited information available. One study of outpatient parenteral antimicrobial therapy in children with osteoarticluar infections found that the rate of infectious complications associated with the catheter was 6.3 per 1000 catheter days and occurred in approximately 10% of patients. The average time to development of infectious complications was 24.5 days.[25]

Approximately 90% of nosocomial bloodstream infections are associated with the presence of a central venous catheter.[3] Coagulase-negative staphylococci account for approximately 40% of the pathogens identified in children with nosocomial bloodstream infections. In neonates, coagulase-negative staphylococci account for an even greater percentage of isolates (50%). Gram-negative aerobic bacilli account for approximately 25% of bloodstream infections, followed by enterococci (11% to 15%) and *Candida* species (6%).[3] The most commonly encountered gram-negative bacilli include *Enterobacter* species, *Pseudomonas aeruginosa*, *Klebsiella pneumoniae*, *Escherichia coli*, *Serratia marcescens*, *Acinetobacter* species, and *Citrobacter* species[3] (Table 71-3). *Candida* species are the fourth most common cause of nosocomial bloodstream infection in the United States.[26] Children with central catheters managed predominantly in home health care settings may be at higher risk for nonendogenous gram-negative pathogens (e.g., from water and other environmental sources) such as *Pseudomonas*, *Acinetobacter*, and *Agrobacterium* species, particularly during the summer months.[7,27]

Although coagulase-negative staphylococci are the most commonly reported isolate from children with nosocomial bloodstream infections, they are also common skin colonizers that frequently contaminate blood cultures. A study using a mathematical model of blood cultures positive for coagulase-negative staphylococci in patients with central venous lines found that the positive predictive value of one positive culture was 55% if only one culture was obtained, 20% if two cultures were performed, and only 5% if three were

Table 71-3 Most Common Pathogens Identified in Patients in Pediatric Intensive Care Units (National Nosocomial Infections Surveillance System, 1992-1997)

Pathogen	Bloodstream Infection (%) (N = 1887)
Coagulase-negative staphylococci	37.8
Enterococcus	11.2
Staphylococcus aureus	9.3
Enterobacter species	6.2
Candida albicans	5.5
Pseudomonas aeruginosa	4.9
Klebsiella pneumoniae	4.1
Escherichia coli	2.9

Table 71-4 Catheter Management in Patients with Central Venous Catheter-Related Infection

Infection Type	Catheter Management
Exit site	Remove CVC if: No longer required; Alternative site exists; Patient is critically ill (e.g., hypotension); Infection is due to *Pseudomonas aeruginosa* or fungi
Tunnel	Remove CVC
Pocket	Remove CVC
Catheter-related bloodstream	Remove CVC if: No longer required; Infection is due to *Staphylococcus aureus*, *Candida* species, or mycobacteria; Patient is critically ill; Bacteremia fails to clear in 48-72 hr; Symptoms of bloodstream infection persist beyond 48-72 hr; Patient has any of the following: Noninfectious valvular heart disease (increased risk of endocarditis), Endocarditis, Metastatic infection, Septic thrombophlebitis

CVC, central venous catheter.

performed. If two of two cultures were positive, the positive predictive value was 98% if both samples were obtained from a peripheral vein, 96% if one sample was obtained through a catheter and the other was obtained through a vein, and only 50% if both samples were obtained through a catheter.[28] Further, the distinction between pathogen and contaminant is affected by the age and underlying condition of the child. Coagulase-negative staphylococci as true pathogens in neonates have been well described, but the issue remains controversial.[29] The identification of coagulase-negative staphylococci often results in clinical intervention, with increased patient exposure to vancomycin. Overuse of vancomycin has implications for the continued increase of vancomycin resistance among gram-positive organisms.[30-32]

Treatment

There are limited data to guide the management of catheter-related bloodstream infections in children, and most of the management recommendations are derived from adult populations. However, even in adults, there are no randomized or controlled studies to address the optimal management of catheter-related bloodstream infections.[1] Empirical therapy in children with suspected catheter-related bloodstream infections should include an antimicrobial agent with activity against gram-positive bacteria, such as nafcillin, oxacillin, or vancomycin, and an agent effective against gram-negative bacteria (including *Pseudomonas*), such as ceftazidime or cefepime with or without an aminoglycoside. The empirical use of both an antipseudomonal β-lactam and an aminoglycoside may be appropriate in severely ill patients or when infection with a resistant gram-negative organism is suspected. In institutions in which methicillin-resistant *Staphylococcus aureus* is common, the use of vancomycin is appropriate. Fluoroquinolones are commonly used in adults but have been approved for only limited indications in children.

Once there is initial identification of an organism from the blood culture (e.g., coccus or bacillus, gram negative or positive, fungal elements), the therapy can be adjusted. Ulti-

mately, the treatment is narrowed as organisms are identified and susceptibilities are determined.

One of the most commonly asked clinical questions with regard to catheter-related bloodstream infections is whether the catheter should be removed (Table 71-4). In adult populations, it is recommended that most nontunneled central venous catheters be removed in cases of catheter-related bloodstream infection.[1] Removal of a catheter may not always be feasible in children because of potential complications associated with reinsertion and limited vascular access sites; therefore, treatment of the bloodstream infection without removal of the catheter is often attempted. In patients with catheter-related bloodstream infections associated with a tunneled catheter or an implanted device such as a port, the decision to remove the catheter is more complicated. However, it is strongly recommended (based on good evidence) that in patients with evidence of a tunnel or pocket infection (the subcutaneous pocket of an implanted device), the catheter should be removed to clear the infection.[1] Once culture data are available, treatment decisions can be tailored to specific organisms. Several studies have reported successful treatment of catheter-related bloodstream infections without catheter removal,[33-36] but this may depend on the pathogen identified.

Few data exist regarding the optimal duration of antibiotic therapy for catheter-related bloodstream infections. It depends in part on the pathogen, whether the catheter is removed, and whether the infection is complicated by septic thrombosis, endocarditis, osteomyelitis, or other metastatic foci of bacteria. For complicated infections, the duration of therapy is based on the time necessary to treat the complication. Further, there are no data to determine the optimal duration of intravenous versus oral antibiotics for the treatment of catheter-related bloodstream infections. Certain antibiotics with excellent oral bioavailability may be considered once the bacteremia has cleared and the patient has shown clinical improvement, the catheter has been removed, and compliance with therapy is ensured. Some pathogen-specific recommendations are provided in the following sections.

Coagulase-Negative Staphylococci

Coagulase-negative staphylococci are considered less virulent than other pathogens that cause catheter-related bloodstream infections. These infections usually present with fever alone or with inflammation of the catheter exit site. Patients rarely develop sepsis or have a poor outcome with this organism. Coagulase-negative staphylococcal infections may resolve with only removal of the catheter, without antibiotic therapy. Some experts recommend a short course of antibiotic therapy (3 to 5 days), however, even after removal of the catheter.[37] If the catheter remains in place, the recommended duration of treatment is 10 to 14 days after a negative blood culture. In neonates with coagulase-negative staphylococcal bacteremia, treatment without removal of the catheter can be attempted; however, once a neonate has three positive blood cultures despite appropriate antimicrobial therapy, the catheter should be removed because of the risk of end-organ damage.[38] The relapse rate in adult patients with coagulase-negative staphylococcal catheter-related bloodstream infections is 20% if the catheter is not removed, compared with 3% if it is removed.[39]

Staphylococcus aureus

Serious complications, including endocarditis and other deep tissue infections, have been reported in association with *S. aureus* catheter-related bloodstream infections.[40] Adult patients with *S. aureus* bacteremia are at significant risk for endocarditis and often have echocardiography as a routine part of management.[41,42] The frequency of infective endocarditis is low in children with *S. aureus* bacteremia and structurally normal hearts, so echocardiography is not commonly performed[43]; however, it should be considered in children with persistent bacteremia while on appropriate antimicrobial therapy or if a new murmur is identified on physical examination. In a prospective study of 51 children with *S. aureus* bacteremia, definite or possible endocarditis was diagnosed in 52% of patients with congenital heart disease but in only 3% of those with structurally normal hearts.[43] Neonates may be more vulnerable to complications of *S. aureus* bloodstream infections than are older infants. Therefore, some researchers recommend catheter removal for neonates with a single positive blood culture for either *S. aureus* or a gram-negative bacillus, because this significantly improves outcome.[38] Two weeks of appropriate antimicrobial therapy, based on sensitivities, is recommended for uncomplicated *S. aureus* catheter-related bloodstream infections.[1] Longer durations of therapy may be necessary for patients with prolonged bacteremia (>3 days), persistent fever, or complicated infections.[44]

Gram-Negative Bacilli

There is a paucity of data addressing whether catheters should be removed in patients with catheter-related bloodstream infections caused by the wide variety of gram-negative bacilli. Some children have been treated successfully without catheter removal,[1] but catheter removal has been shown to be beneficial in the treatment of infections with specific gram-negative bacilli such as *Pseudomonas* species, *Burkholderia cepacia, Acinetobacter baumanni,* and *Stenotrophomonas* species.[1,40] In a recent study of adult patients with catheter-related bloodstream infections caused by gram-negative bacilli, catheter removal was associated with a reduced rate of relapse.[45] In general, antimicrobial therapy should be administered for 10 to 14 days after blood cultures become negative.[1]

Fungemia

Treatment of fungemia without catheter removal has been associated with poor outcomes in both children and adults.[46-48] However, these studies did not account for the confounding effect of illness severity (sicker patients required catheter retention and were also the most likely to die).[49] Failure to remove the catheter promptly may lead to prolonged candidemia, which has been associated with higher rates of disseminated infection. The rate of dissemination (to lung, liver, spleen, eye, brain, heart) from candidemia is reportedly 17%, and the crude mortality rate in children with candidemia is 26%.[50] Interestingly, in one study, 27% of children with candidemia were on a general pediatric or surgery ward at the time of infection, emphasizing the role of the general pediatric hospitalist in the management of this condition. The consensus opinion is that catheters should be removed in patients with candidemia, whenever feasible.[51] Therapy with amphotericin B or fluconazole should be continued for 2 weeks. All patients with candidemia should have an ophthalmologic examination to evaluate for candidal endophthalmitis, preferably after the infection seems to be controlled and further disseminated disease is unlikely.[51]

Consultation

Involvement of the team that prescribed the central catheter is appropriate, such as gastroenterology if the catheter was placed for parenteral nutrition, orthopedics for treatment of osteomyelitis, oncology for chemotherapy, and so forth. Input from an infectious disease specialist is often helpful. Those who actually inserted the catheter (e.g., interventional radiologist or surgeon) may be appropriate to consult, especially if replacement of the line is likely to be necessary.

Admission Criteria

Most patients with catheter-related bloodstream infections are initially managed as inpatients. Hemodynamic instability usually requires transfer to a critical care setting.

Discharge Criteria

- Resolution of the bacteremia.
- Ability to provide ongoing antibiotic therapy in the outpatient setting, if needed.

- Institution of an appropriate plan to continue therapy for the underlying condition that initially warranted placement of the catheter.

Prevention

Advances have been made in the reduction of catheter-related bloodstream infections. Practices associated with a reduced risk of catheter-associated infections include the following:

- Use of maximal sterile barriers during catheter placement.[52]
- Use of chlorhexidine-isopropyl alcohol solution to prepare the skin before placement or during routine care of the catheter.
- Prompt removal of catheters as soon as they are no longer required.
- Strict adherence to appropriate hand hygiene practices.

In studies performed in adult intensive care units, antiseptic-impregnated catheters have been associated with reduced rates of catheter-related bloodstream infection.[53]

In a Nutshell

- Catheter-related infections include local infections at the insertion site, such as exit site cellulitis, pocket infections, and tunnel infections.
- Bacteremia or fungemia associated with an indwelling venous catheter is considered a catheter-related bloodstream infection. These include primary infections of the catheter, coexisting infection of the catheter and a distant site, and infusion of contaminated fluid through the catheter into the bloodstream.
- Differentiating bloodstream infections due to infected catheters from those without catheter infection is a challenge. Useful techniques include quantitative assessments of specimens obtained from the catheter compared with those obtained from peripheral venous sites. Time to positivity of a blood culture also provides some guidance.
- Common pathogens include gram-positive bacteria (e.g., coagulase-negative staphylococci) and gram-negative bacteria. Fungal catheter-related bloodstream infections are most commonly due to *Candida* species.
- Empirical antibiotic therapy should include coverage for gram-positive and gram-negative bacteria, including *Pseudomonas* species.

On the Horizon

- Future research may determine the impact of increased catheter use in non–intensive care hospital settings and in home care. Antibiotic- and antiseptic-impregnated catheters have been shown to reduce catheter-related bloodstream infection in adults. Antibiotic lock therapy involves filling the lumen of the catheter with an antibiotic solution and leaving it there. This method has limited use owing to concerns about increasing antibiotic resistance.

VENTRICULOPERITONEAL SHUNTS

Background

The introduction of the VP shunt in the late 1960s provided significant advantages over the previously used ventriculoatrial shunt and revolutionized the treatment of hydrocephalus.[54] Although VP shunts are associated with significantly less bacteremia than are ventriculoatrial shunts, the shunts themselves frequently become infected, with a reported incidence of 2% to 30%.[54]

Clinical Presentation

The clinical manifestations of shunt-associated infections can be quite varied (Table 71-5), owing to the existence of different locations along the track of the shunt that are prone to infection. These include the lumen of the shunt itself, the extraluminal ventricles, the cranial and distal surgical sites, and the peritoneal cavity.

It is also important to consider the timing of shunt infection in relation to placement of the device. The majority of shunt infections occur within the first 6 months after shunt placement,[55-57] with approximately half occurring within the first 2 weeks.[56,58]

Fever and shunt malfunction are commonly seen in shunt infections but are neither specific nor sensitive. Shunt malfunction usually presents with the clinical features of increased intracranial pressure, such as headache, vomiting, lethargy, or seizures.

Distal shunt infection commonly presents with abdominal pain. A known complication of VP shunts is the development of pseudocysts, pockets of cerebrospinal fluid (CSF) that form at the distal end of the shunt and are often related to decreased peritoneal absorption of CSF. These can be the direct consequence of a shunt infection or may develop in the absence of infection and become secondarily infected. If an infected pseudocyst leaks into the abdominal cavity, patients often present with frank peritonitis. If leakage does not occur, abdominal symptoms may be more indolent.[59]

Patients with wound infections present with incisional erythema and purulence, with or without local collections of CSF.

Differential Diagnosis

Most children with indwelling VP shunts and fever do not have shunt infections; therefore, the full spectrum of causes of fever should be considered. Also, in children presenting with shunt malfunction without fever, mechanical processes are likely responsible, with or without an infectious process. Obstruction may occur proximally, at the intake portion of the device (e.g., clogging, blockage from adjacent tissue), at any point along the tubing (e.g., kinking), or at the point of fluid exit. If the tubing becomes disconnected, flow may cease. Further discussion of shunt function and assessment can be found in Chapters 195 and 213.

Diagnosis

A commonly accepted definition of a shunt infection is isolation of a bacterial pathogen from ventricular fluid, lumbar CSF, or blood, with or without pleocytosis greater than 50 white blood cells/mm^3 and one or more of the

Table 71-5 Percentage of Patients with Clinical Findings of Possible Shunt Infection

Presentation	Odio[58] (N = 59)	Ronan[57] (N = 49)	Kontny[56] (N = 28)	Mancao[55] (N = 29)	Total (N = 165)
Fever	87	72	96	62	77
Shunt malfunction	–	36	50	–	51
Irritability	81	27	25	69*	49
Vomiting	39	24	–	–	31
Meningismus	–	20	21	–	18
Cellulitis	19	15	–	24	18
Abdominal pain	22	15	36	17†	21
Lethargy	–	12	–	–	12

*This percentage represents patients with "neurologic signs," which included vomiting, irritability, bulging fontanelle, or meningismus.
†This percentage represents patients with "abdominal signs," which included abdominal pain, ileus, or diarrhea.

Table 71-6 Pathogens Commonly Found in Shunt Infections

Organism	NUMBER OF PATIENTS (%)						
	Enger[72] (N = 9)	Odio[58] (N = 59)	Ronan[57] (N = 41)	Kontny[56] (N = 28)	Mancao[55] (N = 29)**	McGirt[66] (N = 92)	Total (N = 258)
Staphylococcus epidermidis	7 (78)	27 (46)	7 (17)	16 (57)	14 (48)	49 (53)	120 (47)
Staphylococcus aureus	1 (11)	17 (29)	12 (30)	1 (4)	7 (24)	24 (26)	62 (24)
Gram negatives	–	15 (25)	10 (24)	2 (7)	3 (10)	8 (9)	38 (15)
Viridans streptococcus	–	6 (10)	–	–	–	–	6 (2)
Enterococcus	–	3 (5)	2 (5)	–	–	4 (4)	9 (3)
Mixed	–	–	–	5 (18)	3 (10)	–	8 (3)
Other*	2 (22)	–	–	4 (14)	2 (7)	4 (4)	12 (5)

*Other culture results include *Candida* species (n = 2; Enger), no growth (n = 4; Kontny), *Corynebacterium* (n = 1) and group B streptococcus (n = 1; Mancao), and *Propionibacterium* (n = 4; McGirt).

following: fever, shunt malfunction, neurologic symptoms, or abdominal signs or symptoms.[58] Although cultures of blood and lumbar CSF can be helpful, sampling of the ventricular fluid is critical to make the diagnosis for two main reasons. First, positive blood cultures are commonly seen with ventriculoatrial shunting, in which infected CSF drains directly into the bloodstream.[58] Since VP shunting has become the standard of care, bacteremia has become a relatively uncommon finding in shunt infections. Second, most patients who require CSF shunts often have an underlying impairment or absence of CSF reabsorption into the venous system, which would limit the passage of bacteria into the bloodstream. If the ventricles have little or no communication with the lumbar spinal fluid, it is possible to have a shunt-associated ventriculitis with a normal lumbar puncture. In addition, if a patient has more than one shunt, it is important to culture all of them because they may be draining different collections of CSF that are not in communication.

CSF pleocytosis is a helpful marker, but it alone is not diagnostic of infection. Many shunt infections occur shortly after placement, and it can be difficult to distinguish whether the CSF pleocytosis is caused by postoperative inflammation or infection. In addition, shunt infections can be caused by indolent organisms that do not induce a vigorous immune response. This is exemplified by coagulase-negative staphylococci, the most common organisms cultured from infected shunts. These bacteria produce a biofilm that protects them from the host immune response and enhances adherence to the device. When considered in association with other clinical markers, however, the CSF white blood cell count can be useful. One recent study found that a history of fever and ventricular fluid neutrophilia (>10%) had a specificity of 99% and positive and negative predictive values of 93% and 95%, respectively, for identifying or excluding shunt-related infection.[60] Techniques for sampling CSF from a VP shunt are provided in Chapter 214.

Causes

Table 71-6 summarizes the organisms most commonly found in CSF shunt infections. *Staphylococcus* species are by far the most common species identified, and coagulase-negative staphylococci are the most prevalent organisms.

Various gram-negative organisms have been implicated in shunt infections. Anaerobic bacteria—especially *Propionibacterium*—are also known to cause shunt infections.[61] They have historically been implicated in culture-negative infections, and they can be difficult to grow, especially when CSF is not sent for anaerobic culture. Fungi, predominantly *Candida* species, have been reported rarely.[62]

One study analyzed pathogens isolated from shunt infections in relation to time of infection.[58] Eighty-five percent of infections that occurred within the first 15 days after surgery were caused by staphylococci. In addition, 75% of all *S. aureus* infections occurred in this period. In contrast, gram-negative infections generally occurred a longer time after the initial surgery, and they are thought to arise from ascending infection of enteric organisms that colonize the distal portion of the shunt.[58] Sixty-four percent of infections that occurred more than 15 days after surgery were caused by gram-negative organisms. Another study found an association between shunt infections occurring longer than 30 weeks after shunt placement and *Haemophilus influenzae*,[57] but this study was done before routine vaccination against *H. influenzae*. Finally, a review of 94 shunt infections found that 8 occurred more than 9 months after surgery; none were caused by *S. aureus*.[63] These observations support the common belief that the majority of shunt infections are caused by the introduction of skin organisms at the time of shunt placement.[58,64,65]

Many studies have attempted to define factors that predispose children to shunt infection. Several retrospective studies have suggested that younger patient age, hydrocephalus, and more frequent revisions are correlated with shunt infection. A recent retrospective case-control study of 820 consecutive VP shunt placements identified four independent risk factors for infection. Each year of decreasing age was associated with a 4% increase in the risk of infection. The other risk factors were insertion of a shunt into a premature neonate, use of a neuroendoscope, and shunt insertion after a previous shunt infection.[66]

Treatment

To date, there has been only one prospective, randomized study of the treatment of shunt infection.[67] Nevertheless, it is generally accepted that optimal management of a shunt infection includes removal of the shunt and placement of a temporary ventricular reservoir until the infection resolves. In the retrospective studies that addressed shunt removal, this strategy was clearly associated with better outcomes. An analysis of treatment options for shunt infection that included 17 studies published over 30 years revealed that the combination of shunt removal and antibiotics successfully treated 88% of 244 infections, whereas antibiotic therapy alone was successful in only 33% of 230 infections.[68]

Empirical antibiotic therapy should include broad-spectrum antibiotics that cover the major pathogens associated with shunt-related infections. Because staphylococcal species are the most commonly found pathogens, vancomycin is recommended for gram-positive coverage, especially given the high prevalence of *Staphylococcus epidermidis* and the increasing prevalence of methicillin-resistant *S. aureus*. The array of pathogenic gram-negative organisms is even larger. The report of *P. aeruginosa* in several series and case reports, combined with its propensity to adhere to foreign material, warrants including pseudomonal coverage in empirical therapy. Ceftazidime or a fluoroquinolone has excellent pseudomonal coverage and penetrates the CSF well. Therapy can be further tailored based on the identification and susceptibility of the causative organism. If appropriate systemic therapy fails to eradicate the infection, both vancomycin and aminoglycosides can be given intrathecally. Rifampin, which has better CSF penetration than vancomycin, is often added for gram-positive shunt infections that fail to clear on vancomycin monotherapy; however, there is no strong evidence that this strategy is successful.[69]

Consultation

Neurosurgical services are routinely involved with the evaluation and management of VP shunt infections. Critical care involvement varies with the patient's condition and the particular institution. Infectious disease specialists are often consulted for guidance on evaluation, empirical therapy, and short- and long-term management.

Admission Criteria

The vast majority of patients with shunt infections require hospitalization owing to the complexity of care, including parenteral antibiotic therapy and externalization of the shunt. Externalized shunts require close attention to the rate of drainage, and adjustments in the apparatus may be needed to remain within satisfactory parameters. Also, ongoing assessment of the neurologic and overall clinical status of the patient often requires inpatient care. Transfer to a critical care setting may be appropriate, depending on the clinical status of the patient and the ability to provide close medical support in a non–intensive care environment.

Discharge Criteria

Commonly, discharge is considered when the infection has resolved and a stable CSF drainage management system is in place. Reinsertion of a new CSF drainage device may be delayed, if appropriate (e.g., slow-paced progression to increased intracranial pressure). Close outpatient follow-up is needed to watch for reinfection, malfunction, and signs of raised intracranial pressure.

Prevention

Despite aseptic technique in the operating room, some surgical contamination is inevitable. With that in mind, several studies have examined the benefit of antibiotic prophylaxis for shunt placement surgeries, but the results have been largely inconclusive.[65,70] More recently, VP shunts impregnated with clindamycin and rifampin have been successful in animal models. Two small clinical trials in humans are promising, and this technique warrants further investigation.[64,71]

In a Nutshell

- Children with VP shunt infections present with a range of symptoms, including fever, evidence of increased intracranial pressure, meningismus, or cellulitis at incision sites. Abdominal pain or frank peritonitis is associated with infection at the distal site.
- Shunt infection is confirmed by the isolation of a bacterial pathogen from ventricular fluid, lumbar CSF, or blood, along with a constellation of symptoms and laboratory evaluations. CSF pleocytosis is a helpful marker but is not diagnostic.
- Determining the site of infection is essential, because shunt removal is often required for definitive treatment. Careful evaluation is needed to avoid inappropriate procedures and to provide appropriate therapy.
- *Staphylococcus* species are responsible for many shunt infections, with coagulase-negative staphylococci being the most common pathogen.

On the Horizon

- New technologies such as antimicrobial-impregnated ventricular shunts show promise in reducing the infection rates associated with these devices.

REFERENCES

1. Mermel LA, Farr BM, Sherertz RJ, et al: Guidelines for the management of intravascular catheter-related infections. Clin Infect Dis 2001;32:1249-1272.
2. Neville HL, Lally KP: Pediatric surgical wound infections. Semin Pediatr Infect Dis 2001;12:124-129.
3. Richards MJ, Edwards JR, Culver DH, Gaynes RP: Nosocomial infections in pediatric intensive care units in the United States. National Nosocomial Infections Surveillance System. Pediatrics 1999;103:e39.
4. Wisplinghoff H, Seifert H, Tallent SM, et al: Nosocomial bloodstream infections in pediatric patients in United States hospitals: Epidemiology, clinical features and susceptibilities. Pediatr Infect Dis J 2003;22:686-691.
5. National Nosocomial Infections Surveillance (NNIS) System report: Data summary from January 1992 through June 2004, issued October 2004. Am J Infect Control 2004;32:470-485.
6. Elward AM, Hollenbeak CS, Warren DK, Fraser VJ: Attributable cost of nosocomial primary bloodstream infection in pediatric intensive care unit patients. Pediatrics 2005;115:868-872.
7. Shah SS, Manning ML, Leahy E, et al: Central venous catheter-associated bloodstream infections in pediatric oncology home care. Infect Control Hosp Epidemiol 2002;23:99-101.
8. O'Grady NP, Alexander M, Dellinger EP, et al: Guidelines for the prevention of intravascular catheter-related infections. The Hospital Infection Control Practices Advisory Committee, Centers for Disease Control and Prevention, US. Pediatrics 2002;110:e51.
9. Shah SS, McGowan KL, et al: Time to blood culture positivity in children with central venous catheters. Presented at the Pediatric Academic Societies Annual Meeting, Washington, DC, May 14-17, 2005.
10. Gorelick MH, Owen WC, Seibel NL, Reaman GH: Lack of association between neutropenia and the incidence of bacteremia associated with indwelling central venous catheters in febrile pediatric cancer patients. Pediatr Infect Dis J 1991;10:506-510.
11. Raad II, Luna M, Khalil SA, et al: The relationship between the thrombotic and infectious complications of central venous catheters. JAMA 1994;271:1014-1016.
12. Raad I, Hanna HA, Alakech B, et al: Differential time to positivity: A useful method for diagnosing catheter-related bloodstream infections. Ann Intern Med 2004;140:18-25.
13. Blot F, Nitenberg G, Chachaty E, et al: Diagnosis of catheter-related bacteraemia: A prospective comparison of the time to positivity of hub-blood versus peripheral-blood cultures. Lancet 1999;354:1071-1077.
14. Blot F, Schmidt E, Nitenberg G, et al: Earlier positivity of central-venous-versus peripheral-blood cultures is highly predictive of catheter-related sepsis. J Clin Microbiol 1998;36:105-109.
15. Seifert H, Cornely O, Seggewiss K, et al: Bloodstream infection in neutropenic cancer patients related to short-term nontunnelled catheters determined by quantitative blood cultures, differential time to positivity, and molecular epidemiological typing with pulsed-field gel electrophoresis. J Clin Microbiol 2003;41:118-123.
16. Brun-Buisson C, Abrouk F, Legrand P, et al: Diagnosis of central venous catheter-related sepsis: Critical level of quantitative tip cultures. Arch Intern Med 1987;147:873-877.
17. Maki DG, Weise CE, Sarafin HW: A semiquantitative culture method for identifying intravenous-catheter-related infection. N Engl J Med 1977;296:1305-1309.
18. Li J, Plorde JJ, Carlson LG: Effects of volume and periodicity on blood cultures. J Clin Microbiol 1994;32:2829-2831.
19. Chandrasekar PH, Brown WJ: Clinical issues of blood cultures. Arch Intern Med 1994;154:841-849.
20. Schelonka RL, Chai MK, Yoder BA, et al: Volume of blood required to detect common neonatal pathogens. J Pediatr 1996;129:275-278.
21. Isaacman DJ, Karasic RB, Reynolds EA, Kost SI: Effect of number of blood cultures and volume of blood on detection of bacteremia in children. J Pediatr 1996;128:190-195.
22. Mermel LA, Maki DG: Detection of bacteremia in adults: Consequences of culturing an inadequate volume of blood. Ann Intern Med 1993;119:270-272.
23. Weinstein MP, Murphy JR, Reller LB, Lichtenstein KA: The clinical significance of positive blood cultures: A comprehensive analysis of 500 episodes of bacteremia and fungemia in adults. II. Clinical observations, with special reference to factors influencing prognosis. Rev Infect Dis 1983;5:54-70.
24. Reimer LG, Wilson ML, Weinstein MP: Update on detection of bacteremia and fungemia. Clin Microbiol Rev 1997;10:444-465.
25. Maraqa NF, Gomez MM, Rathore MH: Outpatient parenteral antimicrobial therapy in osteoarticular infections in children. J Pediatr Orthop 2002;22:506-510.
26. Edmond MB, Wallace SE, McClish DK, et al: Nosocomial bloodstream infections in United States hospitals: A three-year analysis. Clin Infect Dis 1999;29:239-244.
27. Smith TL, Pullen GT, Crouse V, et al: Bloodstream infections in pediatric oncology outpatients: A new healthcare systems challenge. Infect Control Hosp Epidemiol 2002;23:239-243.
28. Tokars JI: Predictive value of blood cultures positive for coagulase-negative staphylococci: Implications for patient care and health care quality assurance. Clin Infect Dis 2004;39:333-341.
29. Sohn AH, Garrett DO, Sinkowitz-Cochran RL, et al: Prevalence of nosocomial infections in neonatal intensive care unit patients: Results from the first national point-prevalence survey. J Pediatr 2001;139:821-827.
30. Sinkowitz RL, Keyserling H, Walker TJ, et al: Epidemiology of vancomycin usage at a children's hospital, 1993 through 1995. Pediatr Infect Dis J 1997;16:485-489.
31. Garrett DO, Jochimsen E, Murfitt K, et al: The emergence of decreased susceptibility to vancomycin in *Staphylococcus epidermidis*. Infect Control Hosp Epidemiol 1999;20:167-170.
32. Smith TL, Pearson ML, Wilcox KR, et al: Emergence of vancomycin resistance in *Staphylococcus aureus*. Glycopeptide-Intermediate *Staphylococcus aureus* Working Group. N Engl J Med 1999;340:493-501.
33. Weiner E: Catheter sepsis: The central venous line Achilles' heel. Semin Pediatr Surg 1995;4:207-214.
34. King DR, Komer M, Hoffman J, et al: Broviac catheter sepsis: The natural history of an iatrogenic infection. J Pediatr Surg 1985;20:728-733.

35. Hartman GE, Shochat SJ: Management of septic complications associated with Silastic catheters in childhood malignancy. Pediatr Infect Dis J 1987;6:1042-1047.

36. Flynn PM, Shenep JL, Stokes DC, Barrett FF: In situ management of confirmed central venous catheter-related bacteremia. Pediatr Infect Dis J 1987;6:729-734.

37. American Academy of Pediatrics: Staphylococcal Infections, 26th ed. Elk Grove Village, Ill, American Academy of Pediatrics, 2003.

38. Benjamin DK Jr, Miller W, Garges H, et al: Bacteremia, central catheters, and neonates: When to pull the line. Pediatrics 2001;107:1272-1276.

39. Raad I, Davis S, Khan A, et al: Impact of central venous catheter removal on the recurrence of catheter-related coagulase-negative staphylococcal bacteremia. Infect Control Hosp Epidemiol 1992;13:215-221.

40. Raad II, Bodey GP: Infectious complications of indwelling vascular catheters. Clin Infect Dis 1992;15:197-208.

41. Rosen AB, Fowler VG Jr, Corey GR, et al: Cost-effectiveness of transesophageal echocardiography to determine the duration of therapy for intravascular catheter-associated *Staphylococcus aureus* bacteremia. Ann Intern Med 1999;130:810-820.

42. Fowler VG Jr, Li J, Corey GR, et al: Role of echocardiography in evaluation of patients with *Staphylococcus aureus* bacteremia: Experience in 103 patients. J Am Coll Cardiol 1997;30:1072-1078.

43. Valente AM, Jain R, Scheurer M, et al: Frequency of infective endocarditis among infants and children with *Staphylococcus aureus* bacteremia. Pediatrics 2005;115:e15-e19.

44. Raad II, Sabbagh MF: Optimal duration of therapy for catheter-related *Staphylococcus aureus* bacteremia: A study of 55 cases and review. Clin Infect Dis 1992;14:75-82.

45. Hanna H, Afif C, Alakech B, et al: Central venous catheter-related bacteremia due to gram-negative bacilli: Significance of catheter removal in preventing relapse. Infect Control Hosp Epidemiol 2004;25:646-649.

46. Blumberg HM, Jarvis WR, Soucie JM, et al: Risk factors for candidal bloodstream infections in surgical intensive care unit patients: The NEMIS prospective multicenter study. The National Epidemiology of Mycosis Survey. Clin Infect Dis 2001;33:177-186.

47. Lecciones JA, Lee JW, Navarro EE, et al: Vascular catheter-associated fungemia in patients with cancer: Analysis of 155 episodes. Clin Infect Dis 1992;14:875-883.

48. Eppes SC, Troutman JL, Gutman LT: Outcome of treatment of candidemia in children whose central catheters were removed or retained. Pediatr Infect Dis J 1989;8:99-104.

49. Nucci M, Anaissie E: Should vascular catheters be removed from all patients with candidemia? An evidence-based review. Clin Infect Dis 2002;34:591-599.

50. Zaoutis TE, Greves HM, Lautenbach E, et al: Risk factors for disseminated candidiasis in children with candidemia. Pediatr Infect Dis J 2004;23:635-641.

51. Pappas PG, Rex JH, Sobel JD, et al: Guidelines for treatment of candidiasis. Clin Infect Dis 2004;38:161-189.

52. Hu KK, Lipsky BA, Veenstra DL, Saint S: Using maximal sterile barriers to prevent central venous catheter-related infection: A systematic evidence-based review. Am J Infect Control 2004;32:142-146.

53. Darouiche RO, Raad II, Heard SO, et al: A comparison of two antimicrobial-impregnated central venous catheters. Catheter Study Group. N Engl J Med 1999;340:1-8.

54. Yogev R: Cerebrospinal fluid shunt infections: A personal view. Pediatr Infect Dis 1985;4:113-118.

55. Mancao M, Miller C, Cochrane B, et al: Cerebrospinal fluid shunt infections in infants and children in Mobile, Alabama. Acta Paediatr 1998;87:667-670.

56. Kontny U, Hofling B, Gutjahr P, et al: CSF shunt infections in children. Infection 1993;21:89-92.

57. Ronan A, Hogg GG, Klug GL: Cerebrospinal fluid shunt infections in children. Pediatr Infect Dis J 1995;14:782-786.

58. Odio C, McCracken GH Jr, Nelson JD: CSF shunt infections in pediatrics: A seven-year experience. Am J Dis Child 1984;138:1103-1108.

59. Anderson CM, Sorrells DL, Kerby JD: Intra-abdominal pseudocysts as a complication of ventriculoperitoneal shunts: A case report and review of the literature. Curr Surg 2003;60:338-340.

60. McClinton D, Carraccio C, Englander R: Predictors of ventriculoperitoneal shunt pathology. Pediatr Infect Dis J 2001;20:593-597.

61. Brook I: Meningitis and shunt infection caused by anaerobic bacteria in children. Pediatr Neurol 2002;26:99-105.

62. Chiou CC, Wong TT, Lin HH, et al: Fungal infection of ventriculoperitoneal shunts in children. Clin Infect Dis 1994;19:1049-1053.

63. Baird C, O'Connor D, Pittman T: Late shunt infections. Pediatr Neurosurg 1999;31:269-273.

64. Aryan HE, Meltzer HS, Park MS, et al: Initial experience with antibiotic-impregnated silicone catheters for shunting of cerebrospinal fluid in children. Childs Nerv Syst 2005;21:56-61.

65. Morris A, Low DE: Nosocomial bacterial meningitis, including central nervous system shunt infections. Infect Dis Clin North Am 1999;13:735-750.

66. McGirt MJ, Zaas A, Fuchs HE, et al: Risk factors for pediatric ventriculoperitoneal shunt infection and predictors of infectious pathogens. Clin Infect Dis 2003;36:858-862.

67. James HE, Walsh JW, Wilson HD, et al: Prospective randomized study of therapy in cerebrospinal fluid shunt infection. Neurosurgery 1980;7:459-463.

68. Schreffler RT, Schreffler AJ, Wittler RR: Treatment of cerebrospinal fluid shunt infections: A decision analysis. Pediatr Infect Dis J 2002;21:632-636.

69. Brackbill ML, Brophy GM: Adjunctive rifampin therapy for central nervous system staphylococcal infections. Ann Pharmacother 2001;35:765-769.

70. Pople IK, Bayston R, Hayward RD: Infection of cerebrospinal fluid shunts in infants: A study of etiological factors. J Neurosurg 1992;77:29-36.

71. Govender ST, Nathoo N, van Dellen JR: Evaluation of an antibiotic-impregnated shunt system for the treatment of hydrocephalus. J Neurosurg 2003;99:831-839.

72. Enger PO, Svendsen F, Wester K: CSF shunt infections in children: Experiences from a population-based study. Acta Neurochir (Wien) 2003;145:243-248.

CHAPTER 72

Human Immunodeficiency Virus

Jason Y. Kim

Human immunodeficiency virus (HIV) has led to a worldwide pandemic that has exacted a dramatic toll on children, especially in resource-limited countries. It is estimated that there are approximately 2.1 million children younger than 14 years living with HIV, with the vast majority in sub-Saharan Africa. Worldwide, approximately 700,000 children were infected perinatally with HIV in 2005, and 570,000 children died due to HIV/AIDS (acquired immunodeficiency syndrome) in 2005 (see *www.cdc.gov* and *www.unaids.org*). As of 2003, there were more than 9000 children younger than 13 years living with AIDS in the United States. The vast majority of these children were infected by perinatal transmission. In resource-rich countries, the perinatal infection rate has dropped to less than 2%, and combination antiretroviral therapy (known as highly active antiretroviral therapy, or HAART) has diminished mortality and morbidity associated with HIV disease.[1] The pediatric hospitalist must be familiar with the care of HIV-exposed newborns and HIV-infected children, because the initial diagnosis and management of complications often occur in the hospital setting.

Historically, HIV infection and AIDS were differentiated by the 1987 Centers for Disease Control (CDC) case definition for AIDS surveillance—that is, the presence of opportunistic infections or other so-called AIDS-defining conditions. In 1994 the pediatric classification of the severity of HIV disease was revised to include infection status, clinical status, and immunologic status (Tables 72-1 and 72-2). Children younger than 7 years have higher numbers of CD4$^+$ T cells than adults do; therefore, total CD4$^+$ T-cell count is not an effective marker of immunologic status in these children. The immunologic status is categorized by the lowest percentage of CD4$^+$ T cells relative to total lymphocytes (CD4%) the child has ever had. A CD4% equal to 25% in children younger than 7 years is analogous to a total CD4$^+$ count of 500 cells/mm^3 in adults. A CD4% less than 15% corresponds to a total CD4$^+$ of less than 200 cells/mm^3. Thus, an HIV-infected child with a prior episode of *Pneumocystis jiroveci* pneumonia (previously *Pneumocystis carinii* pneumonia and, by convention, still abbreviated PCP) and a prior CD4% nadir of 5% would be categorized as C3.[2]

CLINICAL PRESENTATION

HIV-Exposed Newborn

On physical examination, there are often no stigmata of vertical HIV infection in the newborn, because the majority of cases of vertical transmission occur intrapartum. It is estimated that less than one third of cases of vertical HIV transmission occur in utero. Thus, the physical examination often reveals no features that would distinguish vertical transmission of HIV from other comorbid conditions such as prematurity, intrauterine illicit drug exposure, or other congenital infections. Premature delivery has been reported in 19% of HIV-infected infants. Children born to mothers who also abuse illicit drugs have smaller head circumferences and lower birth weights.

HIV-Infected Child

Presenting symptoms and signs of HIV infection tend to be more prevalent and more severe in children than in adults, and conditions associated with HIV infection are more common. The pattern of disease associated with HIV infection varies greatly among children, but children with HIV infection tend to have a faster progression to AIDS compared with adults; this is exhibited by more invasive bacterial infections, systemic cytomegalovirus (CMV) infection, lymphocytic interstitial pneumonitis, and HIV encephalopathy. Approximately 25% to 50% of infected children die or have a rapidly progressive course, with presentation of AIDS-defining opportunistic infections within the first year of life, commonly attributed to the infant's immature immune system. These children are known as rapid progressors.

Other children may not show signs of HIV infection or may not develop opportunistic infections until school age. However, a review of the child's past medical history often demonstrates recurrent infections, multiple episodes of invasive bacterial disease, or longer duration of infections than uninfected siblings. Besides infections, children with vertically acquired HIV infection often present with nonspecific conditions such as failure to thrive, generalized lymphadenopathy, or loss of developmental milestones. The age of onset of symptoms predicts long-term survival.

DIAGNOSIS

HIV-Exposed Newborn

In the early years of the HIV epidemic, perinatal transmission of HIV (also termed vertical transmission or mother-child transmission) occurred at rates of 13% to 30%. In the United States, the estimated number of vertically transmitted HIV infections peaked in 1992, at approximately 900 cases. Since then, numerous interventions, including prenatal counseling and testing for HIV, use of antenatal HAART for pregnant women, elective cesarean delivery, zidovudine (ZDV, also known as AZT) infusion during labor, and ZDV prophylaxis for newborns, have been instituted. This has dramatically reduced the vertical transmission rate to about 1% of infants born in the developed world. In 2003, 131 cases of vertically acquired HIV infection were reported to the CDC. In contrast, during the years 2000 to 2003, approximately 27,000 women of childbearing age were newly diagnosed with HIV in the United States. Thus, as the number of women of childbearing age diagnosed with HIV

Table 72-1 HIV Infection Status

Status	Description
Acute HIV infection	Febrile illness with nonspecific symptoms that are self-limited (mononucleosis-like); associated with a high viral load; patients are highly contagious
Seroconversion	Development of anti-HIV antibodies, usually 1-6 mo after exposure
Clinically latent HIV infection	Period of asymptomatic infection that follows acute infection; generalized lymphadenopathy may be present; viral load is usually lower than during acute infection
Early symptomatic HIV infection	Equivalent to class B (see Table 72-2)
AIDS	Presence of AIDS-defining condition (see Table 72-2, class C) or CD4+ count <200/mL

AIDS, acquired immunodeficiency syndrome.

increases, practitioners in the newborn nursery may be required to manage HIV-exposed neonates.

The initial evaluation of an HIV-exposed neonate begins with a detailed prenatal history. In addition to the typical elements (e.g., prenatal laboratory studies, medical complications of pregnancy, alcohol or illicit drug use, mode of delivery), the nursery clinician should determine the following aspects of the prenatal history: when the mother was diagnosed with HIV; the prenatal antiviral regimen, if any; and the most recent maternal viral load and CD4+ T-cell count. The clinician must also verify that the mother received intrapartum intravenous ZDV at the onset of labor. It should be noted that although elective cesarean section is often performed to decrease the risk of vertical transmission, vaginal delivery may be performed when the maternal viral load is less than 1000 copies/mL and intravenous ZDV is administered at the onset of labor.

Immediately following birth, a complete blood count with differential should be performed on the newborn as a baseline, before initiating postpartum antiretroviral prophylaxis. Although there are several effective postpartum antiretroviral prophylaxis regimens, the U.S. Public Health Service recommends ZDV therapy for 6 weeks. Neonates are at higher risk for vertical transmission of HIV-1 in certain situations, such as peripartum seroconversion in a previously undiagnosed woman, high maternal viral load, low maternal CD4+ T-cell count, prolonged rupture of membranes, and precipitous vaginal delivery without intrapartum ZDV. Some experts recommend the use of multiple antiretroviral agents as prophylaxis when the risk of vertical transmission with HIV is high, but this practice is not universal, and there are no data to support such practices.[3]

Initial diagnostic testing should be performed at 48 hours of age. Serologic testing for anti-HIV-1 and anti-HIV-2 immunoglobulin G (IgG) antibodies is not interpretable because of the maternal-fetal immunoglobulin transfusion

that occurs in the third trimester. Therefore, most experts recommend molecular testing of neonates using qualitative DNA polymerase chain reaction (PCR) to detect cases of in utero infection. The infant's serum must be used for the test. Cord blood samples should not be sent for testing because maternal blood may contaminate the sample. Subsequent qualitative DNA PCR tests should be performed at 1 to 2 months and 4 to 6 months of age to diagnose HIV infection. Three negative PCR tests and a negative serologic test done at 12 to 18 months of age exclude HIV infection in an infant.

HIV-Infected Child

The type of test performed for suspected HIV infection depends on the age of the child. An enzyme-linked immunosorbent assay (ELISA) and confirmatory Western blot for anti-HIV-1 and anti-HIV-2 IgG can be performed in children older than 18 months. Those younger than 1 year should have PCR tests for HIV DNA. It should be noted that children born in Africa may be infected with HIV-2, which may be missed by HIV-1 PCR primers. A child younger than 18 months with a positive molecular test for HIV is considered infected, as is an older child with a positive serologic assay.

TREATMENT

HIV Infection

As stated earlier, the treatment of HIV infection consists of HAART. However, the treatment of HIV-infected children requires special considerations. For example, the immunologic status is age specific for children younger than 7 years. In addition, the pharmacokinetic properties of antiretroviral medications differ significantly in children compared with adults. When selecting antiretroviral agents, one must keep in mind the inevitable development of resistance to these agents. An excellent resource that is updated frequently is available at *http://aidsinfo.nih.gov*.

Two independent and complementary pieces of laboratory data are used to determine the status of HIV disease and the prognosis of HIV-infected children: quantitative HIV RNA copies per milliliter of plasma (viral load) and CD4%. The goals of therapy are to maintain undetectable viral loads and to restore normal CD4% while minimizing the adverse effects of the medications.

There are four classes of antiretroviral agents used against HIV:

1. Nucleoside reverse transcriptase inhibitors (NRTIs)
2. Non-nucleoside reverse transcriptase inhibitors (NNRTIs)
3. Protease inhibitors (PIs)
4. Fusion inhibitors

HAART comprises at least three agents from at least two classes. Currently, the recommended HAART regimens have a "backbone" consisting of at least two, and sometimes three, NRTIs; in addition, children receive either a PI or an NNRTI. As with adults, fusion inhibitors are reserved for HIV-infected children with late-stage disease and multiply resistant virus strains.[4]

Adjunctive therapy is sometimes used in children with recurrent invasive bacterial infections. These children often

Table 72-2 Clinical and Immunologic Status of Pediatric HIV Infection

Status	Description
Clinical class	
N: not symptomatic	No signs or symptoms considered to be the result of HIV infection, or the presence of only one condition listed in class A
A: mildly symptomatic	Presence of two or more of the following: Lymphadenopathy Hepatomegaly Splenomegaly Dermatitis Parotitis Recurrent or persistent URI, sinusitis, or otitis media
B: moderately symptomatic	Presence of symptomatic conditions other than those listed in class A or C attributable to HIV infection: Anemia, neutropenia, thrombocytopenia for >30 days Bacterial meningitis, pneumonia, sepsis Candidiasis or thrush for >2 mo Cardiomyopathy Diarrhea (chronic or recurrent) Hepatitis Herpes simplex virus or herpes zoster infection Lymphoid interstitial pneumonia Persistent fever (>1 mo) CMV or toxoplasmosis (onset before 1 mo of age)
C: severely symptomatic	Multiple or recurrent serious bacterial infections: Candidiasis (esophageal or pulmonary) Coccidioidomycosis, cryptococcosis, histoplasmosis Cryptosporidiosis, isosporiasis Encephalopathy, progressive multifocal leukoencephalopathy Malignancy: Kaposi sarcoma, lymphoma Mycobacterial infection *Pneumocystis jiroveci* (formerly *carinii*) pneumonia Wasting syndrome

		CD4⁺ LYMPHOCYTE COUNT (CELLS/µL)		
	CD4%	**Age <12 Months**	**Age 1-5 Years**	**Age 6-12 Years**
Immunologic status				
1	>25	>1500	>1000	>500
2	15-24	750-1499	500-999	200-499
3	<15	<750	<500	<200

CD4%, percentage of CD4⁺ T cells relative to the total number of lymphocytes; CMV, cytomegalovirus; URI, upper respiratory infection.

receive intravenous immunoglobulin infusions every 3 to 4 weeks.

Infections in an HIV-Infected Child

Although the evaluation for possible infection generally warrants greater attention in an HIV-infected child than in an uninfected one, the clinical assessment depends greatly on the patient's current immunologic status. As noted earlier, children younger than 7 years have a higher number of CD4⁺ T cells than adults do; thus, the CD4% is a more accurate marker of immunologic status. A CD4% greater than 25% is considered normal,[4] and the risk of opportunistic infection increases dramatically at a CD4% less than 15%. The most common AIDS-defining infections are PCP, recurrent bacterial infections, *Candida* esophagitis, cytomegalovirus

(CMV) infection, and disseminated *Mycobacterium avium* complex (MAC) infection. When evaluating an HIV-infected child for infection, it is crucial to determine the child's CD4%, total CD4 count, most recent viral load, and HAART regimen.[6] CD4⁺ counts must be interpreted according to age-specific ranges (see Table 72-2).

Acute onset of fever is a common reason for an HIV-1-infected child to be brought to medical attention. The child may be admitted for fever without localizing signs or for fever of unknown origin. As with all children, the majority of fevers are due to common, self-limited infections, such as a viral upper respiratory infection. HIV infection necessitates a more thorough investigation for a focus of infection, however. Children with HIV have a slightly higher incidence of bacteremia and invasive bacterial disease than does the general population, regardless of CD4%. *Streptococcus*

Table 72-3 Causes of Undifferentiated Fever in HIV-Infected Children

Focal bacterial infection (with symptoms and signs obscured)
Salmonellosis
Mycobacterial infection (*Mycobacterium tuberculosis* or
  atypical mycobacteria)
Pneumocystis jiroveci pneumonia
Toxoplasma gondii infection
Herpesvirus infection (Epstein-Barr, cytomegalovirus, herpes
  simplex, varicella-zoster)
Hepatitis
Lymphoma
Drug fever

pneumoniae is the most common cause of invasive bacterial infection, and bacteremia with *Salmonella* species should also be considered in HIV-infected children with fever of unknown origin.

The absence of localizing signs in a child with a fever and a low CD4% dictates a broader, more intensive diagnostic evaluation because of the breadth of potential infectious causes. The compromised immunity caused by advanced HIV disease may obscure the focus of infection, including infection within the central nervous system (CNS). A child whose CD4% is less than 15% may have an infection caused by either typical pathogens (e.g., *S. pneumoniae*, *Staphylococcus aureus*) or opportunistic pathogens (e.g., mycobacteria, fungi). Fever without localizing signs may also be caused by disseminated herpesvirus infections, such as herpes simplex virus, varicella-zoster virus, Epstein-Barr virus, or CMV. The scope and tempo of the evaluation are dictated by the child's immunologic status and the acuity of presentation. A partial list of causes of undifferentiated fever in HIV-infected children is provided in Table 72-3.

In HIV-infected children whose CD4% is greater than 25%, CNS infections are likely caused by the same pathogens as in HIV-uninfected children. In general, children with HIV are at slightly increased risk for bacterial meningitis compared with children without HIV. HIV-infected children whose CD4% is greater than 15% have cerebrospinal fluid findings similar to those in children without HIV.

In children with a CD4% less than 15%, opportunistic pathogens such as *Cryptococcus neoformans*, JC virus, and CMV must be considered, in addition to typical CNS pathogens. Cryptococcal meningitis is a common opportunistic CNS infection. The course of cryptococcal meningitis is often insidious, with a gradual onset of fever, headache, malaise, and emesis. Frank signs of meningismus are often absent. The cerebrospinal fluid findings may be normal, including cell count, glucose, and protein levels.

JC virus causes progressive multifocal leukoencephalopathy, and reactivation of latent JC virus in the CNS can occur with advanced HIV infection (CD4% <15%), leading to progressive demyelination. There have been case reports of adults with normal CD4+ T-cell counts on HAART who developed progressive multifocal leukoencephalopathy. Patients often present with confusion, personality changes, and focal neurologic findings. Progressive multifocal

leukoencephalopathy often leads to death within months of diagnosis; however, survival has increased with the advent of HAART.

Focal CNS lesions, with or without mass effect, may have either infectious or noninfectious causes. Infections that can lead to focal CNS lesions include bacterial brain abscess, cryptococcoma, CNS toxoplasmosis, and tuberculoma, but these opportunistic infections are very rare in HIV-infected children. The noninfectious causes of CNS lesions include acute disseminated encephalomyelitis and lymphoma. Primary CNS lymphoma (usually of B-cell lineage) is considered an AIDS-defining condition.

Children with HIV infection and a CD4% greater than 25% are at no increased risk from typical viral respiratory pathogens such as respiratory syncytial virus, adenovirus, and parainfluenza viruses. The outcomes of influenza A virus infection in these children are similar to those in other high-risk groups (e.g., those with asthma). Consequently, it is recommended that all children with HIV receive the inactivated influenza vaccine annually.

The most common bacterial lower respiratory tract infection among HIV-infected children is pneumococcal pneumonia. Bacterial pneumonia is more common in children with HIV infection than in HIV-infected adults. HIV-infected children are also more likely to become bacteremic as a result of bacterial pneumonia than are other children or HIV-infected adults. In addition, HIV-infected children are more likely to be infected with *S. aureus*, *Haemophilus influenzae* type B, *Klebsiella pneumoniae*, *Pseudomonas aeruginosa*, and *Mycobacterium tuberculosis*.[1,5]

Children with a CD4% lower than 15% are at risk for opportunistic respiratory tract infections. PCP was the most common opportunistic infection before the advent of effective anti-*Pneumocystis* chemoprophylaxis and the widespread use of HAART, and it remains so today. The peak incidence of PCP is at 3 to 6 months of age, and it is seen among infants of undiagnosed HIV-infected mothers. PCP may also be seen in children with a low CD4% (e.g., those poorly adherent to their HAART regimen) or in those who are nonadherent with PCP prophylaxis. PCP may present with a sudden onset of fever, cough, and respiratory distress. The degree of hypoxemia and respiratory distress is usually out of proportion to the relatively nontoxic appearance of the child. The most common radiographic findings are bilateral perihilar interstitial infiltrates (butterfly pattern); however, PCP is renowned for its multiplicity of radiographic presentations, including lobar infiltrates, pneumothorax, and pneumatoceles.[5]

Other opportunistic infections include atypical mycobacteria (although isolated respiratory symptoms are rare in *M. avium* complex), *C. neoformans*, and *Candida* species. Children with AIDS are also at increased risk for extrapulmonary dissemination with endemic mycoses (e.g., *Histoplasma capsulatum*, *Coccidioides immitis*). Undifferentiated fever is the most common presentation for disseminated histoplasmosis.[5]

A noninfectious cause of cough in children with advanced HIV disease is lymphocytic interstitial pneumonitis. The disease has a gradual onset and an indolent course. Cough or wheezing may be associated with disease progression, and generalized lymphadenopathy and clubbing may be present.

A typical reticulonodular pattern may be seen on chest radiographs, with or without hilar lymphadenopathy. The diagnosis of lymphocytic interstitial pneumonitis is made based on clinical symptoms and the persistence of radiographic findings for 2 months in the absence of other identifiable causes.[1,5]

Gastrointestinal symptom complexes can be considered similarly to other infections. Acute, self-limited episodes of diarrhea may occur and have the same causes as in children without HIV infection: rotavirus, adenovirus, *Escherichia coli* (enterotoxigenic), and *Giardia lamblia*. Bloody, dysentery-like diarrheal disease may be caused by *Salmonella* species, *Shigella* species, *Campylobacter jejuni*, *E. coli* (enteroinvasive), and *Entamoeba histolytica*. Children with prolonged diarrhea may be infected with a typical pathogen or may have an opportunistic pathogen such as *Cryptosporidium*, *Isospora*, *M. avium* complex, or CMV. Children with a low CD4% may not be able to recover from diarrhea caused by typical pathogens and are at risk for infection with opportunistic pathogens. HIV itself can cause enteropathy, leading to chronic diarrhea and malnutrition.[5]

Children with advanced HIV disease are prone to episodes of esophagitis. This usually presents with dysphagia and odynophagia, although fever or irritability may be the only presenting signs. The most common cause is *Candida*. Esophageal candidiasis may be associated with oral thrush. Herpes simplex virus and CMV may also cause esophagitis in children with compromised immunity, as well as oropharyngeal ulcers associated with esophagitis.[5]

In general, children with a CD4% greater than 25% present in a manner similar to children without HIV, albeit with a slightly higher risk of invasive bacterial infection. The infectious agents are usually similar to those seen in children without HIV. A lower threshold for obtaining blood culture, urinalysis, urine culture, stool culture, chest radiograph, and lumbar puncture may be appropriate in HIV-infected children, decided on a case-by-case basis.

In general, HIV-infected children with a normal CD4% can be treated the same as immunologically normal children. Appropriate antimicrobial therapy should be instituted as in children without HIV, including oral therapy. The spectrum of activity should be targeted against the most likely bacterial pathogens. Children with neutropenia from HIV infection should have empirical antimicrobial therapy similar to that given to children with neutropenia from other causes (see Chapter 124). Children with a CD4% less than 15% (or older children with a total CD4+ <200 cells) should have broad empirical antimicrobial therapy chosen in consultation with an infectious disease specialist.

DIFFERENTIAL DIAGNOSIS

The cellular immune defects associated with advanced HIV disease predispose patients to different infections. Primary immunodeficiencies may present with similar recurrent infections or opportunistic infections.

Children who have recurrent sinopulmonary infections (e.g., pneumococcal, *S. aureus*) may also have humoral defects, such as hypogammaglobulinemia or X-linked agammaglobulinemia; combined defects, such as hyper-IgM syndrome or severe combined immunodeficiency (SCID); or complement deficiency. Children with phagocytic defects may present initially with recurrent sinopulmonary infections from typical organisms. Lung infections with *Aspergillus* and mycobacteria may be seen with cellular combined and phagocytic defects. For children who present with PCP, hyper-IgM syndrome, or SCID, phagocytic defects and other combined immunodeficiencies should be considered in the differential diagnosis.

Chronic diarrhea may also be seen in children with humoral, cellular, and combined immunodeficiency states. Humoral immunodeficiencies may inhibit the clearance of *Giardia* and other protozoa.[6,7]

A more complete discussion of immunodeficiency states is provided in Chapters 73 and 136.

CONSULTATION

Consultation with an infectious disease specialist is appropriate when the diagnosis of HIV is being considered; when opportunistic infections are suspected or identified; when HIV-infected patients present with fever, especially when no source is identified; and for long-term management. Whenever possible, contact with the physicians involved in the ongoing management of an HIV-infected child is desirable.

If specific organ systems are affected by HIV-related complications, involvement of the appropriate subspecialists is recommended. Their involvement may be necessary for a single event (e.g., biopsy) or for long-term management.

ADMISSION CRITERIA

Febrile HIV-infected children with a CD4% greater than 25% should be admitted according to the same criteria used for HIV-uninfected children. A more thorough evaluation in the emergency department for invasive bacterial infection should be performed, however. Often, HIV-infected children with a CD4% greater than 25% can be discharged while appropriate cultures are incubating in the clinical microbiology laboratory.

All febrile HIV-infected children with a CD4% less than 15% should be admitted for undifferentiated fever. Because of their immunologic compromise, they may not localize infections well, including those in the CNS. Additionally, such children are at risk for rapid decompensation of clinical status. For these reasons, many experts recommend admission of HIV-infected children with a CD4% between 15% and 20%, depending on the patient's past history. For example, if the CD4% exceeds 15% due to the recent initiation of HAART, extra caution should be taken. In addition, if the patient has a history of recurrent bacterial infections, cryptococcal meningitis, or disseminated *M. avium* complex, a lower threshold for admission may be appropriate.

Any child with HIV infection and CNS symptoms and signs (usually with the exception of mild headaches) should be admitted for evaluation. The cause of CNS findings may be infectious, neoplastic, or vasculitic and may present irrespective of CD4%. Progressive, worsening headache should be evaluated more intensively than in a child without HIV.

DISCHARGE CRITERIA

- Completion of empirical therapy that cannot be administered outside the hospital.
- Stabilization of clinical condition (e.g., resolution of hypoxemia) or institution of increased support at home to accommodate the new condition (e.g., home oxygen therapy).
- Ability to continue therapy at home.
- Establishment of appropriate outpatient follow-up, including physician appointments, laboratory testing, and medical imaging.

PREVENTION OF OCCUPATIONAL TRANSMISSION OF HIV

Transmission of HIV to health care personnel due to occupational exposure has been reported since the beginning of the AIDS epidemic. The U.S. Public Health Service guidelines were first drafted in 1996 and were updated in 2005. Health care personnel are defined as all paid and unpaid personnel who work in a health care setting and are at risk for exposure to HIV-infected body fluids or contaminated material. An occupational exposure is defined as any percutaneous injury (e.g., needle stick) or contact of a mucous membrane or nonintact skin with a potentially infectious fluid or substance, including blood and bloody bodily fluids. The risk of transmission from the following fluids has not been studied epidemiologically, but they should be considered infectious: cerebrospinal, pericardial, pleural, ascitic, vaginal, seminal, and amniotic fluids. Other fluids, such as tears and saliva, should not be considered infectious unless they are visibly contaminated with blood.

The risk for acquisition of HIV due to a percutaneous injury with a visibly contaminated sharp object is approximately 0.3% (95% confidence interval [CI], 0.2 to 0.5). The risk resulting from a mucous membrane exposure with blood is approximately 0.09% (95% CI, 0.006 to 0.5). Factors associated with an increased risk for transmission of HIV to health care personnel include a sharp object visibly contaminated with blood, a procedure involving the placement of an intravascular device, a deep injury, and a source patient with end-stage AIDS. However, the viral load of the source patient has not been verified as an independent risk factor, so even patients with low viral loads should be considered a risk for HIV transmission to health care personnel.

The administration of postexposure prophylaxis (PEP) depends on two factors: the exposure source (Table 72-4) and the type of exposure (Table 72-5). A suggested approach to PEP based on exposure risk category and HIV status of the source is shown in Table 72-6.

PEP should be initiated within hours after the exposure whenever possible. PEP is not recommended if the exposure

Table 72-4 Risk of HIV Transmission Based on HIV Status of Exposure Source

HIV Status of Exposure Source	Risk of HIV Transmission
Not HIV infected	No risk
Known not to be infected with HIV*	No risk
HIV infection status unknown or unknown source	Unquantified
HIV infection status unknown; HIV risk status unknown	Unquantified
HIV infection status unknown; low risk	Low
HIV infection status unknown; known not to have risk factors[†]	Low
HIV infection status unknown; high risk	Intermediate
HIV infection status unknown; known to have one or more risk factors[†]	Intermediate
HIV infected	High
Known to be infected with HIV[†]	High

*Absence of HIV infection is identified by laboratory documentation of negative HIV antibody or negative HIV DNA polymerase chain reaction (PCR) assay results from a specimen collected close to the time of exposure and in the absence of interval high-risk behavior or symptoms compatible with acute retroviral infection syndrome.

[†]Risk factors for HIV infection include male homosexual activity, injection drug use, blood transfusion or blood product infusion before 1985, and sexual activity with a member of a high-risk group. Some persons who have sex with members of a high-risk group do not identify themselves as at risk because they are unaware of the risk history of their sexual partners. Their risk of HIV infection is related to the prevalence of HIV infection in the immediate community.

[†]HIV infection is documented by the presence of specific antibody to HIV in persons older than 18 months and by positive plasma HIV RNA PCR assay results, positive cell-associated HIV DNA PCR assay results, or detection of plasma HIV p24 antigen in persons of any age.

Adapted from Havens PL, Committee on Pediatric AIDS: Postexposure prophylaxis in children and adolescents for nonoccupational exposure to human immunodeficiency virus. Pediatrics 2003;111:1475-1489.

Table 72-5 Risk of HIV Transmission Based on Exposure Type

Exposure Type	Risk of HIV Transmission
Cutaneous exposure	
Fluid on intact skin	No risk identified
Bite without break in skin	No risk identified
Skin with compromised integrity (eczema, chapped skin, dermatitis, abrasion, laceration, open wound)	Low to intermediate
Traumatic skin wound with bleeding in donor and recipient*	High
Mucous membrane exposure	
Kissing	No risk identified
Oral sex	Low
Human milk: single ingestion	Low
Splash to eye or mouth	Low
Receptive vaginal sex without trauma	Intermediate
Receptive anal intercourse	High
Traumatic sex with bleeding (sexual assault)	High
Percutaneous exposure†	
Superficial scratch with sharp object, including a needle found in the community	No risk identified
Puncture wound with solid needle	Low
Puncture wound with hollow needle without visible blood	Low
Body piercing	Low
Bite with break in skin	Low
Puncture wound with hollow needle with visible blood	Intermediate
Puncture wound with large-bore hollow needle with visible blood on needle, or needle recently used in source patient's artery or vein	High

*For example, during a fight, a blow to the mouth might break a tooth and lacerate the first, both of which bleed. If there is mixing of blood, both persons may be at risk.
Adapted from Havens PL, Committee on Pediatric AIDS: Postexposure prophylaxis in children and adolescents for nonoccupational exposure to human immunodeficiency virus. Pediatrics 2003;111:1475-1489.

Table 72-6 Approach to Postexposure Prophylaxis Based on Exposure Risk Category and HIV Status of Source

Exposure Risk Category	HIV Infection Status of Source	Suggested Approach
No risk identified	Any status	No PEP
Any risk category	Not HIV infected	No PEP
Low, intermediate, or high risk	Unknown	Consider PEP
Low or intermediate risk	HIV infected	Consider PEP
High risk	HIV infected	Recommend PEP

PEP, postexposure prophylaxis.
Adapted from Havens PL, Committee on Pediatric AIDS: Postexposure prophylaxis in children and adolescents for nonoccupational exposure to human immunodeficiency virus. Pediatrics 2003;111:1475-1489.

occurred more than 72 hours before presentation, if the exposed person refuses PEP, or if the exposed person is unwilling or unable to commit to 28 days of therapy and appropriate follow-up. The recommended PEP regimens are outlined in Table 72-7.

Rapid testing for HIV with Food and Drug Administration–approved kits (e.g., OraQuick) should also be performed on health care workers to determine their baseline status. Because PEP is associated with toxicity, it may be dis-continued if the source patient is determined to be HIV-negative. Institutions should have personnel responsible for responding to occupational exposure to HIV available 24 hours a day, as well as procedures for HIV testing and PEP administration. Other resources include the PEPline at *www.ucsf.edu/hivcntr/PEPline/index.html* (or call 888-448-4911) and the HIV Antiretroviral Pregnancy Registry at *www.apregistry.com*, for questions regarding pregnant health care workers and PEP.[7]

Table 72-7   Postexposure Prophylaxis for Occupational HIV Exposure

Basic Regimen

Recommended for low-severity percutaneous injury with source patient HIV status 1 or large-volume mucous membrane exposure with source patient HIV status 1. Also, may be considered for low-volume mucous membrane exposure with source patient HIV status 1.

Basic regimen (dual NRTIs): Combivir (ZDV, 3TC), ZDV + 3TC, tenofovir + 3TC, or Truvada (FTC, tenofovir)

Alternatives: 3TC + d4T, FTC + d4T, FTC + DDI, 3TC + DDI

Expanded Regimen

Recommended for all percutaneous exposures with source patient HIV status 2, severe percutaneous exposure with source patient HIV status 1, large-volume mucous membrane exposure with source patient HIV status 2.

Expanded regimen: basic regimen + the following:

    Kaletra (lopinavir, ritonavir), or
    Fosamprenavir, or
    Atazanavir
    Nelfinavir
    Efavirenz (NNRTI)

DDI, didanosine; d4T, stavudine; FTC, emtricitabine; NNRTI, non-nucleoside reverse transcriptase inhibitor; NRTI, nucleoside reverse transcriptase inhibitor; 3TC, lamivudine; ZDV, zidovudine.

Adapted from Havens PL, Committee on Pediatric AIDS: Postexposure prophylaxis in children and adolescents for nonoccupational exposure to human immunodeficiency virus. Pediatrics 2003;111:1475-1489.

IN A NUTSHELL

- HIV infection in children is almost exclusively acquired through vertical transmission.
- The diagnosis of HIV is established through molecular testing of neonates using either qualitative DNA PCR or quantitative RNA PCR to detect cases of in utero infection. This testing is performed at 48 hours of age.
- In children older than 18 months, the HIV ELISA and confirmatory Western blot may be performed to determine infection.
- HIV-infected children with a CD4% greater than 15% are not at increased risk for opportunistic infections; however, their risk for bacterial infection (including bacteremia) is higher than in a child without HIV infection.
- Although the risk for HIV transmission through occupational exposure is low, it does occur. Extra care must be taken with regard to PEP and its associated toxicity.

ON THE HORIZON

- Ongoing trials include pharmacokinetic studies designed to optimize HAART in infants and children.
- Trials are also under way to determine efficacious salvage therapy in HAART-experienced patients.
- Phase I and II trials are planned for pharmacologic inhibitors of HIV infections (e.g., a CCR5 analogue).
- Therapeutic and preventative HIV vaccines are an ongoing arm of clinical research.

SUGGESTED READING

Burns DM, Mofensen LM: Pediatric HIV infection. Lancet 1999;354:S111-S116.

King SM, Committee on Pediatric AIDS, American Academy of Pediatrics, Canadian Paediatric Society: Clinical report: Evaluation and treatment of the human immunodeficiency virus-1-exposed infant. Pediatrics 2004;114:497-506.

Mofenson LM, Oleske J, Serchuck L, et al: Treating opportunistic infections among HIV-exposed and infected children: Recommendations from CDC, the National Institutes of Health, and the Infectious Diseases Society of America. MMWR Recomm Rep 2004;53(RR-14):1-92.

Panlilo AL, Cardo DM, Grohskopf LA, et al: Updated US Public Health Service guidelines for the management of occupational exposures to HIV and recommendations for postexposure prophylaxis. MMWR Recomm Rep 2005;54(RR-9):1-17.

Working Group on Antiretroviral Therapy and Medical Management of HIV-Infected Children: Guidelines for the use of antiretroviral agents in pediatric HIV infection. Available at *http://aidsinfo.nih.gov/* (rev June 25, 2003).

REFERENCES

1. Burns DM, Mofensen LM: Pediatric HIV Infection. Lancet 1999;354:S111-S116.
2. Revised classification system for human immunodeficiency virus infection in children less than 13 years of age. MMWR Recomm Rep 1994;43(RR-12):1-10.
3. King SM, Committee on Pediatric AIDS, American Academy of Pediatrics, Canadian Paediatric Society: Clinical report: Evaluation and treatment of the human immunodeficiency virus-1-exposed infant. Pediatrics 2004;114:497-506.
4. Working Group on Antiretroviral Therapy and Medical Management of HIV-Infected Children: Guidelines for the use of antiretroviral agents in pediatric HIV infection. Available at *http://aidsinfo.nih.gov/* (rev June 25, 2003).
5. Mofenson LM, Oleske J, Serchuck L, et al: Treating opportunistic infections among HIV-exposed and infected children: Recommendations from CDC, the National Institutes of Health, and the Infectious Diseases Society of America. MMWR Recomm Rep 2004,53(RR-14):1-92.
6. Bonilla FA, Geha RS: Primary immunodeficiency diseases. J Allergy Clin Immunol 2003;111:S571-S581.
7. Panlilo AL, Cardo DM, Grohskopf LA, et al: Updated US Public Health Service guidelines for the management of occupational exposures to HIV and recommendations for post-exposure prophylaxis. MMWR Recomm Rep 2005;54(RR-9):1-17.

CHAPTER 73

Infections in Special Hosts

Keith Mann

As new therapeutic options for previously untreatable illnesses become available, a growing number of children are undergoing procedures and protocols that place them at greater risk of infection. This chapter focuses on the infection-related issues among children who are immunocompromised owing to solid organ or bone marrow transplantation or splenic dysfunction (complications among patients who are immunocompromised because of chemotherapy for malignancy are discussed in Chapter 124). These special hosts may present for the evaluation of fever or other signs of infection and often require hospitalization, especially for initial evaluation and management.

SOLID ORGAN TRANSPLANT RECIPIENTS

Solid organ transplantation was revolutionized in the early 1980s with the introduction of the immunosuppressant cyclosporine. Heart, kidney, liver, lung, and small bowel transplants have become acceptable therapies for end-organ disease. Although these procedures allow improved survival, infectious complications are among the leading causes of morbidity and mortality in the solid organ transplant population. The pediatric hospitalist should have a basic understanding of the immunosuppressive medications used in these patients and should be able to formulate a plan for evaluating and diagnosing a patient with fever at various stages post transplant.

The two most important variables when evaluating a solid organ transplant recipient with fever are the type of organ transplanted and the amount of time since transplantation. Other considerations include the patient's age, preoperative risk factors such as malnutrition, donor and recipient serostatus for Epstein-Barr virus (EBV) and cytomegalovirus (CMV), intraoperative complications, and postoperative immunosuppressive regimen.

Immediately after transplantation, bacterial pathogens predominate as the cause of infection. The source of bacterial infection is typically related to the type of organ transplanted or the presence of an indwelling catheter.[1] Immunosuppression is a key factor in infection that occurs after the immediate postoperative period. Most children are given a calcineurin-based immunosuppressive regimen with either cyclosporine or tacrolimus. These medications inhibit the production, proliferation, and activation of cytotoxic T cells. This effectively inhibits the cellular immune response and predisposes transplant patients to infectious complications, particularly viral and fungal infections. Other factors predisposing to fungal infection include disruption of anatomic barriers by surgery, fungal colonization enhanced by broad-spectrum antibiotic therapy, and presence of indwelling catheters.

Differential Diagnosis

In the immediate postoperative period, infections are more commonly due to bacteria. Intra-abdominal infections predominate in the first 30 days after liver transplantation, whereas children with kidney transplants commonly have urinary tract infections in the first 30 days postoperatively. Similar to liver transplant patients, small bowel transplant recipients are at risk for intra-abdominal infectious complications. Bacterial pneumonia predominates in heart and lung transplant recipients. The initial diagnostic evaluation during the first month after transplant should be tailored to these organ-specific complications. Peripheral blood, indwelling catheter, and, in renal transplant patients, urine cultures are essential.

Fungal infections, predominantly caused by *Candida* species, also occur early after transplantation. The incidence varies by type of organ transplanted; lung and liver transplants involve a higher incidence of fungal infection than do kidney transplants. Particularly problematic is fungal pneumonia after lung transplantation, because colonization is frequent and difficult to distinguish from infection.[2] Infection with *Aspergillus* species, although less common than *Candida* infection, is associated with a high mortality.

Between 30 and 180 days post transplantation, viral causes of infection predominate.[3] During this time, opportunistic infections and post-transplant lymphoproliferative disorders (PTLDs) must also be considered. Certain organ transplantations are associated with specific infectious concerns, such as bacterial and fungal pneumonia in lung transplant patients and recurrent bacterial cholangitis in liver transplant patients with biliary strictures. However, CMV, EBV, adenovirus, varicella-zoster virus (VZV), and the childhood respiratory viruses must be considered in all solid organ transplant patients with fever during this period.

Opportunistic infections are relatively rare following pediatric solid organ transplantation. Because trimethoprim-sulfamethoxazole prophylaxis has been incorporated into treatment regimens, infection with *Pneumocystis jiroveci* (previously *Pneumocystis carinii*) has been almost eliminated. *Toxoplasma gondii* infection should be considered in seronegative heart transplant recipients, especially if the donor was seropositive.

Late infections, typically occurring 180 days or longer after transplantation, include many of the same viral illnesses that occur in the immunocompetent population. Particular attention should be paid to varicella, influenza, and adenovirus infection, because these can be particularly severe in transplant recipients. EBV-associated PTLDs can also occur during this period. In lung transplant patients, bacterial (including gram-negative bacilli) and fungal pneumonia remains a concern.

Diagnosis and Treatment

Bacterial Infections

This section concentrates on bacterial infections that can occur after liver and kidney transplantation, the two most common transplant surgeries in pediatrics. Infections are common immediately after liver transplantation, and most are associated with either central venous line or abdominal infections. There are several factors that predispose to infection, including previous abdominal surgery, prolonged operating time, hepatic artery thrombosis, and biliary strictures. Prolonged operating time and previous surgery increase the risk for bowel perforation and subsequent infection with *Enterococcus* species or gram-negative bacilli.[4] Biliary strictures and hepatic artery thrombosis predispose to cholangitis and hepatic abscesses with similar organisms.[5] Postoperative cholangitis is particularly difficult to differentiate from acute cellular rejection, and a biopsy is often warranted to help choose the appropriate therapy. Empirical antimicrobial coverage for suspected bowel perforations should include enterococci, gram-negative rods, anaerobes, and *Candida* species. Therapeutic options include the combination of piperacillin-tazobactam and fluconazole, or the combination of cefepime, metronidazole, and fluconazole. Patients receiving calcineurin inhibitors in conjunction with fluconazole require frequent monitoring of the serum levels of calcineurin inhibitor, because fluconazole inhibits P450 metabolism and can cause a patient's calcineurin inhibitor level to rise.

Postoperative bacterial infections in renal transplant patients are similar to those of any postoperative patient and include pneumonia, wound infection, central venous catheter infection, and urinary tract infection. However, uncomplicated urinary tract infection, pyelonephritis, and urosepsis all occur with increased frequency in this population.[3] Infections with gram-negative bacilli predominate, and antibacterial coverage should include an antipseudomonal penicillin or cephalosporin, especially in the first month after transplantation. Historically, one third of renal transplant patients developed recurrent urinary tract infections in the first 6 months after transplantation, but this number is now lower owing to increased use of prophylactic antibiotics.[6] Bacterial pneumonia is another important infection and can be due to gram-negative bacilli or gram-positive cocci; thus, broad-spectrum antibiotic coverage is warranted.

If a site of infection is identified, antimicrobial coverage should be targeted toward the likely offending pathogens (Table 73-1).

Viral Infections

Unlike bacterial infections, viral infections tend to be less organ specific because they are usually related to the immunosuppressive regimen. Transmission can occur through reactivation of a latent virus, transmission via the transplanted organ, or person-to-person spread. The herpesviruses are a major source of post-transplant morbidity and mortality, especially CMV, EBV, and VZV. Other important viral infections in solid organ transplant patients include adenovirus, parvovirus, influenza virus, and respiratory syncytial virus (RSV).

Cytomegalovirus

Despite various prophylactic regimens with antiviral agents and CMV-specific immune globulin, CMV remains a common cause of morbidity in the transplant population. Primary infection, whereby a CMV-naïve (seronegative) recipient receives an organ or blood products from a CMV-infected (seropositive) donor, is the most severe. This mechanism of infection occurs more frequently in children than in adults because a greater proportion of children are CMV naïve at the time of transplant. Reactivation of a previously acquired (latent) CMV infection or infection with a different strain of CMV usually results in less severe disease.[7] In addition to CMV naivete, high doses of immune suppression (especially antilymphocyte therapy used for rejection) and EBV coinfection (due to the immune-modulating effects of EBV) increase the risk for CMV disease.

CMV infection can present as a nonspecific viral syndrome, termed CMV syndrome, or it can present with end-organ involvement. CMV syndrome, which can also be caused by other herpesviruses (e.g., human herpesvirus 6, 7, or 8), usually involves several of the following symptoms: fever, malaise, weakness, myalgia, arthralgia. There is often an accompanying myelosuppression. End-organ CMV disease often affects the transplanted organ, with hepatitis in liver transplant patients[8] and pneumonitis in lung transplant patients being the most common associations. The gastrointestinal tract can be affected regardless of the organ transplanted, and lower gastrointestinal bleeding in a transplant patient should raise the suspicion of CMV colitis.

Diagnosis of CMV disease is difficult. Urine shell vial assay, tissue culture, pp65 antigen detection, and nucleic acid detection via polymerase chain reaction (PCR) all have a role in diagnosing CMV. Preemptive antiviral therapy is now being initiated at many centers based on elevated CMV DNA levels detected by PCR. The drug of choice for CMV is ganciclovir, which inhibits CMV DNA polymerase. An oral form, valganciclovir, is now available and is being used increasingly in pediatric transplant patients.[9]

Epstein-Barr Virus

Primary infection, from an infected donor to a naïve recipient, represents the most common and severe form of EBV infection in post-transplant patients. Children are particularly prone to infection owing to the relatively high incidence of EBV-naïve recipients. EBV accounts for more than 90% of cases of PTLD; other pathogens include human herpesvirus 8 and human lymphotrophic virus type 1.

Following primary infection, EBV, like other herpesviruses, persists for the lifetime of the host despite the presence of a strong humoral and cell-mediated immune response. Ongoing low-grade viral replication normally occurs in the oropharynx simultaneously with a predominantly latent infection of B cells in the peripheral blood and lymphoid tissues. In cases of severe immunosuppression (e.g., following hematopoietic stem cell or solid organ transplantation), the equilibrium is disrupted in favor of the virus. The uncontrolled proliferation of EBV-infected B cells that occurs in this context may result in a spectrum of PTLDs. Although the proliferation is initially polyclonal in nature, certain clones may experience a selective growth advantage, thus transforming a polyclonal lesion into an

Table 73-1   Infections in Solid Organ Transplant Recipients

| INFECTION | | COMMON ORGANISMS | | |
Site	Disease Process	Bacteria	Viruses	Fungi
General symptoms	CMV syndrome		CMV EBV	
Central nervous system	Meningitis	Streptococcus pneumoniae Group B Streptococcus Listeria monocytogenes Salmonella spp. Pseudomonas aeruginosa Escherichia coli	HSV Varicella EBV CMV HHV 6	Cryptococcus Aspergillus Candida Nocardia Toxoplasma
Oropharynx	Painful ulcers Tonsillar hypertrophy		HSV EBV CMV	
Respiratory tract	Pneumonia	S. pneumoniae Staphylococcus aureus Haemophilus influenzae Legionella Pseudomonas Acinetobacter Burkholderia	Influenza Adenovirus RSV CMV EBV HSV Varicella	Candida Aspergillus Pneumocystis
Gastrointestinal tract	Esophagitis		CMV HSV	Candida
	Colitis	Clostridium difficile C. difficile	CMV EBV	
	Diarrhea	Salmomella Shigella E. coli	CMV EBV Rotavirus	Giardia Cryptosporidium
Liver	Hepatitis		CMV HSV Varicella EBV HHV 6, 7, 8	
	Cholangitis/abscess	Enteric gram-negative rods Enterococcus spp. Anaerobes		Candida Aspergillus
Skin	Cellulitis/abscess	S. aureus Streptococcus pyogenes		
	Chickenpox/zoster Warts		Varicella Human papillomavirus	
Hematologic	Cytopenia	Any bacteria causing sepsis	CMV EBV Parvovirus	Candida Aspergillus

CMV, cytomegalovirus; EBV, Epstein-Barr virus; HHV, human herpesvirus; HSV, herpes simplex virus; RSV, respiratory syncytial virus.

oligoclonal or monoclonal one. Ongoing proliferation can lead to the development of cytogenetic abnormalities within the lesion and malignant transformation. Thus, the spectrum of PTLDs ranges from self-limited polyclonal proliferation to true malignancies containing clonal chromosomal abnormalities.[10]

Factors associated with increased risk for PTLD include younger patient age, intestinal or multivisceral transplants,[11] antigenic differences between donor and recipient, more intense immune suppression, and coinfection with other pathogens. Antigenic differences between the donor and recipient may induce polyclonal B-cell proliferation, predisposing to the development of PTLD. The cumulative intensity of immunosuppression also increases the risk of PTLD. The specificity of calcineurin inhibitors and antilymphocyte antibodies for the T-cell limb of the immune response may explain in part the higher frequency of PTLD associated with the use of these agents. Coinfection with other herpesviruses such as CMV and human herpesvirus 8 also increases the risk of PTLD.

The clinical presentation of PTLD can be variable, ranging from a benign illness with self-limited lymphoproliferation to fulminant disease that presents with localized nodules, multifocal disease, or a sepsis-like picture. The most common presentation in children is similar to that of mononucleosis, with vague constitutional symptoms of fever, fatigue, and myalgias accompanied by a sore throat, cervical lymph node hypertrophy, and tonsillar enlargement. Gastrointestinal involvement can present with bleeding, weight loss, constipation, diarrhea, hypoalbuminemia, or intussusception. Pulmonary involvement can present with respiratory distress or lung nodules on the chest radiograph.

Diagnosis is best made by taking a tissue sample of the affected lymph node. Similar to CMV, nucleic acid PCR for EBV is an invaluable tool in the early adjustment of immune suppression.[12] Reduction in immune suppression alone is often successful in treating PTLD limited to the allograft. If reduction of immune suppression is ineffective, or if the patient presents with advanced disease, there are several other treatment options. Although ganciclovir is effective only in the lytic phase and may be less effective for numerous latent EBV-infected B cells, it should still be considered as initial therapy. There is a fairly high incidence of coinfection with CMV, and this alone may be enough reason to consider its use. Treatment with rituximab, a monoclonal antibody to CD20-positive B cells, can be added.[13] Other chemotherapeutic agents, such as cyclophosphamide, also have a role in individual cases.[14]

Varicella-Zoster Virus

Most children are either exposed to varicella before adolescence or immunized at 1 year of age. Children who receive organs before being either exposed or immunized are at risk for severe varicella infection, although herd immunity and the rapid decline in the incidence of varicella lessen that risk somewhat. Less commonly, reactivation of a latent virus can produce severe disease.

Patients with varicella are infectious for 48 hours before and approximately 5 days after the onset of the rash, or until new lesions stop appearing. Transplant patients are at high risk for visceral involvement. If an unimmunized, immunosuppressed transplant patient comes in contact with a VZV-infected patient during this period, immune globulin therapy should be administered within 72 hours of the exposure. A VZV-specific immune globulin preparation (VariZIG) is available through a new investigational drug protocol and can be requested by calling FFF Enterprises (800-843-7477); nonspecific intravenous immunoglobulin (IVIG) can be administered if this product is unavailable. If clinical disease develops, either primary infection or reactivation (herpes zoster), patients should receive intravenous acyclovir in the hospital setting.[15] Some centers have had success with outpatient management of herpes zoster (in the absence of visceral dissemination) with oral acyclovir.

Adenovirus

Adenovirus is the third most common viral cause of morbidity in the solid organ transplant population.[16] Adenovirus is a common cause of pneumonia in all transplant recipients, regardless of the organ transplanted. Risk factors for severe infection are similar to those for other viruses and include extremes of age, infection within 1 month of trans-

plantation, and high levels of immunosuppression. EBV, CMV, and other viruses cause a similar spectrum of disease regardless of the type of organ transplanted; in contrast, adenovirus is more likely to affect the transplanted organ directly. Different adenovirus serotypes have a propensity to infect different organs, leading to specific clinical manifestations. For example, liver transplant recipients tend to develop hepatitis or gastroenteritis from serotypes 1, 2, and 5. In contrast, lung transplant recipients develop pneumonitis and obliterative bronchiolitis, and renal transplant recipients often develop hemorrhagic cystitis or prolonged urinary tract infections caused by serotypes 11, 34, and 35. Detection of adenovirus by culture, antigen detection, or PCR suggests infection only in the context of compatible clinical symptoms. The diagnosis can be difficult to confirm, because patients may shed adenovirus asymptomatically for prolonged periods. The role of antiviral agents is unclear. Both IVIG and cidofovir have been used therapeutically, with anecdotal reports of success in severe infections[17]; however, the drug's nephrotoxicity limits its use in patients with severe renal dysfunction.

Parvovirus

Parvovirus B19 was first recognized as a cause of red cell aplasia in sickle cell patients. It has also been identified as a cause of aplastic anemia and, to a lesser extent, pancytopenia in the transplant population. The aplasia can occur with or without systemic signs of fatigue, malaise, fever, and arthralgias. Treatment is with IVIG, although a standard dose has yet to be determined.[18]

Influenza Virus

Influenza virus has significant morbidity and mortality in both immunocompetent and immunocompromised populations. Morbidity in transplant patients increases with lung transplantation, extremes of age, high levels of immunosuppression, and occurrence of infection immediately post transplant.[19] The Centers for Disease Control and Prevention has long recommended vaccination before influenza season and chemoprophylaxis during outbreaks for immunocompromised patients.[20] If a transplant patient presents with signs and symptoms compatible with influenza, early diagnosis with a rapid antigen assay and treatment with oral antiviral therapy are warranted. Oseltamivir is preferred owing to its efficacy against both influenza A and B, and it is approved in patients as young as 1 year.

Respiratory Syncytial Virus

RSV causes a wide range of symptoms in transplant patients. The risk factors for severe disease are similar to those for influenza: lung transplantation, extremes of age, greater immune suppression, and infection early after transplantation. Unlike influenza, however, there is no proven therapy. Ribavirin should be considered in severe cases. There are insufficient data to determine whether palivizumab is effective in treating RSV pneumonia in solid organ recipients.

Fungal Infections

Candidal infections are diagnosed using site-specific cultures, such as blood cultures from indwelling intravascular catheters, urinary cultures, and peritoneal cultures. *Candida* identified from tracheal or bronchial cultures usually represents colonization rather than true infection. Patients with candidemia should undergo evaluation for disseminated candidiasis. Ophthalmic evaluation of the retina should be performed; abdominal ultrasonography is useful to demonstrate candidal lesions in the liver, spleen, or kidney; and echocardiography can reveal fungal endocarditis. Antifungal agents for candidal infections include amphotericin B, lipid formulations of amphotericin B, and fluconazole. The echinocandins (caspofungin, micafungin, anidulafungin) are a new class of antifungal with good activity against all *Candida* species.

Infection with *Aspergillus* species is diagnosed by culturing these organisms from a sterile body site (e.g., cerebrospinal fluid) or biopsy specimen (e.g., lung tissue). The identification of *Aspergillus* from nonsterile body fluids (e.g., sputum) must be interpreted with caution, because colonization is common among transplant patients. The drug of choice for the treatment of invasive aspergillosis is voriconazole. Alternative agents include amphotericin B, lipid formulations of amphotericin B, itraconazole, and caspofungin.

BONE MARROW TRANSPLANT RECIPIENTS

Neutropenia, defects in cell-mediated immunity, and altered antibody-mediated immunity occur at predictable times in bone marrow transplant patients. Management principles for patients who have undergone hematopoietic stem cell transplantation overlap with those of patients experiencing neutropenia with fever and solid organ transplant recipients.

The pre-engraftment period begins with conditioning therapy that eradicates or reduces the patient's burden of abnormal or malignant cells to below detectable levels and suppresses the patient's immunity to prevent the rejection of donor cells. This period, which extends until approximately 30 days after transplantation, is complicated by neutropenia, lymphopenia, and mucositis. Patients react similarly to those with neutropenia from other forms of chemotherapy (see Chapter 124). Bacterial and fungal infections commonly can gain entry through indwelling venous catheters or through mucosal breakdown along the gastrointestinal tract. If initial conditioning therapy includes agents directed at T cells, the patient is predisposed to an earlier onset of viral infection, particularly EBV and CMV. Reactivation of herpes simplex virus (HSV) may also occur, making acyclovir prophylaxis part of standard therapy during the pre-engraftment period.[21]

The post-engraftment period begins with marrow recovery and extends to 100 days after transplantation, when functional lymphocyte recovery is apparent. This is a time of impaired cellular immunity due to graft-versus-host disease (GVHD) and the use of calcineurin inhibitors, which blunt T-lymphocyte reconstitution via their inhibitory effect on interleukin-2. CMV, EBV, and VZV are frequent causes of infection during this time. Bacterial infections from indwelling catheters and fungal infections, both *Candida* and *Aspergillus* species, continue to be a problem as well. Other opportunistic infections, such as *P. jiroveci* and *T. gondii*, also occur during this period.

The late phase begins 101 days after transplantation. Impaired cellular immunity persists, and GVHD can become a chronic problem. In addition to CMV and EBV, reactiva-tion of VZV often occurs during this phase. The presence of chronic GVHD also predisposes to late-onset infections with encapsulated organisms, particularly pneumococci.

Differential Diagnosis
Bacterial Infections

Bacteremia and serious bacterial infections caused by gram-positive organisms are common after bone marrow transplantation. Mucositis and indwelling catheters in the pre-engraftment period and chronic GVHD in the late phase predispose to such infections. Mucositis and indwelling catheters predispose to infections with *Staphylococcus epidermidis*, *Staphylococcus aureus*, *Streptococcus pneumoniae*, *Streptococcus viridans*, *Streptococcus pyogenes*, and *Enterococcus* species. Viridans streptococci usually gain access to the bloodstream via mucositis and can cause a sepsis syndrome with multiorgan dysfunction in the early pre-engraftment period.[22] Infection with *S. pneumoniae* continues to be a problem in patients with chronic GVHD,[23] despite the use of prophylactic penicillin or trimethoprim-sulfamethoxazole in many centers.

Although not as common, gram-negative organisms can present with a more fulminant, devastating course. *Enterobacter*, *Pseudomonas*, *Stenotrophomonas*, and *Acinetobacter* species, in addition to enteric gram-negative rods such as *Escherichia coli* and *Klebsiella* species, can all cause bacteremia and sepsis in bone marrow transplant recipients.

Viral Infections

HSV 1 is the most common viral infection following bone marrow transplantation and often occurs fairly early in the pre-engraftment or conditioning phase. HSV 1 usually presents with oral or perianal vesicular or ulcerative lesions but occasionally progresses to systemic disease with hepatitis or encephalitis. Marked reduction in the incidence of HSV has been achieved with the use of prophylactic acyclovir.[24]

CMV is a significant cause of morbidity and mortality in bone marrow transplant recipients. Pretransplant exposure with documented immunoglobulin G levels is a risk factor for recurrence after transplantation due to reactivation of latent disease. End-organ disease from CMV can include pneumonitis, hepatitis, enteritis, and retinitis.

VZV can cause illness as a primary infection or after reactivation. Reactivation is much more common and typically occurs several months after transplantation. Patients may have typical painful vesicular lesions in a dermatomal distribution, or the lesions may be atypical with a less obvious pattern. Dissemination can occur with primary infection (rarely with reactivation) and can result in significant end-organ disease, including hepatitis and pneumonitis. As in solid organ transplant recipients, adenovirus can cause significant disease in bone marrow transplant recipients as well, but it seems to be more common in patients with GVHD. Clinical manifestations include hemorrhagic cystitis, pneumonitis, nephritis, and hepatitis. Diagnosis is difficult owing to prolonged viral shedding.[25]

Fungal Infections

Although the use of prophylactic fluconazole has decreased the overall incidence of fungal infections, they remain a relatively common cause of morbidity due to the

Table 73-2   Initial Diagnostic Evaluation in Bone Marrow Transplant Patients with Fever

Site of Infection	Predominant Symptom	Diagnostic Tests to Consider
No obvious source	Fever	Bacterial cultures of all venous catheters Bacterial blood cultures

Central nervous system	Meningitis	CSF analysis
		   Opening pressure
		   Cell count and differential
		   Glucose and protein
		   Gram stain and bacterial culture
		   Viral culture and PCR for HSV 1 and 2, VZV, CMV, EBV, HHV 6, enterovirus
		   India ink, fungal culture, cryptococcal antigen
		   Cytology

Oropharynx	Painful ulcers	HSV culture
Respiratory tract	Pneumonia	Chest radiograph Blood culture Sputum bacterial culture if child is able Urine legionella antigen BAL with Gram stain, bacterial culture, viral culture, fungal staining, PAS staining, and histology
Gastrointestinal tract	Dysphagia	CMV PCR Urine CMV shell vial assay HSV culture of any oral ulcers Endoscopy with proper staining for fungus, HSV culture
	Diarrhea ± hematochezia	CMV PCR EBV PCR Urine CMV shell vial assay Stool viral culture Stool bacterial culture Stool for *Clostridium difficile* toxin Stool for ova and parasites, *Giardia* and *Cryptosporidium* antigen Endoscopy or colonoscopy and biopsy may be warranted

BAL, bronchoalveolar lavage; CMV, cytomegalovirus; CSF, cerebrospinal fluid; EBV, Epstein-Barr virus; HHV, human herpesvirus; HSV, herpes simplex virus; PAS, periodic acid–Schiff; PCR, polymerase chain reaction; VZV, varicella-zoster virus.

emergence of resistant strains of *Candida* species[26] and the presence of *Aspergillus* species. Risk factors include mucositis, neutropenia, early GVHD, the need for corticosteroid therapy, and construction in the vicinity of the hospital. Late-onset infection with *Aspergillus* species occurs almost exclusively in patients with chronic GVHD.[27] Diagnosis is made with peripheral blood cultures and cultures of any suspicious lesions, particularly those seen on computed tomography of the chest.

Diagnosis and Treatment

The evaluation of a bone marrow transplant patient with fever or possible infection should begin with a thorough history and physical examination, attempting to localize the symptoms to a specific location or organ system. Table 73-2 lists common diagnostic tests that should be considered based on the presenting symptoms, but the time frame after transplant should also be considered when beginning this assessment.

Bacterial Infections

Bacteremia from gram-positive and gram-negative organisms occurs in this population for a variety of reasons, including immune suppression, mucosal breakdown, and frequent central venous catheterization. Resistant organisms are being seen with increasing frequency. *S. viridans* is a particular problem for bone marrow transplant patients. It is isolated in approximately 15% of adult transplant patients with mucositis and neutropenia in the weeks following transplant. It can present with fever alone or with overwhelming sepsis.[28]

Typical empirical broad-spectrum antibiotic coverage should include an antipseudomonal agent such as cefepime, piperacillan-tazobactam, or carbapenem, either alone or in combination with an aminoglycoside. Vancomycin is often added for the following indications:

- Patients with mucositis and neutropenia
- Hypotension or other evidence of cardiovascular dysfunction, particularly in the presence of a central venous catheter
- Known colonization with an organism resistant to penicillins and cephalosporins (e.g., methicillin-resistant *S. aureus*, some *Enterococcus* species)
- Growth of a gram-positive organism from the blood with pending susceptibilities
- Recent parenteral antibiotic use

Viral Infections

Even with improved preventive strategies, CMV continues to be the most worrisome viral pathogen in transplant centers. As in solid organ transplants, the immune-modulating properties of CMV link it to graft rejection. More unique to bone marrow transplantation, however, is its occurrence in conjunction with GVHD. Several methods have been used in an attempt to decrease the incidence of CMV reactivation in seropositive patients after transplantation. Although there is currently no consensus regarding prophylaxis or prevention, most centers use either prophylactic ganciclovir until post-transplant day 100 or serial antigenemia or CMV DNA PCR-guided early ganciclovir therapy to prevent severe disease.[21] CMV end-organ disease is treated with intravenous ganciclovir for 6 weeks.

As in those who undergo solid organ transplantation, EBV infection and PTLDs are complications among bone marrow transplant patients. The clinical presentation, diagnosis, and management of CMV and EBV are similar for both bone marrow and solid organ transplant recipients (see earlier).

HSV reactivation appears to be more common in bone marrow than in solid organ transplant recipients and has led to the universal use of prophylactic acyclovir for all seropositive patients.[29] If oral vesicles occur, diagnosis is achieved when HSV is detected by PCR, direct fluorescent antibodies, or viral culture of the vesicle. Dissemination can occur with primary infection and, less commonly, with reactivation and can result in significant end-organ disease, including hepatitis and pneumonitis. Patients with suspected HSV infection should receive intravenous acyclovir empirically while awaiting diagnostic confirmation. If the diagnosis is confirmed, acyclovir should be continued.[6] Early conversion to oral acyclovir may be considered for those with uncomplicated infections, once new lesions have ceased to appear.

Adenovirus infection causes problems similar to those seen in solid organ transplant patients. Among bone marrow transplant patients, it is increasingly recognized as a cause of pneumonitis, hemorrhagic cystitis, and sepsis. Treatment is usually supportive, but recent data suggest a role for cidofovir.[17]

Fungal Infections

Routine prophylaxis with fluconazole has led to an overall decrease in the number of fungal infections; however, there appears to be an increase in the number of fluconazole-resistant *Candida* species and continued concern about *Aspergillus*. Antifungal coverage with amphotericin is often added for bone marrow transplant patients with fever for longer than 3 to 5 days with no identifiable source; if *Aspergillus* infection is a possibility, based on an identifiable site of infection (sinusitis, pneumonia); or in high-risk patients, such as those with GVHD.

ACQUIRED AND FUNCTIONAL ASPLENIA

The spleen is an important organ in the defense against infection. It produces antibodies, and macrophages within the spleen engulf bacteria and eliminate them from the circulation. Patients who are asplenic or have functional asplenia are at risk for a variety of severe infections, particularly with encapsulated bacterial organisms. *S. pneumoniae, Neisseria meningitidis*, and *Haemophilus influenzae* are three encapsulated organisms that commonly cause infection. *Salmonella*, although not an encapsulated organism, is also a common cause of infection, particularly in patients with functional asplenia associated with sickle cell disease. Intracellular organisms that cause babesiosis and malaria also cause disease in asplenic patients. Although the risk of bacterial infection with asplenia is highest in the first several years after the spleen is removed (or functionally absent), the risk of infection is lifelong. The risk is greater in children than in adults owing to the relative lack of protective antibodies against such organisms.

Strategies to prevent infection are important in patients who are at risk of becoming asplenic and in those without splenic function. All patients should receive immunization with meningococcal, pneumococcal, and *H. influenzae* type B vaccine, preferably before the onset of asplenia. Patients scheduled to undergo an elective procedure to remove the spleen should receive immunization with the heptavalent pneumococcal conjugate vaccine (PCV7) and the tetravalent meningococcal polysaccharide vaccines several weeks before the surgery. The *H. influenzae* type B conjugate vaccine should be administered immediately to any unvaccinated or undervaccinated child. The 23-valent pneumococcal polysaccharide vaccine should be administered at 24 months of age and then again 3 to 5 years later. In children older than 24 months, the 23-valent pneumococcal polysaccharide vaccine can be administered as soon as 8 weeks after the last dose of PCV7. To reduce the risk of infection, antibiotic prophylaxis with penicillin, amoxicillin, amoxicillin-clavulanate, trimethoprim-sulfamethoxazole (Bactrim), or cefuroxime is standard therapy for the first several years after splenectomy, although the optimal duration of prophylaxis is not known. Education about infection and the use of a medical alert bracelet are also important measures.

Overwhelming infection is a great concern among asplenic patients. Hypotension, shock, multiorgan dysfunction syndrome, and disseminated intravascular coagulation can rapidly follow a short prodrome of fever, malaise, and headache. Mortality is extremely high. Although gram-negative rods are occasionally implicated, encapsulated organisms are the most common cause of infection. Asplenic patients with suspected bacterial infection should be admitted to the hospital and placed on broad-spectrum antibiotic therapy, typically with a third-generation cephalosporin.

IN A NUTSHELL

- The risk of infection in solid organ transplant recipients is related to the type of organ transplanted, the amount of time since transplantation, the immune suppression regimen, the patient's age, and the patient's immune status against key viruses such as EBV and CMV.
- Bacterial causes of infection predominate during the first 30 days after solid organ transplantation; viral causes are most common between 30 and 180 days after transplantation.
- EBV infections can cause a range of illnesses called post-transplantation lymphoproliferative disorders, including malignant transformation of B lymphocytes.

- Infection in bone marrow transplant patients is related to the conditioning therapy and the time since transplantation and engraftment.
- Before bone marrow engraftment, infections are related to the degree of neutropenia, lymphopenia, and mucositis.
- The presence of GVHD increases the risk of infection, especially with encapsulated bacteria and *Aspergillus* species.
- Asplenic patients and patients with functional asplenia are at increased risk for overwhelming infection, especially secondary to encapsulated bacteria.
- Strategies to prevent infection in patients with splenic dysfunction include proper immunization and prophylactic therapy.

ON THE HORIZON

- The more frequent use of quantitative PCR-based assays to detect viral pathogens, especially CMV and EBV.
- More frequent use of "expanded criteria donors"—those historically associated with worse clinical outcomes—will expand the pool of donor organs and potentially change the epidemiology of post-transplant infections.
- Decreased use of corticosteroids for immunosuppression in some organ transplant recipients (e.g., renal and liver transplants).
- Use of new immunosuppressive agents such as alemtuzumab, a monoclonal antibody that binds to CD52 to deplete lymphocytes.
- Increased awareness of transfusion-associated infections (e.g., West Nile virus) occurring in solid organ and bone marrow transplant patients.

SUGGESTED READING

Bowden RA, Ljungman P, Paya C: Transplant Infections, 2nd ed. Philadelphia, Lippincott Williams & Wilkins, 2003.

Dykewicz CA, Jaffe HW, Kaplan JE: Guidelines for preventing opportunistic infections among hematopoietic stem cell transplant recipients: Recommendations of CDC, the Infectious Diseases Society of America, and the American Society of Blood and Marrow Transplantation. MMWR Recomm Rep 2000;49(RR-10):1-128.

Green M, Michaels MG: Infectious complications of solid-organ transplantation in children. Adv Pediatr Infect Dis 1992;7:181-203.

Hughes WT, Bodey GP, Brown AE, et al: Guidelines from the Infectious Diseases Society of America: 1997 guidelines for the use of antimicrobial agents in neutropenic patients with unexplained fever. Clin Infect Dis 1997;25:551-573.

Orudjev E, Lange BJ: Evolving concepts of management of febrile neutropenia in children with cancer. Med Pediatr Oncol 2002;39:77-85.

Serody JS, Shea TC: Prevention of infections in bone marrow transplant recipients. Infect Dis Clin North Am 1997;11:459-477.

REFERENCES

1. Dummer JS, Hardy A, Poorsattar A, Ho M: Early infections in kidney, heart, and liver transplant recipients on cyclosporin. Transplantation 1983;36:259-267.

2. Paya CV: Fungal infections in solid organ transplantation. Clin Infect Dis 1993;16:677-688.

3. Green M, Michaels MG: Infectious complications of solid organ transplant recipients. Adv Pediatr Infect Dis 1992;7:181-203.

4. George DL, Arnow PM, Fox A, et al: Patterns of infection after liver transplantation. Am J Dis Child 1992;146:924-929.

5. Kusne S, Dummer JS, Ho M, et al: Infections after liver transplantation: An analysis of 101 consecutive cases. Medicine 1988;67:132-143.

6. Bowden RA, Ljungman P, Paya C: Transplant Infections, 2nd ed. Philadelphia, Lippincott Williams & Wilkins, 2003.

7. Breinig MK, Zitelli B, Starzl TE, Ho M: Epstein-Barr virus, cytomegalovirus, and other viral infections in children after liver transplantation. J Infect Dis 1987;156:273-279.

8. Paya CV, Hermans PE, Wiesner RH, et al: Cytomegalovirus hepatitis in liver transplantation: Prospective analysis of 93 consecutive orthotopic liver transplantations. J Infect Dis 1989;160:752-758.

9. Clark BS, Chang IF, Karpen SJ, et al: Valganciclovir for the prophylaxis of cytomegalovirus disease in pediatric liver transplant recipients. Transplantation 2004;77:1480.

10. Cao S, Cox K: Epstein-Barr virus lymphoproliferative disorder after liver transplantation. Clin Liver Dis 1997;1:453-468.

11. Preiksaitis J, Keay S: Diagnosis and management of post-transplant lymphoproliferative disorder in solid-organ transplant recipients. Clin Infect Dis 2001;33(Suppl 1):S38-S46.

12. Lee TC, Savoldo B, Rooney CM, et al: Quantitative EBV viral loads and immunosuppression alterations can decrease PTLD incidence in pediatric liver transplant recipients. Am J Transplant 2005;5:2222-2228.

13. Ganne V, Siddiql N, Chang C, et al: Humanized anti-CD20 monoclonal antibody treatment for post-transplant lymphoproliferative disorder. Clin Transplant 2003;17:417-422.

14. Orjuela M, Gross T, Cheung Y, et al: A pilot study of chemoimmunotherapy (cyclophosphamide, prednisone, and rituximab) in patients with post-transplant lymphoproliferative disorder following solid organ transplantation. Clin Cancer Res 2003;9(Suppl):3945s-3953s.

15. McGregor RS, Zitelli BJ, Urbach AH, et al: Varicella in pediatric orthotopic liver transplant recipients. Pediatrics 1989;83:256-261.

16. Michaels M, Green M, Wald ER, Starzl TE: Adenovirus infection in pediatric orthotopic liver transplant recipients. J Infect Dis 1992;165:170-174.

17. Muller WJ, Levin MJ, Quinones R, et al: Clinical and in vitro evaluation of cidofovir for treatment of adenovirus infection in pediatric hematopoietic stem cell transplant recipients. Clin Infect Dis 2005;41:1812-1816.

18. Nour B, Green M, Michaels M, et al: Parvovirus B19 infection in pediatric transplant patients. Transplantation 1993;56:835-838.

19. Vilchez RA, Fung J, Kusne S: The pathogenesis and management of influenza virus infection in organ transplant recipients. Transplant Infect Dis 2003;4:177-182.

20. Harper SA, Fukuda K, Uyeki T, Bridges CB: Prevention and control of influenza: Recommendations of the Advisory Committee on Immunization Practice. MMWR Recomm Rep 2004;53(RR-06):1-40.

21. Dykewicz CA, Jaffe HW, Kaplan JE: Guidelines for preventing opportunistic infections among hematopoietic stem cell transplant recipients: Recommendations of CDC, the Infectious Diseases Society of America, and the American Society of Blood and Marrow Transplantation. MMWR Recomm Rep 2000;49(RR-10):1-128.

22. Steiner M, Villablanca J, Kersey J, et al: Viridans streptococcal shock in bone marrow transplantation patients. Am J Hematol 1993;42:354-358.

23. Engelhard D, Cordonnier C, Shaw PJ, et al: Early and late invasive pneumococcal infection following stem cell transplantation: A European Bone Marrow Transplantation survey. Br J Haematol 2002;117:444-450.

24. Serody JS, Shea TC: Prevention of infections in bone marrow transplant recipients. Infect Dis Clin North Am 1997;11:459-477.

25. Wasserman R, August CS, Plotkin SA: Viral infections in pediatric bone marrow transplant patients. Pediatr Infect Dis J 1988;7:109-115.

26. Diekema DJ, Messer SA, Brueggemann AB, et al: Epidemiology of candidemia: 3-year results from the emerging infections and the epidemiology of Iowa organisms study. J Clin Microbiol 2002;40:1298-1302.

27. Wald A, Leisenring W, van Burik JA, Bowden RA: Epidemiology of *Aspergillus* infections in a large cohort of patients undergoing bone marrow transplantation. J Infect Dis 1997;175:1459-1466.

28. Villablanca JG, Steiner M, Kersey J, et al: The clinical spectrum of infections with viridans streptococci in bone marrow transplant patients. Bone Marrow Transplant 1990;5:387-393.

29. Boeckh M: Current antiviral stretegies for controlling cytomegalovirus in hematopoetic stem cell transplant recipients: Prevention and therapy. Transplant Infect Dis 1999;1:165-178.

Pulmonology

Apparent Life-Threatening Event, Infant Apnea, and Pediatric Obstructive Sleep Apnea Syndrome

Craig C. DeWolfe and Aaron S. Chidekel

Infants are often brought for urgent or emergent medical assessment owing to abnormal breathing patterns or worrisome respiratory episodes. Often the episode resolves before the patient arrives for initial evaluation and does not recur. However, some infants with respiratory episodes have significant underlying medical conditions or even life-threatening events. Many of these infants are hospitalized for monitoring, diagnostic testing, and management despite a stable appearance at presentation, and there is wide variation in the evaluation and management of these episodes. This chapter addresses those respiratory episodes categorized as apparent life-threatening events (ALTEs) and briefly discusses central apnea of neonates and young infants. It also examines pediatric obstructive sleep apnea.

APPARENT LIFE-THREATENING EVENT

ALTE refers to a complex of symptoms that present unexpectedly in an infant, are of concern to the observer, and cannot be easily characterized by the health care provider.[1,2] Numerous studies have reported on the epidemiology of ALTEs either prospectively or retrospectively, and it is estimated that up to 1% of infants have an ALTE, with the most common age at presentation ranging from 6 to 10 weeks.[3-5] The pediatric hospitalist may be called on to clarify the features of the presentation, stabilize the infant, and reassure the caregivers. If admission is considered, the hospitalist must diagnose and treat the precipitating cause (if one is determined), educate the caregivers, and render a disposition.

Background

In September 1986 the National Institutes of Health (NIH) convened an expert panel to review the literature and discuss the relationship of infantile apnea, ALTE, and sudden infant death syndrome (SIDS). These experts standardized the definition of ALTE by describing it as "an episode that is frightening to the observer and that is characterized by some combination of apnea (central or occasionally obstructive), color change (usually cyanotic or pallid but occasionally erythematous or plethoric), marked change in muscle tone

(usually marked limpness), choking, or gagging." They also proposed eliminating the terms "near miss SIDS" and "aborted crib death" because no causal link could be found between ALTE and SIDS.[1] The relationship among ALTE, infant apnea, and SIDS is still unclear, and there is increasing evidence that these disorders are unrelated.[3,6,7]

Owing to the breadth of the definition, ALTE has been attributed to everything from normal physiologic events to life-threatening illnesses.[5,8-10] Therefore, it must be stressed that the symptoms of ALTE may represent a normal physiologic occurrence and be of no clinical significance. Although the majority of ALTEs are benign, health care providers must be able to distinguish events that are frightening, potentially clinically significant, and truly life threatening.

Pathophysiology and Clinical Presentation

The potential underlying abnormalities of ALTE are myriad; therefore, the pathophysiology is dependent on the diagnosis. The differential diagnosis in ALTE is extremely broad; a partial listing is provided in Table 74-1, and further discussion is found in the corresponding section of this chapter.

Pathologic apnea is defined as an event associated with physiologic compromise, as indicated by changes in oxygenation, color, or tone or bradycardia. Apneic events may be obstructive, central, or mixed. Obstructive apnea, even of brief duration (<10 seconds), is considered abnormal. Central respiratory pauses are generally considered abnormal when they last 20 seconds or longer. Shorter central episodes are considered abnormal when they are accompanied by physiologic compromise. Mixed apnea combines the features of central and obstructive episodes in the same respiratory event (usually defined by an epoch of time). Central apnea results from the lack of brainstem-mediated respiratory effort, as can be seen in premature infants. Obstructive apnea results from attempts to breathe against a blocked airway, as can be seen in laryngomalacia.

Color changes result from decreased oxygenation or differential blood flow to a portion of the body. Transient plethora may result from hyperemia and localized vasodila-

Table 74-1   Differential Diagnosis of Apparent Life-Threatening Events, with Estimates of Frequency

Gastrointestinal: 33%
  Gastroesophageal reflux
  Gastroenteritis
  Dysphagia
  Surgical abdomen
  Laryngeal chemoreflex apnea
  Vomiting

Neurologic: 15%
  Seizure
  Intracranial hemorrhage
  Central apnea or hypoventilation syndromes
  Hydrocephalus
  Brain tumor
  Vasovagal reflex
  Meningitis, encephalitis
  Myopathy
  Congenital malformation of the brainstem

Respiratory: 11%
  Respiratory syncytial virus
  Pertussis
  Aspiration pneumonia
  Foreign body
  Other lower or upper respiratory tract infections

Otolaryngologic: 4%
  Laryngomalacia
  Subglottic stenosis

Cardiac: 1%
  Cardiac arrhythmia (prolonged Q-Tc)
  Congenital heart disease
  Cardiomyopathy
  Myocarditis

Metabolic or endocrine
  Electrolyte disturbance
  Hypoglycemia
  Inborn error of metabolism

Other infections
  Sepsis
  Urinary tract infection

Child maltreatment syndromes
  Shaken baby syndrome
  Intentional suffocation
  Munchausen syndrome by proxy

Other
  Physiologic event (periodic breathing, acrocyanosis)
  Breath-holding spell
  Unintentional smothering
  Anemia
  Toxin ingestion
  Hypothermia
  Overfeeding syndrome

Idiopathic apnea of infancy: 23%

tion (often venous), whereas pallor may result from vasoconstriction. Both tend to be mediated by autonomic activity. Cyanosis is a consequence of hemoglobin desaturation and can result from impaired oxygen exchange or distribution. Differentiating the ruddy appearance of plethora from cyanosis is often difficult and can result in confusion for the caregiver and health care provider. Central cyanosis is most reliably identified by blue or purple discoloration or darkening of the lips or tongue. Acrocyanosis and circumoral cyanosis are not necessarily signs of a central cyanotic state or abnormal gas exchange. Acrocyanosis in newborns is common and may be due to vasomotor instability or vasoconstriction due to heat-retention efforts. Circumoral cyanosis often presents as a circular blue or purple discoloration in the perioral area, not involving the lips or tongue. It is more easily recognized in fair-skinned infants, especially with crying, breath holding, or other Valsalva-type efforts. It is likely related to congestion of the superficial venous plexus in this region.

Altered muscle tone may result from neuronal activity that is centrally or peripherally mediated, as can be seen in seizures or clonus. Choking results in impaired respiration from compression or obstruction of the larynx or trachea. This may be due to laryngospasm, bronchospasm, regurgitation of gastric contents, or aspiration of a foreign body. Gagging is often manifest by retching.

Differential Diagnosis

Because ALTE is a description rather than a diagnosis, the hospitalist must consider the underlying cause (see Table 74-1). Many of the diagnoses associated with ALTE are easy to differentiate on the basis of history and physical examination. For example, an ALTE in a young infant with significant apnea associated with viral respiratory symptoms during the winter is likely due to a viral infection, most commonly respiratory syncytial virus (RSV).[11,12] Interestingly, both central (especially in newborns) and obstructive events can be observed with RSV infection.[13,14] An ALTE in an infant with choking and gagging in association with feeding or regurgitation likely represents underlying gastroesophageal reflux (GER) or dysphagia.[8,15] An ALTE in an infant associated with respiratory irregularity and abnormal repetitive movements likely represents a seizure.[8,16,17]

Other cases are generally less well defined than these examples, presenting challenges in the evaluation and management of infants with ALTEs. The sudden, irreproducible nature of the event may make coordinating the investigation difficult. Often, the history is incomplete or inaccurate because the caregiver is distracted by fear or unaware of the timing or duration of the event. In addition, the infant may appear normal on examination. Clinical judgment must guide the evaluation, and the hospitalist must consider the potential for harm and the expense when ordering a battery of insensitive or nonspecific tests.

Evaluation and Diagnosis

The key to the investigation of an ALTE is a thorough history from the primary witness and a careful physical examination. Key features of the history are detailed in Table 74-2. The history should be individually tailored and specific enough to categorize the episode as an exaggerated normal physiologic response, such as an isolated choking episode or acrocyanosis, or either a complicated or uncomplicated ALTE. Characteristics that differentiate a complicated from an uncomplicated ALTE are listed in Table 74-3.

The evaluating physician must not be confined to a minimum or maximum number of tests, although many experts recommend some level of testing and advocate a standardized approach.[8,10] The sheer number of possible tests makes the detection of some abnormality likely, but this may result in a diagnosis that is misleading because of a coexistent but not causative condition or an abnormal test result that is spurious.[18] For an ill-appearing infant, the hospitalist should rapidly evaluate and stabilize the patient according to his or her clinical condition rather than adhering to a strict algorithm. In an infant presenting with an ALTE while on a home cardiorespiratory monitor or because of frequent alarms, expedited monitor download should be conducted to determine whether true apnea or bradycardia occurred.[6,7,19]

In an uncomplicated ALTE associated with a normal physical examination and a benign history, further testing may not be indicated. However, a limited set of screening tests in such a situation may include standard hematologic and biochemical indices. Routine cultures should be obtained as clinically indicated, and a period of observation undertaken. This may include a period of monitored observation in the outpatient setting or admission to the hospital.[9] Infants who may be considered for early discharge include those with an uncomplicated ALTE in whom a reassuring course of events or underlying diagnosis can be determined. The health care team and parents must also be comfortable with the infant's clinical status, safety, and medical follow-up.[7]

Many infants with uncomplicated ALTEs are admitted to the hospital for observation, clinical monitoring, testing, and discharge planning. In some infants, this period of medical observation and clinical monitoring is the most important part of the assessment. Even in a well-appearing child with an unclear diagnosis, a period of observation and cardiorespiratory monitoring with pulse oximetry is reasonable to assist in the detection of additional episodes and define any associated events of clinical significance. A tailored diagnostic evaluation can proceed, especially if there are evolving symptoms or physical examination findings. Caregivers need to be provided with information, reassurance, and instruction in cardiopulmonary resuscitation. If no underlying cause is found after a thorough history, physical examination, and pointed evaluation, and if the child has no further clarifying events or features during the period of observation, the diagnosis of idiopathic ALTE is offered, and discharge may be considered.

Table 74-2 Focused History for Infants with Apparent Life-Threatening Events

Chief complaint
Presence of apnea or respiratory effort (including duration)
Type of color change and its distribution
Any change in tone and its distribution
Choking, gagging
Duration of the episode
Vomiting
Relationship to feedings
Eye deviation
Loss of consciousness
Fever
History of trauma
State of alertness before the event
Place where the event occurred
Caretaker during the episode
Type of resuscitation needed, and who performed it
Review of the prehospital (emergency medical services) record, if available
Current condition of the child, in the caretaker's opinion
Presence of a monitor
Medicines taken by the child or by the breastfeeding mother
History of ALTE in the past, and type of evaluation
Past medical history, including prematurity
Family history, including SIDS
Social history

ALTE, apparent life-threatening event; SIDS, sudden infant death syndrome.

Table 74-3 Characteristics of Complicated and Uncomplicated Apparent Life-Threatening Events

Feature	Uncomplicated	Complicated
Duration	Brief (<20-30 sec)	Prolonged (≥20 sec)
Pattern of events	Single or infrequent recurrences	Recurrent or clustered episodes
Intervention required	None or minimal stimulation	Moderate or vigorous stimulation, rescue breathing, or CPR
Physical examination	Normal	Abnormal or cardiorespiratory instability
Nature of respiratory event		
Obstructive pattern	Associated with feeding, congestion, or breath-holding spell	No clear association; persistent stridor or retractions at rest
Central pattern	<20 sec and no physiologic compromise	>20 sec or associated with physiologic compromise
Screening laboratory evaluation	If obtained, no acidosis, anemia, or evidence of infection	Abnormalities present

CPR, cardiopulmonary resuscitation.

In complicated ALTE, admission to the hospital is indicated. The diagnostic evaluation must be guided by the history and clinical status to avoid an excessive number of tests that could lead to confounding false-positive results. Specialized testing that may be required for infants with complicated ALTEs includes metabolic and toxicologic screens; microbiologic studies of blood, urine, cerebrospinal fluid, and respiratory secretions; medical imaging studies of the respiratory, gastrointestinal, and neurologic systems; electroencephalograms; and sleep studies. A list of clinical findings that may prompt diagnostic testing or consultation is provided in Table 74-4.

Infants who demonstrate recurrent apnea or ALTEs during the initial evaluation, especially if the events require intervention (e.g., stimulation, supplemental oxygen, ventilatory assistance), need close monitoring. This may best be accomplished in an intensive care setting. Ventilatory support with either noninvasive methods or endotracheal intubation may be necessary until the child stabilizes.

The role of polysomnography in the evaluation of infants with ALTEs is somewhat controversial. Recent studies suggest that polysomnography is not routinely indicated in uncomplicated ALTE, but other authors disagree and suggest that detailed cardiorespiratory testing and infant pneumograms are important components of the evaluation for many infants.[2,18,20] The decision to perform polysomnography usually requires subspecialty consultation and should be individualized. Polysomnography or pneumocardiography provides a snapshot of cardiorespiratory control and by itself is not predictive of future events or the occurrence of SIDS.[7,21,22]

Treatment and Discharge Planning

The medical treatment of ALTE is directed at any underlying cause. Occasionally, an infant with a history of prematurity presents with ALTE caused by anemia during the physiologic nadir of hemoglobin production and requires transfusion. An infant with ALTE due to RSV or some other viral respiratory infection may require significant respiratory support through the acute illness. Apnea associated with these illnesses has an excellent prognosis, however, and is not associated with an increased risk of recurrence or SIDS.[12] An infant with ALTE due to a severe infection such as pertussis or sepsis also requires supportive respiratory care, along with treatment of the acute infectious process. More complicated presentations, such as ALTE associated with underlying metabolic, neurologic, or cardiac conditions, usually require subspecialty consultation. In addition, an infant with idiopathic but complicated or recurrent episodes may require a multidisciplinary team approach. Most often, however, ALTE is attributed to GER or feeding difficulties, conditions that may require evaluation and management in an otherwise well infant (see Chapter 101). Although GER and dysphagia can certainly present with symptoms compatible with ALTE, the strength of the relationship between acidic GER and apnea in young infants has recently been called into question.[23-27]

The role of home cardiorespiratory monitors designed to detect central apnea and bradycardia in patients with ALTEs remains a topic of debate in the medical literature and among practitioners. It is important to remember that home monitors detect breathing through chest wall motion; therefore, obstructive events are not detected unless they are sufficiently severe or sustained to cause bradycardia. The

original 1986 NIH consensus statement, in the absence of supporting literature, suggested that monitors were indicated for ALTEs requiring vigorous stimulation for resuscitation.[1] A 2003 publication by the Committee on the Fetus and Newborn of the American Academy of Pediatrics offered more specific indications (updated in 2005; Pediatrics 116:5).[7] The committee suggested that monitors might be used to alert the family of events in patients with known airway instability, abnormal respiratory control, or symptomatic and technology-dependent chronic lung disease. Although the committee did not specifically address the source of ALTEs, one can infer that if they result from any of the previously mentioned conditions, a monitor might be justified. However, parents should be counseled that monitoring cannot always prevent sudden death from significant underlying conditions, particularly those associated with airway instability, and that monitoring should not be used to prevent SIDS.

Practitioners must be familiar with the current limitations in monitor technology, including its efficacy in managing ALTEs and its inability to prevent SIDS. In appropriate situations, the parents should participate in the decision whether to employ a home monitor. Some caregivers feel more comfortable with a monitor, whereas others find it intrusive or more worrisome in the event of false alarms (commonly due to loose leads or movement artifact). Because the majority of monitor alarms are false or clinically insignificant, the parents should be counseled to use their own assessment of the child in the event an alarm sounds.[28] If the child appears well or active, the alarm is likely malfunctioning. A cardiorespiratory monitor should have an event recorder and should be set with age-appropriate physiologic parameters (Table 74-5).[29]

Caregivers should also be trained in appropriate resuscitation techniques in the event of a future ALTE. Specifically, they should be instructed in proper assessment of an infant, recognition of events that warrant intervention, appropriate stimulation techniques, and cardiorespiratory resuscitation. Reinforcing the fact that an infant should never be shaken is critical. Moreover, caregivers should be counseled on the evidence-based ways to minimize the risk of SIDS, including positioning the infant on his or her back, using a firm crib mattress, avoiding excessive blankets, and avoiding exposure to environmental tobacco smoke.

Pharmacologic therapies for the treatment of pathologic apnea are controversial, particularly in term infants. In preterm infants, however, there is strong evidence that methylxanthines are effective in reducing the number of apneic events and the need for mechanical ventilation. Caffeine was identified as the methylxanthine associated with the least toxicity.[30-33] Continuous positive airway pressure is occasionally used in infants ill enough to require additional respiratory support, in an attempt to maintain gas exchange and avoid the need for invasive mechanical ventilation.[32] In term infants, the efficacy of caffeine in the prevention of clinically significant apnea lacks convincing data. Supplementation with oral carnitine or creatine is ineffective.[34-36]

Course of Illness

The literature on the natural history of infants who present with ALTE is incomplete. However, the vast majority of infants never have a subsequent ALTE and develop

Table 74-4 Evaluation of Apparent Life-Threatening Event Based on Clinical Presentation

System	Signs or Symptoms	Tests*	Consultation*
Gastrointestinal			
Gastroesophageal reflux disease	Relatively effortless emesis associated with discomfort (e.g., arching, crying, writhing) or choking following feedings, or feeding refusal	pH or impedance probe Upper gastrointestinal radiographic imaging with contrast Esophagoscopy	Gastroenterology for infants who remain symptomatic despite initial therapy
Dysphagia	Choking, gagging, snorting, or excessive sloppiness during feeding	Fluoroscopic modified barium swallow (often performed with speech therapist)	Speech therapy
Respiratory			
Apnea (central)	Undetectable breathing effort with central cyanosis, pallor, or limpness	Cardiorespiratory monitoring with pulse oximetry Polysomnography	Apnea team[†] Neonatology Pulmonology
Airway obstruction	Stridor, snoring, wheezing, hoarse cry, retractions, episodes of respiratory effort without detectable air movement, hemangioma (especially in the beard distribution), circumstances suggestive of foreign body aspiration	Polysomnography Radiologic esophagram Chest radiograph (with bilateral decubitus views if nonradiopaque foreign body is a concern) Nasopharyngolaryngoscopy	Apnea team[†] Neonatology Pulmonology Otolaryngology
Cardiovascular			
Cardiac dysfunction (e.g., congenital heart disease, arrhythmia)	Feeding intolerance (e.g., diaphoresis, fatigue), pathologic heart murmur, abnormal peripheral pulses, hepatomegaly, oxygen desaturation not fully correctable with 100% inspired oxygen	Four-extremity blood pressure measurements Preductal and postductal pulse oximetry Chest radiograph Electrocardiogram Echocardiogram	Cardiology
Neurologic			
Seizure	Abnormal movements, especially facial twitching or repeated jerking movements of extremities	Electroencephalogram Brain imaging	Neurology
Neuromuscular abnormality	Hypotonia, spasticity, asymmetrical reflexes, developmental delay, syndromic appearance	Brain imaging Metabolic evaluation Chromosomal evaluation	Neurology Metabolism Genetics
Endocrinologic, metabolic, genetic			
Hypoglycemia	Diaphoresis (especially after prolonged feeding delay), macrosomia, macroglossia, syndromic appearance	Bedside blood glucose monitoring (scheduled or with symptoms) Evaluation for abnormalities of glucose homeostasis	Endocrinology Genetics
Electrolyte abnormalities (e.g., calcium, sodium)	Hypotonia, hyperreflexia, seizure, arrhythmia, polyuria, history of inadequate or excessive free water intake	Serial evaluations of serum electrolytes Urinalysis, electrolytes Evaluation of thyroid and cortisol-adrenal function and bone metabolism	Endocrinology Nephrology
Metabolic acidosis	Hyperpnea, failure to thrive, hypotonia, syndromic appearance	Arterial blood gas evaluations Evaluation for inborn errors of metabolism Review of newborn screen	Metabolism Genetics

Table 74-4 Evaluation of Apparent Life-Threatening Event Based on Clinical Presentation—cont'd

System	Signs or Symptoms	Tests*	Consultation*
Hematologic			
Anemia	Pallor, large hematoma, tachycardia	CBC, RBC indices, reticulocyte count, blood smear, direct Coombs test Stool and urine heme testing Review of newborn screen, hemoglobin electrophoresis	Hematology
Polycythemia	Plethoric or ruddy appearance	CBC, blood smear Serum bilirubin level	Hematology
Infectious			
Viral respiratory illness	Rhinorrhea; coryza; cough (especially "barky"); new-onset hoarseness, wheezing, or rhonchi; increased work of breathing	Detection of respiratory virus by rapid testing or viral culture	
Sepsis, meningitis	Fever or temperature instability, toxic appearance, bulging fontanelle, meningismus, intense irritability, lethargy, petechiae, mottling, hypotension	Blood cell count and culture Cerebrospinal fluid culture, chemistry analysis, cell count, and (if appropriate) viral studies Urine culture and analysis	Infectious diseases
Infant botulism	Constipation, hypotonia (usually bulbar initially), weak cry, poor feeding, areflexia, nontoxic appearance	Stool for botulinum toxin	Neurology Critical care
Behavioral			
Breath-holding spells	Crying episodes following distressing event; usually follows prolonged expiration; central cyanosis, pallor, limpness, or (rarely) seizure activity can ensue, especially if infant is upright		Neurology
Trauma			
Accidental or nonaccidental	History of trauma, unexplained injuries, history of sibling with SIDS	Brain imaging Radiographic skeletal survey Retinal examination	Trauma surgery Child abuse specialist
Munchausen syndrome by proxy	Recurrent events, often uncorroborated, without identifiable cause despite extensive evaluation; failure to disclose previous evaluations	Contact with primary care clinician and other medical facilities where previous evaluations may have been performed Consider long-term in-hospital cardiorespiratory or video monitoring	Social services Child abuse experts
Medication or toxic exposure			
Medication	History of maternal drug use or abuse, dosing of prescribed medication, symptoms suggestive of NAS	Urine or serum toxicology testing of infant, mother, or both	Toxicology Social services
Environmental	History of smoke inhalation or environmental accident, suspected or confirmed contaminated formula or water source	Targeted analysis for specific toxin exposure (e.g., carbon monoxide exposure warrants co-oximetry)	Toxicology

*This table is not exhaustive; the tests and consultations should be considered but are not required.
†Consultation pattern depends on expertise and availability in a given community
CBC, complete blood count; NAS, neonatal abstinence syndrome (see Chapter 56); RBC, red blood cell; SIDS, sudden infant death syndrome.

Table 74-5 Age-Appropriate Cardiorespiratory Monitor Settings

Condition and Age	Setting Threshold
Apnea	
Preterm infants	15 sec
Term infants	20 sec
Bradycardia	
Premature infants	
PCA <40 wk	100 BPM
PCA 40-44 wk	80 BPM
PCA >44 wk	Use full-term threshold with corrected age in months
Full-term infants	
<1 mo	80 BPM
1-3 mo	70 BPM
3-12 mo	60 BPM
>12 mo	50 BPM

BPM, beats per minute; PCA, postconceptional age.

Table 74-6 Conditions Associated with Pediatric Obstructive Sleep Apnea Syndrome

Adenotonsillar hypertrophy
Allergic rhinitis
Obesity
Trisomy 21
Craniofacial syndromes
Skeletal dysplasia syndromes
Neuromuscular disorders
Cerebral palsy
Sickle cell disease

normally.[5] In those infants with ALTEs secondary to an underlying diagnosis, that condition and its treatment define the course. For example, an infant with ALTE secondary to epilepsy is at risk for recurrent events, whereas an infant with ALTE secondary to RSV infection is not. If no underlying diagnosis can be determined in an infant with recurrent ALTEs, a careful social evaluation should be undertaken, because apnea or ALTE may be the presenting complaint among infants who are victims of abuse or Munchausen syndrome by proxy.[17,37-42]

PATHOLOGIC CENTRAL APNEA IN INFANCY

Central apnea is defined as the absence of respiratory effort due to either a lack of output from the central respiratory centers or neuromuscular insufficiency. Chest wall movement is absent, and no breath sounds are evident on auscultation of the chest. Significant central apnea is generally defined as cessation of breathing for at least 20 seconds; shorter episodes are considered significant if they are associated with central cyanosis, bradycardia, pallor, or loss of muscle tone. Pathologic apnea is associated with physiologic compromise, whereas apneic events without these changes are considered normal.

When pathologic apnea occurs for the first time in an infant beyond 37 weeks' postconceptual age, it is called apnea of infancy. Apnea of infancy is distinct from apnea of prematurity, which resolves by 37 weeks' postconceptional age.[43] However, in rare cases, apnea of prematurity may persist beyond term, particularly in infants born at less than 28 weeks' gestation.[7]

Periodic breathing is defined as three or more respiratory pauses of greater than 3 seconds' duration with less than 20 seconds of respiration between pauses. Periodic breathing is normal in preterm infants and may persist beyond term in some infants. If periodic breathing is associated with bradycardia or cyanosis, it is considered a pathologic breathing pattern and warrants evaluation for an underlying cause. In

some cases, respiratory stimulants such as caffeine may be indicated for infants with prolonged cardiorespiratory immaturity.

Pathologic central apnea and symptomatic periodic breathing can be considered entities within the category of ALTE. Therefore, the differential diagnosis and approach in an infant with symptomatic apnea are similar to those in an infant with ALTE.

PEDIATRIC OBSTRUCTIVE SLEEP APNEA SYNDROME

Although the diagnosis and management of pediatric obstructive sleep apnea syndrome (OSAS) are generally performed on an outpatient basis, the hospitalist should be aware of specific circumstances. Polysomnography is often performed in an inpatient facility, and a patient who becomes unstable during the study may come to the attention of the hospitalist. Patients with preexisting or previously undiagnosed OSAS may present to an emergency department or be referred for admission with symptoms of acute airway obstruction. This may also occur in the sedation suite or in a hospitalized patient admitted for an unrelated problem when severe snoring, labored breathing, or gas exchange abnormalities become evident during sleep. This is more common in a postoperative patient or a patient recently extubated from endotracheal intubation.

Obstructive apnea is defined as the absence of airflow at the nose or mouth despite continued respiratory efforts. OSAS has been defined as a disorder of sleep consisting of prolonged partial upper airway obstruction or episodic obstructive apnea that affects gas exchange or sleep architecture and quality.[44-47] OSAS occurs in 1% to 3% of preschool children, with a male predominance. The peak incidence is between 2 and 6 years. Adenotonsillar hypertrophy, insufficient airway, and decreased neuromuscular tone are critical to the pathogenesis of pediatric OSAS. In children with obesity, midfacial hypoplasia and micrognathia (commonly seen in craniofacial syndromes), and disorders associated with abnormal muscle tone, the risk of OSAS is even greater (Table 74-6).

Clinical Presentation

As its name implies, OSAS occurs only during sleep. Respiration during wakefulness may be completely normal, although mouth breathing, nasal obstruction, and chronic congestion may be evident. Gas exchange should be normal during wakefulness, even in patients who have significant OSAS and severe gas exchange abnormalities during sleep. Most patients with OSAS have a history of snoring and restless sleep. Children may experience daytime sleepiness or have behavioral or attention problems. Enuresis may be associated with OSAS as well.

In the absence of an underlying craniofacial skeletal dysplasia or neuromuscular syndrome, the physical examination usually reveals adenotonsillar hypertrophy or possibly rhinosinusitis but is otherwise within normal limits. Pectus excavatum in a young child may suggest prolonged and severe upper airway obstruction. Despite the association with adenotonsillar hypertrophy, the absolute size of the tonsils and adenoids does not correlate with the severity of OSAS. Rarely, in severe cases of OSAS, failure to thrive or even cor pulmonale may be evident. Obesity is much more common.

Evaluation, Diagnosis, and Treatment

It is not possible to make the diagnosis of OSAS based on history alone, and the gold standard for diagnosis is polysomnography (see Chapter 80).[20] Simple bedside observation of snoring and obstructed breathing, with or without oxyhemoglobin desaturation, can be highly suggestive of OSAS and may prompt definitive testing. Other tests that might be indicated include anteroposterior and lateral neck radiographs to assess adenotonsillar hypertrophy, anteroposterior and lateral chest radiographs to assess cardiac silhouette, and electrocardiogram. Electrocardiographic findings indicative of cor pulmonale include right atrial and right ventricular hypertrophy. Blood work is usually unremarkable, although hypercapnia due to severe OSAS could theoretically result in elevated serum bicarbonate.

The management of pediatric OSAS includes support of gas exchange and airway function during sleep and treatment of the underlying condition.[48] Weight loss in an obese child is critical. Adenotonsillectomy is usually curative in an otherwise healthy child. Young children and those with severe OSAS or underlying conditions are at risk for postoperative respiratory compromise and should be observed carefully after adenotonsillectomy until adequate upper airway function can be ascertained.[49,50] This may warrant monitoring in an intensive care setting. Continuous or bilevel positive airway pressure administered via a nasal mask can be used acutely or chronically (see Chapter 209).[51] Supplemental oxygen therapy should be used with care, however, because blunting of the hypoxic drive to breathe in a child with carbon dioxide retention due to OSAS can theoretically worsen obstructive hypoventilation.[52] Steroids are not indicated in the treatment of chronic OSAS but may be of some benefit in an acute setting when tonsillar size increases abruptly due to lymphoid hyperplasia.

CONSULTATION

Subspecialty consultation should be considered on a case-by-case basis for infants with technology dependence, complicated or recurrent ALTEs, or evidence of a serious underlying condition. This often facilitates additional testing (e.g., polysomnography), allows the initiation of medical therapy, or results in an evaluation for possible surgical intervention. Subspecialty consultants might include neonatologists, pulmonologists, otolaryngologists, or an "apnea team," depending on the individual patient's clinical situation. Referral patterns vary according to regional practice and availability of subspecialty support.

ADMISSION CRITERIA

- Complicated ALTE.
- Uncomplicated ALTE requiring further evaluation, treatment, or discharge planning.
- Recurrent idiopathic ALTEs.
- Observed episodes of pathologic central apnea.
- Airway instability or abnormal gas exchange.
- Exacerbation of symptoms that compromise management of underlying disorders.
- Evidence of sequelae of untreated and long-standing symptoms of OSAS (e.g., failure to thrive, cor pulmonale).
- Inability to ensure patient safety or adequate medical follow-up

DISCHARGE CRITERIA

- Documented medical and airway stability.
- Adequate initiation of therapy for any treatable underlying disorder identified.
- Adequate parental education and training in airway management.
- Plan in place for medical follow-up.

IN A NUTSHELL

- ALTE is characterized by some combination of apnea (central or occasionally obstructive), color change (usually cyanotic or pallid, but occasionally erythematous or plethoric), marked change in muscle tone (usually limpness), choking, or gagging.
- ALTE and apnea of infancy are common, potentially serious, but usually benign entities. They represent a heterogeneous group of disorders with many possible causes.
- Providing education, training, and anticipatory guidance to concerned caregivers is key to the effective management and discharge planning for these infants.
- OSAS is a sleep disorder consisting of obstructive apnea or prolonged partial upper airway obstruction that affects gas exchange and sleep quality or architecture.
- Adenotonsillar hypertrophy, obesity, and diminished neuromuscular tone are common underlying conditions in OSAS.

ON THE HORIZON

ALTE and apnea of infancy are difficult to study. New strategies are needed to elucidate the true nature of these episodes and their significance in a prospective fashion. Areas of particular interest include the following:

- Differentiating features of the presenting event that can predict subsequent morbidity or mortality.
- Understanding the significance of 20- to 30-second apnea in healthy and at-risk infants.
- Clarifying the role of GER in ALTE and apnea.
- Identifying patients for whom home cardiorespiratory monitoring may be efficacious.
- Adding to the body of knowledge surrounding normal breathing during sleep.
- Improving the understanding of the anatomic and neuromuscular pathophysiology of airway obstruction during sleep.
- Quantifying the health-related consequences of sleep, such as its impact on growth, development, and behavior.

REFERENCES

1. Infantile Apnea and Home Monitoring. Bethesda, Md, National Institutes of Health, 1986.
2. Silvestri JM, Weese-Mayer DE: Respiratory control disorders in infancy and childhood. Curr Opin Pediatr 1996;8:216-220.
3. Kiechl-Kohlendorfer U, Hof D, Peglow UP, et al: Epidemiology of apparent life threatening events. Arch Dis Child 2005;90:297-300.
4. Stratton SJ, Taves A, Lewis RJ, et al: Apparent life-threatening events in infants: High risk in the out-of-hospital environment. Ann Emerg Med 2004;43:711-717.
5. Davies F, Gupta R: Apparent life threatening events in infants presenting to an emergency department. Emerg Med J 2002;19:11-16.
6. Ramanathan R, Corwin MJ, Hunt CE, et al: Cardiorespiratory events recorded on home monitors: Comparison of healthy infants with those at increased risk for SIDS. JAMA 2001;285:2199-2207.
7. Apnea, sudden infant death syndrome, and home monitoring. Pediatrics 2003;111:914-917.
8. McGovern MC, Smith MB: Causes of apparent life threatening events in infants: A systematic review. Arch Dis Child 2004;89:1043-1048.
9. De Piero AD, Teach SJ, Chamberlain JM: ED evaluation of infants after an apparent life-threatening event. Am J Emerg Med 2004;22:83-86.
10. Kahn A: Recommended clinical evaluation of infants with an apparent life-threatening event: Consensus document of the European Society for the Study and Prevention of Infant Death, 2003. Eur J Pediatr 2004;163:108-115.
11. Kneyber MC, Brandenburg AH, de Groot R, et al: Risk factors for respiratory syncytial virus associated apnoea. Eur J Pediatr 1998;157:331-335.
12. Church NR, Anas NG, Hall CB, Brooks JG: Respiratory syncytial virus-related apnea in infants: Demographics and outcome. Am J Dis Child 1984;138:247-250.
13. Rayyan M, Naulaers G, Daniels H, et al: Characteristics of respiratory syncytial virus-related apnoea in three infants. Acta Paediatr 2004;93:847-849.
14. Pickens DL, Schefft GL, Storch GA, Thach BT: Characterization of prolonged apneic episodes associated with respiratory syncytial virus infection. Pediatr Pulmonol 1989;6:195-201.
15. Chidekel A, Hershberger M, Levine J, Smith C: Cardiorespiratory characteristics of infants with and without dysphagia who present with an apparent life threatening event. Am J Respir Crit Care Med 2000;161:A341.
16. Nunes ML, Appel CC, da Costa JC: Apparent life-threatening episodes as the first manifestation of epilepsy. Clin Pediatr (Phila) 2003;42:19-22.
17. Samuels MP, Poets CF, Noyes JP, et al: Diagnosis and management after life threatening events in infants and young children who received cardiopulmonary resuscitation. BMJ 1993;306:489-492.
18. Brand DA, Altman RL, Purtill K, Edwards KS: Yield of diagnostic testing in infants who have had an apparent life-threatening event. Pediatrics 2005;115:885-893.
19. Poets CF: Apparent life-threatening events and sudden infant death on a monitor. Paediatr Respir Rev 2004;5(Suppl A):S383-S386.
20. Standards and indications for cardiopulmonary sleep studies in children: American Thoracic Society. Am J Respir Crit Care Med 1996;153:866-878.
21. Monod N, Plouin P, Sternberg B, et al: Are polygraphic and cardiopneumographic respiratory patterns useful tools for predicting the risk for sudden infant death syndrome? A 10-year study. Biol Neonate 1986;50:147-153.
22. Southall DP, Richards JM, Rhoden KJ, et al: Prolonged apnea and cardiac arrhythmias in infants discharged from neonatal intensive care units: Failure to predict an increased risk for sudden infant death syndrome. Pediatrics 1982;70:844-851.
23. Arad-Cohen N, Cohen A, Tirosh E: The relationship between gastroesophageal reflux and apnea in infants. J Pediatr 2000;137:321-326.
24. Greenfeld M, Tauman R, Sivan Y: The yield of esophageal pH monitoring during polysomnography in infants with sleep-disordered breathing. Clin Pediatr (Phila) 2004;43:653-658.
25. Molloy EJ, Di Fiore JM, Martin RJ: Does gastroesophageal reflux cause apnea in preterm infants? Biol Neonate 2005;87:254-261.
26. Poets CF: Gastroesophageal reflux: A critical review of its role in preterm infants. Pediatrics 2004;113:e128-e132.
27. Wenzl TG, Schenke S, Peschgens T, et al: Association of apnea and nonacid gastroesophageal reflux in infants: Investigations with the intraluminal impedance technique. Pediatr Pulmonol 2001;31:144-149.
28. Weese-Mayer DE, Brouillette RT, Morrow AS, et al: Assessing validity of infant monitor alarms with event recording. J Pediatr 1989;115:702-708.
29. Silvestri JM, Weese-Mayer DE, Hunt CE: Home monitoring during infancy: What is normal? Paediatr Respir Rev 2002;3:10-17.
30. Erenberg A, Leff RD, Haack DG, et al: Caffeine citrate for the treatment of apnea of prematurity: A double-blind, placebo-controlled study. Pharmacotherapy 2000;20:644-652.
31. Henderson-Smart DJ, Steer P: Methylxanthine treatment for apnea in preterm infants. Cochrane Database Syst Rev 2001;CD000140.
32. Henderson-Smart DJ, Subramanian P, Davis PG: Continuous positive airway pressure versus theophylline for apnea in preterm infants. Cochrane Database Syst Rev 2000;CD001072.
33. Steer PA, Henderson-Smart DJ: Caffeine versus theophylline for apnea in preterm infants. Cochrane Database Syst Rev 2000;CD000273.
34. Kumar M, Kabra NS, Paes B: Role of carnitine supplementation in apnea of prematurity: A systematic review. J Perinatol 2004;24:158-163.
35. Kumar M, Kabra NS, Paes B: Carnitine supplementation for preterm infants with recurrent apnea. Cochrane Database Syst Rev 2004;CD004497.
36. Bohnhorst B, Geuting T, Peter CS, et al: Randomized, controlled trial of oral creatine supplementation (not effective) for apnea of prematurity. Pediatrics 2004;113:e303-e307.
37. Altman RL, Brand DA, Forman S, et al: Abusive head injury as a cause of apparent life-threatening events in infancy. Arch Pediatr Adolesc Med 2003;157:1011-1015.
38. Mitchell I, Brummitt J, DeForest J, Fisher G: Apnea and factitious illness (Munchausen syndrome) by proxy. Pediatrics 1993;92:810-814.
39. Pitetti RD, Maffei F, Chang K, et al: Prevalence of retinal hemorrhages and child abuse in children who present with an apparent life-threatening event. Pediatrics 2002;110:557-562.
40. Southall DP, Plunkett MC, Banks MW, et al: Covert video recordings of life-threatening child abuse: Lessons for child protection. Pediatrics 1997;100:735-760.

41. Stanton AN: Sudden unexpected death in infancy associated with maltreatment: Evidence from long term follow up of siblings. Arch Dis Child 2003;88:699-701.

42. Truman TL, Ayoub CC: Considering suffocatory abuse and Munchausen by proxy in the evaluation of children experiencing apparent life-threatening events and sudden infant death syndrome. Child Maltreat 2002;7:138-148.

43. Baird TM: Clinical correlates, natural history and outcome of neonatal apnoea. Semin Neonatol 2004;9:205-211.

44. Chan J, Edman JC, Koltai PJ: Obstructive sleep apnea in children. Am Fam Physician 2004;69:1147-1154.

45. Erler T, Paditz E: Obstructive sleep apnea syndrome in children: A state-of-the-art review. Treat Respir Med 2004;3:107-122.

46. Marcus CL: Sleep-disordered breathing in children. Am J Respir Crit Care Med 2001;164:16-30.

47. Schechter MS: Technical report: Diagnosis and management of childhood obstructive sleep apnea syndrome. Pediatrics 2002;109:e69.

48. Messner AH: Treating pediatric patients with obstructive sleep disorders: An update. Otolaryngol Clin North Am 2003;36:519-530.

49. Nixon GM, Kermack AS, McGregor CD, et al: Sleep and breathing on the first night after adenotonsillectomy for obstructive sleep apnea. Pediatr Pulmonol 2005;39:332-338.

50. McColley SA, April MM, Carroll JL, et al: Respiratory compromise after adenotonsillectomy in children with obstructive sleep apnea. Arch Otolaryngol Head Neck Surg 1992;118:940-943.

51. Friedman O, Chidekel A, Lawless ST, Cook SP: Postoperative bilevel positive airway pressure ventilation after tonsillectomy and adenoidectomy in children—a preliminary report. Int J Pediatr Otorhinolaryngol 1999;51:177-180.

52. Marcus CL, Carroll JL, Bamford O, et al: Supplemental oxygen during sleep in children with sleep-disordered breathing. Am J Respir Crit Care Med 1995;152:1297-1301.

CHAPTER 75

Asthma

Meredith Heltzer and Jonathan M. Spergel

Almost 5 million children in the United States have asthma,[1] and it is the most common reason for admission to pediatric hospitals.[2] Each year, asthma results in 10 million school absences,[2] 5500 deaths,[3] and 500,000 hospitalizations.[4,5] Appropriate asthma treatment prevents hospital admissions and emergency room visits, reduces the risk for death, and improves the quality of life for children with asthma.[4,6,7] The hospitalist is ideally situated to have a major impact on asthma by treating its acute manifestations, by implementing effective long-term therapy when indicated, and by diagnosing and managing any comorbidity that accompanies or exacerbates asthma (or both).

Asthma results from airway inflammation and smooth muscle dysfunction. It is defined by the National Heart, Lung, and Blood Institute (NHLBI) and World Health Organization as follows:

"A chronic inflammatory disorder of the airways in which many cells play a role, in particular, mast cells, eosinophils, and T lymphocytes. In susceptible individuals this inflammation causes recurrent episodes of wheezing, breathlessness, chest tightness, and cough, particularly at night and in the early morning. These symptoms are usually associated with widespread but variable airway obstruction that is often reversible either spontaneously or with treatment. The inflammation also causes an associated increase in the existing bronchial hyperresponsiveness to a variety of stimuli."[4]

PATHOPHYSIOLOGY OF ASTHMA

The underlying cause of asthma is unknown, and the course of pediatric asthma is dynamic. Early in the course of the disease, airway inflammation, bronchial hyperreactivity, and loss of lung function are evident. Atopy and a family history of asthma are strongly correlated with asthma in childhood. Exposure to allergens activates mast cells and promotes inflammation and infiltration of the airway with neutrophils, eosinophils, and lymphocytes.[8] Whatever the cause, the inflammation results in airway hyperresponsiveness, which causes bronchoconstriction, edema, and mucous plugging, all of which contribute to bronchial obstruction. Chronically, collagen deposition below the epithelial basement membrane results in narrowing of the airway secondary to remodeling

ASTHMA EXACERBATIONS

An asthma exacerbation refers to an increase in a patient's respiratory symptoms above baseline as a result of increased airway obstruction. Status asthmaticus is continued or progressive airway obstruction despite bronchodilator therapy that results in sustained or worsening respiratory distress.[4]

Acute asthma exacerbations can be triggered by infectious respiratory illness, exposure to environmental allergens or irritants, exercise, cold air, or a combination of these factors. An asthma exacerbation involves either a slow onset of symptoms or a rapid decline in respiratory status. Persistent or acute allergen or irritant exposure promotes inflammation, bronchoconstriction, and airway hyperresponsiveness on an ongoing basis. Allergen exposure triggers a biphasic response. The "early response" occurs within minutes of allergen exposure and results in rhinorrhea, sneezing, itching of the eyes and nose, and bronchospasm secondary to release of histamine and other preformed mediators of inflammation. The "late-phase response" peaks 6 to 8 hours after allergen exposure with the development of eosinophilic inflammation and T-cell infiltration of the airway. During an exacerbation of asthma as a result of allergen exposure, both phases must be treated with medications to treat the symptoms of the early phase, as well as the subsequent inflammation of the late phase.[9]

Viral infections cause asthma symptoms by promoting eosinophilic or neutrophilic airway inflammation.[4] Viral-induced asthma exacerbations are common in children, and in fact a majority of acute asthma admissions are associated with viral infections in children and adults.[10,11] The risk for exacerbation of asthma can be modified by a patient's underlying inflammatory state and level of airway hyperreactivity. A patient with reduced airway inflammation because of adequate controller therapy is less likely to have a severe asthma flare when exposed to offending agents.

CLINICAL PRESENTATION

The presentation of acute asthma may vary, but all patients experience worsening airflow obstruction associated with respiratory distress. Patients often complain of shortness of breath, chest tightness, and wheezing. Some patients describe chest pain, cough, or fatigue. Caregivers may report observations of breathlessness, trouble speaking, decreased activity, retractions, rapid breathing, wheezing noises, or relentless cough.[12]

On physical examination, tachypnea is present, often accompanied by tachycardia. Pulse oximetry may reveal decreased oxygen saturation. There is evidence of increased respiratory effort, such as intercostal, supraclavicular, or subcostal retractions. Infants and young children may demonstrate nasal flaring or head bobbing. Paradoxical motion of the thoracoabdominal wall (i.e., expansion of abdominal girth with inspiration) is another useful sign of increased work of breathing. Auscultation of the chest frequently reveals wheezing and a prolonged expiratory phase. Rales or crackles are often heard and may shift in location over a period of minutes to hours ("migratory atelectasis"). Assessment of air movement is determined by the loudness of breath sounds in various areas of the chest and may also vary over time. Patients with poor air movement may have minimal wheezing because the passage of air through the airway is what generates wheezing sounds. As air exchange improves, wheezing may become more pronounced. Conversely, patients with a deteriorating clinical course may have diminishing wheezing indicative of worsening air movement and perhaps respiratory insufficiency. Agitation and somnolence are worrisome signs and may indicate hypoxemia or hypercapnia with impending respiratory failure.

Some patients present without significant wheezing but with prominent cough as their manifestation of asthma, often referred to as "cough-variant" asthma. It is believed that the pathophysiology and response to treatment are similar to that for classic asthma.

DIFFERENTIAL DIAGNOSIS

Many conditions result in acute or chronic respiratory symptoms that mimic an asthma syndrome. Some of these conditions are discussed in the following text.

Anatomic abnormalities should be considered in young children with frequent episodes of cough or wheezing. Inhaled foreign bodies are most common in toddler-aged children (Chapter 79). These problems may manifest as cough, stridor, or wheezing. In all age groups, gastroesophageal reflux can mimic or contribute to underlying asthma (Chapter 101).[13,14] Cystic fibrosis is a genetic disorder that can also present with chronic cough or recurrent episodes of wheezing (Chapter 78).

Viral infections often cause wheezing in childhood as well. Respiratory syncytial virus is the most common cause of infantile bronchiolitis, but other respiratory viruses such as rhinovirus, parainfluenza virus, coronavirus, adenovirus, and influenza viruses are also common infectious agents.[15] Viral bronchiolitis is associated with edema, bronchospasm, and increased mucus production of the smaller airways, features that overlap with asthma (Chapter 66). Because these respiratory viral infections are known to precipitate asthma exacerbations, it may be difficult to determine whether the wheezing represents an isolated episode of bronchiolitis or an asthma exacerbation triggered by the respiratory virus.

Atypical respiratory infections with agents such as *Mycoplasma*, *Chlamydia pneumoniae*, and *Bordetella pertussis* or *parapertussis* can present with chronic cough. Coughing associated with these infections can persist for several months.

Functional disorders can coexist with or mimic asthma and include vocal cord dysfunction (VCD) and psychogenic cough. VCD usually presents in adolescence with upper airway (laryngeal) inspiratory or expiratory stridor, or both, which may be difficult to distinguish from lower airway wheezing. The diagnosis of VCD is confirmed by laryngoscopy demonstrating paradoxical adduction of the vocal cords during inspiration.[16-19] Psychogenic cough is a habitual cough that can also persist for months, and it often occurs after an acute respiratory illness.[20] Habitual cough has a characteristic sound described as barky or honking. The cough is exaggerated by stress or attention to the cough and disappears with sleep.[20] These features help distinguish this entity from cough-variant asthma. A key feature of VCD and psychogenic cough is lack of response to asthma therapy.[16-20] In addition, they are not associated with hypoxia.

Table 75-1 **Questions to Ask Patients Who Present with Wheezing**

Types of Symptoms
Cough
Wheeze
Shortness of breath
Chest tightness
Sputum production

Frequency of Symptoms
Daily, weekly, none
Perennial, seasonally
Do they have a night cough?
Do they cough with activity?
How often do they use their albuterol?

Severity of Symptoms
How often do they have flares of their asthma? How many times in the last year?
How many times have they used oral steroids? How many times in the last year?
How many emergency room visits?
How many visits to the hospital?
Have they ever been in the intensive care unit?

Table 75-2 **Features That Place Patient at Risk for Severe Asthma**

History of respiratory failure with asthma
Recent or multiple emergency department visits or hospitalizations (<6 months)
Daily oral steroid use at the time of exacerbations
Comorbid psychosocial conditions that interfere with administration of medications

EVALUATION

The initial evaluation of a patient presenting with an asthma exacerbation should include assessment of the acute respiratory symptoms, signs or symptoms of coexisting or precipitating conditions, and treatments initiated before presentation. A history should be obtained of the characteristics of the patient's asthma symptoms, the pattern and frequency of the symptoms, and any precipitating or aggravating factors, as well as features indicative of the severity and level of control of the asthma (Tables 75-1 and 75-2).[4]

The physical examination provides clues to the severity of the current illness, as well as the presence of comorbid conditions. Important physical parameters include the respiratory rate, work of breathing, air entry, wheezing, and oxygen saturation. Work of breathing refers to the use of accessory muscles of respiration and involves nasal flaring, abdominal retractions, and depth of respiration.

During an exacerbation of asthma, physical findings may vary and evolve with treatment or progression of the acute condition. A quiet or silent chest is a worrisome sign because poor movement of air can be associated with respiratory insufficiency or failure. Asymmetry of auscultatory findings may indicate other conditions. Unequal breath sounds can be found with pneumonia, pleural effusion (especially in dependent regions of the lung), or atelectasis. Unilateral breath sounds may indicate an aspirated foreign body or pneumothorax on the side with diminished breath sounds[4] and may be accompanied by hyperresonance on that side, especially if significant air trapping is present.

Chest radiographs are not typically needed for patients with known asthma and a straightforward asthma exacerbation.[21] Typical radiographic findings include hyperinflation, peribronchial thickening, and atelectasis (Fig. 75-1). Chest radiographs may be helpful when there is concern for pneumonia, pleural effusion, pneumothorax, pneumomediastinum, or foreign body aspiration.

A classification system for determining the severity of an asthma exacerbation in children 5 years of age or older is provided in Table 75-3. Patients in mild distress typically have slightly increased respiratory rates, may not use accessory muscles of respiration, and have end-expiratory wheezes with good air entry. Patients in severe distress are working hard to breathe, with inspiratory and expiratory wheezing, and are often hypoxic. Signs of impending respiratory failure are provided in Table 75-4. For infants and children younger than 5 years of age, clues to breathlessness include difficulty or reluctance to feed and changes in crying pattern (e.g., softer or shorter). Changes in vital signs in these younger patients must be interpreted in the context of normal values for the age range. Interestingly, paradoxical thoracoabdominal movement, a sign associated with severe respiratory distress in older children, may be seen in young children and infants, even in states of mild or moderate respiratory distress.

Objective measures for evaluation of acute asthma include pulmonary function testing, pulse oximetry, and arterial blood gases. Patients with exacerbations of asthma are at risk for hypoxemia. As a result, patients require frequent monitoring to ensure adequate oxygenation. Continuous pulse oximetry is recommended during a severe exacerbation, whereas intermittent oximetry may be acceptable as the clinical course improves.

Arterial blood gas parameters are typically obtained in critically ill patients and those with clinical deterioration or signs of respiratory insufficiency or failure. Arterial blood gases may reveal hypoxemia from ventilation-perfusion mismatch and respiratory alkalosis with hypocapnia secondary to hyperventilation. A normal or elevated partial pressure of carbon dioxide ($Paco_2$) may be the harbinger of respiratory failure[22] and may be associated with decreased blood pH because of respiratory acidosis.

Pulmonary function tests can be used to assess lung function even during an asthma exacerbation. Spirometric indices such as forced expiratory volume in 1 second (FEV_1) or the peak expiratory flow rate (PEFR) are most useful to assess the severity of asthma. However, because spirometry is often not readily available in the acute care setting, PEFR can be used instead. The hand-held peak flowmeter measures PEFR, and normal values have been established according to age, gender, and height[23] (Table 75-5). PEFR provides a measure of large-airway flow by measuring the rate of airflow in liters per minute. As a flare or asthma exacerba-

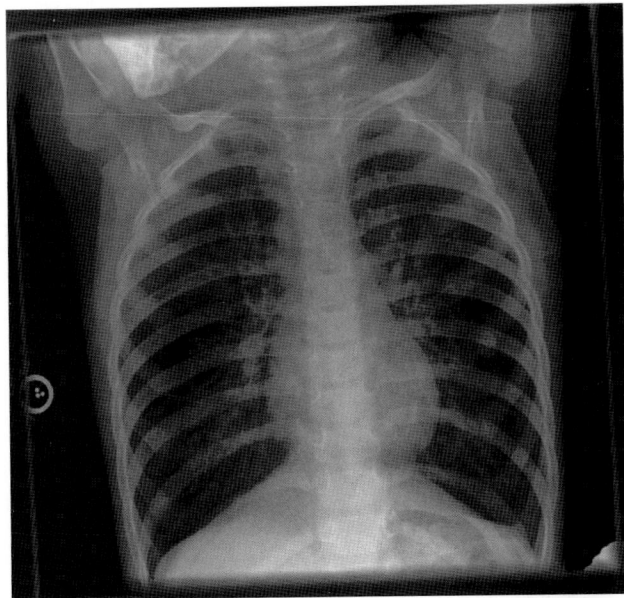

A

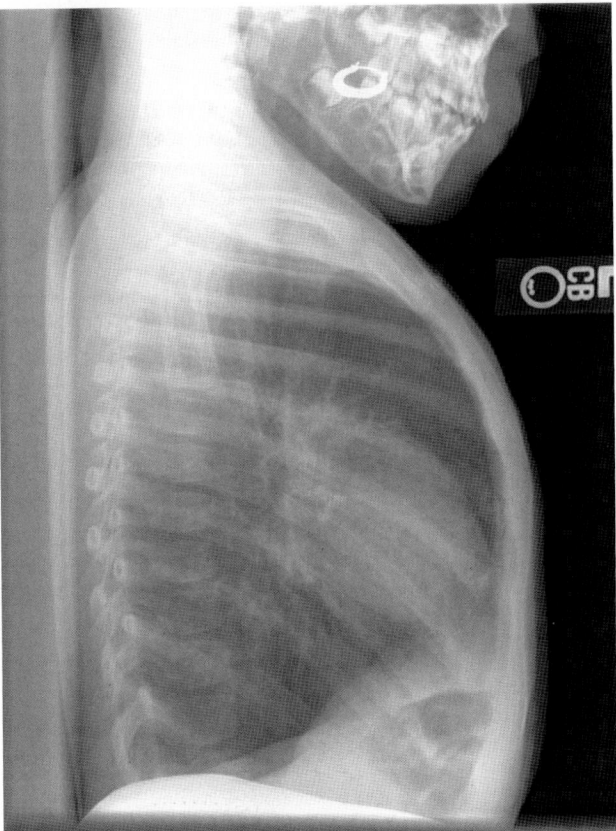

B

Figure 75-1 Typical radiographic findings of hyperinflation and peribronchial thickening in a patient with an acute asthma exacerbation. Flattening of the diaphragms is prominent in both the anteroposterior (A) and lateral (B) view. The lateral view demonstrates a widened anteroposterior diameter and increased prominence of the retrocardiac space.

Table 75-3   Clinical Classification of Severity for Asthma Exacerbation

	SEVERITY OF EXACERBATION			
	Mild	*Moderate*	*Severe*	*Impending Respiratory Failure*
Symptoms				
Breathlessness	While walking	While talking (infants: softer, shorter cry; difficulty feeding)	While at rest (infants: stop feeding)	
Positioning	Can lie down	Prefers sitting	Sits upright	
Speaks in	Sentences	Phrases	Words	
Alertness	May be agitated	Usually agitated	Usually agitated	Drowsy or confused
Signs				
Respiratory rate	Increased	Increased	Often >30/min	
Use of accessory muscles, suprasternal retractions	Usually not	Commonly	Usually	Paradoxical thoracoabdominal movement
Wheezing	Moderate, often only end expiratory	Loud, throughout exhalation	Usually loud, throughout inhalation and exhalation	Absence of wheezing
Pulse/min	<100	100-120	>120	Tachycardia or bradycardia
Pulsus paradoxus	Absent (<10 mm Hg)	May be present (10-25 mm Hg)	Often present (>25 mm Hg for an adult, 20-40 mm Hg for a child)	Absence suggests respiratory muscle fatigue
Functional Assessment				
PEF, % predicted or % personal best	80%	≈50%-80%	<50% of predicted or personal best	
PaO_2 (on room air)	Normal (test not usually necessary)	>60 mm Hg (test not usually necessary)	<60 mm Hg, possible cyanosis	
And/or $PaCO_2$	<42 mm Hg	<42 mm Hg	>42 mm Hg, possible respiratory failure	
SaO_2 (on room air) at sea level	>95%	91%-95%	<91%	

Asthma exacerbation usually includes several parameters, but not necessarily all. These parameters serve only as general guidelines because many have not been systemically studied.

Adapted from Moss MH, Gern JE, Lemanske RF Jr: Asthma in infancy and childhood. In Adkinson NF Jr, Yunginger JW, Busse WW, et al (eds): Middleton's Allergy Principles and Practice, 6th ed. Philadelphia, CV Mosby, 2003.

Available at *http://www.nhlbi.nih.gov/guidelines/asthma/asthgdln.pdf.p107.*

Table 75-4   Indicators of Impending Respiratory Failure

Poor air movement or silent chest in combination with increased respiratory effort, decreased respiratory rate, or disorganized breathing pattern

Inability to speak

Inability to lie supine

Deteriorating mental status, lethargy, or agitation

Diaphoresis

Respiratory or cardiac arrest

tion worsens, PEFR typically becomes lower than baseline and may reflect the severity of the exacerbation. In patients presenting to an emergency room with an asthma exacerbation, FEV_1 is typically 30% to 35% of normal[24] and PEFR is less than 50% of normal. Monitoring PEFR can also assist in tapering medication during the recovery phase of an acute hospitalization. PEFR is effort and technique dependent, and therefore reliability remains a concern. It should be used in conjunction with other parameters of severity for assessment of patients (see Chapter 80).

TREATMENT

Exacerbations of asthma are treated with a combination of supportive therapy and pharmacologic interventions. Treatment is tailored to the severity of symptoms and adjusted according to the patient's response to therapy. Adequate hydration should be established and maintained either

Table 75-5 Predicted Average Peak Expiratory Flow (L/min): Normal Children and Adolescents

HEIGHT			HEIGHT			HEIGHT		
in	*cm*	Males and Females	*in*	*cm*	Males and Females	*in*	*cm*	Males and Females
43	109	147	51	130	254	59	150	360
44	112	160	52	132	267	60	152	373
45	114	173	53	135	280	61	155	387
46	117	187	54	137	293	62	157	400
47	119	200	55	140	307	63	160	413
48	122	214	56	142	320	64	162	427
49	124	227	57	145	334	65	165	440
50	127	240	58	147	347	66	168	454

This table is a guideline. National Heart, Lung, and Blood Institute guidelines suggest using a personal best as baseline values.
From Polgar G, Promahcat V: Pulmonary Function Testing in Children. Techniques and Standards. Philadelphia, WB Saunders, 1971.

orally or with intravenous fluids. Physiologic monitoring should include vital signs and pulse oximetry. Oxygen supplementation is provided to maintain oxygen saturation in a safe range. This range is widely debated, but most agree that levels greater than 91% are needed, and many target levels to greater than 93% to 95%.

Adrenergic Agonists

This class of medications works by stimulating the β_2-adrenergic receptor and causing activation of adenyl cyclase, which increases the production of cyclic 3′,5-adenosine monophosphate (cAMP). This increase in cAMP, depending on the site of stimulation, results in relaxation of bronchial smooth muscle, stimulation of skeletal and cardiac muscle, and inhibition of the release of inflammatory mediators through stabilization of the mast cell membrane. Albuterol is one of the short-acting β_2-adrenergic agents used as first-line therapy for an acute asthma exacerbation because of its ability to rapidly open the airways. Albuterol can be administered by nebulizer, either continuously or intermittently, or by metered-dose inhaler (MDI) with a spacer device. Studies have compared the amount of medication delivered to the lungs when given by MDI with spacer versus nebulizer.[25-27] The two modes are considered equivalent if the patient can use proper technique with the MDI-spacer method of delivery. Dosing information is provided in Table 75-6.

Paradoxical and transient worsening of hypoxia because of increased ventilation-perfusion mismatching can be seen with the administration of albuterol. The medication causes increased cardiac output, which leads to increased perfusion of unventilated lung.[28] Other side effects include sinus tachycardia, tremor, palpitations, headache, agitation, and ventricular irritability (e.g., ventricular premature contractions, ventricular tachycardia). In addition, because frequent or continuous dosing with adrenergic agents can lead to hypokalemia, patients receiving such treatment should have serum potassium levels checked periodically. Nonselective adrenergic agents (e.g., epinephrine) can also cause transient hyperglycemia and elevations in the neutrophil count as a result of demargination.

Albuterol is actually a racemic mixture of *R*-albuterol and *S*-albuterol, with a 50:50 ratio of these two stereoisomers. Levalbuterol (Xopenex) is made up of the *R*-isomer, which is thought to be the active component of the racemic product. However, *S*-albuterol has been found to have some bronchoconstrictive activity in select studies, but not in others, and demonstrates activation of eosinophils in vitro. In addition, *S*-albuterol is cleared much less rapidly, which can cause buildup of this isomer in vivo as opposed to the *L*-isomer. However, the vast majority of clinical studies and in vitro pharmacology data have shown no significant differences in cardiopulmonary side effects and tremor when comparing racemic with *R*-isomer albuterol.[29-31] One study found decreased rates of admission from an emergency department with the use of levalbuterol versus racemic albuterol.[32] Another study showed improved bronchodilation,[33] but these findings have not been confirmed in other studies.[29,30,34]

Terbutaline, a selective β_2-adrenergic agonist, and epinephrine, a nonselective adrenergic agonist, are used in asthmatics not responding to albuterol and corticosteroids or those who are deteriorating. These medications are given by subcutaneous injection or intravenous infusion. Bronchodilation is seen within 5 minutes of administration and can persist for 3 to 4 hours.[35,36] Terbutaline can also be given via continuous intravenous infusion by starting with a bolus and titrating the dose to the desired effect.

Dosing of β_2-adrenergic agonists and other bronchodilators is shown in Tables 75-6 and 75-7.

Corticosteroids

Corticosteroids are indicated for the initial treatment of status asthmaticus. They are potent anti-inflammatory medications that have been shown to hasten recovery, prevent recurrence,[37-41] and prevent hospitalizations.[42] Because of their mechanism of action, the effect of corticosteroids is not immediate. Steroids bind to the intracytoplasmic glucocorticoid receptor and translocate to the nucleus, where they effect RNA transcription in both positive and negative fashion through the transcription factors NF-κB and AP-1.

Table 75-6   Dosages of Bronchodilators Commonly Used for Asthma Exacerbations

Medications	Adult Dose	Child Dose	Onset of Action	Duration	Comments
Inhaled Short-Acting β_2-Agonists					
Albuterol nebulizer 5.0 mg/mL 2.5 mg/3 mL 1.25 mg/3 mL 0.63 mg/3 mL	2.5-5.0 mg every 20 minutes for 3 doses, then 2.5-10 mg every 1-4 hours as needed or 10-15 mg/hr continuously	0.15 mg/kg (minimum dose, 2.5 mg) every 20 minutes for 3 doses, then 0.15-0.3 mg/kg up to 10 mg every 1-4 hours as needed or 0.5 mg/kg/hr by continuous nebulization	15 minutes	3-4 hours	Only selective β_2-agonists are recommended. For optimal delivery, dilute aerosols to minimum of 4 mL at gas flow rates of 6-8 L/min
Albuterol via MDI 90 µg/puff	2-8 puffs every 20 minutes up to 4 hours, then every 1-4 hours as needed	2-8 puffs every 20 minutes for 3 doses, then every 1-4 hours inhalation maneuver. A spacer or holding chamber should be used	15 minutes	3-4 hours	As effective as nebulized therapy if patient is able to coordinate
Levalbuterol via nebulizer 0.31 mg/3 mL 0.63 mg/3 mL 1.25 mg/3 mL	Adults: 0.63 mg 3 times/day, may be increased to 1.25 mg	Children 6-11 years: 0.31 mg 3 times/day every 6-8 hours Children ≥12 years: 0.63 mg 3 times/day, may be increased to 1.25 mg	15 minutes	5-6 hours	0.63 mg of levalbuterol is equivalent to 1.25 mg of racemic albuterol in both efficacy and side effects
Levalbuterol via MDI	1-2 puffs every 4-6 hours as needed	1-2 puffs every 4-6 hours as needed	5-10 minutes	3-6 hours	Children 2-11 years: in a randomized, double-blind, single-dose, crossover study, doses ranging from 0.16 to 1.25 mg were used safely with clinically significant improvements in pulmonary function test values
Anticholinergics					
Ipratropium bromide Nebulizer solution (0.25 mg/mL)	0.5 mg every 30 minutes for 3 doses, then every 2-4 hours as needed	0.25 mg every 20 minutes for 3 doses, then every 2-4 hours	1-3 minutes	3-6 hours	May mix in same nebulizer with albuterol. Should not be used as first-line therapy. Should be added to β_2-agonist therapy
MDI (18 µg/puff)	2-8 puffs as needed	4-8 puffs as needed	1-3 minutes	3-6 hours	Dose in MDI is low and has not been studied in asthma exacerbations

MDI, metered-dose inhaler.
Adapted from National Heart, Lung, and Blood Institute, National Asthma Education and Prevention Program. Expert Panel Report II: Guidelines for the Diagnosis and Management of Asthma (NIH Publication No. 96-4051). Bethesda, MD, U.S. Department of Health and Human Services, National Institutes of Health, 1997, 2002.

In general, steroids lead to down-regulation of inflammatory cytokines. Corticosteroids also activate histone deacetylase, which inhibits DNA transcription.[43] This change in transcription leads to increased expression of the β_2-adrenergic receptor and decreases in airway inflammation and mucus secretion. It can take several hours to reverse airway inflammation, and benefits are typically seen within 4 hours after the administration of corticosteroids.[38,39,44] Studies comparing oral and intravenous corticosteroids have found no sig-

nificant differences in efficacy.[45,46] Oral steroids are typically preferred because intravenous access is not required.[45,47] Suggested dosing of corticosteroids is provided in Table 75-8.

Inhaled Anticholinergic Agents

Anticholinergic agents work by competitively inhibiting acetylcholine at the muscarinic junction to relieve the cholinergic-mediated bronchoconstriction. Nebulized atropine is associated with significant systemic absorption, but

Table 75-7 Systemic (Injected) Bronchodilators for Acute Asthma Exacerbations

Medications	Adult Dose	Child Dose	Onset of Action	Duration	Comments
β₂-Agonists					
Epinephrine 1 : 1000 (1 mg/mL) by IV infusion	0.3-0.5 mg every 20 minutes for 3 doses SC Loading dose: 2-10 μg/kg, followed by continuous infusion of 0.08-0.4 μg/kg/min; titrate dose by clinical response up to 6 μg/kg/min	0.01 mg/kg up to 0.3-0.5 mg every 20 minutes for 3 doses SC	1-3 minutes	30 minutes	No proven advantage of systemic therapy over aerosol
Terbutaline (1 mg/mL) by IV infusion	0.25 mg every 20 minutes for 3 doses SC Loading dose: 2-10 μg/kg followed by continuous infusion of 0.08-0.4 μg/kg/min; titrate dose by clinical response up to 6 μg/kg/min	0.01 mg/kg every 20 minutes for 3 doses, then every 2-6 hours as needed SC Loading dose: 2-10 μg/kg followed by continuous infusion of 0.08-0.4 μg/kg/min; titrate dose by clinical response up to 6 μg/kg/min	SC: 6-15 minutes	SC: 1.5-4 hours	

Table 75-8 Systemic Corticosteroids in the Setting of Asthma Exacerbations

Medication	Adult Dose	Child Dose (≤12 Years Old)	Onset of Action	Duration	Comments
Oral—prednisone/ prednisolone IV— methylprednisolone	120-180 mg/day in 3-4 divided doses for 48 hours, then 60-80 mg/day until PEF reaches 70% of predicted or personal best	1 mg/kg every 6 hours for 48 hours, then 1-2 mg/kg/day (maximum, 60 mg/day) in 2 divided doses until PEF is 70% of predicted or personal best	1-4 hours (variable) 1-4 hours (variable)	12-36 hours	For outpatient burst for 3-10 days: Adult: use 40-60 mg in single or 2 divided doses Children: use 1-2 mg/kg/day with maximum of 60 mg/day
IM methylprednisolone 40 mg/mL 80 mg/mL	240 mg IM once	7.5 mg/kg IM once	1-4 hours (variable)	36-72 hours	IM should be used in place of a short burst of oral steroids in patients who are vomiting or if adherence is a problem

PEF, peak expiratory flow.
Adapted From National Heart, Lung, and Blood Institute, National Asthma Education and Prevention Program. Expert Panel Report II: Guidelines for the Diagnosis and Management of Asthma (NIH Publication No. 96-4051). Bethesda, MD, U.S. Department of Health and Human Services, National Institutes of Health, 1997. Available at *http://www.nhlbi.nih.gov/guidelines/asthma/asthmafullrpt.pdf.*

anticholinergic medications such as ipratropium bromide have fewer side effects and less systemic absorption.[48]

The use of inhaled ipratropium in the initial phase of treatment has been shown to be effective in reducing the need for hospitalization. A few studies have found no benefit in comparison to β₂-agonists alone, whereas others have shown a slight advantage of one to three doses in the initial phase of an acute asthma exacerbation.[49] The role of ipratropium in hospitalized patients is less clear, but an initial study did not show clinical benefit.[50]

Combined administration of anticholinergic and β₂-agonist medications increases bronchodilation, although some controversy about this effect persists.[49,50] Nonetheless, many institutions use a combination of β₂-agonists and anticholinergic medications during the initial phase of acute asthma exacerbations. Studies examining the use of anticholinergic medications as monotherapy have also been controversial. Dosing is listed in Table 75-6.

Nonstandard Therapies

If initiation of the aforementioned standard therapies does not improve the level of respiratory distress or if symptoms progress, additional interventions may be necessary. The clinical experience and expertise available at the particular institution should be considered in such decisions. Safe transfer to a facility able to provide critical care management should be anticipated, and arrangements should be expedited.

Magnesium Sulfate

Magnesium sulfate has been studied as a bronchodilator in severe asthma, with conflicting results.[51-54] Magnesium is thought to inhibit mast cell degranulation and increase bronchial dilation because of a decrease in calcium uptake by bronchial smooth muscle.[55] Its use is considered when a patient fails to improve or worsens despite treatment with continuous inhaled β_2-agonists, systemic corticosteroids, and inhaled anticholinergic agents.

Methylxanthines

Intravenous methylxanthines, such as aminophylline, were commonly used in the past to manage asthma exacerbations because of their ability to act directly on β-adrenergic receptors and relax bronchial smooth muscle. Concern regarding the toxicity and efficacy of this class of medication and the availability of newer agents have limited its use. Methylxanthines may help prevent acute airway hyperresponsiveness but do not appear to produce these effects chronically.[56-58] However, life-threatening events such as cardiac arrhythmia and seizures are associated with toxic levels of theophylline (>30 μg/mL). As a result, methylxanthines are recommended only as adjunctive therapy with close monitoring of serum concentrations and cardiac monitoring.

Studies examining the use of intravenous methylxanthines in children and adults with severe asthma have shown mixed benefit.[59-64] A recent Cochrane review found that theophylline in addition to β_2-agonists and glucocorticoids (with or without anticholinergics) improves lung function within 6 hours of treatment. However, there is no apparent reduction in symptoms, number of nebulized treatments, and length of hospital stay.[65]

Aminophylline requires a loading dose followed by a continuous infusion to reach and maintain a therapeutic level (see Table 75-9). Dosing is titrated according to serum level, clinical efficacy, and side effects.

Heliox

Heliox is a mixture of helium and oxygen used for inhalation. This agent is thought to improve airflow by creating gas with similar viscosity to air but with lower density, which in turn can increase ventilation and decrease work of breathing.[66-68] Heliox is indicated in patients with a refractory exacerbation of asthma in whom respiratory failure is impending. Patients with high oxygen requirements may not be able to tolerate heliox because they need a higher FIO_2 than a helium-oxygen mixture can provide. Heliox can also

lower body temperature because of the high thermal conductivity of the mixture. Therefore, patients need to have their temperature monitored closely.

Dosing of nonstandard therapies is shown in Table 75-9, and adverse effects of medication are listed in Table 75-10.

Initial Treatment

The initial therapy for status asthmaticus has been outlined by the NHLBI guidelines (Fig. 75-2). In brief, patients are first treated with inhaled β_2-adrenergic agonists (e.g., inhaled albuterol), corticosteroids either orally or intravenously, and if needed, oxygen. Inhaled anticholinergics, such as ipratropium bromide, may be added for patients who do not demonstrate prompt improvement. Patients with significant improvement after these initial interventions may not require hospitalization.

Hospitalization is recommended for patients who continue to have moderately severe or severe symptoms after initial intervention. Treatment with inhaled albuterol (either every 1 to 2 hours by nebulizer or MDI with spacer or delivered continuously by nebulizer) and corticosteroid therapy (orally or, if not tolerated, intravenously) should be continued. Continuation of inhaled anticholinergic agents may be considered, although their benefit remains unproven.

If patients continue to deteriorate, they must be monitored for respiratory insufficiency and failure. An arterial blood gas measurement can be used to confirm the condition and should reveal decreased pH, elevated partial pressure of carbon dioxide ($PaCO_2$), and an increased alveolar-arterial oxygen gradient. Pulse oximetry remains a poor monitoring device for early detection of respiratory failure. Oxygen saturation is initially maintained despite a significant degree of hypoventilation, and the addition of supplemental oxygen would further obscure evidence of respiratory failure from this device (Chapter 66). Patients with impending respiratory failure often need mechanical ventilatory support.

Tapering Hospital Therapy

After patients are stabilized and demonstrate improvement, therapies can be gradually reduced and withdrawn. Ongoing assessment of clinical parameters is performed, including the respiratory rate, work of breathing, auscultatory findings, and requirement for supplemental oxygen. If the patient remains comfortable with minimal signs of respiratory distress, the dosing of inhaled β_2-agonists is decreased. For patients receiving continuous inhaled β_2-agonist therapy, the dose may be reduced and then subsequently transitioned to intermittent treatments, usually every 2 hours. As the patient continues to improve, the interval between treatments can be extended. Similarly, the amount of supplemental oxygen is titrated to maintain oxygen saturation above the desired level and eventually discontinued. Systemic corticosteroids are continued throughout the exacerbation and maintained for several days after discharge from the hospital. If inhaled anticholinergic agents have been instituted, they are usually discontinued when albuterol begins to be tapered.

Many hospitals use clinical pathways, which are tools that detail a sequence of assessments and treatments for patients with various conditions.[69] Studies have shown that asthma clinical pathways shorten hospitalization and decrease the

Table 75-9 Nonstandard Therapies for Exacerbations of Asthma

Medication	Adult Dose	Child Dose (≤12 Years Old)	Onset of Action	Duration	Comments
Magnesium sulfate (IV)	1.2-2 g over a 20-minute period	25-50 mg/kg over a 20-minute period Target serum levels, 3.5-4.5 mg/dL	Immediate	30 minutes	
Heliox	Try to deliver at least 60% helium, but 80% ideal	Try to deliver at least 60% helium, but 80% ideal	Immediate	Only while actively inhaling agent	Limited if patient has increased oxygen requirement
Aminophylline*	Loading dose: 6 mg/kg given IV over a period of 20-30 minutes, followed by a maintenance dose of 0.7 mg/kg/hr	Loading dose: 6 mg/kg given IV over a period of 20-30 minutes, followed by a maintenance dose; 6 weeks to 1 year: 0.5-0.7 mg/kg/hour; 1 to 12 years: 0.9-1.2 mg/kg/hour	IV: within minutes	3-5 hours in children, 8-9 hours in adults	No proven advantage over β_2-adrenergic agonists See also comments for theophylline below
Theophylline*	Loading dose: 5 mg/kg given IV over a period of 20-30 minutes or PO†	Loading dose 5 mg/kg given IV over a period of 20-30 minutes or PO†, followed by a maintenance dose; 6 weeks-1 year: 10-18 mg/kg/day; 1-9 years: 20-24 mg/kg/day; 9-12 years: 16 mg/kg/day	IV: within minutes PO: peak serum levels reached within 4 hours	Half-life: premature infants: 57-76 hours; children: 1.2-7 hours; adults: 6-12 hours	Multiple drug interactions Significant interpatient variability of pharmacokinetics Narrow therapeutic ranges; neonate: 5-10 µg/mL (toxic >10 µg/mL); children/adults: 8-15 µg/mL (toxic >20 µg/mL) Must monitor levels

*Doses should be based on lean (ideal) body weight.
†Controlled-release preparations should not be used for the loading dose.
The Pharmacy Handbook and Formulary, Children's Hospital of Philadelphia, Philadelphia, 2006. Klasco RK (ed): DRUGDEX® System. Thomson Micromedex, Greenwood Village, Colorado, edition expires 3/07.

need for readmission for up to 2 weeks after discharge.[70,71] An asthma clinical pathway allows multiple caregivers, including nurses, respiratory therapists, and doctors, to modify treatment based on structured assessments. The NHLBI guidelines (see Fig. 75-2) outline specific criteria that can be used to determine a patient's severity and frequency of therapy. It also provides criteria to assist in weaning treatments.

PEFR measurements may be useful to determine readiness for reduction in medication. If PEFR is at least 70% of baseline before a bronchodilator treatment (see Table 75-5), it is appropriate to space the frequency of the β_2-adrenergic agonist treatments. Technique and effort will affect measurement of PEFR; therefore, it should be used in conjunction with other clinical indicators of improvement.

Therapy after Discharge Home

Patients should be sent home on a regimen of oral corticosteroids, the duration of which depends on the length and severity of illness and the patient's frequency of exacerbations. In general, an isolated exacerbation is treated with oral corticosteroids for 5 days. However, if a patient was admitted to the hospital for an extended period, a prolonged course of corticosteroids will be required, followed by taper-

ing doses. A taper is prescribed to prevent relapse of symptoms, as well as to prevent an addisonian crisis from adrenal suppression. The risk for an addisonian crisis is hypothetical and has not been demonstrated in any study.[72-74] In addition, patients receiving their second course of steroids in a month should undergo prolonged tapering as well. A typical taper involves keeping the patient at a full daily dose of corticosteroids until stable clinical status is achieved and then decreasing the dose by 30% to 50% daily. Patients who required admission to the hospital may not have been on an adequate treatment plan. Thus, hospitalization offers an opportunity to assess the overall treatment regimen. Patients should be evaluated according to the NHLBI guidelines shown in Table 75-11A and B and need their outpatient preventive treatment stepped up. Specific drug choices are outlined in Tables 75-12 through 75-14.

CONSULTATION

Outpatient referral to an asthma specialist (e.g., pulmonologist, allergist) is associated with reduced rates of emergency department visits[75] and is recommended for patients with the following scenarios[76-78]:

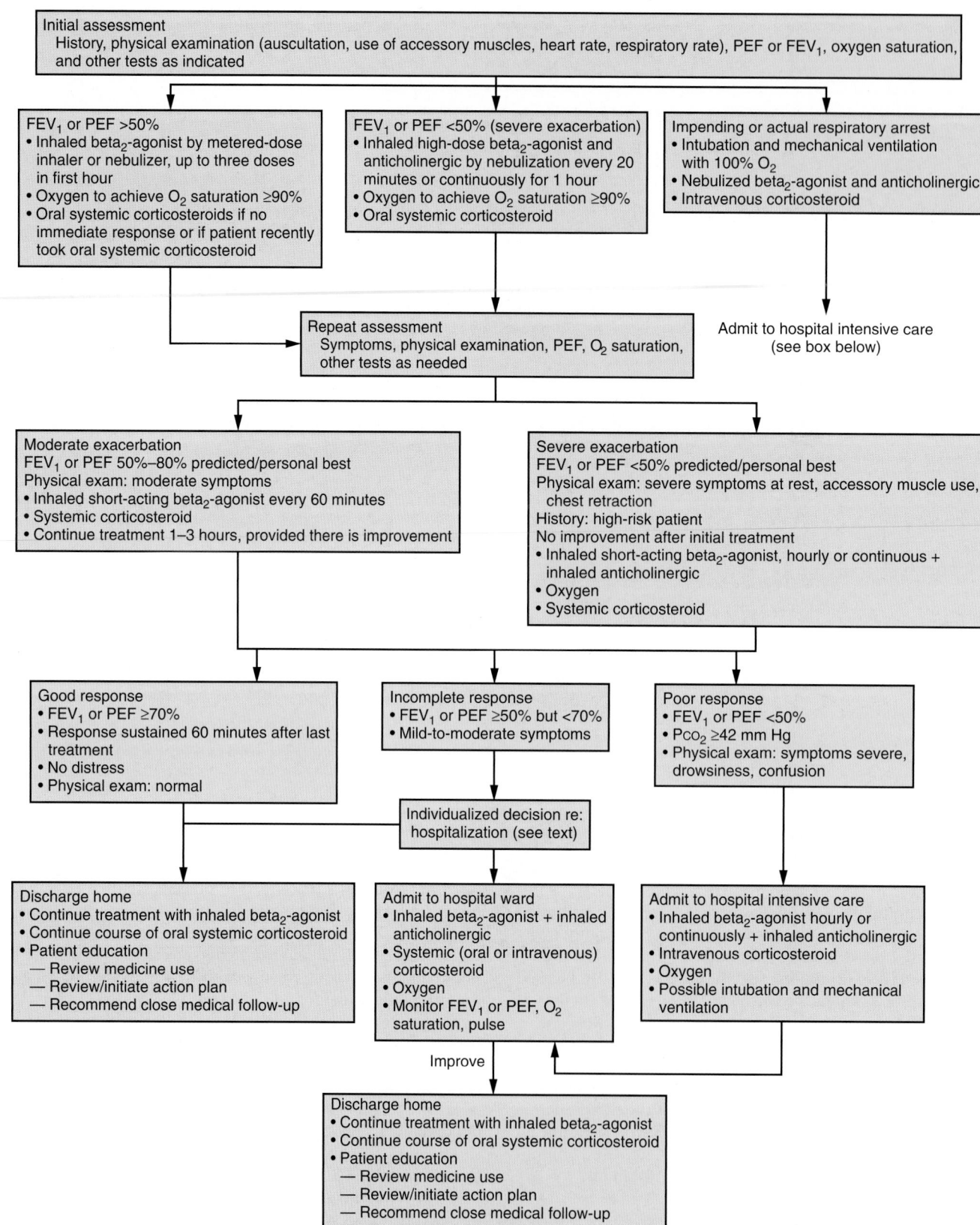

Figure 75-2 NHLBI hospital assessment and management of acute exacerbation. PEF, peak expiratory flow; FEV₁, forced expiratory volume in 1 second. Adapted from National Heart, Lung, and Blood Institute, National Asthma Education and Prevention Program. Expert Panel Report II: Guidelines for the Diagnosis and Management of Asthma [NIH Publication No. 96–4051]. Bethesda, MD, U.S. Department of Health and Human Services, National Institutes of Health, 1997.

Table 75-14 Estimated Comparative Daily Dosages for Inhaled Corticosteroids

| Drug | LOW DAILY DOSE | | MEDIUM DAILY DOSE | | HIGH DAILY DOSE | |
	Adult	*Child**	*Adult*	*Child**	*Adult*	*Child**
Beclomethasone HFA 40 or 80 µg/puff	80-240 µg	80-160 µg	240-480 µg	160-320 µg	>480 µg	>320 µg
Budesonide DPI 200 µg/inhalation	200-600 µg	200-400 µg	600-1200 µg	400-800 µg	>1200 µg	>800 µg
Budesonide inhalation suspension for nebulization (child dose)		0.5 mg		1.0 mg		2.0 mg
Flunisolide 250 µg/puff	500-1000 µg	500-750 µg	1000-2000 µg	1000-1250 µg	>2000 µg	>1250 µg
Fluticasone MDI: 44, 110, or 220 µg/puff	88-264 µg	88-176 µg	264-660 µg	176-440 µg	>660 µg	>440 µg
DPI: 50, 100, or 250 µg/inhalation	100-300 µg	100-200 µg	300-600 µg	200-400 µg	>600 µg	>400 µg
Trlamcinolone acetonide 100 µg/puff	400-1000 µg	400-800 µg	1000-2000 µg	800-1200 µg	>2000 µg	>1200 µg

DPI, dry powder inhaler.

*Children ≤12 years of age.

Modified from National Heart, Lung, and Blood Institute: Executive Summary of NAEPP Expert Panel Report: Guidelines for the Diagnosis and Management of Asthma: Update on Selected Topics (NIH Publication No. 02-5075). Bethesda, MD, US Department of Health and Human Services, National Institutes of Health, 2002.

Table 75-15 Hospital Discharge Checklist for Patients with Asthma Exacerbations

Intervention	Dose/Timing	Education/Advice	MD/RN Initials
Inhaled medications (MDI + spacer/holding chamber) Beta$_2$-agonist	Select agent, dose, and frequency (e.g., albuterol) 2-6 puffs q 3-4 hr prn	Teach purpose Teach technique Emphasize need for spacer/ holding chamber	
Corticosteroids	Medium dose	Check patient technique	
Oral medications	Select agent, dose, and frequency (e.g., prednisone 20 mg bid for 3-10 days)	Teach purpose Teach side effects	
Peak flow meter	Measure AM and PM. PFF and record best of three tries each time	Teach purpose Teach technique Distribute peak flow diary	
Follow-up visit	Make appointment for follow-up care with primary clinician or asthma specialist	Advise patient (or caregiver) of date, time, and location of appointment within 7 days of hospital discharge	
Action plan	Before or at discharge	Instruct patient (or caregiver) on simple plan for actions to be taken when symptoms, signs, and PEF values suggest recurrent airflow obstruction	

Adapted from National Heart, Lung, and Blood Institute, National Asthma Education and Prevention Program. Expert Panel Report II: Guidelines for the Diagnosis and Management of Asthma (NIH Publication No. 96-4051). Bethesda, MD, US Department of Health and Human Services, National Institutes of Health, 1997.

and cigarette smoke, that can cause symptoms and contribute to asthma exacerbations.[80] In addition, other factors, including gastroesophageal reflux, sinusitis, and others that might exacerbate asthma, should be explored and eliminated if possible (Table 75-16). If an allergic component is being considered, further evaluation can be arranged and environmental control measures recommended. Both passive and active cigarette smoking significantly increases the risk

for asthma and worsens asthma symptoms.[81-88] As a result, no smoking should be permitted around asthmatics or in their home or family car. Physicians should provide assistance for caregivers to quit smoking.

Appropriate preventive medications based on daily symptoms and frequency of exacerbations should be maintained on a daily basis. These medications are essential for the prevention of asthma flares. Multiple studies have shown a

Table 75-16   Exacerbating Factors for Asthma and Control Measures

Factors That Worsen Asthma Severity	Control Measures
Animal dander	Remove the animal from the environment At a minimum, remove the pet from the bedroom
House dust mites	Encase mattress and pillows in an allergen-impermeable cover Wash bedding in hot water weekly at >130° F Remove carpets from the bedroom
Cockroaches	Exterminate! Do not leave garbage and food exposed
Pollen	During pollen season, stay indoors with windows closed, especially in the afternoon
Mold	Fix leaks, eliminate water sources Clean moldy surfaces
Cigarette/tobacco smoke	Encourage family members and caregivers to smoke outside and cease smoking
Sinusitis	Promote sinus drainage Antibiotic therapy when appropriate
Gastroesophageal reflux	No eating 3 hr before bedtime Elevate head of bed 6-8 inches Appropriate medications: H_2 receptor antagonist
Medications	No beta-blockers Aspirin and NSAIDs in combination with severe persistent asthma, nasal polyps, and aspirin sensitivity increase the risk for a reaction
Viral infections	Annual influenza vaccination
Irritants	Decrease exposure to wood-burning stoves, fireplaces, unvented stoves or heaters, perfumes, cleaning agents, sprays

NSAIDs, nonsteroidal anti-inflammatory medications.
Adapted from National Heart, Lung, and Blood Institute, National Asthma Education and Prevention Program Expert Panel II: Guidelines for the Diagnosis and Management of Asthma (NIH Publication No. 96-4051). Bethesda, MD, US Department of Health and Human Services, National Institute of Health, 1997.

strong negative correlation between hospital admission for asthma and the use of daily inhaled corticosteroids. Suggested doses and regimens have been established through national and worldwide collaboration between primary physicians, allergists, pulmonologists, and others. An example is seen in Tables 75-12 through 75-14.

Peak flowmeters can be helpful in managing asthma, if used appropriately.[89] However, studies comparing peak flow monitoring with symptom recognition show no benefit of peak flow–based action plans over those based on symptoms alone.[89-91] Peak flowmeters have numeric indicators that allow the creation of green, yellow, and red zones (see Table 75-5). Green represents the "good" or "all clear" zone and is 80% to 100% of a child's personal best. The yellow zone is 50% to 80% of the personal best and indicates a time when the family should be "cautious" because the child may be having or is at risk for asthma symptoms. Asthma reliever medications should be started and contact with the physician considered. The red zone is indicated by a PEFR less than 50% of normal; it is cause for concern and requires a visit to the emergency room or a call to the doctor.[4] Peak flow monitoring is typically helpful for children who are not good at recognizing symptoms of asthma. Current NHLBI guidelines recommend either a symptom-based or peak flow–based management plan.

Additional sources of support for families can include the Asthma and Allergy Foundation of America and Mothers of Asthmatics.

IN A NUTSHELL

- Asthma is a chronic disorder that results in airway inflammation and smooth muscle dysfunction and is manifested as recurrent episodes of wheezing, breathlessness, and chest tightness.
- Exacerbations can be triggered by a variety of stimuli, including respiratory infections, exposure to allergens or irritants, exercise, and cold air.
- Treatment of flares must be directed at decreasing airway inflammation and relieving bronchospasm while providing supportive care.
- The mainstay of pharmacologic therapy includes inhaled short-acting β_2-adrenergic agonist therapy and systemic corticosteroids. Supportive care includes supplemental oxygen if needed and maintenance of hydration.
- Many of the pharmacologic agents have significant side effects, and therefore appropriate monitoring is required.

- Patients with severe symptoms or those with moderately severe symptoms that fail to improve after initial therapy are candidates for admission to an intensive care setting.
- At the time of discharge, patients should have a clear plan for ongoing treatment of the acute exacerbation and transition to maintenance therapy. In addition, an action plan for subsequent exacerbations should be in place.

ON THE HORIZON

- Asthma is a chronic inflammatory disease that affects many Americans, and researchers are actively investigating new drugs and therapies to improve the quality of life of asthmatics. Drugs that modify the immune response are currently under active investigation. An example of one of these drugs is omalizumab, a recombinant humanized anti-IgE antibody. This drug binds circulating free IgE and consequently reduces the level of free IgE in the bloodstream and prevents it from binding to mast cell membrane receptors, thus curtailing the early and late asthmatic responses. Omalizumab has been found to reduce symptoms, exacerbations,[92] and the use of corticosteroids.
- New NHLBI Expert Panel guidelines on the diagnosis and treatment of asthma are expected in late 2006 or early 2007. The new guidelines are expected to emphasize daily symptom control in addition to preventing exacerbations in the management of asthma.

SUGGESTED READING

American Academy of Allergy, Asthma, and Immunology, Inc: Pediatric Asthma: Promoting Best Practice. American Academy of Allergy, Asthma, and Immunology, Milwaukee, 1999.

Lemanske RF, Busse WW: Asthma. J Allergy Clin Immunol 2005;111:S502-S519.

Moss MH, Gern JE, Lemanske RF Jr: Asthma in infancy and childhood. In Adkinson NF, Bochner BS, Yunginger JW, et al (eds): Middleton's Allergy: Principles and Practice, 6th ed. St Louis, CV Mosby, 2003.

National Heart, Lung, and Blood Institute, National Asthma Education and Prevention Program: Expert Panel Report II: Guidelines for the Diagnosis and Management of Asthma (NIH Publication No. 96-405). Bethesda, MD, US Department of Health and Human Services, National Institutes of Health, 1997.

National Heart, Lung, and Blood Institute, National Asthma Education and Prevention Program: Guidelines for the Diagnosis and Management of Asthma (NIH Publication No. 97-4051). Bethesda, MD, US Department of Health and Human Services, National Institutes of Health, 1997.

National Heart, Lung, and Blood Institute, National Asthma Education and Prevention Program: Guidelines for the Diagnosis and Management of Asthma: Update on Selected Topics (NIH Publication No. 02-5075). Bethesda, MD, US Department of Health and Human Services, National Institutes of Health, 2002.

REFERENCES

1. American Lung Association: Trends in asthma morbidity and mortality, 2001.
2. National Heart, Lung, and Blood Institute, National Institutes of Health, National Asthma Education and Prevention Program, 2003.
3. U.S. Department of Health and Human Services (USDHHS), Centers for Disease Control and Prevention, National Center for Health Statistics: Compressed Mortality File, 2005.
4. National Heart, Lung, and Blood Institute: Guidelines for the Diagnosis and Management of Asthma: Expert Panel 2. Bethesda, MD, National Institutes of Health, 1997.
5. National Heart, Lung, and Blood Institute, Data Fact Sheet: Asthma Statistics, 1999.
6. Hartert TV, Windom HH, Peebles RS Jr, et al: Inadequate outpatient medical therapy for patients with asthma admitted to two urban hospitals. Am J Med 1996;100:386-394.
7. Pappas G, Hadden WC, Kozak LJ, Fisher GF: Potentially avoidable hospitalizations: Inequalities in rates between US socioeconomic groups. Am J Public Health 1997;87:811-816.
8. Djukanovic R, Roche WR, Wilson JW, et al: Mucosal inflammation in asthma. Am Rev Respir Dis 1990;142:434-457.
9. Murray CS, Simpson A, Custovic A: Allergens, viruses, and asthma exacerbations. Proc Am Thorac Soc 2004;1:99-104.
10. Johnston S, Pattemore PK, Sanderson G, et al: Community study of role of viral infections in exacerbations of asthma in 9- to 11-year-old children. BMJ 1995;310:1225-1229.
11. Johnston SL, Pattemore PK, Sanderson G, et al: The relationship between upper respiratory infections and hospital admissions for asthma: A time-trend analysis. Am J Respir Crit Care Med 1996;154:654-660.
12. Shim CS, Williams MH Jr: Evaluation of the severity of asthma: Patients versus physicians. Am J Med 1980;68:11-13.
13. Stein MR: Possible mechanisms of influence of esophageal acid on airway hyperresponsiveness. Am J Med 2003;115(Suppl 3A):55S-59S.
14. Nelson HS: Gastroesophageal reflux and pulmonary disease. J Allergy Clin Immunol 1984;73:547-556.
15. Busse WW: The role of respiratory infections in airway hyperresponsiveness and asthma. Am J Respir Crit Care Med 1994;150:S77-S79.
16. Newman KB, Mason UG 3rd, Schmaling KB: Clinical features of vocal cord dysfunction. Am J Respir Crit Care Med 1995;152:1382-1386.
17. Christopher K, Wood RP 2nd, Eckert RC, et al: Vocal cord dysfunction presenting as asthma. N Engl J Med 1983;308:1566-1570.
18. Tilles S: Vocal cord dysfunction in children and adolescents. Curr Allergy Asthma Rep 2003;3:467-472.
19. Wood R, Milgrom H: Vocal cord dysfunction. J Allergy Clin Immunol 1996;98:481-485.
20. Irwin RS, Glomb WB, Chang AB: Habit cough, tic cough, and psychogenic cough in adult and pediatric populations: ACCP evidence-based clinical practice guidelines. Chest 2006;129(1 Suppl):174S-179S.
21. Brooks LJ, Cloutier MM, Afshani E: Significance of roentgenographic abnormalities in children hospitalized for asthma. Chest 1982;82:315-318.
22. Weiss EB, Faling LJ: Clinical significance of PaCO2 during status asthma: The cross-over point. Ann Allergy 1968;26:545-551.
23. Polgar G, Promahcat V: Pulmonary Function Testing in Children. Techniques and Standards. Philadelphia, WB Saunders, 1971.
24. McFadden ER Jr: Clinical physiologic correlates in asthma. J Allergy Clin Immunol 1986;77:1-5.
25. Idris AH, McDermott MF, Raucci JC, et al: Emergency department treatment of severe asthma. Metered-dose inhaler plus holding chamber is equivalent in effectiveness to nebulizer. Chest 1993;103:665-672.
26. Kerem E, Levinson H, Schuh S, et al: Efficacy of albuterol administered by nebulizer versus spacer device in children with acute asthma. J Pediatr 1993;123:313-317.
27. Colacone A, Afilalo M, Wolkove N, Kreisman H: A comparison of albuterol administered by metered dose inhaler (and holding chamber) or wet nebulizer in acute asthma. Chest 1993;104:835-841.
28. Rodriques RR: Gas exchange abnormalities in asthma. Lung 1990;168:s599-s605.

29. Qureshi F, Zaritisky A, Welch C, et al: Clinical efficacy of racemic albuterol versus levalbuterol for the treatment of acute pediatric asthma. Ann Emerg Med 2005;46:29-36.

30. Hardasmalani MD, DeBari V, Bithoney WJ, Gold N: Levalbuterol versus racemic albuterol in the treatment of acute exacerbation of asthma in children. Pediatr Emerg Care 2005;21:415-419.

31. Asmus MJ, Hendeles L: Levalbuterol nebulizer solution: Is it worth five times the cost of albuterol? Pharmacotherapy 2000;20:123-129.

32. Schreck DM, Babin S: Comparison of racemic albuterol and levalbuterol in the treatment of acute asthma in the ED. Am J Emerg Med 2005; 23:842-847.

33. Nelson HS, Bensch G, Pleskow WW, et al: Improved bronchodilation with levalbuterol compared with racemic albuterol in patients with asthma. J Allergy Clin Immunol 1998;102:943-952.

34. Ralston ME, Euwema MS, Knecht KR, et al: Comparison of levalbuterol and racemic albuterol combined with ipratropium bromide in acute pediatric asthma: A randomized controlled trial. J Emerg Med 2005;29: 29-35.

35. Dulfano MJ, Glass P: The bronchodilator effects of terbutaline: Route of administration and patterns of response. Ann Allergy 1976;37:357-366.

36. Nou E: A clinical comparison of subcutaneous doses of terbutaline and adrenaline in bronchial asthma. Scand J Respir Dis 1971;52:192-198.

37. Scarfone RJ, Fuchs SM, Nager AL, Shane SA: Controlled trial of oral prednisone in the emergency department treatment of children with acute asthma. Pediatrics 1993;92:513-518.

38. Rowe BH, Keller JL, Oxman AD: Effectiveness of steroid therapy in acute exacerbations of asthma: A meta-analysis. Am J Emerg Med 1992;10: 301-310.

39. Chapman KR, Verbeek PR, White JG, Rebuck AS: Effect of a short course of prednisone in the prevention of early relapse after the emergency room treatment of acute asthma. N Engl J Med 1991;324:788-794.

40. Fanta CH, Rossing TH, McFadden ER Jr: Glucocorticoids in acute asthma. A critical controlled trial. Am J Med 1983;74:845-851.

41. Harris JB, Weinberger MM, Nassif E, et al: Early intervention with short courses of prednisone to prevent progression of asthma in ambulatory patients incompletely responsive to bronchodilators. J Pediatr 1987;110: 627-633.

42. Littenberg B, Gluck EH: A controlled trial of methylprednisolone in the emergency treatment of acute asthma. N Engl J Med 1986;314:150-152.

43. Didonato JA, Saatcioglu F, Karin M: Molecular mechanisms of immunosuppression and anti-inflammatory activities by glucocorticoids. Am J Respir Crit Care Med 1996;154:S11-S15.

44. Connett GJ, Warde C, Wooler E, Lenney W: Prednisolone and salbutamol in the hospital treatment of acute asthma. Arch Dis Child 1994;70:170-173.

45. Ratto D, Alfaro C, Sipsey J, et al: Are intravenous corticosteroids required in status asthmaticus? JAMA 1988;260:527-529.

46. Szefler SJ: Glucocorticoid therapy for asthma: Clinical pharmacology. J Allergy Clin Immunol 1991;88:147-165.

47. Harrison BD, Stokes TC, Hart GJ, et al: Need for intravenous hydrocortisone in addition to oral prednisolone in patients admitted to hospital with severe asthma without ventilatory failure. Lancet 1986;1:181-184.

48. Weber RW: Role of anticholinergics in asthma. Ann Allergy 1990;65: 348-350.

49. Schuh S, Johnson DW, Calahan S, et al: Efficacy of frequent nebulized ipratropium bromide added to frequent high dose albuterol therapy in severe childhood asthma. J Pediatr 1995;126:639-645.

50. Karpel JP, Schacter EN, Fanta C, et al: A comparison of ipratropium and albuterol vs albuterol alone for the treatment of acute asthma. Chest 1996;110:611-616.

51. Tiffany BR, Berk WA, Todd IK, White SR: Magnesium bolus or infusion fails to improve expiratory flow in acute asthma exacerbations. Chest 1993;104:831-834.

52. Green SM, Rothrock SG: Intravenous magnesium for acute asthma: Failure to decrease emergency treatment duration or need for hospitalization. Ann Emerg Med 1992;21:260-265.

53. Skorodin MS, Tenholder MF, Yettor B, et al: Magnesium sulfate in exacerbations of chronic obstructive pulmonary disease. Arch Intern Med 1995;155:496-500.

54. Kuitert LM, Kletchko SL: Intravenous magnesium sulfate in acute, life-threatening asthma. Ann Emerg Med 1991;20:1243-1245.

55. Skobeloff EM: An ion for the lungs. Acad Emerg Med 1996;3:1082-1084.

56. Hendeles L, Weinberger M, Szefler S, Ellis E: Safety and efficacy of theophylline in children with asthma. J Pediatr 1992;120:177-183.

57. Crescioli S, Spinazzi A, Plebani M, et al: Theophylline inhibits early and late asthmatic reactions induced by allergens in asthmatic subjects. Ann Allergy 1991;66:245-251.

58. Dutoit JI, Salome CM, Woolcock AJ: Inhaled corticosteroids reduce the severity of bronchial hyperresponsiveness in asthma but oral theophylline does not. Am Rev Respir Dis 1987;136:1174-1178.

59. Mitra A: The current role of intravenous aminophylline in acute paediatric asthma. Minerva Pediatr 2003;55:369-375.

60. Yamauchi K, Kobayashi H, Tanifuji Y, et al: Efficacy and safety of intravenous theophylline administration for treatment of mild acute exacerbation of bronchial asthma. Respirology 2005;10:491-496.

61. Yung M, South M: Randomised controlled trial of aminophylline for severe acute asthma. Arch Dis Child 1998;79:405-410.

62. Huang D, O'Brien RG, Harman E, et al: Does aminophylline benefit adults admitted to the hospital for an acute exacerbation of asthma? Ann Intern Med 1993;119:1155-1160.

63. Self TH, Abou-Shala N, Burns R, et al: Inhaled albuterol and oral prednisone therapy in hospitalized adult asthmatics. Does aminophylline add any benefit? Chest 1990;98:1317-1321.

64. Strauss RE, Wertheim DL, Bonaquera VR, Volacer DJ: Aminophylline therapy does not improve outcome and increases adverse effects in children hospitalized with acute asthmatic exacerbations. Pediatrics 1994;93:205-210.

65. Mitra A, Bassler D, Goodman K, et al: Intravenous aminophylline for acute severe asthma in children over two years receiving inhaled bronchodilators. Cochrane Database Syst Rev 2005;2:CD001276.

66. Gluck EH, Onorato DJ, Castriotta R: Helium-oxygen mixtures in intubated patients with status asthmaticus and respiratory acidosis. Chest 1990;98:693-698.

67. Manthous CA, Hall JB, Caputo MA, et al: Heliox improves pulsus paradoxus and peak expiratory flow in nonintubated patients with severe asthma. Am J Respir Crit Care Med 1995;151:310-314.

68. Rivera ML, Kim TY, Stewart GM, et al: Albuterol nebulized in heliox in the initial ED treatment of pediatric asthma: A blinded, randomized controlled trial. Am J Emerg Med 2006;24:38-42.

69. Glauber JH, Farber HJ, Homer CJ: Asthma clinical pathways: Toward what end? Pediatrics 2001;107:590-592.

70. Johnson KB, Blaisdell CJ, Walker A, Eggleston P: Effectiveness of a clinical pathway for inpatient asthma management. Pediatrics 2000;106:1006-1012.

71. Wazeka A, Valacer DJ, Cooper M, et al: Impact of a pediatric asthma clinical pathway on hospital cost and length of stay. Pediatr Pulmonol 2001;32:211-216.

72. Cydulka RK, Emerman CL: A pilot study of steroid therapy after emergency department treatment of acute asthma: Is a taper needed? J Emerg Med 1998;16:15-19.

73. Karan RS, Pandhi P, Behera D, et al: A comparison of non-tapering vs. tapering prednisolone in acute exacerbation of asthma involving use of the low-dose ACTH test. Int J Clin Pharmacol Ther 2002;40:256-262.

74. O'Driscoll BR, Kalra S, Wilson M, et al: Double-blind trial of steroid tapering in acute asthma. Lancet 1993;341:324-327.

75. Zeiger RS, Heller S, Mellon MH, et al: Facilitated referral to asthma specialist reduces relapses in asthma emergency room visits. J Allergy Clin Immunol 1991;87:1160-1168.

76. Shuttari MF: Asthma: Diagnosis and management. Am Fam Physician 1995;52:2225-2235.

77. Mayo PH, Richman J, Harris HW: Results of a program to reduce admissions for adult asthma. Ann Intern Med 1990;112:864-871.

78. Joint Task force on Practice Parameters, representing the American Academy of Allergy, Asthma and Immunology, the American College of Allergy, Asthma and Immunology, and the Joint Council of Allergy, Asthma and Immunology: Practice parameters for the diagnosis and treatment of asthma. J Allergy Clin Immunol 1995;96:707-870.

79. Jarjour NN: Asthma in adults: Evaluation and management. In Adkinson NF Jr, Yunginger JW, Busse WW, et al (eds): Middleton's Allergy: Principles and Practice, 6th ed. Philadelphia, CV Mosby, 2003, p 1269.

80. Eggleston P: Improving indoor environments: Reducing allergen exposures. J Allergy Clin Immunol 2005;116:122-126.

81. Gortmaker S, Walker DK, Jacobs FH, Ruch-Ross H: Parental smoking and the risk of childhood asthma. Am J Public Health 1982;72:574-579.

82. Agudo A, Bardaqi S, Romero PV, Gonzalez CA: Exercise-induced airways narrowing and exposure to environmental tobacco smoke in school-children. Am J Epidemiol 1994;140:409-417.

83. Frischer T, Kuehr J, Meinert R, et al: Maternal smoking in early childhood: A risk factor for bronchial responsiveness to exercise in primary-school children. J Pediatr 1992;121:17-22.

84. Arshad SH, Hide DW: Effect of environmental factors on the development of allergic disorders in infancy. J Allergy Clin Immunol 1992;90:235-241.

85. Leuenberger P, Schwartz J, Ackermann-Liebrich U, et al: Passive smoking exposure in adults and chronic respiratory symptoms (SAPALDIA Study). Swiss Study on Air Pollution and Lung Diseases in Adults, SAPALDIA Team. Am J Respir Crit Care Med 1994;150:1222-1228.

86. Greer JR, Abbey DE, Burchette RJ: Asthma related to occupational and ambient air pollutants in nonsmokers. J Occup Med 1993;35:909-915.

87. Abbey DE, Petersen F, Mills PK, Beeson WL: Long-term ambient concentrations of total suspended particulates, ozone, and sulfur dioxide and respiratory symptoms in a nonsmoking population. Arch Environ Health 1993;48:33-46.

88. Marquette CH, Salnier F, Leroy O, et al: Long-term prognosis of near-fatal asthma. A 6-year follow-up study of 145 asthmatic patients who underwent mechanical ventilation for a near-fatal attack of asthma. Am Rev Respir Dis 1992;146:76-81.

89. Effectiveness of routine self monitoring of peak flow in patients with asthma. Grampian Asthma Study of Integrated Care (GRASSIC). BMJ 1994;308:564-567.

90. Jones KP, Mullee MA, Middleton M, et al: Peak flow based asthma self-management: A randomised controlled study in general practice. British Thoracic Society Research Committee. Thorax 1995;50:851-857.

91. Gibson PG, Powell H, Coughlin J, et al: Self-management education and regular practitioner review for adults with asthma. Cochrane Database Syst Rev 2003;1:CD001117.

92. Soler M, Matz J, Townley R, et al: The anti-IgE antibody omalizumab reduces exacerbations and steroid requirement in allergic asthmatics. Eur Respir J 2001;18:254-261.

CHAPTER 76

Aspiration

Mark I. Neuman

The term *aspiration* encompasses a variety of respiratory syndromes, and many medical conditions can predispose to aspiration. Foreign body inhalation and the aspiration of infectious or noninfectious oropharyngeal secretions and gastric contents are scenarios that may lead to the development of pulmonary symptoms. The clinical circumstances are key to the timely diagnosis of an acute or chronic aspiration syndrome, because highly sensitive and specific diagnostic tests are lacking.

When aspiration leads to acute injury to the airways and lung parenchyma, two specific types of aspiration syndrome can be identified: aspiration pneumonitis and aspiration pneumonia. These aspiration syndromes are distinct entities, but considerable overlap exists. Attempts to distinguish between them may be important, however, because the appropriate evaluation, management, treatment, and prevention strategies differ.

Aspiration pneumonitis occurs after gastric contents, which are typically acidic, are inhaled into the lower respiratory tract. A prompt and intense inflammatory reaction, or pneumonitis, ensues, but bacterial infection is not a significant part of this immediate reaction. Aspiration pneumonia occurs after inhalation of nasal or oropharyngeal secretions, which contain colonizing bacteria, into the lower airways. The infectious process that develops accounts for the clinical features of aspiration pneumonia. The key to either diagnosis is identifying those patients at risk for aspiration, either occasionally or chronically.

PATHOPHYSIOLOGY

Even healthy adults and children may aspirate small amounts of oropharyngeal contents during sleep; however, pulmonary host defense mechanisms usually prevent the development of infection or an inflammatory response.[1] There is a relatively low burden of virulent organisms colonizing the mouth and the naso- and oropharynx in healthy children; thus, aspiration of small amounts of normal flora rarely culminates in a clinically significant pulmonary infection.[2] Additionally, there are protective mechanisms against the development of pulmonary disease at all levels of the respiratory system; these include the anatomic design of the airway, functional gag and cough reflexes, the mucociliary clearance system, and the innate antibacterial and anti-inflammatory properties of surfactant and airway surface liquid (Table 76-1).[3,4] Impairment of any of these protective barriers places a child at risk for the development of an aspiration syndrome.

The association between gastroesophageal reflux (GER) and the development of chronic respiratory symptoms or even aspiration pneumonia is not entirely understood. These disorders coexist, and the influence of this common gas-trointestinal condition on respiratory function, as well as the influence of respiratory conditions on GER, continues to be explored. Some literature suggests that reflux of gastric contents into the esophagus, as measured by pH probe, is associated with respiratory symptoms in children. Chronic microaspiration may explain some chronic respiratory symptoms.[5,6] Further, certain respiratory conditions, including asthma, may worsen the severity of GER.[6] Conversely, between 50% and 80% of children with chronic respiratory disease have abnormal amounts of GER. In addition to asthma, GER commonly accompanies cystic fibrosis and bronchopulmonary dysplasia.[6-8] Other chronic medical conditions that are associated with an increased risk of aspiration syndromes are also associated with GER (Table 76-2).[6]

Although there is clearly a relationship among GER, recurrent aspiration, and respiratory disease, the specific interactions have not been fully elucidated.[6,8] Nevertheless, acute and chronic respiratory disease related to aspiration accounts for much of the morbidity and mortality in children with impaired gastric motility and swallowing disorders, as well as in children with anatomic abnormalities of the aerodigestive tract, including tracheoesophageal fistula.[3,6]

Aspiration Pneumonitis

Mendelson first described the clinical manifestations of the aspiration of gastric contents into the lower respiratory tract in 1946 in a patient who developed pneumonitis after receiving general anesthesia for an obstetric procedure.[9] Any condition that depresses a child's level of consciousness and impairs airway reflexes predisposes to aspiration. This risk factor includes exposure to alcohol, sedatives, paralytic agents, and other anesthetic agents.[10,11] Loss of airway protective reflexes may also occur in children with central nervous system disorders (see Table 76-2).[12,13] Infants and children with dysphagia and even respiratory distress are at increased risk of aspiration as well.

Aspiration pneumonitis may occur after a witnessed episode of vomiting in a patient at risk. In such instances, a sudden change in respiratory status is often noted. However, aspiration pneumonitis may also present in a subacute fashion. It may exacerbate a preexisting condition such as cerebral palsy, or it may complicate a concurrent condition such as tachypnea in an infant with bronchiolitis. Aspiration pneumonitis should also be considered when there is a change in the respiratory status of a patient who is predisposed to aspiration owing to an underlying disorder.[8]

Chemical injury to the lung occurs as a result of the inhalation of gastric acids, which are usually sterile due to their low pH.[5,7] However, children receiving antacids and proton pump inhibitors, as well as children fed through gastrostomy or nasogastric tubes, often have an elevated gastric

Table 76-1 Major Airway Defenses	
Type of Defense	Mechanism
Upper airways	Mechanical trapping of bacteria in nasal passages and larynx, and frequent branching of upper bronchial tree
Mucociliary transport	Prevents most particulate matter in inspired air from reaching lung parenchyma
Cough reflex	Aspiration of large amounts of oropharyngeal material, including flora of the upper respiratory tract, is prevented by cough and laryngeal reflexes
Local immunoglobulin	Immunoglobulin (primarily IgA), complement, and glycoproteins such as fibronectin in airway secretions prevent colonization of the oropharynx by virulent organisms such as *Streptococcus pneumoniae*, *Pseudomonas aeruginosa*, and *Klebsiella pneumoniae*, which can readily cause lower respiratory tract infection after scant aspiration of oropharyngeal contents
Humoral and cellular defenses of lower respiratory tract	Nonspecific antibacterial activity of surfactant and airway surface fluid Immunoglobulin-mediated opsonization Opsonization or direct lysis by complement activation Phagocytosis and intracellular killing by alveolar macrophages Cell-mediated immunity (effector functions of T lymphocytes) Recruitment of polymorphonuclear leukocytes for phagocytosis and intracellular killing

Table 76-2 Risk Factors for Aspiration Syndrome

Anatomic
    Tracheoesophageal fistula
    Gastrostomy or nasogastric enteral tube
    Tracheostomy
    Endotracheal tube
    Cleft palate or other craniofacial syndrome

Pulmonary
    Bronchopulmonary dysplasia
    Bronchiolitis
    Respiratory distress

Impaired airway reflexes (cough, gag)
    Sedation
    General anesthesia
    Toxic ingestion
    Medication
    Neurologic
        Cerebral palsy
        Neuromuscular disease
        Cerebrovascular accident
        Seizure
        Intracranial bleed
        Head injury
        Mass lesions

Miscellaneous
    Impaired gastric motility
    Swallowing disorder, dysphagia
    Poor oral hygiene, gingivitis

pH and may have bacterial colonization of the stomach.[7,14] Lung damage is related to the acidity of the aspirate, with a more pronounced inflammatory response occurring at lower levels of pH.[5] Additionally, aspirates containing large amounts of particulate food matter increase the inflammatory response. With aspiration of acidic gastric contents, the fluid may be sterile, so bacterial infection is not a significant part of the early process.

Aspiration pneumonitis may also occur in children who have ingested mineral oil or hydrocarbons, which can cause severe respiratory compromise. The inhalation may occur during the ingestion or during the regurgitation that often follows. The risk of aspiration and the severity of the lung injury are related to the viscosity (volatility) of the ingested hydrocarbon; higher-viscosity liquids (e.g., oils), which are less volatile, are less dangerous than lower-viscosity liquids (e.g., furniture polishes), which have greater volatility.

Aspiration Pneumonia

Aspiration pneumonia is an infectious process resulting from the inhalation of oropharyngeal secretions that are colonized by pathogenic bacteria. In contrast to aspiration pneumonitis, bacterial colonization and infection of the lower respiratory tract commonly occur. Children with dysphagia and impaired gastric motility, as well as those with poor dental hygiene, are at risk for aspiration pneumonia, as are those with underlying neurologic and neuromuscular disorders.[6,15] GER may predispose to the development of aspiration pneumonia; however, in a neurologically normal child, intact airway defenses such as the gag and cough reflexes usually prevent this complication.[6] Enteral feeding through gastrostomy and nasogastric tubes also increases the likelihood of aspiration pneumonia.[14] Patients with aspiration pneumonia may have either an acute or a gradual onset of symptoms, and the aspiration event is often unwitnessed.

Critically ill children hospitalized in an intensive care setting often have multiple factors that predispose to the development of aspiration pneumonia. Children lying in the supine position for long periods have increased amounts of GER. Endotracheal intubation may also increase the risk of bacterial colonization and transmigration of bacteria from the upper to lower airway. The period immediately following removal of an endotracheal tube is also critical, because patients have depressed or impaired protective airway reflexes in the postextubation period.[10] Finally, gastroparesis and delayed gastric emptying are commonly observed among critically ill patients, including those with burns,

---

Box 76-1   Organisms Causing Aspiration Pneumonia

Gram-positive
  *Streptococcus pneumoniae**
  *Staphylococcus aureus**
  α-Hemolytic streptococci
Gram-negative
  *Haemophilus influenzae**
  Pseudomonas aeruginosa
  Acinetobacter
  Escherichia coli
  Klebsiella pneumoniae
Anaerobic
  Bacteroides
  Peptostreptococcus
  Fusobacterium

---

*Most common community-acquired pathogens.

significant trauma, and sepsis; all these conditions may increase a child's risk of developing aspiration pneumonia.[12]

Much of the literature regarding the microbiologic cause of aspiration pneumonia is based on adult data from the 1970s and involved transtracheal sampling.[16-18] Unlike in patients with community-acquired pneumonia, these studies found a predominance of anaerobic pathogens among adults with aspiration pneumonia. Brook and Finegold in 1980 found that transtracheal aspirates performed in hospitalized children with aspiration pneumonia most commonly yielded multiple pathogens, including both aerobic and anaerobic species.[18] Organisms identified are listed in Box 76-1.[4,19] More recent data, however, suggest that *Streptococcus pneumoniae, Haemophilus influenzae,* and *Staphylococcus aureus* account for most cases of aspiration pneumonia.[4,20] The other influence on upper airway colonization and thereby the pathogens responsible for aspiration pneumonia is the particular patient population. Patients from long-term care facilities or those with frequent or prolonged hospitalization are at greater risk for colonization with gram-negative organisms; *Pseudomonas* has become a particular concern.

DIFFERENTIAL DIAGNOSIS

Community-acquired aspiration pneumonia may be clinically indistinguishable from community-acquired nonaspiration pneumonia; however, an underlying disorder or other risk factor is usually present. Other respiratory processes that overlap clinically with pneumonia, such as bronchiolitis, asthma exacerbation (especially with inciting viral respiratory febrile illness), and bronchospasm unrelated to an underlying asthma condition (e.g., inhaled chemical exposure), should be considered. Aspiration pneumonia is uncommon in otherwise healthy children without predisposing circumstances (e.g., general anesthesia).

CLINICAL PRESENTATION AND EVALUATION

The diagnosis of acute aspiration syndromes is clinical. There are no specific diagnostic tests for aspiration pneumonia or pneumonitis.[21] The diagnosis should be based on new respiratory findings in a patient suspected to be at risk for aspiration.

Aspiration Pneumonitis

Following an aspiration event, there is immediate and direct injury of the airway and alveoli from the acidic fluid, followed by a second phase of intense inflammation. These events typically produce respiratory symptoms within a few hours and include cough, tachypnea, bronchospasm, and respiratory distress. Hypoxemia is common. These respiratory findings in a child with a depressed level of consciousness or another risk factor strongly suggest the diagnosis of aspiration pneumonitis, particularly if a preceding episode of emesis was witnessed or if there is a history of dysphagia or oral motor incoordination. Chest radiography may not be diagnostic, especially early in the illness, and the presence of fever is variable. Multiple factors contribute to hypoxemia, including direct alveolar damage; reflex bronchospasm in response to tracheal irritation; decreased surfactant activity, which leads to atelectasis and ventilation-perfusion mismatch; and intrapulmonary shunting.[3,4,15]

Although this clinical picture is common, the symptoms may range from severe to mild. Additionally, "silent" aspiration can present with hypoxemia and radiographic abnormalities without detectable symptoms. As mentioned earlier, chronic aspiration may produce a subacute picture, with deterioration of the patient's respiratory status over time.

Aspiration Pneumonia

The diagnosis of aspiration pneumonia should be considered when a child at risk for aspiration develops an infiltrate in dependent lung segments. In a supine patient, the dependent portions of the lung are the posterior segments of the upper lobes; in an upright patient, the dependent portions are the basal segments of the lower lobes. Other radiographic findings of aspiration pneumonia include abscess formation or cavitations.[3]

Aspiration pneumonia may be clinically indistinguishable from community-acquired (nonaspiration) pneumonia; both typically present with fever, cough, and tachypnea, and consolidation may be detected on auscultation or chest radiography. However, an underlying disorder or other risk factor for aspiration is usually present with aspiration pneumonia.

ADMISSION CRITERIA

- Hypoxia.
- Severe respiratory distress or airway instability.
- Failure of outpatient management strategies (e.g., home supplemental oxygen or oral antibiotics).
- Inadequate or unsafe nutritional strategy.

TREATMENT

The general treatment of a child with aspiration involves airway support and the maintenance of gas exchange. Airway clearance with inhaled medications such as albuterol, chest physiotherapy, or other devices may be indicated as well. Devices such as cough-assist machines may have particular usefulness in children with underlying neurologic or neuromuscular disorders, in whom airway clearance is impaired under the best of circumstances.[15] These supportive therapies should be individualized to the clinical situation and the diagnosis.

Aspiration Pneumonitis

The treatment of patients with aspiration pneumonitis (including hydrocarbon aspiration) is primarily supportive. Suctioning of the mouth and oropharynx should be performed to remove particulate matter and gastric acid following a witnessed aspiration.[3,4,15] Endotracheal intubation and the use of mechanical ventilation should be considered in any child with severe respiratory distress in the setting of aspiration pneumonitis.

Prophylactic antibiotics are generally not indicated in the initial management of a patient with aspiration pneumonitis. Patients in whom the gastric contents are not likely to be sterile (e.g., those receiving antacids or proton pump inhibitors), as well as patients with recent gastrointestinal surgery, may be more likely to develop infection, so antibiotics are often initiated. Prophylactic antibiotics may increase the risk of infection with more resistant organisms, however. Any patient with significant illness or who fails to improve within 48 hours should be placed on broad-spectrum antibiotics appropriate to the clinical circumstances and the most likely organism. In general, anaerobic coverage is not required. Obtaining bronchoalveolar lavage samples allows for targeted antibiotic therapy, particularly among patients with significant respiratory distress, other comorbidities, or those who fail to respond to initial therapy. There are insufficient data to recommend the use of corticosteroids in children with aspiration pneumonitis.[22]

Aspiration Pneumonia

In contrast to the treatment of aspiration pneumonitis, antibiotics are an important component of therapy for children with aspiration pneumonia. Because pathogens are rarely recovered outside the research setting, antibiotic therapy is usually empirical. There is a paucity of prospective literature comparing antibiotic regimens among children with aspiration pneumonia. One randomized, controlled trial conducted in 1997 found penicillin and clindamycin to be equally effective for the treatment of hospitalized children with aspiration pneumonia.[19] Because more recent studies identify *S. pneumoniae*, *S. aureus*, and *H. influenzae* as the most common pathogens, ampicillin-sulbactam or a third-generation cephalosporin is a good first-line choice for community-acquired aspiration pneumonia, although clindamycin can also be used with success. For patients at increased risk for infection from gram-negative organisms, coverage is extended to include *Pseudomonas*. In this population, piperacillin-tazobactam or ticarcillin-sulbactam is an appropriate choice. Anaerobic coverage is especially important in children with severe periodontal disease and in those with evidence of lung abscess or necrotizing pneumonia on chest radiographs.[2] In these cases, if a third-generation cephalosporin is used, the addition of clindamycin or metronidazole is recommended. The use of corticosteroids for aspiration pneumonia is not supported by the literature.[22]

Treatment of foreign body aspiration requires removal of the foreign body; usually no further treatment is needed.

CONSULTATION

When the clinical picture is uncertain or a significant underlying disorder is contributing to an acute or chronic aspiration syndrome, subspecialty consultation should be considered. Acutely, pulmonology consultation may provide guidance for airway care in a patient with impaired airway clearance, as well as bronchoscopy if the diagnosis is unclear. Foreign body aspiration may require otorhinolaryngology consultation for rigid bronchoscopy. Infectious disease input may be required to tailor antimicrobial therapy. In children with underlying risk factors for aspiration or impaired airway defenses, the subspecialist may recommend a specific plan of airway care and devices to help clear secretions and prevent atelectasis or mucus retention. Finally, in a child with chronic medical risk factors for aspiration or chronic respiratory and gastrointestinal symptoms, a multidisciplinary approach is required to address both the acute and the chronic aspects of the condition.

DISCHARGE CRITERIA

- Respiratory stability.
- Ability to complete the required therapeutic regimens.
- Adequate plan for airway management to minimize the risk of future aspiration episodes:
  - Anticipatory guidance.
  - Airway clearance, if indicated.
  - Safe and adequate nutritional plan.

PREVENTION

Because aspiration syndromes most often occur in patients with temporary or chronic impairment of airway protection, gastrointestinal dysmotility, altered gastric acidification, or swallowing difficulties, a targeted approach should be possible. Optimizing the safe delivery of nutrition and airway clearance should be major clinical goals. Special precautions should be in place in circumstances that increase the risk for aspiration, including postextubation, sedation or general anesthesia, or new neurologic deficits.

IN A NUTSHELL

- Aspiration syndromes represent a diverse group of pediatric lung and airway disorders; the two most common forms are aspiration pneumonitis and aspiration pneumonia.
- Aspiration pneumonitis is a sterile inflammatory process that typically follows inhalation of gastric contents.
- Aspiration pneumonia is a bacterial process that typically follows inhalation of infectious oropharygeal secretions.
- The diagnosis of an aspiration syndrome is generally clinical, with supporting radiographs.
- Treatment is supportive, but antibiotics play a key role in the management of aspiration pneumonia.
- Optimizing airway defenses, careful attention to airway maintenance and clearance, and a safe nutritional strategy may help prevent this condition in susceptible patients.

ON THE HORIZON

- There is a significant need for more sensitive and specific methods of diagnosing pulmonary aspiration. Similarly, evidence-based evaluation of supportive measures, such as inhaled medications and airway clearance devices for patients with chronic aspiration, is lacking.
- Improved diagnostic and therapeutic measures will enable physicians to formulate more efficient and efficacious therapeutic plans for this challenging group of patients.

SUGGESTED READING

Brook I, Finegold SM: Bacteriology of aspiration pneumonia in children. Pediatrics 1980;65:1115-1120.

Marik PE: Aspiration pneumonitis and aspiration pneumonia. N Engl J Med 2001;344:665-671.

REFERENCES

1. Gleeson K, Eggli DF, Maxwell SL: Quantitative aspiration during sleep in normal subjects. Chest 1997;111:1266-1272.
2. Yoneyama T, Yoshida M, Matsui T, Sasaki H: Oral care and pneumonia. Lancet 1999;354:515.
3. Cassiere HA, Niederman MS: Aspiration pneumonia, lipoid pneumonia, and lung abscess. In Baum GL, Crapo JD, Celli BR, Karlinsky JB (eds): Textbook of Pulmonary Diseases, 6th ed, vol 1. Philadelphia, Lippincott-Raven, 1998, pp 645-655.
4. Marik PE: Aspiration pneumonitis and aspiration pneumonia. N Engl J Med 2001;344:665-671.
5. Exarhos ND, Logan WD Jr, Abbott OA, Hatcher CR Jr: The importance of pH and volume in tracheobronchial aspiration. Dis Chest 1965;47:167-169.
6. Orenstein SR, Orenstein DM: Gastroesophogeal reflux and respiratory disease in children. J Pediatr 1988;112:847-858.
7. Bonten MJ, Gaillard CA, van der Geest S, et al: The role of intragastric acidity and stress ulcer prophylaxis on colonization and infection in mechanically ventilated ICU patients: A stratified, randomized, double-blind study of sucralfate versus antacids. Am J Respir Crit Care Med 1995;152:1825-1834.
8. Kikuchi R, Watabe N, Konno T, et al: High incidence of silent aspiration in elderly patients with community-acquired pneumonia. Am J Respir Crit Care Med 1994;150:251-253.
9. Mendelson CL: The aspiration of stomach contents into the lungs during obstetric anesthesia. Am J Obstet Gynecol 1946;52:191-205.
10. de Larminat V, Montravers P, Dureuil B, Desmonts JM: Alteration in swallowing reflex after extubation in intensive care unit patients. Crit Care Med 1995;23:486-490.
11. Kollef MH: Ventilator-associated pneumonia: A multivariate analysis. JAMA 1993;270:1965-1970.
12. Adnet F, Baud F: Relation between Glasgow Coma Scale and aspiration pneumonia. Lancet 1996;348:123-124.
13. Leder SB, Cohn SM, Moller BA: Fiberoptic endoscopic documentation of the high incidence of aspiration following extubation in critically ill trauma patients. Dysphagia 1998;13:208-212.
14. Grant MD, Rudberg MA, Brody JA: Gastrostomy placement and mortality among hospitalized Medicare beneficiaries. JAMA 1998;279:1973-1976.
15. Johnson JL, Hirsch CS: Aspiration pneumonia: Recognizing and managing a potential growing disorder. Postgrad Med 2003;113:99-112.
16. Bartlett JG, Gorbach SL, Finegold SM: The bacteriology of aspiration pneumonia. Am J Med 1974;56:202-207.
17. Lorber B, Swenson RM: Bacteriology of aspiration pneumonia: A prospective study of community- and hospital-acquired cases. Ann Intern Med 1974;81:329-331.
18. Brook I, Finegold SM: Bacteriology of aspiration pneumonia in children. Pediatrics 1980;65:1115-1120.
19. Jacobson SJ, Griffiths K, Diamond S, et al: A randomized controlled trial of penicillin vs clindamycin for the treatment of aspiration pneumonia in children. Arch Pediatr Adolesc Med 1997;151:701-704.
20. Marik PE, Careau P: The role of anaerobes in patients with ventilator-associated pneumonia and aspiration pneumonia: A prospective study. Chest 1999;115:178-183.
21. Krishnan U, Mitchell JD, Vivian T, et al: Fat laden macrophages in tracheal aspirates as a marker of reflux aspiration: A negative report. J Pediatr Gastroenterol Nutr 2002;35:309-313.
22. Bernard GR, Luce JM, Sprung CL, et al: High-dose corticosteroids in patients with the adult respiratory distress syndrome. N Engl J Med 1987;317:1565-1570.

Bronchopulmonary Dysplasia and Chronic Lung Disease of Infancy

Ian MacLusky and Krista Keilty

Bronchopulmonary dysplasia (BPD) is an iatrogenic, chronic lung disorder of infancy that results in persistent respiratory symptoms, medical fragility, and, in most cases, the long-term need for supplemental oxygen. With continuing advances in the care of critically ill neonates, the nomenclature of BPD is evolving, as is its incidence and pathogenesis. Today, BPD is often referred to as chronic lung disease of infancy (CLDI).[1,2] Both BPD and CLDI are chronic pulmonary disorders that result from an acute and often critical respiratory illness in a newborn infant, and there is considerable overlap in their pathogenesis, risk factors, and manifestations. Thus, the two terms are generally considered to be interchangeable.

BPD and CLDI develop in premature infants or critically ill neonates as a consequence of therapeutic maneuvers (oxygen and positive-pressure ventilation) required for survival. The risk of an infant developing CLDI is related to gestational age, the severity of the initial illness, the duration and intensity of oxygen and ventilator therapy, and other factors that are less well characterized. These prognostic factors include variables specific to the infant, such as gender, race, nutritional status, and other complications of newborn intensive care, as well as maternal variables such as cigarette smoking during pregnancy and the presence of amnionitis.[1] These factors often result in significantly different outcomes in infants despite apparently similar care.

The medical fragility associated with BPD and CLDI results in an increased risk of rehospitalization after discharge from the nursery. The pediatric hospitalist will therefore encounter infants with BPD and CLDI and will be called on to address the problems unique to this complex group of patients. Many infants with BPD or CLDI are readmitted to the hospital within the first 2 years of life, with the highest incidence of rehospitalization being in those born most prematurely.[3] Respiratory illness, most notably due to respiratory syncytial virus (RSV) or other viruses, is the most common reason, causing up to two thirds of readmissions, followed by gastroenteritis, feeding difficulties, and seizures.[3] Further, BPD and CLDI often have systemic manifestations that may complicate the respiratory management of these infants. If the extrapulmonary manifestations are not recognized and addressed, they can interfere with lung growth and healing, which are necessary for the resolution of BPD and CLDI. Often the goal of therapy is to reestablish the infant's baseline state or to diagnose and treat a new problem rather than to provide a definitive cure. This requires both skilled medical management and attention to the details of discharge planning.

CLINICAL PRESENTATION

When originally described by Northway and colleagues,[4] BPD occurred primarily in relatively mature infants with an average birth weight of nearly 2 kg and a gestational age of 32 weeks who developed hyaline membrane disease due to surfactant-deficient respiratory distress syndrome. These infants received what would now be considered aggressive therapy consisting of high levels of inspired oxygen and ventilator pressures that are toxic to the lung and result in a specific pattern of lung and airway injury ("classic" BPD).[4] The adverse effects of oxygen and barotrauma impaired primarily the distal airways, resulting in diffuse airway damage and airway obstruction that was either complete (resulting in atelectasis) or partial (resulting in a ball-valve effect and gas trapping).[5] An intense inflammatory reaction ensued, which could hinder lung healing and promote further lung injury. This nonspecific airway injury also resulted in distinctive and evolving radiographic manifestations, with a heterogeneous pattern of focal gas trapping, atelectasis, and interstitial infiltrates followed by fibrosis.[4]

Owing to improvements in neonatal care and medical technology and recognition of the adverse effects of aggressive mechanical ventilation and oxygen therapy, few mature infants with hyaline membrane disease now develop BPD. Concurrently, increasing numbers of infants born at less than 28 weeks' gestation are surviving. In these infants, respiratory failure occurs due to lung immaturity as well as surfactant deficiency, because in extremely premature infants, the alveoli and peripheral airways are unformed. Oxygen therapy and mechanical ventilation necessary for survival cause alveolar growth arrest, resulting in pulmonary hypoplasia in addition to an element of peripheral airway damage and chronic inflammation ("new" BPD).[6] Radiographically, the pattern is more homogeneous.

Evolving medical practice and a better understanding of disease pathogenesis have resulted in altered disease definitions, incidence estimates, and risk factors. Northway originally defined BPD as occurring in any premature infant who still required oxygen past 28 days of age.[5] Although various criteria have been proposed, most authorities agree that an infant should also be at least 36 weeks post conception.[7] A recent consensus conference proposed a severity-based definition of BPD for infants born at less than 32 weeks.[8] Mild BPD was defined as the need for supplemental oxygen therapy for greater than 28 days, but not at the time of discharge or 36 weeks' postmenstrual age (PMA). Moderate BPD was defined as the need for supplemental oxygen therapy for greater than 28 days and treatment with less than 30% fraction of inspired oxygen (FIO_2) at 36 weeks' PMA. Severe BPD was defined as the need for supplemental oxygen therapy for greater than 28 days and treatment with greater than 30% FIO_2, positive-pressure ventilation, or both at 36 weeks' PMA. This definition was recently validated to accurately identify infants at risk for adverse pulmonary and neurodevelopmental outcomes.[9]

The absence of a consistent definition or a standardized BPD severity score makes it difficult to compare changes in incidence over time. Nevertheless, there seems to have been a real change in the incidence of BPD and CLDI. During the 1980s, the decreasing incidence of BPD at any given gestation was offset by an increased survival rate in more premature infants. Further increases in survival rates in the early 1990s resulted in an overall increase in the occurrence of BPD.[10,11] Subsequently, during the latter half of the 1990s and into the early 2000s, there was a plateau; ongoing improvements in neonatal care did not reduce the incidence of BPD, although there appears to have been a reduction in overall severity.[11,12]

BPD and CLDI occur primarily in premature infants (Table 77-1). Any neonate requiring prolonged respiratory support, such as those with sepsis, congenital diaphragmatic hernia, or persistent pulmonary hypertension of the newborn, is at risk for BPD and CLDI. BPD and CLDI are therefore heterogeneous disorders with a wide spectrum of causes, variable patterns, and different degrees of lung damage.[1,2,5] Most critically ill neonates who survive the newborn period are discharged from the nursery, but they may have significant residual lung damage, persistent reduction in pulmonary function, and ongoing disabilities that place them at high risk for repeated hospitalizations in the first 2 years of life, primarily for respiratory illnesses.[13] BPD and CLDI thus constitute a spectrum of diseases with various underlying diagnoses; affected infants range from those with only minimal hypoxemia to infants who require long-term invasive ventilation for survival. The most severely affected infants are at the highest risk for rehospitalization, medical complications (including death), and long-term pulmonary and neurologic sequelae.

Although the degree of hypoxemia is commonly used to assess severity, with an oxygen requirement at 36 weeks' PMA suggested as a standard,[8] other clinical parameters are important as well. Although oxygen saturation is easily measured, it can change significantly from day to day and even from wakefulness to sleep. Therefore, a combination of other parameters may be useful to obtain an overall assessment of an infant's clinical status (Table 77-2). These include growth, arterial carbon dioxide levels (pH corrected), and the actual FIO_2 required to maintain a target oxygen saturation.

TREATMENT

Once the neonatal period is over, the treatment of BPD and CLDI is primarily supportive, aimed at maximizing lung growth and healing over time while preventing any further pulmonary damage.[14] Owing to the heterogeneity of clinical disease in infants with BPD and CLDI, there is no standard therapy. Treatment must be individualized, depending on each infant's pattern and disease severity.

Persistent Hypoxemia

As previously stated, BPD is associated with inflammation and peripheral airway damage, resulting in areas of hyperinflation and atelectasis, as well as alveolar growth arrest. Hypoxemia due to ventilation-perfusion mismatch is a primary feature of BPD and CLDI, making long-term oxygen therapy a mainstay of treatment.[15]

Although there are data supporting the effectiveness of long-term oxygen therapy in improving the outcome in infants with BPD and CLDI, the optimal target saturation is

Table 77-1   Incidence of Bronchopulmonary Dysplasia (BPD) since 1994

Gestation (PMA)	Overall Incidence (%)	Severe BPD (%)
23 wk[6]	57-70	
24 wk	33-89	
25 wk	16-71	
<29 wk[8]	18-34	8-26
≥29 to <33 wk	4-8	2-5

PMA, postmenstrual age.

Table 77-2   Parameters That Determine the Severity of Bronchopulmonary Dysplasia (BPD) and Chronic Lung Disease in Infancy

Parameter	BPD Severity		
	Mild	Moderate	Severe
Oxygen requirement (at 36 wk PMA)[36]	Room air	<30%	≥30% or positive pressure (PPV, nasal CPAP)
Arterial carbon dioxide	≤48 mm Hg	49-59 mm Hg	≥60 mm Hg
Chest radiograph[37]	Normal to faint, hazy opacities	Linear-reticular opacities, extending out from hilum	Increasingly defined cystic lesions
Nutrition	Growth within normal limits	Normal length, decreased weight	Both length and weight reduced, <25th percentile ideal body weight

CPAP, continuous positive airway pressure; PMA, postmenstrual age; PPV, positive-pressure ventilation.

still debated. In general, supplemental oxygen is considered for infants who cannot maintain oxygen saturations greater than 93% during sleep or quiet wakefulness.[16] Infants provided with sufficient supplemental oxygen to maintain arterial saturations around 92% to 94% have better growth and neurologic outcomes and less risk of pulmonary hypertension than do those in whom the saturation goal is less than 90%.[1] Further, sudden death[16] and hypoxic bronchoconstriction[17] may be reduced. Two large studies suggest that maintaining oxygen saturations above 95% may not confer any additional advantage over saturations greater than 89% to 94%[18] or 91% to 94%[19]; rather, this may simply prolong the duration of oxygen therapy.[18,20] It should be noted, however, that both these studies were performed on infants still in the newborn intensive care unit, so it is uncertain whether the findings apply to older infants with established BPD.

Notwithstanding these limitations and the lack of complete data, most authorities use target saturations between 92% and 95%, with no more than 5% of time spent at less than 90% saturation.[15] In the vast majority of infants, this is achievable with oxygen provided in the home, as discussed later.

Hypercapnia

Infants with BPD may have hypercapnia in addition to chronic hypoxemia, reflecting the severity of chronic lung disease and an inability to maintain sufficient alveolar ventilation for normal carbon dioxide levels.[21] With lung growth and repair, carbon dioxide levels return to normal, but until that occurs, any additional stress or insult can result in overt respiratory failure. In the most severely affected infants, long-term invasive ventilation (via tracheostomy) may be required to achieve adequate growth. The decision to initiate long-term invasive ventilation is individualized, based on the infant's clinical status; it is most often considered in those with refractory respiratory failure, failure to thrive, or extreme cardiorespiratory instability.

Airway Hyperreactivity

Infants with BPD and CLDI often have increased nonspecific airway hyperreactivity,[22] the precise mechanism of which is unclear. This results in episodic bronchospasm due to a variety of irritants, with viral respiratory infection being the most common. Contributing to airway hyperreactivity is the residual inflammation associated with BPD and CLDI. Persistent wheezing in infants with BPD and CLDI must be evaluated thoroughly because it may reflect a comorbid condition. Airway hyperreactivity may persist into late childhood.[23]

Many infants with BPD demonstrate a significant bronchodilator response to inhaled β_2-agonist agents.[24] A therapeutic trial of bronchodilators is indicated if there is evidence of persistent or acute bronchospasm and gas trapping. Bronchodilators should not be used routinely in the absence of a therapeutic response.[24]

Airway inflammation is a primary factor in the pathogenesis and persistence of BPD and CLDI. Systemic corticosteroid therapy has been used to prevent the onset of BPD—either before delivery, to stimulate lung maturation, or early after delivery, to minimize subsequent pulmonary inflammation.[25] Recent reports of worse neurologic outcomes in neonates receiving systemic corticosteroids in the first week of life have raised concerns about their use.[26] Although inhaled corticosteroids are frequently used in infants with BPD and CLDI, there is debate about their efficacy as well as potential toxicity. Infants with overt airway hyperreactivity may benefit from long-term inhaled corticosteroids, but their precise role remains unproved.[27] The potential risk of adrenal suppression, hyperglycemia, inhibition of somatic growth, and neurologic insult should limit their use to infants in whom there is a clear therapeutic response.[28]

The differential diagnosis of wheezing in an infant with BPD or CLDI is similar to that of any infant with chronic wheezing. Specific problems that may occur more frequently in this group, however, include tracheobronchomalacia, dysphagia, and gastroesophageal reflux (GER). As with all children, the avoidance of exposure to tobacco smoke is critical.

Respiratory Viruses

Depending on the severity of residual lung disease, infants with BPD may have up to a 50% chance of requiring readmission, usually within the first 2 years of life, and usually owing to viral respiratory tract infection.[29] Infants with BPD are particularly at risk from RSV. Recently, monoclonal antibodies have been developed that provide partial passive immunity. Although not completely effective at preventing RSV infection, they do reduce both the incidence and the severity of RSV infection.[30] Further discussion of bronchiolitis, its management, and the role of monoclonal antibody therapy is provided in Chapter 66. Parents of infants with BPD are advised to minimize exposure to respiratory viruses; this includes rigorous hand washing, obtaining influenza vaccinations for themselves, and avoiding anyone who is potentially infectious. These precautions must be followed during hospitalization as well, owing to the risk of nosocomial infections.

Fluid Intolerance

Infants with BPD and CLDI may demonstrate significant fluid intolerance. Pulmonary edema is common early in the disease process due to lung inflammation with vascular leak, but it persists in many infants. Acute evidence of improved pulmonary mechanics after diuretic administration has led to the use of these drugs,[31] even though their long-term effectiveness remains unproved.[32] The diuretics used most often include thiazides such as hydrochlorothiazide or loop diuretics such as furosemide. Risks associated with diuretic therapy include electrolyte imbalance, which can be addressed by providing salt supplementation, and nephrocalcinosis and renal failure,[33] which are seen more commonly with furosemide. Clinically, infants with BPD and CLDI require careful fluid titration along with diuretic therapy to allow sufficient fluid intake for growth while avoiding pulmonary edema and worsened respiratory mechanics. Ensuring adequate caloric intake (see later) without excessive fluid loading requires daily attention to weight gain or loss and fluid intake and output. A sudden, unexplained weight gain, particularly if associated with respiratory deterioration, may warrant a therapeutic trial of a diuretic. Persistent pulmonary edema may prompt further evaluation of an infant's protein status or testing for occult cardiac disease with pulmonary overcirculation.

Malnutrition

Infants with BPD and CLDI often have some degree of growth failure and malnutrition. The difficulty of providing sufficient caloric intake, as well as frequent illnesses and respiratory exacerbations, complicates the challenge of ensuring adequate nutrition for growth.[34,35] Failure to thrive may prompt admission as a primary diagnosis, or it may be noted during hospitalization for another acute illness.

Feeding difficulties, including dysphagia and unsuspected hypoxia during feedings,[36] may contribute to malnutrition. Malnutrition is further complicated by elevated caloric requirements, up to 130% of normal,[38] owing to the increased work of breathing as well as the need for catch-up growth. Fluid intolerance, GER, and poor oral feeding due to neurologic damage or oral aversion can complicate nutritional management and must be addressed. Infants with BPD and CLDI who cannot grow with oral feedings alone require supplemental feeding via nasogastric tube or percutaneous gastrostomy or gastrojejunostomy tube. Use of concentrated infant formulas (27 to 30 kcal/ounce) and collaboration with nutritionists and feeding specialists can assist in providing sufficient caloric intake to optimize growth.[38] Should poor growth persist despite adequate caloric intake,[39] unsuspected hypoxia or hypercapnia requiring long-term mechanical ventilation should be considered, along with the other causes of failure to thrive seen in children without BPD or CLDI (see Chapter 32).

Gastroesophageal Reflux

GER is common in children born prematurely,[13] although there is a poor correlation between GER and the severity of BPD. GER can compound nutritional difficulties because the regurgitation associated with GER diminishes the net caloric intake, whether the nutrition is delivered orally or directly into the stomach. GER may also be associated with oral aversion and dysphagia. Infants with oropharyngeal incoordination, especially when associated with an inability to protect the airway, are at increased risk of aspiration, which may result in further lung damage.[40] The management of GER in infants with BPD and CLDI should be proactive and aggressive; a more complete discussion is provided in Chapter 101.

Upper Airway Damage

Infants with BPD and CLDI frequently have a history of repeated or prolonged intubation, with the risk of subglottic stenosis complicating lower airway disease.[41] Vocal cord injury, including vocal cord paresis or paralysis, laryngeal webs, and cysts, are other possible postintubation complications. These airway injuries result in partial upper airway obstruction, increase the inspiratory work of breathing, and can interfere with gas exchange. Airway protective mechanisms may be impaired as well. Partial upper airway obstruction also increases the risk for respiratory failure during an acute illness. Persistent upper airway symptoms, dysphonia, or stridor should prompt an evaluation for subglottic stenosis and laryngeal injury. If the upper airway lesion is severe enough, tracheostomy or airway reconstructive surgery may be indicated.

Disordered Sleep and Breathing

Infants with BPD and CLDI are at high risk for disordered sleep and abnormal gas exchange during sleep. Hypoxia during sleep can interfere with growth, and caregivers should be alert for hypoxia during sleep even among infants with acceptable oxygen saturation levels during wakefulness.[36,42] A more complete discussion of obstructive sleep apnea is provided in Chapter 74.

Neurologic Damage

A spectrum of neurologic damage is common among children born prematurely, ranging from subtle intellectual deficits to pronounced neuromotor disease (cerebral palsy) and mental retardation.[43] The degree to which BPD and CLDI contribute to neuromotor disease is unclear, but the two problems frequently coexist. Dysfunction of bulbar muscles increases the risk of swallowing dysfunction[40] and aspiration (see Chapter 101). Seizure disorders may also predispose to this complication. Long-term follow-up of earlier cohorts of infants born with BPD shows an association between BPD and neurocognitive deficits independent of and in addition to the effects of very low birth weight.[44]

Laryngomalacia and Tracheobronchomalacia

These disorders represent abnormal or exaggerated airway collapse due to defects in the cartilaginous rings of the airway. They have various respiratory manifestations but often result in chronic wheezing (tracheobronchomalacia) or stridor (laryngomalacia), with features of increased work of breathing. They may result in partial or intermittent complete airway obstruction, especially during events associated with increased force of breathing, such as crying or a respiratory illness. At worst, this can lead to severe cyanotic episodes with apnea, bradycardia, or both. Airway growth and healing over time lead to an improvement in symptoms and respiratory mechanics. Although tracheobronchomalacia may be congenital, it is usually acquired due to intubation and mechanical ventilation, which cause injury to the compliant, immature neonatal trachea and bronchi.[1,45,46] Tracheobronchomalacia responds poorly to bronchodilator or other medical therapy. Bronchoscopy or airway imaging can be used to diagnose these airway lesions, which, if severe enough, may result in a critical airway requiring tracheostomy and positive-pressure ventilation.

Nonaccidental Injury and Neglect

Premature infants are at increased risk for nonaccidental injury and medical neglect. Neglect may be intentional or unintentional, owing to the complex care required for these children at home. Any infant with medical fragility or technology dependence is thought to be at increased risk. It should be noted, however, that preterm infants with bone disease might have rib fractures that are not due to abuse. Other fractures are highly suspicious and must be treated as such (see Chapter 175).

DIFFERENTIAL DIAGNOSIS

After the initial insult, BPD and CLDI are not progressive disorders. Except for occasional relapses, such as those due to viral infections, infants with BPD and CLDI are expected to show steady, if slow, recovery. Consequently, an alternative explanation must be found for any child who fails to show signs of improvement. Some diagnostic considerations are provided in Table 77-3.

CONSULTATION

Infants with BPD and CLDI often require a team of specialists to manage their care. This is particularly true of infants with technology dependence or chronic medical problems associated with BPD and CLDI (see Chapters 193 and 195). Involving specialists in the care of these medically fragile infants is important and can help the hospitalist facilitate a smoother and potentially earlier transition back

home. Aside from the assistance required for the management of acute issues, consultants can assess newly recognized conditions or reassess ongoing conditions. Common subspecialties include the following:

- Neonatology (many centers have a specific newborn follow-up program)
- Pulmonology
- Neurology
- Otolaryngology
- Gastroenterology
- Developmental medicine
- Nutrition
- Physical, occupational, or speech therapy
- Case management or social work

The primary care physician provides care coordination and is an essential member of the patient care team. Communication with this physician is important throughout the hospital stay.

ADMISSION CRITERIA

Admission criteria for infants with BPD and CLDI are the same as for any patient, but this population is at particular risk for the following:

- Respiratory distress, apnea, or hypoxia secondary to intercurrent respiratory illness
- Failure to thrive
- Dehydration or electrolyte imbalance associated with gastroenteritis or diuretic therapy
- New-onset seizure or change in neurologic status
- Nonaccidental injury or medical neglect

DISCHARGE CRITERIA

Infants with BPD and CLDI constitute a high-risk and high-needs group of patients and place significant burdens on families and caregivers in the home. Careful discharge planning, either after the initial hospitalization or following readmission, ensures that adequate resources are in place for these infants and their families.[15,47] Resolution of the acute events that prompted admission must be achieved before discharge. In addition, short-term or long-term setbacks in the infant's clinical status may require changes in the care

Table 77-3 **Differential Diagnosis of Complications of Bronchopulmonary Dysplasia**

Failure to thrive
Formula intolerance
Protein malabsorption
Short gut
Cystic fibrosis
Inadequate calories
Recurrent pneumonia
Aspiration
Immune deficiency
Cystic fibrosis
Bronchospasm
Fluid intolerance
Occult congenital heart disease
Hypoxemia
Ongoing lung injury
Pulmonary hypertension
Occult congenital heart disease
Pulmonary hypoplasia
Increasing respiratory failure
Pulmonary hypoplasia
Critical airway

Table 77-4 **Additional Signs of Bronchopulmonary Disease and Chronic Lung Disease of Infancy and Their Possible Causes**

Additional Signs	Possible Cause
Failure to thrive, recurrent pneumonia, hypochloremic metabolic alkalosis, distal airway obstruction	Cystic fibrosis
Failure to thrive, bronchospasm, recurring (basal) pneumonia	Aspiration, gastroesophageal reflux, tracheobronchomalacia, hyperreactive airway disease
Apparent diuretic dependency (unable to wean from diuretics without deterioration)	Pulmonary hypertension (first or second degree), partial anomalous pulmonary venous drainage, patent ductus arteriosus
Persisting hypoxemia poorly responsive to oxygen therapy	Congenital cardiac disease
Increasing respiratory failure (hypercapnia)	Pulmonary hypoplasia

plan or the institution of additional resources in the home environment.

Oxygen

Supplemental oxygen therapy is a primary requirement for infants with BPD and CLDI. Oxygen can be provided in the home from compressed gas in tanks, liquid oxygen, or oxygen concentrators. Each system has advantages and disadvantages in terms of the liter flow required, cost, and portability; the system chosen should be based on the needs of the infant as well as the availability of local resources. A proper evaluation of the home environment (e.g., assessment of fire risk and family economic resources) should occur, and the appropriate oxygen source should be established well in advance of discharge.

Pulse oximetry may be appropriate and, with careful guidance, can help in the monitoring and management of infants with BPD and CLDI who are chronically hypoxic or who have developed a need for supplemental oxygen. Pulse oximetry in the absence of home oxygen therapy cannot be recommended. Oxygen saturation is commonly measured during the day. Nocturnal desaturation is frequent, however, and may be unexpected clinically; in addition, nocturnal saturation may correlate poorly with daytime saturation.[36,42] Therefore, overnight oximetry should be performed before nocturnal supplemental oxygen is discontinued.

Apnea Monitoring

Early reports suggested an increased incidence of sudden death among infants with BPD, although the incidence seems to have fallen with the use of long-term oxygen therapy.[39] Given the absence of any proven effect of apnea monitoring on the incidence of sudden infant death syndrome and the stress associated with monitors (due to repeated false alarms), routine use of apnea monitoring in this setting has been questioned[40] (see Chapter 74).

Medical Follow-up

A clear discharge plan with attention to home health care needs, follow-up appointments, and coordination of care through the primary physician is critical for this population.

PREVENTION

The primary treatment of BPD and CLDI is prevention, which involves reducing the incidence of premature births. Surfactant therapy and improved ventilator management are also recognized factors that reduce the severity and incidence of BPD.[48]

IN A NUTSHELL

- BPD and CLDI are iatrogenic lung disorders occurring primarily in premature infants with immature lung development, but also in term or near-term infants requiring prolonged mechanical ventilation.
- Readmission rate among infants with BPD and CLDI is high, especially in those with a history of extreme prematurity.

- Acute respiratory illness, especially viral illness, accounts for the majority of readmissions in this population.
- The lung disease may be associated with persistent hypoxemia, hypercapnia, and hyperreactive airways with bronchospasm.
- Infants with BPD and CLDI may demonstrate fluid intolerance and may require long-term diuretics.
- Providing adequate nutrition is a challenge owing to increased caloric needs and difficulties with oral feeding.
- These infants often have complex medical concerns, both short and long term, that are best served by a multidisciplinary team coordinated by a primary care physician. The hospitalist has a key role in managing acute medical issues and coordinating care during the hospital stay and after discharge.

ON THE HORIZON

- BPD and CLDI are evolving disorders. Advances in neonatal care and technology will continue to affect the outcomes of premature infants with respiratory failure and others with critical respiratory illnesses.
- Therapies on the horizon may include novel anti-inflammatory medications such as superoxide dismutase (SOD), Clara cell secretory protein (CC-10), and lucinactant (Surfaxin), each of which is undergoing active investigation.
- The long-term outcome of infants with BPD and CLDI is evolving as well. Older children with a history of BPD may have an increased risk of asthma, but in the absence of significant neurologic injury, the outcome of this fragile group of infants is quite good.

SUGGESTED READING

Allen J, Zwerdling R, Ehrenkranz R, et al: Statement on the care of the child with chronic lung disease of infancy and childhood. Am J Respir Crit Care Med 2003;168:356-396.

Balfour-Lynn IM, Primhak RA, Shaw BN: Home oxygen for children: Who, how and when? Thorax 2005;60:76-81.

Committee on Fetus and Newborn, American Academy of Pediatrics: Apnea, sudden infant death syndrome, and home monitoring. Pediatrics 2003;111:914-917.

Doyle LW, Ford G, Davis N: Health and hospitalisations after discharge in extremely low birth weight infants. Semin Neonatol 2003;8:137-145.

Gray PH, Rogers Y: Are infants with bronchopulmonary dysplasia at risk for sudden infant death syndrome? Pediatrics 1994;93:774-777.

Jobe AH, Bancalari E: Bronchopulmonary dysplasia. Am J Respir Crit Care Med 2001;163:1723-1729.

Jobe AJ: The new BPD: An arrest of lung development. Pediatr Res 1999;46:641-643.

Parker TA, Abman SH: The pulmonary circulation in bronchopulmonary dysplasia. Semin Neonatol 2003;8:51-61.

Prevention of respiratory syncytial virus infections: Indications for the use of palivizumab and update on the use of RSV-IGIV. American Academy of Pediatrics Committee on Infectious Diseases and Committee of Fetus and Newborn. Pediatrics 1998;102:1211-1216.

Stevens TP, Hall CB: Controversies in palivizumab use. Pediatr Infect Dis J 2004;23:1051-1052.

Weinstein MR, Peters ME, Sadek M, Palta M: A new radiographic scoring system for bronchopulmonary dysplasia. Newborn Lung Project. Pediatr Pulmonol 1994;18:284-289.

REFERENCES

1. Allen J, Zwerdling R, Ehrenkranz R, et al: Statement on the care of the child with chronic lung disease of infancy and childhood. Am J Respir Crit Care Med 2003;168:356-396.
2. Nievas FF: Bronchopulmonary dysplasia (chronic lung disease of infancy): An update for the pediatrician. Clin Pediatr 2002;41:77-85.
3. Doyle LW, Ford G, Davis N: Health and hospitalisations after discharge in extremely low birth weight infants. Semin Neonatol 2003;8:137-145.
4. Northway WH Jr, Rosan RC, Porter DY: Pulmonary disease following respirator therapy of hyaline-membrane disease: Bronchopulmonary dysplasia. N Engl J Med 1967;276:357-368.
5. Northway WH Jr: Bronchopulmonary dysplasia: Twenty-five years later. Pediatrics 1992;89:969-973.
6. Jobe AJ: The new BPD: An arrest of lung development. Pediatr Res 1999;46:641-643.
7. Shennan AT, Dunn MS, Ohlsson A, et al: Abnormal pulmonary outcomes in premature infants: Prediction from oxygen requirement in the neonatal period. Pediatrics 1988;82:527-532.
8. Jobe AH, Bancalari E: Bronchopulmonary dysplasia. Am J Respir Crit Care Med 2001;163:1723-1729.
9. Ehrenkranz RA, Walsh MC, Vohr BR, et al: Validation of the National Institutes of Health consensus definition of bronchopulmonary dysplasia. Pediatrics 2005;116:1353-1360.
10. Hack M, Fanaroff AA: Outcomes of children of extremely low birthweight and gestational age in the 1990s. Early Hum Dev 1999;53:193-218.
11. Horbar JD, Badger GJ, Carpenter JH, et al: Trends in mortality and morbidity for very low birth weight infants, 1991-1999. Pediatrics 2002;110:143-151.
12. Smith VC, Zupancic JA, McCormick MC, et al: Trends in severe bronchopulmonary dysplasia rates between 1994 and 2002. J Pediatr 2005;146:469-473.
13. Smith VC, Zupancic JA, McCormick MC, et al: Rehospitalization in the first year of life among infants with bronchopulmonary dysplasia. J Pediatr 2004;144:799-803.
14. Shah PS: Current perspectives on the prevention and management of chronic lung disease in preterm infants. Paediatr Drugs 2003;5:463-480.
15. Balfour-Lynn IM, Primhak RA, Shaw BN: Home oxygen for children: Who, how and when? Thorax 2005;60:76-81.
16. Poets CF: When do infants need additional inspired oxygen? A review of the current literature. Pediatr Pulmonol 1998;26:424-428.
17. Tay-Uyboco JS, Kwiatkowski K, Cates DB, et al: Hypoxic airway constriction in infants of very low birth weight recovering from moderate to severe bronchopulmonary dysplasia. J Pediatr 1989;115:456-459.
18. Supplemental Therapeutic Oxygen for Prethreshold Retinopathy of Prematurity (STOP-ROP), a randomized, controlled trial. I. Primary outcomes. Pediatrics 2000;105:295-310.
19. BOOST(?)
20. Askie LM, Henderson-Smart DJ, Irwig L, Simpson JM: Oxygen-saturation targets and outcomes in extremely preterm infants. N Engl J Med 2003;349:959-967.
21. Thome UH, Carlo WA: Permissive hypercapnia. Semin Neonatol 2002;7:409-419.
22. Motoyama EK, Fort MD, Klesh KW, et al: Early onset of airway reactivity in premature infants with bronchopulmonary dysplasia. Am Rev Respir Dis 1987;136:50-57.
23. Northway WH Jr, Moss RB, Carlisle KB, et al: Late pulmonary sequelae of bronchopulmonary dysplasia. N Engl J Med 1990;323:1793-1799.

24. De Boeck K, Smith J, Van Lierde S, Devlieger H: Response to bronchodilators in clinically stable 1-year-old patients with bronchopulmonary dysplasia. Eur J Pediatr 1998;157:75-79.
25. Grier DG, Halliday HL: Corticosteroids in the prevention and management of bronchopulmonary dysplasia. Semin Neonatol 2003;8:83-91.
26. Yeh TF, Lin YJ, Lin HC, et al: Outcomes at school age after postnatal dexamethasone therapy for lung disease of prematurity. N Engl J Med 2004;350:1304-1313.
27. Dugas MA, Nguyen D, Frenette L, et al: Fluticasone inhalation in moderate cases of bronchopulmonary dysplasia. Pediatrics 2005;115:e566-e572.
28. Halliday HL: Use of steroids in the perinatal period. Paediatr Respir Rev 2004;5(Suppl A):S321-S327.
29. Kim S, Dueker GL, Hasher L, Goldstein D: Children's time of day preferences: Age, gender, and ethnic differences. Personality Individual Diff 2002;33:1083-1090.
30. Fenton C, Scott LJ, Plosker GL: Palivizumab: A review of its use as prophylaxis for serious respiratory syncytial virus infection. Paediatr Drugs 2004;6:177-197.
31. Kao LC, Warburton D, Cheng MH, et al: Effect of oral diuretics on pulmonary mechanics in infants with chronic bronchopulmonary dysplasia: Results of a double-blind crossover sequential trial. Pediatrics 1984;74:37-44.
32. Brion LP, Primhak RA, Ambrosio-Perez I: Diuretics acting on the distal renal tubule for preterm infants with (or developing) chronic lung disease. Cochrane Database Syst Rev 2000;2:CD001817.
33. Schell-Feith EA, Kist-Van Holthe JE, Conneman N, et al: Etiology of nephrocalcinosis in preterm neonates: Association of nutritional intake and urinary parameters. Kidney Int 2000;58:2102-2110.
34. Abrams SA: Chronic pulmonary insufficiency in children and its effects on growth and development. J Nutr 2001;131:938S-941S.
35. Markestad T, Fitzhardinge PM: Growth and development in children recovering from bronchopulmonary dysplasia. J Pediatr 1981;98:597-602.
36. Garg M, Kurzner SI, Bautista DB, Keens TG: Clinically unsuspected hypoxia during sleep and feeding in infants with bronchopulmonary dysplasia. Pediatrics 1988;81:635-642.
37. Pauwels RA, Pedersen S, Busse WW, et al: Early intervention with budesonide in mild persistent asthma: A randomised, double-blind trial. Lancet 2003;361:1071-1076.
38. Denne SC: Energy expenditure in infants with pulmonary insufficiency: Is there evidence for increased energy needs? J Nutr 2001;131:935S-937S.
39. Huysman WA, de Ridder M, de Bruin NC, et al: Growth and body composition in preterm infants with bronchopulmonary dysplasia. Arch Dis Child Fetal Neonatal Ed 2003;88:F46-F51.
40. Mercado-Deane MG, Burton EM, Harlow SA, et al: Swallowing dysfunction in infants less than 1 year of age. Pediatr Radiol 2001;31:423-428.
41. Hebestreit H: Exercise testing in children—what works, what doesn't, and where to go? Paediatr Respir Rev 2004;5(Suppl A):S11-S14.
42. Moyer-Mileur LD, Nielson DW, Pfeffer KD, et al: Eliminating sleep-associated hypoxemia improves growth in infants with bronchopulmonary dysplasia. Pediatrics 1996;98:779-783.
43. Noble L: Developments in neonatal technology continue to improve infant outcomes. Pediatr Ann 2003;32:595-603.
44. Short EJ, Klein NK, Lewis BA, et al: Cognitive and academic consequences of bronchopulmonary dysplasia and very low birth weight: 8-year-old outcomes. Pediatrics 2003;112:e359.
45. Doull IJM, Mok Q, Tasker RC: Tracheobronchomalacia in preterm infants with chronic lung disease. Arch Dis Child 1997;76:F203-F205.
46. Miller RW, Woo P, Kellman RK, Slagle TS: Tracheobronchial abnormalities in infants with bronchopulmonary dysplasia. J Pediatr 1987;111:779-782.
47. Primhak RA: Discharge and aftercare in chronic lung disease of the newborn. Semin Neonatol 2003;8:117-126.
48. Van Marter LJ: Strategies for preventing bronchopulmonary dysplasia. Curr Opin Pediatr 2005;17:174-180.

CHAPTER 78

Cystic Fibrosis

Marie Egan

Cystic fibrosis (CF) is a multisystem disease affecting the gastrointestinal, respiratory, and reproductive tracts and the sweat glands. It is the most common life-shortening autosomal recessive disorder in the white population, affecting approximately 1 in 2500 live births. However, CF occurs among persons of all races and ethnicities. Although the classic CF triad is chronic obstructive lung disease, exocrine pancreatic insufficiency, and sweat gland abnormalities, CF can mimic many other common pediatric conditions. Its presentation can vary from classic CF with severe manifestations early in life to later presentations with mild or even atypical symptoms.[1-4] Newborn screening for CF is becoming more common,[5-7] and changes in the management strategies for infants and children with CF are resulting in early and aggressive interventions for respiratory and nutritional problems.[8-10] Each of these factors has relevance to the pediatric hospitalist, who is often called on to evaluate and treat patients with chronic respiratory or gastrointestinal symptoms that may include CF in the differential diagnosis or to manage disease-related complications in individuals with known CF.

PATHOPHYSIOLOGY

CF is caused by mutations in a single gene on the long arm of chromosome 7 that encodes for the cystic fibrosis transmembrane conductance regulator (CFTR) protein.[11] More than 1000 disease-causing CFTR mutations have been identified, and six functional classifications have been devised to better understand the implications of specific gene abnormalities (Table 78-1). Despite the sheer number of CFTR mutations that lead to clinical disease (CF), there is a single mutation, ΔF508, that accounts for approximately 70% of affected alleles.[1-4] The ΔF508 mutation results in the deletion of phenylalanine in the 508 position of the CFTR protein and is an example of a class 2 mutation (see Table 78-1).

The CFTR protein functions as a chloride channel in the apical membrane of cells.[12] In addition, it regulates other apical membrane conductance pathways. CFTR is expressed in the cells of affected organs, including the respiratory and intestinal epithelia, pancreatic ducts, hepatobiliary tract, and sweat ducts. It is believed that the loss of function of the CFTR ion channel in CF results in abnormal ion and fluid movement across epithelial membranes, which leads to abnormal secretions in the affected organs.[1-4,13,14] These abnormalities can lead to inspissated mucus and obstruction of glandular ducts, inflammation, and eventual organ destruction. In the lung, this predisposes to specific bacterial infections that promote a cycle of inflammation, abnor-mal secretion, and, over time, lung damage. As a result, individuals with CF universally develop obstructive lung disease, and the majority of CF patients die of pulmonary complications.

CLINICAL PRESENTATION

CF affects multiple organ systems, which means that the presentation can be quite variable and can occur at a variety of ages. However, the classic description of CF is a triad of chronic obstructive lung disease, exocrine pancreatic insufficiency, and sweat electrolyte abnormalities. The majority of individuals with CF are diagnosed in early childhood, by a mean age of 2 years. However, the diagnosis of CF can be made in adolescence and even adulthood.[15-20] The diagnosis should be considered if one or more clinical features of the disease are present (Table 78-2), if there is a history of CF in a sibling, or if there is a positive neonatal screening test.

Failure to thrive and pulmonary manifestations are the most common presenting features. Although gastrointestinal manifestations of the disease may bring a child to medical attention, the pulmonary manifestations usually lead to the eventual decline in a child's health.

DIAGNOSIS

The diagnosis of CF is most often made and confirmed by sweat testing, whereby the chloride concentration of sweat is determined by quantitative pilocarpine iontophoresis. A sweat chloride concentration of greater than 60 mmol/L is consistent with the diagnosis of CF. A second sweat test to confirm the elevated chloride concentration is required. A sweat chloride concentration of less than 40 mmol/L is considered normal and is inconsistent with typical CF. A sweat chloride concentration between 40 and 60 mmol/L is considered borderline; the test should be repeated, and additional testing may be indicated. A number of other tests can be performed to confirm or support the diagnosis, including genotype analysis to directly screen for CF-causing mutations (Table 78-3).[4,17,21]

The role of neonatal screening for CF in the United States is evolving, and it is not universally applied. Further, testing protocols may vary from state to state. The neonatal screening test for CF is not 100% sensitive; therefore, it may be necessary to perform further diagnostic testing in symptomatic infants with negative newborn screens. The hospitalist should be aware of local neonatal screening practices and its limitations.[5,7,22] In addition, prenatal screening of women for carrier status is undergoing expansion.[23,24]

Table 78-1 CFTR Mutations

Class	CFTR Defect	Examples
1	No CFTR protein synthesis	W1282X, G542X
2	Block in processing of CFTR	ΔF508, N1303K
3	Improper regulation of CFTR	G551D, G551S
4	Abnormal conduction through CFTR	R117H, R334W
5	Reduced synthesis of CFTR	A455E
6	Mistargeting of CFTR	Q1412X

Table 78-2 Clinical Features Consistent with Cystic Fibrosis

Respiratory
  Chronic cough and sputum production
  Persistent chest radiograph findings, including atelectasis,
    bronchiectasis, hyperinflation, infiltrates
  Chronic airflow obstruction, which can present as wheezing
    and air trapping
  Persistent airway colonization with organisms such as
    Staphylococcus aureus, Pseudomonas aeruginosa,
    Burkholderia cepacia, and nontypable *Haemophilus*
    influenzae
  Nasal polyps
  Digital clubbing
  Chronic pansinusitis

Gastrointestinal
  Meconium ileus
  Distal ileal obstruction syndrome
  Rectal prolapse
  Focal biliary cirrhosis
  Multilobar cirrhosis
  Pancreatic insufficiency
  Recurrent pancreatitis
  Failure to thrive

Other
  Hypoproteinemia
  Hypoalbuminemia
  Hyponatremic, hypochloremic dehydration
  Chronic metabolic alkalosis (pseudo-Bartter syndrome)
  Male infertility (congenital bilateral absence of the vas
    deferens)

Table 78-3 Additional Tests that Support the Diagnosis of Cystic Fibrosis

Genotyping that demonstrates the presence of mutant CFTR
Computed tomography of the sinuses that demonstrates
  pansinusitis
Abnormal 72-hour fecal fat collection
Sputum or throat culture that demonstrates cystic fibrosis
  pathogens
Abnormal nasal potential difference measurements

Table 78-4 Signs and Symptoms of a Pulmonary Exacerbation of Cystic Fibrosis

Increased cough (duration, frequency, intensity)
Increased or new onset of sputum production
Change in sputum appearance
Increased or new onset of hemoptysis
Increased shortness of breath, wheezing
Decrease in exercise tolerance
Increase in fatigue, weakness, poor appetite, and malaise
Increased work of breathing manifested by use of accessory
  muscles and intercostal retractions
Increased respiratory rate
New findings on chest examination, such as crackles
Air trapping
Weight loss
Decrease in FEV_1 of 10% or more compared with baseline
Chest radiograph changes (increased air trapping, atelectasis,
  infiltrates)
Leukocytosis
Decreased oxygen saturation

FEV_1, forced expiratory volume in 1 second.

COURSE OF ILLNESS

Respiratory

CF is a chronic inflammatory bacterial bronchitis, and early in the course of CF airway disease, the respiratory tract is colonized with bacterial pathogens and subjected to an abnormal inflammatory environment.[25,26] This sets the stage for the development of chronic and progressive obstructive lung disease and the resulting symptoms, morbidity, and mortality.[9] Airway inflammation and infection are the main therapeutic targets for current and future CF therapies.[4]

The airways of CF patients are colonized with a number of unusual but specific pathogens, including *Staphylococcus aureus, Haemophilus influenzae, Pseudomonas aeruginosa, Stenotrophomonas maltophilia,* and *Burkholderia cepacia.*[1-4,13] In addition to chronic airway infection, there is exaggerated and sustained inflammation characterized by neutrophil-dominated inflammation and an abundance of interleukin-8.[25,27] It remains controversial whether the inflammation precedes infection or whether infection is the inciting event. The role of respiratory viruses in the inflammatory response in the CF airway remains an area of interest as well.[28]

CF is an example of a true bacterial bronchitis, and chronic bacterial colonization leads to localized peribronchial and endobronchial infection and inflammation. Over time, the infection and robust inflammatory response in the CF airway result in mucopurulent plugging of small and medium-size bronchioles. Eventually, the persistence of neutrophilic inflammation leads to destruction of the normal integrity of the airways. The airways become dilated and bronchiectatic secondary to proteolysis and chrondrolysis of the support tissues. The combination of mucous plugging of the airways and the loss of airway integrity can result in atelectasis, pneumonia, and eventually respiratory failure.[1,13]

A pulmonary exacerbation is a common reason for hospitalization. Because the baseline condition varies from patient to patient, it may be difficult for a hospitalist to accurately determine an acute or subacute deterioration. Table 78-4 provides guidelines for this assessment. The course of respiratory deterioration in CF is quite variable.[4,13,29] It has been suggested that, on average, there is a 2% to 4% loss in pulmonary function each year.[30] Patients are often referred for evaluation for bilateral lung transplantation once their forced expiratory volume in 1 second (FEV_1) reaches 30% of predicted[31]; however, indications for lung transplantation continue to evolve.[32,33] When patients with CF present with severe respiratory symptoms or acute respiratory failure, admission to the intensive care unit and the implementation of assisted ventilation should be considered on a case-by-case basis.[34] The general philosophy is that even acute CF manifestations in patients with severe disease may be reversible enough to allow for a meaningful return to baseline. This makes the treatment of very sick patients with CF unique and complex. Although palliative care and attention to end-of-life issues are critical for people with CF, many patients are treated for disease manifestations or complications at the same time that comfort care is being provided and pain and dyspnea are being treated.[35,36] Most CF patients die of respiratory failure. Currently, the median survival is 36 years, and CF is becoming an adult disease in many respects.[19] This represents a doubling of life expectancy compared with the average life expectancy of CF patients in 1989.

Gastrointestinal

Gastrointestinal manifestations of CF are common (see Table 78-2). Eighty-five percent of CF patients have exocrine pancreatic insufficiency, and gastrointestinal complaints can range from troublesome symptoms of steatorrhea and irritable bowel syndrome to life-threatening intestinal obstruction, liver disease, and an increased risk for gastrointestinal cancers.[37] In addition, the important relationship between excellent nutrition and the maintenance of lung health makes careful attention to the increased nutritional needs and gut health of CF patients an ongoing priority.[38] The hospitalist needs to be aware of the broad differential diagnosis of gastrointestinal disorders in CF in order to diagnose and manage these CF-related problems efficiently and appropriately.

Gastrointestinal manifestations of CF can begin in utero with meconium ileus, which is thought to be a result of exocrine pancreatic insufficiency. In 10% to 15% of infants with CF, inspissated, tenacious meconium can obstruct the distal ileum in utero, leading to intestinal obstruction in the immediate newborn period. This problem is usually addressed in the special care nursery, and recurrent intestinal obstruction in infancy is uncommon. Exocrine pancreatic insufficiency can also present in the newborn period with symptomatic fat malabsorption resulting in failure to thrive. Other early manifestations include nonspecific feeding difficulties and irritability during feedings. Approximately 50% of infants with CF display signs of pancreatic exocrine insufficiency at birth, and 85% to 90% of individuals with CF develop symptomatic pancreatic insufficiency within the first few years of life.[1-3,39] Poor growth, rectal prolapse, and, rarely, fat-soluble vitamin (A, D, E, K) deficiencies are all signs of fat malabsorption that may prompt an evaluation for CF in an undiagnosed patient; these are also indications of the need for intervention in an individual with known CF.[39]

In addition to exocrine pancreatic insufficiency, CF patients can develop carbohydrate intolerance that can progress to diabetes, most commonly during adolescence, in

Table 78-5 Causes of Abdominal Pain in Cystic Fibrosis

Upper abdominal pain
  Gastroesophageal reflux
  Gastritis
  Gallbladder disease
  Pancreatitis

Mid-abdominal pain
  Obstipation
  Distal ileal obstruction syndrome
  Appendicitis
  Irritable bowel syndrome
  Steatorrhea

Lower abdominal pain
  Irritable bowel syndrome
  Steatorrhea
  Obstipation
  Distal ileal obstruction syndrome
  Antibiotic-associated colitis (*Clostridium difficile*)

Other
  Renal stones
  Fibrosing colonopathy
  Colon cancer
  Rectal prolaspe

Adapted from Yankaskas JR, Marshall BC, Sufian B, et al: Cystic fibrosis adult care: Consensus conference report. Chest 2004;125:1S-39S.

a small percentage of patients.[4,40] CF-related diabetes most often results in nonketotic hyperglycemia and is exacerbated by acute illness and the concurrent use of corticosteroids. CF-related diabetes is also associated with a more rapid decline in lung function and clinical status; therefore, aggressive management, often with insulin therapy, is needed to optimize glycemic control. Further, CF-related diabetes is associated with the same secondary complications as is diabetes mellitus. The management of carbohydrate intolerance in this population can be challenging. A high-fat, high-calorie diet is recommended because these patients have both increased caloric needs owing to chronic illness and increased losses due to malabsorption.

The hepatobiliary tree can also be affected in CF. Focal biliary cirrhosis is characterized by inspissated eosinophilic amorphous secretions in the intrahepatic bile ducts, which can lead to bile duct obstruction followed by proliferation, inflammation, and fibrosis with focal destruction. Approximately 25% of patients develop liver disease. In a small number of patients, the focal biliary cirrhosis can be associated with portal hypertension and its complications, including hypersplenism and variceal bleeding. In some patients, cirrhosis can progress to frank liver failure, requiring evaluation for liver transplantation.[41]

Abdominal pain is common in patients with CF, and the list of causes is broad; some, however, are specific to CF (Table 78-5). Notably, recurrent intestinal obstruction can occur in older patients and is referred to as distal ileal obstruction syndrome.[1-4,17,19,37] This syndrome presents with symptoms of intestinal obstruction, with abdominal pain, vomiting, and distention. Often there is a history of obstipation, but this is not universal. CF patients are also at increased risk for hepatobiliary disease, including cholelithiasis and cholecystitis,[41,42] renal stones,[43,44] pancreatitis,[45] antibiotic-associated colitis, and fibrosing colonopathy.[19]

TREATMENT

Proactive Daily Care

Because there is no approved therapy that treats the underlying genetic defect in CF, the major goal of management is to slow the rate of pulmonary decline and thus preserve respiratory function. A comprehensive multidisciplinary approach to patient care has been instituted at CF centers worldwide. In addition, the Cystic Fibrosis Foundation has established clinical practice guidelines that are followed at most CF centers in the United States. These guidelines emphasize routine quarterly monitoring of the health status of CF patients, as well as patient and family education.

Nutrition

Significant emphasis is placed on the nutritional status of patients with CF owing to the strong link between nutritional health and preservation of pulmonary function. Patients often have much higher daily caloric requirements compared with individuals who do not have CF. These increased needs are believed to be secondary to chronic infection and inflammation and, in some cases, the increased work of breathing. CF patients are encouraged to eat unrestricted high-calorie, high-fat diets. Pancreatic enzyme supplementation is necessary for all pancreatic-insufficient patients. Enzymes are administered as enteric-coated tablets or microspheres, usually given at 500 to 1500 units lipase/kg per meal or snack. Patients are also given vitamin supplements that are high in fat-soluble vitamins A, D, E, and K.[39,46]

Pulmonary Care

To maintain lung health, patients require daily preventive care that is individualized, based on daily symptoms, age, airway microbiology, and pulmonary function.[13,47] Preventive care plans include daily airway clearance maneuvers and an array of medications, such as bronchodilators, mucus-thinning agents, anti-inflammatory agents, and antibiotics. Airway clearance techniques are generally performed twice daily, but this can be tailored to the specific needs and preferences of the patient.[18,48] Inhaled medications such as dornase alfa (Pulmozyme) to thin DNA-laden CF sputum are prescribed routinely.[49] Other medications such as inhaled corticosteroids, nebulized hypertonic saline, and albuterol are also prescribed. Patients who are chronically colonized with *P. aeruginosa* may be treated with inhaled tobramycin (TOBI); less commonly, other inhaled antibiotics such as colistin may be used as well.[50] Azithromycin three times a week was recently shown to be efficacious in patients with chronic *P. aeruginosa* colonization as well, most likely due to its anti-inflammatory activity.[51] Finally, high-dose ibuprofen is used chronically as an anti-inflammatory in some CF patients.[30] These management strategies derive from the pathophysiology of CF as a chronic, inflammatory, suppurative bronchitis and the philosophy that early intervention to preserve lung function will benefit patients when a cure for CF is developed.

Control of airway infection is a mainstay of management. Historically, it was thought that the progression of lung infection in CF began with airway colonization with *S. aureus* and that airway damage due to this organism set the stage for the acquisition of *P. aeruginosa*. However, early acquisition of *P. aeruginosa* has been documented, particularly as more patients are being diagnosed with newborn screening.[52] Prophylactic antibiotic therapy was used with the hope of eradicating or preventing bacterial colonization of the airways with *S. aureus*. Although some regimens were successful at eliminating *S. aureus*, they may have contributed in some cases to the earlier acquisition of *P. aeruginosa*, the major CF pathogen. The role of prophylactic antistaphylococcal antibiotics in CF remains an area of controversy, and the hospitalist may encounter some individuals with CF who have been treated prophylactically with agents such as trimethoprim-sulfamethoxazole, cephalexin, or dicloxacillin.[53,54]

It is widely agreed that infection with *P. aeruginosa* is highly significant and warrants treatment. Initially, patients are colonized with nonmucoid strains of *P. aeruginosa*, and early treatment of such strains can lead to transient eradication of these organisms.[52,55] Many clinicians believe that early, aggressive treatment of nonmucoid *P. aeruginosa* is essential because it may delay or prevent the acquisition of mucoid strains of the bacteria. However, to date, an optimal treatment for the eradication of nonmucoid *P. aeruginosa* has not been established.[13] Mucoid strains, which may be resistant to antimicrobial therapy and hence difficult to eradicate, are associated with progressive chronic infection and inflammation, as well as pulmonary function decline.

Acute Complications

The most notable pulmonary complications of CF are pulmonary exacerbations, hemoptysis, and pneumothorax. Once patients are colonized with organisms, they often have daily symptoms, which can include cough and sputum production. Periodically, however, these daily symptoms increase, leading to a significant decrease in pulmonary function and clinical status, which is referred to as a pulmonary exacerbation (see Table 78-4). The causes of these exacerbations vary and include viral infections, exposure to air pollutants, and reactive airway disease.[13]

Patients with mild pulmonary exacerbations are often treated as outpatients with oral and inhaled antibiotics. In addition, airway clearance therapy, mucolytics, and sometimes anti-inflammatory treatments may be increased to maximize mucociliary clearance of infected secretions. If a patient fails to improve with outpatient management, or if a patient presents with a severe exacerbation, hospitalization and intravenous antibiotics are needed. Standard therapy includes intravenous antibiotics for 14 to 21 days (Table 78-6).[13] In addition, airway clearance treatments, mucolytics, and anti-inflammatory therapy are maximized, and nutritional support is optimized. In the hospital, psychosocial support is offered. Reviewing the patient's daily outpatient health maintenance plan is helpful and often improves adherence once the patient is discharged. Although patients generally require 14 to 21 days of intravenous therapy, once they are demonstrating clinical improvement, the therapy can occasionally be continued at home (Table 78-7). It remains controversial whether home antibiotic therapy is as efficacious as in-hospital care, but it can be effective for some patients.[13,56,57]

Table 78-6   Intravenous Antibiotics to Treat Pulmonary Exacerbations of Cystic Fibrosis

Organism	Medication	Dose (mg/kg/dose)	Dosing Interval (hr)
Staphylococcus aureus	Cefazolin	30	8
	Nafcillin	25-50	6
Haemophilus influenzae	Ampicillin-sulbactam	25-100	6
Pseudomonas aeruginosa	Choose a combination of one β-lactam plus one aminoglycoside		
	β-lactam:		
	Ceftazidime	50	8
	Ticarcillin	100	6
	Piperacillin	100	6
	Imipenem	15-25	6
	Meropenem	40	8
	Aztreonam	50	8
	Aminoglycoside:		
	Tobramycin	3	8
	Amikacin	5-7.5	8
Burkholderia cepacia	Choose a combination of meropenem plus one of the additional medications	40	6
	Meropenem	40	6
	Additional:		
	Minocycline	2	12
	Amikacin	5-7.5	8
	Ceftazidime	50	8
	TMP-SMZ	4-5*	12
MRSA	Vancomycin	15	6

*Based on TMP component.
MRSA, methicillin-resistant *Staphylococcus aureus;* TMP-SMZ, trimethoprim-sulfamethoxazole.
Adapted from Gibson RL, Burns JL, Ramsey BW: Pathophysiology and management of pulmonary infections in cystic fibrosis. Am J Respir Crit Care Med 2003;168:918-951.

Table 78-7   Enteral Antibiotics to Treat Pulmonary Exacerbations of Cystic Fibrosis on an Outpatient Basis

Organism	Medication	Dose (mg/kg/dose)	Dosing Interval
Staphylococcus aureus	Dicloxacillin	6.25-12.5	qid
	Cephalexin	12.5-25	qid
	Amoxicillin-clavulanate	12.5-22.5	bid
	Erythromycin	15	tid
	Clarithromycin	7.5	bid
	Azithromycin	10 (day 1); 5 (days 2-5)	qd
	Clindamycin	3.5-7	tid
Haemophilus influenzae	Amoxicillin-clavulanate	12.5-22.5	bid
Pseudomonas aeruginosa	Ciprofloxacin	10-15	bid
	Inhaled tobramycin	300 mg/dose*	bid
	Inhaled colistin	150 mg/dose*	bid
Burkholderia cepacia	TMP-SMZ	4-5†	bid
	Doxycycline	5 (day 1); thereafter, 2.5	bid
	Minocycline	4 (day 1); thereafter, 2	bid

*Not based on weight.
†Based on TMP component.
TMP-SMZ, trimethoprim-sulfamethoxazole.
Adapted from Gibson RL, Burns JL, Ramsey BW: Pathophysiology and management of pulmonary infections in cystic fibrosis. Am J Respir Crit Care Med 2003;168:918-951.

If a pulmonary exacerbation fails to improve with standard therapy, the differential diagnosis is broadened to include unusual infections such as fungi, atypical mycobacteria, or a different bacterial pathogen. In addition, disease complications such as the development of CF-related diabetes may be associated with an infectious exacerbation that fails to improve.

Hemoptysis is a frightening complication of CF airway disease and can be minor or major in nature. It can accompany a flare of CF bronchitis or occur as an isolated event.[58,59] Massive or major hemoptysis is defined as the expectoration of more than 240 mL of blood in a 24-hour period; it may be life threatening due to asphyxiation or hypotension. Recurrent episodes of significant bleeding over a short period, such as the expectoration of 100 mL/day over several days, is also considered major hemoptysis. Massive hemoptysis is caused by bleeding in the collateral circulation (bronchial arterial vessels), which develops over time in CF lung disease due to pulmonary inflammation and infection. These abnormal vessels are subject to systemic arterial pressures and are prone to brisk bleeding. Massive hemoptysis occurs most commonly with advanced lung disease but may occur in patients with less severe lung disease ($FEV_1 > 50\%$) as well.[58] Detailed discussion of the management of massive hemoptysis is beyond the scope of this chapter; however, it usually involves aggressive anti-infective therapy for a CF exacerbation, supportive respiratory care as indicated, and sometimes specialized interventions such as bronchial artery embolization for unremitting bleeding.[60,61] Minor hemoptysis may occur as blood streaking in the sputum or as the isolated expectoration of a small volume of blood. In contrast to massive hemoptysis, which is a true vascular event, this low-pressure bleeding is usually due to airway inflammation with erosion of the airway wall. It generally resolves spontaneously with treatment of the underlying airway infection.

Pneumothorax in CF occurs due to the rupture of subpleural apical blebs, which form as the emphysematous changes in CF lung disease progress. Pneumothorax occurs more commonly in older CF patients with more advanced lung disease and may manifest acutely as chest pain or shortness of breath.[62] Like hemoptysis, pneumothorax is a frightening complication of CF and is an indication for hospital admission. The management of pneumothorax in CF is similar to the management of spontaneous pneumothorax in non-CF patients (see Chapter 147). Although observation alone may be appropriate for asymptomatic patients, chest tube placement with drainage is often indicated.[63,64] Unfortunately, the occurrence of pneumothorax in an individual with CF is associated with increased morbidity and mortality.[62]

Because patients with CF may be colonized with antibiotic-resistant organisms, infection control measures are required during hospitalization to prevent the nosocomial spread of organisms such as methicillin-resistant *S. aureus* and multiply resistant gram-negative rods to other hospitalized patients with compromised immunity.[47] The choice of antibiotics should be based on recent sputum cultures. Cultures should be obtained during each quarterly outpatient visit to the CF center, and additional cultures should be obtained when symptoms increase. Common pathogens and antibiotic choices are listed in Tables 78-6 and 78-7. Once antibiotics are started, the clinical response needs to be carefully assessed. Patients should experience a decrease in cough, shortness of breath, and sputum production; a change in mucus rheology (mucus should be less tenacious and easier to expectorate); an improvement in pulmonary function; and a decrease in sputum microbial density.[13]

CF patients are also at increased risk for gastrointestinal emergencies. Hospitalization may be warranted for prompt evaluation, close observation, or definitive treatment. These complications (discussed earlier) include acute cholecystitis, pancreatitis, bowel obstruction, and gastrointestinal hemorrhage.

CONSULTATION

Most patients with CF are managed by a CF center, and this team should be involved in the care of any hospitalized patient. If a patient with CF is hospitalized while traveling, consultation with the patient's usual center may be obtained if a local center is unavailable. Other subspecialists involved in the care and management of CF patients include gastroenterologists, infectious disease specialists, endocrinologists, and surgical specialists such as otolaryngologists. In addition to center-based physicians, nutritionists, respiratory therapists, social workers, and physical therapists all serve important roles in the CF care team.

ADMISSION CRITERIA

- New diagnosis of CF in a symptomatic individual
- Pulmonary exacerbation despite appropriate outpatient management
- Hemoptysis
- Pneumothorax
- Intestinal obstruction or other severe gastrointestinal manifestation
- New disease complication, such as diabetes

DISCHARGE CRITERIA

- Control of the acute process
- Return to the baseline condition or institution of an outpatient regimen and follow-up directed at this goal

IN A NUTSHELL

- CF is a common multisystem disorder with various presentations that enters the differential diagnosis in a patient with chronic respiratory or gastrointestinal symptoms.
- Common reasons for the hospitalization of CF patients include pulmonary exacerbation, pneumothorax, and hemoptysis.
- Acute cholecystitis, bowel obstruction, and new-onset diabetes are other complications of CF that warrant hospitalization.
- Infection control measures are important, because highly resistant organisms may colonize some CF patients. Isolation techniques to prevent the transmission of these organisms to other immunocompromised hosts are key.
- CF centers provide primary, extensive, long-term, multidisciplinary care, and these teams should be involved early in the inpatient care of CF patients.

ON THE HORIZON

- A number of future therapeutic strategies are directed toward correcting the basic defect by means of gene replacement, augmentation of the dysfunctional CFTR protein, or bypassing of the dysfunctional CFTR protein.[3,4] Because many of these strategies will be tailored to specific CFTR mutations, patients will need to undergo genotype analysis.[21]
- A number of agents that augment mutant CFTR activity or activate alternative ion channels to normalize airway surface fluid have been identified and are moving to small clinical trials.
- A variety of new anti-inflammatory agents are being developed, as well as new antimicrobial agents.

SUGGESTED READINGS

Gibson RL, Burns JL, Ramsey BW: Pathophysiology and management of pulmonary infections in cystic fibrosis. Am J Respir Crit Care Med 2003;168:918-951.

Mascarenhas MR: Treatment of gastrointestinal problems in cystic fibrosis. Curr Treat Options Gastroenterol 2003;6:427-441.

Orenstein DM, Winnie GB, Altman H: Cystic fibrosis: A 2002 update. J Pediatr 2002;140:156-164.

Saiman L, Siegel J: Infection control recommendations for patients with cystic fibrosis: Microbiology, important pathogens, and infection control practices to prevent patient-to-patient transmission. Am J Infect Control 2003;31:S1-S62.

REFERENCES

1. Davis PB, Drumm M, Konstan MW: Cystic fibrosis. Am J Respir Crit Care Med 1996;154:1229-1256.
2. Sheppard DN, Welsh MJ: Structure and function of the CFTR chloride channel. Physiol Rev 1999;79:S23-S45.
3. Rosenstein BJ, Zeitlin PL: Cystic fibrosis. Lancet 1998;351:277-282.
4. Ratjen F, Doring G: Cystic fibrosis. Lancet 2003;361:681-689.
5. Castellani C: Evidence for newborn screening for cystic fibrosis. Paediatr Respir Rev 2003;4:278-284.
6. Grosse SD, Boyle CA, Botkin JR, et al: Newborn screening for cystic fibrosis: Evaluation of benefits and risks and recommendations for state newborn screening programs. MMWR Recomm Rep 2004;53:1-36.
7. Wilfond BS, Gollust SE: Policy issues for expanding newborn screening programs: The cystic fibrosis newborn screening experience in the United States. J Pediatr 2005;146:668-674.
8. Doring G, Hoiby N: Early intervention and prevention of lung disease in cystic fibrosis: A European consensus. J Cyst Fibros 2004;3:67-91.
9. Rosenfeld M, Gibson RL, McNamara S, et al: Early pulmonary infection, inflammation, and clinical outcomes in infants with cystic fibrosis. Pediatr Pulmonol 2001;32:356-366.
10. Varlotta L: Management and care of the newly diagnosed patient with cystic fibrosis. Curr Opin Pulm Med 1998;4:311-318.
11. Gallati S: Genetics of cystic fibrosis. Semin Respir Crit Care Med 2003;24:629-638.
12. Vankeerberghen A, Cuppens H, Cassiman JJ: The cystic fibrosis transmembrane conductance regulator: An intriguing protein with pleiotropic functions. J Cyst Fibros 2002;1:13-29.
13. Gibson RL, Burns JL, Ramsey BW: Pathophysiology and management of pulmonary infections in cystic fibrosis. Am J Respir Crit Care Med 2003;168:918-951.
14. Boucher RC: New concepts of the pathogenesis of cystic fibrosis lung disease. Eur Respir J 2004;23:146-158.
15. Cystic Fibrosis Foundation Patient Registry. Bethesda, Md, Cystic Fibrosis Foundation, 2002.
16. Orenstein DM, Winnie GB, Altman H: Cystic fibrosis: A 2002 update. J Pediatr 2002;140:156-164.
17. Rosenstein BJ, Cutting GR: The diagnosis of cystic fibrosis: A consensus statement. Cystic Fibrosis Foundation Consensus Panel. J Pediatr 1998;132:589-595.
18. Wagener JS, Headley AA: Cystic fibrosis: Current trends in respiratory care. Respir Care 2003;48:234-245; discussion 246-247.
19. Yankaskas JR, Marshall BC, Sufian B, et al: Cystic fibrosis adult care: Consensus conference report. Chest 2004;125:1S-39S.
20. Rosenbluth D, Goodenberger D: Cystic fibrosis in an elderly woman. Chest 1997;112:1124-1126.
21. Richards CS, Bradley LA, Amos J, et al: Standards and guidelines for CFTR mutation testing. Genet Med 2002;4:379-391.
22. Wagener JS, Sontag MK, Sagel SD, Accurso FJ: Update on newborn screening for cystic fibrosis. Curr Opin Pulm Med 2004;10:500-504.
23. Gregg AR, Simpson JL: Genetic screening for cystic fibrosis. Obstet Gynecol Clin North Am 2002;29:329-240.
24. Mennuti MT, Thomson E, Press N: Screening for cystic fibrosis carrier state. Obstet Gynecol 1999;93:456-461.
25. Chmiel JF, Berger M, Konstan MW: The role of inflammation in the pathophysiology of CF lung disease. Clin Rev Allergy Immunol 2002;23:5-27.
26. Elkin S, Geddes D: Pseudomonal infection in cystic fibrosis: The battle continues. Expert Rev Anti Infect Ther 2003;1:609-618.
27. Heijerman H: Infection and inflammation in cystic fibrosis: A short review. J Cyst Fibros 2005;4(Suppl 2):3-5.
28. Hiatt PW, Grace SC, Kozinetz CA, et al: Effects of viral lower respiratory tract infection on lung function in infants with cystic fibrosis. Pediatrics 1999;103:619-626.
29. Schidlow DV, Taussig LM, Knowles MR: Cystic Fibrosis Foundation consensus conference report on pulmonary complications of cystic fibrosis. Pediatr Pulmonol 1993;15:187-198.
30. Konstan MW, Byard PJ, Hoppel CL, Davis PB: Effect of high-dose ibuprofen in patients with cystic fibrosis. N Engl J Med 1995;332:848-854.
31. Yankaskas JR, Mallory GB Jr: Lung transplantation in cystic fibrosis: Consensus conference statement. Chest 1998;113:217-226.
32. Rosenbluth DB, Wilson K, Ferkol T, Schuster DP: Lung function decline in cystic fibrosis patients and timing for lung transplantation referral. Chest 2004;126:412-419.
33. Aurora P, Wade A, Whitmore P, Whitehead B: A model for predicting life expectancy of children with cystic fibrosis. Eur Respir J 2000;16:1056-1060.
34. Vedam H, Moriarty C, Torzillo PJ, et al: Improved outcomes of patients with cystic fibrosis admitted to the intensive care unit. J Cyst Fibros 2004;3:8-14.
35. Robinson WM, Ravilly S, Berde C, Wohl ME: End-of-life care in cystic fibrosis. Pediatrics 1997;100:205-209.
36. Robinson W: Palliative care in cystic fibrosis. J Palliat Med 2000;3:187-192.
37. Mascarenhas MR: Treatment of gastrointestinal problems in cystic fibrosis. Curr Treat Options Gastroenterol 2003;6:427-441.
38. Konstan MW, Butler SM, Wohl ME, et al: Growth and nutritional indexes in early life predict pulmonary function in cystic fibrosis. J Pediatr 2003;142:624-630.
39. Borowitz D, Baker RD, Stallings V: Consensus report on nutrition for pediatric patients with cystic fibrosis. J Pediatr Gastroenterol Nutr 2002;35:246-259.
40. Moran A, Hardin D, Rodman D, et al: Diagnosis, screening and management of cystic fibrosis related diabetes mellitus: A consensus conference report. Diabetes Res Clin Pract 1999;45:61-73.
41. Sokol RJ, Durie PR: Recommendations for management of liver and biliary tract disease in cystic fibrosis. Cystic Fibrosis Foundation Hepatobiliary Disease Consensus Group. J Pediatr Gastroenterol Nutr 1999;28(Suppl 1):S1-S13.
42. Jebbink MC, Heijerman HG, Masclee AA, Lamers CB: Gallbladder disease in cystic fibrosis. Neth J Med 1992;41:123-126.

43. Gibney EM, Goldfarb DS: The association of nephrolithiasis with cystic fibrosis. Am J Kidney Dis 2003;42:1-11.

44. Chidekel AS, Dolan TF Jr: Cystic fibrosis and calcium oxalate nephrolithiasis. Yale J Biol Med 1996;69:317-321.

45. De Boeck K, Weren M, Proesmans M, Kerem E: Pancreatitis among patients with cystic fibrosis: Correlation with pancreatic status and genotype. Pediatrics 2005;115:e463-e469.

46. Sinaasappel M, Stern M, Littlewood J, et al: Nutrition in patients with cystic fibrosis: A European consensus. J Cyst Fibros 2002;1:51-75.

47. Saiman L, Siegel J: Infection control recommendations for patients with cystic fibrosis: Microbiology, important pathogens, and infection control practices to prevent patient-to-patient transmission. Am J Infect Control 2003;31:S1-S62.

48. Flume PA: Airway clearance techniques. Semin Respir Crit Care Med 2003;24:727-736.

49. Suri R: The use of human deoxyribonuclease (rhDNase) in the management of cystic fibrosis. BioDrugs 2005;19:135-144.

50. Sexauer WP, Fiel SB: Aerosolized antibiotics in cystic fibrosis. Semin Respir Crit Care Med 2003;24:717-726.

51. Saiman L, Marshall BC, Mayer-Hamblett N, et al: Azithromycin in patients with cystic fibrosis chronically infected with *Pseudomonas aeruginosa:* A randomized controlled trial. JAMA 2003;290:1749-1756.

52. Li Z, Kosorok MR, Farrell PM, et al: Longitudinal development of mucoid *Pseudomonas aeruginosa* infection and lung disease progression in children with cystic fibrosis. JAMA 2005;293:581-588.

53. Stutman HR, Lieberman JM, Nussbaum E, Marks MI: Antibiotic prophylaxis in infants and young children with cystic fibrosis: A randomized controlled trial. J Pediatr 2002;140:299-305.

54. Smyth A, Walters S: Prophylactic antibiotics for cystic fibrosis. Cochrane Database Syst Rev 2003;CD001912.

55. Taccetti G, Campana S, Festini F, et al: Early eradication therapy against *Pseudomonas aeruginosa* in cystic fibrosis patients. Eur Respir J 2005;26:458-461.

56. Bosworth DG, Nielson DW: Effectiveness of home versus hospital care in the routine treatment of cystic fibrosis. Pediatr Pulmonol 1997;24:42-47.

57. Thornton J, Elliott R, Tully MP, et al: Long term clinical outcome of home and hospital intravenous antibiotic treatment in adults with cystic fibrosis. Thorax 2004;59:242-246.

58. Barben JU, Ditchfield M, Carlin JB, et al: Major haemoptysis in children with cystic fibrosis: A 20-year retrospective study. J Cyst Fibros 2003;2:105-111.

59. Flume PA, Yankaskas JR, Ebeling M, et al: Massive hemoptysis in cystic fibrosis. Chest 2005;128:729-738.

60. Cipolli M, Perini S, Valletta EA, Mastella G: Bronchial artery embolization in the management of hemoptysis in cystic fibrosis. Pediatr Pulmonol 1995;19:344-347.

61. Barben J, Robertson D, Olinsky A, Ditchfield M: Bronchial artery embolization for hemoptysis in young patients with cystic fibrosis. Radiology 2002;224:124-130.

62. Flume PA, Strange C, Ye X, et al: Pneumothorax in cystic fibrosis. Chest 2005;28:720-728.

63. Baumann MH, Strange C: The clinician's perspective on pneumothorax management. Chest 1997;112:822-828.

64. Baumann MH: Treatment of spontaneous pneumothorax. Curr Opin Pulm Med 2000;6:275-280.

CHAPTER 79

Choking and Foreign Body Aspiration

Aaron S. Chidekel and Natalie Hayes

Choking is defined as the interruption of respiration due to the internal obstruction of the airway. Aspiration is defined as the penetration of foreign material into the trachea, beyond the vocal cords. Airway obstruction relating to the presence of a foreign body may be intraluminal (foreign body within the airway) or extraluminal (foreign body within the esophagus causing airway compression). Children suffering from these conditions may present with cardiorespiratory arrest, impending respiratory arrest, a stable but symptomatic status, or sequelae of a previous choking or aspiration event. These patients often present to hospitalists in the emergency department or inpatient setting, making knowledge of the full range of presentations important.

The death rate from unintentional suffocation in children aged 0 to 4 years, which includes the aspiration or ingestion of food, is estimated at 3 per 100,000; this declines nearly by a factor of 10, to 0.36 per 100,000, for children aged 5 to 9 years.[1] Data from Australia support a similar incidence and trend, with rates of fatal injury being 10 times greater in the first years of life compared with the second decade of life.[2] In the United States, choking on food or other foreign objects is the direct cause of death of several hundred children each year.[3-6] Choking thus remains a major cause of preventable death and morbidity in the United States, although efforts by the federal government and the public health community have made some progress in decreasing its occurrence.

PATHOPHYSIOLOGY

Choking and aspiration involve the interaction between an object and the airway in such a way as to prevent breathing from being fully effective. It may be a reversible event if airway defenses are able to expel the foreign material and clear the airway, or it may result in symptomatic airway obstruction.

If severe enough, airway obstruction leads to oxygen deprivation and death if not rapidly and effectively addressed. If there is partial obstruction of the airway, a subacute process may result in infection, inflammation, and lung injury distal to the lodged object. Another mechanism of choking involves the impaction of foreign material in the esophagus, with resultant airway compression.

Choking results from a complex interaction among the individual, the environment, and the object at hand. Young children are at highest risk for choking owing to their incompletely developed dentition and oral skills, smaller airways, immature swallowing mechanisms, and lack of experience and cognition. Also, they tend to explore the world by bringing objects to their mouths. Children with developmental delay, hypotonia, dysphagia, or anatomic abnormalities

retain this increased risk into their later years (see Chapter 101). In addition, older siblings or playmates may share inappropriate foods or toys with younger siblings. Environmental factors such as lack of supervision, access to an object, and circumstances surrounding meals and snacks are also important. In many published reports, males have a higher risk of choking than do females.[3-7]

Common choking hazards have been well studied and characterized. Object characteristics most commonly associated with choking in children include the following: small, round, smooth, and slippery. Objects of any size with a pliable texture that can conform to the shape of the airway or adhere to the airway mucosa and form a plug represent a hazard as well. If a plug forms and cannot be dislodged in a timely fashion, due to either a lack of adequate response by the child or a supervising adult or the characteristics of the object itself, death will ultimately ensue from asphyxiation. Food and toys are the most common objects involved in accidental choking and foreign body aspiration (Table 79-1).

CLINICAL PRESENTATION

A description of the choking event and the circumstances should be obtained, and any predisposing factors or previous choking episodes should be identified. However, the clinician may not be able to elicit this information, or it may not be available at the time of the initial evaluation. One symptom that is commonly associated with foreign body aspiration is the "penetration syndrome," defined as the sudden onset of choking and intractable coughing, with or without vomiting.[8,9] Patients with acute complete airway obstruction at or above the level of the carina are immediately symptomatic with aphonia, lack of cough, cyanosis, or agitation that can progress to obtundation or cardiopulmonary arrest. Partial airway obstruction may present with a range of symptoms, depending on the degree or level of the obstruction. When the blockage occurs in the extrathoracic airway, physical examination findings may include stridor, cough, or dysphonia. With obstruction of the intrathoracic airway, cough, localized wheezing, or asymmetrical breath sounds may be present. Evidence of increased work of breathing, such as retractions, nasal flaring, or use of accessory muscles, is more prominent with more complete obstruction or involvement of a more proximal airway. In some cases, the physical examination may be normal, especially with more distal airway involvement. Progression from partial airway obstruction to complete obstruction can occur, as can cardiorespiratory failure due to severe or prolonged partial obstruction. Conversely, complete airway obstruction may transition to partial airway obstruction, with subsequent improvement in symptoms; these children may be particularly unstable, however, and deterioration back to complete airway obstruction is a significant concern. Esophageal foreign bodies may present with drooling, odynophagia, gagging, retching, and respiratory distress due to impingement of the esophagus on the membranous posterior wall of the trachea.

In the subacute or chronic setting, patients may present with chronic cough and fever as postobstructive infection develops in the lung parenchyma distal to the aspirated object. Some foreign objects, especially plant and food material, can evoke a particularly intense inflammatory reaction at the site of the foreign body (foreign body reaction).

EVALUATION

A patient presenting with a first episode of wheezing should have a chest radiograph to rule out a foreign body or another unexpected abnormality.[10,11] Children with localized, nonmigratory, or monophonic wheezing; those with a history of a previous choking spell or aspiration event; and those with suspected foreign body ingestion should be imaged as well.

Table 79-1   Common Objects with a High Risk for Causing Choking

Foods
  Hot dogs
  Grapes
  Peanuts
  Other nuts
  Popcorn
  Raw carrots
  Apples

Toys
  Latex balloons
  Small balls
  Marbles
  Toys containing small parts

Other
  Jewelry
  Watch batteries

If a radiopaque foreign body is not identified on the initial anteroposterior and lateral chest radiographs, additional views may be warranted. Inspiratory and expiratory anteroposterior chest radiographs or bilateral decubitus views may indirectly indicate the presence of a radiolucent foreign body. In the acute setting, when a foreign body obstructs a bronchus or bronchiole, air trapping can occur distal to the airway obstruction. During inspiration, the intrathoracic airways are relatively expanded, which allows aeration around an obstructing foreign body. During expiration, there is narrowing of these airways, which can impede flow out of the partially obstructed lung segment, resulting in localized air trapping (ball-valve effect). Children with partial airway obstruction distal to the carina demonstrate inflation throughout both lung fields on an inspiratory chest radiograph. However, on exhalation, hyperinflation or hyperlucency in the lung segment beyond the site of obstruction can be seen.

Bilateral decubitus chest films are used when the patient is too young or otherwise unable to take a deep breath on request. Normally, the dependent lung shows increased density throughout the tissue owing to decreased aeration and increased perfusion, while the nondependent lung remains aerated. With an obstruction, a segment of the involved lung remains aerated when placed in the dependent position, owing to air trapping. In a subacute or chronic setting, lung tissue distal to the point of airway obstruction often appears radiodense. This may be due to postobstructive atelectasis or pneumonia. These radiographic findings are summarized in Table 79-2.

Patients with a clinical history and symptoms of foreign body aspiration may require airway endoscopy if the clinical likelihood or suspicion remains high, even in the presence of unrevealing imaging studies. Computed tomography of the chest may be needed to demonstrate a distal obstruction.

TREATMENT

Stabilization of the airway is the first priority. A child with a tenuous airway who is able to maintain ventilation and oxygenation should have as little intervention as possible until a team is assembled that can secure a definitive airway.

Table 79-2   Typical Chest Radiographic Findings of a Unilateral Intrabronchial Foreign Body

View	ACUTE		SUBACUTE OR CHRONIC	
	Lung with Obstruction	*Lung without Obstruction*	*Lung with Obstruction*	*Lung without Obstruction*
Inspiration	Uniform aeration	Uniform aeration	Persistent segment of atelectasis	Uniform aeration
Expiration	Segment of persistent aeration (hyperlucency)	Decreased aeration throughout lung	Decreased aeration throughout lung	Decreased aeration throughout lung
Decubitus (obstructed lung dependent)	Segment of persistent aeration (hyperlucency)	Uniform aeration	Decreased aeration throughout lung	Uniform aeration
Decubitus (unobstructed lung dependent)	Uniform aeration	Decreased aeration throughout lung	Persistent segment of atelectasis	Decreased aeration throughout lung

This may include anesthesiology, otolaryngology, pulmonology, and respiratory therapy personnel, as well as staff from the operating room or intensive care unit.

Cardiorespiratory and pulse oximetry monitoring should be available during the initial assessment and should continue until the respiratory compromise is resolved. Supplemental oxygen should be provided in the least noxious manner that allows the maintenance of adequate oxygenation. Heliox has been shown to improve gas exchange in patients with upper airway obstruction and acute lung injury.[12]

Consultation with an otolaryngologist or pediatric pulmonologist is required for definitive diagnosis and management of an airway foreign body. In general, otolaryngology is the primary medical specialty involved with the management and retrieval of inhaled foreign bodies. Although airway foreign bodies can be visualized by either flexible or rigid bronchoscopy, the rigid bronchoscope is better suited for the removal of objects from the airway. It allows for ventilation through the bronchoscope and has a greater array of instruments available to facilitate the removal of various types of objects. Removal of foreign objects via flexible bronchoscopy has been reported, however, and in some cases, a combined approach using both flexible and rigid bronchoscopy may be required to fully assess the airways and ensure a good outcome.

If a severe inflammatory reaction or lung injury due to chronic infection has occurred, it may be difficult to retrieve the foreign body, or residual lung or airway damage may occur. In these rare cases, bronchotomy or even lobectomy may be required.

Occasionally, patients are treated with antibiotics or corticosteroids, either inhaled or systemic, when evidence of infection or severe airway inflammation is evident. The choice of antibiotic is based on the results of Gram stain or cultures taken at bronchoscopy. Empirical anaerobic coverage is recommended in the presence of a postobstructive pneumonia or lung abscess due to a retained foreign body. A trial of bronchodilators may be considered and continued in those who respond to them. Most often, however, airway symptoms resolve quickly and without further treatment once the object is removed.

Some practitioners recommend a follow-up airway endoscopy to ensure the absence of a second foreign body that was not visualized during the initial bronchoscopy and to verify complete resolution of any granulation tissue. In general, advances in medical treatment have improved the outcomes of children with retained endobronchial or esophageal foreign bodies who are able to maintain adequate gas exchange and obtain medical assistance before asphyxiation.

Esophagoscopy may be necessary for the removal of esophageal foreign bodies, especially when compression of the airway causes respiratory compromise. This may be performed by either an otolaryngologist or a gastroenterologist.

ADMISSION CRITERIA

- Airway instability, respiratory distress, or hypoxemia
- Suggestive history with supportive clinical features that warrant prompt diagnostic evaluation
- Need for definitive intervention, such as bronchoscopy

DISCHARGE CRITERIA

- Removal of the foreign body
- Resolution of respiratory compromise
- Arrangement for appropriate outpatient follow-up (e.g., appointment with subspecialist for follow-up bronchoscopy)

PREVENTION

In addition to anticipatory guidance, the most effective preventive strategies are specific changes in product design and materials to keep hazardous objects away from small children in the first place. In 1979 the federal Hazardous Substances Act banned toy products with small parts intended for children younger than 3 years.[1] Since 1980 the Consumer Product Safety Commission has required standards for toys intended for this age group. The general standard is determined by a device used to identify those objects that pose a major choking hazard.[13,14] This device, measuring 1.25 inches in diameter by 1 to 2.25 inches in height, is used to evaluate the size and shape of objects that might be able to slip into the posterior pharynx and potentially cause airway obstruction. Any objects that can fit inside the cylinder are deemed to be choking hazards and are banned for children younger than 3 years.[15] One study found that 99% of objects associated with choking fit into this device.[14] To address some residual concerns not covered by these standards, the Child Safety Protection Act of 1995 changed some of the size labeling requirements further, to encompass balls with a diameter of 1.75 inches or less.[16] The Injury Prevention Program sponsored by the American Academy of Pediatrics distributes safety handouts that provide age-appropriate guidance for the prevention of choking and aspiration.

IN A NUTSHELL

- Choking is a serious and potentially life-threatening event that occurs more frequently in toddlers and preschoolers than in older children.
- Inappropriate food, toys, and household items play a major role in pediatric choking events.
- Clinical presentations vary tremendously, based on the degree of airway obstruction and the point along the respiratory tract at which the obstruction occurs.
- Partial airway obstruction near the larynx or in the proximal trachea often presents with coughing, stridor, or dysphonia.
- Obstruction of the intrathoracic airways typically presents with cough, wheezing, or asymmetrical breath sounds.
- Prompt removal of the foreign body is associated with an excellent outcome.

ON THE HORIZON

- Computed tomography virtual bronchoscopy may be useful in determining the presence of an aspirated foreign body in children with normal chest radiographs but worrisome clinical examinations.[17]
- Flexible bronchoscopy is safe for removing aspirated foreign bodies in children and might become a more common method in the future.[8,18]
- Hyperinflation or obstructive emphysema with atelectasis in the same hemithorax and aeration within an area of atelectasis are two newly reported radiologic findings associated with aspirated foreign bodies.[19] These findings may lead to early diagnosis of a foreign body, especially when a history of choking is absent.

SUGGESTED READING

Altmannn A, Nolan T: Non-intentional asphyxiation deaths due to upper airway interference in children 0-14 years. Injury Prevention 1995;1:76-80.

Altmann AE, Ozanne-Smith J: Non-fatal asphyxiation and foreign body ingestion in children 0-14 years. Injury Prevention 1997;3:176-182.

Baker S, Fisher R: Childhood asphyxiation by choking or suffocation. JAMA 1980;244:1343-1346.

Brown JM II, Padman R: Case study of a UFO (unidentified foreign object). Pediatr Asthma Allergy Immunol 2003;16:187-192.

Dikensoy O, Usalan C, Filiz A: Foreign body aspiration: Clinical utility of flexible bronchoscopy. Postgrad Med J 2002;78:399-403.

Harris C, Baker S, Smith G, Harris R: Childhood asphyxiation by food: A national analysis and overview. JAMA 1984;251:2231-2235.

Hayes N, Chidekel A: Pediatric choking. Del Med J 2004;76:335-340.

Panieri E, Bass D: The management of ingested foreign bodies in children: A review of 883 cases. Eur J Emerg Med 1995;2:83-87.

Reilly J, Cook S, Stood D, Rider G: Prevention and management of aerodigestive foreign body injuries in childhood. Pediatr Clin North Am 1996;43:1403-1411.

Reilly J, Walter M, Bests D, et al: Size/shape analysis of aerodigestive foreign bodies in children: Multi-institutional study. Am J Otolaryngol 1995;16:190-193.

Rimell F, Thome A Jr, Stool S, et al: Characteristics of objects that cause choking in children. JAMA 1995;274:1763-1766.

Tarrago S: Prevention of choking, strangulation and suffocation in childhood. WMJ 2000;99:43-46.

Webb W: Management of foreign bodies of the upper gastrointestinal tract. Gastroenterology 1988;94:204-216.

REFERENCES

1. Tarrago SB: Prevention of choking, strangulation and suffocation in childhood. WMJ 2000;99:43-46.
2. Mittleman RE: Fatal choking in infants and children. Am J Forensic Med Pathol 1984;5:201-210.
3. Kosloske A: Respiratory foreign body. In Hilman B (ed): Pediatric Respiratory Disease: Diagnosis and Treatment. Philadelphia, WB Saunders, 1993, pp 513-520.
4. Baker S, Fisher R: Childhood asphyxiation by choking or suffocation. JAMA 1980;244:1343-1346.
5. Gatch G, Myre L, Black RE: Foreign body aspiration in children: Causes, diagnosis, and prevention. AORN J 1987;46:850-861.
6. Rimell F, Thome A Jr, Stool S, et al: Characteristics of objects that cause choking in children. JAMA 1995;274:1763-1766.
7. Reilly BK, Stool D, Chen X, et al: Foreign body injury in children in the twentieth century: A modern comparison to the Jackson collection. Int J Pediatr Otorhinolaryngol 2003;67(Suppl 1):S171-S174.
8. Swanson KL: Airway foreign bodies: What's new? Semin Respir Crit Care Med 2004;25:405-411.
9. Baharloo F, Veyckemans F, Francis C, et al: Tracheobronchial foreign bodies: Presentation and management in children and adults. Chest 1999;115:1357-1362.
10. Gershel JC, Goldman HS, Stein RE, et al: The usefulness of chest radiographs in first asthma attacks. N Engl J Med 1983;309:336-339.
11. Roback MG, Dreitlein DA: Chest radiograph in the evaluation of first time wheezing episodes: Review of current clinical practice and efficacy. Pediatr Emerg Care 1998;14:181-184.
12. Gupta VK, Cheifetz IM: Heliox administration in the pediatric intensive care unit: An evidence-based review. Pediatr Crit Care Med 2005;6:204-211.
13. Fitzpatrick PC, Guarisco JL: Pediatric airway foreign bodies. J La State Med Soc 1998;150:138-141.
14. Rider G, Wilson CL: Small parts aspiration, ingestion, and choking in small children: Findings of the small parts research project. Risk Anal 1996;16:321-330.
15. Trouble in toyland: NYPIRG's 2002 toy safety report. Available at *http://www.nypirg.org/consumer/2002/default.html* (accessed Oct 17, 2005).
16. Child Safety Protection Act fact sheet. Available at *http://www.kidsource.com/CPSC/fact.html* (accessed Oct 17, 2005).
17. Haliloglu M, Ciftci AO, Oto A, et al: CT virtual bronchoscopy in the evaluation of children with suspected foreign body aspiration. Eur J Radiol 2003;48:188-192.
18. Swanson KL, Prakash UBS, Midthun DE, et al: Flexible bronchoscopic management of airway foreign bodies in children. Chest 2002;121:1695-1700.
19. Girardi G, Contador AM, Castro-Rodriguez JA: Two new radiological findings to improve the diagnosis of bronchial foreign-body aspiration in children. Pediatr Pulmonol 2004;38:261-264.

CHAPTER 80

Pulmonary Function Testing

Daniel J. Weiner

Pulmonary function testing encompasses a variety of techniques and tests. The indications for pulmonary function testing include (1) documenting the presence of obstructive or restrictive abnormalities in the course of establishing a diagnosis, (2) monitoring the course of a known pulmonary disease (e.g., cystic fibrosis, asthma), (3) monitoring for pulmonary toxicity related to treatment (e.g., amiodarone, radiation, chemotherapy), (4) monitoring response to therapy, and (5) describing normal and abnormal lung growth.

PULMONARY FUNCTION LABORATORY

The tests described herein require specialized equipment and experienced personnel. The equipment should conform to the standards published by the American Thoracic Society,[1] including daily calibration, biologic controls, and infection control practices. A stadiometer for accurate height measurement is required. The personnel should be patient, have the appropriate credentials, and be comfortable working with children of a variety of ages, who often require different coaching strategies. The space for testing should be quiet and free of distractions. Recently, some primary care physicians have begun to use spirometry in the office setting for patients with asthma or chronic obstructive pulmonary disease. The accuracy of testing in this situation is not well documented.

The values measured in the laboratory are usually normalized with the use of reference equations, most commonly based on the subject's height and gender; some also have corrections for ethnicity and age. With these equations, a predicted value can be calculated for each parameter, and the measured flows can be reported as a percentage of the predicted value or, occasionally, as a standardized deviation score (Z-score). It should be noted that test results from different pulmonary function laboratories should be compared with caution if different reference equations were used.

SPIROMETRY

Spirometry is the measurement of airflow during a maximally forced exhalation. The test is informative because airflow rates are inversely proportional to the fourth power of the radius of the airway; small or obstructed airways result in reduced airflow rates. Indeed, the hallmark of obstructive lung diseases such as asthma and cystic fibrosis is reduced airflow. Further, in small airways, flow limitation usually occurs, necessitating minimal effort to achieve a maximal flow. Many of these tests are fairly reproducible in subjects, making them useful for assessing response to treatment over time. Revised standards for the performance of spirometry have been published.[2]

The subject breathes through a mouthpiece connected to a pneumotachometer while wearing nose clips. After inhalation to total lung capacity, the subject is coached to exhale rapidly and forcefully, for a minimum of 6 seconds, until the lungs have emptied. At least three efforts are required, with two efforts having an exhaled volume within 5% of each other, to meet the criteria for reproducibility.

Several parameters can be calculated from these maneuvers. First, the total exhaled volume is termed the forced vital capacity (FVC). The forced expiratory volume in the first second is the FEV_1. The forced expiratory flow in the midexpiratory phase (i.e., the airflow rate between 25% of the exhaled volume and 75% of the exhaled volume) is the $FEF_{25\%-75\%}$ (or occasionally the maximal midexpiratory flow). Other instantaneous flow rates can also be calculated with reference to a different exhaled volume (e.g., FEF_{50}, FEF_{75}). The patterns of these parameters can suggest an obstructive or a restrictive defect (Table 80-1). The FEV_1/FVC ratio may help distinguish obstructive from restrictive diseases, although measurement of lung volumes is required to accurately diagnose restrictive disease.

When flow is plotted against exhaled volume (Fig. 80-1A), the resultant curve can help locate the site of any flow limitation. Intrathoracic obstructive defects usually result in a curve that is concave to the volume axis (Fig. 80-1B), whereas restrictive defects usually have a normally shaped but narrow curve (Fig. 80-1C). Central airway obstruction can manifest as flattening of the inspiratory limb if the lesion is variable and extrathoracic (e.g., tracheomalacia, paretic vocal cord motion) or flattening of both the inspiratory and expiratory portions of the curve (Fig. 80-1D) if the lesion is fixed in nature.

If an obstructive defect is documented, reversibility can also be assessed using spirometry. A bronchodilator is administered, and the test is repeated in 15 to 20 minutes. Commonly, a 12% increase in the FEV_1 is considered indicative of a significant response. Similarly, in patients with suspected airway hyperreactivity, spirometry can be performed before and after provocative agents such as methacholine, cold air, or exercise.[3]

LUNG VOLUMES

Disease states that affect lung growth would be expected to alter lung volume in addition to airway caliber. These diseases include pulmonary hypoplasia due to severe oligohydramnios or space-occupying lesions (e.g., diaphragmatic hernia, cystic adenomatoid malformation), bronchopulmonary dysplasia, and conditions that alter the growth of the rib cage (thoracic dystrophies, radiation). The volume of gas in the lung can be measured using two techniques: dilution and plethysmography.

Table 80-1 Patterns of Obstructive and Restrictive Lung Disease

Parameter	Obstructive	Restrictive
FVC	Low (may be normal)	Low
FEV$_1$	Low	Low
FEV$_1$/FVC	Low	Normal
FEF$_{25\%-75\%}$	Low	Low

FEF$_{25\%-75\%}$, forced expiratory flow, midexpiratory phase; FEV$_1$, forced expiratory volume in 1 second; FVC, forced vital capacity.

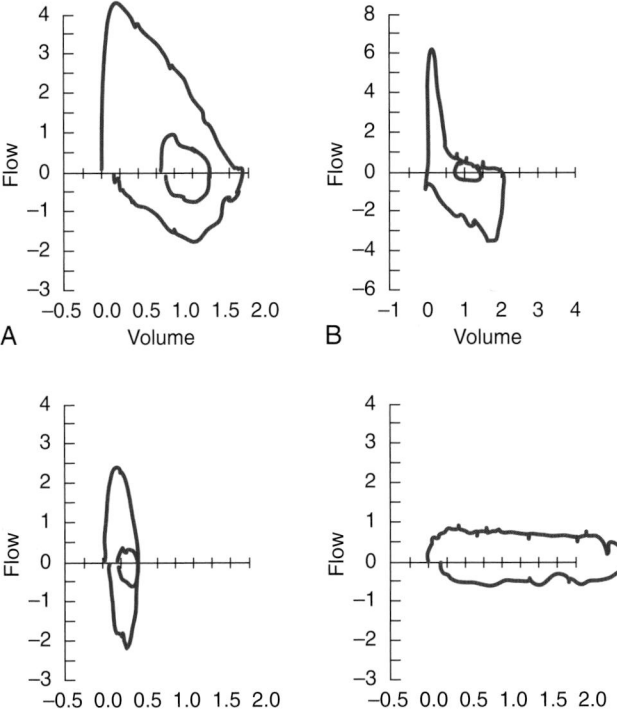

Figure 80-1 Flow-volume curves. The normal curve (*A*) has a smooth, linear decrease in flow from near total lung capacity (to the left) to residual volume (to the right). Note that time is not represented in these curves but is recorded in a separate volume–time curve (not shown). In a patient with obstructive lung disease (*B*), the curve is concave toward the volume access, such that for any given lung volume, measured flow is lower than predicted. Restrictive lung diseases (*C*) result in a curve that has a small exhaled lung volume and is narrow, but without concavity. Fixed airway obstruction (*D*) results in a curve that is flattened in both inspiration and exhalation.

Dilutional techniques use the principle of conservation of mass. That is, the subject breathes through a mouthpiece connected to a closed system into which a known concentration of a marker gas (usually helium) is added. After several minutes to allow for equilibration, the final concentration of the marker gas is measured, permitting calculation of the volume added to the system (the patient's lung volume). One notable limitation of dilutional techniques for measuring lung volumes is that significant obstruction in the airway results in underestimation of the true lung volume, because portions of the lung distal to the obstruction do not participate in the gas mixing and dilution.

Plethysmography uses the principle of Boyle's law: in a closed system, pressure and volume change inversely when temperature is constant. With the subject sitting in a fixed-volume chamber (box) and breathing through a mouthpiece, a shutter is closed in the inspiratory limb of the breathing circuit. The subject makes small panting maneuvers, resulting in small changes in the volume of the lung and corresponding inverse volume changes in the box. Pressures in the box and at the mouth are measured, which allows calculation of the lung volume when the panting efforts began. The subject usually begins the maneuvers at the end of a breath, and this "resting" lung volume is termed functional residual capacity (FRC). One notable limitation of the plethysmographic technique is that in the presence of significant obstruction, lung volume may be overestimated because one assumption of plethysmography—that there is no flow during the occlusion, and alveolar pressure and mouth pressure equilibrate—may not be true. Revised standards for plethysmography have been published.[4]

Lung capacity is the sum of two or more lung volumes; in the case of FRC, it is the sum of residual volume (RV; the amount of gas remaining in the lung after maximal exhalation) and expiratory reserve volume (ERV; the amount of gas exhaled from resting lung volume until the lung is empty). In combination with spirometry, other lung volumes and capacities can be calculated (Fig. 80-2).

The pattern of lung volumes can also assist in diagnosis. Typically, patients with obstructive diseases have an increased RV, especially as a fraction of total lung capacity (TLC). The TLC may be normal or elevated. In contrast, low lung volumes are the hallmark of restrictive lung disease, and these patients have a reduced TLC and RV.

DIFFUSING CAPACITY

The diffusing capacity for carbon monoxide (D$_{LCO}$) is an integrative measurement that describes the transfer of oxygen from the alveolus into the red blood cell. This transfer is (1) proportional to the surface area of the alveolar-capillary membrane, (2) proportional to the pressure gradient for oxygen between the alveolus and the blood, and (3) inversely proportional to the thickness of the alveolar-capillary membrane. The measurement depends on the fact that CO is more soluble in blood than in lung tissue, because it binds rapidly and tightly to hemoglobin in the blood (more than 200 times as quickly as oxygen does). Thus, the partial pressure of CO in the blood remains very low, maintaining a diffusion gradient for the gas. Revised standards for the measurement of D$_{LCO}$ have been published.[5]

In the single-breath technique for measuring D$_{LCO}$, the patient exhales completely to RV and inhales to TLC a gas mixture of 0.3% CO and an inert gas (usually helium or methane). The subject holds his or her breath for 10 seconds, during which CO diffuses into the blood. The uptake of CO (in mL/minute) is divided by the partial pressure gradient for CO (between alveolus and pulmonary capillary) to calculate D$_{LCO}$ (in mL/mm Hg per minute). Alveolar ventilation (VA) is calculated from the inspired and expired concentrations of the inert gas, and this is used to calculate a dilutional factor for the inspired CO concentration and to normalize the D$_{LCO}$ according to the lung volume in which the CO is diluted (D$_{LCO}$/VA in mL/mm Hg per

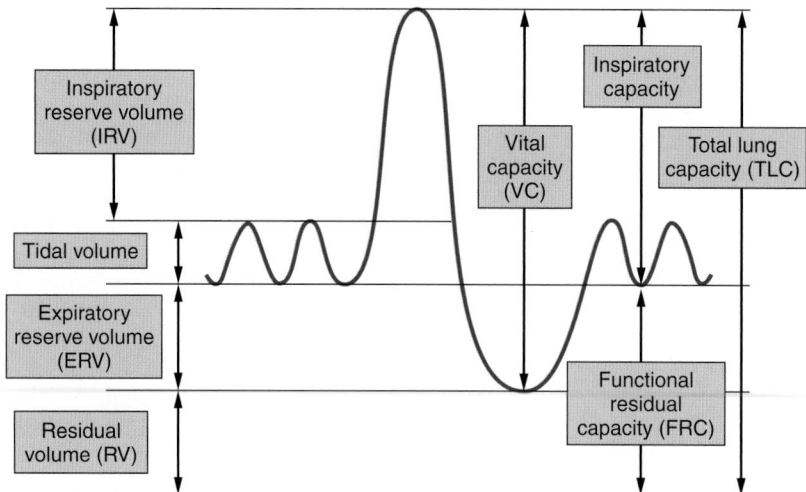

Figure 80-2 Fractional lung volume measurements. After measurement of FRC by dilution or plethysmography, and measurement of FVC and ERV by spirometry, RV (FRC − ERV) and TLC (RV + VC) can be calculated.

minute/L, where VA is the alveolar volume). It is often adjusted for the patient's hemoglobin as well.

Diseases that decrease the surface area for diffusion (emphysema, pulmonary emboli, resection of lung tissue) and diseases that increase the thickness of the alveolar-capillary membrane (fibrosis, pulmonary edema, proteinosis) both decrease the diffusing capacity of the lung. Increased DLCO is much less common but can be seen in patients with alveolar hemorrhage (hemoglobin in the airspace appears to make the uptake of CO very high) or polycythemia or during exercise (via recruitment of more pulmonary capillaries). This test may be useful in evaluating patients with diffuse lung diseases or those with pulmonary vascular obstruction.

RESPIRATORY MUSCLE STRENGTH

The respiratory muscles (the diaphragm, intercostal muscles, and others) contract intermittently 24 hours a day to perform the work of ventilation. Many diseases can affect the strength of these muscles, putting patients at risk for hypoventilation, impaired airway clearance of secretions, and respiratory insufficiency. These conditions include primary muscular disorders (muscular dystrophy, myopathy), conditions affecting nerve transmission to the muscles (neuropathies, disorders of the neuromuscular junction), malnutrition, and stretch of the muscles beyond their optimal length-tension relationship (which can occur in hyperinflation).

Typically, maximum expiratory pressure (PEmax) is measured by having the subject inhale maximally to TLC and blow out as hard as possible into a mouthpiece connected to a pressure transducer with an occluded distal end. Similarly, maximum inspiratory pressure (PImax) is measured by having the subject exhale completely to RV and inhale rapidly against the occluded tube. Usually, several maneuvers are required to elicit the maximal effort. Several sets of standardized values have been published, but they vary considerably.[6]

PULMONARY FUNCTION TESTS IN INFANTS

Most of the tests described here have been adapted to infants, with the obvious challenge being that maximal efforts cannot be elicited voluntarily. Infants are usually sedated with chloral hydrate and placed supine with a mask over the mouth and nose to measure airflow and pressure at the mouth. These techniques require specialized equipment that is not available in most pulmonary function laboratories.

The rapid thoracic compression (RTC) technique has been used to generate maximal expiratory flow by applying positive pressure externally to the chest.[7] This involves placing a plastic jacket around the chest and abdomen of a sedated, supine infant and then rapidly inflating the jacket from a pressure reservoir using a valve controlled manually or by computer. The inflation is timed to occur at end-inspiration, when the infant's lung volume is just above FRC. Expiratory flow and volume are measured via a facemask and pneumotachygraph, and a partial forced expiratory flow-volume curve over the tidal range of breathing can be constructed.

One major limitation of the RTC technique is that flows are dependent on the lung volume at which they are measured, and FRC can vary dramatically in infants from breath to breath; instability of the FRC limits the reproducibility of the flow measurements and may decrease the technique's sensitivity to subtle changes in airway mechanics. Additionally, the flows are measured only over the tidal volume range—a relatively small portion of the infant's lung volume—rather than over the entire range of lung volumes, as they would be in older children and adults.

In the raised volume rapid thoracic compression (RV-RTC) technique,[8] the infant's lung is first inflated to a predetermined pressure (typically 30 cm H_2O). This results in an end-inspiratory lung volume close to TLC (whereas the RTC technique begins measurement close to FRC). At this raised lung volume, the jacket encircling the infant's chest is rapidly inflated from the pressure reservoir, generating a full expiratory flow-volume curve. The resultant curves are

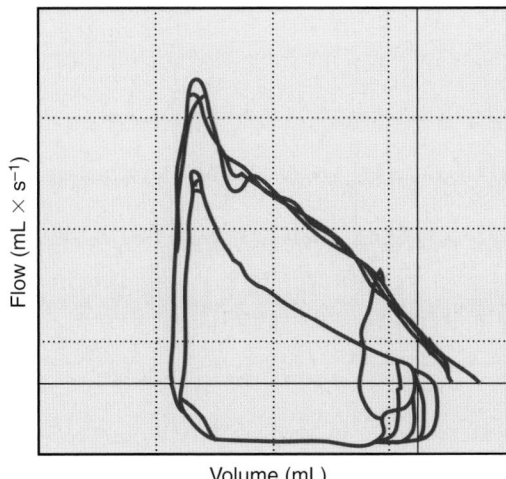

Figure 80-3 Measurement of forced expiratory flow in infants. The largest curves represent maximal flow from a raised lung volume and look very much like curves obtained from cooperative children and adults. The smaller triangular curves represent passive exhalation after inflation to total lung capacity. At the far right (at lower lung volume), a triangular partial expiratory flow-volume curve is superimposed over the even smaller oval-shaped tidal breaths. Note the substantial difference between the partial expiratory flow-volume curve and the maximal flow-volume curve obtained after inflation. (From Stocks J, Sly PD, Tepper RS, Morgan WJ: Infant Respiratory Function Testing. New York, John Wiley & Sons, 1996, pp 393-400.)

highly reproducible, with values being reported as timed volumes (e.g., $FEV_{0.5}$, $FEV_{0.75}$) in addition to instantaneous flow rates (Fig. 80-3). This technique also allows flows to be measured over a larger portion of the vital capacity.

Lung volumes can also be measured by either dilutional or plethysmographic methods.[9] For the latter, the infant is placed in a rigid, closed container. The infant breathes through a facemask connected to an airway pressure gauge and a pneumotachygraph to measure flow and volume. A shutter within the facemask can briefly occlude the infant's airway; continued respiratory efforts alternately compress and rarify the gas within the lung. Because airflow is absent when the shutter occludes the airway, there is no pressure loss from airflow resistance, and the pressure measurements made at the mask (airway opening) are reflective of alveolar pressure. By relating alveolar pressure changes to the volume changes in the plethysmograph (which are equal and opposite to those in the infant's lung), the volume of gas within the lung can be calculated.

PROVOCATIVE CHALLENGE TESTING

A variety of tests have been used in conjunction with spirometry to elicit airway hyperreactivity in patients with suspected asthma.[3] Inhaled methacholine stimulates cholinergic receptors on airway smooth muscle, resulting in contraction and decreased airway caliber. Serial twofold increasing doses of methacholine (0.025 to 16 mg/mL) are delivered until a maximal dose is reached or there is a 20% decrease in FEV_1; this dose is termed the provocative dose required for a 20% decrease (PD_{20}). There is some controversy about what provocative dose constitutes an abnormal response, because even healthy controls may have decreased

flows with high doses of methacholine. Following completion of the challenge, inhaled albuterol is given to document the reversibility of airflow obstruction. Similarly, graded exercise (using a treadmill or cycle ergometer) or hyperventilation with cold air (usually chilled to 4°C) can be used to provoke a bronchospasm response.

INPATIENT APPLICATIONS OF PULMONARY FUNCTION TESTING

A common use of pulmonary function tests in the inpatient setting is to monitor response to therapy. For example, patients with cystic fibrosis receiving intravenous antibiotics for a pulmonary exacerbation of their disease are usually monitored weekly with spirometry. The patient's prior baseline (or previous best) lung function is a helpful target when determining the duration of therapy. Pulmonary function tests may also assist in preoperative planning, such as for patients with restrictive lung disease undergoing scoliosis repair. Additionally, these tests have important uses in the evaluation of respiratory symptoms (shortness of breath, cough, wheeze) when there is no specific diagnosis.

POLYSOMNOGRAPHY

A polysomnograph is a multichannel recording made during sleep to evaluate a variety of symptoms or monitor gas exchange.[10] The variables measured during the study usually include oxyhemoglobin saturation, end-tidal carbon dioxide tension, chest wall and abdominal movement, airflow, and sleep state (determined by electroencephalogram, eye movement, and chin muscle activity). An example of a multichannel polysomnographic recording is provided in Figure 80-4. Studies are usually performed overnight to evaluate the patient during different stages of sleep. The continuous recordings of these variables must then be scored (identification of abnormal events) and interpreted according to age-appropriate standards.[11]

The most common indication for polysomnography is the evaluation of children with suspected airway obstruction during sleep, which may be indicated by snoring, observed apnea, or excessive daytime somnolence. Other abnormalities in the respiratory pattern (central apnea, hypoventilation) can be detected and may suggest disorders affecting the brainstem or respiratory muscles. Specifically, infants experiencing apparent life-threatening events may undergo polysmonography to document their respiratory patterns. Polysomnography can also be used in children with known lung disease or upper airway obstruction to initiate therapy (oxygen, noninvasive ventilation, or mechanical ventilation) and titrate the therapy until gas exchange is improved. This requires technicians with experience in respiratory therapy as well as standard polysomnography.

PULSE OXIMETRY AND CAPNOGRAPHY

Noninvasive pulse oximetry allows for the continuous monitoring of oxygen saturation (SpO_2). This permits a much more rapid detection of changes in clinical status than does intermittent blood gas measurement. The technique is based on light absorption by oxygenated and reduced

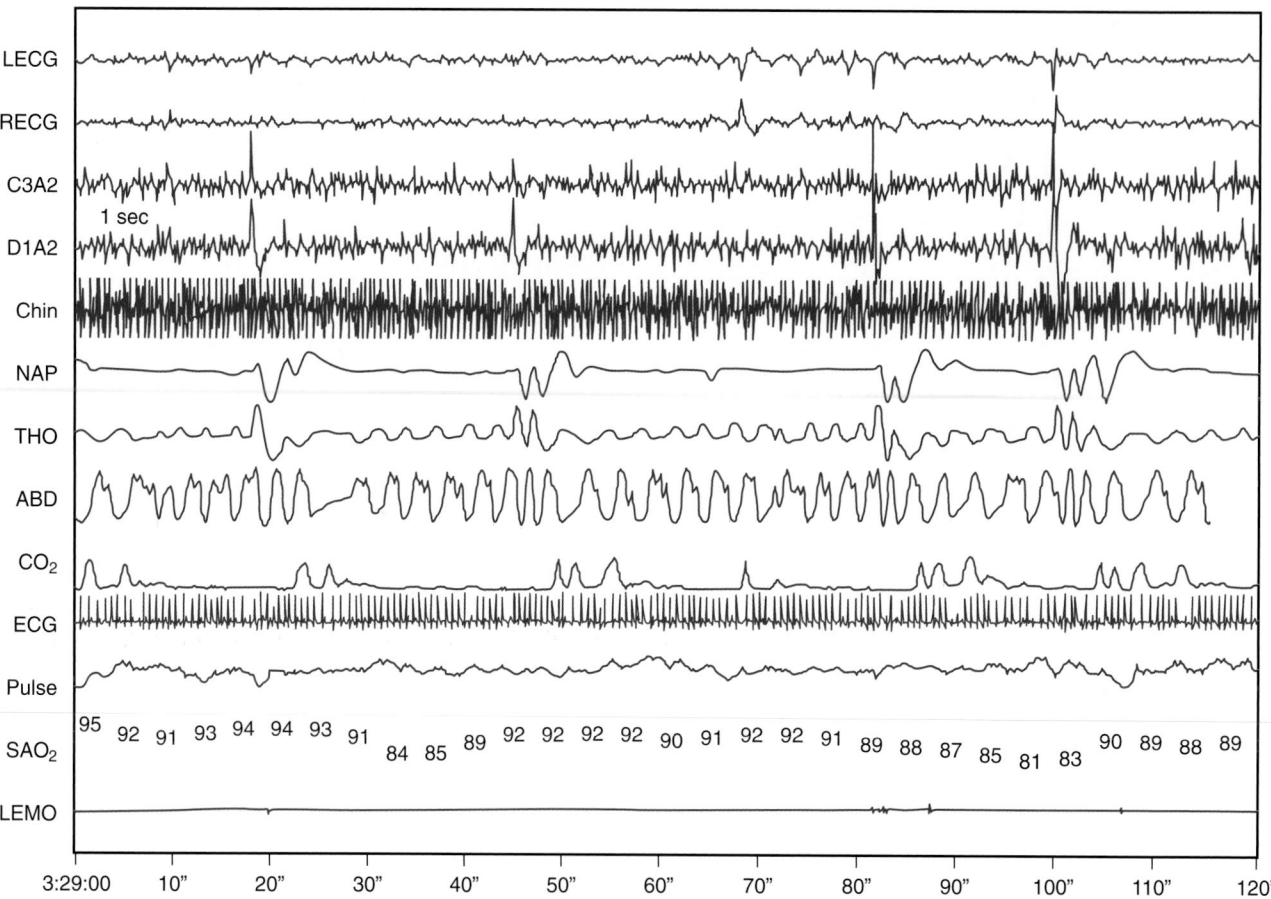

Figure 80-4 Multichannel polysomnographic recording. The tracings (top to bottom) include four electroencephalogram channels, chin movement (submental electromyogram), nasal airflow, thoracic wall movement, abdominal wall movement, end-tidal carbon dioxide, electrocardiogram, pulse oximeter waveform, saturation, and tibial electromyogram. There are multiple episodes of obstructive apnea with associated oxyhemoglobin desaturation depicted in this 2-minute epoch. (From Johnson JT, Gluckman JL, Sanders MH [eds]: Management of Obstructive Sleep Apnea. London, Informa, 2001, p 46.)

hemoglobin at two different (visible and infrared) wavelengths. The oximeter signal depends on detection of a pulsatile waveform, and poor perfusion, edema, or abnormal hemoglobins (e.g., reduced hemoglobin) may interfere with readings. Patient motion is the most common cause of artifactual readings, and a reproducible signal waveform provides one method of determining the accuracy of the reading. Pulse oximetry should be used in all patients requiring supplemental oxygen to determine the adequacy of treatment and as an assessment tool in any patient with respiratory distress.

Normal oximetry values do not ensure normal ventilation. Exhaled gas can be analyzed for carbon dioxide (CO_2) concentrations, and the waveform can be displayed as a capnograph. In the healthy lung, the concentration of CO_2 at the end of a breath (end-tidal CO_2) closely approximates arterial P_{CO_2}. Disease states with increased dead space may dilute alveolar CO_2 with gas devoid of CO_2, and the end-tidal CO_2 could underestimate arterial CO_2. Similarly, leaks resulting in exhaled gas that does not reach the sensor result in an artifactually low end-tidal CO_2. Because of these possible errors, as well as the technical difficulty of measuring humidified gases, the end-tidal CO_2 should be correlated with measured CO_2 in the blood.

CONSULTATION

Consultation with a pediatric pulmonologist is indicated for any test results not consistent with the suspected clinical condition. For example, restrictive lung disease would not be expected in a child with presumed asthma and should prompt an evaluation for other possible diagnoses. Flow-volume curves suggesting a central airway obstruction should prompt consultation with a pulmonologist or otolaryngologist. Consultation with a specialist is often required to obtain specialized testing (e.g., infant lung function testing, polysomnography).

IN A NUTSHELL

- Noninvasive clinical monitoring and the pulmonary function and sleep laboratories offer important tools in the diagnosis and management of a variety of respiratory and nonrespiratory conditions in pediatric patients. The timely and appropriate application of pulmonary diagnostics and clinical monitoring strategies can result in improved diagnostic acumen, patient management, and safety in the inpatient setting.

ON THE HORIZON

* One area of active investigation is the measurement of lung function in preschool-aged children. Children in this age group (3 to 5 years) may be too immature to cooperate with standard techniques but too large for equipment or techniques suitable in infants. Techniques such as inductive plethysmography,[12] which measures the synchrony between the chest and abdomen as an indirect measure of airflow obstruction, and the forced oscillation technique,[13] a method of measuring airway resistance, have been studied. Neither technique requires significant subject cooperation.

SUGGESTED READING

ATS/ERS statement on respiratory muscle testing. Am J Respir Crit Care Med 2002;166:518-624.

Davey M: Investigation of sleep disorders. J Paediatr Child Health 2005;41:16-20.

Miller MR, Crapo R, Hankinson J, et al: General considerations for lung function testing. Eur Respir J 2005;26:153-161.

REFERENCES

1. Miller MR, Crapo R, Hankinson J, et al: General considerations for lung function testing. Eur Respir J 2005;26:153-161.

2. Miller MR, Hankinson J, Brusasco V, et al: Standardisation of spirometry. Eur Respir J 2005;26:319-338.

3. Popa V: ATS guidelines for methacholine and exercise challenge testing. Am J Respir Crit Care Med 2001;163:292-293.

4. Wanger J, Clausen JL, Coates A, et al: Standardisation of the measurement of lung volumes. Eur Respir J 2005;26:511-522.

5. Macintyre N, Crapo RO, Viegi G, et al: Standardisation of the single-breath determination of carbon monoxide uptake in the lung. Eur Respir J 2005;26:720-735.

6. ATS/ERS statement on respiratory muscle testing. Am J Respir Crit Care Med 2002;166:518-624.

7. Morgan WJ, Geller DE, Tepper RS, et al: Partial expiratory flow-volume curves in infants and young children. Pediatr Pulmonol 1988;5:232-243.

8. The raised volume rapid thoracoabdominal compression technique. The joint ATS/ERS working group on infant lung function. Am J Respir Crit Care Med 2000;161:1760-1762.

9. Stocks J, Godfrey S, Beardsmore C, et al: Plethysmographic measurements of lung volume and airway resistance. ERS/ATS task force on standards for infant respiratory function testing. Eur Respir J 2001;17:302-312.

10. Davey M: Investigation of sleep disorders. J Paediatr Child Health 2005;41:16-20.

11. Traeger N, Schultz B, Pollock AN, et al: Polysomnographic values in children 2-9 years old: Additional data and review of the literature. Pediatr Pulmonol 2005;40:22-30.

12. Mayer OH, Clayton RG Sr, Jawad AF, et al: Respiratory inductance plethysmography in healthy 3- to 5-year-old children. Chest 2003;124:1812-1819.

13. Oostveen E, MacLeod D, Lorino H, et al: The forced oscillation technique in clinical practice: Methodology, recommendations and future developments. Eur Respir J 2003;22:1026-1041.

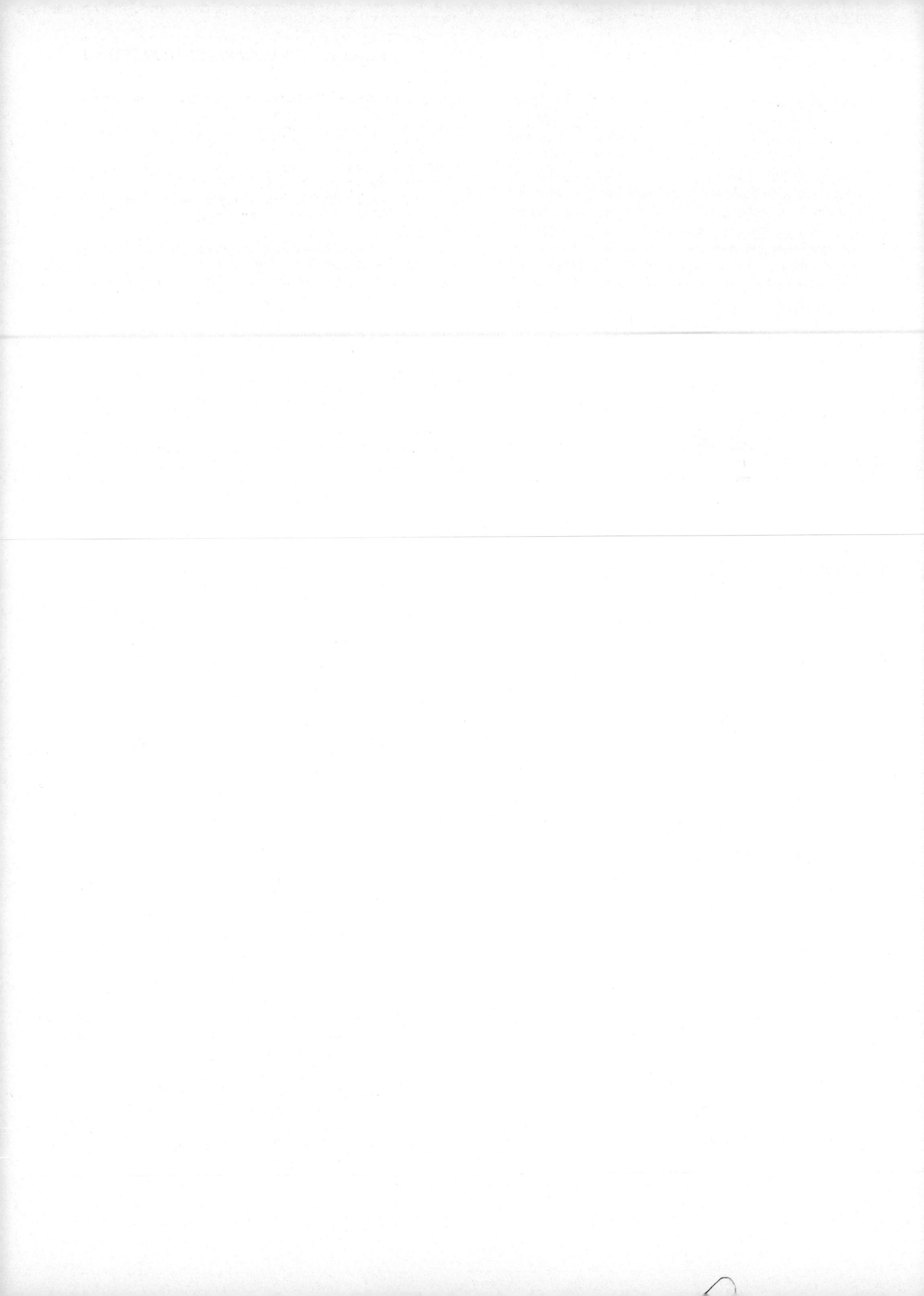

Cardiology

CHAPTER 81

The Cardiac Examination

Robert L. Geggel

Physicians are usually portrayed in the popular media carrying stethoscopes. The term *stethoscope* derives from the Greek word *stethos*, which means "chest," and *scope*, which means "view."[1] The proper use of this tool, initially introduced in 1816 by Laennec,[1] provides information on ventricular pressure, volume, and contractility; valve function; and cardiac anatomy. Unfortunately, the diagnostic auscultation skills of physicians in training are generally poor,[2-4] which is partly the result of the availability of modern imaging techniques, including echocardiography and magnetic resonance imaging. Although such technology has certainly advanced medical care, its appropriate use requires an accurate physical examination that provides a diagnosis or limited differential diagnosis and provides the basis for an efficient patient evaluation.

GENERAL OBSERVATION

Several features of the patient's appearance provide useful clues about the presence of heart disease. Infants with large left-to-right shunts or lesions associated with poor cardiac output can have failure to thrive. Plotting their weight and height measurements on growth curves often demonstrates the crossing of percentiles in a downward direction. In such infants, weight is usually affected before height.

Cyanosis can be caused by cardiac, pulmonary, hematologic, or central nervous system disorders.[5] Because of the characteristics of fetal hemoglobin, which produces higher oxygen saturation for a given oxygen tension, identifying subtle cyanosis in neonates is difficult.[6] Similar challenges are present in patients with darker skin pigmentation.

In patients with congenital heart disease, extracardiac anomalies are present in approximately 20%, and specific syndromes are identified in approximately 8% (Table 81-1).[7,8] Recognition of certain syndromes can lead to the early detection of heart disease, which may not produce murmurs in the neonatal period, when pulmonary vascular resistance is elevated.

VITAL SIGNS

Analysis of the vital signs provides a description of the patient's status and information about the likelihood of a cardiac condition.

Pulse

Various features of the pulse need to be assessed.

Rate and Rhythm

The average resting heart rate varies with the patient's age. For an infant, the value is 125 beats per minute; for a child, it is 100, and for an adolescent, 85.[9] Sinus tachycardia occurs in many conditions, including fever, anemia, anxiety, pain, myocardial dysfunction, cardiac tamponade, hyperthyroidism, sepsis, dehydration, and pulmonary disease. Bradycardia is associated with eating disorders, hypothyroidism, heart block, well-conditioned athletes, and increased intracranial pressure. Atrial tachyarrhythmias in the pediatric age group are most commonly supraventricular tachycardia; in children, the rate of this arrhythmia is typically greater than 220 beats per minute and is too rapid to count.

One common normal variation in heart rate in pediatric patients is sinus arrhythmia, which is characterized by a faster rate during inspiration and a slower rate during expiration. This phasic pattern can sometimes be prominent. The diagnosis is made by identifying the relationship to the respiratory cycle. Premature beats can represent atrial, junctional, or ventricular premature beats. Atrial premature beats that occur during the refractory period are frequent causes of "pauses" in neonates and typically resolve in the first few weeks of life.[10] Atrial flutter or atrial fibrillation can have a variable rhythm, depending on conduction through the atrioventricular node. A specific diagnosis of rhythm can be made by reviewing an electrocardiogram.

Prominence

Prominent bounding pulses are classically associated with moderate or severe aortic regurgitation because of low diastolic pressure and wide pulse pressure. A similar pattern can be present in other lesions that provide aortopulmonary connections (patent ductus arteriosus, aortopulmonary window, truncus arteriosus) or arteriovenous connections (arteriovenous malformation). The pulsatile flow through the capillary bed can be viewed by lightly compressing the nail bed (Quincke's pulse).[11]

Decreased pulses most commonly reflect myocardial dysfunction associated with myocarditis or cardiomyopathy, but they can also be present in cardiac tamponade, constrictive

Table 81-1   Syndromes Commonly Associated with Congenital Heart Disease

Syndrome	Patients with Cardiac Disease (%)	Common Cardiac Lesions
Alagille	85	PPS
DiGeorge	Nearly all	IAA, TrArt, TOF
Holt-Oram	50	ASD
Marfan	Nearly all	MVP, MR, dilated aorta, AR
Noonan	50	PS, PPS, HCMP
Trisomy 21	45	CAVC, VSD, PDA, TOF
Trisomy 13 or 18	>80	VSD, ASD, PDA, CPND
Turner	35	AS, HCMP, CoA
Williams	50	SAS, PPS, CoA
VACTERL	50	VSD, TOF

AR, aortic regurgitation; AS, aortic stenosis; ASD, atrial septal defect; CAVC, complete atrioventricular canal defect; CoA, coarctation of the aorta; CPND, congenital polyvalvular nodular dysplasia; HCMP, hypertrophic cardiomyopathy; IAA, interrupted aortic arch; MR, mitral regurgitation; MVP, mitral valve prolapse; PDA, patent ductus arteriosus; PPS, peripheral pulmonary stenosis; PS, pulmonary stenosis; SAS, supravalvular aortic stenosis; TrArt, truncus arteriosus; TOF, tetralogy of Fallot; VACTERL, vertebral, anal, cardiac, tracheal, esophageal, renal, and limb anomalies; VSD, ventricular septal defect.

pericarditis, or obstructive lesions. Rarely, patients may have Takayasu arteritis, a vasculitis that affects large arteries and which is associated with stenosis or occlusion of the aorta and its branches.[12]

Differential pulse strength is associated with several conditions. The most common is aortic coarctation, which typically occurs in the aortic isthmus, distal to the origin of the left subclavian artery and proximal to the insertion of the ductus arteriosus. The pulse is more prominent in the arm than in the leg. In some patients, the origin of the left subclavian artery is involved in the coarctation, resulting in a difference in pulse strength between the arms. Very rarely, the right subclavian artery arises aberrantly from the descending aorta; in this situation, the carotid pulse is stronger than the pulses in the extremities. Another condition that can produce differential pulses is supravalvular aortic stenosis. In this condition, blood flow can be preferentially directed to the innominate artery, producing asymmetrical pulses in the arms (Coanda effect). Takayasu aortitis can also produce differential pulses if there is variable stenosis of the subclavian and iliac arteries or their branches.

Variation

Respiratory variation in pulse strength is a feature of pulsus paradoxus, a condition associated with a fall in blood pressure greater than 10 mm Hg during expiration. This pattern is a feature of cardiac tamponade but can also be seen in severe respiratory distress. Variation in pulse strength with every other beat is a feature of left ventricular dysfunction and is termed pulsus alternans. A pulse with two peaks separated by a plateau occurs in patients with obstructive left ventricular cardiomyopathy or large stroke volumes and is termed pulsus bisferiens.[11]

Blood Pressure

A cuff of the appropriate size is required for the accurate measurement of blood pressure. The bladder of the inflatable cuff should be wide enough to cover three quarters of the length of the extremity where it is placed, and it should be long enough to fully encircle the extremity.[13] Values may be inaccurately elevated if the cuff is too small or does not fit snugly around the extremity.[11] Falsely elevated values may also occur if the patient is agitated or anxious (white-coat hypertension). If hypertension is detected, it is advisable to repeat the measurement at the end of the examination when the patient may be more relaxed.

For assessment of coarctation of the aorta, measurements are necessary in the upper and lower extremities. As noted earlier, because the left subclavian artery can be involved in the coarctation, it is more useful to measure blood pressure in the right arm. The systolic pressure in the lower extremity is usually 5 to 10 mm Hg greater than that in the upper extremity because of a standing wave effect. If systolic pressures in the arm are more than 10 mm Hg greater than values in the leg, this suggests coarctation.

In most clinics, blood pressure is measured by oscillometric methods. When assessing for pulsus paradoxus, however, the auscultation method is required. The cuff is inflated so that the pressure is approximately 20 mm Hg above the systolic value. The cuff is then slowly deflated. The pressures at which the Korotkoff sound is initially detected intermittently and then consistently are noted. The difference in these values represents the pulsus paradoxus and is normally less than 10 mm Hg.

Respiration

Tachypnea can be present in patients with large left-to-right shunts, cardiac dysfunction, or left-sided obstructive lesions, but it can also occur in patients with sepsis, pulmonary disease, or metabolic acidosis. Tachypnea can be accompanied by retractions at the intercostal or subcostal level, flaring of the alae nasi, or wheezing. Orthopnea implies elevated pulmonary venous pressure, which can occur with obstructive left-sided lesions or cardiomyopathy.

CARDIAC EXAMINATION

Thorough examination of the heart requires attention to detail and adherence to a system so that all aspects of cardiac function are assessed. The evaluation includes three categories: inspection, palpation, and auscultation.

Inspection

Patients with congenital heart disease associated with cardiomegaly may have a more prominent left chest created by compression of the heart against an elastic rib cage.[14] Pectus carinatum can be associated with Marfan syndrome, whereas pectus excavatum can be associated with mitral valve prolapse. A visible apical impulse is associated with left ventricular volume overload lesions (aortic or mitral regurgitation, left-to-right shunts at the ventricular or great vessel level). A visible parasternal impulse is seen in conditions with dilated right ventricles, including tetralogy of Fallot, absent pulmonary valve associated with severe pulmonary regurgitation, or Ebstein's anomaly associated with severe tricuspid regurgitation.

Palpation

Palpation provides information about the ventricular impulse, thrills, and occasionally heart sounds. Normal left and right ventricular impulses have different characteristics in infants, children, and adolescents, so experience in patients with different chest sizes is required to appreciate normal and abnormal impulses. The left ventricular apical impulse is usually located between the fourth and fifth intercostal spaces in the left midclavicular line and is assessed by using the tips of the index and middle fingers. The impulse is located laterally and is more prominent in lesions associated with left ventricular volume overload. Patients with mesocardia have the impulse in the midchest, and those with dextrocardia have the impulse in the right chest. The right ventricular impulse is assessed by placing the heads of the metacarpals parallel to the left side of the sternum. A prominent lift is present in lesions associated with right ventricular pressure or volume overload.

The presence of a thrill indicates a murmur of at least grade 4. By assessing the timing and location of a thrill, a likely diagnosis can be entertained. Systolic thrills at the left lower sternal border are usually caused by a ventricular septal defect; this defect may be small and associated with a high pressure gradient between the ventricles, or it may be large and associated with a significant left-to-right shunt. Occasionally, a thrill in this region is caused by tricuspid regurgitation if right ventricular pressure is elevated. Thrills associated with mitral, aortic, or pulmonary valve disease are located at the apex, right upper sternal border, or left upper sternal border, respectively. Moderate or severe aortic stenosis can also create a thrill in the suprasternal notch or over the course of the carotid artery. This finding helps distinguish aortic from pulmonary valve stenosis. Thrills can also occur in diastole with mitral stenosis, aortic regurgitation, or pulmonary regurgitation, and they are located in the respective valve regions of the precordium.

A palpable S_2 occurs in conditions associated with systemic pressure in the anteriorly positioned great artery. This finding most often indicates the presence of pulmonary artery hypertension, but it can also occur in patients with an anteriorly positioned aorta, such as occurs in transposition of the great arteries. A palpable S_1 can occur in hyperdynamic states.[11]

Auscultation

Thorough auscultation requires a quiet setting without extraneous noises and the use of appropriate equipment. The stethoscope tubing should be no longer than 16 to 18 inches with a bore of $^1/_8$ inch, and there should be no leak from the chest piece to the ear piece.[15] There should be both a bell to detect low-frequency sounds and a diaphragm for high-frequency sounds. In infants and children, a pediatric-sized diaphragm helps localize the point of maximal intensity. Auscultation should be performed with the patient supine, sitting, and occasionally standing, because in many conditions the murmur changes with different positions. Many congenital cardiac lesions produce more than one abnormal heart sound or murmur.

Having a comprehensive system of examination allows the physician to obtain all the available information. One such system is to make a mental list of all potential heart sounds and determine the quality and presence or absence of each one. Components to be evaluated include S_1, S_2, S_3, S_4, opening snap, ejection click, pericardial rub, and murmurs (systolic, diastolic, continuous). Murmurs, especially those occurring in systole, are often the most obvious findings, and by placing them at the bottom of the list, the examiner is reminded to evaluate more subtle features first. By listening to one sound at a time, complex examinations can be "decoded," ensuring that no available data are neglected.

First Heart Sound (S₁)

S_1 is produced by closure of the atrioventricular valves. It correlates with the QRS complex on the electrocardiogram (Fig. 81-1). S_1 is usually a single sound, but in pediatric

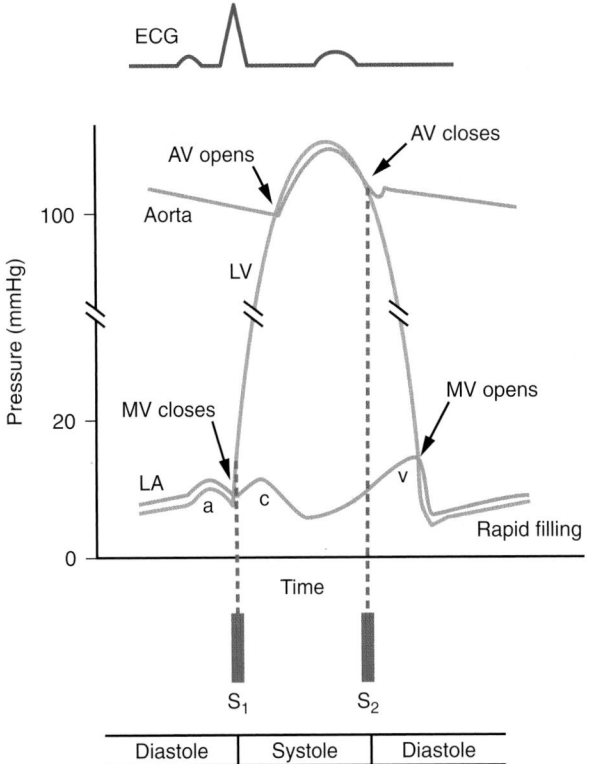

Figure 81-1 The normal cardiac cycle depicted for left-sided chambers. Similar relationships exist for the right-sided chambers (substitute right atrium for left atrium [LA], right ventricle for left ventricle [LV], and pulmonary artery for aorta). The a wave of the atrial pulse coincides with the P wave on the electrocardiogram (ECG). The mitral valve (MV) closes as the left ventricular pressure exceeds atrial pressure and produces the first heart sound (S_1). This coincides with the QRS complex on the ECG. Mitral valve closure increases atrial pressure and produces the c wave on the atrial pressure curve. The aortic valve (AV) subsequently opens as ventricular pressure exceeds aortic pressure. The aortic valve closes during ventricular relaxation and produces the second heart sound (S_2). This roughly coincides with the end of the T wave on the ECG. Atrial pressure rises (v wave) due to filling of the atria while the mitral valve is closed. The mitral valve opens as left ventricular pressure falls below left atrial pressure. (From Marino BS, Goldblatt A: Heart sounds and murmurs. In Lilly LS [ed]: Pathophysiology of Heart Disease. Philadelphia, Lea & Febiger, 1992, pp 18–29.)

patients it may be split due to nonsimultaneous closure of the mitral and tricuspid valves. In this case, the split is usually best appreciated at the left lower sternal border in the tricuspid valve region of the precordium. A split S_1 also occurs in right bundle branch block due to delayed closure of the tricuspid valve. A split S_1 can be difficult to distinguish from an early systolic ejection click created by a bicuspid aortic valve, and echocardiography may be needed for a precise diagnosis.

The intensity of S_1 is increased in conditions associated with increased velocity of leaflet closure (high cardiac output) or greater excursion of the valve leaflet during closure (short P-R interval, mild mitral stenosis). The intensity of S_1 is diminished in conditions associated with poor cardiac contractility, failure of atrioventricular valve coaptation (mitral regurgitation), or diminished valve leaflet excursion (elevated ventricular end-diastolic pressure, prolonged P-R interval, severe mitral stenosis).[16] S_1 has variable intensity in patients with complete heart block.[14]

Second Heart Sound (S₂)

S_2 is produced by closure of the semilunar valves and is coincident with the T wave on the electrocardiogram (see Fig. 81-1). S_2 is best appreciated at the left upper sternal border and varies with the respiratory cycle. During inspiration, the pulmonary valve closes after the aortic valve, creating a split sound; in expiration, the two valves close at the same time. The normal inspiratory split of the components of S_2 is approximately 0.05 second.

The characteristics of S_2 provide information about right ventricular volume and pulmonary pressure. An S_2 that is widely split in both inspiration and expiration (fixed split S_2) is a feature of right ventricular volume overload lesions, most commonly atrial septal defect. This feature can also occur in patients with total or partial anomalous pulmonary venous return or large arteriovenous malformations. In these conditions, the split between the components of S_2 is greater than 0.05 second, occasionally as long as 0.1 second (Fig. 81-2). Wide splitting during inspiration but with normal respiratory variation occurs with right bundle branch block, pulmonary stenosis, idiopathic dilation of

the main pulmonary artery due to delayed activation or prolonged contraction of the right ventricle,[11] or significant mitral regurgitation due to shortened left ventricular ejection time and earlier closure of the aortic valve.[17] Paradoxical splitting (single S_2 in inspiration, split S_2 in expiration) can occur in patients with delayed or prolonged left ventricular contraction associated with left bundle branch block, aortic stenosis, and some forms of Wolff-Parkinson-White syndrome.[11]

The intensity of S_2 depends on the pressure closing the anterior semilunar valve. An analogy would be the amount of noise a door makes when it is gently closed (low pressure in the anterior great artery) or slammed shut (high pressure in the anterior great artery). A loud S_2 usually represents pulmonary hypertension, which can arise from numerous conditions.[18] A loud S_2 can also be present in patients whose aorta is positioned anteriorly, as occurs in transposition of the great arteries and in some patients with tetralogy of Fallot.

S_2 is single in patients with severe pulmonary hypertension, because of earlier closure of the pulmonic component, and in patients with atresia of one of the semilunar valves (pulmonary atresia or hypoplastic left heart associated with aortic atresia). S_2 is narrowly split in patients with mild or moderate pulmonary hypertension.

Third Heart Sound (S₃)

S_3 occurs in early diastole during the rapid filling phase of the ventricle (Fig. 81-3). It is best heard with the bell of the stethoscope. This sound produces a gallop rhythm that can be "fit" to the syllables of "Ken-tuc-ky," with the last component representing S_3.[16] Occasionally this sound is present in normal pediatric patients, but it is usually associated with myocardial dysfunction or volume overload lesions.

Fourth Heart Sound (S₄)

S_4 occurs in late diastole, is associated with atrial contraction, and is coincident with the P wave on the electrocardiogram (Fig. 81-4). It is best heard with the bell of the stethoscope and also produces a gallop rhythm, this time fitting the syllables of "Ten-nes-see," with the first compo-

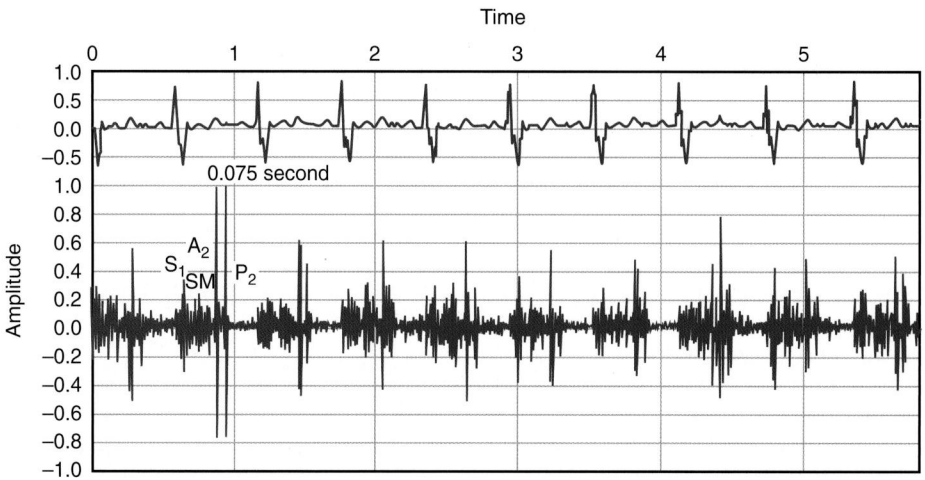

Figure 81-2 Phonocardiogram obtained in a patient with a secundum atrial septal defect. There is a systolic murmur (SM) and a fixed split S_2 interval of 0.075 second.

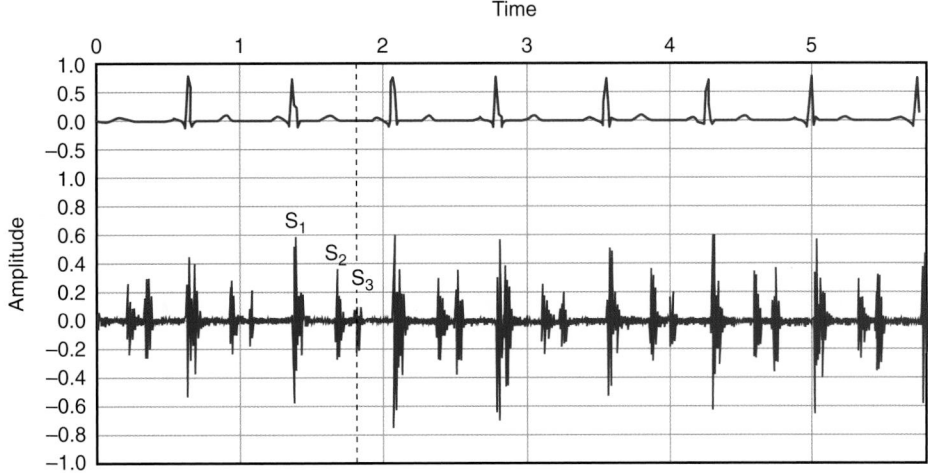

Figure 81-3 Phonocardiogram obtained in a 12-year-old child with S_3 and a structurally normal heart. S_3 occurs in the rapid filling phase of the cardiac cycle, between the T and P waves of the electrocardiogram.

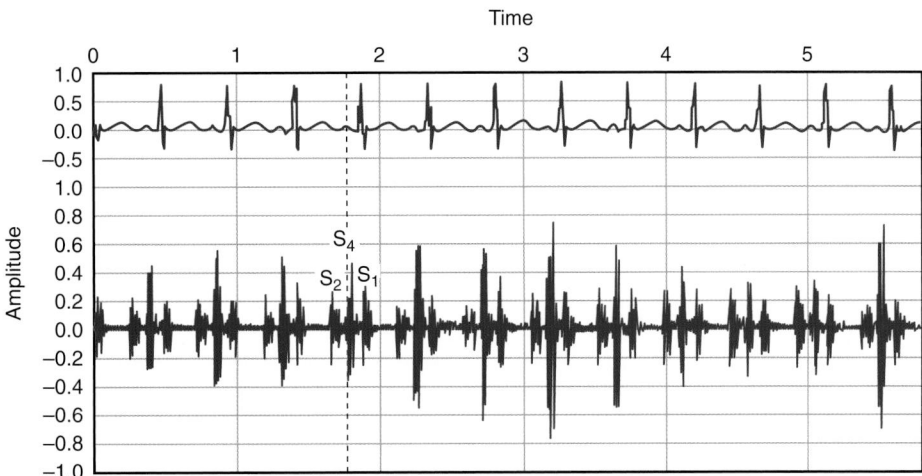

Figure 81-4 Phonocardiogram obtained in an adolescent with severe myocardial dysfunction. The tracing was recorded at the apex. There is an S_4, which is coincident with the P wave on the electrocardiogram.

nent representing S_4.[16] S_4 is abnormal and is associated with myocardial dysfunction caused by myocardial ischemia or ventricular hypertrophy.

If both S_3 and S_4 are present, a quadruple rhythm is created. If tachycardia develops, the extra sounds become superimposed in the shortened diastolic period, and a summation gallop is formed.[16,19,20]

Opening Snap

An opening snap is associated with mitral stenosis (Fig. 81-5). As the degree of mitral stenosis progresses, this high-frequency sound occurs earlier in diastole and becomes softer.

Clicks

Ejection clicks have a quality different from the previously described heart sounds, being sharper and higher in frequency. They are usually produced by abnormal valves. By noting the timing (early versus midsystolic), location, and nature (constant versus variable) of the click, the affected

valve can be determined. A midsystolic, apical, constant click is present in mitral valve prolapse (Fig. 81-6). If there is sufficient prolapse, mitral regurgitation can also be present. An early systolic, apical, constant click is typical of a bicuspid aortic valve (Fig. 81-7). This sound is best heard at the apex rather than the right upper sternal border. It can be difficult to distinguish this sound from the normal variant of a split S_1, and echocardiography may be necessary to make an accurate diagnosis. An early, left upper sternal border, variable click occurs with pulmonary stenosis. This click is louder in expiration (Fig. 81-8).[17] Clicks associated with semilunar valve stenosis become softer as the degree of stenosis increases because of decreased leaflet mobility. An early systolic, left lower sternal border, constant click occurs with Ebstein's anomaly, a rare malformation of the tricuspid valve. A similar click is occasionally produced when the septal leaflet of the tricuspid valve partially closes a membranous ventricular septal defect, forming an "aneurysm."

Clicks occasionally occur in conditions associated with dilation of the great arteries, including idiopathic dilation of the main pulmonary artery, pulmonary hypertension, and

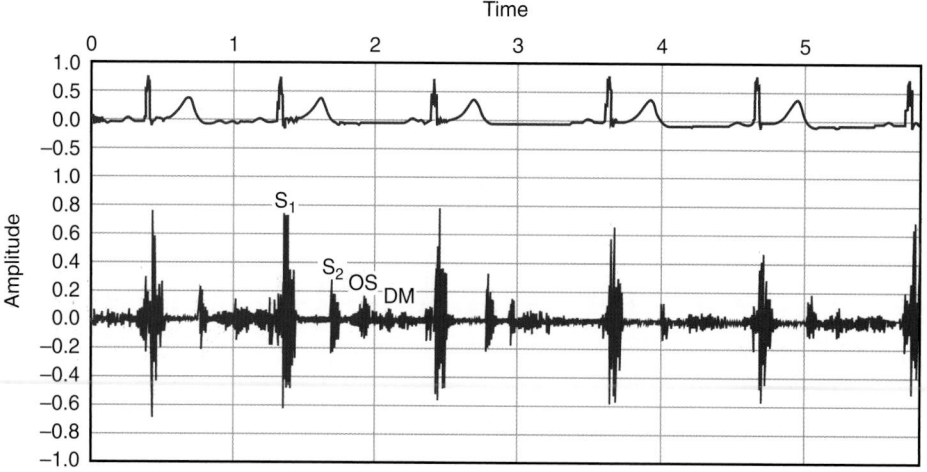

Figure 81-5 Phonocardiogram recorded at the apex in a young adult with rheumatic mitral stenosis. In diastole, there is an opening snap (OS) and a diastolic murmur (DM) that has presystolic accentuation.

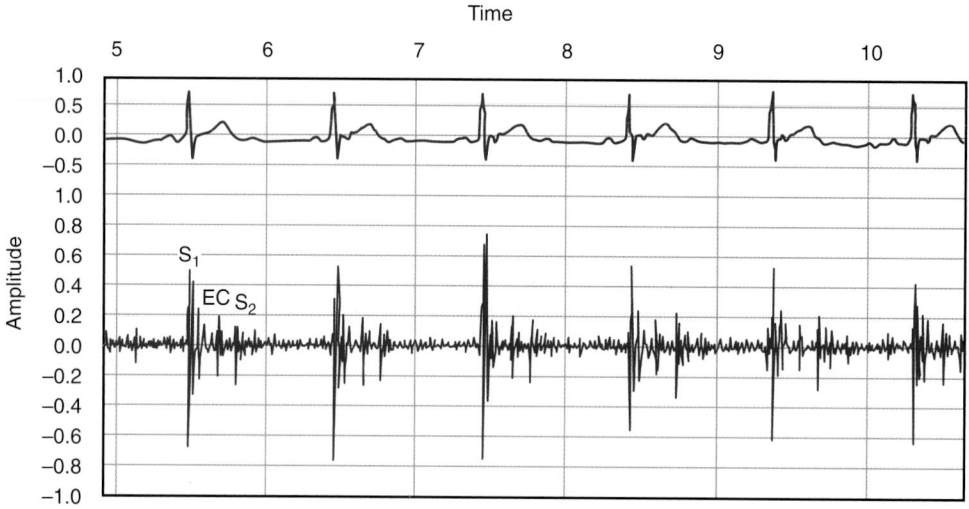

Figure 81-6 Phonocardiogram recorded at the apex with the patient supine, showing a midsystolic ejection click (EC) caused by mitral valve prolapse.

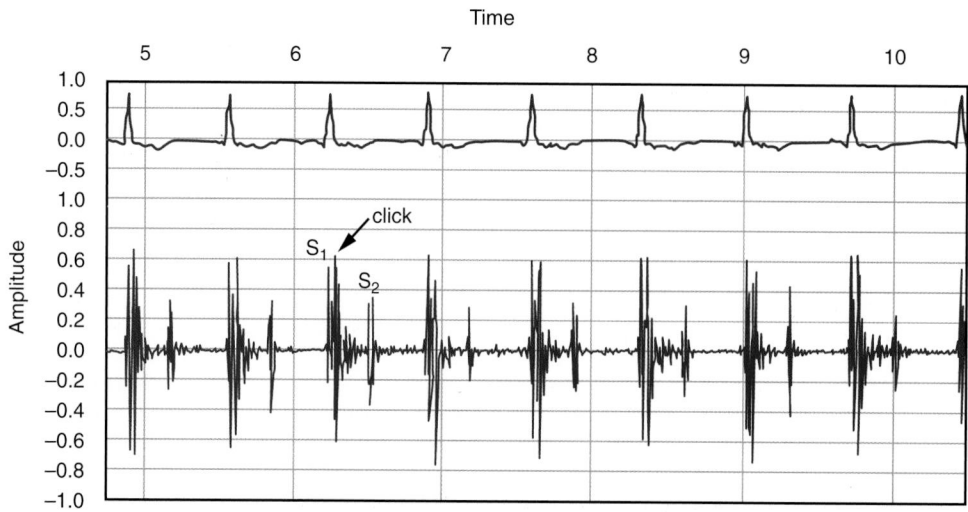

Figure 81-7 Phonocardiogram recorded at the apex in an adolescent with bicuspid aortic valve, demonstrating an early, constant, systolic ejection click (EC).

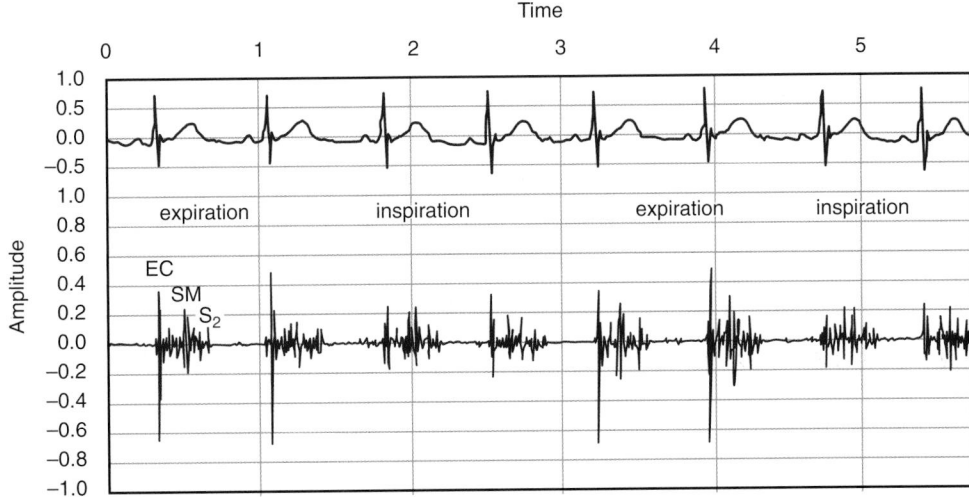

Figure 81-8 Phonocardiogram recorded at the left upper sternal border in a child with valvular pulmonary stenosis and a peak instantaneous Doppler gradient of 45 mm Hg. The tracing shows an intermittent systolic ejection click (EC) that occurs in the expiratory phase of the respiratory cycle and a systolic murmur (SM).

patent ductus arteriosus. In neonates with a compliant main pulmonary artery, left-to-right shunting through a patent ductus arteriosus can produce multiple clicks.

Pericardial Friction Rub

This grating sound is created when the visceral and parietal pericardial surfaces are inflamed and rub against each other. Therefore, it is not present if there is a large pericardial effusion. The rub is accentuated in the sitting position with the patient leaning forward during inspiration, and it may occur in systole, diastole, or continuously. A pericardial rub occurs with pericarditis and after open-heart surgery in which the pericardial space was entered.

Murmurs

Evaluation of a murmur requires an analysis of its intensity, timing, location and radiation, shape, and quality. In the newborn nursery, the age at which a murmur is first detected is useful in predicting a category of diagnosis. Murmurs present in the first 6 hours of life are usually caused by valve stenosis or regurgitation; those detected later often represent shunt lesions that develop findings on cardiac auscultation as pulmonary vascular resistance decreases. The clinician needs to be aware that some patients can have both a valve lesion and a septal defect, as occurs in tetralogy of Fallot.

Intensity

The numerical system used to describe the intensity of a murmur was initially proposed in 1933.[21] Grade 1 describes a faint sound that occasionally is not appreciated by noncardiologists. Grade 2 describes a readily appreciated murmur. Grade 3 is louder than grade 2 but is not associated with a palpable thrill. Grade 4 is a loud sound associated with a thrill. Grade 5 is a loud sound that is audible when the stethoscope is placed lightly on the chest. Grade 6 is a very loud sound that is audible with the stethoscope placed close to the body but off the chest. A thrill is present for murmurs of grade 4 and greater.

The intensity of a sound depends on the pressure gradient across the area of turbulence and the amount of blood flowing across the affected cardiac region. For example, a patient with severe aortic stenosis has a soft systolic murmur if left ventricular contractility is poor and a loud systolic murmur if cardiac function is normal.

Timing

Murmurs can occur in systole, diastole, or continuously. Systolic murmurs are produced in a number of conditions including the following:

- Stenotic semilunar valves
- Stenotic intracardiac lesions (double-chamber right ventricle, subvalvular semilunar valve obstruction)
- Stenotic intravascular lesions (supravalvular semilunar valve obstruction, coarctation, peripheral pulmonary stenosis)
- Regurgitant atrioventricular valves
- Increased flow across normal semilunar valves (tachycardia, anemia)
- Normal cardiac anatomy (innocent murmur)

Diastolic murmurs are produced by regurgitation across semilunar valves or turbulent flow across the atrioventricular valves. The latter situation can represent either true stenosis of the mitral or tricuspid valves or relative stenosis associated with increased blood flow coursing across these structures. The normal human atrioventricular valve can accommodate twice the normal cardiac output during diastole in a nonturbulent manner. Larger blood flows are associated with a murmur. Patients with a large atrial-level shunt can develop relative tricuspid stenosis, whereas those with a large ventricular-level shunt can develop relative mitral stenosis. The presence or absence of a diastolic murmur in these conditions is helpful in determining a bedside estimate of the degree of shunting. Similar diastolic murmurs can be present in moderate or severe tricuspid or mitral regurgitation.

Continuous murmurs begin in systole and extend through S_2 into a portion or all of diastole. They are produced in conditions associated with connections between the systemic and pulmonary circulations (e.g., patent ductus arteriosus, surgically created aortopulmonary shunts), systemic arteries and veins (e.g., arteriovenous malformation), and systemic arteries and cardiac chambers (e.g., coronary arteriovenous fistula) and in conditions associated with disturbed flow in arteries (e.g., collateral circulation associated with coarctation of the aorta) or veins (e.g., venous hum).

Occasionally, patients have two separate conditions—one that produces a systolic murmur, and one that produces a diastolic murmur. Examples include aortic regurgitation associated with either aortic stenosis or a ventricular septal defect, and pulmonary regurgitation associated with pulmonary stenosis. These murmurs do not continue through S_2 and are described as to-and-fro murmurs.

Location and Radiation

The location of maximal intensity and areas of radiation of the murmur are characteristic for each condition. A systolic murmur at the right upper sternal border can represent aortic valve stenosis and typically radiates to the carotids. A systolic murmur at the left upper sternal border can represent pulmonary valve stenosis (see Fig. 81-8), relative pulmonary stenosis associated with increased right ventricular output and an atrial septal defect (see Fig. 81-2), an innocent pulmonary flow murmur, or peripheral pulmonary stenosis. Peripheral pulmonary stenosis usually radiates to and may be best heard in either the axilla or the back. A systolic murmur at the left lower sternal border represents a ventricular septal defect, tricuspid regurgitation, or an innocent Still's murmur. A small muscular ventricular septal defect is usually well localized and occupies only early to midsystole, because the defect is closed as the myocardium contracts. A membranous or moderate to large muscular ventricular septal defect is holosystolic. Tricuspid regurgitation typically increases in intensity during inspiration because of increased blood return to the right side of the heart. An innocent murmur has a characteristic vibratory or musical quality and typically is louder in the supine than the sitting position and becomes louder in high-output states (anxiety, fever, anemia). A systolic murmur at the apex that radiates to the axilla is characteristic of mitral regurgitation.

A diastolic murmur at the left upper sternal border can represent pulmonary or aortic regurgitation. The severity of the regurgitation often correlates with the extent of radiation down the left sternal border: with mild regurgitation, the murmur is limited to the upper sternal border; with moderate, it is audible at the midsternal level; and with severe regurgitation, it extends to the left lower sternal border. A diastolic murmur at the apex usually represents mitral stenosis and is usually best heard with the patient in the left lateral decubitus position (see Fig. 81-5).

A continuous murmur at the left upper sternal border is characteristic of a patent ductus arteriosus. This murmur does not change with body position. The continuous murmur associated with a coronary fistula is usually maximally located lower on the precordium. The continuous murmur associated with a venous hum can be heard at the right or left upper sternal border or in the infraclavicular and supraclavicular regions. The murmur associated with a

venous hum becomes softer or is abolished in the supine position, in the sitting position with rotation or flexion of the neck, or if light pressure is placed over the cervical triangle.

Murmurs can be present in sites other than the precordium. Coarctation can be associated with a systolic murmur on the back between the scapulae and, if significant collateral circulation is present, over the course of the intercostal arteries laterally in the chest. Arteriovenous malformations can create murmurs over the affected body region, over the cranium in patients with vein of Galen malformations, and in the right upper quadrant in patients with a hepatic lesion.

Shape

Systolic ejection murmurs associated with ventricular obstructive lesions or conditions associated with increased flow are diamond shaped. Examples include semilunar valvular, subvalvular, or supravalvular stenosis; coarctation; anemia; hyperthyroidism; fever; and increased flow across the pulmonary valve associated with an atrial septal defect. As semilunar valve stenosis progresses, the murmur peaks later in systole and extends to the component of S_2 of the affected valve. Holosystolic murmurs associated with ventricular septal defects (other than small muscular defects) or atrioventricular valve regurgitation have a plateau shape. Decrescendo diastolic murmurs have maximal intensity early and then become softer; they are characteristic of semilunar valve regurgitation.

Quality

A harsh murmur is typical of obstructive lesions or hyperdynamic states. A blowing murmur is an attribute of semilunar or atrioventricular valve regurgitation. A rumbling feature is present in diastolic turbulence across atrioventricular valves because of the low pressure gradient between the atria and ventricles in this phase of the cardiac cycle. A vibratory or musical quality is associated with an innocent Still's murmur.

CONCLUSION

Knowledge of both cardiac anatomy and physiology, coupled with a thorough cardiac physical examination, should provide a diagnosis or limited differential diagnosis on which to base an efficient patient evaluation.

SUGGESTED READING

Duff DF, McNamara DG: History and physical examination of the cardiovascular system. In Garson A Jr, Bricker TM, Fisher DJ, Neish SR (eds): The Science and Practice of Pediatric Cardiology. Baltimore, Williams & Wilkins, 1998, pp 693-713.

Geggel RL, Armsby LB: Evaluation and initial management of cyanotic heart disease in the newborn. In Rose BD (ed): UpToDate. Wellesley, Mass, UpToDate, 2003.

REFERENCES

1. Abdulla R: The history of the stethoscope [editorial]. Pediatr Cardiol 2001;22:371-372.
2. Gaskin PRA, Owens SE, Talner NS, et al: Clinical auscultation skills in pediatric residents. Pediatrics 2000;105:1184-1187.

3. Mangione S, Nieman LZ: Cardiac auscultation skills in internal medicine and family practice trainees: A comparison of diagnostic proficiency. JAMA 1997;278:717-722.

4. St Clair EW, Oddone EZ, Waugh RA, et al: Assessing housestaff diagnostic skills using a cardiology patient simulator. Ann Intern Med 1992;117:751-756.

5. Geggel RL, Armsby LB: Evaluation and initial management of cyanotic heart disease in the newborn. In Rose BD (ed): UpToDate. Wellesley, Mass, UpToDate, 2003.

6. Rudolph AM: Oxygen uptake and delivery. In Congenital Diseases of the Heart. Armonk, NY, Futura, 2001, p 85.

7. Greenwood RD, Rosenthal A, Parisi L, et al: Extracardiac anomalies in children with congenital heart disease. Pediatrics 1975;55:485-492.

8. Marino BS, Bird GL, Wernovsky G: Diagnosis and management of the newborn with suspected congenital heart disease. Clin Perinatol 2001;28:91-136.

9. Davignon A, et al: Percentile charts—ECG standards for children. Pediatr Cardiol 1980;1:133-151.

10. Marriott HJL: Atrial arrhythmias. In Practical Electrocardiography, 5th ed. Baltimore, Williams & Wilkins, 1975, pp 128-152.

11. Duff DF, McNamara DG: History and physical examination of the cardiovascular system. In Garson A Jr, Bricker TM, Fisher DJ, Neish SR (eds): The Science and Practice of Pediatric Cardiology. Baltimore, Williams & Wilkins, 1998, pp 693-713.

12. Hoffman GS: Takayasu arteritis: Lessons from the American National Institutes of Health experience. Int J Cardiol 1996;54(Suppl): S99-S102.

13. Report of the Second Task Force on Blood Pressure Control in Children—1987. Pediatrics 1987;79:1-25.

14. Fyler DC, Nadas AS: History, physical examination, and laboratory test. In Fyler DC (ed): Nadas' Pediatric Cardiology. Philadelphia, Hanley & Belfus, 1992, pp 101-116.

15. Rappaport MB, Sprague HB: Physiologic and physical laws that govern auscultation, and their clinical application. Am Heart J 1941;21:257-318.

16. Marino BS, Goldblatt A: Heart sounds and murmurs. In Lilly LS (ed): Pathophysiology of Heart Disease. Philadelphia, Lea & Febiger, 1992, pp 18-29.

17. Perloff JK: Heart sounds and murmurs: Physiologic mechanisms. In Braunwald E (ed): Heart Disease: A Textbook of Cardiovascular Medicine, 4th ed. Philadelphia, WB Saunders, 1992, pp 43-63.

18. Geggel RL: Treatment of pulmonary hypertension. In Burg FD, Inglefinger JR, Wald ER, Polin RA (eds): Current Pediatric Therapy, 16th ed. Philadelphia, WB Saunders, 1999, pp 597-601.

19. Wolferth CC, Margolies A: Gallop rhythm and the physiologic third heart sound. Am Heart J 1933;8:441-461.

20. Warren JV, Leonard JJ, Weissler AM: Gallop rhythm. Ann Intern Med 1958;48:580-596.

21. Freeman AR, Levine SA: The clinical significance of the systolic murmur: A study of 1000 consecutive "non-cardiac" cases. Ann Intern Med 1933; 6:1371-1385.

CHAPTER 82

Electrocardiogram Interpretation

Eugene M. Mowad

Despite major technologic advances in the practice of pediatric cardiology, the electrocardiogram (ECG) remains a valuable tool for screening and diagnosing potential cardiac pathology. Detailed and comprehensive reviews of the science and interpretation of pediatric ECGs can be found elsewhere.[1-3] This chapter covers the basic approach to ECG interpretation for hospital clinicians confronted with children with possible cardiac problems.

TYPICAL CARDIAC CYCLE AND WAVEFORMS

One value of the ECG is in localizing problems along the cardiac conduction pathway. In the normal cardiac cycle, an impulse is generated first in the sinoatrial (SA) node. This electrical activity correlates to the P wave on the ECG and results in contraction of the atria. Once the impulse has spread over the atria, it is conducted in a slower fashion to the ventricles. The electrical delay occurs at the atrioventricular (AV) node and results in the PQ segment on the ECG. The QRS complex represents conduction of the electrical impulse through the AV bundles and results in ventricular contraction. Ventricular repolarization occurs during relaxation of the ventricles and is represented by the T wave on the ECG. Figure 82-1 illustrates the important waveforms and intervals seen in a typical cardiogram. Figures 82-2 and 82-3 show normal ECG recordings for patients of different ages.

LEAD ORIENTATION AND OTHER TECHNICAL ASPECTS

A second important aspect of the ECG is that it can provide anatomic information about cardiac structures, such as their relative sizes and locations. This information is obtained by recording the ECG from several different points of view simultaneously. So that information can be easily extracted and generalized, several technical aspects of the ECG are standardized, including the 12 standard leads. Six of the leads are in the frontal plane (bipolar limb leads I, II, and III; augmented unipolar limb leads aV_R, aV_L, and aV_F); the other six leads are in the transverse plane and are known as the precordial leads (V_1 through V_6). Understanding the spatial orientation of the limb leads, as shown in Figure 82-4, is crucial to interpretation of the QRS axis. Note the angular relationships in the frontal plane and the direction that correlates to a positive deflection on the recording from each of these leads. Because many congenital heart lesions affect the right ventricle specifically, pediatric centers may also use specialized leads known as V_{3R} or V_{4R}. These leads are placed over the right chest in mirror-image positions to the V_3 and V_4 leads on the left chest and provide additional assessment of the right ventricle.

In addition to standardized leads, ECG recording speed and sensitivity are standardized, which allows us to use the common interpretation methods discussed later. The standard paper speed for recording is 25 mm/second, and the standard sensitivity equates 1 mV with 10 mm of deflection on the tracing.

HEART RATE

Given the standard recording speed, it follows that each 1 mm on the horizontal axis (one small block on the recording paper) represents 0.04 second of recording, and each 5 mm (one large block) represents 0.2 second of recording. Heart rate can be approximated simply by counting the number of cardiac cycles (or fractions thereof) in a 1-second time frame (five large blocks) and multiplying by 60. A more accurate but more cumbersome method is to divide 60 by the interval in seconds between two successive R waves. Alternatively, an estimate can be obtained by dividing 300 by the number of large blocks between two successive R waves. Heart rates are age dependent; normal values are summarized in Table 82-1.

DURATIONS AND INTERVALS

Using the paper speed as a time reference, durations of the particular waveforms and intervals between them can be calculated. These intervals and durations provide important information about the time course of the cardiac cycle. The P-wave duration is defined as the time elapsed from the beginning of the P-wave deflection until its return to baseline. Normal P-wave durations range up to 0.1 second. The P-R interval is measured from the onset of the P wave to the beginning of the QRS complex. P-R intervals typically range from 0.1 to 0.2 second. The QRS duration is measured from the beginning deflection of the QRS complex until its return to baseline. Normal QRS durations should be less than 0.08 second. QRS duration is prolonged in bundle branch block. The Q-T interval is measured from the beginning of the QRS complex to the end of the T wave. The Q-T interval is influenced by heart rate, and because heart rates in children are so variable, a more useful value is the corrected Q-T interval, or Q-Tc. The Q-Tc is obtained by dividing the measured Q-T interval by the square root of the previous R-R interval, which is the time between the peaks of two successive R waves. Q-Tc intervals should be less than 0.44 second. Excellent, detailed references are available with age-based norms for the durations and intervals discussed here.[3-5]

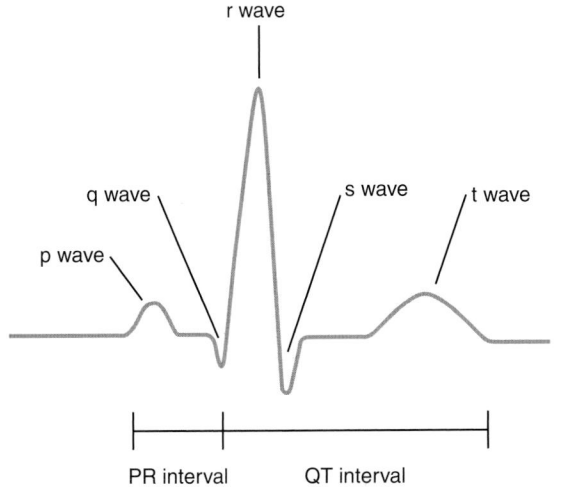

Figure 82-1 Stylized ECG recording of a typical cardiac cycle.

Table 82-1   Heart Rate Norms by Age

Age	Heart Rate Mean (Range)
1-3 days	123 (91-159)
3-6 days	129 (91-166)
1-3 wk	148 (107-182)
1-2 mo	149 (121-179)
3-5 mo	141 (106-186)
6-11 mo	134 (109-169)
1-2 yr	119 (89-151)
3-4 yr	108 (73-137)
5-7 yr	100 (65-133)
8-11 yr	91 (62-130)
12-15 yr	85 (60-119)

Adapted from Gunn V, Nechyba C (eds): The Harriet Lane Handbook. St Louis, Mosby, 2002.

RHYTHM

The typical cardiac rhythm is called normal sinus rhythm. To qualify as normal sinus rhythm, the heart rate must be within age-appropriate norms (see Table 82-1). Additionally, each QRS complex should be preceded by a P wave, and the P-R interval should be constant. If each of these characteristics is met except for a normal heart rate for age, the rhythm is described as sinus tachycardia or sinus bradycardia. Rhythms that originate in the AV node rather than the SA node lack a P wave but retain the characteristic narrow (<0.08 second) QRS complex. A commonly encountered example of a narrow-complex tachyarrhythmia is supraventricular tachycardia (Fig. 82-5). Ventricular rhythms have wide QRS complexes and P waves that have no constant relationship to the QRS complex (Fig. 82-6). It is important to note that some wide-complex rhythms may represent atrial rhythms (atrial premature beats or supraventricular tachycardia) that are conducted aberrantly.

QRS AXIS

The spatial orientation of the electrical forces during the cardiac cycle can be used to determine the electrical axis of ventricular depolarization. The most useful of the electrical axes is the QRS axis, and there are several ways to calculate it. The simplest way is as follows: knowing the orientation of the limb leads, determine the quadrant in which the axis lies. This is usually accomplished by noting the predominant deflection (positive or negative) of the QRS complexes in leads I and aV_F. For example, if the QRS complexes in leads I and aV_F were both positive (see Fig. 82-2), one would locate the axis in the quadrant between 0 and +90 degrees. Once the quadrant is known, a more exact determination of the axis is obtained by locating the limb lead in which the QRS complex is closest to equiphasic (equal positive and negative deflections). The approximated QRS axis lies perpendicular to the equiphasic lead in the quadrant previously determined. Many ECG machines simply calculate the QRS axis as part of the ECG. The QRS axis typically lies between −10 and +110 degrees, but normal newborns have a physiologic rightward shift.

The QRS axis can also provide a clue to the presence of congenital heart disease. Endocardial cushion defects typically have a superior axis, defined as a QRS axis above the horizontal line in Figure 82-4. A primum atrial septal defect is often associated with a QRS axis between 0 and −90 degrees (positive QRS deflection in lead I, negative deflection in lead aV_F). A complete AV canal defect usually produces a QRS axis between −90 and 180 degrees (negative QRS deflection in both leads I and aV_F). In neonates with cyanotic heart disease, relative left axis deviation (QRS axis between 0 and +90 degrees) can occur with severe valvular pulmonary stenosis; a more marked left axis deviation (QRS axis 0 to −90 degrees) is associated with tricuspid atresia and normally related great arteries.

CHAMBER HYPERTROPHY

The ECG can be used to approximate chamber sizes in the atria or to obtain evidence of hypertrophy in the ventricles. Enlargement of the right atrium is associated with tall P waves (>3 mm). The tall P wave of right atrial enlargement is also known as P pulmonale and is typically best seen in lead II (Fig. 82-7). Enlargement of the left atrium is associated with prolongation of the P wave duration beyond 0.1 second. The broad P wave of left atrial enlargement is known as P mitrale (see Fig. 82-7). In addition to having a prolonged duration, the P waves may be notched or biphasic. If both atria are enlarged, the P waves may have both a tall initial deflection and a long duration.

Ventricular hypertrophy is more difficult to determine. The electrical axis of the heart is often shifted toward the hypertrophied ventricle. As previously stated, it is normal for newborns to have a physiologic right axis for the first month of life. After that time, the QRS axis is typically between −10 and +110 degrees. Other criteria used to determine ventricular hypertrophy essentially rely on the fact that a hypertrophied ventricle generates higher voltages on the cardiogram. Criteria for ventricular hypertrophy are listed in Table 82-2, with age-related norms given in Table 82-3. Figures 82-8 and 82-9 show examples of ventricular hypertrophy.

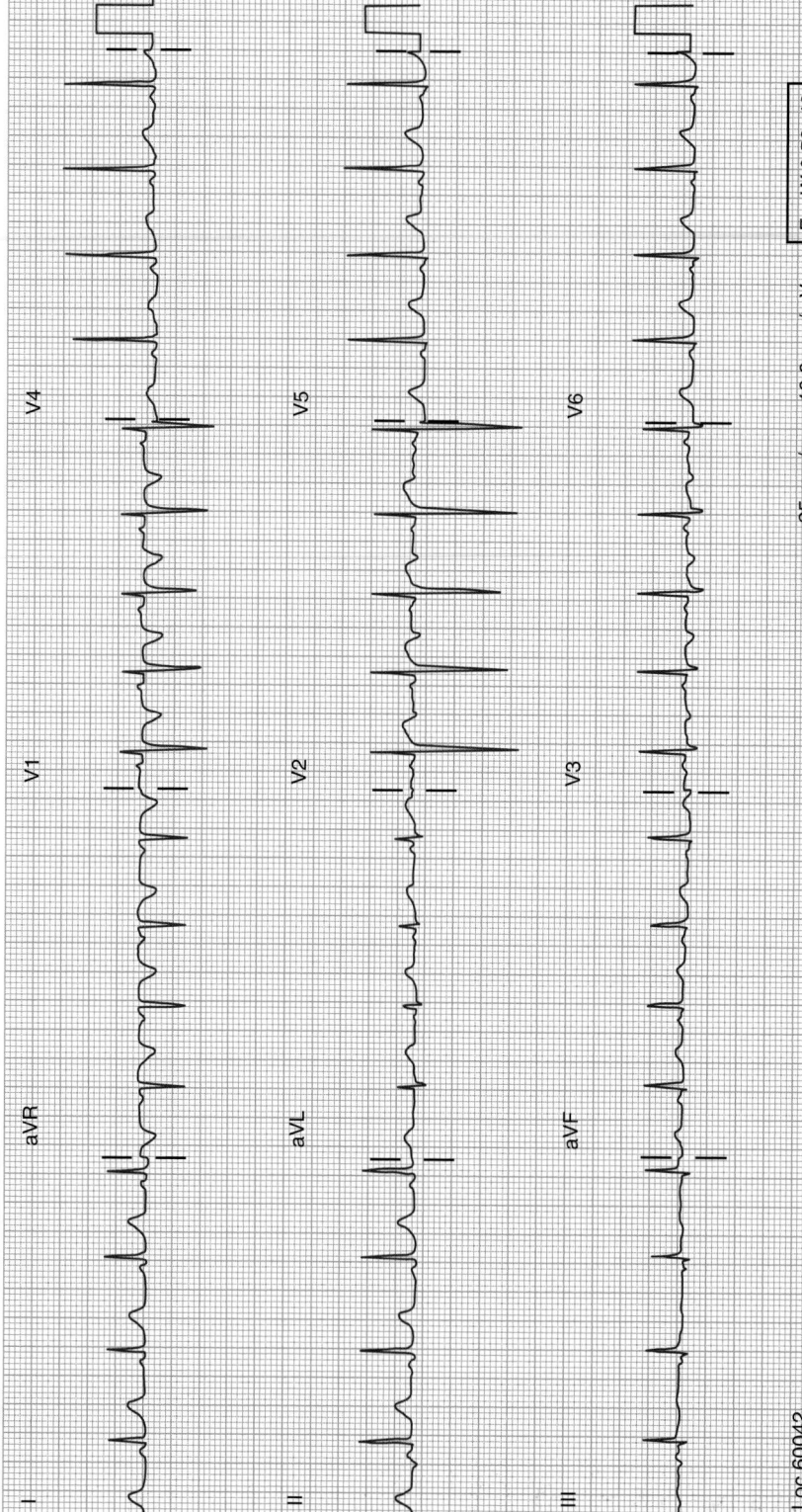

Figure 82-2 Normal ECG from an 8-year-old. Note the upward deflection of the QRS complexes in leads I and aV$_F$, which localizes the axis between 0 and 90 degrees. (Courtesy of Dr. Michael Saalouke, Division of Pediatric Cardiology, Tod Children's Hospital, Youngstown, Ohio.)

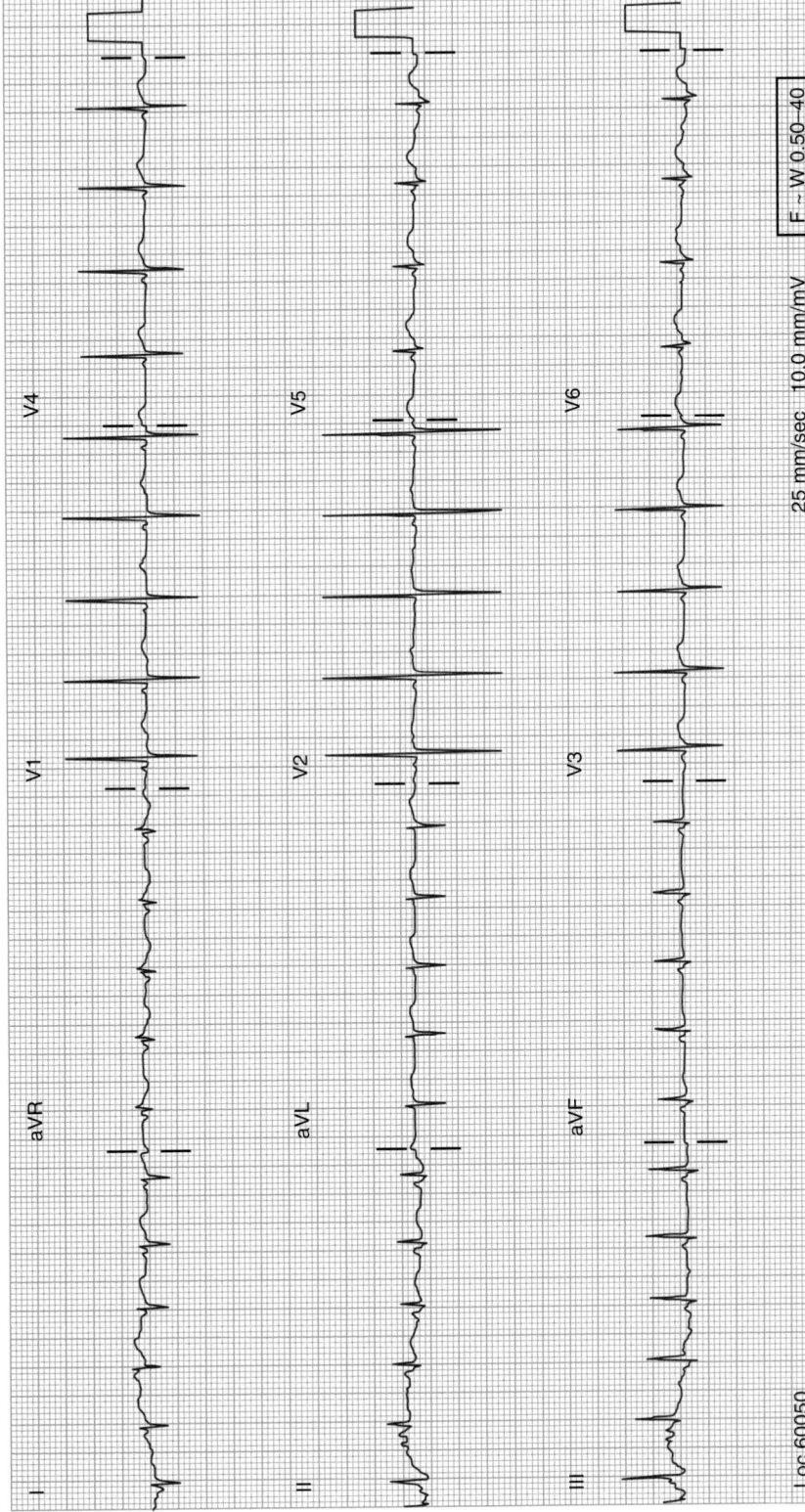

Figure 82–3 Normal newborn ECG. Note the negative QRS deflection in lead I and the positive deflection in lead aV_F, which localizes the axis between 90 and 180 degrees—physiologic for a newborn. At age 2 days, this infant also has a normal upright T wave in lead V_1. (Courtesy of Dr. Michael Saalouke, Division of Pediatric Cardiology, Tod Children's Hospital, Youngstown, Ohio.)

ST-SEGMENT AND T-WAVE CHANGES

The ST segment and T waves relate to ventricular repolarization. Conditions such as myocarditis or ischemia can cause pathologic changes in the ST segment. ST segments are typically on the same baseline as the PQ segment (see Fig. 82-1); however, they may be 1 to 2 mm higher or lower and still be normal. ST segments more than 1 to 2 mm above baseline are termed elevated, and those more than 1 to 2 mm lower than baseline are termed depressed. Elevation or depression alone does not necessarily imply pathology. Early repolarization of the ventricles—a normal variant most commonly seen in adolescents—causes ST-segment elevation in one or more precordial leads. A good rule of thumb is that the combination of an abnormal baseline and a downsloping or flat ST segment is abnormal. A depressed ST segment that slopes upward is often normal.

The T-wave deflection is normally in the same direction as the QRS complex. The T-wave axis can be calculated using the same method described for the QRS axis and should be within 90 degrees of the QRS axis. An abnormal T-wave axis suggests ventricular strain. The T wave normally becomes upright in lead V_6 after 24 to 48 hours of age and in V_5 by 1

Text continued on p. 532.

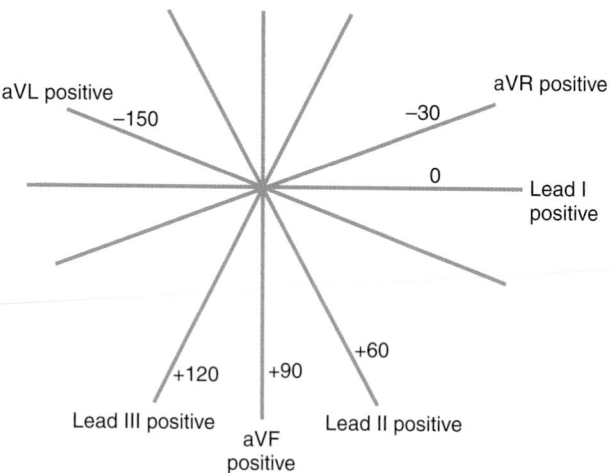

Figure 82-4 Spatial orientation of the limb leads in the frontal plane.

Table 82-2 Criteria for Ventricular Hypertrophy*

Right Ventricular Hypertrophy	Left Ventricular Hypertrophy
R wave in V_1 >98th percentile	R wave in V_6 >98th percentile
S wave in V_6 >98th percentile	S wave in V_1 >98th percentile
Upright T wave in V_1[†]	

Supplemental
  Q wave in V_1
  Right axis deviation
	Supplemental
	  Deep Q wave in V_6
	  Left axis deviation

*At least one criterion must be present to entertain the diagnosis.
[†]In patients between 3 days and 10 years old.
Adapted from Gunn V, Nechyba C (eds): The Harriet Lane Handbook. St Louis, Mosby, 2002.

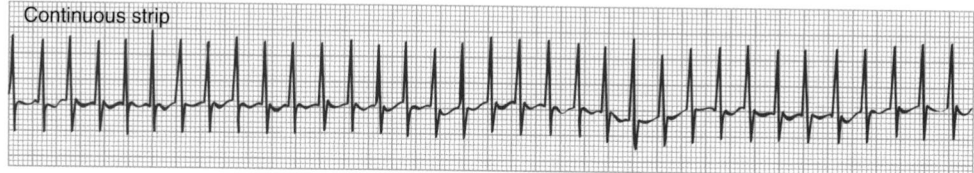

Figure 82-5 ECG showing the narrow QRS complexes and rapid rate seen in a patient with supraventricular tachycardia. (Courtesy of Dr. Michael Saalouke, Division of Pediatric Cardiology, Tod Children's Hospital, Youngstown, Ohio.)

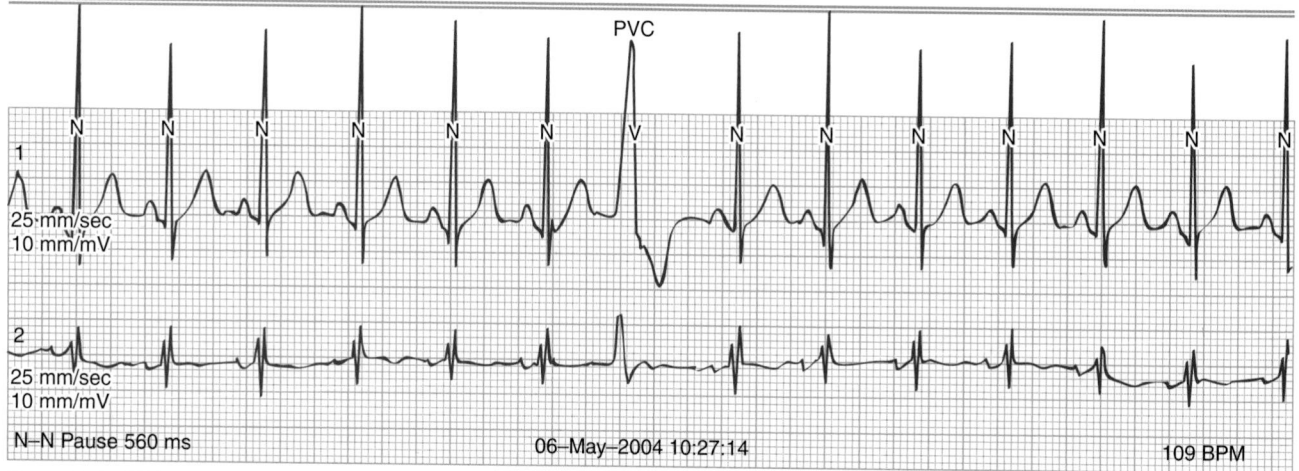

Figure 82-6 Wide QRS complex characteristic of a beat arising in the ventricles. This example represents an isolated premature ventricular contraction (PVC). (Courtesy of Dr. Michael Saalouke, Division of Pediatric Cardiology, Tod Children's Hospital, Youngstown, Ohio.)

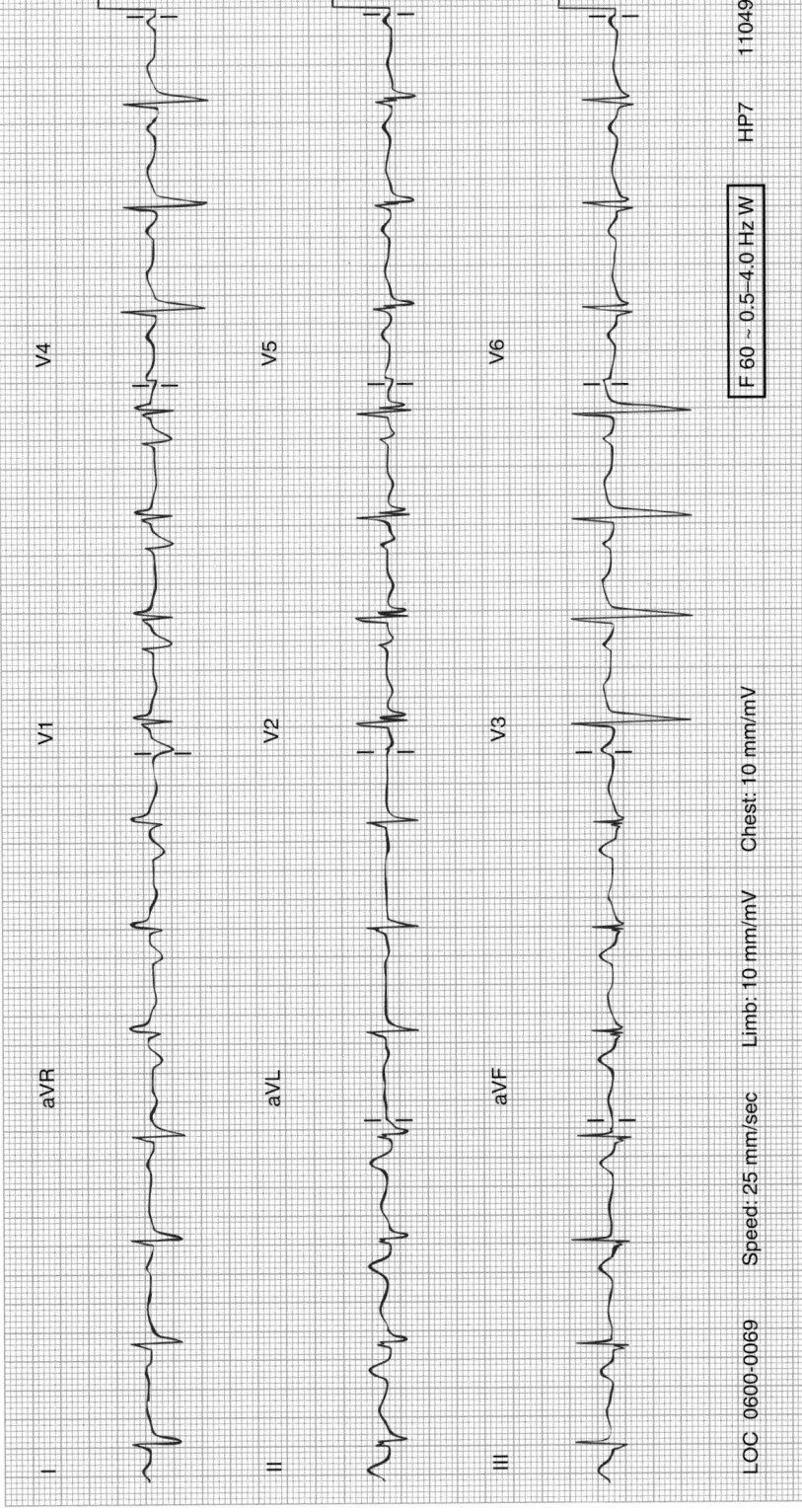

Figure 82-7 ECG showing P mitrale of left atrial enlargement (broad and biphasic P wave seen most readily in lead V₁), P pulmonale of right atrial enlargement (peaked P wave >2.5 mm in lead II), and first-degree heart block (P-R interval 200 msec). (Courtesy of Dr. Michael Saalouke, Division of Pediatric Cardiology, Tod Children's Hospital, Youngstown, Ohio.)

Table 82-3   Normal Pediatric Electrocardiogram Parameters

Age	Heart Rate (bpm)	QRS Axis*	PR Interval (sec)*	QRS Duration (sec)†	LEAD V₁ R-Wave Amplitude (mm)†	LEAD V₁ S-Wave Amplitude (mm)†	LEAD V₁ R/S Ratio	LEAD V₆ R-Wave Amplitude (mm)†	LEAD V₆ S-Wave Amplitude (mm)†	LEAD V₆ R/S Ratio
0-7 days	95-160 (125)	+30 to 180 (110)	0.08-0.12 (0.10)	0.05 (0.07)	13.3 (25.5)	7.7 (18.8)	2.5	4.8 (11.8)	3.2 (9.6)	2.2
1-3 wk	105-180 (145)	+30 to 180 (110)	0.08-0.12 (0.10)	0.05 (0.07)	10.6 (20.8)	4.2 (10.8)	2.9	7.6 (16.4)	3.4 (9.8)	3.3
1-6 mo	110-180 (145)	+10 to +125 (+70)	0.08-0.13 (0.11)	0.05 (0.07)	9.7 (19)	5.4 (15)	2.3	12.4 (22)	2.8 (8.3)	5.6
6-12 mo	110-170 (135)	+10 to +125 (+60)	0.10-0.14 (0.12)	0.05 (0.07)	9.4 (20.3)	6.4 (18.1)	1.6	12.6 (22.7)	2.1 (7.2)	7.6
1-3 yr	90-150 (120)	+10 to +125 (+60)	0.10-0.14 (0.12)	0.06 (0.07)	8.5 (18)	9 (21)	1.2	14 (23.3)	1.7 (6)	10
4-5 yr	65-135 (110)	0 to +110 (+60)	0.11-0.15 (0.13)	0.07 (0.08)	7.6 (16)	11 (22.5)	0.8	15.6 (25)	1.4 (4.7)	11.2
6-8 yr	60-130 (100)	−15 to +110 (+60)	0.12-0.16 (0.14)	0.07 (0.08)	6 (13)	12 (24.5)	0.6	16.3 (26)	1.1 (3.9)	13
9-11 yr	60-110 (85)	−15 to +110 (+60)	0.12-0.17 (0.14)	0.07 (0.09)	5.4 (12.1)	11.9 (25.4)	0.5	16.3 (25.4)	1.0 (3.9)	14.3
12-16 yr	60-110 (85)	−15 to +110 (+60)	0.12-0.17 (0.15)	0.07 (0.10)	4.1 (9.9)	10.8 (21.2)	0.5	14.3 (23)	0.8 (3.7)	14.7
>16 yr	60-100 (80)	−15 to +110 (+60)	0.12-0.20 (0.15)	0.08 (0.10)	3 (9)	10 (20)	0.3	10 (20)	0.8 (3.7)	12

From Gunn V, Nechyba C (eds): Harriet Lane Handbook. St Louis, Mosby, 2002.
*Normal range and (mean).
†Mean and (98th percentile).
bpm, beats per minute.

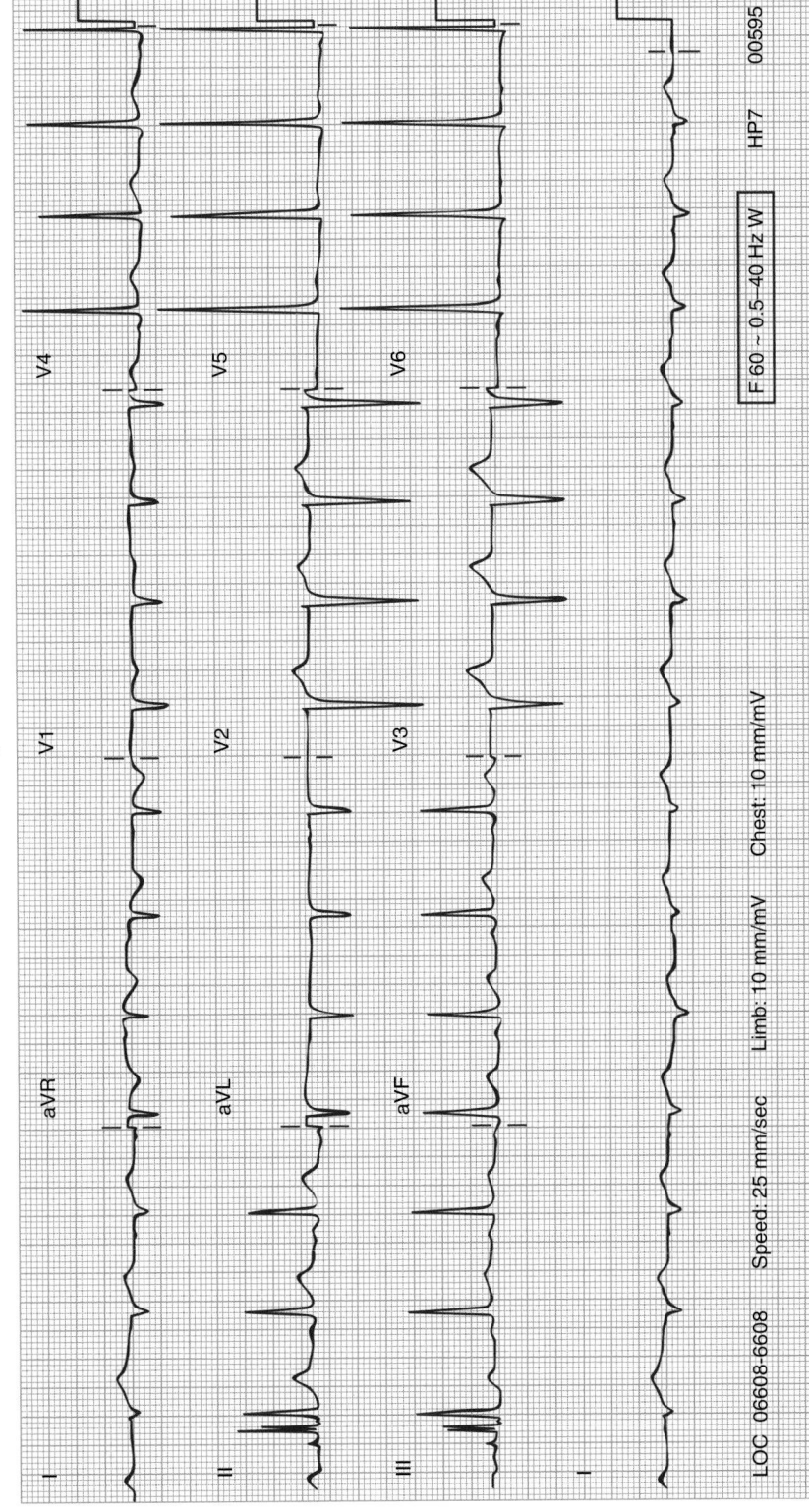

Figure 82-8 ECG demonstrating left ventricular hypertrophy and left ventricular strain. The R wave in V$_6$ is 28 mm, which is above the 98th percentile for this 12-year-old. The T waves are flattened in leads V$_5$ and V$_6$. (Courtesy of Dr. Michael Saalouke, Division of Pediatric Cardiology, Tod Children's Hospital, Youngstown, Ohio.)

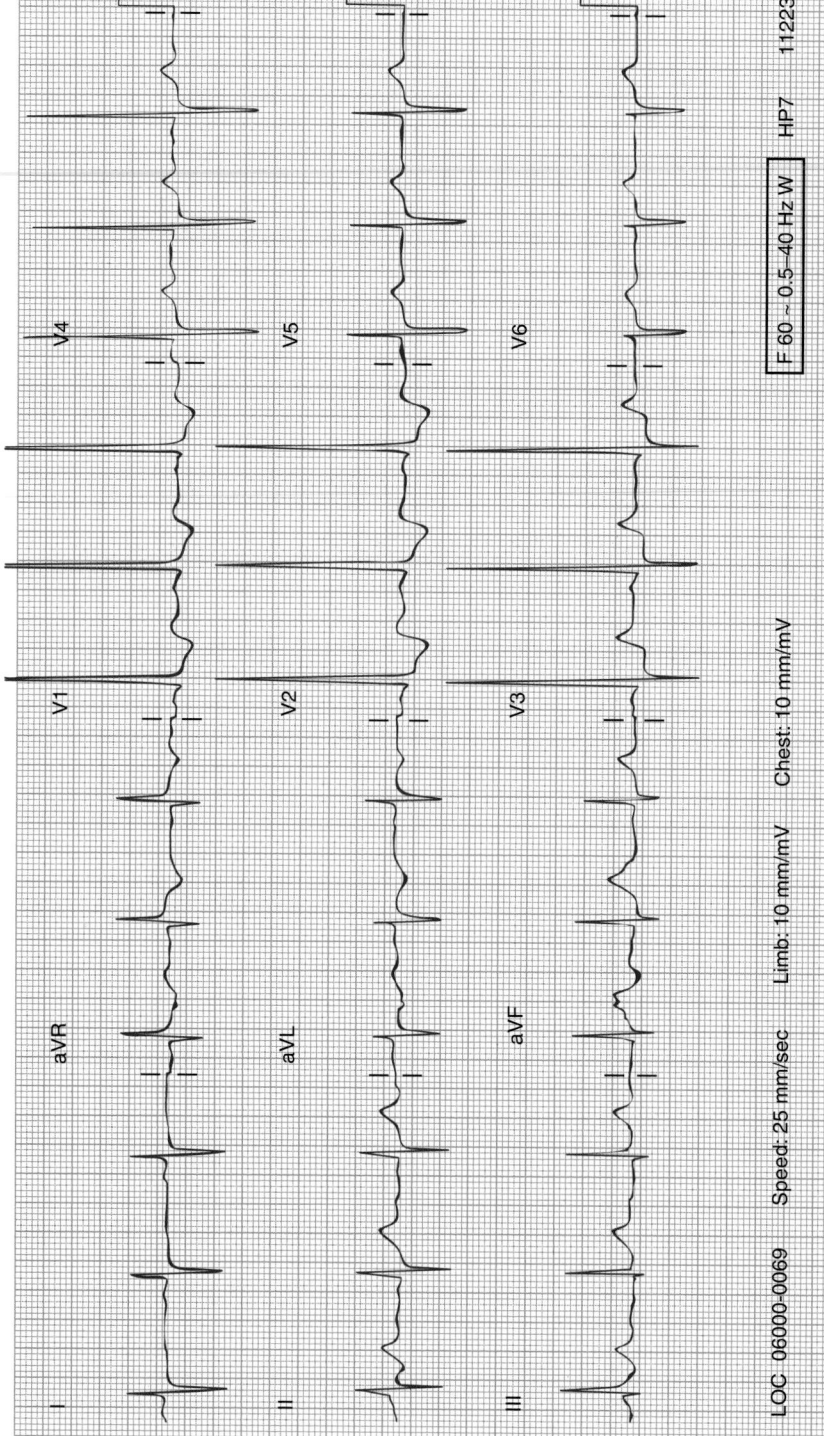

Figure 82-9 ECG demonstrating right ventricular hypertrophy. There is right axis deviation, as evidenced by the predominantly downward deflection in lead I and upward deflection in aV$_F$. The R-wave voltage in V$_1$ and S-wave voltage in V$_6$ are both significantly above the 98th percentile for this 9-year-old. (Courtesy of Dr. Michael Saalouke, Division of Pediatric Cardiology, Tod Children's Hospital, Youngstown, Ohio.)

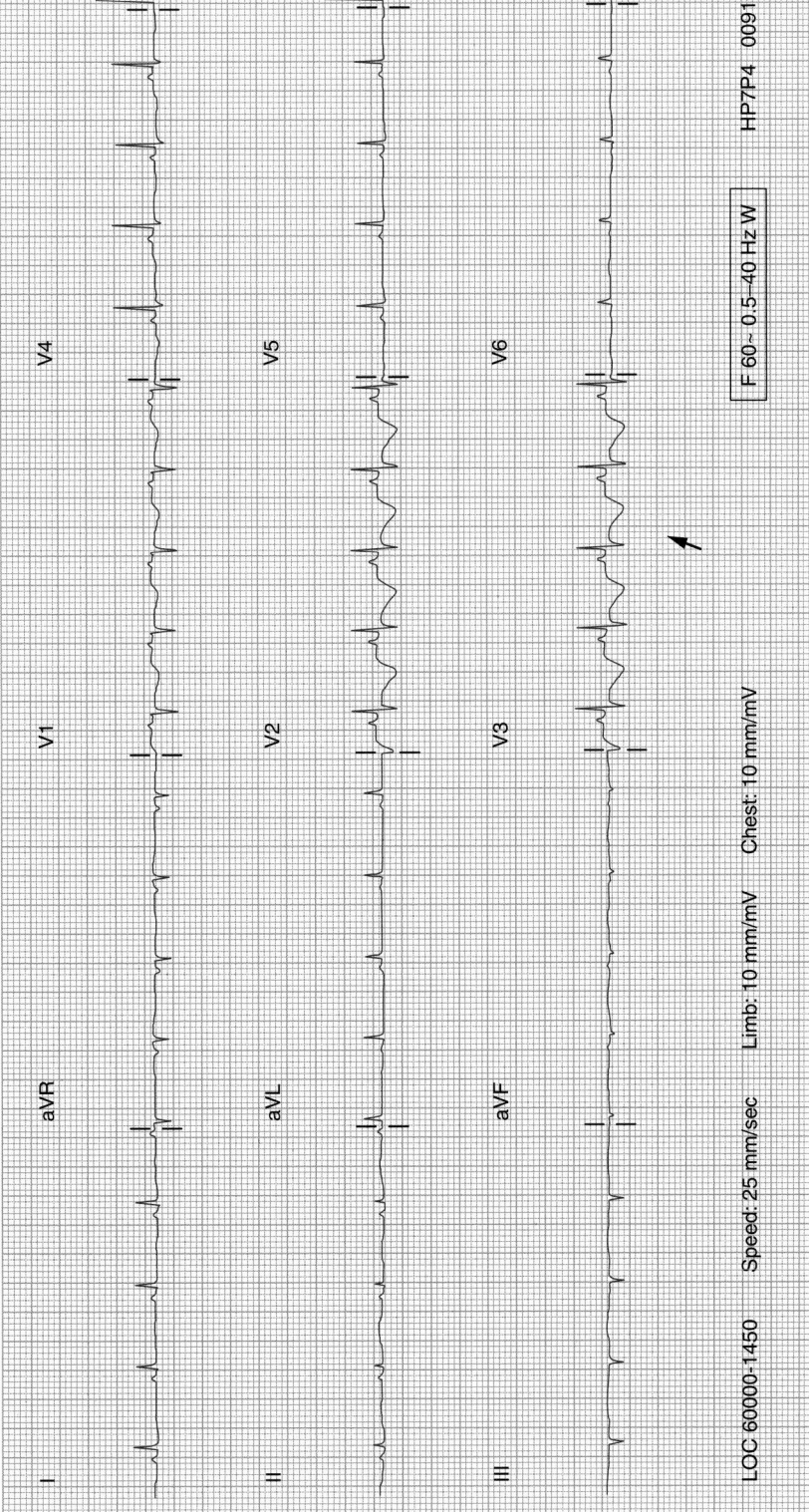

Figure 82-10 ECG demonstrating diminished voltages, ST depression with downward T waves in V_2 and V_3, and flattened T waves in many leads in this patient with myopericarditis. (Courtesy of Dr. Michael Saalouke, Division of Pediatric Cardiology, Tod Children's Hospital, Youngstown, Ohio.)

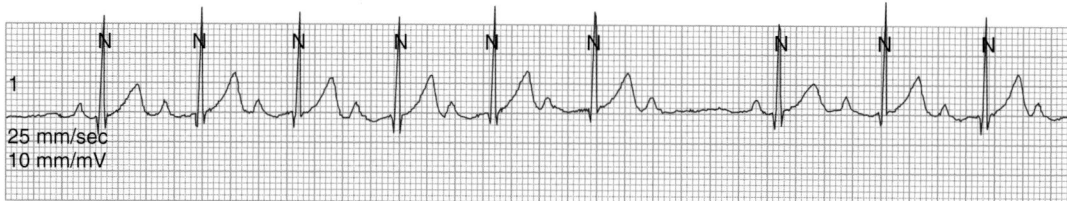

Figure 82-11 ECG demonstrating peaked T waves in a patient with hyperkalemia. There is also gradual prolongation of the P-R interval, with a nonconducted P wave after the sixth QRS complex, consistent with Wenckebach second-degree heart block. (Courtesy of Dr. Michael Saalouke, Division of Pediatric Cardiology, Tod Children's Hospital, Youngstown, Ohio.)

week of age. It then becomes upright sequentially from V_4 to V_1 during childhood, reaching V_1 by early adolescence. The T-wave deflection in V_1 or V_2 can be upright or inverted in normal adolescents or adults. In the first few days of life, the T wave may be upright in V_1 as well. A T wave that is inverted for age is seen in conditions associated with ventricular strain, ischemia, or inflammation (Fig. 82-10). Tall, peaked (tented) T waves may be seen in hyperkalemia (Fig. 82-11) or in patients with ischemia or infarction.

Q-WAVE ABNORMALITIES

Q waves represent the initial phase of ventricular depolarization. They are pathologic if they are abnormally wide (>0.2 second) or abnormally deep (>5 mm). Q waves that are pathologically deep but not wide are often indicators of ventricular hypertrophy. Q waves that are both abnormally deep and wide imply myocardial infarction. Patients with an anomalous origin of the left coronary artery from the pulmonary artery typically develop anterolateral infarction with abnormal Q waves in leads I and aV_L and precordial leads V_4 to V_6 (Fig. 82-12).

P-R AND Q-T INTERVALS

The P-R interval represents the normal conduction time from the sinus node to the onset of ventricular depolarization. It can be prolonged in conditions associated with atrial enlargement, due to a delay in conduction through the atria, or in conditions associated with delay in conduction through the AV node. It is shortened in Wolff-Parkinson-White syndrome, in which case there is a slurring of the upstroke of the QRS complex (delta wave) (Fig. 82-13), or if there is an ectopic atrial pacemaker. The method for calculating the Q-T interval was described earlier. A prolonged Q-Tc is a risk factor for ventricular arrhythmia. Prolonged Q-T intervals are seen as part of the congenital long QT syndrome but may also be acquired and associated with myocarditis, ischemia, electrolyte abnormalities (hypocalcemia or hypomagnesemia), and a variety of medications, including antiarrhythmic agents (quinidine, procainamide, flecainide, amiodarone, sotalol), antibiotics (trimethoprim-sulfamethoxazole), tricyclic antidepressants, and the gastrointestinal agent cisapride.[6]

HEART BLOCK

When sinus impulses are not normally conducted to initiate ventricular responses, an AV block is said to occur. AV block is categorized as first, second, or third degree. In first-degree AV block, there is simply a prolongation of the P-R interval, but each atrial impulse initiates a ventricular response (see Fig. 82-7). The P-R interval varies with age; in adolescents, an interval greater than 0.2 second is prolonged. In second-degree AV block, some but not all atrial impulses are conducted; this results in P waves that are not followed by QRS complexes. In Mobitz type I second-degree heart block (also known as Wenckebach block), the P-R interval of the beats preceding the dropped beat gets progressively longer (see Fig. 82-11). In Mobitz type II second-degree heart block, the P-R interval of the preceding beats is constant. Patients with Mobitz type II heart block are at a higher risk of developing complete, or third-degree, heart block. In third-degree heart block, there is no connection between the atrial rate, as determined by the P-P interval, and the slower ventricular rate, as determined by the R-R interval.

AGE-RELATED ASPECTS OF INTERPRETATION

As discussed previously, heart rate norms vary with age (see Table 82-1), and as heart rates decline, the various waveform durations and intervals consequently increase. There are also several unique features of the newborn cardiogram. Because the right ventricle is the dominant pumping chamber in the newborn heart, newborn cardiograms display a rightward shift of the QRS axis and voltage changes of right ventricular hypertrophy. These changes persist throughout the first 1 to 2 months of life.

CONCLUSION

Interpretation of the ECG can be a complex art; however, some basic principles allow the generalist to understand much of the information to be gleaned from the recording. The most important aspect of ECG interpretation is a consistent approach. First, note the age of the patient and any age-related variations in interpretation that apply. Next, calculate the rate and axis. Evaluate the P waves and QRS complexes for direction and duration, which can point out important changes associated with arrhythmia, chamber enlargement, hypertrophy, ischemia, or infarction. Calculate the P-R and Q-Tc intervals and compare them to norms, especially if arrhythmia is a concern. Evaluate the ST segment and T waves for changes associated with ischemia, infarction, or electrolyte imbalances. The final reading of the ECG should be performed by the attending cardiologist or someone experienced in interpretation.

If the final interpretation is abnormal or diagnostic uncertainty exists, cardiology consultation should be obtained. The patient's clinical condition determines the

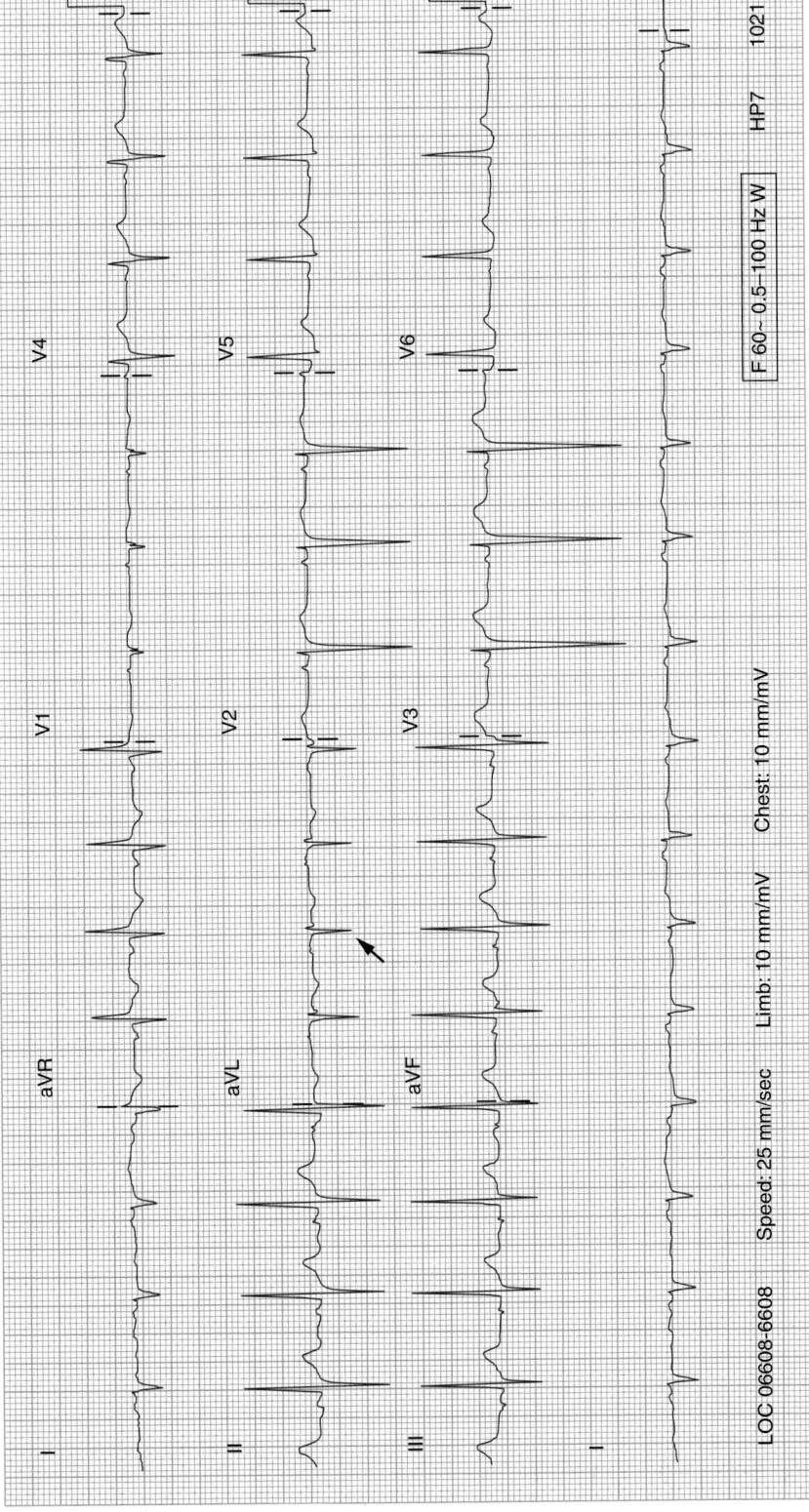

Figure 82-12   ECG demonstrating a pathologic Q wave (8 mm deep) in lead aV$_L$ in this patient with a left coronary artery arising from the pulmonary artery. (Courtesy of Dr. Michael Saalouke, Division of Pediatric Cardiology, Tod Children's Hospital, Youngstown, Ohio.)

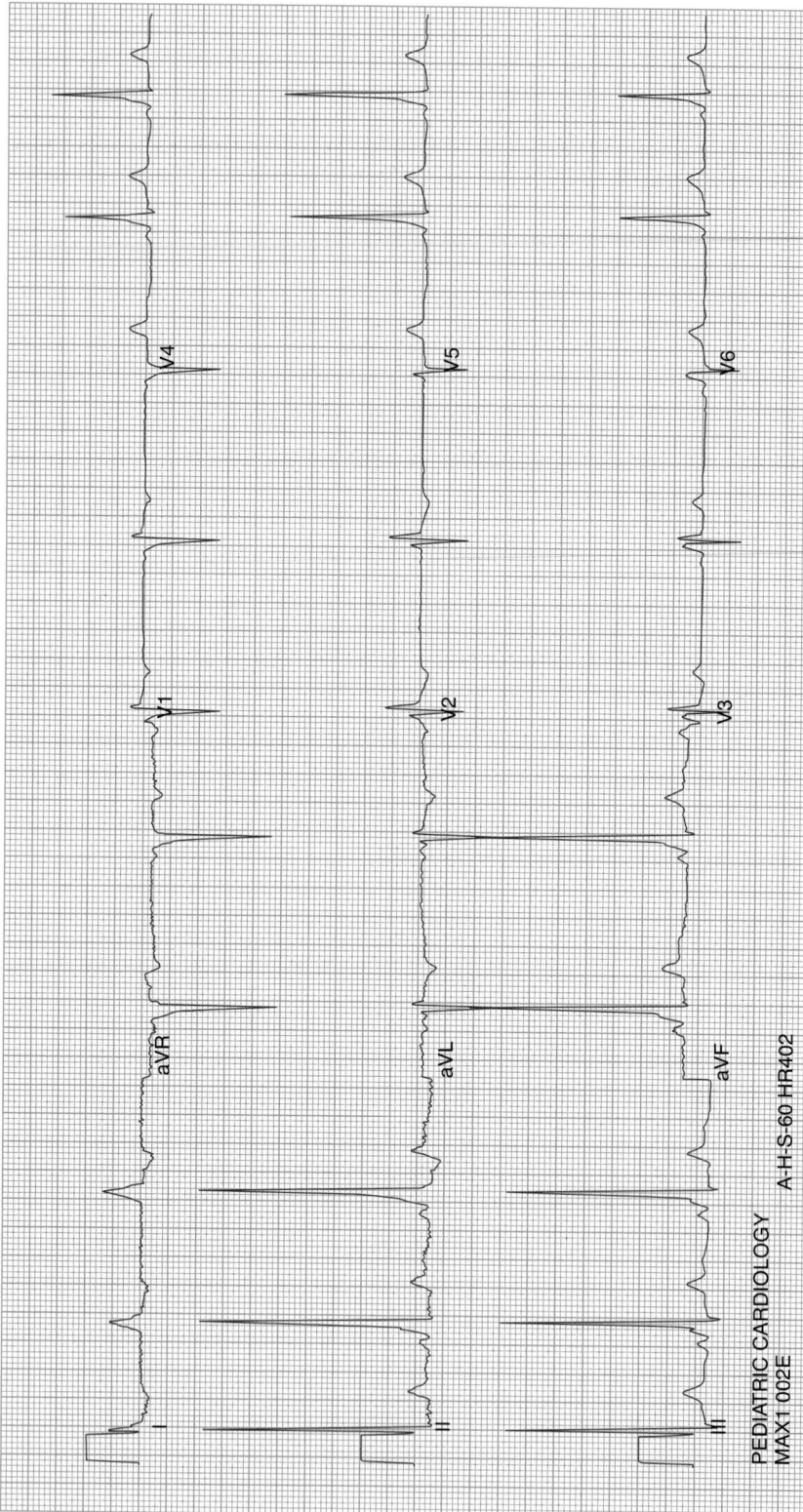

Figure 82–13 ECG demonstrating a delta wave (slurred upstroke of QRS complex) in a patient with Wolff–Parkinson–White syndrome. (Courtesy of Dr. Michael Saalouke, Division of Pediatric Cardiology, Tod Children's Hospital, Youngstown, Ohio.)

urgency of such consultation. Various clinical conditions are discussed in subsequent chapters; however, the following ECG findings alone merit prompt cardiologic intervention:

- Findings suggestive of ischemia or infarction, such as Q-wave and ST-segment abnormalities.
- Rhythms with wide complexes.
- Nonsinus tachy- or bradyarrhythmias.
- Any arrhythmia in a patient with a prolonged Q-Tc.

SUGGESTED READING

Liebman J, Plonsey R, Gillette PC: Pediatric Electrocardiography. Baltimore, Williams & Wilkins, 1982.

Park M, Gunteroth W: How to Read Pediatric ECGs. St Louis, Mosby, 1992.

REFERENCES

1. Park M, Gunteroth W: How to Read Pediatric ECGs. St Louis, Mosby, 1992.
2. Liebman J, Plonsey R, Gillette PC: Pediatric Electrocardiography. Baltimore, Williams & Wilkins, 1982.
3. Gunteroth W: Pediatric Electrocardiography. Philadelphia, WB Saunders, 1965.
4. Davignon A, et al: Normal ECG standards for infants and children. Pediatr Cardiol 1979;1:123-131.
5. Gunn V, Nechyba C (eds): The Harriet Lane Handbook. St Louis, Mosby, 2002.
6. Carboni MP, Garson A Jr: Long QT syndrome. In Deal B, Wolff G, Gelband H (eds): Current Concepts in Diagnosis and Management of Arrhythmias in Infants and Children. Armonk, NY, Futura, 1998, pp 241-265.

CHAPTER 83

Congenital Heart Disease

Barry A. Love

Congenital heart disease is estimated to occur in 0.8% of all children.[1] Fortunately, most of these problems are minor or self-limited and do not require intervention. Congenital heart disease requiring intervention is less common—about 3 to 4 in 1000.[2] For this group of patients with significant heart disease, the second half of the 20th century witnessed remarkable advances in diagnostic and therapeutic techniques. As a result, many children with previously lethal defects can now lead relatively normal lives.

Children with congenital heart disease may be hospitalized at the time of diagnosis if they present with critical heart disease, after cardiac interventions (surgical or transcatheter), or for acute illnesses related or unrelated to their heart conditions. Although some types of congenital cardiac disease involve straightforward anatomy, the hospitalist may be required to care for children with complex cardiac anatomy; these children are typically the ones with comorbid conditions who collectively spend the most time in the hospital. The pediatric hospitalist frequently plays an important role in the care of children with congenital heart disease, especially when it coexists with other disease processes.

CLINICAL PRESENTATION

Congenital heart disease typically presents in one of three time frames: the newborn period, early infancy, or childhood. Most cases of critical congenital heart disease present in the newborn period. These lesions are deemed "critical" because the patient's survival depends on ductal patency or emergent surgical or catheter intervention. Typical clues that suggest critical heart disease in a newborn include cyanosis or signs and symptoms of decreased perfusion. Increasingly, newborns with congenital heart disease already have detailed anatomic diagnoses thanks to prenatal screening by fetal echocardiography. In some centers, more than half of infants born with serious congenital heart disease have been diagnosed antenatally. Antenatal diagnosis allows for appropriate anticipatory management of these infants and has led to improved outcomes for patients with complex heart disease.[3]

A second group of patients with congenital heart disease presents in the weeks after birth as the pulmonary resistance falls to its nadir at 8 to 12 weeks of life. This group may present with murmurs or with symptoms of congestive heart failure (tachypnea, hepatomegaly) if there is significant pulmonary overcirculation. Late presentations associated with closure of the ductus arteriosus may also be seen at this time, with cyanosis, shock, or decreased femoral pulses.

The third common time frame for the diagnosis of congenital heart disease is during childhood. A more subtle heart murmur is often detected between 2 and 5 years of age, when the clinician is able to perform a thorough cardiac examination on a cooperative patient.

In addition to the usual presentations of congenital heart disease, some serious cardiovascular malformations masquerade as more common illnesses such as lung disease or laryngomalacia (Table 83-1).

DIAGNOSIS

The recognition of congenital heart disease rests on the foundation of a good clinical history and physical examination. An electrocardiogram may supplement the assessment of cardiac anatomy and is necessary for the diagnosis of rhythm problems. The diagnosis of congenital heart disease has been revolutionized by two-dimensional echocardiography, which provides a detailed anatomic and physiologic diagnosis of congenital heart disease, is noninvasive, and is easily performed at the bedside. When it is coupled with the Doppler technique, blood velocity can also be assessed, and this can be used to estimate chamber pressures and the presence of heart or great vessel obstruction or valve regurgitation. Because almost all the ultrasound waves are reflected at tissue-air interfaces, echocardiography is limited to views in which the lungs do not obstruct the path between the ultrasound beam and the heart. Factors that limit the usefulness of transthoracic echocardiography include obesity, obstructive lung disease, and certain chest wall deformities. Three-dimensional echocardiography is in the early stages of clinical application and may provide additional anatomic information.

Transesophageal echocardiography has multiple clinical applications. Because the heart sits directly anterior to the esophagus, without intervening lung tissue, excellent echocardiographic images of the heart can be obtained. This modality is well suited to assess cardiac anatomy in patients with poor transthoracic windows; to obtain the highest-quality images of posterior heart structures, such as the atrial septum and left atrium, in larger patients; to aid in interventional catheterization procedures, such as device closure of an atrial septal defect (ASD); or to assess the adequacy of cardiac surgical repair while the patient is still in the operating room. Although cardiologists routinely perform transesophageal echocardiography in lightly sedated adult patients, this is rarely possible in children and adolescents owing to the greater procedure-related anxiety and more pronounced gag reflex in younger patients. Deep sedation or general anesthesia is therefore needed.

Magnetic resonance imaging (MRI) is increasingly being used for the diagnostic evaluation of congenital heart disease. One advantage of cardiac MRI is that it shows excellent anatomic detail that is not limited by lung tissue, making it an especially good modality for imaging the great vessels. Major disadvantages include the relatively long processing and interpretation time and the need for general anesthesia

Table 83-1 Congenital Heart Diseases That Masquerade as Other Diseases

Presenting Symptom or Suspected Diagnosis	Congenital Heart Disease	Clue	Definitive Diagnostic Test
Frequent lower respiratory illnesses, asthma or bronchiolitis, failure to thrive	Ventricular septal defect Patent ductus arteriosus Atrioventricular septal defect Aortopulmonary window with elevated pulmonary vascular resistance	Loud, single second heart sound Abnormal ECG	Echocardiogram
Croup, laryngomalacia, bronchomalacia, feeding difficulties, reflux	Vascular ring	Often right aortic arch on chest radiograph	CT scan MRI Bronchoscopy
Asthma, bronchiolitis	Anomalous left coronary artery from the pulmonary artery Dilated cardiomyopathy	Cardiomegaly on chest radiograph Abnormal ECG	Echocardiogram (looking specifically at origin of coronary arteries)
Primary hypertension	Coarctation of the aorta	Decreased intensity of femoral pulses or radiofemoral delay	Four-extremity blood pressures Echocardiogram MRI
Severe neonatal respiratory distress	Total anomalous pulmonary venous return (with obstruction)	History not suggestive of infant at risk for pulmonary disease	Echocardiogram (complete, but focusing on pulmonary veins)

CT, computed tomography; ECG, electrocardiogram; MRI, magnetic resonance imaging.

in patients too young to remain motionless during image acquisition. Functional assessment of blood flow by MRI is possible and in many instances may be more accurate than echocardiography. MRI is contraindicated in patients with pacemakers. In addition, implanted metal such as surgical clips or embolization coils may cause imaging artifacts in some patients.

Cardiac catheterization with angiography was once considered the gold standard for anatomic diagnosis; however, echocardiography and MRI have now almost completely supplanted catheterization for anatomic diagnosis. Cardiac catheterization remains the gold standard for hemodynamic assessment, and it is increasingly being used as an interventional rather than a diagnostic tool.

TREATMENT

Treatment of congenital heart disease is complex owing to the wide variety of anatomic anomalies, the physiologic changes that happen over time (e.g., fall in pulmonary vascular resistance), and growth. Straightforward heart lesions are approached with surgical or transcatheter techniques that address a single problem (e.g., ASD). More complex forms of congenital heart disease are approached by first deciding whether there are enough cardiac "parts" to immediately or eventually repair the heart in such a way that it is physiologically, if not anatomically, correct.

Complete Repair

A "complete" or "two-ventricle" repair entails separate systemic and pulmonary circuits, each with its own ventricle—one pumping deoxygenated blood to the lungs, and

the other pumping oxygenated blood to the body. Although this type of repair is referred to as "complete," the resulting cardiac anatomy is often very different from normal. When possible, complete repair is the preferred option.

Single-Ventricle Pathway

When the cardiac anatomy does not permit a complete repair, the "single-ventricle" pathway is followed. This option is a type of cardiac palliation that ultimately results in what is generally called a Fontan repair, after the French surgeon who first described this type of operation in 1971 in two patients with tricuspid atresia.[4] Modifications of the technique have taken place, and this type of repair is now used for almost any form of anatomic heart disease not amenable to a complete repair.

The Fontan operation ultimately results in a circulation in which the venous blood return is routed passively to the lungs, without passing though a ventricle, and then returns to a functionally single ventricle that pumps blood to the body. For this type of repair to succeed, the patient must have a relatively competent atrioventricular valve, good systolic ventricular function, unobstructed outflow from the heart, widely patent pulmonary arteries, and low pulmonary vascular resistance. The vascular resistance of the neonatal pulmonary vascular bed is too high to accept the passive pulmonary flow of a Fontan repair, so a series of staged operations is necessary to ultimately achieve this type of palliation.

Stage I

The first stage of the single-ventricle pathway provides for adequate pulmonary blood flow and unobstructed systemic flow in the newborn period (Fig. 83-1). If the original

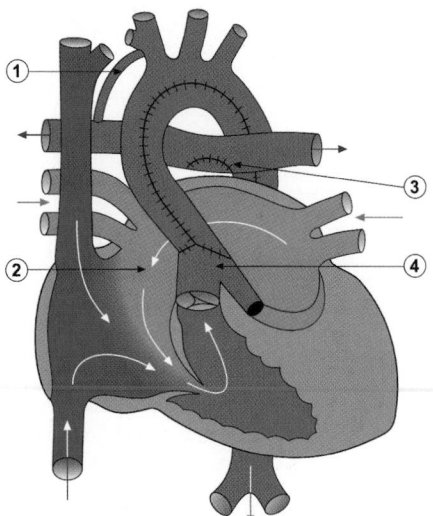

Figure 83-1   Stage I single-ventricle pathway for hypoplastic left heart syndrome (see Fig. 83-8 for unrepaired anatomy). (1) Right modified Blalock-Taussig shunt. (2) Large (surgically created) atrial septal defect. (3) Main pulmonary artery has been detached from branch pulmonary arteries. (4) Unobstructed egress of blood from the heart to the body has been achieved by using the main pulmonary artery and native aorta with additional patch material. (From Biomedical Communications, Health Sciences Center, Winnipeg, Manitoba, Canada.)

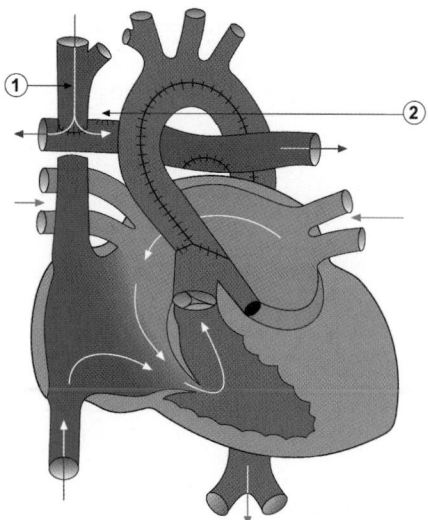

Figure 83-2   Stage II single-ventricle pathway for hypoplastic left heart syndrome. (1 and 2) The right modified Blalock-Taussig shunt that was created during the stage I repair has been removed. The superior vena cava is divided, and the proximal portion is attached directly to the right pulmonary artery, allowing blood from the superior vena cava to flow to both lungs (bidirectional Glenn procedure). "Bidirectional" refers to the superior vena caval blood flowing to both the right and left lungs. (From Biomedical Communications, Health Sciences Center, Winnipeg, Manitoba, Canada.)

cardiac anatomy is such that there is insufficient pulmonary flow, a shunt is surgically placed to provide flow from the systemic circulation to the pulmonary circulation, taking the place of the ductus arteriosus. One of the more common types of shunt is the modified Blalock-Taussig shunt, which is a synthetic tube placed from the subclavian artery to the ipsilateral pulmonary artery. There are many types of shunts and modifications of the technique, depending on the individual anatomy and operator preference.

An infant with an "ideal" physiology following shunt placement has a systemic oxygen saturation of about 80%. Empirically, this saturation has been found to be the best balance between systemic oxygen delivery and pulmonary overcirculation. Because blood circulating to the lungs is already partially saturated, shunt physiology is inefficient, and even with an "ideal" saturation of 80%, there is still about twice as much blood being circulated to the lungs as to the body.

If the original cardiac anatomy dictates a single-ventricle pathway but there is too much pulmonary flow, such that the pulmonary pressures are high or the infant is in congestive heart failure, the first stage in palliation is a pulmonary artery band. A pulmonary artery band is a surgical "noose" placed around the pulmonary artery that creates an artificial stenosis and limits pulmonary flow.

Of great importance in the single-ventricle pathway is the provision of an unobstructed path for systemic blood flow. The proximal pulmonary artery and aorta are often used together to recreate a single unobstructed outflow from the heart in this first stage.

Stage II

At about 4 to 8 months of age, the pulmonary vascular resistance has typically decreased sufficiently to accept a portion of the venous return in a passive manner. The

second step of cardiac palliation for children proceeding down the single-ventricle pathway is the bidirectional Glenn procedure (Fig. 83-2). This involves connecting the superior vena cava directly to the pulmonary arteries and eliminating any previous shunted source of pulmonary blood flow. The arterial saturations are usually about the same before and after the procedure (80%); however, this type of circulation is preferable because it is more efficient. In the shunted scenario, the single ventricle pumps blood to both the body and the lungs, and the blood pumped to the lungs is partially saturated—an inefficient arrangement. After the stage II repair, the heart is pumping blood only to the body, and only desaturated blood is flowing to the lungs, thereby increasing the efficiency.

Stage III

The third stage (Fontan completion) consists of redirecting the blood from the inferior vena cava to the lungs, thereby separating the pulmonary and systemic circuits (Fig. 83-3). The inferior vena cava blood can be directed to the lungs by placing a synthetic tube lateral to the heart (external conduit) or by using part of the right atrium as a wall (lateral tunnel). Often a small communication is left in the tube (fenestration) that can be closed later in the cardiac catheterization laboratory. After closure of the fenestration, these patients have normal oxygen saturations. Stage III is usually performed when the patient is between 2 and 5 years old, depending on center preference and technique.

Postoperative complications in patients with Fontan-type repairs include early problems, such as prolonged pleural effusions, and late problems, such as increased risk for stroke and thrombus formation, arrhythmias (especially atrial flutter), and protein-losing enteropathy.

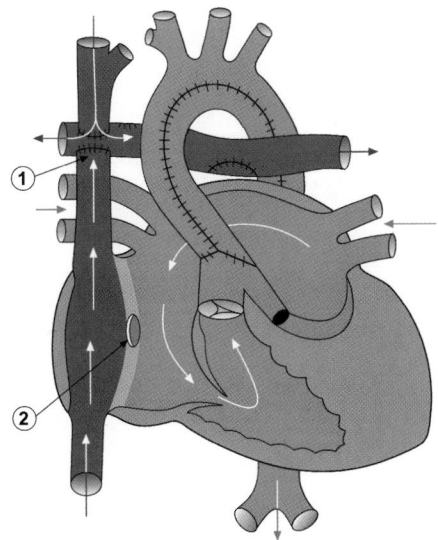

Figure 83-3 Stage III single-ventricle pathway for hypoplastic left heart syndrome. (1) A tube has been placed within the right atrium to direct blood from the inferior vena cava to the pulmonary artery. (2) Fenestration: a small hole is left in the tube to allow some of the venous blood to bypass the lungs. This keeps the venous pressure from rising too high after the Fontan operation but results in some desaturation. Fenestration may be "optional" in some patients, but if desired, it can easily be closed in the cardiac catheterization laboratory later. (From Biomedical Communications, Health Sciences Center, Winnipeg, Manitoba, Canada.)

Table 83-2 Critical Newborn Heart Diseases Dependent on a Patent Ductus Arteriosus (PDA)

PDA required to support pulmonary flow
  Critical pulmonary stenosis
  Pulmonary atresia with intact ventricular septum
  Tricuspid atresia (with normally positioned great arteries)
  Tetralogy of Fallot (some)
  Complex single ventricle with pulmonary stenosis or atresia

PDA required to support systemic flow
  Critical aortic stenosis
  Critical coarctation of aorta, interrupted aortic arch
  Tricuspid atresia (with transposed great arteries)
  Hypoplastic left heart syndrome
  Complex single ventricle with systemic outflow obstruction

PDA increases mixing
  d-Transposition of great arteries

CRITICAL NEWBORN HEART DISEASE

Critical heart disease should be suspected when cyanosis is present without accompanying respiratory distress or when there are signs of decreased systemic perfusion, such as weak or absent femoral pulses or metabolic acidosis (Table 83-2). Another common presentation is an infant who appears to have severe respiratory disease but does not improve with conventional management.

When critical heart disease is suspected in a neonate, diagnostic and empirical interventions need to be performed simultaneously. For diagnosis, consultation with a pediatric cardiologist and a full transthoracic echocardiogram are indicated. With this evaluation, it is possible to diagnose virtually all congenital heart disease presenting in the newborn period. When the index of suspicion for heart disease is lower, a chest radiograph, electrocardiogram, and hyperoxic test should be performed. None of these tests is capable of ruling heart disease in or out with certainty.

In infants suspected of having critical heart disease, empirical therapy with intravenous prostaglandin E_1 should be commenced immediately at a dose of 0.01 to 0.1 µg/kg per minute (usually 0.05 µg/kg/min). Prostaglandin E_1 will reopen a closing ductus arteriosus and restore pulmonary or systemic flow in critical heart disease, temporizing the situation and allowing time for diagnosis and planned intervention. Side effects of prostaglandin include apnea, hypotension, tachycardia, and fever.

Although a complete discussion of all possible heart disease is beyond the scope of this chapter, the more commonly encountered problems are examined, and illustrative examples provided.

Patent Ductus Arteriosus Augments Pulmonary Blood Flow

In this set of lesions, a portion of the normal anatomy supporting pulmonary blood flow (tricuspid valve, right ventricle, pulmonary valve, or pulmonary arteries) is small or absent. The ductus arteriosus provides pulmonary blood flow by shunting systemic blood flow to the lungs. Although d-transposition of the great arteries is included in this section, the physiology of this lesion is somewhat different, as explained later.

Critical Pulmonary Stenosis

In this condition the pulmonary valve leaflets are fused, and there may be only a pinhole for blood to pass to the lungs. Blood returning from the body passes across the atrial septum to the left atrium and ventricle, mixes with the pulmonary venous blood, and is pumped by the left ventricle to the body. The ductus arteriosus provides the source of pulmonary blood flow. The pressure in the right ventricle is usually much higher than that in the left ventricle because it is pumping against the narrow valve opening. As a result, the right ventricle hypertrophies and is often very muscle bound.

Definitive treatment of this condition is usually accomplished in the catheterization laboratory. The pulmonary valve is crossed with a catheter, threaded from the femoral vein, and a balloon is inflated across the valve, tearing the leaflets and enabling it to open more fully. Once this procedure is completed, the prostaglandin infusion can be discontinued, although in some patients it should be continued until the right ventricular hypertrophy regresses sufficiently to accept an adequate amount of pulmonary blood flow. Infants are usually discharged with systemic oxygen saturations greater than 80%. Over time, the systemic saturation rises to normal as the right ventricular relaxation normalizes and right-to-left atrial shunting decreases. For most patients, this is the only procedure required; however, up to one third of infants may require subsequent dilation at an older age.[5]

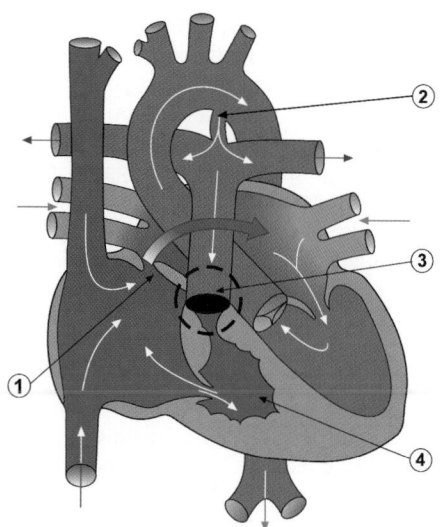

Figure 83-4   Pulmonary atresia with intact ventricular septum. (1) Patent foramen ovale with blood flow right to left. (2) Ductus arteriosus. (3) Atretic pulmonary valve. (4) Hypoplastic right ventricle. (From Biomedical Communications, Health Sciences Center, Winnipeg, Manitoba, Canada.)

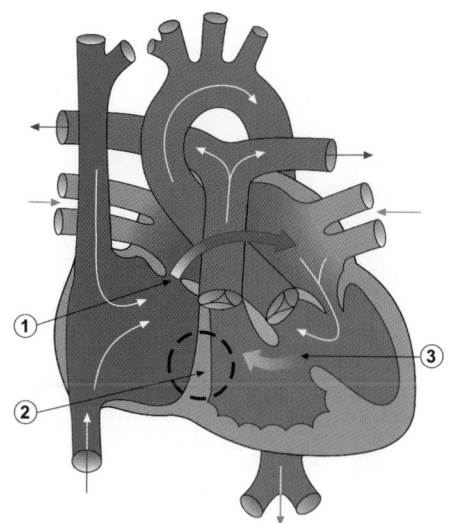

Figure 83-5   Tricuspid atresia (with normal great arteries). (1) Patent foramen ovale with flow right to left. (2) Atretic tricuspid valve. (3) Ventricular septal defect. The size of the VSD and the amount of restriction are variable. (From Biomedical Communications, Health Sciences Center, Winnipeg, Manitoba, Canada.)

Pulmonary Atresia with Intact Ventricular Septum

In this condition, the pulmonary valve is atretic (i.e., completely fused), and the right ventricle has varying degrees of hypoplasia (Fig. 83-4). Like critical pulmonary stenosis, the pressure in the right ventricle is usually much higher than in the left ventricle, and the right ventricle is severely hypertrophied. In the least severe form of this condition, the right ventricle is almost normal sized, and repair can be accomplished by simply opening the pulmonary valve. This procedure can be accomplished surgically or with newly developed transcatheter methods that use radiofrequency energy to create a small hole in the pulmonary valve, thereby "converting" this disease to critical pulmonary stenosis and permitting balloon dilation.[6]

In more severe forms, the right ventricle and tricuspid valve are severely hypoplastic, and part of the coronary blood flow may be dependent on fistulas that develop between the small, hypertensive right ventricle and the epicardial coronary arteries. In the most severe form, the right ventricle cannot be used, and the infant requires a surgically placed systemic–to–pulmonary artery shunt to take the place of the ductus arteriosus. These infants are then managed with the creation of a single-ventricle pathway, as described earlier.[7]

Tricuspid Atresia

The tricuspid valve is atretic in this lesion, and the right ventricle is typically severely hypoplastic (Fig. 83-5). The pulmonary artery arises from the right ventricle, and there may be a ventricular septal defect (VSD). When the VSD is small or the pulmonary artery is hypoplastic, pulmonary blood flow is inadequate, and the ductus arteriosus is required to support it. In some instances, there may be adequate pulmonary flow through the VSD; in other cases, the VSD and pulmonary artery may be so large that the infant has too much pulmonary blood flow.

If the pulmonary flow is inadequate, a systemic–to–pulmonary artery shunt is required. If there is too much pulmonary flow, the infant may require a pulmonary artery band to reduce the amount of pulmonary flow. In some instances, nature provides just enough pulmonary stenosis so that the child is not in congestive heart failure and has adequate systemic saturations. In any case, an infant with tricuspid atresia also follows the single-ventricle pathway described earlier. In some instances, tricuspid atresia is found with transposition of the great arteries. These infants require a repair similar to that for hypoplastic left heart syndrome, because the aortic valve and arch are typically hypoplastic when the great arteries are transposed.

Tetralogy of Fallot

This condition arises when the ventricular septal muscle between the aorta and the pulmonary artery is deviated anteriorly (Fig. 83-6). This causes a stenotic pulmonary outflow area, a special type of VSD under the aorta (anterior malalignment), and alignment of the aorta over the VSD and crest of the ventricular septum (overriding aorta). There is usually accompanying right ventricular hypertrophy, which completes the four parts of the tetralogy. Although this description is simple, there is a huge variation in disease severity, which is largely dependent on the pulmonary artery architecture. When there are well-developed pulmonary arteries and mild or moderate pulmonary stenosis, this lesion is not critical. Systemic oxygen saturations from 80% to 95% are possible, and infants may undergo elective complete repair between 3 and 12 months of age. Surgical repair in these cases involves closing the VSD and relieving the pulmonary obstruction by patching the right ventricular outflow tract, pulmonary valve, and main pulmonary artery as needed.[8]

More severe obstruction at the pulmonary valve and right ventricular outflow tract may lead to more profound cyanosis and ductal dependency. These infants may require a shunt to increase pulmonary flow, in anticipation of a complete repair at an older age, or they may undergo complete repair as infants.

At the extreme, there may be complete atresia of the pulmonary valve and only a threadlike main pulmonary

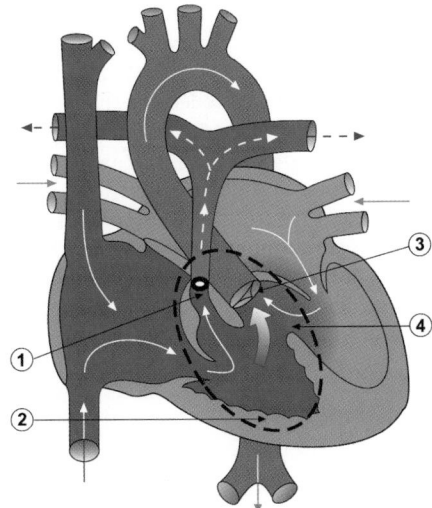

Figure 83-6   Tetralogy of Fallot. (1) Pulmonary valve and subvalvular stenosis. (2) Hypertrophied right ventricle. (3) Overriding aorta. (4) Ventricular septal defect. (From Biomedical Communications, Health Sciences Center, Winnipeg, Manitoba, Canada.)

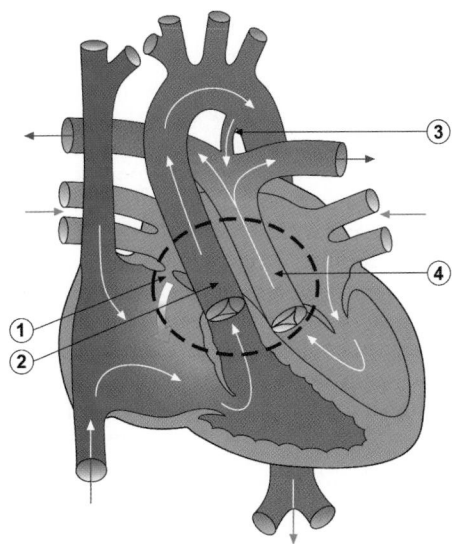

Figure 83-7   d-Transposition of the great arteries. (1) Patent foramen ovale with left-to-right flow. (2) Transposed great arteries. The aorta arises from the right ventricle. (3) Ductus arteriosus with flow from the aorta to the pulmonary artery. (4) Transposed great arteries. The pulmonary artery arises from the left ventricle. (From Biomedical Communications, Health Sciences Center, Winnipeg, Manitoba, Canada.)

artery. Associated with this severe obstruction are downstream architectural abnormalities of the pulmonary arteries, including stenosis or absence of branches, and the presence of collateral vessels from the aorta to the pulmonary arteries that may supply multiple segments of the lung. The presence of these aortopulmonary collateral vessels and small, stenotic pulmonary arteries makes definitive surgical repair a challenge. Repair is thus individualized based on each patient's anatomy, and it usually requires a series of staged operations and cardiac catheterizations for dilation of stenotic pulmonary arteries.[9]

An important concern in infants with tetralogy of Fallot, especially in the presence of pulmonary atresia, is its association with the 22q deletion, velocardiofacial, DiGeorge syndrome complex. Infants with this heart disease should have genetic testing for the 22q deletion, and calcium levels should be monitored in the newborn period. If genetic testing is positive, an immunologic workup and genetic and anticipatory guidance should be provided to patients and families. Another important issue for patients with tetralogy of Fallot is the possibility of experiencing "tet spells," which are sudden episodes of profound desaturation. The classic (but oversimplified) explanation of the pathophysiology of this condition is "spasm" of the muscle under the pulmonary valve, leading to decreased pulmonary flow and increased cyanosis. Tet spells can be treated by increasing the systemic resistance to force more blood across the pulmonary circuit. This can be accomplished mechanically by putting the patient in a knee-to-chest position or pharmacologically by administering intravenous phenylephrine. Supplemental oxygen may be of some benefit, along with the administration of subcutaneous or intravenous morphine as a sedative. Ketamine is an especially useful drug in managing tet spells because it provides both sedation and increased systemic vascular resistance, and it can be administered intravenously or intramuscularly. Patients who have had one or more tet spells should be considered for surgical palliation or repair, because if these spells are prolonged, they are associated with morbidity and mortality.

d-Transposition of the Great Arteries

In this condition, the aorta arises from the right ventricle, and the pulmonary artery arises from the left ventricle (Fig. 83-7). This leads to systemic blood from the body recirculating to the body and pulmonary blood recirculating to the lungs (parallel circulations), with profound cyanosis. Survival depends on mixing of the two circulations at the atrial, ventricular, or great vessel level. Prostaglandin E_1 temporizes this condition by increasing the amount of blood in the pulmonary system, which encourages mixing at the atrial or ventricular level. For prostaglandin to work, there must be an ASD or VSD. If no septal defect is present or if mixing is inadequate, as evidenced by oxygen saturation less than 80%, an ASD may need to be created or enlarged to stabilize the infant in anticipation of corrective surgery. This procedure (balloon atrial septostomy) is accomplished by passing a balloon catheter through the atrial septum, inflating the balloon, and then pulling it back to tear a hole in the atrial septum, thereby creating an ASD. This procedure can be performed at the bedside under echocardiographic guidance alone or in the cardiac catheterization laboratory under fluoroscopic guidance.[10]

Definitive therapy is surgical. Since the mid-1980s the procedure of choice for this lesion has been the "arterial switch," in which the aorta and pulmonary arteries are transected above the valves and reattached to their physiologically correct ventricle. The Achilles heel of this procedure is transfer of the coronary arteries, which must be removed separately and reattached to the aorta. The coronary artery anatomy is variable, making preoperative definition of this anatomy and appropriate surgical planning imperative.[11] Associated lesions, which may include VSD and coarctation of the aorta, are usually corrected at the same surgery. The prognosis for children with d-transposition of the great arteries is generally excellent. Postoperative problems related to coronary artery obstruction can occur, however, as can residual lesions related to the surgical correction.

Patent Ductus Arteriosus Augments Systemic Blood Flow

In this set of lesions, a portion of the normal anatomy supporting systemic blood flow (mitral valve, left ventricle, aortic valve, and aorta) is narrowed, small, or absent. The ductus arteriosus provides systemic blood flow by shunting some of the pulmonary blood to the aorta. Infants with these lesions often present with shock or decreased femoral pulses as the ductus arteriosus closes. Critical aortic stenosis, interrupted aortic arch, and critical coarctation of the aorta are all examples of critical left heart disease that requires prostaglandin to stabilize and temporize, but all are amenable to complete repair. Hypoplastic left heart syndrome is an extreme form of left heart obstructive disease that requires a single-ventricle surgical approach.

Critical Aortic Stenosis

In this lesion, the aortic valve opening is narrowed by partial fusion of the leaflets, and there is severe obstruction to outflow from the left ventricle. Before repair, most of the blood returning from the left atrium passes across the foramen ovale to the right atrium and subsequently to the right ventricle and main pulmonary artery, where a portion of the blood passes across the ductus arteriosus to the body and a portion passes to the lungs. For this lesion to be defined as critical aortic stenosis rather than hypoplastic left heart syndrome, the left ventricle and mitral valve must be of normal size, although left ventricular function is often severely depressed before intervention.

Treatment of this condition usually involves transcatheter balloon dilation of the aortic valve. This procedure relieves the narrowing at the valve sufficiently to permit the recovery of left ventricular function, allowing the left ventricle to pump all the systemic blood. Prostaglandin can be discontinued once the left ventricle has recovered adequately, but this may take several days. There is usually mild to moderate residual aortic stenosis after neonatal dilation, and these patients generally require further interventions for the aortic valve later in infancy or childhood.[12]

Coarctation of the Aorta and Interrupted Aortic Arch

In coarctation of the aorta, the aorta is severely narrowed at or just beyond the origin of the left subclavian artery. In interrupted aortic arch, there is a discontinuity of the aorta at a point between one of the head and neck vessels (usually between the left carotid and left subclavian arteries, called type B interruption). Both lesions typically present with shock or decreased femoral pulses as the ductus arteriosus closes and are temporized by prostaglandin E1, which opens the ductus arteriosus, supplementing systemic blood flow.

The treatment of either lesion is surgical repair in the neonatal period. The surgical repair for critical coarctation usually involves removing the narrowed segment and rejoining the descending aorta to the aortic arch in an unobstructed fashion.[13] The repair can usually be done without cardiopulmonary bypass. Interrupted aortic arch requires a much more complex arch reconstruction and the use of cardiopulmonary bypass. A VSD, associated with the most common type of interrupted aortic arch, is repaired at the same surgery. Interrupted aortic arch type B is also associated with the 22q deletion, DiGeorge complex. As for those with tetralogy of Fallot, these patients should have appropriate calcium monitoring and genetic and immunologic workup.

Hypoplastic Left Heart Syndrome

When the left-sided heart structures (mitral valve, left ventricle, aortic valve, and aortic arch) are too small to support the cardiac output needed for the body, the condition is referred to as hypoplastic left heart syndrome (Fig. 83-8). The mitral or aortic valves may be so small as to be atretic. In the unrepaired state, the right ventricle pumps the combined venous return from the body and lungs to the pulmonary artery, where a portion of the blood passes to the lungs and a portion passes through the ductus arteriosus to supply the body. The degree of cyanosis depends on the proportion of pulmonary to systemic blood flow. As the ductus arteriosus closes, more blood is directed to the lungs and less to the body, leading to higher systemic saturations but signs and symptoms of low cardiac output and, ultimately, shock. Prostaglandin E1 opens the ductus arteriosus and temporizes the situation.

Surgical repair of this condition follows the principles of the three-stage single-ventricle pathway outlined earlier. The first stage is more involved than for most other types of single-ventricle palliation, however, because the main pulmonary artery must be used along with the native (small) aorta and prosthetic patch material to refashion the aortic arch. Pulmonary blood flow is provided by placing a tube graft either from a subclavian artery to the pulmonary artery (modified Blalock-Taussig shunt) or from the right ventricular outflow tract to the pulmonary artery (Sano modification).[14]

Another strategy for managing patients with hypoplastic left heart syndrome is heart transplantation. Despite significant advances in immunosuppresive regimens, the strategy of heart transplantation for hypoplastic left heart syndrome

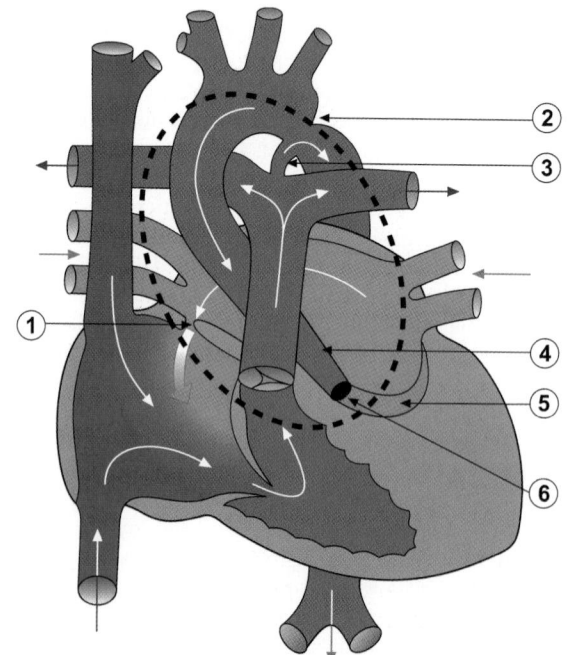

Figure 83-8 Hypoplastic left heart syndrome. (1) Atrial septal defect with left-to-right flow. (2) Coarctation of the aorta. (3) Patent ductus arteriosus with flow from the pulmonary artery to the aorta. (4) Hypoplastic ascending aorta. (5) Small mitral valve—sometimes atretic. (6) Small aortic valve—sometimes atretic. (From Biomedical Communications, Health Sciences Center, Winnipeg, Manitoba, Canada.)

has been limited by a lack of donor organs and late graft failure, which occurs over decades in virtually all transplanted hearts.[15]

Patent Ductus Arteriosus Not Required

Total anomalous pulmonary venous return with obstruction is the classic example of newborn heart disease that is not temporized by prostaglandin E₁. In this lesion, the pulmonary veins do not return to the left atrium but communicate with the systemic veins by means of a supplemental venous channel. This channel may be obstructed, leading to progressive pulmonary edema with "whiteout" on chest radiographs, and an inability to ventilate or oxygenate. This lesion is the one most often mistaken for pulmonary disease in newborns. If a newborn has progressive pulmonary disease and is failing conventional treatment, the diagnosis of congenital heart disease—especially obstructed total anomalous pulmonary venous return—should be entertained and an echocardiogram obtained. Repair consists of reattaching the pulmonary venous chamber to the left atrium.

Complex Congenital Heart Disease

There is a vast array of other complex anatomic combinations of heart disease. Although some of these lesion complexes may be amenable to complete repair, many need to be handled through the single-ventricle route. For the pediatric hospitalist, the exact anatomy is less important than the physiology, because patients with single-ventricle physiology behave fairly comparably at the same level of palliation.

LESIONS PRESENTING WITH CONGESTIVE HEART FAILURE OR MURMUR IN INFANCY

As the pulmonary vascular resistance falls in the first weeks of life, lesions that permit the transmission of high flow or pressure to the lungs become evident. These lesions include VSD, atrioventricular septal defect, and patent ductus arteriosus.

Ventricular Septal Defects

The ventricular septum is a complex anatomic structure dividing the left and right ventricles. Near the aortic valve, the septum is a thin membrane (membranous septum), whereas it is a thick muscle in other parts. A defect in the wall is called a VSD (Fig. 83-9). The most common defects occur in the membranous septum, but they can occur anywhere in the wall and may be multiple. The presentation of VSD is dependent on two factors—the size of the defect and the pulmonary vascular resistance.

Small Defects

A small muscular VSD presents in the first days to weeks of life with a high-pitched, asymptomatic murmur. When the resistance in the pulmonary circulation falls, so does the right ventricular pressure, creating a large pressure difference between the left and right ventricles. A small hole between the ventricles creates a turbulent left-to-right flow jet, and a loud murmur is heard. In this scenario, the total amount of blood recirculated through the lungs and back to the left ventricle is minimal.

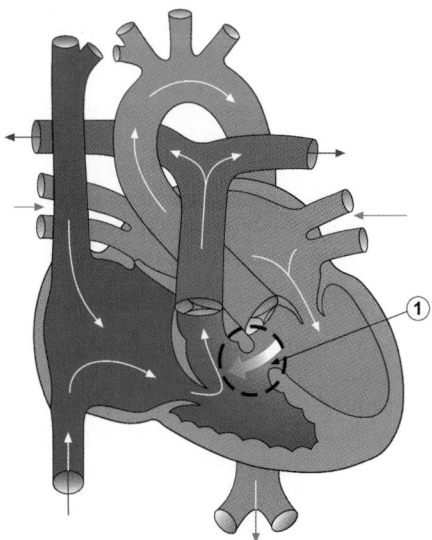

Figure 83-9 Ventricular septal defect. (1) Ventricular septal defect with flow from the left ventricle to the right ventricle. The position of the defect in the ventricular septum determines the type. The more common type is located just underneath the aortic valve (membranous). (From Biomedical Communications, Health Sciences Center, Winnipeg, Manitoba, Canada.)

Moderate Defects

If the VSD is somewhat larger, as the pulmonary resistance falls, the defect may still be small enough to limit the pressure transmitted to the right ventricle but large enough to admit more blood flow. In this circumstance, the amount of extra blood flow to the lungs and recirculating back to the left heart may be significant, and the infant may have respiratory symptoms and perhaps some degree of congestive heart failure. A loud murmur is present because the pressure gradient and flow are high.

Large Defects

At some point, VSDs are too large to limit the pressure transmitted by the left ventricle. As the pulmonary resistance falls, there is more and more blood recirculating to the lungs, but the pressure in the right ventricle and pulmonary artery remains at systemic levels (so-called unrestrictive defects). Because there is little turbulence produced through a large VSD, the murmur may be somewhat less intense than in smaller VSDs. An important caveat, however, is that a large VSD may have relatively little turbulence, resulting in a softer murmur. With excessive pulmonary blood flow, infants typically display failure to thrive. If the defect is left uncorrected for a prolonged period, these infants run the risk of developing irreversible changes called pulmonary vascular obstructive disease, which can progress even after the defect is corrected. Pulmonary vascular obstructive disease can be averted by limiting the pressure to which the lung vasculature is exposed by either closing the VSD or applying downstream resistance to flow by placing a pulmonary artery band. Irreversible pulmonary vascular obstructive disease usually does not develop until after age 1 year, although the time course after that point is remarkably variable. Patients with Down syndrome seem to be at higher risk at an earlier age, and intervention is recommended before age 9 months in this subgroup.[16]

Although most infants with large VSDs and left-to-right shunt present with congestive heart failure as the pulmonary resistance falls, in a small group of patients with unrestrictive VSDs, the pulmonary resistance falls very little or not at all. These infants do not develop congestive heart failure, and if the pulmonary resistance is very high, they may not have much additional pulmonary flow. There is little if any heart murmur because there is no restriction to flow at the ventricular level and not enough increase in pulmonary flow to produce an appreciable flow murmur. The only cardiac sign may be relatively subtle—a single, loud second heart sound. These children typically have frequent respiratory illnesses, which may further limit the ability to clearly auscultate the heart. With no loud murmur demanding attention and the more subtle signs masked by respiratory noise, these children may go undiagnosed for long periods, placing them at high risk of developing pulmonary vascular obstructive disease. The pediatric hospitalist should keep this infrequent presentation of congenital heart disease in mind when assessing and treating infants and young children with frequent respiratory problems.

Surgical closure of a VSD is indicated in infancy (before age 1 year) if there is persistent congestive heart failure or if the pulmonary pressures remain high. Because some VSDs get smaller over time and even close, medical management with anticongestive drugs (e.g., furosemide, digoxin, angiotensin-converting enzyme inhibitors) may be indicated in some infants with moderate and large VSDs. Closure is recommended for VSDs that remain moderate with a pulmonary-to-systemic flow ratio of more than about 2:1. More complex decision making is required for multiple VSDs, especially those located at the apex of the heart. This location is typically difficult to approach surgically. In this instance, a pulmonary artery band may be placed to limit pulmonary flow and pressure until the child is larger. Transcatheter closure devices may be another option in selected children, sometimes combined with a surgical approach.[17]

Transcatheter closure devices for membranous VSDs are in clinical trials. These devices need special design and delivery systems to avoid interfering with the aortic valve, which forms the superior border of the membranous septum.[18]

Atrioventricular Septal Defects

The atrioventricular septal defect is a more complex lesion than simply a combination of both an ASD and a VSD (Fig. 83-10). It involves an incomplete separation of the embryonic common atrioventricular valve into separate tricuspid and mitral components. In addition, there is both a VSD and an ASD in the portion of the septa immediately adjacent to the atrioventricular valve. This lesion is often associated with Down syndrome. The presentation is similar to that of patients with moderate or large VSDs. These defects do not close spontaneously, however, so all patients with atrioventricular septal defects require surgical repair to partition the atrioventricular valve and close the atrial and ventricular defects. Partitioning the atrioventricular valve is surgically challenging, because one must avoid producing mitral stenosis or regurgitation. Most centers perform complete repairs on these children when they are between 3 and 6 months old—waiting until they are somewhat larger but before pulmonary vascular disease has a chance to develop.[19]

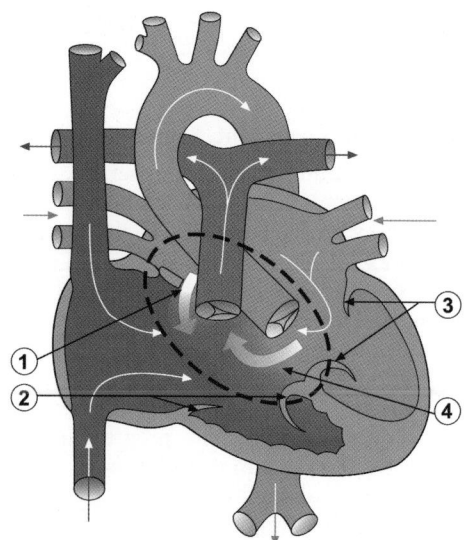

Figure 83-10 Atrioventricular septal defect. (1) Atrial septal defect (ostium primum type). (2) Right side of common atrioventricular valve (incompletely formed tricuspid valve). (3) Left side of common atrioventricular valve (incompletely formed mitral valve). (4) Ventricular septal defect ("inlet" type). (From Biomedical Communications, Health Sciences Center, Winnipeg, Manitoba, Canada.)

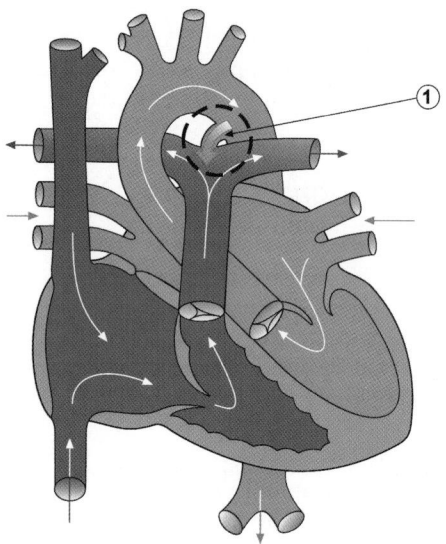

Figure 83-11 Patent ductus arteriosus. (1) Ductus arteriosus with flow from the aorta into the pulmonary artery. (From Biomedical Communications, Health Sciences Center, Winnipeg, Manitoba, Canada.)

Patent Ductus Arteriosus

The ductus arteriosus is the conduit for fetal blood to bypass the lungs in utero. The ductus usually closes in the first days of life. If it does not close, as pulmonary vascular resistance falls, blood shunts from the aorta into the pulmonary artery (Fig. 83-11). Depending on the size of the ductus arteriosus and the pulmonary vascular resistance, the ductus shunts a variable amount of blood (similar to the physiology of a VSD), and this lesion may present with congestive heart failure, if large, or a murmur if the lesion is smaller.

The treatment of a patent ductus arteriosus is surgical or transcatheter closure. Transcatheter closure is now routine in children and infants older than 6 months.[20] Surgical closure is indicated for refractory heart failure in very small infants, premature infants, or those with other heart disease that requires surgical intervention. A small patent ductus arteriosus associated with a murmur—even in the absence of significant shunting—is closed in the catheterization laboratory to prevent the lifelong risk of endarteritis of the ductus, which is estimated at 0.45% per year.[21] Controversy remains whether a small ductus arteriosus found by echocardiography without an associated murmur ("silent ductus") should be closed.

Coarctation of the Aorta

When severe, this lesion presents in the newborn period as a critical newborn heart lesion with shock or cyanosis. Milder lesions may present with a murmur or, more commonly, with an astute pediatrician noting a decreased intensity of the femoral pulses. Repair of this lesion is usually done surgically. Coarctation is sometimes diagnosed later in childhood with the finding of upper extremity hypertension. Therapeutic options later in childhood and through adulthood include surgery or transcatheter balloon dilation with stent placement. Later diagnosis and repair of this lesion may lead to persistent hypertension even after repair.

LESIONS PRESENTING WITH A MURMUR IN CHILDHOOD

Less severe obstructions and shunts typically present with a murmur in childhood. Stenosis of the semilunar valves (aortic stenosis or pulmonary stenosis) and ASDs may present in this time frame.

Pulmonary Stenosis and Aortic Stenosis

When severe, these lesions present as critical heart disease in the newborn period, as previously discussed. Milder lesions present as a murmur. Treatment, which consists of transcatheter balloon dilation of the valve, is undertaken for pulmonary stenosis when the narrowing is moderate to severe. Such intervention is highly effective and typically does not need to be repeated.[22] Treatment is also undertaken for aortic stenosis when the gradient is moderate to severe. The first approach is usually balloon dilation of the valve. The success rate of aortic balloon dilation may be good, but relief of stenosis is often accompanied by the creation of aortic regurgitation. Surgical valve repair, replacement of the aortic valve with the patient's own pulmonary valve (Ross procedure), and prosthetic valve replacement are all options. Prosthetic valve replacement is undesirable in small children because of the limited life span of these valves and growth considerations.

Atrial Septal Defects

The atrial septum divides the right and left atria. A defect in the wall is called an ASD (Fig. 83-12). Blood returning to the left atrium passes from left to right across the ASD and recirculates to the lungs, placing a volume load on the right ventricle, pulmonary vascular bed, and atria. The amount of excess blood flow (or shunt) is determined by both the size of the defect and the balance between the diastolic compliance of the left and right heart. In infancy, the right ventri-

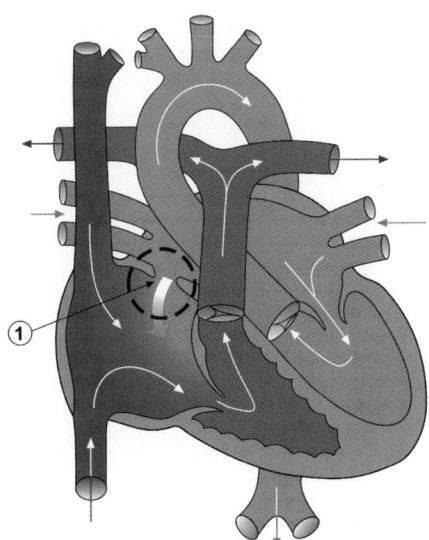

Figure 83-12 Atrial septal defect. (1) Atrial septal defect with flow from the left atrium into the right atrium. (From Biomedical Communications, Health Sciences Center, Winnipeg, Manitoba, Canada.)

cle is relatively noncompliant, and there may be minimal flow across even a large ASD. During childhood, the right ventricle becomes more compliant as the left ventricular compliance decreases, thereby increasing the amount of shunting. The consequences of an unrepaired ASD include right ventricular dysfunction and atrial arrhythmias from chronic volume load; the potentially devastating complication of pulmonary hypertension and pulmonary vascular disease, which may develop in up to 5% to 10% of these patients during adulthood; and the risk of paradoxical embolus.

If there is evidence of right ventricular volume overload by echocardiography, the lesion should be closed. Usually this decision is made after age 2 years, because some ASDs may get smaller. If the defect is of the secundum type, it may be closed in the cardiac catheterization laboratory with a specially designed closure device (Fig. 83-13).[23] If the defect is large or located in other anatomic regions of the atrium, surgery is required for closure.

SPECIAL CONSIDERATIONS

Endocarditis Prophylaxis

Most congenital heart lesions put patients at risk for the development of endocarditis. Children with congenital heart disease should have regular dental care and maintain good oral hygiene. Recommendations for endocarditis prophylaxis should be followed when dental work and other at-risk surgical procedures are planned (see Chapter 84).

Respiratory Syncytial Virus

Respiratory syncytial virus may produce severe disease in children younger than 2 years with cyanotic heart disease, single-ventricle anatomy before or after surgery, dilated or hypertrophic cardiomyopathy, pulmonary hypertension, or significant left-to-right shunts requiring medication to control pulmonary vascular congestion. In such patients, the American Academy of Pediatrics recommends monthly

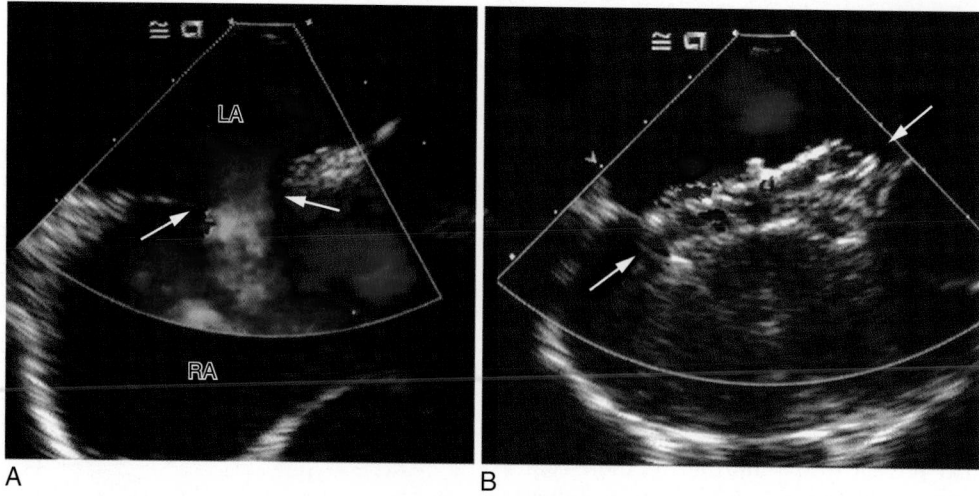

Figure 83-13 Device closure of atrial septal defect. *A,* Transesophageal echocardiogram of atrial septal defect. Blue color demonstrates blood flow from the left atrium (LA) to the right atrium (RA). *B,* Transesophageal echocardiogram after Amplatzer septal occluder is positioned across the atrial septum. Arrows indicate the closure device. Color shows no residual flow across the atrial septum.

passive immunization during the respiratory syncytial virus season with palivizumab.[24] Steps should be taken to minimize the risk from this potentially life-threatening illness. If a congenital heart lesion needs repair, consideration should be given to performing it before the viral season. Appropriate isolation of hospitalized children with heart disease at high risk should be undertaken to prevent nosocomial transmission.

Pacemakers and Implantable Defibrillators

Children with congenital heart disease may have congenital or iatrogenic surgical conduction defects that necessitate pacemaker placement. Pacemakers work by emitting an electrical current that stimulates cardiac depolarization. Although pacemakers are extremely reliable, the interface between the pacemaker and the heart (the leads) is prone to a variety of problems. Extreme physiologic changes (e.g., acidosis) in the patient may also increase the amount of energy needed to depolarize the heart above that set by the pacemaker. In-hospital cardiac monitoring of children with pacemakers is insufficient, because these monitors usually detect the pacemaker impulse even when it is not followed by a cardiac depolarization. A physiologic monitor such as a pulse oximeter or arterial waveform should be used to confirm the heart rate in paced patients. Similarly, during resuscitation, one should not mistake the pacemaker impulse as a cardiac depolarization, and physiologic parameters (e.g., palpation of a pulse) should be used to determine the cardiac rate.

Patients with pacemakers or implantable defibrillators requiring noncardiac surgery may need to have the device reprogrammed before surgery to avoid oversensing, and electrocautery should be avoided. Patients with these devices cannot undergo MRI examinations.

Central Access and Paradoxical Embolization

Central access may be difficult in patients with congenital heart disease because of vein occlusion owing to previous long-term access lines or cardiac catheterization access. Central access in the internal jugular or subclavian veins is usually discouraged in patients who are progressing down the single-ventricle pathway because of the risk of superior vena cava obstruction, making Fontan palliation problematic.

In children with any right-to-left shunting, there is the risk of bubbles or clots introduced into the venous system traveling to the cerebral circulation, causing stroke. Intravenous lines should be meticulously cleared of air before infusion to prevent this potential problem, and indwelling lines should be heparinized.

Feeding and Growth Issues

Infants with congenital heart disease and pulmonary overcirculation have significantly increased caloric needs. Infants with these increased metabolic demands may require more than 160 kcal/kg per day to grow. In addition, infants may be less able to tolerate normal feeding volumes owing to tachypnea. Increased caloric density is usually required, and tube feeding is sometimes necessary to assist these infants.

IN A NUTSHELL

- Congenital heart disease typically presents in three different periods: newborn (as the ductus arteriosus closes), 2 to 4 months of age (as the pulmonary resistance falls), or early childhood (when more subtle findings can be picked up in a cooperative patient).
- Echocardiography and cardiac MRI are the mainstays of diagnosis for congenital heart disease.
- In infants suspected of having critical heart disease, empirical therapy with intravenous prostaglandin E_1 should be commenced immediately.

ON THE HORIZON

- An increasing number of surgical procedures will be complemented or replaced by transcatheter methods. Already in early clinical trials are percutaneous Fontan completion, membranous VSD closure, and pulmonary valve replacement.
- Diagnosis of cardiac defects will continue to improve with real-time, three-dimensional imaging.
- More patients with complex heart disease are living into adulthood. Thus, the long-term implications of these complex repairs will become better defined.

REFERENCES

1. Hoffman JI: Incidence of congenital heart disease. 1. Postnatal incidence. Pediatr Cardiol 1995;16:103-113.
2. Fyler DC: Report of New England Regional Cardiac Program. Pediatrics 1980;65(Suppl):375-461.
3. Kumar RK, Newburger JW, Gauvreau K, et al: Comparison of outcome when hypoplastic left heart syndrome and transposition of the great arteries are diagnosed prenatally versus when diagnosis of these two conditions is made only postnatally. Am J Cardiol 1999;83:1649-1653.
4. Fontan F, Mounicot FB, Baudet E, et al: "Correction" of tricuspid atresia: 2 cases "corrected" using a new surgical technique. Ann Chir Thorac Cardiovasc 1971;10:39-47.
5. Latson LA: Critical pulmonary stenosis. J Interv Cardiol 2001;14:345-350.
6. Justo RN, Nykanen DG, Williams WG, et al: Transcatheter perforation of the right ventricular outflow tract as initial therapy for pulmonary valve atresia and intact ventricular septum in the newborn. Cathet Cardiovasc Diagn 1997;40:408-413.
7. Dyamenahalli U, McCrindle BW, McDonald C, et al: Pulmonary atresia with intact ventricular septum: Management of, and outcomes for, a cohort of 210 consecutive patients. Cardiol Young 2004;14:299-308.
8. Kirklin JW, Ellis FH Jr, McGoon DC, et al: Surgical treatments for the tetralogy of Fallot by open intracardiac repair. J Thorac Surg 1959;37:22-51.
9. Kreutzer J, Perry SB, Jonas RA, et al: Tetralogy of Fallot with diminutive pulmonary arteries: Preoperative pulmonary valve dilation and transcatheter rehabilitation of pulmonary arteries. J Am Coll Cardiol 1996;27:1741-1747.
10. Baylen BG, Grzeszczak M, Gleason ME, et al: Role of balloon atrial septostomy before early arterial switch repair of transposition of the great arteries. J Am Coll Cardiol 1992;19:1025-1031.
11. Mayer JE Jr, Sanders SP, Jonas RA, et al: Coronary artery pattern and outcome of arterial switch operation for transposition of the great arteries. Circulation 1990;82(Suppl):IV139-IV145.
12. Satou GM, Perry SB, Lock JE, et al: Repeat balloon dilation of congenital valvar aortic stenosis: Immediate results and midterm outcome. Catheter Cardiovasc Interv 1999;47:47-51.
13. Backer CL, Mavroudis C, Zias EA, et al: Repair of coarctation with resection and extended end-to-end anastomosis. Ann Thorac Surg 1998;66:1365-1370.
14. Sano S, Ishino K, Kawada M, et al: Right ventricle–pulmonary artery shunt in first-stage palliation of hypoplastic left heart syndrome. J Thorac Cardiovasc Surg 2003;126:504-510.
15. Boucek MM, Edwards LB, Keck BM, et al: The Registry of the International Society of Heart and Lung Transplantation: Sixth official pediatric report—2003. J Heart Lung Transplant 2003;22:636-662.
16. Kawai T, Wada Y, Enmoto T, et al: Comparison of hemodynamic data before and after corrective surgery for Down's syndrome and ventricular septal defect. Heart Vessels 1995;10:154-157.
17. Holzer R, Balzer D, Cao QL, et al: Device closure of muscular ventricular septal defects using the Amplatzer muscular ventricular septal defect occluder: Immediate and mid-term results of a US registry. J Am Coll Cardiol 2004;43:1257-1263.
18. Thanopoulos BD, Tsaousis GS, Karanasios E, et al: Transcatheter closure of perimembranous ventricualr septal defects with the Amplatzer asymmetric ventricular septal defect occluder: Preliminary experience in children. Heart 2003;89:918-922.
19. Murphy DJ: Atrioventricular canal defects. Curr Treatment Opin Cardiovas Med 1999;1:323-334.
20. Pass RH, Hijazi Z, Hsu DT, et al: Multicenter USA Amplatzer patent ductus arteriosus occlusion device trial: Initial and one-year results. J Am Coll Cardiol 2004;44:513-519.
21. Campbell M: Natural history of persistent ductus arteriosus. Br Heart J 1968;30:4-13.
22. Peterson C, Schilthuis JJ, Dodge-Khatami A, et al: Comparative long-term results of surgery versus balloon valvuloplasty for pulmonary valve stenosis in infants and children. Ann Thorac Surg 2003;76:1078-1082.
23. Masura J, Gavora P, Podnar T: Long-term outcome of transcatheter secundum-type atrial septal defects closure using Amplatzer septal occluders. J Am Coll Cardiol 2005;45:505-507.
24. Revised indications for the use of palivizumab and respiratory syncytial virus immune globulin intravenous for the prevention of respiratory syncytial virus infections: American Academy of Pediatrics policy statement. Pediatrics 2003;112:1442-1446.

CHAPTER 84

Infective Endocarditis

Michael H. Gewitz

Although infective endocarditis is a relatively uncommon diagnosis in children, it is an important cause of morbidity and mortality in the pediatric population.[1,2] The incidence of this disease appears to be increasing in patients with known cardiac disease and in other groups as well. For these reasons, the pediatric hospitalist must be well versed in the epidemiology, causative factors, and treatment of this disorder.

Over the past several decades, changes in the epidemiology of childhood cardiac disorders have been reflected in the predisposing factors leading to infective endocarditis. For instance, the decline in rheumatic heart disease has meant a corresponding decline in infective endocarditis resulting from this illness. Conversely, in the United States and other developed nations, an increase in infective endocarditis has occurred in children with congenital heart disease. This includes not only children with untreated cardiac conditions, such as small ventricular septal defects, but also children who have had corrective or palliative surgery, including implanted grafts or patches, prosthetic valves, and conduits. A review of the modern epidemiology of infective endocarditis after surgery for congenital heart disease found that the highest annualized risk was in patients who had had interventions for cyanotic forms of congenital heart disease, including relief of obstructed pulmonary blood flow.[3] Among the acyanotic group, a higher incidence of infective endocarditis occurred in patients who had prosthetic aortic valve placement.

In addition to the rising prevalence of infective endocarditis among survivors of congenital heart disease, the same trend is occurring in children without structural heart disease. As many as 8% to 10% of children with infective endocarditis have no known primary cardiovascular abnormality. This group includes children with chronic indwelling central venous catheters; newborns, particularly premature babies, who are increasingly subjected to invasive procedures; and adolescent intravenous drug abusers.

PATHOPHYSIOLOGY

Studies of animal models confirm that the development of a nidus for endocardial infection requires a locus of denuded endothelium, as well as exposure to bacteria.[4] The disrupted endothelial surface exposes collagen to the bloodstream, which leads to the deposition of fibrin and platelets and the formation of a thrombotic vegetation. Circulating microorganisms, most commonly bacteria, can become embedded in the vegetation, resulting in an endocardial infection. Additional deposits of platelets and fibrin form protective layers that shield the pathogens from host immune defenses. As the process continues, the vegetation grows, creating layers of embedded microorganisms. The organisms sequestered within the vegetation have a great potential for proliferation.

Congenital heart lesions involving high-velocity blood flow jets are most susceptible to vegetation development, owing to the potential for endothelial damage. Adding appreciably to this risk is the presence of foreign material, which itself can offer a site prone to the development of platelet and fibrin plugs. Patients with surgically placed grafts or palliative shunts (e.g., Blalock-Taussig shunts) thus are at high risk for infective endocarditis.[5]

In addition to host factors, a better understanding of virulence factors associated with the organisms themselves has contributed to insight into the pathogenesis of infective endocarditis. Such factors include the ability to produce adhesins that facilitate binding of bacteria, to generate biofilms that cover devices such as prosthetic valves, and to stimulate platelet aggregation, which enhances the propagation of vegetations.[6]

Gram-positive cocci remain the largest single group of organisms associated with infective endocarditis in children. Table 84-1 outlines common causative organisms. After the first year of life, viridans streptococci, including *Streptococcus sanguis* and *Streptococcus mitis*, predominate, with *Staphylococcus aureus* ranking second. *S. aureus* remains the most common cause of endocarditis occurring *acutely* and is the most common agent in children without structural heart disease. Coagulase-negative staphylococci are also causative agents in these children, especially those with chronic indwelling catheters. Gram-positive cocci are often associated with infective endocarditis in newborns.[7] Other less common organisms include enterococci and fungi. Interestingly, children with congenital or acquired immunodeficiency states are *not* at increased risk for infective endocarditis unless other risk factors are present.

The immunologic sequelae of infective carditis are not well understood. The infection results in extensive activation of both the cell-mediated and the humoral immune systems. Especially with long-standing disease, patients are often found to be hypergammaglobulinemic (also represented by elevated rheumatoid factor levels) and to have elevated levels of circulating immune complexes. These immune complexes are thought to play a role in renal disease and may also be involved in some of the secondary symptoms and complications that occasionally arise (e.g., Osler nodes and glomerular nephritis).

CLINICAL PRESENTATION

The presentation of infective endocarditis may be indolent (subacute) or fulminant (acute). The clinical picture relates to the combination of systemic responses to bacteremia or fungemia, the local mechanical impact of the

Table 84-1 Principal Pathogenic Bacterial Agents in Infective Endocarditis

Organism	PERCENTAGE OF PATIENTS IN EACH SERIES		
	Johnson et al (n = 149)	*Martin et al* (n = 76)	*Stockheim et al* (n = 111)
Viridans streptococci	43	38	32
Staphylococcus aureus	33	32	27
Coagulase-negative staphylococci	2	4	12
Streptococcus pneumoniae	3	4	7
HACEK	N/A	5	4
Enterococcus species	N/A	7	4
Culture negative	6	7	5

HACEK, *Haemophilus* species, *Actinobacillus actinomycetemcomitans*, *Cardiobacterium hominis*, *Eikenella* species, and *Kingella kingae*.
From Ferrieri P, Gewitz MH, Gerber MA, et al: Unique features of infective endocarditis in childhood. Circulation 2002;105:2115-2127. (For series references, see original article.)

vegetation, and, in some cases, the deleterious effects of embolic and systemic immunologic responses.

Classically, in subacute bacterial endocarditis, somatic complaints predominate. These nonspecific symptoms include low-grade fever, malaise with weakness and fatigue, anorexia (often with weight loss), intermittent diaphoresis, myalgias, and arthralgias. This group of complaints should raise the suspicion for subactue bacterial endocarditis, especially in the context of a child at risk for infective endocarditis.

In addition to these general complaints, focal signs should be sought. Cardiac manifestations result from either direct valve damage or valvulitis. Thus, new murmurs may appear, such as mitral or aortic regurgitation, and symptoms of congestive heart failure may develop or worsen.

Extracardiac manifestations can also be helpful in establishing the diagnosis, although they occur less frequently in children than in adults. Skin findings such as petechiae, splinter hemorrhages in the nail beds, Janeway lesions (nontender hemorrhagic plaques on the palms and soles), and Osler nodes (tender purplish lesions on the pads of fingers and toes, thenar eminences, and lower arm) may be found on examination. Janeway lesions are thought to represent septic emboli; however, it is unclear whether Osler nodes are attributable to the same phenomenon or are due to an immune vasculitis. Roth spots are pale retinal lesions with areas of hemorrhage usually located near the optic disk. Emboli to any organs, including the heart, kidneys, lungs, brain, spleen, or liver, can cause infarction (thrombotic emboli) or abscess (septic emboli). Emboli to the central nervous system can result in stroke or mycotic aneurysm. Mycotic aneurysms develop when septic emboli cause local arterial infection and inflammation, with resulting occlusion of the vessel. The damage to the muscular wall and increased

pressure cause dilation of the vessel. Despite the name, these aneurysms almost always result from bacterial infection. Splenomegaly is seen in more than half of patients and can be caused by immune system activation. Both focal and diffuse glomerular nephritis have been described, with immune complex deposition noted.

Patients with rapidly progressing acute endocarditis may present in shock, with a clinical picture consistent with overwhelming sepsis. In such circumstances, the classic findings of infective endocarditis may be absent, and suspicion for this disease may be raised only by a history of cardiac lesions and persistently positive blood cultures.

DIFFERENTIAL DIAGNOSIS

Alternative diagnostic considerations are extremely broad and are based on the predominant signs and symptoms. Prolonged fever should prompt evaluation for a fever of unknown origin (see Chapter 61). Neurologic features may suggest a wide range of intracranial conditions, including stroke, epilepsy, and encephalopathy. Rheumatologic and oncologic processes can mimic the nonspecific findings of fatigue, malaise, weight loss, and joint pain.

DIAGNOSIS

The diagnosis of infective endocarditis can be elusive and hinges on a careful assessment of risk factors in the setting of suggestive findings. In an attempt to improve the clinical diagnosis of infective endocarditis, Durack and colleagues developed a scoring system.[8] This was subsequently modified to include a greater emphasis on imaging data.[9] These diagnostic criteria have been tested in pediatric populations and found to be useful.[10,11] Tables 84-2 and 84-3 outline the definitions of and criteria for the diagnosis of infective endocarditis.

Imaging

Echocardiography with Doppler color flow mapping has become the standard diagnostic modality in patients with suspected infective endocarditis. It can identify valvular vegetations (Fig. 84-1) as well as impaired cardiac performance, prosthetic valve dehiscence, disturbed conduit flow, and abscess. Moreover, echocardiography can define the presence of an occult structural abnormality, such as a bicuspid aortic valve, thus identifying a clinically silent risk factor. It has been well established that echocardiography can detect cardiac involvement in patients with otherwise occult infective endocarditis,[12] and this has been confirmed in children.[13]

For infants and children, unlike adults, transthoracic echocardiography is usually sufficient to establish a diagnosis. In certain circumstances, however, transesophageal imaging is required, particularly in children with previous cardiothoracic surgical procedures, pulmonary problems that confound imaging windows, or substantial obesity.

Serial echocardiographic Doppler studies are also useful to gauge the response to therapy and assess for potential complications. For example, vegetation size and mobility may be an indicator of risk for embolization.[14,15] Importantly, in a patient undergoing treatment for infective endocarditis, the diagnosis of myocardial abscess causing a new

---

Table 84-2 Definitions of Criteria for the Diagnosis of Infective Endocarditis (IE)

Major Criteria

Positive blood culture*

    Typical microorganism consistent with IE from two separate blood cultures, as noted below:

        Viridans streptococci, *Streptococcus bovis,* or HACEK group, or

        Community-acquired *Staphylococcus aureus* or enterococci, in the absence of a primary focus

    Microorganisms consistent with IE from persistently positive blood cultures, defined as:

        >2 positive cultures of blood samples drawn >12 hr apart, or

        All of 3 or a majority of >4 separate blood cultures (with first and last samples drawn >1 hr apart)

Evidence of endocardial involvement

    Positive echocardiogram for IE defined as:

        Oscillating intracardiac mass on valve or supporting structures, in the path of regurgitant jets, or on implanted material in the absence of an alternative anatomic explanation, or

        Abscess, or

        New partial dehiscence of prosthetic valve

    New valvular regurgitation (worsening or changing of preexisting murmur not sufficient)

Minor Criteria

Predisposition: predisposing heart condition or IV drug use

Fever: temperature >38°C

Vascular phenomena: major arterial emboli, septic pulmonary infarct, mycotic aneurysm, intracranial hemorrhage, conjunctival hemorrhages, and Janeway lesions

Immunologic phenomena: glomerulonephritis, Osler nodes, Roth spots, and rheumatoid factor

Microbiologic evidence: positive blood culture that does not meet major criteria (see above) or serologic evidence of active infection with organism consistent with IE

Echocardiographic findings: consistent with IE but do not meet major criteria (see above)

*Excludes single positive cultures for coagulase-negative staphylococci and organisms that do not cause endocarditis.
HACEK, *Haemophilus* species, *Actinobacillus actinomycetemcomitans, Cardiobacterium hominis, Eikenella* species, and *Kingella kingae.*
From Durack OT, Lukes AS, Bright DK: New criteria for diagnosis of infective endocarditis: Utilization of specific echocardiographic findings. Am J Med 1994;96:200-209.

Table 84-3 Clinical Criteria for the Diagnosis of Infective Endocarditis (IE)

Definite IE

Pathologic criteria

    Microorganisms: demonstrated by culture or histology in a vegetation that has embolized or in an intracardiac abscess, or

    Pathologic lesions: vegetation or intracardiac abscess present, confirmed by histology showing active endocarditis

Clinical criteria (as defined in Table 84-2)

    2 major criteria, or

    1 major criterion and 3 minor criteria, or

    5 minor criteria

Possible IE

Findings consistent with IE that fall short of "definite" but not "rejected"

Rejected

Firm alternative diagnosis for manifestations of endocarditis, or

Resolution of manifestations of endocarditis with antibiotic therapy for >4 days, or

No pathologic evidence of IE at surgery or autopsy, after antibiotic therapy for >4 days

From Durack OT, Lukes AS, Bright DK: New criteria for diagnosis of infective endocarditis: Utilization of specific echocardiographic findings. Am J Med 1994;96:200-209.

---

arrhythmia or progressive aortic root enlargement could suggest the need for a shift in treatment, including surgical intervention.

Laboratory Studies

Blood cultures are required in all patients with suspected infective endocarditis. This includes any patient with a history of fever without an obvious explanation who has known heart disease or who has had endocarditis previously. Multiple cultures (three to five) are best, with 1 to 3 mL/culture in infants and 5 to 7 mL/culture in older children usually being sufficient. In children who have been on antibiotics, greater numbers of cultures over an extended period may be required. It is useful to notify the laboratory that infective endocarditis is suspected so that prolonged (>2 weeks) incubation of culture specimens will be done.

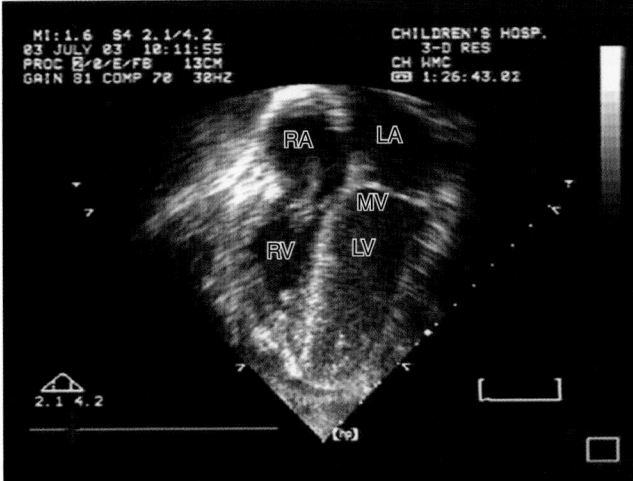

Figure 84-1 Two-dimensional echocardiogram from a child with tricuspid valve vegetation (outlined). LA, left atrium; LV, left ventricle; MV, mitral valve; RA, right atrium; RV, right ventricle.

In addition to cultures, testing for antibiotic susceptibility is extremely important for clinical management. Measurement of the minimum inhibitory concentration of the particular antibiotic chosen is the standard guide to therapeutic efficacy. The minimum bactericidal concentration is no longer universally employed, but it may be of use in particular situations, based on the advice of an infectious disease specialist.

Other laboratory markers of infection and inflammation can be useful, serially, as guides to therapy. Elevated acute phase reactants (erythrocyte sedimentation rate and C-reactive protein) and hypergammaglobulinemia are usually present. Rheumatoid factor may initially be elevated and can be followed as confirmation of response to therapy. Although the presence of leukocytosis (white blood cell count >15,000) is variable, increased segmented neutrophils or other immature forms (bands) are typical. Thrombocytopenia and mild anemia can be present. Abnormal liver function tests are less common without heart failure or hepatic emboli, but abnormalities in urinary sediment are frequently present. Hematuria may represent either an embolic process or glomerular nephritis. Signs of an immune complex nephritis can include proteinuria, red cell casts, and abnormal renal function measures, including creatinine and blood urea nitrogen. Low serum complement levels support the diagnosis of glomerular nephritis, but this is not definitive.

TREATMENT

Antibiotic Regimens

Owing to the tenacious nature of these infections, a prolonged course of parenteral antibiotics is required. Several factors contribute to the difficulty of eradicating the source of the infection. As described earlier, the microbial organisms are layered within elements of the vegetation, which sequesters them from the immune system and antibiotic exposure. Organisms with limited antibiotic susceptibilities may also require prolonged treatment for eradication. Tables 84-4 to 84-6 outline antibiotic regimens for childhood infective endocarditis in a variety of settings.[16]

In most cases, bacteremia resolves within a few days of treatment with appropriate antibiotics. *S. aureus* may persist in the blood for longer periods—up to 5 to 10 days after therapy. It is advisable to wait until bacterial cultures are negative before placing a long-term central venous catheter.

In approximately 5% to 7% of cases, a vegetation is visualized on echocardiograph, but no specific organism grows in the laboratory from blood cultures. In this situation, empirical treatment is required. Consultation with an infectious disease specialist can be helpful in guiding the laboratory in the search for uncommon or fastidious organisms. Most commonly, therapy in children is still aimed against staphylococci or streptococci, but the HACEK organisms (*Haemophilus* species, *Actinobacillus actinomycetemcomitans*, *Cardiobacterium hominis*, *Eikenella* species, and *Kingella kingae*) should also be considered. For valvular endocarditis in the culture-negative setting, the combination of ceftriaxone and gentamicin is frequently employed,[17] with an additional β-lactamase-resistant penicillin drug if there is a chance of staphylococcal involvement. Sometimes, clinical information can suggest microbial suspects in culture-negative endocarditis (Table 84-7).

Complications

Despite an ever-increasing armamentarium of powerful antibiotics for the treatment of infective endocarditis, a high proportion of patients suffer some type of complication.[18] These complications are usually the result of mechanical obstruction by the vegetation or emboli; cardiac dysfunction, including arrhythmias and heart block; or systemic infectious or immunologic issues (Table 84-8).

Urgent surgical intervention in patients with at least moderate congestive heart failure improves survival and quality of life.[19] Table 84-9 reviews the circumstances indicating an increased risk for the development of complications, and Table 84-10 reviews the factors related to the need for surgery. Although it is preferable to administer a prolonged course of antibiotics before proceeding with surgery, it is important not to delay surgery in the face of a changing clinical picture. It is incumbent on the hospitalist, as the leader of the management team, to consider cardiothoracic surgical consultation at an early stage and on a continuing basis when caring for patients with infective endocarditis.

CONSULTATION

- Discussion with a cardiovascular specialist is crucial in managing these patients, particularly when there are concerns about complications.
- Close consultation with an infectious disease specialist may be helpful in determining the optimal antibiotic regimen.
- Early involvement of cardiothoracic surgery is important when managing patients who develop complications that may warrant surgical intervention.

ADMISSION CRITERIA

- Newly diagnosed infective endocarditis
- Newly recognized untreated intracardiac vegetation, even if asymptomatic

Table 84-4 Treatment Regimens for Native Valve Infective Endocarditis Caused by Viridans Streptococci, *Streptococcus bovis,* or Enterococci

Organism	Antimicrobial Agent	Dosage (per kg/24 hr)*	Frequency of Administration	Duration (wk)
Penicillin-susceptible streptococci (MIC ≤0.1 µg/mL)	Penicillin G[†] or	200,000 U IV	q4-6h	4
	Ceftriaxone	100 mg IV	q24h	4
	Penicillin G[†] or	200,000 U IV	q4-6h	2
	Ceftriaxone plus	100 mg IV	q24h	2
	Gentamicin	3 mg IM or IV	q8h[†]	2
Streptococci relatively resistant to penicillin (MIC >0.1-0.5 µg/mL)	Penicillin G[†] or	300,000 U IV	q4-6h	4
	Ceftriaxone plus	100 mg IV	q24h	4
	Gentamicin	3 mg IM or IV	q8h[†]	2
Enterococci,[§] nutritionally variant viridans streptococci, or high-level penicillin-resistant streptococci (MIC >0.5 µg/mL)	Penicillin G[†] plus	300,000 U IV	q4-6h	4-6[¶]
	Gentamicin	3 mg IM or IV	q8h[¶]	4-6[¶]

*Dosages are for patients with normal renal and hepatic function. Maximum dosages per 24 hr are as follows: penicillin, 18 million U; ampicillin, 12 g; ceftriaxone, 4 g; gentamicin, 240 mg. The 2-wk regimens are not recommended for patients with symptoms of infection lasting >3 mo, an extracardiac focus of infection, myocardial abscess, mycotic aneurysm, or infection with nutritionally variant viridans streptococci (*Abiotrophia* species).
[†]Ampicillin 300 mg/kg per 24 hr in 4-6 divided dosages may be used as alternative to penicillin.
[†]Studies in adults suggest that the gentamicin dosage may be administered in single daily dose. If gentamicin is administered in 3 equally divided doses over 24 hr, adjust the dosage to achieve peak and trough concentrations in serum of ≈3 and <1 µg of gentamicin per mL, respectively.
[§]For enterococci resistant to penicillin, vancomycin, or aminoglycosides, treatment should be guided by consultation with an infectious disease specialist. Cephalosporins should not be used to treat enterococcal endocarditis regardless of in vitro susceptibility.
[¶]Adjust gentamicin dosage to achieve peak and trough concentrations in serum of ≈3 and <1 µg of gentamicin per mL, respectively.
MIC, minimum inhibitory concentration.
From Ferrieri P, Gewitz MH, Gerber MA, et al: Unique features of infective endocarditis in childhood. Circulation 2002;105:2115-2127.
[¶¶]Studies in adults suggest that 4 wk of therapy is sufficient for patients with enterococcal infective endocarditis with symptoms of <3 mo duration; 6 wk of therapy is recommended for patients with symptoms of infection lasting >3 mo.

Table 84-5 Treatment Regimens for Infective Endocarditis Caused by Viridans Streptococci, *Streptococcus bovis,* or Enterococci in Patients Unable to Tolerate β-Lactams

Organism	Antimicrobial Agent	Dosage (per kg/24 hr)*	Frequency of Administration	Duration (wk)
Native valve (no prosthetic material)				
Streptococci	Vancomycin	40 mg IV	q6-12h	4-6
Enterococci[†] or nutritionally variant viridans streptococci	Vancomycin plus	40 mg IV	q6-12h	6
	Gentamicin	3 mg IM or IV	q8h[†]	6
Prosthetic devices				
Streptococci	Vancomycin plus	40 mg IV	q6-12h	6
	Gentamicin	3 mg IM or IV	q8h[†]	2
Enterococci[†] or nutritionally variant viridans streptococci	Vancomycin plus	40 mg IV	q6-12h	6
	Gentamicin	3 mg IM or IV	q8h[†]	6

*Dosages are for patients with normal renal function. Maximum dosage of gentamicin per 24 hr is 240 mg.
[†]For enterococci resistant to vancomycin or aminoglycosides, treatment should be guided by consultation with an infectious disease specialist.
[†]Dosage of gentamicin should be adjusted to achieve peak and trough concentrations in serum of ≈3 and <1 µg of gentamicin per mL, respectively.
From Ferrieri P, Gewitz MH, Gerber MA, et al: Unique features of infective endocarditis in childhood. Circulation 2002;105:2115-2127.

Table 84-6 Treatment Regimens for Endocarditis Caused by Staphylococci

Organism	Antimicrobial Agent	Dosage (per kg/24 hr)*	Frequency of Administration	Duration
Native valve (no prosthetic materials)				
Methicillin susceptible	Nafcillin or oxacillin with or without	200 mg IV	q4-6h	6 wk
	Gentamicin[†]	3 mg IM or IV[‡]	q8h	3-5 days
β-Lactam allergic	Cefazolin[§] with or without	100 mg IV	q6-8h	6 wk
	Gentamicin[†]	3 mg IM or IV[‡]	q8h	3-5 days
	or			
	Vancomycin	40 mg IV	q6-12h	6 wk
Methicillin resistant	Vancomycin	40 mg IV	q6-12h	6 wk
Prosthetic device or other prosthetic materials				
Methicillin susceptible	Nafcillin or oxacillin or	200 mg IV	q4-6h	≥6 wk
	Cefazolin[§] plus	100 mg IV	q6-8h	≥6 wk
	Rifampin[‖] plus	20 mg PO	q8h	≥6 wk
	Gentamicin[†]	3 mg IM or IV[‡]	q8h	2 wk
Methicillin resistant	Vancomycin plus	40 mg IV	q6-12h	≥6 wk
	Rifampin[‖] plus	20 mg PO	q8h	≥6 wk
	Gentamicin[†]	3 mg IM or IV[‡]	q8h	2 wk

*Dosages are for patients with normal renal and hepatic function. Maximum dosages per 24 hr are as follows: oxacillin or nafcillin, 12 g; cefazolin, 6 g; gentamicin, 240 mg; rifampin, 900 mg.
[†]Gentamicin therapy should be used only with gentamicin-susceptible strains.
[‡]Dosage of gentamicin should be adjusted to achieve peak and trough concentrations in serum of ≈3 and <1 μg of gentamicin per mL, respectively.
[§]Cefazolin or other first-generation cephalosporins in equivalent dosages may be used in patients who do not have a history of immediate-type hypersensitivity (urticaria, angioedema, anaphylaxis) to penicillin or ampicillin.
[‖]Dosages for rifampin are based on results of studies conducted in adults and should be used only with rifampin-susceptible strains.
From Ferrieri P, Gewitz MH, Gerber MA, et al: Unique features of infective endocarditis in childhood. Circulation 2002;105:2115-2127.

- Any evidence of significant change in cardiac status or evidence of potential distant complications (e.g., embolic complication, worsening cyanosis) in a patient at risk for infective endocarditis

DISCHARGE CRITERIA

- Resolution of clinical signs of active infection after initiation of treatment
- Stable cardiac status
- Decreasing vegetation size
- Confirmed ability to maintain full treatment course after discharge

PREVENTION

The significant morbidity and potential for mortality associated with infective endocarditis make its prevention of significant interest. Unfortunately, prophylaxis regimens have not been very successful. In fact, recent information indicates that dental procedures are no more likely to result in infective endocarditis than are other medical procedures,[20] and prophylaxis regimens in general may not be effective when applied to specific populations.[21] Also, there are many circumstances in which bacteremia occurs spontaneously (e.g., mastication, routine oral hygiene maneuvers) and for which antibiotic prophylaxis is not feasible. The current recommendations of the American Heart Association are outlined in Tables 84-11 to 84-13.[22]

IN A NUTSHELL

- In spite of current prophylaxis guidelines, the incidence of endocarditis is steady or increasing.
- Gram-positive bacteria represent the largest subgroup of causative organisms in infective endocarditis, although infections with gram-negative bacteria and fungi do occur.
- Echocardiography with Doppler color flow mapping is the standard diagnostic modality in patients with suspected infective endocarditis; it is also used to assess the effectiveness of therapy.
- Complications of infective endocarditis can be severe and include mechanical obstruction by vegetations or emboli; cardiac dysfunction, including arrhythmias and heart block; and systemic infection.

Table 84-7 Possible Causative Organisms in Culture-Negative Endocarditis

Clinical Factor	Microorganism
Indwelling cardiovascular device	*Staphylococcus aureus* Coagulase-negative staphylococci Aerobic gram-negative organisms *Corynebacterium* species
Chronic skin disorders	*S. aureus* β-hemolytic streptococci
Poor dentition	Viridans streptococci HACEK organisms "Nutritionally variant" streptococci
Dog or cat exposure	*Bartonella* species *Pasteurella* species
Gastrointestinal lesions	*Streptococcus bovis* *Enterococcus* species *Clostridium septicum*
Early (<1 yr) post open heart surgery	Coagulase-negative staphylococci *S. aureus* Aerobic gram-negative organisms *Legionella* species Fungi

HACEK, *Haemophilus* species, *Actinobacillus actinomycetemcomitans*, *Cardiobacterium hominis*, *Eikenella* species, and *Kingella kingae*.
Modified from Baddour LM, Wilson WR, Bayer AS, et al: Infective endocarditis: Diagnosis, antimicrobial therapy, and management of complications. Circulation 2005;111:e394-e434.

Table 84-8 Complications of Infective Endocarditis

Congestive heart failure
Embolic events Cerebral Pulmonary Renal Coronary
Periannular extension of abscess
Arrhythmia development
New heart block
Prosthetic device dysfunction
Valvular dehiscence
Graft or shunt occlusion
Persistent bacteremia or fungemia
Metastatic infection; mycotic aneurysm
Glomerulonephritis, renal failure

From Ferrieri P, Gewitz MH, Gerber MA, et al: Unique features of infective endocarditis in childhood. Circulation 2002;105:2115-2127.

Table 84-9 Risk Factors for Complications of Infective Endocarditis (IE)

Previous IE
Prosthetic cardiac valves
Left-sided IE
Staphylococcus aureus IE; fungal IE
Cyanotic congenital heart disease
Systemic-to-pulmonary shunts
Poor clinical response to antimicrobial therapy or prolonged symptoms

Modified from Ferrieri P, Gewitz MH, Gerber MA, et al: Unique features of infective endocarditis in childhood. Circulation 2002;105:2115-2127.

Table 84-10 Clinical and Echocardiographic Features Suggesting the Need for Surgical Intervention

Vegetation features Persistent vegetation after systemic embolization Anterior mitral leaflet vegetation, particularly >10 mm* >1 embolic event during first 2 wk of antimicrobial therapy* >2 embolic events during or after antimicrobial therapy* Increase in vegetation size after 4 wk of antimicrobial therapy†
Valvular dysfunction Acute aortic or mitral insufficiency with signs of ventricular failure† Heart failure unresponsive to medical therapy† Valve perforation or rupture†
Perivalvular extension Valvular dehiscence, rupture, or fistula† New heart block† Large abscess or extension of abscess despite appropriate antimicrobial therapy†

*Surgery may be required because of risk of recurrent embolization.
†Surgery may be required because of risk of embolization, heart failure, or failure of medical therapy.
‡Surgery may be required because of heart failure or failure of medical therapy.
From Bayer A, Bolger AF, Taubert KA, et al: Diagnosis and management of infective endocarditis and its complications. Circulation 1998;98:2936-2948.

Table 84-11 Endocarditis Prophylaxis Recommendations Based on Specific Cardiac Conditions

Endocarditis Prophylaxis Recommended
High-risk category
   Prosthetic cardiac valves, including bioprosthetic and homograft valves
   Previous bacterial endocarditis
   Complex cyanotic congenital heart disease (e.g., single ventricle states, transposition of the great arteries, tetralogy of Fallot)
   Surgically constructed systemic pulmonary shunts or conduits
Moderate-risk category
   Most other congenital cardiac malformations (other than above and below)
   Acquired valvular dysfunction (e.g., rheumatic heart disease)
   Hypertrophic cardiomyopathy
   Mitral valve prolapse with valvular regurgitation or thickened leaflets

Endocarditis Prophylaxis Not Recommended
Negligible-risk category (no greater risk than the general population)
   Isolated secundum atrial septal defect
   Surgical repair of atrial septal defect, ventricular septal defect, or patent ductus arteriosus (without residua beyond 6 mo)
   Previous coronary artery bypass graft surgery
   Mitral valve prolapse without valvular regurgitation
   Physiologic, functional, or innocent heart murmurs
   Previous Kawasaki disease without valvular dysfunction
   Previous rheumatic fever without valvular dysfunction
   Cardiac pacemakers (intravascular and epicardial) and implanted defibrillators

From Dajani AS, Taubert KA, Wilson W, et al: Prevention of bacterial endocarditis: Recommendations by the American Heart Association. JAMA 1997;277:1794-1801.

Table 84-12 Endocarditis Prophylaxis Recommendations for Dental Procedures

Endocarditis Prophylaxis Recommended*
Dental extractions
Periodontal procedures, including surgery, scaling and root planing, probing, and recall maintenance
Dental implant placement and reimplantation of avulsed teeth
Endodontic (root canal) instrumentation or surgery only beyond the apex
Subgingival placement of antibiotic fibers or strips
Initial placement of orthodontic bands but not brackets
Intraligamentary local anesthetic injections
Prophylactic cleaning of teeth or implants where bleeding is anticipated

Endocarditis Prophylaxis Not Recommended
Restorative dentistry† (operative and prosthodontic) with or without retraction cord‡
Local anesthetic injections (nonintraligamentary)
Intracanal endodontic treatment; post placement and buildup
Placement of rubber dams
Postoperative suture removal
Placement of removable prosthodontic or orthodontic appliances
Taking of oral impressions
Fluoride treatments
Taking of oral radiographs
Orthodontic appliance adjustment
Shedding of primary teeth

*Prophylaxis is recommended for patients with high- and moderate-risk cardiac conditions.
†This includes restoration of decayed teeth (filling cavities) and replacement of missing teeth.
‡Clinical judgment may indicate antibiotic use in selected circumstances that may create significant bleeding.
From Dajani AS, Taubert KA, Wilson W, et al: Prevention of bacterial endocarditis: Recommendations by the American Heart Association. JAMA 1997;227:1794-1801.

Table 84-13 Endocarditis Prophylaxis Recommendations for Medical and Surgical Procedures

Endocarditis Prophylaxis Recommended
Respiratory tract
   Tonsillectomy or adenoidectomy
   Surgical operations that involve respiratory mucosa
   Bronchoscopy with a rigid bronchoscope
Gastrointestinal tract*
   Sclerotherapy for esophageal varices
   Esophageal stricture dilation
   Endoscopic retrograde cholangiography with biliary obstruction
   Biliary tract surgery
   Surgical operations that involve intestinal mucosa
Genitourinary tract
   Prostatic surgery
   Cystoscopy
   Urethral dilation

Endocarditis Prophylaxis Not Recommended
Respiratory tract
   Endotracheal intubation
   Bronchoscopy with a flexible bronchoscope, with or without biopsy[†]
   Tympanostomy tube insertion
Gastrointestinal tract
   Transesophageal echocardiography[†]
   Endoscopy with or without gastrointestinal biopsy[†]
Genitourinary tract
   Vaginal hysterectomy[†]
   Vaginal delivery[†]
   Cesarean section
   In uninfected tissue:
      Urethral catheterization
      Uterine dilation and curettage
      Therapeutic abortion
      Sterilization procedures
      Insertion or removal of intrauterine devices
Other
   Cardiac catheterization, including balloon angioplasty
   Implanted cardiac pacemakers, implanted defibrillators, and coronary stents
   Incision or biopsy of surgically scrubbed skin
   Circumcision

*Prophylaxis is recommended for high-risk patients; optional for medium-risk patients.
[†]Prophylaxis is optional for high-risk patients.
From Dajani AS, Taubert KA, Wilson W, et al: Prevention of bacterial endocarditis: Recommendations by the American Heart Association. JAMA 1997;227:1794-1801.

ON THE HORIZON

- Enhanced understanding of the virulence factors associated with common bacteria will likely lead to novel improvements in treatment capabilities.
- Substantial modifications of the existing recommendations for prophylaxis can be expected. This review process has already begun in other countries, as indicated by the publication of new recommendations.[23]

SUGGESTED READING

Baddour LM, Wilson WR, Bayer AS, et al: Infective endocarditis: Diagnosis, antimicrobial therapy, and management of complications. Circulation 2005;111:e394-e434.

Ferrieri P, Gewitz MH, Gerber MA, et al: Unique features of infective endocarditis in childhood. Circulation 2002;105:2115-2127.

REFERENCES

1. Martin JM, Neches WH, Wald ER: Infective endocarditis: 35 years of experience at a children's hospital. Clin Infect Dis 1997;24:669-675.
2. Baltimore RS: Infective endocarditis. In Jenson HB, Baltimore RS (eds): Pediatric Infectious Diseases: Principles and Practice. Norwalk, Conn, Appleton & Lange, 1995.
3. Morris CD, Reller MD, Menashe VD: Thirty year incidence of infective endocarditis after surgery for congenital heart defect. JAMA 1998; 279:599-603.
4. Tunkel AR, Scheld WM: Experimental models of endocarditis. In Kaye D (ed): Infective Endocarditis, 2nd ed. New York, Raven Press, 1992, pp 37-56.

5. Sainas L, Prince A, Gersony WM: Pediatric infective endocarditis in the modern era. J Pediatr 1993;122:847-853.

6. Baddour LM, Bettmann MA, Bolger AF, et al: Nonvalvular cardiovascular device-related infections. Circulation 2003;108:2015-2031.

7. Millard DD, Shulman ST: The changing spectrum of neonatal endocarditis. Clin Perinatol 1988;15:587-608.

8. Durack OT, Lukes AS, Bright DK: New criteria for diagnosis of infective endocarditis: Utilization of specific echocardiographic findings. Am J Med 1994;96:200-209.

9. Li JS, Sexton OJ, Mick N, et al: Proposed modifications to the Duke criteria for the diagnosis of infective endocarditis. Clin Infect Dis 2000;30:633-638.

10. Stockheim JA, Chadwick EG, Kessler S, et al: Are the Duke criteria superior to Beth Israel criteria for diagnosis of infective endocarditis in children? Clin Infect Dis 1998;27:1451-1456.

11. Del Poat JM, DeCicco LT, Vartalis C, et al: Infective endocarditis in children: Clinical analysis and evaluation of two diagnostic criteria. Pediatr Infect Dis J 1995;14:1079-1086.

12. Fowler VG, Li JS, Corey GR, et al: Role of echocardiography in evaluation of patients with *Staphylococcus aureus* bacteremia. J Am Coll Cardiol 1997;30:1072-1078.

13. Valente AM, Jain R, Scheurer M, et al: Frequency of infective endocarditis among infants and children with *Staphylococcus aureus* bacteremia. Pediatrics 2005;115:e15-e19.

14. Sanfilippo AJ, Picard MH, Newell JB, et al: Echocardiographic assessment of patients with infectious endocarditis: Prediction of risk for complications. J Am Coll Cardiol 1991;18:1191-1199.

15. DiSalvo G, Habib G, Pergola V, et al: Echocardiography predicts embolic events in infective endocarditis. J Am Coll Cardiol 2001;37:1069-1076.

16. Ferrieri P, Gewitz MH, Gerber MA, et al: Unique features of infective endocarditis in childhood. Circulation 2002;105:2115-2127.

17. Berkowitz FE: Infective endocarditis. In Nichols DG, Cameron DE, Greeley WJ, et al (eds): Critical Heart Disease in Infants and Children. St Louis, Mosby-Year Book, 1995, pp 961-986.

18. Cobell CH, Lerakis S, Selton-Sutty C, et al: Cardiovascular risk factors and outcomes in patients with definite endocarditis: Findings from 1024 patients in the ICE prospective cohort study [abstract]. Circulation 2003;108:IV-432.

19. Stinson EB: Surgical treatment of infective endocarditis. Prog Cardiovasc Dis 1979;22:145-168.

20. Strom BL, Abrutyn E, Berlin JA, et al: Risk factors for infective endocarditis: Oral hygiene and nondental exposures. Circulation 2000;102:2842-2848.

21. Vander Meer JT, Thompson J, Valkenbury HA, et al: Epidemiology of bacterial endocarditis in the Netherlands. II. Antecedent procedures and use of prophylaxis. Arch Intern Med 1992;152:1869-1873.

22. Dajani AS, Taubert KA, Wilson W, et al: Prevention of bacterial endocarditis: Recommendations by the American Heart Association. JAMA 1997;277:1794-1801.

23. Gould FK, Elliott TSJ, Foweraker J, et al: Guidelines for the prevention of endocarditis: Report of the Working Party of the British Society for Antimicrobial Chemotherapy. J Antimicrob Chemother 2006;10:1093-1121.

ACKNOWLEDGMENTS

The author appreciates the assistance of MaryAnn Dickman in the preparation of this chapter.

CHAPTER 85

Myocarditis and Cardiomyopathy

Robert N. Vincent and Kenneth J. Dooley

Myocarditis is a pathologic process characterized by inflammation of the myocardium leading to cellular necrosis and myocardial dysfunction. Although it is often thought of as a viral or postviral process, the causes of myocarditis are numerous and include both infectious (viruses, bacteria, fungi, yeasts, rickettsiae, protozoa, and parasites) and noninfectious (toxins, drugs, autoimmune diseases, Kawasaki disease) entities.

Cardiomyopathy is a general term referring to diseases of the myocardium. Clinically and pathologically, cardiomyopathy can be divided into dilated, hypertrophic, and restrictive types. Because myocarditis is a precursor to and one of the causes of dilated cardiomyopathy, the two are considered together in this chapter.

MYOCARDITIS AND DILATED CARDIOMYOPATHY

Pathophysiology

Although there are a variety of causes of dilated cardiomyopathy (DCM), the final common pathway is one of cellular necrosis within the cardiac muscle. This damage causes decreased ventricular contractility and impaired diastolic filling, which leads to diminished cardiac output. Compensatory mechanisms to improve cardiac output are triggered, including up-regulation of the sympathetic nervous system and the renin-angiotensin axis. Stimulation of these pathways results in volume expansion and vasoconstriction, as well as increased contractility and heart rate (Fig. 85-1).

Initially, these compensatory mechanisms help by enhancing myocardial performance and improving perfusion of vital organs. Unfortunately, both the hormonal up-regulation and the sympathetic stimulation produce a progressive rise in preload and afterload, which eventually results in ventricular dilation and a dwindling cardiac output (Fig. 85-2). The spherical ventricular cavity also causes the papillary muscles to be pulled apart, causing mitral regurgitation and resulting in more inefficient cardiac function.

Clinical Presentation

The presentation of DCM depends on the age of the patient and the rapidity of disease progression. Aggressive, acute viral myocarditis may cause a rapid decline in cardiac function over a very short period. The rate of deterioration may exceed the capacity of the physiologic compensatory mechanisms, resulting in sudden cardiovascular collapse and cardiac arrest.

Other causes of DCM, and occasionally myocarditis, may have a more progressive, subacute course. A slow decrease in ventricular function over many months or years allows partial compensation, and the child may remain relatively asymptomatic; however, such a patient has little cardiac reserve, and an unrelated illness such as an upper respiratory infection may result in cardiac decompensation. Therefore, a history of an antecedent viral infection in a child presenting with new-onset DCM does not necessarily confirm the diagnosis of viral myocarditis, because it is quite possible that the viral illness merely unmasked the chronic compensated form of DCM.

Whether the onset is rapid or chronic, the usual presentation of DCM is congestive heart failure and low cardiac output. Signs and symptoms of heart failure and low cardiac output in newborns and infants include fussiness, poor appetite, poor feeding, fever, listlessness, diaphoresis, and respiratory distress. Physical examination often reveals tachypnea, tachycardia, cardiomegaly, hepatomegaly, and pallor or an ashen appearance. Older children or adolescents may complain of poor appetite and abdominal pain due to hepatic congestion, lethargy, exercise intolerance, malaise, and fever. Jugular venous distention and rales are additional signs of heart failure in older children. Muffled heart sounds or muffled breath sounds may indicate the presence of pericardial effusion or pleural effusion, respectively.

Differential Diagnosis

The differential diagnosis of DCM is based on age (Table 85-1). All attempts should be made to diagnose treatable causes of cardiomyopathy such as structural heart disease, underlying arrhythmias, and vitamin deficiencies. Although structural heart defects and arrhythmias are not truly diseases of the myocardium, they may present similarly to DCM and must be considered in the evaluation of these children.

Evaluation

Table 85-2 lists the studies that may be performed in the evaluation of a patient with newly diagnosed DCM. The extent of the evaluation is guided by the history, clinical findings, and initial screening tests. For example, a history of doxorubicin (Adriamycin) administration, which has well-established cardiotoxicity, would limit the need for a broader search for a cause. When identifiable causes are excluded or the history points to a familial or inherited disorder, family screening is important.

A chest radiograph is often obtained for the evaluation of respiratory symptoms such as tachypnea, dyspnea, or cough (all of which can be manifestations of DCM), and it may reveal radiographic findings of DCM such as cardiomegaly, increased pulmonary venous markings, pulmonary edema, or pleural effusion.

An electrocardiogram (ECG) may reveal nonspecific changes, including decreased QRS voltages and low-voltage or inverted T waves in myocarditis. Q waves in leads I and aVL due to myocardial infarction are suggestive of an

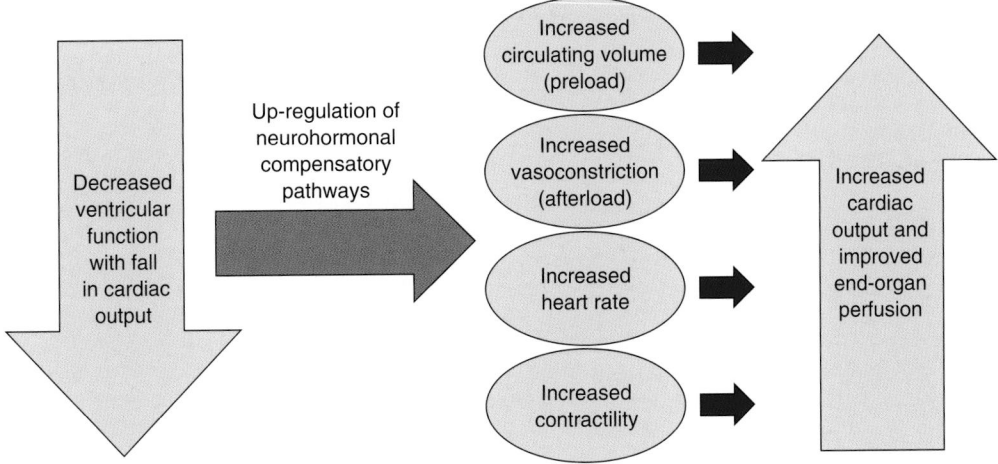

Figure 85–1   The role of neurohormonal mechanisms in compensating for decreased cardiac output in dilated cardiomyopathy.

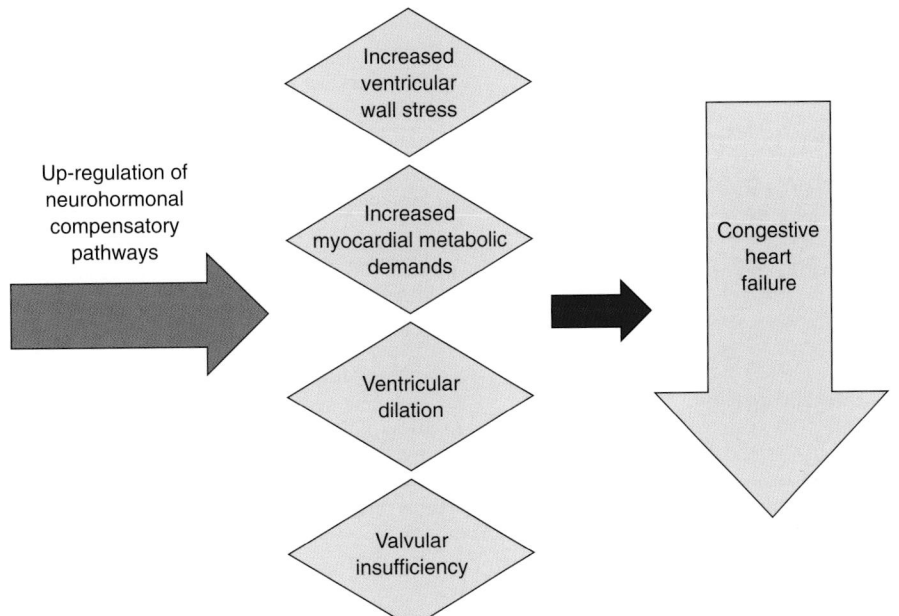

Figure 85–2   Detrimental effects of ongoing neurohormonal compensation in dilated cardiomyopathy.

anomalous origin of the left coronary artery from the pulmonary artery. Ectopic beats should raise the suspicion of poorly controlled supraventricular tachycardia and ventricular arrhythmias, although in severe cardiac dysfunction, ventricular arrhythmias may occur secondary to myocardial disease.

An echocardiogram establishes the presence of a dilated, poorly contracting left ventricle while excluding most structural causes of this dysfunction, such as left ventricular outflow tract obstruction. A few treatable structural anomalies may not be excluded with certainty, such as anomalous origin of the left coronary artery from the pulmonary artery, necessitating further diagnostic testing. The evaluation should also search for the presence of a thrombus in the left atrium or ventricle.

Doppler cardiography often demonstrates mitral as well as tricuspid insufficiency. Right ventricular size and function

may be spared early on, but the right ventricle may also dilate and demonstrate poor contractility. There may be secondary pulmonary hypertension arising from left ventricular dysfunction.

Although not routinely necessary, cardiac catheterization can be used to perform an endomyocardial biopsy, exclude structural diseases not eliminated by echocardiography, and obtain baseline hemodynamic information. This information may be useful for developing a short-term prognosis and predicting response to medical therapy. Endomyocardial biopsy is important in making the diagnosis of myocarditis. A positive biopsy using the Dallas criteria establishes the diagnosis,[1] whereas a negative biopsy does not exclude it. Because myocarditis is a patchy, nonhomogeneous infiltrate, it may be missed on random sampling of the right ventricle.[2,3] Polymerase chain reaction testing for viral genomes, if positive, can also establish the diagnosis.[4]

Table 85–1   Differential Diagnosis of Dilated Cardiomyopathy Based on Age

Fetus	Selenium deficiency
Arteriovenous malformation (vein of Galen)	Anomalous left coronary artery from pulmonary artery
Myocarditis	Kawasaki disease
Severe outflow obstruction	Supraventricular tachycardia
Severe valve insufficiency	Drug toxicity (doxorubicin)
Tachyarrhythmia	β-Ketothiolase deficiency
Severe anemia (immune hydrops)	Ipecac toxicity
Bradyarrhythmia (congenital complete heart block)	Systemic lupus erythematosus
	Polyarteritis nodosa
	Hemolytic uremic syndrome
Newborn to 1 Year Old	Mitochondrial cardiomyopathy
Myocarditis	Nemaline myopathy
Endocardial fibroelastosis	Minicore-multicore myopathy
Barth syndrome	Myotubular myopathy
Carnitine deficiency	
Selenium deficiency	**Older Than 10 Years**
Anomalous left coronary artery from pulmonary artery	Familial dilated cardiomyopathy
Kawasaki disease	X-linked dilated cardiomyopathy
Critical aortic stenosis	Myocarditis
Supraventricular tachycardia	Supraventricular tachycardia
Arteriovenous malformation (especially vein of Galen)	Congenital heart disease (e.g., Ebstein's)
Calcium deficiency	Postoperative congenital heart disease
Hypoglycemia	Mitochondrial cardiomyopathy
Left ventricular noncompaction	Chagas disease
Mitochondrial cardiomyopathy	Arrhythmogenic right ventricular dysplasia
Nemaline myopathy	Eosinophilic cardiomyopathy
Minicore-multicore myopathy	Drug toxicity (doxorubicin)
Myotubular myopathy	Pheochromocytoma
	Duchenne or Becker muscular dystrophy
1 to 10 Years Old	Emery-Dreifuss muscular dystrophy
Familial dilated cardiomyopathy	Hemochromatosis
Barth syndrome	Limb-girdle muscular dystrophy
Myocarditis	Myotonic dystrophy
Arrhythmogenic right ventricular dysplasia	Peripartum cardiomyopathy
Endocardial fibroelastosis	Alcoholic cardiomyopathy
Carnitine deficiency	

Adapted from personal communication from Jeffrey A. Towbin, MD, chief of pediatric cardiology, Texas Children's Hospital, and professor of pediatrics (cardiology), Baylor College of Medicine.

Course of Illness

Patients with viral myocarditis may deteriorate rapidly, follow a chronic course, or have progressive resolution. The old adage that a third of patients get worse, a third stay the same, and a third get better is still fairly true today. Patients with DCM of familial, idiopathic, or untreatable causes may have some improvement in left ventricular function and symptoms with medical therapy, but they generally experience a progressive deterioration over many years or may deteriorate rapidly to the point that medical therapy is no longer effective.

Treatment

Treatment for DCM consists of therapy directed at the myocarditis itself and therapy for congestive heart failure and its sequelae. The treatment of the underlying myocarditis varies by the cause.

Because the cellular inflammation in myocarditis resembles that seen in cardiac transplant rejection, physicians have

hypothesized that immunosuppression might be beneficial. Despite numerous case reports on the treatment of myocarditis with immunosuppression, including steroids, there are no longitudinal data to support this form of therapy. However, based on a small study that did not reach clinical significance,[5] many pediatric centers accept the concept that intravenous immunoglobulin (IVIG) has a benefit and routinely use it (1 to 2 g/kg over 12 to 24 hours). If IVIG is going to be used and the child may require cardiac transplantation, all laboratory samples should be drawn before the IVIG is given. For noninfectious myocarditis, specifically autoimmune disease, immunosuppression may be beneficial.[6]

The second aspect of therapy is targeted at improving cardiac output, blood pressure, and organ perfusion, in addition to treating the side effects of heart failure (e.g., hypoxemia, sodium retention, pulmonary congestion). Most therapy is aimed at improving myocardial function by increasing contractility (inotropy), improving diastolic relaxation and filling of the ventricles (lusitropy), decreasing

Table 85-2 Evaluation of Newly Diagnosed Dilated Cardiomyopathy

Chest radiograph

Electrocardiogram

Echocardiogram (including relatives and tissue Doppler imaging)

Urine
  Organic acids, including 3-methylglutaconic acid
  Urinalysis
  Amino acids

Blood
  Lactic acid
  Pyruvate
  Basic metabolic panel
  Glucose
  Calcium
  Magnesium
  Selenium
  Complete blood count with differential
  Creatine kinase (total and fractionated MM and MB)
  Troponin T or I
  Liver enzymes
  Albumin
  Coagulation profile
  Carnitine
  Acylcarnitine profile
  Cholesterol
  Thyroid function studies
  Plasma for amino acids
  Erythrocyte sedimentation rate
  Viral serologies, including adenovirus

Cytogenetics

Skeletal muscle biopsy
  Histology
  Electron microscopy
  Mitochondrial respiratory chain analysis, acyl-CoA dehydrogenase analysis

Endomyocardial biopsy (with hemodynamic catheterization and angiographic evaluation of structural lesions)
  Histology
  Electron microscopy
  Polymerase chain reaction for viral genome

Mitochondrial respiratory chain analysis

Genetics consultation, including comprehensive metabolic-enzymatic evaluation

Adapted from personal communication from Jeffrey A. Towbin, MD, chief of pediatric cardiology, Texas Children's Hospital, and professor of pediatrics (cardiology), Baylor College of Medicine.

volume expansion and vasoconstriction, and minimizing the increased metabolic demand of the heart.

When initiating and adjusting the various pharmacologic regimens, it is important to closely monitor the patient. Although all these medications are intended to improve cardiac output, the myocardium does not always respond favorably. Therefore, close monitoring and reevaluation are essential.

Sympathomimetic inotropic agents (also known as adrenergic agonists), such as dobutamine and dopamine, serve to improve cardiac contractility and cardiac output. In general, these medications are administered by continuous intravenous infusion during the acute phase of illness. Of note, epinephrine is typically not used because of its potential adverse effects on the myocardium; the exception is a child in cardiovascular shock who has shown no improvement with other medications. Many patients remain on chronic oral digoxin to improve heart function.

Milrinone acts as a positive inotropic agent with vasodilatory and lusitropic effects aimed at improving cardiac output by improving systolic contractility and diastolic ventricular filling.[7] The pharmacologic effect is rapid with an initial loading infusion and occurs within 30 minutes of starting a continuous infusion without a loading dose.[7] It is important to note that milrinone has a relatively long half-life that is even longer in children with severe heart failure. Even if the myocardium does not respond favorably to this medication, the vasodilatory effects may linger, causing concern about cardiovascular instability.

Nesiritide, a brain (B-type) natriuretic peptide, has been shown to cause arterial and venous dilation, enhanced sodium excretion, and suppression of the renin-angiotensin-aldosterone and sympathic nervous systems.[8] It is effective in the treatment of heart failure in adults,[8,9] and preliminary evidence has been encouraging in pediatric patients.[10] For chronic oral therapy, angiotensin-converting enzyme (ACE) inhibitors are recommended in adults and children with heart failure.[11,12]

Despite the negative inotropic effects of β-adrenergic antagonists (beta-blockers), numerous well-controlled studies have demonstrated their effectiveness in reducing symptoms and improving survival when added to ACE inhibitors in adults.[13,14] The positive outcomes associated with this class of drugs are thought to be related to shielding of the myocardium from excessive catecholamines, suppressing arrhythmias, and reducing myocardial oxygen demand. Chronic oral therapy is beneficial in children as well as adults.[13-16] Carvedilol, a nonselective third-generation beta-blocker, has α-adrenergic antagonist activity as well, which provides some vasodilatory effect.[17] The additional benefit of decreasing afterload improves left ventricular systolic performance and diastolic filling.[18] Carvedilol improves survival in adults,[13,19] and based on the experience in adults and early results in children, many cardiology practices are using carvedilol in infants and children.[16,17,20,21]

Diuretics such as furosemide, chlorothiazide, and bumetanide are used in combination with sodium and fluid restriction to treat symptoms of pulmonary and hepatic congestion. Spironolactone, an aldosterone antagonist and weak diuretic with potassium-sparing properties, has been shown to reduce mortality and morbidity in heart failure patients.[22,23] However, when it is used with ACE inhibitors (which are also potassium-sparing diuretics), serum potassium should be monitored carefully for hyperkalemia.

For patients with progressive deterioration, mechanical assistance may be indicated, including intra-aortic balloon pump, left ventricular and biventricular assist devices, or, in younger patients, extracorporeal membrane oxygenation.

The goal of ventricular assistance therapy is to provide time for cardiac recovery or to act as a bridge for those children who are candidates for cardiac transplantation.

When left ventricular dysfunction is severe, there is risk of mural thrombus formation due to severe wall motion abnormalities and atrial dilation. Anticoagulation with heparin or warfarin (Coumadin) is indicated to prevent or treat thromboembolic complications.

Other general supportive measures include maintaining adequate oxygenation and careful attention to fluid, electrolyte, and acid-base status. In addition, adequate caloric support is particularly important, because children with congestive cardiac failure have high-energy needs and often have poor oral intake.

Consultation

Pediatric critical care specialists are routinely involved in the initial management and whenever cardiorespiratory stability is a concern. Pediatric cardiology services should be involved throughout the patient's hospitalization and after discharge.

Admission Criteria

A symptomatic patient with a new diagnosis of DCM and poor left ventricular function should be admitted to the hospital for medical therapy and observation. The severity and course of the illness can be determined and close monitoring can be provided during the initiation of pharmacotherapy. An intensive care setting may be the best initial location until the stability of the patient's condition can be established.

Discharge Criteria

Patients who remain stable in the hospital and can be switched to oral medication are ready for discharge. Newborns and infants must be able to feed and show adequate caloric intake with minimal symptoms of congestive heart failure. Older children and adolescents should be ambulatory and stable for several days on chronic medication. Any ongoing arrhythmia should be well controlled.

HYPERTROPHIC CARDIOMYOPATHY

Hypertrophic cardiomyopathy (HCM) is a heterogeneous, usually familial, disorder of cardiac muscle that affects sarcomeric proteins, resulting in myocyte and myofibrillar disorganization and fibrosis. HCM has an autosomal dominant pattern of inheritance, although morphologic evidence of disease may be absent in 20% of carriers.[24-31] Mutations in any of 10 genes that code for sarcomeric proteins may result in HCM; some mutations are relatively benign, whereas others are associated with early death.[32]

Pathophysiology

Although various parts of the ventricle can undergo myocytic hypertrophy, involvement of the anterior ventricular septum is the most common pattern, accounting for more than 80% of cases of HCM (Fig. 85-3). Characteristically, this results in a stiff left ventricle with impaired diastolic filling.[33] This may lead to left atrial enlargement and

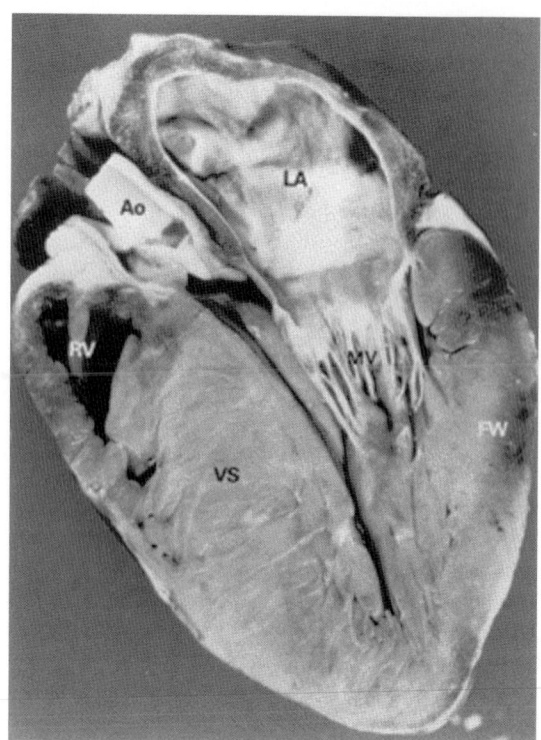

Figure 85-3 Hypertrophic cardiomyopathy. Heart sectioned in a cross-sectional plane shows that left ventricular (LV) wall thickening is asymmetrical, confined primarily to the ventricular septum (VS), which bulges prominently into LV outflow tract. The LV cavity appears small. Ao, aorta; FW, left ventricular free wall; LA, left atrium; MV, mitral valve; RV, right ventricle. (From Maron BJ: Hypertrophic cardiomyopathy. Lancet 1997;350:127-133.)

pulmonary venous engorgement, producing congestive symptoms. In addition, the cellular disarray and hypertrophy can cause electrical instability and arrhythmias.

About 25% of patients with HCM develop outflow tract obstruction when there is systolic anterior motion of the mitral valve against the hypertrophied ventricular septum. In this situation, outflow obstruction increases with high outflow velocities. Thus, lowered systemic vascular resistance or hypovolemia may increase the obstruction, whereas interventions such as intravascular volume expansion or increased systemic vascular resistance may lessen the obstruction. Young children may also demonstrate fixed right ventricular outflow tract obstruction.

Changes also occur in the coronary arteries, such as thickening of the walls with collagen in the intimal and medial areas.[34,35] Mismatch between myocardial mass and coronary circulation leads to episodes of ischemia, cell death, and replacement with scar tissue.

Clinical Presentation

Common features associated with HCM can be traced to the pathologic changes discussed earlier. Chest pain may result from impairment of myocardial perfusion. Arrhythmias can cause palpitations, syncope, or sudden death. Left-sided failure produces dyspnea and exercise intolerance. Syncope with exercise has a high correlation with disease severity. Patients may also present with the onset of a new murmur (usually a medium-pitched systolic ejection murmur). Many asymptomatic patients are found on screening after identification of a family member with HCM.

The estimated overall annual mortality is 1% when HCM is diagnosed in adults[36]; it is higher (2%) in children and adolescents.[37] Sudden death is more common in children than in adults and risk is highest if HCM is diagnosed before 1 year of age.

Differential Diagnosis

Hypertrophic phenotypes similar to but distinct from HCM are found in patients with Noonan syndrome, mitochondrial myopathies, and metabolic disorders, such as infants of diabetic mothers and Pompe disease.

Evaluation

The 12-lead ECG is abnormal in 90% to 95% of patients with HCM,[38] but the changes are not specific to this disorder. Common abnormalities include increased R-wave voltages in V_5 and V_6 and abnormal T waves and Q waves in the lateral precordial leads due to septal hypertrophy. Young children with subpulmonic obstruction may demonstrate changes of right ventricular hypertrophy. Abnormal ECG findings may be present before diagnostic echocardiographic features.

Echocardiography can reveal abnormal hypertrophic areas of the myocardium as well as define outflow tract obstruction and abnormalities of systolic and diastolic function. Up to 40% of carriers may not have diagnostic criteria until later in life. For individuals with a positive family history, screening and follow-up screening are generally not recommended for children younger than 12 years unless there is a high-risk family history or the child participates in intensive competitive sports.[39] In children aged 12 to 18, screening is recommended yearly, because this is the age group that is most likely to demonstrate abnormal findings.

Treatment

The goals of treatment include relief of symptoms, control of complications, and prevention of sudden death.

Beta-blockers reduce left ventricular contractility and heart rate and therefore myocardial wall stress, oxygen requirements, and outflow gradients, all of which may improve symptoms of chest pain and pulmonary congestion.[32] Verapamil, a calcium channel blocking agent, has been demonstrated to improve exercise capacity in adults with or without obstruction.[40] There is no evidence that the combined use of a beta-blocker and verapamil is better than either alone, and there are no data to support medical therapy of asymptomatic individuals to prevent congestive symptoms or obstruction.

Relief of left ventricular outflow obstruction is indicated in symptomatic patients with significant obstruction (gradient >50 mm Hg). The most common procedure performed is surgical myotomy-myectomy, which involves resection of the basal septum.[41] Although relief of obstruction results in symptomatic improvement in 70% of patients, it does not prolong life and therefore should not be performed in asymptomatic or mildly symptomatic individuals.[32] Attempts have been made to relieve outflow tract obstruc-

Table 85-3   Risk Factors for Sudden Death in Hypertrophic Cardiomyopathy
Definite
Family history of premature sudden death related to hypertrophic cardiomyopathy
Prior cardiac arrest or spontaneously occurring and sustained ventricular tachycardia
Identification of a high-risk genotype
Syncope or near syncope (non-neurocardiogenic), particularly recurrent and exercise related
Multiple episodes of nonsustained ventricular tachycardia (Holter monitor)
Abnormal blood pressure response with exercise
Left ventricular wall thickness >30 mm
Possible
Tunneled left anterior descending coronary artery in children (consider surgical unroofing)
Outflow gradient >50 mm Hg

tion by changing the pattern of ventricular contraction through dual-chamber pacing[42-44] and, more recently, radiofrequency ablation. Alcohol septal ablation is effective in reducing the outflow gradient in adults by causing a myocardial infarct in the septum.[45] However, the scar it produces may be proarrhythmogenic, and this procedure is not recommended in children.

Atrial fibrillation occurs in 20% to 25% of patients (usually adults) and is associated with left atrial enlargement. Treatment includes pharmacologic rate control, cardioversion, and anticoagulation to prevent complications, which include stroke and heart failure.

Sudden death is often the first symptom of HCM, and HCM is the most common cause of sudden death in children and adolescents.[32] It is thought to be due to ventricular arrhythmia. Sudden death is rare before age 10 years; it commonly occurs at rest but may occur with vigorous exercise. Therefore, any patient at high risk of sudden death (Table 85-3) should be disqualified from competitive sports. Insertion of an implantable cardioverter defibrillator is recommended.[39,46] Chronic therapy with amiodarone may be effective if two or more risk factors exist,[47] but the potential side effects (thyroid dysfunction, cataracts, pulmonary fibrosis) make this a less attractive option in children.[32]

In end-stage HCM, the cardiac muscle can become "burned out," resulting in DCM; in this case, it is managed as outlined in the previous section. Patients with outflow obstruction or valvular disease require prophylaxis against endocarditis (see Chapter 84).

Consultation

A pediatric cardiologist should be involved with the evaluation and management of children with suspected or confirmed HCM. First-degree family members of patients with HCM should be referred as well.

Admission Criteria

Hospitalization may be warranted to expedite diagnostic studies and establish cardiovascular stability, but patients can often be evaluated as outpatients.

Discharge Criteria

Discharge is appropriate when the patient has demonstrated clinical stability and outpatient follow-up has been established.

RESTRICTIVE CARDIOMYOPATHY

Restrictive cardiomyopathy is the least common form of cardiomyopathy. Patients with restrictive cardiomyopathy have abnormal diastolic function as the noncompliant ventricular myocardium impedes ventricular filling, resulting in decreased cardiac output. Systolic function is relatively unimpaired. Although restrictive disease is often idiopathic, known causes include endomyocardial fibrosis, infiltrative disorders (amyloidosis, hemochromatosis, sarcoidosis), carcinoid syndrome, systemic sclerosis, and radiation therapy to the chest.

Clinical Presentation

Early on, patients with restrictive cardiomyopathy are asymptomatic. With advanced disease, exercise intolerance is a frequent complaint caused by an inability to increase cardiac output during exercise.[47] Weakness and shortness of breath are common, and chest pain occasionally occurs.[48] In advanced cases, signs of right heart failure may be evident, with elevated central venous pressure, peripheral edema, ascites, and anasarca. On physical examination, jugular venous distention along with an S_3 or S_4 gallop may be present; occasionally, systolic murmurs of atrioventricular valve insufficiency may be heard.

Differential Diagnosis

An important entity with a remarkably similar presentation is constrictive pericarditis. This is a treatable condition that is managed with surgical removal of the pericardium.

Evaluation

A 12-lead ECG often shows evidence of left and right atrial enlargement, which occurs secondary to high diastolic pressures within the stiff ventricles. An echocardiogram characteristically demonstrates enlarged left and right atria with normal ventricular systolic function and decreased diastolic function due to ventricular wall noncompliance.

Catheterization defines the hemodynamics and helps differentiate restrictive from constrictive disease. Characteristic hemodynamic findings at cardiac catheterization include a deep and rapid early decline in ventricular pressure at the onset of diastole, with a rise to a plateau phase (the square root sign) similar to that seen in constrictive pericarditis.[49] Both left and right atrial pressures are elevated, although the left atrial pressure is generally higher than the right; in contrast, in constrictive pericarditis, the right and left atrial pressures are usually identical.[48]

Endomyocardial biopsy is useful in evaluating patients with restrictive cardiomyopathy due to amyloidosis and other specific causes (e.g., metabolic storage disease, hemochromatosis, sarcoidosis).[50] Findings of fibrosis in the absence of other specific causes suggests the diagnosis of restrictive disease; however, a normal biopsy does not exclude it.

Treatment

Once restrictive cardiomyopathy becomes symptomatic, it is usually progressive. Occasionally, the disease process can be slowed with treatment, especially if the underlying cause can be determined and is amenable to therapy. For example, for patients with hemochromatosis, therapy aimed at iron binding may be beneficial to slow ongoing iron deposition and resultant damage to the myocardium.

Symptomatic treatment generally involves the use of diuretics to treat high atrial pressures and the congestive symptoms they cause. The diastolic relaxing effects of carvedilol may offer some therapeutic benefit. Eventually, cardiac transplantation may be required.

IN A NUTSHELL

- There are three main forms of cardiomyopathy: dilated, hypertrophic, and restrictive.
- DCM is commonly a postviral process, but it can also be caused by other infectious agents as well as by toxins, drugs, autoimmune disorders, or Kawasaki disease.
- Echocardiography is critical in the diagnosis and monitoring of all forms of cardiomyopathy.
- The management of all forms of cardiomyopathy is directed at assisting cardiac function and preventing complications. Although some cardiomyopathies are amenable to pharmacologic treatment, some patients inevitably require cardiac transplantation.

ON THE HORIZON

- With research in the pharmacologic management of DCM, new beta-blocking drugs will enter the field of pediatric cardiology.
- Immnunosuppression for myocarditis is an area of active study, including the use of steroids, IVIG, cyclosporine, azathioprine, and OKT3.
- Immunoadsorption therapy to remove autoimmune antibodies and cytokines may prove beneficial in postponing or avoiding heart transplantation for patients with nonmyocarditis DCM.

SUGGESTED READING

Maron BJ: Hypertrophic cardiomyopathy. In Allen HD, Gutgesell HP, Clark EB, Driscoll DJ (eds): Moss and Adams' Heart Disease in Infants, Children and Adolescents, 6th ed. Philadelphia, Lippincott Williams & Wilkins, 2001, pp 1167-1186.

Oakley CM: Clinical recognition of the cardiomyopathies. Circ Res 1974; 34/35(Suppl 11).

REFERENCES

1. Aretz HT, Billingham ME, Edwards WD, et al: Myocarditis: A histopathologic definition and classification. Am J Cardiol 1978;41:887-892.
2. Grogan M, Redfield MM, Bailey KR, et al: Long-term outcome of patients with biopsy-proven myocarditis: Comparison with idiopathic dilated cardiomyopathy. J Am Coll Cardiol 1995;26:80-84.

3. Chow LH, Radio SJ, Sears TD, et al: Insensitivity of right ventricular biopsy in the diagnosis of myocarditis. J Am Coll Cardiol 1989;14:915-920.

4. Martin AB, Webber S, Fricker FJ, et al: Acute myocarditis: Rapid diagnosis by PCR in children. Circulation 1994;90:330-333.

5. Druker NA, Colan SD, Lewis AB, et al: Gamma-globulin treatment of acute myocarditis in the pediatric population. Circulation 1994;5:65-69.

6. Noutsias M, Pauschinger M, Poller WC, et al: Immunomodulatory treatment strategies in inflammatory cardiomyopathy: Current status and future perspectives. Expert Rev Cardiovasc Ther 2004;2:37-51.

7. Baruch L, Patacsil P, Hameed A, et al: Pharmacodynamic effects of milrinone with and without a bolus loading infusion. Am Heart J 2001;191:266-273.

8. Colucci W, Elkayam U, Horton D, et al: Intravenous nesiritide, a natriuretic peptide, in the treatment of decompensated congestive heart failure. N Engl J Med 2000;343:246-253.

9. Silver MA, Horton D, Ghali J, Elkayam U: Effect of nesiritide versus dobutamine on short-term outcomes in the treatment of patients with acutely decompensated heart failure. J Am Coll Cardiol 2002;39:798-803.

10. Marshall J, Berkenbosch J, Russo P, Tobias J: Preliminary experience with nesiritide in the pediatric population. J Intensive Care Med 2004;19:164-170.

11. Hunt SA, Baker DW, Chin MH, et al: ACC/AHA guidelines for the evaluation and management of chronic heart failure in the adult: Executive summary. A report of the American College of Cardiology/American Heart Association Task Force on Practice Guidelines (Committee to Revise the 1995 Guidelines for the Evaluation and Management of Heart Failure). Circulation 2001;104:2996-3007.

12. Lewis AB, Chabot M: The effect of treatment with angiotensin-converting enzyme inhibitors on survival of pediatric patients with dilated cardiomyopathy. Pediatr Cardiol 1993;14:9-12.

13. Yancy CW: Clinical trials of ß-blockers in heart failure: A class review. Am J Med 2001;110:7S-10S.

14. Packer M: Beta-blockade in heart failure: Basic concepts and clinical results. Am J Hypertens 1992;11:23S-37S.

15. Shaddy R, Tani L, Gidding S, et al: Beta-blocker treatment of dilated cardiomyopathy with congestive heart failure in children: A multi-institutional experience. J Heart Lung Transplant 1999;18:269-274.

16. Williams R, Tani L, Shaddy R: Intermediate effects of treatment with metoprolol or carvedilol in children with left ventricular systolic dysfunction. J Heart Lung Transplant 2002;21:906-909.

17. Azeka E, Ramires JA, Valler C, Bocchi E: Delisting of infants and children from the heart transplantation waiting list after carvedilol treatment. J Am Coll Cardiol 2002;40:2034-2038.

18. Palazzuoli A, Carrera A, Calabria P, et al: Effects of carvedilol therapy on restrictive diastolic filling pattern in chronic heart failure. Am Heart J 2004;147:E2.

19. Packer M: COPERNICUS (Carvedilol Prospective Randomized Cumulative Survival Trial). Data presented at 22nd Congress of the European Society of Cardiology, Amsterdam, Aug 2000.

20. Giardini A, Formigar R, Bronzetti G, et al: Modulation of neurohormonal activity after treatment of children in heart failure with carvedilol. Cardiol Young 2003;13:333-336.

21. Bruns L, Chrisant MK, Lamour J, et al: Carvedilol as therapy in pediatric heart failure: An initial multicenter experience. J Pediatr 2001;138:505-511.

22. Rousseau M, Gurne O, Duprez D, et al: Beneficial neurohormonal profile of spironolactone in severe congestive heart failure. J Am Coll Cardiol 2002;40:1596-1601.

23. Pitt B, Zannad F, Remme J, et al: The effect of spironolactone on morbidity and mortality in patients with severe heart failure. N Engl J Med 1999;341:709-717.

24. Thierfelder L, Watkins H, MacRae C, et al: α-Tropomyosin and cardiac troponin T mutations cause familial hypertrophic cardiomyopathy: A disease of the sarcomere. Cell 1994;77:701-702.

25. Charron P, Dubourg O, Desnos M, et al: Clinical features and prognostic implications of familial hypertrophic cardiomyopathy related to the cardiac myosin-binding protein C gene. Circulation 1998;97:2230-2236.

26. Coviello DA, Maron BJ, Spirito P, et al: Clinical features of hypertrophic cardiomyopathy caused by "hot spot" in the alpha tropomyosin gene. J Am Coll Cardiol 1997;29:635-640.

27. Niimura H, Bachinski LL, Sangwatanaroj S, et al: Mutations in the gene for human cardiac myosin-binding protein C and late-onset familial hypertrophic cardiomyopathy. N Engl J Med 1998;338:1248-1257.

28. Watkins H, McKenna WJ, Thierfelder L, et al: Mutations in the genes for cardiac troponin T and α-tropomyosin in hypertrophic cardiomyopathy. N Engl J Med 1995;332:1058-1064.

29. Moolman JC, Corfield VA, Posen B, et al: Sudden death due to troponin T mutations. J Am Coll Cardiol 1997;29:549-555.

30. Morgensen J, Klausen IV, Pedersen AK, et al: α-Cardiac actin is a novel disease gene in familial hypertrophic cardiomyopathy. J Clin Invest 1999;103:R39-R43.

31. Charron P, Dubourg O, Desnos M, et al: Diagnostic value of electrocardiography and echocardiography for familial hypertrophic cardiomyopathy in a genotyped adult population. Circulation 1997;96:214-219.

32. Maron BJ: Hypertrophic cardiomyopathy. In Allen HD, Gutgesell HP, Clark EB, Driscoll DJ (eds): Moss and Adams' Heart Disease in Infants, Children and Adolescents, 6th ed. Philadelphia, Lippincott Williams & Wilkins, 2001, pp 1167-1186.

33. Nihoyannopoulos P, Karatasakis G, Frenneaux M, et al: Diastolic function in hypertrophic cardiomyopathy: Relation to exercise capacity. J Am Coll Cardiol 1992;19:536-540.

34. Maron BJ, Wolfson JK, Epstein SE, et al: Intramural ("small vessel") coronary artery disease in hypertrophic cardiomyopathy. J Am Coll Cardiol 1986;8:545-557.

35. Tanaka M, Fujiwara H, Onodera T, et al: Quantitative analysis of narrowings of intramyocardial small arteries in normal hearts, hypertensive hearts, and hearts with hypertrophic cardiomyopathy. Circulation 1987;75:1130-1139.

36. Maron BJ, Spirito P: Impact of patient selection biases on the perception of hypertrophic cardiomyopathy and its natural history. Am J Cardiol 1993;72:970-972.

37. Maron BJ, Casey SA, Poliac LC, et al: Clinical course of hypertrophic cardiomyopathy in a regional United States cohort. JAMA 1999;281:650-655.

38. Lemery R, Kleinebenne A, Nihoyannopoulos P, et al: Q waves in hypertrophic cardiomyopathy in relation to the distribution and severity of right and left ventricular hypertrophy. J Am Coll Cardiol 1990;16:368-374.

39. Maron BJ, McKenna WJ: American College of Cardiology/European Society of Cardiology clinical expert consensus document on hypertrophic cardiomyopathy. J Am Coll Cardiol 2003;42:1-27.

40. Rosing DR, Condit JR, Maron BJ, et al: Verapamil therapy: A new approach to the pharmacologic treatment of hypertrophic cardiomyopathy. III. Effects of long-term administration. Am J Cardiol 1981;48:545-553.

41. Morrow AG, Reitz BA, Epstein SE, et al: Operative treatment in hypertrophic subaortic stenosis: Techniques and the results of pre- and postoperative assessments in 83 patients. Circulation 1975;52:88-102.

42. Nishimura RA, Trusty JM, Hayes DL, et al: Dual-chamber pacing for hypertrophic cardiomyopathy: A randomized, double-blind cross-over study. J Am Coll Cardiol 1997;29:435-441.

43. Maron BJ, Nishimura RA, McKenna WJ, et al: Assessment of permanent dual-chamber pacing as a treatment for drug-refractory symptomatic patients with obstructive hypertrophic cardiomyopathy: A double-blind cross-over study (M-PATHY). Circulation 1999;99:2927-2933.

44. Linde C, Gadler F, Kappenberger L, et al: Placebo effect of pacemaker implantation in obstructive hypertrophic cardiomyopathy. Am J Cardiol 1999;83:903-907.

45. Seggewiss H, Gleichmann U, Faber L, et al: Percutaneous transluminal septal myocardial ablation in hypertrophic obstructive cardiomyopathy: Acute results and 3-month follow-up in 25 patients. J Am Coll Cardiol 1998;31:252-258.

46. Maron BJ, Shen WK, Link MS, et al: Efficacy of the implantable cardioverter-defibrillator for the prevention of sudden death in hypertrophic cardiomyopathy. N Engl J Med 2000;342:365-373.

47. Oakley CM: Clinical recognition of the cardiomyopathies. Circ Res 1974;34/35(Suppl 11).

48. Meaney E, Habetai R, Bhargana V, et al: Cardiac amyloidosis, constrictive pericarditis and restrictive cardiomyopathy. Am J Cardiol 1978; 38:547.

49. Hansen AT, Eskildsen P, Gotzsche H: Pressure curves from the right auricle and right ventricle in chronic constrictive pericarditis. Circulation 1951;3:881.

50. Schoenfield MH, Supple EW, Dec GW Jr, et al: Restrictive cardiomyopathy versus constrictive pericarditis: Role of endomyocardial biopsy in avoiding unnecessary thoracotomy. Circulation 1987;75:1012-1017.

CHAPTER 86

Pericarditis
Timothy Cornell

Pericarditis is the inflammation of the pericardium, the two-layered sac that covers the heart and portions of the great vessels. The inflammatory process can be acute, subacute, or chronic and has a variety of etiologies (Table 86-1). The pediatric hospital physician must be familiar with the clinical presentation, differential diagnosis, evaluation, and management of pericarditis because prompt recognition and treatment may be lifesaving.

CLINICAL PRESENTATION

Acute pericarditis can present anywhere along a spectrum from fever and malaise to severe hemodynamic compromise and shock, but there are common features in most cases. For example, most patients with acute pericarditis have fever, tachypnea, and tachycardia. Chest pain has been reported in 15% to 80% of cases and is less common in younger children.[1] When chest pain is present it usually is pleuritic, worsens with inspiration, and improves when the child sits up and leans forward. Abdominal pain can occur in association with chest pain, but has also been reported as an isolated complaint in acute pericarditis.[2]

A pericardial friction rub heard during auscultation is pathognomonic for acute pericarditis. A rub is a high-pitched scratching sound that has been likened to the sound of crinkling paper. It is usually heard best with the diaphragm of the stethoscope pressed firmly against the chest wall along the second to fourth intercostal spaces between the left lower sternal border and the apex, but it may be heard throughout the chest. Although it is important to listen for a friction rub, a rub may not be present in all cases of pericarditis[3] and may disappear as the pericardial effusion becomes larger.

The clinical presentation may be helpful in determining the cause of the pericarditis. Children with viral pericarditis usually present with a history of upper respiratory or gastrointestinal illness 10 days to 2 weeks prior to the onset of symptoms of pericarditis. They commonly have fever and chest pain but appear less toxic than children with purulent pericarditis. Patients with viral pericarditis rarely develop large effusions or cardiac tamponade. The clinical course of viral pericarditis is usually benign and the symptoms resolve over 3 to 4 weeks.

In contrast to viral pericarditis, purulent pericarditis has a quicker onset and affected children appear more toxic than children with viral pericarditis. Over half of the cases of purulent pericarditis occur in children less than 2 years of age. Most cases of purulent pericarditis result from either direct or hematogenous spread of an ongoing infection. The most common site for the source of the infection is the lung,

followed by bone and joint, central nervous system, and skin.[1,4] It is important to suspect purulent pericarditis in any patient being treated for an infection or sepsis who develops an enlarged cardiac silhouette. Patients who are immunocompromised are also at risk for developing purulent pericarditis with opportunistic organisms.

The two serious complications of acute pericarditis are constrictive pericarditis and pericardial effusion. Constrictive pericarditis is a rare complication of acute pericarditis and is most commonly seen following tuberculous pericarditis. It is characterized by a thickened pericardium.[5] This thick pericardium is noncompliant and inhibits ventricular filling. The limited diastolic filling leads to symptoms of fatigue, weakness, and dyspnea as a result of low cardiac output. On physical examination, a precordial knock is pathognomonic of pericardial constriction. Jugular venous distention, hepatomegaly, and diminished heart sounds without cardiomegly in a patient with a history of pericarditis should raise the suspicion of constrictive pericarditis.

The more common complication of acute pericarditis is pericardial tamponade. The inflammatory process in acute pericarditis frequently causes a pericardial effusion. As the pericardial effusion enlarges, the compliance of the pericardium allows for its expansion, and diastolic filling continues to occur normally. However, as the pericardial space fills with fluid and the pericardium reaches its elastic limit, diastolic filling of the ventricles is inhibited. As right ventricular pressures increase, the intraventricular septum is displaced into the left ventricle, and right ventricular filling is maintained at the expense of left ventricular filling (ventricular interdependence), with a resulting fall in cardiac output (Fig. 86-1). If pericardial effusion develops over a long period of time, the pericardium is able to expand without compromising diastole, but rapid expansion of a pericardial effusion can quickly lead to pericardial tamponade.

One of the early signs of tamponade is pulsus paradoxus, which is an exaggeration of the variation of blood pressure during the respiratory cycle (Fig. 86-2). During inspiration there is an increase in venous return to the right atrium. At the same time a greater increase in the capacity of the pulmonary vascular bed occurs. The increase in the capacity of the pulmonary bed causes a decrease in the left-sided filling volume and thus decreases cardiac output (Fig. 86-3). This phenomenon is clinically seen as a difference in systolic blood pressure between inspiration and expiration. Pulsus paradoxus is present when there is a difference of more than 10 mm Hg between the systolic blood pressure of inspiration and that of expiration. Pulsus paradoxus may

Table 86-1 Common Causes of Acute Pericarditis
Idiopathic (85%–90%)*
Infectious (6%)*
Bacterial *(Staphylococcus aureus, Streptococcus, Neisseria,*
Mcyobacterium tuberculosis)
Viral (coxsackievirus, echovirus, adenovirus)
Fungal *(Candida, Aspergillus)*
Protozoal
Connective Tissue/Autoimmune Disorders (3%–5%)*
JRA
SLE
Rheumatic fever
Medications (<1%)*
Renal failure
Postpericardiotomy syndrome
Hypothyroidism
Malignancy
Trauma

*Percentages of estimated incidence of each category.[6]

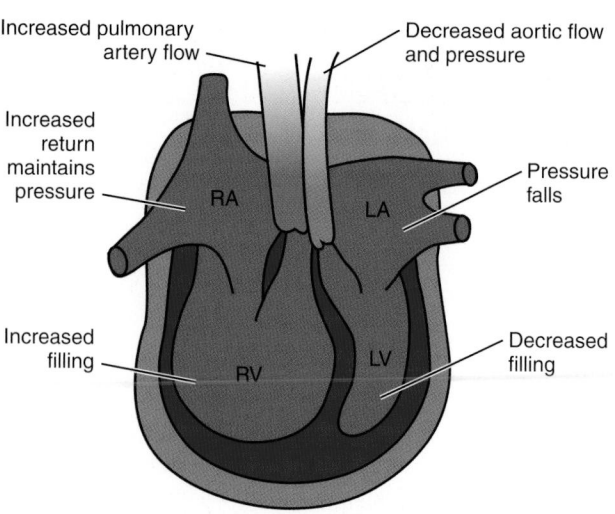

Figure 86-1 Physiology of pericardial tamponade. The presence of pericardial fluid limits outward expansion of the right ventricle. Therefore, the intraventriclular septum is displaced into the left ventricle, resulting in decreased cardiac output. There is an early increase in venous return to maintain pressure, which eventually worsens the shift of the intraventricular septum. (Adapted from Rheuban KS: Pericardial diseases. In Allen HD, Clark EB, Gutgesell HP, Driscoll DJ (eds): Moss and Adams' Heart Disease in Infants, Children and Adolescents, Including the Fetus and Young Adult, 6th ed. Philadelphia: Lippincott Williams & Wilkins. 2001, p 1288.)

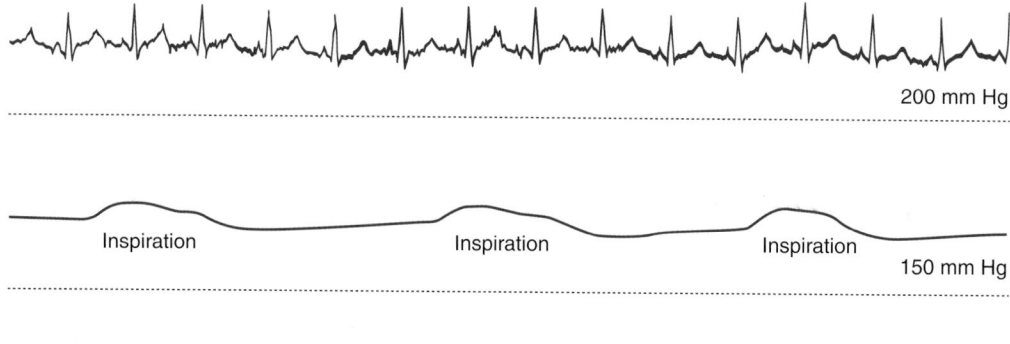

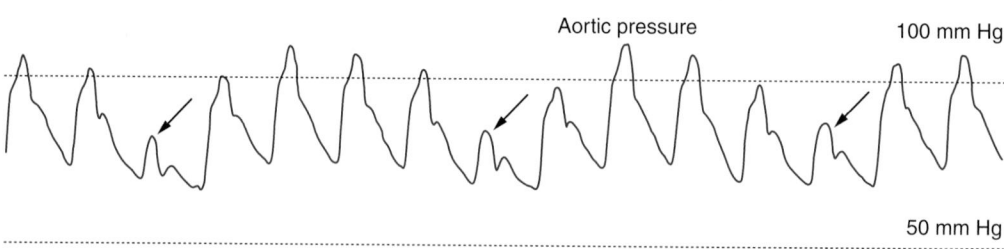

Figure 86-2 Hemodynamic changes with inspiration resulting in pulsus paradoxus. (Adapted from Wu LA, Nishimura RA: Pulsus paradoxus. N Engl J Med 2003;349:666.)

be present in diseases other then pericardial tamponade (Table 86-2).

During evaluation for pulsus paradoxus the patient should be sitting in a comfortable position and a manual blood pressure cuff should be placed on the patient's arm. The cuff should be inflated until the radial pulse is no longer palpable. The cuff pressure should be released until the first Korotkoff sound is heard over the brachial artery only during expiration. Once this systolic pressure is noted, the cuff pressure should be slowly lowered until the first Korotkoff sound

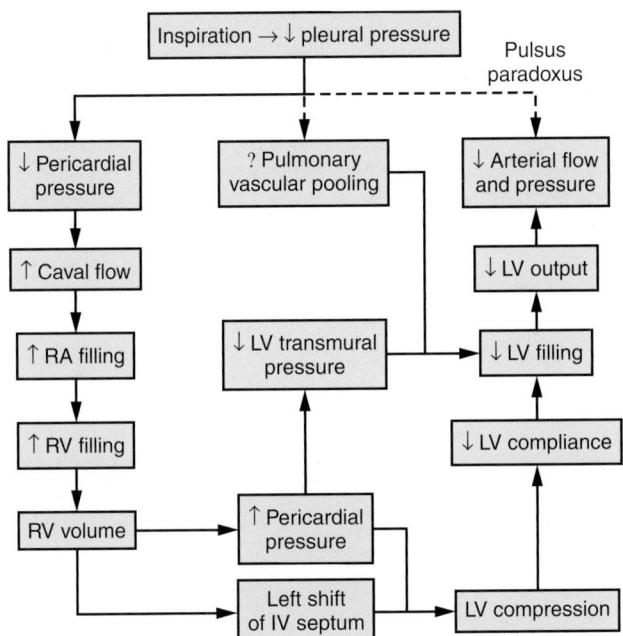

Figure 86-3 Physiology of pulsus paradoxus. IV, intraventricular. (Reprinted from Swami A, Spodick DH: Pulsus paradoxus in cardiac tamponade: A pathophysiologic continuum. Clin Cardiol 2003;26: 215-217.)

Table 86-2	Causes of Pulsus Paradoxus
Pericardial tamponade	
Pulmonary embolism	
Asthma	
Chronic obstructive lung disease	
Restrictive cardiomyopathy	
Tense ascites	
Right ventricular infarct	

is heard throughout the respiratory cycle. If the difference between these two points is greater than 10 mm Hg, pulsus paradoxus is present.

DIFFERENTIAL DIAGNOSIS

Viral pericarditis accounts for the majority of acute pericarditis and is rarely life threatening. Pericarditis can result from the direct infection of the pericardium by the virus, most commonly adenovirus or coxsackievirus. A secondary immune-mediated inflammation of the pericardium has also been observed following viral infections and may account for many cases of idiopathic pericarditis.

Purulent pericarditis, also called bacterial pericarditis, has a high mortality rate if not recognized early. Purulent pericarditis can be an isolated occurrence but usually results from either direct or hematogenous spread from other primary sites of infection. The lung is the most common

Table 86-3	Medications Reported to Cause Pericarditis
Hydralazine	
Procainamide	
Daunorubicin	
Isoniazid	
Anticoagulants	
Cyclosporine	
Methysergide	
Phenytoin	
Dantrolene	
Mesalazine	

primary site of infection, but pericarditis has also been associated with osteomyelitis and meningitis. *Staphylococcus aureus* is the most common organism recovered from purulent pericarditis.

Tuberculous pericarditis is a special type of purulent pericarditis and is seen mainly in developing countries. It develops from contiguous spread from the lungs or thoracic lymph nodes. The course may be insidious and other symptoms of tuberculosis may be more prominent. However, tuberculous pericarditis may develop rapidly and become life threatening. There is also a high association with the development of constrictive pericarditis. The early identification and treatment of tuberculous pericarditis reduce the risk of development of constrictive pericarditis. This identification may require pericardial biopsy.

Pericarditis can also be a manifestation of connective tissue disorders. Clinically apparent pericarditis is seen in up to 25% of children with juvenile rheumatoid arthritis and systemic lupus erythematosus. Up to 50% of patients with connective tissue disorders may have a clinically silent pericardial effusion during a flare. Several medications have been implicated as causing pericarditis as part of a lupus-like syndrome (Table 86-3). Most cases of pericarditis caused by connective tissue disorders resolve with treatment of the underlying illness and never progress to life-threatening complications.

Uremic pericarditis is seen in about 10% of patients with end-stage renal disease. Pericardiocentesis may be necessary to distinguish uremic pericarditis from bacterial pericarditis. Uremic pericarditis usually resolves with dialysis and rarely causes complications.

Postpericardiotomy syndrome is a situation in which pericarditis develops 1 to 3 weeks following cardiac surgery. It occurs in up to 30% of cases of open-heart surgery where the pericardium has been opened, but it is rare in children younger than 2 years of age. In children, postpericardiotomy syndrome presents as fever, irritability, and a friction rub and responds well to symptomatic treatment.

Pericarditis is occasionally associated with malignancy, hypothyroidism, and trauma but is rarely an isolated finding in these illnesses.

EVALUATION

Echocardiograhy is the standard test for detecting evidence of pericarditis. Echocardiograms are quick and noninvasive and can identify the presence, size, and location of a pericardial effusion (Fig. 86-4), but they require technical expertise to obtain and interpret the images. A chest radiograph and an electrocardiogram are helpful in determining the need for an echocardiogram. The chest radiograph in a child with acute pericarditis may show an enlarged cardiac silhouette if the pericardial effusion is moderate to large (more than 250 mL), but the presence of a normal chest radiograph does not rule out pericarditis (Fig. 86-5).[6] The electrocardiogram in pericarditis may also be normal but commonly has ST-segment, PR-segment or T-wave abnormalities. The electrocardiogram changes seen in pericarditis are described in four stages. Stage I consists of ST-segment elevation and PR-segment depression. In stage II the ST-segment returns to baseline and PR-segment depression resolves. Stage III is characterized by T-wave inversion, and stage IV appears like a normal electrocardiogram (Fig. 86-6). Classically, the changes on the electrocardiogram

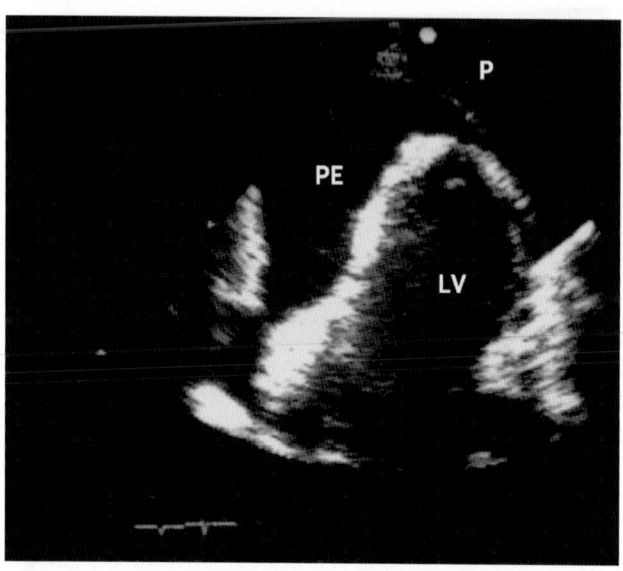

Figure 86-4 Echocardiogram showing pericardial effusion.
LV, left ventricle; P, pericardium; PE, pericardial effusion. (Adapted from Spodick DH:. Acute cardiac tamponade. N Engl J Med 2003;349: 684-690.)

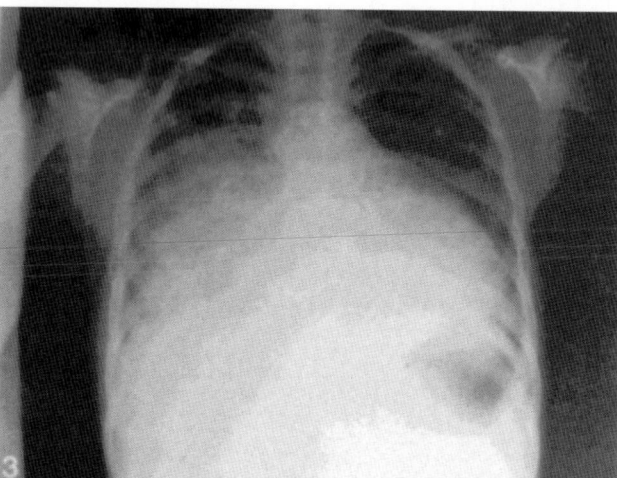

Figure 86-5 Chest radiograph showing severe cardiomegaly due to pericardial effusion. (Adapted from Roodpeyma S, Sadeghian N: Acute pericarditis in childhood: A 10-year experience. Pediatr Cardiol 2000; 21:363-367.)

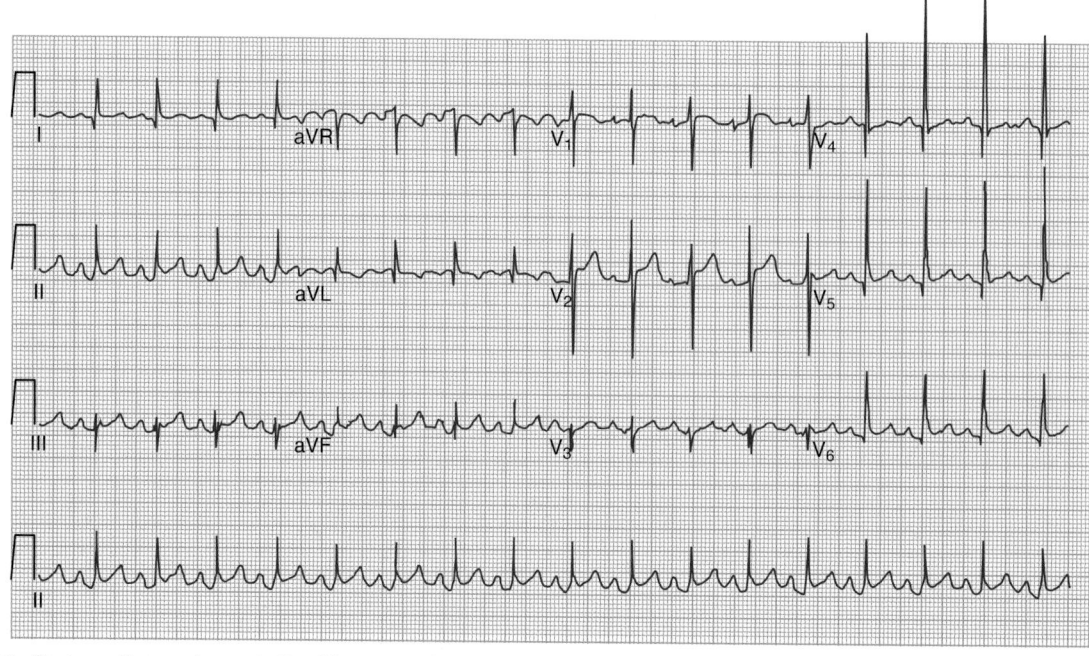

Figure 86-6 Electrocardiogram demonstrating ST-segment elevation and PR-segment depression seen in pericarditis. (Adapted from Lange RA, Hills LD: Acute pericarditis. N Engl J Med 2004;351:2195-2202.)

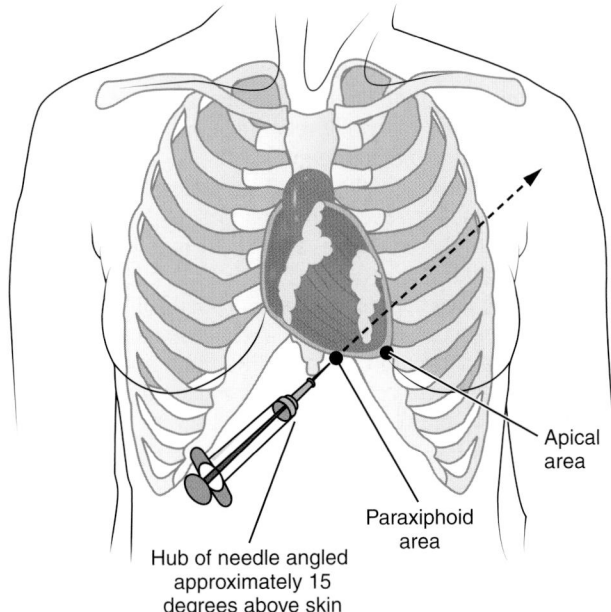

Figure 86-7   Sites of needle insertion for pericardiocentesis. (Adapted from Spodick DH: Acute cardiac tamponade. N Engl J Med 2003; 349:684-690.)

Apical area

Paraxiphoid area

Hub of needle angled approximately 15 degrees above skin

Table 86-4   Complications of Pericardiocentesis

Arrhythmias
Laceration of the coronary arteries or veins
Pneumothorax
Myocardial puncture
Hemopericardium
Liver laceration
Aortic injury
Laceration of the internal mammary artery

Table 86-5   Studies to Perform on Pericardial Fluid

Cell count with differential count
Gram stain
Aerobic and anaerobic cultures
Cultures for *Mycobacterium tuberculosis*, fungi, and viruses
Acid-fast bacilli stain
Viral polymerase chain reaction
Triglyceride level
Protein level
Lactate dehydrogenase

progress from stage I to stage IV depending on the length of time the pericarditis has been present, but the progression of electrocardiographic changes in children with pericarditis is highly variable.

If the cause of the pericarditis cannot be definitively determined by the clinical presentation, pericardiocentesis may need to be performed to obtain pericardial fluid for appropriate diagnostic studies. Pericardiocentesis is also useful for quickly removing pericardial fluid in a patient with tamponade and allowing for improved diastolic filling of the ventricles. Pericardiocentesis involves inserting a needle in the subxiphoid area and advancing it into the pericardial space (Fig. 86-7). Because of the complications associated with pericardiocentesis (Table 86-4) it should be performed by an experienced physician, in a controlled situation, preferably using imaging guidance. The pericardial fluid should be sent for the studies listed in Table 86-5.

MANAGEMENT

The hemodynamic stability of a patient with pericarditis should be addressed prior to seeking a cause for the pericarditis. If a patient with pericarditis presents with tamponade, volume replacement is of utmost importance until pericardiocentesis can be performed. Augmentation of the heart rate with isoproterenol (0.05 to 0.1 µg/kg/min) may also be needed to provide adequate cardiac output. Once the pericardial fluid is removed and the patient is hemodynamically stable, subsequent therapy should address the cause of the pericarditis.

Purulent pericarditis, unlike viral pericarditis, necessitates immediate and extensive treatment. All children with purulent pericarditis require surgical drainage and antibiotics. Empirical antibiotics should consist of a penicillinase-resistant penicillin (nafcillin or oxacillin, 200 mg/kg/day

divided into three doses) or vancomycin (40 to 60 mg/kg/day divided into four doses) plus cefotaxime (200 to 300 mg/kg/day divided into three doses) or ceftriaxone (100 mg/kg/day given in one or two doses). Once an organism is identified, the most specific antibiotic agent should be administered intravenously for a total of 3 to 4 weeks.

Patients with tuberculous pericarditis require multidrug treatment with isoniazid, pyrazinamide, rifampin, and streptomycin for 9 to 18 months. Steroids remain controversial in the treatment of tuberculous pericarditis,[7] but the limited studies suggest there may be benefit by reducing the inflammatory response and enhancing the resolution of the effusion.

Extensive work-up or treatment may not be needed for the previously healthy child who appears nontoxic with a viral syndrome, typical chest pain, and a pericardial friction rub. Close observation is warranted for the first few days, and treatment is aimed at symptomatic relief. The symptoms and effusions resolve in 1 to 3 weeks with bed rest and nonsteroidal anti-inflammatory agents (NSAIDs).

The treatment of pericarditis from causes other than infection has two steps. First, it is necessary to identify and treat the underlying illness that is the cause of the pericarditis. Second, symptomatic treatment with NSAIDs should be started. If a prolonged course of NSAIDs over 2 to 3 weeks is unsuccessful, steroids should be considered as the next step in treatment.

CONSULTATION

Consultation with a pediatric cardiologist is required for all children with pericarditis. Cardiologists are needed not only for appropriate interpretation of the echocardiography studies but also to assist in initial and long-term treatment of the children. Their expertise will also be needed if image-guided pericardiocentesis is necessary.

Guidance from infectious diseases specialists may be appropriate, especially if purulent or tuberculous pericarditis is a consideration.

ADMISSION CRITERIA

Children with newly diagnosed pericarditis should be admitted to the hospital because of the potential for hemodynamic instability.

DISCHARGE CRITERIA

Patients are safe for discharge when symptoms have resolved or when they demonstrate hemodynamic stability and resolving symptoms. If a pericardial effusion is present, it should be resolving with treatment. Once discharged, close follow-up with a pediatric cardiologist is warranted.

IN A NUTSHELL

- Pericarditis is a rare disease that results from a variety of causes that lead to inflammation of the pericardium.
- Most cases of pericarditis in children are viral in origin and benign in clinical course and resolve with symptomatic treatment.
- The recognition of pericardial tamponade is important in reducing the mortality of pericarditis. The clinical presentation, including the hemodynamic stability, appearance, presence or absence of pulsus paradoxus, as well as the appropriate tests (chest radiograph, electrocardiogram, echocardiogram), helps the hospital physician determine the rapidity with which treatment must be initiated.

ON THE HORIZON

- Although recurrence is more common in the adult population, prevention of recurrent pericarditis is an active area of study, especially regarding the use of corticosteroids and pericardiotomy.
- Empirical antibiotic therapy of suspected purulent pericarditis should reflect the changes in the spectrum of causative organisms and their rapidly changing susceptibilities.
- With the increasing prevalence of methicillin-resistant *Staphylococcus aureus*, the most common bacterial cause of pericarditis, the initial antibiotic choices should take into consideration the bacterial resistance patterns in the community.

SUGGESTED READING

Lange RA, Hillis LD: Clinical practice. Acute pericarditis. N Engl J Med 2004;351:2195-2202.

Roodpeyma S, Sadeghian N: Acute pericarditis in childhood: A 10-year experience. Pediatr Cardiol 2000;21:363-367.

Spodick D: Acute pericarditis: Current concepts and practice. JAMA 2003;289:1150-1153.

REFERENCES

1. Kaplan SL, Friedman RA: Infectious Pericarditis. In Feigin RD, et al (eds): Textbook of Pediatric Infectious Diseases. Philadelphia, Saunders, 2004, pp 380-390.
2. Donnelly LF, Kimball TR, Barr LL: Purulent pericarditis presenting as acute abdomen in children: Abdominal imaging findings. Clin Radiol 1999;54: 691-693.
3. Roodpeyma S, Sadeghian N: Acute pericarditis in childhood: A 10-year experience. Pediatr Cardiol 2000;21:363-367.
4. Levy PY, et al: Etiologic diagnosis of 204 pericardial effusions. Medicine 2003;82:385-391.
5. Myers RD, Spodick DH: Constrictive pericarditis: Clinical and pathophysiologic characteristics. Am Heart J 1999;138(2 Pt 1):219-232.
6. Lange RA, Hillis LD: Clinical practice. Acute pericarditis. N Engl J Med 2004;351:2195-2202.
7. Mayosi BM, Burgess LJ, Doubell AF: Tuberculous pericarditis. Circulation 2005;112:3608-3616.

CHAPTER 87

Acute Rheumatic Fever

David R. Fulton

Acute rheumatic fever (ARF) is an inflammatory condition manifested by the nonsuppurative sequelae of a preceding group A β-hemolytic streptococcal (GAS) pharyngitis. ARF involves the heart, central nervous system, joints, and skin and is the most common cause of acquired heart disease in many regions of the world. Historically, the relationship between streptococci and rheumatic fever was not evident; however, investigation over the past several decades has shown that only GAS infections are associated with ARF. Diagnosis of the disease relies on the identification of major and minor criteria that include both clinical observations and laboratory data, an approach that has been modified occasionally since its introduction in 1944 by Jones.[1] The greatest impact of the illness lies in its potential to cause progressive valvular heart disease, which is more likely with recurrent episodes of ARF. Antibiotic prophylaxis is therefore important to minimize the likelihood of recurrent GAS pharyngitis.

EPIDEMIOLOGY AND PATHOGENESIS

It is well accepted that the frequency of ARF has declined in part because of the use of antibiotics to treat pharyngitis. Investigations have shown that appropriate antimicrobial therapy has led to fewer episodes of ARF in the United States,[2-4] although the prevalence remains high in many parts of the world, especially in crowded populations of lower socioeconomic status.[5,6] Nevertheless, sporadic outbreaks have been identified in the United States among populations not thought to be at risk for such events.[7-11]

Only GAS pharyngitis is rheumatogenic,[12] and certain types of group A streptococci predispose to the development of ARF, based on the virulence of the organism. Group A streptococci with high concentrations of M protein, a component of the cell wall, are believed to be the most virulent strains and therefore the most likely to cause ARF. These types of streptococci often form mucoid-appearing colonies in culture. The number of M serotype GAS infections decreased in association with a similar decline in the incidence of ARF.[13]

The actual pathogenetic mechanism by which GAS pharyngitis leads to ARF is still somewhat speculative. The organism adheres to the pharyngeal mucosa, with subsequent destruction of epithelial cells. The immune reaction to this interaction results in both a humoral and a cell-mediated response to streptococcal antigens of the cell membrane. These antigens mimic those of cardiac tissue, whereas M proteins have similar antigenicity to myosin and sarcolemma,[14,15] as well as cartilage and synovium.[16] The cross-reactivity may result in damage to these target tissues. In addition, the GAS carbohydrate components mimic antigens of cardiac valves, a possible explanation for valvular involvement in ARF.[17] Cell-mediated involvement in the pathogenesis is supported by the presence of CD4+ helper cells in heart valves.[18] It is possible that the M protein and streptococcal pyrogenic exotoxins may act as superantigens in the immune response.[19]

PATHOLOGY

The initial pathologic lesion in ARF is edema of the ground substance in connective tissue, with accompanying cellular infiltration of T and B lymphocytes. Degenerative deposition of eosinophils in these regions is described as fibrinoid necrosis. Although these pathologic findings are present early in the process, with the administration of anti-inflammatory therapy, they regress. This stage of inflammation is followed by the more chronic and pathognomonic change known as the Aschoff body.[20] This pathologic lesion is characterized by an area of central necrosis encircled by mononuclear and polynuclear cells. Most observers link this lesion to connective tissue; however, at least one investigator has postulated that the Aschoff body is located in myocardial cells.[21] Some have posited that the lesion is the result of endothelial disruption of cardiac lymphatics.[22] Pathologic changes can be found in all layers of the heart. Myocarditis is seen microscopically in ARF, with inflammatory cells noted in perivascular regions as well as near areas of Aschoff bodies.[23] Though these changes are subclinical in many patients, other affected individuals may have pronounced heart failure in the acute phase of the disease. Pericardial inflammation is manifested as a serofibrinous reaction with pericardial fluid production. Although adhesions can ensue, constrictive changes are unlikely. Valvular inflammation is well described, involving primarily the aortic and mitral valves. Deposition of platelet fibrin collections is seen on the valve leaflets in the acute phase. Over many years, the leaflets may develop progressive fibrosis and contraction, as do the chordae tendineae of the mitral valve. These changes limit excursion of the valves, manifested as stenosis or a lack of coaptation of the leaflets and resulting regurgitation. The tricuspid and pulmonic valves are involved infrequently.

Joint inflammation is common in ARF, leading to the clinical manifestation of arthritis. Pathologically, a serous effusion is seen in the joint space, with inflammation of the articular surfaces; however, long-standing arthritis is not a sequela of the disease. Sydenham chorea is characterized pathologically by cellular infiltration and neuronal loss of the basal ganglia,[24-26] supported by findings of focal striatal enlargement by magnetic resonance imaging.[27] Anti–basal ganglia antibodies have been demonstrated in the sera of patients with Sydenham chorea in both acute and chronic settings.[28] Subcutaneous nodules are located over the extensor surfaces of the large joints, typically the elbows and knees, and are composed of fibrinoid necrosis similar to that seen in Aschoff bodies. These nodules are rarely seen clinically in this era.

CLINICAL PRESENTATION

The onset of ARF occurs after a variable latent period—typically, 10 to 30 days—following streptococcal pharyngitis; however, many patients give no history of a preceding pharyngitis. In particular, when the primary manifestation of the illness is chorea, the latent period from the streptococcal infection can be as long as 6 months. The diagnosis is established by meeting the criteria established by Jones[1] and modified in 1992[29] (Table 87-1).

Early in the disease, complaints may center on a migratory polyarthritis involving the large joints, including the knees, wrists, elbows, and ankles. Fever between 38°C and 39°C is often an accompanying sign. The cardiac examination is notable for tachycardia at rest exacerbated by the fever, but the heart rate is also generally elevated in afebrile patients who have carditis. The precordium is hyperdynamic in the face of the fever-associated tachycardia, myocardial dysfunction, moderate mitral or aortic regurgitation, or the additive effects of mitral and aortic regurgitation producing left ventricular volume overload. The most common murmur is a blowing pansystolic regurgitant murmur heard best at the apex and left lower sternal border with radiation to the axilla. When the regurgitation is moderate or greater, the diastolic rumble of relative mitral stenosis (Carey

Coombs murmur) is present at the apex; this is sometimes best heard with the patient rotated in the left lateral recumbent position and by using the bell of the stethoscope. High-frequency murmurs of aortic regurgitation are heard best using the diaphragm of the stethoscope with the patient seated and leaning forward, with the breath held in expiration. In patients with heart failure, S_3 gallops are present, heard best at the apex with the bell. A three-component pericardial friction rub is heard in the presence of serofibrinous pericarditis, although the sound may be muted when a moderate to large effusion is present. Cardiac tamponade is extremely rare in ARF. Pulses and perfusion are well maintained, except in the unusual case of severe myocardial decompensation.

Erythema marginatum is a serpiginous, salmon-colored eruption characterized by lesions with clear centers over the extremities and trunk. It is evanescent, noted more frequently during febrile episodes or after a bath or shower. Although subcutaneous nodules were once a classic part of the description of ARF, they are now infrequent findings. When present, they are nontender, knobby lesions palpated over the extensor surfaces of the elbows or knees.

Sydenham chorea is a purposeless, involuntary movement disorder of the extremities and face that is exacerbated during periods of stress. Irritability and emotional outbursts are common. The onset may be gradual, but the symptoms may persist for many months, making speech or writing difficult and thereby limiting attendance at school. Carditis and arthritis are generally not noted in combination with chorea. The neurologic signs resolve without long-term sequelae.

Table 87-1　Guidelines for the Diagnosis of Rheumatic Fever

Major Manifestations
Carditis
Polyarthritis
Chorea
Erythema marginatum
Subcutaneous nodules

Minor Manifestations
Clinical findings
  Arthralgia
  Fever
Laboratory findings
  Elevated acute phase reactants
  Elevated erythrocyte sedimentation rate
  Elevated C-reactive protein
  Prolonged P-R interval

Supporting Evidence of Antecedent Group A Streptococcal Infection
Positive throat culture or rapid streptococcal antigen test
Elevated or rising streptococcal antibody titer

If supported by evidence of a preceding group A streptococcal infection, the presence of two major manifestations or one major and two minor manifestations indicates a high probability of acute rheumatic fever

Adapted from Guidelines for the diagnosis of rheumatic fever: Jones criteria, 1992 update. Special Writing Group of the Committee on Rheumatic Fever, Endocarditis and Kawasaki Disease in the Young of the American Heart Association. JAMA 1992;268:2069.

EVALUATION

The diagnosis of ARF relies on criteria derived from the physical examination and laboratory findings. In the setting of a preceding GAS infection, patients with two major manifestations (carditis, polyarthritis, chorea, erythema marginatum, subcutaneous nodules) or one major manifestation and two minor manifestations (see Table 87-1) meet the criteria for the diagnosis of ARF. Because the index of suspicion is higher in an individual with previous ARF, the diagnosis of recurrent ARF is accepted if, in the presence of a preceding streptococcal infection, one major or two minor manifestations are present.

Fever is present in virtually all patients with ARF and should be documented carefully during hospitalization as a marker of the inflammatory process. In addition, the erythrocyte sedimentation rate and C-reactive protein level, nonspecific indicators of inflammation, are elevated in ARF. In a patient with chorea, however, both values might be normal, because that condition can follow the inciting event by a number of months. In the setting of severe heart failure, the erythrocyte sedimentation rate may be within the normal range, but the C-reactive protein is usually elevated. Both values improve after the institution of anti-inflammatory therapy and are useful for following the course of the acute illness.

Laboratory tests that support the likelihood of a preceding streptococcal infection are important for establishing the diagnosis of ARF. All patients should have throat cultures to identify the presence of a GAS infection. Because throat cultures are often negative after patients have been treated, however, and because signs of ARF may not appear until some time after the streptococcal infection, streptococcal antibody tests are useful to establish a recent infection.[30] The antistreptolysin test (ASO) identifies the presence of an antibody to streptolysin O, an extracellular product of β-hemolytic streptococci. ASO titers less than 250 Todd units are considered normal; titers of 500 Todd units or more are considered positive. Values falling between 250 and 500 units are supportive but not diagnostic of a preceding infection. Elevated titers of other serologic tests, including anti-deoxyribonuclease B (anti-DNAase B), antihyaluronidase, and antistreptokinase, suggest a preceding streptococcal infection and may be helpful when ASO titers are not definitive. In the setting of chorea, these tests are often normal, given the latent period between streptococcal exposure and the onset of neurologic signs.

Cardiac testing for ARF historically included an electrocardiogram, which can show prolongation of the P-R interval or higher degrees of atrioventricular block, providing evidence of conduction system inflammation. Echocardiography plays a pivotal role in the assessment of a patient with presumed carditis because it can confirm the presence of mitral or aortic regurgitation by color flow Doppler interrogation of the valves. In the presence of a single major manifestation, aortic or mitral insufficiency not evident by physical examination can be identified, thus adding a second major manifestation. Such testing has not been incorporated into the modified Jones criteria, however, given the variability in the interpretation of physiologic versus pathologic degrees of valvular leak.[31] In addition, the frequency of valvular regurgitation in the setting of other febrile illnesses in children has not been determined.

DIFFERENTIAL DIAGNOSIS

The differential diagnosis of ARF is wide, given the systemic nature of its manifestations. Arthritis is present in many acute illnesses, including juvenile idiopathic (rheumatoid) arthritis, poststreptococcal arthritis, Lyme disease, septic arthritis, infective endocarditis, leukemia, and sickle cell disease. These diseases can be identified by careful consideration of the constellation of history, physical findings, and laboratory tests, including complete blood count with smear, blood cultures, and joint aspiration. Some consider poststreptococcal arthritis to be a separate entity from ARF, but others consider these two disorders to be different presentations of a common disease. Implications for the prevention of recurrence make this an important but controversial point of distinction (see Chapter 106). Children who present with prolonged fever have other diagnostic considerations, which are discussed in Chapter 61.

TREATMENT

All patients with the presumptive diagnosis of ARF should be hospitalized for observation and treatment until their condition stabilizes. Components of the appropriate management of patients diagnosed with ARF are provided in Table 87-2.

The therapy for ARF is supportive and nonspecific. The goal is to reduce inflammation and treat underlying carditis

Table 87-2 Pharmacologic Treatment of Acute Rheumatic Fever (ARF)

ARF Episode and Complications
Inflammation*: aspirin, corticosteroids
Cardiac: diuretics, angiotensin-converting enzyme inhibitors, digoxin
Chorea: haloperidol, valproic acid, diazepam

Antibacterial
Primary prophylaxis*: penicillin, erythromycin, first-generation cephalosporin
Secondary prophylaxis*: penicillin, sulfadiazine, erythromycin
Subacute bacterial endocarditis prophylaxis: see American Heart Association recommendations†

*For all patients with ARF.
†Dajani AS, Taubert KA, Wilson W, et al: Prevention of bacterial endocarditis: Recommendations by the American Heart Association. JAMA 1997;277:1794-1801.

if it is hemodynamically significant. Most clinicians continue to use aspirin as the drug of first choice to reduce fever and control the pain associated with arthritis. Aspirin is administered at a dose of 60 to 100 mg/kg daily divided every 6 hours to achieve a therapeutic salicylate serum level of 10 to 20 mg/dL. The response to aspirin is often dramatic, occurring within 1 to 2 days. The medication is continued over several weeks and then tapered slowly. Nonsteroidal anti-inflammatory medications have not been studied rigorously in this disease. Despite the availability of steroid therapy for the past 50 years, its superiority over aspirin in reducing rheumatic heart disease has not been firmly established. An extensive meta-analysis of the treatment of rheumatic carditis failed to show a convincing superiority of steroids over aspirin for the reduction of rheumatic heart disease a year after the acute illness.[32] With regard to the treatment of acute myocarditis, intravenous gamma globulin infusion has not proved to be of benefit in ARF.[33]

In the setting of carditis, individuals with symptoms of heart failure should be treated with diuretics but rarely require inotropic support or afterload reduction therapy. Restraint from physical activity is mandatory; in fact, complete bed rest for several weeks to months was the rule for many decades. Although these restrictions are somewhat less stringent today, individuals with acute carditis should remain at home and abstain from exertion and sports until the clinician is confident that the ventricular dysfunction or the degree of aortic or mitral regurgitation has stabilized. Restriction from physical activity is warranted for at least 1 month, with relaxation of the limitations based on echocardiographic reassessment at frequent intervals. Given the extended period needed for resolution, home-based tutoring should be implemented for school-aged children.

In rare circumstances, acute rheumatic carditis does not respond to conventional diuretics, aggressive anticongestive measures, anti-inflammatory therapy, and rest. Heart failure is usually the result of marked left ventricular dysfunction with accompanying mitral or aortic regurgitation. In these refractory cases, cardiac surgical intervention with mitral or aortic valve replacement, or both, may be necessary.

Table 87-3 Recommended Doses* of Antibiotics to Prevent Rheumatic Fever

Indication and Antibiotic	Route	Dose in Children (≤27 kg)	Dose in Adolescents and Adults	Frequency	Duration
Treatment of GAS tonsillitis or pharyngitis (primary prophylaxis)					
Phenoxymethylpenicillin (penicillin V)	Oral	250 mg	500 mg	Twice daily	10 days
Benzathine penicillin G	IM	450 mg (600,000 U)	900 mg (1.2 million U)	NA	Single dose
Erythromycin[†]	Oral	20 mg/kg (max 250 mg)	250 mg	Twice daily	10 days
Prevention of rheumatic fever recurrences (secondary prophylaxis)					
Benzathine penicillin G	IM	900 mg (1.2 million U)	900 mg (1.2 million U)	Every 4 wk[‡]	5 yr since last episode or age 21 yr (whichever is longer)
Phenoxymethylpenicillin (penicillin V)	Oral	250 mg	250 mg	Twice daily	To age 40 yr or for life if heart disease present
Erythromycin[†]	Oral	250 mg	250 mg	Twice daily	

*Recommended by the American Heart Association.
[†]Erythromycin should be used only if the patient is allergic to penicillin.
[‡]If possible, dosing every 3 wk provides superior protection.
GAS, group A streptococcal; NA, not applicable.
From Cohen J, Powderly WG: Infectious Diseases, 2nd ed. St Louis, Mosby, 2004.

Continued intense medical therapy is required postoperatively until the underlying hemodynamic derangement improves.

All patients with ARF should receive treatment for GAS infection, whether proved by culture or presumed by serologic testing, as well as long-term therapy to prevent the recurrence of infection (Table 87-3). With regard to long-term prophylaxis, the intramuscular administration of benzathine penicillin every 3 to 4 weeks is preferred, although penicillin twice daily is an acceptable alternative.[34] The risk of a first episode of ARF following untreated streptococcal pharyngitis is 1% to 3%; however, the risk of recurrent attacks of ARF with subsequent streptococcal infections increases dramatically to as high as 50%. Individuals manifesting carditis with the first attack of ARF are at significant risk for recurrent carditis during subsequent episodes, so prophylaxis is particularly critical in this group. Recommendations regarding the duration of prophylaxis have changed over the past half century. Initially, all patients were advised to take penicillin prophylaxis for life; however, many clinicians now suggest discontinuing such therapy after age 21 years if there was no carditis during the episode of rheumatic fever. If carditis was present but there is no residual heart disease, prophylaxis is recommended for 10 years or well into adulthood, whichever is longer. If carditis was present and there is residual heart disease, prophylaxis is recommended for at least 10 years after the last episode or until age 40 years; lifetime prophylaxis may be recommended if the individual is regularly exposed to populations with a high prevalence of streptococcal infections, such as teachers or day-care workers.[35] In individuals with a recurrence of ARF, these boundaries for prophylaxis should be extended, and the frequency of benzathine penicillin administration may need to be increased to every 3 weeks.[36]

In patients with valve disease, prophylaxis for endocarditis should be instituted before they undergo dental or genitourinary tract surgery or other procedures associated with a significant risk of bacteremia. The American Heart Association provides details regarding appropriate chemoprophylaxis regimens.[37]

RECURRENT ACUTE RHEUMATIC FEVER

The Jones criteria are intended for the diagnosis of a first attack of ARF. The diagnosis of a recurrent bout of ARF is straightforward when the Jones criteria are met; however, the diagnosis may be elusive, given the presence of residual mitral or aortic valve disease from the first episode. In these cases, using carditis as a manifestation may not be possible in the presence of a febrile illness. In such situations, polyarthritis along with a minor criterion should be considered diagnostic, as should the presence of chorea. Another confounding issue is the diagnosis of poststreptococcal reactive arthritis, which tends to follow streptococcal pharyngitis by 3 to 14 days. The arthritis can be nonmigratory, persisting longer than that seen with ARF. Often the arthritis does not respond to salicylates, unlike the response generally seen in ARF. When the Jones criteria are met, the patient should be considered to have ARF. For individuals who do not meet the criteria, treatment should occur if all other diagnoses have been considered and ruled out.

CONSULTATION

Cardiology subspecialists are routinely involved in the initial evaluation and management. They are also part of the long-term follow-up of patients after discharge.

ADMISSION CRITERIA

All patients with the presumptive diagnosis of ARF or recurrent ARF should be hospitalized.

DISCHARGE CRITERIA

- Establishment or elimination of the diagnosis of ARF.
- Completion of an observation period to confirm that the course of the illness has stabilized.
- Completion of diagnostic testing to identify the severity of illness, especially cardiac involvement.
- Initiation of appropriate treatment for the primary GAS infection and for ARF symptoms and signs.
- Education of the patient and caregivers regarding endocarditis prophylaxis.
- Institution of a secondary prophylaxis regimen for the prevention of subsequent GAS infection.
- Establishment of follow-up with primary care clinician and appropriate subspecialists.

PREVENTION

The prevention of ARF is based on the prompt treatment of GAS pharyngitis, the only infection known to cause ARF. Positive throat swabs for rapid antigen testing or culture for GAS in patients with pharyngitis indicate the need for antibiotic therapy. In developed countries, where the prevalence of ARF is low, a 10-day course of oral penicillin V is the routine treatment of documented GAS pharyngitis. A single intramuscular injection of benzathine penicillin is recommended in areas with a high prevalence of rheumatic fever to ensure compliance (Table 87-3 provides dosing information). Mass prophylaxis has been implemented at military bases, successfully aborting outbreaks of ARF.[38-40]

Repeat throat culture is not necessary in patients who have received adequate treatment. Despite completion of appropriate therapy, approximately 20% of patients with resolved pharyngitis may continue to test positive for group A streptococci in the throat. However, the strains present lose M proteins and virulence after treatment. In areas where rheumatic fever is not present, the colonization that persists is not considered a threat to the population.[40]

IN A NUTSHELL

- Although less common than in previous decades, ARF continues to affect children, despite the availability of therapy that could eliminate the presumed inciting agent.
- The diagnosis of ARF requires application of the modified Jones criteria, after which treatment of the streptococcal disease is instituted.

- Anti-inflammatory therapy ameliorates the arthritis associated with ARF, but the superiority of steroids over aspirin in decreasing the frequency of rheumatic heart disease has not been established.
- Rest and anticongestive medications are the mainstays of treatment for aortic or mitral carditis, which often persists for several months.
- Long-term penicillin prophylaxis is mandatory to prevent recurrent streptococcal pharyngitis and the likelihood of additional episodes of ARF. Successful reduction of recurrent ARF minimizes the risk for hemodynamically significant rheumatic heart disease in the ensuing 2 to 3 decades.

ON THE HORIZON

- The Committee on Rheumatic Fever, Endocarditis, and Kawasaki Disease of the American Heart Association meets regularly to review the Jones criteria and any new developments associated with ARF and GAS infections. At the meeting held in 2000, the committee considered adding two-dimensional and Doppler echocardiography to the modified Jones criteria as a modality for the diagnosis of carditis and valvulitis. It was concluded, however, that no revision to the criteria was necessary.
- Small outbreaks of ARF were reported in the United States in the last 2 decades of the 20th century,[10,41-44] and the incidence remains high among children of Polynesian descent in Australia, Hawaii, and New Zealand.[45,46] The committee will continue to explore the worldwide impact of ARF and review the diagnostic criteria as new tests become available.
- Efforts continue to create a vaccine that targets the rheumatogenic strains of group A streptococci.

SUGGESTED READING

Bonow RO, Carabello B, de Leon AC Jr, et al: ACC/AHA guidelines for the management of patients with valvular heart disease: A report of the American College of Cardiology/American Heart Association Task Force on Practice Guidelines (Committee on Management of Patients with Valvular Heart Disease). J Am Coll Cardiol 1998;32:1486.

Guidelines for the diagnosis of rheumatic fever: Jones criteria, 1992 update. Special Writing Group of the Committee on Rheumatic Fever, Endocarditis and Kawasaki Disease of the Council on Cardiovascular Disease in the Young of the American Heart Association. JAMA 1992;268:2069.

Lue HD, Wu MH, Wang JK, et al: Long-term outcome of patients with rheumatic fever receiving benzathine penicillin G prophylaxis every three weeks versus every four weeks. J Pediatr 1994;125:812.

REFERENCES

1. Jones TD: The diagnosis of acute rheumatic fever. JAMA 1944;126:481.
2. Denny FW, Wannamaker LW, Brink WR, et al: Prevention of rheumatic fever: Treatment of the preceding streptococcal infection. JAMA 1950;143:151.
3. Gordis L: Effectiveness of comprehensive-care programs in preventing rheumatic fever. N Engl J Med 1973;289:331.
4. Markowitz M, Kaplan EL: Reappearance of rheumatic fever. Adv Pediatr 1989;36:39.

5. Padmavati S: Epidemiology of cardiovascular disease in India. I. Rheumatic heart disease. Circulation 1962;25:703.

6. Abdin ZH: Rheumatic fever and rheumatic heart disease in Egyptian children. Gaz Egypt Pediatr Assoc 1960;8:282.

7. Kaplan EL: Global assessment of rheumatic fever and rheumatic heart disease at the close of the century. Circulation 1993;88:1964.

8. Veasy LG, Hill HR: Immunologic and clinical correlations in rheumatic fever and rheumatic heart disease. Pediatr Infect Dis J 1997;16:400.

9. Congeni B, Rizzo C, Congeni J, Sreenivasan VV: Outbreak of acute rheumatic fever in northeast Ohio. J Pediatr 1987;111:176.

10. Veasy LG, Weidmeier SE, Orsmond GS, et al: Resurgence of acute rheumatic fever in the intermountain area of the US. N Engl J Med 1987;316:421.

11. Wald ER, Dashefsky B, Feidt C, et al: Acute rheumatic fever in western Pennsylvania and the tri-state area. Pediatrics 1987;80:371.

12. Wannamaker LW: Differences between streptococcal infections of the skin and of the throat. N Engl J Med 1970;282:23.

13. Stollerman GH, Siegel AC, Johnson EE: Variable epidemiology of streptococcal disease and the changing pattern of rheumatic fever. Mod Concepts Cardiovasc Dis 1965;34:45.

14. Dale JB, Beachey EH: Protective antigenic determinant of streptococcal M protein shared with sarcolemmal membrane protein of human heart. J Exp Med 1982;156:1165.

15. Dale JB, Beachey EH: Epitopes of streptococcal M proteins shared with cardiac myosin. J Exp Med 1985;162:583.

16. Baird RW, Bronze MS, Kraus W, et al: Epitopes of group A streptococcal M protein shared with antigens of articular cartilage and synovium. J Immunol 1991;146:3132.

17. Goldstein I, Halpern B, Robert L: Immunologic relationship between streptococcal A polysaccharide and structural glycoproteins of heart valve. Nature 1967;214:44.

18. Raizada V, Williams RC, Chopra P, et al: Tissue distribution of lymphocytes in rheumatic heart valves as defined by monoclonal anti-T cell antibodies. Am J Med 1983;74:90.

19. Marrack P, Kappler J: The staphylococcal exotoxins and their relatives. Science 1990;248:705.

20. Gross L, Ehrlich JC: Studies on the myocardial Aschoff body. II. Life cycle, sites of predilection and relation to the clinical course of rheumatic fever. Am J Pathol 1934;10:489.

21. Murphy GE: Nature of the rheumatic heart disease with special reference to myocardial disease and heart failure. Medicine 1960;39:289.

22. Wedum BG, McGuire JW: Origin of the Aschoff body. Ann Rheum Dis 1963;22:127.

23. Coombs CF: The myocardial lesions of the rheumatic infection. BMJ 1907;2:1513.

24. Sydenham T: On St Vitus Dance: The Works of Thomas Sydenham, MD, vol 2. London, Sydenham Society, 1850, p 257.

25. Colony HS, Malamud N: Sydenham's chorea: A clinicopathologic study. Neurology 1956;6:672.

26. Greenfield JG, Wolfsohn JM: The pathology of Sydenham's chorea. Lancet 1922;2:603.

27. Giedd JN, Rapoport JL, Kruesi MJ, et al: Sydenham's chorea: Magnetic resonance imaging of the basal ganglia. Neurology 1995;45:2199.

28. Church AJ, Cardoso F, Dale RC, et al: Anti-basal ganglia antibodies in acute and persistent Sydenham's chorea. Neurology 2002;59:227.

29. Guidelines for the diagnosis of rheumatic fever: Jones criteria, 1992 update. Special Writing Group of the Committee on Rheumatic Fever, Endocarditis and Kawasaki Disease of the Council on Cardiovascular Disease in the Young of the American Heart Association. JAMA 1992;268:2069.

30. Widdowson JP, Maxted WR, Notley CM, et al: The antibody responses in man to infection with different serotypes of group A streptococci. J Med Microbiol 1974;7:483.

31. Ferrieri P, for the Jones Criteria Working Group: Proceedings of the Jones criteria workshop. Circulation 2002;106:2521.

32. Albert DA, Harel L, Karrison T: The treatment of rheumatic carditis: A review and meta-analysis. Medicine 1995;74:1.

33. Voss LM, Wilson NJ, Neutze JM, et al: Intravenous immunoglobulin in acute rheumatic fever: A randomized controlled trial. Circulation 2001;103:401.

34. Wood HF, Feinstein AR, Taranta A, et al: Rheumatic fever in adolescents: A long-term epidemiologic study of subsequent prophylaxis, streptococcal infections and clinical sequelae. III. Comparative effectiveness of three prophylaxis regimens in preventing streptococcal infections and rheumatic recurrences. Ann Intern Med 1964;60(Suppl):31.

35. Bonow RO, Carabello B, de Leon AC Jr, et al: ACC/AHA guidelines for the management of patients with valvular heart disease: A report of the American College of Cardiology/American Heart Association Task Force on Practice Guidelines (Committee on Management of Patients with Valvular Heart Disease). J Am Coll Cardiol 1998;32:1486.

36. Lue HD, Wu MH, Wang JK, et al: Long-term outcome of patients with rheumatic fever receiving benzathine penicillin G prophylaxis every three weeks versus every four weeks. J Pediatr 1994;125:812.

37. Dajani AS, Taubert KA, Wilson W, et al: Prevention of bacterial endocarditis: Recommendations by the American Heart Association. JAMA 1997;277:1794.

38. Stollerman GH: The nature of rheumatogenic streptococci. Mt Sinai J Med 1996;653:144.

39. Centers for Disease Control: Acute rheumatic fever among army trainees—Fort Leonard Wood, Missouri, 1987-1988. MMWR Morb Mortal Wkly Rep 1988;37:519.

40. Stollerman GH: Rheumatic fever. Lancet 1997;349:935.

41. Hoffman TM, Rhodes LA, Pyles LA, et al: Childhood acute rheumatic fever: A comparison of recent resurgence areas to cases in West Virginia. W V Med J 1997;93:260.

42. Veasy LG, Tani LY, Hill HR: Persistence of acute rheumatic fever in the intermountain area of the United States. J Pediatr 1994;124:9.

43. Westlake RM, Graham TP, Edwards KM: An outbreak of acute rheumatic fever in Tennessee. Pediatr Infect Dis J 1990;9:97.

44. Hosier DM, Craenen JM, Teske DW, Wheller JJ: Resurgence of acute rheumatic fever. Am J Dis Child 1987;141:730.

45. McDonald M, Currie BJ, Carapetis JR: Acute rheumatic fever: A chink in the chain that links the heart to the throat? Lancet Infect Dis 2004;4:240.

46. Pope RM: Rheumatic fever in the 1980s. Bull Rheum Dis 1989;38:1.

Endocrinology

CHAPTER 88

Diabetes Mellitus and Hyperglycemia

Mary Pat Gallagher and Sharon E. Oberfield

Diabetes mellitus is a common disorder in which hyperglycemia results from abnormal insulin production, abnormal insulin action, or both. Patients with hyperglycemia often have a history of polyuria, polydipsia, polyphagia, weight loss, and fatigue. Depending on the duration of illness and the underlying pathophysiology, the patient may or may not have ketosis or acidosis. Although more common in autoimmune diabetes mellitus (type 1), ketosis and acidosis can also occur in type 2 diabetes mellitus and reflect an insulin-deficient state.

Children with newly diagnosed diabetes mellitus may present to the hospital in advanced stages of metabolic decompensation because the symptoms of hyperglycemia were not recognized. Treatment of diabetic ketoacidosis (DKA) in childhood requires strict attention to fluid balance and neurologic status because of the risk for cerebral edema in the pediatric population.

DIFFERENTIAL DIAGNOSIS

The cause of hyperglycemia is not always apparent at initial presentation. The differential diagnosis includes type 1 diabetes mellitus (autoimmune), type 2 diabetes mellitus, maturity-onset diabetes of the young, "stress hyperglycemia" from illness, pancreatitis, other pancreatic dysfunction (e.g., cystic fibrosis), and drug effect (glucocorticoids, antipsychotics, etc.). Less commonly, hyperglycemia may be seen in the setting of other endocrine illnesses such as endogenous glucocorticoid, growth hormone, or catecholamine excess.

Type 1 diabetes mellitus is an autoimmune disorder in which destruction of pancreatic islets causes an absolute insulin deficiency. Approximately 90% of patients with autoimmune diabetes have measurable serum antibodies against islet cells, glutamic acid decarboxylase (GAD), or insulin.[1] Most patients with autoimmune diabetes present before the age of 30 years, and for this reason the condition had been termed "juvenile-onset" diabetes by some. It is now clear, however, that autoimmune diabetes may develop at any age.

Type 2 diabetes mellitus is a disorder characterized by insulin resistance and relative insulin deficiency secondary to an inability of the patient's beta cells to adequately compensate for the level of insulin resistance. Patients may experience a period of absolute insulin deficiency at the time of diagnosis and present with ketosis. Obesity and acanthosis nigricans should raise the possibility that a child has type 2 diabetes mellitus, even in the setting of ketoacidosis. These patients do not have antibodies against islet cells, GAD, or insulin. This form of diabetes had previously been thought of as "adult-onset" diabetes. However, the incidence of type 2 diabetes in the pediatric population is increasing rapidly.[2]

Maturity-onset diabetes of the young is a group of disorders of insulin secretion and glucose disposal. They vary in their severity and presentation. Each is caused by a single gene mutation and is inherited in an autosomal dominant pattern. Insulin resistance and obesity are not features of these disorders.[3]

DIAGNOSIS AND EVALUATION

Physical examination with careful attention to vital signs, neurologic status, and clinical signs of dehydration are key to initial evaluation of a patient with hyperglycemia. Specific attention should be paid to temperature, heart rate, respiratory rate, blood pressure, weight, extent of dehydration, level of consciousness, funduscopic examination, presence of Kussmaul respirations, and any possible focus of infection. The patient's body mass index and the presence or absence of acanthosis nigricans (thickening and darkening of the skin in flexural areas such as the axillae and posterior of the neck) may provide insight into the underlying pathophysiology.

Initial laboratory evaluation should include venous or arterial blood gas analysis, stat electrolytes (including glucose, sodium, potassium, calcium, ionized calcium, phosphorus, blood urea nitrogen [BUN], and creatinine), liver function tests, lipase, amylase, acetone, preserved glucose, insulin, C peptide, hemoglobin A_{1c}, GAD-65 antibodies, islet cell antibodies, and insulin autoantibodies. Urine should also be assessed at the bedside for the presence of glucose and ketones. In patients with significant electrolyte abnormalities, an electrocardiogram (ECG) should be obtained.

The history should include the duration of illness; precipitating factors such as infection, trauma, or stress; the patient's previous weight; and any prescription or nonprescription drugs that the patient may have taken. If diabetes has previously been diagnosed, it is helpful to know the current insulin regimen, the time of the last insulin dose, and the patient's compliance with treatment. If this is the patient's first presentation with hyperglycemia, any family history of autoimmune disease, type 1 or 2 diabetes mellitus, and gestational diabetes should be elicited.

Initial Assessment

Hyperglycemia with ketoacidosis (venous pH <7.3, glucose >200 mg/dL, HCO_3 <15 mM/L, and urine with large ketones): Consider admission to an intensive care unit (ICU) or setting where the patient can be closely monitored and have frequent laboratory evaluation performed.

Hyperglycemia with ketosis without ketoacidosis (venous pH >7.3, glucose >200 mg/dL, HCO_3 >15 mM/L, and urine with large ketones): If the patient has a history of diabetes, it is possible to consider emergency department management and discharge home if there is a good response to intravenous fluids and insulin. If the patient has new-onset diabetes, most centers admit for initiation of insulin therapy and diabetes education (see the section Treatment).

Nonketotic hyperosmolar hyperglycemic state (hyperosmolar state with elevated sodium, elevated BUN, serum osmolality >320 mOsm, glucose >300 mg/dL, venous pH >7.3, HCO_3 >15 mM/L, urine with small to moderate ketones): Admission to an ICU is indicated, particularly if there is evidence of altered mental status.

Mixed nonketotic hyperosmolar hyperglycemic state and ketoacidosis (hyperosmolar state with elevated sodium, elevated BUN, serum osmolality >320 mOsm, glucose >300 mg/dL, venous pH <7.3, HCO_3 <15 mM/L, and urine with moderate to large ketones): Admission to an ICU is indicated, particularly if there is evidence of altered mental status.

TREATMENT

Rapid evaluation of the patient should be quickly followed by initiation of treatment. The aim is to reverse the metabolic disturbance and restore and maintain intravascular volume. However, fluid and insulin management must be titrated carefully because rapid changes in glucose and osmolality may contribute to the development of complications.[4]

Treatment of Diabetic Ketoacidosis

This section is not intended as a rigid protocol but is offered as a guideline. Each case should be assessed individually and frequently reassessed during the course of treatment.

Fluids

Emergency fluid resuscitation is determined by evaluation and assessment of the patient's hydration status (perfusion, heart rate, and blood pressure). A bolus of 5 to 10 mL/kg of normal saline (NS) over a 1-hour period is typically used in a mildly to moderately dehydrated patient. The bolus can be repeated if necessary. A conservative approach to fluids is warranted unless contraindicated (i.e., shock requires rapid intravascular repletion to maintain perfusion). The aim is to

replace the fluid deficit evenly over a minimum of 48 hours. Maintenance fluids should be given in addition to replacement of the patient's fluid deficit. The patient's ongoing losses must also be monitored, and if excessive, these losses may require replacement as well. Fluid management must be reassessed at a minimum of every 4 hours. Slower fluid replacement should be considered in a patient who is very young, has had a prolonged prodrome, has severe acidosis, has an elevated corrected sodium (corrected sodium = measured sodium + 1.6 [(serum glucose − 100)/100]), or has significantly elevated serum osmolality (>300 mOsm). The patient should remain without oral intake during the initial stabilization. Adequacy of fluid therapy should be reevaluated frequently. Inadequate hydration will contribute to persistent acidosis, and there is evidence to suggest that rapid hydration may contribute to the development of symptomatic cerebral edema.[4,5]

Maintenance fluid requirements are calculated as follows:

- 100 mL/kg for first 10 kg of body weight
- 50 mL/kg for the second 10 kg of body weight
- 20 mL/kg for each additional kilogram of body weight over 20 kg

Maintenance fluids can usually be given as $^1/_2$NS. However, the sodium content of the fluid may need to be adjusted, depending on the patient's age, serum osmolality, and serum electrolytes.

Replacement of deficit is calculated as follows:

- 5% dehydration = 50 mL/kg
- 10% dehydration = 100 mL/kg

If serum osmolality is less than 300 mOsm, aim to replace the deficit over a 48-hour period.

If serum osmolality is 300 mOsm or greater or dehydration is greater than 10%, aim to replace the deficit over a 48-hour period or longer.

$$\text{Estimated serum osmolality} = 2(Na) + (Glucose/18) + (BUN/2.8)$$

NS should be given for replacement of the deficit. The volume of the initial resuscitation fluid should be subtracted from the total deficit when calculating the volume that should be replaced over the following 48 hours.

Ongoing losses are not generally replaced unless they are excessive (urine output >4 mL/kg/hr); such losses include urine, vomiting, and Kussmaul respirations.

Potassium

Because there is a marked depletion of total body potassium, it should be added to the intravenous fluids as soon as the following criteria have been met: serum K^+ is less than 5.0 mEq/L, the patient has voided, and the ECG demonstrates an absence of peaked T waves. Timely addition of potassium will help avoid the development of life-threatening arrhythmias that can occur if hypokalemia develops with correction of the acidosis and insulin therapy.

Phosphorus

Total body phosphorus is also depleted in patients who present with DKA. However, symptomatic hypophosphatemia is extremely rare, and intravenous replacement of phosphorus is controversial. Phosphate supplementation may be considered if there has been a prolonged period of illness or if an extended period of fasting is anticipated. Potassium phosphate can be used along with potassium chloride in this instance to provide both potassium and phosphorus intravenously. The major risk with phosphate administration is the development of hypocalcemia and arrhythmia. Calcium levels must be monitored carefully, and if hypocalcemia develops, the phosphate infusion should be discontinued immediately.

Bicarbonate

Administration of bicarbonate should be undertaken with extreme caution. Bicarbonate may be appropriate in certain situations, but it is important to consider that there is evidence that sudden correction of blood pH can paradoxically lower cerebrospinal fluid pH. It is also important to be aware that endogenous production of bicarbonate will occur as ketones are metabolized. For this reason, the usual calculation for correction of acidosis will overestimate the bicarbonate required to correct acidosis in patients with DKA. The effect of bicarbonate administration on serum potassium must also be considered, and additional potassium administration may be required.

Insulin

Administration of insulin via an intravenous drip allows for rapid insulin action and dose adjustment. Ideally, an insulin infusion should be initiated within the first 2 hours of treatment of DKA. To ensure good flow of insulin into the patient, we recommend mixing the insulin drip in NS at a concentration of 0.1 U/mL (50 units of regular insulin in 500 mL of 0.9% NS). If this solution is infused at a rate equal to the child's weight in kilograms, the insulin will be infused at a rate of 0.1 U/kg/hr. Priming the intravenous tubing with 50 mL of solution before beginning the infusion of insulin is recommended at some centers. The insulin infusion must be regulated with a pump and should be included when calculating total fluids.

The response to insulin therapy is measured by resolution of ketosis and a rise in the serum bicarbonate level. The insulin infusion rate should be maintained or increased until the ketosis has markedly improved or resolved. Because insulin will lower blood sugar before resolution of the ketosis and acidosis, dextrose will need to be added to the intravenous fluids at some point to avoid a rapid decline in serum glucose or frank hypoglycemia, or both. Generally, dextrose is added to the fluids when serum glucose levels approach 250 mg/dL. The usual infusion rate is 3 to 5 g of dextrose per unit of insulin infused over the same period.

After initial fluid management and initiation of insulin therapy, you should anticipate a decrease in glucose by 100 mg/dL/hr. A larger decrease may be seen with initial fluid resuscitation, depending on the patient's hydration status. The goal is to maintain the corrected serum sodium and to see an increase in the measured serum sodium as the blood glucose level falls. If marked hyperosmolality is present (glucose >1200, serum osmolality >300 mOsm), the therapeutic goals should be adjusted to replace the fluid deficit over a period of 48 to 72 hours and, after an initial period of rehydration, to lower the blood glucose infusion rate to 50 mg/dL/hr.

Continued Monitoring and Reevaluation

After initial therapy for DKA has been instituted, monitor blood pH and electrolytes every 1 to 2 hours until the patient is improving (pH >7.2) and then every 2 to 4 hours. Check serum glucose levels every hour via finger stick (or preserved glucose if too high for the glucose monitor). Neurologic status should be evaluated every 1 to 2 hours. Urine output should be recorded and overall input and output reviewed frequently. A flow sheet is extremely helpful to track changes in fluid balance, vital signs, electrolytes, urine ketones, and blood sugar.

It is important to monitor for problems associated with DKA: hypoglycemia, hypokalemia, hypocalcemia, hypernatremia, fluid overload with edema, acute respiratory distress syndrome, and symptomatic cerebral edema. Symptoms of cerebral edema include any change in sensorium, headache, increased drowsiness, deepening coma, and cranial nerve abnormalities. Cushing's triad (increased blood pressure, decreased heart rate, decreased mental status) may be seen in the setting of increased intracranial pressure. This is a neurosurgical emergency, and the ICU and neurosurgery teams should be involved in the management of these patients. It is important to have mannitol available when a patient is admitted with DKA in the event of the development of symptomatic cerebral edema. If the team concurs that mannitol is indicated as part of the management, the recommended dose is 0.5 to 1 g/kg administered intravenously over a period of 15 to 30 minutes.

Conversion to Subcutaneous Insulin

The criteria for switching from an intravenous insulin infusion to subcutaneous insulin injections include the ability to eat, normal mental status, negative to small urine ketones, improved hydration, and glucose levels less than 250 mg/dL. The first dose of subcutaneous insulin should be given 30 to 60 minutes before stopping the intravenous infusion to prevent the reappearance of ketosis once the drip has been discontinued. It is optimal to convert to a subcutaneous regimen just before a meal. To determine an initial daily dose, it is necessary to consider the patient's age and clinical presentation. A typical starting dose for a patient with newly diagnosed diabetes is approximately 0.5 U of insulin per kilogram of body weight per 24 hours. Younger patients are likely to be more insulin sensitive, whereas adolescents and patients with an underlying illness are likely to be more insulin resistant. A quarter of the estimated total daily dose can then be given as short-acting insulin before the initial meal. The blood sugar level after the first meal will then help determine the patient's insulin sensitivity and create a long-term insulin regimen. Treatment needs to be individualized for each patient and should be discussed with a pediatric endocrinologist. Patients with previously diagnosed diabetes can usually be started on their home insulin regimen.

Treatment of the Hyperosmolar Hyperglycemic State

A hyperosmolar hyperglycemic state may be seen in type 1 diabetes mellitus, although it is more common in type 2 diabetes mellitus. Management of this disorder is outside the scope of this chapter and should involve the ICU team. It is important to know, however, that the underlying pathophysiology involves severe dehydration and requires that

Table 88-1 Insulin Preparations Available for Subcutaneous Therapy

Type of Insulin	Name	Onset of Action	Peak Action	Duration of Action
Rapid acting	Lispro (Humalog) Aspart (NovoLog)	15 min	45 min	3-5 hr
Short acting	Regular	30 min	2-5 hr	5-8 hr
Intermediate acting	NPH	1-3 hr	6-12 hr	10-12 hr
Very long acting	Glargine (Lantus) Detemir (Levemir)	4-6 hr 4-6 hr	None Dose dependent	24 hr 24 hr

adequate fluid administration precede insulin administration to avoid cardiovascular collapse. Gram-negative infections are often a precipitating factor in the development of hyperosmolar hyperglycemia, and initial evaluation of the patient should include appropriate cultures.[5]

Treatment of Hyperglycemia without Acidosis

If the initial workup reveals only hyperglycemia or hyperglycemia with mild to moderate ketosis, it may be possible to manage the patient with oral rehydration and subcutaneous insulin therapy. This approach is not appropriate in patients with hyperosmolality, nausea or vomiting, or another issue precluding oral intake. Electrolyte imbalance is less frequently seen and can usually be corrected with oral therapy. The approach to insulin management is similar to that described in the previous section.

Patients who present without signs of insulin resistance (increased body mass index or acanthosis nigricans, or both) and without ketones are often very insulin sensitive. Conservative management of these patients should be undertaken, with starting doses of 0.25 U/kg/day of insulin given in divided doses. A number of different regimens are possible, and therapy should be tailored to the patient's needs. Newer insulin analogues have made it possible to create insulin and meal regimens that are much more flexible (Table 88-1).

CONSULTATION

- Pediatric endocrinologist
- Possible: Pediatric critical care

ADMISSION CRITERIA

- Hyperglycemia accompanied by ketosis and acidosis
- Altered mental status
- Any patient receiving insulin who is unable to tolerate sufficient oral intake to prevent hypoglycemia
- Pediatric patients with newly diagnosed type 1 diabetes if intensive education is not immediately available on an outpatient basis

DISCHARGE CRITERIA

- Include both clinical criteria and educational criteria
- Normal electrolytes and hydration status
- Able to tolerate food

- It is *not* necessary to obtain perfect glucose control before discharge; insulin doses will require modification after discharge and on an ongoing basis
- For a patient being discharged on insulin therapy, it is necessary to ensure that the family has been educated regarding the following:

Definition and pathophysiology of the different types of diabetes
Insulin action
Signs and symptoms of hypoglycemia
Treatment of hypoglycemia
Glucagon administration
Proper technique in using the glucometer
Proper technique in drawing up and administering insulin
Consequences of poor glycemic control

IN A NUTSHELL

- Hyperglycemia often presents in the inpatient setting and may be a result of type 1 (autoimmune) diabetes mellitus, type 2 diabetes mellitus, illness, or drug effect.
- Any history of polyuria, polydipsia, polyphagia, and weight loss should be noted.
- The presence or absence of ketosis and acidosis at initial presentation does not necessarily differentiate type 1 from type 2 diabetes. If ketosis is present, it does suggest an absolute insulin deficiency at the time of presentation.
- Physical examination should focus on vital signs, neurologic status, and clinical signs of dehydration during initial evaluation of a patient with hyperglycemia.
- Initial laboratory evaluation should include venous or arterial blood gas analysis, stat electrolytes (including glucose, sodium, potassium, calcium, ionized calcium, phosphorus, BUN, and creatinine), liver function tests, lipase, amylase, acetone, preserved glucose, insulin, C peptide, hemoglobin A_{1c}, GAD-65 antibodies, islet cell antibodies, and insulin autoantibodies. Urine should also be assessed at the bedside for the presence of glucose and ketones. In patients with significant electrolyte abnormalities, an ECG should be obtained.
- In patients with DKA, a flow sheet is critical to track changes in fluid balance, vital signs, electrolytes, urine ketones, and blood sugar.

- Management of patients with DKA is individualized and aimed at correcting the underlying insulin deficiency, ketosis, and acidosis, as well as replacing the fluid deficit over a 48-hour period or longer if clinically indicated.
- In hyperglycemia without metabolic decompensation, management is focused on determining the appropriate insulin dose and educating the patient and family members.

ON THE HORIZON

- The incidence of hyperglycemic hyperosmolar nonketotic syndrome in adolescents continues to increase. A subset of this population is being recognized in which the mortality rate is quite high. Hyperthermia and rhabdomyolysis have developed in these subjects after the initiation of insulin therapy. The cause of this syndrome is unclear, but therapy with dantrolene has been reported to be beneficial in these subjects.[6]
- Several new injectable agents have been approved for use in adults with type 1 and type 2 diabetes. They may prove beneficial to the pediatric population as well. They are modeled after the human incretin hormone glucagon-like peptide-1 (GLP-1) and are therefore called incretin mimetics. GLP-1 is secreted in response to food intake and has multiple effects on the stomach, liver, pancreas, and brain.[7]
- Exenatide (Byetta) is being used for adults with type 2 diabetes. It augments insulin release, delays gastric emptying, and suppresses glucagon secretion, which results in a decrease in food intake and less hyperglycemic excursions.
- Pramlintide (Symlin), a synthetic amylin analogue, also decreases glucagon secretion and delays gastric emptying. It results in less glycemic excursion and facilitates weight reduction without causing hypoglycemia.

SUGGESTED READING

Arslanian S: Type 2 diabetes in children: Clinical aspects and risk factors. Horm Res 2002;57(Suppl 1):19-28.

Fajans SS, Bell GI, Polonsky KS: Molecular mechanisms and clinical pathophysiology of maturity-onset diabetes of the young. N Engl J Med 2001;345:971-980.

Kukreja A, Maclaren NK: Autoimmunity and diabetes. J Clin Endocrinol Metab 1999;84:4371-4378.

REFERENCES

1. Kukreja A, Maclaren NK: Autoimmunity and diabetes. J Clin Endocrinol Metab 1999;84:4371-4378.
2. Arslanian S: Type 2 diabetes in children: Clinical aspects and risk factors. Horm Res 2002;57(Suppl 1):19-28.
3. Fajans SS, Bell GI, Polonsky KS: Molecular mechanisms and clinical pathophysiology of maturity-onset diabetes of the young. N Engl J Med 2001;345:971-980.
4. Glaser N: Cerebral edema in children with diabetic ketoacidosis. Curr Diab Rep 2001;1:41-46.
5. Chiasson JL, Aris-Jilwan N, Belanger R, et al: Diagnosis and treatment of diabetic ketoacidosis and the hyperglycemic hyperosmolar state. Can Med Assoc J 2003;168:859-866.
6. Kilbane BJ, Mehta S, Backeljauw PF, et al: Approach to management of malignant hyperthermia–like syndrome in pediatric diabetes mellitus. Pediatr Crit Care Med 2006;7:169-173.
7. Jeha GS, Heptulla RA: Newer therapeutic options for children with diabetes mellitus: Theoretical and practical considerations. Pediatr Diabetes 2006;7:122-138.

CHAPTER 89

Disorders of Thyroid Hormone

Natasha Leibel and Mary Pat Gallagher

Disorders of thyroid hormone are not encountered frequently in the inpatient setting, but it is important for the hospitalist to have an understanding of the hypothalamic-pituitary-thyroid axis, the presentation of hypo- and hyperthyroid states, and the medications used to treat these conditions.

BACKGROUND

Thyrotropin-releasing hormone is produced in the hypothalamus and stimulates the production and secretion of thyroid-stimulating hormone (TSH) in the anterior pituitary gland. TSH stimulates the release of the thyroid hormones thyroxine (T_4) and triiodothyronine (T_3) from the thyroid gland. The majority of T_3, which is the metabolically more potent of the two hormones, is produced by peripheral conversion of T_4 by the enzyme 5-deiodinase.[1] Reverse T_3 (rT_3) is also produced by an isoenzyme of 5-deiodinase (5'-deiodinase). In times of illness, the ratio of T_3 to rT_3 production may shift because of the differing activity of these isoenzymes. Reverse T_3 has no known metabolic effects and does not influence TSH production or secretion. Increased rT_3 is commonly seen in the fetus and in severely ill patients, particularly those who have decreased T_3 production due to catabolic states.

Thyroid hormone circulates in both free and bound forms. The majority of hormone is bound to serum proteins, predominantly thyroid-binding globulin. The remainder circulates in the free form, which is the metabolically active form.

The effects of thyroid hormone on the body are many.[1] Thyroid hormone plays an essential role in growth and development, as well as in central nervous system development, heat production, and regulation of metabolism of carbohydrates, lipids, and proteins. The maturity level of the hypothalamic-pituitary-thyroid axis must be considered to correctly interpret thyroid function tests in newborns and children. In the fetus, this axis is complex and only partially characterized.[2] In the second half of gestation, thyroid hormone production increases, as does the secretion of TSH; both increase to their peak values at term. When a full-term infant is born, there is an acute surge in TSH in response to exposure to the extrauterine environment, which peaks at about 30 minutes of life and then remains elevated for 3 to 5 days after birth. This is correlated with a marked increase in free T_4 and T_3 levels as well, which gradually decline. During childhood, there is a progressive decrease in TSH secretion and T_4 production (Table 89-1).

CLINICAL PRESENTATION

Hypothyroidism

The clinical appearance of a newborn with congenital hypothyroidism is generally normal. The classic signs and symptoms of an untreated infant—large tongue, coarse facies, hoarse cry, umbilical hernia, prolonged jaundice, wide posterior fontanelle, constipation, lethargy, and irritability—are rarely seen because newborn screening identifies infants before these signs and symptoms become apparent. However, any of these findings in a newborn should trigger a consideration of hypothyroidism, and thyroid function tests should be performed before receiving the results of the newborn screen.

Hashimoto thyroiditis is the most common cause of acquired hypothyroidism in children.[1] The presentation is variable, and the child may be euthyroid, hypothyroid, or transiently hyperthyroid at diagnosis. Typically, the laboratory tests demonstrate an elevated TSH, low T_4, and normal T_3. The clinical signs and symptoms of hypothyroidism may not appear until the disease is severe, and growth failure may be the only sign. Occasionally a child may complain of cold intolerance or constipation and may have bradycardia and delayed reflexes on examination. Usually the thyroid is symmetrically enlarged and firm on palpation. Contrary to popular belief, hypothyroidism generally does not cause obesity.

Hashimoto thyroiditis tends to run in families, with a positive family history present in 30% to 40% of patients. There is also a female predominance. It is important to remember that because Hashimoto thyroiditis is an autoimmune disease, it can be associated with other autoimmune disorders, particularly diabetes mellitus and adrenal cortical insufficiency (Addison's disease). Autoimmune thyroiditis is also more common in patients with certain chromosomal disorders, such as Down syndrome, Klinefelter syndrome, and Turner syndrome.

Hyperthyroidism

Neonatal thyrotoxicosis is a rare disease, but it can be life threatening. It occurs because of transplacental passage of TSH receptor-stimulating antibodies from a mother with Graves disease (even if the disease is inactive in the mother).[2] The higher the titer of antibody in the mother during the third trimester, the more likely the infant is to develop the disease. Antithyroid medication taken by the mother during gestation crosses the placenta as well, inhibiting fetal thyroid hormone production. This may result in goiter and hypothy-

Table 89-1 Normal Values* for Thyroid Function Tests

Age	TSH (μU/mL)	T₄ (μg/dL)	Free T₄ (ng/dL)	T₃ (ng/dL)	Reverse T₃ (ng/dL)
Premature infants (26-32 wk): 3-4 days of life	0.8-6.9 (2.3)	2.6-14.0 (6.4)	0.4-2.8 (1.5)	24-132 (65)	
Full-term infants: 1-3 days of life		8.2-20.0 (14.6)		89-405 (273)	90-250[†]
Full-term infants: 3-7 days of life	1.3-16.0 (4.9)	6.0-15.9 (12.0)	2.0-4.9 (3.5)	91-300 (190)	
1-12 mo of life	0.9-7.7 (2.9)	6.1-14.9 (9.8)	0.9-2.6 (1.6)	82-250 (175)	
Prepubertal	0.6-5.5 (1.9)	1-3 yr: 6.8-13.5 (9.3) 3-10 yr: 5.5-12.8 (8.6)	0.8-2.2 (1.6)	119-218 (168)	10-50
Pubertal	0.5-4.8 (1.6)	4.9-13.0 (8.0)	0.8-2.3 (1.5)	80-185 (116)	10-50

*Range of values, with mean in parentheses.
[†]Levels decline to the adult range by 1 wk of life.
TSH, thyroid-stimulating hormone; T₃, triiodothyronine; T₄, thyroxine.
Modified from Esoterix.

roidism in the fetus or newborn. Generally, neonatal hypothyroidism induced by maternal medication resolves within 1 week, and no treatment is indicated. Transplacental passage of maternal medication may delay the onset of clinical symptoms of neonatal thyrotoxicosis.

The clinical presentation of thyrotoxicosis can include fetal tachycardia. In a newborn, a multitude of problems can be seen, including irritability, tachycardia, hypertension, jaundice, poor weight gain, and exophthalmos. High-output cardiac failure can occur. Affected infants need to have close monitoring of vital signs and frequent thyroid function tests. Long term, these infants may develop advanced bone age, craniosynostosis, learning problems, and mental retardation.

In children, the most common cause of hyperthyroidism is Graves disease, an autoimmune disorder in which TSH receptor antibodies or thyroid-stimulating immunoglobulins are present and cause the overproduction and secretion of thyroid hormone.[1] Laboratory studies generally demonstrate a markedly suppressed TSH with an elevated total T₄, free T₄, and T₃. Symptoms may include palpitations, fatigue, weight loss, increased bowel movements, and inability to concentrate. On examination, the thyroid is generally diffusely enlarged, and the patient may be tachycardic and hyperreflexic. Ophthalmopathy may occur in children, but less commonly than in adults.

Thyroid storm is a rare complication of hyperthyroidism, but it is a medical emergency. It consists of acute hyperthermia and tachycardia in a patient with hyperthyroidism and may be accompanied by confusion or coma. Heart failure can result from the tachycardia. Thyroid storm may be precipitated by infection or surgery. It has also been reported following treatment with radioactive iodine.

DIFFERENTIAL DIAGNOSIS

Hypothyroidism

Congenital hypothyroidism can be permanent or transient and can be classified as primary (an inherent defect of the thyroid gland or thyroid hormone production or secretion), secondary (pituitary hypothyroidism), or tertiary

(hypothalamic hypothyroidism).[2] Permanent primary hypothyroidism is most common and is usually caused by thyroid gland dysgenesis. The gland may be ectopically located, hypoplastic, or absent. In some parts of the world, iodine deficiency is an important cause of congenital hypothyroidism (cretinism); however, this condition is almost nonexistent in the United States.

Transient congenital hypothyroidism is rare but can be caused by fetal exposure to medications, such as antithyroid drugs taken by the mother (this is generally apparent from the history); iodine deficiency or excess in the mother; or maternal TSH receptor-blocking antibodies that cross the placenta and prevent fetal TSH from attaching to the TSH receptor on the fetal thyroid gland.

A low T₄ and low TSH are indicative of pituitary or hypothalamic dysfunction. Central hypothyroidism should be suspected in children with a history of central nervous system disease, such as hydrocephalus, hemorrhage, brain tumor, or meningitis, or central nervous system malformations. In any patient with central hypothyroidism, it is important that other pituitary hormone deficiencies be investigated, such as deficiencies of adrenocorticotropic hormone, growth hormone, gonadotropins, and vasopressin.

Nonthyroidal illness, also known as sick euthyroid syndrome, is common in many patients who either are acutely ill or have a prolonged illness, particularly if the patient is malnourished.[1] Starvation appears to inhibit the deiodination of T₄ to T₃, which may or may not be an adaptive physiologic response to decrease the metabolism. If the illness progresses, often both T₄ and T₃ levels decrease, but the TSH level remains normal or low. In mild cases, free T₄ levels remain normal. Reverse T₃ levels are generally elevated, because conversion of T₄ to rT₃ is not impaired, and the degradation of rT₃ is reduced. A very low total T₄ level (<4 μg/dL) is associated with a high risk of mortality (about 50%). T₄ levels below 2 μg/dL increase the risk of mortality to 80%.[3]

Certain medications can also cause hypothyroidism.[4] Drugs that down-regulate the release of TSH from the pituitary include glucocorticoids and dopamine. Usually, total T₄, free T₄, and T₃ levels are also low in patients being treated with these medications. Glucocorticoids appear to inhibit the peripheral conversion of T_4 to T_3. Drugs that affect thyroid hormone synthesis and release include amiodarone, iodine, and lithium. Amiodarone, used to treat cardiac arrhythmias, contains a large amount of iodine and can cause hypothyroidism. Although iodine is essential for proper thyroid function, large amounts can actually block the release of preformed thyroid hormone and the synthesis of new hormone. This is known as the Wolff-Chaikoff effect. Iodine-induced hypothyroidism can also be seen in infants or children who receive large amounts of cutaneous iodine in the hospital. This can occur at any age but may be more common in premature infants, because iodine is absorbed more readily through their skin than that of older children. Lithium carbonate, often used to treat manic depression, inhibits thyroid hormone release.

Antiepileptics, particularly phenytoin and carbamazepine, cause an up-regulation of hepatic metabolism and therefore an increased clearance of total T_4 and free T_4. Generally, TSH and T_3 levels are normal, and an increased TSH level may be indicative of hypothyroidism.

Hyperthyroidism

In addition to Graves disease, other causes of hyperthyroidism include autonomously functioning thyroid nodules, infections of the thyroid, McCune-Albright syndrome, and TSH-secreting adenomas.[1] Amiodarone may cause hyperthyroidism in some patients. This is more common in those with underlying goiters or thyroiditis, but the drug can also cause a thyroiditis-type syndrome in patients without pre-existing thyroid disease.

EVALUATION

Newborn screening for congenital hypothyroidism has dramatically reduced the risk of mental retardation in affected infants. The more rapid the initiation of therapy (the first weeks of life), the better the neurologic outcome for the child; children who are not treated before 3 months of age almost universally have some impairment of cognitive abilities.[2] The newborn screen is based on the measurement of T_4 or TSH (or both) in a dried blood filter paper sample obtained during the first days of life. Ideally, the infant should be at least 3 to 5 days of age to avoid false-positive results. However, given that infants are often discharged 2 days after birth, this is not always possible. If T_4 is being measured, infants with a T_4 level below a specific cutoff point have their TSH measured as well. This method can miss subclinical hypothyroidism, however—that is, infants with normal T_4 but elevated TSH levels. If the primary screening measures TSH, the cutoff for an elevated TSH level is 20 to 25 μU/mL in most programs. Although measuring TSH has a slightly higher detection rate for congenital hypothyroidism, there are more false-positives owing to the early screening. Also, this method misses infants with secondary and tertiary hypothyroidism (who have low TSH levels).

When a newborn has been identified by screening as possibly having hypothyroidism, thyroid function tests should be performed to confirm the diagnosis in a timely manner. At a minimum, thyroid function testing should include TSH and free T_4; if possible, total T_4 and T_3 should also be obtained. Ideally, a newborn with apparent hypothyroidism should be cared for at a tertiary medical center with a pediatric endocrinologist on staff. If laboratory tests confirm elevated TSH and decreased T_4 levels, additional information can be obtained from a technetium thyroid scan and a bone-age radiograph of the knee. The technetium scan can rapidly establish whether there is an ectopic or hypoplastic thyroid, athyreosis, or a goiter indicative of dyshormonogenesis. The radiograph is helpful in term infants because absent or hypoplastic epiphyseal centers at the distal femoral or proximal tibial sites suggest prolonged hypothyroidism in utero. Obtaining the technetium scan should not delay the initiation of treatment, because L-thyroxine therapy will not affect the results of the scan if it is obtained within 14 days of starting treatment. If no thyroid gland is seen on the scan, this is usually indicative of thyroid agenesis; however, it could also be due to thyroid receptor blockade by TSH receptor-blocking antibodies. A thyroid ultrasound study is useful in this situation.

Low thyroid hormone in the setting of a low or normal TSH level is suggestive of secondary hypothyroidism and hypopituitarism. An infant with this presentation should be monitored carefully for hypoglycemia and immediately evaluated for deficiencies of cortisol and growth hormone. In males, microphallus is also a common finding. It is imperative that this evaluation be done in a timely manner, and replacement thyroid hormone in this setting should *never* be given until an adequate cortisol level has been documented. Thyroid hormone supplementation increases cortisol clearance from the circulation and could precipitate cardiovascular collapse in patients with glucocorticoid insufficiency.

Evaluation of older children with suspected hypothyroidism should include, at a minimum, TSH and free T_4 levels; preferably, total T_4 and T_3 levels should also be obtained. Most patients with Hashimoto thyroiditis have circulating antithyroid antibodies. Antithyroid peroxisomal and antithyroglobulin antibodies are most prevalent and are used most frequently to make the diagnosis. Low thyroid hormone levels with a low or normal TSH can also be seen with an inherited deficiency of thyroid-binding globulin. The free T_4 level should be normal in this condition, and treatment is not indicated.

The initial laboratory tests for the evaluation of hyperthyroidism should include TSH, free T_4, and total T_3 levels. The TSH is usually markedly suppressed. Measurements of antithyroid peroxisomal and antithyroglobulin antibodies, TSH receptor antibodies, and thyroid-stimulating immunoglobulins should be obtained to assist in differentiating between Graves disease and other causes of hyperthyroidism. If a child has hyperthyroidism and a TSH level that is persistently greater than 1 μU/mL, an evaluation for a TSH-secreting pituitary tumor should be done, although this is rare.[1]

TREATMENT

Hypothyroidism

The goal of treatment for congenital hypothyroidism is to adequately replace the thyroid hormone as early as possible to maximize the chances for normal neurologic development.[2] Levothyroxine (T_4) is the accepted treatment. The starting dose is generally 10 to 15 μg/kg in one daily dose.

The medication can be given as a crushed tablet in a small amount of milk or water (1 mL); soy milk should not be used because soy impedes absorption of the medication. The goal is to achieve a T_4 level in the upper range of normal. The TSH level may take some time to completely normalize. Overtreatment with thyroxine can lead to advanced bone age, craniosynostosis, and osteoporosis. In infants with congenital hypothyroidism who have not been treated for months, it is advisable to work up to a full replacement dose over a week or two to avoid precipitating the rapid mobilization of fluid. Infants with presumed transient hypothyroidism generally do not require treatment unless the low T_4 and elevated TSH levels persist beyond 2 weeks. If the hypothyroidism is due to TSH receptor-blocking antibodies from the mother, treatment is usually needed for 2 to 5 months, with adjustments based on the T_4 level. Infants should be seen frequently until 12 months of age; after that, they should be seen every 3 months until age 3 years, after which they should be seen every 6 months. This presupposes that the parents are compliant with treatment; obviously, if there is any concern in this regard, the child should be seen more frequently.

Treatment of a child with hypothyroidism due to Hashimoto thyroiditis should begin slowly, particularly if the child was profoundly hypothyroid.[1] Rapid correction of the hypothyroidism may result in pseudotumor cerebri or accelerated skeletal maturation, compromising final adult height. By starting treatment with levothyroxine at a dose of approximately 2 µg/kg per day, the TSH level should come close to the normal range and the T_4 level should normalize within 2 months. The usual total daily dose for acquired hypothyroidism in childhood through adolescence is 50 to 100 µg/day. Central hypothyroidism is also treated with levothyroxine. Because TSH levels cannot be used to monitor treatment in central hypothyroidism, measurement of free T_4 levels is suggested.

Whether to treat patients with nonthyroidal illness is controversial. It is not clear that treatment is beneficial; however, it has not been proved harmful. Mild cases are generally not treated. Some experts agree that if the T_4 level is less than 4 µg/dL, thyroid hormone administration—both T_4 and T_3—should be considered; administration of only T_4 may lead to an increase in rT_3 only.[3] However, treatment must be evaluated in the context of the underlying illness. Particularly in cardiac patients, thyroid replacement must be initiated very slowly and under the observation of an endocrinologist and an intensivist. Thyroid levels have to be monitored frequently, and as serum T_3 levels increase, administration of T_3 can be decreased. It is important to remember, however, that there is no clear evidence that treatment will be beneficial to the patient.

Certain agents affect the absorption of thyroid hormone. Soy, calcium carbonate, and ferrous sulfate all interfere with thyroid hormone absorption from the gut. Therefore, patients on thyroid hormone replacement should be instructed to take their medication separately from these agents.

Hyperthyroidism

Treatment of congenital hyperthyroidism generally includes antithyroid medications (propylthiouracil [PTU] 5 to 10 mg/kg per day or methimazole [MMI] 0.5 to 1 mg/kg per day) and beta-blockers as needed (propranolol 1 mg/kg per day).[2] Frequent reevaluation and monitoring are mandatory. As the TSH receptor-stimulating antibodies are cleared from the infant's circulation, spontaneous recovery begins; medication can generally be weaned between 3 and 6 months.

The first-line treatment for Graves disease is antithyroid drug therapy with PTU 5 to 10 mg/kg per day in two to three divided doses or MMI 0.5 to 1 mg/kg per day in one to three divided doses.[1] These medications inhibit thyroid hormone formation but not its release, so it may take a number of weeks until circulating thyroid hormone levels begin to decrease. A beta-blocker such as propranolol may also be used to control tachycardia. By 4 to 6 weeks, the dose of PTU or MMI can generally be reduced if the patient's thyroid hormone levels are normalizing. PTU and MMI can have significant side effects, including elevated liver enzymes, leukopenia, granulocytopenia, arthritis, and rashes. Serious complications include agranulocytosis, which is generally reversible if the medication is stopped, and severe hepatitis, which may not be reversible. Hepatotoxicity is more frequent with PTU than MMI.

Treatment of thyroid storm may include propranolol (2 to 3 mg/kg per day, divided every 6 hours) to control the tachycardia; dexamethasone (1 to 2 mg every 6 hours) to reduce conversion of T_4 to T_3; and intravenous sodium iodide (125 to 250 mg/day) or Lugol's solution (concentrated iodide; 5 drops by mouth every 8 hours) to decrease the release of thyroid hormone from the thyroid gland. PTU (6 to 10 mg/kg per day; maximum 200 to 300 mg/day) or MMI (0.6 to 0.7 mg/kg per day) should be started, although the effect will not be seen for several days.

Remission rates after treatment with drug therapy are generally less than 30%, although treatment is usually continued for at least 2 to 4 years to try to attain remission. Some children require more definitive treatment, such as thyroidectomy or radioiodine therapy.

CONSULTATION

A pediatric endocrinologist should always be consulted for evaluation of a patient with possible thyroid storm. Whenever possible, a pediatric endocrinologist should be consulted to evaluate any neonate born to a woman with a history of Graves disease, even if the mother was euthyroid during her pregnancy. Thyroid-stimulating immunoglobulins may persist many years after therapy with radioactive iodine. These can be passed transplacentally and cause fetal or neonatal thyroid disease, despite a maternal euthyroid state. If thyroid function tests are performed on a hospitalized patient, a pediatric endocrinologist should be consulted to interpret the results, because interpretation of such tests obtained during periods of illness can be challenging. This situation frequently occurs during the management of newborn infants and in patients with sick euthyroid syndrome. Most often, thyroid disorders are diagnosed and managed in the outpatient setting.

ADMISSION CRITERIA

- Neonatal thyrotoxicosis
- Thyroid storm

- Congenital hypothyroidism or severe hypothyroidism in an older child if there is any suspicion that the family is not administering the medication properly

DISCHARGE CRITERIA

- Resolution of acute symptoms of neonatal thyrotoxicosis or thyroid storm and improving thyroid function tests on medication.
- For any child with thyroid disease, the family must understand proper dosing and administration of medication, and thyroid function tests should be improving.

IN A NUTSHELL

- Normal thyroid function is critical for proper growth and development in children.
- Neonatal hypo- or hyperthyroidism is a medical emergency and needs to be treated without delay to prevent long-term deleterious consequences.
- Thyroid storm (hyperthermia, tachycardia, confusion, coma) is a medical emergency and can result in heart failure if not treated aggressively.
- Evaluation of a patient with suspected thyroid disease should include TSH and free T_4 levels, at a minimum; total T_4 and T_3 levels, if possible; and thyroid antibodies if autoimmune thyroid disease is suspected.
- A pediatric endocrinologist should be involved in the care of infants and children with thyroid disease, if possible.

ON THE HORIZON

- Studies continue to provide evidence that early treatment of congenital hypothyroidism and a rapid normalization of thyroid function in infants is essential for optimizing neurologic development.[5]
- Pharmacologic therapies have traditionally been used as first-line treatments for children with Graves disease. However, some centers now favor radioactive iodine as the initial therapy because of the potential adverse effects of PTU and MMI and the frequent need for long-term medical therapy.[1]
- There does not appear to be any increase in thyroid cancer or congenital abnormalities in the offspring of women treated with radioactive iodine; however, more long-term data are needed.

SUGGESTED READING

DeGroot LJ: Dangerous dogmas in medicine: The nonthyroidal illness syndrome. Clin Endocrinol Metab 1999;84:151-164.

Fisher DA: Disorders of the thyroid in the newborn and infant. In Sperling MA (ed): Pediatric Endocrinology. Philadelphia, WB Saunders, 2002, pp 161-186.

Fisher DA: Thyroid disorders in childhood and adolescence. In Sperling MA (ed): Pediatric Endocrinology. Philadelphia, WB Saunders, 2002, pp 187-209.

Foley TP Jr: Acquired hypothyroidism during infancy, childhood, and adolescence. In Braverman LE, Utiger RD (eds): Werner and Ingbar's The Thyroid. Philadelphia, Lippincott, 1996, pp 994-999.

MacGillivray MH: Congenital hypothyroidism. In Pescovitz OH, Eugster EA (eds): Pediatric Endocrinology: Mechanisms, Manifestations, and Management. Philadelphia, Lippincott, 2004, pp 490-507.

Rivkees SA: Hypothyroidism and hyperthyroidism in children. In Pescovitz OH, Eugster EA (eds): Pediatric Endocrinology: Mechanisms, Manifestations, and Management. Philadelphia, Lippincott, 2004, pp 508-521.

REFERENCES

1. Fisher DA: Thyroid disorders in childhood and adolescence. In Sperling MA (ed): Pediatric Endocrinology. Philadelphia, WB Saunders, 2002, pp 187-209.

2. Fisher DA: Disorders of the thyroid in the newborn and infant. In Sperling MA (ed): Pediatric Endocrinology. Philadelphia, Saunders, 2002, pp 161-186.

3. DeGroot LJ: Dangerous dogmas in medicine: The nonthyroidal illness syndrome. Clin Endocrinol Metab 1999;84:151-164.

4. Rivkees SA: Hypothyroidism and hyperthyroidism in children. In Pescovitz OH, Eugster EA (eds): Pediatric Endocrinology: Mechanisms, Manifestations, and Management. Philadelphia, Lippincott, 2004, pp 508-521.

5. Selva KA, Harper A, Downs A, et al: Neurodevelopmental outcomes in congenital hypothyroidism: Comparison of initial T_4 dose and time to reach target T_4 and TSH. J Pediatr 2005;147:775-780.

CHAPTER 90

Disorders of Pituitary Function

Mary Pat Gallagher and Sharon E. Oberfield

The pituitary gland has been called the "master gland" because of its role in the regulation of endocrine target organs, such as the adrenal gland, ovary, testis, and thyroid gland. Disorders of the pituitary and hypothalamus may therefore result in disruption of any of these hypothalamic-pituitary–target organ axes. Abnormalities in end-organ hormone release caused by pituitary dysfunction are considered "secondary," and those caused by a hypothalamic abnormality are considered "tertiary." For example, abnormal thyroid function caused by a decrease in thyrotropin-releasing factor from the hypothalamus is "tertiary hypothyroidism." Failure of growth and failure of sexual maturation are two common presentations of hypothalamic-pituitary disease in the pediatric population. These disorders may be genetic or acquired.

The hypothalamus secretes releasing factors that travel via the portal circulation to the anterior pituitary gland. These factors stimulate or inhibit release of the six peptide hormones produced by the anterior pituitary gland: growth hormone, prolactin, thyroid-stimulating hormone, adrenocorticotropic hormone (ACTH), follicle-stimulating hormone, and luteinizing hormone.

The posterior pituitary gland releases arginine vasopressin, also known as antidiuretic hormone (ADH), and oxytocin. The neurons that produce vasopressin originate in the hypothalamus. For this reason, diabetes insipidus (DI) will occur with hypothalamic disease, but it may not always occur with pituitary disease, even if the stalk has been transected (depending on the level of transection).

GENETIC CAUSES OF PITUITARY HORMONE DEFICIENCY

Several genetic causes of multiple pituitary hormone deficiency have been described (Table 90-1). Congenital malformations involving the midline of the central nervous system (CNS) are associated with pituitary deficiencies. Findings on magnetic resonance imaging may include a small or absent anterior pituitary gland, an absent or ectopic posterior pituitary "bright spot," or a transected pituitary stalk.[1]

ACQUIRED CAUSES OF PITUITARY HORMONE DEFICIENCY

Mass-occupying lesions in the hypothalamic area may result in disruption of pituitary function. Tumors such as craniopharyngioma and, less commonly, germinoma and astrocytoma may first present during childhood with growth failure, DI, or visual complaints (or any combination). Hypothalamic hamartomas and pineal tumors are associated with precocious pubertal development during childhood.

Pituitary adenomas are rare in childhood and may or may not actively produce peptide hormones. When active, they most often secrete prolactin (50%) or growth hormone (20%). Adenomas that secrete other types of anterior pituitary hormones are extremely rare.[2]

Langerhans cell histiocytosis is a rare disorder that most often presents with DI, but it may also affect the production of other pituitary hormones. Inflammatory, postinfectious, and traumatic lesions of the CNS may cause hypopituitarism as well. CNS irradiation predisposes to the loss of pituitary function, depending on the dose received. Higher doses may precipitate precocious pubertal development.

DIABETES INSIPIDUS

DI is defined as an inability to concentrate urine despite increasing serum osmolality as a result of inadequate secretion of ADH (central DI) or unresponsiveness of the kidney to ADH (nephrogenic DI).

Differential Diagnosis

- Osmotic diuretics (mannitol, high glucose, intravenous contrast)
- Hypercalcemia or hypokalemia (can cause ADH unresponsiveness)

Diagnosis and Evaluation

To establish the diagnosis of DI, it is necessary to confirm that urinary osmolality remains inappropriately low during a period when serum osmolality has increased to an abnormally high level. This requires fluid restriction and careful monitoring of the clinical status of the patient. Fluid restriction in a patient with true DI can result in metabolic derangement and should take place only in a setting in which the patient can be monitored intensively and metabolic derangement can be corrected immediately. This is not recommended in infants.[3]

If conditions allow for this procedure to be undertaken safely, the following regimen is suggested to demonstrate the presence or absence of DI:

Limit intravenous fluids to insensible loss (40% maintenance or 400 to 600 mL/m^2/day) plus hourly replacement of urine output greater than 4 mL/kg/hr.

Urine output should be replaced as 5% dextrose in water (D5W) if urine osmolality is low and urine specific gravity is less than 1.005.

Monitor input and output hourly.

Monitor urine and serum electrolytes every 2 hours.

Monitor urine and serum osmolality every 6 hours.

If polyuria (>4 mL/kg/hr) persists and urine remains dilute (low urine sodium, low osmolality, low specific gravity)

Table 90-1 Genetic Causes of Multiple Pituitary Hormone Deficiencies

Gene	Hormones	Inheritance	Other
POU1F1 (PIT1)	GH, Prl, TSH	AR, AD	
PROP1	GH, Prl, TSH, LH, FSH, and sometimes ACTH	AR, X-linked	
HESX1	Variable, including AVP	AR	Associated with septo-optic dysplasia
LHX3	Variable, including GH, Prl, TSH, LH, FSH	—	

ACTH, adrenocorticotropic hormone; AD, autosomal dominant; AR, autosomal recessive; AVP, arginine vasopressin; FSH, follicle-stimulating hormone; GH, growth hormone; LH, luteinizing hormone; Prl, prolactin; TSH, thyroid-stimulating hormone.

despite climbing serum sodium and serum osmolality (>295 mOsm/kg), the diagnosis of DI is likely. Blood should be sent at this time for measurement of ADH to determine whether the DI is central or nephrogenic.

Once the diagnosis of diabetes insipidus is established, two methods can be used as guides for fluid management:

Method 1: Give maintenance intravenous fluids as normal saline (NS) or $^1/_2$NS. Replace urine output in excess of 4 mL/kg/hr with D5W or D5/$^1/_4$NS, depending on the serum sodium level.

Method 2: Give intravenous fluids for insensible loss of 400 to 600 mL/m^2/day as NS or $^1/_2$NS. Replace all urine output with D5W or D5/$^1/_4$NS, depending on the serum sodium level.

The second method ensures that the fluids will be adjusted for urine output and protects against overhydration if a change in the patient's status is anticipated. Serum glucose needs to be monitored closely with both methods because patients may become hyperglycemic, which can worsen the polyuria. For glucose levels higher than 250 mg/dL, an insulin drip may be required (starting dose, 0.03 U/kg/hr).

Treatment

Treatment with ADH can be initiated if serum sodium is greater than 145 mEq/L and serum osmolality is greater than 195 mOsm. The dose should be titrated according to the patient's response to the initial dose. The most flexible regimen is an aqueous pitressin drip. Its extremely short half-life enables rapid changes in dose.

Aqueous pitressin as an intravenous drip:

- Aqueous pitressin is manufactured as 20 U = 1 mL.
- Add 0.1 mL to 20 mL NS, and then add 5 mL of that solution to 500 mL NS so that 1 mL = 1 mU aqueous pitressin.
- The usual starting dose is 0.10 mU/kg/hr. The dose can be adjusted every 30 minutes until the desired trend in serum sodium is noted. Doses higher than 0.8 mU/kg/hr are not likely to increase the antidiuretic effect.

Subcutaneous aqueous pitressin (20 U/mL) can also be used. It has a half-life of 3 to 6 hours.

- The suggested starting dose is 0.05 to 0.1 U/kg per dose subcutaneously (SC)
- Examples:
  1 U SC every 4 to 6 hours for infants
  2.5 U SC every 4 to 6 hours for toddlers

5 U SC every 4 to 6 hours for children
Maximum of 10 U SC every 4 to 6 hours for adults.

Parenteral desmopressin acetate (DDAVP) (0.1 mL = 0.4 μg) has a half-life of 6 to 12 hours (or longer).

- The suggested starting dose is 0.01 to 0.03 μg/kg per dose intravenously (IV) or SC daily or twice daily
- Examples:
  0.05 mL SC or IV every 12 hours for infants
  0.1 mL SC or IV every 12 hours for toddlers
  0.15 mL SC or IV every 12 hours for children
  Up to 0.5 mL SC or IV every 12 hours for adults

Nasal DDAVP (0.1 mL = 10 μg) has a half-life of 6 to 24 hours.

- Nasal dose of 5 to 20 μg/day (0.05 to 0.2 mL) divided twice daily or daily as needed
- 1 spray = 10 μg or 0.1 mL = 10 μg
- The nasal dose is 10 times the parenteral dose in micrograms

Oral DDAVP (0.1- and 0.2-mg tablets)

- Dose of 0.025 to 0.4 mg orally every 8 to 24 hours

Important Points To Remember

- DI may be transient.
- Posttraumatic or postoperative DI may be followed by the syndrome of inappropriate ADH secretion (SIADH), which may be followed by recurrence of DI (triphasic pattern of DI/SIADH/DI).
- Avoid hyponatremia, which can exacerbate posttraumatic cerebral edema.
- In general, always start with the lowest recommended dose of DDAVP or aqueous pitressin and adjust the dosage as necessary based on ongoing laboratory evaluations.

SYNDROME OF INAPPROPRIATE ANTIDIURETIC HORMONE SECRETION

SIADH is an uncommon cause of hyponatremia in the inpatient setting. Hyponatremia (Na <130 to 135 mEq/L) is more often explained by an underlying disease process. However, it is important to consider the diagnosis of SIADH in a patient in whom hyponatremia with decreased urine output develops. The presence of CNS disease or pulmonary disease predisposes to the development of this disorder. By definition, the patient needs to be euvolemic or hypervolemic for the secretion of ADH to be considered "inappropriate."[4]

Differential Diagnosis

- Intravascular volume depletion, hyponatremic dehydration
- Congestive heart failure
- Inadequate free water excretion secondary to ACTH/cortisol deficiency or thyroid hormone deficiency
- Hyperglycemia, hypertriglyceridemia (factitious)
- Other forms of salt loss (GI)
- Salt wasting via the kidney (should be accompanied by *increased* urine output)

Diagnosis and Evaluation

The diagnosis of SIADH should be considered when a patient has decreased urine output and low serum sodium. The evaluation should include strict measurement of input and output, measurement of serum sodium and osmolality, and measurement of urine sodium and osmolality. Findings should include the absence of edema or dehydration on physical examination, and there should be evidence of intravascular volume expansion (low blood urea nitrogen, low hematocrit, low uric acid) on laboratory evaluation. Causes of factitious hyponatremia (hypertriglyceridemia, hyperglycemia) and other hormonal deficiencies that may interfere with free water excretion (hypothyroidism, glucocorticoid insufficiency) should be ruled out.

Treatment

- Restriction of fluid to 400 to 600 mL/m^2/day (40% of maintenance) or less (not <25% of daily maintenance)
- Strict input and output; monitor urine specific gravity
- Frequent measurement of serum sodium levels
- If acute life-threatening symptoms are present or if the development of hyponatremia is acute and the sodium level is less than 120 mEq/L with symptoms of neurologic deterioration or brain swelling:

  Replace urine Na and K losses with 3% saline and appropriate amounts of K.
  Give 0.5 to 1 mg/kg furosemide by intravenous push, followed by hourly determinations of urine Na and K.

- If necessary, hypertonic (3%) saline can be used to raise serum sodium to 125 mEq/L (3% saline = 0.5 mEq Na/mL; must be given slowly) by using the following formula:

$$(125 - \text{Present serum Na}) \times 0.6 \, (\text{Na space}) \times \text{Wt (kg)}$$

Examples

If you wish to raise serum Na by 10 mEq,

$$10 \times 0.6 \, \text{kg} = 6 \, \text{mEq/kg} = 12 \, \text{mL 3\% saline/kg}$$

If you wish to raise serum Na by 5 mEq,

$$5 \times 0.6 \, \text{kg} = 3 \, \text{mEq/kg} = 6 \, \text{mL 3\% saline/kg}$$

CONSULTATION

- Pediatric endocrinologist
- Pediatric neurosurgeon, as needed
- Pediatric intensivist, as needed

ADMISSION CRITERIA

- Electrolyte imbalance
- Altered sensorium
- Vasomotor instability

DISCHARGE CRITERIA

- Input and output can be monitored at home, a caregiver can administer medication as needed, and the patient is clinically stable
- Regular follow-up for monitoring of serum electrolytes and the underlying disease is arranged

IN A NUTSHELL

- Regulation of water balance is critical and depends on appropriate release of ADH, thyroid hormone, and cortisol.
- DI is most often secondary to congenital abnormalities of the posterior pituitary or disturbance of the pituitary stalk in the setting of a CNS tumor or surgery, or both.
- If DI is secondary to surgery, it may be transient and part of the "triphasic" response of DI, followed by SIADH, followed by DI.
- Hyponatremia in childhood is rarely secondary to SIADH but is more often seen in the setting of dehydration.

ON THE HORIZON

- Missense mutations that alter the folding of proteins may result in failure to deliver cell membrane proteins to the cell surface. This has been reported in mutations of the vasopressin 2 receptor in cases of congenital DI. The development of "pharmacochaperones," or membrane-permeable antagonists that restore the cell surface expression of receptors, may play a role in the management of some forms of congenital DI in the future.[5]

REFERENCES

1. Parks JS: Genetic forms of hypopituitarism. In Finberg L, Kleinman RE (eds): Saunders Manual of Pediatric Practice. Philadelphia, WB Saunders, 2002, pp 840-843.
2. Rosenfeld R: Disorders of growth hormone and insulin like growth factor and action. In Sperling MA (ed): Pediatric Endocrinology. Philadelphia, WB Saunders, 2002, pp 118-169.
3. Maghnie M, Cosi G, Genovese E, et al: Central diabetes insipidus in children and young adults. N Engl J Med 2000;343:998-1007.
4. Muglia LJ, Majzoub JA: Disorders of the posterior pituitary. In Sperling MA (ed): Pediatric Endocrinology. Philadelphia, WB Saunders, 2002, pp 289-322.
5. Wuller S, Wiesner B, Loffler A, et al: Pharmacochaperones post-translationally enhance cell surface expression by increasing conformational stability of wild-type and mutant vasopressin V2 receptors. J Biol Chem 2004;279:47254-47263.

CHAPTER 91

Disorders of Calcium Metabolism

Chhavi Agarwal, Mary Pat Gallagher, and Sharon E. Oberfield

Calcium is the most abundant mineral in the body. It is required for proper functioning of numerous intracellular and extracellular processes, including muscle contraction, nerve conduction, hormone release, and blood coagulation. Calcium also plays a unique role in intracellular signaling and is involved in the regulation of enzyme activity. Maintenance of calcium homeostasis is therefore critical.

Calcium absorption and regulation involve a complex interplay between multiple organ systems and regulatory hormones. There are three major targets for calcium regulation: bone, kidney, and the intestine. Parathyroid hormone (PTH) and the activated form of vitamin D act at bone, intestine, and the kidney to increase serum calcium levels. Calcitonin plays a minor role in decreasing serum calcium levels via its effect on bone and the kidney.

The majority of total body calcium exists as bone mineral, with serum calcium representing less than 1% of total body calcium. Although total serum calcium levels are routinely measured, it is the ionized fraction that is biologically active. Total serum calcium levels include both ionized and bound calcium. The ionized calcium level reflects changes in albumin, serum pH, serum phosphate, serum magnesium, and serum bicarbonate. Ionized calcium may be reduced by exogenous factors such as citrate from transfused blood or free fatty acid from total parenteral nutrition. At physiologic pH, 40% of total serum calcium is bound to albumin; 10% is complexed with bicarbonates, phosphate, or citrate; and the remaining 50% exists in the ionized form.

HYPOCALCEMIA

The definition of hypocalcemia is age dependent. Hypocalcemia is generally defined as a total serum calcium level of less than 8.5 mg/dL (ionized calcium <4.6 mg/dL) in children and adolescents, less than 8 mg/dL (ionized calcium <4 mg/dL or 0.98 mmol/L) in term neonates, and less than 7 mg/dL (ionized calcium <5.2 mg/dL or 1.2 mmol/L) in preterm neonates. Individual laboratory norms should be used when available.[1]

Clinical Presentation

Hypocalcemia is frequently observed in the inpatient setting, and incidentally noted biochemical hypocalcemia is often asymptomatic. Symptomatic hypocalcemia occurs in response to a rapid decrease in calcium concentration, as well as in response to the absolute calcium level. Symptoms tend to be more severe if hypocalcemia develops acutely.

The predominant clinical symptoms and signs in children and adolescents include perioral paresthesias, tingling of the fingers and toes, spontaneous or latent tetany, carpopedal spasms, and seizures.[2] In neonates, manifestations of hypocalcemia are more nonspecific and include jitteriness, feeding intolerance, lethargy, apnea, and seizures. Physical examination may reveal hyperreflexia, a positive Chvostek sign (twitching of facial muscles after tapping the facial nerve anterior to the ear), or the Trousseau sign (carpopedal spasm after maintaining a blood pressure cuff above systolic blood pressure for 3 to 5 minutes). Less often seen are cataracts, papilledema, rachitic deformities, and abnormal dental development. Chronic mucocutaneous candidiasis and other ectodermal abnormalities in the setting of hypoparathyroidism may suggest familial autoimmune polyendocrinopathy type 1, whereas typical physical findings may suggest pseudohypoparathyroidism (PHP) type 1a or DiGeorge syndrome[3] (Table 91-1).

Differential Diagnosis of Hypocalcemia

The differential diagnosis of hypocalcemia differs slightly with the age of the patient. Clinically important categories of pediatric hypocalcemia are listed in Table 91-2.

Early Neonatal Hypocalcemia

In infants presenting with hypocalcemia within 48 to 72 hours of birth, the differential diagnosis includes prematurity, birth asphyxia, and maternal diabetes. In preterm infants, hypocalcemia is essentially due to a deficient increase in PTH secretion along with a relative resistance to calcitriol. In addition, premature infants have limited intake of milk, which contributes to hypocalcemia.[4] In infants of diabetic mothers, magnesium deficiency may also play an important role in the development of early neonatal hypocalcemia.[5] Whenever neonatal hypocalcemia occurs in absence of these three risk factors, the diagnosis of congenital hypoparathyroidism must be considered.

Late Neonatal Hypocalcemia

Late neonatal hypocalcemia presents clinically at 5 to 10 days of life in healthy full-term infants. The three major causes of late neonatal hypocalcemia are phosphate loading, hypoparathyroidism, and magnesium deficiency. Historically, infant formulas with a high phosphorus content have contributed to the development of late neonatal hypocalcemia, but this is seen less commonly with current infant formulas. Phosphate-induced hypocalcemia should be differentiated from congenital hypoparathyroidism. In both situations serum calcium is low and serum phosphorus is high. PTH is appropriately elevated in phosphate-induced neonatal hypocalcemia, however, and the hypocalcemia resolves spontaneously when the neonate is placed on a low-phosphorus formula such as PM 60/40.[6]

Childhood Hypocalcemia

Causes of hypocalcemia in children include PTH deficiency, vitamin D deficiency, and resistance to the biologic effects of these calcium-regulating hormones. The differential diagnosis includes vitamin D deficiency, vitamin D resistance, other abnormalities in vitamin D metabolism, hypoparathyroidism, PHP, metabolic bone disease, and drug effect. Abnormalities in vitamin D metabolism can be seen

Table 91-1   Diagnostic Workup for Hypocalcemia

Detailed history documenting diet, lifestyle, and family and drug history

Examination focusing on skin, nails, teeth, skeleton, and cardiovascular system

Laboratory examination
  Blood
    Calcium (total and ionized)
    Phosphorus
    Alkaline phosphatase
    Electrolytes and creatinine
    Bicarbonate
    Parathyroid hormone
    Magnesium
    Vitamin D—25-hydroxyvitamin D and 1,25-
      dihydroxyvitamin D
    Save serum
  Urine
    Calcium
    Phosphorus
    Creatinine
  Others—depending on the suspected cause
    Hand and wrist radiography
    Electrocardiography
    Renal ultrasonography
    Karyotype
    Autoantibody screen
    Maternal vitamin D status
    Thyroid function

with renal disease and liver disease. In patients with renal failure, 1α-hydroxylation of 25-hydroxyvitamin D (25[OH]D) is impaired, and as a consequence the stored form of vitamin D (25[OH]D) cannot be converted to the biologically active form 1,25-dihydroxyvitamin D (1,25[OH]$_2$D). Hyperphosphatemia may further aggravate hypocalcemia in renal failure and lead to secondary hyperparathyroidism and renal osteodystrophy.

Vitamin D Deficiency

Vitamin D deficiency may be a primary nutritional deficiency or may be secondary to malabsorption. Conditions predisposing to malabsorption of vitamin D include celiac disease, cystic fibrosis, pancreatic insufficiency, intestinal bypass, and laxative abuse. Biochemical features of rickets are often seen with vitamin D deficiency, including secondary hyperparathyroidism, low serum phosphorus, phosphaturia, high serum alkaline phosphatase, and low 25(OH)D. Radiographic evidence of rickets may also be present on radiographs if fusion of the epiphyses has not yet occurred.

Hypoparathyroidism

Hypoparathyroidism may be secondary to surgery, polyglandular autoimmune disease, infiltrative disease, neck irradiation, or an idiopathic process. The diagnosis of hypoparathyroidism is suggested by low calcium levels, high phosphorus levels, and absence of bone disease on radiographs. Hypomagnesemia may be a causative factor in the development of hypoparathyroidism. Severe hypomagnesemia will suppress PTH secretion, and mild hypomagnesemia will interfere with PTH activity.[7]

Pseudohypoparathyroidism

PHP results from peripheral resistance to PTH secondary to a G-protein mutation in the PTH receptor. Type 1 PHP is inherited in an autosomal dominant pattern and is therefore found in one parent. It may occur with or without the

Table 91-2   Clinically Important Categories of Hypocalcemia

Category	Phosphorus	25(OH)D	1,25(OH)$_2$D	PTH	Comments
Neonate					
Early hypocalcemia	N	N	N or L	N or L	Prematurity, IUGR, birth asphyxia, diabetic mother
Late hypocalcemia	H	N	L	L	Low GFR, intake of high-phosphate milk
Older Child					
Congenital hypoparathyroidism	H	N	L	L	DiGeorge syndrome
Autoimmune hypoparathyroidism	H	N	L	L	Part of polyendocrinopathy syndrome, type 1
Pseudohypoparathyroidism	H	N	L	H	Peripheral resistance to PTH
Vitamin D deficiency	L, N, or H	L	L, N, or H	H	Exclusively breastfed with maternal vitamin D deficiency, sunlight avoidance, fat malabsorption
Vitamin D dependent	L	N	H	H	Caused by loss-of-function mutation of 1α-hydroxylase gene
Critical illness	N	N	N	L	PTH dysfunction and increase in cortisol
Magnesium deficiency	H	N	N/L	L	May be part of Bartter syndrome, malabsorption, renal disease
Renal disease	H	N	L	H	Abnormal renal function, metabolic acidosis

GFR, glomerular filtration rate; H, high; IUGR, intrauterine growth retardation; L, low; N, normal; 25(OH)D, 25-hydroxyvitamin D; 1,25(OH)$_2$D, 1,25-dihydroxyvitamin D; PTH, parathyroid hormone.

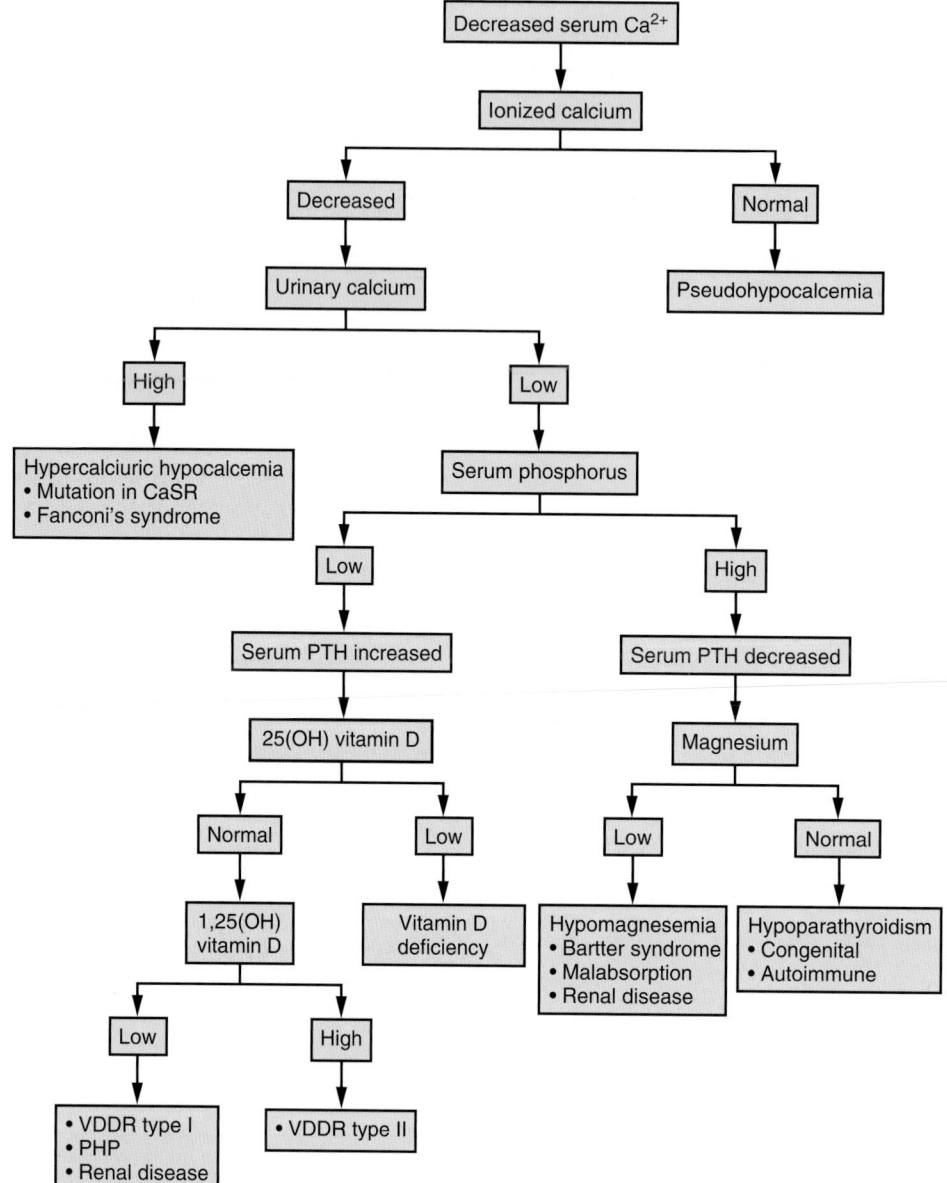

Figure 91-1 Flow chart for diagnosing the cause of hypocalcemia. CaSR, calcium-sensing receptor; PHP, pseudohypoparathyroidism; PTH, parathyroid hormone; VDDR, vitamin D–dependent rickets.

phenotypic features of Albright hereditary osteodystrophy. PTH will not stimulate the production of cyclic adenosine monophosphate (cAMP) or phosphaturia in type 1 PHP. In type 2 PHP, cAMP increases after PTH administration, but phosphaturia does not occur.[8]

A diagnostic schematic to narrow the differential diagnosis in patients with hypocalcemia is shown in Figure 91-1.

Evaluation

The diagnosis of hypocalcemia should be based on the total serum calcium concentration corrected for albumin or ideally on measurements of ionized calcium (if the appropriate tools are available for rapid processing). The phosphate level will aid in narrowing the differential. A high phosphate concentration indicates a deficiency of PTH action, whereas a low phosphate concentration favors

increased PTH effect. The algorithm shown in Figure 91-1 will assist in diagnosis.

Treatment of Hypocalcemia

Although mild hypocalcemia may not require therapy, any neonate with a serum calcium less than 7.5 mg/dL or an older child with a serum calcium of less than 8 to 8.5 mg/dL should be treated to prevent tetany and other symptoms. Oral therapy is preferable whenever possible.

In acute symptomatic hypocalcemia (tetany, seizures), intravenous therapy is required. Calcium gluconate 10% solution (9.4 mg elemental calcium/mL) can be given by slow intravenous push.[9] A cardiac monitor must be used because rapid injection can cause serious cardiac dysrhythmias. All calcium salts are locally toxic and can lead to tissue damage if accidental extravasation occurs. A freely running intravenous line should be used to avoid extravasation. When symptoms of hypocalcemia resolve, serial calcium determinations will determine the need for and the route of further therapy. Because serum calcium levels may fall gradually after the initial infusion, ongoing treatment may be necessary. Mildly symptomatic patients who are unable to take calcium enterally may need calcium gluconate by slow intravenous infusion (every 6 to 8 hours, depending on subsequent calcium levels).

In the absence of tetany or seizures, oral therapy will suffice. Calcium glubionate is the most suitable agent for infants and young children because it is dispensed as a palatable syrup. The usual dose is 115 mg elemental Ca/kg/day given in three or four divided doses. In older children, tablets of calcium gluconate, carbonate, or lactate can be given. A dosage of 50 mg elemental calcium/kg/day is generally prescribed.

Depending on the cause of the hypocalcemia, vitamin D supplementation may be required as well. Calcitriol may be used if the patient is unable to produce $1,25(OH)_2D$ because of renal disease or severe hypoparathyroidism. However, calcitriol bypasses the body's ability to regulate vitamin D activity and therefore carries the risk of hypercalcemia and hypercalciuria. It has a short half-life and persists in the body for only 1 to 2 days. Because calcitriol will not replenish vitamin D stores, $25(OH)D$ should be given if a true deficiency of vitamin D is suspected. The usual dosage of calcitriol is 0.25 μg/day but varies with body weight and the disorder for which it is being used. The dosage may be adjusted until calcium levels have improved.

Individualization of therapy is essential. It is crucial to monitor serum and urinary calcium and creatinine levels frequently to adjust the doses of medications. The goal is to maintain eucalcemia and avoid hypercalcemia and hypercalciuria. Annual renal sonography is also recommended to detect nephrocalcinosis.

Consultation

- Pediatric endocrinologist
- Geneticist

Admission Criteria

- Symptomatic hypocalcemia (unless the diagnosis is hyperventilation)
- Severe hypocalcemia, specifically, a serum calcium level less than 7 to 7.5 mg/dL
- Any newborn with hypocalcemia should be monitored in the neonatal intensive care unit (NICU)

Discharge Criteria

- Asymptomatic and clinically stable patient
- Arrangements made for regular follow-up to monitor the serum calcium concentration and the underlying disorder

HYPERCALCEMIA

Hypercalcemia is less common in childhood than hypocalcemia is and is frequently discovered incidentally on a routine chemistry profile. The most common association is dehydration. Because of the potential clinical significance of a slight elevation in serum calcium levels, it is important to obtain an accurate measure by taking the serum albumin concentration and acid-base status into account.

Pathophysiology

Because serum calcium regulation is dependent on PTH, vitamin D, calcium intake, and renal calcium excretion, derangements in any of these systems can produce hypercalcemia. It is useful to separate the causes into two broad categories: hypercalcemia with inappropriate PTH secretion and hypercalcemia despite adequate PTH suppression.

The normative values for calcium are age dependent. A total serum calcium level of greater than 9.2 mg/dL (ionized Ca >5.8 mg/dL or 1.42 mmol/L) in a premature infant, greater than 10.4 mg/dL (ionized Ca >5.0 mg/dL or 1.22 mmol/L) in a full-term infant, and greater than 10.8 mg/dL (ionized Ca >5.0 mg/dL or 1.22 mmol/L) in a child or adolescent is considered elevated.

Clinical Presentation

Symptoms of hypercalcemia vary little with age. Lethargy, weakness, inability to concentrate, and depression may develop. Many patients have nausea, vomiting, anorexia, constipation, and weight loss. Patients may become hypertensive with extreme elevations in calcium. Neonates may manifest symptoms of gastroesophageal reflux, lethargy, poor weight gain, and a decrease in linear growth. Elevations in extracellular calcium impair the ability of the distal tubule of the nephron to respond to ADH. Therefore, hypercalcemic patients may present with polyuria, dehydration, and azotemia. In addition to general signs of hypercalcemia, affected children may manifest signs and symptoms of the underlying disease process.[10]

Differential Diagnosis of Hypercalcemia

The differential diagnosis of hypercalcemia in childhood, along with associated biochemical findings, is summarized in Table 91-3.

Idiopathic Infantile Hypercalcemia (Williams Syndrome)

Characteristic elfin facies, congenital cardiovascular anomalies, and cognitive impairment are often accompanied by transient infantile hypercalcemia in Williams syndrome. The hypercalcemia may be severe and is exacerbated by dietary vitamin D supplementation. However, the hypercalcemia usually remits between 9 and 18 months of age. Affected hypercalcemic infants have been found to have increased intestinal absorption of calcium and associated elevations of $1,25(OH)_2D_3$ that normalize as calcium levels return to normal.[11] The hypercalcemia often responds to a low-calcium diet and to the administration of corticosteroids.

Familial Hypocalciuric Hypercalcemia

Familial hypocalciuric hypercalcemia, an asymptomatic condition of parathyroid insensitivity to the normal suppressive effect of calcium on PTH secretion, is due to a mutation in the calcium-sensing receptor (CaSR). It is inherited as an autosomal dominant condition, and therefore one of the parents will be affected. A homozygous CaSR mutation is characterized by severe and often lethal neonatal hyperparathyroidism.[12]

Table 91-3 Classification of Hypercalcemia in Childhood

Type	Serum Phosphorus	Serum Calcidiol	Serum Calcitriol	Serum PTH	Urinary Ca	Notes
Idiopathic (Williams syndrome)	N	N	N	N	H	Deletion in 17q11.23. Cognitive impairment, elfin facies, aortic stenosis
Primary hyperparathyroidism	L	N	H	H	H	Rare in children. Part of MEN types I and II
Secondary hyperparathyroidism (secondary to renal insufficiency)	H	N	L	H	H	Can lead to tertiary autonomous hyperparathyroidism
Familial hypocalciuria	N	N	N	N	L	Loss-of-function mutation (generally heterozygous) in CaSR
Hypervitaminosis D	N/L	H	N/H	N	H	Overdose of vitamins, fad megavitamin diets
Increased 1α-hydroxylation of 25-hydroxyvitamin D	N	N	H	N	N	Granulomatous diseases, subcutaneous fat necrosis, neoplasm
Immobilization	N	N	L	L	H	Increased resorption and decreased bone formation
Malignancy	N	N	N	L	H	Release of bone-resorbing substances: PTH-rp
Adrenal insufficiency	N	N	N/L	L	N	Increased GI calcium absorption
Hyperthyroidism	N	N	N/L	L	N	Active bone turnover and enhanced resorption

CaSR, calcium-sensing receptor; GI, gastrointestinal; H, high; L, low; MEN, multiple endocrine neoplasia; N, normal; PTH, parathyroid hormone; PTH-rp, PTH-related protein.

Hyperparathyroidism

Hyperparathyroidism is very rare in childhood. Affected children are hypercalcemic because of increased calcium resorption from bone. Serum phosphorus is usually reduced but may be normal. The skeletal erosion is best evidenced in the phalanges and clavicle. Sporadic cases may result from either a parathyroid adenoma or chief cell hyperplasia.

Any child with hyperparathyroidism should be evaluated for multiple endocrine neoplasia (MEN) syndromes. The autosomal dominant nature of MEN-I and MEN-II inheritance requires examination of both parents and siblings. Ninety percent of patients with MEN-I have parathyroid hyperplasia along with a pituitary adenoma or a pancreatic tumor (or both). In MEN-IIA, medullary thyroid carcinoma and pheochromocytoma are the main features, and chief cell hyperplasia is sometimes associated.[13]

Hypercalcemia of Malignancy

Hypercalcemia may be caused by an elevation of PTH-related protein (PTH-rp) in patients with malignancies. PTH-rp is secreted by many types of malignant tumors, most notably leukemia, lymphoma, rhabdomyosarcoma, and Ewing sarcoma. Hypercalcemia results from activation of the PTH receptor by PTH-rp.[14]

Hypervitaminosis D

Vitamin D intoxication is uncommon but can arise from chronic overdosage of vitamin D given for therapeutic purposes or self-administration of vitamin preparations. The resultant hypercalcemia can be severe and prolonged because of storage of vitamin D in fat. Specific therapy includes discontinuation of vitamin D and ingestion of a low-calcium diet. Glucocorticoids are especially useful because they inhibit the action of vitamin D on both bone and intestine.

Hypervitaminosis A

Excessive intake of vitamins may result in vitamin A excess in addition to vitamin D excess. Excess amounts of the fat-soluble vitamin A also increase bone resorption and cause hypercalcemia.

Immobilization

Hypercalcemia of immobilization occurs more commonly in children and adolescents than in adults because of a higher rate of bone remodeling at this age. It is seen most frequently after leg fractures, spinal cord injuries, and burns. Hypercalciuria and substantial bone loss are more common than hypercalcemia. PTH and 1,25(OH)$_2$D are suppressed, and bone biopsy specimens show increased resorption of bone and decreased formation of bone.[15]

Thiazide Diuretics

Thiazides may cause hypercalcemia as a result of increased renal resorption of calcium and increased calcium binding protein levels.

Other Endocrine Abnormalities

Adrenal insufficiency and hyperthyroidism may be associated with hypercalcemia. Hyperthyroidism induces bone resorption and causes hypercalcemia with suppressed PTH. Hypothyroidism may also be accompanied by elevated calcium levels, possibly as a result of increased sensitivity to vitamin D.

Evaluation

The diagnostic approach to a hypercalcemic patient is strongly influenced by the clinical setting in which the patient is being evaluated and the clinical presentation of the patient. The presence of hypercalcemia should be confirmed by direct measurement of ionized calcium when possible. In patients with mild hypercalcemia, it is advisable to repeat total and ionized calcium measurements before undertaking a costly workup. The diagnostic workup for hypercalcemia involves a detailed history, examination, and investigation, as listed in Table 91-4. A diagnostic algorithm is provided in Figure 91-2.

Treatment of Hypercalcemia

Appropriate management of a patient with hypercalcemia depends on the severity and cause of the hypercalcemia. When the calcium concentration is less than 12 mg/dL in an asymptomatic subject, treatment may be delayed until the cause of the hypercalcemia is known. If the total serum calcium concentration exceeds 12 mg/dL or the child is symptomatic, efforts to lower calcium levels should be instituted to prevent the adverse effects of hypercalcemia while awaiting the laboratory results.

Volume Repletion

The mainstay of initial therapy for acute symptomatic hypercalcemia is vigorous hydration with normal saline. Twice the maintenance infusion rate is recommended initially, if tolerated. Urine output must be closely monitored, and any net fluid deficit should be replaced on an ongoing basis. The goal is to maintain an increased urinary rate and to have input exceed urinary output.

Diuretics

Once adequate hydration has been achieved, furosemide (1 to 2 mg/kg) may be administered intravenously to increase urinary calcium excretion if the serum calcium level is not improving.

After initial stabilization, attention should turn to treatment of the underlying cause of the hypercalcemia.

Glucocorticoids

Oral glucocorticoids decrease calcium, principally by decreasing absorption from the intestine. They also have a role in treating hypercalcemia that arises from granulomatous disease by treating the underlying disease.

Table 91-4 Diagnostic Workup for Hypercalcemia

Detailed history documenting diet, lifestyle, and family and drug history

Examination focusing on growth parameters, hydration status, vital signs, and features associated with specific causes of hypocalcemia (subcutaneous fat necrosis, elfin facies, congenital heart lesions)

Laboratory examination
  Blood
    Calcium (total and ionized)
    Phosphorus
    Alkaline phosphatase
    Electrolytes and creatinine
    Bicarbonate
    Parathyroid hormone
    Magnesium
    Vitamin D—25-hydroxyvitamin D and 1,25-dihydroxyvitamin D
    Save serum
  Urine
    Calcium
    Phosphorus
    Creatinine
  Others—depending on the suspected cause
    Radiographs of the chest, hands, and long bones
    Electrocardiography (shortened QTc interval, bradycardia)
    Renal ultrasonography
    Karyotype
    Thyroid function
    Serum and urine Ca, P, Cr
    Serum parathyroid hormone–related protein
    Screen for occult malignancy

Phosphates

Oral phosphate may be used to bind calcium in the intestine, but its efficacy is limited and its use may result in nausea, abdominal cramps, and diarrhea.

Calcitonin

In cases of severe hypercalcemia, calcitonin (2 to 4 U/kg) via subcutaneous injection can be given every 6 to 12 hours as needed, but rapid tachyphylaxis to this medication is common and limits its utility.[16]

Bisphosphonates

Bisphosphonate therapy should be reserved for refractory cases in which the underlying cause of hypercalcemia is not amenable to other therapies. These agents act via inhibition of osteoclastic bone resorption. Pamidronate (0.5 to 1 mg/kg per dose) may be given intravenously over a period of 4 to 5 hours. The peak effect will not be seen for 48 hours or longer. Other electrolyte imbalances are frequently seen with bisphosphonate therapy, and patients must therefore be monitored for hypocalcemia, hypophosphatemia, hypomagnesemia, and hypokalemia.[17] If renal failure coexists, bisphosphonate therapy is not recommended, and renal dialysis may be necessary to decrease calcium levels in severe cases.

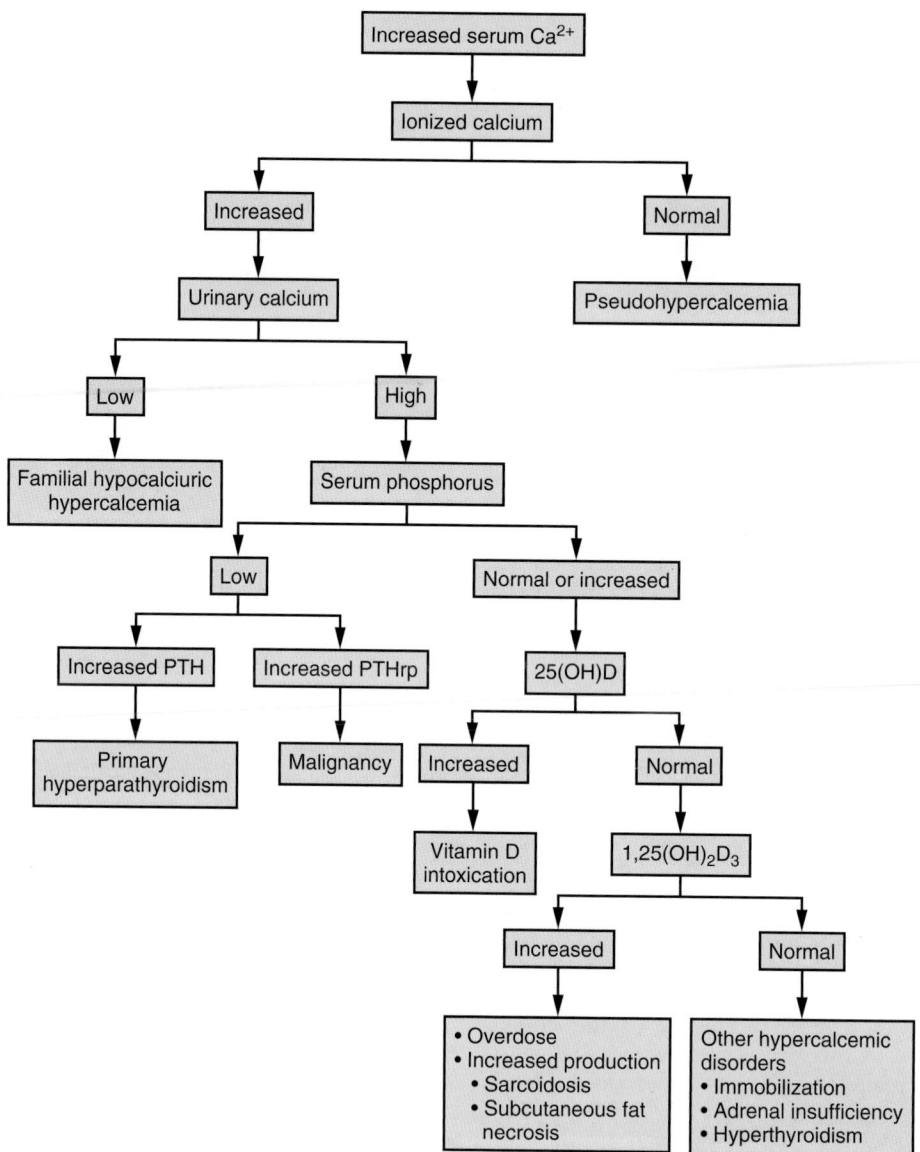

Figure 91-2 Flow chart for diagnosing the cause of hypercalcemia. PTH, parathyroid hormone; PTHrp, PTH-related protein.

If malignancy-derived PTH-rp is the cause of hypercalcemia, treatment of the underlying malignancy is the treatment of choice.

Consultation

- Pediatric endocrinologist
- Pediatric nephrologist
- Geneticist

Admission Criteria

- Symptomatic hypercalcemia
- Severe hypercalcemia, specifically, serum calcium greater than 12 mg/dL (except familial hypocalciuric hypercalcemia)
- Any newborn with hypercalcemia should be monitored in the NICU

Discharge Criteria

- Asymptomatic and clinically stable patient
- Arrangements made for regular follow-up to monitor the serum calcium concentration and the underlying disease

IN A NUTSHELL

- The concentration of calcium in serum is modulated through a delicate interplay between PTH and vitamin D via their actions on target organs such as bone, kidney, and the gastrointestinal tract.
- Pediatric reference ranges should be used to interpret levels of total serum calcium, ionized calcium, and phosphorus because levels differ significantly with age.

- Pediatric units should have a protocol for the diagnostic workup of patients with hypercalcemia and hypocalcemia.
- PTH and vitamin D levels should be checked before any intervention.
- Hypocalcemia may develop as a result of decreased calcium intake or absorption; excessive urinary loss of calcium; abnormal parathyroid gland development; destruction of the gland by antibodies or surgical procedures; synthesis of an abnormal form of PTH; impaired cellular responsiveness to PTH; restricted exposure to sunlight; or abnormal intake, absorption, or activity of vitamin D and its metabolites.
- Hypercalcemia in children can occur when there is increased resorption of calcium from bone (excessive secretion of PTH or PTH-rp), when the intestinal rate of calcium absorption exceeds renal excretory capacity (vitamin D intoxication), or when there is augmented renal tubular absorption of calcium (thiazide diuretics).
- Treatment of hypocalcemia is mainly calcium replacement (intravenously or orally, depending on the severity of symptoms). Concurrent administration of vitamin D may be required, depending on the cause of the hypocalcemia.
- Treatment of hypercalcemia typically begins with saline administration to produce volume expansion and increase urinary calcium excretion. Correction of the underlying cause should be the next focus, but administration of bisphosphonates to reduce bone resorption may be considered in certain severe cases.
- Drugs acting on the CaSR may play an important role in the management of primary and secondary hyperparathyroidism in the future.

ON THE HORIZON

- The CaSR is a G protein–coupled cell surface receptor that belongs to family 3 of the GPCR superfamily.[18]
- The extracellular CaSR on the parathyroid cell surface inhibits PTH secretion. Activation of CaSR by small changes in the extracellular concentration of ionized calcium decreases PTH secretion and secondarily decreases bone turnover. Recent studies have demonstrated that the activity of this receptor maintains steady-state plasma calcium concentrations in humans by regulating key elements in the calcium homeostatic system.
- CaSR agonists (calcimimetics) and antagonists (calcilytics) have been identified and have provided both current and potential therapies for a variety of disorders.[19]
- Calcimimetics can effectively reduce PTH secretion in all forms of hyperparathyroidism. They are likely to become a major therapy for secondary hyperparathyroidism associated with renal failure and for treatment of certain patients with primary hyperparathyroidism.
- Calcilytics, which decrease CaSR function and increase secretion of PTH, might allow the anabolic effects of PTH on bone to be used for the prevention and treatment of osteoporosis.[20]

SUGGESTED READING

Bilezikian JP: Management of acute hypercalcemia. N Engl J Med 1992;326: 1196-1203.

Gertner JM: Disorders of calcium and phosphorus metabolism. Pediatr Clin North Am 1990;37:1441-1465.

Shane E: Hypocalcemia: Pathogenesis, differential diagnosis, and management. In Favus MJ (ed): Primer on the Metabolic Bone Diseases and Disorders of Mineral Metabolism, 4th ed. Philadelphia, Lippincott Williams & Wilkins, 1990, pp 223-230.

Shane E: Hypercalcemia: Pathogenesis, differential diagnosis, and management. In Favus MJ (ed): Primer on the Metabolic Bone Diseases and Disorders of Mineral Metabolism, 4th ed. Philadelphia, Lippincott Williams & Wilkins, 1999, pp 183-187.

REFERENCES

1. Gertner JM: Disorders of calcium and phosphorus metabolism. Pediatr Clin North Am 1990;37:1441-1465.
2. Tohme JF, Bilezikian JP: Hypocalcemic emergencies. Endocrinol Metab Clin North Am 1993;22:363-375.
3. Root AW, Diamond FB Jr: Disorders of calcium and phosphorus metabolism in adolescents. Endocrinol Metab Clin North Am 1993;22:573-592.
4. Tsang RC, Chen IW, Friedman MA, Chen I: Neonatal parathyroid function: Role of gestation and postnatal age. J Pediatr 1973;83:728-738.
5. Mimouni F, Tsang RC, Hertzberg VS, Miodovnik M: Polycythemia, hypomagnesemia and hypocalcemia in infants of diabetic mothers. Am J Dis Child 1986;140:798-800.
6. Venkataraman PS, Tsang RC, Greer FR, et al: Late infantile tetany and secondary hyperparathyroidism. Am J Dis Child 1985;139:664-668.
7. Anast CS, Mohs JM: Evidence for parathyroid failure in magnesium deficiency. Science 1972;177:606-608.
8. Levine MA: Clinical spectrum and pathogenesis of pseudohypoparathyroidism. Rev Endocr Metab Disord 2000;1:265-274.
9. Shane E: Hypocalcemia: Pathogenesis, differential diagnosis, and management. In Favus MJ (ed): Primer on the Metabolic Bone Diseases and Disorders of Mineral Metabolism, 4th ed. Philadelphia, Lippincott Williams & Wilkins, 1990, pp 223-230.
10. Shane E: Hypercalcemia: Pathogenesis, differential diagnosis, and management. In Favus MJ (ed): Primer on the Metabolic Bone Diseases and Disorders of Mineral Metabolism, 4th ed. Philadelphia, Lippincott Williams & Wilkins, 1999, pp 183-187.
11. Garabedian M, Jacqz E: Elevated plasma 1,25-dihydroxyvitamin D concentrations in infants with hypercalcemia and an elfin facies. N Engl J Med 1985;312:948-952.
12. Khosla S, Ebeling PR: Calcium infusion suggests a "set-point" abnormality of parathyroid gland function in familial benign hypercalcemia and more complex disturbances in primary hyperparathyroidism. J Clin Endocrinol Metab 1993;76:715-720.
13. Marx SJ, Simmonds WF: Hyperparathyroidism in hereditary syndromes: Special expressions and special managements. J Bone Miner Res 2002;17(Suppl 2):N37-N43.
14. Pandian MR, Morgan CH: Modified immunoradiometric assay of parathyroid hormone–related protein: Clinical application in the differential diagnosis of hypercalcemia. Clin Chem 1992;38:282-288.
15. Stewart AF, Alder M: Calcium homeostasis in immobilization: An example of resorptive hypercalcemia. N Engl J Med 1982;306:1136-1140.
16. Hosking DJ, Gilson D: Comparison of the renal and skeletal actions of calcitonin in the treatment of severe hypercalcaemia of malignancy. Q J Med 1984;53:359-368.
17. Bilezikian JP: Management of acute hypercalcemia. N Engl J Med 1992;326:1196-1203.
18. Hebert SC: Therapeutic use of calcimimetics. Annu Rev Med 2006;57: 349-364.
19. Urena P, Legoupil N: Calcimimetics, mechanisms of action and therapeutic applications. Presse Med 2005;34:1095-1100.
20. Steddon SJ: Calcimimetics and calcilytics—fooling the calcium receptor. Lancet 2005;365:2237-2239.

CHAPTER 92

Disorders of the Adrenal Gland

Mary Pat Gallagher and Sharon E. Oberfield

BACKGROUND

The adrenal gland is composed of an outer cortex and an inner medulla. The cortex is divided histologically and functionally into three sections: the zona glomerulosa, the zona fasciculata, and the zona reticularis. Production of mineralocorticoid takes place primarily in the zona glomerulosa, production of glucocorticoid in the zona fasciculata, and production of androgen mostly in the zona reticularis. Mineralocorticoid production is predominantly controlled by the renin-angiotensin system. Glucocorticoid production is dependent on secretion of adrenocorticotropic hormone (ACTH) from the pituitary gland and therefore on secretion of corticotropin-releasing hormone (CRH) from the hypothalamus as well. The adrenal medulla is the site of catecholamine production, and abnormalities in medullary function can result in catecholamine excess.

Hypothalamic–Pituitary–Adrenal Axis

CRH from the hypothalamus stimulates pituitary ACTH secretion. CRH is secreted in a pulsatile manner, which leads to pulsatile ACTH release. ACTH regulates adrenal glucocorticoid secretion. Diurnal cortisol secretion is secondary to the varying amplitude of ACTH pulses. It is highest at the time of waking, low in afternoon to evening, and lowest at midnight, or 2 hours after sleep. ACTH acts by binding to the cell surface receptor on adrenal cortical cells, which leads to activation of adenylate cyclase. The increase in cyclic adenosine monophosphate stimulates cholesterol release and transport into mitochondria, where it binds to cytochrome P-450scc, and newly synthesized pregnenolone is released. The long-term effects of ACTH include increased transport of low-density lipoprotein cholesterol into adrenal cells and increased formation of steroidogenic enzymes. Negative feedback on the synthesis and secretion of ACTH and CRH is provided by cortisol.

Adrenal Cortex

Glucocorticoids are both catabolic, increasing protein degradation (muscle, skin, adipose tissue), and anabolic, enhancing the ability for gluconeogenesis. Synthetic analogues are available with varying anti-inflammatory/gluconeogenic activity, as well as varying salt-retaining properties. Androgens promote the growth of pubic and axillary hair. Dehydroepiandrosterone sulfate is the most abundant androgen in the circulation. Mineralocorticoids maintain electrolyte equilibrium and stabilization of blood volume and blood pressure. They control sodium reabsorption in the distal tubule of the kidney.[1]

Renin–Angiotensin–Aldosterone System

Renin is the major regulator of aldosterone synthesis and secretion, although increased potassium causes aldosterone secretion as well. Renin is produced in the juxtaglomerular apparatus of the kidney and reacts with renin substrate to produce angiotensin I. Angiotensin-converting enzyme converts angiotensin I to angiotensin II, which is cleaved to angiotensin III. Angiotensin II and III are potent stimulators of aldosterone synthesis and secretion. A decrease in sodium, blood volume, arterial pressure, and renal blood flow activates the juxtaglomerular apparatus and leads to an increase in renin and aldosterone. Potassium directly increases aldosterone secretion by the adrenal cortex. Both potassium and angiotensin act via intracellular signal transduction to stimulate synthesis of pregnenolone from cholesterol.

Adrenal Medulla

The medulla produces catecholamines such as dopamine, norepinephrine, and epinephrine. Synthesis of catecholamines also occurs in the brain and sympathetic nerve endings and in chromaffin cells outside the medulla. The metabolites found in urine include vanillylmandelic acid (VMA) and metanephrine.[2]

ADRENAL INSUFFICIENCY

Clinical Presentation

The clinical manifestations and age at onset of adrenal insufficiency depend on its cause. Presentation at birth or soon after is seen with adrenal hypoplasia, defects in steroidogenesis, and pseudohypoaldosteronism. Patients present with symptoms of salt wasting and failure to thrive, vomiting, lethargy, anorexia, and dehydration. Adrenal insufficiency caused by Addison's disease presents in older children with muscle weakness, lassitude, anorexia, weight loss, wasting, hypotension, and abdominal pain.

An adrenal crisis may present with cyanosis, cold skin, and a weak, rapid pulse. It can be fatal. In disorders associated with excess ACTH (congenital adrenal hypoplasia, congenital adrenal hyperplasia [CAH], Addison's disease, adrenoleukodystrophy, and ACTH resistance), there is increased skin pigmentation secondary to increased ACTH that does not occur in patients with corticotropin deficiency or pseudohypoaldosteronism. Hypoglycemia with ketosis is also associated with adrenal insufficiency.

The clinical features of CAH are determined by the specific enzyme deficiency and include female pseudohermaphroditism (21-hydroxylase and 3β-hydroxysteroid dehydrogenase [3β-HSD] deficiencies) and male pseudoher-maphroditism (cholesterol desmolase and 3β-HSD deficiencies). 11-Hydroxylase and 17-hydroxylase deficiencies may present with ambiguity of the genitalia but not with adrenal insufficiency.

Differential Diagnosis

The causes of adrenal insufficiency include a wide variety of lesions of the hypothalamus, pituitary, and adrenal cortex (Table 92-1). Hypothalamic and pituitary deficiencies are discussed in a separate chapter. Familial glucocorticoid deficiency, or ACTH resistance, is an autosomal recessive disorder in which there is an isolated deficiency of glucocorticoid. Aldosterone production is normal and there is no salt wasting. ACTH resistance may occur in association with achalasia and alacrima (Allgrove syndrome).

Inborn defects of steroidogenesis are also responsible for adrenal insufficiency. The most common cause of adrenocortical insufficiency is salt-losing CAH, or 21-hydroxylase deficiency. Lipoid adrenal hyperplasia and 3β-HSD deficiency are rarer forms of CAH that also cause adrenal insufficiency. There is deficiency of cortisol and aldosterone. Isolated deficiency of aldosterone is a rare autosomal recessive disorder.

Pseudohypoaldosteronism occurs when there is target organ unresponsiveness to aldosterone. It can be limited to the kidney or may involve multiple target organs (sweat glands, salivary glands, and colon). Both autosomal dominant and autosomal recessive inheritance has been reported.

Addison's disease causes destruction of the adrenal cortex. It is most often secondary to autoimmune destruction by anti–adrenal cytoplasm antibodies, but it can also be secondary to infectious destruction, as with tuberculosis.[3] The cortex is destroyed but the medulla remains intact. Addison's disease frequently occurs with other endocrinopathies, such as type 1 autoimmune polyendocrinopathy-candidiasis-ectodermal dystrophy, which includes mucocutaneous candidiasis, hypoparathyroidism, and Addison's disease. Gonadal failure, alopecia, vitiligo, enamel hypoplasia, intestinal malabsorption, chronic acute hepatitis, and hypothyroidism are also seen. Type 1 autoimmune polyendocrinopathy is caused by an autosomal recessive mutation on chromosome 21q22.3. Addison's disease can also occur in type 2 autoimmune polyendocrinopathy, which includes autoimmune thyroid disease, type 1 diabetes mellitus, gonadal failure, vitiligo, alopecia, and atrophic gastritis. It is associated with HLA-DR3 and HLA-DR4 markers, and multiple generations can be affected.

Adrenoleukodystrophy is caused by the accumulation of very long chain fatty acid in peroxisomes, results in adrenal cortical failure and central nervous system demyelination, and is associated with progressive mental retardation. It is most often X-linked, and more than a hundred mutations in the gene, which has been mapped to Xq28, have been described. It can also be transmitted by an autosomal recessive gene.

Table 92-1   **Differential Diagnosis of Adrenal Insufficiency**

Category	ACTH	Aldosterone	Comments
Congenital			
Congenital adrenal hyperplasia	H	N or L	May see virilization in female neonates; may have salt wasting
Congenital adrenal hypoplasia	H	N	Severe salt wasting always present
ACTH unresponsiveness	H	N	May be associated with alacrima and achalasia (triple A syndrome)
ACTH/CRH deficiency	L	N	May occur with other pituitary hormone deficiencies
Adrenoleukodystrophy	H	N or L	Patients have elevated levels of VLCFA
Wolman disease	N	N or L	Lysosomal storage disease
Aldosterone deficiency	N	L	Deficiency of aldosterone synthase
Neonatal hemorrhage	H	N	Often asymptomatic
Acquired			
Autoimmune	H	N or L	May be associated with other autoimmune endocrinopathies
Trauma or surgery	H	N or L	
Infiltrative	H	N or L	Metastatic malignancies, hemochromatosis, sarcoidosis, amyloidosis
Infectious	H	N or L	Tuberculosis, coccidioidomycosis, histoplasmosis, and so on
HIV associated	H	N	
Acquired ACTH/CRH deficiency	L	N	May be secondary to CNS tumor or trauma
Drugs directly interfering with steroid synthesis	H	N or L	May be seen with ketoconazole, etomidate, aminoglutethimide, etc.
Drugs suppressing the HPA axis	L	N	Steroids
Critical illness	H	N	Probably an inability to keep up with production of steroid in the setting of continuous high demand

ACTH, adrenocorticotropic hormone; CNS, central nervous system; CRH, corticotropin-releasing hormone; H, high; HIV, human immunodeficiency virus; HPA, hypothalamic-pituitary-adrenocorticotropic; L, low; N, normal; VLCFA, very long chain fatty acid.

Diagnosis and Evaluation

Laboratory data will reveal low serum sodium, high potassium, acidosis, low blood glucose, increased plasma renin, increased urine excretion of sodium and chloride, decreased urine potassium, and increased eosinophils. Abdominal radiographs may show calcification of the adrenal gland secondary to infection or hemorrhage. Abdominal ultrasound may reveal enlarged adrenals bilaterally in CAH. Glucocorticoid deficiency is confirmed by a low basal and ACTH-stimulated cortisol level. Isolated defects in aldosterone are associated with increased aldosterone precursors. ACTH levels are increased in primary adrenal insufficiency and decreased in secondary and tertiary insufficiency. Renin levels are increased and aldosterone levels are decreased in salt-wasting CAH, isolated defects in aldosterone synthesis, adrenal hypoplasia, and Addison's disease. Both renin and aldosterone levels are increased in pseudohypoaldosteronism. Elevation of adrenal steroid precursors and androgens is found in CAH.

Treatment

Treatment of adrenal insufficiency includes both acute and chronic therapy. Adrenal crisis requires immediate and vigorous treatment with dextrose and normal saline to correct hypoglycemia and salt loss. A water-soluble form of hydrocortisone is given intravenously in stress doses. Chronic treatment includes oral hydrocortisone two to three times daily and the mineralocorticoid fludrocortisone (Florinef) once daily. Sodium chloride supplementation is often required. Plasma renin levels may be used to monitor the adequacy of mineralocorticoid replacement. Increased doses of hydrocortisone need to be given during periods of stress (e.g., fever, illness, surgery). Mineralocorticoid replacement is not necessary in patients with corticotropin deficiency or ACTH resistance (isolated glucocorticoid deficiency).

Glucocorticoid therapy for CAH not only replaces the deficient cortisol but also suppresses the excessive ACTH secretion, which results in a decrease in adrenal androgen secretion. Controversial treatments include adrenalectomy and therapy with antiandrogens and aromatase inhibitors, in addition to hydrocortisone.

Consultation

- Pediatric endocrinologist
- Geneticist, as indicated

Admission Criteria

- Vasomotor instability
- Electrolyte imbalance

Discharge Criteria

- Asymptomatic and clinically stable patient
- Regular follow-up arranged for monitoring serum electrolytes and the underlying disease

HYPERADRENAL STATES

Clinical Presentation

Features of glucocorticoid excess include central adiposity, hypertension, moon facies, plethora, capillary fragility, violaceous striae, dorsal and supraclavicular fat pads, acne, and possible associated signs of abnormal virilization. In addition, impaired growth velocity and short stature may be present, as well as pubertal delay and amenorrhea. Osteoporosis and renal stones are also consequences of chronic glucocorticoid excess.[4]

Patients with hyperaldosteronism have moderate or severe hypertension, hypokalemia, weakness, tetany, growth failure, and intermittent paralysis.

In children with pheochromocytoma, the symptomatology of catecholamine excess is somewhat different from that seen in adults. In children, more than 90% of hypertension is sustained rather than the paroxysmal hypertension seen in adults. The most common complaints are headache, sweating, nausea, abdominal pain, and palpitations, which may occur in paroxysmal fashion. The following symptoms have been reported at higher frequency in children than in adults: sweating, visual changes, nausea and vomiting, weight loss, polyuria, and polydipsia. Pallor (and infrequently flushing), weight loss, weakness, and fatigue may also be reported. Symptoms may be precipitated by exercise, Valsalva maneuvers, alcohol ingestion, and intubation. Drugs such as beta-blockers, nicotine, and tricyclic antidepressants can also precipitate symptoms. If the catecholamine excess has been long-standing, cardiac examination may reveal left ventricular hypertrophy or even cardiomyopathy, and there may be changes on funduscopic examination. Fasting plasma glucose levels and glucosuria have been reported.

Patients with neuroblastoma may present with an abdominal mass, weight loss, bone pain, anemia, flushing, headache, and hypertension.

Differential Diagnosis

The most common cause of glucocorticoid excess (Cushing's syndrome) in older children is bilateral adrenal hyperplasia. Girls and boys are affected equally. It may be due to hypersecretion of ACTH from the pituitary gland (Cushing's disease), ectopic ACTH secretion, or exogenous ACTH or glucocorticoid administration. Excess cortisol production may also be caused by adrenocortical nodular dysplasia and adrenal tumors, including carcinoma and adenoma. Tumors are the most common cause of glucocorticoid excess in infants, and there is a female preponderance of 3:1.

Primary hyperaldosteronism can be caused by an aldosterone-secreting adenoma, which mainly affects girls, or by bilateral micronodular adrenocortical hyperplasia, which affects older children. A rare form of low-renin hypertension is glucocorticoid-remediable hyperaldosteronism. Primary hyperaldosteronism is independent of the renin-angiotensin-aldosterone system (RAAS) and is rare in children. Apparent mineralocorticoid excess syndrome is a form of low-renin hypertension with exceedingly low levels of mineralocorticoids. The causes of secondary hyperaldosteronism include an activated RAAS,[5] which may be seen in renovascular hypertension. Renin production can also be enhanced in response to sodium loss or volume depletion and in edematous states such as congestive heart failure, cirrhosis, and nephrotic syndrome.

The three catecholamines that are produced in humans are dopamine, norepinephrine, and epinephrine. They are synthesized in the sympathetic neurons, chromaffin tissue (including, but not limited to, the adrenal medulla), and brain. The source of excessive catecholamine production is most often the adrenal medulla. Tumors of the adrenal medulla include pheochromocytoma, neuroblastoma, and ganglioneuroma. All three have been reported to produce catecholamines in excess and to occur as "silent tumors" without any of the enzyme activity required to elaborate catecholamines from tyrosine.[2] Pheochromocytoma is a rare tumor seen uncommonly in childhood. The tumors most often involve the adrenal medulla but may occur at the site of extra-adrenal chromaffin tissue. Extra-adrenal pheochromocytomas are also called paragangliomas. Children with pheochromocytoma are more likely than adults to have bilateral tumors, multiple tumors, and tumors at extra-adrenal sites. Extra-adrenal tumors are usually within the abdominal cavity.[5] Neuroblastoma is the second most common malignant solid tumor in childhood. Some 35% arise from adrenal neuroectoderm and can spontaneously regress in infants younger than 6 months.

Evaluation

Laboratory evaluation of glucocorticoid excess reveals elevated midnight serum cortisol and 24-hour urinary free cortisol levels. Polycythemia, lymphopenia, and decreased eosinophils can be present. Patients may have abnormal glucose tolerance or diabetes, as well as hypokalemia. A two-step or overnight dexamethasone suppression test can aid diagnosis. In normal children, administration of dexamethasone at 12 AM will usually suppress the next 8 AM cortisol level to less than 5 mg/dL. In patients with pathologic excess of cortisol, levels will not be suppressed in response to an overnight dexamethasone suppression test. In the absence of suppression after a test, a two-step (low-dose and high-dose) suppression test should be performed. In the low-dose test, 30 µg/kg/day is administered in four divided doses for 2 days. The high-dose test consists of administration of 120 µg/kg/day in four divided doses for 2 days. In patients with Cushing's disease, cortisol levels will not be suppressed with low-dose but will be with high-dose dexamethasone.[4] A computed tomography (CT) scan or magnetic resonance imaging (MRI) of the abdomen can rule out an adrenal tumor, and MRI of the head can help rule out an ACTH-secreting pituitary tumor.

Patients with primary hyperaldosteronism have hypokalemia, suppressed plasma renin activity, and increased plasma and urinary aldosterone levels. Dexamethasone, 0.25 mg every 6 hours, will suppress aldosterone and normalize blood pressure in glucocorticoid-responsive hyperaldosteronism only. If a tumor is suspected, abdominal CT or MRI and adrenal vein catheterization can help localize the tumor. Patients with secondary hyperaldosteronism are often normotensive and may have hypokalemic alkalosis and hyperreninemia.[5]

The catecholamines or their metabolites may be elevated in serum or urine in a ratio that is dependent on the enzyme activity of each individual tumor. Dopamine is metabolized to homovanillic acid (HVA), norepinephrine to normetanephrine, and epinephrine to metanephrine. Metanephrine and normetanephrine are then further metabolized to VMA. The diagnosis of pheochromocytoma can be very difficult to make because the tumors may secrete cate-

cholamines episodically. Catecholamine levels may also be spuriously elevated by medications or elevated in response to other stressful stimuli. A 24-hour urine collection for catecholamines is recommended as the initial screening test. Total metanephrines may be the most sensitive *single test*, but evaluation of a 24-hour urine collection for fractionated catecholamines (norepinephrine, epinephrine, and dopamine) and VMA increases diagnostic sensitivity.

Determination of plasma catecholamines may be helpful if it is possible to draw a sample from a catheter that has been in place for more than 30 minutes in a patient who is able to cooperate by remaining supine for this 30-minute period. However, this provides only a fraction of the information that can be gained by an integrated measurement of catecholamine release and metabolism, which can be obtained from a 24-hour urine collection. Recently, plasma-free metanephrines have been reported to have superior sensitivity in diagnosing pheochromocytomas in adults.[6] Although promising as a potentially more accurate and less labor-intensive method of diagnosis, this approach will require that adequate norms for the pediatric population be developed.

If only mild to moderate elevations are found in urine catecholamines, the biochemical abnormality should be confirmed by a second 24-hour urine collection before any radiologic or nuclear imaging is undertaken. If a high index of suspicion is present, normal results from a single 24-hour urine collection are not sufficient to rule out the diagnosis. The patient may need to have repeated measurements of urine catecholamines to document an abnormality. Provocative tests should be avoided because they may be dangerous, and suppression tests are not usually helpful.

If significant elevations of catecholamines or their metabolites (or both) are found, radiographic localization with a CT scan or MRI of the abdomen or total body ^{131}I-metaiodobenzylguanidine (^{131}I-MIBG) scintigraphy should be undertaken. Extra-adrenal pheochromocytomas may take up ^{131}I-MIBG less avidly than adrenal pheochromocytomas.

Children with pheochromocytoma should be screened for the genetic disorders with which pheochromocytomas are associated, including multiple endocrine neoplasia IIA and IIB, von Hippel-Lindau disease, and neurofibromatosis. As in adults the majority are benign lesions, but approximately 10% behave in a malignant fashion. Malignancy can be defined only by metastasis to an area of the body that lacks chromaffin tissue because there is no gross or microscopic pathologic finding that reliably predicts malignant behavior.

VMA and HVA spot urine tests are useful screening tests for neuroblastoma. CT of the abdomen can detect and localize a tumor, and a bone scan can indicate the extent of bone involvement and metastases.

Treatment

Treatment of glucocorticoid excess is based on its cause. A benign cortical adenoma is treated by surgical removal of the tumor. Adrenocortical carcinoma will frequently have metastasized at the time of diagnosis. Surgical resection, plus chemotherapy when indicated, is the current treatment. Cushing's disease is often treated with transsphenoidal pituitary microsurgery. These patients require perioperative and postoperative steroid treatment until their hypothalamic-pituitary-adrenal (HPA) axis recovers.

Treatment of mineralocorticoid excess involves correction of hypokalemia and underlying renin and aldosterone abnormalities. Definitive therapy may include aldosterone antagonists, glucocorticoids, or surgery, depending on the cause.

Pheochromocytomas must be surgically removed after adequate alpha-blockade to inhibit catecholamine synthesis. Classically, alpha-blockade of 1 to 3 weeks' duration has been recommended before surgery, although shorter courses have been reported in the literature. Phenoxybenzamine is considered the drug of choice for alpha-blockade. Beta-blockade should never be implemented unless adequate alpha-blockade has been established first. Beta-blockade in the absence of alpha-blockade can exacerbate hypertension by blocking the action of vasodilating β_2-receptors without blocking the action of the vasoconstricting α_1-receptors. In general, beta-blockade is used as an adjunctive therapy only in cases in which alpha-blockade has induced severe tachycardia or tachyarrhythmias. All patients with the diagnosis of pheochromocytoma require lifelong follow-up.

Children with neuroblastoma may require surgical excision of the primary lesion, chemotherapy, and bone marrow transplantation.

Consultation

- Pediatric endocrinologist
- Pediatric surgeon, as needed
- Pediatric oncologist, as needed

Admission Criteria

- Electrolyte imbalance
- Vasomotor instability

Discharge Criteria

- Asymptomatic and clinically stable patient.
- Regular follow-up arranged for monitoring serum electrolytes or blood pressure (or both) and the underlying disease

IN A NUTSHELL

- The adrenal cortex is stimulated by the release of ACTH from the pituitary, which controls the production of glucocorticoids and androgens, and by the activity of plasma renin, which controls the production of mineralocorticoid.

- ACTH/glucocorticoid deficiency can result in cardiovascular instability but does not cause salt wasting or hyperkalemia.
- Deficiency of mineralocorticoid results in salt wasting, dehydration, and hyperkalemia.
- CAH must always be considered in the evaluation of a newborn with ambiguous genitalia. Failure to recognize and treat this disorder can be life threatening.
- Potential suppression of the HPA axis by exogenous steroid administration is a common issue that arises in hospitalized patients. Patients who have received more than 7 days of supraphysiologic doses of glucocorticoid should be considered at risk for HPA suppression.
- The adrenal medulla manufactures catecholamines that can cause hypertension, nausea, headache, and pallor when produced in excess.

ON THE HORIZON

- Measurement of plasma-free metanephrines may eliminate the need to perform cumbersome 24-hour urine collections for the diagnosis of catecholamine excess. This test has been found to be sensitive and specific in the adult population, and pediatric norms are being developed.

REFERENCES

1. Miller WL: The adrenal cortex. In Sperling MA (ed): Pediatric Endocrinology. Philadelphia, WB Saunders, 2002, pp 385-438.
2. Miller WL: The adrenal gland. In Rudolph CD, Rudolph AM (eds): Rudolph's Pediatrics. New York, McGraw-Hill, 2002, pp 2028-2055.
3. Miller WL: Addison disease. In Finberg L, Kleinman RE (eds): Saunders Manual of Pediatric Practice. Philadelphia, WB Saunders, 2002, pp 905-912.
4. Chrousos GP: Cushing syndrome and Cushing disease. In Finberg L, Kleinman RE (eds): Saunders Manual of Pediatric Practice. Philadelphia, WB Saunders, 2002, pp 909-911.
5. Oberfield SE, Gallagher MP, Levine LS: Endocrine hypertension. In Finberg L, Kleinman RE (eds): Saunders Manual of Pediatric Practice. Philadelphia, WB Saunders, 2002, pp 912-915.
6. Ilias I, Pacak K: Diagnosis and management of tumors of the adrenal medulla. Horm Metab Res 2005;37:717-721.

Gastroenterology and Nutrition

CHAPTER 93

Pediatric Biliary Disease

Amethyst C. Kurbegov

The biliary tree includes the ducts that drain bile from the liver and coalesce into the right and left hepatic ducts; the cystic duct and gallbladder; and the common bile duct that drains bile from the gallbladder, through the pancreas, and into the duodenum. Biliary tract diseases can present at any age and have become increasingly recognized in pediatric practice as diagnostic tests have improved. The range of diseases that can involve the biliary system is broad and varies by patient age (Table 93-1).

CLINICAL PRESENTATION

Jaundice is the primary sign of biliary disease, indicating significant obstruction to bile flow. In neonates and infants, this is the most likely reason for the child's being brought to medical attention. Complete or near-complete obstruction of bile flow can result in acholic stools that are light yellow to clay in color. Occasionally, stools may have a hint of pigment on the exterior surface due to sloughing of enteric cells, but once this layer is removed, the clay-colored stool inside is apparent.[1]

Careful attention is required when evaluating jaundice in neonates, because approximately 60% of term neonates and 80% of preterm infants develop physiologic jaundice in the first days of life.[2] This can lead to complacency and delays in diagnosing more serious liver and biliary diseases. Any infant with new or persistent jaundice beyond the first 2 weeks of life requires further evaluation that includes measurement of fractionated serum bilirubin. Physiologic jaundice, breast milk jaundice, and hemolytic diseases are all associated with unconjugated hyperbilirubinemia; in contrast, extrahepatic biliary atresia (EHBA) and other cholestatic hepatobiliary diseases result in an elevated conjugated bilirubin.[1,3,4] These latter conditions require prompt and aggressive evaluation and management.

Biliary disease may present with poor growth and weight gain as a consequence of inadequate bile salts in the intestinal lumen, which leads to fat malabsorption. In addition, symptoms or physical findings indicative of fat-soluble vitamin deficiencies may be found. Specific findings include hemorrhage or hematoma (vitamin K deficiency), rickets (vitamin D deficiency), night blindness and corneal xeroph-

thalmia (vitamin A deficiency), and peripheral neuropathy (vitamin E deficiency).[5]

Biliary disease in older children usually presents with jaundice as well. They often have other symptoms indicating biliary obstruction or inflammation, such as right upper quadrant pain, vomiting, postprandial pain (particularly with fatty foods), light-colored stools, dark urine, and possibly fever if infection is present. Physical signs can include a positive Murphy sign (right upper quadrant tenderness during inspiration), scleral icterus and jaundice, epigastric pain if pancreatitis is present, and right upper quadrant mass. Systemic illnesses such as scarlet fever, Kawasaki disease, and leptospirosis can lead to hydrops of the gallbladder, with subsequent findings of right upper quadrant pain (93%) and mass (55%), but evidence of the broader systemic disease is usually present as well.[6] In patients with infection of the biliary tree or cholangitis, Charcot's triad of fever, right upper quadrant pain, and jaundice may be seen.[4,7-9] Bacterial cholangitis can progress to bacteremia and sepsis, especially if obstruction is present.

Hepatosplenomegaly is not typically associated with primary biliary tract conditions. However, the cholestasis of chronic biliary disease results in hepatocellular injury, which may lead to liver fibrosis and portal hypertension. Thus, the presence of hepatosplenomegaly may indicate the presence of advanced chronic disease due to progressive liver dysfunction.

EVALUATION

Although the evaluation for possible biliary tract disease should be tailored to the individual patient, the initial steps are usually similar (Table 93-2). Thereafter, certain studies may be selected on the basis of clinical suspicion, feasibility, and invasiveness. Evaluation of neonates and young infants with jaundice should be prompt and efficient, because timely intervention is required if EHBA is found. Management of conditions detected during diagnostic evaluation is addressed in the discussions of each specific illness.

The first and most fundamental step in evaluating jaundice is fractionation of the serum bilirubin.[1,3] Biliary tract disease is associated with a direct or conjugated hyperbiliru-

---

Table 93-1   Differential Diagnosis of Biliary Tract Disease by Age

Infancy
Extrahepatic biliary atresia
Choledochal cyst
Gallstone, sludge
Spontaneous perforation of common bile duct
Bile duct paucity
   Syndromic (Alagille syndrome)
   Nonsyndromic
      Hypothyroidism
      Panhypopituitarism
      Congenital infection
Cystic fibrosis

Childhood
Gallstone
Choledochal cyst
Acalculous cholecystitis
Hydrops of gallbladder
Primary sclerosing cholangitis
Common bile duct stricture
Malignancy
Biliary helminthiasis
Graft-versus-host disease

Table 93-2   Evaluation of Suspected Biliary Tract Disease

All Patients
History and physical examination
Laboratory studies
   Fractionated bilirubin
   Aspartate transaminase, alanine transaminase,
      γ-glutamyltransferase, alkaline phosphatase
   Albumin, prothrombin time
   Complete blood count, blood culture (in presence of fever)
Abdominal ultrasonography

Further Options
Hepatobiliary iminodiacetic acid scan
Liver biopsy
Sweat test
Endoscopic retrograde cholangiopancreatography
Magnetic resonance cholangiopancreatography
Genetic testing
Thyroid function tests

---

binemia, as opposed to the elevated indirect or unconjugated bilirubin found in various hemolytic and abnormal liver conjugating conditions such as breast milk jaundice and Crigler-Najjar syndrome. An elevated conjugated bilirubin is associated with obstruction of bile flow from the liver due to either congenital or acquired lesions. Conditions of hepatic dysfunction can also be associated with elevated bilirubin without extrahepatic obstruction, such as occurs in viral hepatitis A, which causes intracellular disruption of bile flow.

In addition to a fractionated bilirubin, a broader laboratory assessment of liver inflammation and function should be pursued in all patients with suspected biliary disease. These include alanine transaminase (ALT), aspartate transaminase (AST), alkaline phosphatase, γ-glutamyltransferase (GGT), total protein, and albumin levels and prothrombin time (PT). ALT and AST are markers of hepatocyte inflammation and breakdown and may be elevated if biliary tract obstruction is severe enough to generate secondary inflammation in the liver. Alkaline phosphatase and GGT are more specific for the biliary tract and are usually elevated, possibly 10 times normal or more, with acute obstruction or inflammation of the biliary tree.[1,4] Albumin and PT are indicators of liver synthetic function and are less likely to be abnormal in an acute biliary process. Although not common, liver failure can be seen with some biliary tract diseases, including EHBA and unrelieved acute obstruction such as untreated common bile duct cholelithiasis.[3,10] In patients with fever, a complete blood count and blood culture should be obtained, given the possibility of cholangitis.

Ultrasonography is the most useful imaging study for assessing biliary tract disease.[1,4,11] A carefully performed ultrasound study can detect stones in the gallbladder, common bile duct, or elsewhere in the biliary tree. Dilation of bile ducts, either intra- or extrahepatic, can indicate obstruction. Congenital malformations of the biliary tree, primarily choledochal cysts, are typically detected by ultrasonography. Although EHBA cannot be definitively diagnosed by ultrasonography, an absent gallbladder or the presence of a "triangular cord" in the porta hepatis is suggestive.[1,3,11,12] Conversely, it is important to note that the presence of a gallbladder does not rule out EHBA. Finally, abdominal ultrasonography allows the evaluation of other abdominal organs that can be affected by or associated with biliary disease, such as gallstone pancreatitis or polysplenia in association with EHBA.[11]

For a young infant presenting with cholestasis, the initial evaluation should include the blood work discussed earlier and ultrasonography. The presence of a choledochal cyst should lead to surgical consultation for repair. If such a definitive finding is absent, further investigation to rule out EHBA should be undertaken, particularly in patients with acholic stools. A hepatobiliary scintigram can be performed to look for excretion of the radioactive tracer from the liver into the gut, which would confirm the patency of the biliary tree.[3,11] Lack of excretion into the gut means that EHBA may be present. This study is not available at all institutions, however, and an abnormal study does not always distinguish extrahepatic obstruction from intrahepatic causes of cholestasis, such as Alagille syndrome or cystic fibrosis. A liver biopsy may be helpful in these patients to distinguish among several causes of jaundice, including neonatal hepatitis, bile duct paucity syndromes such as Alagille, and EHBA (which is characterized by bile duct proliferation on biopsy).[1,3] Because of the possible overlap in the appearance of these cholestatic conditions on biopsy, if there is ongoing clinical concern about EHBA, surgical consultation for an intraoperative cholangiogram should be obtained. The cholangiogram is the most definitive study for EHBA.

A few other studies may be appropriate in selected patients. Because hypothyroidism, either alone or in conjunction with panhypopituitarism, can stunt intrahepatic bile duct formation, jaundiced infants should have thyroid function tests performed.[13,14] Infants with cystic fibrosis can also develop jaundice due to thick, inspissated bile plugging of both intra- and extrahepatic bile ducts, so patients in this age group should have a sweat test performed.[15,16]

Older children presenting with jaundice, abdominal pain, and elevated GGT or alkaline phosphatase in the absence of gallstones may be suffering from primary sclerosing cholangitis, an autoimmune condition of the biliary tree. This condition requires imaging with either endoscopic retrograde cholangiopancreatography (ERCP) or magnetic resonance cholangiopancreatography (MRCP) to show the characteristic areas of alternating stricture and dilation, giving the intrahepatic and extrahepatic ducts a beaded appearance.[4,17,18] Characteristic findings are also present on liver biopsy. A history of inflammatory bowel disease, particularly ulcerative colitis, in the patient or the family should raise the suspicion for primary sclerosing cholangitis and lead to consultation with a pediatric gastroenterologist for a full evaluation.

SPECIFIC DISEASES AND THEIR TREATMENT

This section discusses in greater depth the pathophysiology and management of those biliary diseases most likely to be encountered by the pediatric hospitalist. EHBA and choledochal cysts are typically diagnosed in infancy, although the latter may rarely present in older children and adults. Cholelithiasis and cholangitis are more likely to be found in older children.

Extrahepatic Biliary Atresia

EHBA is the most common cause of chronic cholestasis in infants, occurring in 1 in 8000 to12,000 births, and it is the leading indication for pediatric liver transplantation worldwide.[1,3,19,20] In this condition, all or part of the extrahepatic bile ducts are destroyed or absent, leading to early cholestasis and rapidly progressive liver disease. Without surgical correction, death occurs in the first 1 to 2 years of life; even with therapy, timing and surgical expertise are crucial to patient outcome.

Prolonged neonatal jaundice and the development of acholic stools are the typical presenting symptoms, and EHBA should be considered and ruled out in any infant who is jaundiced past 14 days of life. The physical examination reveals jaundice and possibly malnutrition due to fat malabsorption from inadequate bile secretion into the stools. Laboratory studies reveal an elevated conjugated bilirubin, and liver enzymes are often mildly elevated. Abdominal ultrasonography frequently fails to identify a gallbladder, although the presence of a gallbladder does not rule out EHBA. Radioisotope studies with technetium cholescintigraphy can be helpful in distinguishing between neonatal hepatitis and EHBA as causes of jaundice. Classically, tracer is taken up well by the liver but is not excreted into the bowel in EHBA, whereas the opposite is true in neonatal hepatitis and other nonobstructive lesions. Excretion of the tracer makes EHBA very unlikely, but other causes of chronic cholestasis, such as cystic fibrosis, Alagille syndrome, and α_1-antitrypsin deficiency, may also have nonexcretion of tracer, so an abnormal study by itself is not diagnostic of EHBA.[1,3,4,11,21]

The definitive diagnosis of EHBA is made by liver biopsy or intraoperative cholangiogram. Liver biopsy shows proliferation of intrahepatic bile ductules, diffuse cholestasis, and often fibrosis without the degree of hepatocyte inflammation seen in neonatal hepatitis. If the biopsy is suggestive of obstruction, an intraoperative cholangiogram should be performed before surgical correction to confirm the diagnosis and determine the degree of anatomic involvement. When suspicion of EHBA is high, proceeding directly to operative cholangiogram and open liver biopsy should be considered. A Kasai procedure (hepatoportoenterostomy) should follow if EHBA is confirmed. The goal of this surgery is to reestablish bile flow from the remaining patent ductules in the liver to a jejunal limb attached to the porta hepatitis via a Roux-en-Y anastomosis. The timing of surgery is crucial, with correction before 60 days of life vastly improving outcome. The procedure is initially successful in approximately 80% to 90% of patients if it is performed during this time frame; the success rate drops to less than 20% in patients 90 days or older at the time of surgery.[3,22] Unfortunately, despite initial improvement in bile flow after surgery, only 30% of patients have long-term survival with a Kasai procedure alone. The remainder of patients develop progressive liver disease and require transplantation; however, their survival and outcome after transplantation are often greatly improved owing to their growth and improved nutritional status during the months of functional bile flow.

Choledochal Cysts

Choledochal cysts are congenital cystic dilations of the biliary tree; they may be extrahepatic, intrahepatic, or both. The incidence of cysts varies worldwide, occurring in about 1 in 13,000 to 15,000 births in Western countries but as frequently as 1 in 1000 births in Japan. There is a 4:1 female predominance. Patients usually present in infancy but may occasionally present as late as 10 years of age.[3,4] Cysts are diagnosed in up to 2% of infants presenting with obstructive jaundice.[3,23]

Patients with choledochal cysts most commonly present with jaundice, although vague right upper quadrant pain, cholangitis, and, rarely, recurrent pancreatitis may also be present. The classic triad of intermittent abdominal pain, jaundice, and a right upper quadrant mass occurs in only 20% of patients.[3,4,24] Infants present similarly to those with EHBA, including jaundice and acholic stools. Diagnosis is usually made by ultrasonography, and intraoperative cholangiogram reveals the full anatomy and presence of intrahepatic disease.[3,4,11] Preoperative MRCP can provide a better assessment of the lesion.[11,25]

Treatment consists of complete surgical excision of the cyst and creation of a Roux-en-Y choledochojejunostomy proximal to the most distal lesion.[3,4,24] The goals of surgery are good bile drainage and complete cyst removal to reduce the risk of future malignancy. Biliary adenocarcinoma rates are 20 times higher in patients with choledochal cysts than in the general population, and carcinoma has been reported in up to 26% of patients left with residual cystic tissue after surgery.[24,26,27] With successful radical excision of the cyst and Roux-en-Y formation, long-term outcomes are excellent. However, patients should be followed by a pediatric gastroenterologist after surgery to monitor for recurrent cholangitis, pancreatitis, and malignancy.[4,24,27,28]

Cholelithiasis

Cholelithiasis, or gallstones, is a frequent condition in adults, occurring in up to 10% of the adult population in North America.[29] The incidence and prevalence in children are less well studied, but the prevalence in Italian children in a 1989 study was 0.13% (0.27% in females) in children 6 to 19 years old screened with ultrasonography.[30] Cholelithiasis in children is frequently associated with known predisposing conditions such as obesity, hemolytic disease, ileal disease, total parenteral nutrition (TPN), prolonged fasting, and pregnancy, although recent studies show that up to half of infants and a quarter of older children with gallstones have no identifiable underlying condition.[31,32] Pigmented stones are most common in children younger than 6 years and in patients with hemolytic processes; cholesterol stones predominate in school-age children and adolescents.[33]

Infants with symptomatic cholelithiasis present with jaundice, sepsis, or abdominal pain, although asymptomatic gallstones may be identified incidentally, particularly in infants requiring prolonged fasting and support with TPN. Epigastric and right upper quadrant abdominal pain, vomiting, and jaundice are common presenting symptoms in older children and adolescents, and pancreatitis may be a complication of gallstones in 5% to 10% of patients.[4,31-33] Laboratory studies may be normal in asymptomatic patients, but liver enzymes, GGT, alkaline phosphatase, and conjugated bilirubin may all be elevated in the presence of ductal obstruction or infection. Ultrasonography is the best initial study for identifying both gallstones and dilation of the biliary tree.[4,11] Stones and sludge may be identified in the gallbladder, and a thickened gallbladder wall indicates inflammation.

Asymptomatic stones found incidentally generally do not require therapy. In adults, long-term follow-up studies have shown that less than 5% of patients with silent stones go on to require nonelective cholecystectomy.[34] Longitudinal studies of children with silent stones have not been completed, but complications are not believed to occur more commonly in children than in adults. Dissolution of stones less than 2 cm in size with ursodeoxycholic acid has been effective in 60% of adult patients with small cholesterol stones, although the recurrence rate of stones after cessation of therapy is 10% per year.[35] Pediatric patients with hemolytic diseases are at particular risk for gallstone formation, with 30% to 60% of patients with sickle cell disease developing stones in the first 14 years of life.[4,36] These patients may require ERCP to accurately identify common bile duct stones, and they may benefit from cholecystectomy at the time of silent stone identification, given the risks of cholecystitis and pancreatitis associated with continued stone formation.[37,38]

For symptomatic stones, the definitive therapy is cholecystectomy, usually done laparoscopically. In acute cholecystitis, urgent or even emergent gallbladder removal may be warranted, but in those patients without infection or obstruction, surgery can usually be delayed for a few days to a month or more to allow for convenient timing.[10] Acute cholecystitis, or infection of the gallbladder, is usually associated with cholelithiasis and cystic duct obstruction. It presents with right upper quadrant pain, fever, and vomiting, and approximately half of patients are jaundiced.[32] Treatment includes intravenous antibiotics with gram-negative and anaerobic bacterial coverage, fluid resuscitation, and cholecystectomy.

For stones obstructing the common bile duct, therapeutic ERCP has become popular in older children and adolescents.[39-41] This procedure can identify stones in the common duct and allow their removal via sphincterotomy and clearance techniques. Whether this procedure is required in patients with suspected common bile duct stones is controversial, and some authors argue for intraoperative cholangiography at the time of cholecystectomy, reserving ERCP for patients whose duct cannot be cleared at the time of surgery.[42] Not all centers have an endoscopist skilled in ERCP in children, and in such circumstances, an intraoperative procedure may be preferable to therapeutic ERCP.[43]

Cholangitis

Cholangitis is a bacterial infection of the biliary tree, encompassing the extra- or intrahepatic ducts or both. Cholecystitis is infection of the gallbladder without involvement of the ducts leading to or from it. Patients at risk for bacterial cholangitis are those with biliary tree anomalies and those with acute biliary obstruction. Patients with choledochal cysts, cholelithiasis, biliary atresia following a Kasai portoenterostomy, and strictures of the biliary tree (e.g., primary sclerosing cholangitis) are all at risk for cholangitis.[4,9] Charcot's triad of right upper quadrant abdominal pain, fever, and jaundice is common in older children and adults, and infants may present with fever and acholic stools as well as jaundice.

Up to half of patients with bacterial cholangitis have positive blood cultures, and in those cases, cultures can help direct and narrow antibiotic choices. The most common bacteria identified on culture are *Escherichia coli, Klebsiella* species, *Bacteroides,* enterococci, *Enterobacter,* and *Pseudomonas.*[7-9,44] Mixed aerobic and anaerobic flora commonly occur. Therapy includes relief of obstruction, fluid resuscitation, and intravenous antibiotics. The combination of a penicillin and an aminoglycoside has been standard; however, newer broad-spectrum antibiotics such as piperacillin-tazobactam and meropenem are used as single agents.[7,44,45] Duration of antibiotic therapy is usually 21 days, although the entire course need not be parenteral.

In patients with biliary obstruction, the timing of decompression depends on the stability of the patient. Toxic patients often need emergent endoscopic or operative decompression, whereas most stable patients can wait until they are afebrile for 24 to 48 hours before undergoing therapeutic interventions.[45] Therapy usually involves ERCP with removal of a stone or stenting of a stricture. In patients with cholelithiasis, a cholecystectomy should be performed once the patient has recovered from the acute illness. Duration of antibiotic administration following ERCP and decompression has been debated, but a recent study found no significant difference in outcomes when adult patients were treated with intravenous antibiotics for either 3 or 5 or more days, provided the patient was doing well and had defervesced after surgery.[46]

Acalculous Cholecystitis

Acalculous cholecystitis is an acute distention and inflammation of the gallbladder in the absence of gallstones and is typically due to infection or systemic illness. Prolonged fasting and TPN use, episodic ischemia, and the use of opiates in critically ill or postoperative patients may contribute to its development, resulting from gallbladder stasis and bacterial infection in these circumstances.[4,10] Several systemic illnesses have also been associated with acalculous cholecystitis, including streptococcal and gram-negative sepsis, leptospirosis, Rocky Mountain spotted fever, typhoid fever, ascariasis, and *Giardia lamblia* infection. Parasitic, candidal, and viral infections have been identified in immunocompromised patients.[10,47,48] Anatomically, the cystic duct that drains the gallbladder is narrowed due to a congenital anomaly, edema, or lymph node compression; this leads to inadequate drainage of the gallbladder and subsequent bile stasis and infection.

Clinically, patients present with right upper quadrant abdominal pain, nausea, vomiting, fever, and possibly a palpable gallbladder on examination. Diagnosis of acalculous cholecystitis is most often made via ultrasonography and nuclear medicine imaging.[11] Increased gallbladder wall thickness on ultrasonography is an inconsistent finding, although progressive thickening of the wall in serial examinations may be suggestive.[49,50] Other ultrasound findings include an absence of calculi, gallbladder distention, and poor contraction in response to cholecystokinin, although these can also be seen in hydrops of the gallbladder. Radioisotope studies with technetium cholescintigraphy are sensitive for detecting cystic duct obstruction that is suggestive of acalculous cholecystitis.[11,51] Findings include good hepatic uptake and intestinal excretion of isotope without gallbladder filling. In the event of gallbladder perforation, tracer extrudes into the abdominal cavity.

Therapy for acalculous cholecystitis includes treatment of any underlying condition, intravenous antibiotics, and surgical removal of the gallbladder.[4,10] Cholecystectomy is frequently necessary to avoid progression to gallbladder necrosis and possible perforation with bile peritonitis.

Hydrops of the Gallbladder

Hydrops is the acute distention and poor contractility of the gallbladder without concomitant inflammation or infection of the organ. The lack of gallstones, infection, or anatomic abnormality of the biliary system distinguishes this condition from those previously mentioned.[52] It is associated with several systemic illnesses, including Kawasaki syndrome; it is found in up to 20% of these patients.[53,54] Other associated conditions include staphylococcal or streptococcal infection, leptospirosis, sepsis, TPN administration, and mesenteric adenitis (often with a preceding viral syndrome).[55,56]

Hydrops is a self-limited condition that usually does not require surgical intervention. Symptoms can include abdominal pain and vomiting in addition to those symptoms associated with the underlying disease. Ultrasonography reveals a distended, acalculous, and unthickened gallbladder, and serial examinations can confirm a return to normal size and function. The rare need for surgery arises only if hydrops has led to insufficient gallbladder perfusion, with subsequent gangrene or perforation of the organ. Failure of the hydrops to resolve may also warrant surgical investigation, because clinical and radiographic findings may not reliably distinguish hydrops from acalculous cholecystitis, and laparoscopic investigation may be necessary.[10,11,52]

CONSULTATION

Subspecialty consultation is appropriate in the following circumstances:

- Hepatosplenomegaly: pediatric gastroenterology
- Biliary tree anomaly: pediatric surgery and pediatric gastroenterology
- Obstructive cholelithiasis: pediatric surgery and pediatric gastroenterology
- Liver synthetic dysfunction: pediatric gastroenterology
- Cystic fibrosis: pediatric pulmonology and pediatric gastroenterology
- Dysmorphism or associated congenital anomalies: pediatric genetics and pediatric gastroenterology

ADMISSION CRITERIA

Hospitalization of a child with biliary disease may be indicated for the following reasons:

- Infant with direct hyperbilirubinemia (evaluate for EHBA, choledochal cyst, or other surgical or genetic causes of jaundice)
- Jaundice accompanied by fever (intravenous antibiotics for treatment of cholangitis and evaluation of underlying cause of infection)
- Biliary tree obstruction (surgical or endoscopic relief of obstruction)
- Biliary tree anomaly in the presence of jaundice or fever (intravenous antibiotics and surgical correction of anomaly)
- Evidence of liver failure (vitamin K administration, intensive support and monitoring, correction of underlying cause)

DISCHARGE CRITERIA

Overall, patients may be discharged when the diagnosis has been established or when serious or life-threatening disorders are no longer being considered. Further diagnostic evaluation may proceed after discharge, as appropriate. Treatment should be completed or should be able to be continued or completed after discharge. Appropriate ongoing monitoring and follow-up should be in place.

IN A NUTSHELL

- Diseases of the biliary tract range from those that need urgent surgical correction, such as biliary atresia or septic cholangitis with obstruction, to genetic conditions that require lifelong subspecialist management.
- Jaundice, abdominal pain, and fever are the most frequent presenting signs of biliary disease, and a basic evaluation includes a complete blood count, fractionated bilirubin, hepatic enzymes, liver function tests, and abdominal ultrasonography.
- The basic evaluation often indicates whether the disease is a primary liver disorder or one limited to the biliary tract.

ON THE HORIZON

- The first multicenter longitudinal studies on biliary atresia in North America are currently under way by the Biliary Atresia Research Consortium, with results expected in the near future.
- Therapeutic ERCP is gaining importance in the acute management of obstructive gallstones in the pediatric population, and this represents an important area of study for the future.

SUGGESTED READING

D'Agata ID, Balistreri WF: Evaluation of liver disease in the pediatric patient. Pediatr Rev 1999;20:11.

Gubernick JA, Rosenberg HK, Ilaslan H, et al: Ultrasound approach to jaundice in infants and children. Radiographics 2000;20:1.

Heubi JE, Lewis LG, Pohl JF: Diseases of the gallbladder in infancy, childhood, and adolescence. In Suchy FJ, Sokol RJ, Balistreri WF (eds): Liver Disease in Children. Philadelphia, Lippincott Williams & Wilkins, 2001, pp 343-362.

McEvoy CF, Suchy FJ: Biliary tract disease in children. Pediatr Clin North Am 1996;43:1.

REFERENCES

1. D'Agata ID, Balistreri WF: Evaluation of liver disease in the pediatric patient. Pediatr Rev 1999;20:11.
2. Stoll BJ, Kliegman RM: Digestive system disorders. In Behrman RE (ed): Nelson Textbook of Pediatrics, 17th ed. Philadelphia, WB Saunders, 2004, pp 588-599.
3. Balistreri WF, Bove KE, Rychman FC: Biliary atresia and other disorders of the extrahepatic bile ducts. In Suchy FJ, Sokol RJ, Balistreri WF (eds): Liver Disease in Children. Philadelphia, Lippincott Williams & Wilkins, 2001, pp 253-274.
4. McEvoy CF, Suchy FJ: Biliary tract disease in children. Pediatr Clin North Am 1996;43:1.
5. Vitamins. In Kleinman RE (ed): Pediatric Nutrition Handbook, 5th ed. Chicago, American Academy of Pediatrics, 2004, pp 339-359.
6. Shaffer EA: Gallbladder disease. In Walker WA, Durie PR, Hamilton JR, et al (eds): Pediatric Gastrointestinal Disease, 3rd ed. Hamilton, Ontario, BC Decker, 2000, pp 1291-1311.
7. Lipsett PA, Pitt HA: Acute cholangitis. Surg Clin North Am 1990;70:6.
8. Carpenter HA: Bacterial and parasitic cholangitis. Mayo Clin Proc 1998;73:5.
9. Ecoffey C, Rothman E, Bernanrd O, et al: Bacterial cholangitis after surgery for biliary atresia. J Pediatr 1987;111:824.
10. Heubi JE, Lewis LG, Pohl JF: Diseases of the gallbladder in infancy, childhood, and adolescence. In Suchy FJ, Sokol RJ, Balistreri WF (eds): Liver Disease in Children. Philadelphia, Lippincott Williams & Wilkins, 2001, pp 343-362.
11. Gubernick JA, Rosenberg HK, Ilaslan H, et al: Ultrasound approach to jaundice in infants and children. Radiographics 2000;20:1.
12. Choi SO, Park WH, Lee JH, et al: "Triangular cord": A sonographic finding applicable in the diagnosis of biliary atresia. J Pediatr Surg 1996;31:3.
13. Herman SP, Baggenstoss MD, Cloutier MD: Liver dysfunction and histologic abnormalities in neonatal hypopituitarism. J Pediatr 1975;87:6.
14. Sheehan AG, Martin SR, Stephure D, et al: Neonatal cholestasis, hypoglycemia, and congenital hypopituitarism. J Pediatr Gastroenterol Nutr 1992;14:4.
15. Valman HB, France NE, Wallis PG: Prolonged neonatal jaundice in cystic fibrosis. Arch Dis Child 1971;46:250.
16. Gaskin KJ: The liver and biliary tract in cystic fibrosis. In Suchy FJ, Sokol RJ, Balistreri WF (eds): Liver Disease in Children. Philadelphia, Lippincott Williams & Wilkins, 2001, pp 549-563.
17. Debray D, Pariente D, Urvoas E, et al: Sclerosing cholangitis in children. J Pediatr 1994;124:49.
18. Siegel MJ: Pediatric liver magnetic resonance imaging. Magn Reson Imaging Clin North Am 2002;10:2.
19. Whitington PF, Balistreri WF: Liver transplantation in pediatrics: Indications, contraindications, and pretransplant management. J Pediatr 1991;118:169.
20. Karrer FM, Lilly JR, Stewardt BA, et al: Biliary atresia registry, 1976 to 1989. J Pediatr Surg 1990;254:10.
21. Muraji T, Nishijima E, Hagashimoto Y, et al: Biliary atresia: Current management and outcome. Tohoku J Exp Med 1997;181:1.
22. Rothenberg SS, Schroter GP, Karrer FM, et al: Cholangitis after the Kasai operation for biliary atresia. J Pediatr Surg 1989;24:8.
23. Brough AJ, Bernstein J: Conjugated hyperbilirubinemia in early infancy. Hum Pathol 1974;5:507.
24. Todani T: Choledochal cysts and pancreatobiliary malfunction. In Balistreri WF, Ohi R, Todanti T, et al (eds): Hepatobiliary, Pancreatic and Splenic Disease in Children: Medical and Surgical Management. Amsterdam, Elsevier Science, 1997, pp 231-260.
25. Irie H, Honda H, Jimi M, et al: Value of MR cholangiopancreatography in evaluating choledochal cysts. AJR Am J Roentgenol 1998;171:5.
26. Stain SC, Guthrie CR, Yellin A, et al: Choledochal cysts in the adult. Ann Surg 1995;222:2.
27. Stringer MD, Chawan A, Davenport M, et al: Choledochal cysts: Lessons from a 20 year experience. Arch Dis Child 1995;73:6.
28. Chijiiwa K, Koga A: Surgical management and long-term follow-up of patients with choledochal cysts. Am J Surg 1993;165:2.
29. Friedman GD, Kannel WB, Dawber TR: The epidemiology of gallbladder disease: Observations in Framingham study. J Chron Dis 1966;19:3.
30. Palasciano G, Portincasa P, Vinciguerra V, et al: Gallstone prevalence and gallbladder volume in children and adolescents: An epidemiological ultrasonographic survey and relationship to body mass index. Am J Gastroenterol 1989;84:11.
31. Debray D, Pariente D, Gauthier F, et al: Cholelithiasis in infancy: A study of 40 cases. J Pediatr 1993;122:3.
32. Reif S, Sloven DG, Lebenthal E: Gallstones in children: Characterization by age, etiology, and outcome. Am J Dis Child 1991;145:1.
33. Friesen CA, Roberts CC: Cholelithiasis: Clinical characteristics in children. Clin Pediatr 1989;28:7.
34. Gracie WA, Ransohoff DF: The natural history of silent gallstones: The innocent gallstone is not a myth. N Engl J Med 1982;307:13.
35. O'Donnell LD, Heaton KW: Recurrence and re-recurrence of gallstones after medical dissolution: A long-term follow up. Gut 1988;29:5.
36. Leuschner U, Guldutuna S, Hellstern A: Pathogenesis of pigment stones and medical treatment. J Gastroenterol Hepatol 1994;9:1.
37. Ware RE, Kinney TR, Caseye JR, et al: Laparoscopic cholecystectomy in young patients with sickle hemoglobinopathies. J Pediatr 1992;120:1.
38. Ware RE, Schultz WH, Filston HC, et al: Diagnosis and management of common bile duct stones in patients with sickle hemoglobinopathies. J Pediatr Surg 1992;27:5.
39. Varadarajulu S, Wilcox CM, Hawes RH, et al: Technical outcomes and complications of ERCP in children. Gastrointest Endosc 2004;60:3.
40. Pfau PR, Chelimsky GG, Kinnard MF, et al: Endoscopic retrograde cholangiopancreatography in children and adolescents. J Pediatr Gastroenterol Nutr 2002;35:5.
41. Poddar U, Thapa BR, Bhasin BK, et al: Endoscopic retrograde cholangiopancreatography in the management of pancreaticobiliary disorders in children. J Gastroenterol Hepatol 2001;16:8.
42. Waldhausen JH, Graham DD, Tapper D: Routine intraoperative cholangiography during laparoscopy cholecystectomy minimizes unnecessary endoscopic retrograde cholangiopancreatography in children. J Pediatr Surg 2001;36:6.
43. Prasil P, Laberge JM, Barkun A, et al: Endoscopic retrograde cholangiopancreatography in children: A surgeon's perspective. J Pediatr Surg 2001;36:5.

44. Chang WT, Lee KT, Wang SR, et al: Bacteriology and antimicrobial susceptibility in biliary tract disease: An audit of 10-years' experience. Kaohsiung J Med Sci 2002;18:5.

45. Bornman PC, van Beljon JI, Krige JE: Management of cholangitis. J Hepatobiliary Pancreat Surg 2003;10:6.

46. van Lent AU, Bartelsman JF, Tytgat GN, et al: Duration of antibiotic therapy for cholangitis after successful endoscopic drainage of the biliary tract. Gastrointest Endosc 2002;55:4.

47. Walker DH, Leseske HR, Varma VA, et al: Rocky Mountain spotted fever mimicking acute cholecystitis. Arch Intern Med 1985;45:12.

48. Reid MR, Montgomery JC: Acute cholecystitis in children as a complication of typhoid fever. Johns Hopkins Hosp Bull 1920;347.

49. Patriquin HB, DiPietro M, Barber FE, et al: Sonography of thickened gallbladder wall: Causes in children. AJR Am J Roentgenol 1983;141:1.

50. Jeffrey RB Jr, Sommer FG: Follow-up sonography in suspected acalculous cholecystitis: Preliminary clinical experience. J Ultrasound Med 1993;12:4.

51. Swayne LC: Acute acalculous cholecystitis: Sensitivity in detection using technetium-99m iminodiacetic acid cholescintigraphy. Radiology 1986; 160:1.

52. Rumley TO, Rodgers BM: Hydrops of the gallbladder in children. J Pediatr Surg 1983;18:2.

53. Suddleson EA, Reid B, Wooley MM, et al: Hydrops of the gallbladder associated with Kawasaki syndrome. J Pediatr Surg 1987;22:10.

54. Slovis TL, High DW, Philippart AI, et al: Sonography in the diagnosis and management of hydrops of the gallbladder in children with mucocutaneous lymph node syndrome. Pediatrics 1980;5:4.

55. Strauss RG: Scarlet fever with hydrops of the gallbladder. Pediatrics 1969;44:5.

56. Blood RA, Swain VA: Non-calculous distension of the gallbladder in childhood. Arch Dis Child 1966;41:219.

CHAPTER 94

Constipation

Laura K. Brennan

Constipation is a common pediatric disorder, affecting anywhere from 0.3% to 28% of children.[1,2] It accounts for 3% of visits to outpatient general pediatric offices and up to 25% of visits to pediatric gastroenterologists.[1-6] It is generally defined as infrequent or difficult passage of hard stool, frequently associated with pain and straining. Normal stooling patterns vary greatly among individuals and by age.[2-7] Average stooling frequencies at different ages have been defined (Table 94-1).

Constipation can occur at any age but is particularly common in toddlers and elementary school–age children. In infants and toddlers, males and females are equally affected,[7] but by school age, constipation is more common in males.[3]

The causes of constipation can be divided into anatomic, physiologic, and functional categories. Anatomic causes of constipation include Hirschsprung disease, imperforate anus, and bowel obstruction. Physiologic causes include a number of processes that alter bowel motility, such as hypothyroidism and spinal cord defects. Functional constipation, which results from voluntary stool withholding, is the most common cause of constipation (90% to 97% of cases)[1,2,7] and is often a self-perpetuating condition that starts with an episode of pain on defecation, a battle over toilet training, or toilet phobia.

Functional constipation may progress to encopresis, defined as repeated expulsion of normal stool, whether involuntarily or intentionally, in inappropriate places in a child at least 4 years of age. It can involve the leakage of stool around more distal hard, impacted stool and is thought to result from chronic constipation secondary to functional fecal retention. Encopresis occurs in 1% to 3% of children and is two to nine times more likely in boys.[2,5,6]

CLINICAL PRESENTATION

Constipation does not always present with the obvious history of infrequent or hard stools. Children may have regular, even daily, bowel movements but incomplete evacuation with each episode, leading to progressive stool retention. The presenting complaint is often abdominal pain or discomfort, which can be intermittently severe but is usually low grade and difficult for the child to describe. The location of the pain is usually periumbilical, and on examination there is no focal tenderness, rebound, or guarding. Other manifestations of constipation can include abdominal distention, anorexia, flatulence, pain with defecation, blood-streaked stools, nausea, and vomiting. The presenting complaint in children with encopresis may be diarrhea.

DIFFERENTIAL DIAGNOSIS

Constipation is often diagnosed easily and with specificity by the presence of infrequent or hard stools. However, there is a large differential diagnosis of underlying disorders that can lead to constipation (Table 94-2). Although functional constipation is the most common type, it is important to keep other disorders in mind, especially in children with complex medical needs, recurrent constipation, or severe symptoms necessitating hospitalization.

DIAGNOSIS AND EVALUATION

The diagnosis and evaluation of constipation rests on a thorough history and physical examination. Besides stool texture and frequency, the history should include time to passage of the first meconium stool, age at onset of symptoms, details of toilet training, and associated symptoms of rectal pain and bleeding, abdominal pain, and incontinence.

The history alone can often differentiate those children with an organic cause of constipation from those with functional constipation (Table 94-3). A history of delayed passage of the first stool in the neonatal period raises the suspicion of Hirschsprung disease, because most of these patients fail to pass stool in the first 48 hours after delivery; this suspicion would be supported by a family history of Hirschsprung disease or other causes of constipation. A history of any associated symptoms such as vomiting, fever, abdominal distention, blood in the stool, or poor weight gain should also be elicited, because these suggest an underlying organic disorder. A history of stool withholding or of constipation associated with toilet training or toilet phobia is strongly suggestive of functional constipation.

A careful and thorough physical examination can help identify any underlying disorder. Height and body weight are important to rule out a malabsorptive disorder. The abdominal examination is particularly important, with attention paid to bowel sounds, presence or absence of distention, location and quality of tenderness, and thorough palpation for stool. A digital rectal examination should be performed to assess rectal tone and determine whether impacted stool is present in the rectal vault. With functional constipation, it is common to find large amounts of hard stool in the rectum. Hirschsprung disease is often suggested by an empty, nondistended rectum or by expulsion of gas and stool following a digital rectal examination. An absent anal wink may be a sign of a neurologic cause of constipation. The lumbosacral area of the spine should be examined for signs of myelodysplasia

Table 94-1   Normal Stooling Patterns

Age Group	Average Frequency of Stools
Infants: first week of life*	>4/day
Infants: 16 wk old*	2/day
Toddlers: up to age 4 yr	1-2/day
Adults	3/day to 3/wk

*Breastfed infants initially have more stools, but by age 16 weeks, stooling frequency is equal to that of formula-fed infants.[5]

Table 94-2   Differential Diagnosis of Constipation

Functional
    Toilet phobia
    Coercive toilet training
    School bathroom avoidance
    Sexual abuse

Anatomic
    Hirschsprung disease
    Imperforate anus
    Anal stenosis
    Anteriorly displaced anus
    Bowel obstruction, pseudo-obstruction
    Tethered cord

Physiologic
    Hypothyroidism
    Hypercalcemia
    Diabetes mellitus
    Cystic fibrosis
    Bowel motility disorders
    Spinal cord abnormalities
    Neuropathic conditions
    Drugs (opiates, anticholinergics, lead, iron, antidepressants)
    Poor fluid or fiber intake
    Depression
    Connective tissue disorders (scleroderma, systemic lupus erythematosus, Ehlers-Danlos syndrome)
    Infant botulism

Table 94-3   Historical Factors of Importance in the Evaluation of Constipation

Constipation history
    Timing of first stool in neonatal period
    Quality of stool
    Frequency of stool
    Duration of symptoms

Family history
    Hirschsprung disease
    Other causes of constipation
    Other systemic disease (e.g., thyroid, cystic fibrosis, inflammatory bowel disease)

Diet
    Amount of fluid
    Amount of fiber
    General nutrition
    Recently weaned off formula

Recent events
    Toilet training
    New school
    Family or social stressors
    Sexual abuse

Behavior
    History of withholding behavior
    Toilet phobia

Medications, ingestions, or exposures
    Narcotic use or ingestion
    Previous medication for constipation
    Any other ingestions
    Lead exposure

Associated symptoms
    Abdominal pain
    Nausea
    Vomiting
    Weight loss
    Diarrhea
    Pain with defecation
    Blood in stool
    Fever

General medical history
    Neuropathic disorder
    Cerebral palsy
    Spina bifida

or sacral agenesis, and a thorough neurologic examination, particularly of the lower extremities, should be performed to elicit findings that suggest an occult spinal cord lesion. A careful thyroid examination should also be done.

If the examination is limited by body habitus or the diagnosis is still in doubt, a simple flat-plate abdominal radiograph to look for the presence of stool can be helpful. Laboratory studies or additional imaging are necessary only if, based on the history or physical examination, there is concern about an underlying organic cause of the constipation. If an underlying metabolic disease is suspected, initial laboratory studies should include thyroid function tests (thyroxine and thyroid-stimulating hormone), calcium, glucose, lead level, and celiac panel. If the patient presents with abdominal pain or urinary complaints, a urinalysis and urine culture may be indicated, because constipation significantly increases the risk of a urinary tract infection. A sweat test to rule out the possibility of cystic fibrosis may be considered, especially in the presence of accompanying failure to thrive or pulmonary symptoms. Spinal magnetic resonance imaging and colonic transit time may be warranted if there is concern about an occult spinal abnormality or neuropathy. A barium enema can be useful to evaluate for Hirschsprung disease or other anatomic disorders. Other more sophisticated testing, such as anorectal manometry or rectal biopsy, may be recommended by and performed in consultation with a pediatric gastroenterologist or surgeon if there is still concern about an underlying anatomic or motility disorder.

COURSE OF ILLNESS

Constipation is frequently a chronic problem that requires long-term follow-up and management. In the inpatient setting, acute impaction can often be relieved and the patient discharged home in 1 to 2 days. However, maintenance therapy with stool softeners may be indicated for months, along with behavioral and toileting modification. Constipation can persist for years, and relapses during childhood and adolescence are common.[2,5,6]

Long-term complications are generally related to loss of normal colonic size and tone and the development of encopresis. In severe cases, chronic anorexia and failure to thrive can also result. Also, psychosocial functioning can be severely affected in children with chronic constipation, leading to poor self-esteem, poor school performance, and family stress and conflict.[1,2]

TREATMENT

Most patients with a clear diagnosis of functional constipation can be managed without hospitalization if close outpatient follow-up is available. After the initial diagnosis and initiation of therapy, reassessment of the frequency and character of stools and observation for new symptoms or findings are necessary. Patients should be followed at regular intervals until the child is having regular soft stools with no evidence of stool withholding or fecal soiling.

The successful treatment of functional constipation and encopresis requires a multipronged approach. Acutely, the child must be disimpacted (Table 94-4). Although either the oral or the rectal route can be effective,[4] the rectal route is faster and is often preferred for hospitalized patients. For these patients, disimpaction is often initiated by the administration of pediatric-size enemas, which can be repeated as needed until no hard stool is present in defecation or rectal effluent. The patient should be adequately hydrated prior to initiation of therapy to avoid sudden shifts in fluids and electrolytes. Evaluation of serum electrolytes should be considered after two enema administrations. Recommended enemas include saline, sodium biphosphate (Fleet), or milk and molasses enemas. Soapsuds, water, or magnesium enemas should not be used because of the potential toxicity and risk of electrolyte imbalance.[4] Often, more proximal stool must be evacuated via an oral (or nasogastric) polyethylene glycol–electrolyte solution or mineral oil. If the impaction is not severe, an enema may not be required, and evacuation may be achieved with only an oral solution. Occasionally, stool is impacted to such a severe degree that the impaction is refractory to pharmacologic therapy. In this case, manual disimpaction should be considered. Of note, manual disimpaction should be done only with the patient under adequate sedation, with appropriate airway and vital sign monitoring.

Once disimpaction is successful, a maintenance plan must be established. Patients should be started on stool softeners, laxatives, or both to keep stools soft and ensure that reaccumulation of hard stool does not occur (Table 94-5). Lubricants such as mineral oil or osmotic laxatives such as polyethylene glycol or magnesium hydroxide have been studied in long-term use and are effective and safe.[4,7] Stimulant laxatives, such as senna or bisacodyl, are best used only on a short-term or intermittent basis as "rescue" therapy to prevent ongoing or recurrent stool retention.

Consumption of an appropriate and healthy diet is also an important part of maintenance therapy. Increased intake of fluids and fiber can help soften stools. Carbohydrates—especially sorbitol, which is found in apple, pear, and prune juices—can also help soften stools.[4,5] A balanced diet consisting of whole grains, fruits, and vegetables is recommended for all children as part of constipation treatment.[4]

Additionally, if functional constipation is the diagnosis, behavioral factors must be addressed. Families must be instructed to initiate regular toileting times and durations. On average, a child should be put on the toilet for 5 to 10 minutes once or twice a day, ideally after meals.[2,5,6] With younger or smaller children, attention should be paid to proper foot support to permit 90 degrees of hip and knee

Table 94-4 Disimpaction Guidelines		
Method	**Dosage**	**Comments and Side Effects**
Enemas		
Milk and molasses (mixed 1:1)	<3 yr: 240 mL total ≥3yr: 500 mL total	
Sodium biphosphonate (Fleet)	2-5 yr: $^1/_2$ Fleet Enema for Children (1.125 fluid oz) 6-12 yr: 1 Fleet Enema for Children (2.25 fluid oz) >12 yr: 1 Fleet Enema (4.5 fluid oz)	Do not use in children younger than 2 yr Watch for electrolyte imbalances (hyperphosphatemia, hypernatremia) if there is megacolon or renal impairment
Glycerin suppository	<6 yr: 1 pediatric suppository (1 g) ≥6 yr: 1 adult suppository (2 or 3 g)	Anal irritation
Oral solutions		
Mineral oil	15-30 mL per year of age (max 240 mL) once or twice a day for 3 days	Do not use in infants younger than 12 mo or in those at risk for aspiration
Polyethylene glycol–electrolyte solution (GoLYTELY)	Children ≥6 mo: 25-40 mL/kg/hr for 4-10 hr, until rectal effluent is clear Adults: 240 mL (8 oz) every 10 min, until 4 L are consumed or rectal effluent is clear	Watch children younger than 2 yr carefully for electrolyte abnormalities Rapid drinking of each portion is preferred to drinking small amounts over a period of time

Table 94-5 Stool Softener and Laxative Guidelines

Method	Mechanism	Dosage	Comments and Side Effects
Mineral oil	Lubricant	>12 mo: 1-3 mL/kg/day	Do not use in children younger than 12 mo or in those at risk of aspiration Can cause anal leakage Long-term use (>1-2 yr) can cause fat-soluble vitamin deficiency
Polyethylene glycol 3350 (MiraLax)	Osmotic laxative	0.8 g/kg/day (max 17 g) of powder dissolved in 4-8 oz of water once daily	Can be mixed in any juice or liquid Do not use for more than 2 wk Can cause loose stools
Magnesium hydroxide (milk of magnesia)	Osmotic laxative	<2 years: 0.5 mL/kg/dose 2-5 yr: 1-3 tsp once a day 6-11 yr: 1-2 tbsp once a day ≥12 yr: 2-4 tbsp once a day	Can cause hypermagnesemia Use with caution in those with renal failure

Senna	Stimulant laxative	2-6 yr: Start with $\frac{1}{2}$ tablet at bedtime, or 2.5 mL syrup at bedtime
		7-12 yr: Start with 1 tablet or 5 mL syrup once a day at bedtime
		>12 yr: Start with 2 tablets or 10-15 mL at bedtime
			Forms: 8.6 mg tablet, 15 mg/5 mL granules, 8.8 mg/5 mL syrup
			Start as suggested, monitor effect, and increase dose as needed to maximum doses, as follows:
			  2-6 yr: 1 tablet, or 3.75 mL syrup twice a day
			  7-12 yr: 2 tablets, or 7.5 mL syrup twice a day
			  ≥12 yr: 4 tablets or 15 mL twice a day
			Can cause abdominal cramps

Bisacodyl oral	Stimulant laxative	≤12 yr: 5-10 mg daily >12 yr: 5-15 mg daily	Do not use for more than 1 wk Can cause abdominal cramping
Bisacodyl rectal	Stimulant laxative	6 mo-2 yr: 5 mg suppository daily 3-11 yr: 5-10 mg suppository daily ≥12 yr: 10 mg suppository daily	Do not use for more than 1 wk Can cause abdominal cramping
Lactulose	Osmotic laxative	Children: 5 g/day (7.5 mL) after breakfast Adults: 15-30 mL/day, increased to 60 mL/day in 1-2 divided doses if necessary	Can cause abdominal cramping and flatulence

flexion.[5] Children should not be punished if they fail to produce stool, but they should be encouraged to attempt to do so. The purpose of regular toileting routines is to resensitize the body to the gastrocolic reflex, and parents should explicitly be told not to make this process a source of anxiety for the child. Some children with severe emotional disorders or psychological avoidance of stool production benefit from psychological evaluation and therapy.

Children younger than 1 year should be managed more carefully. For this age group, emphasis is placed on increased intake of fluids and juices containing sorbitol (prune, pear, or apple). Other treatment may include corn syrup or lactulose. Mineral oil is not recommended owing to the risk of aspiration. Stimulant laxatives are not recommended either. Although enemas should generally be avoided, rectal glycerin suppositories may be helpful for rectal disimpaction.

CONSULTATION

Subspecialty consultation should be considered if the initial workup raises concern for any of the following:

- Chronic or refractory constipation, possible bowel motility disorder: gastroenterology
- Hirschsprung disease, bowel obstruction, acute abdomen: general surgery
- Hypothyroidism: endocrinology
- Spinal dysraphism, spina bifida, neuromuscular disorders: neurology
- Severe toilet phobia: psychiatry

ADMISSION CRITERIA

Hospitalization is indicated for any of the following reasons:

- Unclear cause, with concern about potentially life-threatening conditions or those that require presumptive inpatient evaluation and treatment (e.g., cystic fibrosis, bowel obstruction)
- Severe abdominal pain
- Nasogastric electrolyte solution administration for bowel clean-out
- Persistent vomiting or inability to tolerate oral intake
- Lack of appropriate outpatient support or follow-up

DISCHARGE CRITERIA

- Successful evacuation of stool
- Ability to tolerate oral or enteral fluids and nutrition
- Stable or resolving symptoms and issues that the family can manage at home
- Reliable outpatient follow-up with primary pediatrician and, if indicated, pediatric gastroenterologist or other specialist

PREVENTION

Eating a well-balanced diet with plenty of fruits, vegetables, and water can help prevent constipation, as can regular physical activity. Most important, hospitalization can usually be prevented by educating parents about the importance of appropriate toileting regimens. It is also important to deal with any behavioral issues early, before severe constipation and encopresis result.

Special consideration should be given to children with cerebral palsy, other neuromuscular disorders, or severe medical problems. These children are at greater risk for the development of constipation because of their relative inactivity, decreased muscle use and tone, and low-fiber diets. Therefore, efforts should be made to prevent constipation in these children by the routine use of stool softeners and maintenance therapy, and physicians should increase this therapy or begin disimpaction promptly if stools become more infrequent or hard.

IN A NUTSHELL

- Constipation can present with infrequent passage of hard stool and a variety of other symptoms, including abdominal pain, abdominal distention, pain with defecation, and nausea.
- Frequent liquid stools from encopresis may lead the family to report diarrhea.
- Functional constipation may require hospitalization if symptoms are severe or require close monitoring or intervention, and postdischarge follow-up is critical for preventing repeat episodes.

ON THE HORIZON

- Recent advances in pharmacotherapy, such as tegaserod (Zelnorm), a serotonin 5-HT$_4$ receptor agonist, and other new promotility agents, show promise in the management of constipation.
- Continuing research on the pathophysiology of impaired colonic transit may shed more light on the underlying cause of idiopathic constipation.

SUGGESTED READING

Baker S, Liptak G, Colletti R, et al: Constipation in infants and children: Evaluation and treatment. J Pediatr Gastroenterol Nutr 1999;29:612-626.

Benninga MA, Voskuijl W, Taminiau J: Childhood constipation: Is there new light in the tunnel? J Pediatr Gastroenterol Nutr 2004;39:448-464.

Croffie J, Fitzgerald J: Hypomotility disorders: Idiopathic constipation. In Walker W, Durie P, Hamilton J, et al (eds): Pediatric Gastrointestinal Disease: Pathophysiology, Diagnosis, Management, 3rd ed. Hamilton, Ontario, BC Decker, 2000, pp 830-844.

Loening-Baucke V: Prevalence, symptoms and outcome of constipation in infants and toddlers. J Pediatr 2005;146:359-363.

Wenner W: Constipation and encopresis. In Altschuler S, Liacouras C (eds): Clinical Pediatric Gastroenterology. Philadelphia, Churchill Livingstone, 1998, pp 165-168.

REFERENCES

1. Sauvat F: Severe functional constipation in child: What is the solution? J Pediatr Gastroenterol Nutr 2004;38:10-11.
2. Benninga M, Voskuijl W, Taminiau J: Childhood constipation: Is there new light in the tunnel? J Pediatr Gastroenterol Nutr 2004;39:448-464.
3. Arce D, Ermocilla C, Costa H: Evaluation of constipation. Am Fam Physician 2002;65:2283-2290.
4. Baker S, Liptak G, Colletti R, et al: Constipation in infants and children: Evaluation and treatment. J Pediatr Gastroenterol Nutr 1999;29:612-626.
5. Croffie J, Fitzgerald J: Hypomotility disorders: Idiopathic constipation. In Walker W, Durie P, Hamilton J, et al (eds): Pediatric Gastrointestinal Disease: Pathophysiology, Diagnosis, Management, 3rd ed. Hamilton, Ontario, BC Decker, 2000, pp 830-844.
6. Wenner W: Constipation and encopresis. In Altschuler S, Liacouras C (eds): Clinical Pediatric Gastroenterology. Philadelphia, Churchill Livingstone, 1998, pp 165-168.
7. Loening-Baucke V: Prevalence, symptoms and outcome of constipation in infants and toddlers. J Pediatr 2005;146:359-363.

CHAPTER 95

Dyspepsia

David J. Rawat and Denesh K. Chitkara

Children often experience symptoms of epigastric discomfort or dyspepsia either as a presenting complaint or during hospitalization. The challenge to the hospitalist is to identify the cause based on nonspecific complaints, a relatively limited ability to examine the affected organ, and laboratory and radiographic evaluations that are rarely diagnostic.

CLINICAL PRESENTATION

Nausea, vomiting, heartburn, oral regurgitation, early satiety, postprandial abdominal bloating or distention, excess gas with or without belching or flatulence, queasiness, fullness, and retching are all common presentations of gastric dysfunction. These symptoms overlap with the discussions of other disorders such as abdominal pain (Chapter 26), gastrointestinal (GI) bleeding (Chapter 34), failure to thrive (Chapter 32), and feeding difficulties (Chapter 101).

Dyspepsia is defined as chronic or recurrent pain or discomfort centered in the upper abdomen characterized by nausea, vomiting, bloating, and early satiety and usually exacerbated by food intake.[1] In a community-based study, 5% to 10% of otherwise healthy adolescents reported dyspeptic symptoms of nausea, heartburn, and acid brash within the previous year,[2] and the prevalence of dyspepsia is nearly 45% among school-age children in Italy.[3]

There is often a temporal relationship between food intake and symptoms. Pain attributable to gastric ulceration often peaks when the stomach is empty, whereas pain associated with functional dyspepsia usually develops immediately after eating and may persist for 3 to 4 hours.

DIFFERENTIAL DIAGNOSIS

Many disorders can cause dyspepsia, including functional, mucosal, and anatomic abnormalities of the stomach or extragastric GI system. In addition, extra-GI disorders, such as genitourinary or psychiatric dysfunction, can have prominent dyspeptic symptoms (Table 95-1).

DIAGNOSIS AND EVALUATION

The broad differential diagnosis and the subjective nature of these symptoms can present a challenge, and a standard approach or algorithm for evaluation is difficult to establish. A reasonable initial laboratory workup might include a complete blood count, measurement of the erythrocyte sedimentation rate and C-reactive protein, chemistry profile (including liver and renal function tests), stool testing for ova and parasites, urinalysis, and screening for *Helicobacter pylori*. The best noninvasive test for *H. pylori* is a ^{13}C urea breath test (sensitivity and specificity up to 95%). If this is not readily available, a locally validated serologic test for *H. pylori* with a sensitivity and specificity of at least 90% or a stool antigen test should be obtained. These laboratory investigations may raise concerns about the possibility of inflammatory bowel disease, *H. pylori* gastroenteritis, eosinophilic gastroenteritis, chronic hepatitis, chronic renal disease, or parasitic disease. An upper GI series with small bowel follow-through is indicated in children with severe abdominal pain and recurrent vomiting to evaluate for an anatomic disorder or inflammatory bowel disease. Serum amylase, lipase, and ultrasonography are indicated for discrete acute episodes of pain triggered by a meal or localized to the right upper quadrant. Ultrasonography or computed tomography of the abdomen can identify gallstones, pancreatic disease, hydronephrosis, retroperitoneal masses, and bowel wall thickening. Esophageal pH monitoring may be useful to detect atypical or unrecognized gastroesophageal reflux disease (GERD). Hydrogen breath tests may be a useful diagnostic tool for the evaluation of clinically suspected bacterial overgrowth and lactose or carbohydrate malabsorption.

An upper endoscopy should be strongly considered in patients presenting with symptoms such as weight loss, recurrent vomiting, bleeding, anemia, dysphagia, and jaundice and in those taking nonsteroidal anti-inflammatory drugs (NSAIDs). Upper endoscopy is usually indicated in patients with severe or persistent symptoms and is the best way to identify peptic ulcers, erosive esophagitis, *H. pylori* gastritis, and eosinophilic esophagitis.

Patients with severe chronic symptoms may need to be referred for further evaluation of motility of the stomach and small intestine by GI transit or emptying studies, barostat to investigate gastric accommodation or visceral sensation, or manometry to better delineate motor abnormalities.

TREATMENT

Treatment should be directed at the specific disorder, if one is identified. Frequently, however, no obvious cause is found, yet the patient has persistent symptoms. In the case of nondebilitating, chronic dyspeptic symptoms, empirical management is warranted. This usually hinges on measures that reduce gastroesophageal reflux and on the avoidance of triggers (Table 95-2). Traditionally, the initial therapy for patients with dyspepsia is empirical acid blockade with antacids, H_2 receptor antagonists, or proton pump inhibitors.[4-10] Prokinetic agents may also be considered, depending on symptoms. Therapy should usually be started before completion of the diagnostic workup. There is rarely reason to withhold therapy while awaiting endoscopy results.

For patients who test positive for *H. pylori*, treatment should be directed specifically at this infection. There are

Table 95-1 Differential Diagnosis for Dyspepsia

Functional disorders
  Functional dyspepsia
  GERD-predominant symptoms
  Rumination syndrome
  Postviral gastroparesis
  Abdominal migraine

Inflammatory or mucosal disorders
  GERD
  Helicobacter pylori gastritis
  Peptic ulcer
  NSAID ulcer
  Eosinophilic gastroenteritis
  Infection: *Giardia, Blastocystis hominis, Dientamoeba fragilis*
  Bacterial overgrowth
  Inflammatory bowel disease (Crohn's disease)
  Ménétrier disease
  Varioliform gastritis
  Celiac disease
  Lactose or carbohydrate malabsorption or intolerance
  Henoch-Schönlein purpura

Anatomic disorders
  Malrotation with or without volvulus
  Duodenal web

Psychiatric disorders
  Psychogenic vomiting
  Depression
  Somatization
  Anxiety
  Panic disorders
  Conversion reactions
  Anorexia nervosa

Other disorders
  Chronic pancreatitis
  Chronic hepatitis
  Ureteropelvic junction obstruction
  Biliary dyskinesia
  Intestinal pseudo-obstruction
  Lymphoma, carcinoma

GERD, gastroesophageal reflux disease; NSAID, nonsteroidal anti-inflammatory drug.

Table 95-2 Management and Therapeutic Options for Dyspepsia

Diet
  Timing of meals
  Small, frequent meals
  Solid vs liquid diet

Pharmacology
  H_2 agonists (e.g., famotidine, ranitidine)
  Proton pump inhibitors (e.g., omeprazole, esomeprazole, lansoprazole, pantoprazole)
  Prokinetic agents (e.g., metoclopramide, erythromycin, tegaserod)
  Serotonin-1 agonists (e.g., sumatriptan, buspirone)
  Tricyclic antidepressants (e.g., amitriptyline)

Surgery
  Fundoplication for GERD (may exacerbate ulcer-like and dysmotility-like dyspepsia)
  Gastrostomy or jejunostomy for nutritional supplementation

Alternative therapy
  Hypnotherapy
  Behavioral therapy
  Psychotherapy
  Acupuncture

many regimens to treat *H. pylori*, but a 14-day course of amoxicillin, clarithromycin, and a proton pump inhibitor is a good choice in children and is associated with a greater than 90% success rate.[11]

The pharmacologic choices for dysmotility symptoms are relatively limited. Prokinetic agents can be considered in patients with predominant symptoms of fullness, bloating, or early satiety. Metoclopramide (a central and peripheral dopamine-2 antagonist) is helpful for treating nausea, fullness, and bloating but may have neurologic side effects.[12] A low dose of erythromycin (a motilin agonist) increases gastric emptying but also decreases gastric accommodation, so it may increase dyspeptic symptoms in some patients. In addition, erythromycin has a high occurrence of tachyphylaxis after 3 to 4 weeks of therapy.[12] Tegaserod (a serotonin-4 agonist) can influence gastric and small bowel transit, but its efficacy in dyspepsia is unproved.[12] The nonpharmacologic therapies listed in Table 95-2 can be helpful and should be included in treatment plans. Conservative measures such as changes in diet (e.g., reducing fat, avoiding caffeine and carbonated beverages, decreasing meal size) and in the timing of meals (e.g., eating breakfast, avoiding bedtime snacks) may be especially helpful in patients with dysmotility symptoms.

If symptoms persist after a trial of at least 4 weeks of therapy, a change in treatment should be considered. Failure of multiple therapies is usually an indication for referral for endoscopy. If upper endoscopy identifies mucosal disease, treatment can be directed to the specific cause. In patients with functional dyspepsia that is resistant to therapy, the diagnosis should be reevaluated periodically. It is important to provide reassurance and to set realistic expectations, such as acknowledging that symptoms may not be completely eliminated. Alternative therapies such as hypnotherapy and acupuncture may also be considered.

Recent studies suggest a potential role for tricyclic antidepressants, which seem to relieve visceral hyperalgesia.[13] In addition, medications that increase the gastric accommodation reflex such as sumatriptan and buspirone (serotonin-1 agonists) are being evaluated for efficacy, but their general use for dyspepsia cannot be recommended at this time.[14,15]

The need for nutritional support may be an indication for gastrostomy or jejunostomy. Fundoplication may be considered if symptoms are due to typical GERD, but it is usually not recommended in patients with chronic dyspepsia (even if nausea and vomiting are predominant symptoms) because it can result in complications. This is thought to be due to alterations in the gastric accommodation reflex.[16]

CONSULTATION

Input from pediatric gastroenterologists is often helpful if patients continue to experience symptoms despite initial therapy, further diagnostic evaluation is needed, or symptoms are severe.

ADMISSION CRITERIA

Persistent vomiting, severe abdominal pain, hematemesis, bilious emesis, dehydration, persistent weight loss, and significant hematochezia or melena all indicate the need for inpatient evaluation and management.

DISCHARGE CRITERIA

Once patients are able to tolerate adequate oral intake, the remainder of the evaluation can usually be completed on an outpatient basis. It is also important to ensure adequate follow-up, because these problems are often chronic and may recur if they are not managed appropriately.

IN A NUTSHELL

- Dyspepsia can represent gastric, intestinal, or extra-GI disorders.
- Symptomatic relief is often warranted and can be initiated before completion of the diagnostic evaluation.
- Gastric acid blockade and prokinetic agents, as well as modification of the diet, are standard elements of empirical therapy.
- Upper endoscopy should be considered in dyspeptic patients presenting with weight loss, recurrent vomiting, bleeding, anemia, dysphagia, or jaundice; patients taking NSAIDs; and patients with severe or persistent symptoms.

ON THE HORIZON

- Trials are under way to assess the safety of new medications (rabeprazole, pantoprazole) for the treatment of GERD in the pediatric population.
- A major prospective study of the natural history of GERD in children and adolescents is ongoing and may help clarify the lifelong implications of this disease.

SUGGESTED READING

Chitkara DK, Delgado-Aros S, Bredenoord AJ, et al: Functional dyspepsia, upper gastrointestinal symptoms, and transit in children. J Pediatr 2003;143:609-613.

Talley NJ, Stanghellini V, Heading RC, et al: Functional gastroduodenal disorders. Gut 1999;45(Suppl 2):II37-II42.

REFERENCES

1. Talley NJ, Stanghellini V, Heading RC, et al: Functional gastroduodenal disorders. Gut 1999;45(Suppl 2):II37-II42.
2. Hyams JS, Burke G, Davis PM, et al: Abdominal pain and irritable bowel syndrome in adolescents: A community-based study. J Pediatr 1996;129: 220-226.
3. De Giacomo C, Valdambrini V, Lizzoli F, et al: A population-based survey on gastrointestinal tract symptoms and *Helicobacter pylori* infection in children and adolescents. Helicobacter 2002;7:356-363.
4. Talley NJ: Dyspepsia: Management guidelines for the millennium. Gut 2002;50(Suppl 4):IV72-IV78.
5. Hyams JS, Davis P, Sylvester FA, et al: Dyspepsia in children and adolescents: A prospective study. J Pediatr Gastroenterol Nutr 2000;30:413-418.
6. Tack J, Bisschops R, Sarnelli G: Pathophysiology and treatment of functional dyspepsia. Gastroenterology 2004;127:1239-1255.
7. Chitkara DK, Camilleri M, Zinsmeister AR, et al: Gastric sensory and motor dysfunction in adolescents with functional dyspepsia. J Pediatr 2005;146:500-505.
8. Chitkara DK, Delgado-Aros S, Bredenoord AJ, et al: Functional dyspepsia, upper gastrointestinal symptoms, and transit in children. J Pediatr 2003;143:609-613.
9. Rasquin-Weber A, Hyman PE, Cucchiara S, et al: Childhood functional gastrointestinal disorders. Gut 1999;45(Suppl 2):II60-II68.
10. Talley NJ, Lauritsen K: The potential role of acid suppression in functional dyspepsia: The BOND, OPERA, PILOT, and ENCORE studies. Gut 2002;50(Suppl 4):IV36-IV41.
11. Gold BD, Colletti RB, Abbott M, et al: *Helicobacter pylori* infection in children: Recommendations for diagnosis and treatment. J Pediatr Gastroenterol Nutr 2000;31:490-497.
12. Galligan JJ, Vanner S: Basic and clinical pharmacology of new motility promoting agents. Neurogastroenterol Motil 2005;17:643-653.
13. Mertz HPD, Smith S, Morgan V: Amitriptyline reduces visceral sensitization and limbic activation induced by stress in IBS and improves symptoms. Gastroenterology 2002;122:A-310.
14. Tack J, Piessevaux H, Coulie B, et al: Role of impaired gastric accommodation to a meal in functional dyspepsia. Gastroenterology 1998;115: 1346-1352.
15. Chial HJ, Camilleri M, Burton D, et al: Selective effects of serotonergic psychoactive agents on gastrointestinal functions in health. Am J Physiol Gastrointest Liver Physiol 2003;284:G130-G137.
16. Bouras EP, Delgado-Aros S, Camilleri M, et al: SPECT imaging of the stomach: Comparison with barostat, and effects of sex, age, body mass index, and fundoplication. Gut 2002;51:781-786.

CHAPTER 96

Disorders of Gastric Emptying

Richard J. Noel

Passage of the alimentary bolus from the stomach to the duodenum constitutes an important anatomic and functional transition point in the digestive process. The stomach functions as both a digestive organ and a temporary reservoir. Muscular contractions propel the stomach contents across the pylorus into the duodenum, where it is mixed with biliary and pancreatic secretions to aid in further nutrient digestion and absorption. Abnormal gastric emptying into the duodenum may result in symptoms that require hospitalization for supportive care, diagnostic evaluation, and therapeutic procedures. In this chapter, the term *gastroparesis* refers to delayed gastric emptying, whereas *dumping* encompasses all causes of accelerated gastric emptying.

CLINICAL PRESENTATION

It is difficult to differentiate disorders of delayed from those of accelerated gastric emptying by the history alone. Furthermore, as in many pediatric disorders, a child's description of symptoms may not be accurate or medically useful, and the presenting complaint may not be more specific than a "feeding disorder."

Gastroparesis can present dramatically with persistent vomiting that should prompt consideration of small bowel obstruction. However, more often, symptoms are vague and can include nausea, epigastric fullness, early satiety, pyrosis, and belching. Typically, vomiting does not occur during or immediately after ingesting a meal, a pattern more suggestive of rumination syndrome.

Rapid gastric emptying may also cause nausea, vomiting, epigastric fullness, and early satiety. Rapid emptying results in the classic dumping syndrome in a minority of patients, characterized by pallor, diaphoresis, or syncope. The cause of this syndrome is thought to be rapid release of hyperosmolar fluid into the small bowel and resultant fluid shifts into the bowel. Patients have sudden shifts in blood sugar, characterized initially by hyperglycemia and then followed by hypoglycemia as a result of persistently elevated insulin levels when substrate absorption from the intestine rapidly declines.

DIFFERENTIAL DIAGNOSIS

Gastroparesis

Gastric outlet obstruction must be considered in the differential diagnosis of gastroparesis, particularly in younger children, who may have the initial presentation of a congenital or acquired anatomic anomaly (see Chapter 138). Most frequent among these entities is hypertrophic pyloric stenosis (HPS), which is the most common condition requiring operative correction in young infants.[1] Infants typically present with "projectile" vomiting and variable degrees of toxicity, depending on hydration and nutrition. Less impressive is the vomiting that may be seen with antral and duodenal webs. These membranes are fenestrated, mucosal diaphragms that obstruct gastric outflow as a function of the diameter of the fenestrations.[2] Much less commonly, outlet obstruction may occur in association with ectopic pancreatic tissue,[3] pyloric duplication cysts,[4] polypoid tissue,[5] or intermittent duodenogastric intussusception.[6] In patients with poor nutritional status, superior mesenteric artery syndrome may occur. In this condition it is thought that weight loss leads to loss of a key fat pad with resultant obstruction of the duodenum by this vessel as it traverses this section of bowel. Hyperplastic gastric folds have been known to obstruct antral outflow in conditions such as lymphocytic gastritis or viral infection (Ménétrier disease).[7] Bezoars, when of sufficient size, may result in partial gastric outlet obstruction and delayed gastric emptying.[8] These concretions may include lactobezoars, trichobezoars, pharmacobezoars, and phytobezoars. Theoretically, large bezoars may also cause dumping if their main effect is a decrease in fundic compliance.

Gastric dysmotility can accompany hepatitis or pancreatitis whether the cause is infectious, toxic, inflammatory, or traumatic. Direct mechanical trauma (e.g., accidental injury, surgery) can cause a hematoma in the gastric wall or duodenum (or both), which can also alter gastric emptying.

Metabolic problems may result in ineffective gastric emptying as well. Hypothyroidism can decrease antroduodenal motility, and function will return to normal with restoration of the euthyroid state.[9] Acid-base and electrolyte disturbances can disrupt gastrointestinal neuromuscular function and result in impaired motility and delayed gastric emptying. This cause must be considered in settings such as diabetes mellitus or renal insufficiency.[10] Note that metabolic alterations such as hypokalemia may be aggravated by recurrent vomiting, as may be found in HPS, and produce a vicious cycle of worsening gastric function.

Medications may have profound untoward effects on the ability of the stomach to empty properly. Examples include opiates,[11] anticholinergics,[12] and tricyclic antidepressants.[13] Case reports and animal studies have also implicated benzodiazepines, anesthetics (propofol),[14] and some chemotherapeutic agents (cisplatin).[15]

Diseases that affect the neuromuscular components of the gastrointestinal tract can have a significant effect on gastric emptying. Such diseases might include primary central nervous system disease, vagotomy (planned or inadvertent), visceral myopathy, autonomic dysfunction (Riley-Day syndrome), systemic lupus erythematosus, myotonic dystrophy, or chronic idiopathic pseudo-obstruction. Anorexia nervosa and bulimia are frequently associated with gastroparesis that improves with nutrition.[16]

Infectious diseases that result in gastroparesis include viral gastritis and exposure to endotoxin from gram-negative bacteria.[17] The term *postviral gastroparesis* is used when delayed gastric emptying persists after resolution of the other symptoms of acute viral illness, usually a viral gastroenteritis.[18] Duodenal tuberculosis can be a rare cause of gastric outlet obstruction.[19]

Dumping

Dumping syndrome is most commonly seen in postsurgical states in which the normal proximal compliance or distal tone of the stomach has been affected. In children, by far the most likely procedure to result in dumping syndrome is fundoplication.[20] Pyloroplasty is occasionally performed with a fundoplication and can potentially result in more severe dumping.

DIAGNOSIS AND EVALUATION

Although the history alone may not always be specific, especially in young children, attention to key details can be helpful in guiding subsequent evaluation. In patients with recurrent, forceful vomiting, understanding the specific frequency, amounts, and contents of the emesis can help distinguish small bowel obstruction from a problem of gastric emptying. Prenatal or early postnatal exposure to erythromycin[21,22] has been associated with HPS. Infants in whom prostaglandin E_1 has been infused for maintenance of a patent ductus arteriosus are susceptible to the development of obstructing antral hypertrophy.[23] A history of abdominal or thoracic operative procedures in which vagal injury could have occurred should raise suspicion of altered gastric emptying.

Physical examination should initially focus on determination of clinical hydration and general toxicity of the patient. Specific to HPS is a palpable tumor that may be noticed along with strong, ineffective peristaltic gastric contractions. Palpation of this mass may be facilitated by feeding the infant clear liquid, which is then aspirated via nasogastric tube.

A complete electrolyte panel is key in the diagnosis of metabolic disturbances that may either cause or be exacerbated by dysfunctional gastric emptying. A hepatic panel and pancreatic enzymes may help uncover a cause of vomiting such as hepatitis, cholestasis, or pancreatitis. A complete blood count should be performed to assess for anemia. In cases in which dumping is suspected, a glucose tolerance test or a hydrogen breath test may be diagnostic.

Radiographic studies may be the most helpful in making a specific diagnosis. An upper gastrointestinal series has been shown to be the most cost-effective study in a vomiting infant and has the added benefit of diagnosing anomalous rotation and other causes of small bowel obstruction.[1] In young infants, ultrasonography is the test of choice for HPS now that diagnostic criteria for length of the pyloric channel and thickness of the muscle have been established.[24] The imaging modality can also determine the position of the mesenteric vessels, which can indicate intestinal malrotation. In nonemergency situations, radionuclide studies may provide an objective measure of gastric emptying.[25] Studies

of liquid emptying are performed in infants, whereas studies of solid emptying are generally more useful in older children and adults.

Endoscopy may be performed to assess for mucosal inflammation secondary to infection and may also be therapeutic in conditions in which tissue masses (ectopic pancreas or polyps) impede antroduodenal outflow. In addition, endoscopy may be used to place catheters for antroduodenal motility studies, which may be useful in characterizing primary motility disorders.[26] Although not widely available, electrogastrography may help diagnose primary disorders of gastric pacing. This technique has demonstrated the therapeutic efficacy of supplemental thyroxine in hypothyroid adults.[9] However, the value of this diagnostic test in discriminating between patients with gastric and nongastric causes of nausea and vomiting is unclear.

TREATMENT

Patients ill enough to require hospitalization will probably have derangements in fluids and electrolytes or nutrition (or both), and initial clinical management should be directed toward identifying and correcting these problems.

Fluids and Electrolytes

Either impaired or accelerated gastric emptying may result in marked alterations in fluid status and electrolytes. The recurrent vomiting seen in HPS leads to losses of sodium, potassium, and chloride with resultant hypochloremic metabolic alkalosis. This is accentuated by the paradoxical aciduria that results from renal mechanisms to retain sodium and intravascular fluid. The metabolic alterations may be profound and must be corrected before anesthesia and surgery. Patients with severe dumping syndrome may also present with intravascular fluid depletion and hypoglycemia. The former is the result of rapid passage of hyperosmolar fluid into the small bowel. The latter is due to overcompensation to early hyperglycemia.

Nutrition

Severe gastroparesis can limit food intake and lead to malnutrition. Until definitive treatment is available, patients should be given small frequent meals and liquid supplements, which may be better tolerated. For persistent symptoms, use of a nasojejunal tube to bypass the stomach may be successful (although if vomiting persists, the tube may be displaced). If transpyloric feedings are successful and other pharmacologic therapies are unsuccessful, placement of a surgical jejunostomy can be considered. Parenteral nutritional support may be needed in cases of severe malnutrition or if symptoms are intractable.

Once acute fluid and nutritional problems have been addressed, attention should be directed toward identifying the specific cause of the gastric emptying disorder. Obstructive causes should be identified or eliminated from consideration as a first priority.

Pharmacologic therapies for gastroparesis are limited. Metoclopramide, a dopamine receptor antagonist, is most commonly used, but it is not consistently efficacious.[27] This agent can cause dystonia or irritability, or both, in infants. Erythromycin is sometimes used for its prokinetic action on the stomach, but tachyphylaxis to this effect limits the utility of this drug.[28] In cases of idiopathic gastroparesis, direct gastric electrical pacing has been investigated in adults; the results have been promising, but still inconclusive, with symptom improvement despite a lack of objective improvement in gastric emptying.[29]

Initial treatment of dumping syndrome should also be dietary, with smaller, more frequent meals and decreased intake of simple carbohydrates. For more severe dumping symptoms, the use of octreotide (somatostatin) has been shown to provide relief in adults.[30] Additionally, adding acarbose, cornstarch, or glucomannan to the diet may reduce the osmotic load and symptoms.[31,32]

CONSULTATION

- General pediatric surgery if surgical conditions are strong considerations
- Gastroenterology if endoscopy or long-term nutritional management is required

ADMISSION CRITERIA

- Toxic appearance or signs of severe dehydration
- Malnutrition apparent on physical examination or laboratory analysis
- Feeding intolerance related to poor control of pain or hypoglycemia
- Possible mechanical bowel obstruction

DISCHARGE CRITERIA

- Resolved surgical concerns
- Demonstration of a successful feeding regimen that can be continued after discharge and provides adequate nutrition and hydration with control of symptoms

IN A NUTSHELL

- Disorders of gastric emptying may present with symptoms severe enough to warrant hospitalization.
- Symptoms of delayed or accelerated gastric emptying may be nonspecific and have overlapping features.
- Hospital management should initially be directed at correction of fluid and electrolyte abnormalities and identification of acute surgical problems.
- Effort is directed at determining the type of motility disorder, identifying a cause, treating reversible causes, and establishing an effective feeding regimen.

ON THE HORIZON

- There are currently few approved pharmacologic options for the treatment of gastroparesis. 5-HT$_4$, dopamine, and motilin receptors may be stimulated by cisapride (agonist), domperidone (antagonist), and erythromycin (agonist), respectively, and result in prokinetic effects. However, each of these drugs has side effect profiles that may preclude their use in the treatment of gastroparesis.[33-35] Tegaserod (5-HT$_4$ agonist) has been approved for use in patients with chronic constipation and irritable bowel syndrome, but its utility in treating gastroparesis requires further study.

SUGGESTED READING

Milla PJ: Motor disorders including pyloric stenosis. In Walker WA, Goulet O, Kleinman RE, et al (eds): Pediatric Gastrointestinal Disease, 4th ed. Hamilton, Ontario, BC Decker, 2004, pp 551-560.

Parkman HP, Hasler WL, Fisher RS: American Gastroenterological Association medical position statement: Diagnosis and treatment of gastroparesis. Gastroenterology 2004;127:1589-1591.

Sigurdsson L, Flores A, Putnam PE, et al: Postviral gastroparesis: Presentation, treatment, and outcome. J Pediatr 1997;130:751-754.

REFERENCES

1. Hernanz-Schulman M: Infantile hypertrophic pyloric stenosis. Radiology 2003;227:319-331.
2. Noel RJ, Glock MS, Pranikoff T, Hill ID: Nonobstructive antral web: An unusual cause of excessive crying in an infant. J Pediatr Gastroenterol Nutr 2000;31:439-441.
3. Ormarsson OT, Haugen SE, Juul I: Gastric outlet obstruction caused by heterotopic pancreas. Eur J Pediatr Surg 2003;13:410-413.
4. Patel MP, Meisheri IV, Waingankar VS, et al: Duplication cyst of the pylorus—a rare cause of gastric outlet obstruction in the newborn. J Postgrad Med 1997;43:43-45.
5. Wakhlu A, Sharma AK: Gastric outlet obstruction due to solitary gastric polyp in a neonate. Indian Pediatr 1994;31:1299-1300.
6. Osuntokun B, Falcone R, Alonso M, Cohen MB: Duodenogastric intussusception: A rare cause of gastric outlet obstruction. J Pediatr Gastroenterol Nutr 2004;39:299-301.
7. Morinville V, Bernard C, Forget S: Foveolar hyperplasia secondary to cow's milk protein hypersensitivity presenting with clinical features of pyloric stenosis. J Pediatr Surg 2004;39:E29-E31.
8. DuBose TM 5th, Southgate WM, Hill JG: Lactobezoars: A patient series and literature review. Clin Pediatr (Phila) 2001;40:603-606.
9. Gunsar F, Yilmaz S, Bor S, et al: Effect of hypo- and hyperthyroidism on gastric myoelectrical activity. Dig Dis Sci 2003;48:706-712.
10. Ravelli AM: Gastrointestinal function in chronic renal failure. Pediatr Nephrol 1995;9:756-762.
11. Asai T: Effects of morphine, nalbuphine and pentazocine on gastric emptying of indigestible solids. Arzneimittelforschung 1998;48:802-805.
12. Bridges JW, Dent JG, Johnson P: The effects of some pharmacologically active amines on the rate of gastric emptying in rats. Life Sci 1976;18:97-107.
13. Woodhouse KW, Bateman DN: Delayed gastric emptying with dothiepin. Hum Toxicol 1985;4:67-70.
14. Inada T, Asai T, Yamada M, Shingu K: Propofol and midazolam inhibit gastric emptying and gastrointestinal transit in mice. Anesth Analg 2004;99:1102-1106.
15. Sharma SS, Gupta YK: Reversal of cisplatin-induced delay in gastric emptying in rats by ginger (*Zingiber officinale*). J Ethnopharmacol 1998;62:49-51.
16. Benini L, Todesco T, Dalle Grave R, et al: Gastric emptying in patients with restricting and binge/purging subtypes of anorexia nervosa. Am J Gastroenterol 2004;99:1448-1454.
17. Spates ST, Cullen JJ, Ephgrave KS, Hinkhouse MM: Effect of endotoxin on canine colonic motility and transit. J Gastrointest Surg 1998;2:391-398.
18. Sigurdsson L, Flores A, Putnam PE, et al: Postviral gastroparesis: Presentation, treatment, and outcome. J Pediatr 1997;130:751-754.
19. Moirangthem GS, Singh NS, Bhattacharya KN, et al: Gastric outlet obstruction due to duodenal tuberculosis: A case report. Int Surg 2001;86:132-134.
20. Di Lorenzo C, Orenstein S: Fundoplication: Friend or foe? J Pediatr Gastroenterol Nutr 2002;34:117-124.
21. Cooper WO, Griffin MR, Arbogast P, et al: Very early exposure to erythromycin and infantile hypertrophic pyloric stenosis. Arch Pediatr Adolesc Med 2002;156:647-657.

22. Cooper WO, Ray WA, Griffin MR: Prenatal prescription of macrolide antibiotics and infantile hypertrophic pyloric stenosis. Obstet Gynecol 2002;100:101-106.

23. Peled N, Dagan O, Babyn P, et al: Gastric-outlet obstruction induced by prostaglandin therapy in neonates. N Engl J Med 1992;327:505-510.

24. Spinelli C, Bertocchini A, Massimetti M, Ughi C: Muscle thickness in infants with hypertrophic pyloric stenosis. Pediatr Med Chir 2003;25:148-150.

25. Mariani G, Boni G, Barreca M, et al: Radionuclide gastroesophageal motor studies. J Nucl Med 2004;45:1004-1028.

26. Zangen T, Ciarla C, Zangen S, et al: Gastrointestinal motility and sensory abnormalities may contribute to food refusal in medically fragile toddlers. J Pediatr Gastroenterol Nutr 2003;37:225-227.

27. Ponte CD, Nappi JM: Review of a new gastrointestinal drug—metoclopramide. Am J Hosp Pharm 1981;38:829-833.

28. Dhir R, Richter JE: Erythromycin in the short- and long-term control of dyspepsia symptoms in patients with gastroparesis. J Clin Gastroenterol 2004;38:237-242.

29. Abell TL, Minocha A: Gastroparesis and the gastric pacemaker: A revolutionary treatment for an old disease. J Miss State Med Assoc 2002;43:369-375.

30. Scarpignato C: The place of octreotide in the medical management of the dumping syndrome. Digestion 1996;57(Suppl 1):114-118.

31. Zung A, Zadik Z: Acarbose treatment of infant dumping syndrome: Extensive study of glucose dynamics and long-term follow-up. J Pediatr Endocrinol Metab 2003;16:907-915.

32. Kneepkens CM, Fernandes J, Vonk RJ: Dumping syndrome in children. Diagnosis and effect of glucomannan on glucose tolerance and absorption. Acta Paediatr Scand 1988;77:279-286.

33. Tonini M, De Ponti F, Di Nucci A, Crema F: Review article: Cardiac adverse effects of gastrointestinal prokinetics. Aliment Pharmacol Ther 1999;13:1585-1591.

34. Drolet B, Rousseau G, Daleau P, et al: Domperidone should not be considered a no-risk alternative to cisapride in the treatment of gastrointestinal motility disorders. Circulation 2000;102:1883-1885.

35. Ray WA, Murray KT, Meredith S, et al: Oral erythromycin and the risk of sudden death from cardiac causes. N Engl J Med 2004;351:1089-1096.

CHAPTER 97

Liver Failure

Scott A. Elisofon and Maureen M. Jonas

Liver failure, or hepatic failure, is a clinical condition that results from significant hepatocyte dysfunction or death. It differs from hepatitis in that patients must have uncorrectable coagulopathy in addition to hepatocyte injury, with or without encephalopathy. Hepatic failure is an acute process and should be differentiated from the acute decompensation of chronic liver disease.

The strict criteria for acute or fulminant liver failure in adults include encephalopathy, coagulopathy, and evidence of hepatic dysfunction without prior evidence of liver disease, occurring within 8 weeks of the first symptoms of illness. Because encephalopathy is uncommon and difficult to identify in infants and young children, most clinicians use uncorrectable coagulopathy and hepatic dysfunction as clinical criteria for liver failure in this age group.

Recognition and management of hepatic failure and its associated metabolic disturbances (Table 97-1) are crucial so that supportive therapy can be provided until recovery or liver transplantation. Hepatic failure accounts for up to 15% of pediatric liver transplants in the United States each year.

CLINICAL PRESENTATION

Neonates and Infants

Neonates and young infants can present with various symptoms, depending on the disease. Some infants are quite ill immediately after birth with coagulopathy and acidosis. This presentation is highly suggestive of hypoxic or ischemic injury, neonatal hemochromatosis, neonatal enteroviral infection, or some other intrauterine or perinatal insult. Laboratory tests can be significant, with elevated transaminases in the high hundreds to thousands (ischemia) and hyperbilirubinemia. Hypoglycemia may also be significant. Clinical symptoms suggestive of sepsis, including hypotension and poor perfusion, may occur as well. Encephalopathy is identified in only one third of these infants.[1] Infants with neonatal hemochromatosis present with intrauterine growth retardation, coagulopathy, hypoalbuminemia, ascites, mild transaminase elevation, and varying degrees of renal insufficiency.

Children and Adolescents

Children with acute hepatic failure may present with a wide variety of symptoms. Those with infectious hepatitis may present with fever, malaise, nausea, jaundice, and possibly right upper quadrant pain. They may have been discharged from the emergency department or physician's office with a diagnosis of hepatitis and elevated transaminases, jaundice, and a normal prothrombin time (PT). Many children improve (especially those with hepatitis A), but some return with worsening jaundice, petechiae, bruising, or bleeding. Mental status changes may include reversal of day-night sleeping, uncooperative behavior, delirium, stupor, or coma. The physical examination may reveal a shrunken liver.

Patients with hypoxia or drug- or toxin-related injury may present with very high transaminase levels. Metabolic diseases typically present with high transaminase levels and hypoglycemia. Wilson disease presenting as acute hepatic failure is often accompanied by Coombs-negative hemolytic anemia.

DIFFERENTIAL DIAGNOSIS

It is important to remember that acute liver failure differs from acute hepatitis, in that the former involves an uncorrectable coagulopathy, with or without encephalopathy. A greater percentage of patients present clinically with hepatitis—elevated alanine transaminase (ALT), with or without jaundice, and usually normal synthetic function (normal PT, albumin)—but this condition can progress to acute liver failure. The causes of acute hepatitis are almost identical to those of acute liver failure. They include infections, metabolic and autoimmune diseases, and toxic injuries (Table 97-2). Infectious hepatitis is most frequently viral, with hepatitis A and Epstein-Barr virus being the most common. In the United States, hepatitis B and C are uncommon causes of acute hepatitis in children.

In addition to those with acute liver injury, patients with underlying liver disease may present with increasing transaminases, jaundice, and coagulopathy, with or without encephalopathy. This is referred to as an acute decompensation of chronic liver disease. Diseases that involve significant liver fibrosis, such as α_1-antitrypsin deficiency, autoimmune hepatitis, primary sclerosing cholangitis, and Wilson disease, can present in this fashion. These patients need to be evaluated thoroughly, because many have clinical findings that are similar to those in acute liver failure. In addition, many have portal hypertension with thrombocytopenia. These two conditions can contribute to a higher risk of bleeding from esophageal varices, portal hypertensive gastropathy, or mucosal surfaces.

In most cases of hepatic failure in children, the cause is unknown. The most common identifiable causes are infections, toxins (including drugs), metabolic diseases, and vascular or cardiac disease. Infections and toxins, especially acetaminophen, are thought to account for a large proportion of cases in the United States.[2] Natural herbs, such as pennyroyal and kava, can also cause acute liver failure. The causes of fulminant hepatic failure are age dependent, as outlined in Table 97-2.

DIAGNOSIS AND EVALUATION

Liver failure presents differently according to age and cause. A careful history is always important to determine a time course of symptoms; identify exposures, such as infections, chemicals, or drugs; and uncover a family history of liver disease. In the case of ill infants, questions should focus on maternal infections (hepatitis B, human immunodeficiency virus, herpes simplex virus, enterovirus) and a family history of genetic or metabolic diseases.

The physical examination may direct the physician to specific investigations. Splenomegaly, ascites, or cutaneous spider angiomas may suggest an underlying chronic liver disease that has worsened. Splenomegaly may be present in acute processes, such as atypical viral infections or vascular events (e.g., hepatic vein thrombosis), but it is usually more suggestive of portal hypertension from chronic liver disease. Vesicles may suggest a systemic infection with agents such as herpes simplex virus. The liver may be enlarged, normal, or shrunken; a shrunken liver is worrisome for significant hepatic necrosis. If Wilson disease is suspected, the patient should undergo a slit-lamp ophthalmic examination for Kayser-Fleischer rings.

All patients should undergo careful monitoring of liver synthetic and metabolic function (Table 97-3). Patients with hepatic failure usually have a PT greater than 18 to 20 seconds (international normalized ratio [INR] >1.5 to 2). Transaminases may be quite elevated, and hyperbilirubinemia is variable.

Ultrasonography of the abdomen with Doppler interrogation of the vessels can provide information about the size and consistency of the liver, patency of the biliary tree, presence of ascites, and patency of the hepatic veins to rule out hepatic vein thrombosis (Budd-Chiari syndrome).

COURSE OF ILLNESS

Most children who develop hepatic failure are extremely ill and require careful monitoring, sometimes in an intensive care setting. Children may remain confused or slightly drowsy but have the potential to rapidly develop worsening encephalopathy, including coma. Children with early encephalopathy (within 7 days) after the first laboratory evidence of liver disease have a better prognosis than do patients with late encephalopathy.[3] Close monitoring of

Table 97-1 **Complications of Acute Hepatic Failure**

Metabolic
 Hypoglycemia
 Hypokalemia
 Hypophosphatemia
 Hyponatremia

Neurologic
 Encephalopathy
 Cerebral edema
 Intracranial hemorrhage

Acid-base imbalance
 Respiratory alkalosis
 Metabolic acidosis

Hematologic
 Coagulopathy
 Disseminated intravascular coagulation
 Aplastic anemia

Multiorgan dysfunction
 Gastrointestinal hemorrhage
 Ascites
 Pancreatitis
 Renal failure (hepatorenal syndrome)
 Shock
 Sepsis
 Respiratory failure
 Pulmonary hemorrhage

From Squires R: Liver failure. In Rudolph CD, Rudolph AM, Hostetter MK, et al (eds): Rudolph's Pediatrics. New York, McGraw-Hill, 2002, p 1513.

Table 97-2 **Causes of Acute Hepatic Failure in Children**

Cause	Perinatal Period	Infancy	Childhood
Infectious	Herpes simplex virus Echovirus Adenovirus Hepatitis B	Hepatitis A Hepatitis B Epstein-Barr virus Non-A–E hepatitis	Hepatitis A Hepatitis B Hepatitis D Epstein-Barr virus Non-A–E hepatitis
Metabolic	Tyrosinemia Galactosemia Neonatal hemochromatosis	Tyrosinemia Hereditary fructose intolerance Fatty acid oxidation defects Mitochondrial disorders Autoimmune hepatitis	Wilson disease Autoimmune hepatitis
Toxic		Medications Herbs	Medications Herbs
Miscellaneous	Congenital heart disease Cardiac surgery Severe asphyxia	Congenital heart disease Cardiac surgery Severe asphyxia	Ischemia Budd-Chiari syndrome Malignancy

Table 97-3 Laboratory Evaluation in Acute Hepatic Failure

Test	Description
Hematology	Complete blood count with platelets; differential; PT, PTT, INR
Chemistry	AST, ALT, bilirubin (total, direct), alkaline phosphatase, GGTP, total protein, albumin, glucose, blood urea nitrogen, creatinine, electrolytes, ammonia
Infectious evaluation	HAV, HBV, HCV, Epstein-Barr virus Herpes simplex culture, fluorescent antibody of scraped vesicle or PCR (neonates) Enteroviral culture or PCR (neonates) Maternal hepatitis B serologies (neonates)
Other studies	
Neonates and infants	Ferritin, lactate, pyruvate, plasma amino acids, urine succinylacetone (tyrosinemia), urine organic acids, urine ketones, urine reducing substances (galactosemia)
Children	Antinuclear, anti–smooth muscle, anti-liver-kidney microsomal antibody; copper, ceruloplasmin, 24-hr urine copper, toxicology screen, acetaminophen level

ALT, alanine transaminase; AST, aspartate transaminase; GGTP, γ-glutamyl transpeptidase; HAV, hepatitis A virus; HBV, hepatitis B virus; HCV, hepatitis C virus; INR, international normalized ratio; PT, prothrombin time; PTT, partial thromboplastin time; PCR, polymerase chain reaction.

mental status is crucial, because advanced stages of encephalopathy (stupor or coma) are associated with higher mortality.

The cause of liver failure is important in terms of prognosis. Patients with acetaminophen overdose or hepatitis A virus infection have a much higher survival rate than do those with hepatitis B or liver failure with an unknown cause.

Before the advent of liver transplantation, the mortality rate of acute hepatic failure was at least 60% to 70%. With transplantation, mortality has decreased to 20% to 40%.[4] Mortality is usually due to the complications of hepatic failure. Cerebral herniation secondary to cerebral edema is the most common cause of death in children. Infection, either bacterial or fungal, is also a significant contributor. Bleeding, especially gastrointestinal, is less common in children, unless there is underlying chronic liver disease with esophageal or gastric varices from portal hypertension.

In some cases, with or without specific therapy, the INR and mental status begin to improve as transaminase values decrease. However, falling transaminases with a rising INR and bilirubin suggest worsening hepatic necrosis. These patients often require liver transplantation.

TREATMENT

Patients with isolated transaminase elevation and jaundice with no other signs of acute hepatic failure can be managed as outpatients with close follow-up. Any patient with dehydration secondary to vomiting or poor oral intake should be admitted for hydration, and any child with coagulopathy or mental status changes should be admitted and rapidly transferred to a tertiary center that has a pediatric intensive care unit and liver transplantation service.

Even with a known cause of liver failure, many cases are irreversible at the time of diagnosis. Exceptions are toxic ingestions, especially acetaminophen, and autoimmune hepatitis. Treatment is mostly supportive. The key concepts in management are correction of metabolic abnormalities

and prevention of lethal complications such as bleeding, multiorgan failure, and cerebral edema. Major treatment strategies include the following:

- All noncritical medications and herbal supplements should be considered as possible causes and discontinued. Patients with known acetaminophen ingestion should receive N-acetylcysteine. Infants with suspected galactosemia should have galactose-containing formulas withheld.
- If hypoxia or ischemia from cardiac surgery or cardiac insult is suspected, prompt recovery and maintenance of normal blood pressure and oxygenation are crucial.
- Metabolic abnormalities, such as hypoglycemia, hypokalemia, and hypophosphatemia, should be corrected. Many children require infusions of 10% dextrose to remain euglycemic. Once dehydration is corrected, fluids should be restricted to approximately 75% maintenance to prevent fluid overload or contribution to cerebral edema. Renal function and urine output should be closely monitored.
- Coagulopathy should be treated initially with vitamin K, 1 mg/year of age up to 10 mg parenterally each day for 3 days. Products to improve clotting (fresh frozen plasma, cryoprecipitate, platelets) should be given only for significant bleeding or invasive procedures, because excess blood products can contribute to fluid overload, and artificial correction of INR can make clinical assessment difficult. If the patient is having significant gastrointestinal bleeding and has evidence of portal hypertension (splenomegaly, ascites, spider angiomas), octreotide should be considered.
- Blood counts must be monitored closely, because some children with acute hepatic failure develop aplastic anemia. This may occur at the same time as the acute liver disease, as the liver disease is improving, or after a liver transplant.
- Patients should receive intravenous gastric acid suppressants to prevent gastrointestinal bleeding.

- Encephalopathy must be monitored with frequent neurologic examinations. Sedatives, such as benzodiazepines, should be strictly avoided because they can alter the patient's mental status examination. Enteral lactulose may be used if fluid status is stable and electrolytes are normal.
- Patients with hepatic failure are susceptible to bacterial infections. A sepsis evaluation should be performed and antibiotics provided if the patient develops fever or other clinical signs of infection, such as hypotension. Any infant or child with suspected herpes simplex virus infection should receive intravenous acyclovir.
- Some medications should be avoided or adjusted in patients with significant liver injury.

ADMISSION CRITERIA

- Dehydration or the inability to tolerate liquids by mouth
- Encephalopathy or any mental status changes
- Coagulopathy
- Bleeding complications (most importantly, gastrointestinal bleeding)

DISCHARGE CRITERIA

- Steadily improving coagulopathy
- Normal mental status
- Improving transaminases and bilirubin

PREVENTION

There is no single preventive strategy for acute hepatic failure. All infants should be immunized for hepatitis B, and all patients with chronic liver disease should be immunized for hepatitis A, because acute infection may precipitate hepatic decompensation. If a virus is suspected, all caretakers should wear protective gowns, gloves, and masks. Any prescription or over-the-counter medication should be considered potentially hepatotoxic and discontinued promptly if evidence of significant hepatic dysfunction develops.

IN A NUTSHELL

- The majority of cases of acute liver failure have no identifiable cause.
- Infants or children with liver failure present with abnormal transaminases, jaundice, uncorrectable coagulopathy, and possibly mental status changes or hypoglycemia.
- Management of liver failure is largely supportive, including correction of metabolic disturbances, attention to coagulopathy, and rapid referral to tertiary care center for further evaluation and treatment.

ON THE HORIZON

- A multicenter study is currently evaluating the frequency and causes of acute liver failure and the outcomes of the patients in the study.
- A multicenter study using *N*-acetylcysteine for all acute liver failure patients is currently being conducted.

SUGGESTED READING

Squires R: Liver failure. In Rudolph CD, Rudolph AM, Hostetter MK, et al (eds): Rudolph's Pediatrics. New York, McGraw-Hill, 2002, pp 1511-1513.

Treem WR: Hepatic failure. In Walker WA, Durie PR, Hamilton JR, et al (eds): Pediatric Gastrointestinal Disease. Hamilton, Ontario, BC Decker, 2000, pp 179-225.

Whitington PF, Soriano HE, Alonso EM: Fulminant hepatic failure in children. In Suchy FJ, Sokol RJ, Balistreri WF (eds): Liver Disease in Children. Philadelphia, Lippincott Williams & Wilkins, 2001, pp 63-88.

REFERENCES

1. Sundaram SS, Alonso EM, Hynan LS, et al: Characterization of acute liver failure in the neonate. Hepatology 2004;40:467A .
2. Whitington PF, Soriano HE, Alonso EM: Fulminant hepatic failure in children. In Suchy FJ, Sokol RJ, Balistreri WF (eds): Liver Disease in Children. Philadelphia, Lippincott Williams & Wilkins, 2001, pp 63-88.
3. O'Grady JG, Schalm SW, Williams R: Acute liver failure: Redefining the syndromes. Lancet 1993;342:273-275.
4. Treem W: Hepatic failure. In Walker WA, Durie PR, Hamilton JR, et al (eds): Pediatric Gastrointestinal Disease. Hamilton, Ontario, BC Decker, 2000, pp 179-225.

CHAPTER 98

Inflammatory Bowel Disease

Michael C. Stephens and Subra Kugathasan

Crohn's disease (CD) and ulcerative colitis (UC), collectively known as inflammatory bowel disease (IBD), are idiopathic, lifelong, destructive inflammatory conditions of the gastrointestinal tract that typically present during late childhood and adolescence.[1] The burden of these chronic relapsing diseases and their devastating effects imposed on affected children and teenagers may be considerable.

Categorization of IBD into CD and UC is based on clinical characteristics, although 5% to 24% of patients do not clearly fit into either category and are considered to have indeterminate colitis.[2] Chronic inflammation in CD can involve any part of the gastrointestinal tract and is characterized by discontinuous inflammation with intervening areas of normal mucosa (skip lesions) and transmural inflammation, which can result in fistulas, perforations, and strictures. The presence of noncaseating granulomas histologically in the mucosa is a hallmark of CD. Intestinal involvement of UC is limited to the colon and typically begins distally in the rectum and extends proximally. Inflammation in UC is not transmural and is limited to the mucosal layer.

The pathogenesis of IBD has been linked to a combination of genetic and environmental factors, but the exact cause remains elusive.[3] Current thinking suggests that an immune-mediated response to an environmental trigger develops in patients with a genetically determined predisposition and leads to chronic dysregulated inflammation.[4]

Population-based studies suggest that IBD is unevenly distributed throughout the world and that the highest disease rates occur in Western countries.[5] Epidemiologic surveys have also suggested that IBD incidence rates have changed over the second half of the 20th century, with both UC and CD gradually increasing.[6-8] Recently, an epidemiologic study was completed in which all children in Wisconsin with a new diagnosis of IBD were evaluated within a 2-year period between 2000 and 2001.[9] The incidence of IBD was found to be 7 per 100,000 in children younger than 18 years. Additionally, an equal incidence of IBD was noted among all ethnic groups, and children from sparsely as well as densely populated counties were equally affected. The vast majority (89%) of new IBD diagnoses were nonfamilial. The low frequency of patients with a family history, the equal distribution of IBD among all racial and ethnic groups, and the lack of a modulatory effect of urbanization on the incidence of IBD suggest that the clinical spectrum of IBD is still evolving and the various contributing factors are not well understood.

CLINICAL PRESENTATION

Patients with IBD can present with a diverse constellation of signs and symptoms. The clinical presentation of CD varies with the anatomic location of involvement.[1,9] In UC the clinical presentation is typically more predictable because intestinal involvement is limited to the colon. In both conditions, the severity of inflammation usually but not always correlates with the severity of the clinical presentation. It is likely that a primary care provider taking care of adolescents will be faced with a diagnosis of IBD one to three times a year and that as many as one case per week will be diagnosed in a busy hospital-based pediatric gastroenterology practice.[10] Recognition of the various clinical presentations of IBD can aid in early diagnosis and initiation of therapy.

Symptoms in a patient presenting with IBD can include abdominal pain, hematochezia, diarrhea, anorexia, nausea, weight loss, fatigue, and oral ulcerations.[9,11] Signs can include abdominal tenderness, perianal skin tags or fistulas, other fistulas, delayed puberty, short stature, iron deficiency anemia, hypoalbuminemia, and signs of extraintestinal complications. Laboratory abnormalities frequently include an elevated erythrocyte sedimentation rate (ESR) and C-reactive protein (CRP). IBD is a systemic disease and may present with extraintestinal manifestations before development of the more common intestinal symptoms (Table 98-1).

DIFFERENTIAL DIAGNOSIS

The diagnosis of IBD should be suspected from the clinical findings and initial laboratory evaluation, which can lead to a definitive diagnosis with endoscopic or radiologic procedures (or both). Exclusion of intestinal infections that can cause rectal bleeding, such as enteric pathogens (*Salmonella, Shigella, Campylobacter, Yersinia,* and *Escherichia coli* O157:H7) and *Clostridium difficile,* is imperative. Other considerations in adolescents with abdominal pain and rectal bleeding include Henoch-Schönlein purpura,[12] Behçet's disease,[13] hemolytic uremic syndrome,[14] and systemic vasculitis. When an abdominal abscess is found during the investigation of abdominal pain, in addition to CD, a perforated appendix, trauma, and gynecologic diseases must be considered.

DIAGNOSIS AND EVALUATION

The diagnosis of IBD is usually confirmed by a combination of clinical observations and laboratory, radiographic, endoscopic, and histologic findings.[1] A detailed history and physical examination remain the most important aspects in the evaluation of a child with possible IBD. The most appropriate diagnostic approach often includes a complete blood count, ESR, CRP, albumin, and stool specimens to rule out bacterial and protozoal pathogens. Endoscopic examinations (upper endoscopy and colonoscopy) with mucosal biopsies to directly examine the mucosa are key components to confirm the diagnosis. An upper gastrointestinal series with

Table 98–1 Extraintestinal Manifestations of Inflammatory Bowel Disease

Skin
Erythema nodosum
Pyoderma gangrenosum
Perianal disease

Joints
Arthralgia
Arthritis
Ankylosing spondylitis

Eye
Uveitis
Episcleritis
Conjunctivitis

Liver
Primary sclerosing cholangitis
Hepatitis
Cholelithiasis

Bone
Osteoporosis

Mouth
Cheilitis
Stomatitis
Aphthous ulcerations

Blood
Iron deficiency anemia
Anemia of chronic disease
Thrombocytosis
Autoimmune hemolytic anemia

Vascular
Vasculitis
Thrombosis

Kidney
Nephrolithiasis
Obstructive hydronephrosis
Enterovesical fistula
Urinary tract infection
Amyloidosis

Pancreas
Pancreatitis

Lung
Pulmonary vasculitis
Fibrosing alveolitis

Growth
Delayed growth
Delayed puberty

Table 98–2 Diagnostic Evaluation of a Child with Suspected Inflammatory Bowel Disease

Laboratory Studies
Complete blood count with differential, reticulocyte count
Sedimentation rate
Total protein, albumin
Aminotransferases, alkaline phosphatase, bilirubin
Serum iron, ferritin

Stool Cultures
For bacteria (including *Escherichia coli* O157:H7)
Clostridium difficile
Stool for ova and parasites

Radiologic
Upper gastrointestinal series with small bowel follow-through
Abdominal and pelvic computed tomography scan if an abscess is suspected
White blood cell scan if small bowel disease is suspected

Endoscopy
Upper endoscopy
Colonoscopy, ileoscopy, and biopsies

may have occult small bowel CD include enteroclysis, magnetic resonance imaging, and white blood cell scanning.[17-19] Capsule endoscopy, a new technique, may prove to be the most sensitive way to assess the small bowel.[20-22] The use of capsule endoscopy requires careful consideration because there is a risk of impaction of the instrument in patients with narrowing of the intestines, which could necessitate surgery. This concern is particularly important in a smaller child, and capsule endoscopy is currently approved by the Food and Drug Administration only for patients older than 10 years. Serologic testing for markers (perinuclear antineutrophil antibody [pANCA], anti–*Saccharomyces cerevisiae* antibody [ASCA], and outer membrane protein C [OmpC]) associated with IBD may be helpful in the evaluation of patients with suspected IBD,[23,24] but the sensitivity of these markers is not adequate to "rule out" IBD and they do not replace the need for definitive examinations such as endoscopy or radiologic evaluation. Table 98-2 describes the suggested initial diagnostic evaluation in a child with suspected IBD.

TREATMENT

Initial management of a patient hospitalized with IBD must be tailored to the degree of illness. Primary interventions should be directed toward stabilizing the patient and ensuring that emergency surgical intervention is not required while the evaluation proceeds. Intravenous fluids or transfusions, or both, may be required in a dehydrated or anemic patient. Careful attention to hydration status is especially important in a patient with significant hypoalbuminemia. Until appendicitis or other surgical emergencies are eliminated from the differential diagnosis, it is prudent to withhold oral intake and administer intravenous broad-spectrum antibiotics that cover intestinal flora (e.g., ampicillin plus an aminoglycoside plus metronidazole). In less ill patients, oral intake can be permitted while the evaluation proceeds.

small bowel follow-through may be helpful as well. However, in a hospitalized patient, a computed tomography scan[15] may be an important early step to rule out other important diseases such as appendicitis and can reveal other signs that may suggest CD[16] (e.g. "creeping fat" in the mesentery). Other tests that have shown usefulness in selected patients who

Diet may need to be tailored to the patient's individual needs. Patients with upper intestinal CD can have a secondary disaccharidase deficiency[25] and require a low-carbohydrate/lactose-free diet. In patients with significant intestinal narrowing from either inflammation or stricture, a liquid diet may be better tolerated.[26,27] Attention to nutritional status is often necessary in managing IBD in children, more often with CD than UC. Quantifying caloric intake can help the physician determine the best intervention.[28,29] Enteral nutrition is preferable to parenteral, but the route is dictated by the degree of illness.

Recent advances in medical therapy have revolutionized the management of IBD and reduced the need for hospitalization.[30] As with any chronic disease, a cooperative approach between the subspecialist and primary care physician is critical. Because there is no cure for IBD, the goal of therapy is to induce and maintain sustained remission from disease activity. Corticosteroids are typically reserved only for short-term, acute therapy to control symptoms and are avoided for maintenance therapy because of their long-term side effects.[31-33] In the United States, corticosteroids are frequently used to alleviate symptoms in a hospitalized patient presenting with IBD or in a known patient with an acute flare. Budesonide, a newer-generation corticosteroid that may have fewer adverse effects, is effective in CD involving the distal ileum and proximal colon.[34] Nutritional therapy using an exclusive elemental or polymeric formula, often administrated by nasogastric tube as the primary source of nutrition, has been shown to reduce inflammation and is the "front-line" therapy of choice in many Canadian and European IBD centers.[28,29,35] Because children tend to oppose the use of a liquid diet as the only source of calories and because daily use of a nasogastric tube is difficult, this treatment modality has not gained popularity in pediatric practice in the United States.

Many maintenance therapies are available, and it is important to be familiar with the side effects and toxicities associated with them. Table 98-3 provides a partial list of the common agents and side effects. Options include 5-aminosalicylate (5-ASA) agents such as mesalamine; antibiotics such as metronidazole; and immunomodulating agents such as thiopurines (azathioprine or 6-mercaptopurine), methotrexate, infliximab (a monoclonal antibody that binds free and receptor-bound tumor necrosis factor-α), cyclosporine, tacrolimus, and mycophenolate. Because 5-ASA agents provide a sustained remission in only a minority of patients,[36,37] thiopurine analogues such as azathioprine or 6-mercaptopurine are now the drugs of choice for maintenance of remission.[38] Common side effects of thiopurines include bone marrow suppression, hepatotoxicity, pancreatitis, and hypersensitivity.[39] It has been recognized that patients with genetic polymorphisms in thiopurine methyltransferase can be at greater risk for bone marrow suppression.[40] Many IBD centers screen patients for these defects before starting thiopurine therapy. Patients taking immunomodulating medications may be at increased risk for infections or malignancy.[41,42] In an immunosuppressed patient the threshold for imaging must be low in the face of a benign abdominal examination because of the high risk for significant asymptomatic intra-abdominal sepsis in these situations.

Surgical management remains an important component of IBD therapy. Colectomy must be considered in a patient

Table 98-3 Common Side Effects/Adverse Reactions to Drugs for Inflammatory Bowel Disease	
5-Aminosalicylates	Allergic reactions Interstitial nephritis Colitis exacerbation Agranulocytosis
Corticosteroids	Adrenal suppression Cushingoid features Diabetes Hypertension Osteoporosis Cataracts Mood effects Growth retardation
Thiopurines (6-mercaptopurine, azathioprine)	Bone marrow suppression Hepatitis Pancreatitis Allergic reactions
Methotrexate	Bone marrow suppression Hepatitis Nausea
Infliximab	Infusion reactions Autoantibody formation Anti-infliximab antibody formation Invasive infections Reactivation of quiescent tuberculosis Lupus-like reaction Central nervous system vasculitis
Metronidazole	Neuropathy Yeast infections Coated tongue
Cyclosporine	Renal toxicity Anaphylaxis Seizures Hypertension Hirsutism Gum hyperplasia

with colitis unresponsive to medical management, a patient who is steroid dependent, or one with long-standing disease given the risk for malignancy.[43] Emergency colectomy may be necessary in patients in whom toxic megacolon develops. A patient with severe colitis is at increased risk for toxic megacolon after colonoscopy. Surgery may be required in patients with CD in whom strictures, fistulas, abscesses, or intestinal perforation develops. There is a high risk of recurrence after surgery for CD, and medical therapy should not be discontinued after a surgically created state of remission.[44]

CONSULTATION

- Patients in whom either CD or UC is suspected should be evaluated by a gastroenterologist.
- Surgical consultation is warranted in a patient with colitis unresponsive to medical management. Toxic megacolon,

strictures, fistulas, abscesses, and intestinal perforation also require surgical management.

- Nutritional consultation may be helpful both in managing bowel and in optimizing the growth of children with IBD.

ADMISSION CRITERIA

Indications for hospitalization include

- Unclear diagnosis or alternative considerations requiring surgery, intravenous antibiotics, or other therapy that is best started in an inpatient setting
- Active disease refractory to outpatient oral therapy
- Anemia with a potential need for transfusion
- Inability to maintain hydration orally

DISCHARGE CRITERIA

- Ability to tolerate an oral/nasogastric diet and maintain hydration and positive nutritional balance
- Stable or improving signs and symptoms of active disease (e.g., hemoglobin, stool output)
- Reliable outpatient follow-up and family able to manage therapy and recovery at home

IN A NUTSHELL

- The presenting symptoms of IBD will vary with the location of involvement but can include abdominal pain, hematochezia, diarrhea, anorexia, nausea, weight loss, fatigue, and oral ulcerations.[12,14]
- Initial evaluation should include a complete blood count, ESR, CRP, albumin, and stool specimens to rule out bacterial and protozoal pathogens. Endoscopic and radiologic examinations may be required as well.
- Because there is no cure for IBD, the goal of therapy is to induce and maintain sustained remission from disease activity.

ON THE HORIZON

- It is hoped that recent genetic advances will aid in understanding the interaction between environmental and genetic factors in this disease.
- New "humanized" biologic therapies are being designed to target the production of cytokines and cellular adhesion molecules, and agents that modulate tissue architecture are in development.
- As with multiple sclerosis, bone marrow ablation and stem cell transplantation for severe Crohn's disease are being studied, and preliminary results are currently awaited.

SUGGESTED READING

Cho JH: The Nod2 gene in Crohn's disease: Implications for future research into the genetics and immunology of Crohn's disease. Inflamm Bowel Dis 2001;7:271-275.

Escher JC, Taminiau JA, Nieuwenhuis EE, et al: Treatment of inflammatory bowel disease in childhood: Best available evidence. Inflamm Bowel Dis 2003;9:34-58.

Fiocchi C: Inflammatory bowel disease: Etiology and pathogenesis. Gastroenterology 1998;115:182-205.

Griffiths AM, et al: Inflammatory bowel disease. In Walker WA, Goulet O, Kleinmar RE, et al (eds): Pediatric Gastrointestinal Disease: Pathophysiology, Diagnosis, Management. Hamilton, Ontario, BC Decker, 2000, pp 613-651.

Griffiths AM, Nguyen P, Smith C, et al: Growth and clinical course of children with Crohn's disease. Gut 1993;34:939-943.

Heyman MB, Kirschner BS, Gold BD, et al: Children with early-onset inflammatory bowel disease (IBD): Analysis of a pediatric IBD consortium registry. J Pediatr 2005;146:35-40.

Kirschner BS: Safety of azathioprine and 6-mercaptopurine in pediatric patients with inflammatory bowel disease. Gastroenterology 1998;115:813-821.

Kugathasan S, Judd RH, Hoffmann RG, et al: Epidemiologic and clinical characteristics of children with newly diagnosed inflammatory bowel disease in Wisconsin: A statewide population-based study. J Pediatr 2003;143:525-531.

Podolsky DK: Inflammatory bowel disease. N Engl J Med 2002;347:417-429.

Shashinder H, Integlia MJ, Grand RJ: Clinical Manifestations of Pediatric Inflammatory Bowel Disease. Philadelphia, WB Sanders, 2000.

REFERENCES

1. Shashinder H, Integlia MJ, Grand RJ: Clinical Manifestations of Pediatric Inflammatory Bowel Disease. Philadelphia, WB Sanders, 2000.
2. Geboes K, De Hertogh G: Indeterminate colitis. Inflamm Bowel Dis 2003;9:324-331.
3. Fiocchi C: Inflammatory bowel disease: Etiology and pathogenesis. Gastroenterology 1998;115:182-205.
4. Podolsky DK: Inflammatory bowel disease. N Engl J Med 2002;347:417-429.
5. Binder V: Epidemiology of IBD during the twentieth century: An integrated view. Best Pract Res Clin Gastroenterol 2004;18:463-479.
6. Sonnenberg A, McCarty DJ, Jacobsen SJ: Geographic variation of inflammatory bowel disease within the United States. Gastroenterology 1991;100:143-149.
7. Barton JR, Gillon S, Ferguson A: Incidence of inflammatory bowel disease in Scottish children between 1968 and 1983; marginal fall in ulcerative colitis, three-fold rise in Crohn's disease. Gut 1989;30:618-622.
8. Calkins BM, Mendeloff AI: Epidemiology of inflammatory bowel disease. Epidemiol Rev 1986;8:60-91.
9. Kugathasan S, Judd RH, Hoffmann RG, et al: Epidemiologic and clinical characteristics of children with newly diagnosed inflammatory bowel disease in Wisconsin: A statewide population-based study. J Pediatr 2003;143:525-531.
10. Fish D, Kugathasan S: Inflammatory bowel disease. Adolesc Med Clin 2004;15:67-90, ix.
11. Heyman MB, Kirschner BS, Gold BD, et al: Children with early-onset inflammatory bowel disease (IBD): Analysis of a pediatric IBD consortium registry. J Pediatr 2005;146:35-40.
12. Ballinger S: Henoch-Schönlein purpura. Curr Opin Rheumatol 2003;15:591-594.
13. Kasahara Y, Tanaka S, Nishino M, et al: Intestinal involvement in Behçet's disease: Review of 136 surgical cases in the Japanese literature. Dis Colon Rectum 1981;24:103-106.
14. Del Beccaro MA, Brownstein DR, Cummings P, et al: Outbreak of *Escherichia coli* O157:H7 hemorrhagic colitis and hemolytic uremic syndrome: Effect on use of a pediatric emergency department. Ann Emerg Med 1995;26:598-603.
15. Johnson GL, Johnson PT, Fishman EK: CT evaluation of the acute abdomen: Bowel pathology spectrum of disease. Crit Rev Diagn Imaging 1996;37:163-190.
16. Siegel MJ, Evans SJ, Balfe DM: Small bowel disease in children: Diagnosis with CT. Radiology 1988;169:127-130.

17. Antes G: Enteroclysis in children with Crohn's disease. Eur Radiol 2001;11:2341-2342.

18. Charron M: Pediatric inflammatory bowel disease imaged with Tc-99m white blood cells. Clin Nucl Med 2000;25:708-715.

19. Guidi L, Minordi LM, Semeraro S, et al: Clinical correlations of small bowel CT and contrast radiology findings in Crohn's disease. Eur Rev Med Pharmacol Sci 2004;8:215-217.

20. Kornbluth A, Legnani P, Lewis BS: Video capsule endoscopy in inflammatory bowel disease: Past, present, and future. Inflamm Bowel Dis 2004;10:278-285.

21. Seidman EG, Sant'Anna AM, Dirks MH: Potential applications of wireless capsule endoscopy in the pediatric age group. Gastrointest Endosc Clin North Am 2004;14:207-217.

22. Mow WS, Lo SK, Targan SR, et al: Initial experience with wireless capsule enteroscopy in the diagnosis and management of inflammatory bowel disease. Clin Gastroenterol Hepatol 2004;2:31-40.

23. Dubinsky MC, Ofman JJ, Urman M, et al: Clinical utility of serodiagnostic testing in suspected pediatric inflammatory bowel disease. Am J Gastroenterol 2001;96:758-765.

24. Ruemmele FM, Targan SR, Levy G, et al: Diagnostic accuracy of serological assays in pediatric inflammatory bowel disease. Gastroenterology 1998;115:822-829.

25. Pfefferkorn MD, Fitzgerald JF, Croffie JM, et al: Lactase deficiency: Not more common in pediatric patients with inflammatory bowel disease than in patients with chronic abdominal pain. J Pediatr Gastroenterol Nutr 2002;35:339-343.

26. Sakurai T, Matsui T, Yao T, et al: Short-term efficacy of enteral nutrition in the treatment of active Crohn's disease: A randomized, controlled trial comparing nutrient formulas. JPEN J Parenter Enteral Nutr 2002;26:98-103.

27. Korelitz BI: The role of liquid diet in the management of small bowel Crohn's disease. Inflamm Bowel Dis 2000;6:66-67; discussion 68-69.

28. Forbes A: Review article: Crohn's disease—the role of nutritional therapy. Aliment Pharmacol Ther 2002;16(Suppl 4):48-52.

29. Griffiths AM: Enteral nutrition in children. Nestle Nutr Workshop Ser Clin Perform Programme 1999;2:171-183; discussion 183-186.

30. Rutgeerts P, Feagan BG, Lichtenstein GR, et al: Comparison of scheduled and episodic treatment strategies of infliximab in Crohn's disease. Gastroenterology 2004;126:402-413.

31. Griffiths AM, Nguyen P, Smith C, et al: Growth and clinical course of children with Crohn's disease. Gut 1993;34:939-943.

32. Stein RB, Hanauer SB: Comparative tolerability of treatments for inflammatory bowel disease. Drug Saf 2000;23:429-448.

33. Tripathi RC, Kipp MA, Tripathi BJ, et al: Ocular toxicity of prednisone in pediatric patients with inflammatory bowel disease. Lens Eye Toxic Res 1992;9:469-482.

34. Kundhal P, Zachos M, Holmes JL, Griffiths AM: Controlled ileal release budesonide in pediatric Crohn disease: Efficacy and effect on growth. J Pediatr Gastroenterol Nutr 2001;33:75-80.

35. Ruemmele FM, Roy CC, Levy E, Seidman EG: Nutrition as primary therapy in pediatric Crohn's disease: Fact or fantasy? J Pediatr 2000;136:285-291.

36. Sutherland LR: Prevention of relapse of Crohn's disease. Inflamm Bowel Dis 2000;6:321-328; discussion 329.

37. Sutherland L, Roth D, Beck P, et al: Oral 5-aminosalicylic acid for maintenance of remission in ulcerative colitis. Cochrane Database Syst Rev 2002;4:CD000544.

38. Markowitz J, Grancher K, Kohn N, Daum F: Immunomodulatory therapy for pediatric inflammatory bowel disease: Changing patterns of use, 1990-2000. Am J Gastroenterol 2002;97:928-932.

39. Kirschner BS: Safety of azathioprine and 6-mercaptopurine in pediatric patients with inflammatory bowel disease. Gastroenterology 1998;115:813-821.

40. Paerregaard A, Schmiegelow K: Monitoring azathioprine metabolite levels and thiopurine methyl transferase (TPMT) activity in children with inflammatory bowel disease. Scand J Gastroenterol 2002;37:371-372.

41. Markowitz JF: Therapeutic efficacy and safety of 6-mercaptopurine and azathioprine in patients with Crohn's disease. Rev Gastroenterol Disord 2003;3(Suppl 1):S23-S29.

42. Kirschner B: Malignancy and aneuploidy: Prevention and early detection. Inflamm Bowel Dis 1998;4:216-220.

43. Escher JC, Taminiau JA, Nieuwenhuis EE, et al: Treatment of inflammatory bowel disease in childhood: Best available evidence. Inflamm Bowel Dis 2003;9:34-58.

44. Baldassano RN, Han PD, Jeshion WC, et al: Pediatric Crohn's disease: Risk factors for postoperative recurrence. Am J Gastroenterol 2001;96:2169-2176.

CHAPTER 99

Malnutrition

Jennifer Maniscalco

Malnutrition refers to any disorder of nutritional status resulting from a deficiency or excess of nutrient intake, imbalance of essential nutrients, or impaired nutrient metabolism.[1] It is a pathologic state of varying severity and variable clinical presentation. Despite significant advances in prevention and treatment worldwide, malnutrition continues to have a substantial negative impact on child morbidity and mortality. The prevalence of malnutrition among hospitalized children in the United States is thought to be as high as 45%, but it varies considerably by age and disease state.[2-4] In hospitalized adults, malnutrition has been associated with an increased risk of adverse clinical events, prolonged length of stay, and increased hospital costs[5,6]; it is reasonable to assume that children, who have growth needs as well, suffer similar ill effects. This chapter deals specifically with the issues of malnutrition, focusing on problems relating to inpatient care. Chapter 32 addresses failure to thrive.

CLINICAL PRESENTATION AND CLASSIFICATION

Physical examination findings in children with malnutrition are variable and related to the chronicity, severity, and type of nutrient imbalance. Table 99-1 lists some of the findings associated with deficiencies of both macro- and micronutrients. Abnormal growth ultimately occurs in all patients with ongoing malnutrition, and in some cases, it may be the only objective marker of poor nutritional status. Careful anthropometric measurements can assess growth cross-sectionally (e.g., triceps skin-fold thickness) or longitudinally (length or height) and may indicate the presence of malnutrition.

Historically, physical findings and anthropometry have been used to divide patients with malnutrition into two broad categories: marasmus and kwashiorkor.[7] Marasmus develops after chronic and severe calorie deprivation, resulting in weight loss and marked wasting of fat and muscle stores. Because visceral protein stores are generally preserved, edema does not develop. Although both height and weight measurements are abnormally low, weight is often decreased out of proportion to height. Kwashiorkor develops in acute or chronic situations when protein deficits exceed caloric deficits. Decreased visceral protein stores result in muscle wasting, edema, and changes in the skin and hair. Although some degree of growth failure is likely, weight may appear normal for height due to fluid retention.

More recently, the term *protein-energy malnutrition* has been used to describe states of malnutrition in which there are interrelated deficiencies in carbohydrates, proteins, and fat, as well as vitamins, minerals, and trace elements.[8] As a consequence of these multinutrient imbalances, children may have a combination of physical signs. In addition, protein-energy malnutrition results in compromised immune function, malabsorption and other impairments of gastrointestinal (GI) tract function, suboptimal response to medical or surgical therapy, and abnormal cognitive and behavioral development.[2]

Excessive intake of nutrients from overfeeding or unbalanced dietary intake can also result in abnormal physical examination findings, such as increased subcutaneous fat stores. In the United States in 2000, the prevalence of overweight among children and adolescents aged 6 to 19 years has risen to nearly 16% since the 1960s.[9] Abnormal dietary intake contributes to this trend, placing a substantial number of children and adolescents at risk for both malnutrition and the medical complications of overweight and obesity.

DIAGNOSIS AND EVALUATION

The causes of malnutrition can be divided into two broad categories.[2] Primary malnutrition results from inadequate quantity or quality of nutrient consumption. Secondary malnutrition results from excessive nutrient requirements or abnormal nutrient metabolism. Malnutrition has been associated with pathologic conditions of every major organ system and many infectious diseases.

Nutrition screening is a process to identify individuals who are malnourished or at risk for malnutrition to determine whether a more detailed assessment of nutrition is indicated.[2] Although few formal screening tools have been studied and validated in hospitalized pediatric patients,[4] several risk factors for malnutrition have been identified (Table 99-2). The presence of one or more of these risk factors should prompt a comprehensive evaluation using the history, physical examination, anthropometric measurements, and laboratory data to define nutritional status and develop an appropriate nutrition care plan.

An appropriate history includes a complete review of systems; a medication and dietary history, including the use of any dietary supplements; and a psychosocial history. Special emphasis should be placed on conditions or medications that impair the ability to ingest and absorb food or result in high metabolic demands. The dietary history should focus on the type and preparation of food or formula, the amount and frequency of feedings, and the route of feeding. A 3- to 5-day diet diary can provide an objective and accurate method of assessing dietary intake in the home setting.[10] Important psychosocial factors include adequacy of resources to purchase, store, and prepare food; level of parental knowledge and skills; drug and alcohol use or mental illness among caregivers; and potential child abuse or neglect.

A thorough physical examination and precise anthropometric measurements provide convenient and noninvasive methods for evaluating the acute and chronic nutritional status. Common measurements include weight, height (for children aged 2 years or older) or recumbent length (for

Table 99-1 Physical Examination Findings Associated with Macro- and Micronutrient Deficiencies

Finding	Nutrient Deficiency
General	
Short stature	Calorie
Decreased subcutaneous fat	Calorie
Muscle wasting	Protein, calorie
Muscle tenderness	Thiamine, biotin
Edema, ascites	Protein, thiamine
Hepatosplenomegaly	Protein
Hair	
Alopecia or sparse hair	Protein, zinc, biotin, copper
Easy pluckability	Protein
Flag signs (bands of light and dark hair)	Protein
Skin	
Follicular hyperkeratosis	Vitamins A, C
Dermatitis	Niacin, zinc, biotin, vitamin B_6
Poor wound healing	Protein, zinc, vitamins A and C
Dry, xerosis	Essential fatty acids
Petechiae, purpura	Vitamins C, K
Nails	
Koilonychia (spoon shaped)	Iron
Transverse ridging	Protein
Dry, brittle	Essential fatty acids
Eyes	
Xerophthalmia, Bitot spots (conjunctival spots), night blindness	Vitamin A
Angular palpebritis	Riboflavin
Oropharynx	
Dental caries	Fluoride
Cheilosis	Riboflavin, niacin, vitamin B_6
Glossitis	Riboflavin, niacin, pyridoxine, folate, vitamin B_{12}
Angular stomatitis	Riboflavin, niacin, iron, vitamins B_6 and B_{12}
Hypogeusia (reduced ability to taste)	Zinc
Bleeding gums	Vitamin C
Bone	
Craniotabes, rachitic rosary, bowing of legs	Vitamin D
Bone tenderness	Vitamin C
Nervous system	
Neuropathy (weakness, paresthesias)	Niacin, thiamine, copper, vitamins B_6, B_{12}, and E
Dementia	Niacin
Seizures	Vitamin B_6
Miscellaneous	
Goiter	Iodine

Table 99-2 Risk Factors for Malnutrition

Recent unintentional weight loss of >10%

Weight 20% over or under ideal body weight

No oral intake for >7 days

Any medical condition resulting in the following:
  Inadequate intake (e.g., oromotor or swallowing dysfunction, anorexia)
  Malabsorption (e.g., cystic fibrosis, short gut syndrome)
  Increased metabolic needs (e.g., CHD, BPD, trauma, burns)
  Protracted nutrient losses (e.g., vomiting, diarrhea, skin wounds)

Medications with catabolic properties (e.g., steroids, chemotherapy)

BPD, bronchopulmonary dysplasia; CHD, congenital heart disease.

Table 99-3 Waterlow Criteria for the Classification of Malnutrition

Weight for height: $\dfrac{\text{Actual weight}}{\text{50th percentile weight for height}} \times 100$

Height for age: $\dfrac{\text{Actual height}}{\text{50th percentile height for age}} \times 100$

Category	Acute Malnutrition (Weight for Height, % Median)	Chronic Malnutrition (Height for Age, % Median)
Normal	>90	>95
Mild	80-90	90-95
Moderate	70-80	85-90
Severe	<70	<85

Adapted from Waterlow JC: Classification and definition of protein-calorie malnutrition. BMJ 1972;3:566-569.

those younger than 2 years), and head circumference (children younger than 3 years). Body mass index (BMI) is the best measure of adiposity and is commonly used to define underweight, overweight, and obesity in children older than 2 years. It is calculated by the following formula:

$$BMI = \frac{\text{Weight (in kg)}}{\text{Height (in m)}^2}$$

Reference values for these measurements are available on the updated growth charts published by the National Center for Health Statistics.[11] Reference values for children with special health care needs are also available.

The weight-for-height value is the ratio of the patient's actual weight to the ideal weight for the patient's height. When acute medical conditions result in short-term nutritional deprivation, the body weight is depleted out of proportion to length (or height), and the weight-for-height value is low. Conversely, chronic malnutrition affects both weight gain and linear growth, resulting in a small child with a body weight that is more proportional to length. The Waterlow criteria use the weight-for-height value and a similar measure, the height-for-age value, to differentiate and classify acute and chronic malnutrition (Table 99-3).[12]

Although there is no single laboratory test for malnutrition nor a standard panel of tests, several common blood tests can provide important information about nutritional status. The initial evaluation usually includes the following:

- Complete blood count
- Liver function tests
- Electrolyte panel (including calcium, phosphorus, and magnesium)
- Albumin
- Prealbumin
- Prothrombin time

Further testing may be indicated based on abnormalities identified through the initial evaluation. Depletion of electrolyte stores or metabolic bone disease may result in abnormal chemistry and mineral profiles. A number of vitamin and mineral deficiencies can result in lymphopenia and thrombocytopenia, as well as hemolytic, microcytic, or megaloblastic anemia. Vitamin K deficiency often leads to a prolonged prothrombin time.

Serum protein levels often reflect the degree of malnutrition, but they must be interpreted with caution because they can be influenced by the presence of systemic disease as well as the body's response to trauma, infection, and inflammation. Because albumin has a half-life of 14 to 20 days and undergoes shifts in body stores with changes in acute nutritional status, it is a more effective marker of chronic malnu-

trition.[13] Other proteins synthesized by the liver have shorter half-lives and more accurately reflect acute changes in protein stores and metabolism.[14] These include transferrin (half-life 8 days), prealbumin (half-life approximately 2 days), and retinol binding protein (half-life 12 hours).

If renal function is normal, urine studies can provide additional information about total-body protein reserves and turnover. The creatinine-height index evaluates lean muscle mass by comparing the patient's 24-hour urinary creatinine excretion with the predicted urinary excretion for a child of similar height. Nitrogen balance compares 24-hour protein intake with 24-hour urinary urea nitrogen and reflects the rate of protein turnover. A positive nitrogen balance indicates an anabolic state, and a negative nitrogen balance indicates a catabolic state.

TREATMENT

Hospitalized patients who are malnourished or at risk for malnutrition need a formal nutrition care plan that clearly states the nutritional goals and monitoring parameters, the most appropriate route of administration of nutritional support and method of nutrition access, and the anticipated duration of therapy. An interdisciplinary approach is often necessary to ensure that the nutritional needs of the patient are adequately addressed and integrated into the medical and surgical treatment plans. Figure 99-1 presents

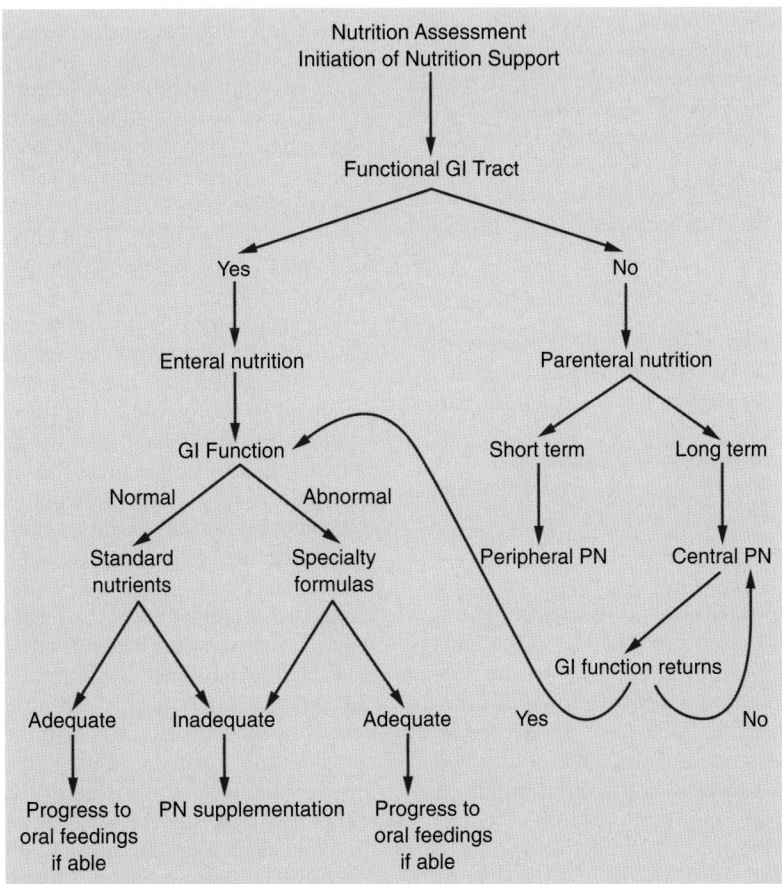

Figure 99-1 Route of administration of specialized nutritional support. GI, gastrointestinal; PN, parenteral nutrition. (Adapted from the ASPEN Clinical Pathways and Algorithms for Delivery of Parenteral and Enteral Nutrition Support in Adults.)

Table 99-4 Recommended Daily Allowance for Calories and Protein by Age

Age	Calories (kcal/kg/day)	Protein (g/kg/day)
0-6 mo	108	1.5
7-12 mo	98	1.5
1-3 yr	102	1.1
4-6 yr	90	0.95
7-10 yr	70	0.95
11-14 yr		
Girls	47	0.95
Boys	55	0.95
15-18 yr		
Girls	40	0.85
Boys	55	0.85

From Dietary Reference Intakes for Energy, Carbohydrates, Fiber, Fat, Fatty Acids, Cholesterol, Protein, and Amino Acids. National Academy of Sciences, 2002-2005. *http://nap.edu.*

Table 99-5 Indications for Enteral Nutrition

Category	Example
Inadequate oral intake	Disorders of sucking or swallowing Congenital anomaly of upper airway or GI tract
Abnormal function of GI tract	Inflammatory bowel disease Gastroesophageal reflux Hirschsprung disease Chronic liver disease
Increased metabolic demands	Cystic fibrosis Congenital heart disease Chronic pulmonary or renal disease
Growth failure or chronic malnutrition	Anorexia nervosa Nonorganic failure to thrive

GI, gastrointestinal.

an algorithm for determining the optimal route of nutritional support when oral intake is not sufficient or not possible.[15]

Total caloric needs can be estimated by several methods that incorporate various factors that may be relevant in individual circumstances. Activity level (e.g., bed rest versus active), stress level (e.g., well versus postoperative), and weight (e.g., obese versus underweight) all influence total caloric needs for adequate nutrition. Often basic caloric needs are determined by the patient's age (Table 99-4) and then adjusted for factors that may increase or decrease the need.

Daily caloric needs for infants and toddlers who are in need of catch-up growth is often estimated using the following formula:

$$120 \text{ kcal/kg/day} \times \text{Expected weight for height}$$

The expected weight for height is the 50th percentile weight (in kilograms) for the child's current height. This estimate is most useful when the patient's height has not fallen from the growth curve significantly.

Routine protein needs are provided in Table 99-4 and can be adjusted for catch-up growth using the expected weight for height.

Enteral Nutrition

Enteral nutrition—the provision of nutrients by tube directly into the GI tract—is indicated when an individual is unable to ingest or absorb a sufficient amount of nutrition orally to meet his or her requirements. Specific indications for enteral nutrition are listed in Table 99-5. Severe pancreatitis, peritonitis, bowel obstruction, intractable vomiting or diarrhea, and other disease processes that severely impair the function of the GI tract are contraindications to enteral nutrition.[10] Therapy for oral motor stimulation should be provided to all patients for the duration of enteral nutritional support to avoid the development of oral aversion and food refusal.

Selection of the appropriate delivery device and method of administration for enteral nutrition is dependent on the anticipated duration of nutrition support, the anatomy and function of the GI tract, and associated medical conditions.[16,17] Common routes of administration include nasogastric, nasoduodenal, nasojejunal, gastrostomy, and jejunosotomy tubes. Generally, nasoenteric tubes are used for short-term enteral nutrition (<3 months), and tube enterostomies are used for long-term enteral nutrition.

Gastric feedings are more physiologic and are preferred in children who require short-term nutritional support, have intact gag and cough reflexes, and have normal function of the GI tract. Gastric feedings may exacerbate underlying gastroesophageal reflux or gastroparesis and increase the risk for aspiration. These patients, as well as those with known tracheal aspiration, gastric outlet obstruction, and congenital anomalies of the upper GI tract, usually require transpyloric feedings.[10,16] See Chapter 195 for more information on enteral tubes.

The age, nutritional requirements, and medical condition of the patient determine the selection of formula. In most cases, enteral feedings are started at a continuous rate and advanced by increasing either the concentration or the rate of the infusion. A feeding pump can be used to control the rate at which formula enters the GI tract. Patients receiving transpyloric feedings or patients with impaired absorption typically remain on continuous feeding. The total duration of continuous feeding can be shortened in some patients, such as 20 or 18 hours a day, allowing periods when the patient is not attached to the feeding pump. Other patients may advance to bolus feedings once tolerance to full continuous feeding has been demonstrated. Bolus feedings involve the delivery of a specific amount of formula in a short period, as occurs with the consumption of meals. They more closely mimic normal feeding patterns and therefore provide more physiologic stimulation of the GI tract. Feeding intolerance is manifested by nausea, pain, persistent regurgitation, malabsorption, dumping syndrome, and aspiration.[10,16]

Compared with parenteral nutrition, enteral nutrition is better at maintaining the physiologic and immunologic integrity of the GI tract. In addition, the administration of

Table 99-6   Complications of Enteral Nutrition

Category	Complication
Feeding tube related	Clogging of tube
	Dislodgment of tube
	Nasopharyngeal ulceration or necrosis
	Hoarseness and vocal cord paralysis
	Bowel perforation
	Bowel obstruction
	Hemorrhage
	Stomal leakage
Infectious	Sinusitis and otitis media
	Aspiration pneumonia
	Cellulitis
Gastrointestinal	Vomiting
	Diarrhea
	Abdominal cramping or bloating
	Dumping syndrome
Metabolic	Electrolyte abnormalities

Table 99-8   Complications of Parenteral Nutrition

Category	Complication
Catheter related	Malposition of catheter
	Occlusion of catheter
	Pneumothorax, hemothorax, hydrothorax
	Cardiac arrhythmia
	Brachial plexus injuries
	Air or catheter embolus
	Vascular injury
	Thrombophlebitis
Infectious	Line infection
	Sepsis
Metabolic	Glucose abnormalities
	Electrolyte and mineral abnormalities
	Acid-base imbalance
	Hypertriglyceridemia
	Biliary and hepatic dysfunction
	Metabolic bone disease
	Refeeding syndrome

Table 99-7   Indications for Parenteral Nutrition

Prematurity and low birth weight

Congenital gastrointestinal anomalies

Necrotizing enterocolitis

Short bowel syndrome

Intestinal obstruction

Severe motility disorders

Intractable diarrhea

Severe pancreatitis

Severe trauma or burns

Severe protein-energy malnutrition

enteral nutrition is easier, more economical, and results in fewer metabolic and infectious complications.[10] The complications of enteral nutrition are listed in Table 99-6.

Parenteral Nutrition

Parenteral nutrition—the provision of nutrients intravenously—is indicated when an individual is unable to meet ongoing nutritional needs with either oral or enteral nutrition. Specific indications for parenteral nutrition are listed in Table 99-7. Relative contraindications include short anticipated duration of nutritional support and probability of imminent death.

Parenteral nutrition can be administered peripherally via a standard intravenous catheter if the duration of nutritional support is not expected to exceed 1 to 2 weeks. However, peripheral veins are not tolerant of highly osmotic solutions, and it is often difficult to provide adequate calories, protein, and electrolytes in this manner. Central venous access, via either a peripherally inserted central catheter or a semiper-

manent catheter, allows for the provision of nutrients at a greater concentration. See Chapter 195 for more information on central venous catheters.

The composition of a parenteral nutrition solution is determined by the patient's age, weight, nutritional and medical needs. Solutions are typically infused over 24 hours in hospitalized patients, but in those receiving long-term parenteral nutrition solutions may be cycled over 10 to 20 hours. Several resources exist for determination of the normal requirements for energy, fluid and electrolytes, protein, carbohydrates, lipids, and micronutrients for pediatric patients.[18-20]

Complications of parenteral nutrition are listed in Table 99-8. Catheter-related complications can be reduced by minimizing the frequency of catheter manipulation and encouraging the use of advanced aseptic techniques. Hepatic dysfunction tends to occur in young patients or neonates, and the severity of liver involvement has been inversely related to the degree and duration of enteral starvation.[21] The risk of hepatic dysfunction decreases with the early introduction of enteral feedings, which stimulate bile flow and the production of GI hormones. In all cases, transition to oral or enteral feedings should ensue when GI function returns.

Refeeding Syndrome

Refeeding syndrome refers to the metabolic and physiologic consequences of rapid electrolyte repletion, fluid resuscitation, and changes in glucose metabolism in a patient with chronic caloric deprivation.[22] Any patient who is categorized as severely malnourished according to the Waterlow criteria is at risk for the fluid and electrolyte imbalances and vitamin deficiencies that can occur with refeeding. As carbohydrates are reintroduced, there is a switch back to the use of glucose as the predominant fuel, with a resultant high demand for the production of phosphorylated intermediates of glycolysis (i.e., adenosine triphosphate and 2,3-diphosphoglycer-

Table 99-9   Monitoring Schedule for Hospitalized Patients Receiving Nutritional Support

Parameter	FREQUENCY	
	Initiation Phase of Support	*Maintenance Phase of Support*
Weight	Daily	Weekly
Length and head circumference	Weekly	Weekly
Serum electrolytes	Daily, then 3 times/wk	Weekly
Serum calcium, magnesium, phosphorus	Daily, then 3 times/wk	Weekly
Serum glucose*		
Liver function tests	Weekly	Weekly
Prealbumin	Weekly	Weekly
Albumin	Monthly	Monthly
Triglycerides	Daily until lipid dose is stable	Weekly
Copper, ceruloplasmin, manganese	Monthly	Monthly

The frequency and duration of serum glucose monitoring are dependent on the occurrence of hyperglycemia or hypoglycemia and the individual clinical scenario.

ate), causing a drop in the serum level of phosphorus. Hypophosphatemia is considered the hallmark of refeeding syndrome, although other imbalances may occur as well, including hypokalemia and hypomagnesemia.[23] Carbohydrate infusion can result in sodium and water retention and lead to rapid expansion of the extracellular fluid compartment. Cardiac decompensation is precipitated by the stress of increased circulatory volume on the already depleted cardiac muscle. Carbohydrate infusion can also lead to hyperglycemia, which may result in osmotic diuresis and dehydration. Vitamin deficiencies are common among malnourished patients, and there is increasing awareness of thiamine deficiency occurring during the refeeding period, possibly related to carbohydrate refeeding.

The earliest indicators of impending refeeding syndrome can be picked up with close electrolyte monitoring, but clinical symptoms may be noticeable as well. Neurologic changes, including paresthesias, weakness, mental status changes, or seizures, can occur when serum levels of phosphorus fall to less than 1 to 1.5 mg/dL. Cardiac dysfunction or diaphragmatic weakness can result in circulatory and respiratory failure. Low levels of adenosine triphosphate in red blood cells may result in impaired oxygen delivery, and low levels of potassium and magnesium may result in electrocardiographic changes. Delirium can occur in the second week of refeeding and may be related to hypophosphatemia and other electrolyte abnormalities; thiamine deficiency is another suspected cause, because some of the features overlap with Wernicke encephalopathy or Korsakoff syndrome.[24]

The refeeding syndrome can occur in patients receiving all forms of specialized nutritional support, especially during the first week of treatment.[25] Although it is commonly associated with the administration of parenteral nutrition, the risk is more closely linked to the degree of malnutrition. Refeeding syndrome is more likely to occur with more severe malnutrition, more rapid weight loss, and more recent weight loss. Careful correction of electrolyte derangements

and circulatory volume should precede refeeding.[24] Slow advancement of nutritional support toward goal levels can greatly reduce the risk of refeeding syndrome. Some experts recommend starting feeds at a rate of 20 kcal/kg per day,[24] with small daily increments as tolerated. Frequent monitoring of laboratory parameters is imperative; this often involves checking electrolytes at least daily in the first week of carbohydrate supplementation. Repletion of electrolytes is the cornerstone of management of refeeding syndrome. It may also be necessary to severely limit the rate of glucose infusion until electrolytes have stabilized. Owing to the need for electrolyte replacement and frequent monitoring, some patients may require an intensive care setting.

Monitoring

A monitoring schedule to ensure the efficacy of supplemental nutritional support and to screen for complications is shown in Table 99-9. Aggressive monitoring is indicated for patients with severe protein-energy malnutrition, patients at risk for refeeding syndrome, and patients receiving parenteral nutrition.

SPECIAL CONSIDERATIONS IN SEVERE MALNUTRITION

Severe malnutrition (as defined by the Waterlow criteria; see Table 99-3) leads to a process of reductive adaptation to conserve energy and affects the functional capacity of every major organ system in the body.[26] These changes place severely malnourished children at increased risk of mortality from four main causes: hypoglycemia, hypothermia, cardiac failure, and infection. Guidelines for the management of the child with severe malnutrition have been published by the World Health Organization.[27] These treatment protocols discourage the use of intravenous fluid resuscitation in the absence of shock, promote the judicious repletion of fluids and nutrients over time, and recommend empirical treatment with antibiotics. The implementation of these protocols results in a substantial reduction in mortality rate.[28]

CONSULTATION

Dieticians can provide valuable guidance in the evaluation and management of malnourished children. Gastroenterologists can offer help during hospitalization and may be key to proper follow-up and ongoing management after discharge.

For patients with evidence of cardiac dysfunction, conduction abnormalities, arrhythmia, or hemodynamic instability, input from cardiologists may be useful.

Critical care consultation is appropriate when cardiodynamic stability is a concern or when the level of monitoring or frequency of intervention needed exceeds the capacity of a non–critical care setting.

ADMISSION CRITERIA

- Physical examination or anthropometric evidence of severe protein-energy malnutrition.
- Significant dehydration or electrolyte abnormalities.
- Inability to meet nutritional needs with a standard oral diet.
- Failure of outpatient management.
- Lack of safe or stable home environment or appropriate outpatient follow-up.

DISCHARGE CRITERIA

- Treatment of underlying or associated medical and surgical conditions is completed.
- Ability to ingest adequate oral nutrients or to tolerate discharge regimen of enteral or parenteral nutrition has been demonstrated.
- Fluid and electrolyte status has been stabilized, and pertinent laboratory parameters have improved.
- Adequate weight gain on the discharge nutrition regimen has been documented.
- There is a safe and stable home environment, and home medical assistance and follow-up have been arranged, as needed.

PREVENTION

Early recognition of patients at risk for malnutrition, as well as those with existing disorders of nutritional status, is imperative. Prompt institution of nutritional support can prevent the development of malnutrition and its sequelae.

IN A NUTSHELL

- Malnutrition refers to any disorder of nutritional status and has variable clinical presentations and severity. Abnormal growth ultimately occurs in all patients with ongoing malnutrition.
- A detailed history and physical examination, with supportive laboratory evidence, are sufficient to make the diagnosis of malnutrition. Anthropometric measurements are useful for the classification of malnutrition.
- Enteral or parenteral nutritional support is indicated until the patient is able to ingest adequate oral nutrients; enteral support is preferred whenever possible.
- Laboratory parameters and anthropometric measurements must be carefully monitored to assess the efficacy of treatment and screen for complications.
- Refeeding syndrome is a complication of malnutrition that occurs with the introduction of increased nutrition. Hypophosphatemia, hypokalemia, and hypomagnesemia are the typical electrolyte abnormalities seen. Cardiac decompensation can occur secondary to volume expansion and increased demands on the malnourished cardiac muscle. Delirium can occur, which may be related to thiamine deficiency.

ON THE HORIZON

- There is growing interest in the role of organ damage in malnutrition and the possible relationship to a shortage of cysteine.
- The bioavailability of many micronutrients in common foods is unclear. Several trials are under way to assess the absorption of specific vitamins from everyday foodstuffs.
- Progress is being made in the delivery of certain essential nutrients (e.g., iron sprinkles) to enhance compliance with home supplementation.

SUGGESTED READING

Acra SA, Rollins C: Principles and guidelines for parenteral nutrition in children. Pediatr Ann 1999;28:113-120.
Hendricks KM, Duggan C, Gallagher L, et al: Malnutrition in hospitalized pediatric patients: Current prevalence. Arch Pediatr Adolesc Med 1995;149:1118-1120.
Kraft MD, Btaiche IF, Sacks GS: Review of the refeeding syndrome. Nutr Clin Pract 2005;20:625-633.
Serrano M, Mannick EE: Consultation with the specialist: Enteral nutrition. Pediatr Rev 2003;24:417-423.

REFERENCES

1. American Society for Parenteral and Enteral Nutrition Board of Directors: Standards for hospitalized pediatric patients. Nutr Clin Pract 1996;11:217-228.
2. American Society for Parenteral and Enteral Nutrition Board of Directors and Clinical Guidelines Task Force: Guidelines for the use of parenteral and enteral nutrition in adult and pediatric patients. JPEN J Parenter Enteral Nutr 2002;26(1 Suppl):1SA-138SA.
3. Hendricks KM, Duggan C, Gallagher L, et al: Malnutrition in hospitalized pediatric patients: Current prevalence. Arch Pediatr Adolesc Med 1995;149:1118-1120.
4. Sermet-Gaudelus I, Poisson-Salomon AS, Colomb V, et al: Simple pediatric nutritional risk score to identify children at risk of malnutrition. Am J Clin Nutr 2000;72:64-70.
5. Reilly JJ, Hull SF, Albert N, et al: Economic impact of malnutrition: A model system for hospitalized patients. JPEN J Parenter Enteral Nutr 1988;12:372-376.

6. Correia MI, Waitzberg DL: The impact of malnutrition on morbidity, mortality, length of hospital stay and costs evaluated through a multivariate model analysis. Clin Nutr 2003;22:219-220.

7. Classification of infantile malnutrition [editorial]. Lancet 1970;2:302-303.

8. Allen SJ: Malnutrition. In Walker WA, Goulet O, Kleinman RE, et al (eds): Pediatric Gastrointestinal Disease: Pathophysiology, Diagnosis, Management, 4th ed. Hamilton, Ontario, BC Decker, 2004.

9. Ogden CL, Flegal KM, Carroll MD, Johnson CL: Prevalence and trends in overweight among US children and adolescents, 1999-2000. JAMA 2002;288:1728-1732.

10. American Academy of Pediatrics, Committee on Nutrition: Pediatric Nutriton Handbook, 5th ed. Elk Grove Village, Ill, American Academy of Pediatrics, 2004.

11. 2000 CDC Growth Charts: United States. *http://www.cdc.gov/ growthcharts/* (accessed May 30, 2005).

12. Waterlow JC: Classification and definition of protein calorie malnutrition. BMJ 1972;3:566-569.

13. Kumar S, Olson DL, Schwenk WF: Malnutrition in the pediatric population. Dis Mon 2002;48:703-712.

14. Golden MH: Transport proteins as indices of protein status. Am J Clin Nutr 1982;35:1159-1165.

15. American Society for Parenteral and Enteral Nutrition: Clinical Pathways and Algorithms for Delivery of Parenteral and Enteral Nutrition Support in Adults. Silver Spring, Md, American Society for Parenteral and Enteral Nutrition, 1998.

16. Serrano M, Mannick EE: Consultation with the specialist: Enteral nutrition. Pediatr Rev 2003;24:417-423.

17. Forchielli M, Bines J: Enteral nutrition. In Walker WA, Watkins JB, Duggan C (eds): Nutrition in Pediatrics: Basic Science and Clinical Applications, 3rd ed. Hamilton, Ontario, BC Decker, 2003.

18. Acra SA, Rollins C: Principles and guidelines for parenteral nutrition in children. Pediatr Ann 1999;28:113-120.

19. Falcone RA, Warner BW: Pediatric parenteral nutrition. In Rombeau JL, Rolandelli RH (eds): Clinical Nutrition: Parenteral Nutrition, 3rd ed. Philadelphia, WB Saunders, 2001.

20. Koo WWK, Cepeda EE: Parenteral nutrition in neonates. In Rombeau JL, Rolandelli RH (eds): Clinical Nutrition: Parenteral Nutrition, 3rd ed. Philadelphia, WB Saunders, 2001.

21. Shattuck KE, Klein GL: Hepatobiliary complications of parenteral nutrition. In Rombeau JL, Rolandelli RH (eds): Clinical Nutrition: Parenteral Nutrition, 3rd ed. Philadelphia, WB Saunders, 2001.

22. Marinella MA: The refeeding syndrome and hypophosphatemia. Nutr Rev 2003;61:320-323.

23. Solomon SM, Kirby DF: The refeeding syndrome: A review. JPEN J Parenter Enteral Nutr 1990;14:90-97.

24. Crook MA, Hally V, Panteli JV: The importance of the refeeding syndrome. Nutrition 2001;17:632-637.

25. Hearing SD: Refeeding syndrome is underdiagnosed and undertreated, but treatable. BMJ 2004;328:908-909.

26. Ashworth A: Treatment of severe malnutrition. J Pediatr Gastrenterol Nutr 2001;32:516-518.

27. World Health Organization: Management of Severe Malnutrition: A Manual for Physicians and Other Senior Health Workers (1999). *http:// whqlibdoc.who.int/hq/1999/a57361.pdf* (accessed May 30, 2005).

28. Ashworth A, Chopra M, McCoy D, et al: WHO guidelines for management of severe malnutrition in rural South African hospitals: Effect on case fatality and the influence of operational factors. Lancet 2004;363: 1110-1115.

CHAPTER 100

Pancreatitis

Patricia V. Lowery and J. Rainer Poley

Pancreatitis is an inflammatory process that occurs acutely or can progress to a chronic condition when relapses of acute episodes lead to irreversible destruction of the pancreas. Pancreatitis can result in varying degrees of pancreatic insufficiency. Childhood pancreatitis is uncommon but is being diagnosed with increased frequency, perhaps related to increased vigilance and an increased understanding of molecular genetics. With the development of advanced procedural and imaging techniques, management and interventional strategies continue to improve. Further elucidation of the underlying genetics and cell biology may allow tailoring of management to the specific cause.

The causes of childhood pancreatitis differ from those in adults.[1] The most common causes of childhood acute pancreatitis are trauma, systemic diseases such as viral infections and metabolic disorders, anatomic and structural abnormalities, medications and ingestion of toxic substances, and hereditary disorders. Abdominal trauma accounts for up to a third of cases of pancreatitis in pediatric patients (Table 100-1). However, the cause remains unknown in up to 25% of cases. In contrast, the leading causes in the adult population are alcoholism and biliary tract disease, and there is now evidence that genetic predisposition can contribute to the development of chronic pancreatitis. Acute pancreatitis is the most common pancreatic disorder in childhood.[2]

Relapsing, acute pancreatitis leading to chronic pancreatitis is most often secondary to trauma, underlying congenital anomalies of the biliary or pancreatic system, and genetic causes. Recurrent attacks of acute pancreatitis, particularly as seen in familial, hereditary pancreatitis, can lead to the development of chronic inflammatory changes with fibrosis and calcifications within the pancreatic ductal system severe enough to decrease the number and function of islet cells and result in insulin-dependent diabetes.[3,4] Several susceptibility genes with mutations of their gene products have been described, including mutations of cationic trypsinogen (PRSS 1), serine protease inhibitor Kazal type 1 (SPINK 1), and cystic fibrosis transmembrane conductance regulator (CFTR).

Chronic/relapsing pancreatitis occurs as a result of persistent and usually progressive inflammation. Histologically, acinar destruction predominates, with islet sparing until later in the disease course, at which point progression to insufficiency may occur. Common causes include hereditary pancreatitis, an autosomal dominantly inherited disease in which mutation of trypsinogen genes mapped to chromosome 7q35 appears to render trypsin and trypsinogen resistant to autolysis and permanent inactivation. A second common cause is idiopathic chronic pancreatitis (ICP), which is the most common cause of chronic pancreatitis in children and nonalcoholic adults. CFTR mutations might predispose to ICP; the cystic fibrosis carrier status increases the risk for ICP by fivefold.

CLINICAL PRESENTATION

Children with acute pancreatitis present similarly to adults, with an acute onset of abdominal pain, persistent vomiting, anorexia, and fever. The pain, described as sharp, steady, and worsened by eating, may be epigastric, periumbilical, generalized, or located in the right upper quadrant and may radiate to the back or flanks. The patient is restless and visibly uncomfortable; frequently, patients are most comfortable when assuming an antalgic position by lying on their side or sitting upright with the hips and knees flexed. Vomiting begins as the pain, caused by pancreatic autodigestion and stretching of the pancreatic capsule, increases within the first 24 to 48 hours. Hypoactive bowel sounds, abdominal tenderness, distention, and guarding are often seen as ileus, or signs of peritonitis may develop.[5] Simple, uncomplicated pancreatitis is most often of viral etiology (enterovirus, influenza, Epstein-Barr, varicella), is probably underdiagnosed in children, and carries a favorable prognosis. Although more common in adults, gallstones and gallstone pancreatitis do occur in children (see Chapter 93).

Even though severe acute pancreatitis is infrequent in children, it must be considered in the setting of severe persistent vomiting, abdominal pain, fever, and toxicity. The abdomen may be distended and ascites may occur. An epigastric mass or left pleural effusion may be appreciated on examination. The Cullen sign (periumbilical ecchymosis) and Grey Turner sign (bluish discoloration in the flank region) are seen in cases of hemorrhagic pancreatitis. The systemic inflammatory response syndrome may occur with multiple organ involvement and is manifested as shock, coagulopathy, hemorrhage, acute respiratory distress syndrome, renal failure, and secondary infections.[6]

The clinical manifestations and severity of acute pancreatitis may have individual variations that are determined by modifier genes such as MCP-1, which confers an increased risk for severe pancreatitis, and GSTT-1A, which is associated with mild disease.[7]

Chronic pancreatitis usually causes persistent abdominal pain with episodic exacerbations of pain; however, some patients experience no pain. With progressive scarring and worsening insufficiency of pancreatic exocrine and endocrine function, symptoms of insulin-dependent diabetes mellitus and malabsorption can develop. Jaundice (secondary to obstruction of the common bile duct), ascites, or pleural effusion can also be seen.

DIAGNOSIS AND EVALUATION

After obtaining a history and performing a physical examination that is suggestive, the diagnosis of acute pancreatitis is most commonly made by determination of pancreatic amylase, lipase, and proteases. Elevation of serum amylase

Table 100-1   Causes and Conditions Associated with Pancreatitis

Trauma
Accidental blunt trauma
Burns
Child abuse
Endoscopic retrograde cholangiopancreatography
Surgical trauma

Infections
Viral
　Cytomegalovirus
　Epstein-Barr virus
　Enterovirus (Coxsackie)
　Hepatitis A and B
　Human immunodeficiency virus
　Influenza A and B
　Measles
　Mumps
　Rubella
　Rubeola
　Varicella
Bacterial
　Campylobacter
　Escherichia coli
　Leptospirosis
　Mycoplasma
　Yersinia
Parasitic
　Ascaris lumbricoides (obstructive)
　Clonorchis sinensis (obstructive)
　Malaria

Systemic Diseases
α_1-Antitrypsin deficiency
Celiac disease
Collagen vascular disorders (lupus, polyarteritis nodosa)
Cystic fibrosis
Diabetes mellitus
Envenomation (scorpion, spider)
Head trauma
Hemochromatosis
Henoch-Schönlein purpura
Hemolytic uremic syndrome
Hyperalimentation
Hypercalcemia
Hyperparathyroidism

Hyperlipidemia (see Metabolic disorders/inborn errors of metabolism)
Hypertriglyceridemia (see Metabolic disorders/inborn errors of metabolism)
Inflammatory bowel disease
Intracranial tumors
Kawasaki's disease
Malnutrition (starvation, eating disorders)
Metabolic disorders/inborn errors of metabolism
　Acute intermittent porphyria
　Apolipoprotein C-II deficiency
　Apolipoprotein lipase deficiency
　Branched-chain ketoaciduria (maple syrup urine disease)
　Cystinuria
　Familial hypertriglyceridemia and chylomicronemia
　Glycogen storage disease
　Hereditary lipoprotein lipase deficiency
　Homocystinuria
　Lysinuric protein intolerance
　Organic aciduria (3-hydroxy-3-methylglutaryl-coenzyme A lyase deficiency)
　Pyruvate kinase deficiency
Renal failure
Sarcoidosis
Sepsis
Shock (multiorgan dysfunction syndrome, systemic inflammatory response syndrome)
Sickle cell disease (vaso-occlusive)
Transplantation (bone marrow, heart, kidney, liver, pancreas)

Anatomic/Obstructive
Annular pancreas
Biliary tract malformations
Choledochal cyst
Cholelithiasis and choledocholithiasis
Duplication cyst
Endoscopic retrograde cholangiopancreatography complication
Pancreas divisum
Pancreatic ductal abnormalities
Pancreatic pseudocyst
Perforated duodenal ulcer
Sphincter of Oddi dysfunction
Tumors

Drugs and Toxins (see Table 100-2)

occurs within hours, but it can return to normal within 48 to 72 hours, even if symptoms persist. The sensitivity of serum amylase is between 70% and 95%, which means that 5% to 30% of patients with pancreatitis have normal or minimally elevated amylase values.[1,6] The test also lacks specificity inasmuch as many other conditions may be associated with elevated amylase, including salivary sources (infection, obstruction, and trauma), diabetic ketoacidosis, pregnancy, burns, and macroamylasemia. Pancreatic amylase may be elevated in bowel injury (obstruction, appendicitis, mesenteric ischemia, peptic ulcer disease) because of enhanced absorption of amylase from the intestinal lumen resulting in

hyperamylasemia. Serum lipase is more specific but may not be elevated until about 72 hours after the onset of symptoms. It remains elevated up to 14 days longer than total serum amylase does and may be particularly useful when amylase is normal. Increased pancreatic enzymes have been reported in approximately 25% of patients with celiac disease.[8] Lipase can also be elevated in other diseases; the clinical presentation should dictate interpretation of any laboratory values. Finally, it is important to note that levels of amylase and lipase do not necessarily reflect the severity of disease. Particularly in cases of chronic pancreatitis, the pancreatic enzymes may be normal as the gland "burns out."[3]

There is an immunoassay for urinary cationic trypsinogen that is both sensitive and specific for pancreatitis, but cost and test availability limit use of this test to the setting of diagnostic uncertainty. Its utility in the pediatric population is still under study. Currently, urinary trypsin activation peptide may be the most sensitive diagnostic test for determining the severity of an episode of acute pancreatitis. This test peaks much earlier and should be obtained within the first 12 to 24 hours after the onset of acute symptoms for prognostic predictive value.

Nonspecific laboratory findings may include leukocytosis, hemoconcentration, increased liver enzymes (particularly elevated γ-glutamyltransferase and bilirubin, which should prompt evaluation for gallstones), decreased calcium and magnesium levels, metabolic alkalosis (as a result of vomiting) or acidosis (severe pancreatitis), hyperglycemia, and evidence of disseminated intravascular coagulation or hypercoagulability.

Radiographic evaluation can include plain films, ultrasound (conventional and endoscopic), computed tomography (CT), magnetic resonance imaging (MRI), endoscopic retrograde cholangiopancreatography (ERCP), and magnetic resonance cholangiopancreatography (MRCP). Plain films of the abdomen may demonstrate nonspecific findings such as a "sentinel loop" (distention of a loop of small bowel in proximity to the pancreas), dilated transverse colon with the "cutoff" sign (absent colonic gas distal to the transverse colon), paralytic ileus, a diffuse haziness indicative of ascites, calcification of the pancreas, blurring of the left psoas margin, pseudocyst formation, or in cases of severe disease, the presence of extraluminal air. Chest radiography may reveal atelectasis, basilar infiltrates, pleural effusions (usually left sided), or pulmonary edema. Abdominal ultrasound remains a cornerstone of diagnosis of pancreatitis and allows determination of pancreatic dimensions; ductal anatomy; the presence of gallstones or dilated bile ducts; hypoechogenicity and sonolucency, which suggest edema; calcification in the setting of recurrent or chronic pancreatitis; and complications such as pancreatic masses, cysts, or abscesses. Endoscopic ultrasound may also provide definition of ductal anatomy, but this is not used in the acute setting and is not widely available in pediatric practice. When ultrasound evaluation is technically suboptimal, CT or MRI may provide additional information regarding the ducts and surrounding organs and can be helpful in further delineation of previously mentioned complications. CT should probably be avoided in the acute phase of severe pancreatitis because a contrast load may exacerbate pancreatic ischemia. Findings on imaging studies may appear normal in up to 20% of children with pancreatitis.[2]

Recurrence suggests underlying pathology and warrants a more thorough investigation, including evaluation for hyperlipidemia, hypercalcemic states, parasite infection, and autoimmune disorders. Cystic fibrosis testing and other genetic testing should be performed.

In the setting of disease recurrence or chronic disease, ERCP is generally indicated to determine the presence of pancreatic and biliary ductal anomalies. This procedure can be both diagnostic and therapeutic (sphincterotomy, stone extraction, biliary stent placement, pseudocyst drainage). Relative contraindications include active acute disease (in the absence of evidence of ductal obstruction), pseudocyst, and abscess. Disadvantages of this study include a requirement for general anesthesia and the risk associated with excessive radiation exposure. It should be noted that pancreatitis is also a potential complication of ERCP.[9,10] Abnormalities in the ductal system may be evaluated with MRCP as a noninvasive alternative to ERCP. MRCP may supplement or replace ERCP as the study of choice for evaluating the anatomy of the ductal system, especially if the need for therapeutic ERCP is thought to be low. Experience with both these procedures is rapidly increasing in the pediatric population.[11]

Chronic pancreatitis can cause endocrine and exocrine dysfunction when the disease has caused significant destruction of pancreatic tissue. Elevations of fasting blood glucose or abnormalities in glucose tolerance testing are indicative of diabetes mellitus. Random ("spot") stool samples for fecal fat (e.g., Sudan III stain or acid steatocrit) and fecal elastase-1 can be used to identify patients with malabsorption.

TREATMENT

Management of pancreatitis is generally supportive, although identification and control of any underlying treatable causes should be pursued. Bowel rest, fluid replacement and management, nutritional support, and pain control are central to supportive care.

Eliminating oral or gastric intake is usually sufficient for bowel rest. However, bowel decompression via nasogastric suction may be needed for patients with persistent vomiting. Fluid replacement and correction of electrolyte imbalances are key in the initial phase. In severe or necrotizing pancreatitis, tremendous amounts of fluid can accumulate in and around the inflamed pancreas and lead to requirements for large amounts of intravenous fluid. Careful monitoring of hemodynamic status, urine output, and serum electrolytes is warranted.

Total parenteral nutrition (TPN) should be initiated if enteral feeding is expected to be withheld for more than 3 to 5 days. Studies suggest that intrajejunal feeding is as safe and as well tolerated as TPN in acute pancreatitis. Such enteral feeding may moderate the acute phase response and thereby decrease the risk for septic complications or the systemic inflammatory response syndrome. Intestinal barrier integrity is better maintained, which results in decreased bacterial translocation when the gut is fed. In addition, placement of a central venous catheter can often be avoided. A low-fat elemental formula (e.g., Vivonex TEN) should be used when feeding is directly into the jejunum.

Pain control can be provided with hydromorphone hydrochloride (Dilaudid), which is preferred over morphine. Morphine is believed to produce contraction of the sphincter of Oddi and therefore has the potential to interfere with drainage of biliary and pancreatic secretions.

Treatable causes of pancreatitis should be identified and addressed. This could include the discontinuation of potentially toxic drugs such as valproic acid or other antiepileptic drugs, chemotherapeutic agents, estrogens, corticosteroids, or diuretics (Table 100-2). Metabolic causes of pancreatitis, such as hypertriglyceridemia, hyperlipidemia, and hypercalcemia, should be addressed and treated.

Table 100-2 Drugs Associated with Pancreatitis

Acetaminophen (overdose)
Alcohol
Amphetamines
Anticoagulants
L-Asparaginase
Azathioprine (Imuran)
Carbamazepine
Cimetidine
Cholestyramine
Cisplatin
Clonidine
Corticosteroids
Cyclophosphamide
Didanosine
Enalapril
Erythromycin
Estrogen
Furosemide
Heroin
Histamine
Isoniazid
Lamivudine
6-Mercaptopurine
Mesalamine
Methotrexate
Methyldopa
Metronidazole
Nitrofurantoin
Penicillin
Pentamidine
Procainamide
Ranitidine
Rifampin
Salicylates
Sulfonamides
Sulindac
Tetracycline
Valproic acid
Vincristine
Vitamin D

A sudden rise in pancreatic enzymes, persistent elevation, or worsening/persistence of symptoms suggests the development of a pseudocyst. Pseudocysts complicate the course in approximately 10% of patients unless associated with abdominal trauma, in which case they occur in more than 50% of patients. Serial ultrasound often reveals evidence of pancreatitis not identified at presentation or earlier in the disease course. In all but the mildest self-limited cases, it is advisable to repeat an ultrasound after approximately 4 weeks to evaluate for possible pseudocyst formation because they usually become evident 2 to 3 weeks after the acute attack. Pseudocysts are most often (85%) located in the body or tail of the pancreas. Most frequently associated with trauma, pseudocysts generally resolve spontaneously, and medical management with several weeks of TPN or jejunal feeding may be necessary. Surgical, endoscopic, or image-guided percutaneous drainage should be undertaken if the pseudocyst is increasing in size or continuing to produce pain.

Surgical intervention should be avoided in the acute setting unless intervention for obstruction of biliary or pancreatic ducts is deemed necessary. ERCP with sphincterotomy, balloon dilation, or stent placement may be an option in this setting. Usually, correction of anatomic defects should be scheduled electively after recovery from the acute episode. Partial pancreatectomy or pancreaticojejunostomy may be indicated in patients with intrapancreatic ductal strictures.[12,13]

Bacterial superinfection is a serious complication of pancreatitis and is more likely to occur in the setting of necrosis of pancreatic tissue and more commonly later in the clinical course. Strategies to prevent pancreatic infection include enteral administration of nonabsorbable antibiotics to decontaminate the gut lumen and prophylactic systemic antibiotics. Although promising, studies using these modalities in adults have yielded conflicting results. However, some experts recommend administration of prophylactic intravenous antibiotic therapy to patients with proven necrotizing pancreatitis. Because coverage of enteric gram-negative organisms is the goal, piperacillin-tazobactam and imipenem are good choices.

The timing of reintroducing oral (or gastric) feeding is not absolute, and it is not necessary to wait for normalization of pancreatic enzymes. Reintroduction of oral feeding may be considered when pain and ileus have resolved and the patient regains an appetite. A clear liquid diet can be started and advanced with reintroduction of fat from 10 to 20 g/kg daily as tolerated. A low-fat diet may be prescribed until complete recovery of acute pancreatitis, but this restriction does not appear to affect the progression of chronic pancreatitis and may contribute to malnutrition if used chronically. In chronic pancreatitis, it is advisable to administer pancreatic enzyme supplementation with each meal to reduce digestive stress on the pancreas. In children, the amount of replacement enzyme should not exceed 2000 U lipase/kg to avoid complications such as fibrotic strictures of the colon, particularly in chronic pancreatitis. Complete correction is not readily achieved. Proton pump inhibitors should be administered as long as pancreatic enzyme supplements are given to prevent acid-induced inactivation of lipase in the stomach and duodenum.[2]

The Ranson criteria (Table 100-3) and other systems, such as the APACHE III (Acute Physiology and Chronic Health

Table 100-3 Ranson Criteria for Determining the Prognosis of Acute Pancreatitis

Present on Admission
Age older than 55 years
White blood cell count greater than 16,000/μL
Blood glucose greater than 200 mg/dL
Serum lactate dehydrogenase greater than 350 IU/L
Serum glutamic-oxaloacetic transaminase (aspartate transaminase) greater than 250 IU/L

Developing during the First 48 Hours
Hematocrit fall greater than 10%
BUN increase greater than 8 mg/dL
Serum calcium less than 8 mg/dL
Arterial oxygen saturation less than 60 mm Hg
Base deficit greater than 4 mEq/L
Estimated fluid sequestration greater than 600 mL

Scoring
1 point for each criterion present
Ranson score of 0-2, minimal mortality
Ranson score of 3-5, 10%-20% mortality
Ranson score >5, more than 50% mortality and associated with more systemic complications

IN A NUTSHELL

- The diagnosis of pancreatitis should be entertained in a pediatric patient with persistent vomiting, abdominal pain, and anorexia.
- Bowel rest, fluid and electrolyte management, and pain control are the mainstays of therapy.
- Although complete recovery is usual in children, recurrence suggests underlying pathology, which mandates evaluation for an underlying cause.
- Diagnostic imaging may begin with plain films of the abdomen, which may reveal pancreatic calcifications or findings suggestive of pancreatitis as previously discussed. Ultrasound and CT are the preferred studies to diagnose and monitor the course of pancreatitis and pseudocysts.
- A pseudocyst complicates the course in approximately 10% of patients unless associated with abdominal trauma, in which case pseudocysts occur in more than 50% of patients.
- ERCP may allow endoscopic therapeutic intervention for pancreatitis. MRCP affords anatomic definition of the pancreas while avoiding radiation exposure.

ON THE HORIZON

- Advances in the understanding of genetic mutations that either produce or predispose an individual to pancreatitis should allow diagnostic insight, provide the framework for interventional strategies, and result in tailoring of management to specific underlying molecular causes. Tests for activation peptides of trypsinogen and carboxypeptidase B will probably improve diagnostic sensitivity and the ability to predict severity of acute pancreatitis in children.[9] Pediatric risk stratification systems to assist the clinician in assessing the severity of acute pancreatitis are being developed and evaluated.

Evaluation) scoring system, have been used to predict the prognosis in adults. They have not been evaluated in pediatric patients, and pediatric risk stratification systems need further study.[14]

CONSULTATION

Collaboration plus consultation with a pediatric gastroenterologist regarding the acute management and follow-up of patients with pancreatitis is prudent. Surgical consultation may be necessary in cases of confirmed or suspected trauma, pancreaticobiliary anomalies, or stones as potential causes of pancreatitis. The interventional radiologist may also provide valuable guidance and assistance when radioimaging is being considered. The pain service, where available, may assist with pain management, particularly in the acute setting. A genetics consultation should be part of the evaluation of recurrent pancreatitis or in a child with a family history of hereditary pancreatitis.

ADMISSION CRITERIA

All pediatric patients with acute or recurrent pancreatitis should be admitted for bowel rest and fluid and electrolyte management.

DISCHARGE CRITERIA

When the child is tolerating adequate intake to sustain hydration and nutrition without pain, discharge home may be considered. Plans for follow-up, including any repeat imaging, should be in place.

SUGGESTED READING

Lerch MM, Zenker M, Turi S, Mayerle J: Developmental and metabolic disorders of the pancreas. Endocrinol Metab Clin North Am 2006;35:219-241.
Mony B, Weizman Z: Acute pancreatitis in childhood: Analysis of literature data. J Clin Gastroenterol 2003;37:169-172.
Morinville V, Whitcomb DC: Recurrent acute and chronic pancreatitis: Complex disorders with a genetic basis. Gastroenterol Hepatol 2005;1:195-205.
Whitcomb DC: Acute pancreatitis. N Engl J Med 2006;354:2142-2150.
Whitcomb DC, Lowe ME: Pancreatitis: Acute and chronic. In Walker WA, Goulet O, Kleinman RE, et al (eds): Pediatric Gastrointestinal Disease: Pathophysiology, Diagnosis, Management, 4th ed. Hamilton, Ontario, BC Decker, 2004, pp 1584-1597.

REFERENCES

1. McPhee S: Disorders of the exocrine pancreas. In McPhee S, Ganong WF (eds): Lange Pathophysiology: An Introduction to Clinical Medicine, 4th ed. New York, McGraw-Hill, 2004, pp 430-455.
2. Werlin S: Exocrine pancreas. In Behrman RE, Kleigman RM, Jenson HB (eds): Nelson Textbook of Pediatrics, 17th ed. Philadelphia, WB Saunders, 2004, pp 1298-1303.

3. Miqdady M, Kitagawa S: Clinical manifestations and diagnosis of chronic pancreatitis in children. 2004 UpToDate Online 11.3. Available at *www.uptodate.com*.

4. Miqdady M, Kitagawa S: Etiology of chronic pancreatitis in children. 2004 UpToDate Online 11.3. Available at *www.uptodate.com*.

5. Hebra A, Adama SD, Thomas PB: Pancreatitis and pancreatic pseudocyst. Available at *www.emedicine* from WebMD. Last Updated 6/12/06.

6. Guzman D, Abramo TJ: Pediatric surgical emergencies, sorting out problems manifested by peritoneal irritation. Clin Pediatr Emerg Med 2002;3:22-32.

7. Morinville V, Perrault J: Genetic disorders of the pancreas. Gastroenterol Clin North Am 2003;32:763-787.

8. Carroccio A, Prima LD, Scalici C, et al: Unexplained elevated serum pancreatic enzymes: A reason to suspect celiac disease. Clin Gastroenterol Hepatol 2006;4:455-459.

9. Adler DG, Baron TH, Davila RE: ASGE guideline: The role of ERCP in diseases of the biliary tract and the pancreas. Gastrointest Endosc 2005;62:1-8.

10. Hsu RK, Draganov P, Leung JW, et al: Therapeutic ERCP in the management of pancreatitis in children. Gastrointest Endosc 2000;51:396-400.

11. Lowe ME: Pancreatitis in childhood. Curr Gastroenterol Rep 2004;6:240-246.

12. Weber TR, Keller MS: Operative management of chronic pancreatitis in children. Arch Surg 200l;136:550-554.

13. Holterman AL, Adams KN, Seeler RA: Surgical management of pediatric hematologic disorders. Surg Clin North Am 2006;86:427-439.

14. DeBanto JR, Goday PS, Pedroso MR, et al: Acute pancreatitis in children. Am J Gastroenterol 2002;97:1726-1731.

CHAPTER 101

Feeding Issues

Beth D. Gamulka

Feeding difficulties are frequent comorbid conditions in infants and children with both acute and chronic illnesses and can alert the clinician to an underlying condition. In fact, feeding problems can precede the diagnosis of cerebral palsy in 60% of children with both cerebral palsy and oromotor dysfunction.[1] Decreased oral intake can lead to nutritional deficiencies, failure to thrive, and dehydration. The ability of infants and children to feed and grow relies on safe oromotor coordination, endurance while feeding, adequate caloric intake, an appropriate food source, and positive feedback with respect to the feeding experience. Although poor feeding may be associated with many other pediatric illnesses, by far the most common feeding-related issues are gastroesophageal reflux (GER) and gastroesophageal reflux disease (GERD). Dysphagia and feeding aversion are two other distinct feeding-related diagnoses that will be addressed. Complications related to feeding aversion and to aspiration are also often concomitant diagnoses in medically complex children.

The hospitalist may be involved in the initial evaluation or management of these feeding disorders, a complication of the disorder in a patient with underlying dysfunction, or a comorbid process in a child hospitalized for an unrelated problem.

Aspiration is a serious complication of feeding disorders, whether an acute event or chronic condition. Aspiration may occur with abnormalities of antegrade feeding (e.g., swallowing disorder) or retrograde flow of food from the stomach or esophagus (e.g., gastroesophageal reflux). Through either route, failure to protect the airway can result in an aspiration event. Aspiration pneumonitis and pneumonia are discussed in Chapter 76.

DYSPHAGIA

Dysphagia is the term often used to refer to a swallowing abnormality, which frequently leads to an effect on eating. Swallowing can be divided into three phases: oral, pharyngeal, and esophageal. Problems at any stage of swallowing can affect eating to some degree. During the oral phase, an infant forms a bolus of fluid after creating suction with the lips, tongue, and palate. The bolus is then moved to the posterior pharynx. Older infants (older than 3 to 4 months) and children are able to complete the oral phase of swallowing with more mature tongue movements and are able to move boluses of food of different consistencies by chewing and tongue movements. The oral phase depends on normal oral anatomy, normal sensation and sensory feedback, strong sucking (in infants), and normal oral muscular function (in children).

The pharyngeal phase of swallowing is an involuntary action that is initiated when the bolus touches the posterior pharyngeal wall. The nasal cavity is sealed by the pharynx and soft palate, and pharyngeal muscular contractions propel the bolus toward the esophagus. During this phase, respiration ceases as the vocal cords close, the larynx elevates, and the upper esophageal sphincter relaxes to allow the bolus to enter the esophagus. In children with poor oral muscular coordination, early entry of the bolus into the pharynx before vocal cord closure may allow aspiration into the trachea. Similarly, delay in relaxation of the upper esophageal sphincter allows food to pool above or penetrate the larynx and increases the risk for aspiration when the vocal cords open again.

The esophageal phase of swallowing, also involuntary, requires normal esophageal mucosa, caliber, and motility to allow the bolus to enter the stomach. Esophageal inflammation, stricture, dysmotility, and obstruction can all contribute to dysphagia.

Abnormalities in swallowing are most common in premature infants and children with neurologic abnormalities or airway anomalies, such as laryngeal clefts, vocal cord palsy, and tracheoesophageal fistula. Disorders of swallowing in children differ from those in adults because of the anatomic relationships of airway structures in children and variations in neurologic maturity. The most common disorders of swallowing in infants relate to immature sucking, inefficient sucking, and difficulty coordinating the suck-swallow-breathe rhythm. Less commonly, incoordination of swallowing may be due to an anatomic or neuromuscular abnormality that impairs one or several phases of swallowing. Swallowing incoordination may cause aspiration into the respiratory tract and lead to acute pneumonitis or pneumonia (see Chapter 76) or to nonspecific airway inflammation. In many children, chronic aspiration can also lead to poor nutritional intake and feeding aversion.

Although the majority of children who aspirate are known to have neurodevelopmental delay or airway anomalies, aspiration can occur as an isolated phenomenon in neurologically normal infants. Two studies of term infants presenting with swallowing dysfunction suggest that the prognosis is excellent, with most babies showing improvement in swallowing by 3 to 9 months and more than 77% successfully exclusively feeding orally by 37 months.[2,3] Theories about the cause of isolated dysphagia in healthy infants include delayed neuromuscular coordination and esophageal dysmotility.[2,3]

Clinical Presentation

The most common symptoms associated with dysphagia are coughing, choking, and "blue" spells with feeding. Blue spells may be actual hypoxic events caused by impaired minute ventilation or aspiration of oral contents into the airway and may be more marked in children who already have underlying cardiorespiratory compromise (e.g., congenital heart disease, bronchopulmonary dysplasia). Parents or caregivers may also report stridor, wheezing, and vomiting. Symptoms may vary in severity and quality depending on the feeding position, feed consistency, and type of feeding apparatus. The symptoms may occur exclusively during feeding (e.g., blue spells, choking, or sputtering), linger after completion of feeding (e.g., cough or stridor), or persist between feedings (increased secretions, wheeze). Some children have a history of pneumonia or a previous diagnosis of reactive airways disease (which may really reflect a previous aspiration event or chronic aspiration). A chest radiograph may show a focal infiltrate or chronic changes.

A larger proportion of children than adults aspirate silently, that is, without associated symptoms and no evidence of protective cough. Silent aspiration is also more common in patients who aspirate more than once during a swallow.[4] It should be considered in children with an anatomic or neuromuscular disorder, a report of slow feeding, chronic respiratory symptoms, or recurrent pneumonia.

Children with cleft palate or cardiorespiratory illnesses (e.g., chronic lung disease, congenital heart disease, or acute infectious respiratory illnesses) may become tachypneic, cyanotic, or diaphoretic and may have difficulty coordinating the suck-swallow-breathe cycle. These infants may suffer a significant reduction in minute ventilation while swallowing that leads to hypoxia. Infants with cleft palate need extra assistance with control of the flow of liquid into the pharynx to prevent aspiration and may have difficulty organizing the swallow at the end of the oral phase.

Healthy infants with recent lower respiratory tract infections, such as bronchiolitis, may also be at increased risk for laryngeal penetration, tracheal penetration, and aspiration into the lower airways. These abnormalities can normalize within 2 to 4 weeks after the infection.[5] Infants with underlying dysphagia would experience worsening of their swallowing dysfunction and a further increase in their risk for aspiration.

Differential Diagnosis

The symptoms and signs that suggest dysphagia warrant consideration of the underlying abnormalities that may contribute to the disorder, including esophageal dysmotility, GERD, and anatomic, sensory, or motor abnormalities of the oropharynx.

Evaluation

Clinical assessment of feeding is a bedside evaluation that is performed by an experienced occupational therapist or speech-language pathologist. It involves observation and assessment of tone, feeding position, sucking, tongue and jaw movements, bolus formation, and bolus manipulation. Observation of changes in respiratory status (coughing, choking, increased secretions, increased adventitious sounds on auscultation) is also important. In addition, assessment includes an evaluation with various food thicknesses and textures, depending on the age of the child. Clinical assessment should be considered for any child with an underlying condition that predisposes to dysphagia and aspiration or a child who exhibits unexplained respiratory symptoms, evidence of recurrent pneumonia, or difficulty feeding. One

community study found that 90% of children with cerebral palsy had some degree of oromotor dysfunction[1]; therefore, these children often warrant clinical evaluation. Children with feeding aversion behavior may also benefit from clinical assessment, as would otherwise healthy infants with symptoms suggestive of aspiration. Clinical assessment is important for evaluation of the caregiver-infant feeding relationship and feeding safety and serves as a guide for the need for additional diagnostic testing (e.g., videofluoroscopic feeding study [VFS]). Clinical assessment of swallowing of liquids and solids at the bedside has a sensitivity of 90% and a specificity of 56% for risk for aspiration[6] and is therefore a useful screening test to determine the need for radiographic evaluation.

VFS is considered the gold standard for assessment of feeding function. Radiographic contrast material is mixed with foodstuff of variable consistency (age appropriate) to visualize its dynamic passage from the mouth to the stomach. The nature and severity of specific abnormalities of function can be identified, including inefficient bolus formation, abnormal movement of the bolus to the posterior pharynx, pooling above the larynx, penetration of the bolus into the trachea (Fig. 101-1), or direct aspiration into the lungs. There is a relationship between the severity of laryngeal penetration and aspiration risk, particularly with thin liquids. Eighty-five percent of children with evidence of deep laryngeal penetration on VFS also aspirate thin liquids on VFS.[7] One review of infants referred for evaluation of dysphagia suggests that more than 50% will show evidence of laryngeal penetration, aspiration, or nasopharyngeal backflow on VFS.[8] Swallowing appears to become more dysfunctional after multiple swallows in infants, thus suggesting that longer assessments with videofluoroscopy are most useful.

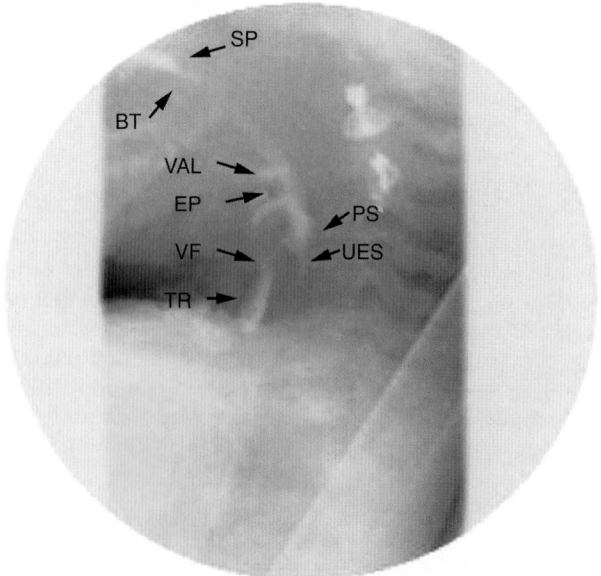

Figure 101-1 Videofluoroscopic study demonstrating laryngeal penetration and tracheal aspiration. In this image of a modified barium swallow, barium (appears white) is seen filling the vallecula (VAL), penetrates the vocal folds (VF), and is aspirated into the trachea (TR). BT, base of tongue; EP, epiglottis; SP, soft palate; PS, piriform sinus; UES, upper esophageal sphincter.

However, because VFS requires radiation exposure, alternatives have been explored, including fiberoptic endoscopic evaluation of swallowing (FEES). This method allows direct visualization of baseline swallowing, as well as observation of swallowing with liquid or solid boluses. In one study of FEES in children who also underwent VFS, there was 100% agreement between the results of both modalities.[9] Although a relatively new technology for evaluation of swallowing in children, FEES has the added benefit of enabling assessment of baseline swallowing without requiring the introduction of oral liquids or solids in high-risk children.

Salivagrams and milk scans are both nuclear medicine tests that have been used to assess swallowing and the presence of aspiration. During a salivagram, a child is placed supine and a radiopharmaceutical tracer is instilled into the mouth close to the salivary glands. Images are acquired in two planes over a 2-hour period. Aspiration is detected when radioactivity is seen in the lung fields. The benefits of this type of study include its ability to assess small boluses in the supine position (which may be better at assessing the risk for aspiration of oral secretions in neurologically impaired children) and the length of observation of the test. Because the salivagram collects information over a 2-hour period, it may be more likely than VFS to capture abnormal swallowing.

Similarly, a milk scan uses a radiopharmaceutical added to milk and swallowed by the child or introduced into the stomach via a nasogastric or gastric catheter. Images are then obtained over a period of 2 hours, and aspiration is seen when radioactivity is noted in the lungs. It has the added benefit of assessing for retrograde aspiration from GER when radioactivity is seen in the lungs in later images but not seen during the dynamic acquisition of images during the swallow itself.

However, there are drawbacks to nuclear scintigraphy in the assessment of swallowing. Unlike VFS, neither type of nuclear medicine scan has the resolution to assess tracheal penetration. One study of children with cerebral palsy and presumed aspiration showed poor agreement between VFS, milk scans, and salivagrams (κ less than 0.2), thus suggesting that these investigations are not interchangeable and that perhaps the salivagram is best (but not ideal) for assessing aspiration.[10]

Delineation of the swallowing disorder directs the clinician toward necessary feeding interventions or limitations. It may also help identify or clarify a condition for which dysphagia is only part of the clinical picture.

Treatment

After completion of the diagnostic investigation, the goal of management is to establish feeding regimens that are safe and improve the efficiency and enjoyment of feeding.

Children with oromotor incoordination may benefit from an ongoing oral stimulation therapeutic program led by a speech pathologist or occupational therapist. It is vital to maintain positive oral experiences and reassess the safety of oral feeding clinically and radiographically, particularly in infants and young children, because there is a potential for improvement and maturation of the swallow mechanism. Without ongoing oral stimulation, feeding aversion may develop in children whose dysphagia improves.

Intervention for children who aspirate depends on which food consistency, if any, is found to be safe. Foods that are associated with aspiration are restricted. Children who are safe only with pureed consistencies often require another method of feeding to receive adequate fluids. Depending on the cause of dysphagia and the likelihood of improvement, nasogastric or gastrostomy tube feedings are indicated. Children who are found to aspirate all consistencies require admission to the hospital to establish tube feeding and to either teach parents how to administer nasogastric feeding or facilitate insertion of a gastrostomy tube.

FEEDING AVERSION

Multiple factors can influence the enjoyment of eating and lead to food refusal in infants and children. Chronic discomfort from abnormal gastrointestinal motility, chronic esophagitis, chronic aspiration, and force-feeding can all lead to persistent feeding aversion, decreased oral intake, and poor nutrition and growth. Stressed feeder-child interactions around mealtime can also influence and exacerbate aversion behavior. Feeding aversion is particularly important in the inpatient setting for children who have prolonged illness. One study suggests that feeding refusal in children may stem from visceral hyperalgesia, often as a result of previous painful experiences such as prolonged neonatal care, multiple painful procedures, and chronic gastritis and esophagitis.[11]

Evaluation

Evaluation of feeding aversion requires a thorough review of a child's health, feeding, growth, and development. It is important to identify experiences that may have contributed to traumatically acquired feeding disorders. Parental reports and mealtime observation are also helpful to evaluate feeding behavior and identify feeder-child interaction problems.[12] Feeding questionnaires and structured observation tools are also available to assist in the evaluation of feeding aversion.[12]

Treatment

The key to management of feeding aversion is a comprehensive multidisciplinary approach. Although some children may require tube feeding to maintain adequate nutrition with ongoing ambulatory support, others may benefit from admission to the hospital to observe multiple meals and introduce specific behavioral feeding techniques. It is often quite difficult to wean children with feeding aversion off enterostomy tube feeding. Behavioral therapy in the hospital, although effective in helping reinstate hunger cues and reducing the fear of swallowing, often requires prolonged hospitalization. One study of outpatient behavioral intervention using extinction along with nutritional counseling over a 7-week period led to successful exclusive oral feeding in 50% of children.[13]

Consultation

- Speech pathologist or occupational therapist
- Otolaryngologist if abnormal anatomy is suspected as a cause of dysphagia
- Consider a psychologist or psychiatrist with experience in feeding behavior
- Clinical dietitian

Admission Criteria

- Dehydration or weight loss in children with feeding aversion
- Risk of aspiration with all consistencies, which requires initiation of nasogastric feeding and caregiver education on nasogastric tube feeding
- Admission for evaluation of feeding behavior and intensive behavioral intervention
- In many instances, dysphagia is identified during admission for respiratory symptomatology caused by aspiration pneumonitis

Discharge Criteria

- A safe enteral feeding program has been established.
- Caloric and fluid intake goals are being met.
- Respiratory symptoms, if present, have been treated.
- An outpatient therapeutic plan and key individuals (dietitian, speech-language pathologist or otolaryngologist, primary physician) have been identified. Frequently, reevaluation of swallow or ongoing support for behavioral interventions, or both, are required. Referral to a pediatric outpatient rehabilitation program may be helpful.

GASTROESOPHAGEAL REFLUX AND GASTROESOPHAGEAL REFLUX DISEASE

GER is a normal physiologic process whereby gastric contents involuntarily pass into the esophagus. The predominant mechanism is transient relaxation of the lower esophageal sphincter.[14] Most episodes of GER in infants, children, and adults are asymptomatic. Regurgitation of gastric contents into the oral cavity is often a normal process in healthy thriving infants that resolves by the second year of life. Factors that influence the incidence of GER include lower esophageal sphincter pressure, angle of insertion of the esophagus into the stomach, gastric volume and emptying, intra-abdominal pressure, esophageal innervation, and motility.[15,16]

GERD is a group of symptoms or complications of GER, which are detailed in Table 101-1.[17-19] Overt regurgitation of

Table 101-1 Gastroesophageal Reflux Disease

Symptoms/Signs	Complications
Recurrent vomiting	Apnea
Failure to thrive	Esophagitis
Irritability	Esophageal stricture
Hematemesis	Anemia
Dysphagia	Aspiration pneumonia
Feeding refusal	Tracheal stenosis
Apparent life-threatening event	Sinusitis
Wheezing	Laryngitis
Stridor or hoarseness	Asthma
Chronic cough	Bronchiectasis
Sandifer syndrome*	

*Sandifer syndrome is a constellation of symptoms associated with gastroesophageal reflux that include arching, torsional spasms of the neck, crying, extension of the extremities, and irritability.

food is not always present. GERD is common in neurologically abnormal children and those with esophageal anomalies, but it is often found in otherwise healthy infants and children. Although GER is quite common in premature infants, there is insufficient evidence to suggest GER is a cause of apnea in premature infants.[15]

Evaluation

The diagnosis of GERD is most often entertained in the presence of vomiting, but there is quite a broad differential for vomiting in an infant or young child, including anatomic abnormalities, infection, central nervous system tumors or bleeding, and metabolic derangements such as diabetes mellitus and inborn errors of metabolism. The evaluation depends on the age and presentation of the child. In most infants with vomiting and in older children with heartburn and regurgitation, a history and physical examination are usually sufficient to exclude other diagnoses, support the diagnosis of GER or GERD, and differentiate between them.[17]

An upper gastrointestinal series (contrast fluoroscopic evaluation of the esophagus, stomach, and duodenum) is not a useful test to rule in or rule out GER because of its low sensitivity and specificity,[20] but it may be helpful in detecting other anatomic abnormalities that may present with vomiting, such as malrotation, pyloric stenosis, duodenal web, and duplication.

Warning signs that suggest an alternative diagnosis include bilious vomiting, gastrointestinal bleeding, projectile vomiting, onset of vomiting after 6 months of age, failure to thrive (although this may occur as a consequence of severe GERD), diarrhea, constipation, fever, lethargy, hepatosplenomegaly, bulging fontanelle, macrocephaly or microcephaly, seizures, abdominal distention or tenderness, and genetic disorders known to be associated with other diagnoses that cause vomiting.[17]

Pyloric stenosis is an important alternative or concomitant diagnosis to consider. Important differences in their presentation are provided in Table 101-2. This entity is discussed in Chapter 138.

Intraesophageal pH monitoring (pH probe) is useful for objective quantification of acid GER and identification of associated symptoms, but it has limitations. It is easily affected by changes in diet and posture[21] and does not detect non-acid reflux. Overall, esophageal pH monitoring is most helpful in correlating acid reflux episodes with other symptoms, as well as evaluating the efficacy of acid suppressant therapy.[17]

Endoscopy and biopsy are useful in evaluating children with severe GERD for detection of strictures or Barrett esophagitis (metaplasia of the mucosa), as well as the severity of esophagitis. Biopsy is also an important tool when other differential diagnoses are being considered, such as infectious or eosinophilic esophagitis.[16] The risks associated with the procedure, which usually requires general anesthesia or deep sedation in children, must be weighed against a trial of therapy in each case.

As mentioned previously, milk scan is another mode of evaluation of GERD, but its role in the pediatric population is unclear because of the absence of age-specific norms.[17]

Table 101-2 Presentation of Gastroesophageal Reflux (Disease) and Pyloric Stenosis

	Gastroesophageal Reflux	Pyloric Stenosis
Age at onset	Any age	Early infancy (2 weeks to 3 months)
Nature of vomiting		
Forcefulness	Nonforceful	Forceful, "projectile"
Presence of bile	Nonbilious	Nonbilious
Course of vomiting severity	Nonprogressive	Progressive
Timing	May occur at variable times between feedings	Promptly after feeding
Signs of discomfort* (e.g., arching, irritability)	Common	Rare
Feeding aversion*	Occasionally	None. Usually eager to feed promptly after emesis
Dehydration/electrolyte derangements	Rare	Eventually if not recognized early in the course
Anemia	Occasionally (with GERD)	Rarely

*Associated with GERD.
GERD, gastroesophageal reflux disease.

Table 101-3 Comparison of Gastrointestinal Studies for Vomiting

Study	Diagnostic Utility	Advantages	Disadvantages
Upper GI series*	Assesses for malrotation, presence of stenosis or stricture	Readily available	Not useful in diagnosing GERD
pH probe	Objective quantification of acid GER	Helps assess effectiveness of PPI therapy; may help correlate other symptoms (discomfort, apnea, arching) with GER	Cannot evaluate non-acid reflux; invasive
Milk scan	Able to detect aspiration into the lungs from GERD	Noninvasive	May not identify GERD in the absence of aspiration to the lungs
Abdominal ultrasound	Helps rule out other causes of vomiting; assesses the presence of pyloric stenosis in infants and cholelithiasis in older children (or in any child prone to stone formation, such as those with hemolytic diseases)	Noninvasive	Cannot evaluate GER/GERD
Gastric emptying scan	May be helpful in identifying children with delayed emptying who would benefit from motility agents or from pyloroplasty with fundoplication	Noninvasive	Cannot evaluate GER/GERD

*Contrast fluoroscopic evaluation of the esophagus, stomach, and duodenum.
GER, gastroesophageal reflux; GERD, GER disease; GI, gastrointestinal; PPI, proton pump inhibitor.

The utility of various gastrointestinal studies is provided in Table 101-3.

Treatment

Although appropriate assessment of growth and parental reassurance are often all that is required in the management of GER, any vomiting infant with irritability, feeding refusal, disturbed growth or sleep, apnea, or other respiratory symptoms warrants consideration of a broader differential diagnosis and appropriate diagnostic evaluation. Because of the invasiveness of endoscopy and biopsy and the lack of evidence to support standard investigations for GERD, a trial of empirical therapy is often chosen for this diagnosis. Management options can be categorized as nonpharmacologic, pharmacologic, and surgical.

In an attempt to ameliorate the regurgitation of patients with GER, many nonpharmacologic interventions have been used, including positioning, formula change, pacifier use, and changes in feeding. A systematic review of these interventions identified key studies that provide guidance regarding their efficacy.[22]

Placing an infant in an infant seat after feeding to provide a more upright position was associated with increased reflux in comparison to the supine position.[23] Elevating the head of the bed offered no benefit.[23] Prone positioning is associated with lower reflux scores, but sleeping prone to reduce GERD is not recommended because the risk for sudden infant death syndrome is greater than the potential benefits of prone sleeping.[17]

Non-nutritive sucking (e.g., pacifier use) after feeding was also found to offer no benefit.[24] Because some infants with cow's milk protein intolerance may present with GERD, there is evidence to support a 1- or 2-week trial of a hydrolyzed hypoallergenic formula.[17] However, it is unclear whether removal of cow's milk from the diet of a breast-feeding mother or a trial of a soy-based formula in formula-fed infants has any effect on vomiting.

Thickening of feeds with cereal or using a prethickened formula does not improve reflux scores, as measured by pH probe. However, both methods of thickening decrease the number of episodes of vomiting. Prethickened formulas that flow through a standard nipple without requiring widening have been shown to reduce regurgitation and choke-gag-cough patterns after feeding, as well as improve sleep.[24] Prethickened formulas with carob bean gum are more successful in reducing reflux symptoms than formula thickened with rice cereal.[22]

Pharmacologic therapy for GERD includes histamine H_2 receptor antagonists (H_2 blockers), proton pump inhibitors (PPIs), and prokinetic agents. Whereas H_2 blockers are effective for mild esophagitis, PPIs are more effective for severe gastritis and esophagitis. PPIs and H_2 blockers interact with the cytochrome P-450 system and can affect the metabolism of other drugs, particularly those with narrow therapeutic ranges.[25] PPI dosing in children can vary and usually requires higher per-kilogram dosing than in adults. One study showed that therapeutic omeprazole doses in children aged 1 to 16 years range from 0.7 to 3.5 mg/kg/day.[26] PPIs decrease the volume and acidity of gastric fluid, thereby decreasing the frequency of GER and allowing esophagitis to heal. Potential concerns of chronic long-term acid suppression from PPI use include intestinal metaplasia and bacterial overgrowth. For children with nasogastric or gastrostomy tubes, serial measurement of gastric pH may help in dose titration of PPIs.

The current recommendations from the North American Society for Pediatric Gastroenterology and Nutrition for the treatment of GERD include a "step-up" or "step-down" approach. Step-up therapy begins treatment with an H_2 blocker and then switches to a standard-dose PPI if no improvement occurs, with the dose increased if necessary. The step-down approach begins with higher-dosage PPI therapy for 8 to 12 weeks and decreases to a standard dose once symptoms are controlled.[17] H_2 blockers are then used for maintenance. There are no clear guidelines regarding the recommended length of overall therapy, which may be dependent on the age of the patient and the presence of comorbid conditions.

Prokinetic agents, including cisapride, metoclopramide, and domperidone, have been used as a way of enhancing gastric emptying. However, there is no clear evidence that

Table 101-4 Indications for Surgical Intervention for Gastroesophageal Reflux Disease

Life-threatening complications
Aspiration
Laryngospasm
Apnea
Peptic strictures with persistent reflux symptoms
Barrett esophagus
Congenital heart disease with prominent regurgitation/ vomiting and poor growth
Disabling side effects of medical therapy
Unwillingness to continue long-term medication therapy

From Gold BD: Gastroesophageal reflux disease: Could intervention in childhood reduce the risk of later complications. Am J Med 2004;117(5A):23S-29S.

these agents are effective in the treatment of GERD. Although concern over prolongation of the Q-T interval has led to the discontinuation of cisapride production in North America, similar cardiac effects have been postulated with domperidone.[27] Caution should be exercised when using these medications because many believe that the risks outweigh the benefits.

In children who remain symptomatic despite maximal pharmacologic therapy, surgical therapeutic options are often considered. However, with the increased success of pharmacologic therapy with PPIs, the indications for surgery have narrowed.[28] A list of indications for surgical intervention is presented in Table 101-4. Surgical approaches to treat GERD include fundoplication, gastrostomy, or gastrojejunostomy (GJ) tube insertion. Another less common surgical approach is esophagogastric dissociation, which involves surgical disconnection of the esophagus and stomach, thereby preventing refluxate from entering the esophagus. Although it has not been well evaluated in children, one series suggests that it may lead to fewer complications in neurologically impaired children than is the case with fundoplication.[29]

Gastrostomy tube insertion has been used for infants and children who cannot maintain adequate growth with oral feeding because of GERD. It is also commonly used in neurologically impaired children, who may have both oromotor difficulties and GERD. When a gastrostomy tube is inserted without fundoplication, GERD can worsen, particularly in neurologically impaired children. Although the mechanism is not understood, the incidence of new or worsening GERD in neurologically impaired children after gastrostomy tube insertion may be as high as 20% to 25%.[30-33]

Fundoplication, which can be performed by open means or laparoscopically, may be accompanied by pyloroplasty for children with slow gastric emptying. In addition, it is often paired with gastrostomy tube insertion for children who also aspirate with oral feeding or who cannot feed enough orally to maintain hydration or achieve or maintain adequate weight.

The concerns about fundoplication revolve primarily around complication rates in neurologically impaired children. One large retrospective series of mostly open fundoplications found a higher success rate (95% versus 84%) in neurologically normal children than in neurologically impaired children.[34] Major complications, such as wrap disruption, increased dysphagia, respiratory deterioration, gas bloating syndrome, intestinal obstruction, and death, are more common in neurologically impaired children.[34,35] Laparoscopic fundoplication performed by an experienced surgeon appears to have a lower postoperative complication rate and shorter hospitalization than open procedures do.[36] There are reports of increased retching in neurologically impaired children after fundoplication, which is most likely related to inappropriate activation of the emetic reflex and persistence of gastric muscle dysrhythmias.[36,37]

Placement of GJ tubes is intended to provide postpyloric feeding. No randomized controlled trials have evaluated fundoplication with gastrostomy versus GJ tube insertion. GJ tubes may be inserted percutaneously under fluoroscopic guidance, which can be performed with sedation rather than general anesthesia. Two retrospective reviews comparing the two procedures in neurologically impaired children suggest that GJ tubes in this population are associated with fewer major but more minor complications.[38,39] Late complications after GJ tube placement include tube breakage and blockage, superficial stoma infection, dislodgement, intussusception, and small bowel obstruction. These complications need to be carefully considered when a patient lives far from a regional center with an interventional radiologist.

Consultation

Treatment of GERD and decision making regarding treatment options are best approached by a multidisciplinary team, which may vary from one pediatric center to the next. Inpatient pediatricians, gastroenterologists, pediatric surgeons, clinical dietitians, and the child's primary care physician may all participate in establishing the diagnosis, choosing appropriate investigations (if any), optimizing nutrition, and optimizing medical management while minimizing symptoms. For children who fail medical and nutritional intervention, surgical options should be assessed by the team and discussed with the family to weigh the risks of the procedure with its expected benefits.

Admission Criteria

- Moderate to severe aspiration pneumonia secondary to GERD
- Dehydration or failure to thrive secondary to GERD
- Cyanotic or apneic spells related to vomiting

Discharge Criteria

- Medical management has been established and surgical intervention has been discussed and evaluated.
- Caloric and fluid intake goals are being met.
- Respiratory symptoms, if present, have been treated.
- An outpatient therapeutic plan and key individuals (dietitian, primary physician, gastroenterologist) have been identified.

IN A NUTSHELL

- Feeding issues in children are multifaceted. Careful history taking and observation of feeding are crucial to making an accurate diagnosis.
- Early diagnosis of dysphagia or GERD and institution of an appropriate intervention may help avoid secondary feeding aversion.
- Admission to the hospital for recurrent respiratory illness, vomiting, or failure to thrive may not at first glance be related to feeding problems. Inpatient pediatricians have an opportunity to further explore feeding during admission to identify such problems.

ON THE HORIZON

- New preparations of PPIs that are more easily dissolved and easier to administer by tube or in suspension form will be available in the near future. The clinical utility of fundoplication versus GJ tube placement for neurologically impaired children with GERD has been difficult to evaluate in the absence of strong evidence. A randomized controlled trial comparing the two procedures would help health care providers counsel parents in the future.

SUGGESTED READING

Arts-Rodas D, Benoit D: Feeding problems in infancy and early childhood: Identification and management. Paediatr Child Health 1998;3:21-27.

Carroll AE, Garrison MM, Christakis DA: A systematic review of nonpharmacological and nonsurgical therapies for gastroesophageal reflux in infants. Arch Pediatr Adolesc Med 2002;156:109-113.

Rudolph CD, Mazur LJ, Liptak GS, et al: Pediatric GE reflux clinical practice guidelines. J Pediatr Gastroenterol Nutr 2001;32(Suppl 2):S1-S31.

Veroff V: The Feeding Frenzy: When Children Can't Eat. Montreal, Ross, 2002.

REFERENCES

1. Reilly S, Skuse D, Poblete X: Prevalence of feeding problems and oral motor dysfunction in children with cerebral palsy: A community survey. J Pediatr 1996;129:877-882.
2. Sheikh S, Allen E, Shell R, et al: Chronic aspiration without gastroesophageal reflux as a cause of chronic respiratory symptoms in neurologically normal infants. Chest 2001;120:1190-1195.
3. Heuschkel RB, Fletcher K, Hill A, et al: Isolated neonatal swallowing dysfunction: A case series and review of the literature. Dig Dis Sci 2003;48:30-35.
4. Smith CH, Logemann JA, Colangelo LA, et al: Incidence and patient characteristics associated with silent aspiration in the acute care setting. Dysphagia 1999;14:1-7.
5. Khooshoo V, Edell D: Previously healthy infants may have increased risk of aspiration during respiratory syncytial viral bronchiolitis. Pediatrics 1999;104:1389-1390.
6. Tohara H, Saitoh E, Mays KA, et al: Three tests for predicting aspiration without videofluorography. Dysphagia 2003;18:126-134.
7. Friedman B, Frazier JB: Deep laryngeal penetration as a predictor of aspiration. Dysphagia 2000;15:153-158.
8. Newman LA, Keckley C, Petersen MC, et al: Swallowing function and medical diagnoses in infants suspected of dysphagia. Pediatrics 2001;

108(6):e106-e107. Available at *http://www.pediatrics.org/cgi/content/full/108/6/e106.*

9. Leder SB, Karas DE: Fiberoptic endoscopic evaluation of swallowing in the pediatric population. Laryngoscope 2000;110:1132-1136.

10. Baikie G, South MJ, Reddihough DS, et al: Agreement of aspiration tests using barium videofluoroscopy, salivagram, and milk scan in children with cerebral palsy. Dev Med Child Neurol 2005;47:86-93.

11. Zangen T, Zangen S, Di Lorenzo C, et al: Gastrointestinal motility and sensory abnormalities may contribute to food refusal in medically fragile toddlers. J Pediatr Gastroenterol Nutr 2003;37:287-293.

12. Arts-Rodas D, Benoit D: Feeding problems in infancy and early childhood: Identification and management. Paediatr Child Health 1998;3:21-27.

13. Benoit D, Wang EE, Zlotkin SH: Discontinuation of enterostomy tube feeding by behavioral treatment in early childhood: A randomized controlled trial. J Pediatr 2000;137:498-503.

14. Davidson G: The role of lower esophageal sphincter function and dysmotility in gastroesophageal reflux in premature infants and in the first year of life. J Pediatr Gastroenterol Nutr 2003;37(Suppl):S17-S22.

15. Poets CF: Gastroesophageal reflux: A critical review of its role in preterm infants. Pediatrics 2004;113:e128-e132. Available at *http://www.pediatrics.org/cgi/content/full/132/2/e128.*

16. Vandenplas Y, Hassall E: Mechanisms of gastroesophageal reflux and gastroesophageal reflux disease. J Pediatr Gastroenterol Nutr 2002;35:119-136.

17. Rudolph CD, Mazur LJ, Liptak GS, et al: Pediatric GE reflux clinical practice guidelines. J Pediatr Gastroenterol Nutr 2001;32(Suppl 2):S1-S31.

18. Milla P, Cucchiara S, DiLorenzo C, et al: Motility disorders in childhood: Working Group Report of the First World Congress of Pediatric Gastroenterology, Hepatology, and Nutrition. J Pediatr Gastroenterol Nutr 2002:35(Suppl 2):S187-S195.

19. El-Serag HB, Gilger M, Kubeler M, et al: Extraesophageal associations of gastroesophageal reflux disease in children without neurologic deficits. Gastroenterology 2001;121:1294-1299.

20. Al-Khawari HA, Sinan TS, Seymour H: Diagnosis of gastro-oesophageal reflux in children. Comparison between oesophageal pH and barium examinations. Pediatr Radiol 2002;32:765-770.

21. Orenstein SR: Tests to assess symptoms of gastroesophageal reflux in infants and children. J Pediatr Gastroenterol Nutr 2003;37(Suppl):S29-S32.

22. Carroll AE, Garrison MM, Christakis DA: A systematic review of nonpharmacological and nonsurgical therapies for gastroesophageal reflux in infants. Arch Pediatr Adolesc Med 2002;156:109-113.

23. Orenstein SR, Whitington PF, Orenstein DM: The infant seat as treatment for gastroesophageal reflux. N Engl J Med 1983;309:760-763.

24. Vanderhoof JA, Moran JR, Harris CL, et al: Efficacy of a pre-thickened infant formula: A multicenter, double-blind, randomized, placebo-controlled parallel group trial in 104 infants with symptomatic gastroesophageal reflux. Clin Pediatr (Phila) 2003;42:483-495.

25. Scaillon M, Cadranel S: Safety data required for proton-pump inhibitor use in children. J Pediatr Gastroenterol Nutr 2002;35:113-118.

26. Hassall E, Israel D, Shepherd R, et al: Omeprazole for treatment of chronic erosive esophagitis in children: A multicenter study of efficacy, safety, tolerability and dose requirements. J Pediatr 2000;137:800-807.

27. Drolet B, Rousseau G, Daleau P, et al: Domperidone should not be considered a no-risk alternative to cisapride in the treatment of gastrointestinal motility disorders. Circulation 2000;102:1883-1885.

28. Gold BD: Gastroesophageal reflux disease: Could intervention in childhood reduce the risk of later complications. Am J Med 2004;117(5A):23S-29S.

29. Gatti C, Federici di Abriola G, De Angelis P, et al: Esophagogastric dissociation versus fundoplication: Which is best for severely neurologically impaired children? J Pediatr Surg 2001;36:677-680.

30. Fonkalsrud EW, Ashcraft KW, Coran AG, et al: Surgical treatment of gastroesophageal reflux in children: A combined hospital study of 7467 patients. Pediatrics 1998;101:419-422.

31. Samuel M, Holmes K: Quantitative and qualitative analysis of gastroesophageal reflux after precutaneous endoscopic gastrostomy. J Pediatr Surg 2002;37:256-261.

32. Mollitt DL, Golladay S, Seibert JJ: Symptomatic gastroesophageal reflux following gastrostomy in neurologically impaired patients. Pediatrics 1985;75:1124-1126.

33. Isch JA, Rescorla FJ, Scherer LRT, et al: The development of gastroesophageal reflux after percutaneous endoscopic gastrostomy. J Pediatr Surg 1997;32:321-323.

34. Pearl RH, Robie DK, Ein SH, et al: Complications of gastroesophageal antireflux surgery in neurologically impaired versus neurologically normal children. J Pediatr Surg 1990;25:1169-1173.

35. Allal H, Captier G, Lopez M, et al: Evaluation of 142 consecutive laparoscopic fundoplications in children: Effects of the learning curve and technical choice. J Pediatr Surg 2001;36:921-926.

36. Richards CA, Andrews PL, Spitz L, et al: Nissen fundoplication may induce gastric myoelectric disturbance in children. J Pediatr Surg 1998;33:1801-1805.

37. Richards CA, Milla PJ, Andrews PL, et al: Retching and vomiting in neurologically impaired children after fundoplication: Predictive preoperative factors. J Pediatr Surg 2001;36:1401-1404.

38. Albanese CT, Towbin RB, Ulman I, et al: Percutaneous gastrojejunostomy versus Nissen fundoplication for enteral feeding of the neurologically impaired child with gastroesophageal reflux. J Pediatr 1993;123:371-375.

39. Wales PW, Diamond IR, Dutta S, et al: Fundoplication and gastrostomy versus image-guided gastrojejunal tube for enteral feeding of neurologically impaired children with gastroesophageal reflux. J Pediatr Surg 2002;37:407-412.

Rheumatology

CHAPTER 102

Kawasaki Disease

Moussa El-hallak

Kawasaki disease (KD), initially called mucocutaneous lymph node syndrome by Kawasaki in 1967 because of its characteristic presentation, is an acute, self-limited systemic necrotizing vasculitis affecting small and medium-size arteries. KD is most common in boys between 2 and 5 years of age, preferentially affecting Asian children. Nonetheless, KD has been reported in all ethnic groups and is now the most common cause of acquired heart disease in children throughout the industrialized world. Although an infectious cause is suspected, extensive investigations have failed to identify a single responsible agent. As a result, the disease must be identified clinically, with no single test available to confirm the diagnosis.

CLINICAL PRESENTATION

The disease is classically described as occurring in three phases. The first is an acute febrile period lasting about 10 to 14 days and associated with rash, edema, mucous membrane changes, conjunctivitis, lymphadenopathy, and myocarditis. The second, or subacute, phase may last 2 to 8 weeks and is characterized by resolution of the fever, desquamation of the rash, findings of arthritis or arthralgia, and the development of coronary artery aneurysms. The final convalescent phase can last many months, during which many of the clinical symptoms resolve and the laboratory findings normalize. During this third phase, coronary aneurysms or other cardiac dysfunction may develop, persist, or resolve.

Most children with KD come to medical attention with complaints of acute-onset rash and fever. Typically, the fever ranges between 38°C and 40°C, is intermittent and spiking, and is minimally responsive to antipyretic agents. The rash is polymorphous and often maculopapular. Occasionally the rash is purpuric or petechial and may be coalescent in areas, but it is rarely bullous or vesicular. The rash generally begins in the perineum and spreads throughout the trunk, extremities, and sometimes the face. Extremity changes, including erythema and edema of the hands and feet, appear toward the end of the first week of fever, evolving into a characteristic periungual desquamation during the next week. Ocular involvement includes bilateral, primarily bulbar conjunctival injection, with anterior uveitis evident on slit-lamp examination in about 75% of cases. A bilateral and nonexudative conjunctivitis is one of the most common features

of the disease. Erythema, cracking and bleeding of the lips, and "strawberry tongue" characterize the mucositis of KD. Oral ulcerations and exudates are generally not seen. Erythema at the urethral meatus, sometimes with complaints of dysuria, is another manifestation of mucosal involvement. Cervical lymphadenopathy is the least common feature of KD, observed in approximately 50% of patients; the other features are estimated to occur in 90% or more of cases. Lymphadenopathy is usually unilateral, with at least one firm and slightly tender lymph node at least 1.5 cm in diameter that typically underlies the sternocleidomastoid muscle. Overlying erythema is not typical, and the node is nonfluctant.

A number of typical manifestations of KD are not included in the diagnostic criteria but may support the diagnosis. Cardiovascular manifestations, including tachycardia and a gallop rhythm due to myocarditis, or rub due to pericarditis, are most prominent. Abdominal pain and fullness in the right upper quadrant may be caused by intrahepatic obstruction or hydrops of the gallbladder. At least 20% of children develop frank arthritis, and a greater proportion develop arthralgia. Aseptic meningitis is thought to be a common complication and is likely responsible for the characteristic extreme irritability noted in patients with KD. Table 102-1 lists the clinical and laboratory findings characteristic of KD.

The incidence of KD in the United States varies by ethnicity. The incidence is highest in children of Asian or Pacific Island descent, second highest among non-Hispanic blacks, third highest among children of Hispanic descent, and lowest among whites. In the United States, a seasonality is also noted, with more occurrences in the winter and early spring.[1,2] Living near a standing body of water is another risk factor.[3]

DIAGNOSIS AND DIFFERENTIAL DIAGNOSIS

In the absence of a specific test, Kawasaki disease is diagnosed clinically, based on the characteristic history and physical findings. Internationally accepted criteria require the presence of fever for at least 5 days and at least four of five manifestations of mucocutaneous inflammation (see Table 102-1). Infectious, immunologic, and rheumatologic illnesses must be excluded to meet these clinical criteria

Table 102-1 Clinical and Laboratory Features of Kawasaki Disease

Epidemiologic Case Definition (Classic Clinical Criteria)
Fever persisting at least 5 days*
Presence of at least 4 of 5 principal features†
    Changes in extremities
        Acute: erythema of palms, soles; edema of hands, feet
        Subacute: periungual peeling of fingers, toes in weeks 2 and 3
    Polymorphous exanthem
    Bilateral bulbar conjunctival injection without exudate
    Changes in lips and oral cavity: erythema, cracking of lips, strawberry tongue, diffuse injection of oral and pharyngeal mucosa
    Cervical lymphadenopathy (>1.5 cm diameter), usually unilateral
Exclusion of other diseases with similar findings‡

Other Clinical and Laboratory Findings
Cardiovascular findings
    Congestive heart failure, myocarditis, pericarditis, valvular regurgitation
    Coronary artery abnormalities
    Aneurysms of medium-size noncoronary arteries
    Raynaud phenomenon
    Peripheral gangrene
Musculoskeletal findings
    Arthritis, arthralgia
Gastrointestinal findings
    Diarrhea, vomiting, abdominal pain
    Hepatic dysfunction
    Hydrops of gallbladder
Central nervous system findings
    Extreme irritability
    Aseptic meningitis
    Sensorineural hearing loss
Genitourinary findings
    Urethritis, meatitis
Other findings
    Erythema, induration at bacille Calmette-Guérin (BCG) inoculation site
    Anterior uveitis (mild)
    Desquamating rash in groin

Laboratory Findings in Acute Kawasaki Disease
Leukocytosis with neutrophilia and immature forms
Elevated erythrocyte sedimentation rate
Elevated C-reactive protein
Anemia
Abnormal plasma lipids
Hypoalbuminemia
Hyponatremia
Thrombocytosis after week 1§
Sterile pyuria
Elevated serum transaminases
Elevated serum γ-glutamyl transpeptidase
Pleocytosis of cerebrospinal fluid
Leukocytosis in synovial fluid

*Patients with fever for at least 5 days and <4 principal criteria can be diagnosed with Kawasaki disease when coronary artery abnormalities are detected by two-dimensional echocardiography or angiography.
†In the presence of ≥4 principal criteria, the diagnosis of Kawasaki disease can be made on day 4 of illness. Experienced clinicians who have treated many Kawasaki disease patients may establish the diagnosis before day 4.
‡See Table 102-2.
§Some infants present with thrombocytopenia and disseminated intravascular coagulation.
From Newburger JW, Takahashi M, Gerber MA, et al: Diagnosis, treatment, and long-term management of Kawasaki disease: A statement for health professionals from the Committee on Rheumatic Fever, Endocarditis and Kawasaki Disease, Council on Cardiovascular Disease in the Young, American Heart Association. Circulation 2004;110:2747-2771.

Table 102-2   Differential Diagnosis of Kawasaki Disease

Infections
  Viral infections (e.g., measles, adenovirus, Epstein-Barr virus)
  Staphylococcal scalded skin syndrome
  Scarlet fever
  Toxic shock syndrome
  Rocky Mountain spotted fever

Drug reactions
  Stevens-Johnson syndrome
  Serum sickness
  Mercury toxicity

Rheumatic diseases
  Systemic-onset juvenile rheumatoid arthritis
  Polyarteritis nodosa
  Reiter syndrome

Adapted from Newburger JW, Takahashi M, Gerber MA, et al: Diagnosis, treatment, and long-term management of Kawasaki disease: A statement for health professionals from the Committee on Rheumatic Fever, Endocarditis and Kawasaki Disease, Council on Cardiovascular Disease in the Young, American Heart Association. Circulation 2004;110:2747-2771.

(Table 102-2). Unfortunately, the criteria are neither sensitive nor specific. Many children who do not fulfill the diagnostic criteria nonetheless develop coronary artery aneurysms, so-called incomplete or atypical KD. Use of the term *atypical* is less accurate, because the features present may be typical of KD, but some of the features necessary to meet the clinical definition may be lacking. Incomplete KD is more common in young infants, in whom the disease manifestations are typically subtle if they are recognizable at all.[4] Clinicians must also be alert to the possibility of KD causing prolonged fever in adolescents, another population in whom the presentation is more likely to be incomplete. The entire clinical picture—including ethnicity, family history, signs and symptoms, associated laboratory findings, and imaging studies—contributes to the ultimate diagnosis of KD.

EVALUATION

There are no specific laboratory tests to confirm a diagnosis of KD. Laboratory findings generally reflect systemic inflammation manifested by the elevation of acute phase reactants (Fig. 102-1). The C-reactive protein and erythrocyte sedimentation rate are often dramatically increased. The complete blood counts show a leukocytosis and increased numbers of neutrophils and band forms. Eosinophilia (>350 cells/mm³) is more common among children with KD than in febrile age-matched controls (36% versus 4%). Within 2 weeks of illness, 69% of children with KD develop eosinophilia.[5] A mild anemia may be seen. Platelet counts may be low, normal, or increased at presentation; however, half of affected children have platelet counts greater than 450,000 /mm³ by day 5 of the fever, and more than 95% have thrombocytosis, with counts of 650,000 to 2 million/mm³, by day 10. Urinalysis usually shows a mild to moderate number of white blood cells. Because the pyuria is due to noninfectious mucositis of the urethra, voided specimens are needed; catheterization bypasses the urethra and would thus

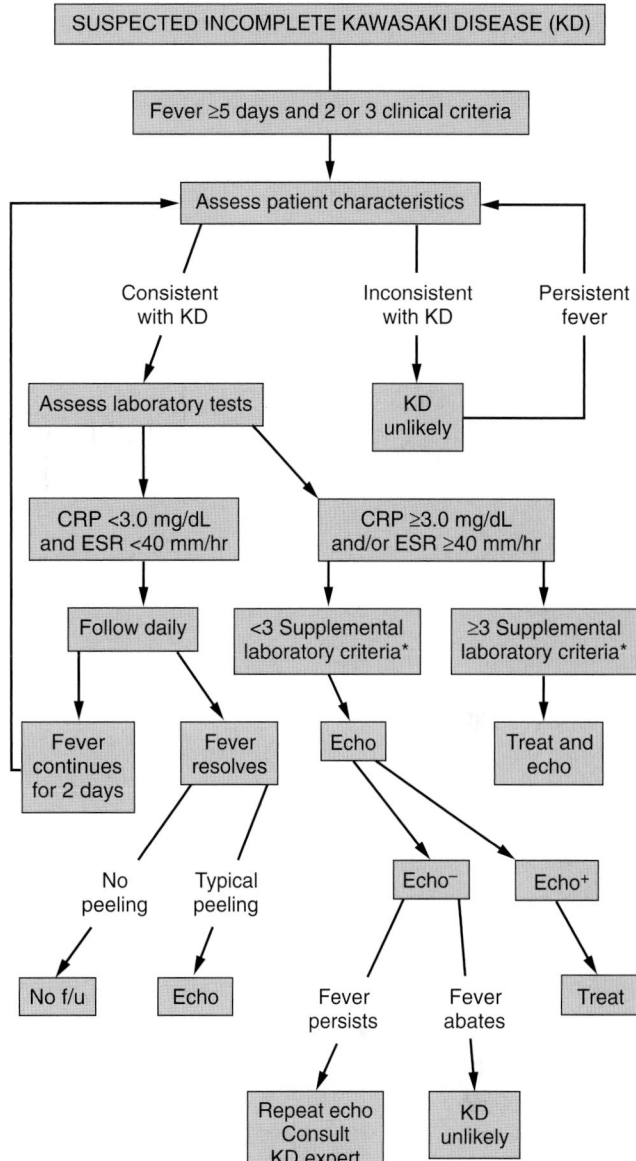

Figure 102-1 Algorithm for the treatment of Kawasaki disease. CRP, C-reactive protein; ESR, erythrocyte sedimentation rate; f/u, follow-up. *Supplementary laboratory criteria include albumin ≤3.0 g/dL, anemia for age, elevation of alanine aminotransferase, platelets after 7 days ≥15,000/mm³, and urine ≥10 white blood cells/high powered field. (From Newburger JW, Takahashi M, Gerber MA, et al: Diagnosis, treatment, and long-term management of Kawasaki disease: A statement for health professionals from the Committee on Rheumatic Fever, Endocarditis and Kawasaki Disease, Council on Cardiovascular Disease in the Young, American Heart Association. Circulation 2004;110:2747-2771.)

fail to detect white blood cells. Analysis of cerebrospinal fluid reveals monocyte-predominant pleocytosis with a negative Gram stain and culture consistent with aseptic meningitis. The glucose and protein levels from the cerebrospinal fluid are usually normal. Arthrocentesis of an arthritic joint typically finds white blood cell counts of 100,000 to 300,000 cells/mm³, with normal glucose levels and negative Gram stain and culture.[6]

Elevations of γ-glutamyl transpeptidase are found in 67% of patients,[7] although elevations of other liver enzymes are elevated in less than 40% of patients.[8] Hypoalbuminemia, another nonspecific indicator of inflammation, is often present. An electrocardiogram done in the acute phase of the illness may show changes in the P-R, QRS, and ST intervals and in the T wave. An echocardiogram is indicated in all patients with suspected KD. In addition, when the diagnosis is uncertain, echocardiography may provide information supporting a diagnosis of KD.[9] Although most children do not develop aneurysms in the first 10 days of illness, coronary artery ectasia, increased coronary artery echogenicity, pericardial effusions, and aortic root dilation are more common in KD than in illnesses that mimic the condition. Ultrasonography may reveal acalculous cholecystitis when hydrops of the gallbladder is present.

COURSE OF ILLNESS

The vast majority of children have an excellent prognosis after KD. Outcomes are determined largely by the extent of cardiac involvement, highlighting the importance of early, effective treatment. Cohorts followed in Japan have no excess morbidity or mortality unless they have persistent dilation of the coronary arteries. Those with giant coronary artery aneurysms (internal diameter >8 mm) have up to a 35% risk of myocardial infarction; those with smaller abnormalities have approximately a twofold greater risk of death by the 25-year follow-up.[10] Most small coronary artery changes resolve within several months of the acute episode, and these patients have no known increase in disease-related morbidity. Risk factors for coronary artery aneurysms, even in the absence of complete diagnostic criteria, include age younger than 12 months or older than 6 years,[11] persistent fever, elevated acute phase reactants (e.g., erythrocyte sedimentation rate, C-reactive protein), anemia, and low sodium and albumin levels.[12]

Recurrence of KD is estimated at 3%, and risk factors for recurrence include age younger than 3 years, male gender, and coronary involvement with the first episode of illness. Recurrent episodes have a higher risk of coronary involvement.[13-15]

Repeeling of the skin is a recognized phenomenon that occurs in approximately 11% of patients with KD. The desquamation occurs as an isolated process (i.e., without other stigmata of KD) and therefore does not represent a recurrence. These repeeling episodes can occur months to years after recovery from the initial illness. Viral upper respiratory tract infections have been associated with some episodes of repeeling. No episodes of repeeling occurred longer than 7 years after the initial illness, and there were no long-term sequelae. No specific therapy is needed for the self-limited skin process. It is important to evaluate patients carefully, however, to differentiate the isolated entity of repeeling from a recurrence of KD so that proper treatment can be rendered.

TREATMENT

Intravenous immunoglobulin (IVIG) is the treatment of choice for patients with KD and should be given promptly once the diagnosis of complete or incomplete KD is established. Aggressive medical treatment is critical in this disease, and the prevention of coronary artery abnormalities is highly dependent on the IVIG dose and the timing of administration. When IVIG is administered within the first 10 days of illness, the risk of coronary artery abnormalities decreases from 20% to 25% down to less than 5%. Although the efficacy may be reduced, IVIG appears to provide some benefit even after the 10th day of illness. These favorable effects extend beyond the heart; besides reducing the risk of coronary artery abnormalities and improving heart contractility, timely administration also decreases signs and symptoms of inflammation and normalizes serum lipid profiles. Patients are hospitalized and treated with IVIG 2 g/kg in a single dose given over 8 to 12 hours. Aspirin therapy is also initiated at the time of diagnosis to provide an additional anti-inflammatory effect; the initial dose is 80 to 100 mg/kg per day, divided every 6 hours.[16] Once the patient has been afebrile for 48 hours, aspirin is administered in antiplatelet doses, 3 to 5 mg/kg per day, until all inflammatory markers return to normal or for at least 8 weeks in patients with normal coronary arteries. In patients with coronary artery abnormalities, the duration of antiplatelet therapy, restriction of activity, and need for cardiology follow-up (including coronary angiography) vary, depending on the severity of the disease.

Of note, during the influenza season, inactivated influenza virus vaccine (subcutaneous) should be administered to reduce the theoretical risk of Reye syndrome. In addition, vaccination with live viruses, such as measles-mumps-rubella, varicella, and influenza (intranasal form), should be deferred for at least 11 months after treatment with IVIG.

Approximately 10% to 15% of children still have fever 48 hours after treatment with IVIG. These patients appear to benefit from an additional infusion of IVIG. If fever persists after the second dose of IVIG, consultation with a referral center experienced in the diagnosis and treatment of KD is advised. Additional anti-inflammatory treatments, such as intravenous methylprednisolone or the biologic tumor necrosis factor inhibitor infliximab, may be beneficial in such cases. For example, IVIG and aspirin plus intravenous methylprednisolone resulted in faster resolution of fever, faster improvement in inflammatory markers (C-reactive protein), and shorter length of hospital stay in patients with acute KD.[17] Some institutions treat refractory fever in KD with continued oral corticosteroids until fever is completely resolved.

Patients with no evidence of coronary artery involvement or transient dilation usually require no treatment beyond the subacute or convalescent phase. Those with persisting aneurysms often continue anticoagulation therapy. Patients with a diagnosis of KD are followed by cardiologists indefinitely, because KD is thought to be an independent risk factor for the development of atherosclerosis. At follow-up visits, guidance for a heart-healthy lifestyle is offered. Specific guidelines for long-term follow-up are available from the American Heart Association.[18]

Ongoing evaluation of the coronary vessels is warranted, whether abnormalities are detected at the time of diagnosis or not. Echocardiography is obtained when KD is suspected; this serves as the baseline evaluation and, in some cases, may help determine the diagnosis. Repeat echocardiography is routinely performed 6 to 8 weeks after the initial study, or sooner if clinically indicated. In patients without evidence of coronary abnormalities or with only minor vessel wall changes, an additional echocardiogram is obtained 6 to 12 months after the illness.

CONSULTATION

Early consultation with a pediatric cardiologist is indicated for patients with KD. In addition to the development of coronary artery aneurysms, pancarditis and generalized myocardial dysfunction may complicate the clinical course. Baseline echocardiogram and electrocardiogram findings are needed for the long-term follow-up of these patients, because even those without evidence of coronary artery abnormalities can develop aneurysms over time. A rheumatologist can offer additional insights and management strategies for vasculitis. Other manifestations of the disease, such as hydrops of the gallbladder, hepatosplenomegaly and jaundice, arthritis, and uveitis, may require evaluation by other appropriate specialists.

ADMISSION CRITERIA

- Need for evaluation and clinical observation to establish the diagnosis.
- Need for cardiology evaluation, including echocardiogram.
- Parenteral IVIG therapy and evaluation of response to therapy.
- Subspecialty evaluation for complications.

DISCHARGE CRITERIA

- Diagnosis has been established and appropriate inpatient therapy completed. Patients who defervesce after IVIG therapy are usually kept as inpatients until they demonstrate a period of 36 to 48 hours without recrudescence of fever.
- No need for additional parenteral therapy is anticipated.
- Patient is clinically stable and able to take adequate oral diet and medications.
- Outpatient follow-up is firmly established.

IN A NUTSHELL

- Kawasaki disease, a necrotizing vasculitis, is the leading cause of acquired heart disease in industrialized countries and should be suspected in children with prolonged fever and signs of mucocutaneous inflammation. The diagnosis of KD can be established by meeting the diagnostic criteria or through a consideration of the complete clinical picture, including KD features and supportive findings on laboratory tests, echocardiogram, and slit-lamp examination.
- The incidence of coronary artery aneurysms in KD is reduced by IVIG therapy within the first 10 days of illness, coupled with retreatment in the face of persistent fever. Aspirin therapy is standard, initially at high doses but then reduced to low doses after defervescence.
- Infants and children are more likely to present with incomplete KD and are at increased risk for the development of coronary aneurysms.

ON THE HORIZON

- Improved accuracy in the diagnosis of KD based on clinical and laboratory assessment coupled with the measurement of novel biomarkers.
- Additional evaluation of the efficacy of parenteral corticosteroids as an adjunct to IVIG and aspirin therapy.
- More effective treatment of children who fail to respond to IVIG using immunosuppressants and biologic response modifiers such as anti-tumor necrosis factor-α monoclonal antibodies or cytotoxic agents such as cyclophosphamide.
- Greater understanding of the long-term implications of KD for cardiovascular health and the development of new tools to monitor coronary artery outcome.

SUGGESTED READING

Burns JC, Mason WH, Glode MP, et al: Clinical and epidemiologic characteristics of patients referred for evaluation of possible Kawasaki disease. J Pediatr 1991;118:680-686.

Japan Kawasaki Disease Research Committee: Diagnostic Guideline of Kawasaki Disease. Tokyo, Japan Kawasaki Disease Research Committee, 1984.

Kawasaki T, Kosaki F, Okawa S, et al: A new infantile acute febrile mucocutaneous lymph node syndrome (MLNS) prevailing in Japan. Pediatrics 1974;54:271-276.

Newburger JW, US Multicenter Kawasaki Study Group: A single infusion of intravenous gamma globulin compared to four daily doses in the treatment of acute Kawasaki syndrome. N Engl J Med 1991;324:1633-1639.

REFERENCES

1. Holman RC, Curns AT, Belay ED, et al: Kawasaki syndrome hospitalizations in the United States, 1997 and 2000. Pediatrics 2003;112:495-501.
2. Chang RK: The incidence of Kawasaki disease in the United States did not increase between 1988 and 1997. Pediatrics 2003;111:1124-1125.
3. Rauch AM, Kaplan SL, Nihill MR, et al: Kawasaki syndrome clusters in Harris County, Texas, and eastern North Carolina: A high endemic rate and new environmental risk factor. Am J Dis Child 1988;142:441-444.
4. Burns JC, Wiggins JW Jr, Toews WH, et al: Clinical spectrum of Kawasaki disease in infants younger than 6 months of age. J Pediatr 1986; 109:759-763.
5. Terai M, Yasukawa K, Honda T, et al: Peripheral blood eosinophilia and eosinophil accumulation in coronary microvessels in acute Kawasaki disease. Pediatr Infect Dis J 2002;21:777-780.
6. Hicks RV, Melish ME: Kawasaki disease. Pediatr Clin North Am 1986;33:1151-1175.
7. Ting EC, Capparelli EV, Billman GF, et al: Elevated gamma-glutamyl transferase concentrations in patients with acute Kawasaki disease. Pediatr Infect Dis J 1998;17:431-432.
8. Burns JC, Mason WH, Glose MP, et al: Clinical and epidemiologic characteristics of patients referred for evaluation of possible Kawasaki disease. United States Multicenter Kawasaki Disease Study Group. J Pediatr 1991;118:680-686.
9. Newburger JW, Takahashi M, Gerber MA, et al: Diagnosis, treatment, and long-term management of Kawasaki disease: A statement for health professionals from the Committee on Rheumatic Fever, Endocarditis and Kawasaki Disease, Council on Cardiovascular Disease in the Young, American Heart Association. Circulation 2004;110:2747-2771.
10. Fukushige J, Takahashi N, Ueda K, et al: Long-term outcome of coronary abnormalities in patients after Kawasaki disease. Pediatr Cardiol 1996;17:71-76.

11. Muta H, Ishii M, Sakaue T, et al: Older age is a risk factor for the development of cardiovascular sequelae in Kawasaki disease. Pediatrics 2004;114:751-754.

12. Falcini F: Kawasaki disease. Curr Opin Rheumatol 2006;18:33-38.

13. Hirata S, Nakamura Y, Yanagawa H: Incidence rate of recurrent Kawasaki disease and related risk factors: From the results of nationwide surveys of Kawasaki disease in Japan. Acta Paediatr 2001;90:40-44.

14. Nakamura Y, Yanagawa H, Ojima T, et al: Cardiac sequelae of Kawasaki disease among recurrent cases. Arch Dis Child 1998;78:163-165.

15. Nakamura Y, Oki I, Tanihara S, et al: Cardiac sequelae in recurrent cases of Kawasaki disease: A comparison between the initial episode of the disease and a recurrence in the same patient. Pediatrics 1998;102:e66.

16. Sundel RP: Update on the treatment of Kawasaki disease in childhood. Curr Rheumatol Rep 2002;4:474-482.

17. Sundel RP, Baker AL, Fulton DR, Newberger JW: Corticosteroids in the initial treatment of Kawasaki disease: Report of a randomized trial. J Pediatr 2003;142:611-616.

18. Dajani AS, Taubert KA, Takahashi M, et al: Guidelines for long-term management of patients with Kawasaki disease: Report from the Committee on Rheumatic Fever, Endocarditis, and Kawasaki Disease, Council on Cardiovascular Disease in the Young, American Heart Association. Circulation 1994;89:916-922.

CHAPTER 103

Henoch-Schönlein Purpura

Steven J. Spalding and Paul Rosen

Henoch-Schönlein purpura (HSP) is the most common vasculitis in children. Since it was first described in the 19th century, research has demonstrated that the classic clinical signs and symptoms of HSP are due to an immunoglobulin A (IgA)-mediated small-vessel leukocytoclastic vasculitis affecting the venules, capillaries, and arterioles. The incidence of HSP is estimated to be anywhere from 9 to 20 per 100,000,[1-3] with a slight male predominance. HSP occurs most frequently in children; 80% to 90% of those affected are younger than 10 years. The incidence of HSP varies by season, occurring with increased frequency during fall and winter, but cases can present at any time.

The cause of HSP is unknown, although a variety of stimuli may be capable of inciting the inflammatory process.[4,5] The most frequently recognized triggers of HSP are viral upper respiratory infections. Other causes, including group A streptococci, *Mycoplasma pneumoniae*, hepatitis B, parvovirus B19, and varicella infections and immunizations, have been implicated in the development of HSP. There may also be a genetic predisposition to HSP, because certain human leukocyte antigen haplotypes have been found to be more frequent in individuals who develop the vasculitis.

PATHOPHYSIOLOGY

Immunoglobulin A1 (IgA1), the major subclass of IgA found in the serum, appears to play a central role in the pathogenesis of HSP.[6] Immunohistochemical staining of skin and kidney biopsies reveals IgA1 and complement component C3 deposits in dermal capillaries and mesangial tissues. The associated leukocytoclastic vasculitis is characterized by neutrophilic infiltration, inflammation, and necrosis of vessel walls. Studies have documented elevated levels of interleukin-1, interleukin-6, and tumor necrosis factor in these patients.[7] Antibody-antigen deposition, with resultant complement activation and inflammation, likely explains the typical cutaneous and renal lesions. Glomerulonephritis in HSP ranges in severity from minimal changes to diffuse involvement. Fibrin deposition in Bowman's capsule results in crescent formation. The number of crescents detected on biopsy correlates directly with the degree of renal impairment.

CLINICAL PRESENTATION

Classically, HSP is characterized by the clinical triad of rash, abdominal pain, and arthralgia or arthritis. Virtually all patients develop palpable purpuric lesions (Fig. 103-1), without evidence of thrombocytopenia, during the course of the illness, but it is not always a presenting feature. The rash is central to establishing the diagnosis. It characteristically begins with edema and progresses to clinical evidence of loss of vessel wall integrity and resulting leakage of serum into adjacent tissues. This nonpitting subcutaneous edema is most pronounced in the dependent portions of the body, such as the scalp, periorbital region, dorsum of hands and feet, and scrotum. It tends to be more noticeable in patients younger than 2 years. The rash almost always involves the lower extremities, but in up to 10% of patients, it may involve only the upper extremities. A similar condition largely restricted to young children, acute hemorrhagic edema of infancy, may represent a forme fruste of HSP limited to the skin.

The rash of HSP next progresses to erythematous macules, representing extravasation of erythrocytes into the dermis.[8] These lesions may appear urticarial early in the course of the illness. The macules enlarge, coalesce into patches, and then evolve into palpable purpura, developing a purple color owing to erythrocyte breakdown. Over time, the purpuric lesions fade and turn brown owing to hemosiderin deposition. Lesions tend to appear in crops, so lesions of differing ages may be present at the same time. The rash is usually symmetrical and acral in distribution, with sparing of the trunk. Other less common cutaneous manifestations of HSP include subcutaneous nodules and hemorrhagic, bullous lesions.

Gastrointestinal (GI) system involvement is also a cardinal manifestation of HSP. Overall, almost 80% of children develop GI signs and symptoms at some point during the course of the illness.[9] In up to two thirds of cases, GI symptoms develop within 4 weeks of the onset of rash; in almost one quarter of cases, GI symptoms precede the rash. Colicky abdominal pain, typically periumbilical in location and exacerbated by eating, is the most frequent GI complaint. Abdominal distention, vomiting, melena, ileus, or hematemesis may accompany this pain. Up to 75% of patients have evidence of extravasation of blood into the GI tract (heme-positive stools or hematemesis), reflecting small-vessel vasculitis in the GI tract. This bleeding is usually self-limited and does not require intervention. Less than 5% of children develop clinically significant hemorrhage, perforation, or intussusception. Most cases of intussusception in HSP are ileoileal rather than the ileocolic form seen in most other conditions. Other rare GI complications that have been reported in HSP include fistula formation, late ileal stricture, acute appendicitis, pancreatitis, hydrops of the gallbladder, and pseudomembranous colitis.

The last element in the diagnostic triad of HSP, joint involvement, occurs in up to 82% of cases. It may present with complaints of pain or refusal to walk in young children. The arthritis of HSP is usually symmetrical and nonmigratory and most frequently involves the knees and ankles. Rarely, the arthritis may be asymmetrical and involve the wrists, elbows, and fingers. Periarticular swelling and tenderness without warmth, redness, or effusion may be found on examination. The arthritis usually coincides with the edematous stage of the rash. Joint findings may precede the rash in 25% of cases, and they often recur during disease flares.

Although renal involvement was not included in the initial description of HSP by Neberden in 1801, nephropathy occurs in 50% to 75% of patients within 4 weeks after disease onset. Unlike other organ involvement, renal vasculitis in HSP rarely precedes the onset of rash. Approximately 95% of those who develop nephropathy do so during the first 3 months of the illness. The manifestations of renal disease observed in HSP are listed in Table 103-1.

Microscopic or macroscopic hematuria, with or without proteinuria, is the most common renal finding in children with HSP, reflecting glomerular inflammation and injury. Acute nephritic syndrome, nephrotic syndrome, and renal failure occur less frequently. Risk factors for the development of chronic renal disease due to HSP include age older than 4 years, persistent purpuric lesions, severe abdominal symptoms, nephrotic syndrome or renal failure at onset, low

factor XIII activity, and greater than 50% crescents on the initial renal biopsy.[10-13]

As with all types of vasculitis, virtually any organ system can be involved in HSP. Acute scrotal pain and swelling occur in 10% to 30% of boys and must be differentiated from testicular torsion, sometimes necessitating Doppler ultrasonography.[14] Peripheral edema may also involve the penile shaft and glans. Orchitis, epididymitis, and priapism can also occur. Central nervous system manifestations may include headache, encephalopathy, ataxia, seizure, paresis, coma, subdural hematoma, cortical hemorrhage, stroke, or peripheral neuropathy (Guillain-Barré syndrome). Lung involvement, especially subclinical inflammation, is common. A significant number of children with HSP exhibit impaired lung diffusion capacity, reflecting asymptomatic parenchymal changes.[15] Pulmonary hemorrhage and interstitial pneumonia may also occur rarely. Other potential findings include carditis, uveitis, parotitis, myalgia, and weakness.

DIFFERENTIAL DIAGNOSIS

The differential diagnosis of HSP is broad and includes other causes of purpura, arthritis, and abdominal pain. Infections, oncologic processes, and other vasculitides, such as Wegener granulomatosis and Goodpasture syndrome, have all been mistaken for HSP. Table 103-2 lists other conditions that may present with findings similar to those of HSP.

DIAGNOSIS AND EVALUATION

HSP is a clinical diagnosis and usually requires little laboratory investigation or imaging (Table 103-3). A complete blood cell count and coagulation studies are generally required to rule out thrombocytopenia and coagulopathies as causes of the palpable purpura observed on examination. A urinalysis should be examined for evidence of nephritis (hematuria or proteinuria). Blood urea nitrogen and creatinine levels should also be obtained to evaluate renal function. Table 103-4 illustrates characteristic laboratory values for patients with HSP. Radiographic imaging is not

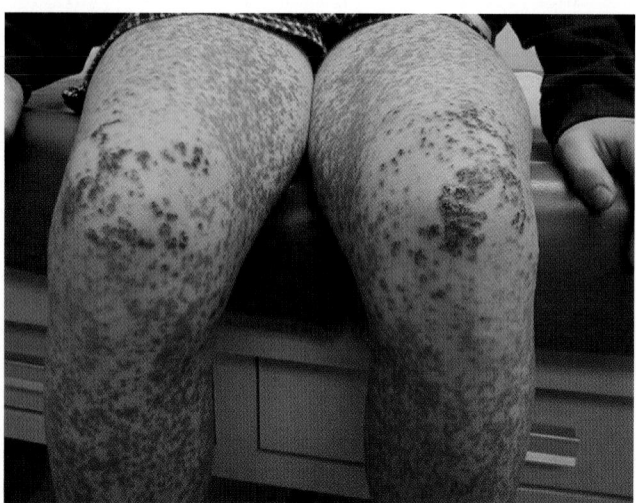

Figure 103-1 Male patient with Henoch-Schönlein purpura and severe skin involvement of the lower extremities.

Table 103-1	Renal Disease in Henoch-Schönlein Purpura		
Feature	Present at Diagnosis	Clinical Findings	Progression to Renal Failure
None	40-50%	Normal urinalysis	<1%*
Asymptomatic nephritis	40-50%	Microscopic or macroscopic hematuria with minimal or absent proteinuria; most common finding	<5% 15% with persistent heavy proteinuria
Acute nephritic syndrome	5-10%	Hematuria and hypertension, with or without evidence of renal insufficiency	15%
Nephrotic syndrome	5-10%	Proteinuria >40 mg/m²/hr, serum albumin <2.5 g/dL, generalized edema, elevated serum levels of cholesterol and triglycerides	40%
Nephritic-nephrotic syndrome	<5%	Combination of findings in acute nephritic and nephrotic syndromes	>50%

*Children without evidence of nephritis at the time of presentation may go on to develop active nephritis within 3 months of the appearance of other symptoms.

Table 103-2 Differential Diagnosis of Henoch-Schönlein Purpura

Category	Conditions
Infectious	Viral: Epstein-Barr virus, parvovirus B19, adenovirus, coxsackievirus Bacterial: meningococcal infection, streptococcal infection, Rocky Mountain spotted fever, subacute bacterial endocarditis
Postinfectious	Acute rheumatic fever, acute poststreptococcal glomerulonephritis
Hematologic, oncologic	Idiopathic thrombocytopenic purpura, hemolytic uremic syndrome, leukemia, lymphoma, antiphospholipid antibody syndrome
Gastrointestinal	Crohn's disease, ulcerative colitis
Connective tissue disease	Systemic-onset juvenile arthritis, systemic lupus erythematosus
Vasculitides	Wegener's granulomatosis, Goodpasture disease, polyarteritis nodosa, microscopic polyangiitis, urticarial vasculitis, hypersensitivity or allergic vasculitis

Table 103-3 American College of Rheumatology 1990 Criteria for Classification of Henoch-Schönlein Purpura

Criterion*	Description
Palpable purpura	Slightly raised, palpable hemorrhagic skin lesions, not related to thrombocytopenia
Age	Patient younger than 20 yr at onset of disease symptoms
Bowel angina	Diffuse abdominal pain, worse after meals, or the diagnosis of bowel ischemia, usually including bloody diarrhea
Wall granulocytes on biopsy	Histologic changes showing granulocytes in the walls of arterioles or venules

*For purposes of classification, a patient is considered to have Henoch-Schönlein purpura if at least two of the four criteria are present. The presence of any two or more criteria yields a sensitivity of 87.1% and a specificity of 87.7%.
From Mills JA, Michel BA, Bloch DA, et al: The American College of Rheumatology 1990 criteria for the classification of Henoch-Schönlein purpura. Arthritis Rheum 1990;33:1114-1121.

Table 103-4 Laboratory Studies in Henoch-Schönlein Purpura

Test	Finding
Complete blood count	White blood cell count: normal or elevated Hemoglobin and hematocrit: normal or low Red blood cell indices: normal Platelet count: normal or increased
Serum electrolytes	Usually normal except for children with renal insufficiency or renal failure
Blood urea nitrogen and creatinine	Elevated in dehydration or renal insufficiency
Erythrocyte sedimentation rate and C-reactive protein	Normal or elevated
Transaminases and biliary tree enzymes	Normal or elevated with gallbladder or small bowel involvement
Albumin	Normal or decreased due to inflammation or nephrotic syndrome
Serum lipids	Triglyceride, cholesterol, and very-long-chain fatty acids may all be increased in patients with nephrotic syndrome
Immunoglobulins	May see polyclonal elevation; IgA and IgM elevated in 50% of patients
Antineutrophil cytoplasmic antibody (ANCA), antinuclear antibody, rheumatoid factor	All usually negative; may have "atypical" ANCA due to production of IgA ANCA
Coagulation profile	Prothrombin time, partial thromboplastin time, international normalized ratio all normal; D-dimer, fibrin split products may be increased
Complement	C1q, C3, C4 usually normal; properdin, factor B, CH50 may be decreased
Urinalysis	May contain red blood cells, white blood cells, protein, and casts, depending on degree of renal disease; up to 50% have abnormal urinalysis

Table 103-5	Imaging Abnormalities in Henoch-Schönlein Purpura
Test	Finding
Radiography	Dilated bowel loops, thickening of bowel wall, blurring of bowel folds, scalloping of bowel wall due to erosion
Ultrasonography	Hepatosplenomegaly and thickening of gallbladder wall
Computed tomography	Bowel wall thickening, mesenteric edema, vascular engorgement, nonspecific lymphadenopathy
Endoscopy	Redness, swelling, petechiae, erosions, and ulcerations; lesions anywhere from duodenum to rectum, but more common in proximal gastrointestinal tract; duodenum and small intestine most frequently involved

necessary unless there is concern for a surgical emergency (Table 103-5). Because intussusception, an uncommon complication of HSP, is most often ileoileal, barium enema is not helpful in detecting this condition. Ultrasonography is preferred and offers the advantage of not exposing patients to ionizing radiation. This allows repeated examinations, which may be necessary in patients with recurrent, severe abdominal pain. Skin biopsy may prove helpful in those with an atypical presentation; findings of leukocytoclastic vasculitis with prominent IgA deposits on biopsy of a fresh purpuric lesion support the diagnosis. Renal biopsy is indicated in patients with acute nephritis, nephrotic syndrome, mixed nephritic-nephrotic syndrome, renal insufficiency, or renal failure. The severity of renal involvement on renal biopsy helps determine the prognosis and guide the therapy for children with HSP.

COURSE OF ILLNESS

HSP is a self-limited illness, and its symptoms can be expected to resolve within 4 weeks in two thirds of children. In general, younger patients have a shorter duration of symptoms, and they are less likely to suffer recrudescent symptoms. Up to 40% of children have a recurrence of symptoms within 6 weeks, but symptoms may reappear up to several years later. These exacerbations are usually shorter in duration and the symptoms are generally milder compared with the initial episode. Abdominal pain and rash are most likely to recur.

Nephritis is the one feature of HSP that may become persistent, and the morbidity and mortality of children with HSP hinge on the severity of the renal disease. Up to 60% of patients with HSP have persistent urinary abnormalities, depending on the degree of nephritis. Serial urinalyses are required for at least the first 6 months in those without renal involvement at presentation, because 95% of children with nephritis develop signs within 3 months of the appearance of other symptoms. Frequent examination of the urine is also important in patients with minimal urinary abnormalities, because HSP may cause an asymptomatic but progressive nephritis.

Up to 35% of children who have HSP nephropathy (either nephrotic syndrome or nephritic-nephrotic syndrome) at the time of presentation develop renal failure within 10 years. Fortunately, the vast majority of children with HSP nephropathy experience a good renal outcome (either no disease or minor urinary abnormalities). Overall, less than 5% of patients with any clinical sign of HSP nephropathy progress to end-stage renal disease.[16] Although patients

without renal symptoms have an extremely low incidence of chronic renal disease, renal failure or hypertension can occur up to 10 years after the initial manifestations of the disease. Of note, a patient's first kidney biopsy may not predict outcome, owing to sampling error. Renal biopsy up to 9 years after resolution of disease may demonstrate persistent IgA deposition and chronic glomerular disease.

TREATMENT

Treatment for HSP is mainly supportive, and most children can be safely managed as outpatients. Nonsteroidal anti-inflammatory medications, such as naproxen or ibuprofen, can be safely used for arthralgia or arthritis, provided there is no evidence of renal insufficiency. These drugs do not seem to provoke GI bleeding, despite the presence of GI vasculitis. Patients with hypertension may require temporary pharmacotherapy to control blood pressure. In patients with nephritis, angiotensin-converting enzyme inhibitors may be used to reduce proteinuria. Analgesia with acetaminophen or even narcotics may be necessary for children with severe abdominal pain. Parenteral hydration is indicated when severe abdominal pain prevents adequate fluid intake.

The use of systemic corticosteroids in HSP remains controversial, primarily because of a lack of clinical trials demonstrating efficacy. Although there is little doubt that steroids result in the rapid resolution of arthritis and edema, in most cases, these symptoms are neither severe nor prolonged enough to require therapy. Indications for systemic corticosteroids include severe abdominal complications (intussusception, massive GI bleed, infarction), significant renal disease (rapidly progressive glomerulonephritis or crescentic glomerular disease resulting in nephrotic syndrome, severe nephritis, renal insufficiency or failure), and severe orchitis. Other serious sequelae of HSP, such as pulmonary hemorrhage or central nervous system disease (encephalopathy, seizure, hemorrhage), are also indications for parenteral steroid therapy. Regimens reported in the literature use daily oral steroids, up to 2 mg/kg per day, for 1 to 2 weeks, followed by an extended taper or pulse therapy with 30 mg/kg per day methylprednisolone or equivalent, with similar results. Cytotoxic agents, such as cyclophosphamide and cyclosporine, are often used in conjunction with systemic corticosteroids to control severe renal manifestations. There are also reports describing the use of azathioprine, mycophenolate mofetil, thalidomide, and plasmapheresis for the treatment of refractory renal disease. Methotrexate and intravenous immunoglobulin have been used to control the extrarenal manifestations of HSP.

More controversial is the role of steroids in patients with mild to moderate GI and renal disease. Patients with significant abdominal pain or evidence of GI bleeding without evidence of severe GI complications may benefit from steroids over the first 48 hours, but one study suggests that this improvement is lost after 72 hours. The potential role of steroids in the prevention of both renal and GI complications is also controversial, and there is currently no strong clinical evidence that supports the prophylactic use of steroids to prevent GI or renal disease in patients with HSP. Similarly, there is no evidence that steroids alter the fundamental immunopathology of HSP. Rather, they seem to minimize the inflammation incited by circulating immune complexes. Once started, steroids should be tapered slowly—typically over 1 to 2 months—to avoid precipitating a flare of symptoms.

CONSULTATION

Consultation with a pediatric nephrologist is recommended when HSP nephropathy is identified. The nephrologist can help assess the severity of the renal disease and provide management and ongoing follow-up if needed. A rheumatologist may offer guidance in the management of recalcitrant, recurrent, or steroid-resistant HSP or those cases with severe joint involvement. Other severe manifestations of HSP, such as hypertension or central nervous system disease, should prompt the use of appropriate consultative services.

ADMISSION CRITERIA

- Uncertain diagnosis requiring further evaluation and monitoring.
- Symptoms that prevent enteral hydration or nutrition (e.g., severe abdominal pain).
- Intractable abdominal or joint pain unresponsive to conventional outpatient analgesia.
- GI complications such as hemorrhage or intussusception.
- Uncontrolled hypertension.
- Complication involving the central nervous system.
- Lack of appropriate outpatient support or follow-up.

DISCHARGE CRITERIA

- Clinically stable patient.
- Adequate pain control on outpatient medications.
- Sufficient family education regarding the outpatient treatment plan and necessary follow-up.

IN A NUTSHELL

- HSP is the most common vasculitis of childhood, affecting 1 child in 5000.
- The classic triad of symptoms is palpable purpura, abdominal pain, and joint pain. These symptoms may not present simultaneously, and the characteristic rash may appear after the other presenting symptoms.
- The prognosis of children with HSP is excellent, although up to 50% experience recurrences during the first 6 months after the initial illness.

- Long-term sequelae are largely restricted to renal complications, most often affecting children who develop both hematuria and proteinuria early in the course of the illness.
- Steroids are recommended for the management of active disease, but they are unproved in terms of preventing GI or renal sequelae.

ON THE HORIZON

- Prediction of children likely to develop HSP, with the goal of creating a primary prevention strategy.
- Identification of novel serum markers or the development of models to predict those at risk for severe renal disease.
- Controlled clinical trials to clarify the role of steroids and other agents in the treatment and prevention of GI and renal disease in HSP.

SUGGESTED READING

Allen DM, Diamond LK, Howell DA: Anaphylactoid purpura in children (Schönlein-Henoch syndrome). Am J Dis Child 1960;99:833-854.

Goldstein AR, White RHR Akuse R, Chantler C: Long term follow-up of childhood Henoch-Schönlein nephritis. Lancet 1992;339:280-282.

Huber AM, King J, McLaine P, et al: A randomized placebo-controlled trial of prednisone early in Henoch-Schönlein purpura. BMC Med 2004;2:7.

Mollica F, LiVolti S, Garozzo R, Russo G: Effectiveness of early prednisone treatment in preventing the development of nephropathy in anaphylactoid purpura. Eur J Pediatr 1992;151:140-144.

Saulsbury FT: Henoch-Schönlein purpura in children. Medicine 1999;78:395-409.

REFERENCES

1. Gardner-Medwin JM, Dolezalova P, Cummins C, Southwood TR: Incidence of Henoch-Schönlein purpura, Kawasaki disease and rare vasculitides in children of different ethnic origins. Lancet 2002;360:1197-1202.
2. Dolezalova P, Telekesova P, Nemcova D, Hoza J: Incidence of vasculitis in children in the Czech Republic: 2-year prospective epidemiology survey. J Rheumatol 2004;31:2295-2299.
3. Yang YH, Hung CF, Hsu CR, et al: A nationwide survey on epidemiological characteristics of childhood Henoch-Schönlein purpura in Taiwan. Rheumatology 2005;44:618-622.
4. Chave T, Neal C, Camp R: Henoch-Schönlein purpura following hepatitis B vaccination. J Dermatol Treat 2003;14:179-181.
5. Askhenazi S, Mimouni M, Varsano I: Henoch-Schönlein vasculitis following varicella. Am J Dis Child 1985;139:440-441.
6. Rostoker G, Rymer JC, Bagnard G, et al: Imbalances in serum proinflammatory cytokines and their soluble receptors: A putative role in the progression of idiopathic IgA nephropathy (IgAN) and Henoch-Schönlein purpura nephritis, and a potential target of immunoglobulin therapy? Clin Exp Immunol 1998;114:468-476.
7. Besbas N, Saatci U, Ruacan S, et al: The role of cytokines in Henoch-Schönlein purpura. Scand J Rheumatol 1997;26:456-460.
8. Nussinovitch M, Prais D, Finkelstein Y, Varsano I: Cutaneous manifestations of Henoch-Schönlein purpura in young children. Pediatr Dermatol 1998;15:426-428.
9. Choong CK, Beasley SW: Intra-abdominal manifestations of Henoch-Schönlein purpura. J Paediatr Child Health 1998;34:405-409.

10. Kawasaki Y, Suzuki J, Sakai N, et al: Clinical and pathological features of children with Henoch-Schoenlein purpura nephritis: Risk factors associated with poor prognosis. Clin Nephrol 2003;60:153-160.

11. Sano H, Izumida M, Shimizu H, Ogawa Y: Risk factors of renal involvement and significant proteinuria in Henoch-Schönlein purpura. Eur J Pediatr 2002;161:196-201.

12. Schärer K, Krmar R, Querfeld U, et al: Clinical outcome of Schönlein-Henoch purpura nephritis in children. Pediatr Nephrol 1999;13:816-823.

13. Kaku Y, Nohara K, Honda S: Renal involvement in Henoch-Schönlein purpura: A multivariate analysis of prognostic factors. Kidney Int 1998;53:1755-1759.

14. Ben-Sira L, Laor T: Severe scrotal pain in boys with Henoch-Schönlein purpura: Incidence and sonography. Pediatr Radiol 2000;30:125-128.

15. Cazzato S, Bernardi F, Cinti C, et al: Pulmonary functions abnormalities in children with Henoch-Schönlein purpura. Eur Respir J 1999;13:597-601.

16. Stewart M, Savage JM, Bell B, McCord B: Long term renal prognosis of Henoch-Schönlein purpura in an unselected childhood population. Eur J Pediatr 1988;147:113-115.

CHAPTER 104

Juvenile Dermatomyositis

Laura J. Mirkinson

Juvenile dermatomyositis is a multisystem disease of unknown cause characterized by a nonsuppurative inflammation primarily of striated muscle, skin, and the gastrointestinal (GI) tract. A well-recognized set of clinical features, resulting from an underlying small-vessel vasculitis, includes dramatic proximal muscle weakness, characteristic skin findings, and laboratory abnormalities. The onset and overall clinical course are variable. The vasculopathy, thought to be immune mediated, may involve arterioles, capillaries, and venules. Juvenile dermatomyositis is an uncommon disease with a recent estimated incidence of 2.5 to 4.1 per million.[1] The average age of onset is about 7 years. It is more common in girls than boys, with a ratio of approximately 2.3:1. Juvenile dermatomyositis is distinct from the adult disease polymyositis.

CLINICAL PRESENTATION

The onset of juvenile dermatomyositis may be acute but is more often subacute, with the gradual appearance of weakness and fatigue often associated with fever and rash. Typically affected are proximal muscle groups such as the shoulders, neck, and hip girdle muscles. Abdominal muscles are also characteristically affected. Parents may note that their children have increasing difficulty climbing the stairs or riding a bicycle. The classic Gower sign refers to the manner in which patients with proximal lower extremity muscle weakness rise from a seated position by climbing up their legs with their hands. Standardized childhood myositis assessment scales are useful to follow a patient's clinical course.[2] Typical findings of muscle weakness are noted in Table 104-1.

Severely affected patients may have a nasal, muffled voice; demonstrate difficulty swallowing; or have problems with coughing, choking, reflux, or aspiration. A significant number of patients have arthralgia or arthritis. Other affected organ systems may include cardiac (pericarditis, myocarditis), GI (bowel ulceration or infarction), and respiratory (pneumonitis, interstitial lung disease). Classic skin manifestations include a facial rash, Gottron papules, nailfold capillary loop abnormalities, skin ulcers, and calcinosis (Table 104-2). Similar to systemic lupus erythematosus, juvenile dermatomyositis is a photosensitive disease; sun exposure is associated with the exacerbation of symptoms.

DIFFERENTIAL DIAGNOSIS

The differential diagnosis of juvenile dermatomyositis includes postinfectious myositis, particularly acute myositis associated with influenza A and B or coxsackievirus infection; neuromuscular diseases, such as muscular dystrophy; and inflammatory myositis associated with other connective tissue diseases, such as scleroderma. Neuromuscular disorders associated with myopathy also include metabolic disorders, such as glycogen storage diseases; genetic disorders; trauma; and spinal and peripheral nerve abnormalities.

DIAGNOSIS AND EVALUATION

Abnormalities in a number of muscle-derived enzymes, including creatine kinase, lactate dehydrogenase, aspartate transaminase, and aldolase, are seen in juvenile dermatomyositis. In any individual patient, one, several, or all of these enzymes may be abnormal. Of interest, creatine kinase does not necessarily correlate well with the degree of disease activity. Aspartate transaminase and lactate dehydrogenase are better at reflecting the overall activity and predicting flares of disease. Nonspecific indicators of inflammation, such as the erythrocyte sedimentation rate and C-reactive protein, may be elevated or normal. The antinuclear antibody is typically positive, and the rheumatoid factor is negative. In 1975, when specific diagnostic criteria for juvenile dermatomyositis were first published,[3] an electromyography and muscle biopsy were recommended to establish the diagnosis. The electromyogram shows denervation and inflammatory myopathy. The results of a muscle biopsy, which should demonstrate inflammation or fiber necrosis and small-vessel vasculitis, may be affected by the site chosen for sampling. Recently, magnetic resonance imaging has largely replaced electromyography and biopsy. T1-weighted magnetic resonance images of the thigh muscles demonstrate fibrosis, atrophy, and fatty infiltration; T2-weighted images with fat suppression demonstrate active inflammation.

COURSE OF ILLNESS

The course of juvenile dermatomyositis is variable. Some patients experience complete recovery, and others require prolonged courses of steroid therapy and experience occasional flares of disease. Recurrence of disease can occur after long periods of remission. Long-term disability is often related to calcifications and flexion contractures. All these sequelae can be prevented by complete control of the inflammation underlying the disease.

TREATMENT

Early, aggressive therapy of juvenile dermatomyositis is associated with a better long-term outcome, and corticosteroids are the mainstay of therapy. Once the diagnosis is confirmed, prednisone is started at an initial dose of 2 mg/kg (maximum 60 to 80 mg) divided two or three times daily. Traditionally, therapy at this dose was continued for at least several months, and it was not uncommon for patients with juvenile dermatomyositis to be on corticosteroid therapy for 1 or 2 years. This often led to severe corticosteroid toxicity,

Table 104–1 Clinical Findings of Muscle Weakness in Juvenile Dermatomyositis

Affected Muscle Group	Clinical Finding
Neck flexors	Unable to lift head when lying supine
Shoulders	Unable to lift arms above head or maintain arms raised above head
Abdomen	Unable to do a sit-up
Hip flexors	Difficult to go from a standing to a sitting position on the floor without support Unable to go from a prone to an all-fours position Unable to rise from a chair, step up onto a stool, or bend over and pick up a pencil off the floor

Table 104–2 Typical Skin Manifestations of Juvenile Dermatomyositis

Finding	Description
Facial rash	Fine, erythematous, scaly malar rash associated with heliotrope discoloration and edema of the upper eyelids; occasionally confused with the rash of systemic lupus erythematosus
Gottron papules	Scaly, thick papules over the extensor surfaces of the joints, including the MCP and PIP joints of the hands, elbows, knees, and ankles; may initially appear erythematous and later atrophic and pale; sometimes mistaken for atopic dermatitis or psoriasis
Nails	Periungual erythema; hypertrophied cuticles; and thickened, tortuous nail-bed capillary loops, with dropout areas of surrounding vessels
Skin ulcers	Vasculitic ulcerations often occur over pressure points (elbows, knuckles); painful ulceration of superficial tissues can be associated with calcinosis; gingival, buccal, and gastrointestinal ulcerations can also occur
Calcinosis	Small to large calcific deposits in the skin, primarily in areas susceptible to pressure (e.g., elbows) or trauma; calcinosis can affect subcutaneous tissues and muscles or develop within fascial planes; it may be limited or widespread

MCP, metacarpophalangeal; PIP, proximal interphalangeal.

and involvement of the GI tract meant that absorption of oral medications could be unreliable. Alternatives to daily corticosteroid therapy may include adding weekly or consecutive daily doses of pulsed intravenous methylprednisolone (30 mg/kg per day; maximum 1 g) or steroid-sparing agents (methotrexate, azathioprine, cyclophosphamide, cyclosporine, intravenous immunoglobulin) earlier in the disease course in an attempt to minimize the long-term sequelae of both the disease itself and the steroids used to treat it. Medications are tapered once patients demonstrate substantial or complete clinical and laboratory improvement.

Children with juvenile dermatomyositis may be very photosensitive and should be advised to wear protective clothing and sunscreen daily. Hydroxychloroquine appears to ameliorate the rash and modulate the effects of sun exposure. Early in the disease course, when there is acute muscle inflammation, strenuous physical activity is avoided. Supportive care includes maintenance of range of motion and prevention of flexion contractures, as well as support of other affected organ systems. Patients should be watched for the development of complications such as skin ulcers, calcinosis, and aspiration, as well as the recognized sequelae of long-term steroid therapy. Up to 35% of children with chronically active myositis develop calcinosis. There is currently no specific therapy for calcinosis other than treatment of the local infection and attention to the effects of calcific deposits on the range of motion of affected muscles, but expeditious control of the disease appears to lower the risk considerably.

CONSULTATION

A rheumatologist can assist with diagnosis and management, as well as long-term follow-up. If complications develop, consultation with other subspecialists may be appropriate. A gastroenterologist can offer guidance with complications such as swallowing dysfunction, malabsorption due to intestinal involvement, or GI bleeding. Surgeons are helpful when gallbladder or mesenteric complications arise. A full range of services, including nutrition, occupa-

tional therapy, physical therapy, and speech therapy, should be included in the overall management plan. Periodic ophthalmic evaluation is indicated for patients on long-term corticosteroid therapy.

ADMISSION CRITERIA

- Patients may require admission to expedite the initial evaluation.
- Close observation and support may be required in the presence of significant symptoms such as severe muscle weakness or difficulty swallowing either at the onset of disease or during a flare-up.
- Parenteral antibiotic therapy may be required for the complications of secondary infection of skin ulcerations due to calcinosis.
- GI symptoms such as significant abdominal pain, bloody stool, or emesis require immediate evaluation.

DISCHARGE CRITERIA

- Resolution of significant symptoms of disease, including severe weakness, inability to ambulate or perform tasks of daily living, and difficulty swallowing.

- Establishment of revised short-term and, if needed, long-term management plan, with appropriate outpatient follow-up.

IN A NUTSHELL

- Juvenile dermatomyositis is a multisystem vasculitis that affects primarily muscles, skin, and the GI tract.
- The diagnosis is made when muscle weakness and rash are noted, along with laboratory evidence of myositis such as elevated creatine kinase, lactate dehydrogenase, aspartate transaminase, or aldolase. Magnetic resonance imaging is useful to demonstrate edema and inflammation in the affected muscles.
- Management centers on early, aggressive control of muscle inflammation, including corticosteroids.
- Common complications include contractures, skin ulcers, and calcinosis. They can be minimized or avoided by rapid and complete disease control.

ON THE HORIZON

- Expect studies that compare treatment regimens for early juvenile dermatomyositis, including the role of intravenous versus oral corticosteroids and the role of biologic agents such as rituximab (anti-CD20 monoclonal antibody).
- Look for research on the immunogenetics of juvenile dermatomyositis. Also being studied are the role of antigens, cytokines, and tumor necrosis factors and the genetic control of the immune response.
- Clinical scores for the measurement of disease activity and assessment of muscle damage are being tested for reliability and validity.

SUGGESTED READING

Ansell BM: Juvenile dermatomyositis. Rheum Dis Clin North Am 1991;17:931-942.

Cassidy JT, Petty RE: Juvenile dermatomyositis. In Cassidy JT, Petty RE (eds): Textbook of Pediatric Rheumatology, 4th ed. Philadelphia, WB Saunders, 2001, pp 465-504.

Ramanan AV, Feldman BM: Clinical features and outcomes of juvenile dermatomyositis and other childhood onset myositis syndromes. Rheum Dis Clin North Am 2002;28:833-857.

Rennebohm R: Juvenile dermatomyositis. Pediatr Ann 2002;31:426-433.

REFERENCES

1. Mendez EP, Lipton R, Ramsey-Goldman R, et al: US incidence of juvenile dermatomyositis 1995-1998: Results from the National Institute of Arthritis and Musculoskeletal and Skin Diseases Registry. Arthritis Rheum 2003;49:300-305.
2. Lovell DJ, Lindsley C, Rennebohm R, et al: Development of validated disease activity and damage indices for the juvenile idiopathic inflammatory myopathies—the Childhood Myositis Assessment Scale (CMAS): A quantitative tool for the evaluation of muscle involvement. Arthritis Rheum 1999;42:2213-2219.
3. Bohan A, Peter JB: Polymyositis and dermatomyositis. N Engl J Med 1975;292:344-347.

CHAPTER 105

Juvenile Idiopathic Arthritis

Sampath Prahalad

Arthritis is inflammation of synovial tissue within a diarthrodial joint. Infection-related arthritides are discussed in Chapter 106, but idiopathic athritides constitute another group. Because the pathogenesis of the idiopathic forms is not completely understood, a variety of schemes have been devised to classify childhood arthritides according to the pattern of involvement, associated symptoms, and genetic factors. For clarity, this chapter adheres to the classification of the American College of Rheumatology, using the term *juvenile idiopathic arthritis* (JIA), which was previously known as juvenile rheumatoid arthritis. Based on the number of inflamed joints and extra-articular features, three subtypes are recognized: pauciarticular, polyarticular, and systemic onset (Table 105-1). It should be noted that the term JIA as used here differs from that proposed by the International League of Associations for Rheumatology, which includes other subtypes of juvenile arthritis, including enthesitis-related arthritis, psoriatic arthritis, and unclassified arthritis.

The diagnosis of JIA is clinical, defined as joint swelling or effusion or at least two of three signs of joint inflammation: limitation of range of motion, tenderness or pain on motion, and joint warmth. These signs must be present consistently for at least 6 weeks in a patient younger than age 16 years. The annual incidence of JIA is estimated at 10 per 100,000 children, and the prevalence of JIA in the United States is about 1 in 1000 children younger than 16 years. Estimates of the actual number of American children with JIA vary between 70,000 and 100,000, including both active and inactive cases. Nationally, in 2000, JIA accounted for 872 of the estimated 6.3 million hospital discharges of children younger than 17 years in the Kids Inpatient Database (0.01%). The mean length of stay was 5 days, and the total cost of hospitalization was estimated at $13 million.[1]

CLINICAL PRESENTATION

Children with arthritis typically demonstrate stiffness after prolonged periods of inactivity, such as upon arising in the morning or after naps, long car rides, or sitting in class at school (the so-called theater sign). Conversely, children with arthritis typically feel better after a warm bath or several minutes of activity. Cold, damp weather or swimming in cool water tends to be more difficult for children with arthritis, whereas warm weather generally relieves symptoms. Thus, a child with arthritis may suffer joint stiffness in the

Supported in part by grants from the National Institute of Arthritis and Musculoskeletal and Skin Diseases (AR-50177), National Center for Research Resources (RR-00064); the Val A. Browning Charitable Foundation; the Primary Children's Medical Center Foundation; and the Children's Health Research Center, Salt Lake City, Utah.

morning but may be quite comfortable exercising strenuously later in the day. Pain is an unusual complaint in a child with JIA, and nighttime awakening is uncommon as well.[2]

Systemic-onset JIA, or Still disease, accounts for about 10% to 15% of all children with JIA. This is the subtype of JIA that most closely resembles an infectious disease. Although systemic-onset JIA can occur at any age, the peak age of onset is between 1 and 6 years. Boys and girls are equally affected. As its name implies, this is a systemic illness characterized by fever, rash, and arthritis. These children are often admitted to the hospital for evaluation of fever of unknown origin. The fever of systemic-onset JIA is described as double quotidian; children typically have one or two spikes of fever greater than 39°C at about the same time every day. In between episodes of fever, the temperature returns to the baseline level or lower. The fever must be present for at least 2 weeks to be considered a diagnostic criterion.

The rash of systemic-onset JIA is salmon pink, transient (lasting minutes to a few hours), nonpruritic, and migratory. It consists of discrete macules 2 to 5 mm in size, mostly on the trunk and proximal extremities. The rash often accompanies fever spikes, and it is typically seen after a shower. Rubbing or lightly scratching the skin elicits erythema (Koebner phenomenon) and might be followed by the appearance of transient macular lesions. Fever and rash are found in systemic-onset JIA but are not part of the clinical picture of pauciarticular arthritis and are rarely present in the polyarticular form. These symptoms may precede the onset of arthritis by days to months. Most children with systemic-onset JIA develop chronic polyarthritis over time. Joint involvement is variable at disease onset, with anywhere from no joints to numerous joints being involved. Children with systemic-onset JIA also have laboratory evidence of systemic inflammation. The white blood cell count is usually elevated, with a predominance of neutrophils, accompanied by anemia and thrombocytosis; the erythrocyte sedimentation rate (ESR) is moderately to significantly elevated. Hepatosplenomegaly, lymphadenopathy, and serositis can also be seen in systemic-onset JIA.

Polyarticular JIA is characterized by the presence of arthritis of at least 6 weeks' duration in five or more joints. Polyarticular JIA accounts for 30% to 40% of cases of JIA and typically affects more girls than boys. Two distinct subtypes are recognized, based on the presence or absence of rheumatoid factor (RF). If the onset occurs during the first peak, at age 1 to 3 years, patients are generally RF negative. Girls affected during the second peak, just before puberty, have a disease that is more like adult rheumatoid arthritis, are RF positive, and have early erosions and often subcutaneous nodules. In all types of polyarticular JIA, the onset is generally insidious, with children gradually accruing additional swollen joints over time. Typically, the arthritis is symmetrical above and below the waist and between the left and

Type	Peak Age of Onset	Typical Features
Pauciarticular		Arthritis of ≤4 joints in the first 6 mo
		Few or no complaints of pain, but swelling is noticeable, especially in large joints
		Morning limp or refusal to walk
Early onset	<6 yr	Predominantly girls
Later onset	≥6 yr	Predominantly boys
		Often positive for HLA-B27
		Some go on to develop spondyloarthropathy
Polyarticular	First peak: 1-3 yr	Girls > boys
	Second peak: prepubertal	Arthritis of ≥5 joints for at least 6 wk
		Insidious onset of joint symptoms
		Symmetrical distribution
		Small joints of hands and feet are commonly involved
		Fatigue, malaise, anorexia
RF negative	Usually first peak	
RF positive	Usually second peak	Early joint erosions
		Subcutaneous nodules
Systemic onset	1-6 yr	Girls = boys
		Double quotidian fever
		Transient, salmon-colored rash
		Onset of systemic symptoms often precedes arthritis

Table 105-1 Types of Juvenile Idiopathic Arthritis

HLA, human leukocyte antigen; RF, rheumatoid factor.

right sides, and it often involves the small joints of the hands and feet. Fever is generally absent or low grade, but children may complain of fatigue, malaise, and anorexia. Polyarticular JIA may be accompanied by mild anemia and a modest elevation of the ESR. Synovitis in multiple joints may lead to chronic joint changes and bony erosions. Up to 50% of those with polyarticular JIA show radiographic abnormalities within 2 years of onset if not treated aggressively.

Pauciarticular JIA, the most common type, accounts for about 50% of all children with JIA. It is characterized by the presence of arthritis in four or fewer joints during the first 6 months of disease. Two clinical subgroups of pauciarticular JIA are observed. The early-onset type is common in girls younger than 6 years. The other occurs in an older group of boys who are often positive for HLA-B27; a proportion of these children go on to develop spondyloarthropathy later in life. In younger children, pauciarticular JIA often presents insidiously with refusal to walk or a limp in the morning that typically improves as the day goes on. Children seldom complain of pain, although parents may notice swelling of a knee or other large joint. This type has relatively few systemic signs such as fever, and it is the least likely of the three types to be a diagnostic or management challenge.

COMPLICATIONS

Macrophage activation syndrome (MAS) is rare, but it is the one complication of systemic JIA that is most likely to cause significant morbidity or mortality. MAS appears to be a subtype of hemophagocytic lymphohistiocytosis, which occurs both as a familial form and as a result of genetic abnormalities in natural killer T lymphocytes. It also occurs sporadically as a complication of malignancy or infection.[3] In systemic-onset JIA, MAS most commonly occurs during the first 6 months of disease, during periods of active systemic inflammation that are often associated with a change in medication. MAS manifests as unremitting fever, unlike the spiking fevers of the underlying illness. Children may demonstrate bruising and mucosal bleeding from the consumptive coagulopathy seen in MAS, as well as mental status changes, hepatosplenomegaly, and diffuse lymphadenopathy. Activation of macrophages results in phagocytosis of erythrocytes, platelets, and leukocytes, so MAS should be suspected when patients with JIA present with a sudden drop in platelets, hematocrit, and white blood cells, accompanied by an elevation of hepatic transaminases. Laboratory studies also demonstrate elevated triglycerides, ferritin, D-dimers, prothrombin time, and partial thromboplastin time, and a fall in fibrinogen, ESR, and serum albumin. Pauciarticular and polyarticular JIA are not usually associated with MAS.

Pericarditis is seen in about 3% to 9% of children with JIA, almost always in association with systemic-onset JIA. Older children are more likely to develop pericarditis, which may present as precordial chest pain, dyspnea, or discomfort referred to the back, shoulder, or neck, or it may be noted incidentally on chest imaging. Physical examination findings include tachycardia, cardiomegaly, or a pericardial friction rub at the lower left sternal border (see Chapter 86). Cardiac tamponade is a rare but serious complication of constrictive pericarditis. It is characterized by venous distention, hepatomegaly, and peripheral edema. Urgent evaluation and management are necessary to avoid progressive cardiovascular instability. JIA seldom causes parenchymal lung disease, but pleuritic chest pain due to a pleural effusion may accompany pericarditis or occur in isolation.

Anterior uveitis, or iridocyclitis, is a well-recognized and potentially serious complication of JIA. Uveitis in JIA is usually asymptomatic and chronic; it is most common in children with pauciarticular JIA (approximately 10%) and, to a lesser extent, polyarticular JIA. A younger age, female gender, and positive antinuclear antibody (ANA) test increase the risk of iritis in most studies, although boys are at risk as well. Uveitis is rare in systemic-onset JIA, occurring in less than 1% of cases. Acute uveitis, accompanied by pain and redness, may be associated with spondyloarthritis but is not typically seen in children with JIA. The detection of acute uveitis in a child suspected of having systemic-onset JIA should prompt a consideration of other causes of fever and rash, such as Kawasaki disease and acute viral infections.

Children with long-standing polyarticular or systemic-onset JIA may develop involvement of the joints of the cervical spine. This can result in instability or fusion of the posterior elements, so care should be exercised when these children undergo procedures that require sedation or anesthesia. Preoperative flexion and extension views of the cervical spine may aid in the detection of cervical involvement and the avoidance of subluxation and injury to the spinal cord or brainstem with hyperextension.

DIFFERENTIAL DIAGNOSIS

JIA is a clinical diagnosis made by history and physical examination. Care must be exercised in labeling a child with JIA before symptoms have been present for more than 6 weeks, because infectious arthropathies may be prolonged but ultimately transient. Conversely, although chronic inflammatory synovitis is seldom an emergency, acutely dangerous conditions must be excluded urgently in all cases. Thus, a child with an acute febrile monoarthritis must be considered to have septic arthritis or osteomyelitis until proved otherwise, especially in the presence of elevated inflammatory markers (see Chapter 70). A new monoarthritis in an otherwise healthy-appearing child may represent an acute postinfectious arthritis (see Chapter 106). Common causes of postinfectious arthritis include parvovirus B19, group A streptococcus, and *Borrelia burgdorferi* (Lyme disease).

Systemic-onset JIA may be difficult to distinguish from severe infections, particularly when children present with fever before the onset of arthritis. The fevers of infectious diseases are usually hectic and spike less predictably than the fevers of systemic-onset JIA, and the fever often does not return to baseline between spikes. Additional studies are essential in most cases to exclude other causes of prolonged unexplained fever such as infections, malignancies, and inflammatory bowel disease (see Chapter 61). When migratory arthritis and arthralgias accompany fever, acute rheumatic fever (Chapter 87), and serum sickness should be

considered. Cutaneous and cardiac manifestations usually allow these conditions to be distinguished, although echocardiography may be necessary to exclude rheumatic fever. Children with either dermatomyositis or systemic lupus erythematosus can present with polyarthritis and fevers, but additional clinical or laboratory features of the underlying disease are typically present (see Chapters 104 and 107).

Vasculitides such as Kawasaki disease and Henoch-Schönlein purpura often include arthritis among their symptoms (see Chapters 102 and 103). Other entities to consider are transient synovitis of the hip, slipped capital femoral epiphysis, and traction apophysitides (e.g., Osgood-Schlatter syndrome).

EVALUATION

Laboratory tests may help rule out alternative diagnoses and classify the form of arthritis, but they are insufficient to confirm a diagnosis. Expected results from the complete blood count, ESR, and ANA are provided in Table 105-2. A positive ANA increases the risk for chronic uveitis. Rheumatoid factor is seen in about 5% to 10% of children with JIA, primarily in adolescent girls with polyarticular JIA.

In healthy-appearing patients with a new monoarthritis, parvovirus B19 and Lyme titers and antistreptococcal antibodies are generally included in the initial evaluation. Evaluation for a septic joint is pursued if clinically indicated.

At disease onset, imaging studies are usually normal, or they can show soft tissue swelling or effusions. Periarticular demineralization, narrowing of joint spaces, subchondral cysts, or bony erosions on plain radiographs are indicative of long-standing inflammatory arthritis. Plain radiographs are also helpful for identifying children with cervical spine abnormalities. Imaging is particularly useful when other diagnoses must be excluded. For example, lucent metaphyseal bands in the long bones of a child older than 2 years suggests a diagnosis of leukemia, especially when unexpectedly severe anemia or thrombocytopenia is also present. A radionuclide bone scan may be helpful when osteomyelitis or malignancy is suspected, although the incidence of false-positive results owing to minor trauma, altered weight bearing, and normal growth centers can significantly limit its utility. Similarly, magnetic resonance imaging is usually not necessary in a child with arthritis, although a contrast-enhanced scan may confirm the presence of subtle synovitis that is not clearly demonstrable on physical examination. When periarticular disorders are under consideration, magnetic resonance imaging may be useful because it provides clear images of adjacent soft tissues and bone.

Table 105-2 Key Laboratory Features of Juvenile Idiopathic Arthritis			
Type	CBC	ESR	Likelihood of Positive ANA (%)
Pauciarticular	Normal	Normal or mildly elevated	70
Polyarticular	Mild anemia, mild thrombocytosis	Normal or mildly elevated	40
Systemic onset	Leukocytosis, anemia, thrombocytosis	Elevated	5-10

ANA, antinuclear antibody; CBC, complete blood cell count; ESR, erythrocyte sedimentation rate.

Arthrocentesis can be helpful in diagnosing JIA and excluding other causes of arthritis. Typically, synovial fluid in JIA is yellowish and cloudy, with white blood cell counts between 15,000 and 20,000 and a predominance of neutrophilic forms (75%). In septic arthritis, the fluid is usually serosanguineous and turbid, and the cell count is higher, often between 50,000 and 300,000, with more than 75% neutrophilic forms. Unlike in JIA, in septic arthritis the fluid has a low glucose level, and bacteria may be observed on Gram stain.

COURSE OF ILLNESS

All three types of JIA tend to be characterized by remissions and relapses. Further, it is not unusual for children with JIA to experience a flare of symptoms as a result of intercurrent infection. Systemic-onset JIA may follow a systemic course in which the fever, rash, and laboratory abnormalities persist. More commonly, it follows a polyarticular course, with arthritis persisting after resolution of the other systemic symptoms.[4]

Polyarticular JIA usually follows a chronic course over several years. In 30% to 50% of children with pauciarticular JIA, the disease evolves and follows a polyarticular course in which more than four joints are involved. The management and prognosis for this group of children are similar to those for children with polyarticular-onset disease. All three types of JIA have the potential to develop erosions or joint space narrowing after 2 to 5 years of persistent synovitis. Active synovitis can be detected in 30% to 55% of children with JIA 10 years after disease onset. Estimates of mortality in JIA range from 0.29 to 1.1 per 100 patients, severalfold higher than the standardized mortality rate for a similarly aged U.S. population.

TREATMENT

Children with JIA are best served by a comprehensive interdisciplinary team of health care providers that includes the primary care provider, pediatric rheumatologist, rheumatology nurse, social worker, and physical and occupational therapists. The aims of management in all types of JIA are to control pain, prevent and restore loss of motion in affected joints, improve overall functioning, and minimize the effects of inflammation on normal growth and development.[5] Nonpharmacologic modalities such as moist heat can be especially helpful for relieving morning stiffness.

The first line of pharmacologic management for all forms of JIA traditionally has been a nonsteroidal anti-inflammatory drug (NSAID). Naproxen is preferred by most rheumatologists for its ease of administration and pediatric labeling. It is usually administered at a dose of 10 to 20 mg/kg per day in two to three divided doses; as with all NSAIDs, 2 to 4 weeks of therapy is necessary before a child's response to naproxen can be assessed. Alternative NSAIDs include ibuprofen, sulindac, tolmetin, and indomethacin. All should be administered with food to minimize gastrointestinal side effects such as abdominal pain, nausea, heartburn, or anorexia. Surveillance for gastrointestinal side effects of NSAIDs is extremely important, and H$_2$ blocker or proton pump inhibitor therapy is often used in conjunction with NSAID therapy. Naproxen is associated with pseudoporphyria (small blisters that scar) or skin fragility in up to 10% of children; fair skin and blue or gray eye color are reported to be risk factors. Other NSAIDs are associated less often with increased skin fragility. Bruising or bleeding can also be seen with NSAIDs. In patients with systemic JIA, indomethacin can be particularly helpful to treat fever and pericarditis. Patients should be cautioned not to use other over-the-counter NSAIDs while on naproxen or a similar agent. However, acetaminophen can be used occasionally for fever or extra pain relief. Children on NSAIDs need a complete blood count, urinalysis, and levels of serum liver transaminases, blood urea nitrogen, and serum creatinine checked every 3 to 6 months and at baseline.

It is important to note that all forms of JIA may progress to a polyarticular course and may require additional therapy beyond the use of NSAIDs. Medical management frequently requires aggressive escalation of therapy using multiple agents.

Corticosteroid therapy is often used as an adjunct to anti-inflammatory therapy in patients with JIA. The high frequency of side effects and lack of objective evidence that corticosteroids alter the long-term articular outcome weigh against the prolonged use of systemic corticosteroids in JIA. However, oral corticosteroids used at the lowest possible doses to minimize side effects may be useful in children with systemic-onset disease and significant and persistent systemic features such as fever. Because corticosteroids can mask other diagnoses and worsen infections, they should be used only after the diagnosis has been clearly established. Intra-articular steroid therapy, in the form of triamcinolone hexacetonide, is often effective in treating polyarticular and pauciarticular JIA, especially early in the illness. It is used in select cases when a single joint is considered amenable to local corticosteroid therapy. Topical corticosteroid ophthalmic preparations are used in the treatment of uveitis.

Second-line or disease-modifying antirheumatoid drugs are generally instituted by pediatric rheumatologists or others experienced in their use. However, the hospitalist is likely to encounter patients with an established diagnosis of JIA who are on these medications and are hospitalized for a flare of arthritis or other unrelated conditions. The following is a brief synopsis of some of the more commonly used medications.

Methotrexate, a folate antagonist, is the most commonly used disease-modifying antirheumatoid drug to treat polyarticular or systemic-onset JIA. Methotrexate is administered weekly by oral or subcutaneous routes; the latter is associated with better absorption and fewer gastrointestinal adverse effects. Although well tolerated in the majority of children, methotrexate may be associated with headache, nausea, or fatigue, usually within 1 or 2 days of administration. Oral mucosal ulcers are common unless children receive concurrent folic acid. More serious but less frequent side effects of methotrexate include leukopenia, hypersensitivity pneumonitis, elevation of transaminases, and hepatic fibrosis. These side effects may require modification of the dose or discontinuation of the drug. Of interest, methotrexate is also used as therapy for persistent uveitis in patients with and without overt arthritis.

Older second-line medications such as hydroxychloroquine and sulfasalazine are used infrequently because more effective agents are available. The availability of biologic agents in particular has increased the therapeutic options for children with JIA. The most frequently used are anti–tumor necrosis factor (TNF) agents. TNF is a proinflammatory cytokine known to be elevated in children with JIA. Although TNF is central to the development of synovitis, it is also important for immune surveillance. Thus, all anti-TNF agents increase the risk of infection, including viral illnesses, severe bacterial infections, and reactivation of latent tuberculosis. A tuberculosis skin test should be performed before initiating treatment with an anticytokine agent and repeated annually. Anti-TNF agents can also exacerbate other serious bacterial or opportunistic fungal infections. Hence, if a serious infection is suspected in a child on an anti-TNF agent, the medication should be withheld until the child is evaluated and appropriate antimicrobial treatment has been instituted.

Etanercept (Enbrel) is a soluble TNF receptor that binds TNF, thereby blocking its binding to cell surface receptors. It is given by subcutaneous injection once or twice weekly. The most frequent side effects are injection site reactions. Usually these are mild, manifesting as erythema, and do not warrant discontinuation of etanercept. Infliximab (Remicade) is a chimeric anti-TNF monoclonal antibody that binds to TNF, thereby neutralizing its biologic activity. The antibody is administered by intravenous infusion every 1 to 2 months. These infusions may be accompanied by fever, chills, myalgia, or headache. Premedicating with acetaminophen and diphenhydramine is often helpful. Adalimumab (Humira) is a fully humanized anti-TNF antibody given subcutaneously every other week. The most common adverse effect is a mild injection site reaction manifested by a self-limited red rash or swelling. Cold compresses can be helpful in providing symptomatic relief. Other biologic agents being considered for use in children with JIA include interleukin-1 receptor antagonists (anakinra, IL-1 TRAP), inhibitors of T-cell costimulation (anti-CTLA4-Ig), and anti-CD20 monoclonal antibodies (rituximab).

Ongoing pediatric rheumatology evaluation is important in the care of children with JIA. When this is not routinely available, intermittent rheumatology evaluation is extremely helpful. In addition, periodic evaluation by an ophthalmologist is needed to detect and treat chronic anterior uveitis. Uveitis in patients with JIA is often silent; they do not complain of eye pain and rarely present with a red eye. If undetected and untreated, uveitis can result in significant and irreversible loss of vision. For this reason, there is a recommended schedule of screening for uveitis based on type of JIA, age of onset, and ANA status. These guidelines should be strictly adhered to and can be found in the published policy statement of the American Academy of Pediatrics.[6] Generally, children with JIA do well at school, and arthritis per se seldom accounts for absences. Rather, truancy is a warning sign of psychosocial difficulties. Nonetheless, children with significant arthritis might need special accommodations at school. Usually there is no need to restrict physical activity, apart from avoiding direct trauma to joints, but children should be allowed to limit their activities as needed. Follow-up with a physical or occupational therapist should also be arranged to initiate a home exercise program to aprevent or treat contractures or for splints.

JIA is a chronic illness, and families often have many concerns about the long-term consequences of the disease. The term *arthritis* may evoke images of crippled digits or wheelchairs, which are fortunately rare with today's therapeutic options. The treatment of JIA should include education that addresses important issues such as peer relations, family dynamics, social adjustment, and vocational planning. Young adults with JIA treated by comprehensive multidisciplinary teams can surpass community standards in terms of level of schooling and professional attainment. The American Juvenile Arthritis Organization, a branch of the Arthritis Foundation, is an excellent source of information for newly diagnosed patients with JIA and their families; its link can be found at the Arthritis Foundation website (*www.arthritis.org*). Other sources of information include the National Institute of Arthritis, Musculoskeletal and Skin Diseases at the National Institutes of Health. (*www.niams.nih.gov/*) and the American College of Rheumatology (*www.rheumatology.org*).

CONSULTATION

Although a diagnosis of JIA can be straightforward, this is ultimately a clinical diagnosis that requires the exclusion of other causes of acute and chronic arthritis. The long-term management of children with JIA can be challenging, often involving the use of medications that require monitoring for adverse effects. Consultation with a pediatric rheumatologist, when available, can facilitate an early diagnosis and the prompt institution of appropriate medical management.

Following are some of the common indications for other types of consultation:

- Pediatric infectious disease: for the evaluation of patients when fevers secondary to infectious disorders are suspected.
- Cardiology: for the evaluation and management of chest pain, pericarditis, and pericardial effusions.
- Hematology-oncology: for the evaluation of MAS or when malignancy is suspected.
- Orthopedics: when there is a high index of suspicion for a septic joint or osteomyelitis.
- Physical and occupational therapy: to preserve and improve range of motion and strength.
- Ophthalmology: to screen for chronic (and clinically silent) anterior uveitis.
- Social services: to help in locating financial, educational, and social assistance.
- Mental health services: to assist in the management of affective disorders associated with chronic disease and to improve coping skills needed to manage a chronic disease and long-term medication therapy.

ADMISSION CRITERIA

- Evaluation of patients with suspected systemic-onset JIA for persistent fever, potential malignancy, or serious infection.
- Management of serious flares of disease associated with pain, disability, or nonarticular organ system complications.
- Evaluation and teaching for patients with chronic disease and poor compliance with therapeutic regimens.

DISCHARGE CRITERIA

- Completion of evaluation for possible malignancy or serious infection.
- Resolution of fever and evidence of improving inflammatory markers.
- Establishment of a therapeutic regimen, including medication, physical or occupational therapy, ophthalmology, and social services.
- Discharge planning, including patient and family education and general pediatric and pediatric rheumatology follow-up.
- If on steroids, a plan for tapering the medication and monitoring for side effects, including measuring blood pressure and following urinalyses for glycosuria, should be considered.

IN A NUTSHELL

- JIA is among the most prevalent chronic diseases of childhood, affecting 1 in 1000 children younger than 16 years.
- Children with arthritis typically complain of joint swelling or morning stiffness; pain is unusual and suggests a mechanical rather than an inflammatory process.
- Aggressive treatment of synovitis with disease-modifying agents such as methotrexate and biologic agents such as anti-TNF monoclonal antibodies effectively controls arthritis and prevents long-term complications in most children.
- Periodic ophthalmic evaluation is an essential component of the care of children with JIA.

ON THE HORIZON

- Further refinement of biologic response modifiers, including targeted B- and T-cell monoclonal antibodies, will continue to improve the safety and efficacy of therapy for JIA.
- Identification of genetically determined disease subsets will allow therapy to be individualized.
- Improved understanding of the pathophysiology of systemic-onset JIA may necessitate its reclassification as an autoinflammatory rather than an autoimmune disorder.

SUGGESTED READING

Cassidy JT, Petty RE: Textbook of Pediatric Rheumatology, 5th ed. Philadelphia, WB Saunders, 2005.

Cron RQ: Current treatment for chronic arthritis in childhood. Curr Opin Pediatr 2002;14:684-687.

Foster CS: Diagnosis and treatment of juvenile idiopathic arthritis-associated uveitis. Curr Opin Ophthalmol 2003;14:395-398.

Jarvis JN: Juvenile rheumatoid arthritis: A guide for pediatricians. Pediatr Ann 2002;31:437-446.

Lovell DJ: Juvenile rheumatoid arthritis and juvenile spondyloarthropathies. In Klippel JH (ed): Primer on the Rheumatic Diseases, 12th ed. Atlanta, Arthritis Foundation, 2001, pp 534-542.

Murray KJ, Lovell DJ: Advanced therapy for juvenile arthritis. Best Pract Res Clin Rheumatol 2002;16:361-378.

Prahalad S, Glass DN: Is juvenile rheumatoid arthritis/juvenile idiopathic arthritis different from rheumatoid arthritis? Arthritis Res 2002;4(Suppl 3):303-310.

Reiff AO: Developments in the treatment of juvenile arthritis. Expert Opin Pharmacother 2004;5:1485-1496.

Schneider R, Passo MH: Juvenile rheumatoid arthritis. Rheum Dis Clin North Am 2002;28:503-530.

Weiss JE, Ilowite NT: Juvenile idiopathic arthritis. Pediatr Clin North Am 2005;52:413-442.

REFERENCES

1. Cassidy JR, Petty RE: Chronic arthritis in childhood. In Textbook of Pediatric Rheumatology, 5th ed. Philadelphia, WB Saunders, 2005, pp 206-260.
2. McGhee JL, Burks FN, Sheckels JL, Jarvis JN: Identifying children with chronic arthritis based on chief complaints: Absence of predictive value for musculoskeletal pain as an indicator of rheumatic disease in children. Pediatrics 2002;110:354-359.
3. Grom AA: Natural killer cell dysfunction: A common pathway in systemic-onset juvenile rheumatoid arthritis, macrophage activation syndrome, and hemophagocytic lymphohistiocytosis? Arthritis Rheum 2004;50:689-698.
4. Oen K, Malleson PN, Cabral DA, et al: Early predictors of longterm outcome in patients with juvenile rheumatoid arthritis: Subset-specific correlations. J Rheumatol 2003;30:585-593.
5. Hashkes PJ, Laxer RM: Medical treatment of juvenile idiopathic arthritis. JAMA 2005;294:1671-1684.
6. Section on Rheumatology and Section on Ophthalmology: Guidelines for ophthalmologic examinations in children with juvenile rheumatoid arthritis. Pediatrics 1993;92:295-296.

CHAPTER 106

Postinfectious Arthritis

James A. Nard and Laura J. Mirkinson

Acute arthritis resulting from infection is typically categorized as septic, reactive, or postinfectious. Septic arthritis is diagnosed when any infectious agent is recovered from synovial fluid (see Chapter 70). Reactive arthritis is an autoimmune response to an infectious agent that is remote from the joints. Unlike in septic arthritis, pathogens are not recoverable from the synovial space. In postinfectious arthritis, which is often considered a form of reactive arthritis, a preceding or concurrent infection triggers an immune response, causing inflammation of the joints. There is clearly some overlap between the syndromes of acute reactive arthritis and postinfectious arthritis. In addition, aspects of the relationship between these infectious entities and chronic arthritis in children are still evolving. For the purposes of this chapter, reactive and postinfectious arthritis are considered together. Although these entities by themselves rarely require hospitalization, hospitalists are often confronted with diagnostic challenges involved in their presentation. Patients presenting with joint disease may have a limb- or life-threatening process, or the joint disease may be just one aspect of a complex clinical picture.

CLINICAL PRESENTATION

Patients may present with an isolated articular process or with coexisting extra-articular findings (Table 106-1). Characteristics of the joint complaints should be pursued, including duration, nature, severity, limitations of function, and factors that relieve or exacerbate the symptoms. Questions regarding nonarticular symptoms, malaise, weight loss, precedent or concomitant illnesses (especially diarrheal or upper respiratory tract infections), or infectious exposures should be included. If there is a history of fever, the pattern of fever should be determined. Rashes are also an important focus for the history. The patient should be prompted to recall rashes that may have preceded the presentation of the arthritis by days (e.g., erythema marginatum of acute rheumatic fever), weeks, or months (e.g., erythema migrans of Lyme disease).

The physical examination may reveal joint swelling, erythema, decreased range of motion, or pain on active or passive motion of the joints. Joint involvement may be limited to a single joint (monoarticular), four or fewer joints (pauciarticular), or more than four joints (polyarticular). *Migratory arthritis* is the term used when there is sequential involvement of single joints over time, usually days to weeks. At times, distinguishing between large and small joint involvement is helpful in making the diagnosis and guiding further evaluation. The term *arthralgia* is used when the patient localizes pain to a joint, with or without motion, but the examiner does not detect swelling or redness. Arthralgia may coexist in joints other than the presenting arthritic joint.

If acute rheumatic fever is a diagnostic consideration, important physical findings such as nodules on the extensor surfaces, erythema marginatum, and a pathologic murmur should be sought.

DIFFERENTIAL DIAGNOSIS

The main task of the clinician is to differentiate postinfectious or reactive arthritis from the more chronic arthritides such as juvenile inflammatory (rheumatoid) arthritis, juvenile psoriatic arthritis, and spondyloarthropathy. Table 106-2 lists some of the entities that should be considered. The chronicity of the symptoms and other clinical, laboratory, and radiographic findings usually allow the clinician to distinguish these chronic conditions from postinfectious arthritis. The differential diagnosis of new-onset childhood arthritis should include malignancies.

Viral arthritides are often migratory and polyarticular and may include a prominent component of arthralgia. Viral entities to consider include Epstein-Barr, hepatitis B, parvovirus B19, and rubella (almost exclusively vaccine-related in immunized communities). Respiratory infections due to atypical bacteria (e.g., *Mycoplasma pneumoniae*, *Chlamydia pneumoniae*) and gastrointestinal infections due to bacterial agents such as *Yersinia enterocolitica* and *Salmonella* species are also associated with postinfectious arthritis. Aside from the septic arthritis that can complicate bacteremia, bloodstream infections with *Neisseria meningitidis*, *Neisseria gonorrhoeae*, or *Haemophilus influenzae* can cause sterile, reactive arthritis.[1]

Periarticular processes such as overlying cellulitis, fractures, or destructive bone lesions can mimic joint disease. Adjacent osteomyelitis can cause an inflammatory intra-articular synovitis that may be sterile.

Some of the arthritides associated with specific diseases are discussed in the following section.

SPECIFIC INFECTIOUS CAUSES

Parvovirus B19

Parvovirus B19 is the infectious agent that causes erythema infectiosum, also known as fifth disease. During the stage of viremia, patients may present with a nonspecific febrile illness or may be asymptomatic. Infection of red blood cell precursors may lead to reticulocytopenia. The viremia resolves with the appearance of immunoglobulin M (IgM) antibodies, but this may herald the appearance of the postinfectious rash, arthritis, or arthralgia. Typical cutaneous findings include facial erythema ("slapped cheek") and a reticular, lacy rash on the trunk and extremities. The joint abnormalities can either accompany or follow the rash;

Table 106-1 Clinical Findings Suggestive of Infection-Related Arthritis

Acute onset
Migratory arthritis
Systemic symptoms
Para-articular swelling
Redness or discoloration out of proportion to swelling
Hip involvement
Painful or erythematous symmetrical polyarticular PIP or MCP involvement with limited swelling (common in viral arthritis)
Intermittent monoarthritis (suggestive of Lyme disease)

MCP, metacarpophalangeal joint; PIP, proximal interphalangeal joint.
From Rose CD, Eppes SC: Infection-related arthritis. Rheum Dis Clin North Am 1997;23:677-695.

Table 106-2 Differential Diagnosis of Reactive Arthritis

Infectious
Viral arthritis
Lyme disease
Septic arthritis
Diseases possibly related to infection
Transient synovitis of the hip
Kawasaki disease
Behçet disease
SAPHO syndrome
Orthopedic and pain syndromes
Legg-Calvé-Perthes disease
Osgood-Schlatter disease
Idiopathic pain syndromes*
Trauma (effusion, hemarthrosis, bursitis, fracture)
Malignancy
Neuroblastoma
Leukemia
Lymphoma
Idiopathic arthritides
Juvenile chronic arthritis
Spondyloarthropathies
Psoriatic arthritis
Inflammatory bowel disease

*Includes complex regional pain syndrome (previously known as reflex sympathetic dystrophy) and fibromyalgia.
SAPHO, synovitis, acne, pustulosis, hyperostosis, and osteomyelitis.
Adapted from Burgos-Vargas R, Vázquez-Mellado J: Reactive arthritis. In Cassidy JT, Petty RE (eds): Textbook of Pediatric Rheumatology, 4th ed. Philadelphia, WB Saunders, 2001, p 685.

Table 106-3 Comparison of Poststreptococcal Reactive Arthritis (PSRA) and Acute Rheumatic Fever (ARF)

	PSRA	ARF
Antecedent GABHS infection	Yes	Yes
Onset of arthritis after infection	<2 wk	2-3 wk
Migratory arthritis	No	Yes
Axial arthritis	Yes	No
Cardiac involvement	6%	50%
Response to ASA	Not dramatic	Dramatic

ASA, acetylsalicylic acid; GABHS, group A β-hemolytic streptococcal.
Adapted from Ahmed S, Ayoub EM, Scornick JC, et al: Poststreptococcal reactive arthritis: Clinical characteristics and association with HLA-DR alleles. Arthritis Rheum 1998;41:1096-1102.

Table 106-4 Prophylaxis for Poststreptococcal Reactive Arthritis (PSRA) and Acute Rheumatic Fever (ARF)

Diagnosis	Associated Findings	Duration of Prophylaxis
PSRA	No carditis	5 yr, or until age 21
ARF	No carditis	5 yr, or until age 21
ARF	Carditis	10 yr, or well into adulthood
ARF	Carditis, residual heart disease	10 yr, and at least until age 40

indicated by an elevated IgM parvovirus titer. In contrast, IgG antibodies appear after IgM and remain detectable for life, making them less useful in distinguishing recent from past infection. A specific polymerase chain reaction test is now available and may aid in making the diagnosis.

Poststreptococcal Reactive Arthritis and Acute Rheumatic Fever

Acute rheumatic fever (ARF) was one of the first well-documented forms of postinfectious arthritis. Some consider poststreptococcal reactive arthritis (PSRA) to be a distinct entity from ARF, whereas others consider them to be two points on a spectrum of noninfectious sequelae of group A β-hemolytic infection (Table 106-3). A more complete discussion of ARF can be found in Chapter 87.

The arthritis of ARF is exquisitely painful and migratory. PSRA has a more acute onset and a more prolonged course (several weeks to several months) than the arthritis of ARF and commonly affects the knees, ankles, and hands. It can be monoarticular or polyarticular, tends to be asymmetrical, and is not commonly migratory. Some believe that the distinction between PSRA and ARF is important with regard to prognosis and long-term therapy; however, both require long-term antibiotic prophylaxis (Table 106-4).[2]

Lyme Disease

The spirochete *Borrelia burgdorferi*, the cause of Lyme disease, is transmitted via the deer tick. This arachnid vector is classically found in woodland areas in the temperate

they can also occur in the absence of rash. The form of arthritis may be polyarticular, pauciarticular, or occasionally monoarticular. Large joints such as the hips and knees, as well as the small joints of the hands, are more commonly affected. Younger children tend to have an asymmetrical pattern, whereas older children and adults are more likely to develop symmetrical joint involvement. A positive antinuclear antibody titer is not uncommon. Recent infection is

Table 106-5 Stages of Lyme Disease
Early Localized
Erythema migrans
Early Disseminated
Cardiac
Atrioventricular block
Myocarditis
Nervous system
Meningitis
Optic neuritis
Cranial neuropathy
Radiculopathy
Peripheral neuritis
Mononeuritis multiplex
Cerebellar ataxia
Myelitis
Cutaneous
Disseminated multiple erythema migrans
Ocular
Uveitis
Iritis
Late
Arthritis
Encephalitis, encephalopathy

regions of the Northern Hemisphere, but the geographic area of Lyme disease is continually expanding.

Clinical features of Lyme disease form the basis for its staging (Table 106-5). The early localized phase is characterized by the appearance of erythema migrans; this may be accompanied by influenza-like symptoms. Erythema migrans is pathognomonic of Lyme disease and appears days to weeks after the tick bite; however in 30% of patients, it is never identified. Frequently, the serology is negative at this stage. The early disseminated stage occurs weeks to months after the initial infection and is characterized by extra-articular manifestations involving the heart, eyes, and central and peripheral nervous systems.[3-5]

The arthritis of late disseminated Lyme disease occurs in 60% to 70% of untreated patients. The onset is typically months to years into the illness and presents as a monoarticular process involving the knee in approximately 70% of childhood cases.[3-5] Classically, the knee findings include marked edema and effusion but limited erythema. The range of motion is limited mostly by the magnitude of the effusion. Typically, the physical findings are more dramatic than the pain.

A migratory polyarticular pattern can develop over time, and the joint involvement often becomes more prolonged and chronic. The knees, elbows, wrists, hips, shoulders, and ankles are most often affected. Diagnostic testing is complicated by the considerable variability in the sensitivity and specificity of serologic tests. For this reason, an enzyme-linked immunosorbent assay (ELISA), which has a high false-positive rate, needs to be confirmed by Western blot testing. Detection of *B. bergdorferi* by polymerase chain reaction from sterile fluids is not reliable for diagnosis.

Transient Synovitis of the Hip

Transient synovitis of the hip, also known as toxic synovitis or irritable hip syndrome, is a commonly diagnosed but poorly understood entity. It may actually reflect several entities, and many believe that it is a postviral reactive arthritis. This self-limited condition typically occurs in children 3 to 10 years of age; they present with joint pain with motion or ambulation, limp, or refusal to bear weight or walk.[6,7] The symptoms usually resolve within 1 week. A small number of children with transient synovitis go on to develop Perthes disease, but a causal relationship has not been well established.[8] The major challenge is distinguishing this benign entity from septic arthritis. Recent publications have created validated prediction models for differentiating them.[9]

EVALUATION

The evaluation of postinfectious arthritis is based on a thorough history, physical examination, and limited laboratory studies. Screening laboratory tests often include a complete blood count; inflammatory markers such as C-reactive protein and erythrocyte sedimentation rate can be helpful but are generally nonspecific. Many physicians are reassured by normal values for serum uric acid and lactate dehydrogenase when there is concern about malignancy. An elevated white blood cell count, especially with a predominance of neutrophils (segmented or band forms), is suggestive of an acute infectious process such as septic arthritis and is less typical of reactive arthritis. Chronic inflammation can be associated with elevations in erythrocyte sedimentation rate, platelet count, and anemia, but these laboratory abnormalities are nonspecific and overlap with other entities such as malignancy.

The laboratory evaluation for reactive or postinfectious arthritis should be targeted. It can be guided by the clinical picture, infectious exposures, and the need for treatment of either the primary arthritis or the nonarthritic component of the illness. Tests may include IgM titers for parvovirus B19 and serologic studies for Lyme disease, Epstein-Barr virus, hepatitis B, and group A β-hemolytic streptococcus (antistreptolysin O, anti-DNAase B). Although the postinfectious arthritis associated with gastrointestinal infection often follows the diarrheal illness, stool cultures may yield the pathogens (e.g., *Salmonella, Campylobacter, Yersinia*). If there are symptoms of urethritis, urinalysis reveals white blood cells secondary to an inflammatory (e.g., Behçet disease) or infectious process. Urine culture, urethral swab for culture, and urine antigen (e.g., *Chlamydia*, gonococcus) studies may be indicated, depending on the overall clinical picture. Nonspecific studies such as antinuclear antibody, rheumatoid factor, and HLA-B27 may be positive but are usually not helpful in achieving a diagnosis.

Prompt joint aspiration is warranted if a septic joint is a consideration. This diagnostic procedure may be helpful in distinguishing other intra-articular processes. Studies of the fluid should include cell count with differential, Gram stain, culture, and glucose level (see Chapter 70).

Radiographic evaluation other than plain films is rarely needed. Plain films of abnormal joints may show soft tissue swelling and osteopenia, but erosions are rarely seen. Magnetic resonance imaging of the affected joint can further

Table 106-6 Recommended Antimicrobial Therapy Regimens for Patients with Lyme Disease

Recommendation, Drug	Dosage for Adults	Dosage for Children
Preferred oral		
Amoxicillin	500 mg tid	50 mg/kg/day divided into 3 doses (maximum, 500 mg/dose)
Doxycycline	100 mg bid*	Age <8 yr: not recommended
		Age ≥8 yr: 1-2 mg/kg bid (maximum, 100 mg/dose)
Alternative oral		
Cefuroxime axetil	500 mg bid	30 mg/kg/day divided into 2 doses (maximum, 500 mg/dose)
Preferred parenteral		
Ceftriaxone	2 g IV once daily	75-100 mg/kg IV per day in a single dose (maximum, 2 g)
Alternative parenteral		
Cefotaxime	2 g IV tid	150-200 mg/kg/day IV divided into 3 or 4 doses (maximum, 6 g/day)
Penicillin G	18-24 million units IV/day divided into doses given q4h†	200,000-400,000 units/kg/day, divided into doses given q4h† (maximum, 18-24 million units/day)

*Tetracyclines are relatively contraindicated for pregnant or lactating women.
†The penicillin dosage should be reduced for patients with impaired renal function.
From Wormser GP, Nadelman RB, Dattwyler RJ, et al: Practice guidelines for the treatment of Lyme disease. The Infectious Diseases Society of America. Clin Infect Dis 2000;31(Suppl 1):1-14.

delineate the arthritis and accompanying tendon abnormalities (enthesitis) and identify bony and soft tissue abnormalities adjacent to the joint.

Chronic forms of childhood arthritis, such as juvenile rheumatoid arthritis and juvenile psoriatic arthritis, carry a risk of eye inflammation, so if these diagnoses are being considered, ophthalmologic evaluation, including a slit-lamp examination, is appropriate. Echocardiography may be helpful if there is concern for valvular dysfunction, which is sometimes seen in ARF.

TREATMENT

Most forms of reactive arthritis are self-resolving over weeks to months and rarely require hospitalization once an acute infectious process has been excluded. For the most part, reactive arthritides and transient synovitis of the hip are well managed with nonsteroidal anti-inflammatory drugs, which provide pain relief and may limit the inflammatory process.[9] If there is a poor response, treatment with glucocorticoids may be necessary.

Other infections associated with extra-articular involvement, such as ARF (see Chapter 87), hepatitis, gonorrhea, *Chlamydia,* and *Salmonella,* have their own specific therapeutic regimens.

Treatment of Lyme disease is based on the stage and the patient's specific condition at presentation. The Infectious Diseases Society of America has created specific guidelines for therapy (Tables 106-6 and 106-7). Success of therapy cannot be measured by antibody titers, because these levels are lifelong. In addition, these are nonprotective antibodies, meaning that reinfection is possible.

Close follow-up as an outpatient should include a thorough evaluation of ongoing inflammatory signs and symptoms, the ability to participate in normal activities, and the potential side effects of therapy. Outpatient physical therapy may be beneficial in maintaining a full range of motion in the involved joints.

CONSULTATION

- Orthopedics: for assistance with the aspiration of joint fluid for diagnostic studies. In the case of septic arthritis, an orthopedic surgeon may be needed for immediate surgical intervention.
- Rheumatology: for assistance in determining the cause of arthritis, initial management, or ongoing outpatient involvement.
- Cardiology: for the diagnosis or management of ARF with carditis.
- Ophthalmology: for the evaluation or management of ocular involvement, such as uveitis.
- Oncology: for assistance with the evaluation or management of malignancy.

ADMISSION CRITERIA

Hospitalization should be considered for the following reasons:

- A diagnosis that requires expeditious evaluation and treatment (e.g., septic arthritis, malignancy).
- ARF with significant carditis or congestive heart failure.
- Pain control that requires parenteral medications.

DISCHARGE CRITERIA

- Exclusion of conditions that require inpatient therapy.
- Adequate control of pain and inflammation.
- Ability to tolerate oral medications.
- Reliable outpatient follow-up with a primary care physician and, if indicated, appropriate subspecialist.

Table 106-7 Recommended Therapy for Patients with Lyme Disease

Indication	Treatment	Duration (days)
Tick bite	None recommended; observe	
Erythema migrans	Oral regimen*,†	14-21
Acute neurologic disease		
Meningitis or radiculopathy	Parenteral regimen*,†	14-28
Cranial nerve palsy	Oral regimen*	14-21
Cardiac disease		
First- or second-degree heart block	Oral regimen*	14-21
Third-degree heart block	Parenteral regimen*,§	14-21
Late disease		
Arthritis without neurologic disease	Oral regimen*	28
Recurrent arthritis after oral regimen	Oral regimen* or parenteral regimen*	28
		14-28
Persistent arthritis after 2 courses of antibiotics	Symptomatic therapy	
Central or peripheral nervous system disease	Parenteral regimen*	14-28
Chronic Lyme disease or post-Lyme disease syndrome	Symptomatic therapy	

*See Table 106-6.

†For adult patients who are intolerant of amoxicillin, doxycycline, and cefuroxime axetil, alternatives are azithromycin (500 mg orally daily for 7-10 days), erythromycin (500 mg orally 4 times per day for 14-21 days), or clarithromycin (500 mg orally twice daily for 14-21 days [except during pregnancy]). The recommended dosages of these agents for children are as follows: azithromycin, 10 mg/kg daily (maximum, 500 mg/d); erythromycin, 12.5 mg/kg 4 times daily (maximum, 500 mg/dose); clarithromycin, 7.5 mg/kg twice daily (maximum, 500 mg/dose). Patients treated with macrolides should be closely followed.

‡For nonpregnant adult patients intolerant of both penicillin and cephalosporins, doxycycline (200-400 mg/d orally [or IV if oral medications cannot be taken], divided into 2 doses) may be adequate.

§A temporary pacemaker may be required.

From Wormser GP, Nadelman RB, Dattwyler RJ, et al: Practice guidelines for the treatment of Lyme disease. The Infectious Diseases Society of America. Clin Infect Dis 2000;31(Suppl 1):1-14.

IN A NUTSHELL

- Postinfectious arthritis is a common condition that may be caused by parvovirus B19, group A streptococcus, and Lyme disease. It can also be caused by myriad other known and unknown infectious agents.
- Postinfectious arthritis must be distinguished from septic arthritis and malignancy.
- Whenever possible, a specific diagnosis is desirable, because this may affect therapy, the duration of the arthritis, and the need to evaluate other organ systems.
- Diagnosis is usually accomplished with a thorough history, physical examination, and selective laboratory evaluation.
- Management consists mainly of nonsteroidal anti-inflammatory drugs. Rarely, patients require hospitalization and aggressive anti-inflammatory therapies.

ON THE HORIZON

- Identification of additional infectious causes of reactive arthritis.
- Evaluation of chemokines and chemokine receptors in reactive arthritis.
- Potential therapy for pain and synovial inflammation with immunomodulatory agents.

SUGGESTED READING

Ayoub E: Acute rheumatic fever and poststreptococcal reactive arthritis. In Cassidy JT, Petty RE (eds): Textbook of Pediatric Rheumatology, 4th ed. Philadelphia, WB Saunders, 2001, pp 690-705.

Rose CD, Eppes SC: Infection-related arthritis. Rheum Dis Clin North Am 1997;23:677-695.

Sigal LH: Pitfalls in the diagnosis and management of Lyme disease. Arthritis Rheum 1998;41:195-204.

Steere AC: Lyme disease. N Engl J Med 2001;345:115-125.

REFERENCES

1. Rose CD, Eppes SC: Infection-related arthritis. Rheum Dis Clin North Am 1997;23:677-695.
2. Poststreptococcal reactive arthritis: Clinical characteristics and association with HLA-DR alleles. Arthritis Rheum 1998;41:1096-1102.
3. Shapiro ED, Gerber MA: Lyme disease. Clin Infect Dis 2000;31:533-542.
4. Sigal LH: Pitfalls in the diagnosis and management of Lyme disease. Arthritis Rheum 1998;41:195-204.
5. Steere AC: Lyme disease. N Engl J Med 2001;345:115-125.
6. Haueisen DC, Weiner DS, Weiner SD: The characterization of "transient synovitis of the hip" in children. J Pediatr Orthop 1986;6:11-17.
7. Briggs RD, Baird KS, Gibson PH: Transient synovitis of the hip joint. J R Coll Surg Edinb 1990;35:48-50.
8. Landin LA, Danielsson LG, Wattsgard C: Transient synovitis of the hip joint: Its incidence, epidemiology, and relation to Perthes' disease. J Bone Joint Surg Br 1987;69:238-242.
9. Kermond S, Fink M, Graham K, et al: A randomized clinical trial: Should the child with transient synovitis of the hip be treated with nonsteroidal anti-inflammatory drugs? Ann Emerg Med 2002;40:294-299.

CHAPTER 107

Systemic Lupus Erythematosus

Stacey E. Bernstein

Systemic lupus erythematosus (SLE) is a chronic multi-system disease characterized by diffuse vasculitis and inflammation of connective tissues that may lead to widespread organ damage affecting the kidneys, brain, and joints. SLE is an autoimmune condition marked by abnormalities of B and T lymphocytes and the complement system. The hallmark of the disease is the production of autoantibodies against nuclear and cytoplasmic antigens that cause tissue damage through the deposition of antigen-antibody complexes, complement activation, and direct antibody- and cell-mediated cytopathicity. Current pathogenic models indicate that the disease evolves through the complex interplay of immune, genetic, infectious, hormonal, and environmental factors.

SLE is more common in adults than in children, with only 20% of cases presenting during childhood and adolescence. In the pediatric population, the illness typically manifests during adolescence and rarely presents before age 5 years. SLE is predominantly a disease of women and girls, with an overall female preponderance of 4.5:1. Female susceptibility increases during the childbearing years and peaks in the third decade of life, when 90% of those with SLE are women. Nonetheless, major organ involvement is increased in children and adolescents when compared with adults. At all ages, the disease can affect people of any ethnic background, but it is more common in African Americans, Asians, and Hispanics.

Neonatal lupus may present owing to the transplacental transfer of immunoglobulin G (IgG) autoantibodies (anti-Ro, anti-La) in pregnant woman with undiagnosed or known connective tissue disorders such as SLE or Sjögren syndrome. Manifestations may include congenital heart block and photosensitive, annular, erythematous cutaneous lesions on the face and scalp. Other less common findings include hepatitis and cytopenia. Most symptoms resolve over 6 months without treatment as the autoantibodies disappear. Only the heart block is permanent and may require cardiac pacing.

CLINICAL PRESENTATION

In 1997 the American College of Rheumatology revised and updated the criteria for the classification of SLE (Table 107-1).[1] The patient must serially or simultaneously have at least 4 of the 11 following features: malar rash, discoid rash, photosensitivity, oral or nasopharyngeal ulcers, arthritis, nephritis, neuropsychiatric symptoms or encephalopathy, serositis, cytopenia, positive immunoserology, and positive antinuclear antibody. These criteria have a sensitivity and specificity of 96% in adults, and they are applied without modification in children even though their use in this population has not been validated. These criteria are by no means exhaustive, and children with SLE may have many other signs and symptoms, varying from alopecia and malaise to hepatosplenomegaly, fever, and hemoptysis.

SLE is variable in its presentation, and symptoms may develop acutely or insidiously. A recent retrospective study of military recruits found that patients developed autoantibodies a mean of 33 months before SLE was recognized and manifested their first symptoms an average of 18 months before diagnosis.[2] In children, cutaneous, renal, hematologic, and musculoskeletal systems are most commonly affected, but any organ may be involved.

DIFFERENTIAL DIAGNOSIS

Owing to the multiorgan involvement and the wide range of clinical presentations, many illnesses must be considered in children manifesting signs or symptoms of SLE. In general, other inflammatory conditions such as juvenile rheumatoid arthritis, acute rheumatic fever, systemic vasculitides, mixed connective tissue diseases, infections (especially Epstein-Barr virus, parvovirus B19, and human immunodeficiency virus [HIV]), and malignancies (leukemia, lymphoma) must be excluded before a diagnosis of SLE can be confirmed. Drug-induced lupus can be precipitated by certain medications such as hydralazine, anticonvulsants, and antibiotics (isoniazid, penicillin, sulfonamides). The symptoms are usually self-limited and resolve when the drug is discontinued.

EVALUATION

Tables 107-2 and 107-3 outline the investigations to consider when diagnosing and evaluating a patient with suspected SLE.

COURSE OF ILLNESS

SLE is a chronic disease with an often unpredictable remitting and relapsing course. In general, lupus that presents during childhood tends to have multisystem involvement, a more severe onset, and a more aggressive clinical course than does adult SLE. After the first 1 to 2 years of disease, new organs tend not to be involved, with the exception of the central nervous system. Chronic, daily symptoms of fatigue, anorexia, arthralgia, and arthritis are common complaints among patients with SLE. Hair loss, Raynaud phenomenon, oral ulcers, and dermatitis are other frequent manifestations of this insidious disease.

The long-term prognosis is related to renal disease and central nervous system involvement, which are the main causes of morbidity. Poor renal outcomes are associated with hypertension, impairment of renal function at diagnosis,

Table 107-1 American College of Rheumatology Criteria for the Diagnosis of Systemic Lupus Erythematosus

Criterion	Distinguishing Characteristics
Malar rash	"Butterfly" rash—red, flat or raised, symmetrical rash that covers the nasal bridge and cheeks but spares the nasolabial folds; photosensitive; rarely scars; most common skin manifestation
Discoid rash	Asymmetrical erythematous raised patches with scales and follicular plugging on the face, scalp, and limbs; photosensitive; scars; isolated discoid lupus is rare in childhood
Photosensitivity	Any rash with an unusually dramatic reaction to sunlight
Oral lesions	Typically shallow, painless ulcers of the hard palate, oral mucosa, or nose
Arthritis	Generally symmetrical synovitis of two or more joints (both large and small), especially the fingers, wrists, and knees; permanent deformities and erosions are uncommon
Serositis	Serosal inflammation and effusions of the pleura or pericardium
Renal disorder	Proteinuria >0.5 g/day, cellular casts, hematuria, hypertension, nephrotic syndrome, renal failure; seen in 85%-100% of patients, often during the first year following diagnosis
Neurologic disorder	Seizures and psychosis define the classification criterion, but there may be a broad array of peripheral and central nervous system pathology (e.g., headache, chorea, stroke, transverse myelitis, mononeuritis multiplex)
Hematologic disorder	Autoimmune hemolytic anemia, leukopenia, lymphopenia, or thrombocytopenia
Antinuclear antibody	Antibodies to nuclear antigens seen in close to 100% of cases, but also seen in many other infectious and inflammatory conditions
Immunologic disorder	Anti-DNA, anti-Smith antigen, or antiphospholipid antibodies (anticardiolipin, lupus anticoagulant, false-positive test for syphilis for 6 mo)

Adapted from Tan EM, Cohen AS, Fries JF, et al: The 1982 revised criteria for the classification of SLE. Arthritis Rheum 1982;25:1271-1277.

and specific renal biopsy findings such as diffuse proliferative lupus nephritis (Table 107-4). Although serologic markers do not generally correlate with disease activity, high titers of anti-double-stranded DNA and falling complement levels are potential markers for worsening disease.

The 2-year mortality of SLE approached 100% in the early 1960s. With the use of immunosuppressive treatments and improved management of chronic renal failure, mortality dropped to 15% in the 1980s. These increased survival rates are accompanied by greater morbidity secondary to the side effects of medications, end-organ damage, and the development of comorbid conditions. In fact, children with lupus are at particularly high risk for accelerated atherosclerosis, cerebrovascular accident, and myocardial infarction as they age. Risk factors include prolonged use of steroids, coronary vasculitis, obesity, hypertension, lupus nephritis, hyperlipidemia, lupus anticoagulant, and family history of cardiac disease.

Overwhelming infection is the most frequent cause of mortality among children with SLE, and those with active disease are at the greatest risk of developing an infection.[3] Children with SLE are immunocompromised by the disease itself (neutropenia, hypocomplementemia, functional asplenia) as well as by the immunosuppression of steroids and other cytotoxic agents (e.g., cyclophosphamide). High-dose steroids may mask the signs of a serious infection, so children with SLE and fever should generally receive broad-spectrum antibiotics while physicians attempt to distinguish between a lupus flare and an acute infection. Other major causes of mortality include nephritis, central nervous system disease, pulmonary hemorrhage, and myocardial infarction.

TREATMENT

Early diagnosis and treatment can significantly improve the prognosis of children with SLE. Goals of therapy include optimizing disease control and reducing irreversible end-organ damage while remaining mindful of the morbidity associated with the treatments themselves. Consistent and close monitoring of patients is critical for long-term management. Early detection and treatment of flares of disease and ongoing counseling and education can help patients maintain their normal lifestyle and activities.

Corticosteroids are the cornerstone of treatment. High-dose steroids (prednisone 1 to 2 mg/kg per day) and intravenous pulse methylprednisolone are used for acutely ill patients. As with all patients on prolonged glucocorticoid therapy, during periods of physiologic stress (e.g., surgery, fever), increased doses of corticosteroids are required owing to the chronic hypophyseal-pituitary axis suppression. Steroids have numerous undesirable side effects, including avascular necrosis, osteoporosis, psychosis, proximal muscle weakness, hyperlipidemia, gastritis, glucose intolerance, cataracts, and growth failure. The cosmetic complications of acne, hirsutism, striae, cushingoid facies, and obesity are particularly distressing to adolescents, who may be noncompliant with the medical regimen.

Immunosuppressive drugs are used when glucocorticoids alone are insufficient to control the disease and for their steroid-sparing effect. These medications are also used for severe organ involvement, with the goal of preventing morbidity and mortality. The most common indications are acute lupus nephritis (especially diffuse proliferative

Table 107-2 Investigations to Consider in the Evaluation and Diagnosis of Systemic Lupus Erythematosus

Investigation	Significance
ESR, CRP, C3 and C4	ESR, CRP, complement elevated as nonspecific measures of inflammation; hypocomplementemia reflects active nephritis
Autoantibodies, immunoglobulins, Coombs test, CBC with differential, smear, reticulocyte count	See Table 107-3 for a list of autoantibodies; immunoglobulins are elevated due to polyclonal activation of B lymphocytes
INR, PTT, PT	Prolongation of the PTT is the screening test for the lupus anticoagulant, which in vivo causes a hypercoagulable state
Cholesterol, triglycerides, HDL, LDL	Dyslipidemia associated with disease and treatment
Liver function tests	Abnormality more likely due to medication toxicity than to SLE
Urinalysis, urea, creatinine, albumin, total protein; 24-hr urine collection for protein and creatinine clearance; renal biopsy	Almost all children with SLE have some degree of renal involvement, which should be characterized with a renal biopsy before therapy is initiated; the extent and severity of nephritis is quantified according to the World Health Organization classification system (see Table 107-4)
Chest radiograph, pulmonary function tests	Asymptomatic pneumonitis may be present at diagnosis, or pulmonary hemorrhage may develop during the course of the disease
Radiograph of involved joint	Diagnostic joint aspiration rarely necessary unless there is concern about infection
Echocardiogram, ECG	Cardiac disease associated with SLE (serositis) and complications of disease (infection, atherosclerosis)
Bone marrow biopsy	May be required to rule out malignancy or infection that could mimic manifestations of SLE
Neuroimaging: CT; MRI, MRA, MRV; single-photon emission computed tomography (SPECT) Lumbar puncture (LP) Electroencephalogram (EEG)	No consensus on imaging for evaluation of CNS disease; CT or MRI to rule out structural anomalies and assess for infarction; SPECT to evaluate neuropsychiatric symptoms; LP to rule out infection (primary, opportunistic); EEG for patients with seizures

CBC, complete blood count; CNS, central nervous system; CRP, C-reactive protein; CT, computed tomography; ECG, electrocardiogram; ESR, erythrocyte sedimentation rate; HDL, high-density lipoprotein; INR, international normalized ratio; LDL, low-density lipoprotein; MRA, magnetic resonance angiography; MRI, magnetic resonance imaging; MRV, magnetic resonance venography; PT, prothrombin time; PTT, partial thromboplastin time; SLE, systemic lupus erythematosus.

glomerulonephritis), pulmonary hemorrhage, and severe neuropsychiatric disease. Specific drugs include cyclophosphamide, azathioprine, methotrexate, cyclosporine, and newer agents such as mycophenolate mofetil. Monthly intravenous cyclophosphamide is one of the major factors contributing to improved outcomes among children with SLE nephritis today, even though it is a particularly toxic medication that increases the risk of malignancy, infection, and infertility. Immunosuppressive medications are also used as steroid-sparing agents to facilitate the tapering of glucocorticoids. They should be considered in patients with chronic active disease when the daily dose of prednisone cannot be weaned to less than 0.5 mg/kg per day after 6 months or when the steroid side effects become intolerable to the patient or the family.[4] The benefits of these medications must always be weighed against their significant potential for toxicity, including hair loss, nausea, infection, malignancy, and irreversible gonadal dysfunction.

Hydroxychloroquine, an antimalarial drug, is a disease modifier that can prevent relapses.[5] It is also beneficial for the rashes and arthritis of SLE and improves patients' dyslipoproteinemia. Hydroxychloroquine is contraindicated in patients with glucose-6-phosphate dehydrogenase (G6PD) deficiency, and it has specific retinal toxicity. Patients must be tested for G6PD before starting hydroxychloroquine, and a biannual ophthalmic examination is required for patients taking this drug.

Other treatments are useful for specific problems. Arthritis in SLE usually responds well to medications aimed at treating other organ-specific disease. Isolated joint involvement can be managed with nonsteroidal anti-inflammatory drugs, although patients with SLE are at increased risk for hepatotoxic side effects from this class of medication. Physiotherapy is important for the treatment of arthritis and muscle weakness. Antipsychotics and anticonvulsants may be necessary as adjunctive therapy to control neuropsychiatric lupus. Hypertension must be treated aggressively because it accelerates the development of renal failure due to lupus nephritis. Vasodilators can be used to treat Raynaud phenomenon, and intravenous immunoglobulin can be beneficial in patients with autoimmune thrombocytopenia.

Preventive management is critical. This includes avoiding sun exposure, which is one of the triggers of lupus flares. Patients are advised to use the highest SPF, water-resistant, ultraviolet A and B protective sunscreen available. It is essential to promote a healthy lifestyle by discouraging smoking

Table 107-3 Autoantibodies in Systemic Lupus Erythematosus

Autoantibodies	Significance
Antinuclear antibody	Sensitive (almost universally positive) but not specific (also positive in infection, malignancy, other inflammatory conditions in the normal population); high negative predictive value when screening for SLE (if negative, SLE is unlikely)
Anti-double-stranded DNA	Specific but not sensitive: positive in 50%-70% of children at the time of presentation with SLE and in a higher percentage during the course of the illness; may correlate with disease activity (especially nephritis)
Antiphospholipid antibodies	Seen in 65% of children with SLE, with higher titers correlating with increased morbidity; associated with venous or arterial thrombosis, recurrent fetal loss, thrombocytopenia, transverse myelitis, and Libman-Sacks endocarditis; assays for detection of antiphospholipid antibodies include PTT with mixing studies, Russell viper venom time, kaolin clotting time, VDRL, ELISA for cardiolipin or phospholipid binding protein
Anti-Ro (Anti-SS-A) Anti-La (Anti-SS-B)	Seen in 20%-30% of adults with SLE, as well as in Sjögren syndrome and neonatal lupus erythematosus, in which it is associated with heart block
Anti-Sm (Smith)	Very specific but not sensitive: positive in <50% of children with SLE
Anti-RNP	Characteristic of mixed connective tissue disease; when seen in SLE, correlates with myositis, esophageal dysmotility, Raynaud phenomenon, interstitial lung disease, sclerodactyly
Antihistone	Typical of drug-induced lupus (e.g., anticonvulsants, sulfonamides, hydralazine)
Antiribosomal P, antineuronal antibodies	Seen in CNS disease of various causes, including SLE, schizophrenia, rheumatic fever
Rheumatoid factor	Positive in 15%-30% of adults with SLE; uncommon in children.

CNS, central nervous system; ELISA, enzyme-linked immunosorbent assay; PTT, partial thromboplastin time; SLE, systemic lupus erythematosus.

Table 107-4 World Health Organization Histopathologic Classification of Renal Disease

Class	Description
I	Normal
II	Mesangial nephritis
III	Focal proliferative lupus nephritis
IV	Diffuse proliferative lupus nephritis
V	Membranous nephritis

and encouraging exercise, weight control, and a balanced diet. Patients should wear medical alert bracelets. Adolescent females must be counseled about the adverse effects that the disease and immunosuppressive medications may have on pregnancy, as well as the increased risks to pregnant women with active SLE. Patients should receive inactivated vaccines, including immunizations against *Pneumococcus,* hepatitis B, and influenza. Live vaccines should not be administered to patients with active disease or those on high-dose steroids or immunosuppressive agents. Vitamin D and calcium should be administered to patients on steroids who lack a well-rounded diet or sufficient calcium intake, to prevent osteoporosis. Bone density can be monitored with dual-energy x-ray absorptiometry scans. Osteoporosis prophylaxis with bisphosphonates is controversial in pediatric patients, although these medications may be included in regimens for the treatment of fractures. Patients with positive antiphospholipid antibodies are treated with low-dose acetylsalicylic acid. Patients with a history of thrombosis should receive anticoagulation.

As with any complex systemic disease, children with SLE must be followed closely by an interdisciplinary team composed of physicians, dieticians, occupational or physical therapists, social workers, psychologists, and nurses. This is important for many reasons, including the following:

- To monitor for disease flares and follow markers of disease activity.
- To assess and minimize end-organ damage.
- To review medications, reinforce drug compliance, wean steroids, and watch for medication-related complications.
- To monitor growth and development, which may be adversely affected by the underlying disease, the treatment (e.g., steroids), and comorbid conditions such as autoimmune hypothyroidism.
- To perform longitudinal neurocognitive function testing to follow school performance and optimize access to special programs.
- To assess quality of life and how the patient and the family are coping with this chronic disease.

CONSULTATION

- Rheumatology: to provide follow-up by a subspecialist experienced in the recognition and management of the diverse manifestations of SLE.
- Nephrology: to monitor and treat renal involvement.

- Hematology: to treat significant cytopenias or investigate the cause of hematologic abnormalities.
- Neurology: to assist in distinguishing neurologic signs of SLE from toxic manifestations of medications.
- Ophthalmology: to treat retinal vasculitis and scleritis (which may be manifestations of the underlying disease) and to monitor for complications of specific treatments, such as steroids (cataracts, glaucoma) and hydroxychloroquine (retinal damage).
- Coagulation: to treat hypercoagulability due to antiphospholipid antibodies.
- Psychiatry: to evaluate and treat psychosis due to neuropsychiatric lupus.

ADMISSION CRITERIA

Hospitalization of a child with SLE may be necessary for any of the following reasons:

- Investigations at presentation if the diagnosis is unclear or the patient is unwell.
- Discrimination between lupus flare and acute or opportunistic infection.
- Active disease that cannot be managed on an outpatient basis.
- Treatment of target organ damage, such as pulmonary hemorrhage, cerebrovascular accident, psychosis.

DISCHARGE CRITERIA

- Diagnostic workup is complete, subspecialty consultations are obtained, and treatment is initiated.
- Any acute infection, lupus flare, or new end-organ involvement is stabilized and treated.
- Patient and family have been instructed regarding the disease, medications, and diet.
- Follow-up appointments have been arranged.

IN A NUTSHELL

- SLE is a chronic multisystem autoimmune disease with widespread manifestations.
- Diagnosis is made when a patient serially or simultaneously meets at least 4 of the 11 established classification criteria.
- The prognosis of SLE is improving, but children with lupus continue to suffer significant morbidity and mortality related to infection and renal and central nervous system disease.
- Steroids and immunosuppressive steroid-sparing agents are the mainstays of treatment.

ON THE HORIZON

- Well-designed studies allowing the development of consensus treatment protocols for childhood lupus.
- Development of new agents to improve the risk-benefit ratio of treatment by enhancing the specificity of immunosuppression, including monoclonal anticytokine antibodies (e.g., anti-IL-10 antibodies), biologic response modifiers targeting lymphocyte costimulatory molecules (e.g., abetacept, anti-CTLA4-Ig), and small immunoregulatory molecules (e.g., abetimus sodium).
- Autologous stem cell transplantation for patients with intractable SLE.

SUGGESTED READING

Arbuckle MR, McClain MT, Rubertone MV, et al: Development of autoantibodies before the clinical onset of systemic lupus erythematosus. N Engl J Med 2003;349:1526-1533.

Cervera R, Khamashta MA, Font J, et al: Morbidity and mortality in systemic lupus erythematosus during a 10-year period: A comparison of early and late manifestations in a cohort of 1000 patients. Medicine (Baltimore) 2003;82:299-308.

Klein-Gitelman M, Reiff A, Silverman ED: Systemic lupus erythematosus in childhood. Rheum Dis Clin North Am 2002;28:561-577.

Lee T, von Scheven E, Sandborg C: Systemic lupus erythematosus and antiphospholipid syndrome in children and adolescents. Curr Opin Rheumatol 2001;13:415-421.

Tan EM, Cohen AS, Fries JF, et al: The 1982 revised criteria for the classification of systemic lupus erythematosus. Arthitis Rheum 1982;25:1271-1277.

Tucker LB: Controversies and advances in the management of systemic lupus erythematosus in children and adolescents. Best Pract Res Clin Rheumatol 2002;16:471-480.

REFERENCES

1. Tan EM, Cohen AS, Fries JF, et al: The 1982 revised criteria for the classification of systemic lupus erythematosus. Arthitis Rheum 1982;25:1271-1277.

2. Arbuckle MR, McClain MT, Rubertone MV, et al: Development of autoantibodies before the clinical onset of systemic lupus erythematosus. N Engl J Med 2003;349:1526-1533.

3. Lacks S, White P: Morbidity associated with childhood systemic lupus erythematosus. J Rheumatol 1990;17:941-945.

4. Lehman TJ, Onel K: Intermittent intravenous cyclophosphamide arrests progression of the renal chronicity index in childhood systemic lupus erythematosus. J Pediatr 2000;136:243-247.

5. Canadian Hydroxchloroquine Study Group: A randomized study of the effect of withdrawing hydroxychloroquine sulfate in systemic lupus erythematosus. N Engl J Med 1991;324:150-154.

CHAPTER *108*

Acute Renal Failure

Melissa J. Gregory

Acute renal failure (ARF) is a sudden decline in renal function with associated increases in metabolic waste products such as blood urea nitrogen (BUN) and serum creatinine. It can occur with or without changes in urine output. *Oliguria*, defined as either urine output less than 1 mL/kg/hr in infants and younger children or daily urine output less than 200 mL/m^2/24 hr in older children, occurs in approximately 25% of hospitalized children with ARF.[1] *Anuria*, or complete absence of urine output, is less common and occurs in 15% of hospitalized children with ARF. Non-oliguric renal failure accounts for the majority of cases of pediatric ARF.

PATHOPHYSIOLOGY

There are multiple causes of ARF in children. Classically, the causes are grouped into three main categories: prerenal, intrinsic, and postrenal, which is also referred to as obstructive (Table 108-1). Prerenal azotemia is probably the most common overall cause of ARF in children and occurs when renal perfusion is inadequate. Decreased renal perfusion can occur as a result of decreased circulating blood volume, as seen in dehydration and acute blood loss, or as a result of hypotension, as seen in sepsis and congestive heart failure. This decrease in renal perfusion leads to decreased glomerular perfusion and filtration with resultant decreases in urine output and increases in BUN and serum creatinine. Prerenal ARF can quickly be reversed by correction of the primary defect, such as administration of intravenous fluids in the case of dehydration or pressors in the case of hypotension. However, prolonged severe decreases in renal perfusion can lead to acute tubular necrosis and intrinsic renal failure.

Intrinsic renal failure occurs when renal injury from any cause has damaged the kidney such that it is unable to maintain normal function. In hospitalized children, acute tubular necrosis is the most common cause of intrinsic renal failure and has replaced hemolytic uremic syndrome (HUS) as the most common primary renal disease causing ARF in children in industrialized countries. However, other primary renal diseases such as glomerulonephritis, toxins, drugs, and systemic diseases can also cause ARF. In all forms of intrinsic ARF there is a substantial decrease in renal blood flow, although the factors leading to this reduction have not been

clearly defined.[1] Vasoactive compounds such as nitric oxide and endothelin are thought to have a role. In children with multiorgan failure, activation of the inflammatory cascade with subsequent release of a variety of cytokines, oxygen radicals, enzymes, and adhesion molecules is also thought to have a role.

Obstructive causes of renal failure exist when there is distal blockage of the urinary tract. Unilateral obstruction rarely causes ARF because the nonobstructed kidney is usually able to adequately regulate water and electrolyte homeostasis. Posterior urethral valves are the most common cause of congenital obstructive renal failure and may also be associated with varying degrees of intrinsic renal disease. In hospitalized patients, obstruction by an indwelling bladder catheter is the most common cause of postrenal ARF.

CLINICAL PRESENTATION

The clinical presentation of ARF varies, depending on the cause of the renal failure. Patients with prerenal ARF present with a history of either excessive fluid loss, such as diarrhea and vomiting or severe burns, inadequate fluid intake, or loss of effective circulating volume, as seen in congestive heart failure and after major surgery. Neonates with obstructive ARF may have a history of abnormal prenatal ultrasound findings or decreased amniotic fluid during pregnancy. Older children may have a history of nephrolithiasis or complain of either suprapubic pain or flank pain.

The presentation of children with intrinsic ARF is quite variable. Patients with acute tubular necrosis may have a history of severe hypotension or ischemia, or both. They may also have been exposed to nephrotoxic drugs or toxins. HUS presents with a several-day history of bloody diarrhea and abdominal pain with concurrent pallor, bruising, and irritability (see Chapter 111), although some forms of this disease occur without diarrhea. In glomerulonephritis, there is usually gross hematuria and, frequently, edema. A history of a streptococcal infection within the past 2 to 3 weeks suggests postinfectious glomerulonephritis. Headache and visual changes from hypertension may also be present. Pyelonephritis usually presents with fever, dysuria, urgency, frequency, and foul-smelling urine. Pulmonary-renal syndromes such as Wegener granulomatosis and Goodpasture

Table 108-1   Causes of Acute Renal Failure

Prerenal
Dehydration
Hypotension
Congestive heart failure
Severe burns
Sepsis
Gastrointestinal hemorrhage

Renal
Acute tubular necrosis
Hemolytic uremic syndrome
Glomerulonephritis
    Postinfectious glomerulonephritis
    Systemic lupus erythematosus
    Membranoproliferative glomerulonephritis
    IgA nephropathy
    Henoch-Schönlein purpura
Pulmonary-renal syndromes
    Wegener granulomatosis
    Goodpasture syndrome
Acute interstitial nephritis
Nephrotoxins
    Drugs: aminoglycosides, cyclosporine, amphotericin B, cisplatin
    Toxins: ethylene glycol, heavy metals
    Pigments: hemolysis, rhabdomyolysis

Postrenal (Obstructive)
Bladder calculi
Posterior urethral valves
Bladder catheter obstruction
Neurogenic bladder

Table 108-2   Normal Age-Specific Values of Serum Creatinine and Creatinine Clearance

	Serum Creatinine (mg/dL)	Creatinine Clearance (mL/min/1.73 m²)
Preterm infants		
<2 weeks	0.7-1.4	11-28
>2 weeks	0.7-0.9	15-65
Term infants		
<2 weeks	0.4-1.0	17-68
>2 weeks	0.3-0.5	26-86
Infants >1 mo	0.2-0.5	70-100
Toddlers	0.2-0.5	100-120
School-aged children	0.3-1.0	100-120
Adolescents	0.6-1.2	100-120

syndrome are associated with respiratory complaints, including hemoptysis, epistaxis, chronic sinusitis, or cough.

The physical findings in ARF also vary greatly, depending on the cause. Children with prerenal ARF present with symptoms of inadequate intravascular volume: tachycardia, hypotension, and poor perfusion. They can also have decreased skin turgor, sunken eyes, and dry mucosae. With obstructive ARF there is frequently a distended bladder, and there may be a palpable abdominal mass if the ureters and renal pelvis are grossly distended. Children with intrinsic ARF may have periorbital edema and hypertension if they have glomerulonephritis, with the addition of a malar rash and joint abnormalities if they are presenting with lupus nephritis. The physical findings of HUS include marked pallor, petechiae, bruising, and hypertension. Pyelonephritis is associated with fever, costovertebral tenderness, and suprapubic tenderness.

DIFFERENTIAL DIAGNOSIS

The differential diagnosis of ARF is fairly short. Dehydration with appropriately decreased urine output can mimic oliguria. Another cause of decreased urine output without renal failure is the syndrome of inappropriate antidiuretic hormone secretion. These patients also have hyponatremia and an elevated urine specific gravity without

an appropriate response to a fluid bolus. A false increase in serum creatinine can occur in ketoacidosis because of the interference of acetoacetate. Isolated increases in BUN without associated increases in serum creatinine can occur in patients with excessive protein intake or with gastrointestinal bleeding. Chronic renal failure can also present acutely. Findings of nonhemolytic anemia, hyperparathyroidism, rickets, small kidneys on renal ultrasound, or a history of previous renal problems are distinguishing features of chronic renal failure (see Chapter 109).[2]

DIAGNOSIS AND EVALUATION

ARF should be suspected whenever there is a sudden rise in serum creatinine, with or without changes in urine output. Creatinine is widely used as a marker of renal function. It is a byproduct of normal muscle metabolism that is excreted at a steady state by the kidney. Alterations in renal function will decrease the rate of excretion of creatinine and produce a higher steady-state concentration that results in elevated serum creatinine. Normal serum creatinine depends on the patient's muscle mass, which varies with size and development[3] (Table 108-2). For every doubling of serum creatinine, renal function is roughly halved. A more accurate way to measure renal function is by creatinine clearance, which is used as a marker for the glomerular filtration rate (GFR). Creatinine clearance also varies with age and development (see Table 108-2). Creatinine clearance can be measured in two ways. Classically, a 24-hour urine collection is obtained for measurement of creatinine, along with simultaneous serum creatinine, and creatinine clearance is determined via the following formula:

$$Cl_{creat} = (U_{creat}/P_{creat}) \times V/t/1.73 \text{ m}^2$$

where Cl_{creat} is creatinine clearance, U_{creat} is the urine creatinine concentration, P_{creat} is the plasma creatinine concentration, V is the volume of urine (in milliliters), and t is the collection time (in minutes).

Clinically, in children who are acutely ill with suspected renal failure, obtaining a 24-hour urine collection is impractical and cumbersome. Creatinine clearance can be estimated according to the formula provided in Table 108-3.[4] The

Table 108-3 Estimating Creatinine Clearance

kL/P_{Cr} = estimated creatinine clearance
  L   = length (in centimeters)
  P_{Cr} = serum creatinine
  k   = age-dependent constant
      k = 0.33 for low-birth-weight infants during the first year
        of life
      k = 0.45 for term infants during the first year of life
      k = 0.55 for children and adolescent girls
      k = 0.7 for adolescent boys

From Schwartz GM, Brion LP, Spitzer A: The use of plasma creatinine concentration for estimating glomerular filtration rate in infants, children, and adolescents. Pediatr Clin North Am 1987;34:571-590.

Table 108-4 Laboratory Differential Diagnosis of Prerenal versus Intrinsic Acute Renal Failure

	Prerenal	Intrinsic
Urinary Indices		
Fractional excretion of sodium (FE_{Na})*	<1% <2.5% (neonate)	>1% >2.5% (neonate)
Urine specific gravity	>1.020	<1.020
Urine osmolality (mOsm)	>400 >350 (neonate)	<400 <350 (neonate)
Urine and Plasma Indices		
U_{urea}/P_{urea}	>20 >10 (neonate)	<3 <3 (neonate)
U_{creat}/P_{creat}	>40 >30 (neonate)	<20 <10 (neonate)
U_{osmol}/P_{osmol}	>2 >1.5 (neonate)	<1 <1 (neonate)
BUN/P_{creat}	>20	<20

*$FE_{Na} = (U_{Na}/P_{Na}) \times (P_{creat}/U_{creat}) \times 100$.
BUN, blood urea nitrogen; P_{creat}, plasma concentration of creatinine; P_{urea}, plasma concentration of urea; U_{creat}, urine concentration of creatinine; U_{urea}, urine concentration of urea.

constant k varies with age because of the change in muscle mass that occurs with normal development. When interpreting the results of either of these methods in patients with ARF, it is important to bear in mind that the serum creatinine may not yet be in steady state, so the estimated GFR may be significantly inaccurate. A patient should be considered to be in renal failure if serum creatinine is twice the normal value or if the estimated GFR is halved.

It is important to determine whether the cause of ARF is prerenal, intrinsic, or obstructive (Table 108-4). Obstructive causes of ARF can often be determined by placement of a urinary catheter or flushing of an existing catheter, with subsequent resumption of urine output and normalization of renal function. Alternatively, in patients who have obstruction above the bladder outlet or for whom catheter placement is deemed undesirable, renal ultrasound should be performed to look for hydronephrosis or hydroureter, or both. Because ultrasound does not provide a dynamic picture of urine flow, follow-up with a diuretic renal scan or intravenous pyelogram may be indicated. Before performing

either study, nephrology or urology consultation should be obtained to help determine the most appropriate study.

It is more difficult to differentiate prerenal and intrinsic causes of ARF, although a few basic laboratory studies are usually sufficient. A urine specific gravity greater than 1.020 suggests prerenal ARF because injured kidneys are unable to raise the urine concentration much above that of the glomerular filtrate, which has a specific gravity of 1.010. Calculation of the urinary fractional excretion of sodium (FE_{Na}) by using random urine sodium and creatinine with simultaneous serum values of the same is also helpful in differentiating between prerenal and intrinsic ARF. The following formula allows calculation of FE_{Na}:

$$FE_{Na} = (U_{Na}/P_{Na}) \times (P_{creat}/U_{creat}) \times 100$$

where U_{Na} is the concentration of sodium in urine, P_{Na} is the concentration of sodium in plasma, P_{creat} is the concentration of creatinine in plasma, and U_{creat} is the concentration of creatinine in urine.

Neonates have higher FE_{Na} because of tubular immaturity, and results should be interpreted accordingly. Also, diuretics can obscure the results by blocking sodium reabsorption in the renal tubule. A child with an elevated FE_{Na} who has received a diuretic within the past 4 to 6 hours should not be considered to have intrinsic renal failure, although a child with a normal FE_{Na} who has received diuretics can be assumed to have prerenal ARF. Several other formulas may be helpful in differentiating between prerenal and renal ARF, but none have a decided advantage over FE_{Na} (see Table 108-4).

Similar electrolyte disturbances can be seen in both prerenal and intrinsic ARF, although hypernatremia may be more common in prerenal conditions. A disproportionate increase in BUN as compared with serum creatinine suggests prerenal azotemia because with dehydration BUN can be reabsorbed by the renal tubule as the kidney attempts to prevent further water loss, whereas creatinine cannot be reabsorbed. A BUN:serum creatinine ratio greater than 20 suggests prerenal ARF, although interpretation is complicated in conditions that cause elevated BUN, such as gastrointestinal bleeding as seen in HUS.

Once it has been established that a child has ARF secondary to intrinsic causes, diagnosis becomes more difficult. Pyuria and fever suggest pyelonephritis, although systemic lupus erythematosus can present with sterile pyuria and fever. Gross hematuria, with or without proteinuria, especially in association with hypertension, indicates acute glomerulonephritis.

COURSE OF ILLNESS

A variety of classifications exist, but in general there are three classic phases of ARF: the oliguric phase, the diuretic phase, and the recovery phase.[2] The oliguric phase, which will not occur in all patients, may last for a few days or several weeks. The duration depends in large part on the severity of the initial renal injury. The diuretic phase usually begins 7 to 14 days after the oliguric phase. BUN and serum creatinine may continue to rise at the onset of the diuretic phase, even though the kidney has begun to recover. Close monitoring of urine output and fluid status is vital at this point of the illness to prevent further renal injury that might not be recoverable. The recovery phase of ARF may take several weeks or even months for all urinary abnormalities to resolve.

TREATMENT

At the present time, the only treatment of ARF is supportive care. ARF with urine output is much easier to treat than ARF with either anuria or severe oliguria, so it is imperative to try to establish urine output, if possible, early in the course of ARF. In all patients with ARF, regardless of cause, initial treatment should be directed toward restoring intravascular volume. Crystalloid (normal saline) boluses, 10 to 20 mg/kg, are appropriate for all patients without evidence of volume overload and should be repeated until volume is clinically replete. Hypertension is not necessarily an appropriate marker for intravascular volume because of the frequent association of hypertension with renal disease. Heart rate, capillary refill, and peripheral perfusion are all helpful in determining volume status, although tachycardia may be present in patients with significant anemia regardless of volume status. Once intravascular volume has been normalized, the patient should be assessed for resumption of urine output. If the child is unable to void voluntarily because of either age or mental status, a bladder catheter should be placed. If minimal or no urine is produced after normalization of volume status, judicious use of diuretics is indicated. The efficacy of diuretics depends on the renal tubular concentration of diuretic, which in turn is dependent on drug filtration by the glomerulus. In ARF, the percentage of drug filtered can be vastly reduced, thereby leading to a low intratubular concentration of diuretic. Consequently, in ARF one must frequently administer diuretics at high doses to obtain a response. To minimize drug toxicity, it is better to use a single high dose of loop diuretic (i.e., furosemide, 3 to 5 mg/kg per dose) and assess a patient's response than to use repeated lower drug doses. A thiazide may be added to a loop diuretic to further block tubular reabsorption of sodium and maximize diuretic response, a method that anecdotally has been effective. The response to diuretics can be delayed in ARF, and some patients may take more than an hour to show increased urine output. If there is a significant increase in urine output, diuretics can continue to be used to maintain urine output as needed. If there is no urine output in response to this one-time high-dose diuretic, future doses should be withheld.

Therapy for ARF is directed toward maintaining volume status and correcting electrolyte abnormalities. Daily weights and accurate measurement of a patient's daily intake and output are imperative. Frequent adjustments to intravenous fluids may be required to prevent dehydration, especially in very small children. It is critical to remember that traditional methods of calculating pediatric fluids assume normal renal function and are inappropriate in children with renal failure. One method of fluid management involves two intravenous lines running at the same time. One line is for 5% dextrose in water (D5W) to replace insensible water losses, which are estimated at 10 to 15 mL/kg/day for children and adolescents and 15 to 20 mL/kg/day for infants. The other line is for D5 0.45% saline, which is used for replacement of urine output. The rate of this latter line can be adjusted every 4 to 6 hours according to a patient's urine output over the preceding time period. Ongoing losses, if present (i.e., diarrhea), also need

to be replaced with an appropriate intravenous fluid (usually 0.2% to 0.45% saline, depending on sodium losses in stool). Potassium should be left out of intravenous fluids for the first 24 to 48 hours after presentation unless marked hypokalemia is present so that the severity of ARF and its accompanying electrolyte disturbances can be assessed.

Low-dose dopamine (<5 μg/kg/min) has been widely used for ARF in an attempt to improve renal perfusion after a hypoxic insult. Dopamine has been found to both improve renal blood flow by increasing vasodilation and increase urine output by promoting natriuresis.[1] However, randomized controlled trials of the use of low-dose dopamine in critically ill patients have failed to demonstrate its efficacy despite widespread use. Additionally, low-dose dopamine has been associated with suppression of the respiratory drive, alterations in fluid and electrolyte homeostasis, and negative hemodynamic changes.

Electrolyte disturbances associated with ARF include uremia, hyperkalemia, hyponatremia, acidosis, and hypocalcemia. Hyperphosphatemia may also be present, although it is less common. In general, children tolerate higher serum levels of potassium than adults do, and there is usually little reason to treat potassium levels lower than 5.8 mg/dL other than restricting potassium intake. An electrocardiogram should be obtained in patients with a potassium level of 5.8 mg/dL or higher to assess for evidence of abnormal cardiac conductivity (i.e., the presence of peaked t waves) and establish a baseline. Patients with a potassium level greater than 6.0 mg/dL without electrocardiographic (ECG) changes should receive sodium polystyrene sulfonate (e.g., Kayexalate), a sodium resin that can be administered either orally or rectally. Patients with acute ECG changes can be treated with β-agonists, insulin/glucose drips, intravenous calcium, and sodium bicarbonate administration, in addition to sodium resin. In patients with extreme hyperkalemia and ECG changes, dialysis may be necessary. It is important to remember that of the aforementioned measures, only sodium resin and dialysis actually remove excess potassium. The other therapies simply change the cellular distribution of potassium and stabilize the myocardium. The only symptom of severe hyperkalemia is a lethal cardiac arrhythmia, and therefore patients with ARF and hyperkalemia need to be treated aggressively (see Chapter 58).

Hyponatremia occurs in ARF when there has been excessive sodium loss, excessive administration of hypotonic fluids, or both. Volume restriction is required after restoration of intravascular volume. The use of hypertonic saline is rarely appropriate in ARF. Patients with severe hyponatremia may require dialysis. Acidosis frequently accompanies ARF and is easily corrected with the administration of sodium bicarbonate or sodium citrate. The latter requires conversion of citrate to bicarbonate within the liver and should not be given to patients with liver dysfunction. Sodium bicarbonate should be administered at doses of 1 mEq/kg, with reassessment of serum bicarbonate between doses. Intravenous bicarbonate should be used cautiously in hypertensive patients because of the volume expansion that occurs with administration. When acidosis is associated with marked hypocalcemia, the hypocalcemia should be corrected before the acidosis to prevent tetany from the intracellular shift of calcium. Hyperphosphatemia can be treated with non–aluminum-containing phosphate binders such as calcium carbonate or calcium acetate. Aluminum salts should not be used because of their potential for irreversible neurotoxicity.

ARF is often associated with severe hypertension, and aggressive treatment is indicated, especially in children with evidence of hypertensive encephalopathy. Extreme irritability, photophobia, altered mental status, narcolepsy, and seizures are all symptoms of hypertensive encephalopathy (see Chapter 35). Seizures can also be seen in ARF in association with electrolyte abnormalities such as hypocalcemia, hypokalemia, and uremia. Intravenous diazepam should be administered to these patients, in addition to correction of the primary disturbance causing the seizure.

Children with ARF also require close monitoring of their nutritional status. At least 25% of the daily caloric requirement must be supplied to reduce the catabolism associated with ARF.[2] Protein intake should be kept at 1 to 1.5 g/kg/day to minimize uremia. Potassium, phosphorus, and magnesium intake should also be minimal until the patient's serum levels have been stabilized.

Children with ARF may require multiple medications. Because the kidney is responsible for clearance of many drugs, especially antibiotics, care must be taken to avoid overdosing. All medications should be reviewed to determine whether alterations in dosing are needed in children with reduced renal function.

Dialysis may be needed in patients with volume overload, severe electrolyte abnormalities, or prolonged oliguria to allow adequate nutrition. Three forms of dialysis are available: peritoneal dialysis, hemodialysis, and hemofiltration. Determination of the most appropriate form of dialysis for a specific patient should be left to the consulting nephrologist.

CONSULTATION

Any child with suspected intrinsic ARF should have a pediatric nephrology consultation. For intrinsic ARF other than acute tubular necrosis, the long-term prognosis improves dramatically with rapid treatment of the primary disorder, thus making nephrology involvement early in the course of the disease imperative. The presence of suspected obstructive ARF, other than that caused by an obstructed bladder catheter, requires the involvement of a pediatric urologist.

ADMISSION CRITERIA

In general, children with suspected ARF and a calculated creatinine clearance below 50% of normal should be admitted. Additionally, any child with ARF and suspected oliguria or hyperkalemia should be admitted. Patients with mild renal insufficiency (i.e., creatinine clearance >60% of normal) and normal urine output may be monitored closely as outpatients, with hospital admission if any evidence of further deterioration in renal function is noted.

DISCHARGE CRITERIA

Children with ARF may be discharged once the following criteria have been met. First, electrolyte abnormalities have either resolved or are well controlled with medical therapy. However, Kayexalate should not be considered an outpatient medication. Second, if ARF has been determined to be intrinsic in etiology, the cause should be known and therapy, if indicated, initiated. Third, urine output should be normal. Finally, there should be clear evidence of improving renal function. If a child is discharged without complete normalization of renal function, close outpatient follow-up is needed. There are some cases in which ARF becomes chronic; for these patients, discharge should be per nephrology recommendations.

PREVENTION

Because there is currently no treatment of ARF other than supportive therapy, prevention is crucial. Patients with multiple risk factors for ARF (e.g., sepsis, hypotension, use of nephrotoxic drugs) should have close monitoring of urine output, fluid balance, and weight to assist in early recognition of renal dysfunction. Patients with impaired renal function who require exposure to nephrotoxic drugs should be well hydrated before drug administration. Finally, nonsteroidal anti-inflammatory drugs should be avoided in volume-depleted patients because prostaglandin inhibition can lead to ARF.

IN A NUTSHELL

- Currently, the only treatment of ARF is supportive, so prevention is crucial.
- Rapid restoration of intravascular volume is critical in all patients with ARF.
- Serum creatinine is based on muscle mass. The smaller the child, the lower the normal serum creatinine.
- A doubling of serum creatinine roughly corresponds to halving of renal function.
- For most causes of intrinsic ARF, rapid initiation of treatment of the primary disease causing the renal dysfunction is essential for a good long-term prognosis, so involvement of a pediatric nephrologist early in the course of the disease is a crucial step.

ON THE HORIZON

- Research continues on potential therapies to treat ARF.
- Anaritide, or atrial natriuretic peptide, acts to increase GFR by dilation of afferent arterioles. In both animal and human studies, anaritide improves GFR, urine output, and histologic changes, although it has not been found to induce improvement in long-term survival.[1]
- Melanocyte-stimulating factor has been found to prevent ARF in mice and rats, even when given several hours after the primary insult, although human studies have not been performed.
- The use of other growth factors, such as insulin-like growth factor type I, epidermal growth factor, and hepatocyte growth factor, and free radical scavengers after ischemic renal injury also show promise in animal studies.
- Current research into biomarkers predictive of ARF and a new classification system that is being readied for release after validation will add standardized analysis of pediatric ARF and, it is hoped, have an impact on outcomes in pediatric patients.

SUGGESTED READING

Andreoli SP: Acute renal failure. Curr Opin Pediatr 2002;13:183-188.

Chan JCM, Williams DM, Roth KS: Kidney failure in infants and children. Pediatr Rev 2002;23:47.

Sehic A, Chesney RW: Acute renal failure: Diagnosis. Pediatr Rev 1995;16:101-106.

REFERENCES

1. Andreoli SP: Acute renal failure. Curr Opin Pediatr 2002;13:183-188.
2. Chan JCM, Williams DM, Roth KS: Kidney failure in infants and children. Pediatr Rev 2002;23:47-60.
3. Sehic A, Chesney RW: Acute renal failure: Diagnosis. Pediatr Rev 1995;16:101-106.
4. Schwartz GM, Brion LP, Spitzer A: The use of plasma creatinine concentration for estimating glomerular filtration rate in infants, children, and adolescents. Pediatr Clin North Am 1987;34:571-590.

CHAPTER 109

Chronic Renal Failure

Melissa Gregory

Chronic renal failure (CRF) is an irreversible reduction in renal function, or glomerular filtration rate (GFR), with accompanying derangements in biochemical homeostasis. End-stage renal disease (ESRD) is defined as CRF so severe that a form of renal replacement therapy is required. The incidence of CRF in children is low, and the incidence of ESRD is 3 to 6 children per 1 million total population.[1] Unlike adults with CRF, in whom the primary causes are diabetes and hypertension, the overwhelming majority of children with CRF have primary renal disease, usually of congenital origin.[2] This means that the care of children with CRF can deviate dramatically from that of adults.

There have been striking improvements in the treatment of children with CRF and ESRD, with a subsequent increase in the prevalence of CRF in the pediatric population. More than 50% of children with CRF have congenital conditions such as posterior urethral valves or renal dysplasia; frequently, marked polyuria and salt wasting are present, complicating their care. Additionally, children with CRF have the burden of growth and development. Normalization of these parameters is the key to successful treatment. These factors, along with the psychosocial issues specific to childhood, make the treatment of children with CRF exacting, but with meticulous care and attention to detail, these children can reach adulthood with minimal associated morbidity.

PATHOPHYSIOLOGY

There is a wide spectrum of causes of childhood CRF (Table 109-1). Regardless of the cause, the basic pathophysiology is the same: renal injury leads to glomerular scarring, tubular atrophy, and interstitial fibrosis, with an ultimate reduction in normal renal function. The consequences of decreased function are usually not evident until renal function has been reduced to less than 30% to 50%. These consequences can include acidosis, hyper- or (more rarely) hypokalemia, anemia, deranged calcium-phosphorus balance (hyperphosphatemia and hypocalcemia), abnormal bone metabolism, hypertension, short stature, hyponatremia, and disrupted water homeostasis.

CLINICAL PRESENTATION

The clinical presentation of children with CRF varies tremendously due to both the wide range of causes and the different stages of disease at which a child may present. The most universal finding in children presenting with undiagnosed CRF is growth failure. Fatigue, anorexia, malaise, and worsening school performance are also common findings. Renal osteodystrophy can be seen, regardless of the cause of CRF. Signs and symptoms may include bone pain, refusal to walk, valgus deformities of the lower extremities, frontal bossing, and a rachitic rosary. Children with congenital uropathies or nephropathies are likely to present with the symptoms of polyuria and salt wasting: dehydration, emesis, acidosis, hyperkalemia, and either hyper- or hyponatremia, depending on the salt and water balance of the individual patient. This subset of patients rarely has hypertension. Children with juvenile nephronophthisis (a chronic, progressive tubulointerstitial nephritis) can also present with signs and symptoms of polyuria, but they often have accompanying hypertension and ocular abnormalities. Children with reflux nephropathy may present initially with signs and symptoms of pyelonephritis and develop hypertension as the nephropathy progresses. Edema and hypertension are typically found in children with CRF due to a glomerulopathy. Polycystic renal disease and renal tumors may present with abdominal pain, hypertension, and an abdominal mass.

DIFFERENTIAL DIAGNOSIS

The differential diagnosis of CRF is limited to acute renal failure (ARF). It is important to rapidly distinguish between the two because with ARF it may be possible to restore renal function. With CRF, the focus of treatment is correcting the associated derangements and slowing the progression of the primary disease. CRF should be suspected in children with marked nonhemolytic anemia, hyperparathyroidism, small kidneys on renal ultrasonography, or physical findings consistent with rickets. Once a patient has had elevated serum creatinine levels with associated metabolic derangements for 3 months or more, he or she is considered to have CRF.

DIAGNOSIS AND EVALUATION

The early identification of CRF can improve a patient's long-term outcome. The Kidney Disease Outcomes Quality Initiative of the National Kidney Foundation has established standards for the identification and initial evaluation of children with chronic kidney disease to promote early diagnosis.[3] The term *chronic kidney disease* (CKD) incorporates CRF and chronic renal insufficiency, which are considered part of the spectrum of CKD. These standards define CKD as being present in any patient who meets one of two criteria: (1) there is evidence of kidney damage for 3 months or more, as defined by structural abnormalities of the kidney with or without decreased GFR, as evidenced by abnormalities in the composition of blood or urine, abnormalities in imaging tests, or abnormalities on kidney biopsy; (2) the GFR is less than 60 mL/minute per 1.73 m^2 for 3 months or more, with or without any structural changes. GFR is not adequately determined using serum creatinine alone; it should be estimated using a prediction equation such as the Schwartz equation (Table 109-2).[4] A patient with suspected

Table 109-1 Causes of Chronic Renal Failure in Children

Congenital urinary tract malformations
  Renal dysplasia
  Renal hypoplasia
  Obstructive uropathies
    Posterior urethral valves
    Ureteropelvic junction obstruction
  Megaureter

Glomerulopathies
  Focal segmental glomerulosclerosis
  Rapidly progressive glomerulonephritis
  Membranoproliferative glomerulonephritis
  Membranous nephropathy
  IgA nephropathy

Hereditary diseases
  Polycystic kidney disease
  Alport syndrome
  Cystinosis
  Oxalosis
  Nephronophthisis

Systemic diseases
  Systemic lupus erythematosus
  Goodpasture disease
  Wegener granulomatosis
  Polyarteritis nodosa

Vascular diseases
  Hypertension
  Diabetes mellitus

Miscellaneous causes
  Denys-Drash syndrome
  Wilms tumor
  Neuroblastoma

Table 109-2 Estimating Creatinine Clearance

kL/P_{Cr} = Estimated creatinine clearance

k = Age-dependent constant:
  k = 0.33 for low-birth-weight infants during first year of life
  k = 0.45 for term infants during first year of life
  k = 0.55 for children and adolescent girls
  k = 0.7 for adolescent boys

L = Height (cm)

P_{Cr} = Serum creatinine

From Schwartz GM, Brion LP, Spitzer A: The use of plasma creatinine concentration for estimating glomerular filtration rate in infants, children, and adolescents. Pediatr Clin North Am 1987;34:571-590.

CRF presenting to the hospital for the first time will not meet the time criterion but should be evaluated as if CRF were present.

The evaluation of a patient with suspected CRF should be directed toward determining the cause of kidney disease, its severity, comorbid conditions such as hypertension, complications such as renal osteodystrophy, and the risk for further loss of renal function. The initial evaluation to determine the cause of kidney disease should be done with the guidance of a pediatric nephrologist. Important historical information includes previous kidney disease, hypertension, diabetes, abnormal prenatal ultrasonography, or oligohydramnios; the presence of polyuria, dysuria, or gross hematuria; and systemic complaints such as anorexia, fatigue, malaise, fever, or arthralgias. Deteriorating school performance and family history of renal disease are also important elements. Pertinent findings of the physical examination may include short stature, elevated blood pressure, edema, rashes, joint effusions or arthritis, ascites, or evidence of rickets.

Initial laboratory studies should include a complete urinalysis, serum electrolytes (including calcium and phosphorus), albumin, complete blood count, parathyroid hormone, and renal ultrasonography. Children with proteinuria on the initial urinalysis should have a 24-hour urine collection for protein and creatinine or a spot urine protein-creatinine ratio (normal is <0.18) on a first-morning void if 24-hour urine collection is not feasible. Daily weights and accurate monitoring of urine output are also important.

TREATMENT

The focus of treatment in CRF is threefold: correcting biochemical and hematologic disturbances due to CRF, preventing comorbidities associated with CRF, and slowing the progression of CRF. Additionally, for some patients with acquired causes of CRF, treatment of the primary disease is required.

Biochemical Disturbances

Biochemical disturbances associated with CRF include hyperkalemia, acidosis, hyperphosphatemia, hypocalcemia, and sodium derangement. Hyperkalemia results from increased catabolism associated with uremia, coupled with diminished excretion due to both decreased GFR and tubular dysfunction.[1] Acidosis can worsen hyperkalemia by inducing the extracellular shift of intracellular potassium. Hyperkalemia is a potentially life-threatening condition owing to its effect on cardiac conductivity. At levels greater than 7 mEq/L, electrocardiographic abnormalities can be seen, including potentially life-threatening arrhythmias. Acute hyperkalemia can be treated by administering sodium bicarbonate, beta-agonists, kayexalate cation exchange resins, loop diuretics, or dialysis. For acute hyperkalemia with electrocardiographic changes, cardiac stabilization with calcium infusion or intravenous insulin and glucose is also required (see Chapter 58). However, in CRF, the goal is to prevent the need for acute interventions, and central to preventing hyperkalemia is dietary control of potassium intake. In patients with moderate CRF, chronic loop diuretics can be used to increase potassium excretion.

Acidosis is another common abnormality seen in CRF, resulting from the inadequate excretion of ammonium by the kidney. Chronic acidosis results in impaired growth caused by both inadequate caloric intake due to the accompanying anorexia and nausea and abnormal bone formation due to hydrogen ion deposition in bone, which acts as a buffer to maintain normal body pH. Acidosis also induces hyperpnea, which is a compensatory mechanism to remove excess acid via increased ventilation (compensatory respiratory alkalosis). Acidosis is treated by the administration alkali, usually in the form of sodium bicarbonate or sodium citrate, to maintain serum bicarbonate levels above 22 mEq/L.

Hyperphosphatemia results from diminished phosphate excretion. As serum phosphate levels increase, serum calcium levels drop; this stimulates parathyroid hormone excretion, leading to secondary hyperparathyroidism. Hyperphosphatemia also has a direct stimulatory effect on the parathyroid gland. Chronic hyperphosphatemia can be associated with an elevated serum calcium-phosphorus product, leading to metastatic calcifications and increased atherosclerosis. There are two treatments for hyperphosphatemia, both of which are usually necessary: (1) dietary restriction of phosphorus intake, usually to 800 to 1200 mg/day, depending on the age of the child; and (2) administration of phosphate binders with meals to prevent the intestinal absorption of ingested phosphorus. These phosphate binders include calcium salts, such as calcium carbonate and calcium acetate, as well as synthetic polymers, such as sevelamer hydrochloride and lanthanum carbonate. Aluminum salts were once widely used as phosphate binders but are no longer used because of their association with bone deposition and dementia due to aluminum toxicity.

Hypocalcemia occurs as a physiologic response to hyperphosphatemia and as a result of the diminished levels of activated vitamin D that occur with reduced renal function. Activation of vitamin D to calcitriol (1,25-dihydroxymitamin D) normally takes place in the proximal nephron, but with CRF, inadequate production of this active hormone leads to diminished intestinal calcium absorption, diminished release of calcium from bone, and diminished renal tubular calcium reabsorption, all of which contribute to hypocalcemia. Although extreme hypocalcemia may require treatment with calcium supplements, the majority of patients respond to the administration of activated vitamin D metabolites such as calcitriol or dihydrotachysterol.

Sodium derangement can result from both sodium retention and sodium wasting. Glomerular diseases are often associated with impaired sodium excretion, and patients can develop edema and hypertension if they are not placed on a sodium-restricted diet. Congenital causes of CRF, in contrast, are frequently associated with polyuria and renal salt wasting. These patients may present with normal serum sodium levels because of simultaneous intravascular volume depletion, or they may have hyponatremia. In both scenarios, there is often decreased circulating plasma volume, with subsequent renal hypoperfusion. These children frequently need sodium and fluid supplementation.

Comorbidities

Anemia frequently occurs in patients with CRF once the GFR falls to less than 30 mL/minute per 1.73 m^2, mainly due to inadequate erythropoietin production by the kidneys. Although chronic blood transfusions were once a mainstay of treatment, the development of recombinant human erythropoietin means that, for most CRF patients, transfusions can be avoided. Additionally, iron supplementation is required; current recommendations are for a target hematocrit between 33% and 36%.

Renal osteodystrophy results from secondary hyperparathyroidism, which is a result of hypocalcemia and hyperphosphatemia. Additionally, skeletal resistance to parathyroid hormone is present in those with uremia, further contributing to the development of renal osteodystrophy.[5] Treatment is aggressive control of hyperphosphatemia by dietary restriction and the administration of oral phosphate binders and activated vitamin D metabolites. In rare cases, some patients with severe hyperparathyroidism that is nonresponsive to these measures may require parathyroidectomy. Oversuppression of parathyroid hormone is associated with aplastic bone disease, so the goal is not complete normalization of intact parathyroid hormone levels but rather a target level between 150 and 300 pg/mL.

Growth failure is frequently associated with CRF once the GFR has fallen to less than 30 mL/minute per 1.73 m^2, although it may occur earlier. Although acidosis and renal osteodystrophy contribute to the poor growth seen in children with CRF, the major cause of growth failure in those older than 2 years is growth hormone resistance due to decreased tissue expression of insulin-like growth factor (IGF) and increased IGF-binding proteins. The use of recombinant human growth hormone is effective in maintaining normal growth. In contrast, in infants with CRF, poor growth is likely due to inadequate nutrition. These babies benefit from aggressive nutritional management; in those with congenital renal disease, high-volume gavage feedings with sodium supplements may normalize growth.

Cardiac dysfunction is frequently seen in individuals with CRF, although it is less common in children than in adults owing to the different causes of CRF in these two populations. Hypertension is frequently associated with CRF and can result in left ventricular hypertrophy. Severe hypertension can result in congestive heart failure. Patients with oliguria may also develop congestive heart failure due to hypervolemia. With marked uremia, pericarditis and pericardial effusions can occur.

Uremic patients may have increased bleeding due to platelet dysfunction. This can be an especially important issue for menstruating girls or patients requiring surgery. Patients with CRF and uremic bleeding have normal prothrombin times and partial thromboplastin times but an elevated skin bleeding time. Desmopressin, administered intravenously, subcutaneously, or intranasally, can be used acutely to treat uremic bleeding, although it is ineffective for the control of prolonged bleeding due to tachyphylaxis. Cryoprecipitate can be used in patients with prolonged bleeding or in those who are unresponsive to desmopression. Antifibrinolytic agents such as ε-aminocaproic acid are also effective in treating acute hemorrhage.[6] Patients who require prolonged therapy can be treated with conjugated estrogens, although these compounds are not effective in the acute setting.

Renal Replacement Therapy

Some method of renal replacement, either dialysis or transplantation, is needed once the GFR has decreased to less than 15 mL/minute per 1.73 m^2. Some patients may require intervention earlier owing to uncontrolled metabolic complications. Although hemodialysis is the primary modality used in adult patients with ESRD, peritoneal dialysis plays a more predominant role in children. Continuous cycling peritoneal dialysis, in which the child is dialyzed overnight through a peritoneal catheter using an automated cycler, has several advantages. It can be done at home by the child's caregiver, with minimal interference with the patient's schooling. Peritoneal dialysis also allows increased sodium and fluid intake, which makes compliance with dietary restrictions easier. Peritoneal dialysis is frequently complicated by peritonitis and catheter site infection, however. Recurrent infections can result in scarring of the peritoneum, making it unusable for dialysis.

Hemodialysis is an option for patients who do not have an intact peritoneum, those whose caregivers are not capable of performing peritoneal dialysis, or those for whom the presence of a peritoneal dialysis catheter is unacceptable. Chronic hemodialysis is usually performed three times a week in an outpatient setting, although some patients require more frequent dialysis. Dialysis access is a problem in children on hemodialysis, especially in very small children in whom placement of a dialysis fistula or shunt is impractical. The intermittent nature of hemodialysis also requires more severe dietary and fluid restrictions, especially for children with oliguria.

Renal transplantation is the renal replacement modality of choice for children with ESRD. Children receiving kidney transplants from living, related donors have excellent long-term survival rates, and the average half-life of a renal allograft is now 13 years or more.[5] Suspected allograft rejection is one of the most common causes of hospitalization in transplant patients following the initial surgery. Infectious complications, especially viral, are other common reasons for the hospitalization of children with kidney transplants (see Chapter 73). The immunosuppressive agents used in transplant patients may have significant interactions with a variety of drugs, and great care must be used in prescribing additional medications in this patient population.

Special Dosing of Medications

Because the kidneys are responsible for the elimination of many drugs, once renal function drops to less than 50%, many medications require adjustments in dosage, dosing interval, or both. All patients with CRF should have their renal function calculated and their medication lists reviewed on a quarterly basis to determine whether alterations in drug dosing are indicated. Several reference books contain information about which drugs require renal dosing.[7,8] The website *www.pdr.net* also has this information, as do most hospital pharmacists.

CONSULTATION

Any child admitted for suspected CRF requires a pediatric nephrology consultation. Similarly, any dialysis or renal transplant patient who requires hospitalization needs to be followed by a pediatric nephrologist. Other patients with CRF who are hospitalized for reasons unrelated to their kidney disease do not necessarily require nephrology consultation, although it may be helpful, especially when adjustments in medications are necessary to account for abnormal renal function.

ADMISSION CRITERIA

- Initial diagnosis and stabilization.
- Life-threatening electrolyte disturbance.
- Congestive heart failure.
- Severe anemia requiring blood transfusion.
- Malignant hypertension.
- Infection associated with hemodynamic compromise.
- Dialysis access complication.
- Suspected allograft rejection.

DISCHARGE CRITERIA

Children hospitalized for suspected CRF can be discharged once the diagnosis has been confirmed, the cause established, and any electrolyte or volume derangements normalized. Other children with CRF who require hospitalization can be discharged once the condition leading to their hospitalization (e.g., severe hyperkalemia, peritonitis, suspected rejection) has been corrected.

PREVENTION

CRF is usually a progressive disease with an orderly sequence of deterioration. Recently, the National Kidney Foundation proposed a classification system for CKD based on GFR (Table 109-3).[3] This system was designed to identify those patients at risk for progression of disease so that measures to both reduce the risk and slow the progression could be initiated. Interventions that can slow the progression of renal failure include meticulous blood pressure control, proper dietary management, control of proteinuria, reduction of glomerular hyperfiltration, and control of dyslipidemia. In patients with CRF, the goal of antihypertensive therapy should be maintenance of blood pressure below the 90th percentile for age and height. Protein restriction is not as clearly indicated in children as it is in adults, because children have the additional burden of growth; in general, however, infants and toddlers should have a protein intake of 2 g/kg per day, and older children should have 1 to

Table 109-3 **Stages of Chronic Kidney Disease**

Stage	GFR (mL/min/1.73 m²)	Description
1	≥90	Kidney damage with normal or increased GFR
2	60-89	Kidney damage with mild decrease in GFR
3	30-59	Moderate reduction of GFR
4	15-29	Severe reduction of GFR
5	<15	Need for renal replacement therapy

GFR, glomerular filtration rate.
From Hogg RJ, Furth S, Lemley KV, et al: National Kidney Foundation's Kidney Disease Outcomes Quality Initiative: Clinical practice guidelines for chronic kidney disease in children and adolescents: Evaluation, classification and stratification. Pediatrics 2003;111:1416-1421.

1.5 g/kg per day. Angiotensin-converting enzyme inhibitors and angiotensin II receptor inhibitors are both effective in reducing intraglomerular pressure, even without associated systemic hypertension, and their use can slow the progression of CRF. Both drugs can be useful in controlling proteinuria as well.

IN A NUTSHELL

- Congenital kidney disease is the most common cause of CRF in children and, unlike other types of CRF, can be associated with polyuria and salt wasting.
- The evaluation of a patient with suspected CRF should be directed toward determining the cause and severity of kidney disease, identifying comorbid conditions and complications, and assessing the risk for further loss of renal function.
- Comorbidities of CRF include anemia, osteodystrophy, growth failure, cardiac dysfunction, and abnormal bleeding.
- Estimates of GFR can be made using the patient's height and plasma creatinine concentration.
- Many medications require dosage adjustments when administered to children with diminished GFR.
- Slowing the progression of CKD is an important goal of therapy, and effective interventions include control of blood pressure, proteinuria, and dyslipidemia and reduction of glomerular hyperfiltration.

ON THE HORIZON

- More emphasis is being placed on improving the long-term morbidity and mortality of children with CRF. For example, young adults with CRF have a high incidence of cardiovascular complications, and efforts are focused on improving this outcome.
- For some genetic causes of CRF, such as polycystic kidney disease, the genes implicated in the disease have been identified, and research is directed toward interventions to prevent disease development and progression. Scientists have also been successful in identifying some of the genetic aberrations responsible for abnormal fetal kidney development, although we are still far from being able to medically intervene in these patients.
- Improvements in the delivery of dialysis and in the development and use of immunosuppressive agents in renal transplant patients will continue to improve their long-term prognosis.

SUGGESTED READING

Chan JCM, Williams DM, Roth KS: Kidney failure in infants and children. Pediatr Rev 2002;23:47-60.

Hogg RJ, Furth S, Lemley KV, et al: National Kidney Foundation's Kidney Disease Outcomes Quality Initiative: Clinical practice guidelines for chronic kidney disease in children and adolescents: Evaluation, classification and stratification. Pediatrics 2003;111:1416-1421.

REFERENCES

1. Fine RN: Recent advances in the management of the infant, child, and adolescent with chronic renal failure. Pediatr Rev 1990;11:277-283.
2. Harmon WE: Treatment of children with chronic renal failure. Kidney Int 1995;47:951-961.
3. Hogg RJ, Furth S, Lemley KV, et al: National Kidney Foundation's Kidney Disease Outcomes Quality Initiative: Clinical practice guidelines for chronic kidney disease in children and adolescents: Evaluation, classification and stratification. Pediatrics 2003;111:1416-1421.
4. Schwartz GM, Brion LP, Spitzer A: The use of plasma creatinine concentration for estimating glomerular filtration rate in infants, children, and adolescents. Pediatr Clin North Am 1987;34:571-590.
5. Chan JCM, Williams DM, Roth KS: Kidney failure in infants and children. Pediatr Rev 2002;23:47-60.
6. Salman S: Uremic bleeding: Pathophysiology, diagnosis, and management. Hosp Physician 2001;76:45-50.
7. Robertson J, Shilkofski N (eds): The Harriet Lane Handbook: A Manual for Pediatric House Officers, 17th ed. St Louis, Mosby, 2005.
8. Physicians' Desk Reference. Montvale, NJ, Thomson, 2006.

CHAPTER 110

Glomerulonephritis

Melissa J. Gregory

Glomerulonephritis (GN) is not a specific disease, but rather an inflammatory state within the renal glomerulus. This inflammation causes glomerular injury and results in impaired glomerular filtration with subsequent abnormal urinary sediment and possibly decreased renal function. It is often associated with hypertension. Clinically, GN spans a wide spectrum of disease from a fairly benign, self-limited condition such as postinfectious GN (PIGN) to an aggressive systemic disease that if left untreated can lead to rapid loss of renal function and even death, such as Wegener granulomatosis. This chapter focuses on the four common presentations of GN that are most likely to be found in hospitalized patients: asymptomatic hematuria, acute GN, rapidly progressive GN (RPGN), and chronic GN.

CLINICAL PRESENTATION

Asymptomatic Hematuria

Asymptomatic hematuria can be either microscopic or macroscopic and is not associated with hypertension, impaired renal function, or proteinuria. Asymptomatic isolated microscopic hematuria, defined as hematuria unaccompanied by proteinuria or pyuria, can be the result of many different conditions other than GN, including fever, gastrointestinal disturbances, and bladder catheterization. Because this presentation may frequently be misdiagnosed as urinary tract infection, urine culture is imperative. Outpatient follow-up is appropriate in these patients. Asymptomatic gross hematuria is substantially less common than microscopic hematuria and may be secondary to a variety of conditions, not just GN. The combination of hematuria, either microscopic or gross, and proteinuria is concerning for possible GN, and diagnostic evaluation is therefore indicated.

Acute Glomerulonephritis

Acute GN is characterized by an abrupt onset of gross hematuria, azotemia, and hypertension. Proteinuria is common, although rarely is it within the nephrotic range (nephrotic range is >40 mg urinary protein/m²/hr or a urinary protein-creatinine ratio >2.0). Edema is common and usually due to renal sodium retention secondary to an abrupt decrease in renal function, not from hypoalbuminemia. PIGN is the most common cause of acute GN. In its classic presentation, a sudden onset of painless gross hematuria, often described as "tea colored," develops in a child 14 to 21 days after a streptococcal infection. PIGN occurs most frequently in children between 4 and 10 years of age. Physical examination often reveals pallor, mild periorbital edema, and hypertension. The latter is the most common reason for hospitalization and can be severe enough to cause hypertensive encephalopathy and seizures. PIGN is a self-limited disease, with normalization of renal function usually occur-

ring within 3 weeks. RPGN and chronic GN can present as acute GN, but the clinical courses of these illnesses are distinctive. In PIGN, renal function and blood pressure should normalize within 4 weeks, serum complement should normalize within 8 weeks, and proteinuria should disappear within 3 months.[1]

Rapidly Progressive Glomerulonephritis

RPGN is a clinical syndrome that can be due to a variety of forms of GN. RPGN is characterized by the signs of GN (hematuria, either microscopic or gross, and proteinuria); systemic symptoms such as fever, malaise, fatigue, and anorexia; and rapid deterioration in renal function (Table 110-1). Although uncommon in children, RPGN can result in end-stage renal failure in up to 50% of afflicted children and, if untreated, can progress to irreversible renal failure within a number of weeks.[3] Even though RPGN can be the clinical presentation of any form of GN, it is more commonly associated with either pauci-immune GN, small-vessel vasculitis with a positive antineutrophil cytoplasmic antibody (ANCA) test, or immune complex GN, which includes a mixture of diseases associated with extensive glomerular deposition of immune complexes.[1] A less common cause of RPGN is anti–glomerular basement membrane (anti-GBM) disease.

ANCA-associated renal vasculitis is the most common cause of RPGN in children.[1,2] There are three clinical manifestations of this disease: microscopic polyangiitis, which presents with systemic signs and symptoms of vasculitis, in addition to the renal findings; Wegener granulomatosis, which presents with pulmonary or sinus findings (or both), along with kidney disease; and idiopathic crescentic GN, in which the disease process is confined to the kidney.

Immune complex GN consists of a variety of renal diseases characterized by immune complex deposition within the glomeruli, including systemic lupus erythematosus (SLE), membranoproliferative glomerulonephritis (MPGN), and IgA nephropathy. SLE GN presents with systemic signs and symptoms consistent with lupus: arthralgias, joint effusions, fatigue, malaise, leukopenia, anemia, and thrombocytopenia, in addition to hematuria and proteinuria. MPGN and IgA nephropathy tend to be renal-specific diseases, although systemic symptoms are present in patients with RPGN in addition to the findings of GN.

Anti-GBM nephritis is fortunately rare in children. When renal involvement occurs with pulmonary hemorrhage, the disease is referred to as Goodpasture syndrome.[2]

Chronic Glomerulonephritis

Chronic GN can present acutely, but more commonly it presents as persistent hematuria and proteinuria, with or without hypertension or slowly progressive renal failure.

Table 110-1 Clinical Presentation Concerning for Rapidly Progressive Glomerulonephritis

Prodrome of vague systemic symptoms such as fatigue, malaise, and anorexia before the development of glomerulonephritis
Associated systemic symptoms (fever, malaise, arthralgias, myalgias) concurrent with glomerulonephritis
Rapid deterioration in renal function

Chronic GN can be manifested as isolated renal disease, as is seen with IgA nephropathy, MPGN, and renal vasculitis, or as part of a systemic disease, such as SLE, chronic endocarditis, and Henoch-Schönlein purpura. Hospitalization for chronic GN is relatively unusual, although children with chronic GN may be hospitalized after diagnostic or prognostic renal biopsy.

DIFFERENTIAL DIAGNOSIS

The differential diagnosis for GN includes the subtypes outlined earlier. Hematuria has a broad etiology, but the association of proteinuria and other potential systemic manifestations, including hypertension, should direct the clinician to suspect the presence of GN. Without associated proteinuria, the initial evaluation of hospitalized patients with gross hematuria should focus on causes other than GN, including infection, trauma, nephrolithiasis, papillary necrosis, neoplasm, and obstruction. Acute interstitial nephritis may also have a similar presentation, and renal biopsy and consultation with nephrology are required to establish the diagnosis.

DIAGNOSIS AND EVALUATION

All patients with suspected GN require a complete blood count; a comprehensive electrolyte panel, including albumin, phosphorus, and magnesium; complement levels; and serology for antinuclear antibody (ANA) and ANCA. Additionally, urinalysis with microscopy is essential, along with evaluation for proteinuria. Other studies that may be helpful include intact parathyroid hormone, as well as the prothrombin and partial thromboplastin time and viral serology if indicated. Renal ultrasonography is the mainstay of initial imaging and can be of help in identifying medical renal disease accompanying acute GN. In the case of acute GN the kidneys are generally enlarged, whereas with a more chronic process the kidneys may be small.

In acute GN, urinalysis shows hematuria and proteinuria on urine dipstick, with microscopic evaluation revealing dysmorphic red blood cells and red cell casts. Although the presence of red cell casts is diagnostic for GN, their absence does not rule the disease out. Blood tests show evidence of renal dysfunction with elevated blood urea nitrogen (BUN) and serum creatinine and, sometimes, accompanying electrolyte derangements such as hyperkalemia and metabolic acidosis. Immunologic studies show hypocomplementemia in approximately 75% of patients, specifically, depressed CH50 and C3 components. In poststreptococcal GN, antibodies to

group A β-hemolytic streptococci may be detected, with anti–DNAse B antibodies being the most sensitive marker, although antibodies to streptolysin O, streptokinase, and hyaluronidase may be seen. Even though PIGN is most commonly associated with streptococcal infections, it can also be seen in a variety of other bacterial and viral infections.

Rapidly Progressive Glomerulonephritis

On renal biopsy, more than 50% of sampled glomeruli in patients with RPGN show glomerular crescents. ANCA-associated renal vasculitis is pathologically characterized by microscopic polyangiitis involving the glomerular capillaries without associated immune deposits.

Positive ANCA serology is seen in 90% of patients with microscopic polyangiitis, Wegener granulomatosis, or idiopathic crescentic GN. The antibody may be directed toward myeloperoxidase (perinuclear ANCA [p-ANCA]) or proteinase 3 (cytoplasmic ANCA [c-ANCA]). The presence of p-ANCA is more common in patients with microscopic polyangiitis, and c-ANCA is more commonly found in patients with Wegener granulomatosis. However, there is a great deal of overlap between the two subtypes, and a diagnosis cannot be made purely on the result of an ANCA test. Clinical findings, radiologic evaluation for possible sinus or pulmonary involvement (or both), and renal biopsy are all needed to confirm the diagnosis.

Among the immune complex–mediated forms of RPGN, laboratory findings in SLE-associated GN include positive ANA, antibodies to double-stranded DNA, and depressed complement levels (primarily C3 and C4). MPGN is associated with depressed C3 levels and may often be misdiagnosed as PIGN. In children, MPGN is most often a primary disease, although it can be seen in conjunction with hepatitis C and cryoglobulinemia, so appropriate serology and protein studies should be performed. A renal biopsy is sometimes needed to differentiate between SLE and MPGN.

Anti-GBM nephritis is diagnosed by the finding of elevated circulating anti-GBM antibody and linear deposits of IgG in the GBM on renal biopsy. Complement levels are normal, but some patients may have positive ANCA.[2]

TREATMENT

Management of GN is guided by the underlying cause; however, the basic approach for all is similar. Initial treatment focuses on stabilization of blood pressure and strict fluid management. Collection of appropriate laboratory data and imaging should also be high on the priority list of initial management. If the patient's BUN is higher than 80 mg/dL or there is significant electrolyte disturbance, referral for potential dialysis should be considered. Finally, developing a plan to determine the cause is important, for which renal biopsy may be the best option.

Blood pressure control is the most important concern initially. Children with symptomatic hypertension (i.e., headache, mental status changes including irritability, symptoms of congestive heart failure, or papilledema) should be treated as hypertensive emergencies. Potential parenteral therapies include nicardipine, labetalol, and diazoxide. For less urgent situations, diuretics can be helpful, whereas for moderate hypertension, angiotensin-converting enzyme inhibitors (ACEIs) are effective. When using ACEIs in this situation, however, there is a risk of further decreasing the glomerular filtration rate, so this class of drug should be avoided in patients with marked renal insufficiency.

RPGN is a medical emergency, and the long-term prognosis improves dramatically with early initiation of treatment.[4] Treatment should not be withheld in a patient with suspected RPGN because of difficulty obtaining a renal biopsy, nor should it be withheld in patients requiring dialysis because in some patients, especially those with renal vasculitis, substantial recovery of renal function can occur after therapy. Pulse corticosteroid (methylprednisolone, 30 mg/kg/day intravenously, not to exceed 1 g) for three doses is the initial treatment of all forms of RPGN, followed by oral prednisone at 2 mg/kg/day, not to exceed 80 mg/day. Pulse methylprednisolone can be associated with hypertension and gastritis. Careful monitoring of vital signs is important in these patients, and prophylactic use of H_2 blockers or proton pump inhibitors should be considered.

The addition of cyclophosphamide is indicated for patients with ANCA-associated renal vasculitis, anti-GBM disease, and some forms of lupus nephritis. Cyclophosphamide therapy is frequently associated with nausea or emesis, or both, and may be complicated by hemorrhagic cystitis. Antiemetic therapy is often used in these patients routinely. Aggressive intravenous hydration is needed to decrease the risk for hemorrhagic cystitis. Cyclophosphamide also causes neutropenia and thrombocytopenia, and a complete blood count, including a platelet count, is essential before drug administration. Patients with absolute neutropenia or a platelet count lower than 50,000/mm[3] should not receive cyclophosphamide. An exception would be a patient with SLE whose clinical presentation included neutropenia or thrombocytopenia (or both). Plasma exchange may also be helpful in patients with anti-GBM disease. Renal biopsy should be performed as soon as possible once a patient is stabilized to determine whether additional therapy is needed.

Some forms of chronic GN, especially certain types of lupus nephritis, require treatment with pulse methylprednisolone or cyclophosphamide. In some institutions and with certain patients, these therapies are best administered in the hospital. Patients with chronic GN may also be hospitalized because of severe hypertension or, in the case of systemic diseases such as SLE, for nonrenal complications.

Postbiopsy Patients

Care of patients after renal biopsy focuses mainly on preventive measures aimed at decreasing the risk for postprocedural hemorrhage. Many institutions recommend strict bed rest for 6 to 12 hours after the procedure, along with frequent assessment of vital signs for 6 to 8 hours. Serial hematocrit determinations are not generally needed after renal biopsy because tachycardia is a sensitive indicator of significant blood loss and thus makes close monitoring of heart rate trends more helpful. Gross hematuria is common after biopsy and occurs in up to 30% of patients; it usually clears within one or two voids. Microscopic hematuria can persist for several days. Gross hematuria that does not clear or is associated with clots or severe pain, either suprapubic or flank, is concerning and requires urgent nephrology consul-

tation. There is usually minimal postprocedural pain, and for most patients, acetaminophen provides adequate pain control. Ibuprofen and other nonsteroidal anti-inflammatory drugs should be avoided, both for their possible prolongation of bleeding and for their potential nephrotoxic effect. On occasion, patients may experience severe pain after renal biopsy, presumably from subcapsular hematoma. If unaccompanied by tachycardia, these patients may be treated symptomatically with narcotics. Pain unrelieved by narcotics or associated with tachycardia requires further investigation and nephrology consultation. The majority of patients undergoing biopsy require overnight hospitalization and may be discharged within 24 hours with nephrology follow-up.

CONSULTATION

Consultation with pediatric nephrologists can provide assistance with diagnostic evaluation and management of patients with GN. RPGN should be considered a nephrologic emergency, and rapid consultation with a nephrologist is essential. Consultation is warranted in patients with acute GN who do not demonstrate resolution over time, those with recurrent disease, or patients with symptoms that are difficult to control. Methylprednisolone or cyclophosphamide for GN should be administered under the guidance of a nephrologist.

ADMISSION CRITERIA (CONSIDERATION FOR REFERRAL TO PEDIATRIC NEPHROLOGY)

- Acute renal failure (azotemia associated with oliguria/anuria)
- Severe hypertension (blood pressure >15 mm Hg above the 95th percentile for age/height)
- Presentation of GN in patients younger than 2 years or older than 12 years
- Nephrotic-range proteinuria
- Progressive decrease in renal function as measured by serum creatinine or urine output
- Recurrent episodes of acute GN

DISCHARGE CRITERIA

- Stabilization of renal function
- Adequate blood pressure control
- Completion of therapies that require close monitoring or inpatient level of support (e.g., pulse steroids or cyclophosphamide)
- Establishment of appropriate referrals and follow-up

PREVENTION

At this time there are no good preventive strategies to avoid the development of GN. Early detection plus intervention is the best option presently available. Excellent blood pressure control and avoidance of further renal injury through careful fluid and electrolyte control, along with nutritional management, will decrease the morbidity associated with GN. Early and appropriate medical management will also help decrease the morbidity and mortality associated with GN.

IN A NUTSHELL

- GN spans a wide spectrum of disease from self-limited conditions such as PIGN to aggressive systemic disease.
- There are four common presentations of GN: asymptomatic hematuria, acute GN, RPGN, and chronic GN.
- All patients with suspected GN need a complete blood count, a basic metabolic panel, serum complement levels, urinalysis with urine microscopy, and renal ultrasonography.
- Acute management is directed at controlling blood pressure, achieving fluid and electrolyte balance, and providing adequate nutrition.
- Early nephrology consultation should be considered in complex cases, especially if there is evidence of progressive deterioration in renal function, recurrence, or symptoms that are difficult to control.

ON THE HORIZON

- Current strategies at developing urinary and serum biomarkers are under investigation. It is anticipated that identification of disease-specific biomarkers will eventually replace the need for renal biopsy for definitive diagnosis.

REFERENCES

1. Hricik KE, Chung-Park M, Sear JR: Glomerulonephritis. N Engl J Med 1998;339:888-889.
2. Couser WG: Glomerulonephritis. Lancet 1999;353:1509-1515.
3. Hoschek JC, Dreyer P, Dahal S, Walker PD: Rapidly progressive renal failure in childhood. Am J Kidney Dis 2002;40:1342-1347.
4. Madaio MP, Harrington JT: The diagnosis of glomerular diseases. Acute glomerulonephritis and the nephrotic syndrome. Arch Intern Med 2001;161:25-34.

CHAPTER 111

Hemolytic Uremic Syndrome

Amy Holst

Hemolytic uremic syndrome (HUS), which was first described in 1955, is one of the most frequent causes of acute renal failure in children. It consists of an acute gastrointestinal (GI) illness followed by the triad of microangiopathic hemolytic anemia, thrombocytopenia, and acute nephropathy. The incidence of HUS is 2.7 cases per million people per year in the United States.[1] HUS can occur at any age but most often presents between 2 months and 8 years of age, with equal male and female predominance. It has a seasonal peak in the summer and early fall. Classic HUS presents after a prodrome of diarrheal illness and has thus been called D+ HUS (Table 111-1). Other forms of HUS that do not follow a diarrheal prodrome are classified as D– HUS (Table 111-2).

CLINICAL PRESENTATION

Classic HUS presents a few days to 2 weeks after a prodrome of diarrheal illness. The diarrhea is usually bloody or mucoid and is associated with abdominal pain. Just as the child's symptoms of colitis seem to be resolving, he or she presents with pallor, irritability, and oliguria or anuria. Patients commonly have petechiae, edema, dehydration or evidence of fluid overload, hypertension, and electrolyte abnormalities. Minor neurologic findings such as irritability and lethargy often occur. Less commonly, children may have significant neurologic effects such as seizure, coma, or stroke. Other manifestations include pancreatitis, hepatitis, GI bleeding, intussusception, and cardiac involvement such as myocarditis.

DIAGNOSIS AND EVALUATION

The diagnosis can be made based on the history, physical examination, and laboratory findings. As noted, a prodome of diarrheal illness is usually present. Enterohemorrhagic *Escherichia coli* infection with the subtype O157:H7 is one of the most commonly associated causes. Stool cultures may reveal *E. coli* O157:H7, but the yield of positive cultures decreases dramatically after 6 days of illness. The presence of Shiga toxin in the stool, even in the absence of positive stool cultures, is suggestive of enterohemorrhagic *E. coli* infection. Shiga toxin-producing *E. coli* is found in the GI tract of beef cattle and can be isolated from inadequately cooked ground beef. Shiga toxin can also be produced by *Shigella dysenteriae* and may be present in contaminated water. It is active against the vascular endothelium of small blood vessels such as those found in the GI tract and renal glomerulus. As the diarrhea of the acute illness resolves, the child presents with irritability and pallor. The physical examination is notable for signs of volume overload, thrombocytopenia, and anemia.

Laboratory work reveals anemia, with hemoglobin in the range of 5 to 9 g/dL. Red blood cells have the morphology of spherocytes, burr cells, and helmet-shaped forms, all consistent with microangiopathic hemolysis caused by cell trauma from the renal microvasculature. Platelets are decreased in more than 90% of patients due to a consumptive process. Megakaryocytes are normal. Fibrin degradation products are elevated, but coagulation studies are normal, and there is no evidence of disseminated intravascular coagulation. On occasion, if vitamin K levels are decreased due to the diarrheal illness, the child may have a mild coagulopathy. White blood cell counts are often increased, and the reticulocyte count is increased as the marrow attempts to replace hemolyzed red blood cells. A broad range of electrolyte abnormalities can be seen related to the renal dysfunction; most often patients have hyperkalemia, hypocalcemia, and either hypo- or hypernatremia. Both blood urea nitrogen and creatinine are variably elevated, based on the degree of renal involvement, and the urinalysis may reveal microscopic hematuria, proteinuria, and casts. Amylase, lipase, and liver enzymes may be elevated.

Additional studies, including imaging studies, may be useful, depending on the individual presentation. Renal ultrasonography usually reveals nonspecific findings. Echocardiography should be considered in the face of myocarditis or other cardiac dysfunction. Electrocardiography may be considered to evaluate for the effects of hyperkalemia. Computed tomography or magnetic resonance imaging of the brain should be considered when neurologic complications arise. Air or contrast enema can be helpful when GI complications such as intussusception, perforation, stricture, or toxic megacolon are suspected.

DIFFERENTIAL DIAGNOSIS

When present, the constellation of findings in HUS is generally easily recognized. Early in the course, however, diagnosis can be more difficult. Diseases that cause acute renal failure, such as the glomerulonephritides, vasculitides, and overwhelming sepsis, may mimic HUS. Other considerations are early ulcerative colitis, bilateral renal vein thrombosis, systemic lupus erythematosus, and malignant hypertension. Thrombotic thrombocytopenic purpura has a similar presentation to HUS but is usually seen in the adult population and typically has greater central nervous system involvement compared with HUS.

COURSE OF ILLNESS

The course of HUS can be variable in severity and duration, but there is a general pattern to the illness. Patients are diagnosed following the usual clinical course of resolving

Table 111-1   Diarrhea-Associated (D+) Causes of Hemolytic Uremic Syndrome

Aeromonas hydrophila
Bacteroides species
Campylobacter jejuni
Escherichia coli O157:H7
Entamoeba histolytica
Pseudomonas species
Salmonella typhi
Shigella dysenteriae
Yersinia species

Table 111-2   Non-Diarrhea-Associated (D–) Causes of Hemolytic Uremic Syndrome

Drug related
Oral contraceptives
Cyclosporine
Tacrolimus
Chemotherapy
Idiopathic
Infections
Streptococcus pneumoniae
Coxsackievirus
Influenza virus
Epstein-Barr virus
Portillo virus
Human immunodeficiency virus (HIV)
Inherited
Autosomal recessive
Autosomal dominant
Factor H gene mutation
Malignancy
Malignant hypertension
Pregnancy
Transplantation

colitis and the onset of anemia, thrombocytopenia, and renal dysfunction. Over the next hours to days of illness, the patient's general clinical picture worsens, with further decreases in hemoglobin, platelets, and urine output and increasing blood urea nitrogen and creatinine. Patients may progress to renal failure with anuria, requiring dialysis, or may follow a milder course of illness. After this period of decline, there is usually a plateau that lasts for several days or even weeks. The child may remain on dialysis and be transfusion dependent during this time. Eventually, most patients recover, heralded by an increase in platelets. Recovery of other systems follows slowly. Most children survive the acute phase; however, there is a mortality rate of 3% to 5%.

Although the majority of children are thought to have a complete recovery following HUS, some may suffer long-term effects. The long-term sequelae of the illness have not been extensively studied. One Argentinean study divided patients into four general groups based on outcome: there was complete recovery in approximately 60%, only proteinuria with or without hypertension in 18%, reduced creatinine clearance (often with proteinuria and hypertension) in 16%, and end-stage renal failure in 3% to 4%.[2] Some predictors of poor prognosis are severe prodromal illness, increased white blood cell count at presentation, increasing number of days of anuria, multisystem involvement, and prolonged proteinuria.[3]

TREATMENT

Initially, many children can be managed as outpatients, with frequent physical examinations and laboratory evaluations. Supportive care may be all that is necessary, and the illness may resolve rather quickly. However, inpatient treatment is often warranted for more severe or progressive illness. The mainstay of therapy is management of renal dysfunction. Urine output and electrolytes should be monitored closely, and fluids adjusted as necessary. Oliguric patients can be given furosemide to enhance output. Anuric patients should have fluid intake limited to insensible losses (about one third maintenance) plus output.

Despite meticulous management, many children eventually require dialysis. Dialysis is indicated if the patient has hyperkalemia, severe metabolic acidosis, severe uremia, or signs of volume overload. Careful transfusion with packed red blood cells should be used to maintain adequate perfusion and prevent congestive heart failure. Platelets should be given only in the face of active bleeding or the need for an invasive procedure (e.g., dialysis catheter placement, central venous line placement). More liberal use of platelets can actually increase thrombus formation in the renal microvasculature and cause clinical deterioration.

Nutritional support is imperative for recovery, and enteral feeding should be maintained, based on clinical status. If this is not possible, parenteral nutrition should be initiated. Diarrhea should be managed with supportive care, with the avoidance of antimotility agents and antibiotics, which some believe may prolong or increase the severity of HUS.

Hypertension is initially controlled through the careful stabilization of volume status. If hypertension persists, medical management can be initiated. Calcium channel blockers such as nifedipine are frequently used as first-line agents. Potentially nephrotoxic drugs, such as nonsteroidal anti-inflammatory agents, should be avoided. In cases of long-term renal sequelae, such as hypertension and proteinuria, ongoing surveillance and close follow-up are indicated.

CONSULTATION

Specific consultative services are indicated based on the severity of illness and the organ systems involved. Examples include the following:

- Nephrology evaluation for significant renal dysfunction.
- Cardiology consultation for management of hypertension and carditis.

- Hematology evaluation for management of hemolytic anemia and indications for transfusion.
- Gastroenterology or surgical evaluation for complications of colitis.

ADMISSION CRITERIA

- Signs of moderate to severe dehydration.
- Signs of volume overload or electrolyte derangement.
- Rapidly declining renal function.
- Uncontrolled hypertension.
- Severe anemia or thrombocytopenia, evidence of active bleeding, or need for transfusion.
- Mental status changes.

DISCHARGE CRITERIA

- Renal function resolving, and electrolytes stable.
- Platelet count rising.
- Hemoglobin stable or increasing.
- Ability to ingest adequate oral intake for fluid and nutritional needs.
- Hypertension resolved or controlled with medication.

PREVENTION

Because many cases of HUS follow a GI illness, prevention of the inciting illness may lead to the prevention of HUS. This is relevant in the case of infection with *E. coli* O157:H7, because 2% to 13% of infected pediatric patients develop HUS. Reduction in *E. coli* infection can be accomplished by avoiding raw or undercooked ground beef and unpasteurized milk, cheese, or cider. Decreasing levels of O157:H7 in cattle, thereby reducing the risk of humans' acquiring the disease, can be accomplished by modification of the animals' diet before slaughter and by irradiation of meat.

Infection can be associated with exposure to farm and zoologic animals (e.g., petting zoos, farm tours), because many animals shed this organism.[4] Person-to-person transmission is also a concern, especially in places such as daycare centers, where outbreaks might occur. Hand hygiene is an effective tool to reduce transmission, although compliance can be a challenge. In the hospital setting, contact precautions are indicated to limit the risk of transmission.

Routine antibiotic treatment of *E. coli* O157:H7 is not recommended, because antimicrobial therapy of the diarrheal illness neither increases nor decreases the risk of developing HUS.[5]

IN A NUTSHELL

- The presentation of HUS is generally a prodromal GI illness followed by microangiopathic hemolytic anemia, thrombocytopenia, and varying degree of renal failure.
- Diagnosis is made clinically and by laboratory findings.
- Management includes meticulous fluid balance, judicious red cell transfusions, nutritional support, and dialysis when indicated.

ON THE HORIZON

- New therapies for HUS are under investigation. Among these is Synsorb-Pk, a drug that mediates the binding of Shiga toxin and prevents systemic absorption, therefore preventing disease. Also being investigated are a monoclonal antibody to Shiga toxin[6] and vascular endothelial growth factor therapy.[7]

SUGGESTED READING

Trachtman H, Christen E: Pathogenesis, treatment, and therapeutic trials in hemolytic uremic syndrome. Curr Opin Pediatr 1999;11:162-168.

Varade WS: Hemolytic uremic syndrome: Reducing the risks. Contemp Pediatr 2000;17:54-64.

REFERENCES

1. Miller DP, Kaye JA, Shea K, et al: Incidence of thrombotic thrombocytopenic purpura/hemolytic uremic syndrome. Epidemiology 2004;15:208-215.
2. Spizzirri FD, Rahman RC, Bibiloni N, et al: Childhood hemolytic uremic syndrome in Argentina: Long term follow-up and prognostic features. Pediatr Nephrol 1997;11:156-160.
3. Gianviti A, Tozzi A, DePetris L, et al: Risk factors for poor renal prognosis in children with hemolytic uremic syndrome. Pediatr Nephrol 2003;18:1229-1235.
4. National Association of State Public Health Veterinarians, Inc: Compendium of measures to prevent disease associated with animals in public settings, 2005. MMWR Recomm Rep 2005;54:1-12.
5. Safdar N, Said A, Gangnon RE, Maki DG: Risk of hemolytic uremic syndrome after antibiotic treatment of *Escherichia coli* O157:H7 enteritis: A meta-analysis. JAMA 2002;288:996-1001.
6. Tzipori S, Sheoran A, Akiyoshi D, et al: Antibody therapy in the management of Shiga toxin-induced hemolytic uremic syndrome. Clin Microbiol Rev 2004;17:926-941.
7. Kim YG, Suga SI, Kang DH, et al: Vascular endothelial growth factor accelerates renal recovery in experimental thrombotic microangiopathhy. Kidney Int 2000;58:2390-2399.

CHAPTER 112

Interstitial Nephritis

Kevin D. McBryde

Interstitial nephritis was first described histologically nearly 100 years ago in the kidneys of patients dying of scarlet fever or diphtheria in the absence of direct infection of the kidneys. Unlike the glomerulonephritides, interstitial nephritis refers to the histologic demonstration of primary inflammation of the renal interstitium and tubular cells by inflammatory cells, accompanied by interstitial edema or fibrosis and varying degrees of tubular atrophy. More accurately, interstitial nephritis should be termed *tubulointerstitial nephritis* (TIN). *Acute tubulointerstitial nephritis* (AIN) refers to a sudden onset and rapid decline in renal function, whereas *chronic tubulointerstitial nephritis* (CIN) describes a more insidious decline in renal function. In AIN, the acute inflammatory process predominates in the pathologic picture, with inflammation of the renal interstitium, interstitial edema, and tubular epithelial cell damage being present. In contrast, in CIN, the histopathologic picture is one of tubular epithelial damage, interstitial fibrosis, and tubular atrophy.

The true prevalence of TIN in the pediatric population is unknown. According to the 2004 annual report from the North American Pediatric Renal Transplant Cooperative Study, TIN and pyelonephritis account for approximately 1.4% of all identified causes of chronic kidney disease and 1.6% of all causes of end-stage renal disease in the United States.[1] In a single pediatric center experience, AIN was diagnosed by percutaneous kidney biopsy in 7% of biopsy samples obtained in a 3-year period.[2]

PATHOPHYSIOLOGY

Both T-cell and B-cell mechanisms are involved in the development of TIN in humans. Immunohistochemical staining of kidney tissue in TIN may demonstrate anti–tubular basement membrane antibodies, as well as deposition of IgG and complement, along the tubular basement membranes.[3-5] Potential antigens include the tubular basement membrane, Tamm-Horsfall protein, and Heyman nephritis.[3-5] These potential antigens may be internalized, processed, and presented by renal tubular epithelial cells with major histocompatibility complex (MHC) class II antigens to helper T cells, thereby activating cytotoxic T cells or B cells.[3-5] Alternatively, these antigens may be internalized by circulating antigen-presenting cells outside the kidney and stimulate immune activation.[3-5] Finally, an extrarenal antigen may cross-react with a component of the renal tubulointerstitium and lead to an antibody response.[3-5]

In contrast to the relatively uncommon B-cell–mediated causes of TIN, T-cell mechanisms appear to predominate in human TIN.[3-5] The most common clinical manifestation of T-cell involvement in TIN is in the syndrome of TIN with uveitis. T cells infiltrate the tubulointerstitial compartment of the kidney in the absence of demonstrable antibody deposition.[3-5] The T-cell immune response may be mediated by CD8+ T cells recognizing antigens in association with MHC class I antigens.[3-5] This direct cytotoxic effect of CD8+ T cells may explain the tubular cell damage found in AIN. A second mechanism of T-cell–mediated injury in TIN involves delayed-type hypersensitivity. In this instance, CD4+ T cells activate macrophages, which are responsible for the lesions seen in TIN.[3-5] In a delayed-type hypersensitivity reaction causing TIN, the inflammatory cells contain a mixture of CD8+ T cells, CD4+ T cells, natural killer cells, B cells, and macrophages.[3-5] A final mechanism of T-cell–mediated TIN is the formation of antibody-dependent immune responses. This is the mechanism believed to underlie the development of medication-induced TIN. Here, a drug metabolite may bind to the tubular basement membrane and form a hapten complex, thereby stimulating the production of anti–tubular basement membrane antibodies.[3-5]

There are many causes of TIN, including infectious, medication induced, immune mediated, toxic, metabolic, and hereditary. Some specific etiologic agents or disorders are provided in Table 112-1.

CLINICAL PRESENTATION

The most common clinical presentation of TIN consists of nonspecific constitutional symptoms, including fever, abdominal pain, nausea, vomiting, anorexia, weight loss, polydipsia, polyuria, hypertension, headache, and rash.[2,6-10] Some authors have also described a seasonal predilection for the development of TIN in pediatric patients, most commonly occurring between December and June.[6] Laboratory findings include anemia, leukocytosis, eosinophilia, elevated erythrocyte sedimentation rate, acute renal failure, elevated fractional excretion of sodium, proteinuria, hematuria, and sterile pyuria (Table 112-2).[2,6-10] Attention to the temporal relationship of the initiation of medication and the onset of symptoms may be especially helpful in making a diagnosis of medication-induced AIN.

DIFFERENTIAL DIAGNOSIS

The differential diagnosis for AIN is essentially limited to the glomerulonephritides (see Chapter 110). In the face of acute renal failure, the list may be expanded to include a variety of intrinsic causes of renal failure (see Chapter 108). The signs associated with AIN, including hematuria and pyuria, lend themselves to a number of renal and nonrenal disorders, such as trauma, urinary tract infection, renal vein

Table 112-1   Causes of Tubulointerstitial Nephritis

Infections	Drug Reactions	Immune Mediated	Other
Bacterial	**Antibiotics**	**Anti-TBM Antibodies**	**Metabolic**
β-Hemolytic streptococci	Penicillins	Primary anti-TBM nephritis	Oxalate nephropathy
Corynebacterium	Cephalosporins	Secondary anti-TBM nephritis	Hypercalcemic nephropathy
Brucella sp.	Sulfonamides	Anti-GBM disease	Urate nephropathy
Legionella pneumophila	Rifampin	Membranous nephropathy	Cystine nephropathy
Campylobacter jejuni	Ethambutol	**Immune Complex Deposits**	
Mycoplasma sp.	Azithromycin	Primary immune complex nephritis	**Heavy Metal**
Salmonella sp.	Ciprofloxacin	Secondary immune complex nephritis	Lead
Yersinia pseudotuberculosis	Tetracycline	Lupus nephritis	Cadmium
	Vancomycin	Sjögren syndrome	Mercury
Viruses	Erythromycin	MPGN	
Rubeola	Aminoglycosides	Membranous nephropathy	**Hereditary**
Epstein-Barr virus		Mixed cryoglobulinemia	Alport syndrome
HIV	**Anti-inflammatory**		Nephrolithiasis–medullary cystic
Hepatitis viruses	**Drugs**	**T Cell Mediated**	kidney
Cytomegalovirus	Ibuprofen	Tubulointerstitial nephritis with	
Polyomavirus (BK)	Indomethacin	uveitis syndrome	**Miscellaneous**
Hantavirus		Sarcoidosis	Chinese herb nephropathy
Adenovirus	**Diuretics**	Granulomatous tubulointerstitial	Radiation nephritis
	Furosemide	nephritis	Ischemic nephropathy
Fungi	Thiazides		Balkan endemic nephropathy
Candida sp.			
Aspergillus sp	**Other Medications**		
Cryptococcus neoformans	Cimetidine		
Histoplasma capsulatum	Omeprazole		
Coccidioides immitis	Captopril		
Blastomyces dermatitidis	Carbamazepine		
Mucormycosis	Phenobarbital		
	Cyclosporine		
Parasites	Lithium		
Plasmodium sp.	Gold		
Schistosoma sp.	Aspirin		
Filariasis	Azathioprine		

GBM, glomerular basement membrane; HIV, human immunodeficiency virus; MPGN, membranoproliferative glomerulonephritis; TBM, tubular basement membrane.

Table 112-2   Laboratory Abnormalities in Tubular Interstitial Nephritis

CBC	Chemistry	Immunology	Urinalysis
Anemia	Acute renal failure*	Elevated ESR	$FE_{NA} > 2\%$
Leukocytosis	Hypoalbuminemia	Elevated IgG	Proteinuria
Eosinophilia		Hypocomplementemia	Hematuria
		Elevated antistreptolysin O and antihyaluronidase titers	Leukocyturia
		Increased anti-DNase titer	Glycosuria
			Granular casts

*Serum creatinine greater than 3 mg/dL or calculated glomerular filtration rate less than 50 mL/min/1.73 m².
CBC, complete blood count; ESR, erythrocyte sedimentation rate; FE_{NA}, fractional excretion of sodium.

Table 112-3 Key Laboratory Findings in Acute Renal Failure, Acute Glomerulonephritis, and Tubulointerstitial Nephritis

	Prerenal Acute Renal Failure	Acute Glomerulonephritis	Tubulointerstitial Nephritis
Serum creatinine	↑	↔ or ↑	↑
Serum potassium	↑	↔ or ↑	↓
Serum HCO_3^-	↓	↓ or ↔ or ↑	↓
Proteinuria	None	>2 g/24 hr (U_{pr}/U_{cr} > 2.0)	<1 g/24 hr (U_{pr}/U_{cr} < 1.0)
Hematuria	None	↔ or ↑	↔ or ↑
Pyuria	None	↔ or ↑	↔ or ↑
Urine sediment	Hyaline casts	RBC, WBC, granular or hyaline casts	Granular, hyaline, or WBC casts
FE_{NA}	<1%	<2%	>2%

↓, Decreased; ↔, normal; ↑, increased; FE_{NA}, fractional excretion of sodium; RBC, red blood cell; U_{pr}/U_{cr}, urine protein–to–urine creatinine ratio; WBC, white blood cell.

thrombosis, calculi, sickle cell trait, hemorrhagic cystitis, and vasculitis.

DIAGNOSIS AND EVALUATION

Noninvasive studies may be useful in establishing the diagnosis of TIN. As noted previously, the most common laboratory abnormality in TIN (in some cases >90% of patients) is elevated serum creatinine with a decreased calculated or measured glomerular filtration rate.[6-8] Proteinuria is a prominent finding, although it is often less than nephrotic range (see Table 112-3).[6-9] Because different segments of the nephron may be involved in TIN, one may identify evidence of Fanconi syndrome (involving the proximal tubule) or distal renal tubular acidosis (affecting the distal convoluted tubule). Pyuria, in the absence of active infection, may provide a clue to the diagnosis of TIN.

A commonly reported laboratory finding in TIN is the presence of eosinophiluria. Although the majority of cases of eosinophiluria are due to infection of the upper or lower urinary tract, it may be seen in up to 25% of cases of TIN.[11,12] Hansel stain is better for the detection of eosinophiluria than Wright stain.

Most commonly, renal ultrasonography is used to image the kidneys in cases of acute renal failure in which TIN may be in the differential diagnosis. The kidneys often appear larger in width, depth, and length in patients with AIN than in normal, age-matched pediatric patients.[13,14] In addition to nephromegaly, the kidneys appear diffusely echogenic in comparison to the liver and spleen, with increased echogenicity occurring particularly in the renal cortices.[13,14] In contrast, chronic CIN is characterized ultrasonographically by small renal size and diffusely increased echogenicity.

Percutaneous kidney biopsy remains the "gold standard" for the diagnosis of TIN. In one study, more than 50% of pediatric patients in whom AIN was diagnosed by kidney biopsy were not thought to have AIN based on clinical and laboratory evaluations preceding the biopsy.[6] Kidney biopsy can provide accurate diagnosis in the more than half of children who are initially misdiagnosed on clinical grounds. Kidney biopsy may provide invaluable prognostic information as well. The use of a tubulointerstitial score at the time

of biopsy has been reported to be useful in predicting clinical response to corticosteroid therapy, as well as long-term renal function.[15,16]

Table 112-3 provides comparisons of laboratory findings in acute glomerulonephritis, acute renal failure, and TIN.

TREATMENT

Treatment of acute renal failure (ARF) secondary to TIN remains primarily supportive in nature.[2,4,6-10] Potentially offending medications that may be responsible for TIN should be discontinued. If a medication is necessary for treatment of an underlying disorder and an appropriate substitute agent is available, replacement of the suspected medication is justified. If an infectious cause is suspected, prompt medical treatment with appropriate antibiotics, antifungals, or antiviral medications should be initiated. For patients presenting with acute renal failure and indications for dialytic therapy, renal replacement therapy should be provided until the patient's renal function recovers.[2,4,6-10]

For the treatment of AIN that is unresponsive to drug discontinuation in cases of suspected medication-induced TIN or for the treatment of a suspected infection, corticosteroids should be used. Several uncontrolled adult studies have demonstrated faster return to the previous or to a new baseline serum creatinine, as well as a higher percentage of patients returning to their previous serum creatinine and a lower mean serum creatinine in patients receiving corticosteroids than in those not treated with corticosteroids. Few studies of AIN in the pediatric population have been performed, and thus whether corticosteroids induce a similar response is unclear. However, it seems prudent to prescribe prednisone at a dose of 1 to 2 mg/kg/day (maximum of 60 mg/day) as a single dose or in divided doses for approximately 4 weeks.[2,4,6-10] On completion of the course of daily corticosteroids, the patient may be switched to an alternate-day corticosteroid regimen followed by a tapered schedule of the prednisone.

Although recommendations exist for the use of cyclophosphamide or cyclosporine in the treatment of corticosteroid-resistant AIN, there are no controlled studies to support this recommendation.

COURSE OF ILLNESS

The overall prognosis of TIN is rather good, unlike that reported for TIN in adults. Several studies showed that most patients had complete recovery of renal function after supportive therapy or treatment with corticosteroids or cytotoxic agents, even though some patients required hemodialysis.[2,4,9,10] Estimates of time to recovery range from 1 to 10 months.[6,9] TIN plus uveitis in children has a similarly good long-term prognosis.[17]

CONSULTATION

Involving nephrologists in the evaluation process is helpful when AIN is a diagnostic consideration. Consultation should be considered warranted when symptoms persist despite discontinuation of the inciting agent, renal function is compromised, corticosteroid therapy is being considered, and recurrent disease is present.

ADMISSION CRITERIA

- Acute renal failure
- Age younger than 2 years or older than 12 years
- Nephrotic-range proteinuria
- Progressive decrease in renal function as measured by serum creatinine or urine output, or both
- Recurrent episodes of AIN
- Patients failing to respond to symptomatic therapy (i.e., those requiring steroid initiation with or without biopsy)

DISCHARGE CRITERIA

- Stabilization of renal function
- Establishment of appropriate referrals and follow-up

PREVENTION

Prevention of AIN is probably difficult, especially the initial episode. It may be preventable by careful consideration of medications prescribed to pediatric patients. With commonly prescribed antibiotics being one of the primary offenders, early recognition of systemic symptoms and discontinuation of the potential offending medication may circumvent the development of AIN.

IN A NUTSHELL

- TIN is an inflammation of the renal interstitium and tubular cells that can be accompanied by interstitial edema, fibrosis, or tubular atrophy.
- Medication-induced AIN is one type of TIN. Removal of the offending medication is key to management of this disorder.
- The clinical presentation of TIN consists of constitutional symptoms, including rash, fever, abdominal pain, nausea, vomiting, anorexia, weight loss, polydipsia, polyuria, hypertension, and headaches.
- Laboratory findings include anemia, leukocytosis, eosinophilia, an elevated erythrocyte sedimentation rate, elevated fractional excretion of sodium, sterile pyuria, proteinuria, hematuria, and evidence of acute renal failure.
- The prognosis in children is good, with recovery of renal function occurring in most patients with proper treatment.
- Treatment involves support of renal function and, in some cases, corticosteroid therapy and removal of an inciting medication or treatment of a causative infection when such triggers can be identified.

ON THE HORIZON

- Research into the mechanisms underlying AIN is ongoing. In addition to eosinophiluria, other urinary biomarkers are being investigated.

SUGGESTED READING

Greising J, Trachtman H, Gauthier B, Valderrama E: Acute interstitial nephritis in adolescents and young adults. Child Nephrol Urol 1990;10:189-195.

Harris DC: Tubulointerstitial renal disease. Curr Opin Nephrol Hypertens 2001;10:303-313.

Jones CL, Eddy AA: Tubulointerstitial nephritis. Pediatr Nephrol 1992;6:572-586.

Kodner CM, Kudrimoti A: Diagnosis and management of acute interstitial nephritis. Am Fam Physician 2003;67:2527-2534.

REFERENCES

1. North American Pediatric Renal Transplant Cooperative Study: North American Pediatric Renal Transplant Cooperative Study (NAPRTCS) 2004 Annual Report. Boston, NAPRTCS, 2004.
2. Greising J, Trachtman H, Gauthier B, Valderrama E: Acute interstitial nephritis in adolescents and young adults. Child Nephrol Urol 1990;10:189-195.
3. Cavallo T: Tubulointerstitial nephritis. In Jennette JC, Olson LL, Schwartz MM, Silva FG (eds): Heptinstall's Pathology of the Kidney, 5th ed. Philadelphia, Lippincott-Raven, 1998, pp 667-723.
4. Dell KM, Kaplan BS, Meyers CM: Tubulointerstitial nephritis. In Barratt TM, Avner ED, Harmon WE (eds): Pediatric Nephrology, 4th ed. Baltimore, Lippincott Williams & Wilkins, 1999, pp 823-834.
5. Jones CL, Eddy AA: Tubulointerstitial nephritis. Pediatr Nephrol 1992;6:572-586.
6. Ellis D, Fried WA, Yunis EJ, Blau EB: Acute interstitial nephritis in children: A report of 13 cases and review of the literature. Pediatrics 1981;67:862-870.
7. Kobayashi Y, Honda M, Yoshikawa N, Ito H: Acute tubulointerstitial nephritis in 21 Japanese children. Clin Nephrol 2000;54:191-197.
8. Kobayashi Y, Honda M, Yoshikawa N, Ito H: Immunohistological study in sixteen children with acute tubulointerstitial nephritis. Clin Nephrol 1998;50:14-20.
9. Burghard R, Brandis M, Hoyer PF, et al: Acute interstitial nephritis in childhood. Eur J Pediatr 1984;142:103-110.
10. Hawkins EP, Berry PL, Silva FG: Acute tubulointerstitial nephritis in children: Clinical, morphologic, and lectin studies. A report of the Southwestern Pediatric Nephrology Study Group. Am J Kidney Dis 1989;14:466-471.
11. Corwin HL, Korbet SM, Schwartz MM: Clinical correlates of eosinophiluria. Arch Intern Med 1985;145:1097-1099.
12. Corwin HL, Bray RA, Haber MH: The detection and interpretation of urinary eosinophils. Arch Pathol Lab Med 1989;113:1256-1258.

13. Winkler P, Altrogge H: Sonographic signs of nephritis in children: A comparison of renal echography with clinical evaluation, laboratory data and biopsy. Pediatr Radiol 1985;15:231-237.
14. Hiraoka M, Hori C, Tsuchida S, et al: Ultrasonographic findings of acute tubulointerstitial nephritis. Am J Nephrol 1996;16:154-158.
15. Suzuki K, Tanaka H, Ito E, Waga S: Repeat renal biopsy in children with severe idiopathic tubulointerstitial nephritis. Pediatr Nephrol 2004;19:240-243.
16. Foster BJ, Bernard C, Drummond KN, Sharma AK: Effective therapy for severe Henoch-Schönlein purpura nephritis with prednisone and azathioprine: A clinical and histopathologic study. J Pediatr 2000;136:370-375.
17. Vohra S, Eddy A, Levin AV, et al: Tubulointerstitial nephritis with uveitis in children and adolescents. Four new cases and a review of the literature. Pediatr Nephrol 1999;13:426-432.

CHAPTER 113

Nephrotic Syndrome

Melissa J. Gregory

Nephrotic syndrome is one of the most common chronic renal diseases in children. It has an incidence of 2 to 7 per 100,000 population and a prevalence of 16 per 100,000 population, well above the 1 per 1 million incidence of chronic renal failure in children.[1] Before the era of effective treatment and easily available antibiotics, children with nephrotic syndrome had a dismal prognosis, with a mortality rate of up to 50%. With the advent of prednisone, an effective therapy for the majority of children with nephrotic syndrome, and the common availability of broad-spectrum oral antibiotics, the long-term prognosis of childhood nephrotic syndrome is excellent. Nevertheless, even with access to treatment and antibiotics, the mortality rate among those with the most common form of nephrotic syndrome is close to 2%.[2] Most children do not require hospitalization except at diagnosis, and a significant proportion avoid a hospital stay altogether. Hospitalization is more often required for the treatment of complications than for nephrotic syndrome itself.

PATHOPHYSIOLOGY

There are many different types of nephrotic syndrome. The most common histopathologies seen in childhood nephrotic syndrome are minimal change disease, focal segmental glomerulosclerosis, and membranoproliferative glomerulonephritis (Table 113-1).[2] Membranous nephropathy, a common cause of nephrotic syndrome in adults, is rarely seen in children. The basic pathophysiology of all forms of nephrotic syndrome is an abnormal permselectivity barrier, leading to pathologic protein loss across the glomerular basement membrane. This barrier is formed by three structural elements: endothelial cells, glomerular basement membrane, and specialized epithelial cells called podocytes that connect to one another through a network of slit diaphragms.[1] Slit diaphragms are largely responsible for preventing the glomerular filtration of protein. Different forms of nephrotic syndrome are associated with different defects of the permselectivity barrier. The most common form of congenital nephrotic syndrome is due to an abnormal slit diaphragm protein called nephrin. Certain cases of focal segmental glomerulosclerosis are associated with a soluble circulating permeability-modifying factor that can be removed through plasmapheresis. In minimal change disease there is a change in the polarity of the glomerular basement membrane. It is still unclear, other than in clearly genetic forms of nephrotic syndrome, which factors are responsible for the development of disease.

CLINICAL PRESENTATION

The most common presentation of childhood nephrotic syndrome is a young child with a complaint of several weeks of slowly progressive edema, usually periorbital, often fol-

lowing an upper respiratory infection. An initial misdiagnosis of allergic reaction is common, and the correct diagnosis may be delayed until a more generalized edema brings the child back to the physician's office. Ascites is common, as is scrotal and labial edema. In preambulatory children, sacral edema may be present. The development of edema is associated with rapid weight gain, and children may be unable to fit into their usual clothing and shoes.

DIFFERENTIAL DIAGNOSIS

Early in the course of nephrotic syndrome, when the child has mainly periorbital edema, the presentation may be suggestive of environmental allergies. Occasionally, a severe allergic reaction can be associated with hypoalbuminemia as well as edema. As the disease progresses and the edema becomes more generalized, other protein-losing states, such as protein-losing gastroenteropathy, can be confused with nephrotic syndrome before a urinalysis is obtained. Congestive heart failure can rarely present with anasarca, but it is easily distinguished by associated symptoms. Secondary nephrotic syndrome can be caused by multiple systemic diseases but is rarely seen in children. Other forms of renal disease can also present with nephrotic-range proteinuria and need to be considered (Table 113-2).

DIAGNOSIS AND EVALUATION

Nephrotic syndrome of childhood is characterized by the clinical finding of edema and the laboratory findings of hypoalbuminemia, massive proteinuria (>4 mg/m^2 per hour), and hyperlipidemia. There are other possible causes of edema and hypoalbuminemia, and a urinalysis is essential for the diagnosis of nephrotic syndrome, preferably with the addition of a semiquantitative protein assessment by means of a first-morning void (spot) protein-creatinine ratio. A 24-hour urine collection is not required to make the diagnosis of nephrotic syndrome; in fact, it may be nearly impossible to achieve in younger patients and can delay the initiation of treatment. Any child presenting with edema who is found to have elevated lipids (usually cholesterol), a serum albumin less than 2.5 g/dL, and 3 to 4+ proteinuria on urine dipstick should be assumed to have nephrotic syndrome. A spot urine protein-creatinine ratio greater than 2.0 confirms the diagnosis (normal is <0.18).[1]

In children between the ages of 2 and 8 years who present without associated gross hematuria, severe hypertension, systemic symptoms, or acute renal failure, no further laboratory evaluation is needed. For this group of children, there is a 95% likelihood that the cause of nephrotic syndrome is minimal change disease. These patients are likely to respond to prednisone and have an excellent long-term prognosis. Children who fall outside of these parameters may still have

Table 113-1 Causes of Primary Nephrotic Syndrome

Idiopathic
  Minimal change disease
  Focal segmental glomerulosclerosis
  Membranonproliferative glomerulonephritis
  IgM nephropathy
  Membranous nephropathy

Congenital
  Finnish-type congenital nephrotic syndrome
  Denys-Drash syndrome
  Diffuse mesangial sclerosis
  Focal segmental glomerulosclerosis

Table 113-2 Differential Diagnosis of Nephrotic Syndrome

Nonrenal disease
  Protein-losing enteropathy
  Congestive heart failure

Renal disease
  IgA nephropathy
  Membranoproliferative glomerulonephritis
  Acute interstitial nephritis
  Postinfectious glomerulonephritis
  Alport disease

Secondary nephrotic syndrome
  Systemic lupus erythematosus
  Henoch-Schönlein purpura
  Acquired immunodeficiency syndrome (AIDS)
  Cytomegalovirus
  Hepatitis
  Sickle cell disease
  Malaria
  Diabetes mellitus
  Drugs (ibuprofen, heroin)

minimal change disease, but because there is a greater chance of them having a less benign condition, an early nephrology consultation is beneficial.

Children younger than 1 year who present with nephrotic syndrome are more likely to have either congenital or genetic disorders rather than minimal change disease.[1] The care of this subset of children can be complex and requires the expertise of a pediatric nephrologist. For children between the ages of 12 and 24 months, nephrotic syndrome is less commonly due to minimal change disease compared with older children, and the likelihood of congenital and genetic disorders is decreased compared with the infant population. Children older than 8 years with nephrotic syndrome may have minimal change disease, but they are statistically more likely to have a different cause, such as focal segmental glomerulosclerosis or membranoproliferative glomerulonephritis. Because of the increased risk of non–minimal change diseases, older children need an immunologic workup, including antinuclear antibody, C3 complement level, and immunoglobulin A, in addition to the laboratory studies mentioned earlier. These children also need nephrol-

ogy consultation and may require renal biopsy before the initiation of treatment.

TREATMENT

Pharmacologic Therapy

In children with suspected minimal change disease, the initial treatment is prednisone 60 mg/m^2 daily (up to a maximum of 80 mg/day). Anecdotally, divided doses are thought to be more effective in inducing remission, although this has not been substantiated by clinical trials. Although most patients with classic minimal change disease respond to steroids in the first 1 to 2 weeks, it is clear from multiple clinical trials that a prolonged initial course (6 to 8 weeks) of daily prednisone, followed by 4 to 6 weeks of alternate-day prednisone, is superior to a short-term regimen in inducing long-term remission.[3] Thus, prolonged initial treatment should be given regardless of the rapidity of remission. Following initial treatment, the prednisone dose is gradually tapered, usually over 4 to 6 weeks. Subsequent relapses, which occur in almost two thirds of children with nephrotic syndrome, can be treated using a short course of prednisone lasting only a few days past the induction of remission. Children who fail to respond to an initial 8-week course of prednisone, relapse during tapering of prednisone, relapse within a few weeks of stopping prednisone, or have four or more relapses within a 12-month period should be referred to a nephrologist.

There are multiple second-line therapies for children with complicated nephrotic syndrome. Children with frequently relapsing nephrotic syndrome (two or more relapses within 6 months of initial response, or four relapses within a 12-month period) and those with steroid-dependent nephrotic syndrome (two consecutive relapses during prednisone taper or within 14 days of stopping prednisone) often have a good response to alkylating agents such as cyclophosphamide or chlorambucil. The anthelmintic levamisole can also help decrease the number of relapses in children with frequently relapsing nephrotic syndrome. Steroid-resistant nephrotic syndrome is more difficult to treat. Pulse methylprednisolone, with or without cyclophosphamide, and calcineurin inhibitors such as cyclosporine and tacrolimus have been used successfully in these patients. Any of these secondary agents should be administered only with the advice and involvement of a nephrologist.

Edema

The reason for the development of edema in nephrotic syndrome is controversial. The classic theory is that hypoalbuminemia causes decreased intravascular oncotic pressure, leading to the movement of plasma water into the interstitial space. According to this theory, sodium retention is secondary, occurring in response to decreased intravascular volume. However, studies in children with nephrotic syndrome do not show a uniform decrease in intravascular volume; some patients have normal or even increased intravascular volume.[2] In response to these studies, a second theory is that there is a primary defect in sodium excretion in nephrotic syndrome. Regardless of the physiology that causes edema formation, edema is the most common reason for the hospitalization of children with nephrotic syndrome.

Not all children presenting with edema secondary to nephrotic syndrome require hospitalization. Mild to moderate edema can be managed at home with a low-salt diet to prevent the development of further edema, with or without a low-dose thiazide diuretic. Children who are placed on both a low-salt diet and a diuretic also need to limit their fluid intake, because hyponatremia can result from the diuretic-induced natriuresis. For most children, limiting the fluid intake to 1000 mL/day is effective in preventing hyponatremia without imposing a hardship on the child. Children weighing less than 10 kg, however, should be limited to 750 mL/day.

Children with severe edema that impedes ambulation, is painful, or appears to be compromising skin integrity should be hospitalized for diuresis. Children with symptoms of intravascular volume overload (e.g., congestive heart failure, pulmonary edema, severe hypertension) should also be admitted for diuresis. The safest and most effective method of inducing diuresis in severely edematous children is controversial. Protocols vary widely among practitioners, depending largely on personal experience and training, because there are relatively few clinical trials on which to base therapy.

Clearly, a diuretic is needed, and loop diuretics tend to be most effective. Intravenous furosemide 1 to 2 mg/kg is widely used; however, there is no consensus among nephrologists regarding the safety and efficacy of using 25% albumin (the majority of which is rapidly excreted in the urine) along with furosemide. Advocates of using 25% albumin argue that children with nephrotic syndrome are intravascularly depleted at the time of presentation and that aggressive diuretic use without concurrent volume expansion further decreases intravascular volume, potentially leading to intravascular collapse. However, 25% albumin is expensive, and its administration is potentially complicated by fluid overload, including pulmonary edema, hypertension, and congestive heart failure. Practitioners opposing the use of 25% albumin cite the aforementioned risks and point to evidence that children with nephrotic syndrome are not intravascularly depleted and therefore are not at risk for intravascular collapse.

It is difficult to determine appropriate clinical care in the face of two diametrically opposing factions, both of which can cite supporting literature. However, in clinical situations, the following guidelines may be helpful: In patients with obvious signs and symptoms of hypervolemia (tachypnea, chronic nonproductive cough, orthopnea, hepatosplenomegaly, hypertension), intravenous furosemide without an albumin infusion should be prescribed. Conversely, patients with obvious signs and symptoms of hypovolemia (tachycardia, hypotension, orthostatic pulse or blood pressure changes) should receive an infusion of 25% albumin before diuretic administration. For patients without a clear-cut intravascular volume status—that is, the majority of patients—the coadministration of furosemide and 25% albumin may increase the diuresis achieved and decrease the duration of hospitalization. In this subset of patients, one might also attempt diuresis with a diuretic alone and add albumin if there is an inadequate response or if the patient develops symptoms of intravascular depletion.

Guidelines for albumin infusion are not clear-cut either. Generally, 0.5 to 1 g/kg of 25% albumin is given every 12 hours until the findings that led to the patient's hospitalization have resolved. It is not appropriate to use 5% albumin in place of 25% albumin owing to the increased salt and water load with the more dilute solution. The duration of infusion varies among institutions. A too rapid infusion can lead to volume overload as the interstitial fluid translocates to the vascular space. Durations reported in the literature range from 1 to 8 hours, with 4 hours being a good compromise. Furosemide is incompatible with albumin and should be given either immediately before or after completion of the albumin infusion. Close monitoring of vital signs is required during albumin infusion to assess for volume overload. Patients who develop tachypnea, cough, or hypertension during albumin infusion should have the infusion stopped and furosemide administered; once the symptoms resolve, the infusion can be resumed at a slower rate.

Hypertension

For most children with nephrotic syndrome, hypertension is associated with volume overload and can be adequately managed with diuretics. Diuretics are not uniformly successful, however, and in volume-replete patients with normal renal function, angiotensin-converting enzyme inhibitors may be useful. However, this class of medication can induce acute renal failure and should be used only under the guidance of a pediatric nephrologist.

COMPLICATIONS

Infection

Infection was once the leading cause of mortality in children with nephrotic syndrome and is still a significant concern. Children with nephrotic syndrome are at risk for serious infections for several reasons. First, there is impaired complement-dependent opsonization of encapsulated bacteria (e.g., *Streptococcus pneumoniae*, *Neisseria meningitidis*, typeable species of *Haemophilus influenzae*). Also, important immune proteins may be lost in the urine with the massive proteinuria, leading to hypogammaglobulinemia. This increases the risk of infection by encapsulated organisms and *Candida* species. Additionally, edema and ascites provide a rich breeding ground for bacteria. Finally, most children with nephrotic syndrome are on immunosuppressive therapy for their disease.

Spontaneous bacterial peritonitis is a serious infection seen in patients with nephrotic syndrome. Any child with active nephrotic syndrome who presents with severe abdominal pain should be closely evaluated for peritoneal signs such as rebound tenderness and rigidity. Fever may not be present if the child is on steroids. Laboratory evaluation should include a peripheral white cell count and blood culture, along with paracentesis to obtain peritoneal fluid for cell count, culture, protein, and glucose. The peritoneal fluid sample should be obtained quickly—ideally, before antibiotic therapy is started. However, if conditions prevent prompt paracentesis, the administration of antibiotics should not be delayed; they must be started as soon as possible to prevent the development of sepsis. *S. pneumoniae* is the most common organism seen in spontaneous bacterial peritonitis, but initial antibiotic therapy should include coverage for both gram-positive and gram-negative organisms.

Some practitioners recommend prophylactic antibiotics in all patients with active nephrotic syndrome, although this has not been demonstrated to decrease the incidence of peritonitis. The American Academy of Pediatrics recommends pneumococcal vaccination in all patients with nephrotic syndrome.[4]

Cellulitis is another serious infectious complication of nephrotic syndrome. Owing to generalized edema, the normal tissue planes that usually contain superficial cutaneous infections are disrupted, allowing their rapid spread. Thus, any skin infection must be treated aggressively in these patients. Similarly, areas of skin breakdown need to be addressed promptly to both prevent the development of infection and preserve skin integrity. Intensive diuresis may be needed in these patients to reduce edema.

Children with nephrotic syndrome who are being treated with immunosuppressive agents are at increased risk for disseminated viral infections. Infection with varicella-zoster virus is particularly dangerous for these patients. Primary varicella infection (chickenpox) can be life threatening, especially for patients on chronic corticosteroid therapy. Among these children, reactivation of infection (herpes zoster) is more common and more serious, with a greater risk of dissemination of this usually localized process. Children on chronic corticosteroid therapy without protective antibodies (i.e., no history of varicella infection and negative varicella serology) who are exposed to varicella need treatment with immune globulin within 96 hours after exposure. Although VZIG, a varicella-specific product, is no longer available, nonspecific immune globulin therapy can be used. In addition, an investigational varicella-specific product (VariZIG) is available at some institutions. Any child with nephrotic syndrome who is on immunosuppressive therapy and develops varicella or herpes zoster needs prompt antiviral therapy (e.g., acyclovir), preferably parenterally and in a hospital to monitor for dissemination or clinical deterioration. Children on chronic high-dose steroid therapy should not receive the varicella vaccine because it is a live-attenuated virus preparation.

Thrombosis

Thrombosis is another serious complication of nephrotic syndrome. Although it is more common in adults, presumably owing to the greater percentage of non–minimal change disease in adult patients, it is still a significant problem in children, with an estimated occurrence of 1.8% to 5%.[4] Thrombosis in pediatric patients is usually venous, including deep venous thrombosis of the extremities, renal vein thrombosis, pulmonary emboli, and sagittal sinus thrombosis. Factors contributing to the development of abnormal clots include abnormal platelet function, increased blood viscosity, decreased intravascular volume, and abnormal clotting factor concentrations. There are currently no recommendations for prophylactic anticoagulation therapy for children with active nephrotic syndrome, although some pediatric nephrologists prescribe aspirin 81 mg/day to their patients. Any patient who develops thrombosis requires anticoagulation treatment, including prophylactic anticoagulation for 6 months if they remain actively nephrotic. All nephrotic children who develop thrombosis should also be evaluated for a familial coagulation abnormality. If there is no intrinsic coagulation disorder, the risk of thrombosis is eliminated once a patient is no longer nephrotic. For these reasons, the use of diuretics in the face of active nephrotic syndrome should be undertaken with extreme care and diligent follow-up, because the additional decrease in intravascular volume may hasten clot formation.

CONSULTATION

Consider nephrology consultation in the following situations:

- Patients younger than 2 years or older than 8 years.
- Uncontrolled hypertension.
- Evidence of diminished renal function.
- Gross hematuria.
- Systemic symptoms (e.g., fever, malaise, anorexia).
- Presence of thrombosis.
- Infection.
- Disruption of skin integrity.
- Anasarca or recalcitrant edema.
- Family history of nephrotic syndrome.
- Recurrent nephrotic syndrome.
- Need for intensive family education.

Infectious diseases specialists can provide valuable guidance for the management of infections or infectious exposures, especially among nephrotic patients with compromised immunity.

Involvement of hematologists can provide guidance in the evaluation and management of patients with thrombosis.

ADMISSION CRITERIA

The majority of children presenting with nephrotic syndrome can be managed on an outpatient basis, assuming that close follow-up is possible. Hospitalization is indicated for the following reasons:

- Marked hypertension requiring therapy.
- Evidence of diminished renal function (oliguria, elevated serum creatinine).
- Possible coexisting bacterial infection (fever, severe abdominal pain, possible cellulitis).
- Gastrointestinal symptoms that may compromise the administration of prednisone (vomiting, diarrhea).
- Edema that is compromising skin integrity or preventing activities of daily living.
- Pulmonary edema or congestive heart failure.
- Possible thrombosis.
- Need for intensive family education.
- Lack of appropriate outpatient support or follow-up.

DISCHARGE CRITERIA

Children with nephrotic syndrome who require hospitalization can be discharged once the following are achieved:

- Adequate treatment of underlying infection, if present.
- Adequate treatment of thrombosis, if present.
- Restoration of clinically normal intravascular volume (i.e., resolution of symptoms of congestive heart failure or pulmonary edema).
- Ability to maintain normal activities of daily living.

- Restoration of skin integrity.
- Appropriate family and patient education.
- Organization of appropriate follow-up (usually within 1 week of discharge).

PREVENTION

Currently, no preventive strategies are available for nephrotic syndrome; however, early suspicion and diagnosis are the cornerstones to appropriate management and may influence long-term renal outcomes.

IN A NUTSHELL

- The diagnosis of nephrotic syndrome is based on the presence of edema and the laboratory findings of hypoalbuminemia, massive proteinuria (>4 mg/m^2 per hour), and hyperlipidemia.
- Infection is a leading cause of morbidity and mortality in children with nephrotic syndrome.
- Children with nephrotic syndrome are at risk for the development of thromboembolic complications.
- Once proteinuria has been confirmed, children presenting with symptoms of nephrotic syndrome should be evaluated for the presence of secondary kidney disease.
- Any child with nephrotic syndrome who is outside the age range of 2 to 8 years or who has any complication, including hypertension, diminished renal function, thrombosis, or disseminated infection, requires nephrology consultation.

ON THE HORIZON

- Genetic testing may allow differentiation among the various forms of childhood nephrotic syndrome. Distinguishing between minimal change disease and genetic causes of focal segmental glomerulosclerosis may allow therapy to be tailored.
- The investigational drug VariZIG can be requested by calling FFF Enterprises (800-843-7477). Recommendations for its use are delineated in the American Academy of Pediatrics' *Red Book 2006*.

SUGGESTED READING

Eddy AA, Symons JM: Nephrotic syndrome in childhood. Lancet 2003;363: 629-639.

Roth KS, Amaker BH, Chan JCM: Nephrotic syndrome: Pathogenesis and management. Pediatr Rev 2002;23:237-247.

REFERENCES

1. Eddy AA, Symons JM: Nephrotic syndrome in childhood. Lancet 2003;363: 629-639.
2. Roth KS, Amaker BH, Chan JCM: Nephrotic syndrome: Pathogenesis and management. Pediatr Rev 2002;23:237-247.
3. Hiraoka M, Tsukahara H, Matsubara K, et al: A randomized study of two long-course prednisolone regimens for nephrotic syndrome in children. Am J Kidney Dis 2003;41:1155-1162.
4. Overturf GD: American Academy of Pediatrics, Committee on Infectious Diseases, technical report: Prevention of pneumococcal infections, including the use of pneumococcal conjugate and polysaccharide vaccines and antibiotic prophylaxis. Pediatrics 2000;106:367-376.

CHAPTER 114

Renal Tubular Acidosis

Mary B. Garza

Renal tubular acidosis (RTA) refers to a collection of renal disorders that result in nongap metabolic acidosis. RTA may be an isolated disorder or one feature of a more complex disorder, disease, or syndrome. Because RTA can present with life-threatening electrolyte abnormalities, recognizing, diagnosing, and managing these disorders are essential skills for the hospitalist.

RTA is categorized into three types, depending on the location of the tubular dysfunction. Proximal, or type II, RTA refers to disorders involving bicarbonate reabsorption at the proximal tubule. Distal, or type I, RTA encompasses syndromes of defective hydrogen ion transport in the distal convoluted tubule. Type IV RTA also involves the distal tubule but is related to defects in the aldosterone response; it is often referred to as hyperkalemic RTA. What was once called type III RTA is now believed to be a combination of types I and II.

PATHOPHYSIOLOGY

A normally functioning kidney excretes acid at the same rate that metabolic processes generate acid, usually about 1 to 3 mEq/kg per day in children.[1] In RTA, this acid-excreting mechanism is disrupted, resulting in a net surplus of acid. The equation for calculating the anion gap is as follows:

Anion gap = Serum sodium (Na^+) −

[Serum bicarbonate (HCO_3^-) + Serum chloride (Cl^-)]

The normal range of the anion gap is 12 ± 4 mEq/L.[2]

In RTA, the retained acid is in the form of hydrogen ions (H^+) paired with chloride; therefore, the serum chloride is elevated to the same degree that the serum bicarbonate is diminished.[3] Accordingly, the anion gap remains within normal limits.

There are two main ways whereby the kidney excretes acid. One is by tubular reabsorption of bicarbonate in the proximal tubule. When blood is filtered in the kidney, the bicarbonate ends up in the collecting tubule and must be reabsorbed to maintain serum pH. About 85% of this reabsorption occurs in the proximal tubule; therefore, if there are any defects in this process, a large amount of bicarbonate is wasted in the urine, resulting in a net retention of acid.[4] This leads to proximal RTA.

The second way the kidney excretes acid is through the distal collecting tubules. There, prompted by the hormone aldosterone, hydrogen is pumped into the lumen, paired with ammonia (NH_3) to make ammonium (NH_4^+), and excreted in the urine. In a similar fashion, hydrogen ions are paired with other ions, referred to as titratable acids, for excretion.[2] In distal RTA, the mechanism of hydrogen delivery to the lumen is defective.[1] In hyperkalemic or type IV RTA, there is a defect in the hormonal message initiating this distal acid excretion—that is, aldosterone is not sent or received correctly.

Proximal Renal Tubular Acidosis

In the proximal tubule, intraluminal and intracellular carbonic anhydrase facilitates bicarbonate reclamation. This process is supported by an Na^+-H^+ exchanger, which in turn is regulated by Na^+/K^+-ATPase. Any of these three components can be defective, leading to proximal RTA.[1]

Proximal RTA can be primary or secondary. The primary form can be either sporadic or genetically inherited in an autosomal dominant or autosomal recessive manner.[1] Sporadic proximal RTA is usually transient in nature, whereas the inherited forms require lifelong treatment.[2] The secondary forms of proximal RTA are numerous and can be associated with other inherited tubulopathies (e.g., Fanconi syndrome, hereditary fructose intolerance, cystinosis, galactosemia, Wilson disease), drugs and toxins (e.g., ifosfamide, 6-mercaptopurine, valproic acid, carbonic anhydrase inhibitors, outdated tetracycline), and other miscellaneous disorders (e.g., amyloidosis, hyperparathyroidism, vitamin D deficiency, tetralogy of Fallot, osteopetrosis).[5] The prognosis of secondary proximal RTA depends on the underlying condition.

In proximal RTA, the threshold for bicarbonate reabsorption is reset at a lower level than in normal individuals. In normal children, this setpoint keeps serum bicarbonate around 22 mEq/L, whereas in those with proximal RTA, the setpoint is around 15 mEq/L.[2] Patients waste bicarbonate until they reach this new threshold, and then the proximal tubule begins resabsorbing bicarbonate again. Therefore, at the outset of the illness, bicarbonate is wasted in the urine in large amounts, resulting in alkalotic urine (pH >5.5).[6] However, once the serum bicarbonate has reached the new threshold, the proximal tubule begins reabsorbing bicarbonate again, and the urine is acidified distally as normal.[6] Thus, a feature that distinguishes proximal from distal RTA is the ability to make acidic urine (pH <5.5) in the setting of severe acidosis.[5]

Patients with proximal RTA often have hypokalemia because the increased delivery of bicarbonate and sodium to the distal tubule results in increased aldosterone-mediated potassium excretion.[1,5] This phenomenon is aggravated by treatment with alkali supplements, so patients must receive potassium supplementation concurrently.[2]

Distal Renal Tubular Acidosis

In the distal tubule, hydrogen ion excretion is mediated by the H^+-ATP pump on the luminal aspect of the intercalated cells.[1] This function can be impaired in three distinct ways: pump failure, back-diffusion of the ions, and inadequately negative lumen charge (also known as voltage-dependent distal RTA).[2] As a result, a lesser amount of ammonium and titratable acids is excreted, and there is a net acidosis. This acidosis is progressive and can be profound. Unlike in proximal RTA, the urine cannot be acidified to less than 5.5, even in the face of severe systemic acidosis.[1]

Distal RTA can also be primary or secondary, genetic or sporadic. The primary form is more likely to be permanent.[5] Secondary distal RTA can occur in a number of clinical states, including genetic disorders (Ehlers-Danlos syndrome, elliptocytosis, sickle cell disease, Wilson disease, osteopetrosis, Marfan syndrome, systemic lupus erythematosus), hyperglobulinemic states (cryoglobulinemia, polyarteritis nodosa, Sjögren syndrome), drug or toxin exposure (amphotericin, toluene, analgesics, lithium, mercury), renal diseases (transplantation, tubulointerstitial disease, obstructive uropathy, pyelonephritis), endocrine disorders (hyperparathyroidism, congenital adrenal hyperplasia, hypothyroidism), and hyponatremic states (nephrotic syndrome, hepatic cirrhosis).[1,5]

Hyperkalemic Renal Tubular Acidosis

Normally, aldosterone stimulates acid secretion in two ways: it stimulates the H^+-ATP pump that excretes hydrogen ions in the distal tubule, and it generates the ammonia that buffers the hydrogen ions in the collecting duct.[1] Aldosterone also prompts the retention of sodium and the excretion of potassium. Therefore, when the function of aldosterone is impaired, the patient suffers from hyperkalemia and acidosis.

Type IV RTA can occur due to primary mineralocorticoid deficiency (Addison's disease, adrenalectomy, congenital adrenal hyperplasia, treatment with angiotensin-converting enzyme inhibitors), secondary mineralocorticoid deficiency (hyporeninemia, impairment of renin release due to nonsteroidal anti-inflammatory drugs, diabetic nephropathy), and mineralocorticoid resistance (pseudohypoaldosteronism), or when the tubule is transiently nonresponsive to aldosterone (pyelonephritis, obstructive uropathy).[1,4,6] Serum levels of aldosterone and renin are the key to distinguishing among these different types.

CLINICAL PRESENTATION

In children, all three types of RTA share many of the same symptoms: growth failure, anorexia, vomiting, dehydration, polyuria, and constipation.[1,4] Because RTA is often secondary to other illnesses, children frequently present with symptoms of the primary process.

Some symptoms are specific to the type of RTA. For example, children with proximal RTA often have polyuria during the early phase of the disorder due to the diuresis associated with bicarbonate wasting. They can also have metabolic bone disease (osteopenia, osteomalacia) if associated tubulopathy leads to phosphaturia.[1] Hypokalemia is another feature that may be prominent.

Children with distal RTA often have nephrocalcinosis and nephrolithiasis secondary to hypercalciuria and hypocitraturia.[6] Older patients with distal RTA often suffer from myalgia and arthralgia.[6] The majority of patients have hypokalemia due to volume contraction and overstimulation of the renin-aldosterone pathway. This can be profound

and life threatening in children, so it must be monitored closely and corrected before the initiation of alkali therapy.[1] The voltage-dependent type of distal RTA is associated with elevated serum potassium.[5]

Children with type IV RTA can present with potentially life-threatening hyperkalemia in addition to the usual symptoms of RTA.[4] In contrast to those with distal RTA, the urine in patients with type IV RTA can be acidified to less than 5.5 in the setting of systemic acidosis. Type IV RTA patients do not have nephrocalcinosis, nephrolithiasis, or metabolic bone disease.[5]

DIFFERENTIAL DIAGNOSIS

When faced with a patient with a nongap metabolic acidosis, one must consider diarrheal illness, exogenous acid administration (e.g., hyperalimentation), ureterosigmoidostomy, and extensive pancreatic fluid drainage, in addition to RTA. Malnourished patients can appear to have RTA due to acid-generating catabolism and decreased renal filtration.[1] Patients with a *Proteus* urinary tract infection can appear to have RTA because their urine is alkaline secondary to the bacteria's capacity to split urea.[1]

DIAGNOSIS AND EVALUATION

The evaluation begins with a complete history and physical examination, paying particular attention to growth parameters. Baseline serum electrolytes, creatinine, blood urea nitrogen, and urinalysis identify the nongap acidosis and assess overall renal function.

If the patient has a nongap metabolic acidosis, bicarbonate loss from diarrheal illness must be excluded as a cause. It is important to allow a child recovering from gastroenteritis several days to replenish bicarbonate stores before entertaining a diagnosis of RTA.[1,2] If there is concern about acidosis caused by metabolic compensation for primary respiratory alkalosis, arterial blood gas analysis can clarify the diagnosis.[4] Renal ultrasonography can be used to identify nephrocalcinosis or obstruction if the clinical picture is suggestive of such entities.

To distinguish the type of RTA, begin by checking the patient's urinary pH with a formal urinalysis (not a dipstick reading, which is notoriously inaccurate). If it is 5.5 or higher in the face of profound systemic acidosis, the patient most likely has distal RTA.[2] If it is less than 5.5, the patient could have either proximal or type IV RTA. To distinguish between these two, check the urinary anion gap by measuring urinary sodium, potassium, and chloride,[1] as follows:

$$\text{Urinary anion gap} = \text{Urinary } Na^+ + \text{Urinary } K^+ - \text{Urinary } Cl^-$$

If there is a large amount of ammonium in the urine, the urinary anion gap will be negative because the abundance of negatively charged chloride anions matches the positively charged ammonium cations, which are not measured. Both distal and type IV RTA have impaired ammonium excretion in the distal tubule, so a negative urinary anion gap rules out these conditions. Proximal RTA or diarrheal illness is most likely if the urinary anion gap is negative.[2] Table 114-1 presents the distinguishing characteristics of the different types of RTA.

Table 114-1 Distinguishing Features of Renal Tubular Acidosis (RTA) Types

Feature	Proximal RTA	Distal RTA	Type IV RTA
Urinary pH in the presence of profound systemic acidosis	<5.5	>5.5	<5.5
Urinary ammonium	Normal	Decreased	Decreased
Urinary anion gap	Negative	Positive	Positive
Serum potassium	Low	Low*	High
Nephrolithiasis	No	Yes	No

*Except in the voltage-dependent form.

COURSE OF ILLNESS AND TREATMENT

The first phase of treatment is fluid resuscitation and correction of any electrolyte abnormalities. Potassium must be normalized before alkali therapy is initiated, or life-threatening hypokalemia can ensue.[6] Replace bicarbonate over 1 to 2 days using the following formula to calculate the deficit:

Bicarbonate deficit = 0.6 × Body weight in kg ×
[Desired HCO_3 – Measured HCO_3]

Treatment of proximal RTA is primarily with alkali supplementation titrated to maintain normal serum bicarbonate levels. Of all the types, proximal RTA usually requires the most alkali for successful treatment.[6] Occasionally, hydrochlorothiazide can be added to the regimen to decrease the alkali dose, because it enhances proximal tubule bicarbonate reabsorption.[2] As mentioned earlier, potassium levels must be monitored, and potassium supplementation should be administered as needed. Symptoms resolve and growth normalizes with appropriate therapy.

Treatment of distal RTA is with alkali supplementation, usually for life. Citrate is a useful form of alkali, and it also helps curb nephrolithiasis.[2] Most patients also need potassium supplementation at least initially. Treatment generally results in resolution of nephrolithiasis and resumption of normal growth; however, polyuria may persist.[5]

Treatment of type IV RTA consists of alkali therapy and removal of excess dietary potassium. Volume contraction should be treated, and sodium supplementation should be considered. In cases of hypoaldosteronism, mineralocorticoid therapy can be useful.[5] For severe hyperkalemia, furosemide or potassium resins may be helpful.[4] A high-sodium diet can help prevent volume depletion and potentiates potassium excretion.[2]

CONSULTATION

A nephrologist is routinely involved in the initial evaluation, treatment decisions, and long-term follow-up.

ADMISSION AND DISCHARGE CRITERIA

Electrolyte abnormalities, which may be life threatening, warrant hospitalization. Once these are corrected and the patient is stabilized on alkali therapy, he or she can be discharged, with nephrology follow-up.

IN A NUTSHELL

- RTA encompasses a collection of disorders of renal acid excretion that result in nongap metabolic acidosis.
- The typical presentation is a nongap metabolic acidosis in the absence of diarrheal illness, usually accompanied by poor growth and anorexia. RTA is often secondary to other conditions.
- Diagnosis is based on an evaluation of serum and urinary pH and chemistries.
- Treatment consists of alkali replacement, with close attention to potassium status, and consultation with a pediatric nephrologist.

ON THE HORIZON

- Current research focuses on the molecular biology of tubular function and the genetic basis for the various types of RTA.
- A better understanding of the pathophysiology of the disorder may lead to improved diagnosis and treatment for affected patients.

SUGGESTED READING

Dell KM, Avner ED: Renal tubular acidosis. In Behrman RE, Kliegman RM, Jenson HB (eds): Nelson Textbook of Pediatrics, 17th ed. Philadelphia, WB Saunders, 2004, pp 1759-1761.

Herrin JT: Renal tubular acidosis. In Barrett TM, Avner ED, Harmon WE (eds): Pediatric Nephrology. Baltimore, Lippincott Williams & Wilkins, 1999, pp 565-581.

REFERENCES

1. Herrin JT: Renal tubular acidosis. In Barrett TM, Avner ED, Harmon WE (eds): Pediatric Nephrology. Baltimore, Lippincott Williams & Wilkins, 1999, pp 565-581.
2. Johnson V, Perelsteine E: Tubular diseases. In Trachtman H, Gauthier B (eds): Pediatric Nephrology. Amsterdam, Henwood Academic Publishers, 1998, pp 231-239.
3. Postlethwaite RJ: The approach to a child with metabolic acidosis or alkalosis. In Webb N, Postlethwaite R (eds): Clinical Paediatric Nephrology, 3rd ed. Oxford, Oxford University Press, 2003, pp 61-68.
4. Dell KM, Avner ED: Renal tubular acidosis. In Behrman RE, Kliegman RM, Jenson HB (eds): Nelson Textbook of Pediatrics, 17th ed. Philadelphia, WB Saunders, 2004, pp 1759-1761.
5. Rodriguez-Soriano J: Renal tubular acidosis. In Edelman CM (ed): Pediatric Kidney Disease, 2nd ed. Boston, Little Brown, 1992, pp 1737-1775.
6. Dubose TD: Acid base disorders. In Brenner BM (ed): Brenner & Rector's The Kidney, 7th ed. Philadelphia, WB Saunders, 2004, pp 946-960.

CHAPTER 115

Renal Venous Thrombosis

Mary B. Garza

Renal venous thrombosis (RVT) is a condition in which a thrombus forms in the venous drainage system of one or both kidneys. The thrombus can extend from the arcuate renal vessels through the renal vein and as far as the vena cava.[1] The condition is also referred to as renal *vein* thrombosis, but because the thrombus often extends beyond the anatomic boundaries of the renal vein both proximally and distally, the term renal *venous* thrombosis is preferred.[2]

In the pediatric population, the majority of cases of RVT occur in the first week of life.[2] Newborns are commonly affected by elements of Virchow's triad (hypercoagulability, stasis, and vessel wall injury), which puts them at risk for the development of venous thrombosis. Newborns also have increased renal vascular resistance and therefore relatively diminished renal blood flow.[1,2] Polycythemia, either idiopathic or associated with maternal diabetes mellitus or congenital heart disease, leads to sludging and stasis in small vessels.[3] Similarly, acute blood loss, shock, asphyxia, or sepsis can result in hypovolemia and vessel wall injury.[4] Infants with traumatic delivery are at higher risk for RVT than are those delivered uneventfully.[1] Further, central venous catheters, which are frequently needed in the neonatal period, are a well-documented risk factor for venous thrombosis.[3]

RVT occurs less commonly in older infants and children. When it does, there is likely a predisposing condition, and RVT is often triggered by a hyperosmolar state.[4] For example, patients with severe dehydration (e.g., gastroenteritis) have decreased renal blood flow and hemoconcentration, which can increase the risk of thrombus formation.[5] Similarly, radiologic procedures using hyperosmolar intravenous contrast agents can lead to RVT.[2] Health care providers should have a high index of suspicion for RVT in patients with hypercoagulability due to an underlying condition (e.g., cancer, trauma, burns, surgery, congenital heart disease, nephrotic syndrome, pregnancy, lupus) or inherited thrombophilia (e.g., factor V Leiden, homocystinuria, prothrombin mutation).[1,4,5] Certain medications, such as oral contraceptives and steroids, can also cause hypercoagulability.[5] Rarely, trauma can lead to RVT, which may be associated with concurrent renal arterial thrombosis.[5] Children with renal transplants are at risk for RVT, particularly if they are treated with cyclosporine.[5]

CLINICAL PRESENTATION

RVT classically presents with macroscopic hematuria and enlargement of one or both kidneys.[3] Older children often complain of lumbar or flank pain.[5] If both kidneys are affected, the patient will have oliguria and renal insufficiency.[5] If the thrombus extends to the inferior vena cava, it can affect venous return from the lower extremity, in which case the child's leg will be edematous, cool, and cyanotic.[2,3]

DIFFERENTIAL DIAGNOSIS

The differential diagnosis of hematuria is broad, because bleeding can arise anywhere from the glomerulus to the urethral opening. Renal causes include glomerulonephritis, tubular interstitial nephritis, pyelonephritis, polycystic kidney disease, and acute tubular necrosis. Extrarenal causes include trauma, anatomic abnormalities, bleeding disorders, foreign bodies, Henoch-Schönlein purpura, sickle cell disease or trait, endocarditis, and hemolytic uremic syndrome.[4] Artifactual hematuria may occur when the sample is contaminated by menstrual blood or when the urine appears pink owing to urate crystals in a dehydrated newborn.

Similarly, a palpable renal mass can have many causes, including hydronephrosis, renal abscess, polycystic kidney disease, and Wilms tumor.[4]

DIAGNOSIS AND EVALUATION

Urinalysis with microscopy, complete blood count, and serum chemistries are the usual first-line studies for the evaluation of possible RVT. The diagnosis is suggested by microscopic or macroscopic hematuria, proteinuria, and evidence of intravascular coagulation such as microangiopathic hemolytic anemia and thrombocytopenia.[1,2,4] If the thrombus is bilateral, elevated creatinine and uremia may be evident.[1,5]

Confirmation is best obtained with renal ultrasonography with Doppler, which in affected patients reveals increased renal size, renal vein dilation with decreased pulsation, and often direct visualization of the thrombus.[2,3,5] Renal scintigraphy with mercaptoacetyltriglycine shows a lack of function in the affected kidney.[4] Renal venography is generally not indicated, because the contrast material can exacerbate the hyperosmolar state that led to thrombus formation.[2]

If an inherited hypercoagulable state is suspected, a full thrombophilia evaluation should be undertaken, optimally in consultation with a pediatric hematologist (see Chapter 120).

COURSE OF ILLNESS

Owing to the presence of the clot, the affected kidney continues to enlarge over the course of about 1 week. Depending on the degree of obstruction, the kidney may become completely or partially atrophic over the following months.[4,5] Some patients then develop hypertension, renal impairment, and tubulopathy.[4] The prognosis depends on the extent of the initial thrombus, whether it was bilateral or unilateral, and the degree of spontaneous recanalization.[1]

TREATMENT

Supportive care is the mainstay of therapy. Fluids, electrolytes, and renal function must be monitored closely and optimized.[1,2,4] Some advocate anticoagulation with heparin or low-molecular-weight heparin in severe cases (e.g., inferior vena cava obstruction, bilateral disease, renal failure), although this is controversial.[1,2,5] Risks and benefits of such interventions must be carefully assessed, ideally in consultation with a pediatric hematologist. More aggressive treatment, such as thrombolytic therapy or surgery, is not currently indicated.[2,5] Management in consultation with a pediatric nephrologist is advised if renal function is impaired.

As the condition resolves, the patient must be monitored for hypertension and renal insufficiency and treated accordingly. For refractory hypertension despite optimal medical management, nephrectomy may be indicated.[2,4]

ADMISSION AND DISCHARGE CRITERIA

Infants and children with RVT should be admitted to the hospital for prompt diagnostic testing, close monitoring, supportive care, and evaluation and management of any underlying condition. Discharge is appropriate when the condition is stabilized and adequate follow-up can be assured.

PREVENTION

Prevention of RVT hinges on awareness of the predisposing factors. Patients at risk should be hydrated adequately to prevent hyperosmolar states. Further, health care providers must be judicious in the use of hypertonic contrast material in radiographic studies, because this can lead to RVT in a susceptible child.[2]

IN A NUTSHELL

- RVT typcially presents with hematuria, flank mass, and microangiopathic anemia with thrombocytopenia.
- Diagnosis is made by urinalysis, serum chemistries, and renal ultrasonography.
- Treatment consists of supportive care aimed at optimizing fluids, electrolytes, and renal function, as well as long-term monitoring for hypertension.

ON THE HORIZON

- Magnetic resonance venography for the diagnosis of RVT.
- Further study of the safety and efficacy of therapy with anticoagulants (e.g., heparin) and thrombolytics (e.g., tissue plasminogen activator).

SUGGESTED READING

Davis ID, Avner ED: Renal vein thrombosis. In Behrman RE, Kliegman RM, Jenson HB (eds): Nelson Textbook of Pediatrics, 17th ed. Philadelphia, WB Saunders, 2004, pp 1747-1748.

Yudd M, Llach F: Renal vein thrombosis. In Brenner BM (ed): Brenner & Rector's The Kidney, 7th ed. Philadelphia, WB Saunders, 2004, pp 1584-1591.

REFERENCES

1. Guignard JP, Drukker A: Clinical neonatal nephrology. In Barrett TM, Avner ED, Harmon WE (eds): Pediatric Nephrology. Baltimore, Lippincott Williams & Wilkins, 1999, p 1060.
2. Arneil GC, Beattie TJ: Renal venous obstruction. In Edelman CM (ed): Pediatric Kidney Disease, 2nd ed. Boston, Little Brown, 1992, pp 1909-1915.
3. Andrew ME, Monagle P, deVeber G, Chan AKC: Thromboembolic disease and antithrombotic therapy in newborns. Hematology Am Soc Hematol Educ Program 2001;358-374.
4. Davis ID, Avner ED: Renal vein thrombosis. In Behrman RE, Kliegman RM, Jenson HB (eds): Nelson Textbook of Pediatrics, 17th ed. Philadelphia, WB Saunders, 2004, pp 1747-1748.
5. Yudd M, Llach F: Renal vein thrombosis. In Brenner BM (ed): Brenner & Rector's The Kidney, 7th ed. Philadelphia, WB Saunders, 2004, pp 1584-1591.

Hematology

CHAPTER 116

Anemia

Ian J. Davis

The initial evaluation of a child with anemia is a common task for general pediatricians or hospitalists. Defined as insufficient red blood cell (RBC) mass for the age of the patient, anemia can develop acutely or insidiously. In children, when anemia develops gradually over several weeks to months, the resulting anemia can be profound but with little clinical consequence other than obvious pallor. However, if anemia develops acutely, the patient has no time to compensate for decreased oxygen carrying capacity, and symptoms of anemia (ranging from fatigue to cardiovascular collapse) can develop rapidly. Because anemia can result from many disease processes, it is helpful to divide anemia into broad pathophysiologic categories: (1) decreased production of either hemoglobin or RBCs, (2) premature RBC destruction, or (3) blood loss.[1] Fortunately, distinguishing among these processes usually requires only basic, widely available laboratory tests. Once the pathophysiologic category is determined, the differential diagnosis narrows, and the workup becomes much less daunting. This chapter focuses primarily on children with newly recognized anemia in whom the evaluation is often initiated by pediatric hospitalists.

CLINICAL PRESENTATION

Anemia is often discovered incidentally during laboratory screening for other indications in a child who otherwise exhibits no symptoms of anemia.[2] Alternatively, pallor and fatigue, the cardinal symptoms of anemia, may bring the patient to medical attention. Severe anemia (especially when there is a rapid onset) may present with weakness, obtundation, syncope, exertional dyspnea, congestive heart failure, or shock.

The probable causes of anemia can often be predicted by considering the age of the patient and taking a careful history. A directed history should thoroughly review the child's diet, including the amount and type of milk, red meat, fruits, and vegetables consumed daily, as well as a history of pica. Growth and development, blood loss (melena, hematemesis, hemoptysis, or hematuria), and recent illnesses are also important areas of inquiry. Because many causes of anemia are inherited, the family history is critical and should include questions about transfusions,

bleeding, splenectomy, cholelithiasis or cholecystectomy, and prior diagnoses of anemia.

The physical examination should focus on manifestations of anemia and diagnostic clues. Tachycardia, systolic murmur, and pallor suggest a moderate degree of anemia. Severe anemia can be accompanied by symptoms of congestive heart failure and tachypnea, despite children's typically profound and effective cardiovascular compensatory mechanisms. Jaundice or dark urine suggests intravascular hemolysis and rapidly narrows the differential diagnosis. Similarly, hepatosplenomegaly, a physical sign of great importance in the diagnostic evaluation of an anemic patient, suggests extramedullary hematopoiesis (as in chronic hemolytic anemias) or other diagnoses (e.g., storage diseases, bone marrow infiltration, infections).

The initial laboratory evaluation typically includes a basic panel of hematologic studies, followed by selected studies as directed by the presentation and the history. A complete blood count (CBC) with differential white blood cell count, reticulocyte count, and direct and indirect antiglobulin (Coombs) tests are central for initial classification. RBC indices are usually included in the CBC and provide additional clues to the pathophysiology of the anemia (Table 116-1). Examination of the peripheral blood smear should be performed, with particular attention to RBC morphology and evidence of hemolysis (Table 116-2). Some examples of RBC abnormalities that may be seen on the peripheral smear are provided in Figure 116-1.

Evaluation for occult blood loss should include several stool guaiac tests for subclinical gastrointestinal bleeding. Although less common, trauma-related injuries should also be considered, such as femur fracture with major hematoma, hemothorax, or hemoperitoneum. Outside the special population of very premature infants, it is uncommon for intracranial hemorrhage to account for significant anemia, and unless neurologic symptoms or signs accompany the presentation, cranial imaging is not generally indicated.

Subclinical hematuria usually involves only small amounts of blood in the urine and generally does not result in significant anemia in the absence of some other causative factor. However, blood detected by urinalysis is an important finding and requires attention to both the urine dipstick and microscopic analysis. Blood detected by dipstick without a

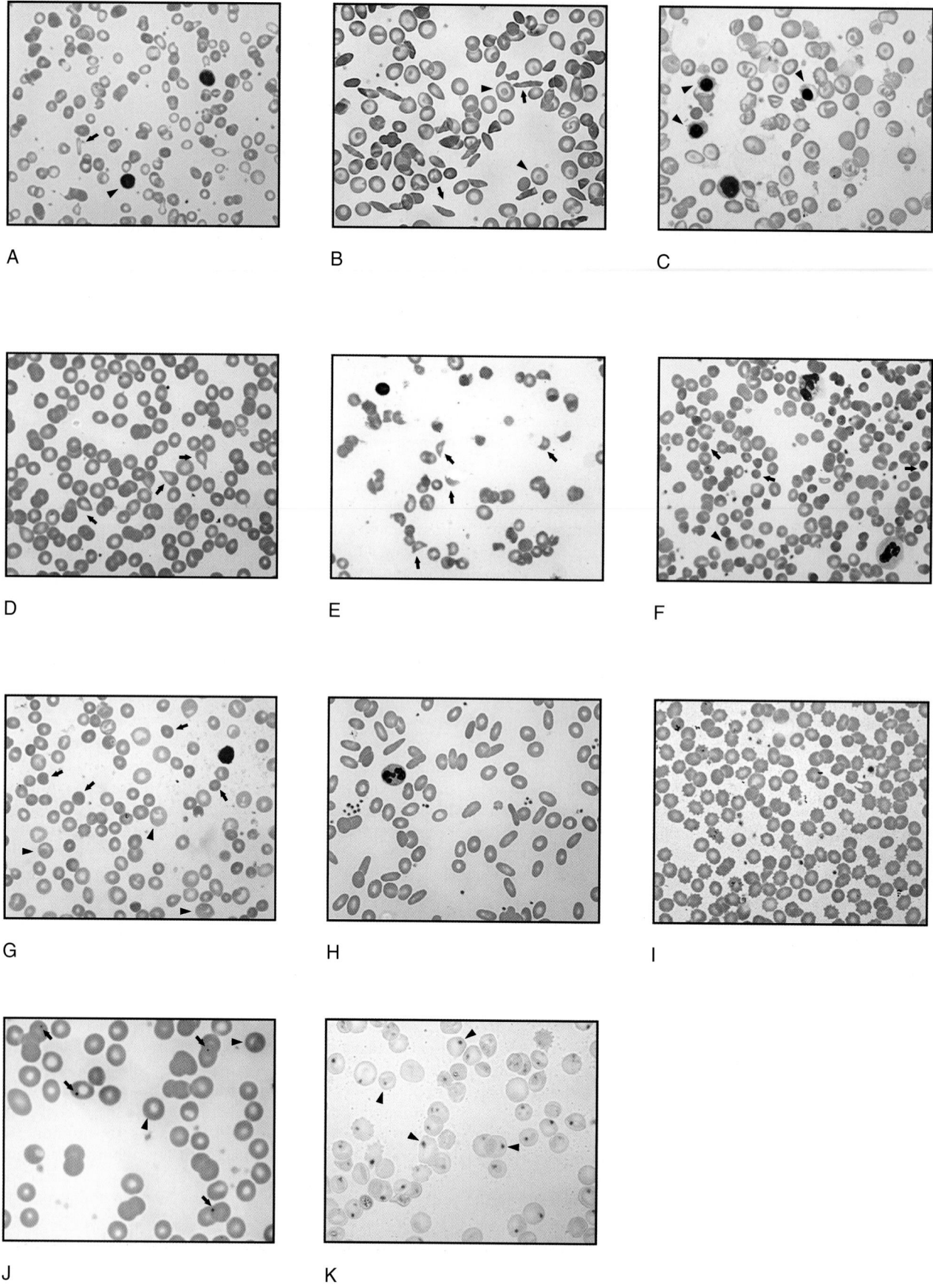

A

B

C

D

E

F

G

H

I

J

K

significant number of RBCs on the microscopic examination indicates the presence of either hemoglobin (suggesting intravascular RBC hemolysis) or myoglobin (due to rhabdomyolysis). Serum concentrations of muscle enzymes (e.g., creatine kinase) or free hemoglobin should help differentiate between myoglobinuria and hemoglobinuria.

Depending on the patient's age and the history and physical examination findings, further evaluation can be tailored accordingly. Iron-deficiency anemia is a common cause of microcytic anemia, and further evaluation includes a serum iron level, total iron binding capacity, and ferritin (see later). Microcytic anemia with risk factors for plumbism should prompt the measurement of serum lead levels (see Chapter 181). Clinical concerns for endocrine, renal, or hepatic disease justify the assessment of hepatic transaminases and thyroid and renal function. Hematologic consultation is often useful if initial efforts fail to yield a definitive diagnosis. Further laboratory studies such as hemoglobin electrophoresis (to investigate hemoglobinopathies) and osmotic fragility studies (to rule out spherocytosis) may be indicated. Bone marrow aspiration and biopsy may be useful in the diagnosis of anemias of unclear cause and to rule out diagnoses such as myelodysplastic syndrome, congenital dyserythropoietic anemias, aplastic anemia, and leukemia. Although occasionally presenting with isolated anemia, myelodysplastic syndrome and leukemia usually result in pancytopenia or the appearance of abnormal (e.g., dysplastic or immature) cells in the peripheral blood.

Comparing current RBC indices with those of previous blood examinations may provide important information, such as the rate and timing of onset of the anemia. In addition, whenever possible, specific laboratory studies should be obtained before transfusion so that they reflect the patient's condition rather than that of the blood donor.

Table 116-1   Red Blood Cell Indices and Anemia-Related Laboratory Studies

Index	What It Measures	What It Tells Us
Hemoglobin	Concentration of hemoglobin in blood	Inclusive quantitation of red cell hemoglobin
Hematocrit	Volume of packed cells (may be calculated from red cell number/red cell volume)	Red cell concentration in plasma
Mean corpuscular volume	Average volume (size) of red cells	Helpful in classifying pathophysiologic mechanisms of anemia
Mean corpuscular hemoglobin (MCH)	Average hemoglobin content per red cell	Low MCH suggests inefficient hemoglobin synthesis
Mean corpuscular hemoglobin concentration	Average concentration of hemoglobin per red cell volume	Elevated values suggest membranopathy (hereditary spherocytosis) or hemoglobinopathy (e.g., hemoglobin C disease)
Red cell count	Direct quantitation of red cell number	Provides insight into red cell production somewhat independently of hemoglobin synthesis
Red blood cell distribution width	Measure of variability of red cell size	Indicates variation in red cell populations; often high in iron-deficiency anemia and low in thalassemias
Reticulocyte count	Quantitation of immature red cells	Increased number demonstrates active bone marrow red cell synthesis
Haptoglobin	Hemoglobin binding plasma protein	Depleted in conditions of intravascular hemolysis
Direct Coombs	Immunoglobulin or complement bound to erythrocytes	Detects the presence of bound autoreactive antibodies
Indirect Coombs	Serum immunoglobulin or complement capable of binding donor erythrocytes	Demonstrates alloantibody development or unbound autoantibodies

Figure 116-1   Erythrocyte morphologic abnormalities. *A,* Microcytosis and hypochromia associated with severe iron-deficiency anemia. Infrequent elliptocytes (pencil cells) can be seen *(arrow).* Note erythrocyte sizes relative to lymphocytes *(arrowhead). B,* Sickle *(arrows)* and target *(arrowheads)* erythrocytes associated with sickle cell anemia. *C,* Target erythrocytes associated with hemoglobinopathy or liver disease. Nucleated red blood cells *(arrowheads)* and polychromasia suggest increased red cell production. *D,* Teardrop-shaped cells *(arrows)* associated with marrow replacement (myelophthisis). Note the otherwise normal erythrocytes. *E,* Schistocytes *(arrows)* associated with microangiopathic hemolytic anemia. Note thrombocytopenia. *F,* Spherocytic erythrocytes *(arrows)* associated with hereditary spherocytosis. Note polychromasia, suggestive of reticulocytosis *(arrowheads). G,* Microspherocytes *(arrows)* and polychromasia from reticulocytosis *(arrowheads)* in autoimmune hemolytic anemia. *H,* Elliptocytes associated with hereditary elliptocytosis. Infrequent elliptocytes can also be seen in other anemias. *I,* Burr cells (echinocytes) may be associated with uremia or may be a laboratory artifact. *J,* Howell-Jolly bodies *(arrows)* associated with impaired splenic function. Note polychromasia from reticulocytosis *(arrowheads). K,* Special stains detect Heinz bodies *(arrowheads),* which are associated with unstable hemoglobins and enzymopathies.

Table 116-2   Red Blood Cell Findings on Peripheral Blood Smear

Finding	Description	Commonly Associated Conditions	Comments
Microcytosis	Small erythrocytes	Iron deficiency Thalassemias Hemoglobinopathies	Interpret in context of age-dependent norms
Macrocytosis	Large erythrocytes	Folate deficiency Vitamin B_{12} deficiency Bone marrow failure	
Hypochromia	Decreased hemoglobin	Iron deficiency	
Spherocytosis	Erythrocytes without central pallor	Hereditary spherocytosis AIHA	Associated with loss of membrane
Schistocytosis (also referred to as burr or helmet cells)	Erythrocyte fragments	Hemolytic uremic syndrome Mechanical or vascular-mediated destruction Thrombotic thrombocytopenic purpura DIC	Microangiopathic hemolysis
Polychromasia	Variability in erythrocyte staining	Hemolytic anemias Recovery from anemia	Reflects mix of reticulocytes with older cells
Target cells	Erythrocytes with central area of hyperchromia	Hemoglobinopathies (especially hemoglobin C disease) Obstructive liver disease	
Basophilic stippling	Punctate pattern in erythrocytes	Lead poisoning Hemoglobinopathies Enzymopathies Infection	
Sickle cells	Crescent-shaped cells	Sickle cell anemia	
Reticulocytosis	Increased number of young erythrocytes	Hemolytic anemias	Can be seen in conditions of elevated red cell destruction or hemorrhage
Howell-Jolly bodies	Fragments of nuclei containing condensed DNA	Asplenia (anatomic or functional)	Associated with impaired splenic function
Heinz bodies	Accumulation of precipitated hemoglobin	Unstable hemoglobin Erythrocyte enzymopathy	Requires special stain

AIHA, autoimmune hemolytic anemia; DIC, disseminated intravascular coagulation.

DIFFERENTIAL DIAGNOSIS

Because anemia is associated with various pathophysiologic abnormalities, functional classification simplifies the initial evaluation. One approach divides anemias into those with microcytic, normocytic, or macrocytic erythrocytes based on the mean corpuscular volume (MCV); another considers whether the anemia results from diminished RBC production rather than increased RBC destruction. Table 116-3 unifies both classification schemes for the common anemias encountered by pediatric hospitalists. It is critical to interpret both the hemoglobin and the MCV based on the child's age, because normal RBC parameters change with age.[3] Multiple concurrent pathophysiologic processes often complicate even straightforward diagnoses. For example, it can be challenging to evaluate anemia in a patient with chronic renal failure and possible nutritional deficiencies who develops subclinical hemorrhage.

DISORDERS OF RED CELL PRODUCTION: THE RETICULOCYTOPENIC ANEMIAS

Microcytic Anemia

Iron-Deficiency Anemia

Iron deficiency is the most common cause of anemia in the pediatric population, displaying a bimodal age of distribution affecting mainly toddlers and female adolescents.[4] Although iron supplementation of infant formula has diminished its incidence, the absence of sufficient iron intake after the depletion of stores deposited in the third trimester commonly results in anemia in older infants and toddlers. Premature infants are also at high risk because of their inability to accumulate sufficient iron stores during the third trimester. Patients with iron-deficiency anemia may also exhibit microscopic stool blood loss from enterocolitis (e.g., cow's milk protein allergy in toddlers). Although reduced

Table 116-3 Functional Classification of Anemias

Anemia Type	Decreased Production	Increased Destruction
Microcytic	Iron deficiency Chronic lead poisoning Chronic inflammation	Thalassemia syndromes
Normocytic	Chronic renal disease Transient erythroblastopenia of childhood Pure red cell aplasia (Diamond-Blackfan anemia) Chronic inflammation	Inherited hemolytic anemias (hemoglobinopathies, enzymopathies, membranopathies) Acquired hemolytic anemia (AIHA, MAHA, DIC) Splenic pooling Hemorrhage
Macrocytic	Vitamin B_{12} or folate deficiency Aplastic anemia Pure red cell aplasia (Diamond-Blackfan anemia) Hypothyroidism Liver disease	Hemolytic anemia accompanied by significant reticulocytosis

AIHA, autoimmune hemolytic anemia; DIC, disseminated intravascular coagulation; MAHA, microangiopathic hemolytic anemia.

intake is the most common cause of iron-deficiency anemia, malabsorption may also result in iron deficiency and should be suspected in patients with duodenal pathology (the site of intestinal iron absorption). In toddlers, iron-deficiency anemia is sometimes accompanied by pica, the involuntary ingestion of inert compounds such as dirt, which can result in lead poisoning (see Chapter 181); this exacerbates iron-deficiency anemia because lead competes with iron for intestinal uptake. In young women, iron deficiency usually results from regular menstrual blood loss. Anemia in this context can be especially severe if associated with a low dietary iron intake.

A nutritional history suggestive of poor iron intake associated with microcytic anemia, a normal to slightly elevated reticulocyte count, an elevated RBC distribution width, and erythroid hypochromasia suggests iron deficiency. Reticulocyte hemoglobin content may be an early indicator of iron deficiency.[5,6] Typical laboratory findings in iron-deficiency anemia are summarized in Table 116-4. Bone marrow examination is rarely required to make this diagnosis. Concurrent causes of microcytic anemia such as α-thalassemia trait can be difficult to diagnose in the context of severe iron deficiency.

A therapeutic trial of oral iron is appropriate for likely iron-deficiency anemia before referral to a hematologist. Mild anemia can be treated with 3 mg elemental iron/kg per day, given once daily. Severe anemia may justify dosing up to 6 mg elemental iron/kg per day, given in divided doses. Because parenteral iron is associated with significant side effects, its use is reserved for children with severe anemia for whom oral intake is insufficient to replenish iron stores. Given the gradual development of iron-deficiency anemia, pediatric patients rarely exhibit significant physiologic consequences necessitating RBC transfusion, despite presenting with profoundly low hemoglobin levels. However, diminishing physiologic compensation for severe anemia (e.g., symptoms of impending congestive heart failure) may justify RBC transfusion.

Effective treatment with iron should result in a rising reticulocyte count within 2 to 3 days and an increasing hematocrit within a few weeks. The absence of a response to iron necessitates further evaluation for other causes of anemia. Treatment should be continued for 3 months to replace iron stores. For toddlers with iron-deficiency anemia caused by excess milk consumption, the intake of all dairy products should be restricted until a rising hematocrit is documented. Small amounts of milk can then be introduced with meals, provided that allergic enterocolitis and occult gastrointestinal bleeding secondary to milk protein allergy have been ruled out.

Anemia of Inflammation

Also called anemia of chronic disease, anemia of inflammation produces a mild normocytic to microcytic anemia. Erythrocytes may be normochromic to slightly hypochromic. Associated with infection, inflammatory disorders, and malignancy, anemia of inflammation results from ineffective hematopoiesis (due to restricted iron availability) along with a slightly decreased erythrocyte life span.[7] Anemia of inflammation is suggested by a clinical history combined with elevated ferritin and C-reactive protein.

Normocytic or Macrocytic Anemia
Transient Erythroblastopenia of Childhood

Transient erythroblastopenia of childhood (TEC) is a relatively common cause of normocytic anemia in young children (aged 6 months to 5 years). Most commonly presenting at age 2 years, TEC is probably an immune-mediated suppression of RBC production that frequently follows mild viral infections (e.g., upper respiratory tract infections), although tests of anti–red cell antibodies (e.g., Coombs tests) are negative as a rule. Although platelets are usually normal in number, there may be associated neutropenia. Hemolysis is not present in TEC; therefore, lactate dehydrogenase, bilirubin, haptoglobin, and urinary bilirubin and hemoglobin are within normal limits. TEC should be strongly suspected in the setting of moderate to severe normocytic anemia with an inappropriately low reticulocyte response, although it is worth noting that reticulocytosis may be

Table 116-4 Studies Pertinent to the Evaluation of Suspected Iron-Deficiency Anemia

Study	Finding in Iron-Deficiency Anemia	Comment
Hemoglobin	Low	Normal level increases with age (refer to age-appropriate standards)
Plasma iron level	Low	Varies with recent iron intake
Serum ferritin level	Typically low	Acute phase reactant that may be falsely elevated with illness; usefulness increased when interpreted in context of C-reactive protein level
Total iron binding capacity (TIBC)	Normal to elevated	A measure of plasma transferrin concentration
Iron/TIBC	Low	Normal value decreases slightly with age
Mean corpuscular volume	Low	Reflects decreased hemoglobin production
Red blood cell distribution width	Increased	Reflects increased variability of cell size due to variable hemoglobin incorporation or increased numbers of reticulocytes
Reticulocyte count	Variable	Expect increase 2-3 days after starting effective iron therapy
Reticulocyte hemoglobin concentration	Low	Provides measure of heme synthesis in youngest erythrocytes and may indicate early iron deficiency

present if TEC is detected during the recovery phase. TEC must be distinguished from Diamond-Blackfan anemia (pure red cell aplasia), an inherited bone marrow failure syndrome that usually presents in the first year of life. TEC resolves over a period of weeks to months, whereas Diamond-Blackfan anemia persists. Infectious causes of bone marrow suppression should also be considered (e.g., parvovirus B19, human herpesvirus 6, Epstein-Barr virus, cytomegalovirus, human immunodeficiency virus). Bone marrow examination may be warranted, especially if reticulocytopenia continues for more than a few weeks, repeated blood transfusions are required, or other hematopoietic lineages are affected. Complete recovery usually occurs in 4 to 8 weeks. Transfusion of RBCs is indicated with clinical decompensation as a result of anemia or when the hemoglobin is less than 6 g/dL in the setting of a poor reticulocyte count (<5%). With or without transfusion, patients should be monitored with weekly blood and reticulocyte counts until they recover.

Inherited Bone Marrow Failure Syndromes

If the anemia is chronic, is present from a young age, or is refractory to treatment, one must suspect an inherited cause, especially if the MCV is normal or slightly elevated. Frequently, inherited marrow failure syndromes are accompanied by physical abnormalities (birth defects), necessitating a careful examination for physical stigmata (e.g., short stature, limb abnormalities, heart defects, pigmentation changes). Some inherited causes of bone marrow suppression are specific to RBCs (e.g., Diamond-Blackfan anemia), whereas others (e.g., Fanconi anemia) affect multiple cell lines, resulting in pancytopenia. Careful attention must be paid to the remainder of the CBC when considering bone marrow failure syndromes. In general, subspecialist consultation is recommended to diagnose and treat these rare patients.

Megaloblastic Anemia

Patients with anemia caused by dietary deficiencies of folic acid or cobalamin (vitamin B_{12}) present with reticulocytopenic macrocytic anemia. The MCV is generally quite elevated (often >100 fL). Other clues to the diagnosis may derive from examination of the peripheral blood smear, most notably hypersegmented neutrophils (>5 nuclear lobes). Folic acid is naturally found in fruits and vegetables and cow's milk, and deficiency is normally limited to those patients with self-imposed dietary restrictions (e.g., consumption of only unfortified goat's milk or a diet devoid of fruits and vegetables). Serum or RBC folate levels can be assayed; the latter is less susceptible to short-term fluctuation and more reflective of tissue stores. Vitamin B_{12} is present in animal products, so a dietary basis for vitamin B_{12} deficiency is usually limited to strict vegans. Vitamin B_{12} and folate deficiencies can also result from malabsorption. In contrast to folate, however, vitamin B_{12} absorption depends on the activity of a gastric-derived cofactor (intrinsic factor); therefore, vitamin B_{12} deficiency can be due to a lack of intrinsic factor (e.g., pernicious anemia) rather than simple dietary deficiency or malabsorption. It is important to differentiate the causes of megaloblastic anemia, because irreversible neuropathy often accompanies vitamin B_{12} deficiency, making timely diagnosis and treatment critical.

DISORDERS OF RED CELL DESTRUCTION: THE HEMOLYTIC ANEMIAS

Hemolytic anemias result from the accelerated destruction of RBCs and should be suspected when there are signs of hemolysis such as jaundice, hyperbilirubinemia, organomegaly, dark urine, and reticulocytosis. RBCs normally survive for 4 months, so any cause of premature destruction can result in anemia, particularly when bone marrow production fails to keep pace with the destructive process. Hemolytic anemias result from factors either intrinsic or extrinsic to the RBC. In general, intrinsic defects are inherited, whereas extrinsic causes are usually acquired.

Inherited Hemolytic Anemias

Inherited hemolytic anemias can be caused by defects in the erythrocyte membrane (e.g., spherocytosis), defects in globin genes (e.g., sickle cell anemia, thalassemia, unstable hemoglobin), or defects in RBC metabolism (e.g., pyruvate kinase deficiency, glucose-6-phosphate dehydrogenase deficiency). A directed family history is critical in the workup of patients with hemolytic anemias, because family members are often affected as well. Such children are usually well compensated hemodynamically and, as demonstrated by persistently elevated reticulocyte counts, tend to rely on chronic overproduction of RBCs to compensate for their premature destruction. These children generally do well clinically unless an intercurrent illness slows bone marrow production of new RBCs. Parvovirus B19, the causative agent of erythema infectiosum (fifth disease), replicates in RBC precursors and can almost completely shut down erythropoiesis for days to weeks, leading to aplastic crisis in children with hemolytic anemias. Often, RBC transfusion is required to maintain homeostasis until erythropoiesis recovers from the infection (typically within 1 month). In general, it is appropriate to involve hematology subspecialists in the diagnosis and long-term management of patients with inherited hemolytic anemias.

Abnormalities of the Red Blood Cell Membrane

The most common genetic RBC membrane abnormality is hereditary spherocytosis, which is usually inherited dominantly and results from defects in membrane proteins that bridge the actin cytoskeleton and the phospholipid bilayer.[8] Defective membrane-protein interactions lead to the loss of small segments of the lipid membrane, resulting in spherocytic red cells that have lost their biconcave discoid shape and have an increased mean corpuscular hemoglobin concentration. Spherocytic cells are less deformable and are cleared rapidly by the spleen, resulting in a much shortened life span. Patients with hereditary spherocytosis usually have mild chronic hyperbilirubinemia and splenomegaly. The disease is diagnosed by osmotic fragility testing because the cells are unusually sensitive to lysis in hypotonic solutions. Other membrane abnormalities associated with hemolysis include hereditary elliptocytosis, hereditary pyropoikilocytosis, and hereditary stomatocytosis.

Disorders of Red Blood Cell Metabolism

To survive normally, the RBC must be replete with the enzymes needed for adenosine triphosphate (ATP) generation and reduced nicotinamide adenine dinucleotide phosphate (NADPH) production. Defective enzymes of the hexose monophosphate shunt or Embden-Meyerhof pathway can result in anemia by limiting the RBCs' energy or antioxidant capabilities, shortening their life span in the circulation. The most common abnormality is X-linked glucose-6-phosphate dehydrogenase (G6PD) deficiency. The enzyme G6PD is important for NADPH regeneration needed to produce reduced glutathione, which protects the RBC from oxidative damage. Cells deficient in G6PD are susceptible to injury from oxidant drugs, infection, acidosis, and

fava bean ingestion. Unlike the more severe Mediterranean and Asian variants, the "A" variant of G6PD, common in African Americans (1 in 10 males is thought to be affected), is mild and usually does not result in severe hemolysis. G6PD deficiency should be suspected in the setting of prolonged jaundice in the neonatal period after alloimmune hemolysis has been ruled out by a normal Coombs test. Supravital staining for Heinz bodies (to detect precipitated hemoglobin) may be positive. G6PD testing can be performed, although the results may be falsely normal soon after a hemolytic event owing to selective hemolysis of cells with the lowest G6PD levels and increased G6PD levels in abundant reticulocytes. Inheritance of pyruvate kinase deficiency, the second most common enzymopathy, is autosomal recessive. Pyruvate kinase deficiency can result in severe anemia, with reticulocytosis and splenomegaly. In general, the management of patients with enzymopathies is supportive (chronic folic acid supplementation), with an emphasis on the avoidance of known oxidative stressors (e.g., medications, foods, environmental exposure).

Hemoglobinopathies

Many abnormal hemoglobin variants result in premature destruction of the RBC by relative insolubility and precipitation of hemoglobin in the red cell cytoplasm. Hemoglobin precipitation somehow leads to less deformable RBC membranes, resulting in accelerated splenic clearance of the affected cells. Hemoglobin defects can result from either unbalanced expression of α- and β-globin genes (thalassemias) or mutations of the globin genes themselves (e.g., sickle cell, hemoglobin C, hemoglobin E, unstable hemoglobins). Although abnormal RBC morphology is a common finding in hemoglobinopathy, hemoglobin evaluation by electrophoresis, sequencing, and other tests, along with Heinz body testing (which detects hemoglobin precipitation in RBCs), is the preferred method of diagnosing this group of hemolytic anemias. Certain hemoglobin disorders such as α-thalassemia trait are difficult to detect even by electrophoresis. Other than detecting a small amount of Bart's hemoglobin at birth, electrophoresis is virtually normal in those with silent α-thalassemia trait and carriers, who are usually diagnosed by genetics or by sequencing the α-globin loci. Owing to its high incidence and special management considerations, sickle cell anemia is discussed separately in Chapter 117.

Treatment of Inherited Hemolytic Anemias

In general, treatment of inherited hemolytic anemias is dictated by the severity of the anemia, the nature of the defect, and its clinical consequences. Patients with mild anemia can be observed, whereas those with severe anemia may require chronic transfusions or splenectomy. In general, patients with chronic hemolytic anemias require only supportive care (e.g., folic acid supplementation) to facilitate chronic compensatory reticulocytosis; such patients probably should be managed in conjunction with a hematology specialist.

Acquired Hemolytic Anemias
Microangiopathic Hemolytic Anemia

The hallmark of microangiopathy is the finding of schistocytes (red cell fragments) on peripheral blood smear analysis. Infection and sepsis can result in microangiopathy through uncontrolled fibrinogenesis and consequent physical disruption of RBCs by shearing forces that occur when blood circulates through vessels clogged with fibrin strands. RBC destruction in this setting can be severe and may be accompanied by thrombocytopenia and coagulation factor consumption, resulting in disseminated intravascular coagulation (DIC). These patients are typically quite ill and often have multiorgan pathology in addition to hemolytic anemia. Microangiopathic anemia also occurs with hemolytic uremic syndrome (HUS) and thrombotic thrombocytopenic purpura (TTP). HUS and TTP exist on a continuum and have in common decreased activity of von Willebrand protease. HUS is far more common in the pediatric population and typically results from infection with enteric bacteria, classically *Escherichia coli* O157:H7, that express the Shiga toxin, which directly interferes with von Willebrand protease.[9] The clinical syndrome of HUS together with neurologic symptoms suggests TTP, an inherited or acquired deficiency of von Willebrand protease,[10,11] and justifies prompt treatment with plasma infusion and plasmapheresis.[12]

Immune-Mediated Hemolytic Anemias

Immune-mediated hemolytic anemias are common causes of acquired hemolytic anemias in the pediatric population. By definition, antibody is produced against one or more antigens on the surface of RBCs, promoting premature destruction by opsonization and subsequent erythrocyte removal by the reticuloendothelial system or by complement-mediated lysis of RBCs in the bloodstream.[13,14] Antibodies may come from the patient (in which case the process is known as autoimmune hemolytic anemia [AIHA]) or from another source (alloimmune hemolytic anemia), such as occurs in hemolytic disease of the newborn. Unlike hemolytic disease of the newborn, which is invariably caused by transplacental maternal immunoglobulin (Ig) G and is a problem only in utero and in the newborn period, AIHA can affect patients of any age and can be caused by either IgM or IgG.

Patients with AIHA often relate a history of previous viral or viral-like illness preceding the development of fatigue and pallor. The presentation of AIHA is usually sudden and may include symptoms of severe anemia. A history of dark urine suggests acute intravascular hemolysis and argues for complement-mediated red cell lysis (see later). Jaundiced sclerae or pruritus suggests hyperbilirubinemia. Mild splenomegaly is occasionally present.

AIHA can result in intravascular or extravascular hemolysis. Intravascular hemolysis is complement mediated and caused by IgM or complement-fixing IgG directed against RBC antigens, resulting in lysis of RBCs directly in the plasma and leading to jaundice or hyperbilirubinemia, elevated lactate dehydrogenase, and low haptoglobin. In contrast, extravascular hemolysis is typically mediated by IgG without complement-fixing characteristics. Extravascular hemolysis may result in little or no increase in lactate dehydrogenase and bilirubin, presumably because RBCs are destroyed in the phagocytic cells of the reticuloendothelial system rather than in the plasma itself. Laboratory evaluation of AIHA reveals a moderate to severe anemia with a brisk reticulocytosis. However, it is important to note that the reticulocyte count may be unexpectedly low if the reactive antibody also results in clearance of young RBCs. Review of the peripheral blood smear may show spherocytosis, poly-

chromasia, and RBC clumping. Urinalysis may show hemoglobinuria in the absence of hematuria. Direct Coombs testing (which tests for antibody bound to the patient's RBCs) is almost always positive in AIHA. Indirect Coombs testing, which tests for free antierythrocyte antibody in the patient's serum, usually detects alloantibodies but may be positive in AIHA when the antibody titer exceeds antigen binding; this can help define which isotype and RBC antigen are involved. If multiple cell lineages are depressed or Coombs testing is negative, examination of the bone marrow should be considered to rule out leukemia or aplastic anemia. Primary AIHA can be divided into three types based on the nature, thermal reactivity, and amplitude of the implicated antibody.

Warm-Reactive Autoimmune Hemolytic Anemia

In warm-reactive AIHA, antibody (usually IgG) binds RBC antigens at 37°C, resulting in opsonization and removal by the reticuloendothelial system. Warm-reactive IgG typically binds common RBC protein antigens, which explains why blood bank testing often demonstrates a pan-reactive pattern. Warm-reactive AIHA tends to behave in a more chronic fashion than cold agglutinin disease and may warrant a more long-term treatment approach.

Paroxysmal Cold Hemoglobinuria

In paroxysmal cold hemoglobinuria (PCH), complement-fixing IgG autoantibody binds RBCs at low temperatures (usually in the extremities in vivo) and then causes complement-dependent intravascular hemolysis at warm temperatures (in central, warmer parts of the body). PCH sometimes follows infection with *Mycoplasma pneumoniae* or other atypical organisms. Testing for the cold-reactive (Donath-Landsteiner) antibody of PCH is performed by maintaining freshly drawn venous blood at 37°C until it is intentionally cooled in the laboratory, permitting antibody binding (if the patient's blood is not kept warm until separation of plasma from RBCs, the antibody may be cleared by binding RBCs in the collection tube, leaving none free to be detected). Erythrocyte-antibody complexes are then warmed, inducing complement activation and hemolysis.

Cold Agglutinin Disease

In cold agglutinin disease, antibody (usually IgM) binds erythrocyte antigens (typically red cell surface polysaccharides) and fixes complement at temperatures below 37°C. In this manner, IgM efficiently results in intravascular hemolysis. Because IgM inefficiently binds antigen at 37°C, unbound antibody can frequently be detected in the plasma. Cold agglutinin AIHA is usually a self-limited process and typically does not respond well to immunosuppressive therapy.

Treatment of Acquired Hemolytic Anemias

Treatment of hemolytic anemias due to extrinsic defects is normally directed toward the underlying problem resulting in hemolysis. Severe anemia may justify RBC transfusion, although the underlying pathophysiologic mechanism will likely destroy the newly transfused cells as well as the patient's own RBCs. Transfusion of other blood products may also be beneficial; however, platelet transfusion should be avoided when TTP is a consideration, given the increased risk of thrombosis.

The appropriate treatment of AIHA depends on the degree of hemolysis and resulting anemia. Children with mild anemia associated with postinfectious antibody development can usually be observed without transfusion. However, children with severe anemia or anemia with physiologic consequences should be promptly transfused with erythrocytes. Determination of the antigenic target of the autoantibody can be helpful in the selection of compatible blood for transfusion. If time permits, blood bank personnel should select the most compatible (or least incompatible) blood available, but emergent transfusion should not be delayed for this purpose.[15] Transfusion in this challenging situation can be facilitated by direct clinician–blood bank interaction. Because incompatible transfused erythrocytes may be rapidly hemolysed, multiple transfusions are often required until more definitive therapy can be instituted. Children with cold reactive antibodies should avoid cold exposure, and blood should be administered with the use of a blood warmer. AIHA is often responsive to immunosuppression, and systemic corticosteroids are particularly effective for patients with warm-reactive IgG.[16]

For life-threatening hemolysis, treatment with methylprednisolone (1 to 2 mg/kg per day intravenously every 6 hours) should be initiated promptly. Response to therapy is characterized by increasingly stable hemoglobin, decreasing reticulocytosis, and diminishing requirement for transfusion. After stabilization, prednisone 1 to 2 mg/kg per day can be substituted for methylprednisolone and, based on response, gradually tapered over several weeks to months. To avoid the side effects of chronic steroid treatment, high-dose therapy should not continue for more than several days, and in the absence of a response, alternative treatments should be considered. Intravenous immunoglobulin has been used to treat AIHA with occasional success, but it should be considered a second-line treatment. Exchange transfusion or plasmapheresis has limited efficacy in AIHA, although plasmapheresis may be marginally more effective for IgM- than IgG-based disease. Splenectomy may be considered for refractory IgG-dependent chronic extravascular hemolysis. Other immunosuppressive drugs such as cyclophosphamide, 6-mercaptopurine, 6-thioguanine, azathioprine, and cyclosporine A may serve as steroid-sparing agents for children with chronic AIHA. Intravenous immunoglobulin may have some efficacy in a limited number of warm-reactive AIHA patients.[17] Treatment with any of these agents should be in consultation with a hematology or immunology specialist.

CONSULTATION

Hematology or oncology consultation should be obtained in cases of unclear diagnosis, persistent or refractory anemia, requirement for bone marrow examination, concern about bone marrow failure syndromes, possible need for immunosuppressive therapy, or blast forms seen on the peripheral blood smear. Such specialists should also be consulted during the diagnostic workup before transfusion and for the long-term management of patients with chronic or refractory anemia.

Transfusion medicine specialists should be consulted when there is a need for plasmapheresis or exchange transfusion, there are difficulties in blood crossmatching due to autoantibody production, or a determination of autoantibody specificity is required.

ADMISSION CRITERIA

- Severe anemia complicated by physiologic changes.
- Ongoing hemolytic process that requires monitoring and possible transfusion.
- Anemia associated with severe neutropenia or thrombocytopenia.
- Lack of appropriate follow-up.

DISCHARGE CRITERIA

- Absence of physiologic manifestations of anemia.
- No evidence of excessive ongoing hemolysis.
- Reliable outpatient follow-up with a pediatric practitioner to evaluate for a durable response to treatment and for recurrence of anemia. Communication of the inpatient treatment and laboratory values at the time of discharge is critical for appropriate posthospital care.
- Follow-up with a hematology or oncology specialist is necessary for children with ongoing hemolysis, unclear diagnoses, bone marrow failure syndromes, or possible neoplastic processes.

IN A NUTSHELL

- The clinical syndrome of anemia can have diverse causes.
- Children with mild anemia are most appropriately evaluated in the outpatient setting. However, children with severe anemia, especially when the cause is uncertain, may require hospitalization for evaluation and treatment. Hospitalization allows the close monitoring of physiologic indicators (heart and respiratory rate) and blood counts, affording the ability to respond rapidly to changes.
- Severe anemia, especially with signs of cardiovascular compromise, should be treated with blood transfusion to enhance oxygen carrying capacity and reverse the associated physiologic changes. It is important to note that transfusion of blood products complicates subsequent laboratory testing by infusing donor cells and plasma. Thus, it is critical to collect samples for laboratory investigation before transfusion, which probably justifies consultation with a hematologist.

ON THE HORIZON

- The use of soluble transferrin receptor levels to evaluate erythropoiesis and iron status.[18]
- Increasing use of antibody-mediated immune suppression for autoimmune cytopenias. For example, rituximab (anti-CD20 monoclonal antibody) has demonstrated efficacy in a subset of children with chronic or refractory AIHA.[19]
- Better understanding of the mutations causing intrinsic hemolytic anemias, together with improvements in gene delivery to hematopoietic stem cells, will result in curative treatments.
- Increased understanding of the mechanisms of HUS and TTP, including congenital or acquired deficiencies of the von Willebrand factor cleaving protease ADAMTS13.

SUGGESTED READING

Ball SE, Gordon-Smith EC: Failure of red cell production. In Lilleyman J, Hann I, Blanchette V (eds): Pediatric Hematology. London, Churchill Livingstone, 1999, pp 65-81.

Gallagher PG, Forget BG, Lux SE: Disorders of the erythrocyte membrane. In Nathan DG, Orkin SH (eds): Nathan and Oski's Hematology of Infancy and Childhood. Philadelphia, WB Saunders, 1998, pp 544-664.

Oski F, Brugnara C, Nathan DG: A diagnostic approach to the anemic patient. In Nathan DG, Orkin SH (eds): Nathan and Oski's Hematology of Infancy and Childhood. Philadelphia, WB Saunders, 1998, pp 375-384.

Ware RE, Rosse WF: Autoimmune hemolytic anemia. In Nathan DG, Orkin SH (eds): Nathan and Oski's Hematology of Infancy and Childhood. Philadelphia, WB Saunders, 1998, pp 499-522.

REFERENCES

1. Oski F, Brugnara C, Nathan DG: A diagnostic approach to the anemic patient. In Nathan DG, Orkin SH (eds): Nathan and Oski's Hematology of Infancy and Childhood. Philadelphia, WB Saunders, 1998, pp 375-384.

2. Kwiatkowski JL, West TB, Heidary N, et al: Severe iron deficiency anemia in young children. J Pediatr 1999;135:514.

3. Dallman PR, Siimes MA: Percentile curves for hemoglobin and red cell volume in infancy and childhood. J Pediatr 1979;94:26-31.

4. Looker AC, Dallman PR, Carroll MD, et al: Prevalence of iron deficiency in the United States. JAMA 1997;277:973-976.

5. Ullrich C, Wu A, Armsby C, et al: Screening healthy infants for iron deficiency using reticulocyte hemoglobin content. JAMA 2005;294:924-930.

6. Brugnara C, Zurakowski D, Di Canzio J, et al: Reticulocyte hemoglobin content to diagnose iron deficiency in children. JAMA 1999;281:2225.

7. Ganz T: Molecular pathogenesis of anemia of chronic disease. Pediatr Blood Cancer 2006;46:554-557.

8. Gallagher PG, Forget BG, Lux SE: Disorders of the erythrocyte membrane. In Nathan DG, Orkin SH (eds): Nathan and Oski's Hematology of Infancy and Childhood. Philadelphia, WB Saunders, 1998, pp 544-664.

9. Tsai HM, Chandler WL, Sarode R, et al: Von Willebrand factor and von Willebrand factor-cleaving metalloprotease activity in *Escherichia coli* O157:H7-associated hemolytic uremic syndrome. Pediatr Res 2001;49:653-659.

10. Furlan M, Robles R, Galbusera M, et al: Von Willebrand factor-cleaving protease in thrombotic thrombocytopenic purpura and the hemolytic-uremic syndrome. N Engl J Med 1998;339:1578.

11. Tsai HM, Lian EC: Antibodies to von Willebrand factor-cleaving protease in acute thrombotic thrombocytopenic purpura. N Engl J Med 1998;339:1585-1594.

12. Furlan M, Robles R, Morselli B, et al: Recovery and half-life of von Willebrand factor-cleaving protease after plasma therapy in patients with thrombotic thrombocytopenic purpura. Thromb Haemost 1999;81:8.

13. Gehrs BC, Friedberg RC: Autoimmune hemolytic anemia. Am J Hematol 2002;69:258.

14. Ware RE, Rosse WF: Autoimmune hemolytic anemia. In Nathan DG, Orkin SH (eds): Nathan and Oski's Hematology of Infancy and Childhood. Philadelphia, WB Saunders, 1998, pp 499-522.

15. Petz LD: A physician's guide to transfusion in autoimmune haemolytic anaemia. Br J Haematol 2004;124:712.

16. King KE, Ness PM: Treatment of autoimmune hemolytic anemia. Semin Hematol 2005;42:131-136.

17. Flores G, Cunningham-Rundles C, Newland AC, Bussel JB: Efficacy of intravenous immunoglobulin in the treatment of autoimmune hemolytic anemia: Results in 73 patients. Am J Hematol 1993;44:237-242.

18. Beguin Y: Soluble transferrin receptor for the evaluation of erythropoiesis and iron status. Clin Chim Acta 2003;329:9-22.

19. Zecca M, Nobili B, Ramenghi U, et al: Rituximab for the treatment of refractory autoimmune hemolytic anemia in children. Blood 2003;101:3857.

CHAPTER 117

Sickle Cell Disease

Matthew M. Heeney

Sickle cell disease (SCD) is an inherited hemolytic anemia that affects approximately 70,000 persons in the United States, mostly among the African American population. It is responsible for lifelong medical complications in most affected individuals. The complications of SCD can be divided into those that are acute and those that are chronic, caused by repetitive vaso-occlusion of the various organ systems (Table 117-1). This chapter focuses on the acute complications that the general hospitalist is likely to encounter.

PATHOPHYSIOLOGY

SCD refers to a group of hemolytic anemias in which hemoglobin S (HbS) is present in either a homozygous state (HbSS) or a compound heterozygous state, such as when combined with hemoglobin C (HbSC) or β-thalassemia (HbS–β-thalassemia). The HbS mutation is the result of an amino acid substitution (valine is substituted for glutamic acid at position 6) in the β-globin of the hemoglobin heterotetramer. The mutation creates a hydrophobic region that, in the deoxygenated state, facilitates a noncovalent polymerization of HbS molecules into rigid strands. These HbS polymers damage the erythrocyte membrane and change the rheology of the erythrocyte in circulation, causing hemolytic anemia and vaso-occlusion.

CLINICAL PRESENTATION

The National Institutes of Health recommends that all infants be screened in the neonatal period for SCD,[1] and currently, all 50 states and the District of Columbia perform universal screening for SCD.[2] For this reason, most children with SCD are identified early, and medical management is started before the usual age of presentation. Because the sickle mutation affects β-globin, a component of adult hemoglobin rather than fetal hemoglobin, affected infants are usually asymptomatic for the first 6 months of life. Anemia and complications from SCD usually present toward the end of the first year of life, after the physiologic switch from fetal to adult hemoglobin.

Although universal newborn screening will diagnose the majority of new pediatric SCD cases, the clinician is advised to consider SCD in the differential diagnosis of patients with non-immune-mediated hemolytic anemia, especially those who are foreign born. Although affected patients are typically quite anemic (hemoglobin between 7 and 9 g/dL), they are generally not overly symptomatic (e.g., weakness, fatigue) because the anemia is chronic and compensated for physiologically. As a result of the markedly shortened red cell survival time, bone marrow production of new erythrocytes is brisk, as indicated by chronically elevated reticulocyte counts (usually 10% to 20%). Patients may be jaundiced or icteric due to chronic hemolysis and may have features of extramedullary hematopoiesis (e.g., maxillary hypertrophy). They may have splenomegaly and skull bone deformities due to extramedullary hematopoiesis.

HEALTH MAINTENANCE

Infants diagnosed by newborn screening should be referred to pediatric hematologists for confirmation of the diagnosis, parental education, genetic counseling, and long-term follow-up. Routine visits to a pediatric hematologist are scheduled every 3 months for the first 2 years of life, then every 6 months until age 4 to 5 years, and annually thereafter. More frequent visits may be required for patients with greater educational needs or accumulated complications or for therapeutic monitoring (e.g., hydroxyurea or chronic transfusion therapy). "Well visits" allow the practitioner to obtain baseline clinical, laboratory, and radiographic data, which are important in the event of an acute complication; they also afford the opportunity for parent and patient education and anticipatory guidance.

TREATMENT AND COMPLICATIONS

Acute and chronic complications are an important part of the management of SCD (see Table 117-1). Although the hematologist manages conditions associated with chronic disease, the generalist may need to consider these complications and their impact when called on to evaluate children with SCD. The following discussion focuses on acute complications.

Fever

Patients with SCD are functionally asplenic by 2 years of age and are therefore at risk for invasive and overwhelming infections caused by encapsulated bacteria (e.g., *Streptococcus pneumoniae, Haemophilus influenzae, Neisseria meningitidis*).[3] Antibiotic prophylaxis should be initiated when the diagnosis of SCD is made (Table 117-2). Children with SCD should receive all routine immunizations, including the *H. influenzae* type B series (HiB), the pneumococcal conjugate vaccine series (Prevnar, PCV7), and a pneumococcal polysaccharide vaccine (Pneumovax, PPV23) at age 2 years, with a booster 3 to 5 years later, to decrease the risk of bacteremia.[4] Influenza vaccines should be administered to all sickle cell patients annually, and the meningococcal polysaccharide vaccine should be administered to patients 2 years of age and older.[5]

Even with antibiotic prophylaxis and complete immunizations, all sickle cell patients should be considered at high risk for bacteremia and overwhelming sepsis. Aggressive

Table 117-1 Medical Complications of Sickle Cell Disease

Acute	Chronic
Vaso-occlusive	Constitutional: decreased stamina
Dactylitis (hand-foot syndrome)	Cardiovascular: pulmonary hypertension, cardiomegaly
Splenic sequestration	Renal: hyposthenuria, hematuria, nocturnal enuresis
Priapism	Ocular: proliferative retinopathy
Pain crisis	Pulmonary: chronic lung disease
Acute chest syndrome	Skin: leg ulcers
Stroke, cerebrovascular accident	Musculoskeletal: osteonecrosis, avascular necrosis
Non-vaso-occlusive	Endocrine: growth failure, delayed puberty
	Neurologic: learning disability, motor deficits
Cholelithiasis, cholecystitis	Psychiatric: poor self-image, depression
Aplastic crisis	
Bacteremia	

Table 117-2 Antibiotic Prophylaxis in Sickle Cell Disease

Age	Dose*
Birth-3 yr	Penicillin VK 125 mg PO bid
3-5 yr	Penicillin VK 250 mg PO bid
>5 yr	Discontinue, except in the case of previous surgical splenectomy, after which antibiotic prophylaxis should be continued indefinitely

*Erythromycin can be substituted in patients with penicillin allergies.

evaluation and empirical treatment of febrile SCD patients are necessary to reduce the mortality and morbidity of sepsis. Children with an obvious source of infection (e.g., otitis, gastroenteritis) should still receive a full evaluation and appropriate treatment. Key to the proper management of febrile SCD patients (or any asplenic patient) are rapid triage and assessment and the administration of empirical parenteral antibiotics within 1 hour of presentation. The focused history, physical examination, and blood work, including blood cultures, should be done promptly. If the patient has a central line or an implanted port, blood cultures must be drawn off this line. A chest radiograph is recommended for most patients, especially those with tachypnea, cough, hypoxemia, thoracic pain, and history of asthma or acute chest syndrome (ACS). Urinalysis and urine culture are recommended for all males younger than 6 months and all females younger than 2 years. Throat culture, cerebrospinal fluid analysis and culture, stool cultures, respiratory viral panels, and other studies should be obtained as clinically indicated.

All febrile patients with SCD require empirical parenteral antibiotic coverage for at least 24 hours. Ceftriaxone is the mainstay of empirical therapy (50 mg/kg intravenously or intramuscularly, to a maximum of 1 to 2 g/day).[6,7] Other third-generation cephalosporins may be used to complete coverage for the first 24 hours, depending on the institu-

tional guidelines or formulary. For patients allergic to cephalosporins, other broad-spectrum possibilities include clindamycin and quinolones (e.g., gatifloxacin, levofloxacin). Vancomycin is usually reserved for those with signs of meningitis, a history of pneumococcal sepsis, or a toxic appearance. Vancomycin should also be considered in areas with a high local prevalence of resistant organisms[8,9] and if a central venous line or port is present. If a central venous line is present, the antibiotics should be administered via this route. If a new infiltrate is identified on the chest radiograph, a macrolide antibiotic should be added to the previously mentioned empirical antibiotics because of the high incidence of pneumonia caused by atypical organisms in this setting.[10]

Admission to the hospital should be considered if there is any indication of possible complications or if any high-risk features are present (Table 117-3).[11-13] If there are no high-risk factors, discharge from the acute care setting can be considered if the patient is stable 1 hour after receiving empirical antibiotics. Patients should be counseled to return immediately in the event of persistent fever, increased respiratory symptoms, dehydration, lethargy, pain, or other worsening symptoms. Clear instructions should also be given for follow-up in 24 hours with the primary care physician or emergency department or by phone so that pending cultures can be tracked.

Cerebrovascular Accident

Stroke is one of the most important causes of disability in the sickle cell population. Sickle cell patients are at increased risk of stroke starting in the late school-age period. Primary vaso-occlusive stroke affects 10% of homozygous sickle cell patients before the end of the second decade of life.[14] Risk factors for primary stroke include previous transient ischemic attack, low baseline hemoglobin, preceding ACS, hypertension, and abnormal transcranial Doppler ultrasound screening. Transcranial Doppler ultrasonography is a reliable screening test to identify patients at highest risk of stroke. These patients are prescribed chronic intermittent transfusion therapy, with the goal of suppressing endogenous erythropoiesis and maintaining the sickle hemoglobin at less than 30%. This has been demonstrated to reduce the risk of both recurrent stroke and primary stroke in children with elevated transcranial Doppler velocities.[15,16]

Any acute neurologic findings such as weakness, altered consciousness, seizure, or language or speech disturbance should prompt an immediate evaluation for cerebral ischemia, although infection, tumor, intoxication, and thromboembolic disease should also be considered. The majority of strokes in children with SCD are caused by nonhemorrhagic vaso-occlusion. Computed tomography findings may be normal in early ischemia. Highly sensitive magnetic resonance diffusion and FLAIR-weighted images remain abnormal for several days after significant cerebral ischemia, and magnetic resonance angiography often reveals static intracranial artery vasculopathy. However, neuroimaging should not delay the initiation of therapy.

Initial stabilization includes fluid hydration with crystalloid while samples are sent for crossmatching in preparation for red blood cell exchange transfusion. The goal of exchange transfusion is to reduce the proportion of sickle hemoglobin

Table 117-3 Admission Considerations for Sickle Cell Disease Patients with Fever

High-Risk Features	Other Considerations for Admission
Age <6 mo	History of noncompliance with medical care
Toxic appearance	Poor likelihood of outpatient follow-up (e.g., no phone, no transportation)
Hypotension or poor perfusion	Incomplete immunizations
History of previous infection with resistant organism	Age <5 yr and not compliant with antibiotic prophylaxis
Inability to maintain oral hydration	Multiple emergency department or clinic visits for same febrile illness
New onset of abnormal neurologic findings (concern for stroke or meningitis)	Unable to deliver initial 24 hr of empirical antibiotic coverage on outpatient basis owing to allergies
Respiratory findings (new hypoxia >3 points below baseline, or <92% if baseline is unknown; new pulmonary infiltrate on chest radiograph; asthma exacerbation)	
Exaggerated hematologic findings (hematocrit ≤18%, or ≥5 points below baseline; white blood cells >40,000 or <5000; platelet count <100,000)	
New splenomegaly suggestive of evolving splenic sequestration	

to less than 30% as measured by hemoglobin electrophoresis. Correction of dehydration plus maintenance hydration alone may quickly reverse symptoms; more aggressive hydration should be avoided, however, to lessen the risk of cerebral edema. Consultation with an experienced pediatric hematologist is important. Automated exchange transfusion by erythrocytapheresis is the preferred method of treatment, but it requires specialized equipment, trained personnel, and central access in most children. Exchange transfusion can also be achieved through manual techniques. Simple transfusion may be a temporizing measure until adequate cross-matched blood and personnel are present to perform the exchange. Patients should be monitored for metabolic or electrolyte disturbances, such as hypocalcemia or hyperkalemia, arising from large transfusions, with prompt treatment provided as necessary.

Other symptoms or signs should also be investigated and treated, such as an electroencephalogram and antiepileptics for seizure activity and antipyretics for fever. Treatments involving tissue plasminogen activator, antiplatelet agents, and hypothermia have not been studied adequately in children and are generally not used.

Acute Chest Syndrome

ACS is a leading cause of morbidity and mortality in children with SCD. It is an acute illness characterized by fever, respiratory symptoms (tachypnea, cough, wheeze, or hypoxemia relative to baseline), and a new infiltrate on the chest radiograph. Risk factors for the development of ACS include low fetal hemoglobin, elevated steady-state white blood cell counts,[10,17] comorbid asthma,[18] preceding vaso-occlusive pain crisis, and general anesthesia. The underlying pathophysiology is unclear, although infection, infarction, and pulmonary fat embolism have been implicated.[10] The infectious agents most often identified are *Chlamydia*,[19] *Mycoplasma*,[20] and viruses, with children showing a seasonal

variation in presentation.[21] Inadequately treated vaso-occlusive pain involving the sternum, ribs, or trunk may lead to splinting respirations, decreased tidal volume, and the development of atelectasis, ventilation-perfusion mismatch, hypoxemia, and progression to ACS. ACS is the most common complication of surgery and anesthesia in patients with SCD,[22] likely related to the risk factors of cold exposure, hypoxia, acidosis, atelectasis, and psychological stress in the perioperative period. Use of incentive spirometry has been shown to decrease the incidence of ACS in patients hospitalized with vaso-occlusive crisis and should be used routinely in all sickle cell patients.[23]

The initial treatment of patients with ACS should include supplemental oxygen for those who are hypoxemic (PaO_2 <75 mm Hg or oxygen saturation <95%) or to achieve a level less than their known baseline. Control of chest pain with frequent incentive spirometry (5 to 10 times/hour) and avoidance of oversedation with analgesics are key to minimizing hypoventilation.[23] Arterial blood gas measurement of the partial pressure of arterial oxygen (PaO_2) and calculation of the alveolar to arterial (A-a) oxygen gradient can serve as a guide to severity and the need for more intense treatment, but they are not routinely recommended. An increasing A-a gradient indicates worsening ventilation-perfusion mismatch.

Judicious fluid replacement should correct deficits but not exceed 100% of maintenance, because rapid or excessive hydration can contribute to pulmonary edema, effusions, and respiratory distress. Fever should be investigated with blood cultures before the institution of empirical broad-spectrum antibiotics (e.g., ceftriaxone, cefuroxime) as well as a macrolide (e.g., azithromycin) for atypical bacterial pathogens. Bronchodilators should be used aggressively in patients with a history of asthma or clinical evidence of wheezing and bear consideration in any patient who is worsening clinically. Systemic corticosteroids have been shown to hasten recovery from ACS but are also associated with rehospitalization from "rebound" vaso-occlusive crisis[24]; if used, corticosteroids should be tapered before discontinuation.

Red blood cell transfusion is the mainstay of therapy for ACS. Simple transfusion should be considered early in an attempt to abort progressive hypoxemia.[20] Various triggers for simple transfusion have been suggested, including greater than 5% drop in arterial oxygen saturation from baseline or PaO_2 less than 70 mm Hg. If simple transfusion is not effective in aborting the progression of respiratory symptoms, exchange transfusion must be considered. Corticosteroids and inhaled nitric oxide are other adjuvant therapies, but they lack proven benefit. If mechanical ventilation is required, frequent therapeutic bronchoscopy with aggressive suction to remove tenacious plastic bronchial casts is often indicated,[25,26] and inhaled mucolytics should be considered.[27]

Vaso-occlusive Pain

Acute vaso-occlusive bone pain is the central clinical manifestation of SCD and is characterized by its recurrent, excruciating, and often unpredictable nature. As fetal hemoglobin wanes in the first year of life, the proportion of HbS increases, and patients with SCD become vulnerable to vaso-occlusive pain episodes. Often, the first manifestation in infants and young children is secondary to infarction of the small bones of the hands and feet, leading to painful swelling referred to as dactylitis or hand-foot syndrome. In older children, vaso-occlusive pain of the long bones (humerus, tibia, and femur, in particular), vertebrae, ribs, and sternum is more common. Warmth, swelling, and decreased range of motion of adjacent joints may occur. Chronic or recurrent vaso-occlusion may lead to osteonecrosis, with the femoral head and humeral head most commonly affected.

Acute vaso-occlusive pain should be considered a medical emergency. Episodes can be mild and transient or intense and of several weeks' duration. Vaso-occlusive pain is the leading cause of acute care visits and hospital admissions for patients with SCD.[28] Parental education and an effective outpatient pain management plan are critical. Rapid assessment and treatment can halt the progression of vaso-occlusion to life-threatening events such as ACS or stroke. Ineffective treatment is often a result of inadequate provider knowledge of SCD, poor pain assessment skills, unfamiliarity or discomfort with the use of opioid analgesics, and poor understanding of concepts of opioid tolerance, dependence, and addiction.

The assessment of sickle cell pain should include standardized assessment tools such as the visual analog scale or the Wong-Baker faces scale. Care must be taken during the assessment to look for comorbid processes that may complicate the pain of SCD (e.g., cholelithiasis, splenic sequestration, appendicitis).

The mainstay of treatment for acute vaso-occlusive pain is pharmacologic therapy. Treatment of mild to moderate pain begins with nonsteroidal anti-inflammatory drugs, either orally (e.g., ibuprofen) or parenterally (e.g., ketorolac). If these agents have already been initiated at home or the pain is severe, clinicians should not hesitate to use parenteral opioid medications. Loading doses equivalent to 0.1 mg/kg morphine are recommended, and reassessment of both the patient's pain and the level of sedation should be performed at the anticipated peak effect of the chosen opioid and at frequent intervals thereafter. If there is inadequate analgesic effect, additional doses (0.025 to 0.05 mg/kg morphine equivalent) should be administered approximately every 30 to 60 minutes, with frequent reassessment until the pain is reduced to at least 50% of the initial score without excessive sedation. Patient-controlled analgesia plays an important role in older children and adolescents.

In addition to diligent pharmacologic pain control, the initial management of a pain crisis should include nonpharmacologic and psychosocial interventions. Important supportive measures include heating pads, distraction with art or music by child life specialists, and adequate oral or parenteral hydration. Correction of fluid deficits with normal saline should be followed by total fluid hydration not exceeding 150% of maintenance. Because of sickle-associated hyposthenuria, the initial maintenance fluid choice should be relatively hypotonic (e.g., 5% dextrose + $\frac{1}{2}$ normal saline + 20 mEq KCl/L) and adjusted based on chemistry results. Many patients find nonpharmacologic approaches such as local heat or massage beneficial. Based on the patient's age and cognitive-developmental stage, progressive muscle relaxation, meditation, guided imagery, or self-hypnosis may prove helpful. In addition, attention should be given to the elimination or diminution of psychosocial stressors that may potentiate pain perception (e.g., educating family members to avoid dysfunctional family interactions).

Discharge can be considered when consistent analgesia is achieved and parenteral opioids can be converted to oral formulations, if needed. Optimal outpatient pain management often involves the use of long-acting controlled-release opioids (e.g., morphine sulfate controlled-release capsules, oxycodone extended-release capsules), along with short-acting immediate-release preparations for breakthrough pain.

Acute Splenic Sequestration

Acute splenic sequestration is a significant cause of mortality in children with SCD.[29] With this event, the hypoxic environment of the spleen promotes acute trapping of sickle erythrocytes, leading to acute anemia and hypovolemia manifested by weakness, pallor, tachycardia, tachypnea, and abdominal distention that can progress to shock. The peak incidence of acute splenic sequestration is most commonly between 6 months and 5 years of age,[30,31] although it has been described in early infancy[32,33] and adulthood.[34] It recurs in approximately half of those who survive the first event, and subsequent mortality may be as high as 20%.[30] Acute splenic sequestration occurs most commonly in homozygous SCD (HbSS), but it also occurs in HbSC and HbS–β-thalassemia disease, often at a later age.

The definition of acute splenic sequestration is a drop of 2 g/dL in steady-state hemoglobin, with evidence of a compensatory marrow response (accentuated reticulocytosis above baseline) and an acutely enlarging spleen. The splenomegaly may be so massive that the splenic tip is found in the right lower quadrant. Parents should be taught how to palpate the infant's spleen and instructed to seek medical attention if it becomes enlarged.

Acute treatment is focused on the emergent correction of hypovolemia with crystalloid or erythrocyte transfusion or both. Improvement of circulating volume is often accompanied by the release of sequestered sickle erythrocytes, leading to an increase in hemoglobin higher than that predicted by the volume of transfused erythrocytes alone. One must take this autotransfusion phenomenon into account when planning the transfusion volume to avoid the hyperviscosity associated with hemoglobin greater than 10g/dL. Although observation may be recommended in adults,[35] the rate of recurrent sequestration is high in children, so they should be considered for short-term serial transfusion[36] or laparoscopic splenectomy once symptoms of the acute episode have waned. Laparoscopic splenectomy appears to be the treatment of choice in a child requiring transfusion support during the acute episode or who has suffered multiple episodes of sequestration. Children with persistent hypersplenism (splenomegaly associated with premature or inappropriate clearance of blood elements from the circulation, resulting in new or accentuated anemia, leukopenia, or thrombocytopenia) are also candidates for splenectomy. Postsplenectomy antibiotic prophylaxis should continue for at least 2 years and likely indefinitely.[37]

Priapism

Priapism is defined as a sustained, painful, and unwanted erection usually unrelated to sexual activity.[38,39] It should be treated as a medical emergency because of the subsequent high incidence of erectile dysfunction and impotence if it is not treated promptly. Priapism can be subclassified as prolonged or stuttering. Prolonged priapism refers to an episode lasting longer than 4 hours, and stuttering priapism refers to recurrent episodes lasting for minutes to less than 3 hours, although stuttering may herald a prolonged event.

Priapism reportedly affects as many as 75% to 89% of males with SCD by the time they reach 20 years of age.[40,41] It may occur in patients as young as 3 years old. Lack of awareness of this sickle-related complication and embarrassment about discussing an acute event represent significant hurdles to appropriate care.

The precise pathophysiology of priapism associated with SCD is unclear, although it is considered a low-flow ischemic state. It is assumed that relative hypoxia in the turgid corpus cavernosum leads to enhanced sickling and obstruction of venous outflow through the dorsal penile vein.[3,40] Recurrent or prolonged priapism can result in corpus cavernosal fibrosis and erectile dysfunction, the incidence of which is correlated to the duration of priapism.[42] Venous stasis leads to further oxygen extraction, acidosis, and a vicious circle of sickling and inflammation that, if not broken, may lead to fibrosis and erectile dysfunction. Triggers for priapism include sexual arousal or intercourse, fever, cold exposure, nocturnal tumescence (during REM sleep), full bladder, dehydration, alcohol, cocaine, and testosterone.[3,40,43,44]

The goal of management is pain relief, detumescence, and preservation of erectile function. Effective treatment of early priapism includes increased fluid intake, urination, oral pain medications, warm baths, gentle exercise, and oral pseudoephedrine.[38,40,41,45] The patient should seek urgent medical attention if priapism is accompanied by inability to void, unusually severe pain, or no improvement with home treatment within 2 hours.

Emergency care includes prompt institution of supportive medical therapy (intravenous fluids, analgesia, oxygen) and catheterization if there is inability to void. *Ice packs should never be used* in SCD, despite their use in nonsickle priapism. Urgent urology consultation is required for adjunctive corporeal aspiration and possible injection of vasoactive drugs if medical therapy is ineffective after 3 to 4 hours.[41,46] The patient is sedated and given local anesthesia, and the urologist irrigates the corpus cavernosum with a dilute epinephrine solution while aspirating until detumescence is achieved. This procedure may need to be repeated, with application of firm pressure for 5 minutes after each irrigation-aspiration. If this fails to produce consistent detumescence, exchange transfusion has been shown to be effective in small series.[47,48] If sustained detumescence is not achieved, surgical shunting between the corpus cavernosum and draining veins may be indicated. Complications of priapism and its surgical treatment include infection, stricture, fistula, and a high risk of impotence. Long-term management of patients with recurrent priapism requires collaboration between hematologists and urologists. The mainstay of chronic medical therapy is pseudoephedrine.[41]

Transient Aplastic Crisis

In hemolytic anemias, erythrocytes have a shortened life span, causing a compensatory increase in the bone marrow erythropoietic rate and peripheral reticulocytosis. Transient suppression of the marrow's response can lead to a rapid and severe decline in hemoglobin, the magnitude of which depends on the underlying rate of hemolysis and the duration of the suppression. Transient aplastic crises generally have an infectious cause, as evidenced by a preceding viral illness; often several family members with underlying hemolytic anemias are affected within days of one another. The typical presentation includes symptoms of exacerbated anemia (fatigue, dyspnea, tachycardia) and a relative reticulocytopenia and anemia compared with baseline values. Suppression of erythropoiesis typically lasts 7 to 10 days, and the convalescent phase is marked by a brisk reticulocytosis and gradual return to baseline hemoglobin levels.

The great majority of aplastic crises in SCD are related to infection with human parvovirus B19,[49] although other viruses have been implicated. Parvovirus B19 has a direct cytolytic effect on primarily erythroid progenitors in the bone marrow, but it may affect several cell lines. Elevated parvovirus B19 immunoglobulin M titers usually occur within 1 to 2 weeks of the acute infection, followed by seroconversion to immunoglobulin G and the "slapped cheek" appearance of erythema infectiosum, or fifth disease. Recurrent parvovirus B19 infection is rare in immunocompetent hosts, suggesting that exposure provides long-term immunity. Approximately one third of school-age children and three quarters of adults in the general population are seropositive,[50] and many have no history of clinical infection or erythroid suppression.[51] Transient aplastic crisis often resolves spontaneously, although some patients may require hospitalization and erythrocyte transfusion until baseline erythropoiesis returns.

Cholelithiasis and Cholecystitis

Any patient with a chronic hemolytic anemia is at risk of developing gallstones because of the precipitation of excessive bilirubin derived from the catabolism of heme released by red blood cells as they die prematurely.[52] Approximately one third of patients with SCD develop cholelithiasis by adulthood. Cholelithiasis is responsible for considerable morbidity, including recurrent abdominal pain mimicking vaso-occlusive pain events, cholecystitis, and choledocholithiasis, with the possible complication of pancreatitis. To avoid these clinical consequences, elective cholecystectomy is often recommended,[53,54] even for those with asymptomatic cholelithiasis[55] or biliary sludge.[56] Others advocate a more conservative approach with serial ultrasonography.[57] Cholecystectomy has become the most common elective surgical procedure performed in the United States for patients with SCD,[58] and the laparoscopic approach is favored in children.[55]

ADMISSION CRITERIA

Admission to the hospital is required for many of the acute complications of SCD, especially if outpatient management is complex or follow-up is not assured. Fever with complicated or high-risk features, new neurologic symptoms, ACS, or vaso-occlusive pain not controlled by the outpatient management plan are absolute indications for admission.

DISCHARGE CRITERIA

Discharge can be considered when the acute complication has been diagnosed and managed. Completion of treatment or transition to continued outpatient treatment should be achieved. This includes the institution of any preventive therapies or follow-up necessary to monitor for possible recurrence.

IN A NUTSHELL

- SCD is an inherited hemolytic anemia with wide phenotypic variation, despite being a single gene disorder.
- Increased risk of infection, especially by encapsulated organisms, is related to functional asplenia.
- Empirical antibiotic therapy is often indicated when patients develop fever, and immunizations are a vital tool in reducing the risk of overwhelming bacterial infection.
- Vaso-occlusion can lead to serious complications that are associated with significant morbidity and mortality. These include cerebrovascular accident, acute chest syndrome, pain crisis, and priapism. Intravenous hydration, analgesics, transfusion, and supplemental oxygen are key interventions.
- Splenic sequestration can lead to hypovolemia, which can progress to shock and significant splenomegaly. Initial treatment focuses on reestablishing intravascular volume with crystalloid or transfusion.
- As with other hemolytic anemias, high red cell turnover can lead to cholelithiasis, which can precipitate acute cholecystis. Dependence on high red cell production also predisposes patients to transient aplastic crisis when there is suppression of erythropoiesis.

ON THE HORIZON

- In addition to the Comprehensive Sickle Cell Centers, the recent establishment of an NIH-funded multicenter Sickle Cell Disease Clinical Research Network will provide an increased number of medical centers to provide education for health care professionals, comprehensive health maintenance, and clinical trials for SCD.
- Hydroxyurea, through the induction of fetal hemoglobin, has proven to be a safe and effective therapy for the prevention of acute complications in affected children and improved mortality in affected adults. Ongoing clinical trials will assess the ability of hydroxyurea to prevent chronic organ damage.
- Hematopoietic stem cell transplantation provides a tantalizing opportunity for cure. There have been great improvements in outcome, and ongoing efforts to identify the ideal recipient and the ideal stem cell source and to minimize the toxicity of current conditioning regimens may lead to more widespread use.
- The National Human Genome Research Institute's recent focus on SCD promises to shed light on why patients with SCD have divergent clinical phenotypes despite having the same single gene disorder. Hopefully these efforts will allow risk stratification of patients, further our understanding of the complex pathophysiology, and lead to innovative treatments.

SUGGESTED READING

The Management of Sickle Cell Disease, 4th ed. National Heart Lung and Blood Institute, 2003. Available at *http://www.nhlbi.nih.gov/health/prof/blood/sickle/sc_mngt.pdf.*

REFERENCES

1. Consensus conference: Newborn screening for sickle cell disease and other hemoglobinopathies. JAMA 1987;258:1205-1209.
2. US National Newborn Screening Status Report. http://genes-r-us.uthscsa.edu/nbsdisorders.pdf.
3. The Management of Sickle Cell Disease, 4th ed. National Heart Lung and Blood Institute, 2003. Available at http://www.nhlbi.nih.gov/health/prof/blood/sickle/sc_mngt.pdf.
4. Adamkiewicz TV, Sarnaik S, Buchanan GR, et al: Invasive pneumococcal infections in children with sickle cell disease in the era of penicillin prophylaxis, antibiotic resistance, and 23-valent pneumococcal polysaccharide vaccination. J Pediatr 2003;143:438-444.
5. Immunocompromised children. In Pickering L (ed): Red Book: 2003 Report of the Committee on Infectious Diseases, 26th ed. Elk Grove Village, Ill., American Academy of Pediatrics, 2003, pp 69-81.
6. Wilimas JA, Flynn PM, Harris S, et al: A randomized study of outpatient treatment with ceftriaxone for selected febrile children with sickle cell disease. N Engl J Med 1993;329:472-476.
7. Williams LL, Wilimas JA, Harris SC, et al: Outpatient therapy with ceftriaxone and oral cefixime for selected febrile children with sickle cell disease. J Pediatr Hematol Oncol 1996;18:257-261.
8. Sakhalkar VS, Sarnaik SA, Asmar BI, et al: Prevalence of penicillin-nonsusceptible *Streptococcus pneumoniae* in nasopharyngeal cultures from patients with sickle cell disease. South Med J 2001;94:401-404.
9. Hongeng S, Wilimas JA, Harris S, et al: Recurrent *Streptococcus pneumoniae* sepsis in children with sickle cell disease. J Pediatr 1997;130:814-816.

10. Vichinsky EP, Neumayr LD, Earles AN, et al: Causes and outcomes of the acute chest syndrome in sickle cell disease. National Acute Chest Syndrome Study Group. N Engl J Med 2000;342:1855-1865.

11. West TB, West DW, Ohene-Frempong K: The presentation, frequency, and outcome of bacteremia among children with sickle cell disease and fever. Pediatr Emerg Care 1994;10:141-143.

12. Rogers ZR, Morrison RA, Vedro DA, Buchanan GR: Outpatient management of febrile illness in infants and young children with sickle cell anemia. J Pediatr 1990;117:736-739.

13. Platt OS: The febrile child with sickle cell disease: A pediatrician's quandary. J Pediatr 1997;130:693-694.

14. Ohene-Frempong K, Weiner SJ, Sleeper LA, et al: Cerebrovascular accidents in sickle cell disease: Rates and risk factors. Blood 1998;91:288-294.

15. Pegelow CH, Adams RJ, McKie V, et al: Risk of recurrent stroke in patients with sickle cell disease treated with erythrocyte transfusions. J Pediatr 1995;126:896-899.

16. Adams RJ, McKie VC, Hsu L, et al: Prevention of a first stroke by transfusions in children with sickle cell anemia and abnormal results on transcranial Doppler ultrasonography. N Engl J Med 1998;339:5-11.

17. Castro O, Brambilla DJ, Thorington B, et al: The acute chest syndrome in sickle cell disease: Incidence and risk factors. The Cooperative Study of Sickle Cell Disease. Blood 1994;84:643-649.

18. Boyd JH, Moinuddin A, Strunk RC, DeBaun MR: Asthma and acute chest in sickle-cell disease. Pediatr Pulmonol 2004;38:229-232.

19. Dean D, Neumayr L, Kelly DM, et al: *Chlamydia pneumoniae* and acute chest syndrome in patients with sickle cell disease. J Pediatr Hematol Oncol 2003;25:46-55.

20. Neumayr L, Lennette E, Kelly D, et al: *Mycoplasma* disease and acute chest syndrome in sickle cell disease. Pediatrics 2003;112:87-95.

21. Vichinsky EP, Styles LA, Colangelo LH, et al: Acute chest syndrome in sickle cell disease: Clinical presentation and course. Cooperative Study of Sickle Cell Disease. Blood 1997;89:1787-1792.

22. Vichinsky EP, Haberkern CM, Neumayr L, et al: A comparison of conservative and aggressive transfusion regimens in the perioperative management of sickle cell disease. The Preoperative Transfusion in Sickle Cell Disease Study Group. N Engl J Med 1995;333:206-213.

23. Bellet PS, Kalinyak KA, Shukla R, et al: Incentive spirometry to prevent acute pulmonary complications in sickle cell diseases. N Engl J Med 1995;333:699-703.

24. Bernini JC, Rogers ZR, Sandler ES, et al: Beneficial effect of intravenous dexamethasone in children with mild to moderately severe acute chest syndrome complicating sickle cell disease. Blood 1998;92:3082-3089.

25. Raghuram N, Pettignano R, Gal AA, et al: Plastic bronchitis: An unusual complication associated with sickle cell disease and the acute chest syndrome. Pediatrics 1997;100:139-142.

26. Moser C, Nussbaum E, Cooper DM: Plastic bronchitis and the role of bronchoscopy in the acute chest syndrome of sickle cell disease. Chest 2001;120:608-613.

27. Manna SS, Shaw J, Tibby SM, Durward A: Treatment of plastic bronchitis in acute chest syndrome of sickle cell disease with intratracheal rhDNase. Arch Dis Child 2003;88:626-627.

28. Platt OS, Thorington BD, Brambilla DJ, et al: Pain in sickle cell disease: Rates and risk factors. N Engl J Med 1991;325:11-16.

29. Manci EA, Culberson DE, Yang YM, et al: Causes of death in sickle cell disease: An autopsy study. Br J Haematol 2003;123:359-365.

30. Topley JM, Rogers DW, Stevens MC, Serjeant GR: Acute splenic sequestration and hypersplenism in the first five years in homozygous sickle cell disease. Arch Dis Child 1981;56:765-769.

31. Emond AM, Collis R, Darvill D, et al: Acute splenic sequestration in homozygous sickle cell disease: Natural history and management. J Pediatr 1985;107:201-206.

32. Pappo A, Buchanan GR: Acute splenic sequestration in a 2-month-old infant with sickle cell anemia. Pediatrics 1989;84:578-579.

33. Airede AI: Acute splenic sequestration in a five-week-old infant with sickle cell disease. J Pediatr 1992;120:160.

34. Moll S, Orringer EP: Case report: Splenomegaly and splenic sequestration in an adult with sickle cell anemia. Am J Med Sci 1996;312:299-302.

35. Powell RW, Levine GL, Yang YM, Mankad VN: Acute splenic sequestration crisis in sickle cell disease: Early detection and treatment. J Pediatr Surg 1992;27:215-218.

36. Rao S, Gooden S: Splenic sequestration in sickle cell disease: Role of transfusion therapy. Am J Pediatr Hematol Oncol 1985;7:298-301.

37. Guidelines for the prevention and treatment of infection in patients with an absent or dysfunctional spleen. BMJ 1996;312:430-434.

38. Mantadakis E, Cavender JD, Rogers ZR, et al: Prevalence of priapism in children and adolescents with sickle cell disease. J Pediatr Hematol Oncol 1999;21:518-522.

39. Miller ST, Rao SP, Dunn EK, Glassberg KI: Priapism in children with sickle cell disease. J Urol 1995;154:844-847.

40. Adeyoju AB, Olujohungbe AB, Morris J, et al: Priapism in sickle-cell disease: Incidence, risk factors and complications—an international multicentre study. BJU Int 2002;90:898-902.

41. Mantadakis E, Ewalt DH, Cavender JD, et al: Outpatient penile aspiration and epinephrine irrigation for young patients with sickle cell anemia and prolonged priapism. Blood 2000;95:78-82.

42. Mykulak DJ, Glassberg KI: Impotence following childhood priapism. J Urol 1990;144:134-135.

43. Conrad ME, Perrine GM, Barton JC, Durant JR: Provoked priapism in sickle cell anemia. Am J Hematol 1980;9:121-122.

44. Jiva T, Anwer S: Priapism associated with chronic cocaine abuse. Arch Intern Med 1994;154:1770.

45. Maples BL, Hagemann TM: Treatment of priapism in pediatric patients with sickle cell disease. Am J Health Syst Pharm 2004;61:355-363.

46. Lane PA, Buchanan GR, Hutter JJ, et al: Sickle cell disease in children and adolescents: Diagnosis, guidelines for comprehensive care and care paths and protocols for management of acute and chronic complications. http://www.dshs.state.tx.us/newborn/pdf/sedonaoz.pdf.

47. Walker EM Jr, Mitchum EN, Rous SN, et al: Automated erythrocytopheresis for relief of priapism in sickle cell hemoglobinopathies. J Urol 1983;130:912-916.

48. Rifkind S, Waisman J, Thompson R, Goldfinger D: RBC exchange pheresis for priapism in sickle cell disease. JAMA 1979;242:2317-2318.

49. Serjeant GR, Serjeant BE, Thomas PW, et al: Human parvovirus infection in homozygous sickle cell disease. Lancet 1993;341:1237-1240.

50. Smith-Whitley K, Zhao H, Hodinka RL, et al: Epidemiology of human parvovirus B19 in children with sickle cell disease. Blood 2004;103:422-427.

51. Zimmerman SA, Davis JS, Schultz WH, Ware RE: Subclinical parvovirus B19 infection in children with sickle cell anemia. J Pediatr Hematol Oncol 2003;25:387-389.

52. Fevery J, Verwilghen R, Tan TG, De Groote J: Glucuronidation of bilirubin and the occurrence of pigment gallstones in patients with chronic haemolytic diseases. Eur J Clin Invest 1980;10:219-226.

53. Stephens CG, Scott RB: Cholelithiasis in sickle cell anemia: Surgical or medical management. Arch Intern Med 1980;140:648-651.

54. Ware R, Filston HC, Schultz WH, Kinney TR: Elective cholecystectomy in children with sickle hemoglobinopathies: Successful outcome using a preoperative transfusion regimen. Ann Surg 1988;208:17-22.

55. Suell MN, Horton TM, Dishop MK, et al: Outcomes for children with gallbladder abnormalities and sickle cell disease. J Pediatr 2004;145:617-621.

56. Al-Salem AH, Qaisruddin S: The significance of biliary sludge in children with sickle cell disease. Pediatr Surg Int 1998;13:14-16.

57. Walker TM, Serjeant GR: Biliary sludge in sickle cell disease. J Pediatr 1996;129:443-445.

58. Haberkern CM, Neumayr LD, Orringer EP, et al: Cholecystectomy in sickle cell anemia patients: Perioperative outcome of 364 cases from the National Preoperative Transfusion Study. Preoperative Transfusion in Sickle Cell Disease Study Group. Blood 1997;89:1533-1542.

CHAPTER 118

Neutropenia

Katherine A. Janeway

The risk of sepsis, fungal infection, and mucositis correlates inversely with the number of circulating neutrophils at any given time. However, because the normal homeostatic state is characterized by an abundance of functioning neutrophils (along with other circulating blood elements), problems involving immunosuppression generally do not arise until the neutrophil count is profoundly suppressed.

Once the immune system has been activated, neutrophils phagocytose bacteria opsonized by either immunoglobulin or complement and then kill bacteria both inside and outside the phagosome by means of enzymatic and oxidative mechanisms. Because neutrophils play such an important role in the killing of bacteria, neutropenic patients often have bacterial infections.

Neutropenia is defined as an absolute neutrophil count (ANC) of less than 1500 cells/μL, calculated as follows:

ANC = White blood cell count ×
(% Segmented neutrophils + % Band forms)

For example, when the white blood cell count is 5000 cells/μL with a differential of 10% segmented neutrophils and 5% band forms, the ANC is 750 cells/μL. Neutropenia can be classified as mild (1000 to 1500 cells/μL), moderate (500 to 1000 cells/μL), or severe (<500 cells/μL).

Neutropenia is caused by a number of different underlying conditions (Table 118-1). The epidemiology, presenting symptoms, risk of infection, clinical course, and management differ, depending on the cause. Congenital forms are the result of production problems in the bone marrow and generally result in lifelong neutropenia, with frequent, severe bacterial infections. Acquired causes of neutropenia are diverse but can be related to either production problems or increased clearance of neutrophils or their precursors. Primary autoimmune neutropenia and alloimmune neonatal neutropenia are typically transient; secondary autoimmune neutropenia, seen in the setting of chronic diseases such as lupus erythematosus, can be lifelong. A number of different drugs can cause neutropenia, usually related to interference with bone marrow production but also, in some cases, due to immune-mediated destruction of neutrophils. Neutropenia can be a complication of viral and bacterial infections because of both production problems and consumption or sequestration in active sites of infection. Any disorder affecting the bone marrow, such as bone marrow failure or bone marrow infiltration, can present with neutropenia, although pancytopenia is more common in these conditions.

CLINICAL PRESENTATION

Neutropenia can present as a laboratory abnormality in an asymptomatic or previously well child. A common clinical scenario is a well child who, in the course of evaluation for an acute illness or during preoperative screening, is found to be neutropenic. In the absence of a personal history of severe infections, and with no family history suggestive of neutropenia or related problems, most of these children have transient neutropenia and are not at increased risk of infection. Alternatively, neutropenia can present in the setting of increased susceptibility to severe, unusual, or frequent bacterial infections. In general, children with mild to moderate neutropenia have only a minimally increased risk of infection, whereas those with severe neutropenia have a significantly increased risk of infection. However, certain types of neutropenia (e.g., benign neutropenia of childhood) can present with profound neutropenia yet have little clinical consequence.

The most common types of infections seen in neutropenic patients are otitis media, skin infections (cellulitis, abscess), gingivitis, pneumonia, bacteremia, and sepsis.[1,2] The bacteria most commonly isolated are listed in Table 118-2. Fungal infections tend to occur when the neutropenia is of long duration or in the setting of concomitant use of corticosteroids or other immunosuppressive agents. In general, increased susceptibility to viral pathogens is not observed (unlike in patients with lymphocyte abnormalities). Beside infections, symptoms that suggest pathologic neutropenia include fever, oral ulcers or stomatitis, and delayed separation of the umbilical cord in infants.

CONGENITAL NEUTROPENIA

Severe Congenital Neutropenia (Kostmann Disease)

Severe congenital neutropenia, or Kostmann disease, is a rare disorder that results in severe neutropenia (ANC <200 cells/μL) that is present from birth. Inheritance can be autosomal recessive or autosomal dominant, and sporadic cases have been described. Patients with severe congenital neutropenia typically present in the first 6 months of life with frequent or severe bacterial infections. Bone marrow biopsy shows maturation arrest at the promyelocyte stage. Before the availability of granulocyte colony-stimulating factor (G-CSF) therapy, the median age of death was 3 years, most commonly due to sepsis or pneumonia.[3] G-CSF therapy corrects neutropenia and significantly reduces the incidence and duration of infectious complications in 90% of patients.[4,5] Bone marrow transplantation is indicated for those patients who do not respond to G-CSF and have matched sibling donors[6] or for those who develop myelodysplastic syndrome or acute myelogenous leukemia, life-threatening complications seen in roughly 10% of patients with severe congenital neutropenia.

Cyclic Neutropenia

Cyclic neutropenia is a rare disease in which 3- to 5-day episodes of severe neutropenia (typically with ANC <200 cells/μL) occur in regular and predictable 19- to 24-day

Table 118-1	Causes of Neutropenia

Congenital
  Severe congenital neutropenia (Kostmann disease)
  Cyclic neutropenia
  Shwachman-Diamond syndrome
  Reticular dysgenesis
  Myelokathexis and WHIM syndrome*

Immune mediated
  Alloimmune neonatal neutropenia
  Primary autoimmune neutropenia
  Secondary autoimmune neutropenia

Drug-induced neutropenia (see Table 118-3)

Infection-related neutropenia (see Table 118-4)

Sequestration (secondary to splenomegaly)

Bone marrow failure

Familial benign neutropenia

*WHIM, warts, hypogammaglobulinemia, infections, and myelokathexis.

Table 118-2	Bacterial Pathogens Isolated in Patients with Neutropenia

Staphylococcus aureus

Pseudomonas species

Escherichia coli and other enteric pathogens

Streptococcus pyogenes

Streptococcus pneumoniae

cycles. Fever, painful aphthous ulcers, pharyngitis, and cervical adenitis often occur during the neutropenic period. Risk of infection is increased during episodes of neutropenia in some patients but not in others. Most infections are mild and easily treated, but death secondary to overwhelming bacterial infection may occur. Therefore, fever and other symptoms must be taken seriously in such patients. Between periods of neutropenia, neutrophil counts are typically greater than 1500 cells/µL, and patients are asymptomatic. Inheritance is autosomal dominant, and penetrance is complete; severity is variable, however, so some affected family members may have near-normal ANCs and no increased risk of infection. Sporadic cases have also been reported.[7] Cyclic neutropenia is diagnosed by monitoring blood counts two to three times a week for 6 to 8 weeks and observing regular and characteristic oscillations in neutrophil counts. Bone marrow biopsy at the time of neutropenia shows maturation arrest or hypocellularity. Treatment with G-CSF often results in an increase in the ANC during neutrophil nadirs, a decrease in the duration of cycles from 21 to 14 days, and a significant decrease in the frequency and severity of infections.[4] Unlike patients with severe congenital neutropenia, those with cyclic neutropenia are not at increased risk for myelodysplasia or leukemia.

Shwachman-Diamond Syndrome

Shwachman-Diamond syndrome is characterized by the coexistence of neutropenia and exocrine pancreatic insufficiency. Other common features of the disease are failure to thrive early in life and short stature later on. Skeletal abnormalities are present in half of patients, although they may not appear until after 6 months of age. The disease is autosomal recessive and has an estimated incidence of 1 in 100,000 live births. The typical age at presentation is 1 year, and the male-female ratio is 1.8:1.[8] The neutrophil count in a single affected individual can vary (though not cyclically, as in cyclic neutropenia) and may even be normal at times. In one series of 80 patients with Shwachman-Diamond

syndrome, physicians reported a history of pneumonia in 24%, sepsis in 8%, abscess in 8%, and osteomyelitis in one patient (1.25%).[9] Pathogenic organisms are the same bacteria that are usually responsible for infection in neutropenic patients (see Table 118-2). Anemia and thrombocytopenia are seen in 40% and 30% of patients, respectively, and patients with Shwachman-Diamond syndrome have a significant risk of progression to myelodysplastic syndrome and acute myelogenous leukemia. G-CSF is effective in increasing neutrophil counts and decreasing infectious complications and can be used in patients with severe neutropenia or severe infection.[4]

Other Congenital Neutropenias

There are several other extremely rare congenital causes of neutropenia that deserve mention. In myelokathexis, bone marrow and sometimes circulating neutrophils are dysmorphic. Some patients with myelokathexis have WHIM (warts, hypogammaglobulinemia, infections, and myelokathexis) syndrome. WHIM is caused by a mutation in chemokine receptor 4 (CXRC4).[10] Patients with reticular dysgenesis have severe neutropenia and lymphopenia, and bone marrow evaluation shows decreased neutrophil precursors. Patients with reticular dysgenesis are treated with bone marrow transplantation because infections occur early in life and can be severe.

ACQUIRED NEUTROPENIA

Immune-Mediated Neutropenia

Primary Autoimmune Neutropenia

Primary autoimmune neutropenia usually occurs in young children between 5 and 15 months of age who develop autoantibodies against neutrophils. Patients who develop autoantibodies for some other reason, such as an underlying autoimmune disease or exposure to an infection or drug known to cause immune-mediated neutropenia, are excluded from this diagnosis. The estimated incidence of primary autoimmune neutropenia is 1 in 100,000, and it is most common in white children. Neutrophil counts are often less than 500 cells/µL but can be between 500 and 1500 cells/µL in up to 30% of children. Neutrophil counts may increase during periods of infection but return to less than 1500 cells/µL after the infection has resolved. The risk of infection is moderate. In a large series of patients with autoimmune neutropenia, 12% had severe bacterial infections, including sepsis, pneumonia, and meningitis.[11]

Diagnosis is made by the identification of antineutrophil antibodies. Testing for antineutrophil antibodies is difficult and should be performed by an experienced laboratory. Both granulocyte immunofluorescence and granulocyte agglutination testing should be performed. Antibodies are not always identified on initial testing, and the results of antibody testing should be interpreted in consultation with a specialist. Repeated testing may be required to make the diagnosis, and the lack of positive antibody testing does not exclude the diagnosis.[2] Bone marrow biopsy, which is not necessary if antibodies are identified, shows hypercellularity and a decreased number of mature myeloid cells, but without maturation arrest.

Almost all patients undergo spontaneous remission. Typically, antineutrophil antibodies disappear and neutrophil counts return to normal within 7 to 24 months of diagnosis. Because neutropenia is transient and the infection risk is only moderate, specific treatment of neutropenia is not required. When treatment of neutropenia is required for severe infection or surgery, G-CSF,[12] steroids, and intravenous immunoglobulin (IVIG) have all been used with moderate success. Prophylaxis with trimethoprim-sulfamethoxazole has been shown to decrease the frequency of infections without significant side effects in a small number of patients.[11,13]

Alloimmune Neonatal Neutropenia

Alloimmune neonatal neutropenia, similar to Rh disease in the newborn, is caused by transplacental passage of maternal immunoglobulin G antibodies directed against fetal cells (neutrophils) bearing paternally derived antigens. This causes an immune-mediated neutropenia that is present at birth. Like Rh disease, alloimmune neonatal neutropenia usually affects the children of multiparous women, likely because maternal exposure to paternal neutrophil antigens occurs during prior pregnancy or childbirth. Neutropenia is typically severe and resolves when maternal antibodies cease to be present in the child's serum, usually between 3 and 28 weeks of life. Risk of infection is increased, but infections tend to be mild, with the skin being affected most commonly; however, more severe infections such as pneumonia have been reported.[14] Delayed separation of the umbilical cord has been described.[15] Diagnosis is made either clinically or by identifying antineutrophil antibodies in both the mother and the infant. As with autoimmune neutropenia, testing for antineutrophil antibodies is difficult and may not yield a positive result, even when antibodies are present. Likewise, bone marrow biopsy shows a hypercellular marrow with a decreased number of neutrophils, suggestive of premature destruction of mature forms rather than bone marrow failure. Treatment with G-CSF,[15] steroids, or IVIG should be reserved for neutropenic patients with infections that are not responsive to antimicrobial therapy.

Secondary Autoimmune Neutropenia

Autoimmune neutropenia can be seen in association with a number of rheumatologic conditions, including systemic lupus erythematous, Sjögren syndrome, and scleroderma; in the setting of malignancy; in certain immunodeficiency states, such as common variable immunodeficiency; and as a consequence of infections and drugs. In general, treatment of the underlying condition or removal of the offending agent (in the case of drug-induced neutropenia) is the most effective means of correcting secondary neutropenia.

Drug-Induced Neutropenia

Drug-induced neutropenia typically occurs 1 to 2 weeks after initiation of the offending agent. Table 118-3 lists commonly used drugs that reportedly cause neutropenia or are associated with a relatively high risk of inducing neutropenia; it is not a comprehensive list of all drugs in which neutropenia is an observed side effect. Drug-induced neutropenia can be mild or severe. Although the precise mechanisms of drug-induced neutropenia are not well understood, in general, the underlying pathophysiology is suppression of myeloid precursor formation in the bone marrow. A direct toxic effect is suspected in the case of sulfasalazine, with neutropenia being more likely in patients with reduced hepatic acetylation activity.[16] In the case of antithyroid agents, antineutrophil antibodies are frequently present, suggesting an immune-mediated mechanism.[17] Symptoms of drug-induced neutropenia are similar to those of neutropenia in general and include fever, mouth sores, and an increased risk of infection. Drug-induced neutropenia should be treated with removal of the offending agent. The neutropenia usually resolves 1 to 2 weeks after the drug is discontinued but can be prolonged in some cases. Deaths related to drug-induced neutropenia, usually due to infection, have been reported.[18]

Neutropenia Secondary to Infection

A number of childhood infections have been reported to result in neutropenia (Table 118-4), although the precise mechanisms are not well characterized. Suggested mechanisms include direct infection of neutrophil precursors or other means of increased destruction of myeloid forms. Parvovirus B19, known for interrupting red cell production in the marrow by replication in (and destruction of) erythrocytic precursors, can also cause a mild neutropenia 10 to 14 days after infection.[19,20] Epstein-Barr virus infection is often associated with mild neutropenia. Antineutrophil antibodies are often present in Epstein-Barr–associated neutropenia, suggesting an immune-mediated mechanism.[21] There are several case reports in the literature of severe neutropenia occurring in conjunction with hepatitis viruses.[22] Infection with human immunodeficiency virus (HIV) has been associated with perturbations in all three hematologic cell lines, with neutropenia being present in as many as 8% of affected patients.[23] Importantly, HIV-related neutropenia is associated with an increase in the frequency and severity of bacterial infections, and treatment with G-CSF can decrease the infection risk.[23] Measles, human herpesvirus 6, varicella, rubella, and influenza have all been reported to cause mild to moderate transient neutropenia in children.[24-27] Bacterial infections associated with neutropenia include typhoid fever, tularemia, and brucellosis.[28-30] Sepsis, particularly in neonates, is frequently complicated by neutropenia. Certain rickettsial diseases, including human granulocytic ehrlichiosis, are known to cause leukopenia and neutropenia, often in association with thrombocytopenia.[31]

DIFFERENTIAL DIAGNOSIS

Bone marrow failure syndromes, including aplastic anemia and Fanconi anemia, and diseases involving bone marrow infiltration, such as malignancy or Gaucher disease,

Table 118-3 Drugs Causing Neutropenia

Drug Class	Specific Agent	Comments
Antimicrobial	Macrolides Trimethoprim- sulfamethoxazole β-Lactams Acyclovir Dapsone	
Antiplatelet	Dipyridamole Ticlopidine	Neutropenia occurs in 0.9% of users[31]
Antiarrhythmic	Digoxin Propranolol Procainamide	Especially sustained-release formulations[33]
Antithyroid	Propylthiouracil Methimazole	Neutropenia usually occurs during first 3 mo of use; seen in 0.5% of users[34]; autoimmune mechanism
Anti-inflammatory	Sulfasalazine Indomethacin Ibuprofen	Neutropenia occurs in <0.1% of users, associated with slow acetylation[16]
Antipsychotic	Clozapine	Neutropenia occurs in 1%-2% of users[35]
Antihistamine	Cimetidine Ranitidine	Rare occurrence of severe neutropenia
Antiepileptic	Phenytoin Carbamazepine	
Miscellaneous	Furosemide	

Table 118-4 Infections Causing Neutropenia

Infectious Agent	Comment
Virus	
Parvovirus B19	Usually mild; rare reports of severe neutropenia
Epstein-Barr virus	Antineutrophil antibodies common
Cytomegalovirus	Rarely causes neutropenia
Human immunodeficiency virus (HIV)	Treatment with G-CSF decreases infection
Measles	Neutropenia usually follows onset of rash
Human herpesvirus 6	Neutropenia occurs with rash, often associated with thrombocytopenia
Hepatitis viruses	Rarely cause severe neutropenia
Varicella	Neutropenia occurs on first few days of rash
Rubella	
Bacteria	
Sepsis due to any cause	Most common in neonates
Tularemia	
Brucellosis	Mild neutropenia, often with concurrent anemia, thrombocytopenia, or both[30]
Salmonella typhi	Neutropenia in a small percentage; mediated by hemophagocytosis
Human granulocytic ehrlichiosis	Neutropenia common

G-CSF, granulocyte colony-stimulating factor.

can initially present with neutropenia. Therefore, isolated neutropenia does not rule out global bone marrow dysfunction. Neutropenia is a complication of several metabolic diseases, particularly glycogen storage disease type IB. Pearson syndrome, a rare disorder in which there is bone marrow failure (typically anemia) and exocrine pancreatic insufficiency, should be considered whenever Shwachman-Diamond syndrome is diagnosed. In some cases, it is not possible to identify the underlying cause of a patient's neutropenia. The term *chronic benign neutropenia* has been used to describe neutropenia with an unclear cause in children with no history of severe or unusual infections.

DIAGNOSIS AND EVALUATION

When evaluating a patient with neutropenia, the history should include questions about a personal history of fevers, mouth sores, and infections, as well as a thorough family history eliciting the presence of any blood disorders and untimely childhood deaths due to infection. Attention should also be paid to medications being taken both presently and in the recent past. The physical examination should take particular note of oral lesions, lymph nodes, and subtle sites of infection. The laboratory evaluation varies, depending on the most likely cause. If immune mechanisms are suspected, the presence of antineutrophil antibodies should be evaluated, although false-negative results are common. Bone marrow aspiration and biopsy should be obtained whenever more than one hematologic cell line is decreased, with the objective of eliminating more sinister diagnoses such as aplastic anemia, leukemia, and myelodysplasia. If neutropenia is associated with a recent infection, tests for entities known to be associated with that infection are warranted.

Given the low risk of serious infection in neutropenic children without a serious illness or a positive personal or family history, it is appropriate to monitor complete blood counts for up to 1 month before referral to a pediatric hematologist,[32] as long as the remainder of the complete blood count is normal and there is no suspicion (by history, physical examination, or laboratory evaluation) of leukemia or aplastic anemia. Complete blood counts should be checked at least weekly to evaluate for cyclic neutropenia and promptly identify the development of abnormalities in other cell lines.

CONSULTATION

Consultation with a pediatric hematologist is indicated whenever there is a personal or family history of severe or frequent infections, when neutropenia is persistent, or when abnormalities in other cell lines are present in the complete blood count.

Infectious disease specialists may assist with the management of infections in neutropenic patients, including guiding the choice of empirical therapy and providing advice when unusual organisms are identified.

TREATMENT AND ADMISSION CRITERIA

Most previously healthy children who present with neutropenia in the absence of a significant illness or a suggestive personal or family history do not have an underlying neutrophil abnormality and will improve without intervention. Neutropenia in children without an underlying disorder can be mild, moderate, or severe; even so, in most of these children, neutrophil counts return to normal, usually within 30 days. Infections are uncommon in this group of children unless neutropenia persists.

Any patient with severe neutropenia and fever should be evaluated for bacterial infection, treated with broad-spectrum antibiotics, and admitted to the hospital. The management of children with neutropenia who present with fever is consistent regardless of the cause (see Chapter 124). Neutropenia in the absence of fever does not require admission to the hospital. Digital rectal examination and any other manipulation of the rectum, such as rectal temperatures and suppositories, should be avoided in neutropenic children because of the risk of promoting gram-negative sepsis.

In many patients with congenital disorders, neutropenia can be corrected with recombinant G-CSF, which may have a role in treating infections in neutropenic patients regardless of the cause. In general, G-CSF therapy should not be used simply to correct the ANC; it should be reserved for patients who have had severe or recurrent bacterial infections as a result of neutropenia.

IN A NUTSHELL

- Neutropenia is defined as an ANC less than 1500 cells/μL. It is classified as mild (1000 to 1500 cells/μL), moderate (500 to 1000 cells/μL), or severe (<500 cells/μL).
- The frequency and severity of infections in neutropenic patients depend on the degree of neutropenia and the underlying cause. Most infections seen in the setting of neutropenia are bacterial (otitis, cellulitis, gingivitis, pneumonia, bacteremia, sepsis). Fungal infections are a greater concern when the neutropenia is prolonged.
- Congenital neutropenias present with lifelong neutropenia complicated by more frequent and severe infections. In many congenital disorders, neutropenia can be corrected with G-CSF. Stem cell transplantation can be curative for congenital neutropenia.
- Immune-mediated causes of neutropenia, with the exception of those secondary to autoimmune disorders, are typically transient.
- All children with severe neutropenia and fever warrant a thorough evaluation and empirical antibiotic therapy tailored to the most likely infection and pathogen.
- Neutropenic children without a significant infectious illness, a worrisome personal or family history, or additional laboratory abnormalities can be monitored with frequent complete blood counts.
- A pediatric hematologist should be consulted for patients with known neutrophil disorders, neutropenia in the setting of a significant illness, prolonged neutropenia, and neutropenia accompanied by anemia or thrombocytopenia.

ON THE HORIZON

- Scientists are moving toward a better understanding of genetic mutations that cause severe congenital neutropenia, cyclic neutropenia, and Shwachman-Diamond syndrome.
- Investigations are under way into the use of pegylated G-CSF, a long-acting formulation for the treatment of non-chemotherapy-related neutropenia.

SUGGESTED READING

Boxer L: Neutrophil abnormalities. Pediatr Rev 2003;24:52.

Dinauer MC: The phagocyte system and disorders of granulopoiesis and granulocyte function. In Nathan DG, Orkin SH, Ginsburg D, Look AT (eds): Hematology of Infancy and Childhood. Philadelphia, WB Saunders, 2003, pp 923-1010.

Palmblad JE, Von Dem Borne AE: Idiopathic, immune, infectious and idiosyncratic neutropenias. Semin Hematol 2002;39:113.

REFERENCES

1. Howard MW, Strauss RG, Johnson RB: Infections in patients with neutropenia. Am J Dis Child 1977;131:788.

2. Dinauer MC: The phagocyte system and disorders of granulopoiesis and granulocyte function. In Nathan DG, Orkin SH, Ginsburg D, Look AT (eds): Hematology of Infancy and Childhood. Philadelphia, WB Saunders, 2003, pp 923-1010.

3. Alter BP, D'Andrea AD: Inherited bone marrow failure syndromes. In Handin RI, Lux SE, Stossel TP (eds): Blood Principles and Practice of Hematology. Philadelphia, Lippincott Williams & Wilkins, 2003, pp 251-253.

4. Dale DC, Bonilla MA, Davis MW, et al: A randomized controlled phase III trial of recombinant human granulocyte colony-stimulating factor (filgrastim) for treatment of severe chronic neutropenia. Blood 1993;81:2496.

5. Dale DC, Cottle TE, Fier CJ, et al: Severe chronic neutropenia: Treatment and follow-up of patients in the severe chronic neutropenia international registry. Am J Hematol 2003;72:82.

6. Zeidler C, Welte K, Barak Y, et al: Stem cell transplantation in patients with severe congenital neutropenia without evidence of leukemic transformation. Blood 2000;95:1195.

7. Dale DC, Bolyard AA, Aprikyan A: Cyclic neutropenia. Semin Hematol 2002;39:89.

8. Smith OP: Shwachman-Diamond syndrome. Semin Hematol 2002;39:95.

9. Ginzberg H, Shin J, Ellis L, et al: Shwachman syndrome: Phenotypic manifestations of sibling sets and isolated cases in a large patient cohort are similar. J Pediatr 1999;135:81.

10. Paolo A, Hernandez RJ, Gorlin JN, et al: Mutations in the chemokine receptor gene CXCR4 are associated with WHIM syndrome, a combined immunodeficiency disease. Nat Genet 2003;34:70.

11. Bux J, Behrens G, Welte K: Diagnosis and clinical course of autoimmune neutropenia in infancy: Analysis of 240 cases. Blood 1998;91:181.

12. Smith MA, Smith JG: The use of granulocyte colony-stimulating factor for treatment of autoimmune neutropenia. Curr Opin Hematol 2001;8:165.

13. Kobayashi M, Sato T, Kawaguchi H, et al: Efficacy of prophylactic use of trimethoprim-sulfamethoxazole in autoimmune neutropenia in infancy. J Pediatr Hematol Oncol 2003;25:553.

14. Bux J, Chapman J: Report on the second international granulocyte serology workshop. Transfusion 1997;37:977.

15. Gilmore MM, Stroncek DF, Korones DN: Treatment of alloimmune neonatal neutropenia with granulocyte colony-stimulating factor. J Pediatr 1994;125:948.

16. Wadelius M, Sternberg E, Wiholm B: Polymorphisms of NAT2 in relation to sulphasalazine-induced agranulocytosis. Pharmacogenetics 2000;10:35.

17. Cooper DS: Antithyroid drugs. N Engl J Med 1984;311:1353.

18. van der Klauw MM, Wilson JHP, Stricker BHC: Drug-associated agranulocytosis: 20 years of reporting in the Netherlands (1974-1994). Am J Hematol 1998;57:206.

19. Mustafa MM, McClain KL: Diverse hematologic effects of parvovirus B19 infection. Pediatr Clin North Am 1996;43:809.

20. Barlow GD, McKendrick MW: Parvovirus B19 causing leucopenia and neutropenia in a healthy adult. J Infect 2000;40:192.

21. Schooley RT, Denson P, Harmon D, et al: Antineutrophil antibodies in infectious mononucleosis. Am J Med 1984;76:85.

22. Nagaraju M, Weitzman S, Baumann G: Viral hepatitis and agranulocytosis. Am J Dig Dis 1973;18:247.

23. Zon LI, Groopman JE: Hematologic manifestations of the human immune deficiency virus. Semin Hematol 1988;25:208.

24. Benjamin B, Ward SM: Leukocyte response to measles. Am J Dis Child 1932;44:921.

25. Hashimoto H, Maruyama H, Fujimoto K, et al: Hematologic findings associated with thrombocytopenia during the acute phase of exanthem subitum confirmed by primary human herpesvirus-6 infection. J Pediatr Hematol Oncol 2002;24:211.

26. Holbrook AA: The blood picture in chickenpox. Arch Intern Med 1941;68:294.

27. Lewis DE, Gilbert BE, Knight V: Influenza virus infection induces functional alterations in peripheral blood lymphocytes. J Immunol 1986;12:3777.

28. Mallouh AA, Rahman S: White blood cells and bone marrow in typhoid fever. Pediatr Infect Dis J 1987;6:527.

29. Pullen RL, Stuart BM: Tularemia. JAMA 1943;129:495.

30. Al-Eissa YA, Assuhaimi SA, Al-Fawaz I, et al: Pancytopenia in children with brucellosis: Clinical manifestations and bone marrow findings. Acta Hematol 1998;89:132.

31. Fritz CL, Glaser CA: Ehrlichiosis. Infect Dis Clin North Am 1998;12:123.

32. Alario AJ, O'Shea JS: Risk of infectious complications in well-appearing children with transient neutropenia. Am J Dis Child 1989;143:973.

33. Ellrodt AG, Murata GH, Riedinger MS, et al: Severe neutropenia associated with sustained-release procainamide. Ann Intern Med 1984;100:197.

34. International Agranulocytosis and Aplastic Anemia Society: Risk of agranulocytosis and aplastic anaemia in relation to use of antithyroid drugs. BMJ 1988;297:262.

35. Alvir JMJ, Lieberman JA, Safferman AZ, et al: Clozapine-induced agranulocytosis. N Engl J Med 1993;329:162.

CHAPTER 119

Thrombocytopenia

Sam Volchenboum

Thrombocytopenia, defined as an absolute platelet count less than 150,000/mm³, is a common cause of bleeding in pediatric patients. A low platelet count can be the result of increased platelet destruction, reduced production, consumption, or sequestration (Table 119-1). This chapter focuses on the major causes of thrombocytopenia and their evaluation and management.

CLINICAL PRESENTATION

Formation of a platelet plug is vital to hemostasis. Regardless of the cause, when platelet numbers are decreased, there can be petechiae, bruising, or bleeding. The body has a remarkable capacity to maintain hemostasis despite low platelet numbers, so symptoms may not become evident until the platelet count is quite low—usually below 50,000/mm³. Patients with moderately decreased platelet counts may be asymptomatic, with the thrombocytopenia being noted incidentally.

Immune-Mediated Thrombocytopenia

Thrombocytopenic Purpura

Presentation and Evaluation

The incidence of idiopathic thrombocytopenic purpura (ITP) in children is about 50 per million per year. A common presentation is an otherwise healthy child with a sudden onset of widespread petechiae or bruising, or both. The typical story often includes a recent viral illness or administration of a live vaccine. A complete blood count demonstrates a normal number of white blood cells and a relatively normal hematocrit. The platelet count is typically extremely low, often less than 10,000/mm³ and frequently as low as 1000/mm³. Although the precise trigger remains unclear, ITP is generally thought to be caused by antiplatelet antibodies, which lead to a drastically shortened platelet survival time by opsonization and enhanced clearance.

For more than 75% of pediatric patients, ITP is a disease with an abrupt onset and a quick and permanent resolution. In the remaining 25% of cases, however, the disease becomes chronic, defined as persistence of thrombocytopenia for 6 months or longer, with or without treatment. The incidence of protracted ITP increases with age and is highest in adolescents.

ITP most commonly affects children between 2 and 6 years of age, an age distribution similar to that of acute leukemia, which may also be present in a young patient with widespread bruising as a result of thrombocytopenia. In the vast majority of cases, the history, physical examination, and review of the complete blood count and peripheral blood smear are all that is required to differentiate ITP from acute leukemia or aplastic anemia (Table 119-2).

In the absence of other complicating factors or causes, the diagnosis of ITP can be based on these findings, and bone marrow examination is not usually necessary. However, one also needs to consider other causes of "secondary immune thrombocytopenia," including drugs, infections, malignancy, and autoimmune disorders (Table 119-3). Systemic lupus erythematosus, rheumatoid arthritis, and human immunodeficiency virus infection, as well as other inflammatory diseases, must be considered while working up children presenting with thrombocytopenia, especially teenagers. Any aberrations in the history, physical examination, or laboratory findings warrant a bone marrow examination to rule out acute leukemia or aplastic anemia as a cause of thrombocytopenia, especially if steroids are being considered as treatment.

Treatment

Despite extremely low platelet counts, children with ITP have less than a 1% incidence of intracranial hemorrhage, and these cases are often complicated by trauma or the use of antiplatelet medications such as aspirin.[1-3] Many physicians opt for close observation alone for a child with ITP who is not actively bleeding, although many care providers and families of patients with ITP feel much more comfortable treating the thrombocytopenia rather than waiting for spontaneous resolution. Therapies may raise the platelet count, but they do not shorten the duration of the disease state. In general, physicians tend to treat ITP under the following circumstances: when the patient has active bleeding, when the platelet count is below 10,000/mm³, or when the patient is prone to trauma (e.g., toddlers).

Treatment of ITP includes corticosteroids, intravenous immunoglobulin (IVIG), anti-Rh₀D therapy (WinRho), rituximab (anti-CD20 monoclonal antibody treatment), and splenectomy (Table 119-4). Steroids are the most cost-effective therapy and are easiest to administer. Before steroids are given, however, the clinician must make absolutely certain that the child does not have leukemia because steroids can induce temporary remission in acute lymphoblastic leukemia and thus make the ultimate diagnosis and treatment more difficult. For ITP, a short course of steroids usually causes a rise in the platelet count in a few days, which is thought to mainly be a result of interference with splenic uptake of antibody-coated platelets. In most children steroids can be tapered quickly, and most will not relapse. In some patients, however, another course of steroids or a slower taper may be needed.

The treatment that results in the most rapid rise in the platelet count is IVIG,[4] which is very expensive and generally involves hospitalizing the patient for the 8- to 12-hour infusion. In addition, many children experience headaches after the infusion, probably related to the increased protein load, and this often leads to unnecessary imaging studies to evaluate for possible intracranial hemorrhage.

The use of anti-Rh$_0$D has increasingly gained popularity as a treatment option for ITP, but it is useful only in patients with an Rh-positive blood type. Administration of anti-Rh$_0$D causes a rise in platelet count with a predictable decline in hemoglobin, perhaps related to saturation of the reticuloendothelial system by opsonized red blood cells, although the precise mechanism remains unknown. Very rarely, a patient with ITP has a concomitant immune-mediated hemolytic anemia at presentation, a constellation of autoimmune processes known as "Evans syndrome." In this setting, addition of more anti–red blood cell antibody to the system would exacerbate the hemolytic anemia. Therefore, before using anti-Rh$_0$D the clinician must ensure a negative Coombs test (direct and indirect antiglobulin tests).

After any of these treatments, the development of new petechiae/purpura should slow, and the platelet count typically rises over the next several days. In general, a platelet count check is recommended in 2 to 3 days and then again in 1 week if stable.

An emerging therapy for chronic ITP (defined as persistence of thrombocytopenia for at least 6 months) is rituximab, a monoclonal antibody that targets plasma cells, the source of the antiplatelet antibodies causative of ITP. Rituximab has been used successfully in adults with ITP,[5,6] and there are case reports of its use in children.[7] The most common side effects are mainly fevers, chills, rigors, hypotension, and bronchospasm. Fortunately, these adverse reactions are usually mild. Importantly, treatment with rituximab will cause hypogammaglobulinemia that can last up to a year or more. Therefore, fevers during this period may require evaluation and prophylactic antibiotics and IVIG. Despite these drawbacks, rituximab is becoming a valuable tool in the treatment of chronic refractory ITP.

In addition to the aforementioned treatment modalities, there are agents that help prevent bleeding in patients with ITP. ε-Aminocaproic acid (Amicar) acts as an inhibitor of fibrinolysis. This medication is often useful as adjuvant therapy in a patient with wet purpura or epistaxis because it

---

Table 119–1 Partial Differential Diagnosis for Thrombocytopenia

Increased Platelet Destruction
Immune thrombocytopenia
  Idiopathic thrombocytopenic purpura (ITP)
  Drug induced
  Neonatal alloimmune thrombocytopenia (NAIT)
  Neonatal ITP (secondary to maternal ITP)
  Systemic lupus erythematosus (SLE)
  Evans syndrome (ITP with another immune-mediated cytopenia)
Nonimmune thrombocytopenia
  Hemolytic uremic syndrome (HUS)
  Thrombotic thrombocytopenic purpura (TTP)
  Kasabach-Merritt syndrome (KMS)
  Drug induced

Decreased Platelet Production
Decreased bone marrow activity
  Drug induced
  Genetic/inherited (Fanconi anemia, thrombocytopenia with absent radii)
  Vitamin B$_{12}$/folate deficiency
  Viral infections
  Aplastic anemia
  Inborn errors of metabolism
Marrow infiltration
  Leukemia and other malignancies
  Storage diseases

Table 119–3 Differential Diagnosis of Thrombocytopenia

Class	Examples
Drugs	Alcohol, heparin, quinine, sulfonamides
Infection	Parvovirus, HIV, rubella, infectious mononucleosis
Malignancy/bone marrow failure	Leukemia, myelodysplasia, aplastic anemia
Pseudothrombocytopenia	Clumping in tube because of EDTA
Vasculitis	TTP/HUS, DIC
Autoimmune	SLE
Other	Pregnancy, hypersplenism secondary to chronic liver disease

DIC, disseminated intravascular coagulation; EDTA, ethylenediaminetetraacetic acid; HIV, human immunodeficiency virus; HUS, hemolytic uremic syndrome; SLE, systemic lupus erythematosus; TTP, thrombotic thrombocytopenic purpura.

Table 119–2 Differentiating between Idiopathic Thrombocytopenic Purpura and Leukemia

	ITP	Leukemia
Review of systems	Otherwise healthy	History of fevers, swollen glands, bone or joint pain, other systemic complaints
Physical examination	Findings limited to petechiae, purpura, and epistaxis	Splenomegaly, hepatomegaly, lymphadenopathy
Complete blood count	Extremely low platelets with normal red and white cell count	Multiple cell lines may be decreased
Blood smear	Paucity of platelets, otherwise normal	Blast forms

Table 119-4 Treatment Options for Idiopathic Thrombocytopenic Purpura

Treatment	Dosage	Pros	Cons
Observation	N/A	Simple	Very small but real incidence of life-threatening bleeding
Steroids	Initially 1-2 mg/kg/day IV/PO, then tapered as platelet count dictates	Inexpensive Easy to administer Fairly rapid response (usually within a week)	Must exclude leukemia first Can cause mood changes acutely and serious side effects when used chronically
IVIG	1-2 g/kg IV; may be repeated q3-4 wk	Very effective Quick response (usually days)	Expensive May require hospital stay May cause headaches Is a blood product
Anti-Rh$_0$D (WinRho)	50-100 µg/kg IV; may be repeated q3-4 wk	Effective Low incidence of side effects Lower incidence of headaches than with IVIG	More expensive than steroids Can cause headaches Patient must be Rh positive
Splenectomy	N/A	Can be curative in chronic refractory patients	Splenectomized patients have a risk for overwhelming sepsis with encapsulated organisms
Rituximab (anti-CD20)	Typically a course of 4 weekly doses	Can be effective for chronic or refractory ITP Low side effect profile	Experimental Expensive Allergic reactions possible Profound depletion of B cells, often requiring subsequent IVIG for agammaglobulinemia
Chemotherapy	Varies	May work for refractory disease	Toxic side effects

IVIG, intravenous immunoglobulin.

can help prevent bleeding until the platelet count rises. Before aminocaproic acid is given, the patient's urine must be examined because hematuria and the risk for urinary obstruction by blood clots in the setting of inhibition of fibrinolysis are considered contraindications to the use of ε-aminocaproic acid.

In the face of any immune-mediated thrombocytopenia, platelet transfusions will raise the count only briefly at best and are reserved for children with acute life- or limb-threatening bleeding. Similarly, splenectomy is generally reserved as an option of "last resort" for chronic ITP after other therapies aimed at interrupting immune destruction of platelets have been exhausted. Although removing the spleen does little to affect the generation of antiplatelet antibodies, the procedure removes the main site of platelet destruction in ITP and often results in a rise in platelet counts, which can improve quality of life significantly.

It is important to keep in mind that patients will occasionally "relapse" after first-line therapy for ITP. Such relapses should not be confused with chronic ITP, which is a prolonged, protracted disease course. Acute ITP is self-limited and lasts a few weeks to a few months. Children with acute ITP may require several courses of therapy to maintain their platelet counts until the disease subsides. This is in contrast to patients with chronic ITP, who will often still respond to standard therapies for ITP, but with only a transient and short-lived response. Their disease does not subside spontaneously and may require more aggressive intervention (rituximab, splenectomy).

Children with platelet counts less than 50,000/mm^3 should refrain from any high-impact activities, including contact sports and situations in which they are at risk for falls and injuries. The lower limit is controversial, but most physicians let their patients participate in sports once their platelet count reaches 50,000/mm^3 and certainly when it is above 100,000/mm^3. Although many families feel reassured by spending a night or two in the hospital, the artificial environment (and hard floors) of the inpatient unit may actually predispose toddlers to falls or accidents. Some centers recommend helmets for children between the ages of 1 and 5.

Neonatal Thrombocytopenia

Presentation and Evaluation

Neonatal immune thrombocytopenia is a relatively common, potentially devastating disorder that necessitates prompt intervention once diagnosed. Unlike older children with very low platelet counts who are at only small risk of intracranial bleeding, the incidence of intracranial hemorrhage in neonates with thrombocytopenia is higher than 20%.[8] Therefore, if diagnosed in utero, cesarean section is often recommended to avoid head trauma during vaginal delivery. A fetus can be exposed to antiplatelet antibodies in two main ways. First, a mother with ITP can pass her antiplatelet antibodies to her child, as evidenced by low platelet counts in both the mother and baby. This disease is usually self-limited, and the child should respond to the same therapies as described earlier for ITP, mainly IVIG and steroids. Serial platelet counts need to be obtained to document a durable response to therapy.

A more serious disorder occurs when the mother's immune system recognizes paternal antigens on fetal platelets and makes immunoglobulin G (IgG) that crosses the placenta and binds to fetal platelets, thereby hastening their destruction. This disorder is known as neonatal alloimmune thrombocytopenia (NAIT). It is similar to Rh disease of the newborn, but unlike Rh disease, antigenic exposure can occur early in gestation and lead to an affected offspring with the first pregnancy. Generalized petechiae can develop within minutes of birth. Intracranial hemorrhage can occur, sometimes in utero, and result in fetal demise. Because future pregnancies are clearly at risk, high-risk obstetric care for the affected mother is essential.

The diagnosis of NAIT can often be made by carefully considering the history, physical examination, and laboratory findings. Unlike neonatal ITP secondary to maternal ITP, the mother's platelet count should be normal in NAIT. Furthermore, the baby should have no evidence of other systemic disease. If a bone marrow study is performed, there should be increased numbers of megakaryocytes, as would be expected when the cause is increased destruction of platelets.

Treatment

As mentioned, thrombocytopenia secondary to maternal ITP is self-limited and usually requires no therapy. However, NAIT requires immediate treatment. The ideal treatment is transfusion of platelets known to not exhibit the offending antigen on their surface. Fortunately, a source of these antigen-negative platelets exists in the mother of the child. Importantly, the mother's platelets should be washed before transfusion (to remove plasma containing maternal antibodies) and irradiated (to eliminate the risk for transfusion-associated graft-versus-host disease). If maternal platelets are not available, the blood bank may be able to obtain platelets lacking the platelet antibody. Random donor platelets may be used, but the benefit will probably be very short lived, and they should be reserved for cases of life- or limb-threatening bleeding. Intravenous gamma globulin and steroids are good options to maintain adequate platelet counts until resolution of the process (typically several weeks). Additionally, a head ultrasound should be performed during the acute phase of the illness to evaluate for intracranial hemorrhage. Finally, once a baby is found to have NAIT, every effort should be made to determine the platelet genotypes of the mother and father because this will be important both for verifying the diagnosis of NAIT and for genetic counseling and obstetric care in future pregnancies.

Thrombocytopenia Secondary to Consumption

Several different states can cause thrombocytopenia by removing platelets from the circulating pool, including disseminated intravascular coagulation (DIC), hemolytic uremic syndrome (HUS), thrombotic thrombocytopenic purpura (TTP), and Kasabach-Merritt syndrome (KMS).

Disseminated Intravascular Coagulation

DIC is generally a consequence of overwhelming sepsis or other systemic illness that results in an imbalance between the clot promotion and clot lysis systems in the body. Its presence always represents another underlying problem (infection, malignancy, major trauma). Activation of the coagulation system leads to a depletion of clotting factors, and platelets are consumed and activated by both thrombin and the underlying process. Screening tests for DIC may include the prothrombin time (PT), partial thromboplastin time (PTT), platelet count, fibrinogen level, and D-dimer level. In DIC, the PT and PTT are usually high, and the platelet count and fibrinogen level are usually low. Treatment of DIC-induced thrombocytopenia is supportive while treating the underlying disease process. It may be helpful to replace clotting factors with fresh frozen plasma and cryoprecipitate or replace platelets, but the consumptive process will continue until the underlying problem is corrected. In addition, there is a risk for volume overload because isotonic products such as fresh frozen plasma are infused in significant amounts.

Hemolytic Uremic Syndrome.

Thrombocytopenia in HUS occurs as a result of platelet aggregates becoming trapped in small vessels. Please see Chapter 111 for details.

Thrombotic Thrombocytopenic Purpura

TTP is more uncommon than HUS in children, has a much higher mortality rate, and can have a remitting/relapsing course. As with HUS, a microangiopathic hemolytic anemia is seen, but unlike HUS, there is no association with microorganisms. Instead, because of the production of specific antibodies, there is no cleavage of high-molecular-weight von Willebrand complexes circulating in the blood, which in turn cause platelet clumping and red blood cell destruction. Treatment of TTP is aggressive daily exchange plasmapheresis with cryoprecipitate-poor plasma. As with HUS, platelet transfusions should be used only in patients with life-threatening bleeding because they will probably worsen the disease.

Kasabach-Merritt Syndrome

KMS, characterized by consumptive coagulopathy and thrombocytopenia, can develop in infants with large vascular tumors. This condition is rare (affecting only 0.3% of infants with hemangiomas) but has a very high mortality rate (30% to 40%). Although the precise mechanism is not known, KMS is thought to arise secondary to platelet trapping by the vascular endothelium. This causes platelet activation and subsequent consumption of clotting factors. The profound thrombocytopenia (sometimes less than 20,000/mm^3) along with the coagulopathy leads to a very high risk for devastating bleeding. Therapy for KMS is aimed first at correcting the bleeding diathesis, which may involve product replacement or systemic treatment with steroids, interferon alfa, or vincristine. Once the patient is stabilized, the focus of treatment can be shifted to management of the lesion. Surgical therapy can be attempted for small cutaneous lesions, but this is not always feasible. Other local therapies include vascular embolization, laser therapy, and radiotherapy.

Hypersplenism

Many conditions (liver disease, infection, malignancy) are associated with an enlarged spleen. As the spleen enlarges, there is greater opportunity for blood cells to be damaged and for platelets to be sequestered. This is purely a physical phenomenon, and splenectomy is often helpful in cases of protracted, chronic thrombocytopenia. Of course, removing the spleen of a young patient carries a significant risk, especially infection with encapsulated organisms. Therefore, splenectomy is only rarely offered as a primary treatment option.

Thrombocytopenia Caused by Decreased Production

Decreased bone marrow production of platelets is a predictable iatrogenic consequence of treatment with cytotoxic drugs that suppress hematopoiesis of all bone marrow elements. In addition to many chemotherapeutic agents, other drugs that can cause thrombocytopenia include ibuprofen, ranitidine, vancomycin (and other antibiotics), and phenytoin.

Thrombocytopenia can also be a prominent feature of bone marrow failure syndromes such as Fanconi anemia, but generally more than one blood cell line will be affected in such cases. The syndrome of thrombocytopenia–absent radii (TAR) presents with signs of thrombocytopenia in infants with upper limb abnormalities. Fortunately, patients with TAR syndrome need only supportive care in the first few years of life, including platelet transfusions, because the thrombocytopenia frequently improves with age. Wiskott-Aldrich syndrome is an X-linked disorder consisting of the triad of atopic dermatitis, immune dysfunction, and thrombocytopenia. Effective treatment of Wiskott-Aldrich syndrome requires stem cell transplantation. Finally, there are rare types of bone marrow failure specific to platelet precursor stem cells, most notably amegakaryocytic thrombocytopenia, that also require stem cell transplantation. As alluded to earlier, one clue to decreased bone marrow production in a child with a low platelet count is the presence of tiny platelets on the blood smear and low mean platelet volume on the complete blood count.

Platelet Dysfunction

Although there are bleeding disorders that result from disorders of platelet function, they are very rare. A bleeding patient with a normal platelet count is much more likely to have another disorder responsible for the bleeding (e.g., coagulopathy). One of the most common causes of platelet dysfunction ("functional thrombocytopenia") is uremia. In this scenario, dialysis may actually be more effective than platelet transfusion. Of course, consultation with a specialist is necessary in such settings. Other disorders of platelet function are much more unusual and usually involve congenital defects in platelet adhesion (Bernard-Soulier syndrome), platelet aggregation (Glanzmann thrombasthenia), or platelet secretion (gray platelet syndrome). These disorders can be difficult to diagnose, and patients require the care of a hematologist.

CONSULTATION

Consultation with a hematologist is recommended in the following circumstances:

- Serious bleeding in the setting of a low platelet count
- Any signs or symptoms suggesting another hematologic process such as leukemia or aplastic anemia

- Any case of neonatal thrombocytopenia
- If TTP is being considered
- Persistent thrombocytopenia, without other symptoms, lasting longer than 6 months

ADMISSION CRITERIA

- Uncertain cause, especially if considering HUS/TTP or DIC
- New diagnosis of leukemia or aplastic anemia (a relative indication for admission)
- Life- or limb-threatening bleeding
- Very young age (<1 month)
- Very low platelet count (5000 to 10,000/mm^3)—although this is controversial and some physicians manage their patient at home regardless of the platelet count

DISCHARGE CRITERIA

- No ongoing, uncontrolled bleeding
- Adequate oral intake
- Parents comfortable with caring for the child at home
- Adequate follow-up plan

IN A NUTSHELL

- Thrombocytopenia can be caused by immune-mediated mechanisms (ITP, NAIT) or consumption (DIC, HUS, TTP, KMS).
- When considering ITP, leukemia and aplastic anemia must be excluded by the history, physical examination, and laboratory studies.
- Once the diagnosis is certain, ITP can usually be managed by close observation only.
- HUS or TTP must be considered in any sick child with thrombocytopenia because failure to make the diagnosis quickly may have devastating consequences.
- Transfusion of platelets is indicated when thrombocytopenia is severe and due to decreased platelet production. Platelet transfusion will often be more harmful than not. Carefully consider the cause of the low platelet count and consider consultation with a hematologist.

ON THE HORIZON

- Preliminary evidence suggests that only a subset of children with ITP will respond to rituximab. Research is being conducted to develop techniques for prospective identification of this population.
- Clinical trials are ongoing to investigate the potential role of prenatal steroids in managing neonatal ITP secondary to maternal ITP.
- There is much interest in oral thrombopoietin receptor agonists as treatment of refractory ITP. A clinical trial of this therapy is under way.

SUGGESTED READING

Blanchette VS, Chir B, Carcao M: Childhood acute immune thrombocytopenia purpura: 20 years later. Semin Thromb Hemost 2003;29:605-618.

Cines DB, Blanchette VS: Immune thrombocytopenic purpura. N Engl J Med 2002;346:995-1008.

Cines DB, Bussel JB, McMillan RB, Zehnder JL: Congenital and acquired thrombocytopenia. Hematology Am Soc Hematol Educ Program 2004;390-406.

Rothenberger S: Neonatal alloimmune thrombocytopenia. Ther Apher 2002;6:32-35.

Sadler JE, Moake JL, Miyata T, George JN: Recent advances in thrombotic thrombocytopenic purpura. Hematology Am Soc Hematol Educ Program 2004;407-423.

REFERENCES

1. George JN, Woolf SH, Raskob GE, et al: Idiopathic thrombocytopenic purpura: A practice guideline developed by explicit methods for the American Society of Hematology. Blood 1996;88:3-40.

2. Iyori H, Bessho F, Ookawa H, et al: Intracranial hemorrhage in children with immune thrombocytopenic purpura. Japanese Study Group on childhood ITP. Ann Hematol 2000;79:691-695.

3. Lilleyman JS: Intracranial haemorrhage in idiopathic thrombocytopenic purpura. Paediatric Haematology Forum of the British Society for Haematology. Arch Dis Child 1994;71:251-253.

4. Rosthoj S, Nielsen S, Pedersen FK: Randomized trial comparing intravenous immunoglobulin with methylprednisolone pulse therapy in acute idiopathic thrombocytopenic purpura. Danish I.T.P. Study Group. Acta Paediatr 1996;85:910-915.

5. Stasi R, Pagano A, Stipa E, Amadori S: Rituximab chimeric anti-CD20 monoclonal antibody treatment for adults with chronic idiopathic thrombocytopenic purpura. Blood 2001;98:952-957.

6. Zaja F, Iacona I, Masolini P, et al: B-cell depletion with rituximab as treatment for immune hemolytic anemia and chronic thrombocytopenia. Haematologica 2002;87:189-195.

7. Pusiol A, Cesaro S, Nocerino A, et al: Successful treatment with the monoclonal antibody rituximab in two children with refractory autoimmune thrombocytopenia. Eur J Pediatr 2004;163:305-307.

8. Johnson JA, Ryan G, al-Musa A, et al: Prenatal diagnosis and management of neonatal alloimmune thrombocytopenia. Semin Perinatol 1997;21:45-52.

CHAPTER 120

Disorders of Coagulation and Thrombosis

Paul Galardy

Disorders involving the systems of coagulation, thrombosis, and thrombolysis are common hematologic complications in hospitalized patients. These disorders represent a spectrum of biochemical and cellular changes in the blood that act in concert and that are not easily separated from one another. In the normal homeostatic situation, procoagulant forces are held in check by anticoagulant mechanisms, and there is no propensity to either bleed or clot inappropriately. This balance is important in terms of normal clotting; without anticoagulant mechanisms in place, normal clotting can become amplified out of proportion, and without significant procoagulant activities in the plasma, excessive bleeding results.

Because coagulopathy (an increased tendency to bleed) and thrombosis (an increased tendency to clot) are opposite ends of the same physiologic spectrum, both are discussed in this chapter. The first two sections on pathophysiology and laboratory testing address issues common to both coagulopathy and thrombosis; these are followed by a discussion of the diagnosis and treatment of specific disorders of bleeding and thrombosis.

PATHOPHYSIOLOGY

Normal hemostasis can be mechanistically separated into four phases: (1) platelet plug formation, (2) fibrin mesh formation, (3) clot maturation, and (4) fibrinolysis. Dysregulation of any phase can result in pathologic bleeding or thrombosis.

The Clotting Process
Platelet Plug Formation

Following an injury to the vessel wall, the first event in hemostasis is the formation of a platelet plug. The most important factor in the initiation of clotting seems to be exposure of subendothelial tissues to blood. Initially, platelets form a single-cell layer covering the wall defect through the process of platelet adhesion. Platelet adhesion results in the activation of platelets, leading to further platelet recruitment and facilitating reactions of the coagulation cascade. The subsequent formation of a multicell network of platelets occurs through a process called platelet aggregation. Platelet adhesion and aggregation depend on the proper functioning of the surface receptors for von Willebrand factor (glycoprotein Ib/V/IX) and fibrinogen (glycoprotein IIb/IIIa). Defects in either of these receptors are known to cause inherited coagulopathic tendencies (Bernard-Soulier syndrome and Glanzmann thrombasthenia, respectively). In addition to acting as the initial patch in a ruptured vessel, the platelet plug provides abundant phospholipid surface on which subsequent fluid phases of coagulation reactions can occur.

Fibrin Mesh Formation

Platelet aggregation is not enough to form a clot; fibrin generation must occur to stabilize the clot. The overall function of the coagulation cascade is to generate fibrin polymers that link platelets together to stabilize clots. The coagulation cascade is a self-amplifying series of reactions that occur in the serum involving the sequential conversion of proenzymes to active serine proteases. Importantly, there are many checks and balances in the cascade to limit clotting to areas of active bleeding.

Blood coagulation was initially thought to occur through two separate pathways: the intrinsic and extrinsic pathways (Fig. 120-1). Although it is still useful to separate these pathways for didactic and diagnostic purposes, the intrinsic and extrinsic clotting cascades actually act in concert in the development of a fibrin mesh, providing a durable seal to vessel wall injuries.

Activation of thrombosis in vivo occurs primarily through the activity of tissue factor, found in the subendothelium and exposed to the serum on disruption of the endothelial layer. Tissue factor forms a complex with factor VII, converting factor VII to factor VIIa. The resulting tissue factor–factor VIIa complex then converts factor X to factor Xa. Factor Xa, together with factor Va, catalyzes the production of thrombin (from prothrombin), which serves as the catalytic enzyme to convert fibrinogen to fibrin, thus stabilizing the platelet plug. Effective generation of factor Xa depends on the activity of a complex between factors VIII and IX (activated by the action of tissue factor–factor VIIa), thus explaining why patients with hemophilia (genetic defects of factor VIII or IX) bleed.

Clot Maturation

Once formed, the meshwork of fibrin must be stabilized to slow its removal through the fibrinolytic pathway. Clot maturation occurs through the action of factor XIII, which generates interchain cross-links, strengthening the meshwork and making it more resistant to the action of plasmin. Consistent with factor XIII's role late in the hemostatic process, deficiencies of factor XIII result in delayed bleeding following injuries.

Fibrinolysis

Once hemostasis has been achieved, the process of fibrinolysis acts to dissolve the clot. This step, along with several previous "checks" in the coagulation cascade, is aimed at limiting the coagulation of blood to areas of disrupted

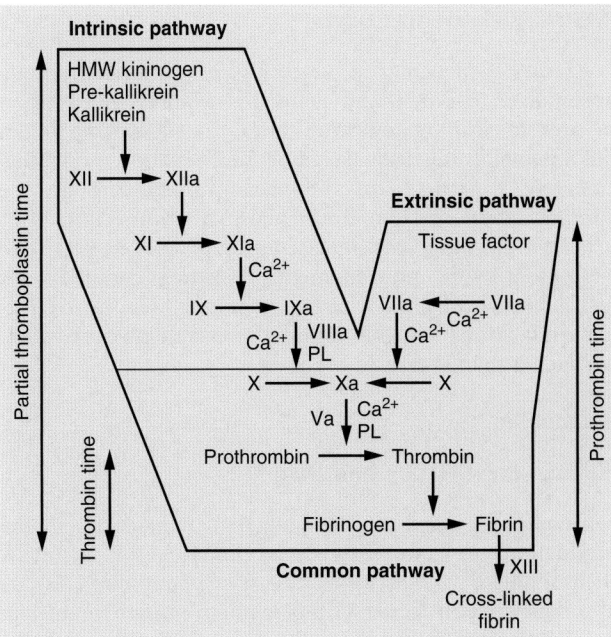

Figure 120-1 Schematic of the coagulation cascade. The factors tested by the partial thromboplastin time, prothrombin time, and thrombin time are shown. HMW, high molecular weight; PL, phospholipid.

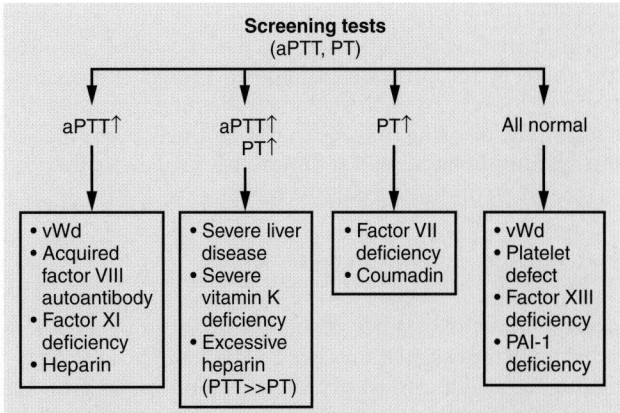

Figure 120-2 Interpretation of initial coagulation screening tests. aPTT, activated partial thromboplastin time; PAI, plasminogen activator inhibitor; PT, prothrombin time; PTT, partial thromboplastin time; vWd, von Willebrand disease. (Modified from Nathan DG, Oski SH: Hematology of Infancy and Childhood, 6th ed. Philadelphia, Saunders, 2003.)

vasculature and allowing resolution of blood flow once the vessel injury is healed.

Natural Anticoagulants

At all stages of thrombus formation, procoagulant activities are rapidly counterbalanced with natural anticoagulant pathways of fibrinolysis. Defects in this system of "checks and balances" often lead to inappropriate clotting (thrombotic disorders). Important factors in this regard are proteins C and S, tissue factor pathway inhibitor, antithrombin III, thrombomodulin, tissue plasminogen activator, and urokinase. Coincident with activation of the normal coagulation cascade, protein C is activated, associates with protein S, and feeds back into the cascade to inactivate factors VIIIa and Va (both of which are important in the activity of factor Xa). Similarly, antithrombin III serves to inactivate thrombin and limit fibrin formation. Normal clotting and clot dissolution occur through the balance of coagulation profactors and antifactors; imbalance in the system leads to either prolonged bleeding or inappropriate clotting, with pathologic consequences.

LABORATORY TESTING

Several screening tests are commonly used to identify bleeding and clotting disorders (Fig. 120-2).

Prothrombin Time

The prothrombin time (PT) tests for the "extrinsic" coagulation cascade. A normal result therefore requires factors VII, X, V, and II (prothrombin) and fibrinogen. Thromboplastins (tissue factor) are mixed with the patient's serum in excess to initiate clotting through this pathway. This test is particularly sensitive to alterations in the vitamin K–dependent clotting factors II, X, and VII and is therefore the primary tool used to monitor the effect of warfarin.

International Normalized Ratio

The international normalized ratio (INR) is designed to standardize the results obtained when PT testing is performed in different laboratories using reagents from different manufacturers. The INR allows the results from any laboratory to be readily compared for therapeutic monitoring of warfarin therapy.

Activated Partial Thromboplastin Time

The activated partial thromboplastin time (aPTT), which measures the extrinsic pathway factors, assays the function of high-molecular-weight (HMW) kininogen; kallikrein; factors XII, XI, IX, and VIII; and the common pathway factors X, II, and fibrinogen. Factor levels (VIII, IX, or XI) below 50% are generally required to prolong the aPTT, making this a reasonable screen for hemophilia (caused by deficiencies in either factor VIII or factor IX). Curiously, however, deficiencies in HMW kininogen, kallikrein, and factor XII (all part of the intrinsic clotting pathway) prolong the aPTT but are not associated with bleeding disorders.

Thrombin Time

The thrombin time test involves mixing the patient's plasma with active thrombin and measuring the conversion of fibrinogen to fibrin. It is prolonged in the setting of low levels of fibrinogen, dysfunctional fibrinogen, or inhibitors to thrombin or fibrinogen.

Mixing Studies

Many times, abnormal (prolonged) PT or aPTT tests are due to soluble factors (usually antibodies) that interfere with the assays themselves but may not be associated with a clinical tendency to bleed. Mixing studies are used to rapidly determine whether a prolonged screening test is due to a circulating inhibitor (drug or antibody) rather than a deficiency of a particular coagulation factor.

Bleeding Time

Although theoretically useful to detect a defect involved anywhere in the processes leading to the generation of a fibrin clot (and particularly good for identifying platelet disorders), the bleeding time test is not routinely performed in our institution because of technical inconsistencies that can make it difficult to interpret the results.

Platelet Aggregation Studies

Sometimes, a tendency to bleed is due to a problem in platelet function rather than thrombocytopenia or a problem in the coagulation cascade. Studies of platelet aggregation detect diminished platelet activation in the presence of various substances known to trigger platelet aggregation. Platelet dysfunction can be either inherited (e.g., Bernard-Soulier syndrome, Glanzmann thrombasthenia, storage pool disorders) or acquired (e.g., drug effect).

Tests of Fibrinolysis

Once a clot is formed, there must be an effective mechanism to limit coagulation and eventually degrade the clot once the vessel rupture has healed. Plasmin acts to cleave fibrin polymers in a process known as fibrinolysis. Fragments of fibrin are released in the process and can be measured as a marker of the activity of the fibrinolytic system. This is the basis of the D-dimer, fibrin degradation product, and fibrin split product tests. The extreme sensitivity of the commonly used D-dimer assay makes this test useful as a negative predictor of thrombosis, unless the sample is drawn through a line. A negative D-dimer test is able to exclude deep venous thrombosis and pulmonary embolism with greater than 98% accuracy. A positive test, however, is less useful because it does not pinpoint the exact pathophysiology behind the fibrinolytic activity. Elevated D dimers are seen in disseminated intravascular coagulation, deep venous thrombosis, pulmonary embolism, and other disease states.

DISORDERS OF BLEEDING

Excessive bleeding is a common condition among hospitalized children and generally requires intervention to prevent volume loss and shock. In the setting of an unknown bleeding disorder, while the evaluation is ongoing, emergent treatment can be accomplished through the administration of fresh frozen plasma, cryoprecipitate, or platelets. Bleeding tendencies due to platelet defects tend to present with mucocutaneous bleeding coupled with petechiae and purpura, whereas coagulopathies due to coagulation factor deficits (hemophilia) present with deep bleeding such as hemarthrosis.

Hemophilia

Clinical Presentation and Diagnosis

Hemophilia results from congenital deficiencies in the production of factor VIII (hemophilia A) or factor IX (hemophilia B, or Christmas disease). Hemophilia C is due to a deficiency in factor XI but is much more benign than hemophilia A or B and is not discussed further. Because the genes encoding factors VIII and IX are located on the X chromosome, hemophilia affects males almost exclusively. The combined incidence of hemophilia is approximately 1 in 5000 live male births, consisting of 80% hemophilia A and 20% hemophilia B.[1]

The severity of clinical bleeding and the age of diagnosis can be predicted based on the level of circulating factor. Severe disease results with less than 1% of the normal level of circulating factor VIII or IX, and moderate hemophilia results from levels between 1% and 5% (Table 120-1). Patients with severe disease are often diagnosed in the immediate neonatal period in the setting of a family history of hemophilia and symptomatic bleeding or an abnormal screening test (aPTT). It is important to point out that the aPTT is normal with as little as 40% to 50% of the normal factor level, making it an insensitive tool to diagnose mild

---

Table 120-1 Relationship between Factor Levels and Symptoms in Hemophilia A or B

Symptom	FACTOR LEVEL DEFICIENCY		
	Severe (<1%)	Moderate (1%-5%)	Mild (5%-20%)
Age at onset	<1 yr	<2 yr	3-14 yr or later
Musculosketeltal bleeding	Spontaneous	Minor trauma	Unusual except with severe trauma
Central nervous system bleeding	3% (mean age, 14 yr)	Less prevalent than with severe	Rare
Postsurgical bleeding	Frank bleeding	Wound hematomas or oozing common	Occasional wound hematomas or oozing
Inhibitor development	15%-20%	<3%	Very rare
Bleeding from trauma	Common with contact sports	Muscle and joint bleeding with contact sports	Significant hematomas; deep bleeding only with significant trauma
Bleeding following dental extraction	Usual	Common	Often; can be persistent
Response to DDAVP	None	Usually <10%	2- to 3-fold increase

cases of hemophilia. Patients with mild or moderate hemophilia may not be diagnosed for years, and mild deficiencies may not present until adulthood. Nearly 60% of patients with factor VIII deficiency have severe disease, compared with only 20% to 45% of patients with factor IX deficiency. Within a family, the severity of disease is usually conserved because of the identical inherited genotype.

Hemophilia should be suspected in the setting of a prolonged aPTT once inhibitors (antibodies that interfere with the aPTT) have been ruled out. Confirmation of hemophilia and determination of the factor deficiency in question are accomplished by measuring the levels of factors VIII and IX.

Deficiency of factor VIII must be differentiated from von Willebrand disease (vWD). Von Willebrand factor (vWF) is a soluble protein that acts as a "carrier" for factor VIII and protects factor VIII from degradation. In the setting of reduced levels of vWF, factor VIII levels can also be low (without any defect in the factor VIII gene). By measuring vWF, true factor VIII deficiency can easily be distinguished from vWD.

Treatment

The goals of treatment for hemophilia constitute a balance between the desire to reverse the hemostatic defect and the desire to avoid the risk of developing inhibitors (antifactor antibodies), the risk of viral transmission from pooled human serum products, and the tremendous financial cost of the regular administration of recombinant clotting factors. Therefore, the amount of factor administration must be appropriate for the clinical scenario, and treatment guidelines have been established.

Mild factor VIII deficiency can often be treated with DDAVP (arginine vasopressin). Administration of 0.3μg/kg of DDAVP intravenously results in a threefold increase in the baseline level of factor VIII. This is usually adequate to achieve effective hemostasis for minor trauma or surgery. The dose can be repeated in 12 to 24 hours, but beyond that time frame, tachyphylaxis occurs as endothelial stores of vWF and factor VIII are depleted. Before using DDAVP in circumstances of hemostatic challenge, the response to DDAVP should be demonstrated with a test dose, measuring factor levels before and after administration. It can be assumed that the response seen with the test dose will be representative of future responses. Patients must be monitored for hyponatremia following the administration of DDAVP, especially those who cannot fully regulate their own thirst mechanisms. Further, hypotonic saline solutions should not be administered, because they may precipitate hyponatremia.

Moderate or severe hemophilia usually requires replacement with clotting factor concentrates.[2,3] Many different factor concentrates are available in the United States and are classified as either plasma derived or recombinant in nature.

Although it is tempting to replace factor levels to 100% with each bleeding episode, it is clear that far less is required for most bleeding events. Besides the financial burden of factor replacement, each exposure to clotting factor concentrates provides an opportunity for the development of antibodies that inactivate coagulation factors (known as inhibitors). Once inhibitors develop, simple factor replacement becomes a less viable option for future bleeding episodes. Therefore, factor should be replaced judiciously. The decision to administer factor and the dosage must take into consideration the degree of bleeding, the location of bleeding, and the potential complications arising from the bleeding.

A general guideline to the replacement of coagulation factors is presented in Table 120-2. One international unit (IU) per kilogram of factor VIII increases the plasma factor level by 2%, whereas 1 IU/kg of factor IX raises the plasma factor level by only 1%. Thus, 50 IU/kg of recombinant factor VIII are needed to replace 100% of factor VIII activity, whereas 100 IU/kg of recombinant factor IX are needed

Table 120-2 Factor Replacement Goals in Hemophilia

Type of Bleeding	Replacement Goal (%)	Replacement Dose Factor VIII (IU/kg/day)	Replacement Dose Factor IX (IU/kg)	Duration (days)
Hemarthrosis	40	20	40	1-2
Intramuscular hematoma	General: 40 Iliopsoas: 30-100	General: 20 Iliopsoas: 15-50	General: 40 Iliopsoas: 30-100	General: 1-2 Iliopsoas: 100% for 3 days, then 30% for 7 days
CNS, life threatening	100	50	100	14 days, trough >50%; then 30% for 7 days
Oral, dental extraction	40	20	40	1 day, then aminocaproic acid for 5-7 days
Surgery	100	50	100	100% for 1 day, 50% for 5-7 days, 30% for 5-7 days
GI bleeding	100	50	100	Continue 1-2 days after stool clears of blood
Compartment syndrome	100	50	100	Days to weeks

CNS, central nervous system; GI, gastrointestinal.
Adapted from Nathan DG, Oski SH: Hematology of Infancy and Childhood, 6th ed. Philadelphia, Saunders, 2003, p 1551.

to replace 100% of factor IX activity. When more than 1 day of inpatient replacement is required, it is common to administer factors by continuous infusion, which avoids the unnecessary peaks and nadirs of bolus therapy. For example, if the target level is 100%, a bolus of 50 IU/kg is given initially, followed by 2 to 3 IU/kg per hour (total daily 100% replacement per 24 hours).

von Willebrand Disease

Inherited vWD is a heterogeneous disorder resulting from a biochemical reduction in the amount of functioning vWF.[4] This disease affects 1% to 2% of individuals, making it the single most common inherited bleeding disorder.

Clinical Presentation and Diagnosis

The clinical presentation of vWD is that of a mild bleeding disorder. Characteristically, patients may experience excessive bruising, epistaxis, menorrhagia, or prolonged bleeding following dental extraction or tonsillectomy. The age at which symptoms come to attention is highly variable. Because the severity of symptoms is only loosely correlated with the plasma levels of vWF, some patients with moderate vWD are asymptomatic into adulthood, especially if they have not undergone significant hemostatic challenges. In severe vWD, which is rare, the near total absence of vWF results in extremely low factor VIII levels.

The diagnosis of vWD is made through the measurement of vWF levels in the plasma, coupled with functional assays to exclude qualitative defects. The three standard tests to screen for vWD include a vWF antigen level, a factor VIII level, and a ristocetin cofactor activity assay. In general, levels of vWF antigen and ristocetin cofactor activity above 60% are considered normal, 40% to 60% is mild or borderline, and less than 40% represents frank deficiency.

Treatment

For the vast majority of patients with vWD, treatment is required only for surgical procedures or trauma. The two principal treatment options include DDAVP and plasma-derived products containing vWF and factor VIII (Humate-P, Alphanate, or Koate-HP. DDAVP at a dose of 0.3 µg/kg intravenously every 24 hours can provide elevated vWF levels for 2 to 3 days, at which point endothelial stores of vWF will likely be depleted. DDAVP is not appropriate for all patients with vWD, especially those with qualitative vWF muations or complete deletion of the vWF gene. For these patients, the only effective treatment is to administer plasma-derived concentrates containing factor VIII and vWF. The dosing of Humate-P, the preparation used most commonly at our institution, is based on the vWF–ristocetin cofactor unit (IU vWF–Rco). In general, a dose of 40 to 80 IU vWF–Rco/kg should be given every 12 hours. The duration of therapy is dictated by the clinical situation, but in most cases, patients should be treated for 24 to 48 hours following trauma or surgical procedures.

Platelet Disorders

Bleeding may occur due to inherited or acquired defects in platelet functioning. Collectively, these are rare disorders, and they are discussed only briefly. (Conditions causing thrombocytopenia are discussed in Chapter 119.) Bernard-Soulier syndrome and Glanzmann thrombasthenia are inherited disorders resulting from deficiencies in the platelet receptors for vWF (glycoprotein Ib/IX) or fibrinogen (glycoprotein IIb/IIIa). Acquired platelet defects involve either insufficient platelet numbers or impaired platelet function.

Coagulopathies Associated with Transfusions

Chapter 121 provides a complete discussion of this issue.

Disseminated Intravascular Coagulation

Disseminated intravascular coagulation (DIC), or consumptive coagulopathy, is characterized by the widespread activation of the coagulation cascade, resulting in the depletion of clotting factors and microvascular thrombin deposition. DIC is not a discrete entity but rather the final result of hemostatic insults from a large number of sources, including (but not limited to) trauma, sepsis, and malignancy.

DIC can be classified as acute or chronic. Acute DIC results from abrupt, often critical, changes in clinical status; chronic DIC may last for years and be associated with relative clinical wellness. Acute DIC is characteristically (but not always) seen in the setting of severe systemic illness and is often associated with multiorgan failure. Patients with DIC may have the paradoxical occurrence of simultaneous bleeding and thrombosis, making management a challenge. Typically, bleeding occurs from mucous membranes, venipuncture sites, entrance tunnels to central venous lines, and bruising.

The laboratory picture seen in DIC is typically one of prolonged PT and aPTT, along with depletion of fibrinogen and elevated D dimers. A microangiopathic hemolytic anemia may occur due to fibrin deposition, and thrombocytopenia may arise due to consumption. When DIC occurs in the setting of severe multiorgan failure, the laboratory picture may be confounded by the coagulopathy resulting from hepatic dysfunction. Although nearly all coagulation factors are produced in the liver, factor VIII is synthesized in the endothelium. If factor VIII deficiency coexists with other factor deficiencies (e.g., factor VII and fibrinogen), DIC is the likely diagnosis. In chronic DIC, laboratory tests may be mostly normal, with the only anomaly being decreased fibrinogen or positive D dimers on repeated testing.

The treatment of DIC must focus on the underlying cause and supportive measures. A hematologist should be consulted for assistance in decision making regarding correction of the coagulopathy. In chronic DIC due to vascular anomalies, low-molecular-weight heparin can be used to slow the production of fibrin, especially if sclerotherapy is planned. Acute DIC management must focus on the clinical picture. If the primary "symptoms" are limited to laboratory anomalies, treatment of the underlying cause without directed coagulopathy treatment typically leads to resolution. Platelet concentrates, fresh frozen plasma, and cryoprecipitate are frequently used to replenish coagulation factors, although many believe that this simply "fuels the fire" of coagulation. In the absence of bleeding, heparin products can be used to slow fibrin generation while fresh frozen plasma and cryoprecipitate replenish factors. Of course, without addressing the primary cause of the coagulopathy, these measures are merely supportive, not curative. Additional therapies that may be given in special instances include antithrombin III and activated protein C.

Vitamin K Deficiency

Vitamin K is a fat-soluble vitamin found in leafy green vegetables and many cooking oils. It is also produced through the activity of enteric flora. In the setting of poor nutrition or prolonged antibiotic use, vitamin K deficiency may lead to a coagulopathy. Neonates are at risk for vitamin K deficiency due to the relatively low passage of vitamin K across the placenta, the sterility of the newborn intestinal tract, and the lack of vitamin K in breast milk. In the era of widespread administration of vitamin K to newborns, however, vitamin K–related hemorrhagic disease is a rare neonatal event. Bleeding may occur at any site, although vitamin K deficiency is frequently discovered in nonbleeding children who are screened with a PT or aPTT. Treatment involves the delivery of 1 mg of parenteral vitamin K, which results in normalization of the PT within 4 to 6 hours and the aPTT within 24 hours.

THROMBOSIS

Epidemiology and Risk Factors

Venous thromboembolic events (VTEs) are estimated to affect approximately 5 of every 10,000 children admitted to the hospital.[5] The role of inherited thrombophilic risk factors in pediatric thromboembolic disease is not clear. Although the prospective rate of VTEs in children with known risks for thrombophilia is low, these children are present in disproportionately high numbers in some, but not all, VTE case series.

Our understanding of thrombosis has increased tremendously through the analysis of mutations associated with thrombophilia. Perhaps not surprisingly, deficiencies in natural anticoagulant proteins are associated with an increased risk of thrombosis. Additionally, polymorphisms in traditionally procoagulant proteins may elevate the risk of thrombosis (Table 120-3).

The most common acquired risk factor (other than central venous catheters) is antiphospholipid antibodies, also known as the lupus anticoagulant. Although the incidence of these antibodies is highest in patients with systemic lupus erythematosus, most patients who develop lupus anticoagulants do not have that disease and never will. The term *anticoagulant* is also a misnomer, because there is no increased risk of bleeding in these patients. Most commonly, lupus anticoagulants are detected through their ability to prolong the aPTT. Despite this effect, lupus anticoagulants actually promote thrombosis and heighten the risk of clotting considerably. In general, however, evidence does not support prophylactic anticoagulation in children with known risk factors unless a VTE has already occurred.

Other acquired risk factors include those outlined by Virchow in the eponymous triad of stasis, endothelial damage, and hypercoagulability. Stasis refers to areas of relatively sluggish blood flow that result from anatomic causes, immobility of the patient, or both. Stasis is a particular hazard to those with coexisting hypercoagulable states; those with prolonged immobility, such as occurs in the intensive care setting; or those permanently restricted to bed or a wheelchair. Endothelial damage is common following surgical procedures and in those with vascular anomalies. Patients with vascular anomalies often experience chronic DIC that predisposes to bleeding and thrombosis simultaneously. In patients with known hypercoagulable states, it is common to prescribe prophylactic low-molecular-weight heparin during times of stasis.

Central Venous Line–Associated Thrombosis

Advances in pediatric care have led to dramatic improvements in the survival of children with previously fatal disorders. One such development is improved technology for secure venous access in children. Although they are critical for the proper care of seriously ill patients, central venous lines (CVLs) are the single greatest risk factor for the development of deep venous thrombosis in children. In a review of the Canadian Thrombosis Registry, the incidence of CVL-associated VTEs was estimated to be 3.5 per 10,000 hospital admissions,[6] representing more than 50% of all pediatric VTEs. The most common sites included the subclavian vein, femoral vein, superior vena cava, jugular vein, and inferior vena cava. Pulmonary embolism occurred in 16% of cases, with approximately one third occurring in the setting of an upper venous system thrombosis and one third with thrombosis of the lower venous system. In this study, nearly 4% of patients died as a result of the CVL-associated VTE. Further, CVL-associated VTE is associated with the development of superior vena cava syndrome, chylothorax, and an increased rate of CVL-associated sepsis. These data are in direct contrast with the commonly held belief that upper venous system VTEs are "safer" than those of the lower system.

The most common symptoms of VTEs associated with CVLs include problems with CVL function (e.g., failure to flush or draw from either lumen of the CVL), swelling of the upper extremity, and prominence of the superficial veins of

Table 120-3	Inherited Thrombotic Risk Factors	
Genetic Risk Factor	Incidence in General Population (%)	Incidence in Children with VTE (%)
Factor V R506Q (factor V Leiden)	4	4.7
Prothrombin G20210A	2	2.3
Protein C or S deficiency	0.6	1.8
Antithrombin III deficiency	0.02	0.02
Elevated lipoprotein (a)	7.5 (influenced by diet)	7.5 (influenced by diet)

VTE, venous thromboembolic event.

the chest and neck. The latter two signs occur late, when the thrombosis is extensive and involves the subclavian and axillary veins. Symptoms of deep venous thrombosis in the lower extremity include swelling, pain, and discoloration. These symptoms are usually unilateral, although obstructive thrombi in the inferior vena cava may produce bilateral symptoms. Extensive involvement of the inferior vena cava may lead to obstructed venous return from the renal system. Thus, renal failure is occasionally a presenting symptom in severely affected patients. In patients with CVLs, there is a high incidence of asymptomatic line-associated thrombi; however, routine screening for thrombosis is not recommended in the absence of symptoms.

The treatment of symptomatic CVL-associated thrombosis involves line removal and anticoagulation. Although it is much debated, the timing of CVL removal has little impact on the incidence of embolization. We recommend early removal followed by low-molecular-weight heparin, transitioned to warfarin, for 3 months, or until the high risk of thrombosis (if one exists) has passed. In the event of extensive upper venous thrombosis with poor resolution on anticoagulants, we often extend anticoagulation for a total of 6 months. In patients with CVLs who are receiving chemotherapy or have poor nutrition, we routinely use low-molecular-weight heparin for the entire course of anticoagulation owing to the difficulty of achieving stable therapeutic warfarin effects in such patients.

Sinovenous Thromboembolism

Thrombosis involving the venous drainage system of the brain is a serious event leading to severe and often irreversible complications.[7] The incidence of sinovenous thromboembolism (SVT) in children is reported to be 0.29 per 100,000 per year, with 45% occurring in the first 3 months of life. Headache is the most common symptom associated with SVT in childhood, and seizures occur in nearly half of patients. Other symptoms include altered mental status (44%), papilledema (12%), and focal neurologic signs (42%). The diffuse nature of the symptoms seen in SVT in children makes a high index of suspicion critical. There is thought to be a complex interplay between genetic and environmental causes. This condition rarely occurs in the absence of predisposing systemic medical illness. Dehydration and head and neck infections account for up to 18% of cases of SVT. Chronic illnesses, including connective tissue disorders, hematologic disorders, and cardiac disease, are present in nearly 60% of affected patients. Supporting an environmental predisposition is the fact that inherited causes of thrombophilia may be identified in up to 40% of affected patients.

The most commonly affected sites are the superior sagittal, lateral, and straight sinuses, with multiple sinuses involved in the vast majority of cases. Cerebral infarcts occur in 41% of patients with SVT, and they are frequently hemorrhagic. The outcome of pediatric SVT is poor, with death occurring in 10% and neurologic deficits in 40% of patients.

Anticoagulation is commonly used to treat SVT, but great care must be taken to avoid anticoagulating those at risk for cerebral hemorrhage. Consultation with specialists in both hematology and neurology is required so that the risks and benefits of anticoagulation can be balanced. Once the decision to anticoagulate has been made, the choice between

unfractionated and low-molecular-weight heparin is important. Although low-molecular-weight heparin has a much more predictable and stable anticoagulant effect, many clinicians prefer the easy on-off control that a heparin drip affords. This is particularly useful in patients who may need urgent or emergent surgical measures. The total duration for anticoagulation is 3 to 6 months, depending on the resolution rate and the severity of the initial event.

Renal Vein Thrombosis

Thrombosis of the renal veins may occur in isolation or in association with extensive inferior vena cava thrombus. Renal vein thrombosis (covered in more detail in Chapter 115) is largely a neonatal complication, with the vast majority of cases occurring within the first month of life.[8] A diagnostic triad of flank mass, hematuria, and thrombocytopenia is occasionally present, but most patients have only one of these signs. Renal function is impaired in some but not all patients, and many patients present with anuria.[9] Associated hemorrhage of the adrenal glands may be seen.

Anticoagulation in the setting of renal vein thrombosis may be extremely challenging if renal embarrassment is significant. Dosing of low-molecular-weight heparin must be adjusted in the setting of renal insufficiency. In patients on hemodialysis, dosing must be performed after dialysis, because the drug is removed by the osmotic process. Following a transition to warfarin (if possible), the total duration of therapy is between 3 and 6 months, depending on the degree of resolution and the extent of the thrombosis.

Pulmonary Embolism

Pulmonary embolism in children is an uncommon event compared with adults. The incidence in hospitalized children is estimated to be 0.86 in 10,000 admissions, although the true incidence is likely much higher owing to the low index of suspicion for this complication in children. However, in children, pulmonary embolisms can be found in 30% to 60% of those with documented deep venous thrombosis and in 18% of those with CVL-associated thrombi. Most of these are small emboli, with only the largest events leading to the classic symptoms of cough, shortness of breath, chest pain, and hemoptysis.

The treatment of pediatric pulmonary embolism is identical to that recommended for other forms of VTEs. Following 7 days of low-molecular-weight heparin, patients can be converted to warfarin and treated for a total of 3 to 6 months.

Diagnosis

The gold standard diagnostic test for VTEs is the venogram, although this modality has been largely replaced by spiral computed tomography scanning and Doppler ultrasonography for the diagnosis of extremity VTEs.

D-dimer testing is useful in the diagnosis of pediatric VTEs. Given the sensitivity of current assays for the detection of D dimers, a negative D-dimer test strongly predicts the absence of acute VTE, with a negative predictive value greater than 98%. Rarely, D dimers may be negative very early in the evolution of VTE. Alternatively, the D-dimer assay may be negative in the presence of a mature "old" VTE. Given that the risk of pulmonary embolism is low in the

Table 120-4 Guidelines for the Initiation, Monitoring, and Adjustment of Unfractionated Heparin

Initiate therapy with a 75 units/kg bolus over 10 min
Initial maintenance dose:
   1 yr or younger: 28 units/kg/hr
   Older than 1 yr: 20 units/kg/hr
Obtain first aPTT 4 hr later, and adjust dosage as follows:

aPTT (sec)	Heparin (U/mL)	Bolus (U/kg)	Hold	Rate	Recheck
<40	0-0.15	50	—	+20%	4 hr
40-50	0.16-0.2	0	—	+20%	4 hr
51-59	0.21-0.29	0	—	+10%	4 hr
60-90	0.3-0.5	0	—	—	24 hr
91-110	0.51-0.7	0	—	−10%	4 hr
111-150	0.71-1	0	30 min	−10%	4 hr
>150	>1	0	60 min	−15%	4 hr

aPTT, activated partial thromboplastin time.
Modified from Michelson AD, Bovill E, Andrew M: Antithrombotic therapy in children. Chest 1995;108:506S-522S.

setting of organized thrombi, it is common to use D-dimer testing to stratify patients into two groups: those who require immediate anticoagulation (radiographic evidence of VTE and positive D dimers) and those who merit further evaluation with imaging studies before making a decision about anticoagulant therapy (negative D dimers).

Treatment

Anticoagulation is the mainstay of VTE management. The three main therapies are discussed in the following sections.

Unfractionated Heparin

Unfractionated heparin has the drawbacks of a narrow therapeutic range; a highly variable pharmacokinetic behavior, necessitating frequent blood draws for monitoring; and the need for continuous infusions to achieve full anticoagulation. The main advantage of heparin is its short half-life, which allows rapid discontinuation of therapy in the event of acute bleeding or the need for surgical procedures. For a recommended dosing algorithm, refer to Table 120-4.

If immediate reversal of heparin effect is required, protamine sulfate can be administered. The dose of protamine administered is based on the amount of heparin present in the plasma: 1 mg of protamine sulfate can reverse 100 units of heparin. The amount of heparin infused can be used in this calculation; however, given the short half-life of heparin, reduced doses of protamine should be given with greater times from the administration of heparin. Thus, approximate doses of protamine sulfate are 0.5 to 0.75 mg/100 units at 30 to 60 minutes and 0.25 to 0.375 mg/100units at longer than 2 hours from the heparin dose.

Low-Molecular-Weight Heparin

The use of unfractionated heparin is quickly being surpassed by the use of low-molecular-weight heparin, which has the potential advantages of more predictable pharmaco-

kinetics, the requirement of less therapeutic monitoring, and a likely reduced risk of heparin-induced thrombocytopenia. Enoxaparin has been studied in children, and dosing guidelines have been established. [10,11] Therapy should be initiated with 1.5 mg/kg subcutaneously every 12 hours for infants younger than 2 months, and 1 mg/kg subcutaneously every 12 hours for infants and children older than 2 months. Heparin levels (anti–factor Xa levels) should be obtained 4 hours after the second dose from a fresh venipuncture site to avoid the presence of contaminating heparin in vascular access devices. The therapeutic range for the treatment of acute VTE has been extrapolated from adult data to be 0.5 to 1 unit/mL. For those at higher risk of bleeding, it may be appropriate to aim for a lower level of 0.4 to 0.6 unit/mL to reduce hemorrhagic complications, although this approach has not been validated prospectively. Particular caution must be used in patients with a recent history of surgery, brain tumor, thrombocytopenia, or any condition that creates an increased risk of bleeding. Dosing must be adjusted in the presence of renal impairment. The dose for prophylaxis of VTE is 0.75 mg/kg every 12 hours for infants younger than 2 months, and 0.5 mg/kg every 12 hours for those older than 2 months. Although monitoring is not necessary for low-risk patients receiving prophylactic low-molecular-weight heparin, those at high risk of bleeding or at risk for altered pharmacokinetics (e.g., renal failure) should have at least one level documented to be within the range of 0.1 to 0.4 unit/mL.

As with unfractionated heparin, the anticoagulant effects of low-molecular-weight heparin can be reversed with protamine sulfate. Within 8 hours of enoxaparin injection, the dose is 1 mg protamine sulfate per 1 mg enoxaparin in the last dose. A second infusion of 0.5 mg protamine sulfate per 1 mg enoxaparin injected may be required, based on the patient's clinical status or the results of a heparin level.

Warfarin

Warfarin is the most common vitamin K antagonist in clinical use. The degree of anticoagulant effect is related to the half-life of the vitamin K–dependent factors. The protein with the shortest half-life is protein C. Therefore, patients experience a period of increased risk of thrombosis early in the course of treatment with warfarin. As a result, warfarin should never be started without concurrent heparin therapy. The risk of thrombotic complications is highest in patients with protein C deficiency, in whom warfarin-induced skin necrosis is classically described.

Most people have a significant store of vitamin K in the body, necessitating a loading dose for the initiation of warfarin therapy. Guidelines for the use of warfarin are provided in Table 120-5. Monitoring of the INR should be performed daily during the first week of therapy, but only weekly thereafter because the long half-life of warfarin leads to long lag times before dosing changes are reflected by changes in the INR.

The anticoagulant effects of warfarin can be reversed emergently in the event of severe bleeding. Fresh frozen plasma should be administered in a dose of 10 mL/kg to replace the depleted coagulation factors. After repeat analysis of the PT and INR, more fresh frozen plasma may be needed for full reversal. Although factors II, IX, and X have long half-lives, factor VII has a short half-life of 3 to 5 hours.

Table 120-5 Protocol for Oral Anticoagulation with Warfarin

Stage	INR	Action
I: day 1	1.0-1.3	0.1-0.2 mg/kg orally (maximum 10 mg)
II: days 2-7	1.1-1.3	Repeat day 1 dose
	1.4-1.9	50% of day 1 dose
	2.0-3.0	50% of day 1 dose
	3.1-3.5	25% of day 1 dose
	>3.5	Hold until INR <3.5, then resume with stage III guidelines
III: maintenance	1.1-1.4	Increase dose by 20%
	1.5-1.9	Increase dose by 10%
	2.0-3.0	No change in dose
	3.1-3.5	Decrease dose by 10%
	>3.5	Hold until INR <3.5, then resume with 20% dose reduction

INR, international normalized ratio.
Modified from Michelson AD, Bovill E, Andrew M: Antithrombotic therapy in children. Chest 1995;108:506S-522S.

Therefore, redosing of fresh frozen plasma may be required as soon as 3 to 5 hours after the initial administration. Vitamin K can be used in addition to fresh frozen plasma, but its effects as a reversal agent are slower, and vitamin K administration makes the subsequent warfarin-based anticoagulation more difficult. For life-threatening bleeding, 5 mg of intravenous vitamin K may be administered; for non-life-threatening bleeding, 0.5 to 2 mg is sufficient. These doses lead to an increase in factor VIII levels initially, but full restoration of the vitamin K–dependent factors can take up to 2 to 3 days. Elective reversal is frequently required before scheduled surgical procedures. For patients whose risk of recurrent thrombosis is relatively low, the warfarin should be stopped 72 hours before the procedure, and the INR should be checked the day of the procedure. If the INR remains elevated, fresh frozen plasma can be administered before the procedure. For patients at high risk of recurrent thrombosis, warfarin should be discontinued 72 hours before the procedure, and the patient should be treated with unfractionated heparin 24 hours before the procedure and continuing until the postprocedure INR has returned to the target range. Heparin should be stopped from 6 hours before the procedure to at least 8 hours after the procedure. It is imperative to coordinate postoperative decisions regarding anticoagulation with the surgical team to avoid bleeding.

Prevention

Because the overall incidence of VTEs is low in the pediatric population, there are few data on the efficacy of prophylactic measures. However, the ever-increasing medical complexity of hospitalized children makes VTE prophylaxis a relevant issue. Borrowing from the adult literature, VTE prophylaxis involves primarily the use of nonpharmacologic measures or heparin. Intermittent pneumatic compression boots are frequently used to prevent VTEs in adults following surgery. Pharmacologic inhibition traditionally involves low doses of unfractionated heparin injected subcutaneously twice daily. The standard adult dose is 5000 units, which does not prolong the aPTT. Alternatively, low doses of low-molecular-weight heparin can be used twice daily. Because there is no easy conversion for the subcutaneous administration of unfractionated heparin to children, we generally recommend low-molecular-weight heparin.

IN A NUTSHELL

- Disorders of the coagulation system are common in hospitalized children.
- Although efficient treatment of bleeding disorders requires an accurate diagnosis, emergent treatment of an unknown bleeding disorder can be accomplished through the administration of fresh frozen plasma, cryoprecipitate, or platelets.
- Hemophilia, an X-linked congenital deficiency in the production of factor VIII (hemophilia A) or factor IX (hemophilia B), can present with life-threatening bleeding episodes. These events can be treated with DDAVP or factor replacement if the diagnosis is known, or with fresh frozen plasma, cryoprecipitate, or platelets if unknown.
- Von Willebrand disease is a heterogeneous disorder resulting from a biochemical reduction in the amount of functioning von Willebrand factor. DDAVP, factor VIIa, and von Willebrand factor are the mainstays of treatment.
- DIC is a severe systemic disorder commonly seen in critically ill patients. Central to its management is treatment of the underlying cause, with blood products or anticoagulant support as needed.
- The main categories of venous thromboembolism are central line associated, sinovenous thrombosis, renal artery thrombosis, general deep venous thrombosis, and pulmonary embolism.
- Patients with central venous lines are at high risk for the development of thrombi and are at risk for embolization.
- Unfractionated heparin, low-molecular-weight heparin, and warfarin are the main treatment options for management of venous thromboembolism.

ON THE HORIZON

- Because most inherited disorders of coagulation involve single gene defects, there is great interest in the application of gene therapy. Intensive investigations are ongoing into gene therapy for hemophilia, although to date, success has been limited in clinical trials.
- It is critical to gain a better understanding of the influence of inherited prothrombotic risk factors on the development of VTEs and the proper post-VTE management strategies in children.
- New anticoagulants that directly inhibit thrombin are currently in phase II or III trials in adults. Argatroban is a direct antithrombin agent that is increasingly used in the anticoagulation of children with heparin-induced thrombocytopenia.

SUGGESTED READING

Andrew M, David M, Adams M, et al: Venous thromboembolic complications (VTE) in children: First analyses of the Canadian Registry of VTE. Blood 1994;83:1251-1257.

Chan AK, Deveber G, Monagle P, et al: Venous thrombosis in children. J Thromb Haemost 2003;1:1443-1455.

Mannucci PM: Treatment of von Willebrand's disease. N Engl J Med 2004;351:683-694.

Mannucci PM, Duga S, Peyvandi F: Recessively inherited coagulation disorders. Blood 2004;104:1243-1252.

REFERENCES

1. Soucie JM, Evatt B, Jackson D: Occurrence of hemophilia in the United States. The Hemophilia Surveillance System Project investigators. Am J Hematol 1998;59:288-294.

2. Manco-Johnson MJ, Riske B, Kasper CK: Advances in care of children with hemophilia. Semin Thromb Hemost 2003;29:585-594.

3. Manco-Johnson M: Hemophilia management: Optimizing treatment based on patient needs. Curr Opin Pediatr 2005;17:3-6.

4. Mannucci PM: Treatment of von Willebrand's disease. N Engl J Med 2004;351:683-694.

5. Andrew M, David M, Adams M, et al: Venous thromboembolic complications (VTE) in children: First analyses of the Canadian Registry of VTE. Blood 1994;83:1251-1257.

6. Massicotte MP, Dix D, Monagle P, et al: Central venous catheter related thrombosis in children: Analysis of the Canadian Registry of Venous Thromboembolic Complications. J Pediatr 1998;133:770-776.

7. deVeber G, Andrew M, Adams C, et al: Cerebral sinovenous thrombosis in children. N Engl J Med 2001;345:417-423.

8. Zigman A, Yazbeck S, Emil S, Nguyen L: Renal vein thrombosis: A 10-year review. J Pediatr Surg 2000;35:1540-1542.

9. Kosch A, Kuwertz-Broking E, Heller C, et al: Renal venous thrombosis in neonates: Prothrombotic risk factors and long-term follow-up. Blood 2004;104:1356-1360.

10. Michelson AD, Bovill E, Monagle P, Andrew M: Antithrombotic therapy in children. Chest 1998;114:748S-769S.

11. Monagle P, Chan A, Massicotte P, et al: Antithrombotic therapy in children: The Seventh ACCP Conference on Antithrombotic and Thrombolytic Therapy. Chest 2004;126:645S-687S.

Transfusion Medicine

Melody J. Cunningham and Kristina A. Cole

Approximately 13 million units of blood are collected each year in the United States,[1,2] and 10 million to 11 million units of packed red blood cells (RBCs) are transfused annually. Nearly 70% are transfused during the perioperative period for acute blood loss.[3] The recognition that human immunodeficiency virus (HIV) and other viruses can be transmitted through transfusions, along with studies evaluating the physiologic response to transfusion, has led to a more conservative approach to transfusion therapy. Consensus statements published by the National Institutes of Health can guide clinicians[3-5]; however, clinical judgment is still the most important factor in the decision to treat with transfusion. Knowledge of the data and guidelines, complications associated with transfusions, and strategies to prevent those complications can aid clinicians in the decision whether to transfuse and the choice of product.

RED BLOOD CELL TRANSFUSIONS

The primary indication for packed RBC transfusion is to ensure adequate oxygen carrying capacity,[6,7] most often because of acute blood loss or chronic anemia in patients with hemoglobinopathies or significant nutritional deficiencies. The normal dose of packed RBCs for transfusion is 5 to 10 mL/kg in children.[8] In general, 5 mL/kg or, in an adult-size patient, one unit of packed RBCs can be expected to increase the hemoglobin by 1 g/dL (or raise the hematocrit by 3 percentage points).[9]

Pretransfusion Testing

Transfused RBCs should be ABO group and Rh type specific to prevent transfusion reactions and to avoid sensitization that would compromise future transfusions and promote alloimmune hemolytic reactions in future pregnancies.[10] Blood typing determines the patient's ABO group and Rh type. The patient's plasma is then screened against a panel of RBCs with known common antigens to ensure that alloantibodies are not present or have not developed since the last transfusion. If the cells used for screening react positively—that is, agglutinate when exposed to the patient's serum, indicating the presence of alloantibodies—the antibody must be identified, and RBCs without that antigen must be transfused to prevent an acute hemolytic transfusion reaction. Once the type and screen have been performed and a unit of blood has been identified for the recipient, a crossmatch is performed. This involves mixing the patient's serum with cells from the donor to ensure that no agglutination occurs.[9]

In most centers, testing for blood type and screening for antibodies are performed before packed RBC transfusions in all patients, with the exception of infants younger than 4 months. Studies have demonstrated that these young infants do not develop antibodies against red cell antigens.[11,12] Therefore, if the initial antibody screen is negative, the baby is transfused with ABO- and Rh-identical or -compatible cells. The screen for alloantibodies can be performed on either the infant's or the mother's serum or plasma, because any antibodies that the baby has were passively acquired from the mother.[13-15]

Emergencies

In emergency situations, when there is insufficient time to type, screen, and crossmatch, the patient may be given blood group O, Rh-negative packed RBCs while the blood bank workup is being performed.[16] As a rule, however, this therapy is reserved for unanticipated acute blood loss and hypovolemic shock, such as might occur in the setting of trauma or neonatal blood loss (e.g., placental abruption).

Preoperative Transfusions

It is unsafe to undergo general anesthesia with a very low hematocrit. In adults, RBC transfusion is almost never indicated with a hemoglobin greater than 10 g/dL and is usually considered necessary with a hemoglobin less than 6 g/dL.[4] Clinical judgment determines the need when the hemoglobin is between these values, taking into consideration factors such as the patient's overall preoperative health, basal hemodynamic state, and nature, length, and expected blood loss of the procedure being performed.[5,17] It must be emphasized that most pediatric patients can tolerate a very low hemoglobin without clinical compromise owing to excellent cardiac capacity, especially if the decrease is gradual.[18] Therefore, the threshold for preoperative transfusion in children may be higher than in adults. Patients with sickle cell disease should probably receive a transfusion preoperatively to increase hemoglobin to 10 g/dL and decrease sickle load to avoid acute chest syndrome and other vaso-occlusive complications of general anesthesia known to occur in sickle cell patients.[19]

Transfusions to Treat Anemia

The amount of packed RBCs to transfuse and the time over which the transfusion should occur depend on the clinical situation. Patients who have developed significant anemia over a long period usually compensate for the anemia by increased oxygen extraction and increased cardiac capacity; in these circumstances, the transfusion rate should be slow and the patient should be carefully monitored to prevent fluid overload or congestive heart failure. Certainly, such patients should not be given crystalloid along with packed RBCs; otherwise, fluid overload may result, manifesting as pulmonary edema and respiratory symptoms. Anemia brought on by nutritional deficiency (e.g., iron) is often chronic and well compensated. Unless there is evidence of impending heart failure from anemia, many children can be effectively managed by nutritional replacement alone without the need for transfusion.[18] In contrast, acute blood loss (e.g., trauma, surgery) with physiologic compromise almost always requires replacement of blood volume with RBCs, and transfusion is often best done more rapidly to correct volume and counteract hypovolemic shock.

Hemoglobinopathies

Transfusion is often indicated in patients with severe hemoglobinopathies, both to provide adequate red cells and to suppress the many chronic and serious sequelae of ineffective erythropoiesis.[20,21] Chronic hemolytic anemias caused by thalassemia or hemoglobinopathies can be accompanied by the disfiguring consequences of expansion of the marrow cavity and the discomfort and health risks of splenomegaly. In the case of thalassemia major (defined as the need for more than eight transfusions per year),[22] the usual regimen is transfusion every 3 to 4 weeks to maintain a trough hemoglobin of approximately 9.5 g/dL.[20,23]

Most patients with sickle cell anemia do not require regular transfusions despite having chronic anemia. In this population, transfusions are reserved for specific clinical situations (e.g., aplastic crisis, splenic sequestration, acute chest syndrome, acute stroke,[24,25] and preoperatively) and are therefore given episodically. Patients who have suffered a stroke or demonstrate a propensity for stroke based on screening studies (e.g., abnormal transcranial Doppler imaging) are managed by chronic, repetitive transfusion therapy, with the goal of suppressing erythropoiesis and reducing hemoglobin S levels.[26,27] It is important to remember that the tendency for vaso-occlusion in sickle cell disease is increased with viscosity; therefore, as a rule, sickle cell patients should not be transfused to a hematocrit greater than 30%.[28,29]

PLATELET TRANSFUSIONS

Indications

A typical dose of platelets for transfusion in pediatric patients is 1 to 2 units per 10 kg of body weight. In general, this dose should raise the patient's platelet count by 40,000 to 100,000/mm^3.[30] Platelet transfusions are indicated for patients with clinical evidence of bleeding who have thrombocytopenia (because of either decreased production or increased clearance of platelets) or poor platelet function (either inherited or acquired). In the clinical situation of bleeding due to decreased platelet number or intrinsic poor platelet function, transfusion of platelets is often effective in ameliorating the bleeding, and patients should be transfused based on clinical bleeding or before planned invasive procedures.[18] In situations in which platelet function or number is abnormal due to an underlying nonmarrow pathophysiology (e.g., immune-mediated platelet destruction, liver disease, uremia, sepsis), transfusion of platelets has limited effectiveness unless the underlying process is treated. In these situations, platelet transfusion is usually reserved for life- or limb-threatening bleeding. A more practical approach is to treat the underlying disease responsible for platelet dysfunction.

Compatibility

ABO-compatible platelets are preferred for transfusion for several reasons. Platelets have ABO antigens present on their surface; thus, ABO-incompatible platelets have a diminished half-life,[31] although this effect is not thought to be particularly significant clinically. However, in pediatric patients, the amount of antibody in the plasma component of the platelet product may be sufficient to cause hemolysis of the patient's native RBCs.[18] Platelets may contain up to 2 mL of RBCs, a sufficient amount of antigen for the development of allosensitization; this is particularly relevant for anti-D (Rh) sensitization in girls because of the future risk of Rh hemolytic disease of the newborn.[32] If an Rh-negative girl receives Rh-positive platelets, she should receive a dose of WinRho (anti-D) within 72 hours of that transfusion to prevent alloimmunization against the D antigen.

Transfusion of Platelet Refractory Patients

The best measure of response to platelet transfusion is cessation of bleeding. In patients who seem to have no response to platelets, a platelet count 10 to 60 minutes after transfusion can be used to determine response. Two consecutive poor responses suggest platelet refractoriness,[33] caused by either an immunologic mechanism (anti-HLA or antiplatelet antibodies) or a nonimmunologic process (e.g., amphotericin B, disseminated intravascular coagulation, hypersplenism). In appropriate situations, HLA-matched platelets can sometimes be beneficial in overcoming platelet refractoriness.[34,35]

ACELLULAR BLOOD PRODUCT TRANSFUSIONS

Fresh Frozen Plasma

Fresh frozen plasma (FFP) contains all labile and stable coagulation factors and is indicated for multiple coagulation deficiencies.[36,37] In general, however, if coagulation tests (prothrombin time, partial thromboplastin time) are less than 1.5 times normal, FFP will not correct the deficit.[17] FFP can be used for the immediate reversal of warfarin therapy[4,37] and for the correction of specific factor abnormalities when a purified product is not available. Specific recombinant factor is generally preferable to FFP when isolated coagulation factor deficiencies exist, because FFP is not virally inactivated. The recommended starting dose of FFP is 10 to 20 mL/kg for pediatric patients,[36] but caution must be used to avoid fluid overload because FFP is isotonic and an effective volume expander.[37]

Cryoprecipitate

Cryoprecipitate represents the components of plasma that precipitate from solution when thawed in the cold (4°C). It contains fibrinogen, fibronectin, von Willebrand factor, factor VIII, and factor XIII. Because cryoprecipitate does not contain all the clotting factors, it should not be used when the patient requires all factors to correct a coagulopathy. It can be used in bleeding patients to replace fibrinogen (when the level is <100 mg/dL) or if the patient has dysfunctional fibrinogen.[36] It can be used to replace factor XIII, von Willebrand factor, or factor VIII when recombinant factor is unavailable.[37]

Intravenous Immunoglobulin

Intravenous immunoglobulin (IVIG) is derived from pooled human plasma and contains immunoglobulin (Ig) G of all subclasses and allotypes but only minimal amounts of IgM and IgA. It can be used in patients with primary and secondary immunodeficiency syndromes and a variety of autoimmune disorders.[38] The dose and frequency of dosing are determined by the disease being treated.[39] IVIG is an acellular blood by-product and therefore does not carry the risk of cell-associated viruses. The product is now virally inactivated with an organic solvent-detergent, which eliminates the risk of lipid-enveloped viruses such as hepatitis B and C, herpesviruses, and retroviruses (including HIV).[39]

Factor VIIa

Activated factor VII (factor VIIa) is a recombinant factor that is indicated for hemophilia patients with inhibitors and for patients with liver disease who produce insufficient coagulation factors and cannot tolerate the necessary volume of FFP.[40] The standard dose is 90 µg/kg every 2 to 3 hours, but it has been used in other clinical situations at doses of 20 to 30 µg/kg.[40]

PRODUCT TREATMENT, TESTING, AND PREVENTION OF COMPLICATIONS

Irradiation

Graft-versus-host disease (GVHD), thought to be a consequence of transfused (donor) lymphocytes responding immunologically to recipient (host) HLA differences, is a reported complication of transfusion, especially in patients with poor lymphocyte function (e.g., neonates, immunocompromised patients, bone marrow transplant recipients). Irradiation is the only accepted method of preventing transfusion-associated GVHD, because leukofiltration does not eliminate the risk.[40] All immunocompromised patients are susceptible to transfusion-associated GVHD and should receive irradiated cellular blood products (including directed donor blood). Irradiated products should be used in infants younger than 1 year, patients with congenital immunodeficiencies, patients with solid organ or bone marrow transplants, HIV-positive patients, and patients on chemotherapy.[41,42]

Leukocyte Reduction

Leukocyte reduction, defined as a product with less than 5×10^6 donor leukocytes in the final transfused volume, is indicated when it is necessary to decrease the risk of cytomegalovirus transmission[43] and decrease rates of alloimmunization due to anti-HLA antibodies.[44] Practitioners are advised to discuss the specific clinical scenario with the blood bank to determine the appropriateness of using leukoreduced products.

Washed Blood Products

Washed packed RBCs or platelets are indicated for patients who have had significant allergic reactions that are not abrogated by the use of pretransfusion antihistamines.[45] Transfusion-associated allergic reactions are most commonly caused by the recipient's reaction to donor plasma proteins. These reactions are idiosyncratic, and a patient may have a relatively severe allergic reaction to one donor's plasma proteins but no subsequent reactions. Washing of RBCs with 1 to 2 L of sterile normal saline removes about 99% of plasma proteins, antibodies, and electrolytes.[46] It is important to point out that because washed products have been manipulated, there is a higher risk of bacterial contamination. RBCs must be used within 24 hours of washing or discarded, because after that time, the risk of bacterial contamination increases significantly.[46] Platelets, which are stored at room temperature and thus have an inherently higher risk of bacterial contamination, must be used within 4 hours of washing.[46]

Viral Transmission

The risk of transmitting viruses through transfusions is one of the most important considerations in deciding which blood product to use. Transfusion-associated viral infections have markedly diminished since the 1980s, and the advent of nucleic acid testing (NAT) for HIV and hepatitis C virus has further diminished the risk of viral transmission.[13,45] Currently, with mandated testing in the United States, the risk of HIV transmission is estimated at 1 in 1.9 million transfused units, and the risk of hepatitis C is 1 in 1.6 million units.[13,47] NAT is not currently performed for hepatitis B, and the risk of hepatitis B transmission is estimated at 1 in 180,000 units.[13,47] Hepatitis B vaccine is universally recommended for all babies born in the United States and for all patients who require chronic blood transfusions.

TRANSFUSION REACTIONS

Although the majority of transfusion reactions are self-limited, some can be life threatening, making it important for the pediatric hospitalist to be able to recognize a potential transfusion reaction. This section briefly describes the pathophysiology, symptoms, laboratory investigations, and treatment of immune-mediated transfusion reactions (Table 121-1). They are divided into acute (<24 hours) and delayed (>24 hours) reactions.

Acute Transfusion Reactions

Acute Hemolytic Transfusion Reactions

Donor-recipient Rh or ABO incompatibility is the most common cause of acute hemolytic transfusion reactions. They are usually caused by human errors such as mislabeling or transfusion of the wrong unit to a patient. Antibodies in the recipient's plasma react to antigens on the donor erythrocytes, causing rapid intravascular hemolysis of donor cells. Signs and symptoms include fever; chills; abdominal, chest, or lower back pain; nausea; vomiting; apprehension; hemoglobinuria; hypo- or hypertension; oliguria or anuria; disseminated intravascular coagulation; and shock. If an acute hemolytic transfusion reaction is suspected, the transfusion should be stopped immediately and therapeutic interventions initiated as necessary. Blood samples should be sent to the blood bank, according to the institution's transfusion reaction protocol. Blood and urine should be sent to the clinical laboratory to evaluate the patient's coagulation profile, hemoglobin, bilirubin, creatinine, and urinalysis, according to the clinical situation. The patient's cardiovascular status

Table 121-1 Acute Transfusion Reactions

Reaction	Signs and Symptoms	Evaluation	Management
Hemolytic transfusion reaction (AHTR)	Fever, chills, chest or back pain, tachycardia, hypotension, hypertension, DIC, oliguria, pallor, hemoglobinuria, shock	Coombs, CBC, creatinine, bilirubin, urinalysis, PT, PTT	Stop transfusion Cardiovascular and airway support (inotropes) Solu-Medrol (1-2 mg/kg/dose IV) Furosemide (1 mg/kg/dose IV) as needed DIC management as needed
Febrile nonhemolytic reaction	Fever >38.5°C, chills	Coombs (to exclude AHTR)	Acetaminophen (15 mg/kg/dose PO)
Minor allergic reaction	Hives, itching		Diphenhydramine (5 mg/kg/day IV or PO)
Anaphylaxis	Hives, chills, wheezing, laryngeal edema, dyspnea, hypotension		Stop transfusion Cardiovascular and airway support Solu-Medrol (1-2 mg/kg/dose IV) Epinephrine (subcutaneously or infusion)
TRALI	Respiratory distress, hypoxia	Chest radiograph, CBC	Respiratory support
Bacterial contamination	Fever (may be >40°C), chills, hypotension	Coombs (to exclude AHTR), blood culture	IV antibiotics Cardiovascular and airway support

AHTR, acute hemolytic transfusion reaction; CBC, complete blood count; DIC, disseminated intravascular coagulation; PT, prothrombin time; PTT, partial thromboplastin time; TRALI, transfusion-related acute lung injury.

and urine output should be closely monitored. Therapy consists of managing hypotension, disseminated intravascular coagulation, and urine output with conventional therapy (intravenous fluids, pressors such as dopamine, and furosemide). Treatment related to the transfusion reaction consists of the administration of 1 to 2 mg/kg of intravenous methylprednisolone (dexamethasone or hydrocortisone can also be used).

Febrile Nonhemolytic Reactions

Cytokines released from leukocytes within a donor product may cause fever during a transfusion. The incidence of febrile nonhemolytic reactions is lower in institutions that require white blood cells to be removed from blood products (leukoreduction). Because fever can also be a sign of acute hemolytic transfusion reaction or bacterial contamination, febrile nonhemolytic reaction is a diagnosis of exclusion. Management includes stopping the transfusion and sending specimens to the blood bank for analysis. If a hemolytic reaction is ruled out, the patient can be treated with acetaminophen and the transfusion resumed at a slow rate. Acetaminophen pretreatment should be given for future transfusions, although this might be required less often in institutions using leukoreduced products.[48]

Allergic Reactions

Mild reactions occur due to patient antibodies against donor plasma proteins. Severe reactions can occur in individuals who have immunoglobulin deficiencies (e.g., IgA deficiency) when they are exposed to donor immunoglobulins; this can occur with the patient's first transfusion (allosensitization is not required). Typical reactions are characterized by hives and itching and are treated with diphenhydramine or other antihistamines. Whether the transfusion is stopped depends on the severity. With more severe allergic reactions, children may have laryngeal edema and bronchospasm, requiring treatment with steroids or epinephrine and respiratory support. In these situations, the transfusion should be stopped, and any future administration of blood products should be done with premedication and close observation.

Transfusion-Related Acute Lung Injury

Transfusion-related acute lung injury (TRALI) is a new-onset lung injury that is temporally related to the transfusion of plasma containing blood products.[49] Within 6 hours of a transfusion, patients with TRALI typically develop bilateral chest infiltrates, respiratory distress, and hypoxia. They may or may not have associated symptoms of a transfusion reaction, such as fever, chills, and hypotension or hypertension. A complete blood count in the earliest phase may demonstrate a transient leukopenia. The pathophysiology is thought to involve the transfer of antileukocyte antibodies and other granulocyte activators from the donor plasma in the transfused blood product; these antibodies interact with the recipient's leukocytes to cause endothelial damage, with resultant capillary leak and pulmonary edema. Unlike many other causes of acute lung injury, TRALI is transient, and most patients recover within 48 to 96 hours of onset. Management includes respiratory support and notifying the blood bank that a suspected TRALI workup should be initiated.

Non-Immune-Mediated Transfusion Reactions

These reactions include coagulopathy associated with dilution of clotting proteins (volume overload), hypothermia, hypo- or hyperkalemia, or hypocalcemia. Many of these conditions are most commonly encountered during a massive blood product resuscitation (e.g., after trauma or during surgical procedures associated with high blood loss).

Delayed Hemolytic Transfusion Reactions

Delayed hemolytic transfusion reactions occur when the recipient develops antibodies against a donor blood product more than 24 hours after the transfusion. There are two types of delayed hemolytic transfusion reactions: primary immunization and amnestic response. Primary immunization occurs weeks after a transfusion and should be suspected when an individual does not get the expected rise in hemoglobin from a previous transfusion; it rarely causes significant hemolysis. An amnestic response occurs in a patient who has been sensitized to minor blood group antigens from prior transfusions; this should be suspected in children requiring chronic or intermittent transfusion therapy, such as sickle cell or thalassemia patients. Patients may present up to 10 days after a transfusion with symptoms similar to those experienced with acute hemolytic transfusion reactions, but milder. They may have profound anemia and hyperbilirubinemia. The diagnosis is made by documenting a positive Coombs test or alloantibody. Management consists mainly of careful typing of any future blood products to avoid exposure to the offending minor antigen. Allosensitization occurs more frequently in the setting of periodic or intermittent transfusions rather than chronic (e.g., monthly) replacement.

IN A NUTSHELL

- Although specific parameters can be used to guide the transfusion of blood products, clinical judgment is paramount.
- The widespread use of NAT has substantially decreased the risk of transmission of HIV and hepatitis C through transfusions.
- Appropriate treatment of blood products before transfusion can minimize some of the risks and reactions associated with transfusion.
- When in doubt about which blood product to use or how to best use the product in a specific clinical situation, consultation with a blood bank specialist is advised.
- Transfusion reactions can be immediate or delayed, and it is important to be aware of the varied and often nonspecific presentations.

ON THE HORIZON

- Research into the development of safe hemoglobin substitutes to function as oxygen carriers is moving forward rapidly.
- Refinement of guidelines for the administration of factor VIIa is a high priority in the hematology community.
- There is a need to expand the blood donor pool in light of stricter donor deferral rules. Progress must be made in finding new ways to recruit donors.

SUGGESTED READING

Goodnough LT, Brecher ME, Kanter MH, AuBuchon JP: Transfusion medicine: First of two parts—blood transfusion. N Engl J Med 1999;340:438-447.

Guidelines for the use of fresh-frozen plasma, cryoprecipitate and cryosupernatant. Br J Haematol 2004;126:11-28.

Stramer SL: US NAT yield: Where are we after 2 years? Transfus Med 2002;12:243-253.

Vichinsky EP: Current issues with blood transfusions in sickle cell disease. Semin Hematol 2001;38(1 Suppl 1):14-22.

REFERENCES

1. Wallace EL, Churchill WH, Surgenor DM, et al: Collection and transfusion of blood and blood components in the United States, 1994. Transfusion 1998;38:625-636.
2. Wallace EL, Sullivan MT: New beginnings: The National Blood Data Resource Center. Transfusion 1998;38:622-624.
3. Consensus conference: Perioperative red blood cell transfusion. JAMA 1988;260:2700-2703.
4. Nuttall GA, Stehling LC, Beighley CM, Faust RJ: Current transfusion practices of members of the American Society of Anesthesiologists: A survey. Anesthesiology 2003;99:1433-1443.
5. Simon TL, Alverson DC, AuBuchon J, et al: Practice parameter for the use of red blood cell transfusions: Developed by the Red Blood Cell Administration Practice Guideline Development Task Force of the College of American Pathologists. Arch Pathol Lab Med 1998;122:130-138.
6. Haller M, Forst H: Red cell transfusion therapy in the critical care setting. Transfus Sci 1997;18:459-477.
7. Stehling L, Simon TL: The red blood cell transfusion trigger: Physiology and clinical studies. Arch Pathol Lab Med 1994;118:429-434.
8. Goodnough LT, Brecher ME, Kanter MH, AuBuchon JP: Transfusion medicine: First of two parts—blood transfusion. N Engl J Med 1999;340:438-447.
9. Brecher ME: Blood transfusion practice. In AABB Technical Manual, 14th ed. Bethesda, Md, American Association of Blood Banks, 2002, pp 451-483.
10. Aygun B, Padmanabhan S, Paley C, Chandrasekaran V: Clinical significance of RBC alloantibodies and autoantibodies in sickle cell patients who received transfusions. Transfusion 2002;42:37-43.
11. Ludvigsen CW Jr, Swanson JL, Thompson TR, McCullough J: The failure of neonates to form red blood cell alloantibodies in response to multiple transfusions. Am J Clin Pathol 1987;87:250-251.
12. Floss AM, Strauss RG, Goeken N, Knox L: Multiple transfusions fail to provoke antibodies against blood cell antigens in human infants. Transfusion 1986;26:419-422.
13. Hume H, Blanchette V, Strauss RG, Levy GJ: A survey of Canadian neonatal blood transfusion practices. Transfus Sci 1997;18:71-80.
14. Levy GJ, Strauss RG, Hume H, et al: National survey of neonatal transfusion practices. I. Red blood cell therapy. Pediatrics 1993;91:523-529.
15. American Association of Blood Banks: Neonatal and Pediatric Transfusion Practice, 14th ed. Bethesda, Md, American Association of Blood Banks, 2003, pp 517-537.
16. Toy P: Red blood cell transfusion and the transfusion trigger, including the surgical setting. In Hillyer CD, Silberstein L, Ness P, Anderson KC (eds): Blood Banking and Transfusion Medicine: Basic Principles and Practice, 1st ed. Philadelphia, Churchill Livingstone, 2003, pp 283-290.
17. Practice guidelines for blood component therapy: A report by the American Society of Anesthesiologists Task Force on Blood Component Therapy. Anesthesiology 1996;84:732-747.
18. Strauss RG: Transfusion of the neonate and pediatric patient. In Hillyer CD, Silberstein L, Ness P, Anderson KC (eds): Blood Banking and Transfusion Medicine: Basic Principles and Practice, 1st ed. Philadelphia, Churchill Livingstone, 2003, pp 335-345.
19. Vichinsky EP, Haberkern CM, Neumayr L, et al: A comparison of conservative and aggressive transfusion regimens in the perioperative

management of sickle cell disease. The Preoperative Transfusion in Sickle Cell Disease Study Group. N Engl J Med 1995;333:206-213.

20. Old JM, Olivieri NF, Thein SL, et al: Management and Prognosis. The Thalassaemia Syndromes, 4th ed. London, Blackwell Science, 2001, pp 630-685.

21. Olivieri NF: The beta-thalassemias. N Engl J Med 1999;341:99-109.

22. Cunningham MJ, Macklin EA, Neufeld EJ, Cohen AR: Complications of beta-thalassemia major in North America. Blood 2004;104:34-39.

23. Cazzola M, Borgna-Pignatti C, Locatelli F, et al: A moderate transfusion regimen may reduce iron loading in beta-thalassemia major without producing excessive expansion of erythropoiesis. Transfusion 1997;37: 135-140.

24. Vichinsky EP: Current issues with blood transfusions in sickle cell disease. Semin Hematol 2001;38(1 Suppl 1):14-22.

25. Ohene-Frempong K: Indications for red cell transfusion in sickle cell disease. Semin Hematol 2001;38(1 Suppl 1):5-13.

26. Adams RJ, Brambilla DJ, Granger S, et al: Stroke and conversion to high risk in children screened with transcranial Doppler ultrasound during the STOP study. Blood 2004;103:3689-3694.

27. Miller ST, Wright E, Abboud M, et al: Impact of chronic transfusion on incidence of pain and acute chest syndrome during the Stroke Prevention Trial (STOP) in sickle-cell anemia. J Pediatr 2001;139:785-789.

28. Eckman JR: Techniques for blood administration in sickle cell patients. Semin Hematol 2001;38(1 Suppl 1):23-29.

29. Schmalzer EA, Lee JO, Brown AK, et al: Viscosity of mixtures of sickle and normal red cells at varying hematocrit levels: Implications for transfusion. Transfusion 1987;27:228-233.

30. Nugent DJ: Platelet transfusion. In Nathan DG, Orkin SH (eds): Hematology of Infancy and Childhood, 5th ed. Philadelphia, WB Saunders, 1998, pp 1802-1817.

31. Aster RH: Effect of anticoagulant and ABO incompatibility on recovery of transfused human platelets. Blood 1965;26:732-743.

32. Menitove JE: Immunoprophylaxis for D– patients receiving platelet transfusions from D+ donors? Transfusion 2002;42:136-138.

33. Askari S, Weik PR, Crosson J: Calculated platelet dose: Is it useful in clinical practice? J Clin Apheresis 2002;17:103-105.

34. Dan ME, Schiffer CA: Strategies for managing refractoriness to platelet transfusions. Curr Hematol Rep 2003;2:158-164.

35. Levin MD, Kappers-Klunne M, Sintnicolaas K, et al: The value of alloantibody detection in predicting response to HLA-matched platelet transfusions. Br J Haematol 2004;124:244-250.

36. Guidelines for the use of fresh-frozen plasma, cryoprecipitate and cryosupernatant. Br J Haematol 2004;126:11-28.

37. Practice parameter for the use of fresh-frozen plasma, cryoprecipitate, and platelets. Fresh-Frozen Plasma, Cryoprecipitate, and Platelets Administration Practice Guidelines Development Task Force of the College of American Pathologists. JAMA 1994;271:777-781.

38. Clinical uses of intravenous immunoglobulin. Clin Exp Immunol 2005; 142:1-11.

39. Strauss RG: Transfusion of the neonate and pediatric patient. In Hillyer CD, Silberstein L, Ness P, Anderson KC (eds): Blood Banking and Transfusion Medicine: Basic Principles and Practice, 1st ed. Philadelphia, Churchill Livingstone, 2003, pp 167-180.

40. Goodnough LT, Lublin DM, Zhang L, et al: Transfusion medicine service policies for recombinant factor VIIa administration. Transfusion 2004;44: 1325-1331.

41. Orlin JB, Ellis MH: Transfusion-associated graft-versus-host disease. Curr Opin Hematol 1997;4:442-448.

42. Weiss B, Hoffmann M, Anders C, et al: Gamma-irradiation of blood products following autologous stem cell transplantation: Surveillance of the policy of 35 centers. Ann Hematol 2004;83:44-49.

43. Preiksaitis JK: The cytomegalovirus-"safe" blood product: Is leukoreduction equivalent to antibody screening? Transfus Med Rev 2000;14:112-136.

44. Seftel MD, Growe GH, Petraszko T, et al: Universal prestorage leukoreduction in Canada decreases platelet alloimmunization and refractoriness. Blood 2004;103:333-339.

45. Buck SA, Kickler TS, McGuire M, et al: The utility of platelet washing using an automated procedure for severe platelet allergic reactions. Transfusion 1987;27:391-393.

46. American Association of Blood Banks: Preparation, Storage, and Distribution of Components from Whole Blood Donations, 14th ed. Bethesda, Md, American Association of Blood Banks, 2003, pp 161-186.

47. Stramer SL: US NAT yield: Where are we after 2 years? Transfus Med 2002;12:243-253.

48. Sanders RP, Maddirala SD, Geiger TL, et al: Premedication with acetaminophen or diphenhydramine for transfusion with leucoreduced blood products in children. Br J Haematol 2005;130:781-787.

49. Sanchez R, Toy P: Transfusion related acute lung injury: A pediatric perspective. PBC 2005;45:248-255.

Oncology

CHAPTER 122

Oncologic Emergencies

Elizabeth A. Mullen

The recognition of an oncologic emergency is a critical task. Both at presentation and during treatment, pediatric cancer patients can develop acute, severe, life-threatening conditions (Table 122-1). Some of these emergent conditions can be generalized to all pediatric patients and are addressed elsewhere in this book. This chapter is an overview of the presentation and initial management of the most common emergent conditions encountered in pediatric cancer patients. Although many of these conditions have general treatment algorithms, the pediatric hospitalist should always be cognizant of the special circumstances of pediatric cancer patients and be prepared to adapt targeted therapies as needed.

Most childhood cancers present with signs and symptoms of invasion of a normal body cavity by malignant cells. This can manifest as pallor and bruising resulting from replacement of the bone marrow by leukemic or metastatic solid tumor cells. Abdominal symptoms such as pain, constipation, or distention can be caused by mass effect from an underlying Wilms tumor, neuroblastoma, sarcoma, or lymphoma. In rare instances, the location of a tumor mass or the degree of tumor burden can cause the sudden onset of life-threatening symptoms. A mediastinal mass can cause compression of the trachea and significant respiratory compromise.[1] Tumors involving the central nervous system can cause increased intracranial pressure (ICP), with the potential for uncal herniation, or symptomatic spinal cord compression. Metabolic derangements from high tumor burden and rapid cell turnover can lead to renal or cardiac dysfunction. Prompt recognition and rapid diagnosis and treatment are essential in these cases.

Once a presentation of cancer has been identified, a pediatric oncologist should immediately be involved in the initial diagnostic and therapeutic management. After stabilization, most pediatric cancer patients benefit from rapid referral to a tertiary care center with a subspecialty pediatric oncology program. The ideal treatment of many oncologic emergencies may involve the initiation of chemotherapy, which should be done in a facility and by physicians experienced with the administration of chemotherapy to children.

METABOLIC EMERGENCIES

Tumor Lysis Syndrome

Tumor lysis syndrome (TLS) is defined by the triad of hyperuricemia, hyperkalemia, and hyperphosphatemia. It results from the release of the intracellular contents of tumor cells. TLS can have high morbidity and can progress to multiorgan failure. It is most often associated with the initiation of therapy for cancers with massive tumor burden or high cell turnover. Patients occasionally have evidence of TLS at presentation, even before the initiation of therapy. This occurs most often in the setting of high-grade non-Hodgkin's (Burkitt's) lymphoma or the acute leukemias.[2-4] Increased lactate dehydrogenase, uric acid, and creatinine and decreased urine output are predictors of increased severity of TLS and increased risk of acute renal and end-organ failure.[2] Recognition of risk and prevention of complications are critical. Treatment should be initiated immediately when TLS is identified (Table 122-2).

Hyperuricemia

Hyperuricemia in TLS results from the breakdown of nucleic acid. Hyperuricemia should be treated with vigorous hydration, forced diuresis, and alkalization with allopurinol or rasburicase. The metabolic pathway of uric acid production is demonstrated in Figure 122-1. Hypoxanthine and xanthine are converted by xanthine oxidase to uric acid. Uric acid precipitates in acidic urine and deposits in the renal tubules. Allopurinol blocks the action of xanthine oxidase and limits the buildup of uric acid (but does not reduce previously formed uric acid). Purine precursors also continue to accumulate, and their excretion is aided by alkalization of the urine.[3] Urate oxidase catalyzes the oxidation of uric acid into allantoin, which is readily excretable. A recombinant form of urate oxidase (rasburicase) has been approved by the Food and Drug Administration for the initial management of pediatric patients with elevated plasma uric acid levels who are receiving anticancer therapy. Several studies in pediatric patients have demonstrated the safety and efficacy of rasburicase, as well as its improved uric acid reduction compared

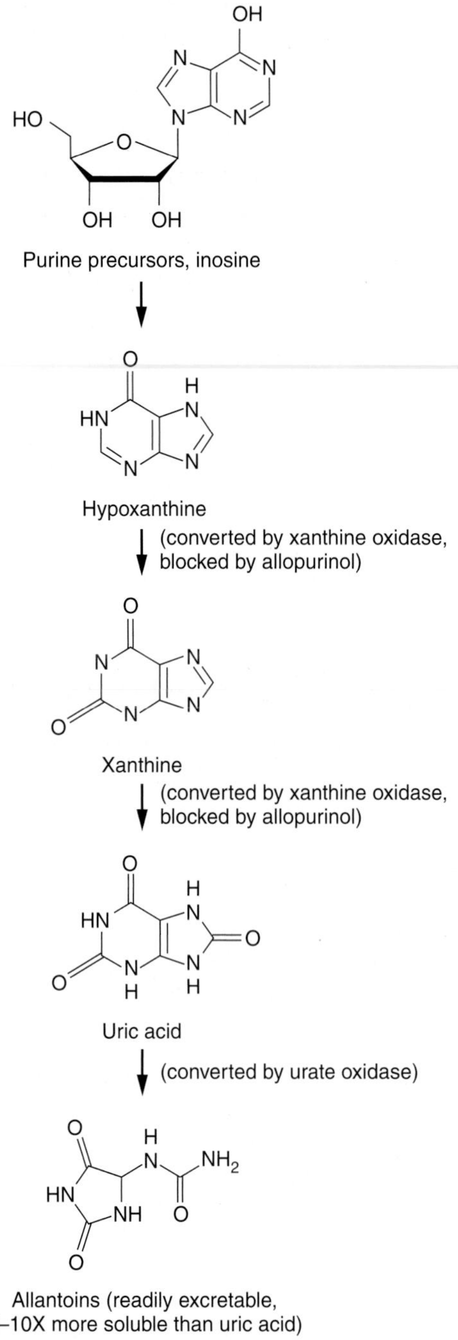

Purine precursors, inosine

↓

Hypoxanthine

↓ (converted by xanthine oxidase, blocked by allopurinol)

Xanthine

↓ (converted by xanthine oxidase, blocked by allopurinol)

Uric acid

↓ (converted by urate oxidase)

Allantoins (readily excretable, 5–10X more soluble than uric acid)

Figure 122-1 Uric acid metabolism.

Table 122-1   Pediatric Oncologic Emergencies
Metabolic emergencies
Tumor lysis syndrome, hyperuricemia
Hypercalcemia
Hyponatremia
Hematologic emergencies
Hyperleukocytosis, leukostasis
Hemorrhage, coagulopathy
Thrombosis
Mechanical emergencies
Superior vena cava syndrome, superior mediastinal syndrome
Spinal cord compression
Increased intracranial pressure
Massive organomegaly
Pleural and pericardial effusions
Cardiac tamponade
Infectious and inflammatory emergencies
Septicemia, shock
Typhlitis
Pneumonitis
Pancreatitis
Other emergencies
Pain
Malignant hypertension
Seizures

with allopurinol.[4,5] However, allopurinol is effective in preventing TLS, is readily available, and is comparatively inexpensive. Thus, the use of rasburicase should be reserved for a select population of patients, particularly those with elevated uric acid levels in combination with other known markers of predicted severe TLS.[6] Guidelines for the administration of allopurinol and rasburicase are given in Table 122-3.

Hyperkalemia, Hyperphosphatemia, and Hypocalcemia

The hyperkalemia, hyperphosphatemia, and hypocalcemia associated with TLS must also be rapidly identified and treated (Table 122-4). Hyperkalemia can be the most life-threatening complication of TLS. Potassium is present in high concentrations intracellularly. Cell lysis and high turnover can lead to a rapid increase in serum levels, particularly when combined with some degree of renal dysfunction. Metabolic acidosis can also contribute to the rapid worsening of hyperkalemia.

Hyperphosphatemia also results from the lysis of tumor cells. Lymphoblasts contain three to four times the amount of phosphorus of normal lymphocytes. With hyperphosphatemia, calcium-phosphate complexes exceed their solubility product, and calcium phosphate can precipitate in the renal tubules and renal microvasculature, causing significant nephropathy. Hypocalcemia results from hyperphosphatemia and must be monitored closely. When it is clinically symptomatic, hypocalcemia must be treated. Clinical symptoms of the metabolic derangements seen in TLS are presented in Table 122-4.

Hypercalcemia

Pediatric cancers can be associated with hypercalcemia, although much less frequently than in adult malignancies. The initial evaluation of a pediatric patient with a new diagnosis of cancer should include screening electrolytes. If hypercalcemia is identified, it should be carefully monitored; if a patient becomes symptomatic or serum levels rise above 12 mg/dL, intervention is required.

Syndrome of Inappropriate Antidiuretic Hormone Secretion and Hyponatremia

Syndrome of inappropriate antidiuretic hormone secretion (SIADH) and hyponatremia are encountered occasionally in pediatric oncology patients. The cause is usually the

Table 122-2 Initial Treatment and Prevention of Tumor Lysis Syndrome

Hydration and alkalization with 3 L/m²/day of D5/¼NS with 75 mEq NaHCO₃/L to maintain urine output >100 mL/m²/hr, specific gravity <1.010, and urine pH 6.5-7.5
  Do *not* alkalinize if giving uric acid oxidase (rasburicase) instead of allopurinol
  May use furosemide (1-2 mg/kg) or mannitol (0.5 mg/kg) to increase urine output if necessary; avoid in hypovolemic patients

Initiate uric acid–reducing therapy—allopurinol or rasburicase (see Table 122-3)*
Monitor strict intake and output; measure weight bid
Take vital signs at least q4h; place on cardiovascular-respiratory monitor if any significant metabolic abnormalities
Monitor lysis laboratory studies q8h, or more frequently if indicated   Electrolytes, blood urea nitrogen, creatinine, uric acid, ionized calcium, magnesium, phosphorus, lactate dehydrogenase, urine pH
Avoid nephrotoxic medications or IV contrast material
Avoid supplemental potassium or phosphorus intake
Monitor for associated hyperkalemia, hyperphosphatemia, and hypocalcemia and treat as clinically indicated (see Table 122-4)
For severe metabolic abnormalities, persistent oliguria, or renal failure, hemofiltration or dialysis may be warranted

*Rasburicase *should not* be used in patients with known or suspected glucose-6-phosphate dehydrogenase deficiency because severe hemolysis can occur, further increasing the likelihood of renal impairment.

Table 122-3 Guidelines for Administration of Allopurinol and Rasburicase

Allopurinol
Begin 24-48 hr before start of cytoreductive therapy
Give with IV hydration at 1.5-2 times maintenance, with NaHCO₃
Follow urine pH, and maintain at 6.5-7.5; avoid excess alkalization, which may cause calcium phosphate precipitation
Administer IV or PO; children often have difficulty with oral administration
  Allopurinol PO 100 mg/m²/dose tid, or 10 mg/kg/day divided bid-tid (maximum dose 800 mg/day)
  Allopurinol IV 200 mg/m²/day in 1-3 divided doses

Rasburicase
Recommended dose: 0.15 or 0.20 mg/kg/day for 5 days
Administer as a single daily dose via IV infusion over 30 min
Chemotherapy should be administered 4 to 24 hr after initial dose of rasburicase
Rasburicase causes continued degradation of uric acid in blood, plasma, and serum samples, which must be processed on ice, according to manufacturer's instructions
Urine should not be alkalinized
IV fluid at 1.5-2 times maintenance should be continued
Do not administer to G6PD-deficient patients; if G6PD deficiency is suspected, status should be confirmed before administration

G6PD, glucose-6-phosphate dehydrogenase.

administration of chemotherapeutic agents, most commonly vincristine or etoposide. Some tumors may be associated with SIADH, particularly tumors of the central nervous system. Full assessment of intake and output, as well as serum and urine electrolytes and osmolality, should be performed. As in all cases of SIADH, fluid restriction is the mainstay of treatment. However, this is sometimes contraindicated in the setting of required hyperhydration during chemotherapy. Consultation with a pediatric oncologist is advised in these situations.

HEMATOLOGIC EMERGENCIES

Leukocytosis and Leukostasis

Leukocytosis is defined as a white blood cell count greater than 100×10^9/L.[7] It has been reported to occur in up to 20% of childhood leukemias. Although it is more common in

acute lymphoblastic leukemia (ALL) than in acute myelocytic leukemia (AML), more significant clinical consequences of leukostasis are observed in AML. Increased blood viscosity, sludging of the circulation, and small-vessel thrombi can occur. The intracerebral and pulmonary circulations are most at risk. Priapism, ischemic cardiac and renal failure, and acute ischemia of digits can also occur.

Prompt administration of intravenous fluid and the institution of tumor lysis prevention are the first steps in the initial management of hyperleukocytosis. Red cell transfusions and diuretics should be avoided if possible, because these increase blood viscosity. Directed antitumor therapy is the most efficient means of decreasing the white blood cell count. It is critical that a pediatric oncologist be consulted to obtain the necessary diagnostic tissue and institute the appropriate course of chemotherapy.

The role of leukapheresis and exchange transfusion in hyperleukocytosis is controversial, and a decision to institute

Table 122-4   Treatment of Metabolic Derangements Associated with Tumor Lysis Syndrome

Disorder	Clinical Features	Treatment
Hyperkalemia	ECG abnormalities: peaked T waves, lengthening of P-R interval, widened QRS complex. Can lead to arrhythmias and cardiac arrest. Paresthesias, paralysis	Avoid any potassium intake. Oral potassium-binding resin (sodium polystyrene sulfonate) 0.25 g/kg q6h. IV furosemide 0.5-1 mg/kg/dose. IV glucose and insulin: 1 g/kg glucose with 0.25 unit/kg insulin. IV sodium bicarbonate 1-2 mmol/kg (dilute 1:10 with 0.9% NaCl if given peripherally, 1:5 if centrally). IV 10% calcium gluconate 0.3-0.5 mL/kg slow bolus; must monitor for bradycardia; use only for severe life-threatening arrhythmias; may cause calcium phosphate precipitation
Hyperphosphatemia	Related to resultant hypocalcemia	Avoid dietary phosphate, phosphate-containing medications. Oral phosphate binder: aluminum hydroxide 50 mg/kg q8h. Forced diuresis (hydration, furosemide, mannitol). IV glucose and insulin (see hyperkalemia above)
Hypocalcemia	Positive Trousseau or Chvostek sign, tetany, seizure, laryngospasm, carpopedal spasm. Prolonged Q-T interval on ECG	Control hyperphosphatemia. Implement seizure precautions. If severely symptomatic, treat with IV 10% calcium gluconate 0.3-0.5 mL/kg slow bolus; must monitor for bradycardia; may cause calcium phosphate precipitation
Hyperuricemia	Clinical symptoms usually associated with levels >10 mg/dL and include lethargy, nausea, vomiting, uric acid calculi, hematuria, oliguria, anuria	Hydration; allopurinol or rasburicase (see Table 122-3)

ECG, electrocardiogram.
Adapted from Cairo MS, Bishop M: Tumor lysis syndrome: New therapeutic strategies and classification. Br J Haematol 2004;127:3-11; Nicolin G: Emergencies and their management. Eur J Cancer 2002;38:1365-1377, and Secola R, Cairo M, Bessmertny O, Bergeron S: Tumor Lysis Syndrome (TLS) Guidelines. COG Nursing Discipline, COG Nursing Clinical Practice Subcommittee, Pharmacology Section, 2002.

these procedures should involve a pediatric oncologist. These procedures are considered for a white blood cell count greater than 100×10^9/L in AML and greater than 500×10^9/L in ALL, as well as for any symptomatic patient. Symptoms depend on the systems involved. Patients with pulmonary leukostasis have tachypnea, desaturation, and respiratory compromise. Patients with intracerebral involvement most commonly have headache but can also present with papilledema, stroke, or seizure.

Hemorrhage and Disseminated Intravascular Coagulation

Severely depressed blood counts are commonly seen in pediatric oncology patients. Cytopenias can result from direct invasion of the marrow and replacement of normal marrow elements, or they can be a consequence of both chemotherapy and radiation therapy. Markedly decreased platelet numbers can lead to symptomatic and severe bleeding or hemorrhage. Particular chemotherapy agents, such as asparaginase, carry the risk of causing hemorrhagic stroke. Some pediatric malignancies, particularly some subtypes of AML (M3, M4, and, less commonly, M5), can present with severe and symptomatic disseminated intravascular coagulation (DIC). DIC is also commonly seen in sepsis (for which pediatric cancer patients are at very high risk) and in some rare patients with widely disseminated solid tumors.

Pediatric oncology patients may present acutely with hemorrhage and DIC requiring emergent management. A complete guide to pediatric oncologic transfusion medicine is beyond the scope of this chapter; however, several principles of transfusion medicine are unique to cancer patients. In general, it is recommended that blood product replacement be discussed with a transfusion medicine specialist or a pediatric hematologist or oncologist.

Although it is often required as part of a cancer treatment program, patient exposure to blood products should be minimized. The threshold for transfusion varies at different centers, but it should be based on a careful weighing of the risks and benefits for each individual patient. In the case of a pediatric patient with hemorrhage or DIC, however, blood product support is clearly indicated. Based on symptoms and blood counts, patients with hemorrhage likely require both platelet and packed red blood cell transfusions. Patients with DIC may require cryoprecipitate for fibrinogen replacement and fresh frozen plasma for correction of prolonged prothrombin time and partial thromboplastin time through factor replacement. As in any clinical situation involving DIC, correction of the underlying cause is imperative. In the case of leukemia-associated coagulopathy, appropriate chemotherapy must be initiated to treat the underlying cause of DIC. Specific leukemia blast cells (such as in acute promyelocytic leukemia) have been shown to cause DIC, and resolution of DIC correlates with clearance of peripheral blast cells.

Correction of both thrombocytopenia and coagulopathy should be achieved before invasive procedures such as surgical placement of indwelling central catheters and lumbar puncture. Bone marrow aspiration, however, usually does not carry a high risk of bleeding complications, even in patients with disrupted coagulation.

Blood products administered to pediatric oncology patients must be selected carefully because of the particular risks inherent in this population. The following general principles should be observed.

- All blood and platelets should be irradiated before administration to prevent the potentially lethal complication of graft-versus-host disease in immunocompromised patients.
- Leukofiltration of blood and platelets is recommended for all pediatric oncologic patients to decrease the risk of alloimmunization and febrile transfusion reactions.
- Nonimmunity to cytomegalovirus (CMV) should be assumed in pediatric oncology patients, and ideally, blood products should be CMV negative. If CMV-negative products are not available and there is an emergent need for the administration of blood products, leukocyte filtration decreases the risk of transmission of CMV.
- Directed donation of blood products from related family members is discouraged in oncology patients who may need bone marrow or stem cell transplantation at some point. Exposure to familial human leukocyte antigens may increase the risk of graft rejection.

Thrombosis

Thrombosis in pediatric oncologic patients is most often related to therapy and usually does not confer a need for lifetime anticoagulant therapy. However, to prevent long-term consequences of thrombosis, prompt and appropriate evaluation and management are crucial and may require timely initiation by a pediatric hospitalist.

The risk of thrombosis is increased in pediatric cancer patients. The most common risk factor is the presence of indwelling central venous catheters. Studies have shown that catheter-associated clots can be found in the majority of pediatric patients with indwelling central lines, although not all clots are symptomatic. Certain medications commonly used in childhood leukemia treatment, such as L-asparaginase, increase the risk of thrombosis. This likely occurs through the depletion of antithrombin III, plasminogen, protein C, and protein S. Although much less common in pediatric cancer patients than in adults, hypercoagulable states can be associated with malignancy.

The clinical presentation of thrombosis is varied but may include extremity or facial swelling, superior vena cava (SVC) syndrome, central venous line malfunction, or new neurologic symptoms. The suspicion for thrombosis should be high in these situations, and an evaluation with the appropriate imaging modality is indicated. The role of testing for D dimers is not clear; they are often elevated in cancer patients, but thrombosis can clearly occur in the absence of increased D dimers.

Once identified, the management of thrombosis in pediatric cancer patients is individualized. The role and choice of anticoagulant therapy are dependent on factors such as clot location, use of chemotherapy agents with inherent throm- botic risk, overall expected degree of myelosuppression, age and activity level of the child, need for central venous access, tolerance of subcutaneous therapy, and other identified prothrombotic risk factors. In patients with thrombosis, anticoagulant therapy with agents such as enoxaparin can allow treatment with L-asparaginase to continue safely. However, for effective anticoagulation with enoxaparin, antithrombin III replacement is often required during asparaginase therapy, owing to decreased production due to decreased protein synthesis.

INFECTIOUS AND INFLAMMATORY EMERGENCIES

The most common infectious and inflammatory emergency for pediatric cancer patients is fever and neutropenia, which is discussed in Chapter 124.

MECHANICAL EMERGENCIES

Anterior Mediastinal Mass

Space-occupying lesions in the thoracic cavity can impinge on vital structures, causing gradual or sudden airway or cardiac compromise. The most common cause of compression of the large airways or pulmonary vessels is the presence of an anterior mediastinal mass. Lymphoid malignancies such as Hodgkin's lymphoma, non-Hodgkin's lymphoma, and acute leukemia (most often T-cell ALL) are the most common causes of anterior mediastinal masses. The differential diagnosis also includes germ cell tumor, Ewing sarcoma, neuroblastoma, rhabdomyosarcoma, thymoma, and thyroid malignancy. The presence of an anterior mediastinal mass can cause two pathophysiologically distinct but often overlapping clinical emergencies: tracheal compression and SVC syndrome.

Tracheal compression in a patient with an anterior mediastinal mass can present with gradual or sudden symptoms of airway obstruction. The clinical symptoms relate to the level, degree, and rate of change of the obstruction. Stridor is usually a manifestation of extrathoracic involvement. Lower obstruction of the trachea or mainstem bronchi can present with wheeze, cough, dyspnea, orthopnea, dizziness, and syncope. Often these symptoms are worse when the patient is in the supine position, so this position should be avoided. Improvement in symptoms can occur when the patient is upright or prone, a maneuver that can be critical in a patient who is in severe distress.

SVC syndrome is caused by intrinsic compression of the superior vena cava, usually from a mass but sometimes from a clot, most often associated with an indwelling catheter. Patients with SVC syndrome present with edema and plethora or cyanosis of the face, neck, or upper extremities. In extreme cases, patients can present with shock due to cardiac compromise caused by decreased venous return and ventricular volume. Rarely, neurologic symptoms from increased ICP can occur due to severely impeded return and venous congestion. Echocardiograms and electrocardiograms are valuable diagnostic tools in patients with SVC syndrome, permitting assessment of the degree of cardiac compromise.

Once a mass has been identified, usually by chest radiograph, caution must be used when planning further diagnostic imaging or biopsy for histologic diagnosis. Placing a child in the supine position for imaging, or the use of sedation or anesthesia, can cause a rapid worsening of symptoms, including the precipitation of cardiorespiratory arrest. Diagnosis should be attempted through the least invasive method. If the blood smear is abnormal, a bone marrow biopsy with local anesthesia may provide a diagnosis. Peripheral lymph node biopsy should be considered if indicated by the physical examination. In a cooperative child, aspiration of pleural fluid may be possible under local sedation in an upright position. Elevated urinary catecholemines can be diagnostic of neuroblastoma; elevated tumor markers such as α-fetoprotein and β-human chorionic gonadotropin may be present if the mass is caused by a germ cell tumor.

If sedation is required for biopsy, the risk to the airway should be assessed. The clinical presence of orthopnea has been associated with a high risk of respiratory collapse. The best radiographic evaluation of the trachea is with lateral films and computed tomography scanning.[8] The risk of anesthesia can be assessed by measuring the cross-sectional diameter of the trachea on computed tomography. Pulmonary function tests, particularly peak expiratory flow rates, are also useful. Patients with a greater than 50% tracheal diameter and a peak expiratory flow rate greater than 50% generally tolerate anesthesia well. If these studies cannot be obtained or if the patient does not meet these criteria, anesthesia and intubation should be avoided, because these procedures can pose a significant risk of death for patients with anterior mediastinal masses. Any attempt at intubation in a child with an anterior mediastinal mass should be coordinated with specialists in pediatric anesthesia, pediatric intensive care medicine, or otolaryngology.

Although tissue diagnosis is needed to implement specific therapy, in some clinical situations, the risk of obtaining tissue is too great, and empirical therapy aimed at reducing the mass must be initiated. Emergent treatment modalities include radiation therapy, steroids, or chemotherapy. A pediatric oncologist should always be involved in this decision. Once treatment is initiated, the opportunity for accurate diagnosis may be lost, because many childhood cancers are extremely chemo- or radiosensitive.

Spinal Cord Compression

Spinal cord compression has been reported to occur in up to 5% of pediatric patients with solid tumors. It occurs most commonly in the terminal phase of widely metastatic cancers but can be the presenting sign of a previously undiagnosed cancer. Cancers associated with spinal cord compression include neuroblastoma, Ewing sarcoma, rhabdomyosarcoma, osteosarcoma, metastatic central nervous system tumors, lymphoma, and AML.[9] Back pain is the most common presenting symptom, but patients may also demonstrate loss of bladder or bowel function, loss of motor function (gait disturbance, weakness), loss of sensory function (paresthesias or dysesthesias), or localized spine tenderness.

Any patient presenting with these complaints or symptoms should have a thorough neurologic examination and consideration of immediate imaging. Magnetic resonance imaging is the optimal modality for imaging the spine. If cord compression is strongly suspected clinically or has been confirmed with imaging, intravenous dexamethasone

should be administered immediately at a dose of 1 mg/kg given over 30 minutes. An urgent decision regarding surgery (laminectomy or laminotomy), chemotherapy, or radiation must be made. A neurosurgeon, oncologist, and radiation oncologist should be involved in this decision. Although the primary goal is to restore neurologic function, the best treatment modality depends on several factors, including the extent of neurologic deficit and the timetable of progression, the ability to make a histologic diagnosis, the tumor type, and the expected response to chemotherapy or radiotherapy.[7]

Cerebral Herniation

The presence of an expanding intracranial mass can result in increased ICP and eventual uncal herniation. This grave complication can occur in pediatric oncology patients from an expanding or obstructive tumor mass or in association with complications of both the primary tumor and therapy. Treatment-related intracranial disasters include thrombosis, hemorrhage, infarction, and abscess. Ventriculoperitoneal shunt malfunction can also be a cause of increasing ICP.

Nausea, emesis, and stiff neck are the most common presenting signs. Abnormal eye findings, including pupil abnormalities, upward gaze limitation, and papilledema, should be carefully sought. Bradycardia, hypertension, and respiratory changes are late and emergent signs of increased ICP.

If increased ICP is suspected, immediate diagnostic and therapeutic measures are required. Computed tomography is the most rapidly available imaging study and can detect the presence of elevated ICP or impending cerebral herniation. After initial management, magnetic resonance imaging may be needed to better define the pathologic process, particularly for tumors in the posterior fossa. Patients with an indwelling ventriculoperitoneal or ventriculoatrial shunt should be assessed by a neurosurgeon immediately. A series of radiographs may be indicated to check shunt placement. Some shunts can also be adjusted externally to better equalize pressure.

As emergent treatment, intravenous mannitol can be administered as a 25% solution at a dose of 0.5 to 2 g/kg over 30 minutes. Hyperventilation (after intubation), with the goal of decreasing P_{CO_2} to 30 to 35 mm Hg, can be effective in the management of severe ICP. Intravenous dexamethasone may also be indicated and can be administered at a dose of 1 mg/kg over 30 minutes. Early consideration of surgical intervention is also critical.

IN A NUTSHELL

- Pediatric cancer is relatively rare, and the overall prognosis is very good. Significant morbidity and mortality still result from expected and unexpected complications of the underlying malignancy and its treatment.
- A pediatric hospitalist must be able to recognize these conditions as life threatening and initiate appropriate emergency treatment. Although early consultation with a pediatric oncologist is critical to the management of pediatric oncologic emergencies, treatment often needs to be instigated by the initial care provider.

- A careful physical examination and history, appropriate radiographic studies, and complete metabolic laboratory evaluation are required in the management of children with malignancies. Laboratory evaluation should include complete blood count, liver function tests, lactate dehydrogenase, uric acid, serum creatinine, and a full electrolyte panel including calcium, magnesium, and phosphorus.
- Intravenous access should be established, and airway management anticipated owing to the possibility of severe cardiac or respiratory compromise resulting from the rapid progression of the tumor.
- A stepwise plan for intervention in the face of progressive symptoms should be available.

ON THE HORIZON

- Numerous new drug therapies are under active study in the pediatric oncology population. Some of the most active research is in the area of targeted therapy, such as specific enzyme inhibitors and antibody therapies. Institution of more targeted therapy may decrease its overall toxicity, be less prone to precipitating metabolic emergencies, and reduce the overall morbidity of therapy.
- Earlier diagnosis and screening for those with realized genetic risks may lead to fewer pediatric cancers presenting as oncologic emergencies.
- Rasburicase is under active study in the pediatric population. Clarification of its safety profile and clear indications for its appropriate use may result in a marked decrease in the morbidity and mortality of severe TLS.

SUGGESTED READING

Adamson PC, Blaney SM: New approaches to drug development in pediatric oncology. Cancer J 2005;11:324-330.

Kelly KM, Lange B: Oncologic emergencies. Pediatr Clin North Am 1997;44:809-830.

Nicolin G: Emergencies and their management. Eur J Cancer 2002;38:1365-1377.

Poplack DG: Introduction: Pediatric oncology. Cancer J 2005;11:253-254.

Reaman GH: Pediatric oncology: Current views and outcomes. Pediatr Clin North Am 2002;49:1305-1318.

REFERENCES

1. Azizkhan RG, Dudgeon DL, Buck JR, et al: Life threatening airway obstruction as a complication to the management of mediastinal masses in children. J Pediatric Surg 1985;20:816-822.
2. Cairo MS, Bishop M: Tumor lysis syndrome: New therapeutic strategies and classification. Br J Haematol 2004;127:3-11.
3. Del Toro G, Morris E, Cairo M: Tumor lysis syndrome: Pathophysiology, definition, and alternative treatment approaches. Clin Adv Hematol Oncol 2005;3:54-61.
4. Goldman SC, Holcenberg JS, Finkelstein JZ, et al: A randomized comparison between rasburicase and allopurinol in children with lymphoma or leukemia at high risk for tumor lysis. Blood 2001;97:2998-3003.
5. Pui CH, Jeha S, Irwin S, Camitta B: Recombinant urate oxidase (rasburicase) in the prevention and treatment of malignancy-associated hyperuricemia in pediatric and adult patients: Results of a compassionate-use trial. Leukemia 2001;15:1505-1509.
6. Holdsworth MT, Nguyen P: Role of IV allopurinol and rasburicase in tumor lysis syndrome. Am J Health Syst Pharm 2003;60:2213-2224.
7. Nicolin G: Emergencies and their management. Eur J Cancer 2002;38:1365-1377.
8. Shamberger RC, Holzman RS, Griscom NT, et al: CT quantitation of tracheal cross-sectional area as a guide to the surgical and anesthetic management of children with anterior mediastinal masses. J Pediatr Surg 1991;26:138-142.
9. Lewis DW, Packer RJ, Raney B, et al: Incidence, presentation, and outcome of spinal cord disease in children with systemic cancer. Pediatrics 1986;78:438-443.

CHAPTER 123

Childhood Cancer

Barbara Degar and Michael Isakoff

Childhood cancer is rare, with approximately 7000 new cases diagnosed each year in the United States.[1] Nonetheless, cancer is the leading cause of disease-related mortality in children younger than 15 years. Pediatricians and general practitioners commonly encounter children with vague symptoms that could signal an undiagnosed cancer. The challenge is to identify those children who warrant an evaluation for malignancy. This chapter reviews the typical presentations of the most common pediatric hematologic and solid tumors and provides guidelines for the initial diagnostic evaluation. A review of current therapies and expected outcomes is beyond the scope of this chapter. However, it can be broadly stated that the majority of children diagnosed with cancer will be cured of their disease.

Cancer results from the uncontrolled proliferation of a clonal cell population, and it can arise in essentially any cell type or organ. In general, children with cancer present with symptoms related to the location and extent of the tumor. Cancers cause symptoms by invading or obstructing tissues locally or by spreading to distant sites, leading to pain, organ dysfunction, or both. During childhood, the incidence of specific malignancies varies dramatically with age. The most common types of cancer in children are hematologic malignancies (leukemias and lymphomas), brain tumors, and extracranial solid tumors, including sarcomas and embryonal tumors.

CAUSE

Because childhood cancer is rare and heterogeneous, the elucidation of its causes is extremely challenging. It is known that certain factors are associated with an increased risk of some types of childhood cancer. For example, in utero exposure to ionizing radiation leads to about a 1.5-fold increased risk of lymphoblastic leukemia. External beam radiation, sometimes used to treat patients with solid tumors, is associated with an increased risk of osteosarcoma within the radiation field. Patients with Down syndrome have a 20-fold increased risk of developing leukemia. Several other genetic syndromes are also associated with an increased risk of developing cancer, including neurofibromatosis, Beckwith-Wiedemann syndrome, and Li-Fraumeni syndrome (Table 123-1). However, in the vast majority of children with cancer, no predisposing factors are identified.

INCIDENCE

The incidence of childhood cancer is highest in the first year of life, declines until about age 9 years, and then gradually increases into adulthood. The peak rates of specific childhood malignancies occur at different ages. In a child with suspected cancer, the age at presentation has a major impact on the differential diagnosis.

Leukemia accounts for approximately one third of cancers diagnosed in childhood. In contrast to adults, acute lymphoblastic leukemia (ALL) occurs relatively more commonly than acute myeloid leukemia (AML). In fact, ALL is the most common childhood malignancy,[2] representing approximately 20% of cancers diagnosed in children younger than 15 years. The peak age at diagnosis of childhood ALL is 2 to 3 years. White children are about two times more likely than black children to be diagnosed with ALL, and boys are affected slightly more commonly than girls. In contrast, the incidence of AML peaks in the first year of life, subsequently decreases, and then gradually increases late in childhood and throughout adulthood. Chronic leukemias are distinctly uncommon in childhood. Chronic myeloid leukemia can occur at any age but accounts for only about 3% to 5% of childhood leukemia cases. Chronic lymphoid leukemia essentially does not occur in children. Non-Hodgkin's lymphomas account for 3% of cancers diagnosed in children, and Hodgkin's disease accounts for about 5%.

Among pediatric solid tumors, neuroblastoma is the most common, representing 8% of childhood cancers and affecting primarily children younger than 5 years. Wilms tumor accounts for 6% of childhood cancers and also occurs primarily in those younger than 5 years. The bone sarcomas, including osteosarcoma and Ewing sarcoma, together represent 5% of childhood cancers. These tumors generally affect older children, with the highest incidence in adolescence and young adulthood. Brain tumors are a diverse group of malignant neoplasms that, taken together, account for approximately 30% of childhood cancers.

HEMATOLOGIC MALIGNANCIES

Leukemia

ALL is the consequence of malignant transformation of lymphocyte precursors in the bone marrow or lymphoid organs. Patients with ALL typically present with symptoms caused by the impaired production of normal blood cells owing to the proliferation of leukemia cells in the bone marrow. Patients may demonstrate fatigue and pallor due to anemia. Decreased numbers of normal white blood cells lead to an increased risk of serious infection. Bruising and petechiae may be present due to thrombocytopenia. Coagulopathy can occur, magnifying the risk of serious bleeding. Patients may complain of bone pain related to infiltration and expansion of the bone marrow space. ALL cells may infiltrate organs such as the lymph nodes, liver, or spleen, resulting in lymphadenopathy or hepatosplenomegaly. Lymphoblasts may form solid masses, especially in the anterior mediastinum, leading to tracheal or vascular compression. Additionally, new-onset ALL uncommonly involves the central nervous system, testicles, and eye. Children with very

Table 123-1 Common Childhood Genetic Syndromes and Associated Malignancies

Genetic Syndrome	Associated Malignancy
Trisomy 21 (Down syndrome)	ALL, AML
Ataxia-telangiectasia	ALL
Familial monosomy 7	AML
Neurofibromatosis type 1	ALL, AML, optic glioma, rhabdomyosarcoma
Tuberous sclerosis	Brain tumors
Beckwith-Wiedemann syndrome	Wilms tumor, hepatoblastoma
Li-Fraumeni syndrome	Osteosarcoma, rhabdomyosarcoma, retinoblastoma
Nevus basal cell carcinoma syndrome	Medulloblastoma, rhabdomyosarcoma, basal cell carcinoma
Klinefelter syndrome	Dysgerminoma

ALL, acute lymphoblastic leukemia; AML, acute myeloid leukemia.

Table 123-2 Differential Diagnosis of Childhood Acute Lymphoblastic Leukemia

Noncancer diagnoses
  Infectious mononucleosis
  Juvenile rheumatoid arthritis
  Systemic lupus erythematosus
  Pertussis
  Immune thrombocytopenic purpura
  Aplastic anemia

Malignant diagnoses*
  Neuroblastoma
  Retinoblastoma
  Rhabdomyosarcoma
  Ewing sarcoma

*With small, round, blue cell morphology similar to acute lymphoblastic leukemia.

large numbers of circulating malignant cells (white blood cell counts >200,000/μL) may experience symptoms of hyperleukocytosis with visual changes or neurologic or respiratory symptoms (see Chapter 122).

AML is an analogous malignant process involving myeloid progenitors.[3] The presentation of childhood AML may be indistinguishable from that of childhood ALL. Fatigue, pallor, and fever are common presenting symptoms. The risk of bleeding in newly diagnosed AML is higher than in ALL, especially with certain histopathologically and molecularly defined AML subtypes. Disseminated intravascular coagulation may be present. Symptoms of hyperleukocytosis can occur in patients with AML at relatively lower white blood cell counts than in ALL. AML blasts may infiltrate tissues such as the gingivae, skin, visceral organs, and central nervous system. Leukemic tumor masses, called chloromas, are seen rarely.

The diagnosis of new-onset leukemia may be obvious or subtle. New-onset leukemia may even be asymptomatic, with an incidental finding of leukemia blasts on peripheral blood smears. Occasional patients present with prominent misleading symptoms, such as localized bone pain or abdominal pain. Often, the differential diagnosis includes benign conditions, including acute viral infection (e.g., Epstein-Barr virus), aplastic anemia, hemophagocytic syndrome, and other rare congenital disorders (Table 123-2).

When leukemia is suspected, the evaluation should begin with a complete blood count. The white blood cell count may be low, normal, or elevated. Leukemia blasts may be seen in the peripheral blood smear. Anemia with reticulocytopenia and thrombocytopenia is usually present but of variable severity. If the suspicion for leukemia is high, it is important to assess renal function and serum electrolytes, including calcium, phosphate, and uric acid. Patients with a large tumor burden and high proliferative rate may present

with features of acute tumor lysis syndrome (see Chapter 122) even before the initiation of cytotoxic therapy. Liver function tests should be performed; marked elevation of lactate dehydrogenase is often seen. Coagulation studies should be obtained, and coagulation abnormalities should be corrected before high-risk invasive procedures are performed, including lumbar puncture and central line placement. Blood cultures should be obtained from patients presenting with fever, and empirical antibiotics should be strongly considered, especially if the neutrophil count is low. A blood sample should be sent to the blood bank in preparation for red blood cell or platelet transfusion. A screening chest radiograph is also recommended.

When the clinician suspects a diagnosis of leukemia, further diagnostic workup should proceed without delay, in consultation with a pediatric hematologist-oncologist. Expert evaluation of the peripheral blood smear is often helpful. Examination of the bone marrow is usually necessary to establish the diagnosis. In addition to morphologic assessment, flow cytometry and cytogenetic studies should be performed on the bone marrow aspirate specimen. These studies have become increasingly important in terms of risk stratification in patients with ALL and AML. In most cases, assessment of the cerebrospinal fluid by lumbar puncture is performed to document the presence or absence of leukemic involvement. At the time of the initial staging lumbar puncture, chemotherapy should be instilled directly into the spinal fluid. Diagnostic lumbar puncture without intrathecal chemotherapy is discouraged.

Lymphoma

Hodgkin's disease is a malignant lymphoma that arises within lymphoid tissues, most commonly in the neck.[4] It is typically an indolent illness characterized by slowly progressive nodal enlargement and spread of tumor to contiguous lymph node groups over time. Involved lymph nodes are usually nontender and may have a firm, rubbery, or matted texture on physical examination. Mediastinal involvement is common and may be demonstrated on chest radiographs. Uncommonly, bulky tumors in the mediastinum may be associated with vascular compression and symptoms of superior vena cava syndrome. Widespread nodal involvement, as well as extranodal spread of tumor to the liver, lung, cortical bone, and bone marrow, occurs in advanced stages of the disease. Some patients, especially those with extensive disease, may experience systemic symptoms, termed "B" symptoms, such as fevers, night sweats, and weight loss. For unclear reasons, occasional patients present with generalized pruritus. Nonspecific markers of inflammation, including the erythrocyte sedimentation rate and C-reactive protein, are often elevated at diagnosis and may be used as markers of response to therapy and as early indicators of recurrence. The diagnosis of Hodgkin's disease is made by biopsy of involved tissue. Many children undergo biopsy after a course of oral antibiotics for presumed lymphadenitis is ineffective. Once the diagnosis of Hodgkin's disease is established, a staging evaluation is performed under the direction of the treating oncologist. Radiologic studies, including computed tomography (CT) scans of the neck through pelvis, gallium scans, and positron emission tomography scans, are usually obtained. Only rarely is surgical staging (i.e., exploratory laparotomy with splenectomy) indicated.

Several different subtypes of non-Hodgkin's lymphoma occur in childhood.[5] The most frequently encountered types demonstrate high-grade histology and aggressive behavior. Lymphoblastic lymphoma is a malignant lymphoma that is indistinguishable from ALL except that the extent of bone marrow involvement is, by definition, less than 25%. Most cases of lymphoblastic lymphoma are of precursor T-cell origin. Commonly, children with lymphoblastic lymphoma present with a mass in the anterior mediastinum. Compression of the airway or vascular structures at or below the thoracic inlet can lead to orthopnea or superior vena cava syndrome. Diagnosis is made by means of biopsy of involved tissue. When a mass is present in the anterior mediastinum, biopsy requires extreme caution owing to the high risk of anesthesia in the setting of tracheal compression.

Burkitt's lymphoma is a high-grade malignancy of mature B-cell origin. In the United States, the disease occurs in a sporadic form, with the majority of tumors presenting in the abdomen. Bone marrow or central nervous system involvement is not uncommon. Because of the extremely rapid growth rate of this tumor, patients are at high risk for the development of hyperuricemia and acute tumor lysis syndrome at presentation and after initiation of treatment.

Large cell lymphomas may be of B-cell, T-cell, or null-cell origin. These tumors arise most commonly in the lymph nodes of the mediastinum and abdomen but may arise in or spread to skin, bone, and soft tissues.

The same laboratory assessment described for leukemia, including measurement of electrolytes, creatinine, and uric acid, is recommended for all patients with suspected or confirmed non-Hodgkin's lymphoma. Diagnosis depends on histopathologic examination of tumor tissue. Sufficient biopsy material should be obtained so that specialized flow cytometric and molecular studies can be performed. These studies may demonstrate specific molecular characteristics that define certain tumor types, such as the t(14;18) in Burkitt's lymphoma. CT of the chest, abdomen, and pelvis; nuclear medicine gallium and/or bone scans; and examination of the bone marrow and cerebrospinal fluid are usually performed to determine the stage of the disease. Because systemic therapy is necessary in nearly all cases of lymphoma,

an attempt at complete surgical resection is usually not warranted.

BRAIN TUMORS

Central nervous system tumors are a diverse group of neoplasms that occur in the brain, brainstem, spinal cord, or ependymal lining of the ventricles. Most brain tumors in children are primary tumors, whereas brain metastases of extra-axial tumors commonly occur in adults.

Pediatric brain tumors can be broadly classified as tumors of glial origin and those of primitive neuroectodermal cell origin. Tumors of glial origin can arise anywhere within the craniospinal axis and are of variable grade. Specific diagnoses in this group range from low-grade astrocytomas to high-grade glioblastoma multiforme and ependymoma.[6,7] The neuroectodermal tumors presumably arise from primitive undifferentiated cells in the central nervous system. Tumors with this histology that arise in the cerebellum are called medulloblastoma.[8]

Depending on their location, pediatric brain tumors come to medical attention because of signs and symptoms of increased intracranial pressure or because of the development of focal neurologic signs. Infratentorial tumors account for more than half of all pediatric brain tumors. Commonly, infratentorial tumors obstruct the flow of cerebrospinal fluid, leading to headache and vomiting (characteristically without nausea, especially in the morning). As symptoms of elevated intracranial pressure progress, patients may experience severe headache, intractable emesis, visual disturbances, abnormal eye movements, and eventually altered mental status. Infants may demonstrate bulging of the anterior fontanelle. Children with cerebellar tumors may demonstrate nystagmus and ataxia. Supratentorial tumors sometimes cause symptoms of increased intracranial pressure but more commonly come to medical attention because of focal seizures, hemiparesis, or visual changes. Vague personality changes, ranging from lethargy to irritability, may be noted.

Imaging of the brain is usually the first step in the evaluation of a patient with a suspected brain tumor. A CT scan may be obtained emergently to demonstrate the mass or associated findings such as hydrocephalus or cerebral edema; however, magnetic resonance imaging (MRI) is the preferred study for the diagnosis and follow-up of pediatric brain tumors because it is more sensitive than CT and does not expose the child to ionizing radiation. In the setting of increased intracranial pressure, lumbar puncture should not be performed because it may precipitate fatal herniation of the cerebellar tonsils.

When a brain tumor is suspected, the patient should be referred to a pediatric neurosurgeon, preferably one who collaborates with an experienced neuro-oncology team that includes a pediatric oncologist and neurologist. Depending on the size, appearance, and location of the tumor, biopsy, subtotal resection, or complete resection may be undertaken. Sometimes biopsy is not recommended because the radiographic appearance of the tumor is characteristic or because its location makes biopsy extremely risky. Patients with optic pathway gliomas (especially those known to have neurofibromatosis) and diffuse intrinsic pontine gliomas are usually not subjected to biopsy.

EXTRACRANIAL SOLID TUMORS

Children with solid tumors may present with a range of signs and symptoms, depending on the size, location, and site of origin of the tumor. In children, malignant solid tumors most often arise in the abdomen and, less commonly, in the thorax, extremities, and head and neck.

Abdominal tumors come to medical attention because of abdominal pain, distention, vomiting, or change in bowel or bladder habits. An abdominal mass may be detected incidentally during routine child care or may come to medical attention when an individual without daily contact with the child notices abdominal distention. Abdominal masses may be difficult to palpate, especially in toddlers. Because abdominal masses in children usually represent malignant disease, expedited evaluation is warranted. In most cases, abdominal ultrasonography is the first study performed to confirm the presence of the mass and to begin to formulate a differential diagnosis. Once a mass is confirmed, the child should be referred to a pediatric oncologist or pediatric surgeon for further evaluation.

Thoracic tumors can emanate from the chest wall or originate in any compartment of the mediastinum. Patients may complain of pain or show signs of respiratory compromise with coughing, wheezing, or shortness of breath. Apical lung or mediastinal tumors may lead to Horner syndrome (unilateral ptosis, miosis, and anhidrosis). A chest radiograph is the initial study of choice.

Extremity tumors are usually accompanied by pain. Soft tissue swelling with or without a palpable mass may be present. A history of trauma or athletic injury to the extremity is frequently reported. Again, plain films are obtained initially. Additional studies such as ultrasonography, CT, or MRI can help narrow the differential diagnosis and direct further diagnostic evaluation.

Neuroblastoma

Neuroblastoma is the most common extracranial solid tumor in children. It is a diverse disease, ranging from a localized tumor with benign behavior to disseminated disease with extremely aggressive features.[9] Neuroblastoma arises from primitive neural crest elements that exist throughout the body. Most tumors arise in the abdomen, especially in the adrenal gland; thoracic tumors also occur, especially in infants. Infants with thoracic tumors may present with incidental findings on chest radiographs or with respiratory distress, wheezing, or facial swelling. Thoracic and retroperitoneal tumors may extend into the spinal canal and lead to spinal cord compression. In these cases, diagnostic evaluation and initiation of treatment must be expedited to minimize the risk of irreversible spinal cord injury. Neuroblastoma may disseminate to cortical bone, bone marrow, liver, or skin (cutaneous involvement is characteristic of infants with metastatic disease). Patients with disseminated disease experience bone pain, irritability, fatigue, pallor, bruising, and fevers. Spread of neuroblastoma to the orbital bones may lead to proptosis and orbital discoloration, a characteristic sign referred to as "raccoon eyes."

Occasionally, neuroblastoma is associated with paraneoplastic syndromes. Secretion of vasoactive intestinal peptide and catecholamines by the tumor may lead to secretory

diarrhea and hypertension, respectively. Up to 5% of children with neuroblastoma develop opsoclonus-myoclonus syndrome ("dancing eyes, dancing feet") secondary to autoantibodies against neural tissue.

Blood tests in children with disseminated neuroblastoma may demonstrate cytopenias as a consequence of bone marrow infiltration. The red blood cell morphology may show "teardrop" forms. Blood levels of lactate dehydrogenase and ferritin may be elevated. Elevated levels of the catecholamines vanillylmandelic acid and homovanillic acid are detectable in the urine in the majority of cases and support the diagnosis of neuroblastoma. Histopathologic examination of the primary tumor or of a metastatic focus is necessary to establish the diagnosis. When neuroblastoma is suspected, sufficient biopsy tissue should be obtained for analysis of *mycn*, ploidy, and cytogenetics, if possible. Evaluation for metastatic disease with CT, bone scan, MIBG imaging, and bone marrow aspirates and biopsies is usually indicated. If there is intraspinal extension of tumor, spinal MRI may be recommended to assess the risk to the spinal cord.

Renal Tumors

The majority of primary renal tumors in children are Wilms tumor; however, several other histologic types do occur.[10] A small but significant fraction of renal tumors occurs in children with congenital anomalies. Abdominal distention, without other symptoms, is the most common presenting feature. Abdominal pain may result from stretching of the renal capsule. Occasionally, patients come to medical attention because of rapid abdominal enlargement and signs of anemia due to intratumoral hemorrhage or tumor rupture. In extreme cases, sudden hemorrhagic shock can occur. Gross or microscopic hematuria may be present, and moderate to severe hypertension is commonly seen. Abdominal ultrasonography is useful to confirm the presence of a mass and may suggest the renal origin of the tumor. CT with contrast may demonstrate the characteristic "claw sign" of preserved renal parenchyma adjacent to the tumor. The contralateral kidney should also be evaluated, because bilateral tumors do occur. Wilms tumor characteristically metastasizes via the renal vein into the inferior vena cava and to the lungs. Doppler ultrasonography of the venous system and a chest radiograph (or chest CT scan) are important for staging the tumor and planning therapy. When feasible, upfront nephrectomy is recommended for unilateral tumors that do not extend into the renal vein. However, in some circumstances, preoperative chemotherapy is preferred.

Bone Tumors

Osteosarcoma is the most common primary malignant bone tumor in children and adolescents, followed by Ewing sarcoma.[11,12] Children older than 10 years are affected more frequently than are younger children. Both types of tumors can arise in any bone, but Ewing sarcoma is relatively more likely to involve the axial skeleton and can arise in soft tissues. A hallmark of bone malignancy is "deep," unrelenting pain that occurs at night and is poorly controlled with analgesics. Typically, these tumors grow relatively slowly, and the pain is chronic and progressive. Pain, swelling, and limitation of range of motion associated with the tumor may be attributed to a sports injury or to trauma for some time before medical attention is sought. Pathologic fracture may precipitate the diagnosis. The blood work is usually normal, but alkaline phosphatase or lactate dehydrogenase is elevated in some cases. Metastatic disease to the lungs and other bones may be present at diagnosis or may develop later. Unlike osteosarcoma, Ewing sarcoma can metastasize to the bone marrow. In patients with disseminated Ewing sarcoma, systemic symptoms such as fever, malaise, weight loss, and an increased sedimentation rate sometimes occur. If a primary bone tumor is suspected, referral to an orthopedic surgeon with experience in the surgical management of bone malignancies is strongly encouraged. In most cases, percutaneous biopsy is performed to establish the diagnosis. Surgical resection or, in some cases, radiation therapy to the primary tumor is often delayed until a course of systemic chemotherapy has been administered.

Other Embryonal Tumors

A variety of other solid tumors of embryonal origin occur in children, including rhabdomyosarcoma, hepatoblastoma, retinoblastoma, and germ cell tumors. The clinical manifestations correspond to the location and extent of the tumor.

Rhabdomyosarcoma is a soft tissue sarcoma with histologic features of primitive muscle development.[13] It can arise anywhere in the body, but the most common sites are the head and neck, genitourinary tract, and extremities; chest wall tumors also occur. In advanced stages, rhabdomyosarcoma can spread to the lungs, bones, and bone marrow.

Hepatoblastoma is a primary tumor of the liver that occurs almost exclusively in children younger than 2 years. Abdominal distention is the most common presenting symptom. In most cases, serum levels of α-fetoprotein are elevated. Children with a history or prematurity and those with Beckwith-Wiedemann syndrome are at increased risk for the development of this tumor.

Retinoblastoma is an uncommon tumor of retinal origin that occurs in young children. Retinoblastoma was the first cancer to be linked to a specific genetic defect—namely, mutation of the *RB* gene on chromosome 13. Individuals with inherited or acquired constitutional mutations involving this genetic locus are at high risk of developing multiple and bilateral tumors. The sporadic (i.e., nongermline) form of the disease accounts for about 60% of cases. Patients with sporadic disease always have unilateral tumors, and they are diagnosed at a slightly older median age. The most common presenting sign of retinoblastoma is leukokoria, or loss of the normal red retinal reflex. If the tumor is large, it may manifest as a painful red eye.

Germ cell tumors are a heterogeneous group of malignant tumors of several different histologic types that, taken together, account for only about 1% of cancers in children. These tumors develop from primordial germ cells that migrate during embryogenesis from the yolk sac to the gonads. Therefore, these tumors may arise in gonadal or extragonadal (usually midline) sites. A mass in the abdomen or pelvis or in the male testis is the usual presenting complaint. Adolescent boys may be reluctant to complain about testicular enlargement, and some patients present with surprisingly large tumors discovered during a thorough physical examination. Several serum markers may be elevated in patients with germ cell tumors, including α-fetoprotein, β-human chorionic gonadotropin, lactate dehydrogenase, and placental alkaline phosphatase. When serum markers are elevated at diagnosis, they may be useful for following response to therapy and identifying disease recurrence.

CONSULTATION AND ADMISSION AND DISCHARGE CRITERIA

- All patients with newly diagnosed leukemia should be admitted to a hospital experienced in the management of children with cancer.
- Patients with a new diagnosis of a solid tumor can be evaluated on an outpatient basis as long as pain is controlled and there is no evidence of superior vena cava syndrome, spinal cord compression, respiratory distress, bleeding, or metabolic derangement.
- The initial management of all childhood cancers is directed by a pediatric hematology-oncology team, with the consultation of other appropriate specialists.
- The primary care provider's support and involvement are needed for the optimal care of the patient and his or her family.
- Discharge criteria are determined by the type of cancer and by the recommendations of the hematology-oncology team and involved subspecialists.

IN A NUTSHELL

- Childhood cancer is a rare disease, and the cause is usually unknown. The majority of children diagnosed with cancer will be cured of their disease.
- The most common childhood malignancy is acute lymphoblastic leukemia.
- The most common pediatric solid tumor is neuroblastoma. Osteosarcoma is the most common primary malignant bone tumor.
- Treatment regimens vary according to diagnosis, staging, and histopathologic and cytogenetic studies.

ON THE HORIZON

- Dramatic progress has been made in elucidating the molecular basis of various types of cancer. The ability to rapidly amplify and sequence disease-associated genes and detect specific chromosomal translocations has enhanced diagnostic precision, risk stratification, and early detection of residual and recurrent disease. These molecular techniques will continue to evolve and gain clinical applications.
- The preliminary cloning of the human genome and other technologic advances have led to the development of microarrays, which are powerful tools that can screen the expression of thousands of genes in a single procedure. Analogous techniques for detecting disease-associated changes on the protein level are under development.

SUGGESTED READING

Arceci RJ: Progress and controversies in the treatment of pediatric acute myelogenous leukemia. Curr Opin Hematol 2002;9:353-360.

Cairo MS, Raetz E, Lim MS, et al: Childhood and adolescent non-Hodgkin lymphoma: New insights in biology and critical challenges for the future. Pediatr Blood Cancer 2005;45:753-769.

Maris JM: The biologic basis for neuroblastoma heterogeneity and risk stratification. Curr Opin Pediatr 2005;17:7-13.

Pui CH, Relling MV, Downing JR: Acute lymphoblastic leukemia. N Engl J Med 2004;350:1535-1548.

Ries LAG, Eisner MP, Kosary CL, et al (eds): SEER Cancer Statistics Review, 1975-2001. Bethesda, Md, National Cancer Institute, 2004. http://seer.cancer.gov/csr/1975_2001/.

Shamberger RC: Pediatric renal tumors. Semin Surg Oncol 1999;16:105-120.

REFERENCES

1. Ries LAG, Eisner MP, Kosary CL, et al (eds): SEER Cancer Statistics Review, 1975-2001. Bethesda, Md, National Cancer Institute, 2004. http://seer.cancer.gov/csr/1975_2001/.

2. Pui C, Relling MV, Downing JR: Acute lymphoblastic leukemia. N Engl J Med 2004;350:1535-1548.

3. Arceci R: Progress and controversies in the treatment of pediatric acute myelogenous leukemia. Curr Opin Hematol 2002;9:353-360.

4. Hudson M, Donaldson SS: Treatment of pediatric Hodgkin's lymphoma. Semin Hematol 1999;36:313-323.

5. Cairo MS, Raetz E, Lim MS, et al: Childhood and adolescent non-Hodgkin lymphoma: New insights in biology and critical challenges for the future. Pediatr Blood Cancer 2005;45:753-769.

6. Finlay J, Zacharoulis S: The treatment of high grade gliomas and diffuse intrinsic pontine tumors of childhood and adolescence: A historical—and futuristic—perspective. J Neurooncol 2005;75:253-266.

7. Watson GA, Kadota RP, Wisoff JH: Multidisciplanry management of pediatric low-grade gliomas. Semin Radiat Oncol 2001;11:152-162.

8. Jakacki R: Treatment strategies for high-risk medulloblastoma and supratentorial primitive neuroectodermal tumors: Review of the literature. J Neurosurg 2005;102(1 Suppl):44-52.

9. Maris J: The biologic basis for neuroblastoma heterogeneity and risk stratification. Curr Opin Pediatr 2005;17:7-13.

10. Shamberger R: Pediatric renal tumors. Semin Surg Oncol 1999;16:105-120.

11. Herzog C: Overview of sarcomas in the adolescent and young adult population. J Pediatr Hematol Oncol 2005;27:215-218.

12. Grier H: The Ewing family of tumors: Ewing's sarcoma and primitive neuroectodermal tumors. Pediatr Clin North Am 1997;44:991-1004.

13. Meyer WH, Spunt SL: Soft tissue sarcomas of childhood. Cancer Treat Rev 2004;30:269-280.

CHAPTER 124

Common Complications of Chemotherapy and Radiation: Mucositis and Febrile Neutropenia

Maureen M. O'Brien and Elizabeth Mullen

The treatment of childhood cancer requires the use of powerful medications that may result in serious side effects. Cytotoxic chemotherapeutic agents are effective because they target cell cycle activity and metabolic processes that are increased in malignant cells. Unfortunately, the therapeutic index of these medications is often quite narrow, and their efficacy in treating cancer is accompanied by toxicity to normal tissues. Static normal tissues with relatively low rates of cell division are generally spared, while those tissues with rapid cell turnover such as bone marrow, the mucosal lining of the gastrointestinal tract, and hair follicles are damaged. For this reason, myelosuppression, mucositis, and alopecia are common secondary effects of many different chemotherapeutic agents. Similarly, radiation therapy causes damage to dividing cells present in normal tissues and mucosal surfaces that fall within the radiation field. The combination of mucositis and myelosuppression predisposes children undergoing therapy for malignancies to significant infectious complications. This increased risk of infection is compounded by the fact that the underlying cancer, especially the lymphoid malignancies, may compromise patients' immune systems to a certain degree.

Although pediatric oncologists direct the treatment of children with malignancies, hospital-based physicians are likely to encounter these children when they develop therapy-induced mucositis or fever and neutropenia. These physicians should be prepared to initiate the evaluation and management of these common complications of chemotherapy and radiation, with the guidance of oncology and infectious disease specialists as needed.

MUCOSITIS

Although many commonly used chemotherapeutic agents may cause mucositis, it is particularly severe with the antimetabolites, such as methotrexate and cytarabine (ara-C), and the anthracyclines, such as doxorubicin and daunomycin. Mucositis commonly develops 1 week after the start of chemotherapy and usually resolves within 3 weeks of chemotherapy administration. Good oral hygiene and frequent diaper changes in infants may help decrease the severity of symptoms. Mucositis can occur in any part of the gastrointestinal tract. Early signs include erythema and edema that may progress to necrosis and ulceration. The severity can be assessed with careful examination of the oropharynx and perianal area. Localized mucositis may develop in the esophagus or other areas due to focal radiation therapy. Severe pain caused by oral ulceration and esophagitis may lead to difficulty speaking or swallowing. Patients may require intravenous fluids, parenteral nutrition,

and pain control ranging from topical lidocaine and oral analgesics to intravenous narcotics.[1,2]

Besides requiring supportive management of pain, hydration, and nutrition, mucositis is a clinical concern because damaged mucosal surfaces promote local and systemic infection. Breakdown of natural mucosal barriers allows endogenous microbial flora to gain access to the bloodstream, resulting in bacteremia and the risk of sepsis. Denuded mucosal surfaces are prone to superinfection with *Candida* species, viral pathogens (e.g., herpesviruses), and bacteria. Mucosal breakdown in the perianal area can result in significant local infection with abscess formation. Mucositis throughout the intestines can result in abdominal pain, diarrhea, and malabsorption and may progress to necrosis, particularly in the setting of concomitant infection. Typhlitis, or necrotizing colitis, is a mixed infection of the gut wall. It typically occurs in the cecum due to translocation and focal invasion of gut flora, particularly anaerobes, in areas of mucosal breakdown. Therapy consists of broad-spectrum antibiotics, including anaerobic coverage, as well as abdominal imaging and surgical evaluation and intervention as needed.[3]

FEBRILE NEUTROPENIA

Mucosal breakdown with alteration of integumentary barriers to pathogens contributes to the risk of serious infection in children undergoing therapy for malignancy. It is compounded by immune dysfunction and myelosuppression, the presence of indwelling venous catheters, alterations in indigenous microflora due to hospital and antibiotic exposure, malnutrition, and local tissue damage from radiation or surgery. Both chemotherapy and the primary malignancy may result in severe neutropenia, placing patients at high risk of infection. In the setting of infection, patients with neutropenia may fail to demonstrate typical signs of inflammation such as pain, erythema, or purulent drainage.[4] As a result, fever may be the only presenting symptom of life-threatening infection and requires urgent evaluation and empirical antibiotic therapy. Severe infection is the most common and serious risk for children undergoing treatment for cancer.[3]

Definition of Fever

From a practical standpoint, fever is defined by the Infectious Diseases Society of America (IDSA) as "a single oral temperature of >38.3°C (101°F) or a temperature of >38.0°C (100.4°F) for greater than one hour."[5] Oral, axillary, or tympanic temperature measurement is recommended. Rectal temperature measurement should not be performed in children with cancer.

Definition of Neutropenia

Many chemotherapeutic agents cause a predictable suppression of blood cell production, with peripheral blood counts reaching a nadir approximately 10 days after chemotherapy administration. Chemotherapeutic agents with the most significant suppressive effects on bone marrow function include the alkylating agents, the anthracyclines, and cytarabine. All cell lines can be affected, and transfusion of red cells or platelets may be required to correct significant anemia or thrombocytopenia. Unfortunately, neutropenia is not easily corrected by transfusion. Recovery of neutrophil production occurs at its own pace and can be accelerated only slightly by the administration of granulocyte colony-stimulating factor (G-CSF). Neutropenia is defined by the IDSA as an "absolute neutrophil count (ANC) <500 cells/mm^3 or <1000 cells/mm^3 with expected nadir <500 cells/mm^3." The ANC can be calculated as follows:

$$ANC = White\ blood\ cell\ count \times$$
$$(\%\ Neutrophils + \%\ Bands)$$

Once a child with cancer is determined to have fever, the ANC is the key factor in predicting the risk of bacterial and fungal infection. The risk of serious infection increases with both the depth and duration of neutropenia. Studies have shown that although children with ANCs less than 1000 cells/mm^3 are at higher risk for serious bacterial infection than normal children, the risk increases most significantly for those with ANCs less than 500 cells/mm^3 and is extremely high with ANCs less than 100 cells/mm^3. Prolonged neutropenia (>5 to 7 days) is also associated with increased risk of infection, particularly with fungal pathogens such as *Candida* and *Aspergillus* species.[5,6]

Bacterial Pathogens

There has been a shift in the pathogens most likely to be isolated from the blood of patients with febrile neutropenia. Historically, the predominant pathogens were enteric gram-negative rods, including *Escherichia coli*, *Klebsiella*, and *Pseudomonas* species that gained access to the bloodstream via mucosal breakdown in the gastrointestinal tract.[7] Although these infections remain a concern and continue to be associated with significant morbidity and mortality, gram-positive bacteria now account for approximately 60% to 70% of cases of documented bacteremia.[5] Factors contributing to this change in the pattern of infection may include an increase in patient colonization with resistant strains, treatment with prophylactic antibiotics, and the widespread use of indwelling vascular-access devices. Many infections, especially those with coagulase-negative staphylococci, are indolent and associated with indwelling lines. However, blood-borne infection with other organisms, including *Staphylococcus aureus*, enterococci, viridans streptococci, and *Streptococcus pneumoniae*, may present with overwhelming sepsis.[8] Of note, certain intensive chemotherapy regimens that cause severe mucositis are associated with an increased risk of sepsis due to viridans streptococci; this condition often presents with fulminant sepsis associated with hemodynamic compromise.[9] Given the range of documented pathogens in febrile neutropenic patients, the initial empirical antibiotic regimen must provide broad coverage for both gram-negative and gram-positive organisms, with attention paid to the institutional nosocomial infection and resistance patterns where the patient is being treated.

Evaluation

The initial evaluation of a child with febrile neutropenia should include a detailed history and careful physical examination, because localizing signs of infection may be subtle. The lack of neutrophils blunts many of the inflammatory signs typically observed in patients with infection. Even in the absence of fever, any neutropenic patient who has signs or symptoms suggestive of infection, including hemodynamic instability, should be managed similarly to a patient presenting with fever.[3]

Important historical data include the underlying diagnosis and recent chemotherapy, infectious exposures, antibiotic usage, surgical procedures, known colonization or prior infection with resistant organisms (e.g., methicillin-resistant *S. aureus*), and prior known infections related to an indwelling catheter. The review of systems should include evaluation for the presence of rash, sore throat, headache, neck stiffness, nasal congestion or discharge, cough, shortness of breath, abdominal pain, vomiting, diarrhea, dysuria, or pain with defecation.

The physical examination should include a rapid general assessment and evaluation for the stability of vital signs and, if necessary, emergent stabilization of the airway, breathing, and circulation. A thorough physical examination should then be performed, with close attention to frequent sites of infection in febrile neutropenic patients, including the following:

- Oropharynx and gingivae: mucositis, periodontal infection, abscess.
- Respiratory tract: sinusitis, pneumonia.
- Abdomen and perirectal area: mucositis, local infection, abscess (an internal rectal examination should *not* be performed, owing to the risk of inciting abscess formation or bacteremia through local mucosal breakdown).
- Gastrostomy or recent surgical incision sites: erythema, tenderness, drainage.

Routine laboratory evaluation should include a complete blood count with differential to determine the presence and degree of neutropenia. Blood cultures (aerobic and anaerobic) should be obtained from each lumen of any indwelling central lines; however, peripheral venipuncture is not generally performed because it rarely contributes significantly to clinical management decisions. Published guidelines generally recommend that urinalysis, routine chemistries, liver function panel, blood urea nitrogen, and creatinine be analyzed to help direct supportive care. The presence of significant renal or hepatic dysfunction may influence antibiotic selection and dosage.[5]

Other specific laboratory and imaging studies should be directed by any localizing signs or symptoms elicited in the history and physical examination.[10] Recommendations include the following:

- Culture of any drainage at a surgical or catheter site.
- Rapid strep test or throat culture for complaints of throat pain or evidence of pharyngeal exudates.

- Clean-catch urine culture when urinary symptoms suggest infection, the urinalysis is abnormal, the patient is at increased risk for urinary tract infection (e.g., recent urinary catheter), or there is a history of urinary tract infections. Urine culture obtained by catheterization should be *considered* in infants or young children, as is routinely recommended in the evaluation of fever of unknown origin.
- Stool cultures for bacterial pathogens and *Clostridium difficile* toxin should be performed if diarrheal symptoms are prominent or there is heme-positive stool. If seasonally appropriate, consider stool viral cultures, particularly rotavirus.
- Chest radiograph should be obtained if there are any respiratory symptoms or abnormal findings on examination (e.g., persistent cough, tachypnea, oxygen saturation <95%, rales) and should be considered for any patient with projected prolonged neutropenia as a baseline examination.
- Nasal washings should be sent for respiratory pathogens (e.g., respiratory syncytial virus, influenza, parainfluenza) if symptoms and epidemiology are appropriate.
- Oral lesions consistent with herpesvirus should be scraped for rapid fluorescence screening and culture. If a patient has a known history of oral herpetic lesions, empirical therapy with antiviral agents may be warranted.
- Tenderness on abdominal examination or vomiting may be an indication for plain radiographs to evaluate for intestinal obstruction or free peritoneal air. Additional laboratory testing consisting of liver function panel and pancreatic enzymes, along with computed tomography to evaluate for abscess, typhlitis, or other focal infection, may be indicated.
- Lumbar puncture may be indicated if there are signs or symptoms of meningismus. Computed tomography of the head should be considered before lumbar puncture to rule out intracranial hemorrhage or increased intracranial pressure. Thrombocytopenia and coagulopathy should be recognized and corrected before lumbar puncture. The presence of a recently placed ventriculoperitoneal shunt (within the past 1 to 2 months) or neurologic symptoms in a patient with a long-standing ventriculoperitoneal shunt are indications for neurosurgical consultation and empirical coverage for possible shunt infection.

Initial Antibiotic Therapy

Empirical broad-spectrum antibiotics should be initiated as soon as possible, preferably within 1 hour of the documentation of fever. Although every effort should be made to obtain relevant cultures, antibiotic therapy should not be delayed. In a patient with suspected sepsis, including a patient with any unstable vital signs, urgent antibiotic administration is the priority. A variety of regimens that cover both gram-negative and gram-positive bacterial pathogens have similar efficacy and safety. Because therapeutic regimens take into consideration local sensitivity and resistance patterns, consultation with oncology and infectious disease specialists at the institution where the patient is being treated is recommended before initiating therapy. Examples of therapeutic regimens include the following[5]:

- Monotherapy with a third- or fourth-generation cephalosporin such as ceftazidime or cefepime 50 mg/kg per dose intravenously (IV) every 8 hours (maximum 2 g/dose).[11]
- Monotherapy with a carbapenem such as meropenem 40 mg/kg per dose IV every 8 hours (maximum 2 g/dose).
- Multidrug regimen with an antipseudomonal cephalosporin or penicillin, including piperacillin-tazobactam (Zosyn) 75 mg/kg per dose IV every 6 hours (maximum 4.5 g/dose piperacillin) combined with an aminoglycoside such as gentamicin 2 to 2.5 mg/kg per dose IV every 8 hours (dosing based on age, creatinine clearance, and monitored drug levels).

In patients who are allergic to penicillin or cephalosporin, alternative regimens include the following[5]:

- Aztreonam 30 mg/kg per dose IV every 6 hours (maximum total daily dose 8 g).
- Vancomycin 15 to 20 mg/kg per dose IV every 8 hours (maximum 1 g/dose) or clindamycin 12 mg/kg per dose IV every 8 hours (maximum 1.6 g/dose).

These empirical recommendations apply to febrile neutropenic patients with no clear source of infection based on the history and physical examination. If localizing signs or symptoms are present, the initial antibiotic regimen should be broadened or tailored as necessary. In particular, the clinician must consider the need for vancomycin, anaerobic, antiviral, or antifungal coverage. For patients with evidence of periodontal, perirectal, or intra-abdominal infections, anaerobic coverage with metronidazole, clindamycin, or extended-spectrum penicillins such as piperacillin-tazobactam should be added.[3,5]

Blood-borne infections with gram-positive bacteria, especially coagulase-negative staphylococci, are common in pediatric cancer patients, and these infections may not be effectively treated with the empirical regimens described. The addition of vancomycin is frequently debated as physicians try to balance the need to treat high-risk patients aggressively against the desire to avoid contributing to the proliferation of resistant organisms.[12] Because infections with coagulase-negative staphylococci tend to be indolent and carry a low risk of tissue seeding and invasion, empirical coverage of this organism with vancomycin is not encouraged.[13] The IDSA's 2002 guidelines recommend that vancomycin not be routinely included in initial regimens; however, it should be available if positive cultures or new clinical findings warrant its use.[5] Specific cases in which empirical vancomycin therapy should be initiated include the following:

- Clinically suspected serious catheter-related or soft tissue infections (e.g., cellulitis, tunnel infections).
- Known colonization with penicillin- and cephalosporin-resistant pneumococci or methicillin-resistant *S. aureus*.
- Positive results of blood culture for gram-positive bacteria before identification and susceptibility testing.
- Hypotension or other evidence of cardiovascular instability.
- Intensive chemotherapy that produces substantial mucosal damage or increases the risk for penicillin-resistant streptococcal infections such as viridans streptococci (e.g., high-dose cytarabine).

- Prophylaxis with fluoroquinolones for afebrile neutropenic patients before the onset of fever.

Antifungal Therapy

Research has demonstrated that in addition to invasive bacterial infections, neutropenic patients, particularly those with prolonged neutropenia (>5 to 7 days), are at risk for invasive fungal infections.[6] Such infections may be primary or may develop secondarily in patients receiving broad-spectrum antibiotic therapy. Therefore, in patients who remain neutropenic and febrile with no cause identified despite 3 to 5 days of empirical antibacterial therapy, empirical antifungal coverage is added. Amphotericin B 0.5 to 1 mg/kg per day is frequently used, although liposomal amphotericin (AmBisome, 3 mg/kg/day) may be preferable because it has a more favorable toxicity profile, especially in the setting of renal impairment. Use of amphotericin requires frequent monitoring of serum potassium, magnesium, and creatinine owing to its nephrotoxicity. After the initiation of empirical therapy, imaging of the head, chest, abdomen, and pelvis should be performed to evaluate for evidence of fungal disease of the sinuses, lungs, liver, spleen, and kidneys. Of note, fungal microabscesses may not be radiologically apparent in the setting of profound neutropenia. Thus, even when initial imaging studies are negative, they should be repeated after neutrophil recovery and before discontinuation of antifungal therapy. Computed tomography is the usual mode of imaging, but magnetic resonance imaging may be more sensitive for evaluating the abdominal viscera. Serum galactomannan levels can be helpful in detecting *Aspergillus* infection, and serum β-glucan levels are often elevated in invasive candidal infections. False-positive results for serum galactomannan can occur in patients receiving piperacillin-tazobactam, so tests should be interpreted with caution.[14]

The newer antifungal agents voriconazole and caspofungin are being evaluated for safety and efficacy for fungal prophylaxis and treatment in the pediatric population.[15,16] Consultation with a pediatric infectious disease specialist and oncologist is recommended to tailor the choice of antifungal agents in pediatric oncology patients with known or suspected fungal infections.

Antiviral Therapy

There is no indication for the empirical use of antiviral medications in febrile neutropenic patients who do not have localizing findings consistent with a viral infection. However, if a neutropenic patient develops skin or mucous membrane vesicular or dermatomal lesions that are consistent with herpes simplex or varicella-zoster infection or reactivation, empirical therapy with IV acyclovir is indicated (10 to 20 mg/kg per dose IV every 8 hours) until all the lesions have crusted. Attempts should be made to obtain immunofluorescence studies or viral cultures from any lesions to document the pathogen.[5] Specific antiviral therapy may be indicated for immunocompromised patients with certain confirmed viral illnesses, such as respiratory syncytial virus or influenza. Consultation with a pediatric infectious disease specialist should be strongly considered in these cases.

Duration of Therapy

In general, febrile neutropenic patients are hospitalized and treated with broad-spectrum intravenous antibiotics until *both* fever and neutropenia have resolved. Patients who defervesce but remain neutropenic should continue broad-spectrum antibiotics until the neutropenia resolves. Once cultures are negative, the patient is afebrile and appears well, and the ANC is greater than 500 cells/mm^3 or greater than 200 cells/mm^3 on 2 consecutive days and rising, empirical antibiotic coverage is discontinued, and the patient may be discharged. Any documented infectious cause (e.g., sinusitis, cellulitis, bacteremia) should be treated with an appropriate course of antibiotics once neutropenia has resolved. For patients who remain persistently febrile and neutropenic, daily reevaluation for focal sources of infection and adjustments to the empirical regimen, such as the addition of vancomycin or antifungal therapy, should be strongly considered.[3,5]

Catheter Removal

The majority of children receiving cancer chemotherapy have indwelling central venous access devices. These catheters, though vital to patient care, increase the risk of bacteremia and fungemia because they act as a nidus for colonization with pathogens and provide such organisms direct access to the bloodstream. Bacteremia in a patient with an indwelling catheter can often be treated without catheter removal. The most common cause of catheter-associated bacteremia is coagulase-negative staphylococci; this infection can typically be cleared with intravenous vancomycin infused through the catheter. Bacteremia due to gram-negative organisms and pneumococci can also be treated without catheter removal. Antibiotic administration should be rotated through all lumens of the catheter, and clearance of the bloodstream and the catheter should be documented by clinical improvement (i.e., resolution of fever) and multiple negative blood cultures from all lumens. Persistent positive blood culture with any organism despite adequate antibiotic coverage for 48 hours is an indication for catheter removal.[3,6]

Other infections, including candidemia and *S. aureus* bacteremia, are significantly more difficult to clear from an infected catheter and have a high incidence of dissemination and subsequent complications. In these cases, catheter removal is almost always necessary for cure. Infection with certain *Bacillus* species, as well as vancomycin-resistant enterococcal infections, may also require catheter removal. In addition, although localized skin infections at the catheter exit site can be treated without catheter removal, the presence of a tunnel infection (cellulitis, fluctuance, or purulent drainage tracking along the catheter) is an indication for catheter removal. Finally, recurrent catheter-related infections with the same organism also necessitate catheter removal.[3,6,17]

CONSULTATION

Pediatric oncology patients undergo specialized therapeutic regimens and are at risk for many common and uncommon infections. Although they may present with signs and symptoms of infection or sepsis at a local health care facility, decisions about their evaluation and treatment should be made in consultation with their primary hematology-oncology team.

ADMISSION CRITERIA

- Suspicion of infection or sepsis suggested by, but not limited to, fever, unstable vital signs, evidence of mucositis, or other localizing findings.
- Need for imaging studies or other extensive investigation for a source of fever or infection.
- Requirement for intravenous antimicrobial therapy.
- Inability to maintain normal hydration and nutrition as an outpatient or to comply with the recommended outpatient medication regimen.

DISCHARGE CRITERIA

- Concerns for infection are resolved and antimicrobial therapy is complete.
- Both fever and neutropenia have resolved.
- Cultures are negative, the patient is afebrile and appears well, and the ANC is greater than 500 cells/mm³ or greater than 200 cells/mm³ on 2 consecutive days and rising.
- Outpatient follow-up is established, and a plan to complete an outpatient course of therapy for a documented infection is in place.

IN A NUTSHELL

- Severe infection is the most common and serious risk for children undergoing treatment for cancer.
- Neutropenic patients with or without fever must be thoroughly evaluated if they present with signs or symptoms suggestive of infection.
- The initial evaluation of a child with febrile neutropenia should include a detailed history and careful physical examination, because localizing signs of infection may be subtle.
- Fever may be the only presenting symptom of life-threatening infection and requires urgent evaluation and empirical antibiotic therapy.
- Prompt evaluation and treatment of pediatric cancer patients with febrile neutropenia are essential and may be lifesaving.
- The directed history, physical examination, and choice of appropriately broad antimicrobial coverage should be based on an understanding of the infectious risks of these severely immunocompromised patients.
- Empirical broad-spectrum antibiotics should be initiated as soon as possible and should not be delayed if relevant cultures are difficult to obtain. In a patient with suspected sepsis, urgent administration of antibiotics is the priority. In specific cases, antiviral and antifungal therapy may be indicated.

ON THE HORIZON

- In the past, all febrile neutropenic patients received intravenous antibiotics and were admitted to the hospital for the duration of therapy. However, recent research (mainly involving adults) suggests that it may be possible to identify a subset of patients with febrile neutropenia who are at relatively low risk for significant morbidity and mortality and can be safely managed with broad-spectrum oral antibiotics and monitored as outpatients.[18] Simplified outpatient regimens would decrease the frequency of hospitalization for these patients, which would be more cost-effective and less disruptive and decrease their exposure to nosocomial pathogens.
- Increasingly intensive chemotherapeutic regimens, the advent of stem cell rescue, and the emergence of resistant bacterial and fungal strains ensure that the approach to cancer patients with fever and neutropenia will continue to evolve.

SUGGESTED READING

Alexander SW, Walsh TJ, Freifeld AG, Pizzo PA: Infectious complications in pediatric cancer patients. In Pizzo PA, Poplack DG (eds): Principles & Practice of Pediatric Oncology, 4th ed. Philadelphia, Lippincott Williams & Wilkins, 2001, pp 1239-1283.

Hughes WT, Armstrong D, Bodey GP, et al: 2002 Guidelines for the use of antimicrobial agents in neutropenic patients with cancer. Clin Infect Dis 2002;34:730-751.

REFERENCES

1. Sonis ST, Elting LS, Keefe D, et al: Perspectives on cancer therapy-induced mucosal injury: Pathogenesis, measurement, epidemiology, and consequences for patients. Cancer 2004;100(9 Suppl):1995-2025.
2. Rubenstein EB, Peterson DE, Schubert M, et al: Clinical practice guidelines for the prevention and treatment of cancer therapy-induced oral and gastrointestinal mucositis. Cancer 2004;100(9 Suppl):2026-2046.
3. Alexander SW, Walsh TJ, Freifeld AG, Pizzo PA: Infectious complications in pediatric cancer patients. In Pizzo PA, Poplack DG (eds): Principles & Practice of Pediatric Oncology, 4th ed. Philadelphia, Lippincott Williams & Wilkins, 2001, pp 1239-1283.
4. Sickles EA, Greene WH, Wiernik PH: Clinical presentation of infection in granulocytopenic patients. Arch Intern Med 1975;135:715-719.
5. Robertson J, Shilkofski N (eds): Harriet Lane Handbook, 17th ed. St Louis, Elsevier/Mosby, 2005, p 611.
6. Pizzo PA: Management of fever in patients with cancer and treatment-induced neutropenia. N Engl J Med 1993;328:1323-1332.
7. Escande MC, Hebrect R: Prospective study of bacteremia in cancer patients. Support Care Cancer 1998;6:273-280.
8. Pizzo PA, Ladisch S, Robichaud K: Treatment of gram-positive septicemia in cancer patients. Cancer 1980;45:206-207.
9. Gassas A, Grant R, Richardson S, et al: Predictors of viridans streptococcal shock syndrome in bacteremic children with cancer and stem-cell transplant recipients. J Clin Oncol 2004;22:1222-1227.
10. Wolff LJ, Ablin AR, Altman AJ, Johnson FL: The management of fever. In Ablin AR (ed): Supportive Care of Children with Cancer, 2nd ed. Baltimore, Johns Hopkins University Press, 1997, pp 23-36.
11. Pizzo PA, Hathorn JW, Hiemenz J, et al: A randomized trial comparing ceftazidime alone with combination antibiotic therapy in cancer patients with fever and neutropenia. N Engl J Med 1986;315:552-558.

12. Blijlevens NM, Donnelly JP, de Pauw BE: Empirical therapy of febrile neu-tropenic patients with mucositis: Challenge of risk-based therapy. Clin Microbiol Infect 2001;7(Suppl 4):47-52.

13. Feld R: Vancomycin as part of initial empirical antibiotic therapy for febrile neutropenia in patients with cancer: Pros and cons. Clin Infect Dis 1999;29:503-507.

14. Martino R, Viscoli C: Empirical antifungal therapy in patients with neu-tropenia and persistent or recurrent fever of unknown origin. Br J Haematol 2005;132:138-154.

15. Herbrecht R, Denning DW, Patterson TF, et al: Voriconazole versus amphotericin B for primary therapy of invasive aspergillosis. N Engl J Med 2002;347:408-415.

16. Mora-Duarte J, Betts R, Rotstein C, et al: Comparison of caspofungin and amphotericin B for invasive candidiasis. N Engl J Med 2002;347:2020-2029.

17. Adler A, Yaniv I, Solter E, et al: Catheter-associated bloodstream infec-tions in pediatric hematology-oncology patients. J Pediatr Hematol Oncol 2006;28:23-28.

18. Orudjev E, Lange BJ: Evolving concepts of management of febrile neu-tropenia in children with cancer. Med Pediatr Oncol 2002;39:77-85.

CHAPTER 125

Stem Cell Transplants

Christine N. Duncan

Hundreds of pediatric stem cell transplants are performed annually in the United States. Transplants are done for malignant conditions, nonmalignant hematologic diseases, immunologic disorders, and some metabolic diseases (Table 125-1). Although the majority of transplants are done at large medical centers, post-transplant patients receive a portion of their care in community hospitals and local oncologists' offices. It is important for the pediatric hospitalist to have a general understanding of the medical issues facing stem cell transplant patients who may present to emergency departments or require admission to inpatient units.

BACKGROUND

Stem cell transplantation most often involves the process of replacing diseased bone marrow with healthy hematopoietic stem cell progenitors. In some pediatric solid cancers, very high-dose chemotherapy regimens are needed to effectively treat the tumor, necessitating reconstitution of the marrow with previously banked autologous stem cells. This type of transplant happens when the patient does not have bone marrow disease.[1]

Stem cells for transplantation come from either the patient (autologous transplant) or another individual (allogeneic transplant). Autologous transplants have several advantages, including their ready availability for current and future transplants, no risk of graft-versus-host disease (GVHD), more rapid engraftment, and lower short-term mortality.[2] Allogeneic transplants also have several benefits. First, there is no risk of residual tumor in the donated cells because the donor is disease free. Second, the donor has not received prior chemotherapy, which carries its own set of complications. Finally, the donor cells may exhibit a graft-versus-leukemia effect, which occurs when the donated cells attack malignant cells in the patient and destroy them.[3] Allogeneic donors may be related or unrelated to the patient. Unrelated allogeneic donors found through a donor search may be less readily available than related donors and may be unavailable for future transplants if needed.

The National Marrow Donation Program is a nonprofit organization in the United States that anonymously matches unrelated stem cell transplant recipients and donors.[4] Human leukocyte antigen (HLA) typing is done to determine the suitability of potential donors. HLAs are genetic markers found on the surface of white blood cells. The genetic composition of these antigens, located on the short arm of chromosome 6, is determined by testing the blood of the recipient and the potential donor.[5] HLAs are inherited, making siblings more likely than unrelated donors or parents to have similar typing. There is a 25% chance of two siblings having matching HLAs. The closer the match between the donor and the recipient, the lower the risk of GVHD.

Sources of stem cells include bone marrow, peripheral blood, and umbilical cord blood. Bone marrow has traditionally been the source of stem cells for pediatric transplants. It has the greatest concentration of stem cells and requires no physical preparation of the donor. Bone marrow is typically harvested while the donor is under anesthesia, which carries some risk. Peripheral blood has a lower concentration of circulating stem cells.[6] Chemotherapy or stimulating factors, used to mobilize stem cells from the bone marrow, are frequently given to autologous donors before peripheral blood stem cell collection. Allogeneic donors may receive granulocyte colony-stimulating factor (G-CSF) or granulocyte-macrophage colony-stimulating factor (GM-CSF) before peripheral blood collection.[7] Peripheral blood stem cells are removed via apheresis through large peripheral intravenous access or a central venous line. For young sibling donors, the need for large intravenous access may preclude the collection of peripheral blood stem cells. Umbilical cord blood can be used when a matched donor cannot be identified. Cord blood is rich in stem cells and is either drained from the placenta or removed via cannulation at delivery.[8] The blood is stored frozen in public or private banks.

TRANSPLANT PROCEDURE

Before receiving stem cells, patients undergo a conditioning regimen of chemotherapy or chemotherapy plus total-body irradiation. Patients are admitted to the hospital for conditioning and remain hospitalized throughout the transplant. The purposes of conditioning are to create marrow space for the transplanted cells, eliminate diseased marrow cells when applicable, and remove host lymphocytes capable of rejecting the transplanted cells. The specific conditioning protocol depends on the disease being treated and the practice of the transplanting institution. Commonly used regimens include cyclophosphamide with total-body irradiation and cyclophosphamide-busulfan. Toxicities common to most conditioning regimens are myelosuppression, nausea, emesis, mucositis (inflammation, irritation, and ulceration of gastrointestinal mucosal cells), alopecia, and infertility. A detailed discussion of specific conditioning agents and their toxicities is beyond the scope of this chapter.

Patients receive supportive care in the form of platelet and packed red blood cell transfusions, antiemetics, analgesics, nutritional supplementation, prophylactic antimicrobial agents, and other therapies targeted at individual toxicities. Select groups of patients also receive growth factors (G-CSF or GM-CSF) after the stem cell infusion.

Once conditioning is completed, stem cells are infused through a central venous line. This can be done by manual injection or by a pump similar to a blood transfusion. The day on which the stem cells are infused is called "day 0." The

Table 125-1 Pediatric Diseases Treated with Stem Cell Transplants

Malignant bone marrow diseases
   Acute myelogenous leukemia
   Acute lymphoblastic leukemia*
   Chronic myelogenous leukemia
   Juvenile myelomonocytic leukemia

Bone marrow failure syndromes
   Aplastic anemia
   Shwachman-Diamond syndrome
   Fanconi anemia
   Diamond-Blackfan syndrome

Hematologic disorders
   Sickle cell anemia
   Thalassemia major
   Hemophagocytic lymphohistiocytosis

Other malignancies
   Neuroblastoma
   Relapsed lymphoma
   Relapsed Wilms tumor
   Certain brain tumors

Immunodeficiencies
   Severe combined immunodeficiency
   Chronic granulomatous disease
   Wiskott-Aldrich syndrome
   X-linked lymphoproliferative disease

Metabolic disorders
   Glycogen storage diseases
   Osteopetrosis
   Niemann-Pick disease
   Lysosomal storage disease

*Stem cell transplantation is not a primary treatment for acute lymphoblastic leukemia.

days before day 0 are referred to as "minus" days, and the days following the transplant are referred to as "plus" days. For example, the day before stem cell infusion is considered day −1, and the day following transplantation is day +1.

The time from stem cell infusion to engraftment can be a medically complicated period. Patients are profoundly immunosuppressed and at risk for severe, potentially life-threatening infections. They may experience mucositis requiring narcotic analgesia. Nausea and emesis remain significant problems during this period, exacerbated by mucositis and the paralytic effects of narcotics on the gastrointestinal (GI) tract. Other less common but important medical issues during this period are veno-occlusive disease of the liver, renal failure, and noninfectious pulmonary complications.

After stem cell infusion, patients remain in the hospital until their stem cells have engrafted, all acute medical issues have resolved, they are tolerating all oral medications, and they are able to maintain adequate hydration at home. The definition of engraftment varies by institution, but it is commonly considered the achievement of an absolute neutrophil count greater than 500 for 3 consecutive days. After discharge, transplant patients require close monitoring and continued treatment and are seen frequently in an outpatient stem cell transplant clinic. The frequency of visits is dictated by the patient's condition.

GRAFT-VERSUS-HOST DISEASE

GVHD is a significant cause of morbidity and mortality in stem cell transplant patients. It can present with either subtle or fulminant symptoms at any time following the transplant. An understanding of the disease and its varied presentations is essential for any health care provider who may care for stem cell transplant patients.

GVHD is a T-cell mediated immunoreactive process in which donor cells react against recipient cells. Tissue damage is caused by direct cytolysis and by the effects of inflammatory cytokines such as tumor necrosis factor-α, interleukin-6, and interleukin-10.[9] Acute GVHD occurs in the first 100 days after the transplant, whereas chronic GVHD occurs after day +100. Risk factors for both acute and chronic GVHD are HLA mismatch between recipient and donor, type of GVHD prophylaxis, older age of donor and recipient, parity in female donors, and presence of T lymphocytes in the stem cell infusion.[10,11] Additional risk factors for chronic GVHD are previous acute GVHD, female donor, and total-body irradiation during conditioning.[12]

Acute and chronic GVHD differ not only in time of onset but also in presentation. The skin and GI system are frequently affected in both types. The rash seen in acute GVHD can have many different appearances. Initially, acute skin GVHD often appears as tender, erythematous patches on the palms, soles, occiput, posterior neck, or face. The patient may then develop diffuse erythroderma. Severe skin GVHD can blister and ulcerate. Chronic skin GVHD typically involves larger areas and presents with a dry, thick, pruritic rash. This can progress to tight, sclerodermatous skin that can interfere with joint mobility.

Oral changes are also seen in both acute and chronic GVHD. In acute GVHD, the oral lesions are often ulcerative and painful. Oral ulceration may also occur in chronic GVHD. Patients with chronic oral GVHD may develop sicca syndrome, characterized by severely dry eyes and mouth and the potential for salivary gland atrophy.

Acute GVHD can affect any portion of the GI tract, as well as the liver. The gold standard for diagnosis is biopsy revealing cellular necrosis, glandular dropout, and apoptosis.[13] However, the condition is often diagnosed clinically. Anorexia, nausea, emesis, and abdominal pain are symptoms of upper GI GVHD. Lower GI GVHD presents with profuse, watery diarrhea, abdominal cramping, and anorexia. Abnormalities in liver function tests can also occur with GVHD. Chronic GI GVHD is less common than the acute type, but it presents with similar symptoms: diarrhea, abdominal pain, nausea, emesis, weight loss, dysphagia, and early satiety. Histologically, chronic GVHD appears more fibrotic, with crypt distortion. Other signs and symptoms of acute and chronic GVHD are listed in Table 125-2.

GVHD prophylaxis is given to all patients undergoing allogeneic stem cell transplantation. Immunosuppression with immunomodulating drugs is the mainstay of GVHD prevention. Methotrexate, cyclosporine, FK-506, mycophenolate mofetil, and corticosteroids are the most commonly used agents. T-cell depletion of the graft before infusion is

Table 125–2   Signs and Symptoms of Graft-versus-Host Disease

Acute
Erythematous rash on palms, soles, occiput, face, and posterior neck
Bullous skin eruption with peeling skin
Oral ulceration
Nausea, vomiting
Anorexia, weight loss
Profuse diarrhea
Liver function abnormalities
Jaundice

Chronic
Dry, pruritic, diffuse rash
Sclerodermatous skin changes with contractures
Sicca syndrome (dry skin, dry eyes) with possible tooth decay and corneal ulceration
Dysphagia
Abdominal pain
Abnormal liver function tests
Premature graying of hair
Patchy alopecia
Pulmonary function changes
Bronchiolitis obilterans with organizing pneumonia

also used in some cases. The prophylactic measures taken depend on the patient's risk factors for GVHD and the practices of the transplanting institution. Immunosuppressant drugs are also first-line treatment for acute and chronic GVHD. Additional treatments are directed at specific symptoms.

Most allogeneic stem cell transplant patients remain on immunosuppressive drug therapy for at least 6 months after transplantation, even if there is no evidence of acute or chronic GVHD. Immunosuppressive drugs are then tapered over a period determined by the clinical situation. Patients with evidence of GVHD may remain on immunosuppressant therapy for years. In these cases, the clinician attempts to maintain the patient on the lowest dose that controls the symptoms. In addition to immunosuppressant therapy, these patients continue to receive prophylactic antimicrobial agents. It is important to monitor patients for complications of immunosuppressant therapy.

INFECTION

Infection is a significant cause of death in stem cell transplant patients. Profound immunosuppression, breakdown of the GI mucosa, indwelling central lines, and disruption of skin integrity contribute to the infectious risk in these patients. During hospitalization, patients are placed on infection prophylaxis. They are isolated either in a hospital room or on the transplant floor, depending on the air filtration system and hospital policy. Antimicrobial prophylaxis is commonly given, but the specific agents used differ among institutions. Antifungal prophylaxis is often accomplished with fluconazole or liposomal amphotericin B. Trimethoprim-sulfamethoxazole and other agents are used for *Pneumocystis* coverage. Acyclovir is commonly given for antiviral

prophylaxis, based on the patient's and donor's cytomegalovirus and herpes simplex virus status. Vancomycinpolymyxin capsules and a low-bacteria diet may be used to achieve decontamination of the GI tract.

FEVER

All fevers or symptoms of potential infection need to be taken seriously both during hospitalization and in the posttransplant period. Patients presenting to an emergency department should be moved to a private examination room as soon as possible; they should not spend time in the waiting room owing to the infectious risk. Reverse precautions should be observed. All febrile stem cell transplant patients must have a meticulous physical examination, with special attention to the skin, perirectal tissue, central venous line site, and neurologic examination. Rectal temperatures and rectal examinations should not be performed because of the increased risk of introducing infection. Blood cultures should be drawn from all central venous lines or peripherally if lines are no longer present. A chest radiograph is recommended for any patient with respiratory symptoms. Broad-spectrum antibiotics should be started as soon as possible—ideally, within 30 to 60 minutes of presentation. Antimicrobial therapy should not be delayed for diagnostic procedures, including blood or urine culture or lumbar puncture, if there is difficulty obtaining the sample.

The need for hospital admission of stem cell transplant patients with fever depends on the time since the transplant and the clinical situation. This should be discussed with the transplant team. Most allogeneic transplant recipients need to be admitted for any episode of fever within a year of transplantation, particularly if they are on immunosuppressive drugs.

VACCINATION

Autologous and allogeneic stem cell transplant recipients lose their immunologic memory responses to most vaccinations. Thus, patients need to be revaccinated after stem cell transplantation. The timing of revaccination differs among institutions. Clinicians evaluating stem cell transplant patients should be aware of their vaccination status and remain alert for unusual infections. Live vaccines should be avoided in any patient receiving immunosuppressive drugs and for a minimum of 2 years after discontinuing therapy.

MEDICATION ISSUES

Stem cell transplant patients are frequently taking multiple medications, and drug interactions can be a significant issue. Immunosuppressants, antimicrobial agents, and antiepileptics often interact with other drugs. Because of the potential for drug interaction, it is important to review drug information with a pharmacist or other credible source before adding any new agent. This is also important when considering a dosage change for a medication a patient is already taking. In addition to interacting with other drugs, some common medications are known to cause decreased blood counts due to either marrow suppression or peripheral destruction. These drugs should be avoided in stem cell transplant patients if possible. The transplant team can provide assistance in choosing appropriate medications for these patients.

CONSULTATION

Transplant patients have a complicated medical history and specialized medical needs. The complexity of their underlying disease, as well as their past and current therapy, necessitates a timely and thorough discussion with the primary oncologist and transplant team. Admission and discharge criteria are guided by the recommendations of these specialists.

ADMISSION CRITERIA

- Any sign or symptom consistent with an infectious process or GVHD.
- Any change in the baseline outpatient status.
- Inability to maintain adequate hydration or nutrition.
- Inability to take prescribed medications.
- Concerns about compliance or social issues that may prevent the patient's adherence to the recommended therapeutic regimen.

DISCHARGE CRITERIA

- Resolution of the infection or other concern that prompted hospitalization.
- Ability to take adequate oral hydration, nutrition, and medications as an outpatient.
- Sufficient outpatient resources to comply with the medical regimen and continue outpatient follow-up with the primary care provider and specialists.

IN A NUTSHELL

- Patients who have undergone bone marrow transplantation are often cared for in community settings afterward. These patients have complex medical histories and require prompt and thorough evaluation and initiation of treatment.
- Transplant patients are at significant risk for common and uncommon infections. They may be on varied antimicrobial prophylactic regimens and have an incomplete immunization status. The index of suspicion for infection (bacterial, fungal, viral, or parasitic) should be very high.
- GVHD is a major cause of morbidity and mortality in this patient population and can present with a variety of signs and symptoms any time after transplantation.
- Rapid and effective communication with a transplant center is crucial for the optimal care of this patient group. The patient's primary transplant team must be included in management decisions.

ON THE HORIZON

- Stem cell transplantation is a rapidly changing field. The focus of clinical development is on reducing the toxicity of the inpatient transplant process. This includes developing and improving nonablative transplants, creating less immunosuppressive treatment strategies for GVHD, and decreasing the length of hospitalization. These and other developments may enable stem cell transplants to be offered to a more diverse patient population.

SUGGESTED READING

Akpek G, Chinratanalab W, Lee LA, et al: Gastrointestinal involvement in chronic graft-versus-host disease: A clinicopathologic study. Biol Blood Marrow Transplant 2003;9:46-51.

Diaz MA, Vicent MG, Gonzalez ME, et al: Risk assessment and outcome of chronic graft-versus-host disease after allogeneic peripheral blood progenitor cell transplantation in pediatric patients. Bone Marrow Transplant 2004;34:433-438.

Gross TG, Egeler RM: Pediatric hematopoietic stem cell transplantation. Hematol Oncol Clin North Am 2001;15:795-808.

Kollman C, Howe CW, Anasetti C, et al: Donor characteristics as risk factors in recipients after transplantation of bone marrow from unrelated donors: The effect of donor age. Blood 2001;98:2043-2051.

Machado C: Reimmunization after bone marrow transplantation: Current recommendations and perspectives. Braz J Med Biol Res 2004;37:151-158.

Snover DC: Graft-versus-host disease of the gastrointestinal tract. Am J Surg Pathol 1990;14:101-108.

Vermylen C: Hematopoietic stem cell transplantation in sickle cell disease. Blood Rev 2003;17:163-166.

Weaver CH, Schwartzberg LS, Hainsworth J, et al: Treatment-related mortality in 1000 consecutive patients receiving high-dose chemotherapy and peripheral blood progenitor cell transplantation in community cancer centers. Bone Marrow Transplant 1997;19:671-678.

Zecca M, Prete A, Rondelli R, et al: Chronic graft-versus-host-disease in children: Incidence, risk factors, and impact on outcome. Blood 2002;100:1192-1200.

REFERENCES

1. Johns A: Overview of bone marrow and stem cell transplantation. J Intraven Nurs 1998;21:356-360.
2. Saba N, Abraham R, Keating A: Overview of autologous stem cell transplantation. Crit Rev Oncol Hematol 2000;36:27-48.
3. Busca A, Amoroso A, Miniero R: Bone marrow transplantation from unrelated volunteer donors: An overview. Panminerva Med 1997;39:71-77.
4. Perkins HA, Hansen JA: The US National Marrow Donor Program. Am J Pediatr Hematol Oncol 1994;16:30-34.
5. McCluskey J, Peh CA: The human leucocyte antigens and clinical medicine: An overview. Rev Immunogenet 1999;1:3-20.
6. Arai S, Klingemann HG: Hematopoietic stem cell transplantation: Bone marrow vs mobilized peripheral blood. Arch Med Res 2003;34:545-553.
7. Cottler-Fox MH, Lapidot T, Petit I, et al: Stem cell mobilization. Hematology Am Soc Hematol Educ Program 2003;419-437.
8. Brunstein CG, Wagner JE: Umbilical cord blood transplantation and banking. Annu Rev Med 2006;57:403-417.
9. Blazar BR, Murphy WJ: Bone marrow transplantation and approaches to avoid graft-versus-host disease (GVHD). Philos Trans R Soc Lond B Biol Sci 2005;360:1747-1767.

10. Ferrara JL, Yanik G: Acute graft versus host disease: Pathophysiology, risk factors, and prevention strategies. Clin Adv Hematol Oncol 2005;3:415-419, 428.

11. Martin PJ, Carpenter PA, Sanders JE, Flowers ME: Diagnosis and clinical management of chronic graft-versus-host disease. Int J Hematol 2004;79:221-228.

12. Klingebiel T, Schlegel PG: GVHD: Overview on pathophysiology, incidence, clinical and biological features. Bone Marrow Transplant 1998;21(Suppl 2):S45-S49.

13. Akpek G, Chinratanalab W, Lee LA, et al: Gastrointestinal involvement in chronic graft-versus-host disease: A clinicopathologic study. Biol Blood Marrow Transplant 2003;9:46-51.

Neurology

CHAPTER 126

Seizures

Annapurna Poduri and Paul E. Manicone

Epilepsy, the presence of recurrent or unprovoked seizures, has a prevalence in childhood of approximately 0.5%.[1] It is estimated that 5% of children will have at least one seizure before the age of 20.[2] Most children who experience a single seizure, which is often provoked by fever or acute illness, do not go on to develop epilepsy.

The evaluation and management of a patient with a seizure should focus on stabilization and rapid assessment for potentially reversible causes of the seizure. Most spontaneous or unprovoked seizures are brief and last less than a few minutes. However, seizures that occur in the setting of a systemic metabolic disturbance, intracranial infection, or intracranial hemorrhage may last longer. Because prolonged seizures may lead to hypoventilation, inadequate respiration, tissue hypoxia, and cerebral edema, prompt evaluation and treatment are essential.

EPILEPTIC SEIZURES

Clinical Presentation

A seizure is the manifestation of abnormally synchronized electrical activity in the brain. The presentation depends on the region of brain involved. Previous classification systems (e.g., the 1981 International Classification of Epileptic Seizures and the 1989 International Classification of Epilepsies, Epileptic Syndromes, and Related Disorders), although widely accepted, were based primarily on the phenomenology of the seizure. In 2001 the International League against Epilepsy (ILAE) published its diagnostic scheme for epileptic disorders and epilepsy, which is based on five axes to allow flexibility in the classification of these disorders (Table 126-1).[3] Axis 1 uses a standardized glossary of terms to describe the ictal semiology (behavior during a seizure). Axis 2 is derived from a list of accepted seizure types (Table 126-2); this includes reflex epilepsy, in which seizures are caused by a specific stimulus (Table 126-3). Axis 3 is based on specific syndromes (Table 126-4). Axis 4 is used when a specific cause is identified, and Axis 5 recognizes impairments secondary to the epilepsy disorder.

A seizure or recurrent seizures lasting more than 30 minutes without a return to baseline are considered continuous. A localization-related (focal or partial) seizure is one that begins in one region of the cortex. For example, a seizure beginning in or rapidly spreading to the left motor strip (left frontal cortex) would likely involve clonic movements of the right arm, leg, or face. A partial seizure arising from the temporal lobe might result in an abnormal psychic experience such as déjà vu. A partial seizure is said to be "simple" if consciousness is preserved and "complex" if consciousness is impaired; impaired consciousness can occur at the onset of the seizure or after a simple partial seizure has begun. A partial seizure can spread to involve the entire cortex and produce generalized seizure activity.

A generalized seizure begins deep in the brain, and the abnormal electrical impulses appear to reach all parts of the cortex at more or less the same time. This produces a loss or impairment of consciousness and may produce tonic activity (stiffening), clonic activity (rhythmic jerking), tonic-clonic activity (stiffening followed by or alternating with rhythmic jerking), atonic activity (loss of tone), myoclonic activity (sudden contraction of muscles), or absence seizures (typically with staring, blinking, and automatisms).

Not all generalized seizures produce noticeable convulsive seizure activity. The stereotypical presentations of partial and generalized seizures are as described earlier, but any change in consciousness or unexplained loss of consciousness can be due to electrical seizure activity without other outward signs. Therefore, seizure—particularly nonconvulsive status epilepticus—must be included in the differential diagnosis of any patient with an altered mental status or altered level of consciousness (see Chapter 28).

Differential Diagnosis

The differential diagnosis of seizure includes a variety of neurologic and non-neurologic conditions (Table 126-5). In a previously normal child, the evaluation of a first seizure should include a careful review of the event itself and its possible precipitating factors. In most cases, a description of the event by the parent or caretaker, or possibly from the child, must suffice in arriving at a working clinical diagnosis.

Diagnosis and Evaluation

The causes of a new seizure in a previously healthy child or an increase in seizure frequency in a child with known seizures should always be investigated. Although an other-

Table 126-1 International League against Epilepsy: Diagnostic Scheme

Axis 1: Ictal phenomenology
    Description of the seizure event

Axis 2: Seizure type (see Table 126-2)
    Self-limited
        Generalized
        Focal
    Continuous
        Generalized status epilepticus
        Focal status epilepticus
    Reflex: ictal events precipitated by sensory stimuli (see Table 126-3)

Axis 3: Syndrome (see Table 126-4)
    Complex of signs and symptoms that define a unique epilepsy condition

Axis 4: Cause
    Based on a specific cause, if known (e.g., diseases frequently associated with epileptic seizures, genetic defects, pathologic substrate)
        Symptomatic: resulting from structural brain lesion (secondary epilepsy)
        Probably symptomatic: believed to be symptomatic but no cause identified (cryptogenic)
        Idiopathic: primary epilepsy with no identified structural brain lesion, presumed to be genetic

Axis 5: Impairment
    Description of disability caused by the epileptic condition

Table 126-2 Epileptic Seizure Types

Self-Limited Seizures
Generalized seizures
    Tonic-clonic seizures (includes variations beginning with a clonic or myoclonic phase)
    Clonic seizures
        Without tonic features
        With tonic features
    Typical absence seizures
    Atypical absence seizures
    Myoclonic absence seizures
    Tonic seizures
    Spasms
    Myoclonic seizures
    Massive bilateral myoclonus
    Eyelid myoclonia
        Without absences
        With absences
    Myoclonic atonic seizures
    Negative myoclonus
    Atonic seizures
    Reflex seizures in generalized epilepsy syndromes
    Seizures of the posterior neocortex
    Neocortical temporal lobe seizures
Focal seizures
    Focal sensory seizures
        With elementary sensory symptoms (e.g., occipital and parietal lobe seizures)
        With experiential sensory symptoms (e.g., temporoparieto-occipital junction seizures)
    Focal motor seizures
        With elementary clonic motor signs
        With asymmetrical tonic motor seizures (e.g., supplementary motor seizures)
        With typical (temporal lobe) automatisms (e.g., mesial temporal lobe seizures)
        With hyperkinetic automatisms
        With focal negative myoclonus
        With inhibitory motor seizures
    Gelastic seizures
    Hemiclonic seizures
    Secondarily generalized seizures
    Reflex seizures in focal epilepsy syndromes

Continuous Seizures
Generalized status epilepticus
    Generalized tonic-clonic status epilepticus
    Clonic status epilepticus
    Absence status epilepticus
    Tonic status epilepticus
    Myoclonic status epilepticus
Focal status epilepticus
    Epilepsia partialis continua (Koshevnikoff epilepsy)
    Aura continua
    Limbic status epilepticus (psychomotor status)
    Hemiconvulsive status epilepticus with hemiparesis

wise healthy child is unlikely to have an occult abnormality, children with known epilepsy may have an underlying infection, such as a urinary tract infection, or other systemic disturbance that has decreased the seizure threshold. Factors that can provoke seizures are listed in Table 126-6. The likelihood of each must be judged on the basis of the entire clinical picture. The same precipitating factors apply to children with epilepsy who are taking antiepileptic medication, along with the additional considerations listed in Table 126-7.

The pace and extent of the diagnostic evaluation depend on the clinical setting. A detailed history and physical examination—with immediate assessment of airway, breathing, circulation, and glucose, followed by a comprehensive general and neurologic examination—should guide the evaluation. Table 126-8 presents several approaches to the diagnostic evaluation of a child with seizures, based on the clinical history and state of the patient.

Little is gained from an extensive laboratory evaluation in a stable, well-appearing, previously healthy child with a brief new-onset seizure and a swift return to baseline. In the emergency department, measurement of glucose, serum electrolytes, and calcium constitutes a comprehensive emergent evaluation. There is evidence that even this limited screen for abnormalities is not compulsory in patients older than 6 months with no history of possible dehydration or gastrointestinal losses who have returned to baseline mental status.[4] The history and clinical judgment must be used to decide whether other tests, such as urine toxicology screening, are

Table 126–3 Precipitating Stimuli for Reflex Seizures
Visual stimuli
Flickering light—color to be specified when possible
Patterns
Other visual stimuli
Thinking
Music
Eating
Praxis
Somatosensory stiumli
Proprioceptive stimuli
Reading
Hot water
Startle

Table 126–4 Epilepsy Syndromes and Related Conditions
Benign familial neonatal seizures
Early myoclonic encephalopathy
Ohtahara syndrome
Migrating partial seizures of infancy*
West syndrome
Benign myoclonic epilepsy in infancy
Benign familial infantile seizures
Benign infantile seizures (nonfamilial)
Dravet syndrome
Hemiconvulsion-hemiplegia-epilepsy (HHE)
Myoclonic status epilepticus in nonprogressive encephalopathies*
Benign childhood epilepsy with centrotemporal spikes
Early-onset benign childhood occipital epilepsy (Panayiotopoulos type)
Late-onset childhood occipital epilepsy (Gastaut type)
Epilepsy with myoclonic absences
Epilepsy with myoclonic-astatic seizures
Lennox-Gastaut syndrome
Landau-Kleffner syndrome
Epilepsy with continuous spike and waves during slow-wave sleep (other than Landau-Kleffner syndrome)
Childhood absence epilepsy
Progressive myoclonic epilepsies
Idiopathic generalized epilepsies with variable phenotypes
Juvenile absence epilepsy
Juvenile myoclonic epilepsy
Epilepsy with generalized tonic-clonic seizures only
Reflex epilepsies
Idiopathic photosensitive occipital lobe epilepsy
Other visual-sensitive epilepsies
Primary reading epilepsy
Startle epilepsy
Autosomal dominant nocturnal frontal lobe epilepsy
Familial temporal lobe epilepsies
Generalized epilepsies with febrile seizures plus*
Familial focal epilepsy with variable foci*
Symptomatic (or probably symptomatic) focal epilepsies
Limbic epilepsies
Mesial temporal lobe epilepsy with hippocampal sclerosis
Mesial temporal lobe epilepsy defined by specific causes
Other types defined by location and cause
Neocortical epilepsies
Rasmussen syndrome
Other types defined by location and cause
Conditions with epileptic seizures that do not require a diagnosis of epilepsy
Benign neonatal seizures
Febrile seizures
Reflex seizures
Alcohol withdrawal seizures
Drug or other chemically induced seizures
Immediate and early post-traumatic seizures
Single seizures or isolated clusters of seizures
Rarely repeated seizures (oligoepilepsy)

*Syndromes in development.

needed. A previously healthy child with a new seizure should have neurologic follow-up within 1 to 2 weeks for a comprehensive evaluation, including electroencephalogram (EEG). Outpatient magnetic resonance imaging (MRI) should be performed after a first-time seizure in children younger than 1 year and in children with an abnormal neurologic history or examination or with EEG abnormalities that do not fall into the category of a benign epilepsy syndrome (e.g., childhood absence epilepsy).[4] Both EEG and MRI can be helpful in assessing the risk of seizure recurrence.

In children who appear ill, were previously abnormal, or have already been admitted to the hospital for other medical reasons, a more exhaustive search for a precipitating factor is warranted. After stabilization and assessment of glucose, additional laboratory studies and computed tomography (CT) of the head should be performed. In the presence of fever and findings that suggest the possibility of meningitis or encephalitis, CT of the head should be followed by lumbar puncture. These tests should not delay the administration of broad-spectrum antibiotics or acyclovir in an ill-appearing febrile child who has had a seizure. If a patient does not return to a normal baseline neurologic status, an EEG is required to evaluate for nonconvulsive status epilepticus.

A child with a history of epilepsy may have seizures that result from the same precipitating factors as in a child without previous seizures. In these patients, particular attention should be given to a history of recent infection, head trauma, or a change in the medication regimen that might lead to increased seizure frequency. Anticonvulsant levels must be interpreted with regard to the timing of last administered dose, and, when possible, those levels should be compared with typical levels for a given patient.

Course of Illness

The clinical course of a patient with seizures depends on the cause of the seizures. An otherwise well child with a brief provoked seizure, such as a febrile seizure, does not have a significantly increased risk of epilepsy, whereas a child with

Table 126-5 Differential Diagnosis of Seizures

Syncope (in which anoxia may also precipitate a provoked seizure)

Cardiac arrhythmia with collapse

Breath-holding spell

Tic

Myoclonus

Gastroesophageal reflux disease (including Sandifer syndrome)

Behavioral event (e.g., nonepileptic staring)

Parasomnia

Migraine variant (complicated migraine)

Conversion disorder (nonepileptic event resembling an epileptic seizure)

Table 126-7 Additional Factors That May Precipitate Seizures in Patients with Epilepsy

Systemic infection (with or without fever)
    Urinary tract infection
    Upper or lower respiratory tract infection
    Sinusitis
    Bacteremia

Other systemic disturbance
    Dehydration

Low level of antiepileptic medication
    Illness causing decreased intake or absorption of antiepileptic medication
    Concurrent use of other medications that lower antiepileptic medication levels
    Noncompliance

Toxic level of antiepileptic medication (e.g., phenytoin, valproic acid)

Table 126-6 Factors That May Precipitate Seizures

Fever

Infection
    Meningitis (bacterial; viral, including herpes simplex virus)
    Encephalitis
    Sepsis (especially in neonates)

Hypoxia or ischemia

Head trauma producing concussion or intracranial hemorrhage

Metabolic disturbance
    Low or high glucose
    Low or high sodium
    Low calcium
    Low magnesium
    Hyperammonemia

Pregnancy or toxemia (usually second or third trimester)

Inborn error of metabolism

Medication (e.g., imipenem, meperidine, cyclosporine)

Medication withdrawal (e.g., benzodiazepines)

Toxin or illicit substance (e.g., cocaine)

a known chronic encephalopathy with seizures has a high likelihood of seizure recurrence.

Most individual seizures are brief and cause no damage to the brain. A fall during a seizure might result in head trauma, and aspiration of gastrointestinal contents or excessive saliva could result in pneumonia, but these are uncommon events.

Treatment

Because most seizures are self-limited, management consists of stabilization of the airway, breathing, and circulation and prompt evaluation of underlying causes of the seizure. Proper monitoring should be established, including cardiorespiratory monitoring and pulse oximetry. Supplemental oxygen should be administered as needed and, whenever possible, intravenous access should be obtained. Reversible causes of the seizure should be appropriately corrected. Hypoglycemia requires rapid correction, and disturbances in sodium balance require judicious, slow correction. Broad-spectrum antibiotics should be given at doses appropriate to treat meningitis until central nervous system or other infection has been excluded in any child with signs of infection; acyclovir should be added if central nervous system herpetic infection is suspected.

It is well established that intervention for a child with continuous or recurrent seizures should begin by 5 minutes into the seizure, because a seizure of that length may evolve into status epilepticus.[5] In a child with a prior history of seizures, a seizure longer than his or her typical seizure should be treated as one that might evolve into status epilepticus. A child at high risk of intracranial pathology with seizure activity lasting more than a few minutes should be considered to have incipient status epilepticus, and pharmacologic treatment should be initiated.[5,6]

After stabilization of the cardiorespiratory status and treatment of any reversible causes of seizure, pharmacologic management to arrest seizure activity should be initiated. Medications used in the acute treatment of seizures are outlined in Table 126-9. Vigilant monitoring of oxygenation, ventilation, and circulatory status is essential during the administration of these medications because of their sedative and potential respiratory and cardiac effects. If the medications listed in Table 126-9 are not effective, suppressive therapy with agents such as pentobarbital, midazolam (by continuous intravenous infusion), or general anesthesia should be administered in an intensive care setting, ideally with continuous EEG monitoring.

The initial treatment of a child with a new diagnosis of epilepsy requires an accurate diagnosis of the particular seizure disorder, as well as an understanding of the wide range of antiepileptic drugs available (Table 126-10). There are limited studies of antiepileptic drugs in children, so some

Table 126-8 Diagnostic Evaluation of a Patient with Seizure

Basic Evaluation

History and physical examination
Blood glucose level
Serum electrolytes and calcium level*
Urine toxicology screen*
Urine pregnancy screen in age-appropriate girls*
If febrile, evaluation for source of fever (e.g., blood culture, urine culture, chest radiograph)

Additional Studies

In well-appearing, previously normal patients who return to baseline after a first seizure
  Outpatient neurologic consultation with EEG
  Possible outpatient MRI
In hospitalized or ill-appearing patients, especially after a first seizure
  CBC with platelets
If the patient has depressed mental status
  Liver transaminases
  Consider blood ammonia level and screening tests for other inborn errors of metabolism
  Consider arterial blood gas
  CT of the head, especially in those with a ventricular shunt, history of recent head trauma, coma, or focal neurologic abnormality
  Lumbar puncture after CT when patient is stable
  EEG if patient does not return to baseline or nonconvulsive status epilepticus is suspected
In patients with a prior history of seizures
  Liver transaminases and blood urea nitrogen level
  Serum ammonia level if taking valproic acid or if comatose
  Consider other screens for inborn errors of metabolism if cause of patient's seizures is not well established
  Consider arterial blood gas
  Appropriate anticonvulsant levels
  CBC with platelets
  CT of the head in those with a ventricular shunt, history of recent head trauma, coma, or focal neurologic abnormality
  EEG if patient does not return to baseline or nonconvulsive status epilepticus is suspected

*Depending on history, at clinician's discretion.
CBC, complete blood count; CT, computed tomography; EEG, electroencephalogram; MRI, magnetic resonance imaging.

drugs may not be approved by the Food and Drug Administration for specific indications. Table 126-11 provides the trade names of antiepileptic drugs used in children and a limited list of their adverse reactions.

Consultation

Consultation with a neurologist is advised for new-onset seizures, especially in the case of a focal neurologic deficit, and for seizures that are not self-limited.

Critical care consultation is required when the patient's cardiorespiratory status is unstable or for intractable status epilepticus that requires cardiorespiratory support (e.g., intravenous infusion sedatives or general anesthesia).

Table 126-9 Medications for the Acute Treatment of Seizures

After 5 min, or sooner if warranted by the clinical situation:
  Lorazepam (Ativan) 0.1 mg/kg IV or IM (maximum dose 8 mg)
  Midazolam (Versed) 0.2 mg/kg IV or 0.5 mg/kg PR (if no IV access)
  Diazepam rectal gel (Diastat): for use in children older than 2 yr
    Children 2-5 yr: 0.5 mg/kg PR
    Children 6-11 yr: 0.3 mg/kg PR
    Children ≥12 yr: 0.2 mg/kg PR
Doses may be repeated every 5 min, but if seizures persist after 10 min, proceed to:
  Fosphenytoin 20 mg phenytoin equivalents/kg IV
  Phenobarbital 20 mg/kg IV
  Valproic acid 15 mg/kg IV*
In neonates or infants with refractory seizures, pyridoxine (vitamin B_6) should be administered, with respiratory and EEG monitoring in consultation with a neurologist

*Use if child is older than 2 years and there is no suspicion of metabolic disease or liver dysfunction.
EEG, electroencephalogram.

Table 126-10 Antiepileptic Drugs for Pediatric Seizures and Epileptic Syndromes

Seizure Disorder	Drugs of Choice
Generalized tonic-clonic seizures	Topiramate Valproic acid Carbamazepine Levetiracetam
Generalized absence seizures	Ethosuximide Valproic acid Lamotrigine
Partial seizures	Carbamazepine Oxcarbazepine Lamotrigine Topiramate
BECTS	Carbamazepine Gabapentin
Juvenile myoclonic epilepsy	Valproic acid Lamotrigine
Neonatal seizures	Phenobarbital Phenytoin
Infantile spasms	ACTH Vigabatrin
Lennox-Gastaut syndrome	Lamotrigine Topiramate Felbamate

ACTH, adrenocorticotropic hormone; BECTS, benign epilepsy of childhood with centrotemporal spikes (also known as rolandic epilepsy).
Adapted from Sankar R: Initial treatment of epilepsy with antiepileptic drugs: Pediatric issues. Neurology 2004;63(Suppl 4):S30-S39.

Table 126-11 Antiepileptic Drugs and Prominent Adverse Effects

Generic Name	Trade Name	Side Effects*
ACTH	Acthar Gel	Insomnia, cataracts, hirsutism, diabetes mellitus
Carbamazepine	Tegretol, Carbatrol	Cardiac arrhythmia and conduction delays, sedation, photosensitivity, SJS, bone marrow suppression, hepatitis, SIADH
Ethosuximide	Zarontin	Sedation, agitation, headache, increase in GTC seizure frequency, GI symptoms, SJS, hiccups, chorea
Felbamate	Felbatol	Ataxia, GI symptoms, aplastic anemia, hepatotoxicity, diplopia
Gabapentin	Neurontin	Sedation, agitation, leukopenia, nystagmus, GI symptoms
Lamotrigine	Lamictal	Dizziness, sedation, photosensitivity, SJS, GI symptoms, nystagmus
Levetiracetam	Keppra	Ataxia, paresthesias, memory difficulties, hallucinations, diplopia
Phenobarbital	Barbita, Luminal, Solfoton	Cardiac arrhythmia, sedation, SJS, GI symptoms, agranulocytosis, megaloblastic anemia, respiratory depression, may reduce serum levels of a wide variety of drugs
Oxcarbazepine	Trileptal	Psychomotor slowing, dizziness, hyponatremia, GI symptoms
Phenytoin	Dilantin	Ataxia, lethargy, folic acid depletion, nystagmus, SJS, hirsutism, gingival hyperplasia, SLE-like syndrome
Topiramate	Topamax	Ataxia, memory difficulties, language regression, hyperchloremic metabolic acidosis, menstrual disorders, GI symptoms, nystagmus
Valproic acid	Depakene, Depakote, Epilim	Ataxia, irritability, thrombocytopenia, GI symptoms, hepatotoxicity, hyperammonemia, carnitine depletion
Vigabatrin	Sabril	Ataxia, fatigue, hyperactivity, visual field defects, nystagmus, GI symptoms

*This is only a partial list. Prescribers should consult pharmaceutical references for complete information.
ACTH, adrenocorticotropic hormone; GI, gastrointestinal; GTC, generalized tonic-clonic; SIADH, syndrome of inappropriate antidiuretic hormone; SJS, Stevens-Johnson syndrome; SLE, systemic lupus erythematosus.

Admission Criteria

- Patient does not return to baseline mental status.
- Identification of the underlying cause of the seizure is not straightforward.
- The cause of the seizure requires inpatient therapy.

Discharge Criteria

- The patient is medically stable, and seizure control is adequate for outpatient management.
- The patient's caretakers are trained in basic cardiopulmonary resuscitation and first aid during seizures. Some caretakers can be instructed in the use of diazepam rectal gel for the initial management of a prolonged seizure.
- Patients who are started on antiepileptic medications are able to take them orally and do not have significant side effects, such as excessive drowsiness, severe nausea, or ataxia.

In A Nutshell

- Most spontaneous or unprovoked seizures are self-limited. Children with underlying metabolic abnormalities, intracranial infection, or trauma are more likely to have prolonged seizures.
- A new classification scheme for seizures has been established that uses multiple approaches to categorize epileptic seizures and epilepsy.
- The evaluation of children with seizures is guided by clinical assessment, including well versus ill appearance, and first seizure versus history of previous seizures.
- Nonconvulsive status epilepticus may present as an altered mental status or altered level of consciousness.
- Initial management includes cardiorespiratory stabilization, correction of metabolic disturbances, treatment of underlying localized or systemic infection, and, if there is ongoing seizure activity, pharmacologic therapy to abort the process.
- Children with known seizure disorders (with or without anticonvulsant therapy) may have a lower seizure threshold in the face of fever, metabolic abnormalities, or infection. When these patients show an increase in their baseline seizure activity, they require the same evaluation as patients without a history of seizures.
- Consultation with a neurologist is recommended when seizure activity is not self-limited, is difficult to control, or includes focal neurologic deficits or if the patient does not return to baseline neurologic status.

On the Horizon

- Advances in diagnostic imaging—including refinements of structural imaging by MRI, functional studies (functional MRI, positron emission tomography [PET], single photon emission computed tomography [SPECT]), and combination techniques such as subtraction ictal SPECT coregistered to MRI (SISCOM)—will improve the identification of children with seizures refractory to medication who are candidates for surgical resection of the cortex generating the seizures. Epilepsy surgery is currently underutilized in children, who are more likely than adults with long-duration epilepsy to experience benefits in cognitive development and quality of life after successful procedures.[7-9]
- The new generation of antiepileptic drugs, introduced in the early 1990s, offers equal or superior efficacy and, in most cases, fewer adverse effects and interactions compared with conventional drugs.[10] Still, we lack drugs to prevent epilepsy or its progression and therapies to address drug-resistant epilepsy. These are important targets for research.[11]

FEBRILE SEIZURES

Febrile seizures are the most common seizures seen in children younger than 5 years. The 1993 ILAE guidelines defined a febrile seizure as an epileptic seizure occurring in children older than 1 month and associated with a febrile illness, excluding those with prior unprovoked or neonatal seizures, acute central nervous system infection, or electrolyte imbalance, and not meeting criteria for other acute symptomatic seizures.[12]

Febrile seizures are classified as simple or complex. Simple febrile seizures, which constitute 85% of all febrile seizures, last for less than 15 minutes, are generalized tonic-clonic seizures, and occur only once in 24 hours. Febrile seizures that last for more than 15 minutes, have focal features (at any time), or recur within 24 hours are considered complex. The majority of febrile seizures are self-limited and last only a few minutes.

Febrile seizures occur in 2% to 5% of all children. The peak age of onset is 14 to 18 months. A strong family history of febrile seizures in siblings and parents suggests a genetic predisposition. Twenty-five percent to 40% of patients have an immediate family member with a history of febrile seizures. If one parent has a history of febrile seizures, a child's risk of having a febrile seizure is greater than four times that of the general population. If both parents have a history of febrile seizures, the risk increases 20-fold over that of the general population. Siblings of a child with febrile seizures have a risk 3.6 times greater than that of the general population. Even the concordance rate in monozygotic twins is higher than that in dizygotic twins.[13]

Cause

The underlying pathophysiology is unknown. Viral infections are frequently associated with febrile seizures, particularly human herpesviruses and influenza A and B. It is estimated that human herpesvirus 6 accounts for one third of first-time febrile seizures in children younger than 2 years, and human herpesvirus 7 is increasingly being recognized as a causative agent as well. There is a clear genetic predisposition, but no specific locus or pattern of inheritance has been described. The mode of inheritance likely varies among families and may be multifactorial.

The rates of serious bacterial infection in patients with febrile seizures are similar to the rates in age-matched febrile children without seizures.[13]

Clinical Presentation

Children with simple febrile seizures are neurologically and developmentally healthy before and after the seizure. Simple febrile seizures often occur with the initial temperature elevation at the onset of illness. The seizure may be the first indication that the child is ill.

The history should address the details of the event to differentiate the seizure as simple or complex. Additional information should focus on the fever's duration, exposures, and associated symptoms. Medications given at home should also be ascertained, especially antibiotics. The possibility of partially treated meningitis in an infant or child with recent or current antibiotic use should be considered.

The physical examination should concentrate on identifying the underlying source of the fever, as well as any generalized or focal neurologic abnormalities. It is important to evaluate the child for signs of meningitis or encephalitis. The child should have a normal neurologic examination or, if presenting in the postictal period, should be observed until the examination is normal. Any prolonged alteration in the child's general appearance or mental status or any finding suggestive of a focal deficit signifies the need for a more aggressive evaluation, such as neuroimaging and lumbar puncture.

Differential Diagnosis

A broad range of entities can present with a febrile seizure, seizure-like activity, or altered mental status (Table 126-12). Convulsive behavior may be a consequence of the fever itself or of the condition that caused the fever.

Diagnosis and Evaluation

When a child presents with a febrile seizure, the evaluation should encompass the seizure component as well as the febrile illness. The evaluation of febrile children is discussed in Chapters 33 and 60. The discussion here focuses on the neurodiagnostic evaluation.

Routine laboratory studies are usually not indicated for patients with simple febrile seizures, with the exception of a whole-blood or serum glucose test. Laboratory studies should be driven by the nature of the underlying illness rather than the presentation of a febrile seizure. For example, patients with dehydration may warrant an electrolyte panel to evaluate for hyponatremia, which can cause convulsions.

Many physicians are faced with the difficult decision of whether to perform a lumbar puncture to rule out meningitis in a patient with a febrile seizure. According to the American Academy of Pediatrics (AAP) 1996 practice parameter for children with a first simple febrile seizure, a lumbar puncture should be strongly considered in infants younger than 12 months, because the signs and symptoms

Table 126-12 Differential Diagnosis of Febrile Seizure

Epilepsy

Intracranial infection
  Meningitis
  Encephalitis
  Brain abscess
  Epidural or subdural infection

Cerebrovascular accident

Epidural or subdural hematoma

Acute disseminated encephalomyelitis

Shivering or rigors

Febrile myoclonus

Febrile delirium

Drug-induced hyperthermia

Table 126-13 Indications to Perform Lumbar Puncture in a Child Younger than 18 Months with a Febrile Seizure

History of irritability, poor feeding, or lethargy

Abnormal mental status beyond the postictal period

Physical signs of meningitis, such as bulging fontanelle, Kernig or Brudzinski sign, photophobia, or inconsolable crying

Febrile seizure with complex features

Pretreatment with antibiotics

of bacterial meningitis may be minimal or absent in this age group. Lumbar puncture should also be considered in children 12 to 18 months old, given the subtle nature of the signs and symptoms of bacterial meningitis (Table 126-13). In children older than 18 months, the decision to perform a lumbar puncture rests on the clinical suspicion of meningitis.[14] It is important to note that patients with simple febrile seizures have the same risk for bacterial illnesses, including meningitis, as those who present with similar febrile illnesses without seizures. The indications for lumbar puncture in Table 126-13 reflect the recommendations for a similarly aged patient with fever but no seizure.

The AAP practice parameter does not recommend neuroimaging (CT or MRI) for the routine evaluation of children with first simple febrile seizures.[14] There are currently no guidelines for complex febrile seizures; however, recent studies have demonstrated that the risk of intracranial pathology requiring emergency neurosurgical or medical intervention is low in children with first complex febrile seizures.[15] This suggests that routine imaging in patients with complex febrile seizures may be unnecessary as well. Neuroimaging should be considered in the following situations: uncertain diagnosis, inability to exclude increased intracranial pressure by physical examination, status epilepticus, persistent focal features, evidence of trauma, or presence of ventriculoperitoneal shunt.

The AAP practice parameter does not recommend an EEG for a neurologically healthy child with a first simple febrile seizure.[14] The EEG does not reliably predict which patients will have recurrent febrile seizures or subsequently develop epilepsy. An EEG might be indicated in patients with evidence of developmental delay or underlying neurologic abnormalities, but this study is rarely needed on an urgent basis in this setting.

Treatment

Several approaches have been investigated in the management and prevention of febrile seizures. These strategies include continuous or intermittent anticonvulsant therapy, prophylactic benzodiazepine therapy, and prophylactic antipyretic therapy.

On the basis of a risk-benefit analysis, neither long-term nor intermittent anticonvulsant therapy is indicated for children who have experienced one or more simple febrile seizures.[16] Phenobarbital is effective in preventing febrile seizures but has serious adverse effects, such as hyperactivity, hypersensitivity reactions, and a risk of cognitive impairment. Valproic acid is similarly effective in preventing febrile seizures but is associated with hepatotoxicity, thrombocytopenia, weight changes, gastrointestinal disturbances, and pancreatitis.

Oral diazepam given at the first sign of a febrile illness is effective in preventing febrile seizures; however, the adverse effects include lethargy, drowsiness, and ataxia. In addition, oral diazepam could mask the evolving signs of a central nervous system infection. In the rare instances where preventing subsequent febrile seizures is essential, diazepam is considered the treatment of choice. The dose is 0.33 mg/kg orally at the onset of fever, then every 8 hours until the child is afebrile.

Antipyretic agents are not effective in preventing recurrent febrile seizures. Although the routine use of prophylactic medications for simple febrile seizures is not indicated, there is insufficient evidence regarding their role in the treatment of complex febrile seizures.

Abortive therapy for future febrile seizures is another important consideration because approximately one in three children with a first febrile seizure will experience at least one recurrence with future febrile illnesses. Rectal diazepam gel (Diastat) has been approved by the Food and Drug Administration for home administration by trained nonprofessional caregivers and is effective in terminating febrile seizures.[17] Because most febrile seizures are brief, abortive therapy is often not necessary. Those children with a history of prolonged seizure activity or multiple seizures, those that live far from medical care, or those with overly anxious caregivers may benefit from this medication. Proper training in use of the drug should occur before the child is discharged from the hospital.

Abortive therapy for children who are actively seizing in the hospital setting is similar to the therapy for ongoing nonfebrile seizure activity. Intravenous or rectal diazepam is a good first choice.

Prognosis

Overall, the prognosis for children with febrile seizures is excellent. One third of all children will experience a recurrent febrile seizure with a subsequent febrile illness. Children

Table 126-14   Risk Factors for Recurrence of Febrile Seizure

Age younger than 18 mo
Family history of febrile seizures or epilepsy
Lower peak fever (<40°C) with prior febrile seizure
Shorter duration of fever with prior febrile seizure
Initial complex febrile seizure

On the Horizon

- Current and future studies will focus on complex febrile seizures: their evaluation and management and the associated risks. A practice parameter for complex febrile seizures will help reduce the wide variation in how this condition is evaluated and managed.
- Ongoing research in the area of genetic mapping will enhance our understanding of the genetic predispositions to febrile seizures.

younger than 12 months at the time of their first simple febrile seizure have a 50% probability of recurrence. After 12 months, the risk decreases to 30%.[13,16] Several risk factors for recurrence have been identified and are listed in Table 126-14.

The development of epilepsy and cognitive impairments are the two most important long-term outcomes that concern physicians and caregivers. In the general population, the risk of developing epilepsy by age 7 years is approximately 1%. Children younger than 12 months when they had their first simple febrile seizure or those who have had multiple simple febrile seizures have a 2.4% risk of developing epilepsy.[13,16] The risk is higher in patients with one or more complex febrile seizures. There is no evidence that children with simple febrile seizures suffer any cognitive impairment.[18-21] The long-term cognitive outcome for children with complex febrile seizures has not been well studied.

Consultation

Input from a neurologist may be warranted, especially if the diagnosis is in question, there are multiple complex features, or outpatient neurologic evaluation or management is needed.

Admission Criteria

Hospitalization is generally not necessary for the evaluation or management of a febrile seizure in a child who meets the criteria for a simple febrile seizure, has a normal neurologic examination, is well hydrated, and has access to appropriate follow-up. The following are indications for hospitalization:

- Prolonged or persistent alteration of mental status.
- Clinical or laboratory evidence of meningitis or encephalitis.
- Multiple complex features requiring further monitoring or workup.
- Inadequate enteral hydration or nutrition due to underlying source of infection.
- Inadequate follow-up or lack of family reliability.

Discharge Criteria

- Normal neurologic examination.
- Reassuring results of cerebrospinal fluid tests if performed.
- Neuroimaging not consistent with any evolving neurosurgical condition (e.g., space-occupying lesion, increased intracranial pressure) or infectious process (e.g., brain abscess) if performed.
- Demonstration of adequate oral hydration and nutrition.

SUGGESTED READING

Bauman RJ, D'Angelo SL: Practice parameter: The neurodiagnostic evaluation of the child with a first simple febrile seizure. American Academy of Pediatrics, Provisional Committee on Quality Improvement, Subcommittee on Febrile Seizures. Pediatrics 1996;97:769-775.

Fenichel GM: Clinical Pediatric Neurology: A Signs and Symptoms Approach, 4th ed. Philadelphia, WB Saunders, 2001.

Hirtz D: Practice parameter: Evaluating a first nonfebrile seizure in children. Neurology 2000;55:616-623.

Shinnar S: Febrile seizures. In Swaiman KE, Ashwal S (eds): Pediatric Neurology: Principles and Practice, 3rd ed. St Louis, Mosby, 1999, pp 676-682.

Swaiman KF, Ashwal S, Ferriero DM (eds): Pediatric Neurology: Principles and Practice, 4th ed. Philadelphia, Mosby, 2006.

Warden CR, Zibulewsky J, Mace S, et al: Evaluation and management of febrile seizures in the out-of-hospital and emergency department settings. Ann Emerg Med 2003;41:215-222.

REFERENCES

1. Cowan LD: The epidemiology of the epilepsies in children. Ment Retard Dev Disabil Res Rev 2002;8:171-181.
2. Hauser WA, Annegers JF, Rocca WA: Descriptive epidemiology of epilepsy: Contributions of population based studies from Rochester, Minnesota. Mayo Clin Proc 1996;71:576-586.
3. Engel J Jr: International League against Epilepsy: A proposed diagnostic scheme for people with epileptic seizures and with epilepsy: Report of the ILAE Task Force on Classification and Terminology. Epilepsia 2001; 42:796-803.
4. Hirtz D: Practice parameter: Evaluating a first nonfebrile seizure in children. Neurology 2000;55:616-623.
5. Leszczyszyn DJ, Pellock JM: Status epilepticus. In Pellock JM, Dodson WE, Bourgeois BFD (eds): Pediatric Epilepsy: Diagnosis and Therapy. New York, Demos, 2001, pp 275-281.
6. Riviello JJ Jr, Holmes GL: The treatment of status epilepticus. Semin Pediatr Neurol 2004;11:129-138.
7. Kaminska A, Chiron C, Ville D, et al: Ictal SPECT in children with epilepsy: Comparison with intracranial EEG and relation to postsurgical outcome. Brain 2003;126:248-260.
8. Sabaz M, Lawson JA, Cairns DR, et al: The impact of epilepsy surgery on quality of life in children. Neurology 2006;66:557-561.
9. Gleissner U, Sassen R, Schramm J, et al: Greater functional recovery after temporal lobe epilepsy surgery in children. Brain 2005;128:2822-2829.
10. French JA, Kanner AM, Bautista J, et al: Efficacy and tolerability of the new antiepileptic drugs. I. Treatment of new onset epilepsy: Report of the Therapeutics and Technology Assessment Subcommittee and Quality Standards Subcommittee of the American Academy of Neurology and the American Epilepsy Society. Neurology 2004;62:1252-1260.
11. Loscher W, Schmidt D: New horizons in the development of antiepileptic drugs: The search for new targets. Epilepsy Res 2004;60:77-159.
12. Commission on Epidemiology and Prognosis, International League against Epilepsy: Guidelines for epidemiologic studies on epilepsy. Epilepsia 1993;34:592-596.

13. Warden CR, Zibulewsky J, Mace S, et al: Evaluation and management of febrile seizures in the out-of-hospital and emergency department settings. Ann Emerg Med 2003;41:215-222.

14. Bauman RJ, D'Angelo SL: Practice parameter: The neurodiagnostic evaluation of the child with a first simple febrile seizure. American Academy of Pediatrics, Provisional Committee on Quality Improvement, Subcommittee on Febrile Seizures. Pediatrics 1996;97:769-775.

15. DiMario FJ Jr: Children presenting with complex febrile seizures do not routinely need computed tomography scanning in the emergency department. Pediatrics 2006;117:528-530.

16. Bauman RJ, Duffner PK, Schneider S: Practice parameter: Long term treatment of the child with simple febrile seizures. American Academy of Pediatrics, Committee on Quality Improvement, Subcommittee on Febrile Seizures. Pediatrics 1999;103:1307-1309.

17. Morton LD, Rizkallah E, Pellock JM: New drug therapy for acute seizure management. Semin Pediatr Neurol 1997;4:51.

18. Verity CM, Greenwood R, Golding J: Long-term intellectual and behavioral outcomes of children with febrile convulsions. N Engl J Med 1998;338:1723-1728.

19. Ellenberg JH, Nelson KB: Febrile seizures and later intellectual performance. Arch Neurol 1978;35:17-21.

20. Chang YC, Guo NW, Huang CC, et al: Neurocognitive attention and behavior outcome of school-age children with a history of febrile convulsions: A population study. Epilepsia 2000;41:412-420.

21. Chang YC, Guo NW, Wang ST, et al: Working memory of school-age children with a history of febrile convulsions: A population study. Neurology 2001;57:37-42.

CHAPTER 127

Headache
Annapurna Poduri

Although headache is a common condition in children and adolescents, patients are rarely admitted solely for the evaluation of headache. When it does occur or when headache develops during hospitalization, it is important to determine whether the headache represents a primary headache disorder, such as migraine or tension headache, or a secondary disorder resulting from a potentially serious intracranial or systemic process.

Epidemiologic studies in large cohorts of children reveal estimated 1-year prevalence rates of 6% to 20% for migraine and 11% to 18% for tension headache.[1-7] In general, post-pubertal girls have the highest prevalence rates of both migraine and tension headache. The most recent classification criteria established by the International Headache Society (IHS) in 2003 (Table 127-1)[8] provide a reliable and useful clinical tool to classify children's headaches.[9]

CLINICAL PRESENTATION

As with most medical and neurologic disorders, evaluation of headache consists chiefly of a careful history and detailed physical examination. Any abnormalities on neurologic examination in a previously healthy child or changes from neurologic baseline in a child with previous abnormalities warrant expeditious evaluation. In the absence of worrisome symptoms and abnormalities in the physical (including neurologic) examination, the majority of headaches in children are not caused by serious pathology. The physician should consider the following key questions during the evaluation:

Do the symptoms fit into the pattern of migraine or other typical headache syndromes?

Are there any warning symptoms or signs suggesting increased intracranial pressure (ICP) or focal neurologic deficit that would necessitate emergency neuroimaging and monitoring of the patient for worsening neurologic status?

Are there any predisposing factors to secondary headaches such as a ventriculoperitoneal (VP) shunt?

Finally, although the majority of headaches in children do not represent life-threatening emergencies, the pain experienced by the child and the ensuing anxiety of the family can be great. Once a patient with headache is deemed stable and relevant secondary causes have been considered and ruled out, the focus should shift to providing symptomatic analgesia and reassurance.

The typical presentations of headaches caused by increased ICP, other secondary headaches, and common primary headache disorders will be reviewed. Familiarity with the constellations of symptoms for each group can aid in differentiating among them by a careful history.

Although less common than primary headaches, secondary headaches are of greater immediate clinical concern, especially for the physician evaluating a child in the emergency department or the inpatient hospital setting. Symptoms and signs that should alert the physician to the possibility of a headache secondary to increased ICP are reviewed in Table 127-2.

Headaches Associated with Increased Intracranial Pressure

The adage that a "first or worst" headache warrants immediate evaluation for the possibility of a mass lesion causing increased ICP can be generally followed, but further historical details may either confirm or mollify this concern. In the setting of acute intracranial hemorrhage caused by spontaneous aneurysmal rupture into the subarachnoid space, a sudden "thunderclap" quality of the headache or the report that it is the "worst headache of my life" may suggest such pathology. A severe headache in the setting of recent head trauma or in a patient with a bleeding diathesis may suggest acute or subacute hemorrhage into the epidural, subarachnoid, or subdural space.

Headaches caused by mass lesions and slowly increasing ICP are often worse in the morning or after a period of lying in the supine position. There may be associated vomiting, visual disturbance (e.g., blurring or enlargement of the blind spot caused by optic nerve swelling), or other complaints reflecting focal neurologic deficits. Children with brain tumors in the posterior fossa, which account for only a small minority of children with headache, may present with ataxia and other symptoms referable to the brainstem, such as diplopia and difficulty swallowing. A child with such symptoms will also most likely have corresponding abnormalities on neurologic examination. The presence of all three features of the Cushing triad (hypertension, bradycardia, and irregular respirations) is a late sign of increased ICP and represents impending coma or a comatose state. One should also consider the possibility of headache secondary to increased ICP in several special circumstances, as listed in Table 127-3. Such circumstances include patients with a known bleeding diathesis or disseminated intravascular coagulation and patients with hypertension. Patients with a tendency toward clotting are at risk for the development of cerebral venous sinus thrombosis. Among such patients are those with a deficiency of factor V Leiden or antithrombin III and patients with secondary coagulopathies as a result of rheumatologic disease (such as systemic lupus erythematosus associated with lupus anticoagulant), inflammatory bowel disease, or cancer. The medications cyclosporine and methotrexate are associated with a posterior leukoencephalopathy syndrome presenting with headache, seizures, cortical blindness, and hallucinations.

Table 127-1 International Headache Society Classification of Headache Disorders

Primary headaches
   Migraine
   Tension-type headache
   Cluster headache and other trigeminal autonomic cephalgias
   Other primary headaches

Secondary headaches associated with one of the following:
   Head and/or neck trauma
   Cranial or cervical vascular disorders
      Examples: stroke, hematoma, subarachnoid hemorrhage, unruptured vascular malformation, arteritis, carotid/vertebral artery pain, hypertension, other vascular disorder
   Nonvascular intracranial disorders
      Examples: high or low cerebrospinal fluid pressure, intracranial infection, inflammatory condition such as sarcoidosis, intracranial neoplasm, intrathecal injection
   Substances or withdrawal
      Examples: opiates, caffeine
   Infection
   Disorders of homeostasis
      Examples: hypoxia, hypercapnia, hypoglycemia, dialysis, lead
      Disorders of the cranium, neck, eyes, ears, nose, sinuses, teeth, mouth, or other facial or cranial structure
   Psychiatric disorder

Cranial neuralgias, central and primary facial pain, and other disorders

From the Headache Classification Subcommittee of the International Headache Society: International Classification of Headache Disorders, 2nd ed. Oxford, Blackwell, 2003.

Table 127-3 Special Circumstances in Which Headache May Be Associated with Increased Intracranial Pressure

Ventriculoperitoneal shunt

Bleeding disorder (including disseminated intravascular coagulation)

Clotting tendency, increasing risk for venous sinus thrombosis
   Primary clotting disorders
   Systemic disease
      Examples: lupus anticoagulant syndrome, inflammatory bowel disease, cancer

Hypertension

Medications—cyclosporine, methotrexate

Table 127-2 Worrisome Symptoms and Signs Suggesting Headache from Increased Intracranial Pressure

Symptoms of Increased Intracranial Pressure
"First or worst" headache
Chronic and progressively worsening headache
Sudden "thunderclap" headache
Early morning headache or headache worse in the morning
Headache worse in the supine position
Change from mental status baseline (including irritability)
Associated loss of vision or other neurologic deficit
Associated vomiting

Other Worrisome Symptoms
Presence of a ventriculoperitoneal shunt
Recent head trauma or neurosurgery

Signs of Increased Intracranial Pressure
Depressed or abnormal mental status
Papilledema
Cranial nerve abnormalities, particularly 3rd nerve palsy (including "blown pupil") and 6th nerve palsy (impaired abduction)
Asymmetry in the motor examination

panying abnormalities may include subtle mood changes or decreased energy. Papilledema and other signs of increased ICP may not be present in the first several hours of presentation. For all these reasons, headache in a patient with a VP shunt should be considered secondary to shunt obstruction until proved otherwise unless it is a typical headache for a given child and there are no other worrisome features in the history or physical examination to suggest otherwise.

Other Secondary Headache Presentations

The history and physical examination are crucial for correctly identifying secondary headaches not associated with increased ICP. For example, headache may be a presenting feature of meningitis, but there are typically other features, such as fever, to suggest this diagnosis.

Headache with or without neck pain in the setting of head or neck trauma, even relatively trivial trauma, can be caused by dissection of the carotid or vertebral arteries. Although uncommon in children, this entity deserves consideration because the clot that forms in response to the dissection can embolize and produce a stroke.

Secondary headaches may herald otherwise occult head and neck conditions, such as dental abscess, otitis media, or sinusitis. Pain may not be well localized in these conditions.

Particularly in the inpatient setting, other causes of secondary headache may include metabolic disturbances (listed in Table 127-1 as disorders of homeostasis), intracranial hypotension (or a "low-pressure" or "lumbar puncture" headache) caused by a cerebrospinal fluid (CSF) leak after lumbar puncture, and opiate withdrawal in patients receiving analgesia for other conditions or for headache itself.

Pseudotumor cerebri, or benign idiopathic intracranial hypertension, is considered a secondary headache, although the underlying cause is often elusive. Patients with this condition have symptoms suggesting increased ICP. They may also report transient visual obscurations or a large blind

Another important feature to elicit from the history is the presence of a VP shunt. Not every headache in a child with a VP shunt represents a neurosurgical emergency, but one must be suspicious of shunt malfunction and increased (or increasing) ICP, especially if the headache is severe, if it is a first or new type of headache for the child, or if there are any other symptoms or signs suggesting increased ICP. Of note, early in the process of VP shunt obstruction, accom-

Table 127-4 Common Features of Migraine (Not All Required)

Unilateral, throbbing headache
Nausea, vomiting
Photophobia, sonophobia
Visual aura (e.g., scintillating scotoma)
Desire for sleep
Family history of migraine

spot. Typical examination findings include papilledema and enlargement of the blind spot. Occasionally, weakness of the lateral rectus muscle is noted as a result of decreased ability to abduct the eye because of pressure on the sixth cranial nerves. Findings on computed tomography (CT) can be normal or small ventricles may be seen, and CSF opening pressure at lumbar puncture is high. Often the patient experiences relief of symptoms transiently after lumbar puncture. Although not a life-threatening condition, pseudotumor cerebri can lead to permanent loss of vision if not treated expeditiously.

Common Headache Disorder Presentations— Migraine Headache

Migraine accounts for about three quarters of all pediatric headaches. The typical constellation of symptoms associated with migraine headaches is listed in Table 127-4. Some modifications have been made to the IHS criteria for migraine to incorporate features more common in children and adolescents.[10] Not all patients with migraine display all of these features, but they serve as a helpful starting place when obtaining the medical history. The word *migraine* is derived from "hemicrania," which is in keeping with the unilateral head pain found in classic migraine. However, children with migraine often report bilateral or holocranial headache. Older children and adults with migraine typically describe a throbbing quality of the headache, but younger children may not be able to characterize or localize their pain. At times, one can elicit a distinction between throbbing and steady pain by holding the child's hand and gently squeezing intermittently to represent throbbing pain and squeezing steadily to represent steady pain. The examiner then asks which handshake is more like the child's own headache. Migraine can occur with or without aura. Atypical aura can include "scintillating scotomas," which are shining, often brightly colored regions of the visual field in which normal vision is transiently obscured. Nausea is typical, and there is also a tendency for patients with migraine to suffer from motion sickness (not necessarily at the same time as their headaches), a feature not often offered in the history because the patient and family may not associate it with headache. The family history is frequently positive for migraine or other related entities, including syncope, recurrent abdominal pain, and motion sickness.

Patients with migraine may have concurrent photophobia and sonophobia, which may be expressed simply by a preference for a dark, quiet room during the episode. Although it is not reflected in the criteria listed in Table 127-4, children with migraine often express the desire to sleep, and most patients with migraine report that sleep can relieve their headaches. Typical migraines last 1 to 2 hours, but they may last longer, sometimes leading the patient to seek medical attention.

Complicated migraines present with focal neurologic deficits such as hemianopia, hemiparesis, or aphasia, which may occur before, during, or after an otherwise typical migraine headache. These symptoms and signs are naturally and appropriately alarming and often warrant emergency evaluation for stroke or the presence of structural lesions. This is especially important with the initial episode of these symptoms. The diagnosis of complicated migraine can be considered after other diagnostic considerations have been excluded.

DIFFERENTIAL DIAGNOSIS

The IHS classification system presented in Table 127-1 offers a general framework for considering the differential diagnosis of headache. The chief distinction lies between primary and secondary headaches, the latter typically requiring more urgent medical attention. A more comprehensive differential diagnosis is included in Table 127-5. This table is organized to depict the most likely diagnoses for patients with headache and normal neurologic findings versus headache with signs of increased ICP or focal neurologic abnormalities.

DIAGNOSIS AND EVALUATION

The history and physical examination form the basis for evaluation of patients with headache. Further evaluation of a secondary headache may be warranted, as dictated by specific circumstances. For example, a patient with symptoms and signs of sinusitis and normal neurologic findings might receive empirical antibiotic therapy and symptomatic pain relief with outpatient follow-up and no further diagnostic testing. In contrast, a child with headache, fever, and meningeal signs might merit a lumbar puncture. Table 127-6 provides an overview of the general principles of diagnosis for headache.

The role of neuroimaging in the evaluation of a child with headache requires clinical judgment. Not every headache in every child warrants CT or magnetic resonance imaging (MRI) of the head, but prudent and judicious use of these modalities clearly has a place in the evaluation of headache. Any patient with headache and symptoms and signs suggesting increased ICP should undergo an emergency CT scan, including patients with the "red flag" items listed in Table 127-2, especially those with the "worst headache of my life," which raises concern for subarachnoid hemorrhage. Although rare in children, it is important to note that CT alone cannot sufficiently rule out subarachnoid hemorrhage and must be followed by lumbar puncture when this diagnosis is suspected and CT findings are normal.[11] This is a cautious approach, but particularly in the emergency department and the inpatient setting, the likelihood of a secondary headache may be higher than in the outpatient setting. The likelihood of identifying a significant abnormality in a patient with headache and normal neurologic findings, especially a patient with recurrent episodic headache suggestive

---

Table 127-5   **Differential Diagnosis of Headache**

Patients with Normal Neurologic Examination and No Concern for Increased Intracranial Pressure

Migraine, tension headache, or other primary headache disorder

Head and neck problems
  Orbital disease
  Sinusitis
  Otitis
  Dental infection
  Temporomandibular joint pain
  Recurrent facial pain syndromes (e.g., trigeminal neuralgia)

Metabolic disturbance
  Hypoglycemia
  Hypoxia
  Hypercapnia
  Dialysis headache

Intracranial hypotension ("post–lumbar puncture" headache)

Ingestions from food—monosodium glutamate, nitrites, individual food triggers

Marijuana

Oral contraceptives

Substance withdrawal
  Analgesics (including those used for headache treatment)
  Opiates
  Caffeine

Patients with Abnormal Neurologic Examination or Concern for Increased Intracranial Pressure

Central nervous system infection
  Meningitis
  Encephalitis
  Brain abscess

Intracranial hemorrhage
  Subarachnoid hemorrhage (presents with "worst headache of my life")
  Epidural hemorrhage, often after trauma and associated with skull fracture
  Subdural hemorrhage, often associated with trauma

Posttraumatic headache without intracranial headache

Cerebral venous sinus thrombosis

Stroke

Complicated migraine, in which stroke must be suspected and ruled out, especially at first presentation

Hypertensive encephalopathy

Carotid or vertebral artery dissection

Ventriculoperitoneal shunt obstruction

Inflammatory disease with central nervous system involvement (e.g., vasculitis)

Brain tumor

Pseudotumor cerebri

Ictal headache (rare) or postictal headache, possibly after an unwitnessed seizure

Conversion—diagnosis of exclusion

Table 127-6   **Diagnostic Evaluation of Headache**

History
With attention to worrisome features, as outlined in Table 127-2

Physical Examination
Focus should be on identifying secondary causes of headache, particularly worrisome causes requiring hospitalization and close observation:
  General examination: temperature, blood pressure
  Head, ears, eyes, nose, and throat examination: palpation of the head and face, sinus percussion, eyes for papilledema, ears and tympanic membranes, neck for tenderness, mouth, throat, teeth
  Neurologic examination
    Mental status
    Cranial nerves
    Motor
    Cerebellar

Computed Tomography of the Head
To evaluate for hemorrhage if headache is first or worst, if mental status is abnormal, or if findings on neurologic examination are focal
To evaluate for a mass lesion causing hydrocephalus and increased intracranial pressure

Magnetic Resonance Imaging of the Brain with Gadolinium Enhancement
If stroke is suspected, MRI with diffusion-weighted images
If venous sinus thrombosis is suspected, MRI and MR venography
If posterior fossa tumor is suspected

Lumbar Puncture
Should be performed after a CT scan if there is any concern for increased intracranial pressure from a mass lesion and after ensuring a platelet concentration $>50 \times 10^9$/L
If the headache is new and severe or the "worst headache of my life" or if the headache is accompanied by focal neurologic abnormalities, head CT may be insufficient to rule out early subarachnoid hemorrhage. LP is needed
If infection is likely (after CT is performed if there is any concern for increased intracranial pressure)
To measure opening pressure to evaluate for pseudotumor cerebri (after CT)
If inflammatory disease is suspected

Laboratory Studies
Glucose, others on a case-by-case basis
Urine human chorionic gonadotropin in girls

Electroencephalography
Only if transient focal neurologic symptoms and signs are present

---

of a primary headache disorder, is extremely low.[12,13] Because the causes of headache are so varied, it is difficult to generalize, but a well-appearing child without worrisome features and with normal results on examination can be observed without neuroimaging.

It is usually more convenient and expeditious to perform a CT scan than MRI; this factor, as well as the fact that CT scans are more sensitive in the evaluation of acute hemorrhage, makes CT the first line of neuroimaging for an acute headache and for most headaches that warrant neuroimaging. A limitation of CT scans is their decreased ability to evaluate the posterior fossa, and MRI is warranted as a first-line study if there is high suspicion of a brain tumor[14] or other lesion in the posterior fossa. In addition, although the ionizing radiation associated with repeat CT scans must be considered, the dose of radiation per scan should be based on the size of the patient in any center that routinely performs these studies in children; fear of ionizing radiation should not preclude the performance of a clinically warranted scan in an acutely ill patient who may require emergency intervention.

Lumbar puncture is indicated for the diagnosis of meningitis or other infections, subarachnoid hemorrhage, and pseudotumor cerebri. When increased ICP is caused by a mass lesion, such as an abscess or tumor, the pressure differential created by lumbar puncture can lead to catastrophic herniation of the brainstem. A CT scan should be obtained before lumbar puncture if there is suspicion of such a mass lesion, even though lumbar puncture is a safe procedure in the majority of cases. The platelet concentration should be at least 50×10^9/L to minimize the risk for epidural hemorrhage.

COURSE OF ILLNESS

The course of a child's headache will depend on its cause. Secondary headaches usually respond to treatment of the associated underlying condition. Primary headache disorders in children, as in adults, are characteristically recurrent and, if particularly frequent or severe, may require prophylactic management.

TREATMENT

Management of the pain of a secondary headache depends on the underlying cause of the headache. During the initial phase of evaluation, when monitoring of the patient's mental status is important and the possibility of intracranial hemorrhage exists, narcotics and nonsteroidal anti-inflammatory drugs (NSAIDs) should be avoided. Acetaminophen is an appropriate alternative that can be given orally or per rectum. Once the patient is deemed stable and the risk for hemorrhage low, NSAIDs may provide additional symptomatic relief while underlying causes are investigated or treated.

In the acute management of migraine, ensuring adequate hydration is important, especially if the migraine has been protracted and has led to decreased oral intake or vomiting, or both. If home medications at appropriate doses have been ineffective or if oral therapy is not tolerated, intravenous fluids and medications should be considered. Ketorolac, an NSAID available for intravenous administration, is a good choice for pain relief, especially if avoiding narcotics is a goal. Some pediatric centers treat severe and intractable migraine in older children and adolescents with dihydroergotamine, often with metoclopramide pretreatment. Some patients experience relief of the migraine symptoms with the premedication dose of metoclopramide, thereby obviating the need for dihydroergotamine. Narcotics often provide reliable pain relief and may help the patient achieve sleep. Concern regarding the chronic use of narcotics for the treatment of migraine, especially with the potential for addiction or promotion of drug-seeking behavior, is a consideration. However, prompt pain relief is a goal of initial management and should be weighed against these concerns.

CONSULTATION

Consider subspecialty consultation for any of the following reasons:

- Neurosurgical consultation for patients with increased ICP who are unstable, patients in whom CT identifies an intracranial hemorrhage, and patients with a VP shunt
- Neurologic consultation for patients with abnormal neurologic findings and a suspected intracranial cause of secondary headache and for patients with known primary headache disorders that have become refractory to standard management
- Ophthalmologic consultation for patients with pseudotumor cerebri to monitor the visual fields

ADMISSION CRITERIA

- Suspected or identified underlying cause that requires prompt investigation, ongoing observation, or intervention (e.g., increased ICP, intracranial mass or hemorrhage, bacterial meningitis)
- Severe pain that cannot be managed with an outpatient regimen

DISCHARGE CRITERIA

- Completion of the urgent diagnostic studies indicated
- Definitive treatment or initiation of therapy for an underlying process
- Pain relief regimen that can be continued after discharge
- Appropriate outpatient follow-up with a primary care clinician and, if needed, a subspecialist

IN A NUTSHELL

- The history and physical examination form the cornerstone of evaluation of headache in the hospital setting.
- Physicians evaluating patients with headache must perform a careful neurologic examination, with particular attention focused on mental status, the optic fundi, horizontal eye movements, and motor symmetry.
- Distinction between primary and secondary headache is important in determining the likelihood of an acute intracranial process that may require emergency or urgent intervention.
- Patients with a history or physical examination findings suggesting possibly raised ICP should undergo emergency neuroimaging, in most cases with CT. This category includes patients with a VP shunt and headache for which medical attention has been sought.
- Patients with signs and symptoms suggesting possibly raised ICP from a posterior fossa lesion should undergo CT acutely and MRI for detailed posterior fossa evaluation.
- Most patients with a history of headache but without "red flag" features worrisome for increased ICP and without abnormalities on neurologic examination do not have serious intracranial pathology. In these cases, headache should be managed symptomatically.

ON THE HORIZON

- Mechanisms invoked for the pathophysiology of migraine include vascular, neurotransmitter-mediated, electrophysiologic, and inflammatory abnormalities. It may be that it is an interplay of several such factors that produces migraine and other severe headache symptoms. In the future, as the underlying mechanisms are better understood, we should be able to develop more specific strategies for treating headache in general.

- Additionally, as for the treatment of many pain syndromes, the addition of complementary and alternative medicine is likely to have a growing role in the management of chronic headache. When patients are admitted for exacerbations of chronic headache conditions, it will be increasingly important to incorporate aspects of nonpharmacologic treatment in keeping with their outpatient treatment strategies.

SUGGESTED READING

Fenichel GM: Clinical Pediatric Neurology: A Signs and Symptoms Approach, 4th ed. Philadelphia, WB Saunders, 2001.

Silberstein SD, Lipton RB, Goadsby PJ: Headache in Clinical Practice. London, Martin Dunitz, 2002.

Swaiman KF, Ashwal S (eds): Pediatric Neurology, Principles and Practice, 3rd ed. St Louis, CV Mosby, 1999.

REFERENCES

1. Fenichel GM: Clinical Pediatric Neurology: A Signs and Symptoms Approach, 4th ed. Philadelphia, WB Saunders, 2001.

2. Laurell K, Larsson B, Eeg-Olofsson O: Prevalence of headache in Swedish schoolchildren, with a focus on tension-type headache. Cephalalgia 2004;24:380-388.

3. Zwart JA, Dyb G, Holmen TL, et al: The prevalence of migraine and tension-type headaches among adolescents in Norway. The Nord-Trondelag Health Study (Head-HUNT-Youth), a large population-based epidemiological study. Cephalalgia 2004;24:373-379.

4. Ayatollahi SM, Moradi F, Ayatollahi SA: Prevalences of migraine and tension-type headache in adolescent girls of Shiraz (southern Iran). Headache 2002;42:287-290.

5. Cheung RT: Prevalence of migraine, tension-type headache, and other headaches in Hong Kong. Headache 2000;40:473-479.

6. Deleu D, Khan MA, Al Shehab TA: Prevalence and clinical characteristics of headache in a rural community in Oman. Headache 2002;42:963-973.

7. Al Jumah M, Awada A, Al Azzam S: Headache syndromes amongst schoolchildren in Riyadh, Saudi Arabia. Headache 2002;42:281-286.

8. Headache Classification Subcommittee of the International Headache Society: International Classification of Headache Disorders, 2nd ed. Oxford, Blackwell, 2003.

9. Ozge A, Bugdayci R, Sasmaz T, et al: The sensitivity and specificity of the case definition criteria in diagnosis of headache: A school-based epidemiological study of 5562 children in Mersin. Cephalalgia 2003;23:138-145.

10. Winner P, Martinez W, Mate L, Bello L: Classification of pediatric migraine: Proposed revisions to the IHS criteria. Headache 1995;35:407-410.

11. Medina LS, D'Souza B, Vasconcellos E: Adults and children with headache: Evidence-based diagnostic evaluation. Neuroimaging Clin North Am 2003;13:225-235.

12. Alehan FK: Value of neuroimaging in the evaluation of neurologically normal children with recurrent headache. J Child Neurol 2002;17:807-809.

13. Maytal J, Bienkowski RS, Patel M, Eviatar L: The value of brain imaging in children with headaches. Pediatrics 1995;96:413-416.

14. Medina LS, Kuntz KM, Pomeroy S: Children with headache suspected of having a brain tumor: A cost-effectiveness analysis of diagnostic strategies. Pediatrics 2001;108:255-263.

CHAPTER 128

Hypotonia and Weakness

Heidi Wolf

Hypotonia and weakness are signs of a variety of systemic, neurologic, and neuromuscular disorders. Information about the age of onset and progressive or static nature of the hypotonia is essential in sorting the diagnostic possibilities. When these signs occur acutely in an otherwise healthy infant or child, they are most commonly the result of severe infection, fluid or electrolyte derangements, toxic ingestion, or trauma. If present at birth, they may be the result of injury to the nervous system. Hypotonia that is progressive may herald the onset of a number of neurologic diseases. It is important that the pediatric hospitalist have a basic understanding of these diagnostic possibilities and their clinical course, pathophysiology, diagnosis, associated morbid conditions, and treatment.

Hypotonia and weakness are signs that may localize to any level of the nervous system (Fig. 128-1). Classically, these disorders have been divided into "upper motor neuron" and "lower motor neuron" diseases (Table 128-1). Upper motor neuron diseases affect the corticospinal tracts at any point from their origin in the cortex to their termination in the spinal cord. Lower motor neuron disorders are further localized to the anterior horn cell, peripheral nerve, neuromuscular junction, or muscle fibers. Overlap occurs in processes that affect central and peripheral myelin, such as metachromatic leukodystrophy, or those that involve multiple tissues, such as oxidative phosphorylation (mitochondrial) defects.

UPPER MOTOR NEURON DISORDERS

A variety of perinatal events can damage the upper motor neuron structures and result in congenital hypotonia, including infections with the TORCH organisms (toxoplasmosis, other [congenital syphilis and viruses], rubella, cytomegalovirus, and herpes simplex virus), abnormal development of brain structures, injury resulting from bleeding, hypoxia, or toxic exposure.

The fetus may be exposed to drugs during pregnancy or at the time of delivery. The mother may be using therapeutic medications such as phenobarbital or warfarin (Coumadin) or abusing drugs such as cocaine. Likewise, magnesium administered during labor may influence the tone of the newborn.

Cerebral palsy is a symptom complex in which the neurologic findings evolve over time. At birth the newborn may have a relatively normal examination, first becoming hypotonic and subsequently evolving to hypertonia (spasticity, rigidity, or both).

Many syndromes present with decreased fetal movements or neonatal hypotonia, in addition to other clinical features that are less apparent at birth. Down, Prader-Willi, Marfan, and Williams syndromes commonly feature hypotonia.

During infancy and childhood the upper motor neurons may be injured by bacterial infections, bilirubin, toxins, tumors, or injury from either accidental or nonaccidental trauma.

Acute disseminated encephalomyelitis (ADEM) is a demyelinating disorder that may affect infants and children of any age. The pathophysiology resembles that of multiple sclerosis (MS), with significant clinical overlap. ADEM typically occurs after febrile illnesses, either viral or, less commonly, after immunizations. Children may present with a variety of symptoms and signs, including acute optic neuritis, hemiparesis, ataxia, seizures, headache, weakness, or dysphagia. Behavioral changes and mental status changes from confusion to coma may also occur. Specific symptoms and their severity may be related to specific viral triggers. Early diagnosis may be challenging but is essential because effective treatments are available. There are no specific diagnostic laboratory findings, and computed tomography of the brain is often normal. Cranial magnetic resonance imaging (MRI) typically makes the diagnosis, although occasionally the appearance of typical lesions may be delayed after the onset of clinical signs. The lesions of ADEM can be distinguished from those of MS by their more peripheral location in white matter (often at the gray-white junction) and the typically widespread changes that far exceed the clinical findings. ADEM is most often monophasic, but relapsing ADEM has been proposed as an entity. Most such cases are eventually diagnosed as MS. It may only be possible to diagnose ADEM rather than a first episode of MS in retrospect. Newer MRI techniques may help clarify these diagnoses.[1] Early treatments with intravenous steroids, intravenous immunoglobulin (IVIG), and even plasmapheresis have all shown some benefit in improving symptoms and possibly shortening the course of illness. In general, ADEM is a self-limited illness, although some studies report fatality rates up to 20%.[2]

MS most commonly begins in adulthood, with only about 2% of cases having their onset before 21 years of age. The proportion of cases beginning in childhood has been steadily rising over the past decade.[3] MS rarely occurs in children younger than 10 years, although it has been reported in an infant aged 10 months.[3] Women are more commonly affected than men, but in younger children the distribution is more equal. Both geographic and genetic factors contribute to the development of this disease. Rates of MS are highest in the northern United States, Canada, northern Europe, New Zealand, and southern Australia.[3] The country of origin of the individual is less important than the country of residence in terms of the development of MS, depending on the age at immigration. Individuals with a sibling or other first-degree relative with MS have a greatly increased lifetime risk for the disease. This finding along with twin and other genetic studies strongly supports genetic susceptibility to MS. The pathophysiology of MS involves the evolution of plaques in the cerebral and spinal white matter through a

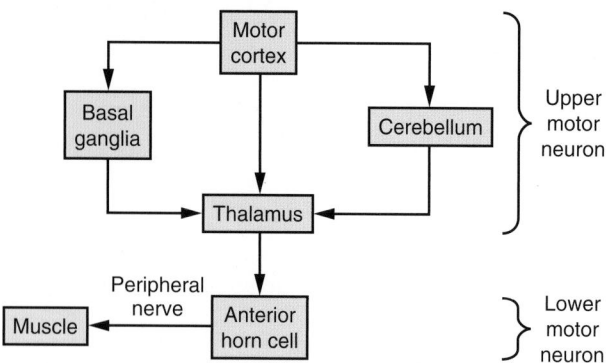

Figure 128-1 Components of the motor system.

Table 128-1 Physical Examination Findings		
	Upper Motor Neuron	Lower Motor Neuron
Deep tendon reflexes	↑	↓
Strength	Normal	↓
Plantar reflexes (Babinski)	Extensor*	Flexor
Clonus	Present	Absent

*May be normal in children younger than 2 years.

process of repeated demyelination, followed by incomplete axonal remyelination. Eventually, axons are lost and scarring and plaque formation follow. The clinical picture reflects the localization of lesions in MS, which has a predilection for the optic nerves, periventricular white matter, cerebellum, and spinal cord.[3] Weakness, ataxia, optic neuritis with visual loss and pain on eye movement, diplopia, and sensory symptoms are common complaints. Advanced disease causes impairment in memory, attention, and other functions. The most common course of MS in children consists of sporadic episodes of neurologic dysfunction alternating with periods of relative quiescence, a "relapsing-remitting" pattern. The best method for establishing the diagnosis is controversial. Some diagnostic criteria rely only on clinical evidence, whereas others require laboratory (cerebrospinal fluid [CSF]) abnormalities and the presence of lesions on MRI. Oligoclonal bands and an increased IgG index in CSF may be found in the majority of patients with MS.[3] MRI findings may initially be normal until disease progression creates the classic inflammatory or scarred plaques of MS. The presence of new plaques scattered in time and space is a hallmark of the disease. Therapy is aimed primarily at relief of symptoms and slowing progression of the disease.[3] Intravenous steroids are the mainstay of treatment of acute MS attacks, although there is little evidence to support their use during asymptomatic periods. Studies with IVIG and immune-modulating drugs are under way and have shown some benefit, but side effects have limited their use. Children may have better clinical outcomes than adults with longer periods of remission and slower progression of disease, although there is great variability. Some children, especially those with seizures, die of MS, whereas others suffer permanent visual impairment, paralysis, and cognitive dysfunction.

Leigh disease (subacute necrotizing encephalopathy) is a neurometabolic disorder that causes spongy degeneration and necrosis of the basal ganglia and cerebellum. Defects in oxidative phosphorylation secondary to mutations in mitochondrial or nuclear DNA underlie most cases.[4] Typically, severe encephalopathy develops in an otherwise normal infant in the first year of life, and the infant dies of respiratory failure or sepsis by the age of 5 years.[4] Other clinical features include hypoventilation, feeding and swallowing difficulties, seizures, clonus, and nystagmus. The diagnosis is supported by the finding of elevated lactate and pyruvate levels in CSF, whereas serum ammonia and glucose are normal, as are urine organic acids. Treatment is primarily supportive, with particular attention to management of feeding and of the airway and ventilation. Biotin, thiamine, and multivitamins are recommended.[4] Dichloroacetate has been shown to be effective at temporarily arresting progression of the Leigh syndrome that is associated with one particular gene mutation.[4] This agent has recently been shown to cause peripheral neuropathy, which has led to termination of a clinical trial for MELAS (mitochondrial encephalopathy, lactic acidosis, and strokelike symptoms).[5]

The leukodystrophies, individually rare genetic disorders, can also cause demyelination or dysmyelination leading to severe hypotonia in the presence of peripheral neuropathy, as occurs in Krabbe disease, metachromatic leukodystrophy, adrenomyeloneuropathy, and peroxisomal disorders such as Zellweger syndrome. Specific genetic defects resulting in abnormal enzyme production have been identified for many of these inborn errors of metabolism. Zellweger (cerebrohepatorenal) syndrome is an autosomal recessive disorder that is generally fatal. There is no effective therapy. The diagnosis is suggested by the characteristic dysmorphic features (high forehead, enlarged fontanelle, and shallow orbits), profound hypotonia, and organomegaly and is confirmed by finding abnormal ratios of very long chain fatty acids in serum and cultured fibroblasts, followed by identification of the specific peroxin defect. Treatment is generally supportive. Morbidity may be favorably influenced by early recognition and treatment of complications of the disease, such as subdural hematoma.[6] Other diseases in this category include Pelizaeus-Merzbacher syndrome, Cockayne syndrome, Alexander disease, Canavan syndrome, Krabbe syndrome, and metachromatic leukodystrophy. These conditions may present in newborns, infants, children, and adults. Early-onset cases are marked by hypotonia and premature death, whereas late-onset variants are usually associated with less severe impairment and prolonged survival.

Gangliosidoses are autosomal recessive lysosomal storage disorders that can present at any time from fetal life (as ascites detected on ultrasound) through adulthood. They are classified according to the predominant stored glycosphingolipid—either GM_1 or GM_2 ganglioside. (GM_3 gangliosidosis is a disputed entity, rarely reported.) Defective activity of lysosomal hydrolases (β-galactosidase in GM_1 gangliosidosis and hexosaminidase A or B in GM_2 gangliosidosis) results in the progressive accumulation of gangliosides and subsequent dysfunction in the brain and peripheral tissues. Infantile GM_1 gangliosidosis is characterized by coarse facial features, frontal bossing, low-set ears, hepatosplenomegaly, and dysostosis; the phenotype is attenuated in later-onset forms. Hypotonia, profound developmental delay, and seizures are common. Hypotonia, progressive macrocephaly, and developmental regression commonly develop in infants with GM$_2$ gangliosidosis beginning at 4 to 6 months of age, with death ensuing in most cases by 2 to 4 years. The form of infantile GM$_2$ gangliosidosis caused by hexosaminidase A deficiency (Tay-Sachs disease) was formerly most frequent in Ashkenazi Jews, but the implementation of a successful screening program has led to a 90% reduction in the frequency of cases in this at-risk population. Similar, albeit much rarer, phenotypes are caused by mutations in different genes causing combined hexosaminidase A and B deficiency (Sandhoff disease) or activator protein deficiency.

Lysosomal enzyme deficiency is easily demonstrated in serum, white blood cells, or fibroblasts, and in the case of Tay-Sachs deficiency, screening for the common Ashkenazi mutations in *HEXA* is available. Amniotic cells and chorionic villus biopsy can be used for prenatal diagnosis in selected cases. Treatment is generally supportive at present. Animal studies of gene therapy, hematopoietic stem cell transplantation, and substrate reduction therapy are in progress.

LOWER MOTOR NEURON DISEASE

Anterior Horn Cell

Spinal muscular atrophy (SMA) type I (Werdnig-Hoffman disease) is the most common inherited cause of death in infancy, with an incidence varying from 1 in 10,000 to 1 in 25,000 in different populations. Later-onset variants are classified as types II to IV. All classic forms of SMA are recessive disorders resulting from mutations (most commonly deletions of exons 7 or 8, or both) in the *SMN* (survival of motor neuron) gene, which is located on the long arm of chromosome 5. SMA-I may present with reduced fetal movements, and in most cases newborn infants are hypotonic and areflexic, with progressive weakness causing paradoxical respiration and impaired swallowing. Characteristic findings include flabby muscles, tongue fasciculations, and a coarse tremor sometimes designated minipolymyoclonus.

In parts of Asia and Africa, anterior poliomyelitis remains an important cause of hypotonia and weakness and should always be considered in a child from an endemic region who presents in this fashion. Acid maltase and hexosaminidase A deficiencies can both lead to lysosomal storage in anterior horn cells and may also cause hypotonia and weakness, although this finding is usually overshadowed by other signs of these diseases. Central cord lesions, such as a syrinx, may impinge on the anterior horns and cause segmental weakness, usually accompanied by other signs of myelopathy.

Peripheral Nerve

Guillain-Barré syndrome (GBS, acute inflammatory demyelinating polyradiculoneuropathy) is the most common peripheral neuropathy that causes hypotonia and diminished or absent reflexes. The incidence is estimated at 0.25 to 1.5 per 100,000. It is preceded by an identifiable acute infectious illness in approximately two thirds of patients.[7] The primary pathology of GBS is demyelination beginning at the nerve roots and extending distally over time. The hallmark of the illness is a symmetrical ascending paralysis that evolves over a period of days to weeks. The diagnosis is primarily clinical. After the first week, CSF shows elevated protein and fewer than 10 white blood cells/mm^3 in approximately 80% of patients.[7] The National Institute of Neurological Disorders and Stroke has defined clinical and electromyographic (EMG) diagnostic criteria for GBS. Vigilant monitoring of ventilatory and autonomic function is essential because failure of these systems may prove fatal. Bradycardia, hypotension, and hypertension can result in significant morbidity and even sudden death. Treatment options in the acute phase include IVIG or plasmapheresis. The mechanism of action of these modalities is incompletely understood. Plasmapheresis is thought to remove antibodies, whereas IVIG is thought to bind and render them inactive. IVIG also binds complement factors thought to contribute to tissue damage and immune system modulation. In 2001, the IVIG Advisory Panel recommended a dose of 0.4 mg/kg/day for 5 days. The overall mortality rate of GBS is 3% to 5%. Ten percent of patients have residual neurologic dysfunction ranging from mild to severe disability. Another 10% may relapse.

Riley-Day syndrome, now referred to as familial dysautonomia or hereditary sensory and autonomic neuropathy type III, is a rare autosomal recessive disorder that affects Ashkenazi Jews almost exclusively. The pathology of this disorder is marked by incomplete development and progressive deterioration of neurons. Clinical features include decreased tearing, absent fungiform papillae on the tongue, and decreased lower extremity reflexes. Ninety-nine percent of affected individuals share a common gene mutation, thus making it possible to diagnose by DNA testing.[8] Before 1960 the prognosis was dismal, with 50% mortality by 5 years, primarily from pulmonary disease.[8] Earlier diagnosis of the disease has allowed physicians to treat the known primary complications of familial dysautonomia, including gastrointestinal, renal, and pulmonary dysfunction, which has greatly increased the overall life expectancy of these patients. An affected infant born today can expect to have a 50% chance of reaching the age of 40 years.[8]

Neuromuscular Junction

Certain medications that impair neuromuscular transmission may cause neonatal hypotonia when administered to mothers in labor or to the newborn infant. Magnesium used to treat preeclampsia may cause apnea, respiratory depression, lethargy, hypotonia, and poor sucking in the newborn. Infantile botulism is a toxin-mediated disease of the neuromuscular junction that commonly strikes later in the first year of life (see Chapter 191).

Myasthenia gravis (MG) describes a group of autoimmune and genetic disorders in which dysfunction of the neuromuscular junction causes hypotonia and fatigable muscle weakness (*mys*, muscle; *asthenia* weakness).[9] Although MG develops in most patients as adults, at least three categories of childhood onset have been described. The transient and juvenile forms of MG are autoimmune disorders in which antibodies directed against epitopes of the acetylcholine receptor (AChR) cause net loss of receptors in the postsynaptic membrane. The transient form results from transplacental passage of maternal antibodies to the fetal circulation. Transient myasthenia complicates pregnancy in as many as

15% of mothers with MG. The symptoms, which may be profound in the newborn,[10] resolve over a period of weeks to months. Juvenile MG shares the symptoms and signs of the later-onset adult disease. Fatigability of voluntary muscles, including the extraocular muscles and those required to articulate, chew, swallow, and breathe, is typical. Specific symptoms and signs include ptosis, diplopia, dysarthria, dysphagia, and dyspnea. The diagnosis of autoimmune MG is confirmed by neurophysiologic studies and assay of serum antibodies directed at components of the neuromuscular junction (anti-AChR or muscle-specific neuromuscular junction [MuSK]).

The congenital myasthenic syndromes are a growing family of genetic disorders that affect specific components of the neuromuscular junction.[9] Most are autosomal recessive, although at least one condition is autosomal dominant. A complete family history may be positive or may reveal an infant death of unknown cause. The prenatal history may include decreased fetal movements, oligohydramnios, or polyhydramnios. The diagnosis is suggested by clinical and neurologic examination findings and confirmed by characteristic EMG findings (a decremental response to repetitive stimuli for postsynaptic disorders, an incremental response from a diminished baseline amplitude in the case of presynaptic disorders). Highly specialized physiologic studies on fresh tissue obtained at muscle biopsy and genetic studies, available only at research centers, are required for specific diagnosis.

Treatment of transient, congenital, and juvenile myasthenia is primarily supportive. Neostigmine, pyridostigmine bromide, and other cholinesterase inhibitors have been shown to be beneficial in preventing severe acute episodes of respiratory and swallowing dysfunction. Immune modulation with prednisone or other immunomodulatory drugs, plasmapheresis, and thymectomy all have a role in the management of autoimmune MG.

The prognosis for transient myasthenia is good, with symptoms resolving in 2 weeks to 2 months. The prognosis for congenital myasthenic syndromes is specific to the defect. Some forms are fatal in childhood, whereas others are compatible with adult survival and reproduction. Children with juvenile MG may become resistant to anticholinergics. The prognosis for MG is compatible with prolonged survival and minimal disability, provided that patients are monitored closely and treated appropriately.

Muscle

Hypothyroidism is common and should be considered in all infants presenting with hypotonia or muscle weakness not explained by systemic illness or intrinsic muscle disease. The prevalence of congenital hypothyroidism is 1 in 4000, and that of acquired hypothyroidism is 1 in 1250. Hypothyroidism is more common in girls than in boys. It causes nonspecific structural and histochemical changes in muscle. An infant with hypothyroidism may be asymptomatic or have mild clinical features in the first days of life. Physical examination may show a large head and large fontanelles. The clinical course may include prolonged jaundice, poor feeding, sluggishness, or sleepiness. Neonatal screening of thyroid function has allowed timely identification and treatment with thyroid hormone.

Myotonic dystrophy is an autosomal dominant progressive muscle and systemic disease. It presents in infants born to mothers with myotonic dystrophy, who may or may not have obvious signs or symptoms of the disease. Inability of the mother to release her handshake (grip myotonia) may be the only clue that she is affected. The prenatal history may reveal spontaneous abortions, decreased fetal movements, polyhydramnios, retained placenta, or postpartum hemorrhage. Presenting signs may include hypotonia, developmental delay, failure to thrive, or respiratory distress. On physical examination the infant may demonstrate facial weakness, a high arched palate, a triple-furrowed tongue, or a patulous anus. The disease is caused by the expansion of a trinucleotide (CTG) sequence in the *MyD* gene on chromosome 19. Subsequent generations may have a greater number of repeats and earlier and more severe expression of the disease (anticipation). Genetic counseling is thus an important aspect of care of the child and family. Treatment is primarily aimed at supporting the weak respiratory musculature; many babies need mechanical ventilation. Twenty-five percent of children with myotonic dystrophy die of respiratory complications before the age of 18 months; 50% of children survive into their fourth decade but are susceptible to hypertrophic cardiomyopathy and, in some cases, sudden death from arrhythmias. There is also an increased prevalence of diabetes mellitus and cataracts in adults with myotonic dystrophy.

Pompe disease is an autosomal recessive lysosomal storage disease that results from deficiency of acid maltase, coded by the *GAA* gene, which is localized to chromosome 17q25.[11] The incidence has been estimated at 1 in 40,000. Lysosomal glycogen accumulates in skeletal, cardiac, and smooth muscle and in anterior horn cells. Infantile-onset Pompe disease presents shortly after birth and is rapidly progressive and fatal before 1 year of age. Hypertrophic cardiomyopathy with cardiomegaly and heart failure is restricted to the infant-onset form.[11] Less severe acid maltase deficiency can present from childhood to adulthood, often as a limb girdle dystrophy or with ventilatory failure. Many such patients are ultimately wheelchair dependent and require artificial ventilation.

Creatine kinase (CK) is generally elevated but is not specific for Pompe disease. Definitive diagnosis requires assay of acid maltase.[11] Some patients who present in childhood may still have up to 10% residual activity.[11] Prenatal testing is available on chorionic villous cells. Treatment of acid maltase deficiency was primarily supportive in the past, but enzyme replacement therapy has proved lifesaving when instituted early. Supportive therapy includes respiratory support, management of cardiomyopathy, nutritional therapy, and physical therapy.

Congenital myopathies are a heterogeneous group of muscle diseases defined by their characteristic structural findings and include the following:

Central core disease
Nemaline myopathy
Centronuclear myopathy
Multicore disease
Congenital fiber-type disproportion
Reducing body myopathy
Fingerprint body myopathy
Cytoplasmic body myopathy

Myopathies with tubular aggregates
Type 1 myofiber predominance

Autosomal dominant, autosomal recessive, and X-linked inheritance patterns have been recognized. Linkage to chromosomes 19, 1, and 2 has been found in certain kindreds, and mutations in specific genes have been identified in some cases. The diagnosis is made by demonstrating characteristic structures on muscle biopsy with special stains and electron microscopy. The CK level is typically normal.

The clinical course of many congenital myopathies may be benign and consist of static muscle weakness and hypotonia. In contrast, cases with facial, ocular, and respiratory muscle involvement may be lethal in infancy. Other complications include cardiomyopathy and malignant hyperthermia. Physical examination features may be mild at birth and become more prominent as the infant grows. Such features include short stature, pes cavus, pectus excavatum, hip dislocation, kyphoscoliosis, and a high arched palate.

Muscular dystrophies feature progressive muscular weakness and wasting with characteristic changes on muscle biopsy. Inheritance may be autosomal recessive, autosomal dominant, or X-linked (as in Duchenne muscular dystrophy [DMD], the most prevalent disorder in this group). Patients with new mutations lack a family history. Nearly 30 different gene loci have been identified. These genes code for a variety of defective or deficient membrane proteins, the most common of these being the absence or deficiency of dystrophin in DMD.

The characteristic findings on muscle biopsy in the dystrophies include fiber splitting and necrosis, variation in fiber size, and progressive replacement of muscle tissue by fat and connective tissue.

Neonates with congenital muscular dystrophy have generalized muscle weakness and hypotonia manifested most strikingly as feeding and swallowing difficulties, with resultant failure to thrive. Arthrogryposis and joint abnormalities are common. Serum CK is elevated. Nerve conduction studies are normal, and electromyography reveals rapidly recruited, brief-duration, small-amplitude action potentials typical of myopathies. When fiber necrosis is prominent, signs of denervation may also be found. The clinical course is variable, depending on the underlying disorder. Some infants die of respiratory failure or other complications of accompanying central nervous system malformations. Most infants will have delayed motor milestones and never learn to walk. They typically survive into the 20s, with a few patients reaching 40 years of age.

DMD affects 1 in 3500 live males.[12] The disease becomes clinically evident in the preschool years, when these boys present with impaired gait or speech delay, or both. The Gower sign (the patient arises from the sitting position by bracing his arms against his thighs and crawling up on his trunk because of trunk, pelvic girdle, and lower extremity weakness) is characteristic, although not pathognomonic. Progressive calf muscle hypertrophy is almost always present. Weakness progresses such that boys are wheelchair bound by 8 to 10 years. Death occurs in the late teens or early twenties as a result of respiratory or cardiac failure. Most patients have normal cognitive function throughout the course of their disease, but the average IQ is lower than predicted because of the expression of dystrophin deficiency in the brain. There is no curative therapy, but steroids have been shown to prolong the duration of walking. Research is focused on correction of the dystrophin deficiency either by transduction of dystrophin to muscle via viral or plasmid vectors or by gene transfer.[12,13] Stem cell transplantation is also under investigation.[13]

HISTORY AND PHYSICAL EXAMINATION

An infant or child presenting with weakness or hypotonia requires a comprehensive history and physical examination. A history of HELLP (hemolysis, elevated liver enzymes, and low platelet count), decreased fetal movement, oligohydramnios or polyhydramnios, fetal ascites, infections during pregnancy, or complicated delivery (breech presentation, cord compression, retained placenta, postpartum hemorrhage) may be helpful in directing further workup. A maternal history of spontaneous abortions suggests an inherited neuromuscular disease. Details about the age and mode of onset (sudden or gradual) and subsequent course (static versus progressive loss of tone or power) should also be elicited.

Tone in an infant is assessed by passive and active maneuvers. The overall resting posture of a hypotonic infant shows decreased flexion in the arms and legs ("frog leg" posture). Passive maneuvers require only gravity to stretch the muscle and include holding the infant prone in one hand while observing the curvature of the spine over the supporting hand. A hypotonic infant supported beneath the axillae will slip through the hands of the examiner unless lateral pressure is exerted. Head lag is increased in a baby with axial hypotonia when the infant is pulled up by the arms from a supine position.

Active maneuvers are those in which the examiner actively stretches the muscle, such as those used to assess immaturity on the Dubowitz scale (heel-to-ear or scarf sign).

Head circumference and shape and other dysmorphic features may help in identifying a cause. Tongue fasciculations, which are associated with denervation, are characteristic of bulbar disorders, including SMA and syringobulbia. A complete neurologic examination with particular attention to deep tendon reflexes, strength, plantar responses, the bulk and consistency of muscles, and sensory findings allows localization to the upper or lower motor neurons (or occasionally both). Clonus, hyperreflexia, and extensor responses signify upper motor neuron dysfunction. Retained primitive reflexes such as the Moro or asymmetric tonic neck reflex may indicate central nervous system immaturity. Strength may be difficult to assess in an infant but can be inferred by a weak cry or poor sucking. In an older child, loss of the ability to run or climb stairs may indicate weakness.

In infants younger than 18 months, both upper and lower motor neuron lesions may present initially as hypotonia as a result of incomplete myelination of the corticospinal tracts. As the child matures, upper motor neuron lesions cause hypertonia. For example, an infant with hyperbilirubinemia resulting in kernicterus is initially hypotonic but becomes hypertonic over time.

Hypotonia in an infant or child with normal strength, reflexes, and development is most likely benign. If CK and thyroid function are normal, benign congenital hypotonia can be diagnosed. Ligamentous laxity produces similar findings and is likewise benign and often familial.

EVALUATION

A diagnostic algorithm is presented in Figure 128-2. The initial step is to differentiate congenital and acquired hypotonia and weakness. The next step is to separate static and progressive disorders and localize the lesion or lesions by history and examination. Subsequent diagnostic testing is outlined in Table 128-2. Specific clinical features, such as the typical dysmorphic facies associated with Down or Prader-Willi syndrome, direct more focused investigation.

Testing

Electromyography can distinguish primary nerve and muscle disorders. In myopathies, the muscle action potentials have reduced duration and amplitude and increased

Table 128-2   Diagnostic Testing for Upper and Lower Motor Neuron Disorders
Upper Motor Neuron
Thyroid function tests (serum)
TORCH titers
Serum and urine toxicology testing
Magnetic resonance imaging of the head
Ophthalmologic examination
Metabolic studies
Chromosomes
DNA probes
Lower Motor Neuron
Thyroid function tests (serum)
Serum electrolytes
Serum creatinine kinase
Chest radiograph
Electromyography
Tensilon test
Muscle biopsy
Genetic testing/DNA probes

TORCH, toxoplasmosis, other (congenital syphilis and viruses), rubella, cytomegalovirus, and herpes simplex virus.

recruitment, in contrast to the prolonged-duration, polyphasic high-amplitude potentials and reduced recruitment seen in chronic denervation. Nerve conduction velocities in axonal disease are normal or mildly slowed, whereas in peripheral nerve disease they are severely slowed. Specific EMG abnormalities occur in myotonic dystrophy and MG.

Muscle biopsy with histologic examination, specific staining techniques, and electron microscopy is essential for morphologic diagnosis, which is required to identify the congenital myopathies. Staining for the muscle membrane protein dystrophin distinguishes DMD (staining absent) from Becker muscular dystrophy (staining reduced).

DNA probes are now available for a variety of syndromes and neuromuscular diseases. A DNA probe is a fragment of DNA that is created to search for a matching abnormal sequence in the patient. Specific DNA sequence abnormalities have been identified for Prader-Willi syndrome, DMD, and myotonic dystrophy, all of which can be detected with the use of DNA probes.

The *Tensilon (edrophonium) test* is a specific test for neuromuscular dysfunction. After administering a test dose to assess tolerance, full-dose edrophonium is given intravenously, with equipment for resuscitation at hand. Edrophonium inhibits acetylcholinesterase, thereby increasing the concentration of acetylcholine in the neuromuscular junction, and increases strength in patients with postsynaptic disorders, including MG. The muscles to be assessed must be identified before the test commences, and ideally the response should be quantifiable (e.g., width of the palpebral fissure, spirometry). It is prudent to closely monitor a patient during the administration of edrophonium because it can precipitate a cholinergic crisis, including bradycardia, hypotension, and bronchospasm. Atropine reverses this reaction. In neonates and young children, neostigmine is a better alternative because its effects last longer and thus allow a prolonged period of observation of involuntary muscle action.

Serum *creatine kinase* is a nonspecific marker of a leaky muscle membrane. CK isoforms occur in the brain (BB),

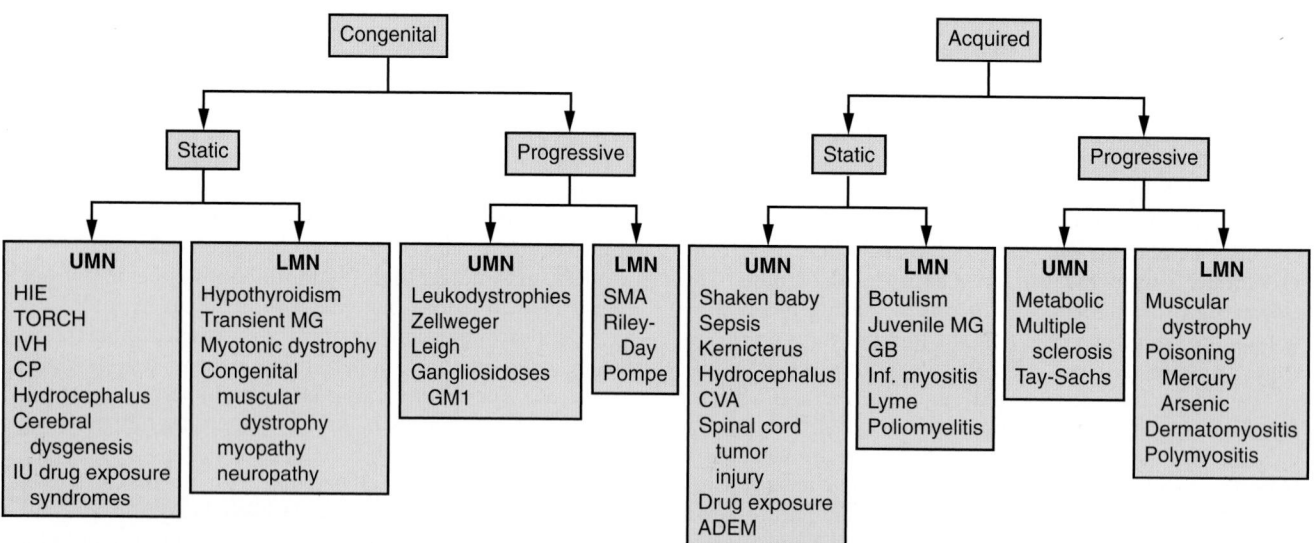

Figure 128-2 Hypotonia algorithm. ADEM, acute disseminated encephalomyelitis; CP, cerebral palsy; CVA, cerebrovascular accident; GB, Guillain-Barré syndrome; HIE, hypoxic ischemic encephalopathy; Inf., infantile; IU, intrauterine; IVH, intraventricular hemorrhage; LMN, lower motor neuron; MG, myasthenia gravis; SMA, spinal muscular atrophy; UMN, upper motor neuron.

heart (MB), and skeletal muscle (MM). It is markedly elevated in Duchenne and Becker muscular dystrophy. Trauma, dermatomyositis, polymyositis, and some neurogenic disorders such as type III SMA may also have elevated CK, but to a much lesser extent.

Metabolic studies may be indicated on samples of serum, urine, or CSF. Such studies include glucose, potassium, CO_2, ammonia, lactate, pyruvate, carnitine, coenzyme Q_{10}, acylcarnitines, and amino and organic acids. Characteristic findings may suggest oxidative phosphorylation defects, glycolytic disorders, and amino and organic acid disorders.

CONSULTATION

Neurology can offer guidance in clinical evaluation, diagnostic testing, and short- and long-term management. The need for other consultants is directed by diagnostic or interventional requirements:

- Pulmonology for respiratory insufficiency
- Otolaryngology for airway obstruction or aspiration
- Orthopedics for joint deformities (e.g., scoliosis, hip dislocation)
- General surgery for feeding-related complications (e.g., fundoplication, insertion of a gastric feeding tube)
- Occupational, physical, and speech therapy services

ADMISSION CRITERIA

Typically, patients are admitted for the evaluation of either new-onset weakness or flare of an underlying disease. Hospitalization is warranted for patients

- Unable to protect their airway from regurgitated stomach contents or oral secretions when feeding by mouth
- With evidence of inadequate ventilation or oxygenation
- Unable to maintain fluid or nutritional needs
- Demonstrating deterioration in their ability to perform activities of daily living
- For whom the family or caretakers are no longer able to provide a safe environment

DISCHARGE CRITERIA

- A safe airway needs to be created and maintained, including protection from aspiration and obstruction.
- Adequacy of ventilation and oxygenation must be established, which may require initiation of noninvasive ventilation, an increased level of support of previous regimens, or the addition of supplemental oxygen. If these noninvasive levels of support are insufficient, patients may require tracheostomy tube placement with mechanical ventilation.
- Means to deliver adequate enteral or parenteral hydration and nutrition have been established.
- Sufficient medical support personnel (home nursing, home health aides, etc.) and equipment (walkers, wheelchairs, assistive devices, etc.) are available to care for the patient in the home environment. Home safety checks should also be performed if a patient's needs have escalated.

IN A NUTSHELL

- The acute onset of hypotonia, in an otherwise healthy infant or child, is most commonly due to severe infection, fluid or electrolyte disturbance, toxic ingestion, or trauma.
- Congenital hypotonia suggests in utero injury to the nervous system.
- A comprehensive history, including conception and gestation, may be helpful in directing the diagnostic workup.
- Dysmorphic features or abnormal movements can be important clues to the diagnosis.
- In an infant younger than 18 months, both upper and lower motor neuron lesions will present initially as hypotonia.
- Physical examination to determine strength, deep tendon reflexes, plantar responses, and clonus may be helpful in localizing the site of pathology to either the upper or lower motor neuron.
- After localizing the lesion as specifically as possible by the history and physical examination, it may be necessary to proceed with diagnostic testing as outlined in Table 128-2.
- Although many of the disease processes have limited or no disease-modifying treatments, early diagnosis allows the physician to anticipate specific complications and intervene to affect overall morbidity and mortality.

ON THE HORIZON

- The focus of current research efforts is directed to early and specific diagnosis, identification, and detection of specific gene abnormalities, and treatment of both the diseases and their complications.
- Existing diagnostic tools such as MRI are being refined to improve specificity in distinguishing ADEM from MS.
- Expanded metabolic screening of newborns is being used by an increasing number of states. It will allow early and automatic identification of infants with these conditions but will require physicians to be familiar with the diseases being screened for and to provide families with appropriate counseling.
- DNA probes and gene identification techniques are becoming more available and less expensive.
- Use of the MitoChip, a high-throughput sequencing tool for reliable identification of mitochondrial DNA mutations, is being evaluated as a clinical test. It will facilitate the diagnosis of mitochondrial diseases in patients with unidentified forms of hypotonia.
- Current treatment methods addressing the associated complications of these diseases are continuing to be evaluated and improved.
- New treatments are being developed to replace or enhance deficient enzymes or correct genetic defects by gene replacement via viral and other vectors.
- The potential role of stem cells in treatment of disease is under investigation.

SUGGESTED READING

Goetz CG, Pappert EJ: Textbook of Clinical Neurology, 2nd ed. Philadelphia, WB Saunders, 2003.

Jones HR, Darras B, De Vivo DC (eds): Neuromuscular Disorders of Infancy, Childhood, and Adolescence: A Clinician's Approach. Philadelphia, Butterworth Heinemann, 2002.

Papazian O, Alfonso I: Adolescents with muscular dystrophies. Adolesc Med 2002;13:511-535.

Younger DS: Peripheral nerve disorders. Prim Care 2004;31:67-83.

REFERENCES

1. Kuker W, Ruff J, Gaertner S, et al: Modern MRI tools for the characterization of acute demyelinating lesions: Chemical shift and diffusion weighted imaging. Neuroradiology 2004;46:421-426.

2. Jones CT: Childhood autoimmune neurologic diseases of the central nervous system. Neurol Clin 2003;21:745-764.

3. Sluder JAD, Newhouse P, Fain D: Pediatric and adolescent multiple sclerosis. Adolesc Med 2002;13:461-485.

4. Fujii T: Dichloroacetate therapy in Leigh syndrome with mitochondrial T8993C mutation. Pediatr Neurol 2002;27:58-61.

5. Kaufmann P, Engelstad K, Wei Y, et al: Dichloroacetate causes toxic neuropathy in MELAS: A randomized, controlled clinical trial. Neurology 2006;66:324-330.

6. Goetz CG: Leukodystrophies. In Goetz CG (ed): Textbook of Clinical Neurology, 2nd ed. Philadelphia, Elsevier, 2003, pp 616-624.

7. Joseph SA, Tsao CY: Guillain-Barré syndrome. Adolesc Med 2002;13:487-494.

8. Axelrod FB: Familial dysautonomia. Muscle Nerve 2004;29:352-363.

9. Vincent A, Newland C, Croxen R, Beeson D: Genes at the junction—candidates for congenital myasthenic syndromes. Trends Neurosci 1997;20:15-22.

10. Zafeiriou DI, Pitt M, deSousa C: Clinical and neurophysiological characteristics of congenital myasthenic syndromes presenting in early infancy. Brain Dev 2004;26:47-52.

11. Kishnani PS, Howell RR: Pompe disease in infants and children. J Pediatr 2004;144:S35-S43.

12. Kapsa R, Kornberg AJ, Byrne E: Novel therapies for Duchenne muscular dystrophy. Lancet Neurol 2003;2:299-310.

13. Papazian O, Alfonso I: Adolescents with muscular dystrophies. Adolesc Med 2002;13:511-535.

CHAPTER 129

Stroke and Aneurysms

Robert H. Fryer

Stroke is defined as the acute appearance of a focal neurologic deficit that lasts longer than 24 hours and shows evidence of infarction on neuroimaging studies. Pediatric stroke can be caused by ischemia secondary to arterial occlusion, hemorrhage of an intraparenchymal blood vessel, or sinovenous thrombosis. Arterial ischemic stroke is the most common type and accounts for more than 80% of pediatric strokes.[1] Neonates have the highest risk for stroke, with an incidence of 28 per 100,000 live births,[1] whereas childhood strokes (1 month to 18 years of age) have an incidence of 2 to 13 per 100,000.[1,2]

Aneurysms in children occur with an incidence of approximately one per million per year and affect males twice as often as females. There is a bimodal age pattern, with a peak at younger than 2 years of age and a second peak in the second decade. Saccular, or "berry," aneurysms are the most common type of aneurysm in children and typically occur in the vessels around the circle of Willis. Approximately 20% of childhood aneurysms are multiple.[3] Mycotic aneurysms are caused by septic emboli and differ from saccular aneurysms in that they are usually located in distal branches of the cerebral arteries rather than around the circle of Willis. Fusiform aneurysms are most commonly caused by atherosclerosis and are therefore rare in children.

CLINICAL PRESENTATION

Transient ischemic attacks are focal neurologic deficits of vascular origin that last less than 24 hours and occasionally presage a stroke. Seizures accompany the stroke in as many as half of all children. Hemiparesis is the most common focal neurologic deficit seen in childhood stroke, but hemisensory loss, aphasias, and hemineglect syndromes also occur. Because stroke is a destructive process, focal brain damage leads to predictable specific impairments in older children and adults. In the developing brain, specific regions have yet to assume their adult function, so pediatric strokes are not always manifested in the same way as adult strokes are. This is particularly evident with regard to prenatal and neonatal strokes. A stroke in the territory of the middle cerebral artery that occurred during the prenatal period is usually clinically silent in the neonatal period and is first recognized when the child presents with hemiparesis between 4 and 8 months of age. This same stroke occurring in the neonatal period typically presents with lethargy or seizures and only rarely with focal signs such as hemiparesis. Only as the child gets older will a stroke in the distribution of the middle cerebral artery typically present with an acute onset of hemiparesis.

Findings on neurologic examination that are consistent with stroke include facial weakness that spares the frontalis muscle and distal greater than proximal weakness of the limbs. Other signs of upper motor neuron lesions include hyperreflexia and a Babinski sign ("up-going" or extensor reflex of the great toe), although these findings may take hours or days to appear after a stroke. Cerebellar strokes in children typically present with acute difficulty walking that is not explained by significant weakness. Rather, the patient has a constellation of cerebellar signs that commonly include a wide-based gait, ataxia, and nystagmus.

Most cerebral aneurysms in children come to clinical attention as a subarachnoid hemorrhage (SAH), although occasionally a giant aneurysm will present with signs of a space-occupying lesion. The clinical manifestations of SAH include an abrupt onset of severe headache, neck stiffness, and vomiting. Alteration of consciousness is commonly seen, and some patients rapidly lapse into coma. Hypertension and seizures are common in patients with SAH.

Traumatic SAH can be distinguished from those caused by a ruptured aneurysm by the history and by evidence of other injuries that are often present.

DIFFERENTIAL DIAGNOSIS

Neuroimaging studies are extremely helpful in narrowing the differential diagnosis and should be pursued early in the evaluation. Cerebral abscess, demyelinating plaque (as seen in multiple sclerosis or acute disseminated encephalomyelitis), and migraine can all produce a strokelike episode. MELAS (mitochondrial encephalomyelopathy with lactic acidosis and strokelike episodes) is a mitochondrial disease and can cause "metabolic strokes." These strokes are probably due to an underlying metabolic abnormality in the brain and do not usually conform to a single vascular territory.

The main consideration in the differential diagnosis of childhood SAH is hemorrhage from an arteriovenous malformation (AVM). It can mimic an aneurysm, although AVM hemorrhages tend to have prominent focal neurologic findings when compared with aneurysmal SAH. Rarely, vertebral artery dissection or a ruptured cavernous malformation causes SAH. Cerebral angiography is the most useful means of distinguishing these entities, although magnetic resonance imaging (MRI) and magnetic resonance angiography (MRA) can also be used.

DIAGNOSIS AND EVALUATION

If stroke or SAH are diagnostic considerations, computed tomography (CT) of the head should be performed promptly (Fig. 129-1). It is an excellent tool for imaging extravascular blood, but it is not useful in the acute phase of ischemic stroke because abnormalities do not generally

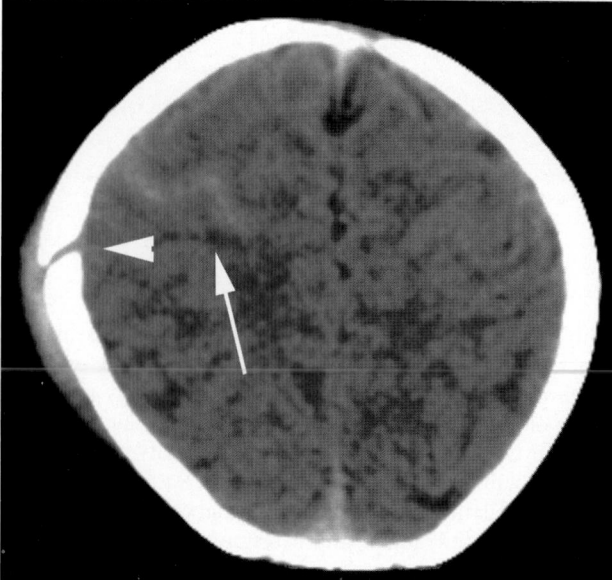

A

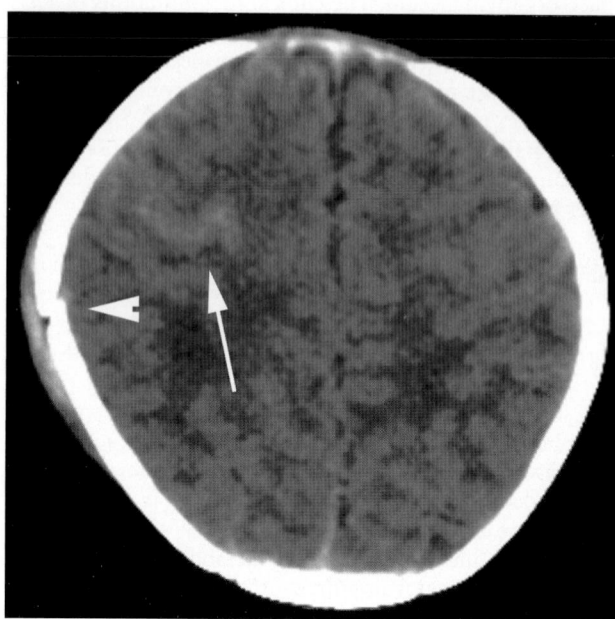

B

Figure 129-1 A and B, Contiguous CT images demonstrate linear increased density conforming to the shape of a sulcus (*arrow*), consistent with subarachnoid hemorrhage in this patient who sustained head trauma. The images also demonstrate an adjacent parietal bone fracture (*arrowhead*).

appear for at least 24 hours after the onset. MRI is the imaging modality of choice for pediatric stroke because abnormalities may be seen early in the process (Fig. 129-2B).

If the diagnosis of stroke is confirmed by neuroimaging studies, the evaluation then shifts to determining the cause of the stroke. The etiology of pediatric stroke is vastly different from that of adult stroke. Risk factors such as atherosclerosis, hypertension, cigarette smoking, and diabetes, which play major causative roles in adult stroke, are virtually absent in pediatric stroke. Common etiologic factors in pediatric stroke include vasculopathies, coagulation disorders, and congenital heart disease (Box 129-1). As a group, the vasculopathies account for as many as 50% of childhood strokes.[4] MRA images blood flow in large and medium-sized cerebral arteries and should be routinely performed during the initial MRI. Focal narrowing of the cerebral arteries suggests an underlying vasculopathy. Cerebral angiography should be considered in all pediatric stroke patients unless a nonvasculopathic cause of the stroke is definite.

Laboratory studies in the workup include a complete blood count, erythrocyte sedimentation rate, antinuclear antibody titer, prothrombin time, partial thromboplastin time, serum homocysteine, protein S, protein C, antithrombin III, factor V Leiden allele, and screening for mutation of the prothrombin gene. For diagnosis of acquired hypercoagulation disorders, studies to detect antiphospholipid antibody syndrome (lupus anticoagulant and anticardiolipin antibodies) should be performed. Transient deficiencies in protein C, protein S, and antithrombin III can be associated with nephrotic syndrome, liver disease, and inflammatory bowel disease.

Because both acquired and congenital heart diseases are risk factors for pediatric stroke, echocardiography should be performed in most cases. Embolic sources in the left side of the heart, including subacute bacterial endocarditis, artificial valves, and atrial myxomas, can cause strokes in children. Other potential cardiac causes of embolism include right-to-left cardiac shunts, which allow thrombi to bypass the pulmonary filtering system and enter the arterial circulation.

If the initial head CT findings are normal, only a lumbar puncture (LP) should be performed. LP can be useful because small hemorrhages or hemorrhages older than 48 hours might not be apparent on head CT. Findings on LP

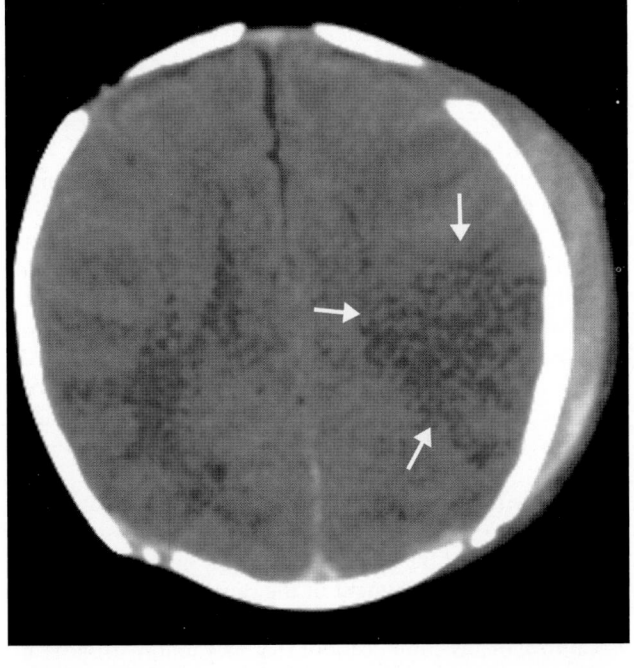

A

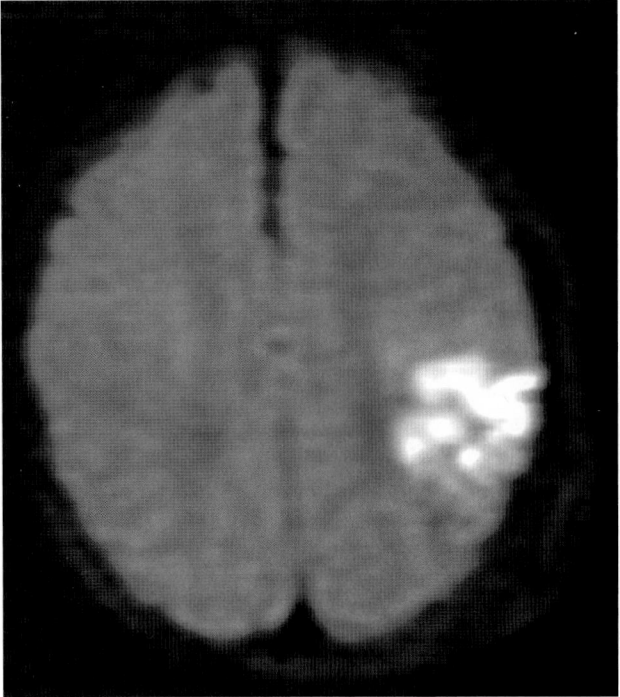

C

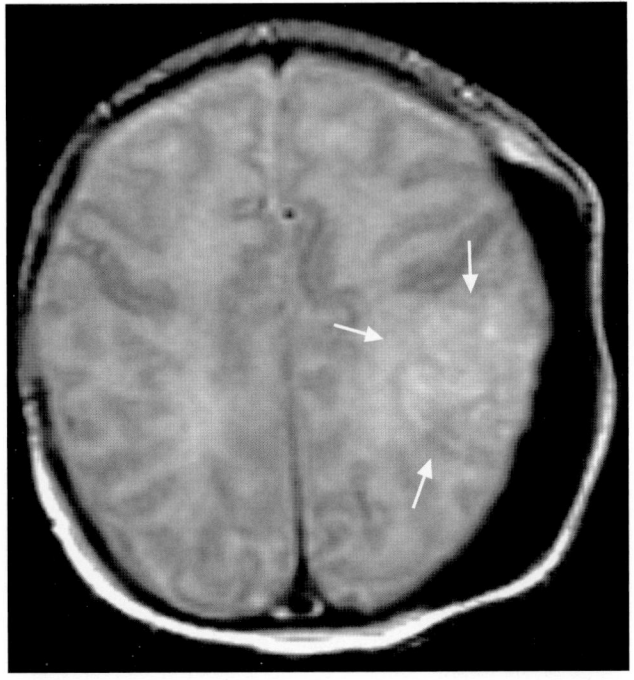

B

Figure 129-2 A, Representative image from the head computed tomography scan in a newborn infant with scalp hematoma from the recent birthing process. In addition, this image shows loss of gray–white differentiation in the left parietal lobe and decreased density in a wedge, shaped configuration (*arrows*), findings consistent with an acute infarct. B, The axial T2 image at a similar level again shows loss of gray–white differentiation and abnormal increased T2 signal in the same region, representing edema from the infarct. C, The diffusion weighted image shows restricted diffusion indicative of an acute infarct in the same location.

consistent with SAH include an elevated opening pressure, elevated red blood cell (RBC) count and protein, and xanthochromia. To help distinguish between a traumatic LP and SAH, an RBC count should be determined from the first and last tubes. With a traumatic LP, the RBC count should be much lower by the last tube. The presence of xanthochromia confirms a previous bleeding episode because it represents breakdown of RBCs. Once the diagnosis of SAH is established, cerebral angiography should be performed as soon as possible to determine the source of the SAH.

COURSE OF ILLNESS

Large ischemic strokes and hemorrhages can cause significant edema with increased intracranial pressure and possible herniation. However, most strokes in children produce focal neurologic deficits that improve gradually with time and therapy. Worsening of symptoms in the hours or days after the stroke should prompt an immediate neurologic evaluation because it could suggest conversion of an ischemic or evolving infarct to a hemorrhagic entity.

More than half of all children with an aneurysmal SAH will have a good outcome, with minimal or no functional impairment. Outcome in childhood SAH is related to the level of consciousness at presentation. Children who are stuporous or in coma with decerebrate posturing will have a poor outcome. Abrupt deterioration during the hospitalization may reflect acute hydrocephalus, vasospasm, or rebleeding. Hydrocephalus may require an external ventricular drain or replacement of an obstructed, previously placed drain. Vasospasm typically occurs between 7 and 21 days after SAH and can result in ischemic stroke. Aneurysmal rebleeding can occur at any time and is a major cause of further morbidity and mortality.

CONSULTATION

- Neurology: Should be consulted in all cases of stroke or aneurysm
- Neurosurgery: Intraparenchymal, intraventricular, or subarachnoid hemorrhage found on head CT
- Cardiology: In cases of pediatric stroke in which a cardiac source of emboli is being considered
- Hematology: In patients with a bleeding diathesis, hypercoagulable disorder, or sickle cell anemia
- Interventional neuroradiology: If endovascular treatment of a vascular malformation is a consideration

TREATMENT AND ADMISSION CRITERIA

All children with an acute stroke should be admitted for evaluation and management and often require stabilization in an intensive care setting. Both antiplatelet agents and anticoagulation have been used in pediatric stroke, but there have been no treatment trials conducted to date. Situations in which heparin anticoagulation should be considered include arterial dissection and cardiac emboli. Heparin should not be used if there is evidence of cerebral hemorrhage or in children with large ischemic infarcts because of the risk for hemorrhagic conversion. In these and many other cases, antiplatelet agents can be used as alternatives. Exchange transfusion should be considered in patients with sickle cell anemia who present with an acute infarct. Moyamoya disease, a progressive cerebral artery occlusive process associated with the development of fine collaterals ("puff of smoke" on arteriography), can be treated surgically with a bypass procedure.

Children with SAH from any cause should be admitted to an intensive care unit for close monitoring with neurosurgical care. A cerebral angiogram should be performed as soon as possible to determine the source of the bleeding. Aneurysms can be treated by endovascular techniques or can be clipped at the aneurysmal neck during open craniotomy. Treatment decisions are based on the size and location of the aneurysm, as well as the child's clinical status. In children with a reasonably good prognosis based on their initial presentation, the goal is to intervene either surgically or endovascularly within a few days of the SAH to prevent rebleeding.

Medical treatment of a child with SAH should include careful management of fluids and electrolytes. Hypotonic intravenous solutions should be avoided because they facilitate a shift of water from the intravascular compartment into the brain and increase intracranial pressure. Current care includes the administration of a calcium channel blocker such as nimodipine, which may act as a neuroprotective agent, and phenytoin as prophylaxis against seizures. If there is evidence of vasospasm and the aneurysm has been repaired, the patient may be a candidate for therapeutic induction of hypertension.

Ischemic stroke or SAH can damage the cranial nerves involved in both the sensory and motor component of swallowing. These children may be at high risk for aspiration, so it is prudent to carefully evaluate the swallowing function of all children with stroke or SAH. Physical and occupational therapy should begin as soon as the patient's condition permits. Long-term sequelae of pediatric stroke and SAH include seizures, which may have to be managed with antiepileptic agents, and spasticity, which can be managed with physical therapy or antispasmodic agents, or both.

DISCHARGE CRITERIA

- Stabilization of the initial hemorrhagic or ischemic injury
- Evaluation and treatment of the cause or any underlying contributing process
- Control of any complications that may follow stroke (e.g., seizures, hydrocephalus, rebleeding, feeding difficulties)
- Referral for any rehabilitation needs, whether as an inpatient (transfer to the rehabilitation unit) or as an outpatient
- Institution of appropriate outpatient follow-up with primary care, subspecialist, or home nursing support

PREVENTION

Prevention of recurrent strokes in children is based on identifying any treatable risk factors during the hospitalization. Surgical bypass procedures for moyamoya disease and hypertransfusion therapy for patients with sickle cell anemia are two treatments that reduce recurrent strokes in these specific patient populations.

There are no interventions known to prevent the formation of aneurysms. In families with more than one first-degree relative with a cerebral aneurysm, screening of unaffected family members by MRA can be performed.

IN A NUTSHELL

- Clinical presentation: Strokes present with an acute, focal neurologic deficit, usually including hemiparesis. Aneurysms generally present with symptoms of SAH, including severe headache, neck stiffness, vomiting, and alteration in consciousness.
- Diagnosis: Clinical features, plus evidence of a vascular origin based on head CT or MRI. Most SAHs can be diagnosed by head CT. Cerebral angiography can then be used to determine the location and size of the aneurysm.
- Treatment: Anticoagulation with heparin or antiplatelet agents is the most common treatment of pediatric stroke. SAH requires neurosurgical and intensive care. Physical and occupational therapy is important in patients with motor deficits.

ON THE HORIZON

• A large, multicenter, international collaboration to study pediatric stroke is being organized. The initial goal of this collaboration will be to identify risk factors for pediatric stroke. Once epidemiologic data have been collected, treatment trials for pediatric stroke can be instituted. For cerebral aneurysms, look for studies on the long-term effectiveness of endovascular treatment of aneurysms versus surgical clipping.

SUGGESTED READING

deVeber G: Stroke and the child's brain: An overview of epidemiology, syndromes and risk factors. Curr Opin Neurol 2002;15:133-138.

Lynch JK, Hirtz DG, DeVeber G, Nelson KB: Report of the National Institute of Neurological Disorders and Stroke workshop on perinatal and childhood stroke. Pediatrics 2002;109:116-123.

REFERENCES

1. deVeber G: Stroke and the child's brain: An overview of epidemiology, syndromes and risk factors. Curr Opin Neurol 2002;15:133-138.
2. Lynch JK, Hirtz DG, DeVeber G, Nelson KB: Report of the National Institute of Neurological Disorders and Stroke workshop on perinatal and childhood stroke. Pediatrics 2002;109:116-123.
3. Punt J: Surgical management of pediatric stroke. Pediatr Radiol 2004;34:16-23.
4. deVeber G: Arterial ischemic strokes in infants and children: An overview of current approaches. Semin Thromb Hemost 2003;29:567-573.

Genetics and Metabolism

CHAPTER 130

Genetic Syndromes Caused by Chromosomal Abnormalities

Matthew A. Deardorff and Elaine H. Zackai

Understanding the influence of genetics on health and disease has been a major goal in scientific research over the last century. The most dramatic result of this initiative is the Human Genome Project, which has sequenced the 3 billion base pairs of DNA to provide a road map for studying the 30,000 to 40,000 human genes.[1]

These advances have been accompanied by an increasing realization that human health—including diseases and conditions associated with pediatric hospitalization—is deeply influenced by genetics. In classic studies, 0.4% to 2.5% of pediatric hospitalizations were attributable to chromosomal abnormalities, and 6% to 8% were attributable to single gene defects; another 22% to 31% of diseases were considered to have a genetic factor.[2,3] Since then, as more diseases have been shown to have genetic components, these numbers have risen. A recent report suggests that 71% of pediatric admissions involve a significant genetic component, and 34% of disorders with a clear genetic basis result in 50% of annual hospital costs.[4]

Here, we review the major pediatric genetic diseases caused by abnormalities that affect a whole chromosome or segment of a chromosome. In addition, clinical situations in which genetic testing should be considered and the types of testing used are discussed.

CLINICAL PRESENTATION

The essential tools that the clinical geneticist uses to diagnose genetic disorders include the following:

- Prenatal, birth, and medical histories.
- Detailed pedigree analysis.
- Careful clinical evaluation, including dysmorphology examination.
- Comprehensive literature searches.
- Cytogenetic and molecular genetic laboratory analyses.

The generalist can also use many of these tools, whereas others may require input from a clinical geneticist.

Some key features of the family history include ethnic origin, consanguinity, related disorders in the family, and pregnancy losses. The dysmorphology examination is intended to reveal and quantify abnormal development of organs or other parts of the body, as outlined in Table 130-1.

A frequent objective of the clinical geneticist is to link a number of findings that relate to an identifiable syndrome to facilitate diagnosis, management, and counseling. To accomplish this, literature searches are useful; typical modalities include textbooks,[5] journals, and the National Library of Medicine online resources (*PubMed.gov*), as well as a number of specialized online resources such as OMIM[6] and GeneTests.[7] The laboratory workup may include cytogenetic analyses or molecular (i.e., gene-based) tests.

CHROMOSOMES

The DNA that makes up the human genome is packaged into 23 pairs of chromosomes. One copy of each pair is inherited from each parent. Most chromosomes contain a short p arm, a long q arm, and a small centromere segment that joins the two arms. The distal ends of the p and q arms are known as telomeres. Each chromosome pair has a distinctive size, centromere position, and banding pattern (Fig. 130-1A) that allows identification and designation by number, typically from largest to smallest, using the International System for Human Cytogenetic Nomenclature.[9] A typical analysis, or *karyotype*, is shown in Figure 130-1B; this normally consists of 46 chromosomes, with 22 pairs of autosomes and one set of sex chromosomes.

Genes are located on chromosomes in fixed positions. With the exception of those on the sex chromosomes, each gene has two copies, or *alleles*. Chromosomal abnormalities that increase or decrease the allele copy number are classic mechanisms that cause genetic disease. Some of these disorders arise due to disruptions of chromosome structure that duplicate or delete multiple genes in a row, known as *contiguous gene syndromes* (see later).

Chromosome Analysis

Karyotype analysis is performed in cells undergoing cell division, or mitosis. Thus, only cells that are rapidly dividing (bone marrow or chorionic villus) or can be stimulated to divide in culture (peripheral blood lymphocytes, skin

Table 130-1   Elements of the Dysmorphology Examination

Category	Subcategory	Examples of Abnormalities
General	Height	Overgrowth
	Weight	Small for gestational age, failure to thrive
	Head circumference	Microcephaly, macrocephaly
Head	Shape	Brachycephaly (disproportionately wide head), turricephaly (cone-shaped head), craniosynostosis (premature closure of one or more cranial sutures)
	Size	Microcephaly, macrocephaly
	Fontanelles	Large, small, third
	Hair distribution	Scalp defects, high or low hairline, hair whorls
Eyes	Shape	Almond
	Eyebrows	Synophrys (meeting at the midline), interruption, absent
	Structures	Colobomas, iris irregularities, blue sclera
	Spacing	Hypertelorism, hypotelorism
	Palpebral fissures	Up-slanted, down-slanted, epicanthal folds
Ears	Placement	Low set
	Rotation	Posteriorly rotated
	Length	Short or long
	Helices	Overfolded
	Preauricular surface	Pits, tags
Nose	Shape of tip	Bulbous
	Alae nasi (sides)	Hypoplastic
	Nares	Anteversion
	Columella	Long or short
	Choana patency	Choanal stenosis
Mouth	Lips	Thin, simple, pits, downturned
	Frenulum	Absent, duplicated
	Teeth	Natal, absent, single front incisor
	Tongue	Protuberant
	Palate	Cleft, high arched
	Uvula	Bifid
Neck	Chin	Retrognathic, micrognathic
	Folds	Excess nuchal folds, webbing
Chest	Cardiac	Murmurs
	Lung	Absent sounds, wheezing
	Sternum	Pectus deformity
	Size	Broad (increased internipple distance–chest ratio)
	Superficial findings	Supernumerary nipple, absent clavicles
Back	Shape	Scoliosis, lordosis, kyphosis
	Sacrum	Dimple, myelomeningocele, hair tuft
Abdomen	Umbilicus	Two-vessel cord, umbilical hernia, omphalocele
	Visceromegaly	Hepatosplenomegaly
Genitourinary	Phallus, clitoris	Hypospadias, chordee, clitoromegaly
	Labia, scrotum	Bifid scrotum, ambiguous genitalia
	Testes	Undescended
Extremities	Limb length	Brachymelia (short limbs), rhizomelia (shortening of proximal limbs), mesomelia (small intermediate segments of long bones), acromelia (shortening of distal limb segments)
	Digit number	Polydactyly (pre- or postaxial), oligodactyly
	Digit fusion	Syndactyly
	Position of digits	Proximally placed thumbs, clinodactyly, camptodactyly
Dermatoglyphics	Digital	Predominance of arches or whorls
	Palmar	Distal triradii, single transverse crease
	Hallucal	Open field
Skin	Pigmentation	Café au lait spots, ash-leaf spots
	Vascular	Hemangioma, telangiectasia
	Hair	Brittle, steely, absent
	Sweat	Absent
Neurologic	Alertness	Lethargic, nonresponsive
	Tone	Hypertonia, hypotonia
	Feeding	Poor
	Movements	Fasciculations, seizures, choreas

Methods for measuring and standard curves are included in reference 8.

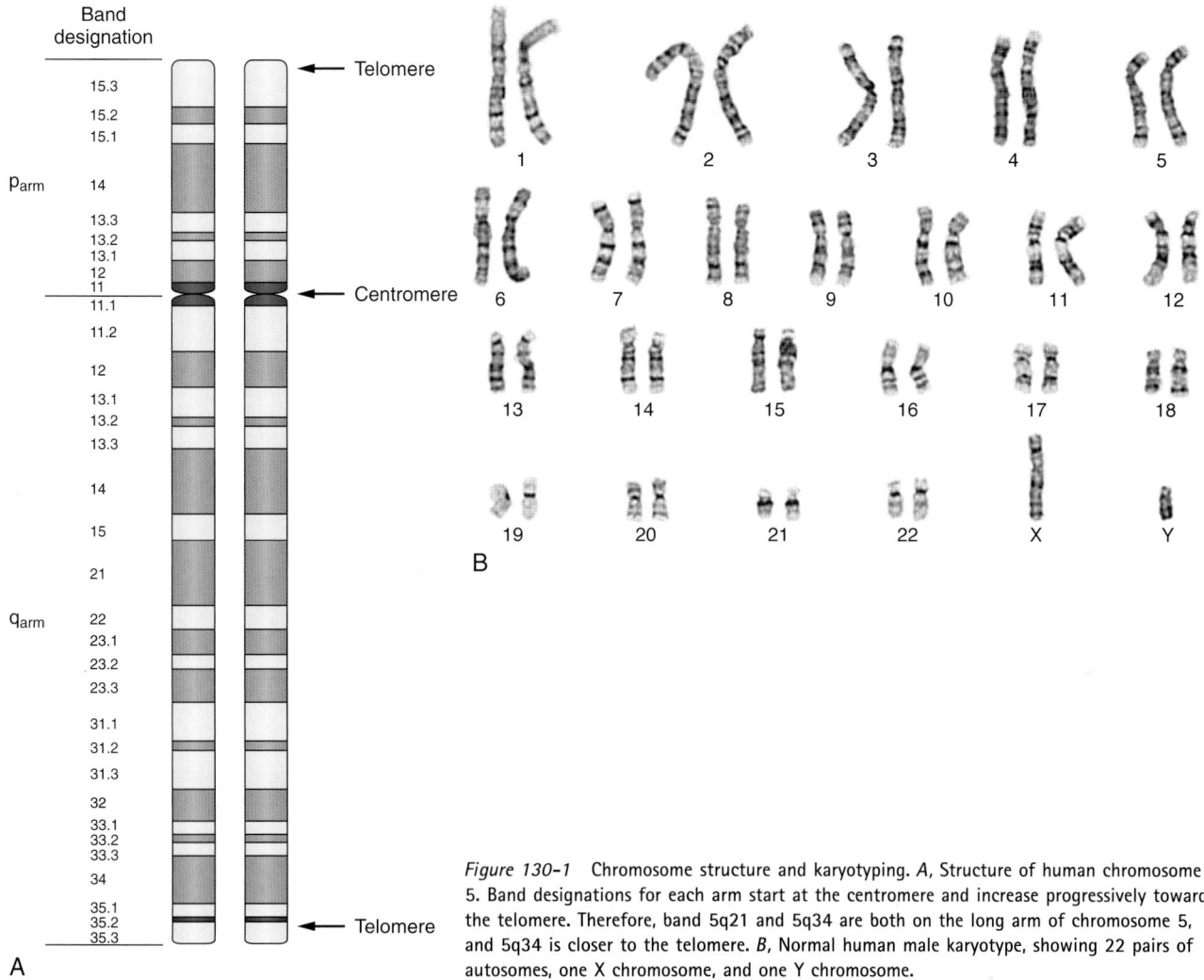

Figure 130-1 Chromosome structure and karyotyping. *A*, Structure of human chromosome 5. Band designations for each arm start at the centromere and increase progressively toward the telomere. Therefore, band 5q21 and 5q34 are both on the long arm of chromosome 5, and 5q34 is closer to the telomere. *B*, Normal human male karyotype, showing 22 pairs of autosomes, one X chromosome, and one Y chromosome.

fibroblasts, and amniocytes) are used. The contemporary method of Giemsa staining (G-banding) allows the resolution of at least 400 to 800 different bands on all chromosomes. However, a single band usually contains 50 or more genes. Therefore, karyotyping is used to detect major structural abnormalities of the chromosomes.

An imbalance of genetic material, known as *aneuploidy*, occurs from a net loss or gain of genetic material during gametogenesis or during the initial zygotic divisions. Classic aneuploidy syndromes include *trisomy* or *monosomy* of a complete chromosome, which often arises from *nondisjunction* or the failure of chromosome separation during meiosis or oocyte formation. In this case, one daughter cell receives both copies of the pair, and the other receives none.

Nondisjunction also occurs during mitosis, when uneven distribution of genetic material occurs during early embryonic cell division. This results in two daughter lines—a trisomic cell line and a monosomic cell line. In most cases, the trisomic line persists and the monosomic line is lost. If the nondisjunction occurs after the first postzygotic division, cells with a normal chromosome complement may coexist with cells containing an aneuploid complement, a condition known as chromosomal *mosaicism.*

Partial aneuploidy, in which only a fragment of a chromosome is deleted or duplicated, occurs in several ways.

Rearrangement of material between nonhomologous chromosomes (e.g., chromosomes 11 and 22) can occur in the gametes of a balanced translocation carrier. The carrier parent has no net loss or gain of genetic material and is usually phenotypically normal. However, offspring are at increased risk for abnormal segregation, resulting in an unbalanced rearrangement and subsequent phenotypic consequences, which may include defects in organogenesis and mental retardation.

Other syndromes are caused by the de novo deletion of a fragment of a chromosome. The location of the breakpoint may be random or may be associated with segmental duplications, which are large repetitive blocks of DNA. These repeats cause misalignment between chromosome pairs and may result in deletion or duplication of contiguous genes, leading to well-recognized syndromes (Fig. 130-2A). The chromosomal abnormalities of many of these syndromes can be easily diagnosed with the use of highly specific fluorescent in situ hybridization (FISH) probes. This technique involves labeling a segment of DNA with a fluorescent tag and allowing it to anneal to its corresponding chromosomal location. When imaged under fluorescence microscopy, two fluorescent signals indicate the presence of both copies of this region. If one chromosome carries a deletion, the FISH probe will anneal only to the normal chromosome, giving

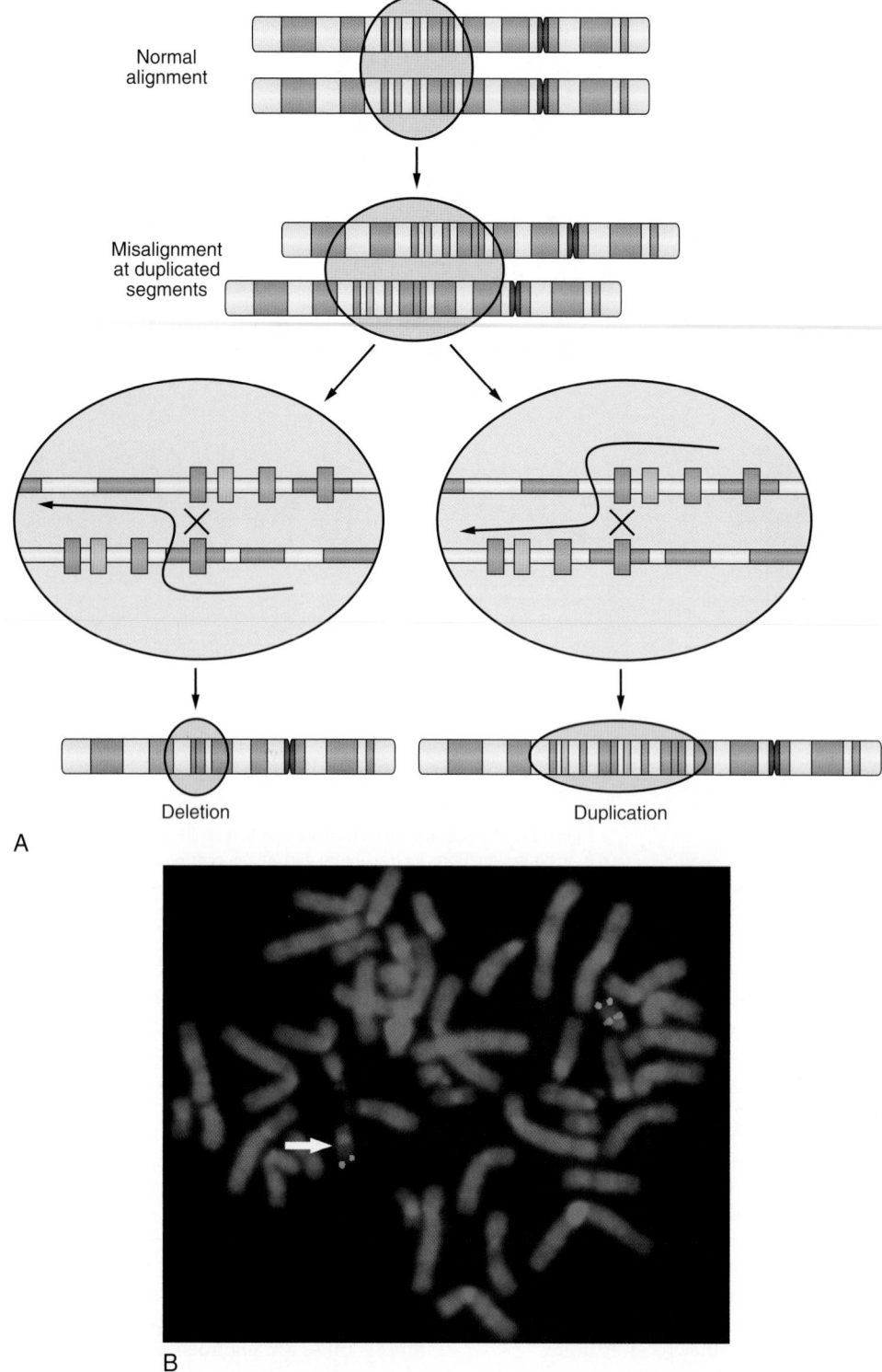

Figure 130-2 Chromosomal rearrangements arising from segmental duplications. *A,* Some genomic regions contain large stretches of repeated DNA (segmental duplications, blue blocks) surrounding nonrepeated sequences (green, orange blocks). During meiosis, the homology between these duplicated segments allows them to align incorrectly. If recombination occurs, the resulting chromosome will contain either a duplication or a deletion of the nonrepeated sequences, causing inappropriate gene dosage and an abnormal phenotype. *B,* Chromosomal deletions can be detected by fluorescent in situ hybridization (FISH). Here, a subtelomeric FISH probe anneals to both chromosomes 22, giving green signals. A 22q11.2 probe detects the presence of the normal chromosome (red signal), but the other chromosome contains a deletion of this region, and the FISH probe does not anneal *(white arrow).*

Table 130-2 Indications for Chromosomal Testing

Indication	High-Resolution Karyotype	FISH
Two or more major malformations, including pre- or postnatal growth failure	Yes	TEL
Mental retardation of unknown cause, with or without accompanying malformations	Yes	TEL
Features of recognized chromosomal syndromes	Yes	SS
Couples with infertility or increased spontaneous abortions	Yes	Not indicated
Parents and children of individuals with known chromosomal translocations	Yes	SS
Sexual malformations or abnormalities of sexual development	Yes	TEL
Patients with various malignancies	Yes	SS

FISH, fluorescent in situ hbridization; SS, syndrome-specific FISH; TEL, subtelomeric FISH.
Adapted from Beaudet AL, Scriver CR, Sly WS, Valle D: Genetics, biochemistry, and molecular bases of variant human phenotypes. In Scriver CR, Sly WS, Childs B, et al (eds): The Metabolic and Molecular Bases of Inherited Disease. New York, McGraw-Hill, 2001, pp 3-48.

one fluorescent signal (Fig. 130-2B). FISH has allowed the identification of small chromosomal deletions that cause common genetic syndromes but are invisible by karyotype analysis. Further, FISH probes in the gene-rich subtelomeric regions enable the identification of rearrangements in these regions, which are difficult to analyze by conventional karyotyping. Subtelomeric FISH has become part of the routine genetic evaluation.

Indications for Chromosomal Testing

Population studies indicate that the frequency of chromosomal abnormalities in all newborn infants is approximately 1 in 200 (0.5%).[10] Several populations of patients have a higher frequency of chromosomal abnormalities, including those with multiple congenital malformations (2% to 20%), infertility and sterility (1% to 10%), mental retardation (1% to 3%), and certain forms of malignancy. Specific indications for cytogenetic testing are summarized in Table 130-2.

RECOGNIZABLE CHROMOSOMAL DISORDERS

Trisomy 21 (Down Syndrome)

Down syndrome is the most common cytogenetically visible autosomal trisomy.[11] The vast majority of cases (>90%) occur secondary to maternal meiotic nondisjunction; this is related to maternal age and results in a 1% risk for women at age 40. Three percent to 5% of cases are due to unbalanced translocations passed from a balanced translocation carrier parent. Mitotic nondisjunction, or mosaic Down syndrome, is seen in approximately 3% of cases, with features ranging from normal to a classic Down syndrome phenotype.

The increased incidence in older mothers has led to the use of prenatal karyotyping for women who will be 35 years or older at the time of delivery. Samples are obtained by amniocentesis after 15 weeks of gestation or by chorionic villus sampling after 10 to 12 weeks. If trisomy 21 is not diagnosed prenatally, most patients are recognized at birth, which prompts karyotype analysis. The clinical features of Down syndrome are summarized in Table 130-3. Because many organ systems can be involved, several clinical investi-

gations are warranted when trisomy 21 is suspected. Routine cardiac, gastrointestinal, ophthalmic, otorhinolaryngologic, cervical spine, and endocrine evaluations are essential for patients with Down syndrome. Of note, the most immediately concerning malformation is congenital heart disease, which occurs in up to 60% and typically requires surgical intervention.[12] Thus, an echocardiogram is indicated in all cases, and medical and surgical intervention for cardiac lesions is routine. Guidelines for the ongoing care of children with Down syndrome have been published by the American Academy of Pediatrics.[13] When counseling the family of a newborn diagnosed with trisomy 21, it is important to explain the severity of each malformation and all the organ systems affected when defining a prognosis. Above all, the wide variability of the phenotype should be emphasized, with a care plan tailored to the individual needs of the patient.

Unless the cause of Down syndrome is a translocation, parental karyotypes are generally not analyzed because they are almost always normal. After having one child with trisomy 21, a mother's risk of having another affected child is approximately 1 percentage point higher than her age-specific risk. For example, a 20-year-old mother's risk increases from 0.2% to 1.2%, while a 45-year-old mother's risk increases from 4.4% to 5.4%. If a de novo translocation resulting in trisomy 21 is found, the risk of recurrence is less than 1%. If the mother carries a balanced Robertsonian translocation involving chromosome 21, the risk for another Down syndrome fetus is about 15% at 15 weeks' gestational age and 10% at birth. However, if the father is the translocation carrier, the recurrence risk is only 1% to 2%.[14]

Trisomy 18 (Edwards Syndrome)

Trisomy 18 occurs in about 1 in 6000 live births and is associated with a high rate of fetal loss. Only 5% of conceptuses with trisomy 18 survive to birth, and 30% of fetuses diagnosed by second-trimester amniocentesis die before the end of the pregnancy.[15] Prenatal and postnatal clinical features are listed in Table 130-3.

Trisomy 18 carries an extremely poor prognosis, with only 5% survival at 1 year. Death is often the result of central apnea, infection, or congestive heart failure. The neonatal

1Table 130–3	Common Autosomal Trisomies		
Feature	Trisomy 21	Trisomy 18	Trisomy 13
Eponym	Down syndrome	Edwards syndrome	Patau syndrome
Live-born incidence	1 in 800	1 in 6000	1 in 12,000
Prenatal	Triple screen: low AFP, low unconjugated estriol, high HCG. Ultrasound: cardiac defects, duodenal atresia, shortened long bones, nuchal translucency, echogenic small bowel	Triple screen: low AFP, low unconjugated estriol, low HCG. Ultrasound: IUGR, oligohydramnios or polyhydramnios, microcephaly, Dandy-Walker malformation, cardiac defects, myelomeningocele, clenched fists, limb anomalies, single umbilical artery	Triple screen: normal. Ultrasound: cardiac anomalies, omphalocele, renal anomalies, pyloric stenosis
Growth	Low-normal at birth (10%-25%), slow postnatal growth velocity	IUGR at birth (1500-2500 g); FTT due to poor feeding, requiring tube feedings	FTT due to feeding difficulties
Tone	Hypotonia	Hypertonia	Hypo- or hypertonia
Cranium, brain	Mild microcephaly, flat occiput, 3 fontanelles	Microcephaly, narrow cranium, prominent occiput, open metopic suture	Microcephaly, anophthalmia, sloping forehead, split sutures, open fontanelles
Eyes	Up-slanting palpebral fissures, epicanthal folds, speckled iris, Brushfield spots (75%), strabismus, cataracts, myopia, glaucoma	Small palpebral fissures, corneal opacity, microphthalmia, coloboma, cataracts	Microphthalmia, hypotelorism, iris coloboma, retinal dysplasia, hamartomatous cartilage "islands"
Ears	Small, low-set, posteriorly rotated, overfolded upper helix; hearing loss (50%)	Low-set, posteriorly rotated, malformed	Low-set, malformed
Nose, mouth	Holds mouth open; prominent tongue; large cheeks; low, flat nasal bridge	Small mouth, micrognathia, choanal atresia	Cleft lip and palate
Neck	Short neck with excess skin, atlantoaxial subluxation		
Skeletal	Brachyclinodactyly of 5th digit, gap between toes 1 and 2, excess nuchal skin, short stature, ligamentous laxity	Clenched hands, overlapping 2nd and 5th digits, absent 5th finger, distal crease, hypoplastic nails, short rocker-bottom feet, prominent heels, convex soles, clubfoot, vertebral anomalies, radial ray limb defects, dorsiflexed great toes	Postaxial polydactyly; hypoconvex fingernails; flexed, overlapped fingers; camptodactyly; rocker-bottom feet
Cardiorespiratory	60% with CHD; AV canal, VSD, ASD, tetralogy of Fallot, PDA	90% with CHD; ASD, VSD, PDA, pulmonic stenosis, aortic coarctation, pulmonary hypoplasia	80% with CHD; VSD, ASD, PDA, dextrocardia
Gastrointestinal	Duodenal atresia (2%-5%); Hirschsprung disease; esophageal atresia, fistulas, and webs	Omphalocele, malrotation, ileal atresia, hernias	Omphalocele, hernias
Genitourinary	Short labial folds	Polycystic kidneys, ureteral anomalies, unilateral renal agenesis, hypospadias, cryptorchidism	Genital anomalies, polycystic kidneys
Endocrine	Hypothyroidism (5%); men almost always infertile, but some women have reproduced	Thyroid and adrenal hypoplasia	

Table 130-3 Common Autosomal Trisomies—cont'd

Feature	Trisomy 21	Trisomy 18	Trisomy 13
Hematologic, oncologic	Neonatal thrombocytopenia, leukemoid reaction, acute nonlymphoblastic leukemia in first 3 yr, ALL	Thymic hypoplasia, increased incidence of hepatoblastoma and Wilms tumor	Increased nuclear projections in neutrophils ("drumstick" appearance), increased risk for malignancy, capillary hemangioma
Dermatoglyphics (skin)	Single palmar crease, plantar crease between 1st and 2nd toes, distal triradii	Excess arch pattern, hypoplastic nails	Occipital scalp defects (cutis aplasia, 50%); single palmar crease; hyperconvex, narrow nails
Neurologic	Seizures (5%-10%), early-onset Alzheimer neurodegeneration	Hypertonia, apnea, seizures	Holoprosencephaly (50%), seizures
Developmental	Language and motor delay, mean IQ 54 (range, 35-65), intensive early intervention critical	Severe psychomotor delay (100%)	Severe delay, many blind and deaf
Survival	Long term; death typically related to heart disease, infection, malignancies	95% die within first year; 1% live to age 10 yr; death often due to apnea, cardiac disease, infection	80% die as neonates; death often related to cardiopulmonary arrest, CHD, pneumonia

AFP, α-fetoprotein; ALL, acute lymphoblastic leukemia; ASD, atrial septal defect; AV, atrioventricular; CHD, congenital heart disease; FTT, failure to thrive; HCG, human chorionic gonadotropin; IUGR, in utero growth retardation; PDA, patent ductus arteriosus; VSD, ventricular septal defect.
Adapted from Epstein CJ: Down syndrome (trisomy 21). In Scriver CR, et al (eds): The Metabolic and Molecular Bases of Inherited Disease. New York, McGraw-Hill, 2001, pp 1223-1256; and Zackai EH, Anyane-Yeboa K, Bergoffen J, et al: Genetics. In Polin RA, Ditmar MF (eds): Pediatric Secrets. Philadelphia, Hanley & Belfus, 2001, p 731.

period is characterized by poor feeding and growth, and patients typically require tube feedings. Poor growth, profound mental retardation, and lack of developmental progress beyond that of a 6-month-old infant have been universally documented. In the few cases attempted, cardiac surgery has not improved the outcome.

Like trisomy 21, the recurrence risk for trisomy 18 is 1 point higher than the maternal age-specific risk for *any* viable autosomal trisomy. Trisomy occurring from a structural rearrangement, such as a translocation, warrants a parental karyotype analysis to assess the risk of recurrence.

Trisomy 13 (Patau Syndrome)

Only 2% to 3% of fetuses with trisomy 13 survive to birth, resulting in a frequency of 1 in 12,500 to 21,000 live births.[15] As with the other trisomies, amniocentesis in cases of advanced maternal age or as indicated by fetal ultrasonographic findings may lead to a prenatal diagnosis of trisomy 13.

Classic features of trisomy 13 include congenital heart disease, cleft palate, holoprosencephaly, renal anomalies, and postaxial polydactyly. Additional findings are noted in Table 130-3. The prognosis for an infant born with trisomy 13 is extremely poor, with 80% mortality in the neonatal period and less than 5% survival at 6 months. Mental retardation is profound, and many patients are blind and deaf.

As with trisomies 21 and 18, recurrence of trisomy 13 in a subsequent pregnancy is rare. The risk is approximately 1 percentage point higher than the maternal age-related risk of any viable autosomal trisomy.

SEX CHROMOSOME ABNORMALITIES: TURNER SYNDROME

In the male, the sex chromosomes consist of an X and a Y chromosome; in the female, there are two X chromosomes, one of which is inactivated, or lyonized, to form a Barr body. Multiple syndromes originate from an abnormal number of sex chromosomes, including Klinefelter (XXY), Turner (XO), and others.

Turner syndrome results from loss of an X chromosome in a female conceptus and occurs in approximately 1 in 2500 female newborns. The 45,XO karyotype, or loss of an entire X chromosome, accounts for roughly half of the cases. Deletions, translocations, and isochromosomes (i.e., a chromosome with two p arms or two q arms) of the X chromosome account for the remainder. Only 0.1% of fetuses with a 45,XO complement survive to term; the vast majority are spontaneously aborted. This underscores the requirement for both X chromosomes during early embryonic development. In approximately 80% of cases, the paternally derived X chromosome is lost.[16]

Approximately one third of Turner syndrome patients are diagnosed at birth based on clinical features. Short stature, webbed neck, craniofacial differences (epicanthal folds and high arched palate), shield chest, renal anomalies, lymphedema of the hands and feet, nail hypoplasia, and congenital heart disease may be noted. Typical cardiac defects include bicuspid aortic valve, coarctation of the aorta, hypoplastic left heart, valvular aortic stenosis, and mitral valve prolapse.

Another one third of patients are diagnosed during childhood and adolescence owing to growth issues, especially short stature. The average adult height of patients with Turner syndrome is 135 to 150 cm without treatment. Growth hormone therapy is routinely considered around age 4 to 5 years.[16] Such therapy can add 6 cm or more to the final adult height, although it may cause insulin resistance and increased blood pressure while the child is taking the hormone. The long-term effects on cardiovascular status, type 2 diabetes, and psychosocial outcomes have not been clarified.[17]

The remaining third of Turner syndrome patients are diagnosed due to primary ovarian failure caused by gonadal dysgenesis or streak gonads.

Turner syndrome patients may demonstrate several additional features. Hypothyroidism is noted in 15% to 30% of patients and should be checked at diagnosis and then annually beginning at age 10. Strabismus is seen in 18% of patients, and cataracts are even more common; for this reason, ophthalmologic evaluation should be considered. Sensorineural hearing loss occurs in 90% of adults with Turner syndrome, so patients should have an auditory examination at diagnosis and annually thereafter. Structural renal malformations are seen in 40% of patients, necessitating renal ultrasonography at diagnosis. In addition, a subset of Turner syndrome patients is mosaic for a population of cells with a Y chromosome, which confers an increased risk of gonadoblastoma.

Approximately 10% of Turner syndrome patients have substantial developmental delays requiring assistance in adult life. Seventy percent of patients have learning disabilities affecting visuospatial and nonverbal perceptual thinking that may predispose to attention-deficit/hyperactivity disorder, which has an increased frequency in Turner syndrome patients. It has been suggested that life expectancy is shorter in patients with Turner syndrome (mean, 30 years; range, birth to 80 years), largely as a result of cardiac disease or diabetes.[17,18]

CONTIGUOUS GENE SYNDROMES CAUSED BY CHROMOSOMAL DELETIONS

Deletion or duplication of a segment or segments of a chromosome frequently leads to recognizable patterns of malformation. Loss of chromosomal fragments has been associated with a number of classic syndromes, presumably due to an inappropriate dosage of crucial genes in the affected genomic segment (Table 130-4).

Cri du Chat Syndrome (5p–)

Partial monosomy of chromosome 5p is seen in approximately 1 in 37,000 live births.[19] It may occur in as many as 1 in 350 children with learning disabilities.[20] The hallmark clinical feature is a high-pitched, monotonous cry that sounds like that of a cat. Other features include low birth weight, microcephaly, hypotonia, dysmorphic facies, and

heart defects. These infants tend to be unsettled and exhibit failure to thrive and pronounced developmental delays. Survival into adulthood is possible, but often with severe mental retardation. Intensive therapy appears to provide some benefit,[21] and sensitive measures of cognition demonstrate that patients' language receptive skills are better than their expressive ability.[22]

Nearly 100 genes are lost when the putative critical region from 5p15.2 to 15.3 is deleted.[23] Approximately 85% of 5p deletions arise de novo in the affected child, so the recurrence risk is minimal (<1%). Approximately 80% of these de novo deletions are paternal in origin.[24] The remaining deletions arise from malsegregation of a balanced translocation in a carrier parent, which is associated with a 10% to 15% risk of an unbalanced karyotype in a future live-born child. Parental karyotype analysis is indicated for proper counseling regarding risk of recurrence.

Wolf–Hirschhorn Syndrome (4p–)

Distal deletions of the short arm of chromosome 4 cause Wolf-Hirschhorn syndrome (WHS), which is estimated to occur in 1 in 50,000 births. Infants with WHS demonstrate characteristic craniofacial features described as a "Greek warrior helmet" appearance, with the bridge of the nose continuing to the forehead. They also have microcephaly, hypertelorism with epicanthal folds, high forehead, prominent glabella, and high arched eyebrows. Prominent low-set ears with pits or tags are also seen. Marked intrauterine growth restriction, followed by failure to thrive with hypotonia and muscle underdevelopment, is observed. Developmental delay and mental retardation of varying degrees are seen in all patients, and seizures occur in 50% to 100%. Other findings include skeletal anomalies (60% to 70%), cleft lip and palate, hearing loss (40%), cardiac septal defects (30% to 50%), structural brain anomalies (33%), and urinary tract malformations (25%).[25] Approximately 20% of WHS infants die in the first 2 years of life. Many patients, however, can live into adulthood, with a mean survival of 34 years in patients with de novo deletions[26]; these patients typically have profound growth and mental retardation.

Conventional karyotype analysis detects a deletion on 4p16.3 in 60% to 70% of patients with WHS. FISH using a probe for the WHS critical region detects 95% of patients. More than 75% of 4p16 deletions arise de novo, with a minimal risk of recurrence. About 12% of patients have an unusual cytogenetic abnormality (such as ring 4), and about 13% of 4p16 deletions result from inheriting an unbalanced parental translocation. Parental karyotypes are necessary to provide appropriate counseling regarding the risk of recurrence.

WAGR Syndrome (11q13–)

The term WAGR refers to Wilms tumor, aniridia, genital anomalies, and mental retardation, a constellation of symptoms seen in patients with a contiguous gene deletion syndrome involving chromosome 11p12-p14, which includes the *WT1* and *PAX6* genes. Mutations or deletions of *WT1* have been implicated in the pathogenesis of Wilms tumor, and the risk of Wilms tumor in WAGR patients approaches 50%. The *WT1* gene has also been implicated in renal and genitourinary abnormalities, including uterine abnormali-

Table 130-4	Contiguous Gene Syndromes			
Syndrome	Locus	Mechanism	Features	Incidence
Monosomy 1p	1p36	Deletion	Developmental delay, seizures, hypotonia, orofacial clefting, dysmorphia, deafness, cardiomyopathy	1 in 5000
Wolf-Hirschhorn	4p16	Deletion	Pre- and postnatal growth retardation, "Greek warrior helmet" facies, developmental delay, skeletal anomalies, cardiac septal defects, hearing loss, urinary tract abnormalities	1 in 50,000
Cri du chat	5p15	Deletion	Catlike cry, SGA, microcephaly, hypotonia, cardiac defects, mental retardation	1 in 50,000
Russell-Silver	7p12	Maternal uniparental disomy (some cases)	Pre- and postnatal growth retardation with sparing of head; triangular facies; limb and facial asymmetry	1 in 100,000
Williams-Beuren	7q11.2	Deletion associated with segmental duplication	"Jowly" facies, cardiac disease (supravalvular aortic stenosis), growth and developmental delay, "cocktail party" personality, infantile hypocalcemia	1 in 25,000
Trichorhinophalangeal, type I	8q24	Deletion	Sparse, thin hair; pear-shaped nose; short metacarpals; small, delayed teeth; infantile hypotonia	Unknown
Langer-Giedion	8q24.1	Deletion	Multiple exostoses; sparse, thin hair; pear-shaped nose; short metacarpals; small, delayed teeth; infantile hypotonia	Unknown
Potocki-Shaffer	11p11.2	Deletion	Multiple exostoses, skull defects, brachycephaly, developmental delay, genital anomalies	Unknown
WAGR	11p13	Deletion	Wilms tumor, aniridia, genitourinary and renal anomalies, mental retardation	Unknown
Beckwith-Wiedemann	11p15.5	Paternal uniparental disomy, imprinting defect	Macrosomia, hemihypertrophy, abdominal wall defects, macroglossia, risk for Wilms tumor and hepatoblastoma	1 in 14,000
Prader-Willi	15q11-13	Paternal deletion, imprinting defect	Newborn hypotonia, hyporeflexia, cryptorchidism, failure to thrive that converts to hyperphagia, behavioral problems, mental retardation	1 in 15,000
Angelman	15q11-13	Maternal deletion, imprinting defect, *UBE3A* mutation	Developmental delay, seizures, exaggerated laughter, repetitive hand movements	1 in 15,000
Smith-Magenis	17p11.2	Deletion associated with segmental duplication	Brachycephaly, flat midface, hoarse voice, brachydactyly, mental retardation, sleep disturbance, hyperactivity, self-destructive behavior	1 in 25,000
Duplication 17p11.2	17p11.2	Duplication associated with segmental duplication	Short stature, mild mental retardation, behavioral difficulties, dental crowding	Unknown
Hereditary neuropathy with pressure palsies	17p12	Deletion associated with segmental duplication	Peripheral weakness and neuropathy from pressure on nerves	Unknown
Charcot-Marie-Tooth type 1A	17p12	Duplication associated with segmental duplication	Distal limb muscle weakness, decreased motor nerve conduction velocities	Unknown

Continued

Table 130-4 Contiguous Gene Syndromes—cont'd

Syndrome	Locus	Mechanism	Features	Incidence
Miller-Dieker	17p13.3	Deletion associated with segmental duplication	Lissencephaly; prominent forehead; bitemporal narrowing; short, upturned nose; protuberant upper lip; small jaw; profound mental retardation	Unknown
Alagille	20p11.23	Deletion, *JAG1* mutation	Chronic cholestasis, triangular facies, peripheral pulmonic stenosis, vertebral anomalies, posterior embryotoxon of eye	1 in 70,000
DiGeorge-velocardiofacial	22q11.2	Deletion associated with segmental duplication	Cardiac conotruncal anomaly, parathyroid hypoplasia, hooded eyelids, bulbous nasal tip, developmental delay	1 in 4000
Cat-eye	22q11.2	Supernumerary marker chromosome	Iris coloboma, anal atresia, down-slanted eyes, ear tags or pits, cardiac or renal malformations	Unknown
Duchenne muscular dystrophy	Xp21	Deletion	Muscular dystrophy	1 in 5000 males
Complex glycerol kinase deficiency	Xp21	Deletion	Glyceroluria, adrenal hypoplasia, ambiguous male genitalia, muscular dystrophy	Unknown
Adrenal hypoplasia congenita	Xp21	Deletion	Adrenal hypoplasia, ambiguous genitalia	Unknown
Dosage-sensitive sex reversal	Xp21	Duplication associated with segmental duplication	Sex reversal and abnormal gonadal development in XY males	Unknown
X-linked ichthyosis	Xp22.3	Deletion associated with segmental duplication	Dark, scaly skin; steryl-sulfatase deficiency	1 in 5000 males
Kallmann	Xp22.3	Deletion	Hypogonadotropic hypogonadism, anosmia	Unknown
Hemophilia A (severe)	Xq28	Inversion associated with segmental duplication	Bleeding diathesis, factor VIII deficiency	1 in 8000 males
Pelizaeus-Merzbacher	Xq22	Duplication, *PLP1* mutation	Progressive neurodegeneration, microcephaly, hypotonia, rotary nystagmus, optic atrophy, head rolling	Unknown

SGA, small for gestational age.
Adapted from Shaffer LG, Ledbetter DH, Lupski JR: Molecular cytogenetics of contiguous gene syndromes: Mechanisms and consequences of gene dosage imbalance. In Scriver CR, Sly WS, Childs B, et al (eds): The Metabolic and Molecular Bases of Inherited Disease. New York, McGraw-Hill, 2001, pp 1291-1324; and Emanuel BS, Shaikh TH: Segmental duplications: An "expanding" role in genomic instability and disease. Nat Rev Genet 2001;2:791-800.

ties, hypospadias, cryptorchidism, ambiguous genitalia, urethral strictures, fused kidneys, ureteric abnormalities, and gonadoblastoma. Patients with WAGR have a 20% to 25% risk of eventual renal failure.[27]

Aniridia is characterized by bilateral aplasia or dysplasia of the iris and optic nerve hypoplasia, leading to visual impairment. Cataracts, glaucoma, and corneal opacification and vascularization can also be seen. These findings are caused by deletion of the *PAX6* gene. The cause of the mild mental retardation seen in WAGR patients is unclear but is likely due to the role of *PAX6* in the developing forebrain.

Many of the deletions in this region are cytogenetically visible, but FISH probes encompassing the *WT1* and *PAX6* locus can be used to distinguish partial phenotypes. Most mutations are de novo and transmitted in an autosomal dominant manner.[23] However, some parents may not exhibit overt ocular phenotypes and should have a detailed ophthalmic examination, as well as cytogenetic analysis to determine the risk of recurrence.

Ongoing care of these patients includes frequent ophthalmic assessment; renal ultrasonography every 3 months until age 8 years; urologic, nephrologic, and endocrine management for gonadal abnormalities; and early cognitive assessment and intervention if developmental delay is noted.

Chromosome 1p Deletion Syndrome (1p36−)

Since the advent of subtelomeric FISH, several new syndromes have been recognized. One of the more common is monosomy for the distal short arm of chromosome 1 (deletion of 1p36). It is estimated to occur in approximately 1 in

5000 births and has been associated with a constellation of clinical findings.[28] The characteristic features include frontal bossing, large anterior fontanelle, deep-set eyes, flattened midface, flat nose, pointed chin, short fifth finger, developmental delay, hypotonia, oropharyngeal dysphagia, and hearing loss. Less frequent features include orofacial clefting (17%), thickened asymmetrical ears (50%), hypermetropia (67%), seizures (48%), hypothyroidism (20%), dilated cardiomyopathy (23%), and dilated aortic root (10%).[29]

Most of these patients (73%) have an isolated terminal deletion in which the subtelomeric sequence of 1p is absent. A number of patients have therefore been diagnosed when subtelomeric FISH screens were performed as part of a general cytogenetic workup. However, 10% of patients have an interstitial deletion that does not extend to the telomere and therefore cannot be detected by the FISH probe. The vast majority of deletions arise de novo, with about 5% attributable to malsegregation of a balanced parental translocation. The size of the deletion varies from 1.5 to greater than 10.5 Mb, and there appears to be a correlation between the size of the deletion and the severity of clinical features.[30] Diagnosis has been made with karyotype analysis, but 50% of patients do not have a cytogenetically visible deletion. FISH studies targeted to this region in patients with suggestive clinical features have uncovered most of the other cases.

Ongoing care of these patients includes yearly hearing screening, monitoring for seizure activity, and thyroid function assessment at birth, 6 months, and then annually. Owing to the presence of oropharyngeal dysfunction, swallow studies should be considered. Ophthalmic examinations and echocardiograms are recommended.

CONTIGUOUS GENE SYNDROMES ASSOCIATED WITH SEGMENTAL DUPLICATIONS

A special category of contiguous gene syndromes includes those caused by chromosomal rearrangements in regions of the genome that contain large blocks of repeated DNA sequences (segmental duplications) flanking a central nonrepeated region. Because of the duplications, such regions are at high risk of misalignment during recombination; this can result in either deletion or duplication of the central region, which usually contains many genes (see Fig. 130-2A). These syndromes are important because they are relatively common and have phenotypes that should be recognized by clinicians. The chromosomal abnormality may be impossible to detect by standard karyotyping, requiring specialized FISH or other testing to confirm the diagnosis.

Williams-Beuren Syndrome (7q11–)

Williams-Beuren syndrome, although variable in spectrum, is characterized by distinct facies, cardiovascular disease, growth and developmental retardation, a "cocktail party" personality, and, occasionally, infantile hypercalcemia. The estimated incidence of Williams-Beuren syndrome is 1 in 20,000 to 50,000 live births.

Neonates with this syndrome demonstrate intrauterine growth restriction and mild microcephaly. Facial features include epicanthal folds with periorbital fullness of subcutaneous tissues, flat midface, anteverted nostrils, long philtrum, full lips, wide mouth, small jaw, and prominent earlobes. Children have full cheeks; small, widely spaced teeth; and stellate irises that may not be observed at birth. Adults typically have gaunt appearance caused by a long face and neck.

Most infants have a cardiovascular anomaly; supravalvular aortic stenosis is the most common, seen in 75% of cases. Any artery may be narrowed, and pulmonary artery stenosis is also encountered. Hypertension may develop from renal artery stenosis. Mesenteric artery stenosis may cause abdominal pain.

Connective tissue abnormalities are caused by deletion of the elastin gene on chromosome 7q11. This causes a hoarse voice, inguinal or umbilical hernia, bowel or bladder diverticula, rectal prolapse, joint limitation or laxity, and soft "doughy" skin.

Severe hypercalcemia occurs in 15% of patients with Williams-Beuren syndrome and may persist through infancy. Other endocrine findings include hypercalciuria (30%), hypothyroidism (10%), and early but not precocious puberty (50%). Infants are usually small for gestational age, and poor linear growth in childhood is sometimes exacerbated by feeding difficulty, pronounced irritability, and "colicky" behavior.

Mild to moderate mental retardation occurs in most patients but can be masked by strengths in language and auditory rote memory; gross motor and visual-motor integration skills are extremely weak. The characteristic personality of a patient with Williams-Beuren syndrome includes overfriendliness, excessive empathy, attention problems, and anxiety. Hyperacusis and fondness for music have also been reported. Attention-deficit disorders, perseveration, and sleep difficulties are common.[31]

Many of the classic features of Williams-Beuren syndrome are not evident in the newborn period, but the diagnosis should be suspected in any child with supravalvular aortic stenosis, hypercalcemia, or facial features consistent with the disorder. The diagnosis is confirmed by FISH, with a probe specific for the deleted region on chromosome 7q11. Because the condition is typically sporadic and most deletions arise de novo, the risk of recurrence in subsequent pregnancies is minimal. An affected adult, however, would pass on the condition in an autosomal dominant manner, with a 50% risk of the disorder in his or her child.

22q11 Deletion Syndrome

DiGeorge syndrome, velocardiofacial syndrome, Shprintzen syndrome, conotruncal anomaly face syndrome, Caylor cardiofacial syndrome, and autosomal dominant Opitz syndrome are members of a clinical spectrum of disorders caused by deletion of chromosome 22q11.2.[32] Estimates indicate that the 22q11 deletion, occurring in approximately 1 in 3000 live births,[33] is the most common microdeletion syndrome in humans. Patients have a variety of anomalies.

Common components of this phenotype include a conotruncal cardiac anomaly (74%), palatal anomalies (70%), and aplasia or hypoplasia of the thymus and parathyroid glands. Most patients diagnosed with a 22q11.2 deletion present as newborns or infants owing to cardiovascular malformations, including tetralogy of Fallot (25%), ventricular septal defect (12%), interrupted aortic arch type B, or truncus arteriosus, along with T-cell abnormalities or hypocalcemia. Facial dysmorphisms may include hooded eyelids, hypertelorism, overfolded ears, bulbous nasal tip, small mouth, and micrognathia.[34] Since the initial report by Lischner and DiGeorge in 1969,[35] the spectrum of associated clinical features has been expanded to include anomalies such as vascular rings, cleft palate, renal agenesis, neural tube defects, and hypospadias.[36] Before the advent of effective medical and surgical management for children with complex congenital heart disease and immune deficiency, this disorder had significant morbidity and mortality.

Developmental delays and learning disabilities occur in 70% to 90% of patients with the 22q11.2 deletion, and a wide range of developmental and behavioral findings have been observed in young children.[37] Preschool-age children are commonly hypotonic and developmentally delayed, with pronounced language and speech difficulties. Severe retardation is uncommon, however, and a few patients function within the average range.

The majority of patients (80% to 90%) have the same large deletion, approximately 3 million base pairs (3 Mb) detected by FISH (see Fig. 130-2B). The deletion remains unchanged within a family; however, the phenotype can be widely variable. Smaller deletions half the size of the common deletion also occur (1.5 Mb) but do not cause milder symptoms. Most 22q11 deletions occur de novo, with less than 10% inherited from an affected parent. The prevalence of these de novo deletions indicates an extremely high deletion rate within this genomic region, which is probably related to the presence of segmental duplications in 22q11.[38]

Prader–Willi Syndrome

Prader-Willi syndrome results from the loss of activity of paternally inherited genes on the long arm of chromosome 15 (15q11). This can occur through deletion or disruption of this region on the paternally inherited chromosome or through the presence of two maternal and no paternal chromosomes (maternal uniparental disomy).[39] This region of chromosome 15 uses genomic imprinting to regulate the level of gene expression based on the parental origin of each chromosome. That is, for some genes, the maternally inherited allele is inactivated (maternally imprinted), and for others, the paternal copy is inactivated (paternally imprinted). Chromosome 15q11 contains both maternally and paternally imprinted genes, so the phenotype resulting from 15q11 deletion depends on which chromosome contains the deletion. Children lacking paternal expression of this region have Prader-Willi syndrome, and those lacking maternal expression have Angelman syndrome.

Newborns with Prader-Willi syndrome have pronounced central hypotonia, weak cry, and hyporeflexia. Consistent with the hypotonia, breech presentation and perinatal insults are more frequent than usual. Poor tone usually manifests as sucking and swallowing difficulties that lead to failure to thrive and the need for gavage feeding during infancy. Facial findings include bifrontal narrowing, almond-shaped eyes, and a small, downturned mouth. Genitalia are often hypoplastic, and cryptorchidism is common in boys. Small hands and feet are usually demonstrated in childhood. Strabismus and hypopigmentation are also common.[40]

The extreme hypotonia improves in the first year of life, as does motor development; nevertheless, developmental delay is the rule, especially with regard to gross motor skills and speech. Feeding difficulties often give way to uncontrollable hyperphagia and obesity beginning in the second year. This and other behavioral problems, including severe temper tantrums, are lifelong. Most patients have mild to moderate mental retardation. Early diagnosis and preemptive implementation of behavioral therapy are essential components of optimal management.

Deletions of the chromosome 15q11 region detectable by FISH have been demonstrated in up to 70% of patients with Prader-Willi syndrome. A small number of patients have a translocation interrupting this region. No single gene in this region has been implicated as the cause of Prader-Willi syndrome. Patients with deletions are more likely to be hypopigmented because this region contains a gene involved in pigmentation, the *p* gene.[41] Risk of recurrence is negligible in cases in which de novo deletions are found.

Approximately 20% to 25% of patients with Prader-Willi syndrome show maternal uniparental disomy, which can be detected by assaying methylation differences between maternal and paternal alleles. A maternal age effect has been demonstrated in cases of uniparental disomy, and recurrence risks in families without deletions are estimated at 1 in 1000.

Angelman Syndrome

Loss of the maternal copy of chromosome 15q11 is associated with Angelman syndrome. After a normal prenatal and perinatal course, patients present with delayed milestones and acquired microcephaly. Facial features may include a protruding jaw, wide mouth, thin upper lip, and widely spaced teeth. Seizures typically begin between 1 and 3 years of age. Ninety percent of children with Angelman syndrome walk, but this is often significantly delayed, with a jerky, ataxic gait. Behavioral features include tongue thrusting, drooling, exaggerated bursts of laughter, sleep disturbance, hyperactivity, proclivity for water, and social-seeking personalities. The mental retardation is most notable for the severe language impairment. The life span of patients with Angelman syndrome is believed to be nearly normal.[42]

Seventy percent to 75% of patients with Angelman syndrome have a deletion of 15q11 detectable by FISH analysis. These patients have more severe disease that correlates with the size of the deletion. Genomic imprinting also regulates Angelman syndrome, and a small percentage of patients (3% to 5%) have evidence of paternal isodisomy of all of chromosome 15, with no apparent maternal chromosome. Further, mutations of an imprinting center locus on chromosome 15 are associated with 1% to 2% of Angelman phenotypes. Angelman syndrome has also been associated with mutations in a single gene, *UBE3A*, in 10% of patients.[43] The vast majority of cases result from a sporadic event, but risk of recurrence is best predicted once a genetic mechanism has been determined.

Beckwith–Wiedemann Syndrome

Beckwith-Wiedemann syndrome (BWS) is another disorder of genomic imprinting that affects about 1 in 14,000 newborns. It typically manifests as an overgrowth syndrome. Characteristic findings are macrosomia, macroglossia, visceromegaly, omphalocele, embryonal tumors, transient neonatal hypoglycemia, and ear creases or pits. BWS babies are large for gestational age, with proportionate weight and length. Advanced bone age, hemihypertrophy due to asymmetrical growth, and visceromegaly of various organs, including the spleen, kidneys, liver, pancreas, and adrenal glands, are often seen. There is an approximately 20% mortality rate in infants with BWS due to complications of omphalocele, macroglossia, neonatal hypoglycemia, and, rarely, cardiomyopathy.[44]

Embryonal tumors seen with BWS include Wilms tumor, hepatoblastoma, neuroblastoma, and rhabdomyosarcoma. The estimated risk of tumor development is 7.5%, and it is higher in patients with hemihypertrophy.[45] The establishment of routine ultrasonographic surveillance at regular intervals is important. Many centers currently perform ultrasonography at 3-month intervals until 8 years of age and annually through adolescence. Measuring serum α-fetoprotein levels at the same intervals to screen for hepatoblastoma has also proved valuable.

Most cases of BWS arise de novo, but up to 15% are familial. In these cases, autosomal dominant transmission with variable penetrance seems to be the mode of inheritance. Additionally, this genomic region (11p15) is significantly regulated by imprinting, with paternal uniparental disomy proving to be the mechanism in up to 20% of sporadic cases. Methylation studies detect approximately 60% of cases. Mutations of the gene *CDKN1C* are detected in 40% of familial cases and 5% of isolated cases. Chromosomal abnormalities are rare.[46] Counseling is most accurate if a precise genetic mechanism can be established.

IN A NUTSHELL

- Chromosomal disorders present with a wide array of clinical phenotypes, some of which are relatively common and are recognized as well-defined syndromes. These disorders pose significant diagnostic challenges and require long-term management and genetic counseling with regard to recurrence risk.
- Children with unexplained mental retardation, multiple congenital malformations, or abnormal sexual development warrant karyotype and subtelomeric FISH analysis. Specific tests for particular disorders may also be available if a phenotype is recognized.

ON THE HORIZON

- Tremendous advances in genomics, led by the Human Genome Project, are facilitating the development of better tools for diagnosing, understanding, and caring for patients and families with genetic disorders. One of the emerging technologies is whole genome array analysis, which enables the detection of deletions and duplications essentially anywhere in the genome that are not visible by karyotype analysis or standard FISH techniques.
- Computational genomics and high-throughput genotyping systems are enabling researchers to begin to dissect the subtleties of common complex genetic disorders such as diabetes, hypertension, and asthma.

SUGGESTED READING

American Academy of Pediatrics: Health supervision for children with Down syndrome. Pediatrics 2001;107:442-449.

Cassidy SB, Dykens E, Williams CA: Prader-Willi and Angelman syndromes: Sister imprinted disorders. Am J Med Genet 2000;97:136-146.

Emanuel BS, McDonald-McGinn D, Saitta SC, Zackai EH: The 22q11.2 deletion syndrome. Adv Pediatr 2001;48:39-73.

GeneTests: Medical Genetics Information Resource (online database). Seattle, University of Washington, 1993-2005. *www.genetests.org.*

Jones KL: Smith's Recognizable Patterns of Human Malformation, 5th ed. Philadelphia, WB Saunders, 1997.

McDonald-McGinn D, Emanuel BS, Zackai EH: 22q11.2 deletion syndrome. Gene Reviews 2003, *www.genetests.org.*

Online Mendelian Inheritance in Man (OMIM). Baltimore, McKusick-Nathans Institute for Genetic Medicine, Johns Hopkins University, and National Center for Biotechnology Information, National Library of Medicine, 2000.

Shuman C, Weksberg R: Beckwith-Wiedemann syndrome. Gene Reviews 2003, *www.genetests.org.*

Sybert VP, McCauley E: Turner's syndrome. N Engl J Med 2004;351:1227-1238.

Zackai EH, Anyane-Yeboa K, Bergoffen J, et al: Genetics. In Polin RA, Ditmar MF (eds): Pediatric Secrets. Philadelphia, Hanley & Belfus, 2001, p 731.

REFERENCES

1. Lander ES, Linton LM, Birren B, et al: Initial sequencing and analysis of the human genome. Nature 2001;409:860-921.
2. Scriver CR, Neal JL, Saginur R, Clow A: The frequency of genetic disease and congenital malformation among patients in a pediatric hospital. Can Med Assoc J 1973;108:1111-1115.
3. Baird PA, Anderson TW, Newcombe HB, Lowry RB: Genetic disorders in children and young adults: A population study. Am J Hum Genet 1988; 42:677-693.
4. McCandless SE, Brunger JW, Cassidy SB: The burden of genetic disease on inpatient care in a children's hospital. Am J Hum Genet 2004;74:121-127.
5. Jones KL: Smith's Recognizable Patterns of Human Malformation, 5th ed. Philadelphia, WB Saunders, 1997, p 861.
6. Online Mendelian Inheritance in Man (OMIM). Baltimore, McKusick-Nathans Institute for Genetic Medicine, Johns Hopkins University, and National Center for Biotechnology Information, National Library of Medicine, 2000.
7. GeneTests: Medical Genetics Information Resource (online database). Seattle, University of Washington, 1993-2005. *www.genetests.org.*
8. Hall JG, Froster-Iskenius UG, Allanson JE: Handbook of Normal Physical Measurements. Oxford, Oxford University Press, 1989.
9. Mitelman F (ed): ISCN: An International System for Human Cytogenetic Nomenclature. Basel, S Karger, 1995.
10. Beaudet AL, Scriver CR, Sly WS, Valle D, et al: Genetics, biochemistry, and molecular bases of variant human phenotypes. In Scriver CR, Sly WS, Childs B, et al (eds): The Metabolic and Molecular Bases of Inherited Disease. New York, McGraw-Hill, 2001, pp 3-48.
11. Hook EB: Ultrasound and fetal chromosome abnormalities. Lancet 1992;340:1109.
12. Epstein CJ: Down syndrome (trisomy 21). In Scriver CR, Sly WS, Childs B, et al (eds): The Metabolic and Molecular Bases of Inherited Disease. New York, McGraw-Hill, 2001, pp 1223-1256.
13. American Academy of Pediatrics: Health supervision for children with Down syndrome. Pediatrics 2001;107:442-449.
14. Zackai EH, Anyane-Yeboa K, Bergoffen J, et al: Genetics. In Polin RA, Ditmar MF (eds): Pediatric Secrets. Philadelphia, Hanley & Belfus, 2001, p 731.
15. Randolph LM: Prenatal cytogenetics. In Gersen SL, Keagle MB (eds): The Principles of Clinical Cytogenetics. Totowa, NJ, Humana Press, 1999, pp 259-315.

16. Willard HF: The sex chromosomes and X chromosome inactivation. In Scriver CR, Sly WS, Childs B, et al (eds): The Metabolic and Molecular Basis of Inherited Diseases. New York, McGraw-Hill, 2001, pp 1191-1211.

17. Sybert VP, McCauley E: Turner's syndrome. N Engl J Med 2004;351:1227-1238.

18. Gravholt CH, Juul S, Naeraa RW, Hansen J: Morbidity in Turner syndrome. J Clin Epidemiol 1998;51:147-158.

19. Higurashi M, Oda M, Iijima S, et al: Livebirth prevalence and follow-up of malformation syndromes in 27,472 newborns. Brain Dev 1990;12:770-773.

20. Niebuhr E: Cytologic observations in 35 individuals with a 5p– karyotype. Hum Genet 1978;42:143-156.

21. Wilkins LE, Brown JA, Wolf B: Psychomotor development in 65 home-reared children with cri-du-chat syndrome. J Pediatr 1980;97:401-405.

22. Cornish KM, Bramble D, Munir F, Pigram J: Cognitive functioning in children with typical cri du chat (5p–) syndrome. Dev Med Child Neurol 1999;41:263-266.

23. Shaffer LG, Ledbetter DH, Lupski JR: Molecular cytogenetics of contiguous gene syndromes: Mechanisms and consequences of gene dosage imbalance. In Scriver CR, et al (eds): The Metabolic and Molecular Bases of Inherited Disease. New York, McGraw-Hill, 2001, pp 1291-1324.

24. Overhauser J, McMahon J, Oberlender S, et al: Parental origin of chromosome 5 deletions in the cri-du-chat syndrome. Am J Med Genet 1990;37:83-86.

25. Battaglia A, Carey JC, Wright TJ: Wolf-Hirschhorn syndrome. Gene Reviews 2004. *www.genetests.org.*

26. Shannon NL, Maltby EL, Rigby AS, Quarrell OW: An epidemiological study of Wolf-Hirschhorn syndrome: Life expectancy and cause of mortality. J Med Genet 2001;38:674-679.

27. Breslow NE, Takashima JR, Ritchey ML, et al: Renal failure in the Denys-Drash and Wilms' tumor-aniridia syndromes. Cancer Res 2000;60:4030-4032.

28. Shaffer LG, Lupski JR: Molecular mechanisms for constitutional chromosomal rearrangements in humans. Annu Rev Genet 2000;34:297-329.

29. Heilstedt HA, Ballif BC, Howard LA, et al: Population data suggest that deletions of 1p36 are a relatively common chromosome abnormality. Clin Genet 2003;64:310-316.

30. Wu YQ, Heilstedt HA, Bedell JA, et al: Molecular refinement of the 1p36 deletion syndrome reveals size diversity and a preponderance of maternally derived deletions. Hum Mol Genet 1999;8:313-321.

31. Cassidy SB, Morris CA: Behavioral phenotypes in genetic syndromes: Genetic clues to human behavior. Adv Pediatr 2002;49:59-86.

32. McDonald-McGinn DM, Tonnesen MK, Laufer-Cahana A, et al: Phenotype of the 22q11.2 deletion in individuals identified through an affected relative: Cast a wide FISHing net! Genet Med 2001;3:23-29.

33. Burn J, Goodship J: Developmental genetics of the heart. Curr Opin Genet Dev 1996;6:322-325.

34. McDonald-McGinn D, Emanuel BS, Zackai EH: 22q11.2 Deletion syndrome. Gene Reviews 2003. *www.genetests.org.*

35. Lischner HW, DiGeorge AM: Role of the thymus in humoral immunity. Lancet 1969;2:1044-1049.

36. McDonald-McGinn DM, LaRossa D, Goldmuntz E, et al: The 22q11.2 deletion: Screening, diagnostic workup, and outcome of results; report on 181 patients. Genet Test 1997;1:99-108.

37. Emanuel BS, McDonald-McGinn D, Saitta SC, Zackai EH: The 22q11.2 deletion syndrome. Adv Pediatr 2001;48:39-73.

38. Emanuel BS, Shaikh TH: Segmental duplications: An "expanding" role in genomic instability and disease. Nat Rev Genet 2001;2:791-800.

39. Nicholls RD, Knoll JH, Butler MG, et al: Genetic imprinting suggested by maternal heterodisomy in nondeletion Prader-Willi syndrome. Nature 1989;342:281-285.

40. Cassidy SB, Dykens E, Williams CA: Prader-Willi and Angelman syndromes: Sister imprinted disorders. Am J Med Genet 2000;97:136-146.

41. Rinchik EM, Bultman SJ, Horsthemke B, et al: A gene for the mouse pink-eyed dilution locus and for human type II oculocutaneous albinism. Nature 1993;361:72-76.

42. Williams CA, Angelman H, Clayton-Smith J, et al: Angelman syndrome: Consensus for diagnostic criteria. Angelman Syndrome Foundation. Am J Med Genet 1995;56:237-238.

43. Lossie AC, Whitney MM, Amidon D, et al: Distinct phenotypes distinguish the molecular classes of Angelman syndrome. J Med Genet 2001;38:834-845.

44. Pettenati MJ, Haines JL, Higgins RR, et al: Wiedemann-Beckwith syndrome: Presentation of clinical and cytogenetic data on 22 new cases and review of the literature. Hum Genet 1986;74:143-154.

45. Wiedemann HR: Frequency of Wiedemann-Beckwith syndrome in Germany; rate of hemihyperplasia and of tumours in affected children. Eur J Pediatr 1997;156:251.

46. Shuman C, Weksberg R: Beckwith-Wiedemann syndrome. Gene Reviews 2003. *www.genetests.org.*

CHAPTER 131

Hyperammonemia

Karen Smith

Ammonia, the nitrogen-containing waste product of protein metabolism, is extremely toxic at high concentrations. Under normal circumstances, blood ammonia is cleared rapidly by the urea cycle, a biochemical pathway of hepatocytes that converts ammonia into water-soluble urea, which is then excreted in urine (Fig. 131-1). This system keeps ammonia levels under 100 μM/L in neonates and generally 20 to 60 μM/L in infants and older children. Elevated blood ammonia levels (hyperammonemia) trigger a variety of neurotoxic consequences that result in aberrant neurotransmitter levels and cerebral edema, causing severe and potentially irreversible injury to the central nervous system.[1]

Hyperammonemia occurs during periods of "nitrogen imbalance," when nitrogen load exceeds the capacity for clearance. Nitrogen load is proportional to circulating amino acid levels, which are the result of both dietary protein intake and breakdown of endogenous protein (e.g., from muscle). Nitrogen clearance depends primarily on the ability of the liver to perform the urea cycle. Therefore, diseases that drastically increase nitrogen load or compromise liver function can result in hyperammonemia, and restoring nitrogen balance is the main goal in treating hyperammonemia. The urea cycle defects (UCDs) are an important category of diseases that present with severe hyperammonemia and are the main focus of this chapter.

CLINICAL PRESENTATION

Symptoms associated with hyperammonemia reflect primarily ammonia's neurotoxicity; therefore, hyperammonemia should be considered in patients with unexplained changes in mental status, encephalopathy, or signs of increased intracranial pressure (Table 131-1). In neonates, symptoms of hyperammonemia may be impossible to distinguish from those of sepsis; they include decreased activity, poor feeding, encephalopathy, and seizure. An important distinguishing characteristic is that neonates with hyperammonemia may have a respiratory alkalosis (average pH 7.5, with a P_{CO_2} of 24) because ammonia stimulates hyperventilation.[2] Further, these children usually fail to improve after fluid resuscitation and antimicrobial therapy; instead, neurologic symptoms may progress, culminating in coma. In such cases, a UCD should be strongly suspected. In older children, hyperammonemia may be even harder to identify because symptoms are either nonspecific (cyclic vomiting, headache, poor appetite) or easily confused with more common problems such as drug abuse or primary psychiatric disease (acute mental status changes, frank psychosis).

The presentation of hyperammonemia in neonates with UCDs is typically that of an unremarkable term-gestation newborn who is well for the first few days of life. However, progressive protein intake leads to nitrogen imbalance and hyperammonemia, usually within the first week of life. A retrospective analysis of 74 infants with ornithine transcarbamoylase (OTC) deficiency, the most common UCD, demonstrated a mean onset of illness at 63 hours of life, with a range of 12 to 240 hours.[2]

Children with most types of UCDs have a lifetime risk of hyperammonemic episodes, which usually occur when a new nitrogen imbalance is introduced. This may be caused by increased dietary protein intake or catabolic stress-induced muscle protein turnover, which occurs during prolonged fasting, fever, or increased exercise. Blood ammonia levels can increase rapidly during these periods, and prompt treatment is critical. Similarly, children with mild forms of UCDs may not suffer an initial hyperammonemic crisis until an illness during infancy or even later in childhood or adolescence, when nitrogen imbalance causes acute mental status changes or other signs of hyperammonemia. In such patients, a thorough history may reveal the cause of the imbalance, such as a sudden increase in dietary protein intake or a dramatic increase in exercise.

DIFFERENTIAL DIAGNOSIS

Although numerous inborn errors of metabolism present in the neonatal period, it is important to remember that many cases of hyperammonemia are due to acquired problems (Table 131-2). Hyperammonemic neonates should be carefully evaluated for treatable problems, especially infection with either bacterial pathogens or herpes simplex virus. In addition, liver function should be evaluated, because hyperammonemia is a complication of liver failure from a variety of causes. Transient hyperammonemia of the newborn (THAN), a phenomenon that generally occurs in premature infants with pulmonary disease, may present similarly to UCDs, causing ammonia levels to rise high enough to induce coma.[3,4] The precise biochemical defect responsible for THAN is not known, and symptoms tend to resolve after initial treatment, often without neurologic sequelae. These children do not have recurrences and tolerate normal amounts of dietary protein.

Metabolic causes of hyperammonemia include diseases that compromise the urea cycle either directly (e.g., UCDs) or indirectly through hepatic toxicity (see Table 131-2). Although a definitive diagnosis of these disorders usually requires metabolic testing, a reasonable differential diagnosis can be established based on the results of common screening tests. For example, the presence of hypoglycemia is more consistent with fatty acid oxidation defects or defects in carbohydrate utilization (e.g., galactosemia, hereditary fructose intolerance) than with a UCD. Although hyperammonemia in UCDs can be associated with respiratory alkalosis, the presence of a metabolic acidosis should raise suspicion for an organic acidemia or a primary lactic acidosis syndrome, such as pyruvate carboxylase deficiency. In

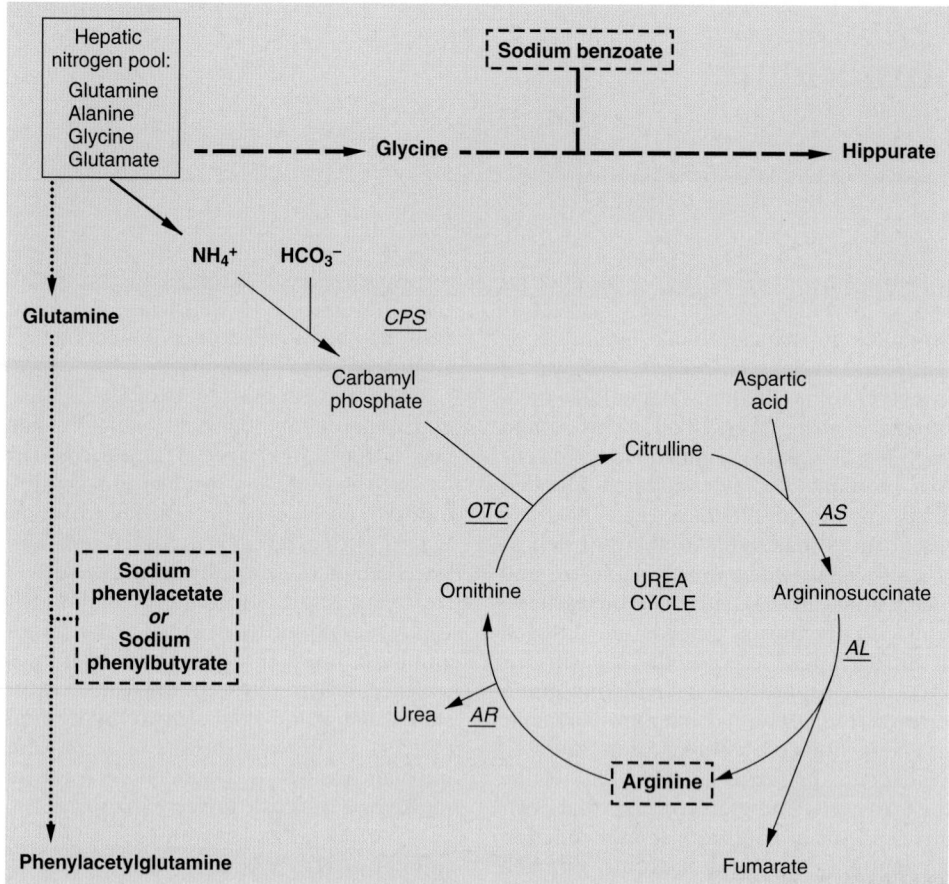

Figure 131-1 The urea cycle. The most common urea cycle defects are underlined and abbreviated as follows: AL, argininosuccinic acid lyase; AR, arginase; AS, argininosuccinic acid synthetase; CPS, carbamoyl phosphate synthetase; OTC, ornithine transcarbamoylase. The scavenger pathway is indicated by dotted lines. Pharmacologic treatments are shown in the dotted boxes.

Table 131-1 Symptoms Associated with Hyperammonemia
Neonates
Decreased activity
Poor feeding
Acid-base disturbance (classically respiratory alkalosis)
Clinical signs of increased intracranial pressure
Emesis
Seizures
May progress to coma if not corrected
Infants and Children
Decreased appetite
Emesis
Headache
Acute or progressive mental status disturbance
Mood lability
Aggression, combativeness
Psychosis
Neurologic deficits
May progress to coma if not corrected

many states, newborn screening programs provide diagnostic information within the first week of life that can rule in or rule out many inborn errors associated with hyperammonemia. In these states, a prompt call to the newborn screening laboratory may allow the physician to establish a tentative diagnosis and proceed with a logical round of confirmatory tests and presumptive treatment.

Collectively, the UCDs have an incidence of roughly 1 in 30,000, with OTC deficiency being the most common disease by far.[3] The UCDs are autosomal recessive disorders, with the exception of OTC deficiency, which is X-linked. As a result, the classic presentation of OTC deficiency in an affected male is overwhelming neonatal hyperammonemia. In females, the severity is determined in large part by the pattern of hepatic X-inactivation; depending on the skew, patients may be essentially asymptomatic or severely affected. In addition, as with most inborn errors of metabolism, phenotype depends on the severity of the mutation and the amount of residual enzyme activity. Therefore, in both boys and girls, a less deleterious mutation can leave a relatively high amount of residual enzyme activity and result in a milder phenotype.

Arginase deficiency differs from other UCDs in that its clinical course is characterized by chronic, progressive neurologic dysfunction rather than catastrophic hyperammonemic crises, although these episodes occasionally occur

Table 131-2 Differential Diagnosis of Hyperammonemia

Acquired Causes
Liver failure (various causes)
Infection
  Sepsis
  Hepatitis
  Infection with urease-positive bacteria
  Herpes simplex virus infection
Iatrogenic
  Valproic acid
  Asparaginase
Severe hypovolemia
Transient hyperammonemia of the newborn
Perinatal depression

Intrinsic Causes (Inborn Errors of Metabolism)
Urea cycle defects
  Ornithine transcarbamoylase deficiency
  Argininosuccinic acid synthetase deficiency (citrullinemia)
  Argininosuccinic acid lyase deficiency
  Carbamoyl phosphate synthetase deficiency
  N-Acetyl glutamate synthetase deficiency
  Arginase deficiency
Organic acidemias
  Methylmalonicacidemia
  Isovalericacidemia
  Propionicacidemia
  Multiple carboxylase deficiency
  Others
Fatty acid oxidation defects
  Medium-chain acyl-CoA dehydrogenase deficiency
  Multiple acyl-CoA dehydrogenase deficiency
  Others
Hyperornithinemia-hyperammonemia-homocitrullinemia
  syndrome
Pyruvate carboxylase deficiency
Hyperammonemia-hyperinsulinemia syndrome
Galactosemia
Hereditary fructose intolerance

Table 131-3 Laboratory Studies for Hyperammonemic Children

Initial laboratory studies
  Electrolytes
  Blood glucose
  Liver enzymes
  Coagulation studies (for liver synthetic function)
  Blood gas (pH, P_{CO_2}, lactate)
  Plasma amino acids
  Urinalysis for ketones and reducing substances
  Urine for organic acids and orotic acid

Studies to consider
  Infectious workup if sepsis is a possibility
  Plasma acylcarnitine profile (for fatty acid oxidation defects)
  Lactate, pyruvate if elevated lactate on blood gas

Table 131-4 Specific Amino Acid Abnormalities in Urea Cycle Defects

Deficiency	Amino Acid Abnormality	Orotic Acid
Ornithine transcarbamoylase	Elevated glutamine Decreased citrulline, arginine	Increased
Argininosuccinic acid synthetase (citrullinemia)	Massively increased citrulline Decreased arginine	Increased
Argininosuccinic acid lyase	Elevated citrulline, argininosuccinic acid Decreased arginine	Increased
Arginase	Elevated arginine, argininosuccinic acid	Increased
Carbamoyl phosphate synthetase	Elevated glutamine Decreased citrulline, arginine	Normal

Modified from Bachman C: Inherited hyperammonemias. In Blau N, Duran M, Blaskovics ME, Gibson KM (eds): Physician's Guide to the Laboratory Diagnosis of Metabolic Diseases, 2nd ed. New York, Springer, 2003.

as well. Symptoms include progressive spastic diplegia or quadriplegia, ataxia, and choreoathetosis.

DIAGNOSIS AND EVALUATION

Table 131-3 outlines the laboratory evaluation that should be considered in hyperammonemic patients. A plasma ammonia level greater than 150 µM with a normal anion gap and normal glucose is particularly concerning for a UCD.[5] Ammonia levels need to be obtained from free-flowing blood, transported immediately to the laboratory on ice, and processed within 15 minutes to ensure accuracy.

In many cases, the initial workup (see Table 131-3) rapidly narrows the differential diagnosis. This is especially true for UCDs, in which the combination of hyperammonemia and amino acid abnormalities is often suggestive of a particular disorder (Table 131-4). Emergent intervention to treat hyperammonemia must begin as soon as an elevated ammonia level is documented (see later); however, the ability to make a strong presumptive diagnosis of a specific UCD

within a few hours allows ongoing treatment to be tailored accordingly.

If the initial workup uncovers metabolic abnormalities in addition to hyperammonemia (e.g., metabolic acidosis with a high anion gap, hypoglycemia), the child could have some other type of inborn error of metabolism. For example, both organic acidemias and fatty acid oxidation defects can present with hyperammonemic crises in neonates and can be diagnosed with additional metabolic tests.

COURSE OF ILLNESS

Infants with neonatal-onset UCDs will most likely suffer some degree of neurologic disability, even if the disease is caught early. Infants not treated early will be severely disabled, and many will not survive the initial presenta-

Table 131–5   Nitrogen Scavenger Therapy for Urea Cycle Defects

Deficiency	Sodium Phenylacetate	Sodium Benzoate	Arginine Hydrochloride*
Children			
Presumed UCD, undiagnosed type	250 mg/kg	250 mg/kg	600 mg/kg
CPS, OTC	250 mg/kg	250 mg/kg	200 mg/kg
AS, AL	250 mg/kg	250 mg/kg	600 mg/kg
Adolescents, adults			
CPS, OTC	5.5 g/m^2	5.5 g/m^2	4.0 g/m^2
AS, AL	5.5 g/m^2	5.5 g/m^2	12 g/m^2

*10% solution.

AL, argininosuccinic acid lyase deficiency; AS, argininosuccinic acid synthetase deficiency; CPS, carbamoyl phosphate synthetase deficiency; OTC, ornithine transcarbamoylase deficiency; UCD, urea cycle defect.

Modified from Summar M: Current strategies for the management of neonatal urea cycle disorders. J Pediatr 2001;138:S30-S34.

tion. Even children with mild disease, such as girls with OTC deficiency, are at risk for neurologic disability, although optimal management is associated with better developmental outcomes.[6]

Intensive parental and patient education on dietary limitations, the early signs of elevated ammonia, and situations likely to result in increased ammonia (e.g., illness with vomiting or poor oral intake) is essential to maximize the child's developmental potential. Parents should be given a written treatment protocol explaining the disease and the appropriate therapy. This document is especially useful when the patient requires treatment in an emergency room or other facility not familiar with UCDs. Health care providers may not be aware that aggressive management is necessary for what may appear to be a minor illness.

TREATMENT

Because of the potential for rapid deterioration and mortality associated with UCDs and other inborn errors of metabolism, a metabolic specialist should be contacted immediately when one of these diseases is suspected. However, management can and should be initiated by the general practitioner. Immediate management of hyperammonemic patients with UCDs should focus on the typical ABCs (airway, breathing, circulation), reversing the nitrogen imbalance by eliminating protein intake and initiating an intravenous dextrose infusion to reverse catabolism (typically twice the maintenance rate with D10), and improving ammonia clearance. The treatment guidelines outlined in this section reflect the recommendations of the 2001 Consensus Conference for the Management of Patients with Urea Cycle Disorders.[5,7]

When patients with hyperammonemia secondary to UCDs present with mental status changes, rapid mobilization of resources and constant monitoring in an intensive care unit are required. Once the patient's respiratory and circulatory status has been stabilized, access should be obtained, and intravenous infusion with a D10-based solution at twice the maintenance rate should be initiated. If nitrogen scavenging agents (see later) are to be used, use D10W or D10/¼NS. No amino acid–containing solutions should be used during this critical period, although intralipids may be useful to boost caloric intake.

Ammonia Clearance

Hemodialysis is the most efficient means of reducing blood ammonia levels in UCD patients. Arrangements for hemodialysis should be made as soon as the patient's condition is recognized. If hemodialysis is not available, hemofiltration or another method of dialysis can be used, but they are less effective. Some authors recommend continuing hemodialysis until the ammonia level falls below 200 μM.[5]

In addition to dialysis, pharmaceuticals that take advantage of scavenger pathways can help reduce blood ammonia. Central intravenous access is recommended for medication administration because of the potential for local tissue necrosis. Recommended doses for scavenging medications are given in Table 131-5. These medications are given as an initial loading dose in D10 over 90 minutes, followed by a continuous infusion of the same dose but given over the next 24 hours. Repeating the loading dose is not recommended, even for patients on hemodialysis, because toxic levels of scavenger drugs can be lethal. Once the serum ammonia level is below 100 μM and stable, intravenous scavenger treatment can be converted to oral supplements by providing sodium butyrate. Depending on the type of UCD, other supplements may also be given, such as citrulline for OTC deficiency and arginine for citrullinemia or argininosuccinic acid lyase deficiency.

Laboratory Monitoring

In the earliest phase of treatment, arterial blood gases should be checked every 4 hours. Sodium should also be checked frequently, because patients on scavenging medications are at risk for sodium overload. Ammonia levels should be checked every hour until they are less than 300 μM. Daily plasma amino acids are also useful for assessing the reversal of metabolic decompensation.

Nutrition

The slow introduction of protein should begin in approximately 24 to 48 hours to provide essential amino acids and prevent ongoing protein turnover. An initial amount of 1 to 1.5 g protein/kg per day is reasonable; this should be coordinated with a nutritionist to ensure that at least 50% of the essential amino acids are provided.[5] Protein intake can be gradually increased toward baseline during the course of hospitalization. Enteral feeding should resume when gastrointestinal and mental status abnormalities have resolved.

CONSULTATION

Metabolic specialists should be involved with the care of children with hyperammonemia or UCDs. They can offer guidance to confirm or refute a diagnosis, and they are essential for the ongoing management of these children, especially for the management of acute decompensation.

ADMISSION CRITERIA

Any patient with a UCD who is unable to take oral nutrition, is vomiting, or has elevated blood ammonia levels should be admitted for intravenous nutrition with an adequate amount of carbohydrate (with or without lipids) to stop or prevent catabolism. Admission or transfer to an intensive care unit is recommended for patients with altered mental status or hemodynamic compromise.

DISCHARGE CRITERIA

- The patient's ammonia level has fallen and stabilized at normal or near-normal values.
- The patient is tolerating a low-protein diet, and the parent is able to obtain the appropriate formula or diet.
- The parent is able to obtain the appropriate medications. (Even some large nationwide pharmacies do not carry these medications, and some may not be able to order them.)
- Appropriate follow-up has been arranged.

IN A NUTSHELL

- Respiratory alkalosis in a newborn with poor feeding and lethargy should prompt an immediate evaluation of ammonia levels and concern for a UCD. In older children, mental status changes out of proportion to the level of illness or frequent episodes of vomiting should raise suspicion of a UCD.
- Testing for inborn errors of metabolism should be done immediately on presentation, because abnormalities often resolve with hydration and therapy.
- If a UCD is suspected, stop protein consumption immediately, and reverse the catabolic state with dextrose and lipids.
- Decrease ammonia levels promptly with hemodialysis and the use of scavenger pathways.
- What is normally a minor illness can be life threatening for a child with a UCD. If a patient cannot tolerate oral nutrition, intravenous dextrose should be started, and the ammonia level should be checked.

ON THE HORIZON

- Several advances may have a significant impact on the diagnosis and treatment of UCDs. Expanded newborn screening using tandem mass spectrometry can diagnose UCDs, including citrullinemia, argininemia, and argininosuccinic acid lyase deficiency.[8] This may allow newborns to be placed on carefully tailored diets before suffering an initial episode of hyperammonemia. Unfortunately, the onset of illness may occur before the results of screening tests are received. If there is suspicion of a UCD in a symptomatic newborn, most laboratories can rush the processing and provide results in 1 to 2 days.
- Liver transplantation is currently performed for severe UCDs and some other inborn errors of metabolism. The 5-year survival rate is 80%.[7] As long-term transplant success increases, this may become the treatment of choice for all children with moderate to severe UCDs.
- Gene therapy may eventually be of significant value to patients with UCDs, but trials have been halted due to the death of a study patient with OTC deficiency in 1999.

SUGGESTED READING

Burton BK: Inborn errors of metabolism in infancy: A guide to diagnosis. Pediatrics 1998;102:E69.

Summar M: Current strategies for the management of neonatal urea cycle disorders. J Pediatr 2001;138:S30-S34.

Summar M, Tuchman M: Proceedings of a consensus conference for the management of patients with urea cycle disorders. J Pediatr 2001;138:S6-S20.

REFERENCES

1. Brusilow SW: Hyperammonemic encephalopathy. Medicine 2002;81:240-249.
2. Maestri NE, Clissold D, Brusilow SW: Neonatal onset ornithine transcarbamylase deficiency: A retrospective analysis. J Pediatr 1999;134:268-272.
3. Summar M, Tuchman M: Proceedings of a consensus conference for the management of patients with urea cycle disorders. J Pediatr 2001;138:S6-S20.
4. Burton BK: Inborn errors of metabolism in infancy: A guide to diagnosis. Pediatrics 1998;102:E69.
5. Summar M: Current strategies for the management of neonatal urea cycle disorders. J Pediatr 2001;138:S30-S34.
6. Maestri NE, Brusilow SW, Clissold DB, Bassett SS: Long-term treatment of girls with ornithine transcarbamylase deficiency. N Engl J Med 1996;335:855-859.
7. Urea Cycle Disorders Conference Group: Consensus statement from a conference for the management of patients with urea cycle disorders. J Pediatr 2001;138:S1-S5.
8. Newborn screening characteristics of state programs. USGAO Report GAO-03-449, 2003.

CHAPTER 132

Hypoglycemia

Neal Sondheimer

In humans, an interlocking set of homeostatic mechanisms maintains blood glucose levels appropriate for survival and growth. Four broad categories of problems contribute to the development of hypoglycemia: loss of homeostatic control; inadequate intake of food; intoxication with a substance that induces low blood sugar; and inborn errors in the utilization, production, or release of sugar. When all systems are operating, there is a balance of supply and demand to maintain normal blood sugar (euglycemia) over a broad range of physiologic settings.

Different organ systems have distinct roles in glucose homeostasis. The liver acts as the most important buffer for blood glucose, storing glucose during times of excess and releasing it during times of fasting. Muscle also produces glucose for local use but cannot release it. Adipose tissue provides energy in the form of fatty acids that can be used during fasting, but it cannot synthesize glucose to be used by other tissues. The brain preferentially uses glucose for energy and is endangered by sudden decreases in blood sugar. As a result, neurologic symptoms are the earliest and most damaging consequences of hypoglycemia.

The blood glucose level is only briefly maintained by sugar obtained from a meal (Fig. 132-1). After a meal, glucose is rapidly converted into other molecules. Some glucose is consumed by glycolysis, which converts 1 mole of glucose into 2 moles of acetyl coenzyme A (acetyl CoA) and provides a modest amount of high-energy phosphates (adenosine triphosphate [ATP]). Acetyl CoA can be used as substrate in the tricarboxylic acid cycle to generate more ATP. Acetyl CoA is also used in the synthesis of other molecules such as fat and cholesterol. Fat serves as a dense, energy-rich storage molecule that can be recovered when the need arises.

Glucose consumed in a meal is also converted to glycogen, a polymer of glucose monomers that serves as the major form of glucose storage. Glycogen storage and release prevent large fluctuations in the blood glucose level after meals and during short fasts, because glycogen can quickly be converted back into free glucose by the liver when necessary. Glycogen is stored primarily in the liver, but there are also some reserves of glycogen in the kidneys as well as in skeletal and cardiac muscle.

Once the supply of glucose and glycogen is exhausted, glucose can be synthesized by the liver using carbon skeletons that are derived largely from the metabolism of amino acids (gluconeogenesis). This process uses many of the same enzymes involved in glycolysis, as well as several unique steps that help keep the body from carrying out glycolysis and gluconeogenesis in the same tissues at the same time, a combination that would be energetically wasteful.

CLINICAL PRESENTATION

Early in hypoglycemia, symptoms such as lethargy, sweating, pallor, and hunger dominate the clinical picture (Table 132-1). The release of adrenergic neurotransmitters causes many of these symptoms as the central nervous system attempts to increase the breakdown of fats and proteins to respond to energy deprivation. Severe or persistent hypoglycemia causes more dangerous complications, such as syncope, seizure, and coma.

When faced with a child who is unresponsive for unknown reasons, hypoglycemia should be suspected immediately. Such a patient may be the victim of accidental or intentional poisoning with hypoglycemic or toxic agents; alternatively, this may be the first presentation of an inborn error of metabolism. A simple blood glucose measurement can reliably guide the diagnostic evaluation.

An accurate determination of clinically significant hypoglycemia combines both clinical observation and laboratory values. In addition, the timing of glucose monitoring has a strong effect on the observed value. For regular monitoring of blood glucose levels, children should be tested before meals rather than on a set time schedule; blood sugar rises rapidly as carbohydrate is absorbed by the intestine and then falls as it is stored for future use as glycogen. Although a perfect numerical definition of hypoglycemia does not exist, values below 40 mg/dL are considered a threshold for immediate treatment.[1] Values from 40 to 55 mg/dL should prompt a reexamination of blood glucose within a short time. It must be stressed that the treatment of symptomatic hypoglycemia—regardless of the actual blood glucose value—is the primary clinical goal.

Neonatal hypoglycemia is a particularly common clinical scenario. After removal from the placental circulation, a newborn has limited reserves of glucose and a brisk metabolic demand, increasing the risk for hypoglycemia. This can be exacerbated by a delay in the initiation of feeding, difficulty with the initial transfer of colostrum, or a cold environment. Because of the neonate's limited ability to show the signs and symptoms of distress, these infants can present with listlessness, vomiting, or poor suck.

Newborn nurseries should have a standard protocol for glucose monitoring that identifies infants at risk for hypoglycemia. Patients who deserve scrutiny include infants who are either small or large for gestational age and infants of diabetic mothers. Small-for-gestational-age infants have low metabolic reserves, and large-for-gestational-age infants and infants of diabetic mothers are often relatively hyperinsulinemic owing to their exposure to high intrauterine glucose levels. Because they cannot immediately down-regulate their high levels of secreted insulin, they are prone to hypoglycemia once the placental glucose supply is interrupted. Infants of diabetic mothers may be large for gestational age, plethoric, or sluggish. These signs and symptoms should raise the suspicion of gestational diabetes even if the mother's history is not available.

In any newborn with hypoglycemia, oral feeding should be attempted immediately. This usually leads to a rapid resolution of symptoms. Serum glucose values of 36 mg/dL in an asymptomatic newborn and 45 mg/dL in a symptomatic newborn are appropriate levels for the initiation of intravenous treatment of hypoglycemia[2] (see Chapter 54). It is extremely important to note that hypoglycemia with neurologic symptoms may be the hallmark of other serious problems, including sepsis and inborn errors of metabolism. Neonates in distress who do not respond to or cannot tolerate oral or gavage feedings with breast milk or formula need rapid administration of intravenous dextrose and a full diagnostic evaluation that includes screening for sepsis and inborn errors of metabolism.

DIFFERENTIAL DIAGNOSIS

Hypoglycemia can be due to extrinsic causes, including toxins and other stresses interfering with normal metabolism, as well as intrinsic causes such as inborn errors of glucose metabolism. A diagnostic scheme for the evaluation of hypoglycemia was created by Saudubray and colleagues (Fig. 132-2).[3]

Extrinsic Causes of Hypoglycemia

Among the extrinsic causes of pediatric hypoglycemia, oral hypoglycemics are among the most frequent culprits (Table 132-2). These medications affect glucose metabolism through several distinct mechanisms. Thiazolidinediones sensitize target cells to insulin so that glucose clearance from the bloodstream is increased, metformin interferes with glucose production by the liver, and sulfonylureas increase insulin secretion. All these medications may lead to hypoglycemia in a normal child, but the effects of sulfonylurea poisoning can be the most severe.

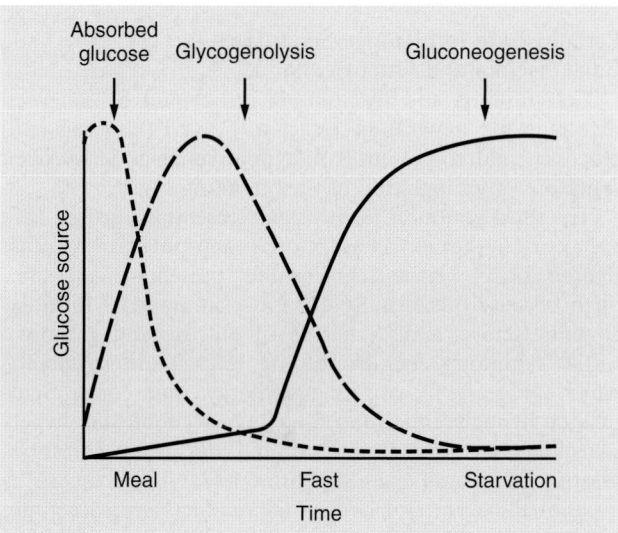

Figure 132-1 Contribution of physiologic processes to blood glucose over time from fast.

Table 132-1 Signs and Symptoms of Hypoglycemia
General
Hunger
Irritability
Neurologic
Headache
Confusion, agitation, combativeness
Lethargy, obtundation, coma
Tremor
Seizure
Syncope
Autonomic
Diaphoresis
Pallor
Palpitations, tachycardia
Jitteriness

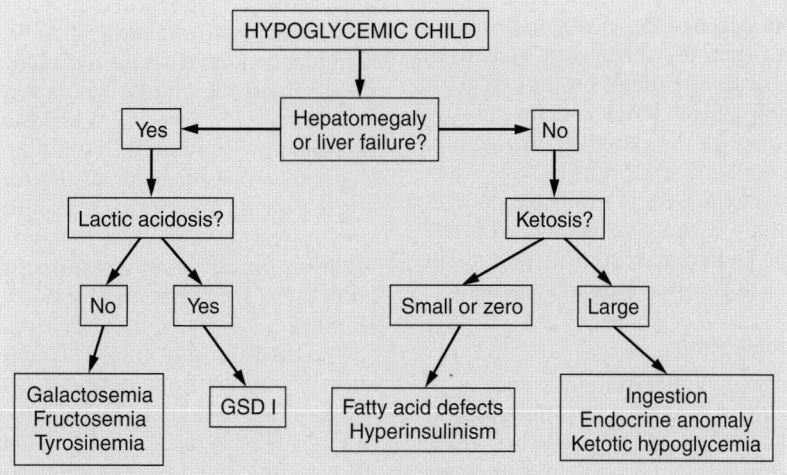

Figure 132-2 Evaluation of a child with hypoglycemia. GSD, glycogen storage disease.

Table 132-2   Drugs and Toxins Causing Hypoglycemia

Oral hypoglycemics
  Thiazolidinediones
    Pioglitazone (Actos)
    Rosiglitazone (Avandia)
  Metformin
  Sulfonylureas
    Glimepiride (Amaryl)
    Glipizide (Glucotrol)
    Glyburide (Micronase)
  Combinations
    Glyburide and metformin (Glucovance)
    Metaglip (glipizide and metformin)

Insulin

Antihypertensives
  Carvedilol
  Atenolol
  Other beta-blockers

Aspirin

Alcohol

Insulin overdose should be suspected in diabetic patients. Accidental overdose, misuse of an insulin pump, iatrogenic error, and Munchausen syndrome are all possible causes. Glucagon kits to be used at home are frequently provided to families with diabetic children.

Other drugs causing hypoglycemia include alcohol and aspirin. Alcohol causes symptoms by blockade of gluconeogenesis, but the actual frequency of alcohol-induced hypoglycemia is quite low.[4] The hypoglycemic effect of alcohol is an important factor in the care of all inebriated children, because they are often unwilling or unable to eat and may have had a prolonged fast by the time they reach medical attention. Salicylate-induced hypoglycemia is quite rare and has been reported only in cases of massive overdose.[5,6]

In certain circumstances, iatrogenic hypoglycemia is therapeutically valuable. Several rare metabolic and neurologic disorders are treated with a diet that induces a state of permanent ketotic hypoglycemia, the so-called ketogenic diet. This diet is a mainstay of therapy for both intractable epilepsy and pyruvate dehydrogenase deficiency. In disorders treated with the ketogenic diet, the therapeutic goal is an unusually low blood glucose level. Patients on the ketogenic diet are adapted to their low glucose levels, and a rapid shift into the normoglycemic range is extremely dangerous. Patients with intractable epilepsy may begin to seize when blood glucose rises, and patients with pyruvate dehydrogenase deficiency can develop lactic acidosis. Appropriate treatment requires specific and accurate information about the typical blood glucose value for the individual patient.

Intrinsic Causes of Hypoglycemia

Intrinsic causes of hypoglycemia include a variety of inborn metabolic defects and deficiencies in counterregulatory hormones. These include disorders of carbohydrate metabolism such as galactosemia and fructosemia, glycogen storage diseases, fatty acid oxidation defects, endocrine disorders, hyperinsulinism, and ketotic hypoglycemia. Crises can be triggered either by illness or by the ingestion of dietary sources that cannot be properly metabolized.

Children with intrinsic metabolic defects tend to present with repeated bouts of hypoglycemia. The degree of hypoglycemia and symptoms may be more severe than expected. The history and physical examination in patients with suspected inborn errors of metabolism may reveal hepatomegaly due to hepatic steatosis or storage of glycogen, abnormal odors, feeding aversions, or unexplained episodes of acidosis during prior illnesses.

A discussion of the numerous inborn errors of metabolism that may present with hypoglycemia is beyond the scope of this chapter. Referral to a specialist in endocrinology or biochemical genetics is required for the diagnosis and management of many of these disorders. However, the principle of immediate treatment in patients with signs and symptoms of hypoglycemia is still useful, even when the underlying disorder is unknown or unfamiliar to the practitioner. The following disease categories provide an overview of the most common and most severe of these disorders seen in children.

Carbohydrate Intolerance Syndromes— Galactosemia and Fructosemia

Galactosemia and fructosemia are caused by inherited defects in the enzymes necessary to convert these sugars to glucose. Children present with hypoglycemia and associated symptoms after ingestion of the offending sugar.

The most common form of galactosemia is caused by a deficiency in the enzyme galactose 1-phosphate uridyltransferase (GALT). Galactosemia usually presents shortly after birth because breast milk and most commercial formulas contain lactose, a disaccharide of glucose and galactose. Initial symptoms include feeding refusal and irritability, which progress to vomiting, lethargy, and coma. Signs include hypoglycemia, unconjugated or conjugated hyperbilirubinemia, elevated prothrombin and partial thromboplastin times, and acidosis. *Escherichia coli* urosepsis is occasionally seen, and congenital cataracts are sometimes present. Galactosemia can be diagnosed on state-mandated newborn metabolic screening by elevated levels of galactose or a deficiency in the measured GALT activity.

Infants with suspected galactosemia based on clinical presentation, or asymptomatic infants with very high levels of galactose 1 (>30 mg/dL), should be switched immediately to non-lactose-containing formula. Most commercial soy formulas contain fructose and sucrose and are safe for use in these infants. Newborns who are determined by screening tests to have low levels of GALT but normal levels of galactose and no symptoms of liver failure should be evaluated by a specialist before changing the formula. Patients who are severely ill on presentation should be treated with intravenous dextrose and may require intensive therapy, including fresh frozen plasma to correct coagulation deficiencies, antibiotics for suspected sepsis, and phototherapy for jaundice.

Fructosemia, also known as hereditary fructose intolerance, is caused by a deficiency in fructose 1-phosphate aldolase (aldolase B) and usually presents when an affected infant is fed fructose-containing items, such as fruit or fruit juice, for the first time. Ingestion of sucrose-containing substances also exposes the infant to fructose as the sucrose disaccharide is hydrolyzed to glucose and fructose. Without adequate enzymes, fructose 1-phosphate is not catalyzed, allowing this toxic substance to accumulate. These infants present with vomiting, lethargy, and hypoglycemia shortly after ingestion. The hypoglycemia may be severe but is often transient, complicating the laboratory diagnosis. Failure to detect this condition can lead to hepatitis, renal failure, and even death if the patient continues to be fed sucrose- or fructose-containing juices or foods. If the condition is not recognized in infancy, most children spontaneously develop food aversions that limit or prevent toxic ingestion, but they continue to be at risk any time a novel food containing fructose or sorbitol is given to them. Diagnosis requires an accurate dietary history. As with galactosemia, treatment involves the avoidance of fructose.

Glycogen Storage Diseases

The glycogen storage diseases are a family of syndromes caused by defects in glycogen synthesis and storage and the degradation and release of glucose. Not all patients with glycogen storage diseases are prone to hypoglycemia; in some disorders, the manifestations are largely limited to muscle. The disorders that cause hypoglycemia can present in a number of different settings, but a common presentation is an infant with hypoglycemic seizures and hepatomegaly. The glycogen storage diseases can affect many tissues, giving children a typical appearance: short stature, rounded face, enlarged abdomen, and wasted extremities. Laboratory studies reflect low glucose in the face of a normal counterregulatory response and brisk increases in circulating ketones at the time of fasting.

In children with glycogen storage diseases, hypoglycemia occurs when glycogenolysis fails to maintain an adequate blood glucose level. Because these children are unable to use glycogen stores efficiently, their blood sugar may fall within a few hours after starting a fast. Proper management of these patients requires that they avoid prolonged fasting, and for many patients, even sleeping through the night without caloric intake is impossible. The use of uncooked cornstarch at pre-bedtime feedings, intermittent overnight feedings, or nasogastric feedings are required for type I glycogen storage disease. These treatments limit the intervals of fasting to ensure adequate energy reserves. There are many long-term complications with all these disorders, including hyperuricemia, hypertriglyceridemia, renal failure, and hepatic adenomas.[7]

Fatty Acid Oxidation Defects

Fatty acid oxidation defects interfere with the ability to convert fatty acids into acetyl CoA, a precursor for oxidative metabolism and ketogenesis. Hypoglycemia occurs because patients are unable to use ketone bodies as an energy source and are overly dependent on glycolysis to produce energy and the substrates for the tricarboxylic acid cycle.

Although many of these disorders exist, medium-chain acyl-CoA dehydrogenase deficiency (MCADD) is the most common, with an incidence of roughly 1 in 10,000. Children with MCADD are developmentally and physically normal and present to medical attention only when a significant illness (usually gastrointestinal) prevents the intake of calories. The most remarkable presenting feature is a lack of urine and serum ketones in the face of serious illness and low blood sugar.

Unfortunately, children can die at this initial presentation if the hypoglycemia is not quickly recognized and treated. They respond very well to infusions of concentrated glucose but are prone to repeat episodes of hypoglycemia with any sustained fast. Parental understanding and awareness are important aspects in the care of these children. Most fatty acid oxidation defects improve as the patient ages and the glycogen reserve increases. Many of these defects, including MCADD, are now detected on newborn metabolic screens that include an acylcarnitine profile.

Hyperinsulinism

Inherited disorders that cause excessive release of insulin from pancreatic beta cells lead to a severe form of hypoglycemia that can be refractory to medical management. In these patients, insulin is continually and inappropriately released, causing the uptake of circulating glucose into the liver and muscle and preventing the breakdown of glycogen. Several genetic defects causing hyperinsulinism have been identified.[8] There is also a common transient form of hyperinsulinism that is not inherited and is related to the hypoglycemia seen in small-for-gestational-age infants. Patients with hyperinsulinism often present shortly after birth with lethargy or seizure, and their hypoglycemia is refractory to feedings and even to peripherally administered dextrose infusions. Clinical suspicion of hyperinsulinism and referral to a specialized center are required for the diagnosis and management of this condition.

Endocrine Causes of Hypoglycemia

Insulin is secreted by the pancreas in response to protein- or carbohydrate-rich meals and increases the conversion of glucose to stored energy forms. In addition, insulin suppresses the endogenous synthesis of glucose by preventing the breakdown of fats, protein, and glycogen. Opposed to the action of insulin are the counterregulatory hormones: glucagon, catecholamines, cortisol, and growth hormone. Generally, these hormones have metabolic effects that lead to increased conversion of glycogen to glucose and the breakdown of fats for use in energy production. Thus, conditions limiting the production or secretion of the counterregulatory hormones can lead to fasting hypoglycemia.

Ketotic Hypoglycemia

Ketotic hypoglycemia is a fairly common phenomenon characterized by reduced fasting tolerance in children who are otherwise healthy. This condition is typically diagnosed in early childhood. Metabolically, these children have a sluggish gluconeogenic response during prolonged fasts or times of metabolic stress. This appears to be due to the inefficient production or utilization (or both) of precursors for gluconeogenesis, particularly the amino acid alanine, which may be decreased in these children. It is important to note that the ketosis is not pathologic per se; rather, it is an exaggeration of normal fasting physiology in which decreased glucose supplies (and therefore decreased insulin levels) promote fatty acid metabolism and ketogenesis. Unlike most well-characterized inborn errors of metabolism, a specific biochemical defect is typically not discovered in these children, and it remains a diagnosis of exclusion. The condition responds well to avoidance of fasting and resolves by adolescence.

EVALUATION

A child with hypoglycemia should be evaluated quickly but carefully by means of a history, physical examination, and laboratory evaluation. Useful information from the history includes the timing of the last meal, the presence of vomiting or diarrhea, the possibility of exposure to toxic substances, and any previous hypoglycemic episodes. A family history of hypoglycemia and unexplained seizures should also be noted. On physical examination, the degree of adiposity, presence or absence of an enlarged liver, and degree of sympathetic tone should all be noted.

Laboratory Evaluation

In an acutely ill hypoglycemic child, laboratory investigations never take priority over the correction of hypoglycemia. However, a blood sample taken during the placement of an intravenous catheter or early in the course of treatment provides important diagnostic information. In children with intrinsic causes of hypoglycemia, biochemical abnormalities often normalize when the hypoglycemia resolves; therefore, the performance of a few "critical" tests during the symptomatic period can go a long way toward establishing a diagnosis. Table 132-3 provides a list of useful laboratory studies in an undiagnosed patient with hypoglycemia. Many clinicians are surprised to learn that in most cases these studies do not require a large amount of blood. Furthermore, urinalysis is indispensable in diagnosing metabolic causes of hypoglycemia, especially in differentiating ketotic from nonketotic forms of hypoglycemia. A simple bag-collected urine specimen is adequate.

Fasting Studies

Often a definitive cause of hypoglycemia cannot be established after the first episode. In such cases, fasting studies are sometimes initiated in the inpatient setting so that the response to hypoglycemia can be evaluated safely. This type of study is especially useful for the diagnosis of inborn errors of metabolism or the failure of hormonal regulation of glucose and to determine the length of fasting that a child can safely tolerate. These tests are usually done in collaboration with a pediatric endocrinology service, and specific protocols are followed that provide guidelines for laboratory testing (see Table 132-4), evaluation of hypoglycemia, and the administration of glucagon.

TREATMENT

In children who are able to take liquids by mouth, replenishment by the oral route is preferred. However, if this is not possible, an intravenous solution of dextrose (the D-isomer of glucose that is nutritionally equivalent to glucose) is indicated. In general, a rapid intravenous infusion of 2 to 4 mL/kg of 10% dextrose (D10W) is administered. If hypoglycemia persists, a continuous infusion of dextrose is indicated. The continuous glucose infusion rate (GIR) should be initiated at 6 to 9 mg/kg dextrose per minute, then titrated to maintain blood glucose levels greater than 80 mg/dL. The GIR can be calculated by the following formula:

$$GIR = (IVR \times \% \text{ Dextrose solution})/6 \times Weight,$$

where the GIR is measured in mg/kg per minute, IVR is the intravenous infusion rate in mL/hour, and weight is expressed in kilograms.

To calculate the initial IVR, the formula can be rearranged as follows:

$$IVR = GIR \times 6 \times Weight/\% \text{ Dextrose solution}$$

If the goal is to deliver a GIR of 8 mg/kg per minute and D10W is used, the formula can be further simplified:

$$IVR = 4.8 \times Weight$$

Table 132-3 Laboratory Evaluation of a Hypoglycemic Child

Test	Analysis
Confirmatory glucose	Confirms presence of hypoglycemia
Insulin, C peptide	Elevated insulin can often (but not always) be documented in hyperinsulinism; insulin level should be very low or undetectable in other types of hypoglycemia C-peptide testing determines whether the excess insulin is endogenous or exogenous in origin
Ketones	Hypoketotic hypoglycemia suggests hyperinsulinism or fatty acid oxidation defects
Free fatty acids	Falling insulin levels normally stimulate lipolysis; low fatty acids suggest hyperinsulinism
Cortisol, growth hormone, epinephrine	These hormones should increase during hypoglycemic episodes; inappropriately low levels suggest hormone deficiency
Lactate	Elevated lactate, especially with elevated fatty acids and uric acid, suggests type I glycogen storage disease; lactate can also be elevated in fatty acid oxidation defects and some rarer metabolic causes of hypoglycemia
Acylcarnitine profile	Profile of fatty acid metabolites; primary method of diagnosing fatty acid oxidation defects
Plasma amino acids	May reveal inappropriately decreased alanine in ketotic hypoglycemia
Urinalysis	Useful screen for ketonuria
Urine reducing substances	Present in galactosemia, fructosemia
Urine organic acids	Quantitation is useful in identifying abnormal metabolites that arise in a variety of disorders, including fatty acid oxidation defects

Table 132–4   Clinical Manifestations and Differential Diagnosis in Childhood Hypoglycemia

Condition	Hypoglycemia	Urinary Ketones (K) or Reducing Sugars	Hepatomegaly	SERUM Lipids	SERUM Uric Acid	EFFECT OF 24-36 HR FAST ON PLASMA Glucose	Insulin	Ketones	Alanine	Lactate	GLYCEMIC RESPONSE TO GLUCAGON Fed	Fasted	GLYCEMIC RESPONSE TO INFUSION OF Alanine	Glycerol
Hyperinsulinemia	Recurrent severe	0	0	Normal or ↑	Normal	↓↓	↑↑	↓↓	Normal	Normal	↑	↑	↑	↑
Ketotic hypoglycemia	Severe with missed meals	Ketonuria +++	0	Normal	Normal	↓↓	↓	↑↑	↓↓	Normal	↑	↓↓	↑	↑
Fatty acid oxidation disorder	Severe with missed meals	Absent	0 to + Abnormal liver function test results	Abnormal	↑	Contraindicated					↑	↓	Not indicated	
Hypopituitarism	Moderate with missed meals	Ketonuria ++	0	Normal	Normal	↓↓	↓	↑↑	↓↓	Normal	↑	↓↓	↑	↑
Adrenal insufficiency	Severe with missed meals	Ketonuria ++	0	Normal	Normal	↓↓	↓	↑↑	↓↓	Normal	↑	↓↓	↑	↑
Enzyme deficiencies Glucose-6-phosphatase	Severe-constant	Ketonuria +++	+++	↑↑	↑↑	↓↓	↓	↑↑	↑↑	↑↑	0	0-↓↓	0	0
Debrancher	Moderate with fasting	Ketonuria ++	++	Normal	Normal	↓↓	↓	↑↑	↓↓	Normal	↑	0-↓↓	↑↑	↑
Phosphorylase	Mild-moderate	Ketonuria ++	+	Normal	Normal	↓↓	↓	↑↑	↓↓	Normal	0-↑	0-↓↓	↓↓	↑↓
Fructose-1,6-bisphosphatase	Severe with fasting	Ketonuria +++	+++	↑↑	↑↑	↓↓	↓	↑↑	↑↑	↑↑	↑	0-↓↓	↑↑	→
Galactosemia	After milk or milk products	0 Ketones(s) +	+++	Normal	Normal	→	↓	↑	→	Normal	↑	↓-↓↓	↑	↑
Fructose intolerance	After fructose	0 Ketones(s) +	+++	Normal	Normal	→	↓	↑	→	Normal	↑	0-↓↓	↑	↑

0, absence; ↑ or ↓ indicates small increase or decrease, respectively; ↑↑ or ↓↓ indicates large increase or decrease, respectively.

For example, a 10-kg child would receive D10W at 48 mL/hour to deliver 8 mg/kg glucose per minute. This formula also conveniently provides maintenance fluid requirements for a child weighing less than 10 kg.

If the patient does not tolerate enteral glucose replenishment and intravenous access is unavailable, glucagon can be administered. The dose of glucagon is 1 mg subcutaneously, regardless of patient size. Response to glucagon should be evaluated and noted within 10 minutes of administration, and blood sugar monitoring should be continued at least hourly until the patient returns to a safe, stable range. Rehydration and sugar replenishment usually lead to a rapid improvement in symptoms such as lethargy or jitteriness.

Management of overdose of oral hypoglycemics is largely supportive. Intravenous or oral glucose is often required until enough of the offending agent is eliminated. Depending on the timing of the exposure and the release form of the medication, activated charcoal can be used to bind unabsorbed medications, especially some of the sustained-release formulations. Communication with poison control centers can provide information on drug half-life and appropriate techniques for detoxification. Octreotide, a long-acting somatostatin analogue, has been used in some cases of sulfonylurea overdose.[9]

Children with metabolic or endocrine abnormalities predisposing them to hypoglycemia require intervention to prevent recurrent crises. Although the particular therapies vary with the underlying disease, a few general guidelines are applicable to many disorders.

In children older than 2 years with early-morning hypoglycemia after an overnight fast, a bedtime snack supplemented with uncooked cornstarch often helps sustain adequate glucose levels overnight. Glucose is slowly released from the starch polymers, mimicking a glucose infusion. If starch snacks are inadequate, gastric feedings may be necessary. Even short periods of fasting pose a significant danger to children at risk for hypoglycemia. When an overnight fast is required (e.g., for anesthesia), the child should be admitted to the hospital and placed on intravenous dextrose during the fasting period.

Measures should be taken to reduce the risk of crisis during other times of stress. For example, febrile illnesses, especially when associated with emesis or diarrhea, often necessitate dextrose infusions. Consider prophylactic antipyretics in these children when they receive immunizations to curtail catabolic periods with increased metabolic demand.

Medical management of hyperinsulinism includes the use of octreotide and diazoxide, which interfere with the release of insulin from the beta cell, and glucagon. Definitive treatment of hyperinsulinism may require subtotal pancreatectomy.

CONSULTATION

Consultation with specialists in endocrinology, metabolism, or neonatology can be helpful in patients with severe, recurrent, or prolonged hypoglycemia. These consultants can also guide the diagnostic evaluation and, when appropriate, follow patients after discharge.

Evaluation by a pediatric or neonatal intensivist is warranted when placement in an intensive care setting is being considered.

Involvement of the diabetes team is needed when a diabetic patient presents with persistent or recurrent hypoglycemia. The team can evaluate the diet, the insulin regimen, and compliance, as well as provide ongoing education, support, and medical management for these patients.

ADMISSION CRITERIA

- Clinical evidence of lethargy, sweating, or pallor; neurologic symptoms such as syncope, seizure, or coma; or unresponsiveness for unknown reasons.
- Persistent or recurrent serum glucose values less than 55 mg/dL.
- Known or suspected ingestion of medications or other toxins that can cause hypoglycemia.
- Known or suspected overdose of insulin.
- For neonates: listlessness, vomiting, poor suck, or serum glucose levels less than 36 mg/dL, particularly infants of diabetic mothers or small- or large-for-gestational-age infants (see Chapter 54).

Admission or transfer to an intensive care unit is appropriate when an infant or child with hypoglycemia requires close observation, frequent laboratory studies and prompt reporting of the results, and rapid adjustments in treatment based on laboratory results and changes in clinical status.

DISCHARGE CRITERIA

- Resolution of laboratory findings of hypoglycemia and the ability to maintain stable serum glucose levels without hospital-level support.
- A clinically stable patient with normal activity, adequate enteral intake, and established medical follow-up after discharge.

IN A NUTSHELL

- Hypoglycemia can present with a broad range of symptoms that are often nonspecific, including changes in mental status or seizure. Owing to the compensatory catecholamine release, findings of diaphoresis, tachycardia, and pallor are often present.
- Evaluation of an infant or child with new neurologic findings or a deteriorating neurologic status should routinely include a blood glucose analysis.
- Neonatal hypoglycemia is a common problem and is especially likely in small- or large-for-gestational-age babies and infants of diabetic mothers.
- Patients with extrinsic causes of hypoglycemia have often been exposed to suspect medications, including oral hypoglycemics.
- Patients with intrinsic causes of hypoglycemia are more likely to have low blood sugar during illnesses and with fasts.
- Immediate treatment of hypoglycemia is far more important than determining the cause. However, blood samples should be obtained if this can be accomplished without delaying the necessary interventions.
- Treatment of hypoglycemia involves the delivery of glucose enterally or intravenously. Ongoing delivery may be needed if the hypoglycemia is severe, recurrent, or persistent.

ON THE HORIZON

- There is intense research into the intrinsic disorders causing hyperinsulinemic hypoglycemia. Recent discoveries include disease-causing mutations in the insulin receptor and the sulfonylurea receptor.[10,11] Both these defects may be inherited in an autosomal dominant fashion, increasing the number of genes associated with familial syndromes of hyperinsulinism.
- In many states, the number of diseases included on newborn metabolic screens has increased. Tandem mass spectrophotometry provides an efficient, low-cost way of detecting fatty acid oxidation defects and organic acidemias.

SUGGESTED READING

Cornblath M, Hawdon JM, Williams AF, et al: Controversies regarding definition of neonatal hypoglycemia: Suggested operational thresholds. Pediatrics 2000;105:1141-1145.

Stanley C, Thornton P, Finegold D, Sperling M: Hypoglycemia in infants. In Sperling M (ed): Pediatric Endocrinology, 2nd ed. Philadelphia, WB Saunders, 2002.

REFERENCES

1. Stanley C, Thornton P, Finegold D, Sperling M: Hypoglycemia in infants. In Sperling M (ed): Pediatric Endocrinology, 2nd ed. Philadelphia, WB Saunders, 2002:135-159.
2. Cornblath M, Hawdon JM, Williams AF, et al: Controversies regarding definition of neonatal hypoglycemia: Suggested operational thresholds. Pediatrics 2000;105:1141-1145.
3. Saudubray JM, Ogier de Baulny H, Charpentier C: Clinical approach to inherited metabolic disease. In Fernandes J, Saudubray JM, Tada K (eds): Inborn Metabolic Diseases: Diagnosis and Treatment, 3rd ed. Berlin, Springer-Verglag, 2000;3-41.
4. Ernst AA, Jones K, Nick TG, Sanchez J: Ethanol ingestion and related hypoglycemia in a pediatric and adolescent emergency department population. Acad Emerg Med 1996;3:46-49.
5. Raschke R, Arnold-Capell PA, Richeson R, Curry SC: Refractory hypoglycemia secondary to topical salicylate intoxication. Arch Intern Med 1991;151:591-593.
6. Arena FP, Dugowson C, Saudek CD: Salicylate-induced hypoglycemia and ketoacidosis in a nondiabetic adult. Arch Intern Med 1978;138:1153-1154.
7. Chen YT: Glycogen storage diseases. In Scriver CR, Sly WS, Childs B, et al (eds): The Molecular and Metabolic Bases of Inherited Disease, 8th ed. New York, McGraw-Hill, 2001.
8. Stanley CA: Advances in diagnosis and treatment of hyperinsulinism in infants and children. J Clin Endocrinol Metab 2002;87:4857-4859.
9. McLaughlin SA, Crandall CS, McKinney PE: Octreotide: An antidote for sulfonylurea-induced hypoglycemia. Ann Emerg Med 2000;36:133-138.
10. Hojlund K, Hansen T, Lajer M, et al: A novel syndrome of autosomal-dominant hyperinsulinemic hypoglycemia linked to a mutation in the human insulin receptor gene. Diabetes 2004;53:1592-1598.
11. Magge SN, Shyng SL, MacMullen C, et al: Familial leucine-sensitive hypoglycemia of infancy due to a dominant mutation of the beta-cell sulfonylurea receptor. J Clin Endocrinol Metab 2004;89:4450-4456.

CHAPTER 133

Metabolic Acidosis

David Adams and Charles P. Venditti

Metabolic acidemia is a common laboratory finding, and most cases are caused by conditions such as hypovolemia, systemic infection, and acute diarrhea. The challenge for the physician is to confirm that the acidemia has a presentation, history, and response to treatment that are consistent with one of these common illnesses rather than a rare metabolic disorder predisposing to acidosis. A careful review of each case should help identify those patients with inborn errors of metabolism. This chapter presents a set of principles by which clinicians can broaden the differential diagnosis to include inborn errors when an acidemia is not adequately explained by the clinical presentation and laboratory workup.

PHYSIOLOGY

The term *acidemia,* or "acid in the blood," is used to denote a state of acidic pH measured by a blood gas analysis or a serum bicarbonate level. The term *acidosis* is reserved for cases in which a specific acidic substance is suspected or has been identified in the blood (e.g., lactic acidosis, ketoacidosis).

Acid Buffering

Buffers in the blood and in the extracellular and intracellular fluid maintain normal body pH. In the blood, both fast-acting mechanisms (buffering by proteins and the bicarbonate-carbonic acid system) and slow-acting mechanisms (modulation of renal bicarbonate reabsorption) contribute to acid-base homeostasis. Quantitatively, proteins, especially albumin and hemoglobin, form the largest reserve of immediate buffer; the bicarbonate-carbonic acid system has the largest capacity to alter its flux in response to an acid challenge. Impairment of any of these mechanisms can decrease the body's ability to respond to a perturbation in acid-base status.

Acid Production and Excretion

Acidemia of any type represents an imbalance between acid production and acid excretion. Physiologic acid production can generally be categorized into volatile (mostly carbon dioxide) and nonvolatile components. The body generates approximately 15,000 mmol of carbon dioxide per day—an amount equivalent to 20 2-L bottles of carbonated beverage.[1,2] Pulmonary ventilation excretes most of this excess carbon dioxide. The majority of nonvolatile acids are generated by dietary acid intake, amino acid catabolism, and fatty acid oxidation (which produces ketones and lactic acid). An adult generates 50 to 70 mEq/day of nonvolatile acid.[3] Most nonvolatile acid secretion occurs through renal mechanisms, including bicarbonate reclamation and ammoniagenesis.[4]

Acidemia Secondary to Bicarbonate Loss

Because the bicarbonate–carbonic acid system is such a critical buffering mechanism, metabolic acidemia may be caused solely by excessive loss of bicarbonate rather than by increased acid production. Bicarbonate losses may be either gastrointestinal or renal. Renal tubular acidosis is a relatively common cause of chronic acidemia and is due to renal tubular dysfunction. The anion gap is usually normal, owing to a compensatory increase in the plasma chloride (Cl^-) concentration (see later). Several inborn errors of metabolism cause bicarbonate loss as part of a profound proximal renal tubular dysfunction that prevents resorption of small molecules, including bicarbonate, glucose, amino acids, phosphate, and urates (renal Fanconi syndrome). Table 133-1 lists inborn errors of metabolism and other conditions associated with such a renal presentation. Metabolic acidosis and other signs of renal dysfunction (e.g., failure to thrive) may be the presenting symptoms in these diseases.

CLINICAL PRESENTATION

Metabolic acidemia causes malaise and a host of end-organ effects. Physiologic effects of acidosis include pulmonary vasoconstriction, decreased myocardial contractility, and a shift of the oxygen-hemoglobin dissociation curve, decreasing oxygen saturation. Air hunger and tachypnea characterize the typical breathing pattern. Patients may be confused, lethargic, or ataxic. Nausea, vomiting, and abdominal pain may also be present. Alcohol poisoning (e.g., methanol) can cause vision changes. Myocardial suppression and cardiac conduction changes can cause chest pain or palpitations. Muscle weakness and bone pain may be described.

Acute decompensation from metabolic acidemia usually presents as a rapidly deteriorating course starting with anorexia, lethargy, and somnolence and progressing to coma. Episodes due to inborn errors of metabolism are usually triggered by an acquired illness, typically a viral infection. Subtle early signs may include worsening of the symptoms associated with the underlying disorder, such as ataxia and an increased maple syrup odor in children with maple syrup disease. Some disorders may lead to characteristic catastrophic events, such as cerebral edema (during diabetic ketoacidosis) or basal ganglia infarction (propionic- and methylmalonicacidemia).

Chronic metabolic acidosis is associated with growth failure and developmental delay. Depending on the underlying mechanism, other clues may emerge over time. Inborn errors causing a renal Fanconi syndrome may eventually cause hypophosphatemic rickets, hypocalcemia, and polyuric renal failure. Neurologic signs such as abnormal tone and ataxia are also common in a number of these conditions.

Table 133-1 Disorders Associated with Renal Fanconi Syndrome

Cystinosis
Galactosemia
Tyrosinemia type I
Lowe syndrome
Glycogen storage disorders, types I and XI
Hereditary fructose intolerance
Wilson disease
Congenital lactic acidosis
Vitamin D metabolism defects
Heavy metal toxicity

Table 133-2 Causes of Non–Anion Gap Acidosis

Gastrointestinal loss of bicarbonate 　Diarrhea 　Surgical drains distal to pylorus 　Cholestyramine
Renal loss of bicarbonate 　Renal tubular acidosis 　Compensation for chronic respiratory alkalosis
Chemicals that alter the measured acid component 　HCl 　NH_4Cl 　Arginine and lysine in parenteral nutrition fluids
Excessive chloride in intravenous fluids
Renal Fanconi syndrome (see Table 133-1)
Carbonic anhydrase inhibitor treatment
Dilution acidosis 　Caused by excessive volume expansion (HCO_3 dilution $\rightarrow$ 　carbonic acid dissociation $\rightarrow$ increased H^+)

DIFFERENTIAL DIAGNOSIS

The differential diagnoses and causes of metabolic acidosis are extensive. These are detailed in Tables 133-1 to 133-4.

EVALUATION

The following steps can guide the clinician toward an accurate diagnosis or referral point:

1. Confirm metabolic acidosis.
2. Differentiate secondary metabolic acidosis due to common illnesses from cases needing further evaluation.
3. Differentiate acid accumulation from bicarbonate loss.
4. If acidic molecules are accumulating, determine what type of acid is being accumulated.

Confirm Metabolic Acidosis

At a minimum, the laboratory studies performed in an acidotic child should include serum electrolytes, renal function tests, and glucose (the basic metabolic panel), as well as a blood gas analysis, preferably arterial. If a particular acid is suspected based on the presentation or a preexisting diagnosis, the initial studies should include the measurement of that acid. In addition, a standard urinalysis is a noninvasive, inexpensive test that should always be done on any patient with an acidosis of unknown cause.

Differentiate Acidosis Due to Common Illnesses from Cases Needing Further Evaluation

An acidemia may not require further evaluation if it presents in the context of a common illness, is an expected consequence of that illness, and resolves in a manner characteristic of that illness. For example, sepsis, diarrhea, and dehydration are at the root of most cases of acidemia seen in the pediatric setting. Severity, chronicity, history, and standard laboratory results can all be used to decide how comprehensive the workup should be. For example, consider a 1-month-old male with severe, frequent vomiting and acidemia. Although pyloric stenosis is an important diagnostic consideration for vomiting in a 1-month-old, it

should present with an alkalosis rather than an acidosis. Therefore, further workup might be required.

Differentiate Acid Accumulation from Bicarbonate Loss

As noted earlier, acidosis may result from increased acid production or abnormal loss of bicarbonate from the kidneys or gastrointestinal tract. Distinguishing between these two possibilities is critical, because effective treatment depends on a correct diagnosis. The history, physical examination, and routine laboratory studies allow some acidemias to be sorted into the bicarbonate-losing category. A typical bicarbonate-losing acidemia is associated with hyperchloremia and a normal anion gap. Causes of nongap metabolic acidemia are listed in Table 133-2. Measurement of urine pH can suggest renal tubular acidosis, but this can be obfuscated by gastrointestinal bicarbonate losses.[5] Clues to the presence of renal Fanconi syndrome include hypophosphatemia, alkaline urine in the setting of acidemia, and the presence of urine reducing substances. A definitive diagnosis should include measurement of urinary amino acids and the excretion of glucose, phosphate, creatinine, and protein.

In contrast, metabolic acidemias caused by the accumulation of acid metabolites generally cause a normochloremic acidosis with an elevated anion gap. Even with an equivocal gap, an unexplained acidemia may warrant additional workup to identify the unknown substance. There are several major categories of accumulated anions that cause acidosis in pediatric patients, and determining which one is elevated is a key step in establishing a definitive diagnosis.

Determine What Type of Acid Is Being Accumulated

Acid accumulation can be caused by stressed normal physiology, toxic ingestion, and inborn errors of metabolism. Table 133-3 lists major causes of gap acidoses. Note that toxins may cause an acidosis by being acidic themselves or by causing secondary metabolic derangements. A good

Table 133-3 Causes of Gap Metabolic Acidosis: MUDPILE	
M:	Methanol (causes accumulation of formic acid) Ethylene glycol and other alcohols
U:	Uremia, renal failure (elevated PO_4, SO_4)
D:	Diabetes (ketoacidosis) Drugs (isoniazid, many others) Diet (high protein, starvation)
P:	Paraldehyde

I:	Inborn errors of metabolism
	    Organic acidemias (e.g., methylmalonicacidemia,
	        propionicacidemia, isovalericacidemia)
	    Secondary acidemias (e.g., ketoacidosis, lactic acidosis
	        due to other primary conditions)

L:	Lactic acidosis (see Table 133-4)
E:	Ethanol (alcoholic ketoacidosis)

Table 133-4   Causes of Lactic Acidosis

States of increased metabolic activity
    Strenuous exercise
    Seizures
    Respiratory distress

States of inadequate oxygen delivery to end organs
    Decreased cardiac output
    Shock (cardiac, septic, hypovolemic)
    Anemia
    Hypoxemia
    Ischemia

Inborn errors of metabolism
    Electron transport chain defects
    Pyruvate dehydrogenase deficiency
    Glycogen storage disease type I
    Pyruvate carboxylase deficiency
    Biotinidase deficiency
    Disorders of gluconeogenesis
    Others

Toxins and drugs   Electron transport chain poisons (cyanide)

example of the latter is the relentless lactic acidosis caused by electron transport chain poisoning with cyanide. Methanol is metabolized to formic acid, which, as an unmeasured anion, increases the anion gap. Other important toxins include toluene, sulfur, iron, isoniazid, ethylene glycol, and salicylates.

Similarly, metabolic disorders can cause acidemia either primarily or secondarily. Propionicacidemia, an organic acidemia (see later), causes a primary acidosis through the accumulation of several organic acids, including propionic acid, lactic acid, and ketone bodies. By contrast, some of the fatty acid oxidation disorders can cause cardiomyopathy, with subsequent decreased tissue perfusion and a secondary lactic acidosis.

Among the types of nonvolatile acids associated with gap acidosis when produced in excess, three categories are particularly important in pediatrics: lactic acid, ketone bodies, and other organic acids that accumulate in specific inborn errors of metabolism.

Lactic Acid

Excess lactic acid is the most common cause of metabolic acidosis in the pediatric population. Table 133-4 lists some of the many causes of lactic acidosis. Lactic acid and pyruvic acid are formed by glycolysis. Lactate and pyruvate are maintained at an approximate 10:1 molar ratio. The normal lactate range varies among laboratories but is generally 0.5 to 2 mEq/L (the alternative unit mmol/L is equal to mEq/L for lactate). Interpretation of a lactate result requires knowledge of the patient's age and fasting or fed state, as well as the conditions under which the sample was obtained. Because glycolysis is the primary energy metabolism pathway when oxygen is in short supply, it is not surprising that most cases of lactic acidosis are due to temporary tissue hypoperfusion and hypoxia. Lactic acidosis may also be a clue to an inborn error of metabolism and can occur due to decreased utilization of pyruvate by downstream enzymes (see Table 133-4). Note that lactic acidosis may be present without frank acidemia or an anion gap. Serum lactate measurement may reveal an elevated lactate level in the context of a normal blood pH and only a mild increase in the anion gap.

A departure from the normal 10:1 ratio of lactate to pyruvate can help narrow the differential diagnosis for lactic acidosis. For example, if a lactic acidosis is due to a respiratory chain defect, lactate and pyruvate should be measured simultaneously and usually have a ratio greater than 10:1. By contrast, pyruvate dehydrogenase deficiency is often associated with increases in both lactate and pyruvate, yielding a normal ratio. Whenever possible, an arterial sample should be collected for lactate and pyruvate measurements. Blood collected distal to the capillary bed often results in a falsely elevated lactate level and lactate-pyruvate ratio. The use of a tourniquet can also cause false-positive results.

Ketones

In the absence of adequate glucose, the body uses fatty acids as an energy source. Partial oxidative metabolism of fatty acids in the liver generates ketones (3-hydroxybutyrate and acetoacetate). These substances are strong acids and can cause a significant elevation of the anion gap and depression in the blood pH when present in millimolar amounts (ketoacidosis), as commonly occurs in diabetes, certain organic acid disorders, and inborn errors of ketone utilization. Specific ketone body concentrations can be measured to confirm that accumulation is contributing to a measured acidemia. Total ketones are usually around 0.1 mM in the nonfasting state but may increase to 2 mM with vigorous exercise. Levels as high as 3 mM can be achieved with a 24-hour fast. Levels in excess of 3 mM or elevation or depression in the setting of a noncongruous history suggests a biochemical disorder.[6]

Other Organic Acids

The organic acidemias are a large group of relatively rare inborn errors of metabolism that share the common feature of generating elevated amounts of nonvolatile acidic metabolic intermediates called organic acids. These non-amino carbon-containing acids are usually derived from aberrant amino acid oxidation. Examples include methylmalonicacidemia, propionicacidemia, and related conditions. Many organic acidemias can be detected, or even diagnosed definitively, by urinary organic acid analysis. Presentations vary from acute to chronic acidemia, with correspondingly dramatic or indolent clinical courses. The presence of an organic acidemia is suggested by a gap metabolic acidemia not adequately explained by the clinical setting or by a profound metabolic ketoacidosis in an otherwise unexpected setting. It is not uncommon for these patients to present with serum bicarbonate concentrations less than 15 mEq/L and a venous pH less than 7.2.

Review of Standard Laboratory Data

Review of routine laboratory data should be performed before specialized tests are considered. Calculations such as the anion gap and delta ratio can be used as adjuncts to interpret the acid-base information provided by a standard electrolyte panel. The anion gap should be determined using the following formula:

$$\text{Anion gap} = Na^+ - (Cl^- + HCO_3^-)$$

The anion gap calculation attempts to determine whether the measured cations and anions are present in proportionate amounts.[7,8] A gap acidosis is present when the concentration of anions is lower than expected. The assumption is that some nonmeasured anion is present in an amount sufficient to satisfy electroneutrality. The anion gap's normal range (12 ± 2 mEq/L) assumes a normal amount of serum protein. Hypoalbuminemia may create a falsely normal anion gap in the presence of a significant amount of unmeasured anion.

The delta ratio is used to determine how much of a metabolic acid is being buffered by bicarbonate,[9] or

$$\text{Delta ratio} = [Na^+ - Cl^- + HCO_3^- - (\text{normal anion gap})]/ \\ [(\text{normal serum bicarbonate}) - HCO_3]$$

Where a "normal" anion gap is typically 12 and a "normal" bicarbonate is typically 24 (all units in mEq/L or mmol/L). This relationship can also be stated as the increase in anion gap divided by the decrease in bicarbonate. The expectation is that one molecule of metabolic acid becomes buffered ($HA \rightarrow H^+ + A^-$) for every molecule of bicarbonate used to accomplish the buffering ($HCO_3^- + H^+ \rightarrow H_2O + CO_2$). If the change in the anion gap (normal gap minus measured gap) is equal to the change in the bicarbonate level (normal bicarbonate minus measured bicarbonate), then the ratio will equal 1, and all the excess metabolic acid and missing bicarbonate will have been accounted for. Any other result indicates a more complicated situation.

A large delta ratio (an anion gap larger than expected for the change in bicarbonate) suggests that excess bicarbonate is present (concurrent metabolic alkalosis or preexisting compensated respiratory acidosis). A small delta ratio suggests hyperchloremia (excess chloride ions are increasing the gap) or a combined gap-nongap metabolic acidosis. The delta ratio should be interpreted with caution for several reasons, including the following:

- The "normal" gap contains a number of substances, such as albumin, that are not always present in normal amounts.

- There is a range of normal anion gaps and bicarbonate levels to choose from.
- Intracellular and extracellular buffering may not be equivalent, and the laboratory values used to measure the delta ratio measure only extracellular ions.

The osmolar gap is calculated according to the following formula:

$$\text{Measured osmolarity} = (2 \times \text{Plasma } [Na^+] + \\ [\text{Glucose}]/18 + \text{Blood urea nitrogen}/2.8)$$

The normal range is 10 to 15.[10] Methanol and ethylene glycol ingestions create an increased osmolar gap by adding osmoles to the blood that are not included in the calculated osmolality equation.

Other diagnostic clues can be gleaned from routine laboratory studies. Creatinine and blood urea nitrogen should be scrutinized to rule out renal impairment. Hyperglycemia may indicate diabetes or, less commonly, an organic aciduria. Hypoglycemia is seen with disorders of gluconeogenesis, fatty acid oxidation disorders, and some organic acidemias. Fatty acid oxidation disorders are usually distinguishable from organic acidemias because the former are typically associated with relative hypoketosis, whereas the latter are associated with ketosis and lactic acidemia. In addition to being useful for categorizing the acid-base imbalance, blood gas and serum bicarbonate measurements may prompt further investigation simply because of the severity of the acidemia. Markedly abnormal serum pH levels (6.9 to 7.2) and serum bicarbonate levels (sometimes below the laboratory's ability to measure) should raise suspicion for an inborn error of metabolism.

Standard urinalysis may provide a wealth of information in the setting of a metabolic acidemia. Inappropriately alkalotic urine in the setting of an acidemia suggests renal tubular acidosis. It should be noted, however, that both gastrointestinal and renal losses of bicarbonate can cause inappropriately alkalotic urine. If the alkalotic urine is caused by gastrointestinal losses, the alkalosis is secondary to ammonium ion secretion from the kidney as opposed to renal tubular dysfunction. Ammonium ion excretion can be estimated using the urine net charge (UNC) calculation:

$$\text{UNC} = Na^+ + K^+ - Cl^-$$

A negative UNC is assumed to be made up of ammonium ions. Importantly, the UNC measurement assumes that no other unaccounted for acid (e.g., an organic acid) is present. Urine ketones are helpful in detecting ketoacidosis and in categorizing inborn errors of metabolism. A positive heme test may be due to the rhabdomyolysis seen in some fatty acid oxidation defects.

Finally, the newborn screening results should be reviewed for every neonatal patient with a septic or catastrophic shocklike presentation. With the increasing use of tandem mass spectrometry, important information may be available from the prenatal panel. If an inborn error of metabolism is suspected and the newborn screening results are not yet available, the state or reference laboratory should be alerted and instructed to process the sample urgently. If a sample was not obtained, it should be done immediately, and always before a transfusion is given.

Table 133-5   Specialized Investigations in Acidotic Children

Test	Utility
Ketones	Verify ketoacidosis
Ammonia	Hyperammonemia occurs in liver failure and in some inborn errors; it can contribute to encephalopathy in acidotic patients
Plasma lactate, pyruvate	Used to identify disorders with primary or secondary elevations in lactate; lactate-pyruvate ratio is sometimes useful in differentiating among lactic acidosis syndromes
Plasma amino acids	Particular patterns of abnormalities suggest specific inborn errors
Plasma carnitine (free and total)	Decreased carnitine occurs in a variety of organic acidemias and fatty acid oxidation defects; carnitine replacement is particularly important in such patients
Plasma acylcarnitine profile	Quantitative acylcarnitine patterns are essentially diagnostic for a variety of organic acidemias and fatty acid oxidation disorders
Urinary amino acids	Global elevations occur in renal Fanconi syndrome, as the proximal renal tubule fails to resorb filtered amino acids
Urinary organic acids	Abnormal elevations of particular metabolites aid in the diagnosis of many inborn errors; excretion of ketones and lactate can also be documented and quantitated
CSF studies	Amino acids, lactate, pyruvate, and organic acids can be measured; if a patient with a suspected inborn error has a lumbar puncture, consider saving a small amount of CSF for metabolic studies

CSF, cerebrospinal fluid.

Specialized Investigations

The specialized investigations used to work up rare causes of acidemia should be performed in consultation with genetics and metabolism staff. The following general principles apply to many specialized metabolic tests. First, make certain that the proper tubes are used (some tests require nonstandard tubes) and that adequate specimens are collected. Some tests, such as serum ammonia and serum lactate, are notoriously susceptible to false-positive results if the samples are drawn or handled incorrectly. Second, samples should be obtained concurrently whenever possible. Biochemical parameters may change rapidly, especially with treatment. Test results obtained from the same blood draw are much more easily compared than are those drawn at different times.

Assuming that standard serum electrolytes and liver enzyme tests, urinalysis, and blood gas measurements have been done, additional tests for a patient with acidosis of an unclear cause include those listed in Table 133-5. A review of the history, preferably with a metabolic specialist, may prompt the inclusion of additional tests.

Plasma amino acid and urinary organic acid analysis may provide pathognomonic or diagnostically important results. A host of conditions can be detected by these analyses, making them critical to the workup of an acidemia of unknown cause. Interpretation requires a biochemical genetics specialist. Some toxic ingestions, such as ethylene glycol, can also be diagnosed by means of amino acid and organic acid analysis.

Serum ammonia elevations are seen in some organic acidemias as well as with hepatic dysfunction. Hyperammonemia can also occur in a number of conditions not associated with acidemia, such as urea cycle disorders (see Chapter 131).

TREATMENT

An algorithm for the treatment of a decompensated child with unexplained severe acidemia is presented in Table 133-6. The general approach is similar to that used for any critically ill child: airway, breathing, and circulation are the initial priorities. Subsequent steps strive to reverse the often precipitous decline in homeostasis that accompanies many metabolic disorders. Fluid resuscitation should be undertaken carefully with 5 to 10 mL/kg boluses of normal saline, followed by reassessment. Overvigorous resuscitation may increase the risk for cerebral edema and fluid shifts. Many patients have coexisting volume losses, which makes sodium and potassium balance important.

Metabolic emergencies are often triggered by fasting physiology. Fatty acid oxidation disorders, for instance, may not cause noticeable disease until glucose stores are low. These patients usually have fasting intolerance and become symptomatic when stressed. Dextrose is administered at a high concentration and rate. Peripheral intravenous access allows a 12.5% dextrose solution to be given at 1.5 times the basal Holliday-Segar fluid rate. For severely ill children, central access should be obtained without delay. Carnitine may be considered because it is beneficial in some disorders and is generally safe over a wide dosage range. The oral dose is 50 to 100 mg/kg/day divided into two or three doses (max 3 g/24 hours). The IV dose is usually 50 mg/kg/24 hours divided into four doses. In addition, children must receive adequate nutrition as soon as possible, especially those with metabolic disorders, even if total parenteral nutrition is necessary. This reverses catabolism and provides for the ongoing anabolic demands of growth.

Correction of the acidosis with bicarbonate, tromethamine (THAM), citrate, or acetate is controversial.[11] The

Table 133-6 Acute Correction Algorithm for Patients Suspected of Having an Inborn Error of Metabolism

1. ABCs (airway, breathing circulation)

2. Cautious fluid resuscitation

3. Dextrose infusion

4. Calculate base deficit and consider correction if severe

   Base deficit (in mEq) = Deficit × 0.3 × Weight (in kg)

   To correct: replace $^1/_2$ deficit and reassess acid-base status
   a. Sodium bicarbonate
      Benefits: readily available
      Watch for: hypercapnia, hypernatremia, fluid overload
   b. Tromethamine (THAM)
      Benefits: useful in setting of poor ventilation or hypernatremia
      Watch for: hypoglycemia
   c. Acetate, citrate
      Benefits: oral preparations available; potassium salts available for inclusion in intravenous infusions
      Watch for: requires functional Krebs cycle in liver; not recommended in ill patients with metabolic disorders

5. Consider carnitine

6. Metabolism consultation

risks of bicarbonate therapy include volume overload, central nervous system acidosis, hypokalemia, and hypercapnia.[12] THAM can cause hypoglycemia and artificially lowers the anion gap by adding unmeasured cations to the acid-base system. As an initial approximation, many clinicians start by giving a one-half deficit replacement and then titrate further therapy based on the change in acid-base status. Serum potassium levels must be followed closely while an acidemia is being corrected.

CONSULTATION

Depending on the underlying cause of the acidosis, the following consultative services may be helpful:

- Genetics—for determination of a specific inborn error of metabolism and assistance in obtaining specialized laboratory tests. Input from a geneticist with training in biochemical genetics is optimal.
- Neurology—for evaluation of the variety of abnormal neurologic findings in patients with metabolic acidosis.
- Nutrition—for assistance in obtaining specialized diets when indicated.
- Nephrology and gastroenterology—for evaluation of patients with suspected primary renal or hepatic disorders.

ADMISSION CRITERIA

For patients with metabolic disorders known to cause rapid deterioration, there is a low threshold for hospital admission. Patients with unknown causes of acidemia should also be worked up aggressively. Criteria for admission include the following:

- Young age, especially neonates.
- Lack of an obvious cause for the acidemia.
- Anion gap acidosis.
- Evidence of systemic decompensation (e.g., altered mentation, coordination, arousal, or respiratory status).

Once the conditions that cause rapid deterioration are excluded, the remainder of the workup can proceed on an outpatient basis.

DISCHARGE CRITERIA

- Stabilization of acid-base balance.
- Establishment of a diagnosis.
- Initiation of appropriate medical or dietary therapy.
- Confirmation of adequate feeding and weight gain.
- Establishment of appropriate follow-up and family education.

IN A NUTSHELL

- Metabolic acidosis can present with a wide variety of signs and symptoms referable to multiple organ systems.
- The differential diagnosis of metabolic acidosis includes moderate to severe infection, inborn errors of metabolism, and chronic hepatic and renal disease.
- Confirmation of metabolic acidosis includes differentiating secondary metabolic acidosis due to common illnesses from more unusual conditions requiring further workup, distinguishing acid accumulation from bicarbonate loss, and determining the type of acid being accumulated.
- In addition to standard laboratory testing, determination of the anion gap, osmolar gap, and urine net charge may be useful in making a diagnosis.

ON THE HORIZON

- Most of the children presenting with metabolic acidosis fall into one of several well-known categories. Thus, many rarer metabolic disorders are not diagnosed until multiple episodes force more complete investigations. The adoption of expanded newborn screening by many states may allow the earlier diagnosis of some inborn errors of metabolism. In addition, screening suggests that mild forms of inborn errors (partial enzyme deficiency) are more prevalent than previously thought. It will become increasingly common for patients to present to general practitioners with preexisting conditions known to predispose them to episodes of metabolic acidosis.

SUGGESTED READING

Clarke JTR (ed): A Clinical Guide to Inherited Metabolic Diseases, 2nd ed. Cambridge, Cambridge University Press, 2002.

Hoffman GF, Nyhan WL, Zschocke J, et al: Inherited Metabolic Diseases. Philadelphia, Lippincott Williams & Wilkins, 2002.

Roth KS, Cohn RM: Biochemistry and Disease: Bridging Basic Science and Clinical Practice. Baltimore, Williams & Wilkins, 1996.

REFERENCES

1. Kellum JA: Determinants of blood pH in health and disease. Crit Care 2000;4:6-14.

2. Seale JL, Conway JM, Canary JJ: Seven-day validation of doubly labeled water method using indirect room calorimetry. J Appl Physiol 1993; 74:402-409.

3. Gluck SL: Acid sensing in renal epithelial cells. J Clin Invest 2004;114: 1696-1699.

4. Levraut J, Grimaud D: Treatment of metabolic acidosis. Curr Opin Crit Care 2003;9:260-265.

5. Oh MS: New perspectives on acid-base balance. Semin Dial 2000;13: 212-219.

6. Hoffman GF, Nyhan WL, Zschocke J, et al: Inherited Metabolic Diseases. Philadelphia, Lippincott Williams & Wilkins, 2002.

7. Maloney DG, Appadurai IR, Vaughan RS: Anions and the anaesthetist. Anaesthesia 2002;57:140-154.

8. Morgan TJ: What exactly is the strong ion gap, and does anybody care? Crit Care Resuscitation 2006;6:155-159.

9. Brandis K: The Delta ratio. *http://www.anaesthesiamcq.com/AcidBase Book/ab3_3.php.*

10. Purssell RA, Lynd LD, Koga Y: The use of the osmole gap as a screening test for the presence of exogenous substances. Toxicol Rev 2004;23:189-202.

11. Gunnerson KJ, Kellum JA: Acid-base and electrolyte analysis in critically ill patients: Are we ready for the new millennium? Curr Opin Crit Care 2003;9:468-473.

12. Adrogue HJ, Madias NE: Management of life-threatening acid-base disorders: First of two parts. N Engl J Med 1998;338:26-34.

Allergy and Immunology

CHAPTER 134

Anaphylaxis
Grace M. Cheng

Anaphylaxis is a serious and acute allergic response that causes a sudden and massive release of mast cell and basophil chemical mediators, triggering multiple system abnormalities. Classically, anaphylaxis involves hypotension of two or more organ systems.

PATHOPHYSIOLOGY

Two forms of anaphylaxis are recognized but are clinically indistinguishable and managed identically: immunoglobulin E (IgE)-mediated anaphylaxis and anaphylactoid reactions. IgE-mediated anaphylaxis occurs when allergen-specific IgE antibodies bind to high-affinity mast cell and basophil IgE FcɛR1 receptors and cross-link these receptors. Typical triggers of IgE-mediated anaphylaxis include foods, Hymenoptera stings, latex, and antibiotics.

Anaphylactoid reactions appear to be caused by direct release of mast cell and basophil chemical mediators. Examples of anaphylactoid triggers include blood product infusions, hyperosmolar radiocontrast dye, vancomycin, and opiates.

Regardless of the initial cause, the mast cells and basophils degranulate and release histamine and other biochemical mediators that cause a multisystem response. Histamine response is mediated through histamine receptors. Vasodilation, tachycardia, and bronchospasm result from H_1 receptors; headache, increased vascular permeability, flushing, and hypotension develop from both H_1 and H_2 receptor responses. Cutaneous pruritus and nasal congestion may be mediated by both H_1 and H_3 receptor pathways.[1] Of note, mast cells also release β-tryptase during anaphylaxis; thus, transiently elevated levels of serum β-tryptase are consistent with anaphylaxis.

EPIDEMIOLOGY

The estimated yearly incidence of anaphylaxis is not known but is estimated at less than 1%. Death from anaphylaxis occurs rarely; a population-based study of mostly adult residents of Olmsted County, Minnesota, demonstrated an average annual incidence rate of 21 per 100,000 person-years and a case-fatality rate of 0.6%.[2] One retrospective chart review of pediatric cases revealed an estimated incidence rate of 10.5 per 100,000 person-years.[3]

The cause of anaphylaxis is not always identified. In the Olmsted County study, a suspected allergen was temporally associated with the anaphylactic reaction in 68% of events, but only 40% of patients in this cohort underwent either skin or in vitro testing. The pediatric study reported that 88% of anaphylactic episodes had a documented cause in the patients' records, but it did not report what percentage of patients had allergy testing.

The most common causes of inpatient anaphylactic reactions are muscle relaxants used during surgical procedures (vecuronium, atracurium, succinylcholine, pancuronium), latex, antibiotics (intravenous penicillin and ampicillin most frequently), blood products, and contrast material.[4] Patients at highest risk for latex allergy are those with a history of multiple surgical procedures (especially patients with spina bifida or urologic abnormalities) and atopic individuals.

The most common causes of outpatient anaphylaxis are food allergy, Hymenoptera stings, medications, and exercise, although many cases have no identifiable trigger. Food allergy accounts for approximately one third of all identifiable cases of anaphylaxis. Eight foods cause more than 90% of allergies: peanuts, tree nuts, fish, shellfish, cow's milk, egg, soy, and wheat. Furthermore, 3% of the U.S. population is sensitive to insect stings. Monoclonal antibody medications and allergen immunotherapy may precipitate anaphylaxis.

CLINICAL PRESENTATION

Most anaphylactic reactions occur within 1 hour of exposure, and more rapid symptom onset usually heralds a more severe reaction. The severity of the anaphylactic reaction depends on the route of exposure, amount of allergen, and constancy of exposure (more frequent exposures may yield less serious reactions with subsequent exposures). Intravenous (IV) exposure typically causes more immediate and more severe reactions, while oral exposure generally results in a more delayed presentation (from minutes to 2 hours), as well as an increased prevalence of gastrointestinal symptoms. Typical organ system reactions are presented in Table 134-1.

The majority of fatalities occur within 30 minutes after antigen exposure, usually from cardiovascular collapse or respiratory failure. In children and adults, 50% to 60% of fatalities are associated with upper airway edema, and 27% to 50% are associated with bronchial obstruction and lung

Table 134–1 Organ System Involvement in Anaphylaxis

Organ	Clinical Findings	Percentage of Patients with Organ Involvement
Skin	Urticaria or angioedema, pruritus, flushing, nonpitting edema	90
Respiratory	Bronchospasm or laryngeal edema, wheeze, cough, dyspnea, hoarseness, hypersalivation, stridor, rhinorrhea, sneeze	70
Cardiovascular	Vasodilation, increased vascular permeability, shock, hypotension, tachycardia, syncope, arrhythmia or arrest, premature atrial or ventricular contractions, ventricular fibrillation, asystole	30
Gastrointestinal	Vomiting, nausea, diarrhea, cramps	30
Other	Sense of impending doom, headache, loss of consciousness, conjunctivitis, urinary incontinence, pelvic pain, uterine contractions	

hyperinflation. In postmortem findings from a U.K. study of fatal cases of anaphylaxis, upper airway edema was more common in deaths associated with food allergens than in those caused by venom or drug reactions.[5] Cardiovascular collapse has been documented in a few patients with anaphylaxis without cutaneous or respiratory symptoms.

Some individuals exhibit a biphasic response, with potentially more severe anaphylactic symptoms recurring after resolution of the initial symptoms. Ninety percent of biphasic reactions occur within 4 hours after the initial symptoms, but they may occur up to 12 hours later. Although the cause of this response is unknown, delayed administration of epinephrine and greater severity of initial symptoms appear to be associated with a higher risk of biphasic reactions. Steroid administration may not reduce the likelihood of a late-phase response.[6]

DIFFERENTIAL DIAGNOSIS

The diagnosis of anaphylaxis requires a manifestation of hypotension or anaphylactic symptoms in two or more organ systems, exposure to an agent known to trigger anaphylaxis, or evidence of an IgE-mediated response to an agent. Other conditions may resemble anaphylaxis and must be considered in the differential diagnosis, including syncope and vasovagal responses, hereditary angioedema, urticaria, asthma, shock from other causes, globus hystericus, and serum sickness. Syncopal or vasovagal events typically lack the bronchospasm and urticaria present in anaphylaxis; additionally, bradycardia and pallor are more likely with a vasovagal response, whereas tachycardia and diaphoresis may be more common in anaphylaxis. Hereditary angioedema often presents in adolescents or, less commonly, in school-aged children with recurrent laryngeal edema, abdominal pain, nausea, vomiting, or diarrhea. Septic and spinal shock may appear clinically similar to anaphylactic shock, but the patient's history aids in the diagnosis. Cardiogenic, hemorrhagic, and hypovolemic shock are all more likely to present with peripheral vasoconstriction, whereas anaphylaxis typically presents with peripheral vasodilation. Patients may present with urticaria in isolation or only with symptoms of asthma, but anaphylaxis should be considered if more than one organ system is involved. Serum sickness may also present with urticaria or angioedema but is typically associated with fever, lymphadenopathy, arthralgia, and

arthritis. Other possible diagnoses include foreign body aspiration, pulmonary embolism, cardiac dysfunction, seizure, mastocytosis, scombroid poisoning, or factitious anaphylaxis.

TREATMENT

Although the mainstay of treatment of anaphylaxis is epinephrine, initial assessment and management of airway, breathing, and circulation (the ABCs) are critical, along with removal of the inciting allergen. In the inpatient setting, cessation of any IV agents and avoidance of latex may be a vital step in preventing the progression of anaphylaxis.

Airway and breathing must be managed with positioning, oxygenation, bag-valve-mask ventilation, and intubation if necessary. Intubation can be complicated by laryngeal edema, and the endotracheal tube size required to manage the airway may be smaller than expected. Consider fiberoptic tracheal intubation or needle cricothyrotomy with a 14- or 16-gauge IV catheter, subsequently connected to the hub of a 2.0 or 3.0 endotracheal tube, for transtracheal ventilation. Specifically, cricothyrotomy may be required if laryngeal edema prevents successful intubation.

Hypotension and shock may occur rapidly, because the increased vascular permeability of anaphylaxis can cause 20% to 50% of the intravascular fluid to diffuse rapidly to the extravascular space. Shock should be managed aggressively with epinephrine and fluid boluses.

Epinephrine is the most important medication for the acute treatment of anaphylaxis. The doses are provided in Table 134-2. Subcutaneous delivery is no longer recommended owing to poorer and slower absorption, particularly if skin manifestations of anaphylaxis are present. The maximum single dose of epinephrine is 0.5 mg. For patients with anaphylaxis, give 0.01 mg/kg of epinephrine intramuscularly (0.01 mL/kg of 1:1000 solution). Repeat doses can be given every 5 minutes. For hypotensive patients or patients who already have intravenous access, consider giving the epinephrine intravenously at the standard cardiac arrest dose of 0.01 mg/kg (0.1 mL/kg of 1:10,000 solution). If hypotension, severe airway compromise, or cardiopulmonary arrest is occurring and IV access is not in place, epinephrine may be administered through intraosseous access at the IV dose. If the patient continues to have an inadequate response to epinephrine, an IV infusion of epinephrine at 0.1 µg/kg per

Table 134-2 Pharmacologic Treatment of Anaphylaxis	
Agent	Dose
Epinephrine	
IM*	0.01 mL/kg of 1:1000 solution[†]
IV or IO*	0.1 mL/kg of 1:10,000 solution[‡]
IV infusion*	0.1 µg/kg/min initially, then titrated up as needed to 1 µg/kg/min
Diphenhydramine PO or IV	1 mg/kg (maximum 50 mg/dose)
Ranitidine or famotidine PO or IV	1-2 mg/kg (maximum 50 mg/dose)
Methylprednisolone IV	1-2 mg/kg (maximum 125 mg/dose
Glucagon[¶]	
IV	≤20 kg: 0.5 mg (or 20-30 µg/kg) >20 kg: 1 mg

*Repeat every 3 to 5 minutes if needed.
[†]Up to 0.5 mL maximum/dose.
[‡]Up to 5 mL maximum/dose.
[¶]Use only if patient is on β-adrenergic antagonist therapy.
IM, intramuscularly; IO, intraosseously; IV, intravenously; PO, orally.

minute, should be initiated and titrated as necessary up to 1 µg/kg per minute.

Delays in giving epinephrine injections have been documented in many witnessed anaphylactic fatalities. In a study comparing fatal to near-fatal anaphylactic reactions to food in children and adolescents, the authors noted that only two of six patients who died of anaphylaxis, versus five of seven who survived, received epinephrine within 1 hour of ingesting the inciting allergen.[7]

Additional therapy for anaphylaxis includes antihistamines, steroids, and albuterol. Diphenhydramine (1 mg/kg intravenously or orally, up to 50 mg/dose) is an H_1 receptor inverse agonist and can help reduce urticaria, angioedema, and pruritus, but it works more slowly than epinephrine and cannot stop anaphylaxis if histamine is already present in large quantities at the histamine receptors. Ranitidine and famotidine (1 to 2 mg/kg [up to 50 mg/dose] intravenously or orally) are H_2 receptor antagonists and may ameliorate persistent hypotension. If the IV route is not readily available, liquid or chewable tablets of any orally administered antihistamine are recommended owing to their faster absorption rate. Methylprednisolone 1 to 2 mg/kg (up to 125 mg/dose) intravenously, or an equivalent dose of another steroid medication, is also recommended. Bronchospasm can be treated with nebulized albuterol, and stridor can be treated with nebulized racemic epinephrine.

Patients on beta-blocker therapy may have persistent hypotension during anaphylaxis despite treatment with epinephrine owing to the predominant α-adrenergic effects of epinephrine in these patients. Glucagon directly activates cellular adenyl cyclase and bypasses the β-adrenergic receptor in stimulating positive inotropic and chronotropic cardiac effects. Among children with anaphylaxis who are taking beta-blockers, the dosage of glucagon is based on the child's weight: for those over 20 kg, give 1 mg IV bolus; for those under 20 kg, give 0.5 mg IV bolus (or 20 to 30 µg/kg).

A subsequent continuous infusion may be necessary to maintain blood pressure.

ADMISSION CRITERIA AND FOLLOW-UP

Indications for admission of a patient with anaphylaxis include hypotension, airway obstruction, prolonged bronchospasm, or poor access to follow-up care. If possible, all patients should be observed for at least 4 hours after the onset of anaphylaxis for signs of late-phase reactions. Prednisone (2 mg/kg per day; 60 mg maximum) and diphenhydramine (5 mg/kg per day divided every 6 hours; maximum 50 mg/dose) are recommended for 3 to 5 days after an anaphylactic reaction. Every patient with anaphylaxis should be prescribed an EpiPen (children ≥22 kg) or EpiPen Jr. (those <22 kg), and the patient and his or her caregivers should be instructed in its use. In one survey, only 30% of individuals with food allergy or their caregivers could demonstrate appropriate use of an autoinjector.[8] The child and family should also be educated on how to avoid allergic triggers. For food allergy, the Food Allergy and Anaphylaxis Network (*www.foodallergy.org*) is a helpful nonprofit resource for food allergy avoidance strategies. Medical alert bracelets should be considered as well. All patients with anaphylactic reactions should be referred to an allergist.

ON THE HORIZON

- Ongoing studies are exploring ways to prevent anaphylaxis, including novel vaccine delivery systems, allergen immunotherapies, and monoclonal anti-IgE therapy.

SUGGESTED READING

Kemp SF: Current concepts in pathophysiology, diagnosis, and management of anaphylaxis. Immunol Allergy Clin North Am 2001;21:611-634.

Leung DY: Effect of anti-IgE therapy in patients with peanut allergy. N Engl J Med 2003;348:986-993.

Sicherer SH, Furlong TJ, Desimone JD, Sampson HA: The US Peanut and Tree Nut Allergy Registry: Characteristics of reactions in schools and day care. J Pediatr 2001;138:560-565.

REFERENCES

1. Simons FER: Advances in H1-antihistamines. N Engl J Med 2004;351: 2203-2217.
2. Yocum MW, Butterfield JH, Klein JS, et al: Epidemiology of anaphylaxis in Olmsted County: A population-based study. J Allergy Clin Immunol 1999;104:452-456.
3. Bohlke K, Davis RL, DeStefano F, et al: Epidemiology of anaphylaxis among children and adolescents enrolled in a health maintenance organization. J Allergy Clin Immunol 2004;113:536-542.
4. Lieberman P: Anaphylactic reactions during surgical and medical procedures. J Allergy Clin Immunol 2002;110:564-569.
5. Pumphrey RSH, Roberts ISD: Postmortem findings after fatal anaphylactic reactions. J Clin Pathol 2000;53:273-276.
6. Lee JM, Greenes DS: Biphasic anaphylactic reactions in pediatrics. Pediatrics 2000;106:762-766.
7. Sampson HA, Mendelson L, Rosen JP: Fatal and near-fatal anaphylactic reactions to food in children and adolescents. N Engl J Med 1992;327:380-384.
8. Sicherer SH: Use assessment of self-administered epinephrine among food-allergic children and pediatricians. Pediatrics 2000;105:359-362.

CHAPTER 135

Drug Allergy

Jordan Scott

Adverse drug reactions are broadly defined by the World Health Organization as "any noxious, unintended, and undesired effect of a drug that occurs at doses used for prevention, diagnosis, or treatment."[1] These reactions can be classified into types A and B.

Type A reactions, which account for most adverse drug reactions, are predictable, dose dependent, and related to the pharmacologic mechanism of the drug. Examples include respiratory depression with the administration of increasing amounts of opiates or cushingoid features with chronic systemic steroid use. Type B reactions are unpredictable, dose independent, and not related to the drug's pharmacologic actions. Allergic reactions to a medication are included in this type. Another example of a type B reaction is drug-induced lupus from minocycline.

Allergic reactions require prior sensitization and typically show signs consistent with an underlying allergic mechanism. They eventually resolve after the implicated drug is discontinued.[2] Nonimmune hypersensitivity reactions, also termed pseudoallergic reactions, are clinically similar to allergic reactions but cannot be proved to be immunologic owing to a lack of detectable drug-specific antibodies or drug-specific T lymphocytes. Many causes for these reactions have been proposed, and they are dependent on the implicated drug. For example, the "allergic reaction" caused by radiocontrast material could be from nonspecific histamine release and complement activation, while the chronic cough seen with angiotensin-converting enzyme inhibitors could be from the accumulation of bradykinin.[3] This chapter focuses primarily on immune-mediated type B reactions.

PATHOPHYSIOLOGY

The immune-mediated reactions are organized according to the Gell and Coombs classification,[1] as follows:

Type I: immediate hypersensitivity reactions (anaphylaxis)
Type II: cytotoxic antibody reactions
Type III: immune complex reactions
Type IV: delayed hypersensitivity reactions

Type I reactions develop when a drug or drug metabolite interacts with preformed specific immunoglobulin E (IgE) antibodies bound to mast cells and basophils. This results in cross-linking of IgE FcɛR1 receptors on mast cells and basophils, leading to cellular degranulation and the release of histamine and leukotrienes. These released chemicals propagate urticaria, bronchospasm, vasodilation, and other manifestations of anaphylaxis (see Chapter 134). Type II reactions involve binding of IgG or IgM antibodies to recognized cell membrane–bound drug antigen. The cells become coated with antibody and are then injured via the complement system. Drug-induced hemolytic anemia is an example of such a reaction. Type III reactions are due to soluble antigen-antibody complexes deposited in the walls of blood vessels, which then activate the complement cascade. This is seen in serum sickness, which consists of fever, urticaria, lymphadenopathy, arthralgias, and a characteristic serpiginous rash at the interfacing dorsal-ventral regions of the hands and feet. Type IV reactions involve antigen-specific T-lymphocyte–mediated reactions, such as those seen in allergic contact dermatitis. Classifying drug hypersensitivities into one of these four categories may not always be possible.

A hapten is a small antigenic determinant that can cause an immune response only when bound to a carrier molecule. Reactive drug metabolites, acting as haptens, may bind to proteins, resulting in the creation of immunogens that may then elicit an immune response. Penicillin, for example, is reactive because of its unstable β-lactam ring, which can open to bind with other proteins.[1,3,4] Penicillin is metabolized to penicilloyl, and, when combined with a protein, it is known as the major determinant. Penicillin can also be metabolized to penicilloate, penilloate, and benzyl-*n*-propylamine. When coupled with proteins, these are known as the minor determinants. Major and minor determinant-specific IgE responses detected on skin testing tend to be associated with urticaria and anaphylaxis, respectively.[3]

EPIDEMIOLOGY

A meta-analysis of 39 prospective studies of hospitalized patients found that serious drug reactions can affect up to 6.7% of hospitalized patients, and the incidence of fatal drug reactions is about 0.3%.[5] Anesthetics, antibiotics, radiocontrast material, and allergen extracts are the medication categories involved most often in fatal reactions.[3] Risk factors for drug allergy include drug type, degree of drug exposure, route of administration, intercurrent viral infection, and allergies to other medications (Table 135-1).[3]

SPECIFIC IMMUNE REACTIONS AND SPECIFIC DRUG CATEGORIES

Penicillin is a frequent cause of anaphylaxis and is still the only antibiotic with reliable predictive values on skin testing for IgE-mediated reactions. Anaphylaxis has never been reported in a patient with a negative penicillin skin test.[6] Morbilliform rashes to penicillins alone are not considered life threatening, but caution is advised if the rash bears any similarity to urticaria. Different penicillins can be cross-reactive owing to the shared β-lactam ring structure as well as side chains.[1] Although positive penicillin skin tests are not more frequent among atopic patients, an atopic history may be a risk factor for a more severe allergic reaction to penicillin.[7] A family history of β-lactam allergy may also increase the risk of sensitization.[8] The risk of an allergic reaction to

Table 135-1 Risk Factors for Drug Allergy Reactions

Drug type: especially antibiotics, anticonvulsants, chemotherapeutic agents, heparin, insulin, biologic response modifiers, latex, neuromuscular depolarizing agents

Degree of drug exposure: multiple but less frequent exposures associated with greater risk than continuous or routine repeated exposures

Route of administration: intramuscular associated with greater risk than intravenous; both pose greater risk than enteral administration

Intercurrent viral infections: risk increases in the presence of a viral illness

Allergies to other medications: risk increases if present

a cephalosporin in a patient with a history of penicillin allergy may be as high as 4.4% in those with a positive penicillin skin test. In patients with a negative penicillin skin test with major and minor determinants, the risk of an adverse reaction to a cephalosporin is no greater than among the general population.[9] Therefore, in those who are skin-test positive to penicillin, an alternative to a cephalosporin should be considered to avoid the small but increased risk of anaphylaxis. Cross-reactivity among cephalosporins, like penicillins, may be due to β-lactam ring structure or side-chain similarities.[1] Penicillins, carbapenems, and first-generation cephalosporins also tend to have cross-reactivity owing to side-chain similarities. The monobactams (e.g., aztreonam) are generally well tolerated in most penicillin-allergic patients. Cross-reactivity has not been demonstrated between monobactams and cephalosporins, except between aztreonam and ceftazidime, which have shared side-chain characteristics.[7] Besides anaphylaxis, numerous other adverse drug reactions have been described with β-lactam antibiotics.

Erythema multiforme, thought to be a lymphocyte-mediated reaction, is characterized by a rash starting distally and progressing proximally that consists of targetoid lesions with a dusky center and a red circumference. Up to 50% of cases are thought to be medication related, starting 1 to 2 weeks after drug exposure.[10] Common associated medications include sulfonamides, penicillins, nonsteroidal anti-inflammatory drugs (NSAIDs), and barbiturates (see Chapter 160).[10] Stevens-Johnson syndrome and toxic epidermal necrolysis can also be medication-induced phenomena that involve a spectrum of blistering mucocutaneous disorders (see Chapter 161).[11]

Anticonvulsant hypersensitivity syndrome, also known as drug reaction with eosinophilia and systemic symptoms (DRESS) syndrome, is seen with aromatic anticonvulsants such as phenytoin, phenobarbital, and carbamazepine.[12] It can also be seen with dapsone, sulfonamides, allopurinol, and minocycline.[10] Anticonvulsant hypersensitivity syndrome consists of fever, a rash that can progress to exfoliative dermatitis, lymphadenopathy, various organ involvement, and eosinophilia.[12] Treatment consists of withdrawing the offending agent, supportive care, and systemic steroids with a slow taper in severe cases to prevent relapses (see Chapter 159).

Red man syndrome is the term used to describe the generalized flushing often seen with intravenous vancomycin administration. It can be elicited in a majority of patients if the medication is given too quickly. Pretreatment with antihistamines and slow infusion times may help avoid this reaction.

Anaphylactoid reactions mimic IgE-mediated reactions clinically, but prior sensitization and specific antibodies cannot be demonstrated. Opiates and radiocontrast material are two common examples. The use of lower-osmolar radiocontrast agents and pretreatment with antihistamines and corticosteroids can help prevent anaphylactoid events when radiographic studies with contrast are critical in those with a prior history of adverse reactions.[3]

Local anesthetics have also been reported to cause allergic symptoms. IgE-mediated sensitivity, however, is not routinely demonstrated. Graded subcutaneous injection challenges at increasing dilutions with different local anesthetics can help determine which ones are tolerated by the patient.[3]

Samter's triad consists of asthma, nasal polyposis, and sensitivity to aspirin or NSAIDs. Patients with these drug sensitivities may experience rhinoconjunctivitis, bronchospasm, urticaria, angioedema, and other manifestations of anaphylaxis when exposed to these medications. Mechanisms of sensitivity, however, are most often cyclooxygenase rather than IgE mediated.[13] The diagnosis of aspirin or NSAID sensitivity can be confirmed only by a graded oral medication challenge. If treatment with an NSAID or aspirin is critical, oral desensitization can be performed.[13]

Adverse reactions have also been associated with other medications. Heparin can cause urticaria, asthma, skin necrosis, and thrombocytopenia.[2] Minocycline and hydralazine have been associated with a lupus-like syndrome.[14] Churg-Strauss syndrome (an allergic granulomatous vasculitis) has been reported with leukotriene receptor antagonists (e.g., montelukast) and macrolide antibiotics.[15,16] Cough and angioedema are adverse reactions to angiotensin-converting enzyme inhibitors.[17] Anaphylaxis caused by neuromuscular blocking agents and latex is more commonly encountered intraoperatively.[18] With the advent of recombinant human insulin, the incidence of insulin-induced allergic reactions has decreased significantly.

DIAGNOSIS AND EVALUATION

The first step to identifying the offending medication in a patient presenting with a probable drug hypersensitivity reaction is a thorough history, including all medication exposures with dates of administration, dose changes, and discontinuation. Concurrent antihistamine exposure is important; besides possibly altering the clinical presentation of drug allergy, it may delay skin-testing opportunities. Constructing a medication time line can be extremely helpful, especially when multiple medications could be associated with a specific reaction. On physical examination, a thorough skin and mucous membrane examination is critical to detect the early onset of potentially life-threatening reactions such as Stevens-Johnson syndrome and toxic epidermal necrolysis. An accurate description of a rash and its relation to drug administration are also important to determine the type of reaction. Dermatographism, lymphadenopathy, hepatosplenomegaly, and joint involvement should be confirmed or excluded. Tryptase, a product of mast cell degranulation, may be transiently elevated in cases of anaphylaxis, but blood specimens for assay must be collected within 4 hours of the reaction. Low complement components C3 and C4 can be seen in serum sickness. Complete blood count with differential, serum chemistries, liver enzymes, and urinalysis can help detect laboratory evidence of organ involvement. For drug-induced hemolysis, a Coombs test may be positive.

Because skin testing and the radioallergosorbent test (RAST) evaluate for IgE-mediated reactions only, they are not helpful in type II, III, or IV hypersensitivities or in other adverse medication reactions such as erythema multiforme, Stevens-Johnson syndrome, toxic epidermal necrolysis, and anticonvulsant hypersensitivity syndrome. RASTs are generally not as sensitive as skin testing.

As previously mentioned, penicillin testing with major and minor determinants has a very reliable predictive value for IgE-mediated sensitivity. Unfortunately, skin-test predictive values for other medications are unknown; thus, negative skin tests in these situations cannot fully exclude an IgE-mediated hypersensitivity to the given medication. This is because the native drug may not carry all the antigenic determinants responsible for the allergic reaction, and the causative antigenic determinants may arise only after the implicated drug is metabolized. Skin testing is performed by first pricking the skin through a drop of medication at a given concentration, usually 1 mg/mL, accompanied by positive (histamine) and negative (saline) controls. If the test is negative for a wheal and flare response after 15 minutes, intradermal testing is initiated at an extremely diluted concentration. The concentration of the intradermal injection is increased at 15-minute intervals until the concentration of the initial skin-prick solution is reached. If the test is still negative, a decision is made whether to perform test dosing or a graded challenge to confirm or exclude the drug allergy. Test dosing involves administering the full therapeutic dose by its expected route, followed by close observation to monitor for adverse reactions. To perform a graded challenge, the medication is administered by its expected route in increasing percentages at selected time intervals toward the full therapeutic dose—for example, at 1%, 10%, and then the remaining 89% of the full dose. The advantage of a graded challenge is that if an allergic reaction occurs sometime during the challenge, less medication will have been given.

Other techniques to measure type I responses include in vitro measurement of leukotriene synthesis, basophil activation, and basophil histamine release. These tests are not standardized at this time. Patch testing can be performed for allergic contact dermatitis.

TREATMENT

Once a drug reaction has been characterized and the medication responsible has been revealed, the offending agent should be avoided. Generally, for immediate hypersensitivity reactions only, if a clinical situation arises in which there is no other suitable therapeutic option, a desensitization procedure can be performed to the sensitizing or potentially cross-reacting medication (Figs. 135-1 and 135-2).[19] Desen-

sitization refers to the process of inducing immunologic tolerance to an antigen in a patient who has developed specific IgE antibodies to that antigen.[20] This term has also been applied to drug challenge procedures that do not involve the neutralization of drug-specific antibodies. Aspirin desensitization and sulfonamide desensitization are two such examples. Desensitization has no benefit and is strictly contraindicated when the causative medication has caused serum sickness reactions, anticonvulsant hypersensitivity syndrome, or desquamating reactions such as Stevens-Johnson syndrome or toxic epidermal necrolysis. The precise immunologic mechanisms of desensitization are still unknown; however, desensitization tends to be antigen specific and does not render a mast cell unable to respond to IgE cross-linking. It has been postulated that a gradual exposure of antigen causes only a gradual cross-linking of IgE on mast cell surfaces, which in turn keeps the intracellular signal of degranulation below a clinical threshold.[20]

In a desensitization procedure, progressively larger doses of the medication to which the patient is allergic are administered at frequent intervals while monitoring for breakthrough reactions, until the full therapeutic dose is reached. Once a patient is desensitized, consistent dosing intervals must be maintained to prevent resensitization. Once the medication is discontinued, the desensitized state will eventually be lost, and if the patient needs to receive this medication in the future, repeat desensitization will be necessary. If a breakthrough reaction occurs during desensitization, depending on its severity and the route of administration (oral versus continuous intravenous infusion), decreasing the infusion to the previously tolerated dose and trying again to reach the full therapeutic dose may be considered. Alternatively, based on the patient's previous reaction history and the severity of the breakthrough reaction, the desensitization protocol may be aborted altogether. Patients should generally not be pretreated with steroids or antihistamines, because this may mask the initial symptoms of anaphylaxis during desensitization.

In addition to discontinuing all medications implicated in serious adverse reactions, monitoring for progressive organ system involvement (other than skin, musculoskeletal, and mucosal involvement) is an important consideration. We recommend a low threshold for hospital admission and laboratory evaluation to more efficiently monitor the clinical course and institute therapy quickly if the patient's clinical status declines. In Stevens-Johnson syndrome, serum sickness, and anticonvulsant hypersensitivity syndrome, if systemic steroids are started, a gradual taper is advised to avoid relapse.

Chapter 134 provides details on the management of anaphylactic reactions.

CONSULTATION

For inpatients with a previous or newly recognized drug allergy that interferes with therapy or diagnostic testing, consultation with an allergist is recommended. Patients admitted for desensitization may warrant consultation with a hospitalist, whether in or out of the intensive care setting. Patients who develop life-threatening allergic reactions at any time in the hospital setting may require a response from a hospitalist.

Antibiotic	Dose (Cystic Fibrosis)	Maximum Dose
Aztreonam	150–200 mg/kg/day ÷ q 6 h	8 g/day
Cefepime	150 mg/kg/day ÷ q 8 h	6 g/day
Ceftazidime	150–200 mg/kg/day ÷ q 8 h	6 g/day
Meropenem	60–120 mg/kg/day ÷ q 8 h	6 g/day
Piperacillin	300–500 mg/kg/day ÷ q 6 h	24 g/day
Piperacillin/Tazobactam	300 mg/kg/day ÷ q 6 h	18 g/day (as pip)

Desensitization doses will be mixed with normal saline (NS). If different fluid needed, please specify _____

Infuse the following drug doses continuously over 30 minutes each Rate = 1.66 mL/min or 100 mL/hour
2 micrograms in 50 mL of NS, then
20 micrograms in 50 mL of NS, then
200 micrograms in 50 mL of NS, then
2 mg in 50 mL of NS, then
20 mg in 50 mL of NS, then
200 mg in 50 mL of NS, then

Aztreonam	Ceftazidime or Cefepime	Meropenem	Piperacillin	Piperacillin/Tazobactam
FTD of _____ mg OR 2 g in 50 mL of NS	FTD of _____ mg OR 2 g in 50 mL of NS	FTD of _____ mg OR 2 g in 50 mL of NS	FTD of _____ mg OR 2 g in 50 mL of NS	FTD of _____ mg OR 2 g in 50 mL of NS
			FTD of _____ mg OR 4 g in 50 mL of NS	FTD of _____ mg OR 4.5 g in 50 mL of NS

Then continue full therapeutic dose (FTD): _____ mg IV Q _____ h after desensitization is complete until discharge.

Verify availability of resuscitation cart and have the following medications at the bedside:
Epinephrine (1:1,000) 0.01 mL/kg × _____ kg = _____ mL (max 0.5 mL/dose) IM × 1
Diphenhydramine 1 mg/kg × _____ kg = _____ mg (max 50 mg/dose) IV × 1
Methylprednisolone 2 mg/kg × _____ kg = _____ mg (max 60 mg/dose) IV × 1
Normal saline bolus 20 mL/kg × _____ kg = _____ mL (max 1000 mL) IV × 1
Albuterol inhalation solution 0.5% 0.03 mL/kg = _____ mL (max 1 mL) in 2 mL NS × 1
PLEASE PAGE ALLERGY FELLOW WITH ANY QUESTIONS:

Signature Allergy Fellow _____ Pager _____
House officer_____ Pager _____

Figure 135-1 Standardized antibiotic desensitization protocol for Children's Hospital, Boston.

ADMISSION CRITERIA

Drug desensitization is often performed in a hospital setting until the full therapeutic dose has been evaluated beyond one dosing interval. This allows ready access to cardiorespiratory monitoring, rescue medications, and other resuscitative measures, particularly emergency airway management. At some institutions, the initial drug desensitization protocol is performed in an intensive care setting.

DISCHARGE CRITERIA

- Completion or termination of the desensitization protocol.
- Stabilization of the patient with a serious allergic reaction.
- Outpatient plan for ongoing therapy or follow-up.

- Training to allow recognition of and appropriate response to serious allergic reactions for patients, families, and other caregivers.
- Education of families, including recommendations for avoiding certain exposures.

IN A NUTSHELL

- Fatal allergic reactions are most often associated with anesthetics, antibiotics, radiocontrast material, and allergen extracts.
- Penicillin is the only antibiotic with reliable predictive values on skin testing for IgE-mediated reactions.
- Up to 4.4% of patients with positive skin testing to penicillin will develop an allergic reaction when exposed to a cephalosporin.

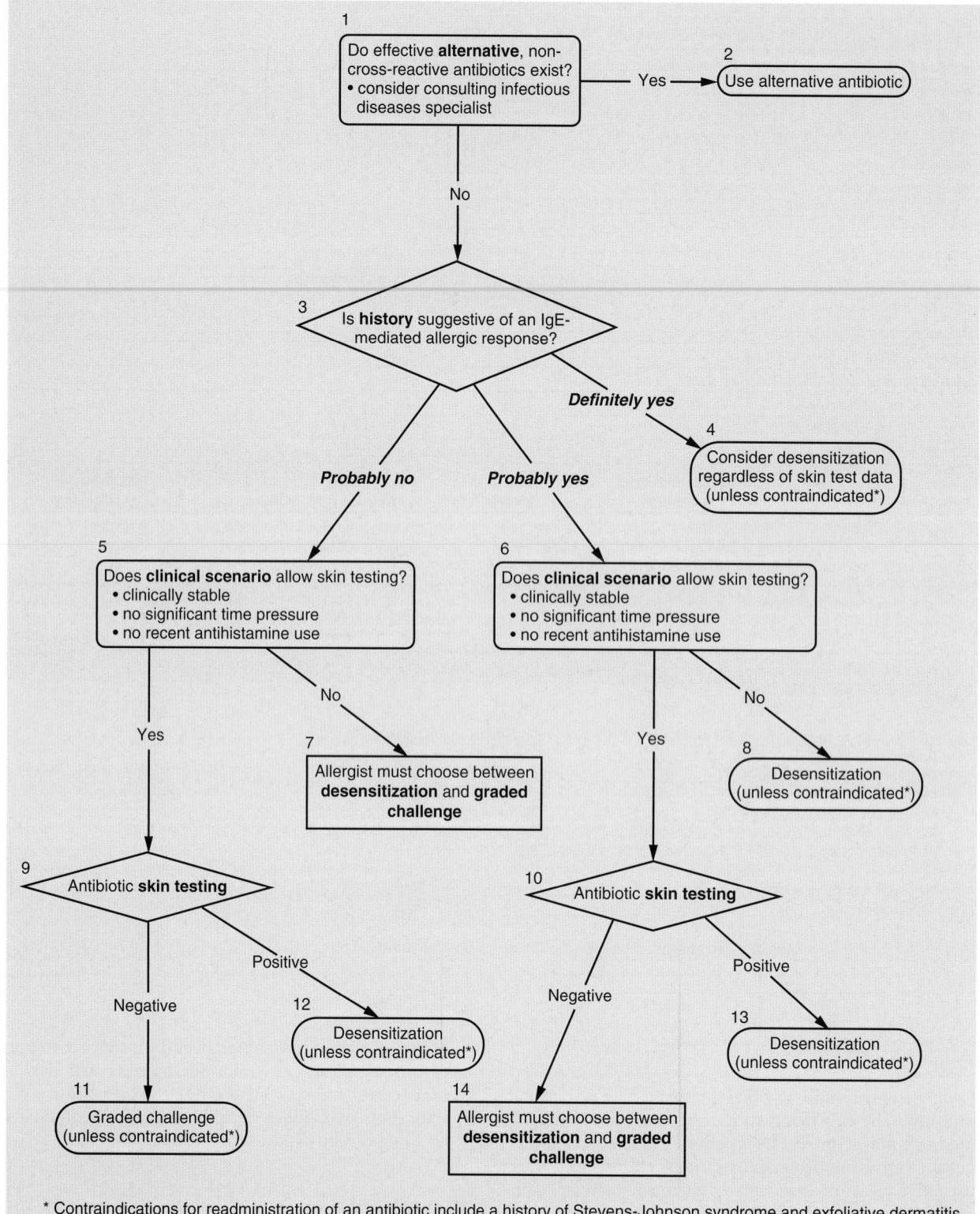

Figure 135-2 A stepwise approach to selecting patients for desensitization to antibiotics other than penicillin. (From Turvey SE, Cronin B, Arnold AD, Dioun AF: Antibiotic desensitization for the allergic patient: 5 years of experience and practice. Ann Allergy Asthma Immunol 2004;92:426–432.)

- Skin testing and RASTs evaluate for IgE-mediated reactions only.
- Desensitization involves the induction of immunologic tolerance to IgE-mediated allergic reactions.
- Once the offending medication is discontinued, desensitization will eventually be lost.

ON THE HORIZON

- Development of strong predictive values and more reliable allergy tests for a wider variety of medications.
- Standardization of desensitization protocols to increase their safety and efficacy.
- Better understanding of the many pathways leading to allergic reactions, thereby offering improved diagnostic and therapeutic opportunities.

SUGGESTED READING

Adkinson NF Jr: Drug allergy. In Adkinson NF Jr, et al (eds): Middleton's Allergy Principles and Practice, 6th ed. St Louis, Mosby, 2003, pp 1679-1694.

Anderson J: Allergic and allergic-like reactions to drugs and other therapeutic agents. In Lieberman P, Anderson J (eds): Allergic Diseases: Diagnosis and Treatment, 2nd ed. St Louis, Mosby, 2000, pp 303-323.

Gruchella R: Drug allergy. J Allergy Clin Immunol 2003;111:548-559.

Solensky R: Drug desensitization. Immunol Allergy Clin North Am 2004;24: 425-443.

Turvey SE, Cronin B, Arnold AD, Dioun AF: Antibiotic desensitization for the allergic patient: 5 years of experience and practice. Ann Allergy Asthma Immunol 2004;92:426-432.

REFERENCES

1. Gruchella R: Drug allergy. J Allergy Clin Immunol 2003;111:548-559.
2. Boguniewicz M: Drug allergy. In Fischer TJ, et al (eds): Allergy and Immunology: Medical Knowledge Self Assessment Program, 3rd ed. Milwaukee, Wis, American Academy of Allergy, Asthma, and Immunology, 2003, pp 209-224.
3. Anderson J: Allergic and allergic-like reactions to drugs and other therapeutic agents. In Lieberman P, Anderson J (eds): Allergic Diseases: Diagnosis and Treatment, 2nd ed. St Louis, Mosby, 2000, pp 303-323.
4. Adkinson NF Jr: Drug allergy. In Adkinson NF Jr, et al (eds): Middleton's Allergy Principles and Practice, 6th ed. St Louis, Mosby, 2003, pp 1679-1694.
5. Lazarou J, Pomeranz BH, Corey PN: Incidence of adverse drug reactions in hospitalized patients: A meta-analysis of prospective studies. JAMA 1998;279:1200-1205.
6. Weiss M, Adkinson NF Jr: Immediate hypersensitivity reactions to penicillin and related antibiotics. Clin Allergy 1988;18:515-540.
7. Solensky R: Hypersensitivity reactions to beta-lactam antibiotics. Clin Rev Allergy Immunol 2003;24:201-220.
8. Kurtz KM, Beatty TL, Adkinson NF Jr: Evidence for familial aggregation of immunologic drug reactions. J Allergy Clin Immunol 2000;105:184-185.
9. Kelkar PS, Li JT: Cephalosporin allergy. N Engl J Med 2001;345:804-809.
10. McKenna JK, Leiferman KM: Dermatologic drug reactions. Immunol Allergy Clin North Am 2004;24:399-423.
11. Abe R, Shimizu T, Shibaki A, et al: Toxic epidermal necrolysis and Stevens-Johnson syndrome are induced by soluble Fas ligand. Am J Pathol 2003;162:1515-1520.
12. Kaur S, Sarkar R, Thami GP, Kanwar AJ: Anticonvulsant hypersensitivity syndrome. Pediatr Dermatol 2002;19:142-145.
13. Szczeklik A, Stevenson DD: Aspirin-induced asthma: Advances in pathogenesis, diagnosis, and management. J Allergy Clin Immunol 2003;111:913-921.
14. Antonov D, Kazandjieva J, Etugov D, et al: Drug-induced lupus erythematosus. Clin Dermatol 2004;22:157-166.
15. Tuggey JM, Hosker HS: Churg-Strauss syndrome associated with monteleukast therapy. Thorax 2000;55:805-806.
16. Hubner C, Dietz A, Stremmel W, et al: Macrolide-induced Churg-Strauss syndrome in a patient with atopy. Lancet 1997;350:563.
17. Morimoto T, Gandhi TK, Fiskio JM, et al: An evaluation of risk factors for adverse drug events associated with angiotensin converting enzyme inhibitors. J Eval Clin Pract 2004;10:499-509.
18. Lieberman P: Anaphylactic reactions during surgical and medical procedures. J Allergy Clin Immunol 2002;110(2 Suppl):s64-s69.
19. Turvey SE, Cronin B, Arnold AD, Dioun AF: Antibiotic desensitization for the allergic patient: 5 years of experience and practice. Ann Allergy Asthma Immunol 2004;92:426-432.
20. Solensky R: Drug desensitization. Immunol Allergy Clin North Am 2004;24:425-443.

CHAPTER 136

Primary Immunodeficiency Diseases

Jerry A. Winkelstein

Although most patients with primary immunodeficiency diseases are cared for in an outpatient setting, they sometimes require inpatient care. This chapter provides an overview of these disorders, with a focus on the circumstances that necessitate hospitalization.

The primary immunodeficiency diseases are a family of disorders characterized by defects intrinsic to the immune system. There are more than 125 primary immunodeficiency diseases affecting virtually every component of the immune system.[1] In some of these diseases, the defect is intrinsic and limited to B cells (e.g., X-linked agammaglobulinemia), T cells (e.g., purine nucleoside phosphorylase deficiency), phagocytic cells (e.g., chronic granulomatous disease), or individual components of the complement system (e.g., C2 deficiency). In other cases, the defects affect more than one component of the immune system (e.g., severe combined immunodeficiency, X-linked hyper-IgM syndrome).

Most of these disorders are genetically determined and inherited as single gene defects. Some are inherited as autosomal recessive traits (e.g., adenosine deaminase deficiency), some as X-linked recessive traits (e.g., X-linked severe combined immunodeficiency), and some as autosomal dominant disorders (e.g., C1 esterase deficiency). However, the two most common, selective immunoglobulin (Ig) A deficiency and common variable immunodeficiency (CVID), are not recognized as being inherited as single gene defects; in most instances, they occur sporadically.

The prevalence of the primary immunodeficiency diseases varies from relatively common to relatively rare. Thus, some occur in as many as 1 in 500 individuals (e.g., selective IgA deficiency),[2] and some occur in 1 in 10,000 (e.g., C2 deficiency)[3]; others are as rare as 1 in 250,000 (e.g., chronic granulomatous disease).[4] However, if they are grouped together as a family of diseases, the primary immunodeficiencies are more common than childhood leukemia and lymphoma.

CLINICAL PRESENTATION

In many instances, the initial clinical presentation of a primary immunodeficiency disease (and, it is hoped, its diagnosis) occurs when an infant or child is admitted to the hospital. There are three general categories of clinical presentation characteristic of the primary immunodeficiency diseases: (1) increased susceptibility to infection, (2) rheumatic or inflammatory disorders, and (3) syndromes specifically associated with primary immunodeficiency diseases. In addition, some patients present without any clinical signs or symptoms and are diagnosed based on family history alone.

Increased Susceptibility to Infection

An increased susceptibility to infection is a cardinal feature of most of the primary immunodeficiency diseases. This usually manifests as an increased number of infections. Thus, recurrent otitis media, sinusitis, or pneumonia is seen fairly often in these patients. Similarly, although single episodes of blood-borne infections such as sepsis, meningitis, osteomyelitis, and septic arthritis are usually not indicative of a primary immunodeficiency disease, patients with recurrent episodes should be evaluated for immunodeficiency. Immunodeficient patients can also have infections that are unusually severe, complicated, or persistent, such as staphylococcal pneumonia with empyema or a pneumatocele. Even though recurrent infections are the most common clinical manifestation of an underlying primary immunodeficiency disease, when an organism of relatively low virulence, such as *Pneumocystis jiroveci*, causes the first infection, primary immunodeficiency must be ruled out.

The kind of infection often provides clues as to the nature of the underlying immunodeficiency. Blood-borne infections indicate difficulty clearing organisms from the bloodstream and are thus characteristic of deficiencies in antibody, complement, or fixed phagocytes of the reticuloendothelial system, such as the spleen. Infections caused by encapsulated bacteria, which require opsonization before ingestion by phagocytic cells, are characteristic of deficiencies in antibody or complement, whereas infections caused by most viruses and fungi are more characteristic of deficiencies in T lymphocytes or natural killer cells. Infections caused by bacteria and fungi that produce catalase and have no net production of hydrogen peroxide cause most of the serious infections in patients with chronic granulomatous disease,[4,5] whereas peroxide-producing bacteria are not more frequent and do not cause severe disease in these patients.

Rheumatic Disorders

Although less prominent than increased susceptibility to infection, patients with primary immunodeficiency diseases can also present with a variety of autoimmune, rheumatic, or inflammatory disorders. These may affect a single cell line or end organ, such as immune thrombocytopenic purpura, or they may affect a variety of organs and organ systems, such as systemic lupus erythematosus (SLE). In some cases, there is clear evidence of an autoimmune process in which autoantibodies or autoreactive T cells can be demonstrated, such as in autoimmune hemolytic anemia; in others, the pathophysiology more closely resembles a systemic inflammatory response, such as in sarcoidosis. In some cases, what appears to be a rheumatic disorder is in fact an infection. For example, the dermatomyositis seen in patients with X-linked agammaglobulinemia is actually a manifestation of a systemic enteroviral infection.[6]

Rheumatic disorders accompany virtually every category of primary immunodeficiency disease. Patients with B-cell defects, such as selective IgA deficiency and CVID, have a relatively high prevalence (10% to 20%) of a variety of rheumatic disorders, including SLE, sicca syndrome, immune thrombocytopenic purpura, and autoimmune hemolytic anemia,[2,7] and a granulomatous inflammatory disorder that resembles sarcoidosis.[7,8] Patients with chronic granulomatous disease often present with inflammatory bowel disease, and either they or female carriers of the X-linked recessive form of the disease may develop a syndrome that resembles SLE.[4] Patients with complement deficiencies frequently develop a lupus syndrome and membranoproliferative glomerulonephritis.[9] Finally, some patients with combined cellular defects, such as those with Wiskott-Aldrich syndrome, can develop systemic inflammatory disorders as they get older.[10]

Syndrome Identification

In some instances, the patient's immunodeficiency is part of a recognized syndrome, in which case the syndrome itself, rather than any specific symptoms referable to immunodeficiency, alerts one to the possibility of immunodeficiency. For example, a newborn with hypocalcemia is diagnosed with DiGeorge syndrome, which in turn brings up the possibility of a T-cell deficiency secondary to thymic hypoplasia. Similarly, a male infant with persistent thrombocytopenia may have Wiskott-Aldrich syndrome, which raises the possibility of an associated hypogammaglobulinemia and T-cell deficiency.

SPECIFIC PRIMARY IMMUNODEFICIENCY DISEASES

Each of the primary immunodeficiency diseases has characteristic clinical features, whether they occur as the initial clinical presentation leading to a diagnosis or are complications arising after diagnosis and treatment (Table 136-1).

Severe Combined Immunodeficiency

Severe combined immunodeficiency is characterized by a severe deficiency in T-cell and B-cell function and is caused by a variety of molecular genetic defects.[11] Most patients have significant lymphopenia and hypogammaglobulinemia.

Patients usually present in the first 6 months of life with infection, malabsorption, or failure to thrive. Although they can present with virtually any kind of infection, *P. jiroveci* pneumonia is often the initial presentation. Chronic or recurrent diarrhea is also very common and can be caused by a variety of viral, bacterial, and parasitic agents.

Early and prompt diagnosis is especially critical, because the success of bone marrow or stem cell transplantation is related to the patient's age: the younger the patient, the more likely a successful outcome.[12] In this regard, lymphopenia is a hallmark of the disease, and any infant who is lymphopenic (<3000 cells/mm^3 for a neonate;

<1500 cells/mm^3 for an infant) should be evaluated for severe combined immunodeficiency.[11]

X-Linked Agammaglobulinemia

This disorder is caused by mutations in a gene (*BTK*) encoding an intracellular tyrosine kinase expressed in B cells.[13] It is characterized by markedly reduced levels of B cells and hypogammaglobulinemia.

X-linked agammaglobulinemia usually presents after the first few months of life,[14] when maternal IgG acquired transplacentally has begun to disappear. In some instances, affected children may not show clinical signs and symptoms until well into the second or third year of life. The most common clinical presentation is infection caused by encapsulated bacteria such as *Pneumococcus, Haemophilus influenzae,* and *Pseudomonas.* Recurrent respiratory infections such as otitis, sinusitis, and pneumonia, and blood-borne infections such as bacteremia, meningitis, osteomyelitis, and septic arthritis, are typical. In addition, these children are susceptible to chronic systemic enteroviral infections,[6,15] although these are much less common.

Early diagnosis is important in X-linked agammaglobulinemia, because treatment with intravenous immunoglobulin before the development of bronchiectasis is critical to long-term survival and quality of life.

Hyper–IgM Syndrome

Hyper-IgM syndrome can be caused by at least four different molecular genetic defects,[16] the most common of which affects the gene on the X chromosome encoding CD40 ligand, a T-cell surface molecule responsible for instructing B cells to switch from IgM to IgG, IgA, and IgE production. Other forms of the disorder involve the autosomal genes *CD40, AID,* and *UNG,* all of which are responsible for B-cell class switching. As the name suggests, all forms of this disorder are characterized by elevated (or normal) IgM levels in the face of reduced levels of IgG and IgA.

The clinical presentation of hyper-IgM syndrome is most commonly related to certain infections.[17] The form caused by a deficiency in CD40 ligand often presents with opportunistic infections such as *P. jiroveci* pneumonia and may be associated with neutropenia. This form of the X-linked hyper-IgM syndrome is also associated with *Cryptosporidium* infections of the biliary tree, leading to sclerosing cholangitis.

Diagnosis is usually prompted by the patient's increased susceptibility to infection. The IgG deficiency can be treated with intravenous immunoglobulin, but in patients with CD40 ligand deficiency, this treatment does not correct the underlying T-cell defect and increased susceptibility to opportunistic infections, prompting the use of stem cell transplantation in these pateints.[17]

Common Variable Immunodeficiency

CVID is characterized by hypogammaglobulinemia and a variable T-cell defect. Its cause and pathogenesis are unknown. Although there are cases in which multiple family members are affected, CVID is usually not inherited as a single gene defect.

There are two peak ages of onset—one in early childhood, and another in adolescence and early adulthood.[7,18] In addi-

Table 136-1   Primary Immunodeficiency Diseases

Disorder	Inheritance	Immunodeficiency	Characteristic Infections	Additional Clinical Features
Severe combined immunodeficiency	XLR, AR	Pan-hypogammaglobulinemia; ↓ T-cell number and function	Severe bacterial, viral, and fungal infections; opportunistic infections	Many different molecular genetic forms; one form (Omenn syndrome) is characterized by hepatosplenomegaly, rash, and eosinophilia
X-linked agammaglobulinemia	XLR	Pan-hypogammaglobulinemia; markedly ↓ B cells	Pyogenic infections caused by encapsulated bacteria; systemic enteroviral infections	
Hyper-IgM syndrome	XLR, AR	↓ IgG and IgA; normal or ↑ IgM; ↓ T-cell response to antigens	Severe bacterial, viral, and fungal infections; opportunistic infections	Many different molecular genetic forms, some of which are associated with neutropenia; one form is associated with anhidrotic ectodermal dysplasia
Common variable immunodeficiency	Unknown	↓ IgG and usually ↓ IgA and ↓ IgM; variably ↓ T-cell number or function	Severe bacterial, viral, and fungal infections; occasional opportunistic infections	May also have a variety of autoimmune, rheumatic, or inflammatory disorders
Wiskott-Aldrich syndrome	XLR	↓ IgM, IgG2; ↓ response to polysaccharide antigens; ↓ T-cell function	Severe bacterial, viral, and fungal infections; opportunistic infections	Associated with eczema and thrombocytopenia; some patients can develop lymphomas
DiGeorge syndrome	AD, sporadic	↓ T-cell number and function	Severe bacterial, viral, and fungal infections; opportunistic infections	Associated with hypoparathyroidism, cardiac defects, and characteristic facies
Ataxia-telangiectasia	AR	↓ IgA, IgG, and IgG2; ↓ T-cell number	Severe bacterial, viral, and fungal infections	Some patients can develop lymphomas
Chronic granulomatous disease	XLR, AR	↓ Intracellular killing by phagocytic cells	Severe bacterial and fungal infections caused by catalase-positive organisms	May also present with gastrointestinal involvement and urinary tract obstruction; some patients can develop systemic inflammatory reactions resembling lupus
Terminal complement component deficiencies	AR	C5, C6, C7, C8, or C9	Systemic neisserial infections	
Hyper-IgE syndrome	AD, AR	Markedly ↑ IgE	Staphylococcal abscesses; fungal infections	Usually associated with eczema; AD form variably associated with a characteristic facies, delayed loss of primary teeth, scoliosis, and fractures

AD, autosomal dominant; AR, autosomal recessive; Ig, immunoglobulin; XLR, X-linked recessive.

tion to recurrent, severe, or unusual infections, about 20% of patients with CVID present with a variety of autoimmune or rheumatic conditions, such as immune thrombocytopenic purpura, autoimmune hemolytic anemia, SLE, or rheumatoid arthritis.[7] A small number of patients with CVID develop granulomatous inflammation of the lungs, liver, and spleen that resembles sarcoidosis.[7,8] Around 10% of patients develop cancer, specifically B-cell non-Hodgkin's lymphoma.

Treatment with intravenous immunoglobulin is the mainstay of therapy for the hypogammaglobulinemia, but it does not appear to improve the autoimmune, inflammatory, or rheumatic manifestations.

Wiskott–Aldrich Syndrome

This disorder is caused by mutations in a gene (*WASP*) expressed in all formed elements of the blood.[19] It is characterized by thrombocytopenia, eczema, and defects in T- and B-cell function.

The clinical presentation of Wiskott-Aldrich syndrome relates to the thrombocytopenia or immunodeficiency.[10] Bleeding, into either the skin or the gastrointestinal tract, is a common presentation in the first year of life, as is recurrent infection, especially otitis.

Diagnosis usually follows recognition of the thrombocytopenia. Interestingly, Wiskott-Aldrich syndrome is the only cause of thrombocytopenia in which platelet volume is decreased rather than increased, and the observation of decreased platelet volume in a male with thrombocytopenia usually prompts the diagnosis and leads to an evaluation for immunodeficiency. Splenectomy for the thrombocytopenia and hematopoietic stem cell transplantation are the two most common forms of therapy.[20]

DiGeorge Syndrome

This syndrome is caused by developmental abnormalities of the third and fourth pharyngeal pouch and is most often associated with chromosomal deletions of 22q11.[21] Patients with DiGeorge syndrome have a variety of clinical manifestations, including hypoparathyroidism and hypocalcemia, cardiac defects, thymic hypoplasia, and characteristic facies. There is a great deal of variation in terms of which organs are affected and the degree to which they are affected. Although the majority of patients have little or no immunodeficiency, some have severe T-cell deficiency. The majority (>90%) of patients have a deletion of 22q11 and can be diagnosed by fluorescent in situ hybridization (FISH).

Patients with DiGeorge syndrome usually present in the neonatal period with hypocalcemia secondary to hypoparathyroidism or with symptoms related to cardiac defects. Although some are identified soon after birth because of their characteristic facies, many patients with DiGeorge syndrome have a normal appearance.

Those patients with severe T-cell deficiency may benefit from the transplantation of cultured thymus epithelium.[22] Intravenous immunoglobulin may be necessary as well.

Ataxia-Telangiectasia

This syndrome is caused by mutations in the *ATM* gene and is inherited as an autosomal recessive disorder.[23] Patients have a variety of clinical manifestations, including ataxia and oculocutaneous telangiectasia, as well as an increased risk for malignancy and a variable immunodeficiency involving both T-cell and B-cell function.[24] The immunodeficiency most often manifests as IgA deficiency, but IgG2 deficiency or a pan-hypogammaglobulinemia can be seen as well.[25] In addition, many patients have decreased numbers of T cells.

Patients with ataxia-telangiectasia usually present with ataxia soon after they learn to walk.[26] The facial telangiectasia usually does not become clinically apparent until age 3 years. These patients may also have an increased susceptibility to upper and lower respiratory infections.[25] Finally, a significant number of patients develop lymphoma. At the current time, there is no specific therapy for ataxia-telangiectasia.

Chronic Granulomatous Disease

Chronic granulomatous disease is caused by a number of molecular defects affecting phagocytic nicotinamide-adenine dinucleotide phosphate oxidase, resulting in a markedly reduced ability of the phagocyte to kill intracellular bacteria and fungi that produce catalase.[5] The most common form of the disease is the result of mutations in phox 91, an integral component of the multimolecular enzyme, that is encoded on the X chromosome.[4,5]

Patients usually present with abscesses, most commonly caused by *Staphylococcus, Serratia,* or fungi, including *Aspergillus.*[4] The abscesses may involve the lymph nodes, liver, spleen, lungs, or skin. In addition, granulomas are common and can cause varying degrees of obstruction of the gastrointestinal or urinary tract. As many as 30% of patients with chronic granulomatous disease develop colitis-like bowel inflammation that may be difficult to manage. Some patients develop a systemic inflammatory disorder characterized by fever and the elevation of acute phase reactants.

Treatment is largely supportive, using prophylactic antibiotics and antifungals. Itraconazole prophylaxis has been studied in this population, and injections of recombinant gamma interferon can be helpful in some cases.[27] Recently, stem cell transplantation has been used to correct the cellular defect.[28]

Deficiencies of Terminal Complement Components

Deficiencies of the individual terminal complement components C5, C6, C7, C8, and C9 are all inherited as autosomal recessive traits[29] and lead to a deficiency of the membrane-attack complex and a lack of serum bactericidal activity. The characteristic clinical presentation is a systemic blood-borne neisserial infection such as meningococcemia.[29] In fact, between 5% and 15% of children who present with an initial episode of meningococcemia or meningococcal meningitis have a genetically determined deficiency in C5, C6, C7, C8, or C9.[29] In those with a previous episode of meningococcemia, a positive family history for meningococcemia, or an uncommon serotype, the percentage is higher, approaching 40%. Thus, screening all patients with blood-borne meningococcal infections for a complement deficiency appears to be warranted.

Early complement component deficiencies, including C2 and C4, are associated with recurrent pyogenic infections and increased susceptibility to autoimmune diseases such as SLE.

Hyper-IgE Syndrome

The cause of hyper-IgE syndrome is unknown, but at least two forms of the disorder exist—one autosomal dominant,[30] and the other autosomal recessive.[31] Although the underlying immunologic defect is not known, there is a characteristic clinical presentation consisting of severe eczema and recurrent staphylococcal skin or lung infections, such as abscesses. Patients characteristically have markedly elevated levels of IgE (>2000 IU/mL) and eosinophilia. In the autosomal dominant form of the disease, there may also be characteristic facies, delayed loss of primary teeth, scoliosis, and frequent fractures.

There is no specific therapy for this condition. Topical immune modulators such as tacrolimus or pimecrolimus can help with the eczema. Patients with significant infections may receive antibiotic prophylaxis.

IN A NUTSHELL

- Primary immunodeficiencies may be due to defects limited to the function of B cells, T cells, phagocytes, or the complement system. They can also be caused by defects in more than one component of the immune system.
- There are three general clinical presentations of the primary immunodeficiencies: (1) increased susceptibility to infection (more frequent, more severe, or caused by opportunistic organisms), (2) rheumatic or inflammatory disorders, and (3) syndromes associated with primary immunodeficiencies.
- Treatment options include antibiotic prophylaxis, intravenous immunoglobulin, and hematopoietic stem cell transplantation.

ON THE HORIZON

- Gene therapy has been used to treat X-linked severe combined immunodeficiency and adenosine deaminase deficiency. Complications include lymphoproliferative disorders.
- Newborn screening for some primary immunodeficiencies is being actively pursued.

SUGGESTED READING

Bonilla FA, Geha RS: Primary immunodeficiency diseases. J Allergy Clin Immunol 2003;111:S571.

Notarangelo L, Casanova JL, Fischer A, et al: Primary immunodeficiency diseases: An update. J Allergy Clin Immunol 2004;114:677.

Segal BH, Leto TL, Mallin JI, et al: Genetic, biochemical and clinical features of chronic granulomatous disease. Medicine 2000;79:170.

Sullivan K, Winkelstein JA: Deficiencies of the complement system. In Stiehm ER, Ochs HD, Winkelstein JA (eds): Immunologic Disorders of Infants and Children, 5th ed. Philadelphia, WB Saunders, 2004.

REFERENCES

1. Notarangelo L, Casanova JL, Fischer A, et al: Primary immunodeficiency diseases: An update. J Allergy Clin Immunol 2004;114:677.
2. Edwards E, Razvi S, Cunningham-Rundles C: IgA deficiency: Clinical correlates and responses to pneumococcal vaccine. Clin Immunol 2004; 111:93.
3. Sullivan KE, Petri M, Schmeckpeper B, et al: The prevalence of a mutation which causes C2 deficiency in SLE. J Rheumatol 1994;21:6.
4. Winkelstein JA, Marino MC, Johnston RB Jr, et al: Chronic granulomatous disease: Report on a national registry of 368 patients. Medicine s
5. Segal BH, Leto TL, Gallin JI, et al: Genetic, biochemical and clinical features of chronic granulomatous disease. Medicine 2000;79:170.
6. Halliday E, Winkelstein JA, Webster AD: Enteroviral infections in primary immunodeficiency: A survey of morbidity and mortality. J Infect 2003; 46:1.
7. Cunningham-Rundles C, Bodian C: Common variable immunodeficiency: Clinical and immunologic features of 248 patients. Clin Immunol 1999; 92:34.
8. Fasano MB, Sullivan KE, Sarpong SB, et al: Sarcoidosis and common variable immunodeficiency: Report of 8 cases and review of the literature. Medicine 1996;75:251.
9. Figueroa JE, Densen P: Infectious diseases associated with complement deficiencies. Clin Microbiol Rev 1991;4:359.
10. Sullivan KE, Mullen CA, Blaese RM, Winkelstein JA: A multi-institutional survey of the Wiskott-Aldrich syndrome. J Pediatr 1994;125:876.
11. Buckley RH, Schiff RI, Schiff SE, et al: Human severe combined immunodeficiency: Genetic, phenotypic and functional diversity in one hundred eight infants. J Pediatr 1997;130:378.
12. Myers LA, Patel DD, Puck JM, Buckley RH: Hematopoietic stem cell transplantation for severe combined immunodeficiency in the neonatal period leads to superior thymic output and improved survival. Blood 2002;99: 872.
13. Ochs HD, Smith CI: X-linked agammaglobulinemia: A clinical and molecular analysis. Medicine 1996;75:287.
14. Lederman HM, Winkelstein JA: X-linked agammaglobulinemia: An analysis of 96 patients. Medicine 1985;64:145.
15. McKinney RE Jr, Katz SL, Wilfert CM: Chronic enteroviral meningoencephalitis in agammaglobulinemic patients. Rev Infect Dis 1987;9: 334.
16. Durandy A: Hyper IgM syndrome: A model for studying the regulation of class switch recombination and somatic hypermutation generation. Biochem Soc Trans 2002;30:815.
17. Winkelstein JA, Marino MC, Ochs H, et al: The X-linked hyper IgM syndrome: Clinical and immunologic features of 79 patients. Medicine 2003;82:373.
18. Conley ME, Park CL, Douglas SD: Childhood common variable immunodeficiency with autoimmune disease. J Pediatr 1986;108:95.
19. Imai K, Nonoyama S, Ochs HD: WASP (Wiskott-Aldrich syndrome protein) gene mutations and phenotype. Curr Opin Allergy Clin Immunol 2003;3: 427.
20. Mullen CA, Anderson KD, Blaese RM: Splenectomy and/or bone marrow transplantation in the management of the Wiskott-Aldrich syndrome: Long-term follow-up in 62 cases. Blood 1993;82:2961.
21. Perez E, Sullivan KE: Chromosome 22q11.2 deletion syndrome (DiGeorge and velocardiofacial syndromes). Curr Opin Pediatr 2002;14:678.
22. Markert ML, Boeck A, Hale LP, et al: Transplantation of thymus tissue in complete DiGeorge syndrome. N Engl J Med 1999;341:1180.
23. Savitsky K, Bar-Shira A, Gilad S, et al: A single ataxia telangiectasia gene with a product similar to PI-3 kinase. Science 1995;268:1749.
24. Crawford TO: Ataxia telangiectasia. Semin Pediatr Neurol 1998;5:287.
25. Nowack-Wegrzyn A, Crawford TO, Winkelstein JA, et al: Immunodeficiency and infections in ataxia telangiectasia. J Pediatr 2004;144:505.
26. Cabana MD, Crawford TO, Winkelstein JA, et al: Consequences of the delayed diagnosis of ataxia-telangiectasia. Pediatrics 1998;102:98.
27. Marciano BE, Wesley R, De Carlo ES, et al: Long-term interferon-gamma therapy for patients with chronic granulomatous disease. Clin Infect Dis 2004;39:692.

28. Horwitz ME, Barrett AJ, Brouwn MR, et al: Treatment of chronic granulomatous disease with nonmyeloablative conditioning and a T-cell-depleted hematopoietic allograft. N Engl J Med 2001;344:926.

29. Sullivan K, Winkelstein JA: Deficiencies of the complement system. In Stiehm ER, Ochs HD, Winkelstein JA (eds): Immunologic Disorders of Infants and Children, 5th ed. Philadelphia, WB Saunders, 2004.

30. Grimbacher B, Holland SM, Gallin JI, et al: Hyper IgE syndrome with recurrent infections—an autosomal dominant multisystem disorder. N Engl J Med 1999;340:692.

31. Renner ED, Puck JM, Holland SM, et al: Autosomal recessive hyperimmunoglobulin E syndrome: A distinct clinical entity. J Pediatr 2004; 144:93.

CHAPTER 137

Intravenous Immunoglobulin

Manish Butte

Intravenous immunoglobulin (IVIG) is a polyclonal mixture of immunoglobulin G (IgG) antibodies that can be administered intravenously. IVIG is used primarily as replacement therapy in a variety of disorders marked by IgG deficiency. In higher doses, IVIG has anti-inflammatory and immune-modulatory functions and plays a role in the treatment of various autoimmune disorders.

There are at least eight licensed IVIG products commercially available in the United States, with more scheduled to be licensed in the near future. IVIG is manufactured from pooled human plasma obtained from large donor groups that are screened for infection with human immunodeficiency virus (HIV) 1 and 2 and hepatitis B and C. Besides donor screening, most IVIG preparations undergo multiple purification steps that further reduce the potential viral risk. These purification steps involve ethanol fractionation followed by chromatography, pasteurization, solvent or detergent treatment, protease treatment, acid treatment, low-salt treatment, or heat exposure. The final product is stabilized with sugars such as sucrose, amino acids such as glycine, or human albumin. All IVIG preparations have trace amounts of IgA antibodies. Although there have been no well-documented cases of HIV transmission from IVIG, more than 200 patients had documented hepatitis C transmission from IVIG in the early 1990s, before screening for hepatitis C became standard.[1]

The mechanisms of action of IVIG are multiple and complex and have not been completely elucidated. Activation of inhibitory Fc receptors and down-regulation of activating Fc receptors, binding to serum complement protein and cytokines, inhibition of pathogenic autoantibodies, and modulation of T- and B-cell function are among the described roles.

APPROVED USES AND DOSING

The U.S. Food and Drug Administration (FDA) has approved six applications of IVIG: primary immunodeficiency, acute immune thrombocytopenic purpura, secondary immunodeficiency due to leukemia, prevention of infection and graft-versus-host disease in bone marrow or stem cell transplant recipients, prevention of infection in pediatric HIV disease, and prevention of coronary sequelae of Kawasaki disease. Dosing recommendations for these approved indications are provided in Table 137-1. There are also many off-label uses, some of which are discussed later.

Primary Immunodeficiency

Antibody replacement for primary immunodeficiency is indicated for patients with hypogammaglobulinemia and increased susceptibility to infection. Disorders in this category include severe combined immunodeficiency, agammaglobulinemia, common variable immunodeficiency, and specific antibody deficiency. In addition, use of IVIG is common in Wiskott-Aldrich syndrome (thrombocytopenia, eczema, frequent infections), hyper-IgM syndrome, hyper-IgE syndrome, nuclear factor essential modulator immunodeficiency, transient hypogammaglobulinemia of infancy, and ataxia-telangiectasia, especially when there are low IgG levels or defective specific antibody responses.

Past studies established the benefit of keeping preinfusion levels above 500 mg/dL to decrease the risk of bacterial and *Pneumocystis* pneumonia.[2,3] Recently, some experts have advocated keeping trough levels greater than 800 mg/dL, although supporting evidence is limited. One recent double-blind crossover trial using a dose of 800 mg/kg every 4 weeks in children resulted in fewer infections and no increase in adverse effects over the usual dosing regimen.[4]

Immune Thrombocytopenic Purpura

Acute immune thrombocytopenic purpura seldom requires treatment, but it is indicated for overt bleeding, surgical procedures, failure of other therapies, and a platelet count below 10,000/mm³. In these situations, use of IVIG has become standard practice in pediatrics. Most patients studied benefit from IVIG, with a rapid increase in platelet counts of 50,000/mm³ or more. Trials using dose regimens other than those recommended (see Table 137-1) or substituting anti-D antibody (WinRho) show slower or less impressive responses in platelet count.

Immunodeficiency with Leukemia

A secondary immunodeficiency can occur with B-cell chronic lymphocytic leukemia. In such patients with hypogammaglobulinemia and a history of infections, IVIG therapy is indicated. Randomized trials have demonstrated a beneficial decrease in infections at recommended doses.[5-9]

Stem Cell Transplantation

In the context of hematopoietic stem cell transplantation, IVIG has many potential roles in preventing infection and decreasing the risk of acute graft-versus-host disease (see Chapter 125). The minimally effective dose is controversial, but most experts recommend standard dosing with adjustments to maintain trough IgG levels of at least 500 mg/dL. There is some evidence that higher doses and higher trough levels reduce the risk and severity of graft-versus-host disease.[10]

Kawasaki Disease

Kawasaki disease is a pediatric vasculitis of unclear cause. Aneurysmal damage to the coronary (or other) arteries is an infrequent but serious sequela. Numerous studies have

Table 137-1   Approved Indications for Intravenous Immunoglobulin Therapy

FDA Indication	Suggested Dose and Regimen
Primary immunodeficiency	400-500 mg/kg every 3-4 wk
Immune thrombocytopenic purpura	0.8-1 g/kg × 1 dose (low dose) or 1 g/kg/day × 2 days or 400 mg/kg/day × 5 days
Chronic lymphocytic leukemia	400 mg/kg every 3-4 wk
Stem cell transplantation	500 mg/kg/wk prn (IgG <500)
HIV infection	400 mg/kg every 4 wk
Kawasaki disease	2 g/kg × 1-2 doses

FDA, Food and Drug Administration; HIV, human immunodeficiency virus; IgG, immunoglobulin G.

demonstrated the benefit of preventing coronary artery aneurysms by using IVIG in the first 7 to 10 days of the disease.[11] A second dose may be necessary after 36 hours if the fever persists.[12] For more information, see Chapter 102.

Human Immunodeficiency Virus Infection

Pediatric HIV infection is marked by frequent viral and bacterial infections. Because of this, the efficacy of IVIG in reducing these infections was studied in large crossover, placebo-controlled, randomized, double-blind trials in the early 1990s. These trials demonstrated conclusive benefits in children with CD4 counts greater than 200 cells/µL.[13,14] In addition to having fewer infections, the CD4 counts of patients receiving IVIG decreased at a slower pace compared with those receiving placebo.

Off-Label Uses

Off-label uses of IVIG include nearly 100 disorders, most with a presumed pathophysiologic basis in immune dysfunction. The role of IVIG in these disorders is controversial and is often not supported by convincing clinical evidence, especially in pediatrics.

Guillain-Barré syndrome is a polyradiculoneuritis with a presumed immune-mediated cause. It typically follows viral respiratory infections and can lead to respiratory failure in children. In adults, numerous trials of IVIG have demonstrated a benefit similar to plasma exchange in hastening the recovery of walking.[15] Consequently, use of IVIG has been incorporated into the latest American Academy of Neurology practice parameters for Guillain-Barré syndrome.[16] The role of IVIG in children is less clear, but small case series have demonstrated improvements in treated patients similar to plasma exchange.[17] The dosing regimen studied in adult trials was 400 mg/kg daily for 5 days.

Chronic inflammatory demyelinating polyneuropathy, which some believe to be a chronic form of Guillain-Barré syndrome, is another neurologic disorder in which IVIG may play a role. Numerous randomized, double-blind, placebo-controlled studies support the use of IVIG in chronic inflammatory demyelinating polyneuropathy.[18] The usual dosing regimen is 1 g/kg daily for 2 days; repeat dosing is frequently required every 2 to 8 weeks.[19]

Isoimmune hemolytic anemia in neonates increases the risk of hyperbilirubinemia and kernicterus, owing to maternal-fetal incompatibility between ABO or D blood groups. In severe cases, exchange transfusion is required—a potentially dangerous procedure. Use of IVIG significantly decreases the need for exchange transfusion, the number of exchanges needed, and the maximum bilirubin level.[20] The IVIG dose is a single infusion of 500 mg/kg. However, the size of the trials and their methodology limit the general applicability of IVIG use for this indication.

Because the majority of IgG in newborns is derived from the mother rather than from the host's adaptive immunity, administration of IVIG is thought to help decrease the morbidity or mortality in suspected or proven infection in these patients. In a recent Cochrane review, use of IVIG was associated with a decrease in mortality in infants who were subsequently shown to have infection.[21] However, this was not the case in neonates with only suspected infection, because of insufficient statistical power. Ongoing trials will help clarify this issue, but for now, there is insufficient evidence to recommend the use of IVIG in this context.

In premature infants, limited third-trimester gestation results in a quantitative decrease in maternally transferred IgG. Prophylactic administration of IVIG may boost immunoglobulin levels enough to prevent nosocomial infections in hospitalized infants. In a recent meta-analysis involving infants weighing less than 2500 g and born at less than 37 weeks' gestation, use of IVIG resulted in a 3% reduction in sepsis and a 4% reduction in serious infection. It was not, however, associated with reductions in other outcomes, including necrotizing enterocolitis, intraventricular hemorrhage, and length of hospital stay. Unfortunately, use of IVIG prophylactically did not decrease overall mortality.[22] With such a modest reduction in sepsis and infection, cost-benefit decisions and local neonatal intensive care unit infection rates need to be considered when using IVIG prophylactically in premature infants. Doses used in the studies ranged from one infusion of 200 mg/kg within 24 hours of birth to 500 mg/kg weekly.

In septic shock, replacing consumed IgG and providing blocking antibodies to endotoxin are two possible goals of IVIG administration. This issue has been the subject of dozens of clinical trials in adults and a few in neonates and premature infants. A recent Cochrane meta-analysis showed a statistically significant reduction in mortality in adult patients, but this was not seen in the limited number of pediatric trials reviewed.[23] Although use of IVIG in septic shock shows promise in adults, the limited evidence in pediatric patients is conflicting. Dosing in reviewed studies ranged from single boluses to continuous infusions, making generalization difficult.

Finally, IVIG may play a role in the treatment of autoimmune disorders such as juvenile dermatomyositis, systemic lupus erythematosus, and antiphospholipid antibody syndrome. Controlled, prospective trials are lacking in children, but retrospective case series suggest a role for high-dose IVIG as an adjuvant therapy in these disorders.

ADVERSE REACTIONS AND OTHER ISSUES

Adverse reactions to IVIG are common, and approximately 15% of patients experience some type of reaction. As with any other blood product, informed consent should be obtained before the administration of IVIG. Special consideration should be given to the infectious risks as well as adverse reactions.

The most common reactions include headache, fever, myalgia, chills, transient urticaria, and flushing during the infusion; these are related to IgG aggregates and complement activation. These effects can be diminished by reducing the rate of infusion, premedicating with diphenhydramine and acetaminophen, decreasing the concentration of the IVIG solution, or changing to a different IVIG product. Hypotension can occur and should be treated with immediate cessation of the infusion, intramuscular epinephrine, and volume expansion based on the usual emergency care guidelines.

True allergic reactions to IVIG are uncommon. Anaphylaxis is extremely rare, and sparse case reports describe a risk of anti-IgA isotype IgE antibodies in patients with absent IgA, although this topic has generated a lot of controversy among experts. In these cases, emergency care for anaphylaxis is instituted. Anaphylaxis associated with IVIG may be diagnosed retrospectively by transiently elevated serum tryptase levels. An IVIG preparation with a low IgA content should be used if IVIG therapy is still necessary.

Renal failure following IVIG is unusual in children but is seen in adults. Osmotic shifts by the sugar stabilizers in the IVIG preparation, especially sucrose, are frequently implicated as the cause. Patients should be well hydrated, preferably with isotonic solutions or those without sucrose, especially in children with underlying renal dysfunction.

Headaches following IVIG administration can be severe and can progress to meningismus. This aseptic meningitis syndrome has been described 6 to 48 hours after administration and is evidenced by papilledema, cerebrospinal fluid pleocytosis, and increased cerebrospinal fluid protein. The cause of this disorder is not known but may be related to cytokines released as a result of the IVIG. In patients with an increased risk of infection, lumbar puncture may be warranted. Usually, only supportive care is needed, and the symptoms typically resolve after 2 to 3 days. Corticosteroid treatment just before the administration of IVIG has been shown to decrease the risk of aseptic meningitis syndrome.[24]

Many other minor reactions have been described. Patients on long-term IVIG may demonstrate asymptomatic elevation in liver enzymes, although the reasons are not clear. Screening for hepatitis infection is recommended in these cases, and it may be necessary to switch products. Because IVIG contains anti-ABO blood group antibodies, transient Coombs-positive hemolytic anemia can been seen. Transient neutropenia following IVIG has been described in case reports.

One relatively recent innovation is the use of subcutaneous immunoglobulin.[25] The limited subcutaneous space necessitates frequent infusions, but because levels are closer to steady state, the total infused dose is generally lower than that administered by the intravenous route. Systemic side effects are significantly reduced, but mild local reactions are common. Another advantage, especially in the pediatric population, is that intravenous access is not required. This alternative may be an important consideration in cases in which central line placement is being considered for the provision of IVIG. Subcutaneous immunoglobulin may not be applicable in children with bleeding disorders.

After a patient has received IVIG, one should avoid giving the measles-mumps-rubella vaccine (or its components) or the varicella live-virus vaccine for 8 to 11 months.[26] There are generally no restrictions to the administration of non–live-virus vaccines following IVIG.

IN A NUTSHELL

- IVIG is a medication consisting of polyclonal antibodies purified from human blood donors. The risk of infection is extremely low, but transfusion reactions are common.
- IVIG plays a major role in pediatric primary immunodeficiencies, Kawasaki disease, HIV infection, and hematopoietic stem cell transplantation and has become a standard off-label therapy for immune modulation in numerous pediatric diseases.

ON THE HORIZON

- A number of new IVIG formulations are currently under evaluation by the FDA. Use of subcutaneous immunoglobulin is growing rapidly, especially in patients with primary immunodeficiencies, because of its fewer adverse effects. Trials of IVIG in many pediatric disorders will conclusively support its use and help standardize dosing.

SUGGESTED READING

Kazatchkine MD, Kaveri SV: Immunomodulation of autoimmune and inflammatory diseases with intravenous immune globulin. N Engl J Med 2001;345:747-755.

Newburger JW, Takahashi M, Gerber MA, et al: Diagnosis, treatment, and long-term management of Kawasaki disease: A statement for health professionals from the Committee on Rheumatic Fever, Endocarditis, and Kawasaki Disease, Council on Cardiovascular Diseases in the Young, American Heart Association. Pediatrics 2004;114:1708-1733.

Oates-Whitehead RM, Baumer JH, Haines L, et al: Intravenous immunoglobulin for the treatment of Kawasaki disease in children. Cochrane Database Syst Rev 2003;CD004000.

REFERENCES

1. Bresee JS, Mast EE, Coleman PJ, et al: Hepatitis C virus infection associated with administration of intravenous immune globulin: A cohort study. JAMA 1996;276:1563-1567.
2. Ochs HD, Fischer SH, Wedgwood RJ, et al: Comparison of high-dose and low-dose intravenous immunoglobulin therapy in patients with primary immunodeficiency diseases. Am J Med 1984;76:78-82.
3. Bonagura VR, Cunningham-Rundles S, Edwards BL, et al: Common variable hypogammaglobulinemia, recurrent *Pneumocystis carinii* pneumonia on intravenous gamma-globulin therapy, and natural killer deficiency. Clin Immunol Immunopathol 1989;51:216-231.

4. Eijkhout HW, van Der Meer JW, Kallenberg CG, et al: The effect of two different dosages of intravenous immunoglobulin on the incidence of recurrent infections in patients with primary hypogammaglobulinemia: A randomized, double-blind, multicenter crossover trial. Ann Intern Med 2001;135:165-174.

5. Molica S: Infections in chronic lymphocytic leukemia: Risk factors, and impact on survival, and treatment. Leuk Lymphoma 1994;13:203-214.

6. Molica S, Musto P, Chiurazzi F, et al: Prophylaxis against infections with low-dose intravenous immunoglobulins (IVIG) in chronic lymphocytic leukemia: Results of a crossover study. Haematologica 1996;81:121-126.

7. Gamm H, Huber C, Chapel H, et al: Intravenous immune globulin in chronic lymphocytic leukaemia. Clin Exp Immunol 1994;97(Suppl 1):17-20.

8. Boughton BJ, Jackson N, Lim S, Smith N: Randomized trial of intravenous immunoglobulin prophylaxis for patients with chronic lymphocytic leukaemia and secondary hypogammaglobulinaemia. Clin Lab Haematol 1995;17:75-80.

9. Dicato M, Chapel H, Gamm H, et al: Use of intravenous immunoglobulin in chronic lymphocytic leukemia: A brief review. Cancer 1991;68: 1437-1439.

10. Winston DJ, Antin JH, Wolff SN, et al: A multicenter, randomized, double-blind comparison of different doses of intravenous immunoglobulin for prevention of graft-versus-host disease and infection after allogeneic bone marrow transplantation. Bone Marrow Transplant 2001;28: 187-196.

11. Oates-Whitehead RM, Baumer JH, Haines L, et al: Intravenous immunoglobulin for the treatment of Kawasaki disease in children. Cochrane Database Syst Rev 2003;CD004000.

12. Newburger JW, Takahashi M, Gerber MA, et al: Diagnosis, treatment, and long-term management of Kawasaki disease: A statement for health professionals from the Committee on Rheumatic Fever, Endocarditis and Kawasaki Disease, Council on Cardiovascular Disease in the Young, American Heart Association. Circulation 2004;110:2747-2771.

13. Mofenson LM, Moye J Jr: Intravenous immune globulin for the prevention of infections in children with symptomatic human immunodeficiency virus infection. Pediatr Res 1993;33:S80-S87.

14. Mofenson LM, Moye J Jr, Korelitz J, et al: Crossover of placebo patients to intravenous immunoglobulin confirms efficacy for prophylaxis of bacterial infections and reduction of hospitalizations in human immunodeficiency virus-infected children. The National Institute of Child Health and Human Development Intravenous Immunoglobulin Clinical Trial Study Group. Pediatr Infect Dis J 1994;13:477-484.

15. Hughes RA, Raphael JC, Swan AV, Doorn PA: Intravenous immunoglobulin for Guillain-Barré syndrome. Cochrane Database Syst Rev 2004; CD002063.

16. Hughes RA, Wijdicks EF, Barohn R, et al: Practice parameter: Immunotherapy for Guillain-Barré syndrome: Report of the Quality Standards Subcommittee of the American Academy of Neurology. Neurology 2003;61:736-740.

17. Abd-Allah SA, Jansen PW, Ashwal S, Perkin RM: Intravenous immunoglobulin as therapy for pediatric Guillain-Barré syndrome. J Child Neurol 1997;12:376-380.

18. Van Schaik IN, Winer JB, De Haan R, Vermeulen M: Intravenous immunoglobulin for chronic inflammatory demyelinating polyradiculoneuropathy. Cochrane Database Syst Rev 2002;CD001797.

19. Ropper AH: Current treatments for CIDP. Neurology 2003;60:S16-S22.

20. Alcock GS, Liley H: Immunoglobulin infusion for isoimmune haemolytic jaundice in neonates. Cochrane Database Syst Rev 2002; CD003313.

21. Ohlsson A, Lacy JB: Intravenous immunoglobulin for suspected or subsequently proven infection in neonates. Cochrane Database Syst Rev 2004;CD001239.

22. Ohlsson A, Lacy JB: Intravenous immunoglobulin for preventing infection in preterm and/or low-birth-weight infants. Cochrane Database Syst Rev 2004;CD000361.

23. Alejandria MM, Lansang MA, Dans LF, Mantaring JB: Intravenous immunoglobulin for treating sepsis and septic shock. Cochrane Database Syst Rev 2002;CD001090.

24. Jayabose S, Mahmoud M, Levendoglu-Tugal O, et al: Corticosteroid prophylaxis for neurologic complications of intravenous immunoglobulin G therapy in childhood immune thrombocytopenic purpura. J Pediatr Hematol Oncol 1999;21:514-517.

25. Radinsky S, Bonagura VR: Subcutaneous immunoglobulin infusion as an alternative to intravenous immunoglobulin. J Allergy Clin Immunol 2003;112:630-633.

26. American Academy of Pediatrics, Committee on Infectious Diseases.: Red Book: Report of the Committee on Infectious Diseases. Elk Grove Village, Ill, American Academy of Pediatrics, 2003.

Surgical Issues

Gastrointestinal Obstruction: Pyloric Stenosis, Malrotation and Volvulus, and Intussusception

Julie Story Byerley and Lesli Taylor

Obstruction of the gastrointestinal (GI) tract can be due to a wide range of causes with many similarities in clinical presentation. Abdominal pain, early satiety or anorexia, and vomiting are common, with abdominal distention being more common with lower tract blockage. Nonbilious emesis is seen in conditions that occur proximal to the sphincter of Oddi or early in the course of abnormalities occurring more distally. Conversely, bilious emesis is seen when obstruction or dysfunction occurs distal to the duodenum.

Obstruction can result from extrinsic compression, intrinsic blockage, or functional abnormalities leading to dysmotility, as detailed in Table 138-1. This chapter focuses on three of the more common causes of GI tract obstruction: pyloric stenosis, malrotation with and without volvulus, and intussusception.

PYLORIC STENOSIS

Pyloric stenosis is one of the most common surgically correctable causes of vomiting in infants. The incidence is about 1 in 250 to 500 with a 4:1 male preponderance; it is seen commonly in white and Hispanic infants and is rare in African, Indian, and Asian infants.[1,2] The familial incidence of pyloric stenosis is remarkable: the highest incidence of pyloric stenosis occurs in the male children of mothers who had pyloric stenosis, and there is a 15-fold increase in siblings of affected patients.[3,4] Traditional teaching has been that it is more common in firstborn males.

Pyloric stenosis results from hypertrophy of the pylorus muscle with associated abnormalities in innervation and obstruction of the lumen with redundant mucosa. Although infectious causes, such as *Helicobacter pylori*, have been speculated because of the finding of leukocytic infiltrates on pathology,[5] the cause of the hypertrophy is unclear. Early exposure to erythromycin has also been considered a factor in the development of this condition.[6]

Clinical Presentation

Most infants with pyloric stenosis present between the ages of 3 and 8 weeks with progressive nonbilious emesis in large quantities, often forceful ("projectile"), after every feeding. If not diagnosed early, severe hypochloremic dehydration with metabolic alkalosis (occasionally along with acidosis) and growth failure will develop. The infant remains eager to feed until the dehydration becomes profound, after which the infant becomes increasingly lethargic. With severe metabolic alkalosis the infant may present with apnea.

Physical examination findings are often normal, but gastric distention, visible peristaltic waves, and a palpable "olive" (the hypertrophied pylorus) may be found. The "olive" is located in the lateral margin of the right rectus muscle just below the liver edge.

Differential Diagnosis

The differential diagnosis often includes gastroesophageal reflux, gastroenteritis, allergy, and other causes of proximal intestinal obstruction such as malrotation and volvulus.

Diagnosis and Evaluation

The hypertrophied pylorus may be apparent on either ultrasound or upper GI series. Ultrasound is considered positive if the pyloric channel is longer than 14 to 16 mm with muscular thickness greater than 3.5 to 4 mm (Fig. 138-1). Upper GI series can show the "string sign," a thin line of barium visible as it passes through a thickened and elongated pylorus, as well as compression of the gastric antrum and evidence of delayed gastric emptying.

Serum chemistry studies reveal hypochloremic metabolic alkalosis when the emesis has been prolonged, and evidence of metabolic acidosis may also be seen when the dehydration is pronounced.

Course of Illness

Nonbilious vomiting usually begins after 3 weeks of age and generally progresses in frequency and severity. Even though pyloric stenosis can resolve spontaneously without intervention, symptoms usually continue to progress and result in fluid loss, electrolyte abnormalities, failure to thrive, and apnea, all of which can be life threatening.

Treatment

Although definitive treatment of pyloric stenosis is surgical, the initial management of pyloric stenosis focuses on correction of the dehydration, electrolyte disturbances, and acid-base abnormalities often present at the time of diagno-

Table 138-1 Causes of Gastrointestinal Obstruction in Children

Differential Diagnosis of GI Obstruction in Neonates
Extrinsic compression
    Malrotation/volvulus
    Incarcerated hernia
    Intussusception
    Annular pancreas
Intrinsic blockage
    Pyloric stenosis
    Gastrointestinal atresia (e.g., duodenal atresia, jejunal
      atresia, imperforate anus)
    Meconium plug
    Meconium ileus
Functional abnormality
    Necrotizing enterocolitis
    Hirschsprung disease
    Gastroparesis
    Ileus

Differential Diagnosis of GI Obstruction in Older Infants and Children
Extrinsic compression
    Malrotation/volvulus
    Incarcerated hernia
    Intussusception
    Adhesions
    Appendicitis
    Tumor
    Hematoma
    Annular pancreas
Intrinsic blockage
    Fecal impaction
    Polyp
    Tumor
    Hematoma
    Stricture (e.g., Crohn's disease)
    Bezoar
    Foreign body
    Meckel's diverticulum
    Parasites
Functional abnormality
    Hirschsprung disease
    Gastroparesis
    Ileus

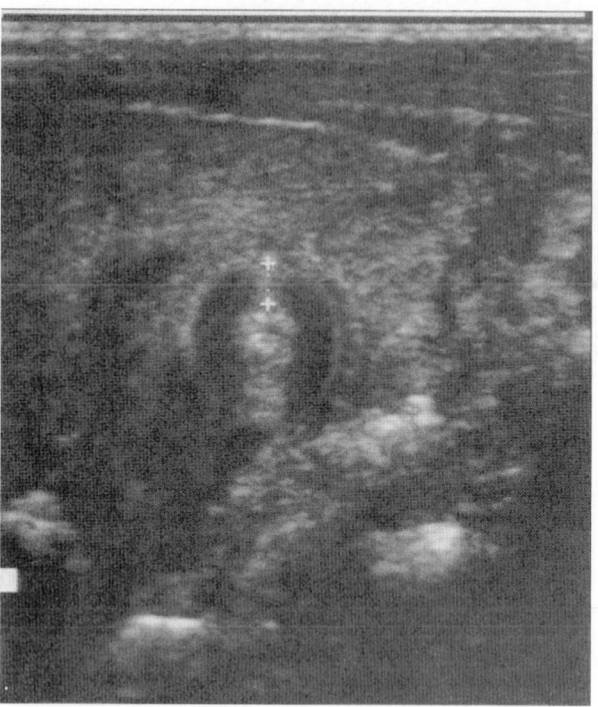

A

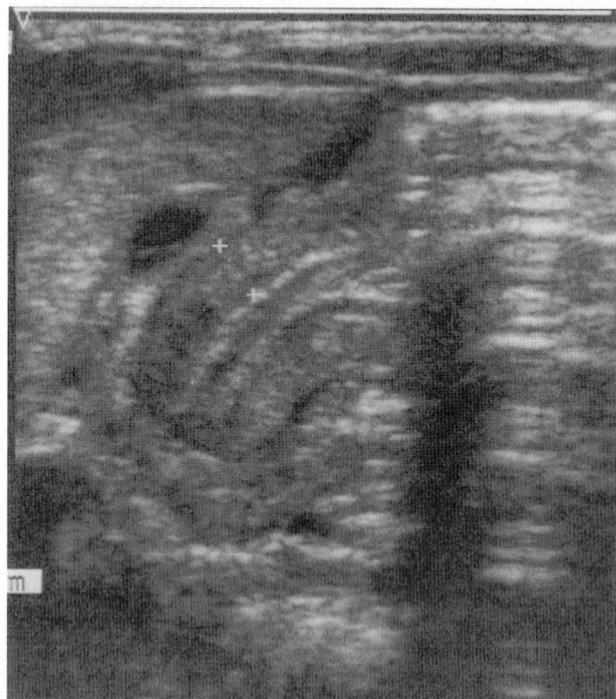

B

Figure 138-1 Ultrasound of pyloric stenosis. (From Wyllie R: Pyloric stenosis and congenital anomalies of the stomach. In Behrman RE, Kliegman RM, Jenson HB [eds]: Nelson Textbook of Pediatrics, 17th ed. Philadelphia, WB Saunders, 2004, p 1230.)

sis. The mainstay of rehydration is intravenous (IV) fluids, initially with the administration of normal saline (20 mL/kg) followed by dextrose-containing maintenance fluids (e.g., 5% dextrose D5/0.45% saline). Serum potassium levels are often normal (but may be low or elevated), but total body potassium is depleted because of gastric losses, alkalosis, and secondary aldosterone effects. In response to the hypovolemia, aldosterone is secreted and causes increases in renal sodium and chloride reabsorption, which consequentially leads to potassium and hydrogen wasting. Therefore, prompt supplementation of maintenance IV fluid with potassium chloride (20 to 40 mEq/L) after the first voiding is recommended. Serial serum electrolyte values are obtained until normalized. Persistence of alkalosis is common and often due to inadequate replacement of chloride. Chloride replacement can be augmented with repeated aliquots of IV normal saline (10 mL/kg).

If IV access is not attainable at first, small volumes of oral electrolyte solution (e.g., Pedialyte) may be tolerated and may sufficiently hydrate the infant to improve the chance of successfully placing a peripheral IV catheter. Central IV access may be necessary if vomiting persists and peripheral IV access is not successful. At times, gastric decompression with a nasogastric tube is indicated preoperatively.

Pyloric stenosis is corrected surgically with a Ramstedt pyloromyotomy after correction of fluid and electrolyte abnormalities and, if needed, decompression of the stomach. Postoperatively, feeding may be restarted within 24 hours. Early refeeding with full-strength formula or breast milk (i.e., without an initial trial of clear oral electrolyte solution) has been demonstrated to be safe and cost-effective and allow more prompt discharge home.[7] Many patients experience some postoperative emesis, thought to be related to postoperative ileus or swelling of the incised portion of the pylorus, or both. Persistent vomiting would not be expected and warrants further investigation. Inadequate pyloromyotomy is rare, but gastritis, gastroesophageal reflux, or previously undiagnosed gastric or intestinal obstruction may be considered.

Consultation

A pediatric generalist often handles the fluid electrolyte abnormalities. Early surgical consultation is recommended for definitive surgical intervention and, if needed, assistance with preoperative diagnostic evaluation.

Admission Criteria

All patients with pyloric stenosis should be admitted to correct fluid and electrolyte abnormalities and prepare them for surgery.

Discharge Criteria

The baby can be discharged once feeding well after surgery, often in 1 to 2 days.

Prevention

Identification of patients with an increased risk for pyloric stenosis may lead to earlier recognition. Newborn exposure to erythromycin has been associated with increased risk, especially if the exposure occurs before 13 days of life. These newborns have an eightfold increased risk. Exposure to erythromycin after 13 days of life or exposure to non-macrolide antibiotics is not believed to be associated with increased risk.[8]

In a Nutshell

- Clinical presentation: Progressive, projectile, nonbilious emesis after feeding in a 3- to 8-week-old infant
- Diagnosis: Clinical, confirmed by ultrasound or upper GI series
- Treatment: Correction of fluid and electrolyte derangements (typically hypochloremic metabolic alkalosis), followed by surgical pyloromyotomy

On the Horizon

- Clarification of the role of genetics in pyloric stenosis
- Consideration of the role of infectious causes of pyloric stenosis
- Discussion about the best surgical approach, including laparoscopic pyloromyotomy, which has been described but not shown to be more beneficial than the conventional open approach
- Discussion of nonsurgical treatment options: atropine, transpyloric feeding until the hypertrophy resolves

MALROTATION AND VOLVULUS

Malrotation results from failure of the intestine to rotate and fix normally during the first trimester of gestation. The midgut (distal duodenum to the transverse colon) extends into the umbilical cord during development and then rotates as it reenters the abdominal cavity. The distal third of the duodenum moves to the left of midline at the ligament of Treitz, whereas the cecum eventually situates itself in the right lower quadrant. At least six different anatomic positions are described as malrotation. Malrotation is reported to occur in up to 1 in 500 births, although the true incidence is uncertain because it can be asymptomatic. The incidence of malrotation is higher in children with other congenital anomalies, especially anomalies of the GI tract.[9]

Volvulus is the term used when twisting the intestines causes GI tract obstruction and ischemia (Fig. 138-2). It is usually associated with malrotation, although adhesions or other pathology can lead to volvulus in a normally rotated GI tract. Most common is midgut volvulus, but gastric or cecal volvulus can occur and may also be associated with intestinal malrotation. Bowel wall ischemia leads to infarction or perforation, or both, which are life threatening.

Clinical Presentation

Malrotation often presents with signs of upper GI obstruction, including bilious vomiting and progressive dehydration. Obstruction can be caused by Ladd's bands compressing the duodenum or from volvulus. Findings on physical examination may be normal early in the course or may reveal a scaphoid abdomen as a result of the proximal obstruction. Volvulus as a complication of malrotation often presents in the first month of life, most frequently in the first week. With volvulus, rapid deterioration occurs and progressive lethargy, tachypnea, grunting, abdominal distention, and shock ensue.

Intermittent volvulus can occur in older children and be confused with cyclic vomiting or abdominal migraine. Chronic symptoms, such as failure to thrive and malabsorption, are often present in these patients.

Differential Diagnosis

Other causes of GI tract obstruction must be considered, including intussusception, obstruction as a result of incarcerated hernia or adhesions, and appendicitis. In neonates, the differential also includes congenital GI malformations (e.g., atresia), gastroesophageal reflux, and gastroenteritis.

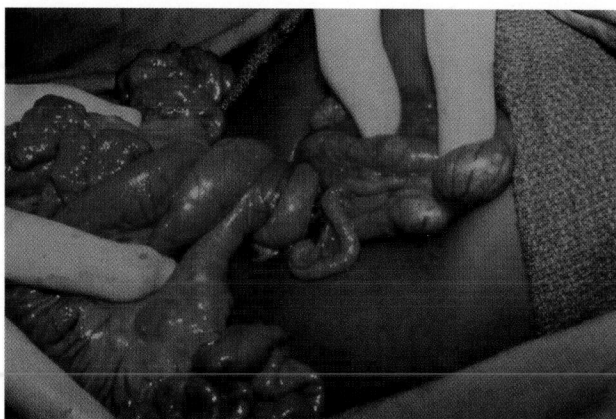

Figure 138-2 Intraoperative appearance of volvulus.

Diagnosis and Evaluation

In normal rotation, the duodenal-jejunal flexure, the marker for the ligament of Treitz, lies to the left of midline under the gastric antrum, usually near the second lumbar vertebra. In malrotation, the duodenum spirals down and the jejunum passes to the right of the vertebral column. Upper GI radiographs reliably demonstrate these findings (Fig. 138-3).

Ultrasonographic diagnosis of malrotation using the "whirlpool" sign, an abnormal relationship between the superior mesenteric artery and vein, is well described but not yet sensitive enough to be standard in all settings. Barium enema may demonstrate malposition of the cecum, which is suggestive, but not reliable for definitive diagnosis.

In the setting of volvulus, it is likely that laboratory tests will show acidosis secondary to lactate from bowel ischemia and dehydration. The white blood count is typically elevated. Occult or gross blood in stool can suggest bowel ischemia or necrosis.

Plain films of the abdomen may show signs of obstruction, including air-fluid levels on upright or lateral decubitus views, whereas free air in the peritoneal cavity would be indicative of perforation. If the obstruction is proximal or incomplete, the film may show only a gasless abdomen or can even be normal. An upper GI series is usually diagnostic of volvulus and reveals the classic "beak" sign or "corkscrewing" at the obstructed point (Fig. 138-4).

Note that when symptoms are severe with an abdominal source clearly identified, some children undergo exploratory laparotomy without awaiting imaging studies.

Course of Illness

Malrotation with unremitting symptoms of upper GI obstruction can lead to dehydration, electrolyte abnormalities, and acid-base disturbances. Forceful and persistent

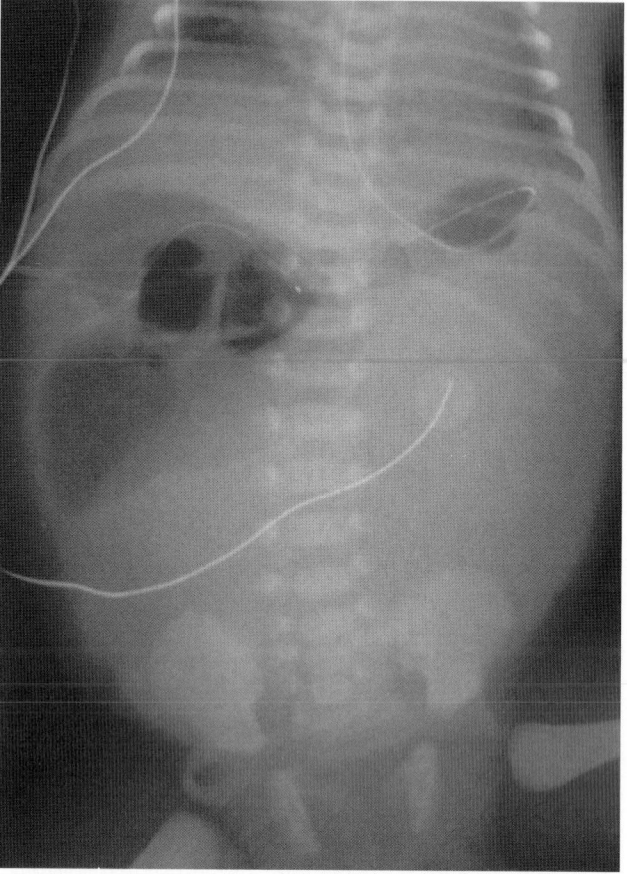

A

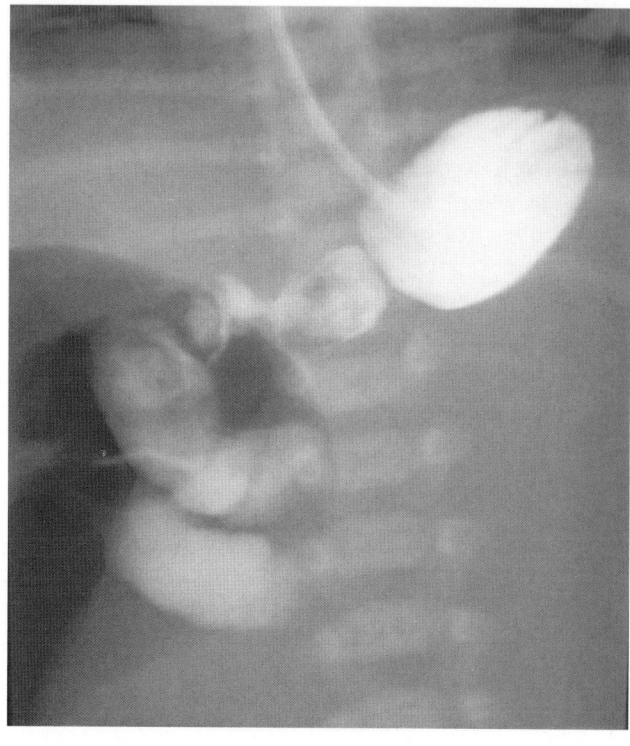

B

Figure 138-3 Radiographic appearance of malrotation. A, A kidney, ureter, bladder (KUB) radiograph from a 2-week-old infant with bilious vomiting shows proximal bowel obstruction, as evidenced by a few dilated bowel loops in the right upper quadrant. B, An upper gastrointestinal radiograph shows that the ligament of Treitz is abnormally located to the right of the spine below the duodenal bulb.

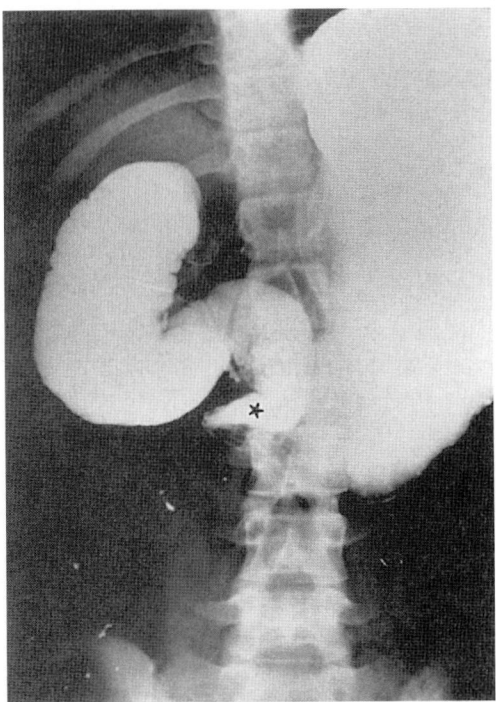

Figure 138-4   Upper gastrointestinal radiograph of volvulus. (From Oldham KT: Pediatric abdomen. In Greenfield LJ, Mulholland M, Oldham KT, et al [eds]: Surgery: Scientific Principles and Practice. Philadelphia, Lippincott-Raven, 1997.)

emesis can result in GI bleeding. Alternatively, a remitting/recurrent course with failure to thrive, abdominal pain, vomiting, malabsorption, or bloody diarrhea may be seen with intermittent obstruction.

Unresolved volvulus generally leads to progressive ischemia, infarction, and necrosis of the bowel wall accompanied by profound acidosis. Perforation with sepsis is another life-threatening complication. Progression can occur in a matter of hours and is associated with significant morbidity and mortality.

Treatment

Malrotation is corrected surgically with a Ladd procedure, which is recommended both for relief of persistent or intermittent symptoms of bowel obstruction and for prevention of subsequent volvulus.

Volvulus is a surgical emergency. Decompression with a nasogastric tube for suctioning, aggressive fluid and electrolyte resuscitation, and administration of antibiotics to cover enteric pathogens are indicated preoperatively. Commonly recommended antibiotic combinations are ampicillin, gentamicin, and metronidazole or a β-lactam/β-lactamase inhibitor with gentamicin to cover gram-negative bacilli, enterococci, and anaerobes. Prompt surgical repair is warranted to reduce the volvulus, restore intestinal blood flow, and resect unsalvageable necrotic gut. Correction of malrotation is performed. Placement of an ostomy may be indicated.

Several postoperative issues need to be considered, especially in patients who require extended periods of bowel rest or who have undergone extensive bowel resection. Parenteral nutrition is often indicated to sustain recovering infants. The amount and location of resected bowel, as well as the functionality of the remaining intestine, determine the ability to eventually feed the child enterally. Infants with greater than 50 cm of remaining small intestine are most likely to tolerate the transition from parenteral to enteral nutrition. Short-gut syndrome is manifested by voluminous or malabsorptive stools and failure to thrive, and children with this condition are at risk for bacterial overgrowth and various nutritional deficiencies. Additionally, long-term parenteral nutrition can induce cholestasis, and there are the attendant risks of long-term IV access.

Postoperative adhesions can be a cause of subsequent bowel obstruction and may occur early or many years after surgery.

Consultation

Generalists are often involved in the diagnosis of malrotation, with subsequent consultation with surgical services. Volvulus requires prompt resuscitative effort and surgical involvement. Intensive care support may also be necessary, especially in children with hemodynamic instability. Postoperative management may be handled collaboratively between the surgical and generalist services. Referral to gastroenterologists is indicated for children requiring prolonged parenteral nutrition or those at risk for short-gut syndrome.

Admission Criteria

Patients with malrotation and persistent vomiting or dehydration require admission. Surgery is often performed at the time of initial diagnosis. All patients with volvulus need admission for access to rapid evaluation, resuscitation, and surgical support.

Discharge Criteria

The patient should be well nourished with adequate enteral or parenteral nutrition, or both.

Prevention

Prevention of volvulus is accomplished by surgical correction of malrotation, whether symptomatic or asymptomatic.

In a Nutshell

- Clinical presentation: Malrotation presents with bilious emesis, often with normal physical examination findings. Volvulus may present similarly initially, but it quickly progresses to abdominal distention, acidosis, and a sepsis-like picture.
- Diagnosis: Malrotation and volvulus may be diagnosed by upper GI imaging (contrast radiography or ultrasonography).
- Treatment: Malrotation requires fluid support and gastric decompression, followed by prompt, but not emergency surgical repair (Ladd procedure). Volvulus requires aggressive fluid resuscitation, rapid diagnosis, perioperative antibiotic coverage, and emergency surgical repair.

INTUSSUSCEPTION

Intussusception is one of the most common causes of small bowel obstruction in the first 2 years of life. Telescoped bowel causes GI obstruction, compression of blood vessels to the gut, and eventually ischemia and necrosis (Fig. 138-5). In young children, intussusception is usually idiopathic, although invagination of the bowel at hypertrophied Peyer patches is frequently implicated. The large majority of cases involve the ileocolic region. In approximately 5% to 8% of cases in children there is a pathologic lead point such as a Meckel diverticulum, hematoma, polyp, or lymphoma.[10] Patients with cystic fibrosis, celiac disease, and Henoch-Schönlein purpura are at increased risk.

Most cases take place in the first year of life, with 80% occurring by 2 years of age. There is a slight male preponderance and an overall incidence of 3 to 5 per 10,000.[11] A temporal association with both rotavirus and adenovirus gastroenteritis has been observed.

Clinical Presentation

The classic signs of intussusception, intermittent abdominal pain ("colic") with vomiting, an abdominal mass, and currant jelly stools, are present concomitantly in less than 50% of patients.[12,13] Currant jelly stools are evidence of bowel ischemia and necrosis, which is a late finding, and the clinician's goal should be to diagnose intussusception before currant jelly stools are produced. Occult blood is demonstrated in 75% of cases at presentation.[14]

Vomiting becomes bilious as the condition progresses; fever can be present but is not predictive. Some children with intussusception will have concurrent diarrhea. An important symptom is lethargy; young children with intussusception can present with intermittent bouts of lethargy and no other identifiable symptoms.

Abdominal examination is best performed between episodes of pain when the abdominal muscles tend to be more relaxed. The Dance sign, palpation of a sausage-shaped mass in the right upper quadrant and absence of bowel gas in the right lower quadrant, is considered pathognomonic of intussusception.

Differential Diagnosis

With symptoms of abdominal pain and vomiting, the differential diagnosis includes appendicitis, gastroenteritis, and other causes of GI obstruction. Ureteral colic secondary to ureteropelvic junction obstruction or ureteral calculus can mimic these symptoms. Pneumonia in children can also present with abdominal pain and vomiting, but it is often accompanied by respiratory symptoms and fever. When lethargy is the sole or predominate feature, the differential diagnosis can be quite broad and includes sepsis, dehydration, nonaccidental trauma, toxic or metabolic abnormalities, central nervous system disorders, and many others.

Diagnosis and Evaluation

Plain films of the abdomen with additional upright or cross-table lateral views are helpful initial studies. Findings strongly suggestive of intussusception include the presence of a soft tissue mass, evidence of bowel obstruction, or identification of intussusceptum, and 80% of patients with these findings have been found to have intussusception. Nonspecific findings of an abnormal bowel gas pattern or normal films do not exclude the possibility of intussusception, but they make it less likely (38% and 9%, respectively).[15]

Contrast enema radiography provides a definitive diagnosis of intussusception, as well as being the therapeutic intervention of choice (Fig. 138-6 and see treatment section). The role of ultrasonography is evolving for diagnosis and therapy. It may be a reasonable intermediate diagnostic step in patients for whom intussusception is a consideration but not a probable diagnosis. It has a sensitivity estimated at 98% to 100%[16,17] for the diagnosis of intussusception, and benefits include its lack of radiation exposure, noninvasive nature, and ability to evaluate other intra-abdominal and pelvic structures not visualized by contrast enema radiogra-

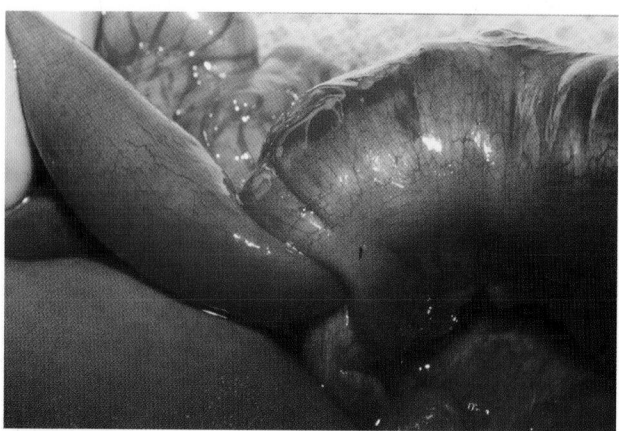

Figure 138-5 Intraoperative appearance of intussusception.

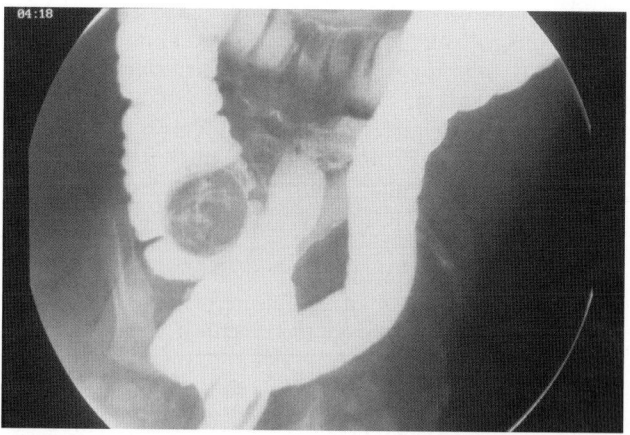

Figure 138-6 Barium enema in a patient with intussusception.

phy. Identification of a lead point may also be accomplished with this technique, which may indicate the need to proceed directly to surgical reduction with excision of the inciting anatomic abnormality. Ultrasound-guided enema reduction is being used with success in some settings and is also performed in some cases as a follow-up study to check for complete success of contrast enema reduction.

Course of Illness

Although intussusception can resolve without intervention, unresolved intussusception will lead to bowel wall ischemia and potentially necrosis, perforation, sepsis, and death. Expectant management is not indicated in a symptomatic patient. A first recurrence of intussusception develops in approximately 10%,[18-20] with an increased risk for subsequent recurrences after the first recurrence.

Treatment

Stabilization, usually fluid resuscitation, and evaluation should proceed until intussusception is suspected or confirmed. Oral or gastric intake should be withheld, and if bowel obstruction is present, nasogastric decompression may be indicated. Although radiologists commonly perform the reduction, surgical involvement is required to provide operative management of unsuccessful reductions, perforation or peritonitis, or clinical deterioration. If there is concern for perforation or prolonged intussusception, antibiotics to cover enteric pathogens should be considered, as detailed earlier in the treatment section for volvulus.

Standard treatment of intussusception has been an air, water-soluble contrast, or barium enema if the patient is clinically stable and has no evidence of perforation, peritonitis, or sepsis. The decision to attempt nonsurgical reduction is made after consensus between the radiologist and surgeon. The success rate for reduction by these techniques is approximately 80%, and the complication rate is reported as less than 4%.[21-25] Longer duration of symptoms, younger age, rectal bleeding, and abnormal radiographic findings have been associated with a decreased rate of success of nonsurgical reduction. Enema reduction can be painful, so analgesia should be provided as needed. Sedation for the procedure is sometimes used but is controversial because it may cloud clinical assessment during and after the procedure.

Consultation

Intussusception is managed through the coordinated efforts of the generalist, surgeon, and radiologist. If the patient is unstable, intensive care involvement may be warranted.

Admission Criteria

Symptomatic intussusception should be treated promptly and is often coordinated in the emergency department, but it may also be managed after admission to an inpatient unit. Patients with unresolved intussusception, an identified lead point, evidence of perforation, or clinical instability should be admitted. Perforation usually occurs at the time of reduction, and symptoms appear within hours in a patient with reliable physical examination findings.

Discharge Criteria

An otherwise well child who has undergone successful reduction of intussusception, shows no signs of perforation, and has no lead point identified can be discharged home after tolerating enteral feeding. Signs and symptoms of recurrence and other complications should be clarified with the caregivers, who should be instructed to return if they develop. There is increasing confidence in early discharge after successful and uncomplicated nonsurgical reduction.[26] Those without adequate follow-up or with abnormal or unreliable postreduction findings warrant more prolonged observation.

Prevention

There is no clear way to prevent intussusception. Use of the first rotavirus vaccine was discontinued because of its epidemiologic association with intussusception.

In a Nutshell

- Clinical presentation: Colicky abdominal pain with evidence of GI obstruction and occult blood in stool. Infants with intussusception may present with only lethargy.
- Diagnosis: Clinical suspicion is confirmed by contrast enema, ultrasound, or surgical evaluation.
- Treatment: Reduction is accomplished by contrast or air enema or by surgery.

On the Horizon

- More on ultrasound-guided reduction of intussusception
- More on repeated attempts at reduction by enema before operative reduction
- Information on the potential use of steroids to prevent recurrence
- Clarification of the role of viral pathogens in the incidence of intussusception

SUGGESTED READING

Daneman A, Navarro O: Intussusception Part 1: A review of diagnostic approaches. Pediatr Radiol 2003;33:79-85.
Daneman A, Navarro O: Intussusception Part 2: An update on the evolution of management. Pediatr Radiol 2004;34:97-108.
Davenport M: ABC of general surgery in children: Surgically correctable causes of vomiting in infancy. BMJ 1996;312:236-239.
McCollough M, Sharieff G: Abdominal surgical emergencies in infants and young children. Emerg Med Clin North Am 2003;21:909-935.
Millar A, Rode H, Cywes S: Malrotation and volvulus in infancy and childhood. Semin Pediatr Surg 2003;12:229-236.

REFERENCES

1. Schechter R, Torfs CP, Bateson TF: The epidemiology of infantile hypertrophic pyloric stenosis. Paediatr Perinat Epidemiol 1997;11:407-427.

2. Mitchell LE, Risch N: The genetics of infantile hypertrophic pyloric stenosis. A reanalysis. Am J Dis Child 1993;147:1203-1211.

3. Finsen VR: Infantile pyloric stenosis—unusual family incidence. Arch Dis Child 1979;54:720-721.

4. Carter CO, Evans KA: Inheritance of congenital pyloric stenosis. J Med Genet 1969;6:233-254.

5. Paulozzi LJ: Is *Helicobacter pylori* a cause of infantile hypertrophic pyloric stenosis? Med Hypotheses 2000;55:119-125.

6. Hauben M, Amsden GW: The association of erythromycin and infantile hypertrophic pyloric stenosis: Causal or coincidental? Drug Saf 2002;25:929-942.

7. Puapong D, Kahng D, Ko A, Applebaum H: Ad libitum feeding: Safely improving the cost effectiveness of pyloromyotomy. J Pediatr Surg 2002;37:1667-1668.

8. Cooper WO, Griffin MR, Arbogast P, et al: Very early exposure to erythromycin and infantile hypertrophic pyloric stenosis. Arch Pediatr Adolesc Med 2002;156:647-650.

9. Forrester MB, Merz RD: Epidemiology of intestinal malrotation, Hawaii, 1986-99. Paediatr Perinat Epidemiol 2003;17:195-200.

10. Navarro OM, Daneman A, Chae A: Intussusception: The use of delayed, repeated reduction attempts and the management of intussusceptions due to pathologic lead points in pediatric patients. AJR Am J Roentgenol 2004;182:1169-1176.

11. O'Ryan M, Lucero Y, Pena Y, Valenzuela MT: Two year review of intestinal intussusception in six large public hospitals of Santiago, Chile. Pediatr Infect Dis J 2003;22:717-721.

12. Simon RA, Hugh TJ, Curtin AM: Childhood intussusception in a regional hospital. Aust N Z J Surg 1994;64:699-702.

13. Kim YS, Rhu JH: Intussusception in infancy and childhood: Analysis of 385 cases. Int Surg 1989;74:114-118.

14. Losek JD, Fiete RL: Intussusception and the diagnostic value of testing stool for occult blood. Am J Emerg Med 1991;9:1-3.

15. Kupperman N, O'Dea T, Pinckey L, Hoecker C: Predictors of intussusception in young children. Arch Pediatr Adolesc Med 2000;154:250-255.

16. Koumananidou C, Vakaki M, Pitsoulakis G, et al: Sonographic detection of lymph nodes in the intussusception of infants and young children: Clinical evaluation and hydrostatic reduction. AJR Am J Roentgenol 2002;178:445-450.

17. Bhisitkul DM, Listernick R, Shkolnik A: Clinical application of ultrasonography in the diagnosis of intussusception. J Pediatr 1992;121:182-186.

18. Ein SH: Recurrent intussusception in children. J Pediatr Surg 1975;10:751-755.

19. Eshel G, Barr J, Heiman E: Incidence of recurrent intussusception following barium vs air enema. Acta Pediatr 1997;86:545-546.

20. Daneman A, Alton DJ, Lobo E, et al: Patterns of recurrence of intussusception in children: A 17-year review. Pediatr Radiol 1998;28:913-919.

21. Ein SH, Palder SB, Alton DJ, Daneman A: Intussusception in the 1990s: Has 25 years made a difference? Pediatr Surg Int 1997;12:474-476.

22. Cohen MD: From air to barium and back to air reduction of intussusception in children. Pediatr Radiol 2002;32:74.

23. Heenan SD, Kyriou J, Fitzgerald M, Adam EJ: Effective dose of pneumatic reduction of pediatric intussusception. Clin Radiol 2000;55:811-816.

24. Hadidi AT, El Shal N: Childhood intussusception: A comparative study of nonsurgical management. J Pediatr Surg 1999;34:304-307.

25. Fecteau A, Flageole H, Nguyen LT, et al: Recurrent intussusception: Safe use of hydrostatic enema. J Pediatr Surg 1996;31:859-861.

26. Bajaj L, Roback MG: Postreduction management of intussuception in a children's hospital emergency department. Pediatrics 2003;112(6, Pt 1):1302-1307.

CHAPTER 139

Abdominal Pain and Acute Abdomen

Eric R. Sundel

Acute abdominal pain is a common problem in pediatrics. Although the spectrum of causes is broad, the most common surgical cause is appendicitis.

Sometime in their lives, about 7% of all people will develop appendicitis.[1] Each year in the United States, about 60,000 to 80,00 children have appendicitis. It is particularly common in the preteen and teen years, with the average age of onset being about 10 years. Before puberty, boys and girls are affected equally; after puberty, there is a slight male predominance.

The appendix, whose function remains unknown, arises from the cecum. Roughly 5% to 15% of people have retrocecal appendixes. In children, the appendix is relatively longer and thinner than in adults, which makes it more susceptible to perforation early in the course of the disease. The greater omentum remains thin, short, and fragile until about 10 years of age. It is therefore less likely to wall off a perforated appendix in a younger child, making generalized peritonitis more common in children than in adults.[2]

The pathogenesis of appendicitis begins with obstruction of the appendiceal lumen. The most common cause of obstruction is enlargement of the lymphoid tissue (Peyer patches) in the wall of the appendix. The lymphoid follicles enlarge probably in response to ingested microorganisms, most likely viruses associated with upper respiratory infections. Fecal material, undigested food, other foreign material, or pinworms may also lead to obstruction. Regardless of the initial trigger, the resultant obstruction causes dilation of the lumen of the appendix and thickening of its wall. Bacterial overgrowth results within the structure, with subsequent bacterial invasion of the appendiceal wall, inflammation, and ischemia. If unchecked, gangrene and eventual appendiceal perforation will occur. As the transmural appendiceal inflammation progresses, so does the local peritoneal inflammation. With perforation, the peritonitis can become widespread.

The responsible bacteria are usual fecal flora, most commonly *Escherichia coli, Peptostreptococcus, Bacteroides fragilis,* and *Pseudomonas* species, and the process is usually polymicrobial.

CLINICAL PRESENTATION

The classic presentation of appendicitis is not hard to recognize and occurs in approximately two thirds of cases. Many preschool-age children, however, present with atypical and challenging clinical pictures.

Typically, a previously healthy child awakes with vague periumbilical pain that is uncomfortable but not debilitating. Shortly after the onset of pain, infrequent nonbilious emesis often develops. Over the next few hours, the poorly localized pain gradually increases in intensity before moving to the right lower quadrant. There is associated anorexia and low-grade fever. A child with appendicitis prefers to remain still, so the jarring and shaking movements during the car ride to the health facility are painful. Diarrhea, if it occurs, is infrequent and consists of small stools caused by irritation of the sigmoid colon by the inflamed appendix. Likewise, bladder irritation may produce dysuria or urgency.

In atypical cases, the pain pattern may be quite different. Young children in particular may not recognize or may be unable to verbalize the change in location of the pain, or they may not develop localized pain. In some, such as those with a retrocecal appendix, the pain may never shift in location, or it may originate in or migrate to the right upper quadrant or flank.

Some children with appendicitis never develop vomiting. Also, although most patients with appendicitis have a low-grade fever, some are afebrile, and an occasional child has a temperature above 39°C. Finally, although anorexia is common, some children report being hungry; if they are actually offered food, however, most but not all patients with appendicitis will decline.

If appendicitis remains unrecognized, perforation will ultimately occur. About one third to one half of children with perforated appendixes have been seen by physicians before the diagnosis of perforation is made.[3,4] With perforation, there is usually temporary relief of the pain, but within hours it classically becomes generalized and progressively more severe as the child develops diffuse peritonitis. However, if the contamination is well localized (walled off) by the omentum, the child develops a discrete abscess and may have localized tenderness without severe pain.

Before examining the child, having him or her ambulate and climb up or down from the parent's lap or examining table can yield helpful clues. A hunched-over posture, tentative gait, limp, and difficulty mounting or dismounting are suggestive of peritoneal irritation. For nonambulatory patients, jarring the examining table may produce evidence of pain.

On physical examination, a patient with appendicitis (nonperforated) usually has a temperature of 38°C to 38.3°C, tachycardia, and a normal respiratory rate and blood pressure. Reliable examination of the abdomen may require accommodations that ease the child's anxiety (e.g., examination on a caregiver's lap). Asking the child to point to the spot that hurts and examining that area last may also facilitate the process. Classically, the abdomen appears flat with normal or hypoactive bowel sounds. Localized and reproducible tenderness at McBurney point (one third the way along a line that would join the umbilicus to the right anterior superior ileac spine) is a useful finding, especially with a normally positioned appendix.

Many techniques are used to elicit signs of peritoneal irritation. For rebound tenderness, the examiner presses down on the tender area slowly, maintains pressure for a few seconds, and then abruptly removes his or her hand. The child experiences pain if there is peritoneal inflammation, but this maneuver may also be uncomfortable for anxious children without peritonitis. Additionally, many experts believe that this test is unduly distressing and recommend finger percussion throughout the abdomen, leaving the right lower quadrant for last. Pain limited to percussion of the right lower quadrant, or pain in the right lower quadrant with percussion of other quadrants, is suggestive of peritonitis (Rovsing sign). In older children, having them stand, lift up onto their toes, and then drop down onto their heels can elicit localized abdominal pain. A prone patient may report right lower quadrant tenderness when the examiner percusses the plantar surface of the heel or the lateral aspect of the pelvis. Any of these maneuvers can produce pain if there is peritoneal irritation.

Voluntary muscle guarding is nonspecific and can be seen with abdominal pain from myriad causes and in ticklish or anxious patients. Involuntary muscle guarding, in contrast, is a powerful finding in a patient with appendicitis but can be subtle and difficult to appreciate.

The previously described signs are common when a normally positioned appendix is inflamed; however, with retrocecal appendicitis, these physical findings may be absent. When the inflamed appendix lies on the psoas muscle, use of this muscle causes pain. The examiner places his or her hand above the knee of the prone patient and asks him or her to raise the thigh against the resistance provided by the examiner. Alternatively, the child lies on his or her left side and the examiner extends the patient's right thigh at the hip. Pain with these maneuvers yields a positive psoas sign.

If the inflamed retrocecal appendix is adjacent to the internal obturator muscle, pain is elicited when it is stretched. With the patient prone, the examiner flexes the right lower extremity at the knee and hip and internally rotates it. If right lower quadrant pain is produced, the obturator sign is positive.

A rectal examination may be helpful. Suggestive findings include tenderness greater on the right side, fullness on the right, and heme-negative stools. Patient cooperation is needed for reliable rectal palpation. Grossly bloody stools are not found with appendicitis, and even occult blood should prompt a consideration of other diagnoses.

DIFFERENTIAL DIAGNOSIS

The condition most commonly confused with appendicitis is gastroenteritis. Many other diseases can simulate appendicitis, including constipation, urinary tract infection, right lower lobe pneumonia, ovarian torsion or cyst, incarcerated inguinal hernia, testicular torsion, intussusception, hemolytic uremic syndrome, diabetic ketoacidosis, and abdominal trauma (Table 139-1). In sexually active female patients, pelvic inflammatory disease and ectopic pregnancy are also considerations.

DIAGNOSIS AND EVALUATION

Appendicitis is often a clinical diagnosis. With rare exceptions, it progresses gradually over several hours, which contrasts with the waxing and waning course of many other

Table 139-1 Appendicitis and Similar Conditions Presenting with Abdominal Pain and Vomiting

Similar Conditions	Distinguishing Characteristics of Appendicitis
Gastroenteritis	Pain precedes vomiting and fever Diarrhea, if it occurs, is small volume
Constipation	Pain progresses in intensity and is typically not fluctuating
Urinary tract infection	Pain usually not suprapubic or flank Urinalysis usually <10 WBCs/hpf
Pneumonia	Cough and tachypnea uncommon Fever typically low grade Abdominal tenderness
Pelvic inflammatory disease	Pain typically localized to right lower quadrant
Ectopic pregnancy	Gradual increase in pain Negative serum β-HCG
Ovarian torsion or ovarian cyst	Gradual increase in pain, which is initially periumbilical Elevated WBCs (>11,000/mm^3)
Incarcerated inguinal hernia or testicular torsion	Normal testicular examination
Intussusception	Progressive, not colicky pain Uncommon in those younger than 2-3 yr Stools typically heme negative
Hemolytic uremic syndrome	Diarrhea, if present, is nonbloody Normal platelets and hemoglobin Normal creatinine
Diabetic ketoacidosis	No polyuria or polydipsia Dehydration usually not severe No hyperglycemia or glucosuria
Abdominal trauma	Negative history of trauma No abdominal wall contusions

β-HCG, β-human chorionic gonadotropin; hpf, high-power field; WBC, white blood cell.

diseases. For equivocal cases, in-hospital observation with serial examinations of the abdomen over a 6- to 12-hour period can be quite useful diagnostically.

A complete blood count is routinely obtained to determine the peripheral white blood cell (WBC) count. In about 75% of cases of nonperforated appendicitis, the peripheral WBC count is greater than 11,000/mm^3 or the neutrophil percentage is greater than 75%. It is unusual in nonperforated appendicitis for the WBC count to be above 20,000/mm^3.

C-reactive protein is increased in more than 85% of patients with appendicitis who have been symptomatic for more than 12 hours.[3] However, elevation in C-reactive protein is nonspecific and therefore of limited value.

Serum β-human chorionic gonadotropin measurement is indicated in all postmenarchal females to rule out pregnancy-related causes.

Urinalysis should be performed to rule out other conditions. Importantly, up to 25% of children with appendicitis have more than 5 white or red blood cells per high-power field, due to urethral or bladder irritation from the inflamed appendix.[5]

Plain radiographs, whether single or multiple (i.e., an obstruction series), are often normal in appendicitis. In approximately 10% of cases, an abdominal plain film shows a calcified appendicolith, which is considered diagnostic.[6] There may be right-sided scoliosis or an indistinct right psoas margin, although these findings are less specific. If a plain film is obtained, the chest should always be included to rule out pneumonia.

The use of ultrasonography (US) to evaluate appendicitis has been studied in nearly 10,000 pediatric patients. Although its specificity (88% to 99%) and accuracy (82% to 99%) are quite good, its sensitivity varies considerably (50% to 100%). Appendiceal visualization rates also vary dramatically, from as high as 98% to as low as 22%.[7] Thus, negative findings by US are not helpful unless an experienced observer unequivocally demonstrates a normal appendix. It should be noted that US is often indicated in females when ovarian torsion or an ovarian cyst is a diagnostic consideration. US is superior to computed tomography (CT) for imaging these gynecologic processes.

CT has become increasingly popular, especially helical CT with rectal contrast. One center using this technique to diagnose appendicitis found that it had 97% sensitivity, 99% specificity, and an overall accuracy of 96%. Colonic administration of contrast material saves time (compared with oral administration) and is well tolerated.[8]

In one study, an imaging protocol of CT following US was used: children with equivocal findings of appendicitis by US went on to have CT with rectal contrast.[9] With this protocol, the perforation rate was reduced, as was the negative appendectomy rate. However, in children younger than 5 years, there was no significant decrease in these rates.

In patients who present late with an abscess or inflammatory mass (phlegmon), CT is helpful in determining whether surgical intervention is warranted in addition to intravenous antibiotics. Although the interpretation of abdominal CT scans is less operator dependent than the interpretation of US, the radiologist's level of experience and comfort with pediatric CT are critical. Also, although an expedient diagnosis is key, radiation exposure should be kept in mind and discussed with families.

Last, a contrast enema may be useful if intussusception and appendicitis are both diagnostic considerations. Smooth and complete filling of the appendix without extrinsic compression of the cecum or terminal ileum is a reliable negative sign and occurs in about 80% to 90% of normal appendixes.[6] Again, radiation exposure is a consideration.

COURSE OF ILLNESS

By 24 hours after pain onset, about 15% of children have perforation. By 48 hours after the initial symptoms, roughly 75% have perforation. A child with pain of 4 days' duration has an approximately 90% risk of perforation. If perforation occurs, the mortality rate increases to as high as 5%, compared with less than 0.1% for nonperforated appendicitis.[1] Those who die are predominantly very young children or those with perforated appendixes and peritonitis who undergo surgery before adequate fluid resuscitation. The morbidity rate also rises appreciably in those with perforation.

TREATMENT

Therapy is dependent on the stage of illness and the certainty of the diagnosis of appendicitis. If the diagnosis of nonperforated appendicitis is equivocal or likely, management includes the following:

- Early consultation with a surgeon skilled in the evaluation and management of children with acute surgical abdomens.
- Nothing by mouth and intravenous fluids as needed.
- In-hospital observation and monitoring with serial examinations, as indicated.
- Imaging studies as needed, depending on the institution's radiologic expertise with children.

To reduce the risk of perforation, many experts recommend that the decision whether to operate be made within 24 to 36 hours of pain onset.

In unequivocal appendicitis, the patient should be prepared to go directly to the operating room. This includes nothing-by-mouth status; assessment of hydration status and administration of appropriate intravenous fluids, including fluid resuscitation, if needed; and antibiotics, which should be administered at least 30 minutes before surgery. Antibiotic prophylaxis can reduce the incidence of wound infection and intra-abdominal abscess. In nonperforated appendicitis, the choice of preoperative antibiotics includes (1) cefoxitin or cefotetan; (2) ampicillin, gentamicin, and either clindamycin or metronidazole; or (3) piperacillin-tazobactam.[10]

Regarding the surgical approach, there are risks and benefits of both laparoscopic and open appendectomy. The choice is the surgeon's and depends on his or her training and experience.

Postoperatively, pain control and adequate hydration are key. Intravenous morphine for the first few hours is often warranted, with a switch to oral pain medications once the patient is drinking well. In nonperforated appendicitis, oral fluids should be allowed when the child awakes postoperatively, and the diet should be advanced as tolerated. If oral intake is poor or if postoperative emesis persists, intravenous fluid support is continued, with attention to maintenance and ongoing replacement needs. Antibiotics are continued only if the appendix was gangrenous or perforated.

The risk of postoperative complications is approximately 15% and is highest in those with a perforated appendix.[10] If the patient has fever or abdominal pain or is unable to tolerate a regular diet by 5 to 7 days postoperatively, consider an intra-abdominal or wound abscess. Wound infections are treated by opening the wound, and most deep abscesses are treated by percutaneous drainage under US or CT guidance. For children unable to tolerate enteral feedings 1 week after surgery, consider parenteral nutrition.

Mechanical small bowel obstruction is an uncommon postoperative complication. Most patients who develop bowel obstruction more than 1 month after appendicitis require laparotomy for lysis of adhesions.

ADMISSION CRITERIA

- Definite appendicitis requiring surgical intervention.
- Abdominal pain of uncertain cause, particularly in pre-school-age children, in whom the diagnosis of appendicitis is more difficult and perforation before diagnosis is more likely.
- Lack of a reliable outpatient observer or inadequate follow-up.

DISCHARGE CRITERIA

Postoperatively, children need to meet the following criteria:

- Afebrile.
- Reassuring abdominal examination.
- Tolerating a regular diet.
- Ambulating with minimal if any discomfort.

PREVENTION

If an incidental appendicolith is found on imaging, most authorities recommend an elective appendectomy.

Diet is postulated but not proved to play a role in the development of appendicitis. This is based on the finding that the rate of appendicitis has been declining in Western countries since the 1980s and increasing in developing ones. Westerners have increased their fiber intake during this period, while those in developing countries have adopted the typical Western diet, resulting in decreased dietary fiber.

IN A NUTSHELL

- The classic presentation of appendicitis is gradually worsening periumbilical pain, followed by infrequent nonbilious emesis. After several hours, the pain shifts to the right lower quadrant. Fever may follow the onset of pain. Atypical presentations are not uncommon.
- Appendicitis is often diagnosed by clinical assessment, with laboratory testing to eliminate other diagnoses or to confirm an inflammatory state. Imaging studies are useful in equivocal cases.
- Inpatient observation and early consultation with a surgeon are recommended for equivocal cases, and appendectomy for confirmed or highly suggestive cases. Preoperative antibiotics are recommended.

ON THE HORIZON

- The development of new and enhanced imaging modalities to aid in the diagnosis of appendicitis.
- Elucidation on whether dietary modification can alter the risk of appendicitis.

SUGGESTED READING

Ashcraft K: Acute abdominal pain. Pediatr Rev 2000;21:363-367.

Garcia Pena BM, Taylor GA, Lund DP, et al: Appendicitis revisited: New insights into an age-old problem. Contemp Pediatr 1999;16:122-131.

Taylor G: Suspected appendicitis in children: In search of the single best diagnostic test. Radiology 2004;231:293-295.

Wesson D: Appendicitis in children. UpToDate 2003. UpToDate.com.

REFERENCES

1. Way LW: Appendix. In Way L (ed): Current Surgical Diagnosis and Treatment, 11th ed. Norwalk, CT, Appleton Lange, 2003.
2. Appendicitis. In Raffensperger J: Swenson's Pediatric Surgery, 5th ed. Norwalk, CT, Appleton Lange, 1990.
3. Garcia Pena BM, Taylor GA, Lund DP, et al: Appendicitis revisited: New insights into an age-old problem. Contemp Pediatr 1999;16:122-131.
4. Hartman G: Acute appendicitis. In Behrman RE, Kliegman R, Jenson HB (eds): Nelson Textbook of Pediatrics, 16th ed. Philadelphia, Saunders, 2000, pp 1178-1181.
5. Perkin R, Swift J, Newton D: Pediatric Hospital Medicine. Philadelphia, Lippincott Willams & Wilkins, 2003.
6. Schnaufer L, Mahlooubi S: Abdominal emergencies. In Fleisher G, Ludwig S: Textbook of Pediatric Emergency Medicine, 3rd ed. Baltimore, Williams & Wilkins, 1993, pp 1309-1313.
7. Taylor G: Suspected appendicitis in children: In search of the single best diagnostic test. Radiology 2004;231:293-295.
8. Mullins ME, Kircher MF, Ryan DP, et al: Evaluation of suspected appendicitis in children using limited helical CT and colonic contrast material. AJR Am J Roentgenol 2001;176:37-41.
9. Pena BM, Taylor GA, Fishman SJ, Mandl KD: Effect of an imaging protocol on clinical outcomes among pediatric patients with appendicitis. Pediatrics 2002;110:1088-1093.
10. Wesson D: Appendicitis in children. UpToDate 2003. UpToDate.com.

CHAPTER 140

Hernias

Peter F. Nichol and Peter Mattei

Hernias are among the most frequent indications for elective surgery in children. In many institutions, patients are admitted onto the hospitalist service (with a surgical consultation). As such, the pediatric hospitalist must be aware of the relevant anatomy, presentation, and treatment options of this common condition.

Hernia refers to any opening, congenital or acquired, in the abdominal musculature or fascia that allows all or part of an abdominal viscus to protrude beyond its usual boundaries; the term may also refer to the protruding viscus itself. Most hernias include an extension of the peritoneum, the *hernia sac,* which encases the herniated viscus and must be excised as part of the surgical repair. *Incarcerated hernias* are those in which the herniated viscus cannot be reduced manually, usually because of edema. *Strangulated hernia* refers to an incarcerated hernia in which the vascular integrity of the herniated viscus is compromised. This usually involves venous and lymphatic congestion of the tissue but can progress to arterial insufficiency, ischemia, and eventually necrosis. Most incarcerated hernias constitute a surgical emergency. *Sliding hernia* refers to a hernia in which the serosa of an intra-abdominal organ forms part of the hernia sac, which can make for a more difficult repair.

The most common hernias in children are indirect inguinal and umbilical hernias. Most hernias in children are congenital defects and are not the result of excessive straining or fascial disruption. Consequently, pain is rarely a symptom of an uncomplicated hernia in children. This also means that pediatric hernias rarely require fascial reconstruction or the use of prosthetic mesh, making the operation more straightforward and less painful than in adults.

Indirect inguinal hernias result from persistence of the processus vaginalis, an embryonic structure that plays a role in testicular descent and is supposed to disappear before birth (Fig. 140-1). Umbilical hernias result from persistence of the umbilical ring, the opening in the fascia that allows passage of the umbilical cord structure and usually closes shortly after birth.

Almost all hernias require operative repair, regardless of location or type. The only exception is an asymptomatic umbilical hernia in a child younger than 3 years, which often resolves spontaneously.[1] No other type of true hernia is known to resolve spontaneously, and all have a small but definite risk of incarceration and subsequent ischemia of the herniated viscus.[2] Most hernias can be repaired electively, depending on the needs and preferences of the family.

Most elective hernia repairs are performed on an outpatient basis. However, admission is indicated for young infants at risk for apnea, some children with complex medical conditions, and those who require emergent operations for complications of the hernia.

INGUINAL AND UMBILICAL HERNIAS

Clinical Presentation

Most pediatric inguinal hernias present as an asymptomatic mass in the inguinal region, usually just lateral to the rectus sheath and just above the pubic bone. In some cases, there is only an asymmetry in the suprapubic fat pad; alternatively, because indirect inguinal hernias can extend into the scrotum, there may be a difference in the size of the scrotal contents. Hernias typically appear or become larger when the patient increases intra-abdominal pressure, such as during the Valsalva maneuver. The classic history is that of a painless bulge that appears during straining; there are usually no other symptoms.

Although some children describe a vague discomfort when the inguinal hernia is "out," the vast majority of uncomplicated hernias in children are painless. Moreover, pain alone is almost never an indication of the presence or imminent development of a hernia. The combination of an apparent hernia and severe pain should raise the suspicion that the herniated viscus has become incarcerated. Young infants with hernias pose a particular challenge because crying for any reason causes the hernia to become larger and more tense, raising the suspicion for incarceration. Parents should be instructed to console the child in the usual way (e.g., rocking, changing the diaper, feeding), but if these fail after 20 to 30 minutes or if other symptoms such as vomiting or fever develop, the infant should be brought urgently to the emergency department. An experienced health care provider should attempt to reduce the hernia if it is in fact incarcerated.

An incarcerated hernia is a true emergency. Fortunately, the presentation is rarely subtle. Children are typically in severe pain and very restless, unable to find a comfortable position. Frequently there is vomiting, either as a reflex secondary to visceral compromise or due to bowel obstruction. Fever, dehydration, and lethargy are usually late signs that suggest bowel ischemia. The hernia itself is usually quite prominent, with overlying erythema; it is very tense and tender on examination. Bluish discoloration is *not* characteristic of a hernia and is more often associated with a hydrocele.

An umbilical hernia presents as a painless bulge at the umbilicus in the newborn period. These hernias are rarely symptomatic and almost never incarcerate. They are more common in African American children but occur in children of every ethnicity.[1] Because most umbilical hernias resolve spontaneously, children younger than 3 years can be safely observed. The size of the herniated contents may appear to enlarge over time, despite the fact that the fascial defect is

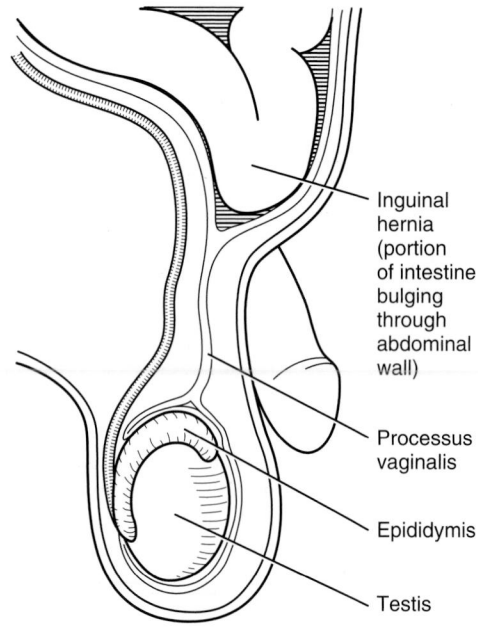

Inguinal hernia (portion of intestine bulging through abdominal wall)

Processus vaginalis

Epididymis

Testis

Figure 140-1   Inguinal hernia.

gradually getting smaller. An incarcerated umbilical hernia is quite rare and is usually evident on presentation: a painful umbilical mass that is tense and tender on examination, sometimes associated with vomiting.

Differential Diagnosis

An asymptomatic bulge in the groin that enlarges with straining and promptly resolves spontaneously or with gentle manual pressure is pathognomonic for hernia. It is sometimes more difficult to distinguish an incarcerated hernia from other, usually more benign, processes (Table 140-1; Fig. 140-2).

Umbilical masses can sometimes be confused with an umbilical hernia. In newborns, a small omphalocele may be difficult to distinguish from a large umbilical hernia. An umbilical mass with granulation tissue, especially if fluid drains from the umbilicus, may represent a patent urachus or omphalomesenteric duct remnant. Any suspicious umbilical lesion, especially in a newborn, should be evaluated by a pediatric surgeon. In older children, there is often residual scar tissue after resolution of an umbilical hernia defect, which can mimic a hernia. If there is no palpable fascial defect and no enlargement with straining, this is usually only of cosmetic importance.

Diagnosis and Evaluation

There is no imaging modality that can reliably confirm or rule out the presence of a hernia. The diagnosis is based solely on the history and physical examination. Ultrasonography or computed tomography is occasionally useful to rule out other diagnoses, but when the imaging studies are equivocal and the diagnosis remains uncertain, surgical consultation should be obtained without delay.

On physical examination, an inguinal hernia is diagnosed by the presence of a bulge that can be manually reduced into the abdomen. An impulse when the patient coughs or strains

Finding	Description and Comments
Hydrocele	Collection of fluid along spermatic cord or in scrotum
	Result of persistence of part of processus vaginalis
	Size changes only gradually
	May be either communicating or noncommunicating with peritoneal cavity
	Distinguished from hernia by normal spermatic cord palpable in inguinal canal above hydrocele
	Ultrasonography or surgery may be required for diagnosis
Lymph node	Enlarges gradually and resolves slowly compared with hernia
	Normal spermatic cord can be palpated separate from lymph node
	Ultrasonography can aid in diagnosis
Tumor	Extremely uncommon in pediatric population
Ovary	May be incarcerated as part of inguinal hernia
	Vascular supply to ovary is narrow, and incarcerated ovary may not produce additional symptoms
	Surgical urgency because of potential for trauma or torsion

Table 140-1   Differential Diagnosis of Groin Mass or Swelling

is not sufficient evidence of a hernia to warrant an operation. It is sometimes difficult to make a hernia appear on request. Infants often strain upon palpation of the abdomen or cry when the diaper is removed. Older children are asked to bear down and have often learned how to make the hernia come out. This can also be accomplished by having them jump up and down or asking them to inflate a nonlatex examination glove.

Umbilical hernias are usually quite evident on examination. The hernia contents should be gently reduced and the fascial defect assessed for size. Tiny umbilical hernias (<4 mm diameter) can probably be safely observed, although there is a small risk that even tiny umbilical hernias may enlarge during pregnancy. As noted previously, all asymptomatic umbilical hernias in children younger than 3 years can be observed as well. All other umbilical hernias should be repaired electively.

Course of Illness

Inguinal hernias never resolve spontaneously. They have a tendency to enlarge and may become more symptomatic over time. There is a small but definite risk of incarceration that is impossible to quantify based on clinical criteria.

Once the diagnosis is confirmed, operative intervention is recommended, preferably within 2 to 3 months. An incarcerated hernia that cannot be reduced manually requires immediate operation. In addition to the complications associated with emergency surgery and the potential for bowel

COMMUNICATING HYDROCELE   NONCOMMUNICATING HYDROCELE

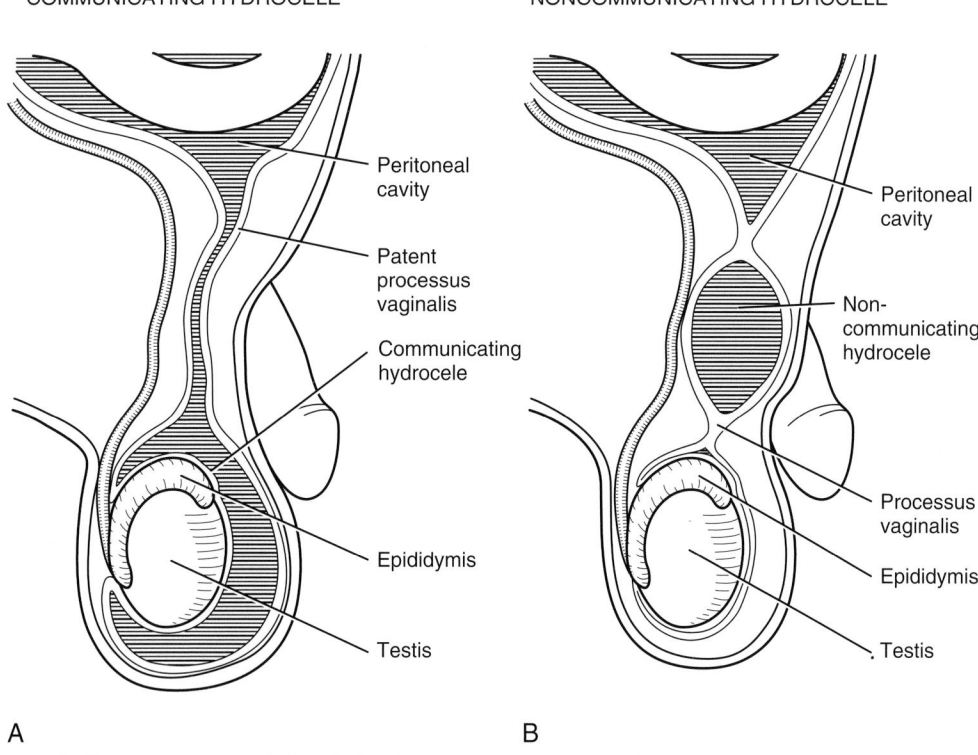

A   B

Figure 140-2 Communicating and noncommunicating hydroceles.

ischemia, there is a risk of testicular ischemia and subsequent atrophy. In girls with incarcerated hernia of the ovary, torsion or injury to the suddenly exposed ovary is also possible.

Because the risk of incarceration is so difficult to predict, guidelines regarding restriction of activities for patients awaiting surgery are difficult to formulate. Mild physical activities do not appear to increase the risk of incarceration for patients with asymptomatic and uncomplicated inguinal hernias. Extreme physical exertion that involves a great deal of straining or the potential for direct injury to the hernia contents should probably be restricted until after surgery. In practice, restrictions are generally based on common sense and the perceived risk of liability for the individual or group (e.g., school officials) making the recommendation.

The natural history of umbilical hernias is that of gradual spontaneous closure within the first few years of life. Those that are larger than 1 cm in diameter at age 3 years are unlikely to close spontaneously.[1] Incarcerated umbilical hernia is thought to be extremely rare in children, but the risk persists throughout life. Umbilical hernias can enlarge significantly during pregnancy and may result in complications requiring urgent operation.

Treatment

All inguinal hernias should be surgically repaired. The current standard is an open operation, although surgeons are in the process of developing a laparoscopic approach for inguinal hernia repair that will likely become the standard of care in the future. Laparoscopy has become popular as a means of identifying the presence of a contralateral hernia during repair of a known hernia. Children who have a history of prematurity, those with a strong family history of inguinal hernia in childhood, and those with left-sided hernias have a higher risk of having one on the contralateral side.[3] Laparoscopic contralateral exploration is usually considered in children younger than 10 years and in any child with risk factors.

If a patient presents with an incarcerated hernia, manual reduction should be attempted, usually after the patient has been given analgesics or mild sedation. The technique involves the application of constant pressure to the herniated bowel with one hand while using the thumb and first two fingers of the other hand to squeeze the neck of the hernia close to where it enters the abdomen. Constant (rather than increasing) pressure for more than 2 minutes is sometimes necessary. This reduces the edema in the herniated bowel and usually allows it to eventually go back in. Multiple attempts in the same session are often necessary, and the hernia is sometimes reduced by a series of small "pops." Hernias that cannot be reduced manually require immediate surgery. Patients whose hernias are reduced with difficulty are usually admitted for observation and hydration. They can then be operated on during the same admission or discharged and readmitted for operation within a week or so. It was thought in the past that ischemic bowel cannot be reduced, but this has been proved wrong on multiple occasions.[4]

Most patients whose hernias are reduced manually are better immediately. They are more alert, their pain is gone, and they are ready to play and eat. In rare cases, the bowel may be reduced "en masse," which means that it is reduced but stays kinked due to adhesions or irreversible injury.

These patients may have persistent symptoms of bowel obstruction and require laparotomy. Not all patients with incarcerated hernias have signs or symptoms of bowel obstruction. In some cases, another organ such as the omentum, ovary, or appendix (Littre hernia) can be involved. Even if the bowel is involved, only one wall rather than the entire lumen may be compromised, a condition known as a Richter hernia. A high index of suspicion and a low threshold for surgery are critical elements of decision making when dealing with a potentially incarcerated hernia.

Umbilical hernias rarely need surgical repair. When they are repaired, it is usually done under general anesthesia on an outpatient basis.

Premature infants whose hernias are diagnosed during a long stay in the neonatal nursery can be managed in one of two ways: operative repair within a few days of anticipated discharge, or follow-up as an outpatient and repair at a later date. The former eliminates the likelihood of incarcerated hernia and its potential sequelae and, with proper planning, should not prolong the hospital stay. The latter approach is preferred by some because of the slightly higher risk of recurrence in infants who undergo repair at such a young age.

Consultation

Surgical consultation is indicated whenever there is suspicion of a hernia. Depending on regional referral patterns and local resources, this might involve a pediatric surgeon, a general surgeon, or a urologist. Any suspicion of an incarcerated hernia calls for immediate surgical consultation. Children with inguinal pain or a questionable history with few physical findings pose a particular challenge for the general practitioner. In general, pediatric surgeons are willing to evaluate any patient with a suspected inguinal hernia in an attempt to resolve the issue.

Admission Criteria

Children whose hernias have been reduced manually should usually be admitted for hydration and observation.

Postoperative admission for monitoring and observation is indicated for newborns who are at risk for apnea during the first 24 hours after general anesthesia. Traditionally, this guideline has been applied to full-term infants younger than 3 months, premature infants less than 60 weeks' postconceptual age, and any child who is on a monitor at home.[5-7] Many centers have liberalized these criteria down to 52 or even 44 weeks' postconceptual age.

Children with other medical conditions requiring inpatient monitoring, such as congenital heart disease, may also require overnight admission.

Postoperative complications, though rare, can sometimes require inpatient therapy:

- Wound infection is uncommon and is usually treated on an outpatient basis with oral antibiotics and, if necessary, incision and drainage of an abscess.
- Infants who are febrile or lethargic may require admission for intravenous antibiotics and hydration.
- Hematomas can form at the surgical site. This is especially common after umbilical hernia repair and in the scrotum after inguinal hernia repair. These usually resolve spontaneously but sometimes require incision and evacuation of the clot if they are painful, enlarging, or infected.
- Uncommon indications for hospital admission after hernia repair include complications of general anesthesia, such as intractable emesis or an airway complication.

Discharge Criteria

Discharge criteria for children who have had surgery under general anesthesia are the same, regardless of the procedure:

- Ability to tolerate a diet.
- Ability to ambulate or safely be moved about.
- Control of pain with oral analgesics.

Patients who are admitted for observation after a difficult manual reduction of an incarcerated hernia can be discharged when they are thought to be out of danger for occult bowel obstruction or visceral ischemia and they are asymptomatic and stable—usually 8 to 12 hours.

Prevention

Because hernias in children are generally congenital, prevention of the hernia itself is not possible. However, some of the complications of hernia are preventable with education and ready access to health care. When a child is suspected of having a hernia, the parents should be advised to obtain a surgical consultation and should be taught to recognize the signs and symptoms of an incarcerated hernia. This applies to all hernias but is especially true for inguinal hernias. Parents should be told that if the child complains of abdominal or scrotal pain and the hernia is visible and tender, they should take no more than 20 to 30 minutes to rule out other more common causes of discomfort and to console the child. If the cause is unclear, they should proceed immediately to the physician's office or the emergency room. Premature newborns with hernias can avoid the complications associated with incarceration by having their hernias repaired before discharge from the newborn nursery.

There is no role for a truss in inguinal hernias or for taping a coin over an umbilical hernia. These measures do not cause resolution of the hernia; in fact, they can cause complications, such as pressure sores and skin breakdown, and delay appropriate therapy.

UNUSUAL HERNIAS

Although hernias can occur anywhere in the abdomen, there are certain locations where they are more common. Epigastric hernia, or epiplocele, is different from other hernias in that it does not have a hernia sac and contains only preperitoneal fat. This type of hernia presents as a small, sometimes rather subtle bulge in the epigastrium anywhere between the umbilicus and the xiphoid process, but always in the midline; they may be multiple. Those that occur just above the umbilicus can be confused with an umbilical hernia. They are usually asymptomatic but have a greater tendency to cause pain in school-aged children and adolescents. They are not reducible, but because they do not contain any intra-abdominal organs, this poses no danger. They are repaired electively under general anesthesia, with excellent results.

Epigastric hernias often occur in the setting of diastasis recti, which is not a true hernia. The linea alba is often wide and lax in infants and young children, so when they strain, the midline fascia bulges forward, sometimes quite dramatically. This is a self-correcting anatomic variant that does *not* require surgical therapy.

Direct inguinal hernias are common in adults but extremely rare in children. These are due to a disruption of the fascia that defines the "floor" of the inguinal canal, producing a bulge or palpable impulse in the inguinal region medial to the epigastric vessels. They may be exacerbated by heavy lifting and chronic straining and are often painful. They can occur concomitantly with indirect inguinal hernias, but the direct component bulges outward on examination and does not communicate with the scrotal contents. These require reconstruction of the fascia using one of several traditional operations, and they are typically reinforced with an artificial mesh material.

Femoral hernias are exceedingly rare in children and present with a bulge below the inguinal ligament. They are due to herniation along the femoral canal and are more common in females. Repair can be difficult and usually requires an extensive inguinal dissection and the use of a mesh.

Spigelian hernias are also rare and present with a bulge at a specific anatomic location: the lower abdomen just lateral to the rectus sheath, at the point where the posterior rectus sheath ends at the arcuate line—where it transitions from being a strong continuation of the lateral abdominal fascia layers to a thin layer of peritoneum. These hernias can be difficult to diagnose but in some cases can be confirmed with CT.

Incisional hernias can occur after any abdominal surgical procedure, including laparoscopy (port-site hernias). Any bulge in an incision that enlarges with straining should be suspected of being an incisional hernia. They occasionally become painful or incarcerated and should therefore be repaired surgically.

IN A NUTSHELL

- Most hernias present as asymptomatic masses that can be evaluated on an outpatient basis and treated electively.
- The most common types are inguinal and umbilical hernias.
- All inguinal hernias require surgical repair in a timely fashion to avoid complications such as incarceration, strangulation, and bowel or testicular ischemia.
- Umbilical hernias are safe to observe in infants; however, those that persist at age 3 years are unlikely

to resolve spontaneously and should be repaired surgically.
- Parents should be educated about the signs and symptoms of an incarcerated hernia and should be instructed to seek appropriate medical attention urgently.

ON THE HORIZON

- Minimally invasive approaches to inguinal hernia repair are being developed. They are used routinely in some centers with acceptable results, but the techniques are not yet broadly applicable.[8] It is likely that a laparoscopic approach to hernia repair will be widely available soon. Despite such advances, we will continue to adhere to the basic principles of hernia repair: high ligation of the hernia sac, protection of adjacent structures, minimal complication rate, and very low recurrence rate.

SUGGESTED READING

Davenport M: ABC of general paediatric surgery: Inguinal hernia, hydrocele, and the undescended testis. BMJ 1996;312:564-567.

Kapur P, Caty MG, Glick PL: Pediatric hernias and hydroceles. Pediatr Clin North Am 1998;45:773-789.

Katz DA: Evaluation and management of inguinal and umbilical hernias. Pediatr Ann 2001;30:729-735.

REFERENCES

1. Cilley RE, Krummel TM: Disorders of the umbilicus. In O'Neill JA, et al (eds): Pediatric Surgery. St Louis, Mosby-Year Book, 1998, pp 1037-1041.
2. Papagrigoriadis S, Browse DJ, Howard ER: Incarceration of umbilical hernias in children: A rare but important complication. Pediatr Surg Int 1999;15:527.
3. Schier F, Danzer E, Bondartschuk M: Incidence of contralateral patent processus vaginalis in children with inguinal hernia. J Pediatr Surg 2001;36:1561.
4. Strauch ED, Voight RW, Hill JL: Gangrenous intestine in a hernia can be reduced. J Pediatr Surg 2002;37:919.
5. Cote CJ, Zaslavsky A, Downes JJ, et al: Postoperative apnea in former preterm infants after inguinal herniorrhaphy: A combined analysis. Anesthesiology 1995;82:809-822.
6. Kurth CD, Spitzer AR, Broennle AM, Downes JJ: Postoperative apnea in preterm infants. Anesthesiology 1987;66:483-488.
7. Kurth CD, LeBard SE: Association of postoperative apnea, airway obstruction, and hypoxemia in former premature infants. Anesthesiology 1991;75:22-26.
8. Prasad R, Lovvorn HN 3rd, Wadie GM, Lobe TE: Early experience with needleoscopic inguinal herniorrhaphy in children. J Pediatr Surg 2003;38:1055-1058.

CHAPTER 141

General Trauma

Anupam Kharbanda

Traumatic injuries are the leading cause of death, disability, and hospitalization among children in the United States. Each year, more than 20,000 children suffer traumatic deaths, resulting in more than 3 million years of potential life lost.[1] In addition, nonfatal injuries in individuals younger than 20 years lead to approximately 10 million emergency department visits, 10 million urgent care visits, and 300,000 hospitalizations each year.[2,3] The annual cost of unintentional injuries to children younger than 14 years is estimated to be $175 billion.[4]

Fatalities from traumatic injury are most commonly caused by head injuries; however, thoracic and abdominal injuries are the direct cause of death in 20% and 10% of pediatric trauma cases, respectively.[5] The majority (85%) of injuries sustained by children and adolescents are from blunt trauma, many of which can be managed nonoperatively.[5,6] Because of their anatomy, children are more vulnerable than adults to blunt trauma. For example, a child's cranial vault is larger and heavier than an adult's, predisposing the brain to injury. In addition, the pediatric brain is less myelinated, making it especially susceptible to shearing forces. The pediatric abdomen is also at high risk of injury secondary to the immature musculoskeletal system and body habitus.[7] Solid organs in children are comparatively larger than in adults, and there is little fat or connective tissue to protect them from injury. Further, owing to a child's smaller size, more force is applied per body surface area, resulting in a higher likelihood of internal injury than in adults.

Because many traumatic injuries in children are managed nonoperatively, it is imperative that the pediatric emergency physician, hospitalist, and intensivist understand the diagnostic approach and management of the most common pediatric injuries. This chapter reviews the most common injury patterns seen in children.

GENERAL ASSESSMENT

The approach to trauma victims is standardized, independent of age. The American College of Surgeons has created the ATLS (Advanced Trauma Life Support) program that outlines the medical and surgical management of trauma. The initial assessment of any trauma patient includes a primary survey, resuscitation, secondary survey, and triage. The goal of the primary survey is to assess the patient's airway, breathing, and circulation (ABCs) while maintaining cervical spine immobilization until that injury can be ruled out. The secondary survey is a systematic assessment of the patient from head to toe to establish the presence of other injuries. Once the patient is stable, he or she may be triaged or transferred to the intensive care unit, general ward, or an outside institution. It is imperative that the receiving medical team perform its own secondary survey, regardless of the injuries found previously; non–

life-threatening injuries such as fractures and lacerations can be missed during the initial assessment.

HEAD AND NECK INJURIES

Head trauma is the most common pediatric injury. Each year there are 600,000 emergency department visits, 95,000 hospitalizations, 7000 deaths, and 30,000 new permanent disabilities due to pediatric head trauma.[8,9] Causes of head trauma vary by age. In children younger than 2 years, the most common causes are falls (40%), followed by injuries suspicious for abuse.[10] In older children, the most common causes are motor vehicle accidents, falls from bicycles, and athletic injuries.[11] Consequences of head injury include intracranial bleeding, cerebral contusion, diffuse axonal injury, skull fracture, concussion, cervical spine injury, and long-term neuropsychological sequelae. In this chapter, the discussion of head trauma is limited to minor head injuries and cervical spine injuries.

Minor Head Injury

Minor closed head injury is defined by the American Academy of Pediatrics as an injury in a previously healthy child aged 2 years or older with normal mental status, no abnormal neurologic findings, and no evidence of skull fracture.[8] In children with minor head injury, the risk of intracranial injury is less than 1%; however, the risk of intracranial injury increases to 1% to 5% if the child also has a history of loss of consciousness, vomiting, or amnesia.[12] Children younger than 2 years have not been as well studied, but those with minor head injury are thought to have a risk of intracranial injury of 3% to 6%.[13]

Clinical Presentation

Children with minor head injury may present with temporary loss of consciousness (<1 minute), vomiting, seizure, headache, or lethargy. Seizures are present in approximately 10% of children with minor head injury, usually occurring at the time of injury. Seizures alone do not predict intracranial injury.[14,15] Skull fracture may also occur in patients with minor head injury; the incidence is highest in those younger than 2 years. Regardless of age, skull fractures are associated with a 15% to 30% risk of intracranial injury.[9] The presence of scalp swelling or hematoma in a young child, especially parietal and temporal lesions, has been linked to the presence of an underlying skull fracture.[16]

Diagnosis and Evaluation

Pediatric patients older than 2 years without loss of consciousness and with a normal neurologic examination can be observed in the emergency department, pediatrician's office, or home. Patients with a brief loss of consciousness should be observed and a computed tomographpy (CT) scan obtained if other historical or physical examination findings are concerning. Patients should be observed in the hospital until signs and symptoms such as amnesia, vomiting, and lethargy clear.

Children younger than 2 years are managed differently from older children because they are at higher risk for intracranial injury. Young children can be divided into those with high, moderate, and low risk for intracranial injury. High-risk patients are those with a depressed mental status, focal neurologic findings, depressed skull fracture, or irritability. It is recommended that these children undergo diagnostic imaging (CT scan) and subspecialty consultation. This group also includes infants younger than 3 months with a history of head trauma. Moderate-risk children present with emesis, a brief loss of consciousness (<1 minute), or lethargy. Observation in the emergency department and CT of the head are strongly encouraged. Low-risk patients have a normal neurologic examination, have a low-risk mechanism of injury, and are older than 12 months. Low-risk patients can be safely discharged without imaging.[13]

Treatment

Patients with a depressed skull fracture, intracranial blood, or cerebral contusion should be managed with the assistance of a neurosurgeon. Patients with amnesia or emesis despite normal imaging normally improve within 24 hours. Goals of inpatient admission are frequent neurologic examinations and hydration.

Consultation

Obtain a neurosurgical consultation for patients with abnormal CT findings, depressed skull fracture, depressed mental status, persistent emesis, or lethargy. Consult a general surgeon if the mechanism of injury is suspicious for occult thoracic or abdominal trauma.

Admission Criteria

- Persistent amnesia, lethargy, irritability, or emesis.
- Inability to tolerate oral intake.
- Focal neurologic deficits.
- Abnormal CT findings.

Discharge Criteria

- Normal mental status.
- Normal neurologic examination.
- Ability to tolerate food or liquid by mouth.

Cervical Spine Injuries

Cervical spine injuries are uncommon in children. They are found in only 1% to 2% of children who sustain blunt trauma.[17] Causes of cervical spine injuries vary by age. In younger children, they are most common after motor vehicle accidents or falls. In older children, sports injuries are the most common cause.[18,19]

Clinical Presentation

Patients with cervical spine injuries often experience focal pain, muscle spasm, and decreased range of motion. Additionally, transient or persistent neurologic findings may be present.[20] Children younger than 8 years are more susceptible to cervical spine injury than adults because of their proportionately larger and heavier heads compared to the rest of their bodies. In addition, young children have less muscle support and more elasticity of ligaments, resulting in more mobility of the upper cervical spine. This leads to the fulcrum of the spine being located at C2-C3 and predisposes children to higher cervical spine injuries.[20] Only 30% of cervical spine injuries in children are below C3. In addition, 25% to 50% of such injuries are spinal cord injuries without radiographic abnormalities (SCIWORA).[21,22]

Diagnosis and Evaluation

Any patient with focal findings or a concerning mechanism of injury should remain immobilized with a cervical collar and undergo radiographic evaluation. This evaluation should include three plain-film views of the cervical spine region: cross-table lateral, anteroposterior, and open-mouth odontoid. The ability of plain films to identify fractures varies by patient age, type of immobilization, and position. In the National Emergency X-Radiography Utilization Study, which evaluated the utility of plain radiography for identifying cervical fractures in adults and children, the three-view series was shown to be 89.4% sensitive.[23,24] The following findings are associated with a low likelihood of cervical fracture: no midline cervical tenderness, no focal neurologic findings, normal mental status, no distracting injury, and no intoxication. These criteria can be safely applied to children older than 8 years.[25] Patients who do not meet these low-risk criteria should undergo radiographic evaluation. Patients with persistent pain despite negative radiographs must remain immobilized.

Treatment

If pain persists despite negative plain radiographs, CT or magnetic resonance imaging should be considered, along with pediatric neurosurgical consultation. The cervical spine can be cleared if the radiographs are negative and the patient is asymptomatic. Patients admitted with cervical immobilization can be cleared once the neurologic examination returns to baseline and they have no midline cervical tenderness and normal cervical radiographs.

Consultation

Neurosurgical consultation should be obtained for patients with abnormal plain radiographs, persistent cervical tenderness, or focal neurologic deficits.

Admission Criteria

- Cervical fractures.
- Focal neurologic deficits.

Table 141-1   Glasgow Coma Scale

Response	Description	Score (points)*
Eye opening	Spontaneous—open with blinking at baseline	4
	Opens to verbal command, speech, or shout	3
	Opens to pain not applied to face	2
	None	1
Verbal†	Oriented	5
	Confused conversation, but able to answer questions	4
	Inappropriate responses, words discernible	3
	Incomprehensible speech	2
	None	1
Motor	Obeys commands for movement	6
	Purposeful movement to painful stimulus	5
	Withdraws from pain	4
	Abnormal (spastic) flexion, decorticate posture	3
	Extensor (rigid) response, decerebrate posture	2
	None	1

*The total score is the sum of the scores in the three categories. Scores range from 3 to 15; patients with scores of 3 to 8 are usually said to be in a coma.
†For children younger than 5 years, the verbal response criteria are adjusted; see Table 141-2.

Table 141-2   Adjustment to Verbal Section of Glasgow Coma Scale for Children Younger than 5 Years

Score	Age 2-5 Years	Age 0-23 Months
5	Appropriate words or phrases	Smiles or coos appropriately
4	Inappropriate words	Cries and consolable
3	Persistent cries or screams	Persistent inappropriate crying or screaming
2	Grunts	Grunts or is agitated or restless
1	No response	No response

THORACIC INJURIES

Children are less likely than adults to experience thoracic trauma. When they do, only a minority of injuries (15%) require surgical intervention beyond a chest tube.[26] Blunt trauma accounts for 85% of thoracic injuries, most commonly secondary to motor vehicle accidents, falls, crush injuries, contact sports, or child abuse.[27, 28] Owing to differences in anatomy, children and adults are predisposed to different types of thoracic injuries. The pediatric chest wall has more elasticity and compliance than the adult thorax. Compressibility of the chest will dissipates the force of impact; therefore, significant force is required to cause rib fractures in children.[27] However, this flexibility, along with the decreased anteroposterior diameter of the chest cavity, predisposes pediatric patients to pulmonary contusions.[29] The mediastinum in children is more flexible, thus reducing the incidence of major vessel and airway injury.[30]

Holmes and coworkers identified several clinical predictors of thoracic trauma: abnormal respiratory rate, low systolic blood pressure, abnormal thoracic examination, abnormal chest auscultation, and Glasgow Coma Scale score less than 15 (Tables 141-1 and 141-2).[31] Plain radiographs of the chest are recommended for patients with any of these findings. Approximately 8% of children undergoing a chest radiograph in the Holmes study had a thoracic injury. The most common injuries were pulmonary contusions (70%), rib fractures (35%), pneumothorax (25%), and hemothorax (10%).[31]

Pulmonary Contusions

Pulmonary contusions occur when injury to the capillary membranes of the lung leads to the collection of blood within the interstitial spaces. This causes alveolar hemorrhage, consolidation, and edema, leading to decreased lung compliance, ventilation-perfusion mismatch, hypoxia, and respiratory distress.[32] Complications of pulmonary contusions include pneumonia, acute respiratory distress syndrome, and, in rare circumstances, death.[33]

Clinical Presentation

The clinical presentation depends on the degree of pulmonary involvement. Children may present with hemoptysis, hypoxemia, tachypnea, or, rarely, respiratory failure.

Diagnosis and Evaluation

Pulmonary contusions should be suspected based on the mechanism of injury. Plain radiographs are diagnostic in more than 85% of cases. CT is useful for differentiating aspiration from pulmonary contusion and for diagnosing other thoracic injuries. Mechanical ventilation of patients with pulmonary contusions may be required, based on the extent of the lung involvement. In a study by Wagner and colleagues, patients with pulmonary contusions involving more than 28% of the lung required mechanical ventilation.[34]

Treatment

Most contusions are small and require only symptomatic treatment. Management techniques include fluid restriction, supplemental oxygen, pain control, and incentive spirometry. Goals of therapy are to reduce atelectasis and prolonged immobilization, both of which can lead to the development of acute respiratory distress syndrome and pneumonia. Respiratory failure may develop several hours after the initial presentation; therefore, patients require serial respiratory examinations.

Consultation

A general surgery consultation is required for placement of chest tubes and for evaluation of other thoracic trauma.

Admission Criteria

- Respiratory distress.
- Oxygen requirement.
- Pain unresponsive to oral therapy.
- Pulmonary contusion associated with other thoracic injuries.
- Need for aggressive pulmonary toilet.

Discharge Criteria

- Stable or resolving symptoms.
- No supplemental oxygen requirement.
- Ability to tolerate oral intake.

Great Vessel and Cardiac Injuries

Injuries to the great vessels and heart are uncommon in children compared with adolescents and adults.[32] When such injuries occur, they are usually secondary to motor vehicle accidents.[35] Aortic injuries are difficult to diagnose and are usually fatal. Blunt cardiac injuries have a reported prevalence of 5%.[36]

Clinical Presentation

Injury should be suspected with any thoracic trauma. Clinical signs and symptoms of blunt cardiac injury include tachycardia, chest wall pain, unexplained hypotension, and elevated cardiac specific enzymes.[36]

Diagnosis and Evaluation

Given the rare occurrence of cardiac/vessel injuries, diagnosis is difficult. Plain radiographs may show a widened mediastinum, deviation of the esophagus, or fractures of the first or second ribs.[32] Diagnosis can be made via CT.[37]

Treatment

Treatment of blunt cardiac injuries is largely supportive. This includes continuous electrocardiography, frequent blood pressure checks, echocardiography, and serial cardiac enzymes. Great vessel or esophageal injuries necessitate immediate general surgical consultation.

Consultation

- General (or thoracic) surgery: for concerning mechanism of injury or a widened mediastinum on plain film
- Cardiology: for evaluation of abnormal rhythms

Admission Criteria

- Tachycardia
- Hemodynamic instability
- Abnormal rhythm on electrocardiography
- Elevated cardiac specific enzymes

Discharge Criteria

- Normal vital signs
- Resolving chest wall pain
- Clearance by cardiology and/or general surgery, including normal or stable finding on cardiac echo

Rib Fractures

Clinical Presentation

Rib fractures are seen in 30% to 50% of children with chest injuries.[38] Physical examination findings consistent with rib fracture are localized pain, palpable deformity, and crepitus. The location of a rib fracture provides information about other injuries the child may have sustained. The upper ribs are well protected by other anatomic structures such as the scapula, humerus, and clavicle; therefore, the middle ribs are most commonly injured. Fractures of the upper ribs should raise the suspicion of intrathoracic or cervical injury.[39] Fractures of the lower ribs are associated with abdominal injuries.[40]

Diagnosis and Evaluation

Diagnosis can be made with plain radiographs. Clinicians must be careful to search for associated injuries such as pneumothorax, clavicular fractures, cervical fractures, and major vascular trauma.

Treatment

Most rib fractures require only symptomatic relief. This can be achieved through analgesics and, rarely, nerve blocks. In addition, incentive spirometry is beneficial.[32] Complications from rib fractures arise if there is impaired ventilation secondary to pain and splinting of the thorax. This can lead to atelectasis and pneumonia from reduced clearance of secretions.

Consultation

General surgery consultation is required for chest tube placement or evaluation of associated injuries.

Admission Criteria

- Flail chest or multiple rib fractures.
- Oxygen requirement.
- Pain not responsive to oral therapy.

Discharge Criteria

- Stable or resolving symptoms.
- No respiratory symptoms.
- Adequate pain control.

ABDOMINAL INJURIES

Abdominal injuries are the third leading cause of death in pediatric trauma patients. Blunt trauma from motor vehicle accidents and falls is the most common mechanism of

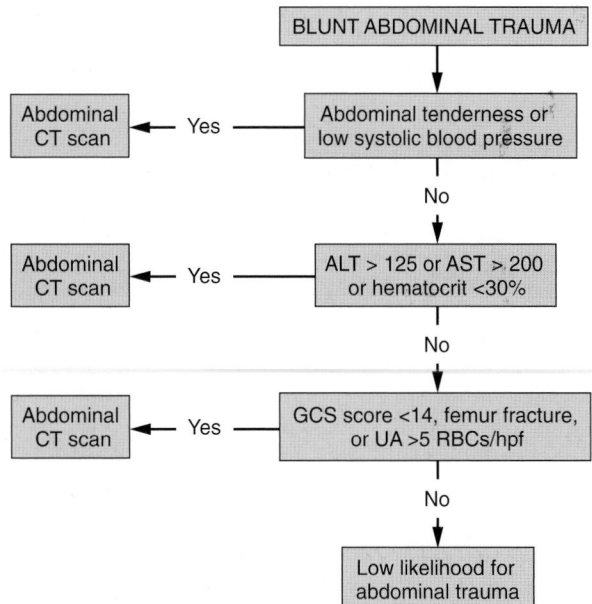

Figure 141-1 Proposed algorithm for the evaluation of intra-abdominal injury. (From Holmes JF, Sokolove PE, Brant WE, et al: Identification of children with intra-abdominal injuries after blunt trauma. Ann Emerg Med 2002;39:500-509.)

Table 141-3 Management of Children with Isolated Spleen or Liver Injury Based on Computed Tomography Grade				
Management	Grade 1	Grade 2	Grade 3	Grade 4
Intensive care unit stay (days)	None	None	None	1
Hospital stay (days)	2	3	4	5
Predischarge imaging	None	None	None	None
Activity restriction (wk)	3	4	5	6

injury.[5] Abdominal trauma often leads to solid organ injury. Nonoperative management is the standard of care for the majority of abdominal injuries, with a greater than 90% success rate.[41]

Trauma to the pediatric abdomen may be overlooked secondary to other injuries and the patient's age (preverbal). Suspicion of trauma should be based on the mechanism of injury and physical examination findings. Taylor and coworkers published indications for CT to evaluate abdominal trauma; these include lap-belt injury, assault, or abuse as the mechanism of injury; abdominal tenderness; gross hematuria; and a trauma score less than 13.[42] More recently, Holmes and colleagues suggested an algorithm to identify patients with intra-abdominal injury (Fig. 141-1).[43]

Splenic Injuries

Clinical Presentation

The spleen is the most commonly injured abdominal organ. Injury often occurs as a result of a direct blow to the left upper quadrant.[7] Patients may complain of diffuse abdominal tenderness, left upper quadrant pain, or left shoulder pain (Kehr sign). The physical examination may reveal left upper quadrant abrasions, abdominal distention, or tenderness.[27]

Diagnosis and Evaluation

Immediate laparotomy is indicated for patients with hemodynamic instability or those requiring more than 40 mL/kg of packed red blood cells to maintain stability. Stable patients with suspected splenic injury should undergo

a CT scan with intravenous contrast to determine the grade of injury and look for other abdominal injuries.[44] Occasionally, plain radiographs are helpful, revealing a medially displaced gastric bubble. The majority of patients with isolated splenic injuries do not require intensive care unit observation, and only 10% to 20% require blood transfusion.[45]

Treatment

Most children with splenic injuries can be managed nonoperatively.[46] Patients with splenic injuries should be hospitalized for serial abdominal examinations, serial hematocrits, and bed rest. The American Pediatric Surgical Association has created guidelines with regard to length of hospital stay and weeks of activity restriction (Table 141-3).[44] One of the major goals of treatment is the preservation of splenic immune function. Patients undergoing splenectomy should receive pneumococcal vaccination before hospital discharge.

Consultation

Consult general surgery for patients requiring laparotomy and interventional radiology for possible splenorrhaphy.

Admission Criteria

- Abnormal vital signs.
- Abdominal tenderness despite negative diagnostic imaging.
- Low hematocrit.
- Evidence of splenic injury on CT.

Discharge Criteria

- Stable or improving abdominal examination.
- Stable hematocrit.
- Ability to tolerate food or liquid by mouth.

Liver Injuries

The liver is the second most commonly injured abdominal organ. The close proximity of the liver to the inferior vena cava and its dual blood supply put patients with liver injuries at risk for severe bleeding after blunt trauma.[7]

Clinical Presentation

Patients with liver injuries may present with abdominal and right shoulder pain. On examination, they exhibit nonspecific abdominal tenderness that is commonly most severe over the right upper quadrant. Liver injuries should raise the suspicion of associated rib fractures or injuries to other abdominal organs.

Diagnosis and Evaluation

In hemodynamically stable patients, elevated transaminases (aspartate transaminase >450; alanine transaminase >250) have been correlated with liver injury.[47] In general, laboratory studies should be used to screen for intraabdominal injuries only in those patients at low risk for abdominal trauma. CT scanning is the gold standard of diagnosis. CT should be obtained to grade the extent of the liver injury and search for associated injuries. However, it should be noted that the grade of liver injury on CT does not correlate with patient outcome.[48]

Treatment

Immediate surgical consultation and operative management are required for patients with hemodynamic instability. Indications for laparotomy include penetrating abdominal trauma, multisystem trauma, and pneumoperitoneum. Most liver injuries (>85%) can be managed nonoperatively. For hemodynamically stable patients, the goals of inpatient admission include fluid resuscitation, serial abdominal examinations, pain control, and evaluation for associated injuries.[44]

Consultation

Consult a general surgeon for any patient with a liver hematoma or laceration.

Admission Criteria

- Abnormal vital signs (tachycardia).
- Inability to tolerate oral intake.
- Evidence of liver trauma on CT.

Discharge Criteria

- Stable or improving abdominal examination.
- Stable hematocrit
- Ability to tolerate oral intake.

Small and Large Bowel

Clinical Presentation

Intestinal injuries are uncommon, and their diagnosis can be challenging. The most common intestinal injury is intestinal perforation of the jejunum.[49] Injuries to the intestines occur following child abuse or motor vehicle accidents, especially from lap-belt injuries.[50] The "seatbelt syndrome" is the triad of abdominal wall bruising, intestinal and mesenteric contusions, and lumbar spine injury (Chance fractures).[51]

Bowel perforation and obstruction may present 24 to 48 hours after a lap-belt injury.[52]

Diagnosis and Evaluation

Serial abdominal examinations are important for diagnosing intestinal injuries.[53] CT may not detect intestinal perforations. The findings of a seatbelt mark, abdominal tenderness, and free fluid in the abdomen (without other organ injury) should raise the suspicion of an intestinal injury.[52] Evaluation of the lumbar spine with plain radiographs is required to ascertain the presence of lumbar spinal fractures.

Treatment

Patients with a concerning history and physical examination should be admitted for inpatient observation and undergo prompt consultation with a pediatric surgeon for possible operative management.

Late Complications

Duodenal hematoma is a rare injury that results from a blunt force trauma to the epigastrium. This injury may present several days after a traumatic event with signs and symptoms consistent with a bowel obstruction. Common clinical findings include abdominal pain, gastric distention, and bilious emesis. The diagnosis can be made by CT scan or an upper gastrointestinal series. Management includes nasogastric decompression and parenteral nutrition.[54]

Consultation

General surgery should be consulted for patients with pneumoperitoneum, persistent abdominal pain, or abnormal CT findings.

Admission Criteria

- Persistent abdominal tenderness despite normal imaging.
- Inability to tolerate food or liquid by mouth.

IN A NUTSHELL

- Traumatic injuries are the leading cause of death in children. Head injuries are most common, followed by injuries to the spleen and liver.
- The evaluation of any trauma patient begins with securing the airway and assessing the breathing and circulation. Hemodynamic instability must be addressed promptly and requires general surgical consultation. CT is the diagnostic test of choice to identify head, thoracic, and abdominal trauma.
- The majority of traumatic injuries experienced by children can be managed nonoperatively. Careful assessment for associated injuries is imperative. Goals of hospitalization are serial examinations, intravenous hydration, pain management, and surgical consultation.

ON THE HORIZON

- Better understanding of risk factors for trauma in children may help decrease the overall incidence of childhood injuries.
- Look for advances in our understanding and management of children with SCIWORA.
- Ultrasonography will play a greater role in the initial evaluation of patients with suspected abdominal or thoracic trauma.
- Patient selection for nonoperative management of splenic and liver lacerations will be refined.

SUGGESTED READING

Baker C, Kadish H, Schunk JE: Evaluation of pediatric cervical spine injuries. Am J Emerg Med 1999;17:230-234.

Bliss D, Silen M: Pediatric thoracic trauma. Crit Care Med 2002;30(11 Suppl):S409-S415.

Cantor RM, Leaming JM: Evaluation and management of pediatric major trauma. Emerg Med Clin North Am 1998;16:229-256.

Committee on Quality Improvement, American Academy of Pediatrics; Commission on Clinical Policies and Research, American Academy of Family Physicians: The management of minor closed head injury in children. Pediatrics 1999;104:1407-1415.

Gaines BA, Ford HR: Abdominal and pelvic trauma in children. Crit Care Med 2002;30(11 Suppl):S416-S423.

Hoffman JR, Mower WR, Wolfson AB, et al: Validity of a set of clinical criteria to rule out injury to the cervical spine in patients with blunt trauma. National Emergency X-Radiography Utilization Study Group. N Engl J Med 2000;343:94-99.

Holmes JF, Sokolove PE, Brant WE, Kuppermann N: A clinical decision rule for identifying children with thoracic injuries after blunt torso trauma. Ann Emerg Med 2002;39:492-499.

Holmes JF, Sokolove PE, Brant WE, et al: Identification of children with intra-abdominal injuries after blunt trauma. Ann Emerg Med 2002;39:500-509.

Newman KD, Bowman LM, Eichelberger MR, et al: The lap belt complex: Intestinal and lumbar spine injury in children. J Trauma 1990;30:1133-1138.

Pang D, Pollack IF: Spinal cord injury without radiographic abnormality in children—the SCIWORA syndrome. J Trauma 1989;29:654-664.

Schutzman SA, Greenes DS: Pediatric minor head trauma. Ann Emerg Med 2001;37:65-74.

Stylianos S: Compliance with evidence-based guidelines in children with isolated spleen or liver injury: A prospective study. J Pediatr Surg 2002;37:453-456.

Stylianos S: Evidence-based guidelines for resource utilization in children with isolated spleen or liver injury. The APSA Trauma Committee. J Pediatr Surg 2000;35:164-167.

Taylor GA, Eichelberger MR, O'Donnell R, Bowman L: Indications for computed tomography in children with blunt abdominal trauma. Ann Surg 1991;213:212-218.

Viccellio P, Simon H, Pressman BD, et al: A prospective multicenter study of cervical spine injury in children. Pediatrics 2001;108:e20.

REFERENCES

1. National Center for Injury Prevention and Control. US Department of Health and Human Services, Centers for Disease Control and Prevention. *http://webappa.cdc.gov/cgi-bin/broker.exe* (accessed July 5, 2004).

2. Hambidge SJ, Davidson AJ, Gonzales R, Steiner JF: Epidemiology of pediatric injury-related primary care office visits in the United States. Pediatrics 2002;109:559-565.

3. CSN-1996. Children's Safety Network Economics and Insurance Resource Center. http://www.edarc.org (accessed July 1, 2004).

4. National Safety Kids Campaign. Childhood Injury 2000. http://www.usa.safekids.org (accessed July 1, 2004).

5. Cooper A, Barlow B, DiScala C, String D: Mortality and truncal injury: The pediatric perspective. J Pediatr Surg 1994;29:33-38.

6. Peterson RJ, Tepas JJ 3rd, Edwards FH, et al: Pediatric and adult thoracic trauma: Age-related impact on presentation and outcome. Ann Thorac Surg 1994;58:14-18.

7. Gaines BA, Ford HR: Abdominal and pelvic trauma in children. Crit Care Med 2002;30(11 Suppl):S416-S423.

8. Committee on Quality Improvement, American Academy of Pediatrics; Commission on Clinical Policies and Research, American Academy of Family Physicians: The management of minor closed head injury in children. Pediatrics 1999;104:1407-1415.

9. Schutzman SA, Greenes DS: Pediatric minor head trauma. Ann Emerg Med 2001;37:65-74.

10. Duhaime AC, Christian CW, Rorke LB, Zimmerman RA: Nonaccidental head injury in infants—the "shaken-baby syndrome." N Engl J Med 1998;338:1822-1829.

11. Lescohier I, DiScala C: Blunt trauma in children: Causes and outcomes of head versus extracranial injury. Pediatrics 1993;91:721-725.

12. Homer CJ, Kleinman L: Technical report: Minor head injury in children. Pediatrics 1999;104:e78.

13. Schutzman SA, Barnes P, Duhaime AC, et al: Evaluation and management of children younger than two years old with apparently minor head trauma: Proposed guidelines. Pediatrics 2001;107:983-993.

14. Quayle KS, Jaffe DM, Kuppermann N, et al: Diagnostic testing for acute head injury in children: When are head computed tomography and skull radiographs indicated? Pediatrics 1997;99:e11.

15. Holmes JF, Palchak MJ, Conklin MJ, Kuppermann N: Do children require hospitalization after immediate posttraumatic seizures? Ann Emerg Med 2004;43:706-710.

16. Greenes DS, Schutzman SA: Clinical significance of scalp abnormalities in asymptomatic head-injured infants. Pediatr Emerg Care 2001;17:88-92.

17. Patel JC, Tepas JJ 3rd, Mollitt DL, Pieper P: Pediatric cervical spine injuries: Defining the disease. J Pediatr Surg 2001;36:373-376.

18. Orenstein JB, Klein BL, Gotschall CS, et al: Age and outcome in pediatric cervical spine injury: 11-year experience. Pediatr Emerg Care 1994;10:132-137.

19. Peclet MH, Newman KD, Eichelberger MR, et al: Patterns of injury in children. J Pediatr Surg 1990;25:85-90.

20. Baker C, Kadish H, Schunk JE: Evaluation of pediatric cervical spine injuries. Am J Emerg Med 1999;17:230-234.

21. Pang D, Pollack IF: Spinal cord injury without radiographic abnormality in children—the SCIWORA syndrome. J Trauma 1989;29:654-664.

22. Kriss VM, Kriss TC: SCIWORA (spinal cord injury without radiographic abnormality) in infants and children. Clin Pediatr (Phila) 1996;35:119-124.

23. Mower WR, Hoffman JR, Pollack CV Jr, et al: Use of plain radiography to screen for cervical spine injuries. Ann Emerg Med 2001;38:1-7.

24. Hoffman JR, Mower WR, Wolfson AB, et al: Validity of a set of clinical criteria to rule out injury to the cervical spine in patients with blunt trauma. National Emergency X-Radiography Utilization Study Group. N Engl J Med 2000;343:94-99.

25. Viccellio P, Simon H, Pressman BD, et al: A prospective multicenter study of cervical spine injury in children. Pediatrics 2001;108:e20.

26. Bender TM, Oh KS, Medina JL, Girdany BR: Pediatric chest trauma. J Thorac Imaging 1987;2:60-67.

27. Cantor RM, Leaming JM: Evaluation and management of pediatric major trauma. Emerg Med Clin North Am 1998;16:229-256.

28. Cooper A: Thoracic injuries. Semin Pediatr Surg 1995;4:109-115.

29. Nakayama DK, Ramenofsky ML, Rowe MI: Chest injuries in childhood. Ann Surg 1989;210:770-775.

30. Sarihan H, Abes M, Akyazici R, et al: Blunt thoracic trauma in children. J Cardiovasc Surg (Torino) 1996;37:525-528.

31. Holmes JF, Sokolove PE, Brant WE, Kuppermann N: A clinical decision rule for identifying children with thoracic injuries after blunt torso trauma. Ann Emerg Med 2002;39:492-499.

32. Bliss D, Silen M: Pediatric thoracic trauma. Crit Care Med 2002;30(11 Suppl):S409-S415.

33. Allen GS, Cox CS Jr: Pulmonary contusion in children: Diagnosis and management. South Med J 1998;91:1099-1106.

34. Wagner RB, Crawford WO Jr, Schimpf PP, et al: Quantitation and pattern of parenchymal lung injury in blunt chest trauma: Diagnostic and therapeutic implications. J Comput Tomogr 1988;12:270-281.

35. Trachiotis GD, Sell JE, Pearson GD, et al: Traumatic thoracic aortic rupture in the pediatric patient. Ann Thorac Surg 1996;62:724-731.

36. Dowd MD, Krug S: Pediatric blunt cardiac injury: Epidemiology, clinical features, and diagnosis. Pediatric Emergency Medicine Collaborative Research Committee: Working Group on Blunt Cardiac Injury. J Trauma 1996;40:61-67.

37. Spouge AR, Burrows PE, Armstrong D, Daneman A: Traumatic aortic rupture in the pediatric population: Role of plain film, CT and angiography in the diagnosis. Pediatr Radiol 1991;21:324-328.

38. Black TL, Snyder CL, Miller JP, et al: Significance of chest trauma in children. South Med J 1996;89:494-496.

39. Logan PM: Is there an association between fractures of the cervical spine and first- and second-rib fractures? Can Assoc Radiol J 1999;50:41-43.

40. Shweiki E, Klena J, Wood GC, Indeck M: Assessing the true risk of abdominal solid organ injury in hospitalized rib fracture patients. J Trauma 2001;50:684-688.

41. Haller JA Jr, Papa P, Drugas G, Colombani P: Nonoperative management of solid organ injuries in children. Is it safe? Ann Surg 1994;219:625-628.

42. Taylor GA, Eichelberger MR, O'Donnell R, Bowman L: Indications for computed tomography in children with blunt abdominal trauma. Ann Surg 1991;213:212-218.

43. Holmes JF, Sokolove PE, Brant WE, et al: Identification of children with intra-abdominal injuries after blunt trauma. Ann Emerg Med 2002;39:500-509.

44. Stylianos S: Evidence-based guidelines for resource utilization in children with isolated spleen or liver injury. The APSA Trauma Committee. J Pediatr Surg 2000;35:164-167.

45. Partrick DA, Bensard DD, Moore EE, Karrer FM: Nonoperative management of solid organ injuries in children results in decreased blood utilization. J Pediatr Surg 1999;34:1695-1699.

46. Stylianos S: Compliance with evidence-based guidelines in children with isolated spleen or liver injury: A prospective study. J Pediatr Surg 2002;37:453-456.

47. Hennes HM, Smith DS, Schneider K, et al: Elevated liver transaminase levels in children with blunt abdominal trauma: A predictor of liver injury. Pediatrics 1990;86:87-90.

48. Hackam DJ, Potoka D, Meza M, et al: Utility of radiographic hepatic injury grade in predicting outcome for children after blunt abdominal trauma. J Pediatr Surg 2002;37:386-389.

49. Sivit CJ, Taylor GA, Newman KD, et al: Safety-belt injuries in children with lap-belt ecchymosis: CT findings in 61 patients. AJR Am J Roentgenol 1991;157:111-114.

50. Rothrock SG, Green SM, Morgan R: Abdominal trauma in infants and children: Prompt identification and early management of serious and life-threatening injuries. Part II. Specific injuries and ED management. Pediatr Emerg Care 2000;16:189-195.

51. Stylianos S: Late sequelae of major trauma in children. Pediatr Clin North Am 1998;45:853-859.

52. Newman KD, Bowman LM, Eichelberger MR, et al: The lap belt complex: Intestinal and lumbar spine injury in children. J Trauma 1990;30:1133-1138.

53. Moss RL, Musemeche CA: Clinical judgment is superior to diagnostic tests in the management of pediatric small bowel injury. J Pediatr Surg 1996;31:1178-1181.

54. Shilyansky J, Pearl RH, Kreller M, et al: Diagnosis and management of duodenal injuries in children. J Pediatr Surg 1997;32:880-886.

CHAPTER 142

Ear, Nose, and Throat

Eric D. Baum

Airway safety is the paramount concern when managing inpatients with head and neck disorders. In addition to ensuring that the breathing passages are large and consistently patent enough for adequate gas exchange, the clinician must take measures to prevent aspiration of blood, food, and secretions.

Head and neck diseases can also cause significant morbidity in other ways as well. Blood loss from a rich vascular supply can be substantial. If prompt and appropriate treatment does not take place, seemingly minor traumatic injuries can lead to notable cosmetic deformities. Localized infections can easily spread to the bloodstream or track through fascial planes to become life threatening. Perhaps most importantly, the intimate relationship between extracranial head and neck structures and the central nervous system is a reminder that otolaryngologic diseases can easily lead to intracranial complications, often with devastating results.

Most patients with complaints referable to the head and neck can be safely and effectively managed as outpatients. Admission is required when there is a significant risk for complications in any of the aforementioned areas. Furthermore, head and neck disorders often arise in already-hospitalized patients, either as a result of iatrogenic intervention or as a complicating factor in patient disease.

EPISTAXIS

Most nosebleeds are self-limited and do not require intervention; however, they are occasionally severe, recurrent, or associated with other symptoms and require medical attention.[1] Epistaxis is rare before the age of 2 years and peaks between the ages of 3 and 8 years.[2]

The blood supply to the nose derives from a lush network of branches of the internal and external carotid artery systems. One particularly vulnerable area is the region of the anterior septum, within 1 cm of the nasal tip, known as Little's area or the plexus of Kiesselbach. More than 90% of nosebleeds can be localized to this small and easily accessible spot.[3]

The differential diagnosis of epistaxis is extensive, but local factors predominate. Minor trauma to the anterior aspect of the nose is common and usually due to nose picking. Any local inflammation, including upper respiratory infections or allergic flares, makes bleeding even more likely.[1] Dry air, especially from home forced air heating systems, plays an important role in promoting epistaxis; one study noted twice as many hospital admissions for management of epistaxis in the coldest month of the year as in the warmest.[4] Nasal steroid sprays, which are increasingly being prescribed for children, can lead to dryness and even perfo-

ration of the septum.[5] Proper spraying technique may reduce the incidence of septal damage.[6]

Although nosebleeds are rarely the single presenting symptom of more serious diseases, a thorough history and physical examination can uncover more unusual causes.[7] Any tumor resulting in obstruction or anatomic changes in the midface can cause epistaxis; this group includes juvenile nasopharyngeal angiofibroma and rhabdomyosarcoma.[8] Hematologic diseases causing severe thrombocytopenia, including malignancies, can be accompanied by nosebleeds as well.[3] Particularly severe and recurrent epistaxis is seen in patients with hereditary hemorrhagic telangiectasia (Osler-Weber-Rendu disease); these patients present at around 12 years of age, and nosebleed may be their first symptom.[9] Other causes of pediatric epistaxis are listed in Table 142-1.

Proper evaluation and management of nosebleeds include interventions that help stop acute bleeding and prevent future occurrences. The importance of removing all coagulated blood from the nasal cavities cannot be overemphasized; whether done by suction or gentle nose blowing, removal of coagulated blood alone can stop bleeding and allows a thorough examination.[1] Careful inspection of Little's area in children rarely requires more than minor upward pressure on the nasal tip,[10] and an actively bleeding or irritated spot can be cauterized with silver nitrate or covered with antibiotic ointment, respectively. Topical oxymetazoline (as drops or spray) is an effective vasoconstrictive agent in this setting. Pinching the nose closed for a full 5 minutes is extremely effective in most cases; interruptions in pressure for a "quick peek" are discouraged.[3]

If bleeding persists, packing may be required. Absorbable packs made from oxidized cellulose or gelatin sponge are preferred and are generally well tolerated. Deep insertion is not required in most cases because most nosebleeds occur in Little's area.[11] In view of the risk for toxic shock syndrome, all packing materials should be covered or impregnated with antibiotic ointment, and patients should receive systemic antibiotics as well. Nonabsorbable packing should be removed as soon as practicable.[12,13]

Most children who require packing are either already inpatients or should be strongly considered for hospital admission. Inpatients with epistaxis are frequently very ill as a result of their primary medical condition and may have anemia, platelet abnormalities, and repeated iatrogenic trauma to the nose because of endotracheal or nasoenteric tube placement. Correction of coagulopathies and removal of indwelling nasal foreign bodies (e.g., nasogastric tubes) should be pursued whenever possible. If administration of oxygen is necessary, it should be aggressively humidified and delivered through an external apparatus (e.g., face tent

Table 142–1 Differential Diagnosis of Epistaxis
Local Predisposing Factors
Trauma (direct or nose picking)
Local inflammation
Acute viral upper respiratory tract infection (common cold)
Bacterial rhinitis (may be blood-tinged discharge)
Foreign body (may be unilateral)
Acute illness associated with nasal congestion
Measles, infectious mononucleosis, acute rheumatic fever
Allergic rhinitis
Nasal polyposis
Furuncle
Telangiectasia (Osler-Weber-Rendu disease)
Juvenile nasopharyngeal angiofibroma (usually teenage boys)
Other tumors
Noninfectious rhinitis
Systemic Predisposing Factors
Hematologic diseases
Idiopathic thrombocytopenic purpura (ITP)
Leukemia
Aplastic anemia
von Willebrand disease
Hemophilia
Sickle cell disease
Vitamin K deficiency
Drugs that cause platelet or clotting dysfunction
Salicylates
Nonsteroidal anti-inflammatory drugs
Warfarin
Coumarins (found in rodenticides)
Hypertension (any cause)

Adapted from Nadel F, Henretig FM: Epistaxis. In Fleisher GR, Ludwig S (eds): Textbook of Pediatric Emergency Medicine, 4th ed. Philadelphia, Lippincott Williams & Wilkins, 2000, pp 227-230.

Table 142–2 Life-Threatening Causes of a Neck Mass in Children
Traumatic hematoma
Cervical spine injury
Vascular compromise
Acute hemorrhage
Late arteriovenous fistula
Subcutaneous emphysema
Airway obstruction
Pulmonary injury
Hypersensitivity reaction
Airway edema
Oral, pharyngeal, or neck space infection
Airway impingement by adenopathy or a mass effect
Sepsis
Hyperthyroidism with thyroid storm
Mucocutaneous lymph node syndrome
Coronary vasculitis
Lymphoma with airway compromise
Mediastinal or cervical adenopathy
Other malignancies associated with a neck mass
Leukemia
Hodgkin's disease
Rhabdomyosarcoma
Langerhans's cell histiocytosis

Adapted from McAneney CM, Ruddy RM: Neck mass. In Fleisher GR, Ludwig S (eds): Textbook of Pediatric Emergency Medicine, 4th ed. Philadelphia, Lippincott Williams & Wilkins, 2000, pp 383-389.

instead of a nasal cannula). Bilateral nasal packing or unilateral posterior nasal packing may rarely lead to iatrogenic sleep apnea, and such patients must be closely monitored if they are not already intubated.[1,14] Nasal packing can also cause sinusitis and nasal injury and can be aspirated if dislodged.[15]

Patients admitted to the hospital primarily because of epistaxis do not necessarily require a more extensive workup for hematologic disorders or other underlying disease. Additional clues from the history and physical examination are better predictors of the presence of such diseases.[7,16] When a bleeding disorder is suspected, initial tests should include a complete blood count, prothrombin time, and activated partial thromboplastin time. von Willebrand disease is the most common disorder found in these cases (see Chapter 120).[17]

Patients with recalcitrant bleeding despite packing and correction of bleeding disorders may require endovascular embolization by an interventional radiologist.[18] Open arterial ligation for epistaxis is rarely required in children.[19]

Regardless of the severity of epistaxis, patients should all be treated with an eye toward prevention. Because local factors—minor trauma, humidity, local infections—play such a prominent role, continued use of emollients, antibi-

otic ointments, and creams plus avoidance of unnecessary manipulation is encouraged.[20,21]

NECK MASS

Neck masses are common in children but require inpatient admission only under select circumstances, including actual or imminent airway compromise, a strong suspicion of malignancy necessitating a complex diagnostic workup, and serious illness associated with the mass (sepsis, blunt or projectile trauma). Life-threatening causes of neck masses are presented in Table 142-2.[22]

The most common cause of a neck mass in a child requiring admission is bacterial cervical adenitis (see also Chapter 65). Common locations of infected lymph nodes include the lateral aspect of the neck, which presents with obvious bulging and tenderness externally, and the deep neck spaces (retropharyngeal and parapharyngeal), which may cause upper aerodigestive tract symptoms. When airway compromise or anorexia occurs in a patient with a neck mass, inpatient admission is required.

Other frequently seen neck masses include congenital anomalies (thyroglossal duct cyst, branchial cleft anomaly), viral lymphadenitis, and benign tumors (lipoma, cystic hygroma, dermoid cyst, hemangioma, vascular malformations). Malignancy is found in fewer than 10% of biopsied neck masses.[23] Even when infected, many of these entities are managed in the outpatient setting.[24]

Patients admitted with airway compromise and poor oral intake require supportive care even before definitive diagnosis. Humidified oxygen, nebulized treatments, and analgesics are administered as needed, but nonsteroidal anti-inflammatory drugs and aspirin are contraindicated in patients with even a small chance of requiring operative treatment. Antibiotics may be used empirically before diagnosis; systemic corticosteroids should be reserved until a suppurative infection or malignant process is ruled out. Bacterial infections in the neck are usually polymicrobial, and standard therapy includes either ampicillin/sulbactam or clindamycin. Because of the frequent presence of resistant and anaerobic organisms, narrowing of coverage is not recommended if patients respond well to the initial antibiotic choice.[25]

Contrast-enhanced computed tomography (CT) is the cornerstone of radiologic diagnosis of infectious neck masses, and it can be useful for operative planning and airway assessment.[26] Because CT requires supine positioning and, in some patients, sedation, it may not be safe when there is concern for airway compromise. CT is reasonably accurate in distinguishing infectious inflammation from an abscess that requires drainage,[27] and it occasionally suggests an alternative diagnosis (nonsuppurative infection, malignancy) that would require further workup.

Large neck abscesses must be surgically drained, but some small abscesses may be successfully treated with antibiotics alone.[26] Physical examination and radiologic findings, along with progression or improvement in patient symptoms, are important elements of the decision-making process, which

should be carried out in conjunction with a head and neck surgeon.[28]

INFANT WITH NOISY BREATHING

The history and physical examination provide the most important clues in the initial management and workup of an infant who presents with noisy breathing. The quality and loudness of the abnormal noise can be misleading; stridor can diminish as the obstruction worsens and airflow decreases. More important is a general survey of the patient's respiratory distress: chest retraction, vital signs, and oxygen saturation. Urgent, controlled securing of the airway by intubation may be required in a tiring infant with severe respiratory distress, but most noisy babies can be safely evaluated and monitored without jumping to this intervention.[29]

Many important clues are gleaned from directed questions to the caregiver and personal observation of the resting child; these clues can often quickly suggest or eliminate many possible causes (Table 142-3).

Screening radiologic studies include a plain chest radiograph and high-kilovolt anteroposterior and lateral neck films. These studies may reveal localized areas of narrowing (e.g., subglottic stenosis, adenotonsillar hypertrophy), foreign bodies, or pulmonary abnormalities.[30] Additional information, especially for anatomic sites below the vocal cords, can be obtained from airway fluoroscopy,[31] magnetic resonance imaging,[32] and CT.[33] Studies to diagnose gastroesophageal reflux disease, an important cause of many airway symptoms, can be helpful as well.[34] Finally, visualization with flexible laryngoscopy may be helpful in assessing the upper airway and vocal cords.

Table 142-3 Signs and Symptoms in a Child with Noisy Breathing

Sign/Symptom	Indicates	Possible Diagnoses
Stertor (snoring sound)	Nasal or pharyngeal obstruction	Rhinitis, snoring
Inspiratory stridor	Laryngeal or subglottic obstruction	Laryngomalacia, subglottic stenosis, vocal cord palsy, high esophageal foreign body
Biphasic stridor	High or mid tracheal obstruction	Tracheomalacia, tracheal stenosis
Expiratory stridor or prolonged expiratory phase	Tracheal or bronchial obstruction	Tracheobronchomalacia, airway foreign body
Cough	Aspiration	Vocal cord palsy, tracheoesophageal fistula, foreign body, reflux, laryngeal cleft
Barking cough	Obstruction with high tracheal lesion	Croup, tracheomalacia
Hoarseness, weak cry	Vocal cord lesion	Vocal cord palsy, laryngeal papillomatosis
Improvement with crying	Nasal obstruction	Choanal atresia, nasal stenosis
Worsening with crying	Increased airflow disturbance	Laryngomalacia, subglottic hemangioma
Acute airway obstruction	Noncongenital cause	Foreign body, infection
Dysphagia, drooling	Pharyngeal obstruction or pain	Tonsillitis, pharyngitis, epiglottitis, deep neck space infection
Worsening during sleep	Pharyngeal obstruction	Adenotonsillar hypertrophy, craniofacial anomaly
Worsening while supine	Posterior laryngeal collapse	Laryngomalacia

Adapted from Albert D, Leighton S: Stridor and airway management. In Cummings CW, et al (eds): Otolaryngology: Head and Neck Surgery, 3rd ed. Philadelphia, Mosby, 2005, pp 285-302.

As previously mentioned, few children with noisy breathing require urgent intubation, but a significant number require hospital admission and supportive care. All such patients should be administered humidified oxygen and put in an appropriately monitored environment that includes continuous pulse oximetry monitoring. Systemic steroids and nebulized medications (racemic epinephrine, budesonide) are also effective in relieving acute airway obstruction.[35] If an infectious cause is suspected, appropriate antibiotic coverage should be initiated.[29] Control of reflux disease may also help.[36]

Children with worsening respiratory distress despite medical management or who are tiring from the work of breathing require endotracheal intubation and ventilatory support. Firm guidelines regarding the timing of intubation and extubation of these patients have not been established; flexible endoscopy may help with the initial decision to secure the airway,[37] and the endotracheal tube "leak test" may be helpful when considering extubation.[38]

RECURRENT RESPIRATORY PAPILLOMATOSIS

Recurrent respiratory papillomatosis (RRP) is a disease in which benign nonkeratinizing squamous papillomas grow in the upper aerodigestive tract, especially at the squamociliary junctions and with a particular predilection for the larynx.[39] There is a strong association with human papillomavirus (HPV) types 6 and 11, which probably accounts for the stubborn and recurrent nature of the disease.[29]

RRP is the most common neoplasm of the pediatric larynx and one of the most frequent causes of hoarseness in children. The disease shows no gender predilection and is generally diagnosed between the ages of 2 and 4 years. The mode of transmission is presumably vertical, although even in the highest-risk cases (vaginal delivery, primigravid mother with visible genital HPV lesions, prolonged labor), RRP develops in only approximately 1 in every 400 instances.[40]

Children with RRP usually present with dysphonia, with or without accompanying stridor. Less typical presenting symptoms include chronic cough, recurrent pneumonia, dyspnea, dysphagia, and rarely, acute airway obstruction. Because lesions are generally slow growing and cause symptoms common to other pediatric airway disorders, diagnosis may be delayed. Visualization of potential airway lesions with flexible laryngoscopy can be of immediate help in evaluating the need for urgent airway intervention and is usually sufficient to make a diagnosis of RRP. A more thorough complete bronchoscopy in which all areas of the upper and lower respiratory tract are evaluated is mandatory.[41]

Although a variety of medical treatments have met with varying degrees of success (photodynamic therapy, interferon alfa, topical cidofovir),[42] most otolaryngologists continue to manage RRP patients with repeated surgical excision of visible lesions.[43] Laryngeal disease alone can cause airway obstruction and death. RRP can also spread to the more distal airways, especially when patients undergo tracheotomy.[44]

Until more durable treatments for RRP emerge, patients will continue to require repeated operative extirpation of lesions. Guidelines are emerging on the optimal time to intervene,[45] and most authors agree that tracheotomy should

be used as briefly and judiciously as necessary because of the increased risk for distal spread.[29]

SUBGLOTTIC HEMANGIOMA

Benign capillary hemangiomas in the subglottic airway typically become symptomatic at 6 weeks of age and almost always present by 6 months. They are more common in whites and females and are associated with similar cutaneous head and neck lesions about half the time. Patients generally present with stridor, but any symptoms associated with airway obstruction (see earlier) may develop. The diagnosis is generally made endoscopically.[29]

Because airway hemangiomas rapidly proliferate until around 1 year of age and then tend to regress over the next 5 to 8 years, they can lead to considerable morbidity if left untreated.[46] A variety of approaches are used, including open surgical excision, laser vaporization, intralesional injection, and systemic corticosteroid treatment, but none has emerged as ideal.[47] Tracheostomy is occasionally required but is used less frequently than in the past.[48]

As with RRP, subglottic hemangioma requires long-term management. Careful attention to airway safety and the side effects of medical interventions is paramount.[49]

VOCAL CORD PALSY

Vocal cord paralysis usually presents within the first month of life. Bilateral disease produces stridor, cyanosis, and apnea, whereas unilateral disease is associated with a weak or hoarse cry. The cause is never identified in about a third of patients.[50] In other cases, it may be due to birth trauma (unilateral, especially in difficult forceps deliveries) or neurologic disease (Arnold-Chiari malformation, hydrocephalus, or meningomyelocele).[51] The prognosis for spontaneous recovery in these cases is generally good,[52] although temporary tracheotomy is still often required, especially with bilateral palsy.[53] Iatrogenic unilateral vocal cord paralysis in children is often due to surgical correction of congenital heart defects or cannulation of large vessels in the neck[54,55]; in these cases the nerve is assumed to have been severed, and function rarely returns.[52] Vocal cord paralysis has also been reported as a complication of endotracheal intubation, with the presumed mechanism being nerve compression by the inflated cuff.[56]

Definitive treatment of vocal cord paralysis is usually deferred until the possibility of spontaneous recovery is exhausted. Surgical intervention attempts to strike a balance between an adequately wide airway and an acceptable voice. Ideally, permanent surgical interventions should be delayed until the patient is old enough to participate in the decision-making process.[29,53]

POSTOPERATIVE CARE OF HEAD AND NECK SURGERY PATIENTS

Many head and neck surgical procedures are performed with the aim of improving the patient's airway in the long term, but edema and other tissue responses may make the airway worse in the immediate postoperative period. Two particular procedures—laryngotracheal reconstruction and adenotonsillectomy—merit specific comment.

Laryngotracheal Reconstruction of Subglottic Stenosis

Open laryngotracheal reconstruction has become more common as both recognition and the absolute incidence of subglottic stenosis have increased in recent years.[57] Patients generally undergo either a multiple-stage or single-stage procedure.

In multiple-stage procedures, the stenotic segment in the larynx or trachea (or both) is either expanded or resected, and the airway is maintained postoperatively with a tracheostomy tube or its functional equivalent. Standard tracheostomy care is appropriate, sometimes with minor modifications, depending on the actual tube used. In addition, changes in laryngeal function because of surgery or placement of laryngeal stents may require that an oral diet be suspended, restricted, or modified.

In single-stage procedures, the airway may require stenting in the immediate postoperative period because of edema and healing. In this case, a standard nasotracheal tube stays in place for up to 2 weeks to perform this function.[58] When the patient is ultimately extubated, there is no artificial airway in place.

In multiple-stage procedures, patients can resume normal ambulatory activity immediately and do not require immobilization or sedation after surgery. Depending on the details of the surgery, patients may not have a sufficient airway superior to the level of the tracheostomy, so particular care must be taken regarding the security and cleanliness of the tracheostomy tube.[59]

In single-stage procedures, there has been an increasing trend against the use of physical and pharmacologic restraints. With a secure nasotracheal tube, patients can be awake and ambulatory, thus avoiding the complications associated with prolonged immobility, sedation, mechanical ventilation, and medication withdrawal.[60] There have even been reports of successful single-stage repair with immediate extubation in the operating room.[61]

Other strategies that are important in the postoperative management of laryngotracheal reconstruction patients include (1) control of gastroesophageal reflux, (2) prophylactic use of broad-spectrum antibiotics against both anaerobic organisms and *Pseudomonas* species, and (3) avoidance of prolonged simultaneous neuromuscular blockage and corticosteroid administration.[62]

Tonsillectomy and Adenoidectomy

Separately or together, tonsillectomy and adenoidectomy are among the most frequently performed surgical procedures in young children, and many studies have reported on the safety of performing these procedures on an outpatient basis.

Most studies of postoperative complications concentrate on patients undergoing removal of the tonsils (with or without removal of the adenoid pad) because it is generally assumed that most of the morbidity arises from the tonsillectomy. For instance, one of the few studies that separately tallied adenoidectomy-only complications noted a postoperative hemorrhage rate of 0.22%, which is substantially lower than published rates for bleeding after tonsillectomy (with or without adenoidectomy).[63]

Important risks in patients undergoing adenotonsillectomy include airway compromise, dehydration, and bleeding,[64,65] and these problems are more likely in certain patient groups: (1) children younger than 36 months[66]; (2) patients with Down syndrome[67] or other congenital disorders,[68] including craniofacial anomalies; (3) former premature babies with bronchopulmonary dysplasia[66]; (4) patients with a history of significant airway obstruction[69]; and (5) morbidly obese children.[70]

Outpatient tonsillectomy can still be performed in many patients who meet these criteria,[71] but it may not be possible to preoperatively identify which patients will require hospital admission.[66] Development of an evidence-based pathway may help reduce length of stay without compromising safety,[72] but early hospital discharge may actually be more expensive than planned overnight admission.[73]

One important complication much more often associated with adenoidectomy than with tonsillectomy is inflammatory atlantoaxial subluxation, also known as Grisel syndrome. Laxity of the transverse spinal ligaments may be due to the use of monopolar cautery in the posterior nasopharynx, a routine and popular technique for achieving hemostasis after removal of the adenoid pad.[74] Patients generally complain of neck pain and have marked torticollis and tenderness over the C1 and C2 vertebral bodies.[75] Patients can rarely present with frank neurologic signs as a result of nerve compression. Appropriate workup includes CT of the cervical spine and orthopedic or neurosurgical consultation. Patients are usually treated conservatively with a soft cervical collar, analgesics, and muscle relaxants and are monitored with flexion-extension plain films of the neck. The prognosis for complete recovery is generally excellent.[76]

After adenotonsillectomy, postoperative nausea and vomiting and subsequent dehydration can be prevented with aggressive antiemetic treatment[77]; a single dose of dexamethasone has been shown to be effective in reducing emesis and improving rapid diet advancement in this patient population.[78] In addition, fever, pain, and fetid breath are reduced with the routine administration of antibiotics,[79] although it is unclear whether there is an advantage to using agents with a broader spectrum than amoxicillin.[80]

ADMISSION CRITERIA

- Concern for airway impingement or impending respiratory collapse
- Epistaxis requiring substantial nasal packing
- Inability to maintain adequate oral intake because of dysphagia or odynophagia
- Infectious process requiring intravenous antibiotics
- Neck mass with a strong suspicion of malignancy requiring a complex diagnostic workup

DISCHARGE CRITERIA

- Respiratory stability, especially while sleeping
- Transition to an enteral regimen ample enough to avoid dehydration
- Stability on an outpatient antibiotic regimen

IN A NUTSHELL

- Epistaxis almost always emanates from the anterior septum within 1 cm of the nasal tip and can usually be controlled with pressure, topical oxymetazoline, cauterization with silver nitrate, or the application of antibiotic ointment. Persistent bleeding may require packing, which necessitates the use of antibiotics and, frequently, admission.
- Contrast-enhanced CT is the cornerstone of radiologic diagnosis of neck masses and is useful in differentiating infectious inflammation from an abscess that requires drainage; it occasionally suggests an alternative diagnosis (nonsuppurative infection, malignancy).
- RRP is a disease in which benign nonkeratinizing squamous papillomas grow in the upper aerodigestive tract with a predilection for the larynx, and it is particularly difficult to treat.
- Subglottic hemangiomas generally present in the first 6 months with stridor and may result in significant airway compromise. If left untreated, they can be deadly.
- Vocal cord paralysis may result from a number of mechanisms. Observation is often the preferred initial management. When treatment is required, surgical intervention is generally recommended.

ON THE HORIZON

- Emerging vaccines against HPV infection may alter the incidence and natural history of RRP.[81]
- Many new techniques for surgically removing the tonsils suggest a decrease in postoperative pain and bleeding, but none has emerged as a substantial improvement over existing methods.

SUGGESTED READING

Albert D, Leighton S: Stridor and airway management. In Cummings CW, Haughey B, Thomas R, et al (eds): Otolaryngology: Head and Neck Surgery, 3rd ed. Philadelphia, Mosby, 2005, pp 285-302.

Derkay CS, Darrow DH: Recurrent respiratory papillomatosis. Ann Otol Rhinol Laryngol 2006;115:1-11.

Gerber ME, O'Connor DM, Adler E, Myer CM: Selected risk factors in pediatric adenotonsillectomy. Arch Otolaryngol Head Neck Surg 1996; 122:811-814.

Torsiglieri AJ Jr, Tom LW, Ross AJ 3rd, et al: Pediatric neck masses: Guidelines for evaluation. Int J Pediatr Otorhinolaryngol 1988;16:199-210.

REFERENCES

1. Manning SC, Culbertson MC: Epistaxis. In Bluestone CD, Stool S, Alper C, et al (eds): Pediatric Otolaryngology, 4th ed. Philadelphia, WB Saunders, 2002, pp 925-931.
2. Juselius H: Epistaxis. A clinical study of 1,724 patients. J Laryngol Otol 1974;88:317-327.
3. Marple BF: Epistaxis. In Cotton RT, Myer CM (eds): Practical Pediatric Otolaryngology. Philadelphia, Lippincott-Raven, 1999, pp 427-448.
4. Nunez DA, McClymont LG, Evans RA: Epistaxis: A study of the relationship with weather. Clin Otolaryngol 1990;15:49-51.
5. Soderberg-Warner ML: Nasal septal perforation associated with topical corticosteroid therapy. J Pediatr 1984;105:840-841.
6. Klimek L, Bachert C, Hormann K: [Steroid sprays in non-infectious rhinitis and sinusitis. Proper and regular spraying does not damage the nasal mucosa] [abstract]. MMW Fortschr Med 2002;144(10):41-43.
7. Brown NJ, Berkowitz RG: Epistaxis in healthy children requiring hospital admission. Int J Pediatr Otolaryngol 2004;68:1181-1184.
8. Enepekides DJ: Recent advances in the treatment of juvenile angiofibroma. Curr Opin Otolaryngol Head Neck Surg 2004;12:495-499.
9. Aassar OS, Friedman CM, White RI Jr: The natural history of epistaxis in hereditary hemorrhagic telangiectasia. Laryngoscope 1991;101:977-980.
10. Potsic WP, Handler SD, Wetmore RF, Pasquariello PS: Nose and paranasal sinuses. In Potsic WP, Handler SD, Wetmore RF, Pasquariello PS (eds): Primary Care Pediatric Otolaryngology, 2nd ed. Andover, NJ, J. Michael Ryan Publishing, 1995, p 64.
11. Koltai PJ: Nose bleeds in the hematologically and immunologically compromised child. Laryngoscope 1984;94:1114-1115.
12. Hull HF, Mann JM, Sands CJ, et al: Toxic shock syndrome related to nasal packing. Arch Otolaryngol 1993;109:624-626.
13. Weber R, Keerl R, Hochapfel F, et al: Packing in endonasal surgery. Am J Otolaryngol 2001;22:306-320.
14. Larsen K, Juul A: Arterial blood gases and pneumatic nasal packing in epistaxis. Laryngoscope 1982;92:586-588.
15. Fairbanks DN: Complications of nasal packing. Otolaryngol Head Neck Surg 1986;94:412-415.
16. Thaha MA, Nilssen EL, Holland S, et al: Routine coagulation screening in the management of emergency admission for epistaxis—is it necessary? J Laryngol Otol 2000;114:30-38.
17. Sandoval C, Dong S, Visintainer P, et al: Clinical and laboratory features of 178 children with recurrent epistaxis. J Pediatr Hematol Oncol 2002;24:47-49.
18. Vokes DE, McIvor NP, Wattie WJ, et al: Endovascular treatment of epistaxis. Aust N Z J Surg 2004;74:751-753.
19. Chandler JR, Serrins A: Transantral ligation of the internal maxillary artery for epistaxis. Laryngoscope 1965;75:1151-1159.
20. Makura ZG, Porter GC, McCormick MS: Paediatric epistaxis: Alder Hey experience. J Laryngol Otol 2002;116:903-906.
21. Burton MJ, Doree CJ: Interventions for recurrent idiopathic epistaxis (nosebleeds) in children. Cochrane Database Syst Rev 2004;1: CD0044661.
22. McAneney CM, Ruddy RM: Neck mass. In Fleisher GR, Ludwig S (eds): Textbook of Pediatric Emergency Medicine, 4th ed. Philadelphia, Lippincott Williams & Wilkins, 2000, pp 383-389.
23. Torsiglieri AJ Jr, Tom LW, Ross AJ 3rd, et al: Pediatric neck masses: Guidelines for evaluation. Int J Pediatr Otorhinolaryngol 1988;16:199-210.
24. Bauer PW, Lusk RP: Neck masses. In Bluestone CD, Stool S, Alper C, et al (eds): Pediatric Otolaryngology, 4th ed. Philadelphia, WB Saunders, 2003, pp 1629-1647.
25. Yellon RF: Head and neck space infections. In Bluestone CD, Stool S, Alper C, et al (eds): Pediatric Otolaryngology, 4th ed. Philadelphia, WB Saunders, 2003, pp 1681-1702.
26. Craig FW, Schunk JE: Retropharyngeal abscess in children: Clinical presentation, utility of imaging, and current management. Pediatrics 2003;111:1394-1398.
27. Vural C, Gungor A, Comerci S: Accuracy of computerized tomography in deep neck infections in the pediatric population. Am J Otolaryngol 2003;24:143-148.
28. Wetmore RF, Mahboubi S, Soyupak SK: Computed tomography in the evaluation of pediatric neck infections. Otolaryngol Head Neck Surg 1998;119:624-627.
29. Albert D, Leighton S: Stridor and airway management. In Cummings CW, Haughey B, Thomas R, et al (eds): Otolaryngology: Head and Neck Surgery, 4th ed. Philadelphia, Mosby, 2005.
30. Tostevin PM, de Bruyn R, Hosni A, Evans JN: The value of radiological investigations in pre-endoscopic assessment of children with stridor. J Laryngol Otol 1995;109:844-848.

31. Rudman DT, Elmaraghy CA, Shiels WE, Wiet GJ: The role of airway fluoroscopy in the evaluation of stridor in children. Arch Otolaryngol Head Neck Surg 2003;129:305-309.

32. Kussman BD, Geva T, McGowan FX: Cardiovascular causes of airway compression. Paediatr Anaesth 2004;14:60-74.

33. Sagy M, Poustchi-Amin M, Nimkoff L, et al: Spiral computed tomographic scanning of the chest with three dimensional imaging in the diagnosis and management of paediatric intrathoracic airway obstruction. Thorax 1996;51:1005-1009.

34. Rudolph CD: Gastroesophageal reflux and airway disorders. In Myer CB, Cotton RT, Shott SR (eds): The Pediatric Airway. Philadelphia, JB Lippincott, 1995, pp 327-358.

35. Cetinkaya F, Tufekci BS, Kutluk G: A comparison of nebulized budesonide, and intramuscular, and oral dexamethasone for treatment of croup. Int J Pediatr Otorhinolaryngol 2004;68:453-456.

36. Yellon RF, Goldberg H: Update on gastroesophageal reflux disease in pediatric airway disorders. Am J Med 2001;111(Suppl 8A):78S-84S.

37. Damm M, Eckel HE, Jungehulsing M, Roth B: Management of acute inflammatory childhood stridor. Otolaryngol Head Neck Surg 1999;121:633-638.

38. Foland JA, Super DM, Dahdah NS, Mhanna MJ: The use of the air leak test and corticosteroids in intubated children: A survey of pediatric critical care fellowship directors. Respir Care 2002;47:662-666.

39. Kashima H, Mounts P, Leventhal B, Hruban RH: Sites of predilection in recurrent respiratory papillomatosis. Ann Otol Rhinol Laryngol 1993;102:580-583.

40. Shah K, Kashima H, Polk BF, et al: Rarity of cesarean delivery in cases of juvenile-onset respiratory papillomatosis. Obstet Gynecol 1986;68:795-799.

41. Derkay CS, Darrow DH: Recurrent respiratory papillomatosis. Ann Otol Rhinol Laryngol 2006;115:1-11.

42. Silverman DA, Pitman MJ: Current diagnostic and management trends for recurrent respiratory papillomatosis. Curr Opin Otolaryngol Head Neck Surg 2004;12:532-537.

43. Schraff S, Derkay CS, Burke B, Lawson L: American Society of Pediatric Otolaryngology members' experience with recurrent respiratory papillomatosis and the use of adjuvant therapy. Arch Otolaryngol Head Neck Surg 2004;130:1039-1042.

44. Valentin G: Prognostic factors of recurrent respiratory papillomatosis spread to lower airway passages [letter]. Int J Pediatr Otorhinolaryngol 2004;68:1589-1590.

45. Derkay CS, Hester RP, Burke B, et al: Analysis of a staging assessment system for prediction of surgical interval in recurrent respiratory papillomatosis. Int J Pediatr Otorhinolaryngol 2004;68:1493-1498.

46. Ferguson CF, Flake CG: Subglottic hemangioma as a cause of respiratory obstruction in infants. Ann Otol Rhinol Laryngol 1961;70:1095-1112.

47. Chatrath P, Black M, Jani P, et al: A review of the current management of infantile subglottic haemangioma, including a comparison of CO_2 laser therapy versus tracheostomy. Int J Pediatr Otorhinolaryngol 2002;64:143-157.

48. Hadfield PJ, Lloyd-Faulconbridge RV, Almeyda J, et al: The changing indications for paediatric tracheostomy. Int J Pediatr Otorhinolaryngol 2003;67:7-10.

49. Pransky SM, Canto C: Management of subglottic hemangioma. Curr Opin Otolaryngol Head Neck Surg 2004;12:509-512.

50. Cohen SR, Geller KA, Birns JW, Thompson JW: Laryngeal paralysis in children: A long-term retrospective study. Ann Otol Rhinol Laryngol 1982;91:417-424.

51. Holinger LD, Holinger PC, Holinger PH: Etiology of bilateral abductor vocal cord paralysis: A review of 389 cases. Ann Otol Rhinol Laryngol 1976;85:428-436.

52. Zbar RI, Smith RJ: Vocal fold paralysis in infants twelve months of age and younger. Otolaryngol Head Neck Surg 1996;114:18-21.

53. Rothchild MA, Bratcher GO: Bilateral vocal cord paralysis and the pediatric airway. In Myer CB, Cotton RT, Shott SR (eds): The Pediatric Airway. Philadelphia, JB Lippincott, 1995, pp 133-150.

54. Salman M, Potter M, Ethel M, Myint F: Recurrent laryngeal nerve injury: A complication of central venous catheterization—a case report. Angiology 2004;55:345-346.

55. Schumacher RE, Weinfeld IJ, Bartlett RH: Neonatal vocal cord paralysis following extracorporeal membrane oxygenation. Pediatrics 1989;84:793-796.

56. Wason R, Gupta P, Gogia AR: Bilateral adductor vocal cord paresis following endotracheal intubation for general anaesthesia. Anaesth Intensive Care 2004;32:417-418.

57. Rothschild MA, Cotcamp D, Cotton RT: Postoperative medical management in single stage laryngotracheoplasty. Arch Otolaryngol Head Neck Surg 1995;121:1175-1179.

58. Cotton RT, Myer CM, O'Connor DM, et al: Pediatric laryngotracheal reconstruction with cartilage grafts and endotracheal tube stenting: The single stage approach. Laryngoscope 1995;105:818-821.

59. McMurray JS, Christopher AJP: Tracheotomy in the pediatric patient. In Cotton RT, Myer CM (eds): Practical Pediatric Otolaryngology. Philadelphia, Lippincott-Raven, 1999, pp 575-593.

60. Jacobs BR, Salman BA, Cotton RT, et al: Postoperative management of children after single-stage laryngotracheal reconstruction. Crit Care Med 2001;29:164-168.

61. Younis RT, Lazar RH: Laryngotracheal reconstruction without stenting. Otolaryngol Head Neck Surg 1997;116:358-362.

62. Yellon RF, Parameswaran M, Brandom BW: Decreasing morbidity following laryngotracheal reconstruction in children. Int J Pediatr Otorhinolaryngol 1997;41:145-154.

63. Windfuhr JP, Chen YS, Remmert S: Hemorrhage following tonsillectomy and adenoidectomy in 15,218 patients. Otolaryngol Head Neck Surg 2005;132:281-286.

64. Tom LW, DeDio RM, Cohen DE: Is outpatient tonsillectomy appropriate for young children? Laryngoscope 1992;102:277-280.

65. Haberman RS, Shattuck TG, Dion NM: Is outpatient suction cautery tonsillectomy safe in a community hospital setting? Laryngoscope 1990:100:511-515.

66. Ross AT, Kazahaya K, Tom LWC: Revisiting outpatient tonsillectomy in young children. Otolaryngol Head Neck Surg 2003;128:326-331.

67. Goldstein NA, Armfield DR, Kingsley LA, et al: Postoperative complications after tonsillectomy and adenoidectomy in children with Down syndrome. Arch Otolaryngol Head Neck Surg 1998;124:171-176.

68. Richmond KF, Wetmore RF, Baranak CC: Postoperative complications following tonsillectomy and adenoidectomy: Who is at risk? Int J Pediatr Otorhinolaryngol 1987;13:117-124.

69. Gerber ME, O'Connor DM, Adler E, Myer CM: Selected risk factors in pediatric adenotonsillectomy. Arch Otolaryngol Head Neck Surg 1996;122:811-814.

70. Spector A, Scheid S, Hassink S, et al: Adenotonsillectomy in the morbidly obese child. Int J Pediatr Otorhinolaryngol 2003;67:359-364.

71. Mitchell RB, Pereira KD, Friedman NR, Lazar RH: Outpatient adenotonsillectomy. Is it safe in children younger than 3 years? Arch Otolaryngol Head Neck Surg 1997;123:681-683.

72. Pestian JP, Derkay CS, Ritter C: Outpatient tonsillectomy and adenoidectomy clinical pathways: An evaluative study. Am J Otolaryngol 1998;19:45-49.

73. Shapiro NL, Seid AB, Pransky SM, et al: Adenotonsillectomy in the very young patient: Cost analysis of two methods of postoperative care. Int J Pediatr Otorhinolaryngol 1999;48:109-115.

74. Tschopp K: Monopolar electrocautery in adenoidectomy as a possible risk factor for Grisel's syndrome. Laryngoscope 2002;112:1445-1449.

75. Boole JR, Ramsey M, Petermann G, Sniezek J: Radiology quiz case. Grisel syndrome with vertebral osteomyelitis and spinal epidural abscess. Arch Otolaryngol Head Neck Surg 2003;129:1247.

76. Yu KK, White DR, Weissler MC, Pillsbury HC: Nontraumatic atlantoaxial subluxation (Grisel syndrome): A rare complication of otolaryngological procedures. Laryngoscope 2003;113:1047-1049.

77. Apfel CC, Korttila K, Abdalla M, et al: A factorial trial of six interventions for the prevention of postoperative nausea and vomiting. N Engl J Med 2004;350:2441-2451.

78. Steward DL, Welge JA, Myer CM: Steroids for improving recovery following tonsillectomy in children. Cochrane Database Syst Rev 2003; 1:CD003997.

79. Telian SA, Handler SD, Fleisher GR, et al: The effect of antibiotic therapy on recovery after tonsillectomy in children. Arch Otolaryngol 1986;112: 610-615.

80. Jones J, Handler SD, Guttenplan M, et al: The efficacy of cefaclor vs amoxicillin on recovery after tonsillectomy in children. Arch Otolaryngol Head Neck Surg 1990;116:590-593.

81. Kahn JA: Vaccination as a prevention strategy for human papillomavirus–related diseases. J Adolesc Health 2005;37(6 Suppl):S10-S16.

CHAPTER 143

Neurosurgical Issues

Christopher C. Stewart

The pediatric hospitalist is bound to encounter neurosurgical issues in everyday practice. The hospitalist may be asked to observe a child who may require neurosurgical intervention or to care for a child with hardware placed by a neurosurgeon. This chapter addresses the most common neurosurgical problems that a hospitalist may encounter: head trauma, hydrocephalus, and increased intracranial pressure (ICP).

HEAD TRAUMA

Pathophysiology

Brain injury from head trauma is a biphasic process. Primary injury as a result of impact or rotational forces can include fractures, hemorrhages, contusions, and axonal injury. Secondary brain injury is a complex process involving cerebral swelling, inflammatory mediators, cerebral microvascular control, programmed cell death, oxidative stress, and other factors that are only now being recognized.

Seizures after head trauma are more common in children than adults and most common in very young children. Postconcussive syndromes, including vomiting, migraine-like syndromes, and transient cortical blindness, can all occur in children after head trauma.[1]

Types of Injuries

Extracranial Hematomas

Subgaleal hematomas are collections of blood in the loose tissue beneath the galea aponeurotica (thus subgaleal) and above the periosteum. They rarely need any intervention. However, these hematomas are in a potential space that can expand, and large hematomas can cause significant anemia and should be monitored carefully with serial checks of blood pressure and hemoglobin, especially in infants. Unlike cephalhematomas, they generally cross suture lines.

Cephalhematomas are collections of blood between the periosteum and the skull and are usually restricted from crossing suture lines. Like subgaleal hematomas, they rarely require intervention, and needle drainage is contraindicated given the risk for infection. Cephalhematomas are more often associated with underlying skull fractures.[2]

Skull Fractures

Skull fractures may be open or closed and may be linear, comminuted, diastatic, depressed, or basilar. Skull fractures can usually be diagnosed by skull radiographs or computed tomography (CT); however, skull fractures apparent on autopsy are sometimes not noted on imaging. CT is less sensitive than plain films for skull fractures, but simple skull radiographs give no information about underlying intracranial injury. When basilar skull fractures are suspected, a thin-section CT scan through the base of the skull is generally necessary to detect them. They may not be visible at all and, in patients with high clinical suspicion, may be assumed to be present in the face of negative CT scans.

Linear skull fractures are responsible for about three fourths of skull fractures in pediatrics. Although most linear skull fractures will have an associated hematoma or soft tissue swelling, this is often not noted on early presentation or is obscured by the presence of hair. Larger hematomas, especially over the parietal or temporal bones, are more likely to be associated with fractures. Studies are conflicting about the significance of skull fractures and the presence of underlying intracranial injury. There is clearly an association of intracranial injuries with skull fractures, with rates as high as 30% in some studies. However, in patients with normal neurologic findings, the clinical importance of these injuries with respect to management and outcome is debatable.[3]

In general, linear skull fractures heal without intervention. Nonetheless, some diastatic fractures (in which the bone edges have been separated by more than 3 mm) can cause what is called a "growing skull fracture" in children usually younger than 3 years. Also called leptomeningeal cysts, they occur over time as a sequela of the diastatic fracture. The brain or meninges pushes through associated torn dura, and pulsations of cerebrospinal fluid (CSF) enlarge the fracture. They can present months to years after the initial fracture as a scalp mass, sclerotic widening fracture on CT or radiography, seizures, or neurologic deficits. These fractures generally need surgical repair. Thus, diastatic fractures larger than 3 mm in a younger child warrant neurosurgical evaluation and follow-up.[4]

Depressed skull fractures are often the result of a more focal impact and have a higher likelihood of intracranial injury than nondepressed fractures do. Open depressed skull fractures (those associated with overlying scalp injury) warrant antibiotic therapy and consultation with a neurosurgeon. In general, closed depressed skull fractures in which the skull fragments are not displaced more than the thickness of the skull do not require surgical intervention. However, those that are displaced greater than the skull thickness should be evaluated by a neurosurgeon because repair or elevation may be necessary to prevent further complications.[4]

Other depressed skull fractures that warrant neurosurgical consultation are (1) those involving the frontal sinuses, (2) those overlying the dural sinuses, (3) those involving tears of the underlying dura, and (4) more complicated depressed skull fractures with possible intraparenchymal bone fragments, even with normal neurologic findings. Cosmetic repair of simple depressed skull fractures may be desired by patients, although there is no evidence that such repair will change the neurologic outcome.[5]

Basilar skull fractures occur in up to 5% of pediatric head trauma. They occur most frequently through the base of the anterior aspect of the skull or the petrous bone in the posterior fossa.[4] They are often associated with clinical findings such as hemotympanum, the Battle sign (ecchymosis of the mastoid region), ecchymosis of the periorbital region, CSF or bloody rhinorrhea or otorrhea, hearing loss, tinnitus, vertigo, or cranial nerve palsies.[4] These findings in the setting of head trauma should raise suspicion for basilar skull fracture.

In basilar skull fractures, leakage of CSF secondary to dural tears usually resolves spontaneously and should not require antibiotic therapy. There should be no attempt to stop the leakage with packing because packing may increase the chance for infection. It can sometimes be difficult to distinguish CSF from mucous discharge initially. Glucose content is often thought to be indicative of CSF, but glucose can be present in mucous drainage as well and thus is not very specific. High chloride levels relative to serum may point to CSF. Persistent leaks lasting longer than a week may need operative intervention.[4]

Meningitis is a possible complication of basilar skull fractures, and a low threshold for workup for meningitis is warranted after the possibility of these types of fractures is evident. Parents should be instructed to pay close attention to the signs and symptoms of possible meningitis before discharge home. Meningitis is more common with CSF rhinorrhea than otorrhea. When meningitis complicates basilar skull fractures, it should be treated initially with broad-spectrum antibiotics to cover common nasal flora such as *Streptococcus pneumoniae* and *Haemophilus influenzae*.[6]

Intracranial Injuries

Epidural hematomas occur in up to 3% of all children hospitalized for traumatic head injury. They usually occur secondary to impact injury from a fall. Epidural hematomas are more common in older children and more frequently have associated skull fractures in older children.[7] After traumatic brain injury, delayed development of symptoms suggesting increased ICP, such as worsening or continued headaches, confusion, lethargy or agitation, or focal neurologic deficits, should be taken very seriously as a possible indication of acute epidural hematoma. Epidural hematomas appear as a lens-shaped or biconcave high-density mass immediately under the skull on CT (Fig. 143-1).

All epidural hematomas warrant neurosurgical evaluation. For epidural hematomas that are large, cause focal neurologic deficits, altered consciousness, or a mass effect, or are located in the temporal or posterior fossa, urgent removal by craniotomy is generally required. The outcome is usually good and strongly correlates with the clinical presentation.[4]

Acute subdural hematomas are more common in infants and younger children. They most often occur as a result of a considerable impact injury such as falls from great heights, motor vehicle accidents, assaults, and child abuse with acceleration-deceleration high-velocity trauma (see Chapters 173 and 175). The subdural bleeding arises from tearing of the cortical bridging veins that drain into the dural venous sinuses. Given the usual mechanism of injury, there are often associated parenchymal contusions or axonal injury.[8] Because of the commonly associated brain injuries, many patients with subdural hematomas are immediately symptomatic. Symptoms may include depressed mental status, focal neurologic deficits, hemiparesis, pupillary abnormalities,

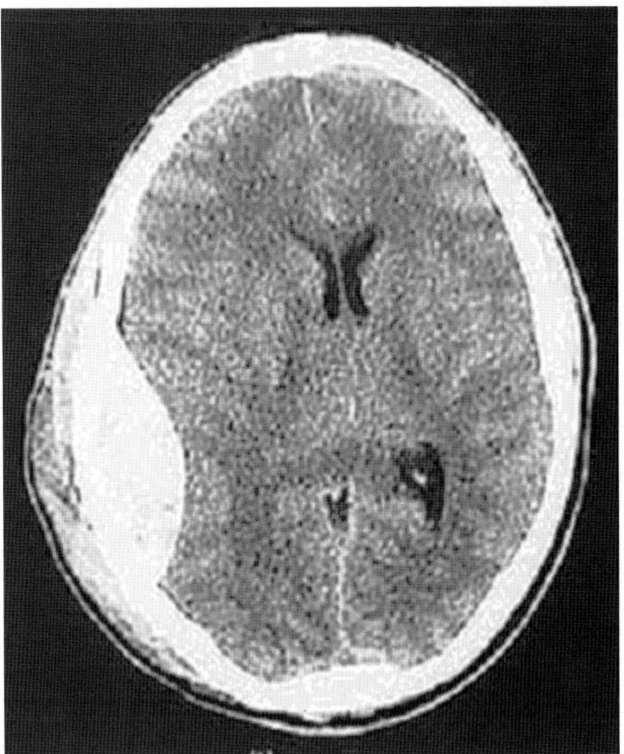

Figure 143-1   Right epidural hematoma with the characteristic lens shape.

and seizures. A CT scan of an acute subdural hematoma reveals a convex high-density collection overlying the brain (Fig. 143-2).

Because of associated brain injuries and complications of secondary injury, the outcome of subdural hematoma is worse than that of epidural hematoma in children.[8] Surgical intervention may be necessary, especially with large subdural hematomas causing a mass effect. Mortality can be high and increases in the setting of increased ICP and diffuse axonal injury. Delay in surgical intervention longer than 4 hours can be a poor prognostic factor. As with epidural hematomas, the neurologic status at presentation is strongly correlated with outcome.[4]

Intraparenchymal hemorrhages may be caused by focal blows or shearing of vulnerable areas against the calvaria; deeper white matter hemorrhages may occur with severe angular forces. Brainstem, basal ganglia, or thalamus injuries may result from these more severe acceleration injuries.[4] Traumatic axonal injuries can also result from rapid acceleration-deceleration forces. Intraventricular hemorrhages may occur and, if large, may cause obstructive hydrocephalus.

Physical Examination

It is important to focus on any external evidence of head injury that might suggest intracranial injuries. The patient should be examined for scalp contusions or lacerations, depressions of the skull, or facial injuries. Basilar skull fractures are suggested by the presence of periorbital or mastoid ecchymoses or swelling, hemotympanum, or clear ear or nasal drainage. In infants, a bulging or tense anterior fontanelle suggests elevated ICP. Although papilledema can

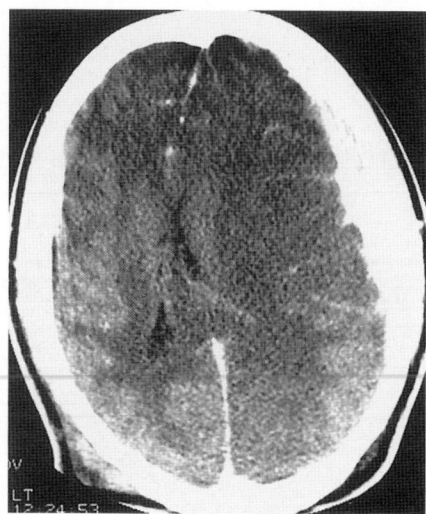

Figure 143-2   Acute subdural hematoma. (From Wilkins RH: Traumatic intracranial hematomas. In Rengachary SS, Wilkins RH [eds]: Principles of Neurosurgery. Philadelphia, CV Mosby, 1994, p 19.5.)

take up to 24 hours to develop in the setting of increased ICP, funduscopic examination can give valuable information about the severity and mechanism of head injury and reveal signs of suspected abusive injury.

Examination of the pupil is an important part of the assessment of patients with head trauma, and changes over time should be carefully noted. Size, shape, and reactivity to light can provide valuable information. Ipsilateral or bilateral dilation (mydriasis), constriction (miosis), and the response to light need to be evaluated. Ipsilateral mydriasis without direct or consensual constriction to light suggests transtentorial herniation with cranial nerve III compromise. Early transtentorial herniation may be manifested as Horner syndrome with ipsilateral miosis, ptosis, and anhidrosis. Ipsilateral miosis may also signal arterial disruption of the carotid on the affected side and would warrant proper imaging studies to evaluate this possibility. Bilateral mydriasis with no response to light is particularly worrisome for global ischemia or anoxia or bilateral cranial nerve III compromise.[4]

Persistent eye deviation may be a sign of cranial nerve compromise, cortical lesions, or seizure activity. Cerebellar or vestibular injury may be revealed by nystagmus.

Motor and sensory function should be assessed to determine the integrity of the spinal cord in a conscious patient. Deep tendon reflexes should be evaluated because symmetrical and hyperactive reflexes could indicate head or spinal cord injury and asymmetric reflexes might suggest a unilateral lesion. The Babinski reflex, or dorsiflexion of the great toe with plantar stimulation, suggests pyramidal tract involvement. This sign may be positive in young infants and thus is not of significance in this population.[5]

Treatment of Mild Head Trauma

Mild head injuries usually require no intervention, and management includes education of the patient or family about what signs and symptoms to look for that would require urgent repeat evaluation. If the parents' ability to come back to the hospital in a timely manner or to properly evaluate their child for worrisome signs and symptoms is in question, inpatient observation may be warranted.[9]

Treatment of Moderate and Severe Head Trauma

The first priority is to evaluate and maintain proper ventilation and hemodynamic status. Secondary brain injury can be prevented by proper identification and stabilization of such compromising conditions as hypotension or hypoxemia. Apnea or hypoventilation may be a result of the brain injury itself and should prompt intubation to ensure adequate oxygen delivery to the brain. Cushing's triad of hypertension, bradycardia, and altered respiration is a late finding and extremely concerning for herniation.

Hypotension must be addressed early and aggressively. There are strong data suggesting a relationship between hypotensive episodes and mortality in pediatric head trauma. Fluid resuscitation with normal saline or hypertonic 3% normal saline is recommended. A serum sodium goal of 145 mEq/L is reasonable, although some centers aim for serum sodium levels in the higher range because there is evidence suggesting that higher serum sodium concentrations are associated with decreases in ICP.[10]

Dextrose-containing fluids should not be used for resuscitation, and in general, high serum glucose levels are associated with worse outcomes.[10] Many centers do not use dextrose in fluids until at least 24 to 48 hours after traumatic brain injury, unless serum glucose levels are decreased. Insulin therapy should be used to treat high serum glucose.

If necessary, coagulation abnormalities should be corrected with fresh frozen plasma or cryoprecipitate. Platelet transfusions may be necessary, and a goal of greater than 100,000/mm^3 platelets is reasonable.

It is critical that pain also be adequately addressed. A short-acting narcotic such as fentanyl titrated upward to achieve adequate pain control is often used. A short-acting benzodiazepine such as midazolam is also often helpful in achieving sedation. High doses are frequently necessary in young children because metabolism of these drugs is increased. Paralysis may be used intermittently or continuously for increased ICP secondary to patient movement after adequate control of pain and agitation is established.

Seizures must be controlled because they will increase ICP. Data suggest that antiepileptic therapy is effective in preventing posttraumatic brain injury seizures for 7 days, but beyond that it has not been demonstrated to be effective. Most neurosurgeons consider a loading dose (20 mg/kg) of phenytoin (Dilantin) and 5 mg/kg/day thereafter for 7 days as prophylaxis for seizures when intracranial injury is significant.[1]

Cervical spine immobilization should be continued until imaging or examination can rule out cervical spine injury, but there are presently no standard protocols for such immobilization. Magnetic resonance imaging (MRI) may be helpful to exclude ligamentous injury. There is some debate regarding the usefulness of flexion and extension radiographs.[10] In general, neurosurgical consultation should be obtained when there is a question of cervical spine injury.

Nutrition should be addressed early, and enteral feeding should be established as early as possible. If nasogastric or jejunal feeding is not possible, parenteral nutrition should be started. Avoidance of hyperglycemia and hypoglycemia, as well as maintenance of proper nitrogen balance, should be achieved.

Attention to urine output and the serum sodium concentration is important after moderate to severe head trauma. The syndrome of inappropriate antidiuretic hormone secretion (SIADH) and cerebral salt wasting are both possible reasons for a decreased sodium concentration. Treatment of SIADH is fluid restriction, whereas treatment of cerebral salt wasting consists of increasing sodium intake. Distinguishing the two can be difficult, especially in the setting of mannitol or other diuretic therapy. Careful determination of overall fluid status can be helpful because SIADH is more often associated with euvolemia, as opposed to hypovolemia with cerebral salt wasting. Urine and serum sodium and osmolarity are also important to evaluate. In addition, diabetes insipidus is a complication of head injury that can occur in close temporal relationship to SIADH or salt wasting, so continued monitoring plus interpretation of electrolytes and fluid status is important.[10]

Postconcussive Syndromes

A number of syndromes can raise concern for intracranial injury after head trauma in children. Seizures can occur in about 10% of children within 24 hours of injury, often after mild trauma. They usually develop on impact or in the first few hours. Seizures are rarely associated with intracranial injury if they are the only abnormality on presentation, and they seldom result in future complications or epilepsy. Seizures either early or late (1 to 7 days or >1 week) after injury are more likely to be associated with obvious intracranial injury and should generally be treated with anticonvulsant medication. Consultation with a neurologist is recommended.[1]

A postconcussive syndrome of irritability, disorientation, lethargy, or even unresponsiveness can occur, often accompanied by vomiting. This syndrome often prompts head imaging, given the symptoms, which can mimic an expanding intracranial lesion. Children recover in a short time, less than a day, and usually need only supportive care inasmuch as CT shows no irregularities.[4]

Migraines can occur after head trauma in children. They are rare and can be associated with aggressive, sometimes violent behavior. Migraines generally resolve after a period of sleep. There is often a personal or family history of migraines; however, headache is not the most noticeable feature of this syndrome. Findings on CT are usually normal. Posttraumatic cortical blindness is another rare occurrence after head injury in children; it can present with partial or complete blindness, with preservation of pupillary responses, and also resolves within a day.[4]

Brain Death

A full discussion of brain death is beyond the scope of this chapter. However, it is important to be aware that the criteria for declaring brain death can be significantly different in children than in adults. Moreover, policies on declaring brain death may differ among hospitals within the same state, so familiarity and strict adherence to hospital policy are important.

In young children, up to 24 hours may be required between two separate examinations to declare brain death, and in infants it can be up to a week. The mechanism of injury and whether hypoxemia/ischemia is a primary cause of brain death may be taken into account in the criteria. Euthermia, absence of sedating medications, and other physiologic criteria are usually required before these examinations. Observation of fixed and dilated pupils unresponsive to light is required, and absence of brainstem function by demonstrating a lack of cold calorics, negative doll's eye reflex, no gag or corneal reflexes, and no response to pain is also necessary. Separate examinations by two different doctors, one a neurosurgeon or neurologist responsible for care of the patient, are generally necessary. Finally, an apnea test demonstrating absence of respiratory effort in the face of rising CO_2 must also be documented.

Posthospital Care

Outcomes for pediatric patients with traumatic head injury are far better than those for adults. For severe head injuries, however, mortality can approach 60%. Patients with severe head trauma who survive are commonly left with focal deficits and learning difficulties, and the majority require rehabilitation after hospital discharge.[5]

Children with moderate to severe traumatic brain injury should be referred for early intervention and rehabilitation services. Families and the child may benefit from psychosocial counseling. In general, after moderate or severe head injury, children should be referred for neuropsychiatric testing, especially when learning difficulties are present.

Prevention strategies for pediatric head injury include education of parents and children about passenger seat belts and air bags, as well as helmet use by children and adolescents during certain sport activities, which may reduce the risk for head trauma. Education on the avoidance of alcohol and drug use can also help in decreasing the incidence of alcohol- and drug-related accidents.

HYDROCEPHALUS

Hydrocephalus is a disturbance in the formation, absorption, or flow of CSF that results in an increased volume of this fluid in the central nervous system. Hydrocephalus can be acute, subacute, or chronic and can occur over a period of days, weeks or months.

Normally, CSF is produced in the choroid plexus and flows from the lateral ventricles, through the foramen of Monro to the third ventricle, then through the aqueduct of Sylvius to the fourth ventricle, and then through the foramina of Luschka and the foramen of Magendie to the subarachnoid space, to the arachnoid granulations, and finally to the dural sinus and into the venous drainage system (Fig. 143-3). Overproduction, blockage, or compromised absorption anywhere along this path can lead to buildup of fluid.

Hydrocephalus can be categorized as either communicating (impaired CSF reabsorption while the ventricles and the subarachnoid space communicate) or noncommunicating (obstructed flow within the ventricular system or its connections to the subarachnoid space). Hydrocephalus can also be classified as congenital or acquired. Some of the more common causes of hydrocephalus are listed in Table 143-1.[11]

Clinical Presentation

The signs and symptoms of hydrocephalus are largely due to increased ICP as a result of increased CSF volume.

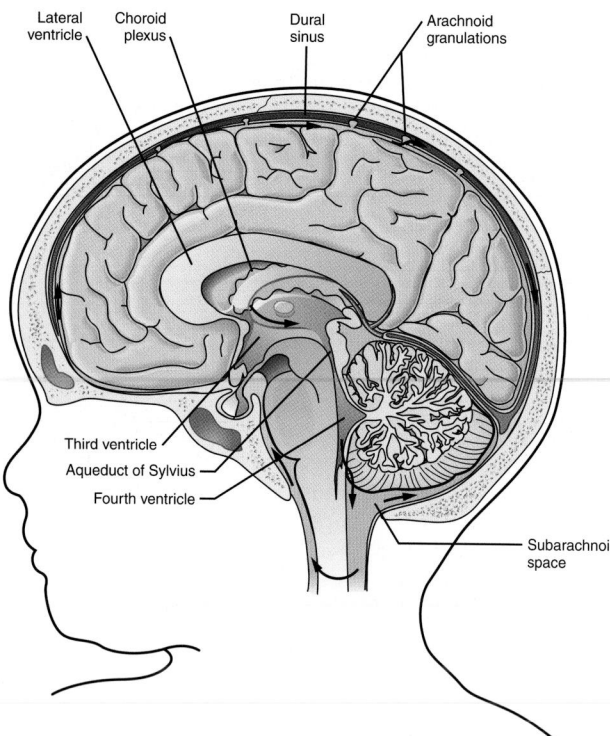

Figure 143-3   Schematic of cerebrospinal fluid flow.

Table 143-1   Causes of Hydrocephalus
Congenital
Myelomeningocele
Idiopathic
Stenosis of the aqueduct of Sylvius (including Bickers-Adams syndrome)
Dandy-Walker malformation
Arnold-Chiari malformation type 1 or type 2
Agenesis of the foramen of Monroe
Infections (toxoplasmosis)
Acquired
Intraventricular hemorrhage
Tumors (astrocytoma, medulloblastoma)
Cerebrospinal fluid infection (meningitis, abscesses, cysticercosis)
Head injury with hematoma
Venous sinus thrombosis
Cysts
Idiopathic

Infants may present with poor feeding, vomiting, irritability, reduced activity, lethargy, coma, or seizures. Common physical examination findings may include

- Hypertension
- Macrocephaly (head circumference greater than the 98th percentile for age)
- Widening of sutures, tense fontanelle, dilated scalp veins

- Increased lower extremity tone or spasticity
- Setting sun sign (downward gaze, upward eyelid retraction revealing the white sclera)

Children usually present with a headache as the earliest symptom, which can initially be worse in the morning. Other symptoms of increased ICP include nausea, vomiting, blurred or double vision (from papilledema and sixth nerve palsy), drowsiness, lethargy or coma, unsteady gait, and seizures. Signs of compromised hypothalamic function may be present.[12] Physical examination findings in children may include

- Hypertension
- Stunted growth or obesity
- Increased head size
- Macewen sign ("cracked pot" sound with percussion of the head)
- Papilledema
- Sixth nerve palsy (inability to gaze upward)
- Ataxia

Evaluation

Imaging can determine the amount of ventricular enlargement and sometimes the cause of the hydrocephalus. Ultrasound is sometimes sufficient for infants when the fontanelle is still open (up to 18 months) and can be used to monitor ventricular size.

CT and MRI are more useful for identifying the underlying cause of hydrocephalus and may well guide management. A baseline CT scan is important for comparison to future studies. When hydrocephalus is diagnosed, consultation with a neurosurgeon is required and should be done urgently if signs or symptoms of increased ICP are present (see later).

Treatment

Particularly in premature infants, nonsurgical management such as acetazolamide to decrease CSF production or repeated CSF removal by lumbar puncture (LP) may be used as a temporizing short-term measure, although long-term management of hydrocephalus usually requires shunt placement or third ventriculostomy if the signs or symptoms of increased ICP do not resolve.[12]

Third ventriculostomy creates a hole in the floor of the third ventricle that allows CSF to flow to the subarachnoid space and bypass the usual flow through the fourth ventricle outlined earlier. Thus, this procedure is used particularly for aqueductal stenosis and is most successful in children older than 6 months.[11]

Shunt placement is the most common treatment of hydrocephalus. The most common shunt is a shunt from one of the ventricles (usually lateral) to the peritoneum, called a ventriculoperitoneal shunt. See Chapters 213 and 214 for a description of shunts, their common complications, and management.

INCREASED INTRACRANIAL PRESSURE

Increased ICP is most frequently due to head trauma and its complications, hydrocephalus, or infections; see Table 143-2 for other causes. According to the Monro-Kellie

Table 143-2 Causes of Increased ICP
Moderate or severe head trauma
Subdural hematoma
Intraventricular hemorrhage
Venous sinus thrombosis
Hypoxemia/ischemia
Brain tumor
Severe hypertension
Meningitis, meningoencephalitis
Lyme disease
Encephalopathy (multiple causes)
Lead poisoning
Reye syndrome
Medications/toxins
Hypervitaminosis A
Diabetic ketoacidosis in response to treatment
Water intoxication
Other electrolyte disturbances (hypernatremia)
Pseudotumor cerebri (idiopathic intracranial hypertension)

principle, the brain is a closed compartment composed of three components: blood, CSF, and brain tissue. These three components are responsible for ICP, which is normally between 8 and 12 mm Hg in children. If any of these components increases in volume, a compensatory decrease in another component must occur or ICP will rise. Increased ICP can cause decreased blood supply to the brain and thereby result in ischemia. Physical compression of the brain leading to a shift across the midline or herniation through the base of the skull can eventually result in death. Increased ICP is an emergency that requires immediate evaluation and management.

Clinical Presentation

Gradual increases in ICP can be tolerated up to a point by children, and thus symptoms from chronic or indolent conditions may not present immediately. Acute increases beyond 20 mm Hg are likely to be symptomatic.

The signs and symptoms of increased ICP in both infants and children are similar to those listed earlier for hydrocephalus. Children usually present with headache, nausea and vomiting, or visual changes, whereas infants can have more nonspecific symptoms such as poor feeding, vomiting, or irritability. Decreased level of consciousness is a reliable and worrisome sign that requires immediate evaluation and management. Careful attention to changes in vital signs, in particular looking for hypertension, bradycardia, and an abnormal breathing pattern, is important.

Evaluation

A thorough physical and a neurologic examination are required. A funduscopic examination to look for papilledema is important, although this sign can take up to 24 hours to develop. Other signs were described earlier.

Brain imaging is almost always necessary when increased ICP is suspected. CT is relatively fast and can diagnose some of the aforementioned causes, although subsequent MRI examination may be necessary. To document increased ICP when a CT scan does not show evidence of any increase, LP may be performed with a manometer. Although the risk of herniation in young children may be overstated, in general it is prudent to obtain imaging before performing LP if increased ICP is suspected. If the CT scan shows signs of increased ICP (increased ventricle size, edema, loss of gray-white matter differentiation), neurosurgery should be consulted before attempting LP.[13]

Treatment

The underlying cause of increased ICP must be addressed and corrected, which may involve surgical evacuation of blood or mass lesions, treatment of infections, correction of electrolyte abnormalities, or removal of exposure to toxins. In general, ICP greater than 20 mm Hg should be managed aggressively, and depending on the situation and age of the patient, lower values may not be tolerated.

Management of increased ICP is focused on ensuring adequate cerebral blood flow. ICP should be managed with attention to positioning of the head; control of temperature, pain, agitation, and seizures; and proper bladder drainage.

To decrease ICP, the head should be elevated 20 to 30 degrees and the head should be midline to promote venous drainage. Hypothermia is common in children with traumatic brain injury, and euthermia should be achieved. Although a promising strategy to reduce or control ICP, at the present time there is no convincing evidence in pediatrics to recommend hypothermia. Temperatures should be kept below 38° C with cooling blankets and acetaminophen because the increased metabolic demands of hyperthermia increase ICP. A goal of 37° C is reasonable. Hypothermia can exacerbate coagulation problems and should be avoided in the setting of coagulopathy, which often accompanies traumatic brain injury.[13]

Osmotic diuretics such as mannitol in doses somewhere between 0.25 and 1 g/kg per dose may be effective in reducing ICP by more than one mechanism: drawing extracellular edema into the vascular space and decreasing blood viscosity, thereby improving cerebral blood flow. Repeat doses are often necessary, but attention to serum osmolarity is important, and mannitol should be used with caution if serum osmolarity is greater than 320. Administration of hypertonic saline to increase serum osmolality and the serum sodium concentration has already been discussed in the management of head trauma earlier in this chapter.

Barbiturates such as pentobarbital may be used, but such treatment is associated with significant risks, including hypotension, hyponatremia, pneumonia, and sepsis. When using barbiturates, proper volume expansion and blood pressure support with medications such as Neo-Synephrine or dopamine are often necessary. Steroids have not been proved to be useful in decreasing edema and secondary brain injury and are not recommended except in the setting of spinal cord injury. Craniectomy, CSF drainage, and continuous lumbar drainage are options to be considered when medical management fails and adequate cerebral perfusion pressure cannot be maintained.[4]

Pseudotumor cerebri, as mentioned earlier, is a condition in which there is increased ICP with a normal CT scan, normal CSF, and normal neurologic findings except for sixth nerve palsies and papilledema.[14] The usual presentation is a headache and sometimes visual disturbances. Visual acuity and visual fields must be evaluated. There can be an association with obesity, anemia, thyroid disease, and medications such as steroids (including birth control pills), acne medicines (tetracycline and isotretinoin), and nitrofurantoin. Evaluation requires a normal examination and brain imaging by either CT or MRI. A complete blood count and determination of cortisol levels may be indicated. Treatment of headache consists of acetazolamide and, if not effective, steroids for a 2-week course and then tapering. Ophthalmologic evaluation and follow-up are necessary because visual loss is a significant complication. Optic nerve sheath fenestration may be required to prevent visual loss.[15]

IN A NUTSHELL

- In the setting of head trauma, understanding the mechanism of injury and performing a careful physical examination are imperative when assessing for the potential for intracranial injury.
- Any neurologic changes distant from the event should raise suspicion of an evolving epidural hematoma.
- Hydrocephalus can be categorized as either communicating (impaired CSF reabsorption) or noncommunicating (obstructed CSF flow).
- Hydrocephalus can be managed pharmacologically, with systems for temporary CSF drainage, or with a shunt.
- Gradual increases in ICP can be tolerated up to a point by children, and thus symptoms from chronic or indolent conditions may not present immediately. Acute increases beyond 20 mm Hg are likely to be symptomatic and require aggressive management.

ON THE HORIZON

- Further studies are needed on the management of increased ICP in children, especially in the setting of head trauma, to evaluate the role of such unproven therapies as hypothermia. Research into improved sedative/anesthetic agents to attenuate posttraumatic hypoperfusion and excitotoxicity, antioxidants with better brain and cellular penetration, and molecular therapies to inhibit endogenous cell death effectors and augment endogenous neuroprotective genes may all yield improvement in the care of these children.

SUGGESTED READING

Dias MS: Traumatic brain and spinal cord injury. Pediatr Clin North Am 2004;51:271-303.

Harwood-Nash DC, Hendrick EB, Hudson AR: The significance of skull fractures in children. A study of 1,187 patients. Radiology 1971;101:151-155.

Kestle JR: Pediatric hydrocephalus: Current management. Neurol Clin 2003;21:883-895.

REFERENCES

1. Dias MS, Carnevale F, Li V: Immediate posttraumatic seizures: Is routine hospitalization necessary? Pediatr Neurosurg 1999;30:232-238.
2. Harwood-Nash DC, Hendrick EB, Hudson AR: The significance of skull fractures in children. A study of 1,187 patients. Radiology 1971;101:151-155.
3. Schutzman SA, Greenes DS: Pediatric minor head trauma. Ann Emerg Med 2001;37:65-74.
4. Dias MS: Traumatic brain and spinal cord injury. Pediatr Clin North Am 2004;51:271-303.
5. Kraus JF, Rock A, Hemyari P: Brain injuries among infants, children, adolescents, and young adults. Am J Dis Child 1990;144:684-691.
6. Goldstein B, Powers KS: Head trauma in children. Pediatr Rev 1994;15:213-219.
7. Luerssen TG: Head injuries in children. Neurosurg Clin North Am 1991;2:399-410.
8. Raimondi AJ, Hirschauer J: Head injury in the infant and toddler. Childs Brain 1984;11:12-35.
9. Committee on Quality Improvement, American Academy of Pediatrics: The management of minor closed head injury in children. Pediatrics 1999:104:1407-1415.
10. Adelson PD, Bratton SL, Carney NA, et al: Guidelines for the acute medical management of severe traumatic brain injury in infants, children, and adolescents. Pediatr Crit Care Med 2003;4(3 Suppl):S1-S75.
11. Kestle JR: Pediatric hydrocephalus: Current management. Neurol Clin 2003;21:883-895.
12. Garton HJ, Piatt JH Jr: Hydrocephalus. Pediatr Clin North Am 2004;51:305-325.
13. Chesnut RM: The management of severe traumatic brain injury. Emerg Med Clin North Am 1997;15:581-604.
14. Friedman DI: Pseudotumor cerebri. Neurosurg Clin North Am 1999;10:609-621.
15. Soler D, Cox T: Diagnosis and management of benign intracranial hypertension. Arch Dis Child 1998;78:89-94.

CHAPTER 144

Ocular Trauma

Jason Levy

Pediatric hospitalists may be called on to manage patients with ocular trauma in many situations, including the emergency department and inpatient units, either as a consultant or primary clinician, and in the preoperative or postoperative period. At times, prompt ophthalmologic consultation is unavailable, and other medical conditions or traumatic injuries may complicate care of the patient. Thus, being able to recognize, evaluate, and provide care for patients with an eye injury may be expected from the hospitalist.

Ocular trauma is second only to amblyopia as a cause of visual loss in the pediatric population. Injuries most commonly occur in adolescent boys while playing sports, the most dangerous being baseball and basketball.[1,2] The approach to a pediatric patient may be different from that of an adult for several reasons. The history is often unreliable or unavailable and the mechanism of injury may be unknown. Examination of an injured eye can be challenging and almost impossible in the face of an inconsolable patient with an injured eye. The visual system is often immature, thus necessitating effort to restore visual development.[3] Four basic principles should be adhered to when caring for a child with ocular trauma: management of life-threatening or central nervous system injury should always take precedence, structural integrity of the eyeball must be ensured, vision should be checked in both the injured and uninjured eye, and ophthalmologic consultation is an important resource.[4]

CLINICAL PRESENTATION

A complete history should be obtained with special attention to the mechanism, time and place of onset of symptoms, and changes in symptoms since the injury. For example, a foreign body sensation occurring near a construction site prompts a search for a different type of object than if symptoms began in a wooded area. Other important historical questions include previous visual status/acuity, the presence of contact lenses, and tetanus status.

PHYSICAL EXAMINATION

Despite the need for a complete examination, the most important goal in the initial assessment is preventing additional injury. If the child is uncooperative or agitated, the chance of further injury is increased and one must weigh the risks and benefits of continuing the examination.

Examination of the eye begins with assessing whether the globe is intact. Most open globe injuries can be diagnosed with simple penlight or flashlight examination. Smaller wounds may require slit-lamp examination for confirmation. If a ruptured globe is suspected, the examiner should

not proceed and the eye should be protected. One should avoid putting pressure on or around the injured eye to prevent extrusion of intraocular contents. For protection, a standard eye shield can be taped to the orbital rim. If a shield is not available, a Styrofoam cup can be cut about 2.5 cm from its base and used for the same purpose. An eye patch should not be used. Antiemetics may be administered to prevent increased intraocular pressure from vomiting.

If the globe has been deemed intact, the examiner should then proceed with the noncontact aspects of the examination first. Visual acuity should be assessed in each eye. Loss of vision is the most serious sequela of any ocular injury, and even in the case of an uncooperative child or an eye that is swollen shut, the examiner should document an attempted visual check. Light perception can still be tested even when the eye remains closed by shining a light source through a closed lid. The patient should be able to perceive the additional light on that side. After visual acuity is tested, the pupils and extraocular movements should be assessed, followed by examination of the lids, periorbital tissue, conjunctiva, sclera, and cornea. Fluorescein staining with examination of the cornea under black light is optimal. Finally, a red reflex should be tested to evaluate for lens abnormalities.[3]

SPECIFIC INJURIES

Injuries to the Lids and Adnexa

About 80% of all pediatric ocular injuries involve the external ocular tissues.[1,5] The most common serious external injuries are eyelid contusions and lacerations.[3] The primary care provider can repair small and uncomplicated lacerations of the eyelid or surrounding tissues, but in general, lid lacerations often warrant ophthalmologic consultation, especially if the lid margin is involved. Special attention should be paid to lacerations involving the medial portion of the eyelid because of their frequent association with canalicular injury. A laterally displaced lid margin punctum indicates tear duct involvement. The eyelid should be everted to look for a conjunctival wound indicating complete perforation and a possible globe-penetrating injury.

Blunt trauma may result in impressive ecchymosis and edema, often with little or no disability. The distribution of hemorrhage, however, can sometimes indicate a serious orbital injury. For example, blood under the superior conjunctiva may suggest an orbital roof fracture, and hemorrhage in the lower lid and inferior orbit may signify an orbital floor fracture. In general, treatment of an uncomplicated "black eye" is cold compresses for 24 hours, followed by warm compresses. The ecchymosis may persist for 2 or

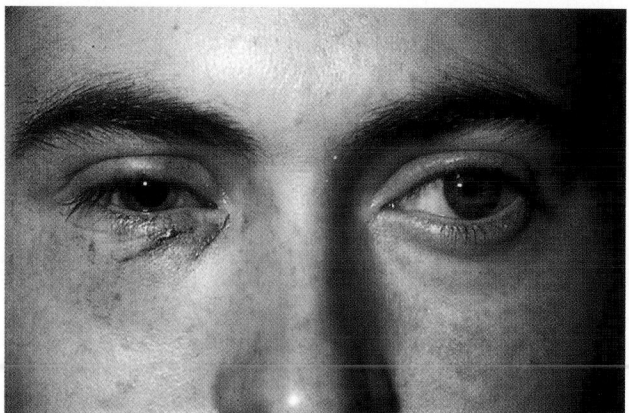

A

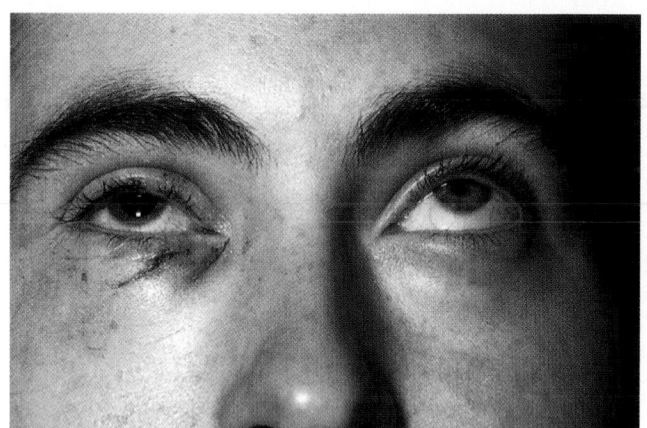

B

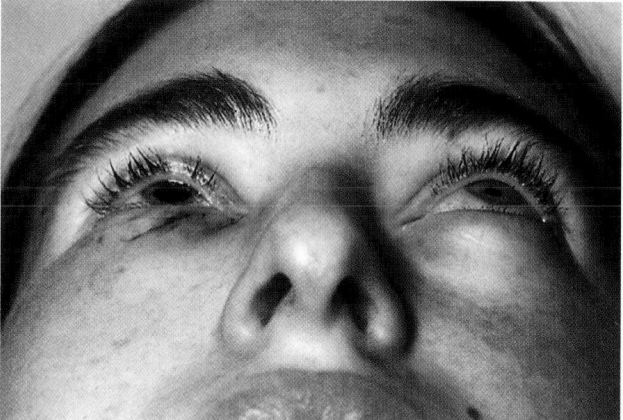

C

Figure 144-1   Right orbital floor blow-out fracture with restricted elevation. (From Kanski JJ: Trauma. In Kanski JJ [ed]: Clinical Ophthalmology: A Systematic Approach. Philadelphia, Elsevier, 2003, p 662.)

more weeks, so appropriate anticipatory guidance is important. Ecchymotic discoloration may track inferiorly and be visible even in the submandibular region.

Blow-Out Fractures

Blow-out fractures, or fractures of the orbital wall, are a result of either increased intraorbital pressure from blunt force leading to compression of the orbital tissue and subsequent fracture or blunt force to the orbital rim resulting in buckling of the orbital floor. They are most common after direct blunt trauma with objects larger than the orbit (such as a baseball) and most commonly involve the medial or inferior wall. Clinical signs of blow-out fractures include lid ecchymosis and edema, epistaxis, decreased sensation of the ipsilateral cheek and lip, and enophthalmos (sunken eye) or exophthalmos. The hallmark sign, however, is restriction of extraocular movement, particularly upward gaze, as a result of entrapment of the extraocular muscles (Fig. 144-1).

Orbital fractures are best diagnosed by computed tomography (CT) (Fig. 144-2) or by plain films with a Waters view if CT is unavailable. Ophthalmologic consultation is almost always warranted inasmuch as 50% of orbital fractures are associated with eyeball injury.[6] Indications for surgical repair are controversial and should be determined in concert with

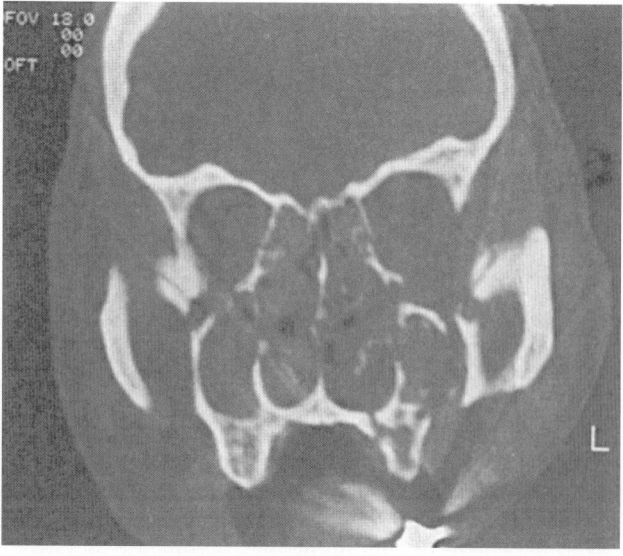

Figure 144-2   Orbital fracture with disruption of the left orbit. (From Yaremchuk MJ, Shore JW: Structural injuries of the orbit. In Albert D, Jakobiec F, Azar DT, et al [eds]: Principles and Practice of Ophthalmology. Philadelphia, WB Saunders, 2000.)

the consulting specialist. Additional therapies in the acute setting include antibiotic prophylaxis, nasal decongestants, ice packs, and instruction to the patient to not blow the nose to avoid creating or worsening orbital emphysema.

Ruptured Globe

A ruptured globe implies laceration or puncture of the cornea or sclera (or both) and is associated with significant visual morbidity in the pediatric population.[7] After injury, the iris or choroid will plug the wound and result in an abnormally shaped pupil (often teardrop), the most apparent clinical sign of a ruptured globe. Other clinical indicators include hyphema, severe subconjunctival hemorrhage, and exposed uveal tissue. If a ruptured globe is suspected, examination of the eye should be discontinued, the eye protected with a shield or cup, and emergency ophthalmologic consultation sought. A patch should never be used in this circumstance. Every attempt should be made to keep the child calm because crying and screaming can result in extrusion of intraocular contents through the rupture. If all else fails, sedation may be indicated.

Hyphema

Hyphema is defined as bleeding into the anterior chamber and is a sign of severe ocular trauma (Fig. 144-3). It is usually the result of blunt injury and subsequent tearing of iris vessels. Hyphemas are graded according to the amount of blood in the anterior chamber, and their size is directly related to morbidity, with larger hyphemas having an increased incidence of secondary glaucoma and a poor visual prognosis. Grade 1 hyphemas have blood that occupies less than a third of the anterior chamber, grade 2 involves filling of a third to half of the anterior chamber, grade 3 is layering greater than half of the anterior chamber, and grade 4 is total filling of the anterior chamber with clotted blood ("black-ball" or "8-ball" hyphema). All cases of hyphema warrant ophthalmologic referral, and hospital admission is recommended in all but the most minor of cases. Factors such as age, probability of noncompliance, and likelihood of complications should be taken into account in any patient in whom outpatient management is being considered.[8]

Treatment is not standardized but is aimed at preventing rebleeding and inflammation and includes restricted activity and bed rest with head elevation. Other management options include cycloplegics, topical corticosteroids, and antifibrinolytics. Rebleeding is the most frequent complication. It usually occurs within the first 5 days, is often of greater magnitude than the original bleeding, and is associated with a worse visual prognosis. Aspirin, ibuprofen, and other anticoagulant analgesics should be avoided. Ophthalmologic follow-up should be undertaken in all children with hyphema within 2 to 4 weeks.[8]

Special consideration should be given to children with sickle cell hemoglobinopathies because they may have poor clearance of the hyphema. All African American children with hyphema should undergo sickle cell testing if their sickle cell status is not known.

IN A NUTSHELL

- The most important goal in the initial assessment of a patient with eye trauma is prevention of further injury.
- If the injury is suspicious for rupture of the globe, the eye should be protected with a shield device. An eye patch should not be used. Further examination of the eye should be deferred.
- Hyphema is usually a result of blunt trauma, and a focus of treatment is prevention of rebleeding.
- Lacerations involving the medial portion of the eyelid may be associated with canalicular injury, especially if the lid margin punctum is displaced. Repair by an ophthalmologic specialist is indicated.
- Orbital fractures, often secondary to blunt trauma, most commonly involve the medial wall or floor of the orbit. Entrapment of the extraocular muscles is a complication and is manifested as limited range of motion, especially with upward gaze.
- Follow-up with an ophthalmologist is often warranted for serious eye injuries, even if the ophthalmologist was not directly involved in the inpatient phase of care.

SUGGESTED READING

Arbour JD, Brunette I, Boisjoly HM: Should we patch corneal erosions? Arch Ophthalmol 1997;115:313-317.

Forbes JR: Management of corneal abrasions and ocular trauma in children. Pediatr Ann 2001;30:465-471.

Levin AV: Eye emergencies: Acute management in the pediatric ambulatory setting. Pediatr Emerg Care 1991;7:367-377.

Levin AV: Direct ophthalmoscopy in pediatric emergency care. Pediatr Emerg Care 2001;17:199-204.

Levine LM: Pediatric ocular trauma and shaken infant syndrome. Pediatr Clin North Am 2003;50:137-148.

Rychwalski PJ, O'Halloran HS, Cooper HM, et al: Evaluation and classification of pediatric ocular trauma. Pediatr Emerg Care 1999;15:277-279.

REFERENCES

1. Cascairo MA, Mazow ML, Prager TC: Pediatric ocular trauma: A retrospective survey. J Pediatr Ophthalmol Strabismus 1994;31:312-317.
2. Danis RP, Neely D, Plager DA: Unique aspects of trauma in children. In Kuhn F, Pieramici D (eds): Ocular Trauma Principles and Practice. New York, Thieme, 2002, pp 307-319.

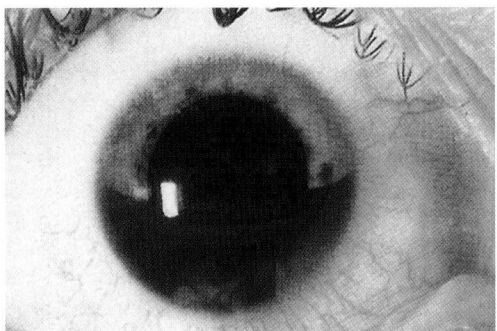

Figure 144-3 Patient with traumatic hyphema and layering of blood in the anterior chamber. (From Hersh PS, Zagelbaum BM, Shingleton BJ, et al: Anterior segment trauma. In Albert D, Jakobiec F, Azar DT, et al (eds): Principles and Practice of Ophthalmology. Philadelphia, WB Saunders, 2000.)

3. Levine LM: Pediatric ocular trauma and shaken infant syndrome. Pediatr Clin North Am 2003;50:137-148, vii.
4. Levin A: Eye trauma. In Fleisher GR, Ludwig S, Henriteg FM (eds): Textbook of Pediatric Emergency Medicine, 4th ed. Philadelphia, Lippincott Williams & Wilkins, 2000, pp 1397-1407.
5. Forbes BJ: Management of corneal abrasions and ocular trauma in children. Pediatr Ann 2001;30:465-472.
6. Hatton MP, Watkins LM, Rubin PA: Orbital fractures in children. Ophthal Plast Reconstr Surg 2001;17:174-179.
7. Rudd JC, Jaeger EA, Freitag SK, Jeffers JB: Traumatically ruptured globes in children. J Pediatr Ophthalmol Strabismus 1994;31:307-311.
8. Lai JC, Fekrat S, Barron Y, Goldberg MF: Traumatic hyphema in children: Risk factors for complications. Arch Ophthalmol 2001;119:64-70.

CHAPTER 145

Orthopedics

B. David Horn and David A. Spiegel

Specialists in pediatric hospital medicine may be involved in the care of patients with a broad variety of orthopedic conditions, including such diverse scenarios as a newborn with congenital anomalies, the postoperative care of patients undergoing elective orthopedic surgery, evaluation of a patient with bone or joint pain (or both), and care of patients with musculoskeletal trauma. A vast spectrum of issues therefore confronts the hospitalist in the evaluation and care of patients with orthopedic conditions. This chapter addresses some of the more common scenarios and diagnoses that are encountered by the pediatric hospitalist and in particular emphasizes the early diagnosis of complications in patients hospitalized with orthopedic conditions.

CONGENITAL CONDITIONS

The pediatric hospitalist frequently evaluates patients with a wide assortment of congenital orthopedic conditions. Although most congenital orthopedic conditions are isolated to the musculoskeletal system, many are associated with anomalies of other organ systems, some of which may be life threatening. All patients with congenital orthopedic conditions therefore require a thorough physical examination not only to define the musculoskeletal issues but also to search for associated or underlying problems.

Developmental Dysplasia of the Hip

Developmental dysplasia of the hip (DDH) may be an isolated finding (so-called typical DDH) or may occur along with syndromes (e.g., arthrogryposis, Larsen syndrome) or neuromuscular diseases (e.g., spina bifida or spinal muscular atrophy). These associated syndromes and diseases typically require further evaluation and treatment from many different specialties, whereas typical DDH can be treated by an orthopedist without further medical evaluation. Nonoperative treatment is usually successful for typical DDH, but surgery is frequently required for the optimal treatment of DDH associated with syndromes or neuromuscular disease.[1]

Congenital Anomalies of the Foot

Congenital anomalies of the foot seen in the newborn include clubfoot, congenital vertical talus, metatarsus adductus, and calcaneal valgus. The clinical appearance of a clubfoot is often confused with metatarsus adductus, whereas a calcaneal valgus foot may be confused with a vertical talus. Clubfoot and metatarsus adductus both appear as a foot with a "C" or bean shape in the midfoot and forefoot, with the lateral border of the foot curved instead of straight. The convexity of this curvature is on the outside. A clubfoot, however, is also characterized by supination of the foot and hindfoot equinus (caused by a contracture of the Achilles tendon and ankle capsule) (Fig. 145-1).[2] This hindfoot equinus is a major finding differentiating clubfoot from metatarsus adductus. In addition, atrophy of the calf will be noted on the affected side in a child with clubfoot. Metatarsus adductus and clubfoot both have a weak association with concomitant DDH. All patients with these conditions should therefore have a thorough hip examination performed and documented. Clubfoot may also be associated with neurologic conditions or other genetic conditions, so a thorough physical examination, including a neurologic assessment, should be performed. Radiographs are not typically needed in the diagnosis and initial treatment of clubfoot. In all cases, orthopedic referral should be made for treatment of a clubfoot. Treatment should ideally begin as early as possible; initial treatment usually consists of serial casts or splints, and typically some type of surgery is needed within the first 6 months of life for further correction.[2] Treatment of metatarsus adductus is generally determined by the flexibility of the foot. Supple metatarsus adductus can usually be treated with stretching exercises. Rigid metatarsus adductus has a less favorable natural history and may require casting for treatment.[3]

Congenital vertical talus is an uncommon foot deformity that consists of dorsal dislocation of the midfoot on the hindfoot, as well as equinus positioning of the hindfoot.[4] Similar to clubfoot, a hallmark of congenital vertical talus is a rigid plantar flexion deformity of the hindfoot. In addition, the midfoot in congenital vertical talus has a rocker-bottom configuration with a convexity on the plantar aspect of the foot. It is bilateral 50% of the time, and about half the time it is associated with other musculoskeletal conditions such as arthrogryposis; neural tube defects; sacral agenesis; neuromuscular disorders; spinal muscular atrophy; trisomy 13, 15, 17, and 18; and Turner syndrome.[4] For this reason an infant with a congenital vertical talus should undergo a genetics evaluation, as well as an orthopedic consultation. Treatment consists of stretching and casts, followed by surgical correction, with surgery generally occurring between 6 and 12 months of age.[4]

Calcaneal valgus deformity of the foot is a positional foot deformity that may be confused with congenital vertical talus. In contrast to congenital vertical talus, the ankle in a calcaneal valgus foot dorsiflexes freely. Calcaneal valgus occurs secondary to intrauterine positioning and is not associated with any other systemic, genetic, or neurologic conditions. Calcaneal valgus is a flexible condition that usually responds well to stretching.[3]

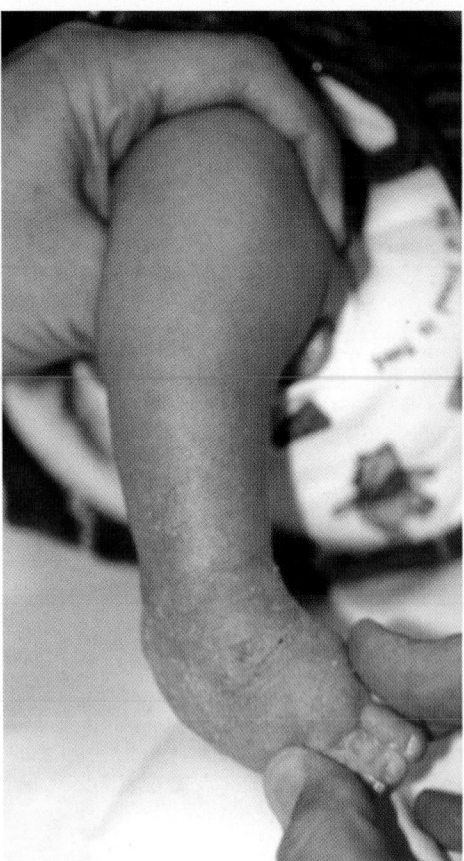

Figure 145-1   Typical appearance of a clubfoot showing calf atrophy and equinus, supination, and adduction of the foot.

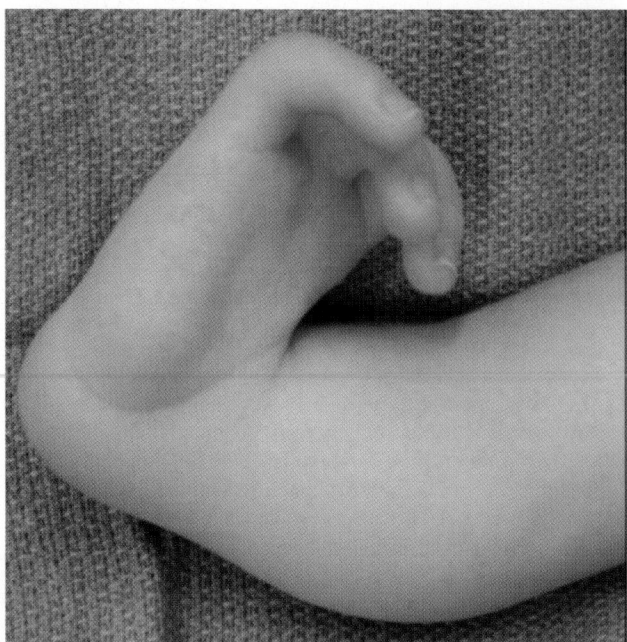

Figure 145-2   Clinical appearance of a radial clubhand with complete absence of the thumb.

Congenital Anomalies of the Upper Extremity

A wide variety of congenital anomalies occur in the upper extremities. Although a detailed discussion of congenital limb differences is beyond the scope of this chapter, it should be noted that most congenital upper extremity anomalies are isolated in nature. There are some notable exceptions to this generalization, however, and these exceptions need to be recognized because some upper extremity anomalies may signal the presence of coexisting life-threatening conditions in other organ systems.

Longitudinal deficiency of the radius (radial clubhand) is one such anomaly that may be accompanied by serious problems in other organ systems.[5] Longitudinal deficiency of the radius describes a spectrum of disease involving abnormal formation of the radius, as well as the radial (thumb) side of the wrist and hand. The term *longitudinal deficiency of the radius* encompasses a wide spectrum of deformity; problems range from a hypoplastic radius or thumb to complete absence of the radius, thumb, and radial side of the hand and wrist (Fig. 145-2). Longitudinal deficiency of the radius is frequently associated with other syndromes, including blood dyscrasias (Fanconi anemia), thrombocytopenia–absent radius (TAR) syndrome, congenital heart anomalies (Holt-Oram syndrome), craniofacial defects, and vertebral anomalies such as the VATER sequence (vertebral defects, imperforate anus, tracheoesophageal fistula, and radial and renal dysplasia).[5] Other nonsyndromic anomalies may also be associated with longitudinal deficiency of the radius,

including DDH, scoliosis, and clubfoot. Patients with congenital upper extremity differences should also have their chest evaluated for chest dysplasia or hypoplasia because the combination of upper extremity anomalies and developmental disruption of the pectoralis major muscle in the chest wall occurs in Poland syndrome. Orthopedic treatment of patients with upper extremity anomalies is individualized for each patient, typically after evaluation by an orthopedic surgeon and an occupational therapist.

Congenital Anomalies of the Spine

There are a wide variety of congenital spine anomalies, including neural tube defects such as spina bifida (which are covered elsewhere in this book) and congenital scoliosis. Most congenital spine disorders result from a developmental defect in formation or differentiation (or both) of the vertebral bodies and occur between the fourth and sixth weeks of in utero development.[6] Because these defects occur early in fetal development, patients with congenital spine anomalies frequently have anomalies of other organ systems. Abnormalities of the genitourinary tract are the most common associated finding and occur in 20% to 33% of patients with congenital scoliosis, whereas congenital cardiac anomalies will be present 10% to 15% of the time.[6] Neurologic conditions such as spinal cord tethering may also coexist with congenital scoliosis. Careful genitourinary, neurologic, and cardiac evaluation should be performed in all patients with congenital scoliosis.[6]

POSTOPERATIVE CARE OF PATIENTS AFTER SPINAL FUSION

Many orthopedic surgeries are now performed as outpatient procedures or with only a 23-hour hospitalization. Postsurgical patients treated as an outpatient or with a brief hospital stay are usually healthy and frequently require only routine care. Some patients, however, undergo pediatric orthopedic procedures that require a prolonged hospital stay. One of the most common of these procedures is spinal fusion with instrumentation, which is typically performed for scoliosis.

In spinal fusion, implants (usually consisting of some combination of rods, hooks, screws, and wires) are used to obtain correction of the scoliosis, stabilize the spine, and facilitate fusion of the spine. Insertion of hardware around the spinal cord and the subsequent manipulation performed to correct the scoliosis may injure the spinal cord. Because of this risk most of these procedures are done with some type of neurologic monitoring (somatosensory evoked potentials or motor evoked potentials). Patients who sustain prolonged or irreversible intraoperative changes to their spinal cord will generally have their surgery halted. The procedure is then usually completed 7 to 10 days after the initial surgery.[7]

Even in uneventful spinal fusions, all patients need to have careful postoperative neurologic monitoring through serial physical examination. Rarely, after spinal fusion and instrumentation patients will experience late neurologic deterioration, possibly related to delayed spinal cord ischemia or compression. In these cases, return to the operating room may be indicated for implant removal and exploration.[7] There is a significant amount of blood loss associated with spinal surgery such as fusion. Despite intraoperative transfusions and the use of cell savers, patients need to have their intravascular volume status monitored closely after spinal fusion.

Other medical complications also occur after spinal fusion and may be encountered by a pediatric hospitalist. Postoperatively patients will have ileus, so patients are restricted from oral intake after surgery until bowel sounds have returned, which commonly occurs 24 to 72 hours after surgery. With prolonged ileus or when there is recurrent or prolonged nausea or vomiting (or both) after initiation of oral intake, other causes must be considered, including gastric hypomotility secondary to narcotic use for pain control, superior mesenteric artery (SMA) syndrome, and pancreatitis.[8,9] SMA syndrome (or cast syndrome) is an upper intestinal obstruction caused by obstruction of the third part of the duodenum by the SMA. The SMA originates from the aorta and crosses over the third part of the duodenum. The duodenum, therefore, is susceptible to compression from the SMA, particularly if there has been a reduction in thoracic kyphosis as a result of either surgery or subsequent casting. SMA syndrome presents with persistent abdominal pain, distention, nausea, and vomiting after the initiation of oral intake. The diagnosis is confirmed with an upper gastrointestinal series demonstrating obstruction of the duodenum. SMA syndrome is treated with placement of a nasogastric tube, intravenous fluid, and gradual resumption of oral intake. Persistent cases may require parenteral hyperalimentation.[8]

Pancreatitis has also been reported after posterior spinal fusion for scoliosis.[9] The cause of the pancreatitis is unclear, but it presents as abdominal pain, nausea, and vomiting after the reinstitution of oral intake. The diagnosis is confirmed by elevated levels of serum lipase and amylase. Treatment of postoperative pancreatitis is restriction of oral intake, nasogastric suction, and if needed, hyperalimentation.

The syndrome of inappropriate antidiuretic hormone secretion (SIADH) has also been reported after spinal fusion for scoliosis.[8] It is diagnosed by decreased urine production, serum hyponatremia, serum hypo-osmolality, and an increase in urine osmolality. Free water retention may also lead to a spurious decrease in the patient's hemoglobin and hematocrit. SIADH is managed by restriction of fluid intake and prevention of fluid overload until the problem spontaneously corrects, which usually occurs within 1 week.

COMPARTMENT SYNDROME

Compartment syndrome is a feared complication of many pediatric injuries and fractures and may not only result in severe, permanent injury but may also be limb or life threatening. Early detection and prompt treatment are key to avoiding complications from compartment syndromes. Risk factors for development of a compartment syndrome include fractures of the tibia, forearm, and elbow; crush injuries; bleeding disorders such as hemophilia; ipsilateral forearm and elbow injuries; and open fractures. Compartment syndrome may arise from both extrinsic and intrinsic causes.[10] Intrinsic causes include crush injury, reperfusion injury, fractures, and intraoperative positioning. Extrinsic causes include compression from a cast or bandages. Any injury may develop into a compartment syndrome, and compartment syndrome may occur after elective surgery as well. There have also been recent reports of compartment syndrome after closed treatment of femur fractures with a spica cast.[11] Patients with altered mental status (such as from a closed head injury) require particularly close evaluation because many of the common signs and symptoms of compartment syndrome will be absent (see later).[10]

Physiologically, compartment syndrome occurs as a result of increased pressure within a muscular compartment of an extremity. Muscle groups in the extremities are contained within fibro-osseous compartments. When there is swelling within the compartment (for example, after an injury, from bleeding, or from reperfusion), the compartment may not be able to expand sufficiently to accommodate the increased volume of the structures residing within the compartment. Consequently, tissue pressure rises within the compartment. Ischemia results when the pressure within the compartment is greater than the opening pressure of the venules traversing through the compartment.[10]

The diagnosis of compartment syndrome is best made on a clinical basis. Its signs and symptoms result from increased tissue pressure and subsequent ischemia. The involved compartments are often swollen to the point at which they are hard and tense. Classically, the diagnosis of a compartment syndrome is made on the basis of the "five p's": pain (particularly pain with passive stretch of muscles contained within the involved compartment), pallor, paresthesias, pulselessness, and paralysis.[10] The earliest and most sensitive clinical finding is pain. Pain from a compartment syndrome is frequently described as severe, unremitting, out of proportion to the initial injury, and poorly controlled by normal levels of analgesics. Intense pain with passive stretch of the muscles in the affected compartment is also a sign of compartment syndrome. Paresthesias, pulselessness, pallor, and paralysis may also be present in compartment syndrome; however, these symptoms usually occur late in the evolution of a compartment syndrome and frequently represent irreversible muscle and nerve ischemia.[10]

Neurologically impaired or very young patients may not exhibit the symptoms of a compartment syndrome or may be difficult to examine. In these situations or when the findings on examination are equivocal, the pressure within a compartment can be directly measured by one of several techniques. Compartment pressures greater than 30 mm Hg or within 20 mm Hg of diastolic blood pressure are considered suggestive of compartment syndrome.[10]

Treatment of compartment syndrome is surgical: a fasciotomy of the affected compartments should be performed to allow muscle swelling and decrease tissue pressure within the compartment. The fasciotomies are left open until the swelling subsides, at which point they are surgically closed. A high index of suspicion, early diagnosis, and prompt treatment are key to successful treatment of this often devastating condition.[10]

BACK PAIN

Although back pain is extremely common in adults, complaints of back pain, especially in the first decade of life, should be taken quite seriously because they can be associated with potentially significant pathology. Still, back pain in the majority of pediatric patients will be due to trauma, stress, or overuse, such as overloaded backpacks in middle- or high-school children, and will be handled on an ambulatory basis.

For patients who are admitted with back pain, several points in the history need to be solicited. Was there any trauma, either acute or chronic/recurrent? Is there fever or other systemic signs of illness, such as weight loss or fatigue? Is there any evidence of extremity weakness or disuse? Are there any changes in bowel or bladder function?

A thorough back and neurologic examination of the patient is essential to assess for any possible spinal cord involvement. The musculature should be evaluated for bulk, tone, and strength. In addition to the deep tendon and Babinski reflexes, anal tone, anal wink, and (in boys) cremasteric reflexes should be evaluated. Sensation to light touch, pin prick, and heat/cold and proprioception should be examined as well. Abdominal reflexes should also be assessed.

Laboratory and radiographic evaluation is based on the clinical presentation. If infection is a possibility, a complete blood count and inflammatory markers (such as an erythrocyte sedimentation rate or C-reactive protein) are helpful. Plain films are a simple and easily obtainable study to initiate the evaluation. However, many cases of back pain will require magnetic resonance imaging to assess for possible intraspinal pathology. A bone scan may help localize areas of involvement if it is not clear from the physical examination.

The most serious causes of back pain can be divided into three major categories: traumatic, infectious, and neoplastic.

Spondylolysis (Fig. 145-3B) is a common cause of back pain in adolescents. It represents a weakening or discontinuity of the pars interarticularis (Fig. 145-3A), which connects the vertebrae at the facet joints. Spondylolysis is most likely due to chronic or recurrent trauma, such as sports that put a great deal of stress on the lower part of the back (e.g., football, wrestling, gymnastics). There is probably a genetic predisposition as well. Spondylolisthesis represents one vertebra slipping forward on the one beneath it, which may result in nerve impingement and may require surgical intervention (Fig. 145-3C).

An epidural hematoma is a very uncommon, but dangerous cause of back pain because the pain may present only shortly before evidence of spinal cord compression. It may be due to trauma, such as from a fall or a blow. It rarely arises as a complication of lumbar puncture.[12] Epidural hematomas may also "spontaneously arise" in patients with a bleeding disorder or coagulopathy.

There are many infectious causes of back pain, and unfortunately, they do not always present with fever. In addition to infections of the spine itself, such as vertebral osteomyelitis (Chapter 70), diskitis, or epidural abscess, paraspinal or retroperitoneal infections may present in a similar fashion and are often ultimately diagnosed through

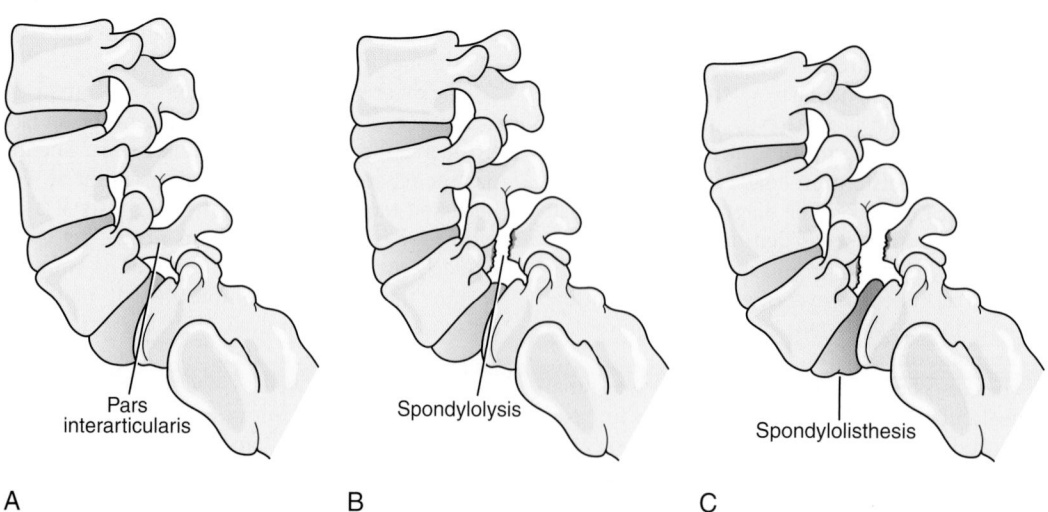

Figure 145-3   Pars interarticularis (A), spondylolysis (B), and spondylolisthesis (C). (Available from http://orthoinfo.aaos.org/fact/thr_report.cfm? Thread_ID=155&topcategory=Spin, 8/17/06.)

imaging. Vertebral osteomyelitis represents approximately 1% to 3% of cases of osteomyelitis.[13] *Staphylococcus aureus* is the most common organism, but other organisms, including *Bartonella henselae* (cat-scratch disease) and *Brucella*, can present as vertebral osteomyelitis. Tuberculous osteomyelitis (Pott disease) or fungal causes (e.g., *Candida* or coccidioidomycosis) should be considered in a patient with persistent fever and symptoms and persistently negative bacterial cultures. Patients with an infection of or around the spine usually require prolonged courses of intravenous antibiotics as compared with other sites of osteomyelitis.

Transverse myelitis is inflammation of a segment or segments of the spinal cord and is occasionally a postinfectious process. Symptoms can develop over a period of several weeks or as rapidly as several hours. Patients usually present with back pain, weakness, sensory disturbance, and bladder or bowel dysfunction. The degree of symptomatology relates to the level of involvement of the spine because weakness and diminution of sensation below the involved segment are hallmarks of the disease. Care of these patients is usually supportive, and recovery can be full, partial, or absent.

Both benign and malignant tumors may present with back pain. Ewing sarcoma can often be mistaken for an infectious process because fever and leukocytosis are common presenting findings. Both leukemia and lymphoma can also present as back pain.

ADMISSION CRITERIA

- Any patient with back pain and neurologic findings must be admitted for evaluation because the prognosis can worsen the longer a patient is symptomatic.

IN A NUTSHELL

- Orthopedists are consulted on a variety of issues that face the pediatric hospitalist—congenital anomalies, postoperative management, and concern for bone or joint infection or injury.
- Congenital anomalies can be treated with a wide range of potential modalities, from simple manipulation exercises to complex reconstructive surgery.
- Careful neurologic assessment is extremely important in the evaluation of an orthopedic patient, particularly those with issues involving the spine.

ON THE HORIZON

- Orthopedists are among the leaders with regard to tissue engineering. Much work has been and continues to be done on developing scientifically engineered bone, ligament, and cartilage substitutes. Ligament reconstruction is performed with the use of scaffolds, cultured cells, and growth factors. Tissue-engineered bone graft substitutes may reduce or eliminate the need for bone graft harvesting and help reduce failure rates when using natural bone alone. Although cartilage has been engineered in a variety of shapes and methods for cosmetic purposes, work continues on the development of weight-bearing articular cartilage to replace injured cartilage in vivo.

REFERENCES

1. Guille JT, Pizzutillo PD, MacEwen GD: Development dysplasia of the hip from birth to six months. J Am Acad Orthop Surg 2000;8:232-242.
2. Roye DP Jr, Roye BD: Idiopathic congenital talipes equinovarus. J Am Acad Orthop Surg 2002;10:239-248.
3. Scherl SA: Common lower extremity problems in children. Pediatr Rev 2004;25(2):52-62.
4. Drennan JC: Congenital vertical talus. Instr Course Lect 1996;45:315-322.
5. Kozin SH: Upper-extremity congenital anomalies. J Bone Joint Surg Am 2003;85:1564-1576.
6. Hedequist D, Emans J: Congenital scoliosis. J Am Acad Orthop Surg 2004;12:266-275.
7. Tolo VT: Surgical treatment of adolescent idiopathic scoliosis. Instr Course Lect 1989;38:143-156.
8. Shapiro G, Green DW, Fatica NS, Boachie-Adjei O: Medical complications in scoliosis surgery. Curr Opin Pediatr 2001;13:36-41.
9. Laplaza FJ, Widmann RF, Fealy S, et al: Pancreatitis after surgery in adolescent idiopathic scoliosis: Incidence and risk factors. J Pediatr Orthop 2002;22:80-83.
10. Elliott KG, Johnstone AJ: Diagnosing acute compartment syndrome. J Bone Joint Surg Br 2003;85:625-632.
11. Large TM, Frick SL: Compartment syndrome of the leg after treatment of a femoral fracture with an early sitting spica cast. A report of two cases. J Bone Joint Surg Am 2003;85:2207-2210.
12. Warren SE: Epidural hematoma from lumbar puncture. Ann Intern Med 1978;89:431.
13. Fernandez M, Carrol C, Baker C: Discitis and vertebral osteomyelitis in children: An 18-year review. Pediatrics 2000;105:1299-1304.

CHAPTER 146

Burns and Other Skin Injuries

Marisa B. Brett-Fleegler

Injuries to skin and adjacent deeper tissues often require the expertise of surgeons, usually with specific training in plastics. However, hospitalists are often involved in the initial evaluation, stabilization, and management of these children when they present to the hospital or require admission. Three major types of injuries are the focus of this chapter: thermal and chemical burns, electrical injuries, and intravenous infiltrates.

THERMAL BURNS

Burns cause significant morbidity and mortality in the pediatric population. An estimated 440,000 pediatric burns occur annually, resulting in more than 20,000 hospitalizations and 1000 deaths.[1] Burns are most common among infants and toddlers, with scald injuries predominating in this age group.[2] Approximately 78% of these burns are accidental injuries caused by the child, 20% are accidental injuries caused by another person, and 2% to 3% are acts of abuse.[3] Burns due to thermal causes (flame, contact, scald, or steam) require similar but distinct management from chemical or electrical burns (discussed later). Careful attention must be paid to both the acute and chronic phases of burn care, because many injuries require long-term rehabilitation and an interdisciplinary approach to minimize their functional, cosmetic, and emotional impact.

Pathophysiology

Following a thermal injury, the body responds locally and systemically. Locally, there are three zones of injury. The zone of coagulation necrosis is an eschar, with irreversible surface tissue injury from the direct heat insult. The zone of stasis is an area of reversible, salvageable cell injury due to a microvascular reaction in the dermis associated with vasoconstriction and thrombosis. Cell damage is not complete, but inflammatory mediators and injured microcirculation put viable tissue at risk. Beyond this is the zone of hyperemia, which lacks direct cell injury but exhibits vasodilation secondary to the surrounding inflammatory cascade. Full recovery in this zone is expected in the absence of additional insults. Systemically, the loss of an effective skin barrier leads to fluid losses, decreased resistance to infection, and the release of vasoactive mediators, affecting hemodynamic status and creating a hypermetabolic state.

Bacterial colonization of burned tissue can cause focal and systemic infection. Vulnerability to infection ensues not only because of disruption of the protective epidermal layer but also because burns are relatively ischemic; thus, defensive elements of the innate immune system, as well as systemic antibiotics, are unable to penetrate burned tissue.

Clinical Presentation

The diagnosis of a thermal injury is usually evident from the history and is obvious on presentation, although the relevant history may be lacking owing to caregiver absence or subterfuge. Thermal injuries are typically divided into first-, second-, and third-degree burns.

First-degree burns are superficial burns involving only the epidermis (Fig. 146-1). They are associated with erythema, mild edema, dryness, and pain; no blistering is seen. Pain typically resolves in 2 to 3 days, and wounds heal in 3 to 6 days. Sunburns are common first-degree burns.

Second-degree burns are partial-thickness burns extending into the dermis, often caused by hot liquids. Superficial second-degree burns involve the epidermis and superficial dermis. Blisters are typically present; the wounds are erythematous, edematous, moist, and extremely painful due to exposed nerve endings. These burns heal in 2 to 3 weeks because the dermal appendages that regenerate epithelial cells are preserved. Deep second-degree burns penetrate deep into the dermal layer. Blisters with weeping exudates are usually present; the wounds are dark red or yellow-white, with a slightly moist surface. These burns are less painful because fewer viable nerve endings are present. They generally require more than 3 weeks to heal and are at risk for hypertrophic scar formation.

Third-degree burns penetrate through the dermis into the subcutaneous fat. They are insensate because cutaneous nerves are destroyed, although there is pain in the surrounding second-degree burns. They appear dry, leathery, and charred and are pearly white or parchment-like; superficial vessel thrombosis may be visible. These burns are often caused by flame or grease. Resurfacing and grafting are required for closure.

Fourth-degree burns refer to burns that extend to underlying muscle or bone.

Differential Diagnosis

As with any injury in a child, vigilance for signs of abuse or neglect is paramount. These include an inconsistent mechanism of injury, variation in historical details, delayed presentation, medical care sought by someone other than the caretaker involved in the incident, or a classic injury pattern. A classic intentional scald injury pattern is buttock injury accompanied by perineal and foot injury that spares the flexion creases, suggestive of defensive posturing. Other intentional injury patterns include scald burns in a stocking or glove distribution and deep local contact burns, such as from a cigarette.

Certain skin conditions such as Stevens-Johnson syndrome or toxic epidermal necrolysis and staphylococcal

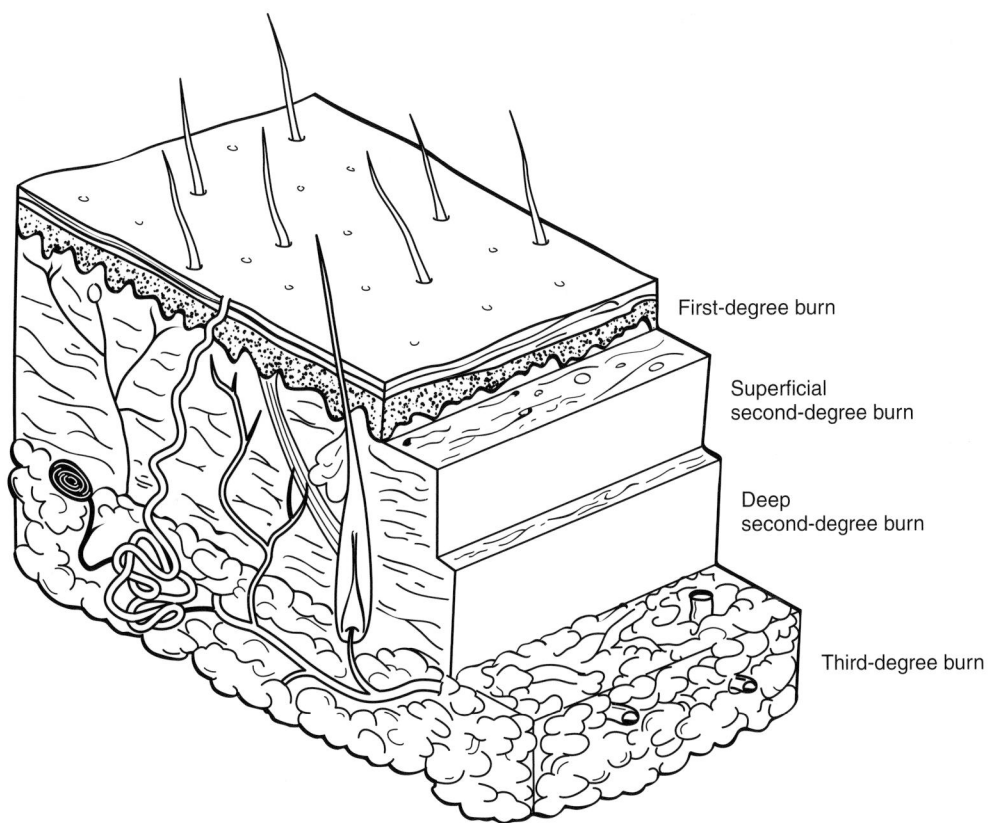

First-degree burn

Superficial
second-degree burn

Deep
second-degree burn

Third-degree burn

Figure 146-1 Depth of burn injury in relation to skin level. First–degree burns involve the epidermis, second–degree burns involve the epidermis and dermis, and third–degree burns penetrate to the subcutaneous tissue. (From Garner WL: Thermal burns. In Achauer BM, Eriksson E [eds]: Plastic Surgery: Indications, Operations, and Outcomes. St Louis, Mosby, 2000, p 361.)

scalded skin syndrome may mimic a diffuse burn injury but should be readily distinguished by the history and overall clinical picture.

Evaluation and Treatment
Initial Stabilization and Management

As with any seriously injured patient, the first management priorities are airway, breathing, and circulation. Careful airway assessment is critical in burn victims because progressive airway involvement may develop. The risk of inhalation injury, with associated airway edema and compromise, is high in victims of an indoor or chemical fire or a hot liquid ingestion. Clinical clues to airway injury include facial burns, hoarseness, stridor, carbonaceous sputum or deposits in the nares, singed eyebrows or facial hair, and shortness of breath. In the case of airway injury, early intubation is preferred because of the likelihood of evolving edema. Intubation may also be required in patients with burns covering a large body surface area because of the associated systemic effects, including pulmonary edema. Consider the possibility of carbon monoxide poisoning, especially in a patient with impaired thinking, syncope, or coma that is otherwise unexplained or if there is a strong exposure history (e.g., kerosene or gas stove, automobile exhaust). Supportive management may include early placement of multiple intravenous lines, which can be inserted through burned tissue if no other sites are available; labora-

tory evaluation; an arterial line; a Foley catheter; and a nasogastric tube.

Initial burn management includes removal of clothing and jewelry to avoid ischemia secondary to swelling and heat conduction. For large burned areas, a clean sheet may be placed to reduce contamination and pain during the initial stabilization. Cold water can be applied to small burn injuries to prevent the spread of heat and decrease pain. Do not use ice, which can cause direct skin injury. Application of cooling measures to large burns should be avoided because of the risk of hypothermia. Treatment rooms should be kept warm to reduce heat loss, especially for small children.

After airway, breathing, and circulation have been stabilized, identification of the burn type and total surface area involved is imperative for appropriate management and disposition. For burn surface area assessment, the "rule of 9s" is typically used in adults and children older than 15 years: each arm represents 9% of the body surface area; the head and neck combined are 9%; 18% each is allocated to the anterior torso, posterior torso, and each leg; and the perineum represents 1%. In younger children, however, this is inaccurate because they have relatively larger heads and a different body size distribution. A pediatric variation allocates 18% for the head and neck, 15% for each lower extremity, 10% for each upper extremity, and 16% each for the anterior and posterior torso. For a rapid estimation, a child's hand (palm plus digits) represents approximately 1% of the

BURN ESTIMATE CHART AND DIAGRAM
Age vs. Area

Area	Birth–1yr	1–4 yr	5–9 yr	10–14 yr	15 yr	Adult	2°	3°	Total	Donor areas
Head	19	17	13	11	9	7				
Neck	2	2	2	2	2	2				
Ant. trunk	13	13	13	13	13	13				
Post. trunk	13	13	13	13	13	13				
R buttock	$2\frac{1}{2}$	$2\frac{1}{2}$	$2\frac{1}{2}$	$2\frac{1}{2}$	$2\frac{1}{2}$	$2\frac{1}{2}$				
L buttock	$2\frac{1}{2}$	$2\frac{1}{2}$	$2\frac{1}{2}$	$2\frac{1}{2}$	$2\frac{1}{2}$	$2\frac{1}{2}$				
Genitals	1	1	1	1	1	1				
R U arm	4	4	4	4	4	4				
L U arm	4	4	4	4	4	4				
R L arm	3	3	3	3	3	3				
L L arm	3	3	3	3	3	3				
R hand	$2\frac{1}{2}$	$2\frac{1}{2}$	$2\frac{1}{2}$	$2\frac{1}{2}$	$2\frac{1}{2}$	$2\frac{1}{2}$				
L hand	$2\frac{1}{2}$	$2\frac{1}{2}$	$2\frac{1}{2}$	$2\frac{1}{2}$	$2\frac{1}{2}$	$2\frac{1}{2}$				
R thigh	$5\frac{1}{2}$	$6\frac{1}{2}$	8	$8\frac{1}{2}$	9	$9\frac{1}{2}$				
L thigh	$5\frac{1}{2}$	$6\frac{1}{2}$	8	$8\frac{1}{2}$	9	$9\frac{1}{2}$				
R leg	5	5	$5\frac{1}{2}$	6	$6\frac{1}{2}$	7				
L leg	5	5	$5\frac{1}{2}$	6	$6\frac{1}{2}$	7				
R foot	$3\frac{1}{2}$	$3\frac{1}{2}$	$3\frac{1}{2}$	$3\frac{1}{2}$	$3\frac{1}{2}$	$3\frac{1}{2}$				
L foot	$3\frac{1}{2}$	$3\frac{1}{2}$	$3\frac{1}{2}$	$3\frac{1}{2}$	$3\frac{1}{2}$	$3\frac{1}{2}$				
						Total				

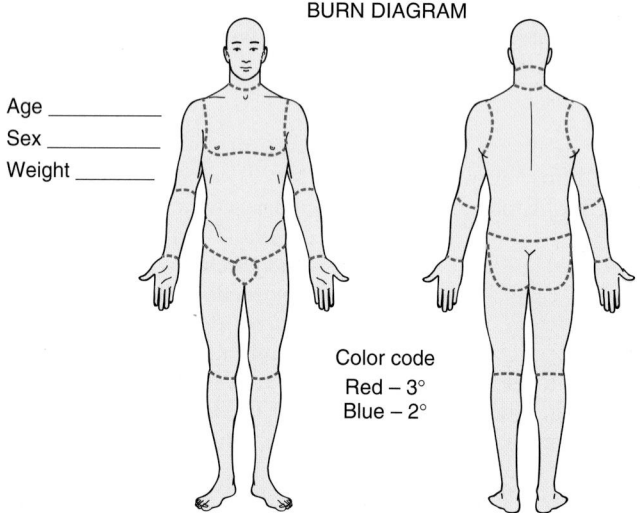

BURN DIAGRAM

Age _____
Sex _____
Weight _____

Color code
Red – 3°
Blue – 2°

Figure 146-2   Lund and Browder burn estimate diagram, as modified by the U.S. Army Institute of Surgical Research. (From Yowler CJ, Fratianne RB: Current status of burn resuscitation. Clin Plast Surg 2000;27:1–10.)

body surface area. For more precise estimates, charts that estimate burn area based on age can be used (Fig. 146-2). First-degree burns are not included in surface area calculations for purposes of fluid resuscitation.

Determine whether any vulnerable areas are involved, specifically the face, hands, feet, genitalia, perineum, and major joints, and evaluate for corneal injury in patients with facial burns. Be vigilant for circumferential burns that may compromise circulation or respiration. In such cases, early escharotomy may be indicated. Chest wall escharotomy incisions are made along the anterior axillary lines, along the costal margins, and across the top of the chest. Extremity incisions should cross the joints because they are particularly vulnerable to constriction owing to the lack of subcutaneous tissue. Consider measuring compartment pressures to assess for compartment syndrome. Pressures in excess of 25 mm Hg suggest the need for escharotomy or compartment decompression. Elevated pressures sufficient to cause muscle necrosis can exist in the presence of palpable pulses.

Patients with burns involving large body surface areas have extensive fluid requirements, and early and aggressive fluid resuscitation is critical. In the first 24 hours, there are large fluid shifts owing to third-spacing of intravascular volume into injured tissue and injury-related histamine release. There is some controversy regarding the use of crystalloid versus colloid, but most providers begin with the former. There are many formulas for calculating these fluid requirements. The Parkland formula calculates estimated fluid requirements in the first 24 hours:

$$4 \text{ mL} \times \text{Body weight (in kg)} \times \text{Total burn surface area} =$$
$$\text{Total fluid replacement in first 24 hours}$$

The first half of the total fluid replacement is given over the first 8 hours, and the second half is given over the next 16 hours.

Most clinicians add maintenance fluids for children younger than 5 years.[4] The goal is a urine output of at least 1 mL/kg per hour; placement of a transurethral bladder (Foley) catheter provides more accurate and continuous measurements.

Do not neglect a complete secondary survey for nonburn-related injuries, particularly if the history involves trauma (e.g., blast injury).

Pain control should be initiated promptly, typically with intravenous narcotics. Tetanus status should be assessed and addressed, and tetanus immunoglobulin should be considered in patients with incomplete or unknown immunization status and large contaminated wounds.

Ongoing Care

After early stabilization and initial management, continuing needs are addressed. Burn patients experience a hyperdynamic state with increased metabolic demands. Calorie requirements are based on burn surface area. Enteral feedings are generally delayed for the first 72 hours owing to gastroparesis and ileus, which are common in severely burned patients.

Ongoing pain management is essential. All but the most minor wounds typically require narcotics for pain control, especially for débridement and dressing changes. Common choices are oral acetaminophen with codeine or oxycodone, and oral or intravenous morphine sulfate. Anxiolytics may also be helpful.

Wound care varies by the depth of the burn injury. For areas of first-degree burns, the skin is kept moist after cleansing. Coverage is optional but may be helpful in reducing friction.

Second-degree burns require cleaning, débriding, and dressing. Ruptured blisters should be débrided to allow healing of viable tissue and to remove a potential growth medium for bacteria. The management of intact blisters is controversial. Some experts recommend leaving them intact as a biologic dressing that provides a moist and sterile environment; others believe that the presence of inflammatory mediators in the blister fluid can increase ischemia. Most providers leave small second-degree burn blisters intact. Larger blisters may not be an effective barrier to bacterial invasion.

After débridement, the mainstay of management for superficial partial-thickness burns is a dressing designed to prevent wound infection and desiccation. This dressing typically consists of a sterile ointment and nonadherent dressing. For minor wounds, bacitracin and silver sulfadiazine (Silvadene) are most commonly used, but some centers

reserve silver sulfadiazine for larger wounds. Avoid this agent in patients with sulfa allergy or glucose-6-phosphate dehydrogenase deficiency and in pregnant women and infants owing to the risk of kernicterus. The primary adverse effect of silver sulfadiazine is leukopenia, which typically resolves with discontinuation of use. Silver nitrate is used in sulfa-allergic patients; it must be kept wet to prevent wound desiccation and has the disadvantage of producing dark discoloration. On the face, consider the use of ophthalmic bacitracin ointment.

In second-degree burns with viable tissue, the use of a skin substitute or occlusive hydrocolloid dressing is an alternative to topical antibiotics and wound dressings. Skin substitutes such as Biobrane (Bertek Pharmaceuticals) and Transcyte (Smith & Nephew) are bilayer materials that mimic the properties of the epidermal and dermal layers and facilitate pain control. The synthetic layer provides protection from mechanical insult and creates a moist environment, and the inner biological layer guides re-epithelialization. It is important to recognize that these dressings do not provide antibiotic coverage and can trap bacteria within a wound. Thus, they should be used only in clean wounds with viable tissue present to promote adherence, and the wound should be examined daily for any purulent drainage. The dressings adhere to the wound within 72 hours and are removed in 7 to 14 days, at which time epithelialization is complete and the dressing has become nonadherent.

Deep second-degree burns similarly require débridement and dressing with topical antibiotics. Because they are at higher risk for infection, scarring, and contractures, these burns should be managed in consultation with a specialist. Early excision and grafting may be indicated. Skin substitutes are not used because of the lack of viable tissue.

Third-degree burns are débrided and treated with a topical antibiotic (e.g., mafenide acetate) that is capable of penetrating eschar. Note that mafenide acetate is painful on application to viable tissue. Full healing is not expected, and the risk of scarring and contractures is high. Surgical excision and grafting are required and may be performed in the first 24 to 48 hours if hemodynamic stability permits. If tissue viability is uncertain, a several-week period of observation may be required.

Dressing changes and wound checks should be performed daily to look for signs of infection. Assessment may be difficult because of the inflammatory changes seen with a healing burn. Burn wound infections are characterized by marked or painful erythema, lymphangitis, focal areas of discoloration within the eschar, discoloration or edema of unburned skin at the wound margin, conversion of partial-thickness wounds to full-thickness wounds, or accelerated separation of eschar. Infections are rare in properly treated partial-thickness burns. In extensive or deep burns, prevention of colonization is generally not achievable. The goal of topical antibiotics is to decrease bacterial colonization and prevent frank infection of the wound, bacteremia, and sepsis.

Most centers reserve systemic antibiotics for systemic spread of infection rather than for prophylactic use. If antibiotics are used, consideration should be given to the common organisms found in burn wounds, including *Streptococcus pyogenes*, *Staphylococcus aureus*, gram-negative organisms (e.g., *Pseudomonas* species), and *Candida* species. Burn wound infection presents a high risk for systemic bacteremia and sepsis and may warrant surgical excision of the infected tissue.

Any substantial burn carries a risk of hypertrophic scar formation and contractures, with resultant functional impairment and disfigurement. Burns involving joints, cosmetically significant areas, and growth regions are managed with a combination of compression and splinting, physical therapy, and surgical skin grafting, tissue expansion, and transposition. Psychological support should be provided early and on an ongoing basis.

Consultation

In general, early consultation with a surgeon is indicated for any significant burn. Depending on community resources, this might be a general, plastic, or burn surgeon. Patients with burns that meet burn center referral criteria who are not transferred require subspecialty consultation. This is especially important for any burns that are potentially disfiguring or have significant functional implications. If time permits, consultation should be sought if escharotomy or compartment decompression is required. Early consultation is also necessary in cases in which excision and grafting may be required; in large or deep wounds, surgery may be indicated as early as 24 hours after injury to decrease the infection risk, facilitate wound care, and decrease metabolic needs.

Admission Criteria

Regional burn centers have evolved in most areas because of the labor-intensive and highly specialized nature of caring for patients with significant burn injuries. Criteria for referral to a specialized burn center, based on American Burn Association recommendations, are listed in Box 146-1. Depending on resource availability, patients meeting these criteria should be transferred to a regional burn center for hospitalization. Additional reasons for hospitalization in patients who do not necessarily require burn center management include the following:

- Full-thickness burns on up to 5% of total body surface area.
- Adequate wound care, including return for follow-up visits, cannot be assured.
- Unsafe home environment.

Discharge Criteria

- Able to take adequate nutrition and fluids by mouth.
- Risk of wound infection is substantially diminished.
- Appropriate wound coverage is in place.
- All wounds of questionable viability have been demarcated.
- Outpatient dressing changes can be accommodated by a combination of caregiver, visiting nurse, and clinic visits.
- A safe home environment is available.
- Ongoing follow-up for both immediate and long-term issues is assured.

Outpatient care instructions should address acute wound care management and safety education. Instructions for

---

Box 146–1 Criteria for Treatment at a Specialized Burn Facility

Second- and third-degree burns over more than 10% body surface area in patients younger than 10 years.
Second- and third-degree burns over more than 20% body surface area in patients of any age.
Second- and third-degree burns posing a serious functional or cosmetic threat to the face, hands, feet, genitalia, perineum, or major joints.
Third-degree burns over more than 5% body surface area in any age group.
Electrical burns, including lightning injury.
Chemical burns posing a serious functional or cosmetic threat.
Concomitant inhalation injury.
Preexisting medical problems that could complicate burn management.
Associated trauma, when the burn injury poses the greater risk.
Injuries that will require long-term rehabilitative support.
Inadequate hospital facilities to provide burn care.

Based on American Burn Association: Hospital and prehospital resources for optimal care of patients with burn injury: Guidelines for development and operation of burn centers. J Burn Care Rehabil 1988;11:98-104.

---

long-term care should include the use of moisturizer and sun block, as well as long-term follow-up.

Prevention

Given the devastating injuries that can result from burns, prevention is key. When an unsafe home environment is suspected, investigation for abuse, neglect, poverty, poor living conditions, and stress should be pursued. Family support and social services intervention should be provided as needed. Anticipatory guidance with regard to home safety should be part of routine health maintenance visits and should be reexplored and reemphasized for any patient with a burn injury.

Water temperature management is key to scald injury prevention. At 130°F, full-thickness burns occur in 30 seconds; at 120°F, full-thickness burns require 10 minutes of contact.[5] The American Academy of Pediatrics recommends that water heaters be set at a maximum of 120°F.[6]

CHEMICAL BURNS

Chemical burns result from exposure to household or industrial products that are categorized as acids, alkalis, and other agents. Injury is usually due to direct chemical injury, but there may also be heat-related injury due to exothermic reactions. Chemical type, concentration, and quantity and the duration, size, and location of contact all influence the severity of a chemical burn. The potential for systemic absorption and toxicity must also be considered with any chemical exposure, especially hydrocarbons or chemicals associated with industrial use. Consider consulting a local poison control center in cases of chemical injury.

The mainstay of therapy for all chemical exposures is rapid and copious irrigation. A litmus paper test documenting a return to normal pH may help guide the duration of irrigation. Neutralization agents are generally not recommended because they may result in exothermic reactions and thermal injury. In cases of ingestion, emetics are not recommended owing to the risk of esophageal injury or aspiration.

Acids are found in household toilet and drain cleaners, as well as in common industrial chemicals. Acids cause coagulation necrosis, thereby avoiding the deeper injury seen with alkali agents. Ingestion causes esophageal injury, and concentration at the pyloric valve may lead to pyloric strictures. Worthy of specific mention is the highly toxic hydrofluoric acid. It causes severe, ongoing injury and systemic hypocalcemia due to ion trapping in cases of extensive tissue involvement. After irrigation, topical calcium gel should be applied to the affected area, and the patient should be monitored and treated as needed for systemic hypocalcemia.

Alkalis such as lye (sodium hydroxide) are found in many household cleaners and detergents, hair relaxants, bleach, cement, and fertilizer. A deeply penetrating liquefaction necrosis causes extensive tissue injury. Irrigation is recommended for extended periods until there is resolution of the soapy feeling representing saponification of fat and oils. In cases of ingestion, severe esophageal injury and perforation may occur, and there is a long-term risk of stricture formation. Early gastroenterology and pulmonary consultation for esophagoscopy and bronchoscopy, respectively, is indicated.

ELECTRICAL INJURY

Electricity traveling through the body meets resistance and generates thermal energy, causing tissue damage. Voltage drop and current flow are related to the cross-sectional area; thus, extremities with small cross-sectional areas are more vulnerable to injury.

Low-voltage injuries (i.e., <1000 volts) are typically from household current. With these injuries, the severe tissue burn limits further flow and minimizes further damage. If contact is sustained, local injury can be substantial. A common electrical injury is the oral commissural injury sustained by a child chewing on an electrical cord. Although this is often managed conservatively with splinting, subspecialty consultation is indicated, because surgical reconstruction is sometimes required. Families should be advised about the possibility of a delayed labial artery bleed occurring before or with eschar separation at 2 to 4 weeks after injury. Systemic consequences are rare with low-voltage injuries, and in many cases, admission is not required if local wound care can be managed at home.[7]

High-voltage injures are those involving electrical currents of 1000 volts or greater, but they also include injuries sustained from contact with high-tension wires (10,000 to 1 million volts). In these injuries, there is no reduction of flow, and a small cutaneous burn may belie significant internal injury. Patients are at risk for cardiac arrhythmia, particularly ventricular fibrillation or asystole, and cardiac monitoring is recommended for 48 hours. Patients are often thrown by the current, so assessment for associated trauma is required. As with other burn injuries, adequate fluid resuscitation is essential; however, because the surface injury may be small, burn surface area calculations are inadequate. Fluid resuscitation should be titrated to a urine output of 1 to 1.5 mL/kg.

Because bone has a high resistance to electrical energy, deeper muscles may sustain greater injury than superficial muscles, and a high index of suspicion must be maintained for necrotic deep tissue. Muscle injury creates a risk for compartment syndrome, which may manifest as tense swelling and decreasing perfusion, with associated pain, pallor, paresthesias, or pulselessness. In these cases, immediate fasciotomy is required. Depending on the nature of the injury and the amount of energy involved, urinalysis, electrocardiogram monitoring, and creatine kinase levels may be considered. Damaged muscle may result in myoglobinuria, with resultant renal injury, especially if fluid resuscitation is inadequate. Alkalization and forced diuresis are indicated and can usually prevent this complication. Muscle injury can also lead to hyperkalemia.

As in third-degree burns, mafenide acetate is often used in electrical burns because of its deeper tissue penetration. Close follow-up is required for all victims of significant electrical injury; late sequelae include neurologic problems such as neuropathy, depression, memory loss, and ophthalmic dysfunction due to cataracts.

INTRAVENOUS INFILTRATES

Infiltration of intravenous fluids or medications is a common complication of peripheral venous catheters; it is estimated to occur in 23% to 78% of patients with such devices.[8] Children's tendency to be mobile leads to a high risk of intravenous line malfunction. Such malfunction may be difficult to detect in children owing to their decreased ability to communicate pain, as well as their flexible subcutaneous tissue, which can distend without increasing infusion pressures and thereby alerting providers to the line malfunction.

A vesicant is a solution capable of causing tissue injury or destruction. Strictly speaking, infiltration is the inadvertent delivery of a nonvesicant solution, such as normal saline, into the subcutaneous tissue. Extravasation is the delivery of a vesicant to this layer. Here, we use the term *infiltration* to refer to both these processes.

Pathophysiology

Infiltration occurs when a catheter dislodges or punctures a vein. Multiple mechanisms of injury have been proposed. Irritation from infusate may lead to vasoconstriction and decreased blood flow, creating an ongoing cycle of less dilution of infusate, increased pressure, and subsequent vessel rupture or exit of fluid from the catheter insertion hole. Alternatively, infiltration of infusate through the catheter insertion hole may occur when the flow becomes obstructed. Additionally, endothelial irritation can damage the vessel intima and allow diffusion of infusate into tissue.

Infusate osmolality, pH, and chemical properties play a role in the vascular injury that predisposes to infiltration, and they can mediate tissue injury after infiltration has occurred. Injury also occurs via ischemia and compression. Certain compounds are especially irritating, including electrolyte solutions (notably calcium, high concentrations of dextrose, and parenteral nutrition), antimicrobials (particularly oxacillin and amphotericin B), contrast media, antineoplastic agents, and pressor agents. Vasoactive medications cause intense vasoconstriction, which can lead to ischemia and necrosis.

Direct tissue damage can result in ulceration and tissue necrosis. Increased compartment pressures can lead to arteriolar compression, vascular spasm, pain, and muscle necrosis. Muscular changes can occur in 4 to 12 hours, and ischemic nerve damage can result in functional loss of an extremity within 24 hours. Finally, long-term complications such as reflex sympathetic dystrophy can develop.

Clinical Presentation and Evaluation

The hallmark of infiltration is edema, but mild edema may be difficult to detect. Comparison to the opposite side— either visually or by measurement—is the most reliable method of assessment. Other markers include induration, tenderness or pain, blanching or discoloration, blistering, temperature change, and decreased range of motion and sensation. Digital pressure at the tip of an intravenous catheter should occlude flow; if solution continues to infuse even with this pressure, the intravenous line is probably infiltrated. The catheter should be assessed for blood return; however, the presence of blood return does not always rule out infiltration, nor does the absence of blood return rule it in, especially in infants.

A small-volume infiltrate may be difficult to defect, but significant damage can occur if a vesicant is involved. With infusion of such an agent, frequent reassessment is needed, and a conservative approach is warranted, including the early removal of any line suspected of being infiltrated. Assessing the severity of injury may be difficult because cutaneous damage may not reflect evolving subcutaneous fat and fascial damage. Edema may resolve or progress to blistering or necrosis.

Differential Diagnosis

Infiltrated intravenous lines should be differentiated from other intravenous line complications such as phlebitis, restrictive taping, venous stasis, and infection.

Treatment

The first step in management is to stop the infusion and attempt to aspirate any remaining drug. Leave the catheter in place if an antidote is indicated; otherwise, remove the line, because the site can no longer be used. Supportive care, including elevation and ice packs, is the mainstay of therapy for most infiltrates; many resolve spontaneously. Although there is some controversy, ice applied for 20 minutes, four times a day, for 24 to 48 hours is often recommended. Warm compresses may be indicated for certain chemotherapy drugs, such as the vinca alkaloids. Close and frequent reassessment is needed.

If an antidote is indicated, inject it through the line if the remaining infusate was aspirated; otherwise, avoid using the line, because that will simply infiltrate the remaining medication. An antidote for dopamine and other pressor agents is phentolamine, an adrenergic blocker. It is used to reverse peripheral ischemia in an attempt to avoid tissue necrosis. Phentolamine is given at a dose of 0.1 to 0.2 mg/kg (to an adult maximum of 5 mg) diluted in 10 mL of normal saline; it is injected through the infiltrate catheter and subcutaneously around the entire area of infiltration with a 25-gauge

needle as soon as the infiltration is detected, or within 12 hours at the latest.[9] For other significant infiltrates, especially when compression is an issue, hyaluronidase may be indicated. It breaks down connective tissue around the area of infiltration, allowing medication reabsorption and decreasing fluid pressures. Hyaluronidase (which is now commercially available again, after being discontinued by its original manufacturer) is administered subcutaneously and intradermally into the infiltration site. It is diluted to a concentration of 15 units/mL; a single 15-unit dose (1 mL) is then divided into five 0.2-mL doses.[9] Other specific antidotes may be indicated for antineoplastic agents.

Consultation

Any vesicant infiltration, particularly one that requires an antidote, necessitates an urgent surgical consultation. Early intervention with wound débridement can minimize the impact of severe infiltrations.

Prevention

Use the smallest catheter possible to avoid restriction of blood flow in the vein. Avoid the administration of vesicants at any site more than 24 hours old or sites that are difficult to immobilize. Vesicants should be administered through central venous access devices whenever feasible.

IN A NUTSHELL

- Initial burn management involves methodical assessment, airway management, fluid resuscitation, and pain control.
- Ongoing burn therapy includes wound débridement, topical antimicrobials, and close observation to detect complications.
- Prompt surgical consultation is indicated for any large surface area burn or any burn with functional or cosmetic significance.
- For infiltration, supportive care is the mainstay of treatment.
- Use vesicants with caution if there is any question about the patency or adequacy of the intravenous access.

ON THE HORIZON

- Allografts and xenografts are currently used for extensive deep second- and third-degree burns. Advances in tissue engineering technology are ongoing, with the development of new products such as bilayer skin substitutes and skin components. These may obviate the need for large donor grafts for the management of burns involving large surface areas.

SUGGESTED READING

American Burn Association: Hospital and prehospital resources for optimal care of patients with burn injury: Guidelines for development and operation of burn centers. J Burn Care Rehabil 1988;11:98-104.

American Burn Association Advanced Burn Life Support Course—Burn resuscitation including children. *http://www.ameriburn.org/ABLSCourse Descriptions.htm.*

Barone CM, Yule GJ: Pediatric thermal injuries. In Bentz ML (ed): Pediatric Plastic Surgery. Stamford, Conn, Appleton & Lange, 1998, pp 595-618.

Drago DA: Kitchen scalds and thermal burns in children five years and younger. Pediatrics 2005;115:10-16.

Finkelstein JL, Schwartz SB, Madden MR, et al: Pediatric burns: An overview. Pediatr Clin North Am 1992;39:1145-1163.

Hadaway LC: Preventing and managing peripheral extravasation. Nursing 2004;34:66-67.

Sheridan RL: Comprehensive treatment of burns. Curr Probl Surg 2001;38: 657-756.

Smith ML: Pediatric burns: Management of thermal, electrical, and chemical burns and burn-like dermatologic conditions. Pediatr Ann 2000;29:367-378.

Weinstein SM: Plumer's Principles and Practice of Intravenous Therapy. Philadelphia, Lippincott Williams & Wilkins, 2001.

Wynsma LA: Negative outcomes of intravascular therapy in infants and children. AACN Clin Issues 1998;9:49-63.

Zubair M, Besner GE: Pediatric electrical burns: Management strategies. Burns 1997;23:413-420.

REFERENCES

1. McLoughlin E, McGuire A: The causes, cost, and prevention of childhood burn injuries. Am J Dis Child 1990;144:677-683.

2. Drago DA: Kitchen scalds and thermal burns in children five years and younger. Pediatrics 2005;115:10-16.

3. Caravajal HF: Burns in children and adolescents: Initial management as the first step in successful rehabilitation. Pediatrician 1990;17:237-243.

4. Finkelstein JL, Schwartz SB, Madden MR, et al: Pediatric burns: An overview. Pediatr Clin North Am 1992;39:1145-1163.

5. Barone CM, Yule GJ: Pediatric thermal injuries. In Bentz ML (ed): Pediatric Plastic Surgery. Stamford, Conn, Appleton & Lange, 1998, pp 595-618.

6. Office-based counseling for injury prevention. American Academy of Pediatrics Committee on Injury and Poison Prevention. Pediatrics 1994; 94:566-567.

7. Zubair M, Besner GE: Pediatric electrical burns: Management strategies. Burns 1997;23:413-420.

8. Pettit J: Assessment of the infant with a peripheral intravenous device. Adv Neonatal Care 2003;3:230-240.

9. Lexi-Comp: Pediatric Lexi-Drugs Online. www.lexi.com.

CHAPTER 147

Pneumothorax and Pneumomediastinum

Joshua Nagler

Pneumothorax and pneumomediastinum are examples of air leak syndromes in which air accumulates in the spaces outside the lung airways and alveoli. Pneumothorax refers to the abnormal presence of air in the pleural space, whereas pneumomediastinum describes accumulation of air in the mediastinum. Air leak can be traumatic, iatrogenic, or spontaneous. Primary air leak occurs in children without clinically apparent lung disease, and secondary pneumomediastinum and pneumothorax refer to those with known underlying pulmonary disease (e.g., asthma, cystic fibrosis) or positive-pressure ventilation.

The exact prevalence and incidence of air leak syndromes in children are hard to determine. The adult literature suggests that primary spontaneous pneumothorax (PSP) occurs in more than 20,000 patients per year, with a slightly higher incidence in men than in women and increased risk in those with a tall, thin body habitus.[1] Similar data are lacking in children; however, studies have shown that secondary pneumothorax occurs in approximately 5% of hospitalized patients with asthma and 10% to 25% of those with cystic fibrosis.[2] Pneumomediastinum has been reported in 0.3% of asthmatic patients in a children's emergency department setting.[3]

PNEUMOTHORAX

Pathophysiology

Although patients with PSP do not have underlying lung disease, computed tomography (CT) and surgical findings show that the majority have subpleural bullae, which may be ipsilateral or contralateral to the pneumothorax. The cause of such bullae is not fully understood, but they probably represent imbalances in protease and antiprotease enzymes leading to emphysema-like changes. Increased intra-alveolar pressure, often from inflammation of small airways, results in tension on the alveolar wall and, ultimately, rupture leading to pneumothorax.

Clinical Presentation

Patients with PSP typically present with an acute onset of pleuritic chest pain, usually described as sharp initially, becoming dull over time, and frequently resolving after 24 hours, even without treatment. Onset frequently occurs while the patient is at rest. Many patients complain of dyspnea. Ipsilateral shoulder pain and dry cough are also common.

Physical examination findings vary depending on the size of the pneumothorax. Patients with small pneumothoraces (i.e., <15% of the hemithorax) may show only tachycardia or have completely normal findings. In those with larger collections, examination findings include decreased chest wall movement and decreased or absent breath sounds on the affected side. Hyperresonance and decreased fremitus may also be appreciated. More severe cases demonstrate accessory muscle use and increased work of breathing. Heart sounds may be decreased, particularly with anterior pneumothoraces. Tachycardia is common, but when accompanied by hypotension, cyanosis, jugular venous distention, or tracheal deviation, it should immediately raise concern for tension pneumothorax with tamponade physiology.

Differential Diagnosis

Cardiovascular, gastrointestinal, pulmonary/pleural, and chest wall disease all cause chest pain, oftentimes with associated respiratory symptoms. The differential for pleuritic chest pain, however, is more limited and includes pneumonia, idiopathic or viral pleurisy, pulmonary embolism, pericarditis, or costochondritis. Decreased breath sounds may be secondary to pneumonia, severe bronchospasm, pleural effusion, foreign body aspiration, or poor respiratory effort. Anxiety disorder is also on the differential for patients with chest pain, tachycardia, and tachypnea. On radiographs, congenital lobar emphysema, skin folds, and overpenetrated films may be mistaken for pneumothoraces.

Diagnosis/Evaluation

Definitive diagnosis is made by chest radiograph. On posteroanterior or portable chest film, a linear shadow of thin visceral pleura is seen, along with absence of lung markings beyond the pleural line (Fig. 147-1). Expiratory films may facilitate the diagnosis of a small apical pneumothorax, but the increased yield is insignificant in most cases and therefore not routinely required.[4] Chest radiographs allow determination of pneumothorax size and may also show the presence or absence of underlying lung disease. In adults, validated formulas can be used to determine the size of pneumothoraces, but they have not been shown to be accurate in children.[5,6] Therefore, pneumothorax sizing in pediatrics is often based on visual approximation.

The role of CT in pediatric patients with pneumothoraces is not well defined. These scans are often able to show underlying blebs and bullae much more accurately than possible with chest radiography. There is some evidence in adults that the presence of blebs greater than 2 cm places a patient at increased risk for recurrence; however, this has not been well studied in children. In addition, scans performed with chest tubes in place or shortly after their removal may show artifact and need to be interpreted cautiously. Many advocate a

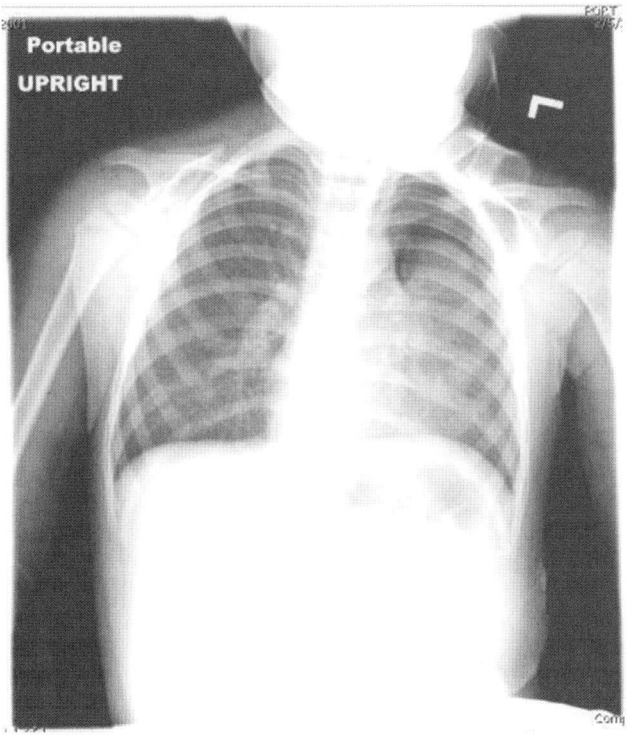

Figure 147-1 Simple pneumothorax. Note the lack of pleural markings in the left apex.

6- to 8-week delay before performing CT in these patients.[5] Further study is needed before more definitive recommendations can be made, especially in children.

Laboratory tests do not aid in the diagnosis or management of PSP. In cases in which clinical circumstances dictate the need for arterial blood gas analysis, an increased alveolar-arterial gradient proportional to the size of the pneumothorax is commonly seen. Hypercapnia is rare in patients with normal underlying lung function. Instead, many patients demonstrate respiratory alkalosis secondary to associated tachypnea.

Treatment

Patients presenting with signs or symptoms consistent with tension pneumothorax require immediate needle thoracostomy without waiting for radiographic confirmation. Such patients may include those with pulseless electrical activity without a clear underlying cause. Tube thoracostomy should follow needle decompression in these patients.

Patients with a clinical presentation consistent with pneumothorax without tension physiology should receive supplemental oxygen with continuous cardiorespiratory and oxygen saturation monitoring as the remainder of the evaluation is completed. Figure 147-2 provides an algorithm of the management options.

The two goals of management of pneumothoraces are to reexpand the affected lung and prevent recurrences. A wide

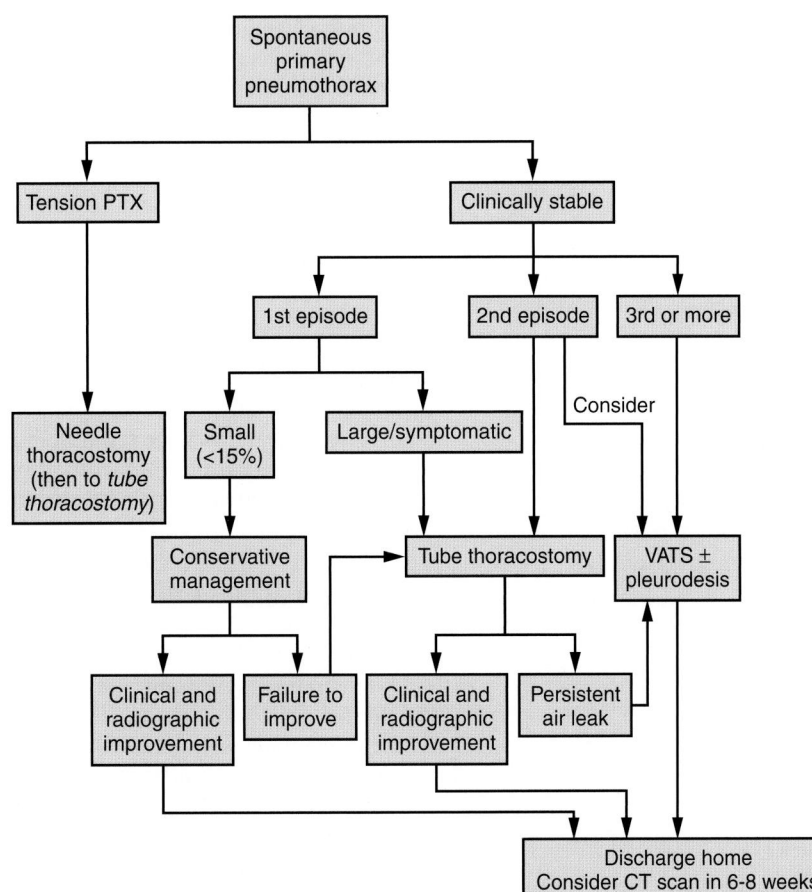

Figure 147-2 Management of pneumothorax. CT, computed tomography; PTX, pneumothorax; VATS, video-assisted thoracoscopic surgery.

variety of therapeutic options exist. In adults, clinical decision making is supported by consensus statements; however, no such guidelines exist in pediatrics.[1] Therefore, management depends on individual practice patterns, available resources, and patient or family preferences.

Observation without intervention is a reasonable approach for first episodes of PSP in otherwise healthy patients with no or minimal symptoms and a small (<15%) pneumothorax by radiograph. Resorption occurs at a rate of approximately 2% per day in patients breathing room air, although it can be increased to nearly 10% per day with supplemental oxygen.[7] Inpatient observation to show clinical and radiographic improvement is recommended.

Patients with more severe symptoms or those with a large (>15%) pneumothorax require active reexpansion of the affected lung. Manual aspiration with a large-bore needle or intravenous catheter is effective in adults, but safety concerns prevent its widespread use in children.[8] Therefore, for larger pneumothoraces, tube thoracostomy is the standard of care. Pigtail (6.5 to 10.5 French) catheters have been shown to be safe and as effective as large-bore surgical thoracostomy tubes (16 to 32 French) for pneumothoraces and are less painful.[9] Low-level wall suction is indicated for patients with underlying lung disease or those who fail to show improvement with a water seal setup alone. Serial chest radiographs should show full reexpansion of the affected lung without a persistent air leak.

Once the affected lung is reexpanded, chest tubes should be clamped and the patient carefully monitored for a minimum of 6 to 8 hours. Patients with reaccumulation of air will probably become symptomatic during this time, although a repeat chest radiograph is recommended before discharge to document improvement.[10]

If tube thoracostomy is not successful in reexpanding the affected lung or the patient has a persistent air leak, surgical repair is indicated. The adult literature shows a benefit of video-assisted thoracoscopic surgery (VATS) over transaxillary minithoracotomy for PSP with the use of numerous outcome variables.[11] VATS has also been demonstrated to be safe and effective in children with pulmonary disease and has therefore become the standard surgical therapy for pediatric PSP.

Consultation

- General surgery: For thoracostomy (chest tube) placement or VATS as indicated
- Interventional radiology: For pigtail catheter placement
- Pulmonology: For patients with secondary pneumothorax or primary pneumothoraces not requiring thoracostomy
- Thoracic surgery: For thoracotomy when clinically indicated

Admission Criteria

Hospitalization is indicated for any of the following reasons:

- Tension pneumothorax
- Hypoxia
- Respiratory distress
- Large (>15% of the hemithorax) primary pneumothorax

- Any secondary pneumothorax (patient with underlying lung disease)

Although adults with small (<15% of the hemithorax) pneumothoraces may be discharged if clinically stable after 3 to 6 hours, pediatric patients are most commonly admitted for overnight observation. Asymptomatic patients with very small air collections are sometimes discharged after a shorter observation period, provided that serial chest radiographs are stable and families have rapid access to medical care.

Discharge Criteria

- Stable or resolving symptoms
- No supplemental oxygen requirement
- For patients being managed without intervention:
  Complete or nearly complete resolution of pneumothorax on serial radiographs
- For patients treated with pigtail or surgical thoracostomy:
  Reexpansion of the affected lung
  No persistent air leak after 6 to 8 hours of observation with the tube clamped
  No recurrence of pneumothorax on chest radiograph 4 to 6 hours after the tube is removed
- For patients with secondary pneumothoraces: Adequate medical/surgical management of the underlying lung disease as well

Prevention

The second goal of treatment of pneumothoraces is prevention of recurrence. Approximately a third of adults with PSP will have a second episode, most commonly within 6 months of the first. Some reports suggest that recurrence rates in children may be twice as high.[12] No currently identified risk factors can reliably identify patients at high risk for recurrence. Even findings of ipsilateral or contralateral blebs on CT have not been shown to predict recurrence in case series.[13] Therefore, no intervention is required to prevent recurrence after first episodes of PSP.

For patients with recurrent disease, however, the efficacy of tube thoracostomy drops off significantly with each subsequent episode.[14] Patients with recurrent disease, large bullae (>2 cm), or both on CT may benefit from surgical therapy. For patients with secondary pneumothoraces, who may be at greater risk for respiratory compromise with even one additional episode of pneumothorax, early, more aggressive interventions to prevent recurrence should also be considered.[13]

PNEUMOMEDIASTINUM

Pathophysiology

Pneumomediastinum most commonly results from rupture of pulmonary alveoli. Although such rupture may occur spontaneously, more commonly a precipitating factor can be identified. Numerous medical and surgical conditions have been shown to lead to pneumomediastinum (Table 147-1). The majority of these conditions result in an increased pressure gradient between the intra-alveolar and interstitial spaces that leads to rupture into the pulmonary interstitium. Air then dissects along the vascular sheaths to

Table 147-1 Conditions Causing Pneumomediastinum and Subcutaneous Emphysema in Children

Airway Obstruction
Bronchial occlusion, foreign body aspiration, space-occupying lesions

Iatrogenic
Adenoidectomy and tonsillectomy, air abrasion device, bronchoscopy, dental procedures, Heimlich maneuver, mechanical ventilation, surgery (abdominal, laparoscopic, thoracic), tracheostomy

Infections
Bacterial and viral pneumonia, laryngitis, *Pneumocystis carinii* pneumonia, retropharyngeal abscess

Obstructive Lung Disease
Asthma, bronchiolitis, bronchiolitis obliterans with organizing pneumonia, cystic fibrosis, lung emphysema

Toxic Effects
Inhaled drug abuse (cocaine, marijuana), paraquat intoxication, toxic gas

Trauma
Barotrauma (diving, flying, nose blowing), oral or blunt cervical trauma, chest trauma, child abuse

Valsalva Maneuvers
Coughing, defecation, postpartum status, vomiting

Weakness of Tissue
Anorexia nervosa, bone marrow transplantation and chemotherapy, dermatomyositis, diabetic hyperpnea, hypersensitivity pneumonitis, lymphangioleiomyomatosis, ulcerative colitis

Idiopathic

From Gesundheit B, Preminger A, Harito B, et al: Pneumomediastinum and subcutaneous emphysema in an 18-month-old child. J Pediatr 2002;141:116-120.

the hilum and mediastinum. In other cases, air from intrathoracic or extrathoracic sources can dissect along fascial planes from the neck, esophagus, or retroperitoneum. Air can also track along these same fascial planes from the mediastinum into subcutaneous tissue in the neck and upper extremities.[15] The most concerning disease progression is rupture of mediastinal air through the adjacent pleura causing an associated pneumothorax.

Clinical Presentation

Most patients with spontaneous pneumomediastinum are asymptomatic. In those with symptoms, chest pain is the most common complaint. The pain is usually pleuritic and retrosternal and often radiates to the back, shoulder, or arms. Some patients will note dyspnea, dysphagia, or neck pain. Occasionally, patients will notice skin changes attributable to subcutaneous emphysema. More commonly, the presenting symptoms are related to the underlying illness (e.g., asthma) and do not result from the air collection in the mediastinal cavity.

On physical examination, precordial crepitus associated with systole, known as the Hamman sign, is pathogno-

monic.[15] Other possible findings include palpable subcutaneous emphysema, neck swelling or torticollis, and in more severe cases, respiratory distress.

Differential Diagnosis

Because patients with pneumomediastinum are generally asymptomatic, the differential focuses on the underlying cause of the air leak, with asthma and esophageal perforation (Boerhaave syndrome) being the most common. See Table 147-1 for a more complete listing. The pericardial friction rub sometimes appreciated with pericarditis can be confused for the Hamman sign.

Diagnosis and Evaluation

Pneumomediastinum may be suspected from the findings on physical examination; however, more often it is found incidentally on a chest radiograph performed to evaluate for chest pain, respiratory complaints, or other clinical concerns. When pneumomediastinum is suspected or confirmed, further review of present and past symptoms should focus on identifying predisposing or triggering factors.

On chest radiograph, pneumomediastinum is seen as a vertical radiolucent line along the left side of the cardiac silhouette (Fig. 147-3). In addition, subcutaneous emphysema can sometimes be seen as streaks or pockets of hypolucency in the soft tissue of the neck, shoulders, and upper extremities (Fig. 147-4). Lateral views may be helpful to document retrosternal air if the diagnosis is in doubt or for other clinical concerns, but they are not otherwise required.[16] Chest radiography may also elucidate an underlying cause, including hyperinflation with asthma or widening of the inferior mediastinum with esophageal perforation. Evaluation for associated pneumothorax is likewise important. Forced expiratory films should be avoided because they may worsen the pneumomediastinum.

Further investigations should be pursued if there is clinical concern or for evaluation of underlying disease, but they are not otherwise required. There are no specific laboratory findings in patients with pneumomediastinum. CT can delineate the anatomic location of the free air, but it is not routinely required. An electrocardiogram may demonstrate a shift in axis and decreased voltage. Concern for foreign body aspiration may be an indication for bronchoscopy or esophagoscopy, or both, whereas pneumomediastinum in the setting of prolonged or violent vomiting requires investigation for Boerhaave syndrome with esophagoscopy or contrast radiography, or both.

Treatment

Unlike air in the pleural space, pneumomediastinum rarely requires intervention. This generally benign condition resolves without sequelae, so conservative management with careful observation is the standard of care. Appropriate analgesia, rest, avoidance of forced expiratory maneuvers (e.g., peak expiratory flow measurement in asthmatics), and careful control of underlying conditions are key to successful resolution.[15] Observation for the development of respiratory compromise or concomitant pneumothorax is recommended, but oftentimes it can be performed at home. Tamponade physiology from mediastinal air has been reported but is exceptionally rare. Time until improvement

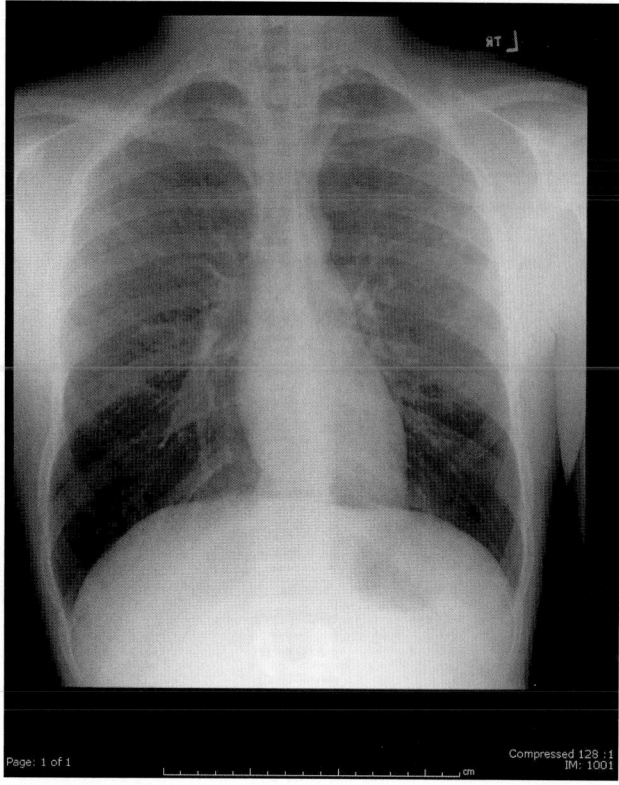 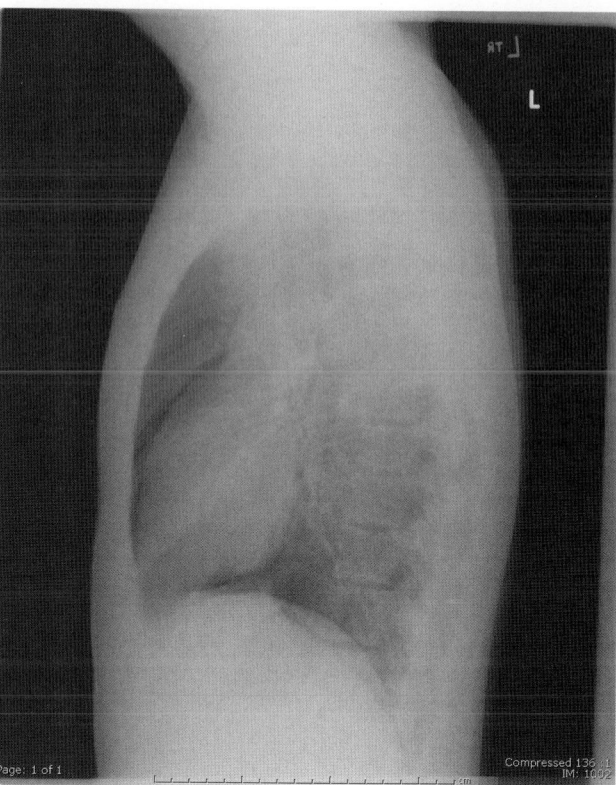

Figure 147-3 Sixteen-year-old patient with an acute exacerbation of asthma. A, On a frontal view of his chest, streaks of air are seen interspersed between the structures of the mediastinum, but in addition, the cardiac silhouette is seen too well, indicative of pneumopericardium. B, On a lateral radiograph, air surrounding the heart and inferior mediastinum is better appreciated.

is dependent on the size of the air collection and the severity of the underlying illness. Most patients require only a few days; however, up to 14 days may be needed in more severe cases. Because of the predictable benign course of this illness and the low incidence of recurrent disease, follow-up radiography is not routinely required in patients with isolated pneumomediastinum without pneumothorax. For clinically tenuous patients or those who fail to improve with conservative therapy, mediastinal drainage and mediastinotomy have been described, but such measures are rarely required.[16]

Consultation

- Pulmonology: For management of severe, underlying lung disease
- Gastroenterology: For evaluation of esophageal perforation by esophagoscopy or esophagography, or both
- Interventional radiology: For mediastinal tube placement (rarely indicated)
- Thoracic surgery: For mediastinal air drainage or mediastinotomy (very rarely indicated)

Admission Criteria

- Symptomatic patients
- Hypoxia
- Associated pneumothorax
- Unclear cause of the air leak
- Medical/surgical management of the underlying illness as indicated

Discharge Criteria

- No respiratory symptoms
- No supplement oxygen requirement
- Stable or resolving air collections
- After adequate management of the underlying medical condition

Prevention

Prevention of pneumomediastinum is best accomplished with adequate management of the underlying disease. In addition, avoidance of maneuvers that may exacerbate the air leak (e.g., peak expiratory flow measurement in asthmatics, forced expiratory radiographs, other Valsalva maneuvers) is important.[17]

IN A NUTSHELL

- Clinical presentation: Pneumothorax frequently presents with acute-onset pleuritic chest pain, oftentimes with associated breathing difficulties. Patients with pneumomediastinum, in contrast, are usually asymptomatic, except for symptoms referable to any underlying illness.
- Diagnosis: Pneumothorax or pneumomediastinum (or both) may be clinically suspected from symptoms or findings on physical examination; however, these diagnoses generally require radiographic confirmation.

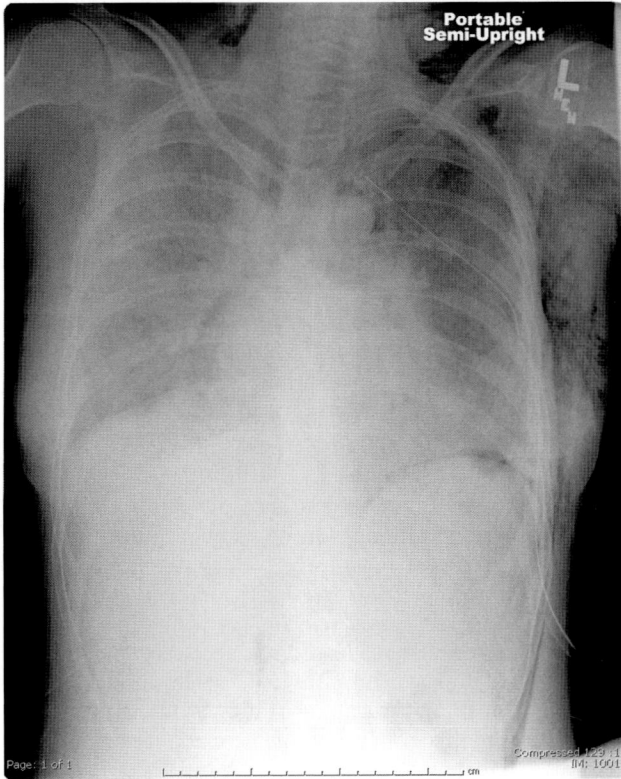

Figure 147-4 An extensive amount of air outlining the left chest wall muscles, extending superiorly into the neck, and crossing over to the right side is noted. Subcutaneous emphysema also extends along the left lateral abdominal wall.

- Treatment: Pneumothorax is usually managed with inpatient observation or intervention, or both. Tension, large primary, or any secondary pneumothoraces are managed by thoracostomy, sometimes with VATS. Management of pneumomediastinum is nearly always conservative, with efforts focused on diagnosing and treating any underlying medical conditions.

ON THE HORIZON

- Look for advances in understanding the pathogenesis of bulla formation.
- Increased experience with VATS in children will probably improve outcomes of pneumothorax in patients requiring surgical intervention.
- Further study into the risk factors for recurrence of pneumothorax will help in assessing who might benefit from prevention interventions.
- Further development of chemical and mechanical pleurodesis techniques may allow more widespread and successful preventive strategies for recurrence.

SUGGESTED READING

Baumann MH, Strange C, Heffner JE, et al: AACP Pneumothorax Consensus Group. Management of spontaneous pneumothorax: An American College of Chest Physicians Delphi consensus statement. Chest 2001;119:590-602.

Chalameau M, LeClainche L, Sayeg N, et al: Spontaneous pneumomediastinum in children. Pediatr Pulmonol 2001;31:67-75.

Gesundheit B, Preminger A, Harito B, et al: Pneumomediastinum and subcutaneous emphysema in an 18-month-old child. J Pediatr 2002;141:116-120.

Sahn SA, Heffner JE: Spontaneous pneumothorax. N Engl J Med 2000; 342:868-874.

Shaw KS, Prasil P, Nguyen LT, Laberge JM: Pediatric spontaneous pneumothorax. Semin Pediatr Surg 2003;12:55-61.

REFERENCES

1. Baumann MH, Strange C, Heffner JE, et al: AACP Pneumothorax Consensus Group. Management of spontaneous pneumothorax: An American College of Chest Physicians Delphi consensus statement. Chest 2001;119:591-602.

2. Orenstein DM: Pneumothorax. In Behrman RE, Kliegman RM, Jenson HB (eds): Nelson Textbook of Pediatrics, 16th ed. Philadelphia, WB Saunders, 2000, pp 1331-1332.

3. Stack AM, Caputo GL: Pneumomediastinum in childhood asthma. Pediatr Emerg Care 1998;12:98-101.

4. Bradley M, Williams C, Walshaw MJ: The value of routine expiratory chest films in the diagnosis of pneumothorax. Arch Emerg Med 1991;8:115-116.

5. Shaw KS, Prasil P, Nguyen LT, Laberge JM: Pediatric spontaneous pneumothorax. Semin Pediatr Surg 2003;12:55-61.

6. Rhea JT, DeLuca SA, Greene RE: Determining the size of pneumothorax in the upright patient. Radiology 1982;144:733-736.

7. Northfield TC: Oxygen therapy for spontaneous pneumothorax. BMJ 1971;4:86-88.

8. Noppen M, Alexander P, Driesen P, et al: Manual aspiration versus chest tube drainage in first episodes of primary spontaneous pneumothorax. Am J Respir Crit Care Med 2002;165:1240-1244.

9. Dull KE, Fleisher GR: Pigtail catheters versus large-bore chest tubes for pneumothoraces in children treated in the emergency department. Pediatr Emerg Care 2002;18:265-267.

10. Pacharn P, Heller DN, Kammen BF, et al: Are chest radiographs routinely necessary following thoracostomy tube removal? Pediatr Radiol 2002; 32:138-142.

11. Ozcan C, McGahren ED, Rodgers BM: Thoracoscopic treatment of spontaneous pneumothorax in children. J Pediatr Surg 2003;38:1459-1464.

12. Davis AM, Wensley DF, Phelan PD: Spontaneous pneumothorax in paediatric patients. Respir Med 1993;87:531-534.

13. Sahn SA, Heffner JE: Spontaneous pneumothorax. N Engl J Med 2000; 342:868-874.

14. Jain SK, Al-Kattan KM, Handy MG: Spontaneous pneumothorax: Determinants of surgical intervention. J Cardiovasc Surg 1998;39:107-111.

15. Gesundheit B, Preminger A, Harito B, et al: Pneumomediastinum and subcutaneous emphysema in an 18-month-old child. J Pediatr 2002; 141:116-120.

16. Chalameau M, LeClainche L, Sayeg N, et al: Spontaneous pneumomediastinum in children. Pediatr Pulmonol 2001;31;67-75.

17. Nounla J, Trobs RB, Bennek J, Lotz I: Idiopathic spontaneous pneumomediastinum: An uncommon emergency in children. J Pediatr Surg 2004;39:23-24.

CHAPTER 148

Urology

Bartley G. Cilento, Jr.

There are a number of urologic conditions that pediatric hospitalists will probably encounter in their care of pediatric inpatients. Primary urologic emergencies such as testicular torsion and urinary obstruction require prompt diagnosis and intervention to limit morbidity. In addition, several medical entities, such as recurrent urinary tract infection (UTI) and vesicoureteral reflux (VUR), may benefit from involvement with urologists, and surgical intervention may be considered in the options for treatment.

TESTICULAR TORSION

Testicular torsion results in compromise of vessels to the testicular parenchyma. Depending on the mechanism and degree of torsion, there is a variable period in which the testis is salvageable. Torsion can occur as a result of two mechanisms: extravaginal torsion and intravaginal torsion, terms referring to the tunica vaginalis, a structure that surrounds the testicle. In some regard this distinction is clinically irrelevant because it cannot be determined clinically, nor does it alter treatment.

Incidence

Although testicular torsion can occur at any age, it has a predominantly bimodal occurrence, namely, the neonatal and pubertal periods. The precise risk for the development of testicular torsion is not clearly established, but the approximate overall risk of testicular torsion developing by 25 years of age is 1 in 160. Testicular salvage rates have increased over the last 40 years, mainly as a result of early recognition and intervention. The undescended testis is also at risk for testicular torsion, presumably because of abnormal mesorchial attachments. Any child with a nonpapable testis and abdominal pain should be evaluated for intra-abdominal testicular torsion.

Diagnosis

Neonatal Torsion

Neonatal torsion is usually the result of extravaginal torsion in which the testicle twists on the spermatic cord or outside the tunica vaginalis; it accounts for 12% of all cases. Neonatal torsion occurs in the prenatal and postnatal period. Such occurrence does not appear to be correlated with prematurity, birth weight, method of delivery, or perinatal trauma. The condition is almost always asymptomatic and discovered on routine examination. The examination generally shows an edematous, erythematous hemiscrotum with a firm testis. The hemiscrotum does not usually transillumi-

nate. Current ultrasound technology is very accurate in determining the presence or absence of testicular blood flow in neonatal torsion.[1] Because of the imprecision of older ultrasound technology, nuclear scans to assess testicular blood flow were common but are now rarely performed. Neonatal torsion is thought to be secondary to the hypermobility of neonatal tissue, which does not firmly fix the testis to the scrotum. Controversy remains over management of the contralateral testis in neonates with torsion. Some believe that contralateral fixation is necessary and cite the occurrence of both synchronous and asynchronous torsion.[2] Others believe that contralateral fixation is not necessary and note that the hypermobility of neonatal tissue quickly resolves and that most cases of neonatal torsion occur within the first 10 days of life. Nevertheless, bilateral testicular torsion does in fact occur, and the surgeon and family must weigh the options of observation versus intervention with regard to the contralateral testis. I prefer and continue to recommend contralateral scrotal fixation.

Pubertal Torsion

In contrast to neonatal torsion, pubertal torsion is symptomatic. Patients experience a sudden onset of hemiscrotal pain, abdominal pain, or both. Nausea is also common. Physical examination usually demonstrates an elevated testicle within the scrotal sac. If palpable, the spermatic cord is thickened or twisted. The cremasteric reflex is generally absent on the affected side. The cremasteric reflex is elicited by stroking the inner aspect of the thigh, which causes the cremaster muscle within the scrotum to contract and thereby elevate the testis and scrotum. It is important to perform this test bilaterally because asymmetry is the key point. Some individuals do not demonstrate this reflex and it is therefore not useful in establishing the diagnosis of testicular torsion in these individuals. In general, manual detorsion should be attempted by a specialist (urologist) and does not preclude surgical intervention. If imaging is deemed necessary to help establish the diagnosis, scrotal ultrasound is the test of choice. Current ultrasound technology is highly sensitive in detecting testicular blood flow (Fig. 148-1).[3] In cases in which the diagnosis is not in question, proceeding directly to surgery is appropriate. The viability of the testis will be determined intraoperatively, and orchiectomy or orchiopexy will be performed. Viability is assessed after manual detorsion and observation for a period. Contralateral scrotal fixation is performed to prevent a similar occurrence on the unaffected side. Some series have reported contralateral torsion in 40% of cases in which contralateral detorsion was not performed.

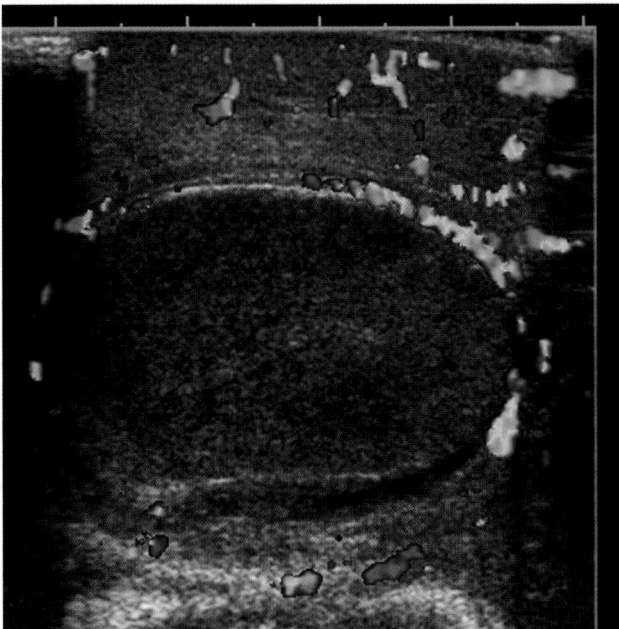

Figure 148-1 Ultrasound of the scrotum in a boy with acute scrotal pain demonstrates no Doppler color flow within the right testicle. The adjacent soft tissues are edematous and hyperemic. At surgery, the patient was found to have acute testicular torsion.

Prognosis

The prognosis refers to testicular salvage and fertility. The duration and degree of ischemia determine testicular salvage. Most of the precise experimental work regarding salvage rates relative to the duration of ischemia has been performed in dogs. Four hours of ischemia kills the germinal epithelium, whereas 8 to 10 hours kills the Sertoli cells (support cells for the germinal epithelium) and Leydig cells (testosterone production). The degree of torsion is also relevant. Intraoperatively, it is seen that some testicles contain one full twist whereas others have three or more twists. Obviously, the extent of torsion will have an impact on the degree of ischemia and the duration of time after which salvage is not possible. Clinically, we use 4 to 6 hours as the time at which testicular salvage becomes questionable.

Torsion of the Testicular Appendages

The small embryologic appendages that occur on the testis and epididymis are subject to torsion. These small appendages serve no function and are vestigial remnants. Torsion of these appendages may cause scrotal pain and swelling. However, there are several characteristics that can help distinguish this diagnosis from testicular torsion. The pain and swelling are usually gradual in onset and are rarely associated with nausea or vomiting. Most boys are able to continue with most of their activities and note discomfort only when the area is touched. It most commonly occurs after the neonatal period but before puberty. Physical examination reveals tenderness of the upper pole of the epididymis or the superior aspect of the testis. The cremasteric reflex is generally intact. Sometimes the necrotic appendage is visible through the scrotum, a finding called the "blue dot" sign. Scrotal ultrasonography rarely identifies the necrotic

appendages, but it does demonstrate normal blood flow to the testis and increased blood flow to the epididymis.[4] This condition is treated conservatively with rest and analgesics. The prognosis is excellent with no known long-term sequelae.

Consultation

- Testicular torsion requires surgical consultation and treatment.

Transfer

- Transfer to a tertiary center is advisable only if anesthetic or surgical services are inadequate for treating the neonate.

In a Nutshell

- Testicular torsion is a surgical emergency.
- Scrotal ultrasonography is highly reliable in determining testicular blood flow.
- Torsion of the appendages warrants conservative management.

HYDRONEPHROSIS

Diagnosis

Early detection of fetal hydronephrosis is commonplace with the widespread use of maternal ultrasonography. Fetal hydronephrosis is detectable at 15 weeks, shortly after the onset of fetal urine production. The internal renal architecture (differentiation between the renal cortex and the medullary pyramids) is best seen at 20 weeks' gestation. Normal findings include sonolucent renal pyramids relative to the renal cortex and a renal cortex that is slightly less echogenic than the liver. It is also important to determine the status of amniotic fluid because polyhydramnios and oligohydramnios have renal origins and implications. Hydronephrosis is the most common finding during prenatal ultrasonography. The differential diagnosis, in order of frequency, includes transient hydronephrosis, VUR, obstruction of the ureteropelvic junction (UPJ), congenital megaureter or obstruction of the ureterovesical junction (UVJ), posterior urethral valves (PUV), ectopic ureter, and ureterocele.[5] The obstructive processes (UPJ obstruction, megaureter, PUV, ectopic ureter, and ureterocele) are discussed in this chapter. The majority of antenatally detected cases are transient or physiologic and resolve spontaneously, particularly mild and moderate degrees of hydronephrosis. Severe prenatal hydronephrosis is more likely to represent a true pathologic entity such as UPJ obstruction or high-grade VUR. Controversy exists over the best method to classify prenatal hydronephrosis. The most common measurement is the anteroposterior (AP) diameter of the renal pelvis in the axial plane. No consensus has been reached on the AP diameter that will identify fetuses in which significant postnatal pathology and need for surgical intervention will ultimately develop. For this reason, others have proposed a qualitative assessment of mild, moderate, and severe hydronephrosis based on the appearance of the renal pelvis, calyces, and renal parenchyma. Hydronephrosis that is most likely associated

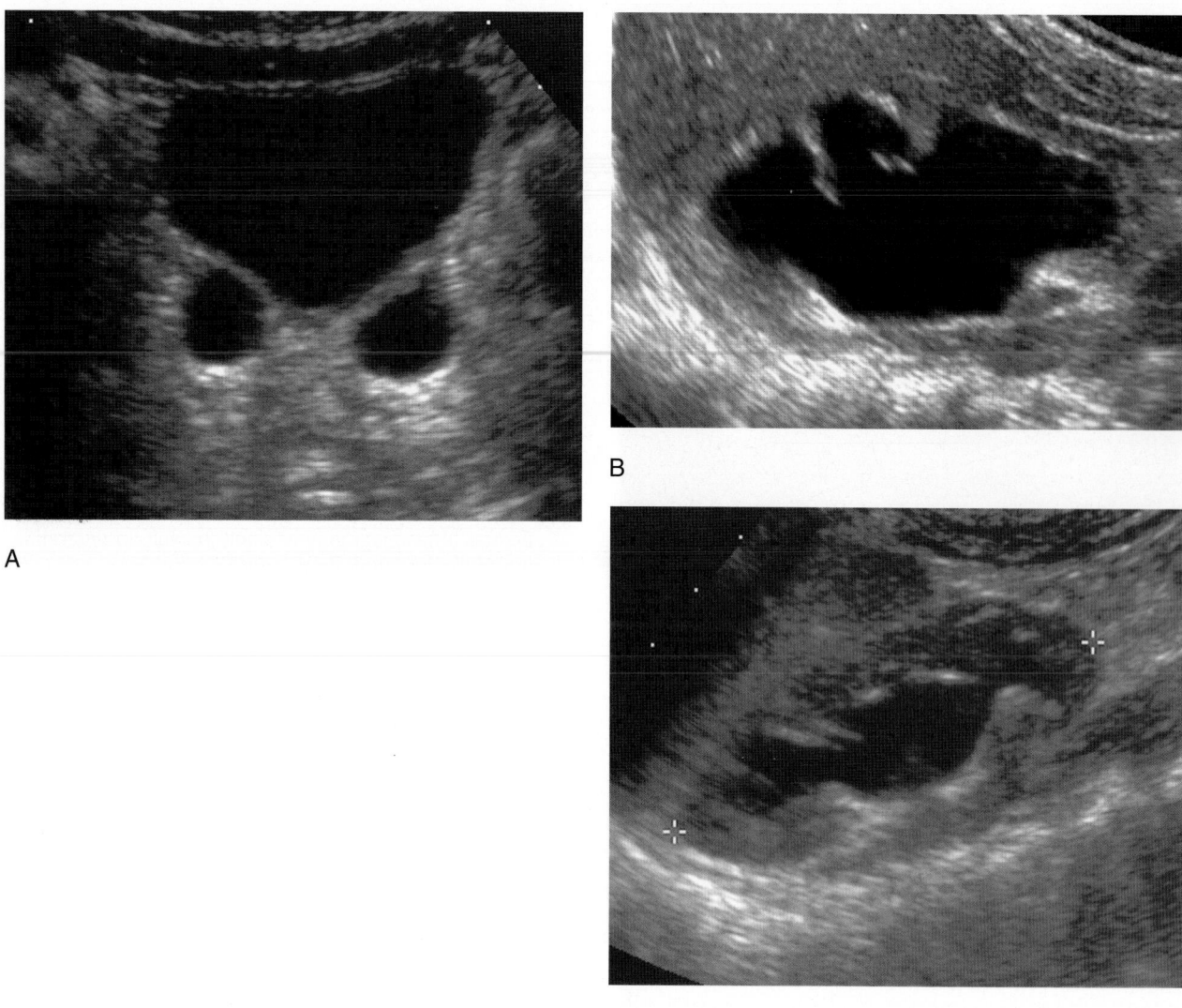

Figure 148-2 A-C, Three ultrasound images from a patient with fetal hydronephrosis demonstrate dilated ureters (behind the bladder) and bilateral hydronephrosis, the right greater than the left. This patient had bilateral primary megaureter.

with significant postnatal pathology is characterized by increasing hydronephrosis through pregnancy, oligohydramnios, increased renal cortical echogenicity, AP diameter greater than 10 mm, and calyceal dilation.

Clinical Presentation

The vast majority of patients with hydronephrosis are asymptomatic. Infants and children rarely present with an abdominal mass. As noted earlier, most children with hydronephrosis are detected antenatally and monitored postnatally. In children not identified in this manner, some will remain undetected, whereas others will present with a febrile UTI or with complaints of episodic abdominal pain. Isolated hematuria is an unusual presentation.

Evaluation

In nearly all cases, prenatal hydronephrosis is monitored by serial ultrasonography until delivery. Postnatal management includes prophylactic antibiotics (amoxicillin, 25 mg/kg/day once daily) and a repeat renal/bladder ultrasound (Fig. 148-2). Renal/bladder ultrasonography is performed after 48 hours because of the relative oliguria that occurs during this period. Voiding cystourethrography (VCUG) is indicated for moderate to severe hydronephrosis and any evidence of bladder wall thickening. In children with mild hydronephrosis, there is debate regarding the necessity for VCUG in the evaluation. Renal scans with mercaptoacetyltriglycine (MAG3) and dimercaptosuccinic acid (DMSA) are used to determine the degree of obstruction and renal scarring, respectively. Consultation with a pediatric urologist is advisable in children with postnatal hydronephrosis.

Consultation

Pediatric urologic consultation is advisable in patients with moderate or greater hydronephrosis, VUR, bladder wall thickening or known PUV, and evidence of renal asymmetry or renal scarring.

OBSTRUCTION

Obstruction is a functional term that encompasses many different urologic conditions, the most common being UPJ obstruction, congenital megaureter or UVJ obstruction, posterior urethral valves (PUV), ectopic ureter, and ureterocele. In most cases, urinary tract obstruction does not involve complete obstruction of urinary flow but is a relative obstructive process that ranges from mild to severe. In most clinical settings, obstruction is inferred by the presence of hydronephrosis on renal ultrasound; however, confirmation by a functional study such as intravenous pyelography (IVP) or a renal radioisotope imaging technique is required. The two most common types of renal scintigraphy are the MAG3 Lasix renal scan and the DMSA renal scan. The MAG3 Lasix renal scan provides information about renal function, from which creatinine clearance can be calculated and the ability of the kidney to drain when stressed. The DMSA scan gives an indication of tubular function but no information regarding drainage. In clinical terms, DMSA is a cortical imaging agent that detects renal scars and determines the percent function of each kidney. The MAG3 Lasix renal scan provides differential percent function, but in addition it is excreted by the kidney and can help determine the presence or absence of obstruction to urine flow. In large part, renal scanning has supplanted IVP as a means of assessing renal function and drainage. Advantages of renal scan include reduced exposure to radiation and avoidance of a potential allergic reaction to the iodinated contrast material.

Clinical Presentation

The vast majority of patients with obstruction are asymptomatic. Infants and children rarely present with an abdominal mass. As noted earlier, most children with hydronephrosis are detected antenatally and monitored postnatally. In children not identified in this manner, some will remain undetected, whereas others will present with a febrile UTI or complaints of episodic abdominal pain. Isolated hematuria is an unusual presentation.

Evaluation

Infants and children with hydronephrosis, which has generally been determined by ultrasonography, need further evaluation to determine the presence or absence of obstruction. VCUG is performed to assess for VUR, PUV, or other anomalies such as a bladder diverticulum. A MAG3 renal scan (or less commonly IVP) is used to evaluate for the presence or absence and the degree of obstruction. Prophylactic antibiotics are generally started in infants and children, pending completion of the workup. In general, 25% of the normal antibiotic dose is used on a daily basis. Higher doses may lead to the development of bacterial resistance by exposing the intestinal bacteria to higher serum concentrations of the antibiotic.

Treatment

Treatment depends on the diagnosis established. Many UPJ and UVJ obstructions improve with time. However, patients with clinically significant obstruction as determined by functional imaging studies or the clinical course require surgery. Pyeloplasty is used to repair UPJ obstruction, whereas ureteral reimplantation is used to correct congenital megaureter or UVJ obstruction. Surgical intervention is required in nearly all cases of PUV, ectopic ureter, and ureterocele because they are fixed anatomic anomalies that do not resolve with time. Cystoscopy plus valve ablation is required in patients with PUV. An ectopic ureter is treated by ureteral reimplantation into the bladder. Treatment of ureterocele is varied and complex. In general, cystoscopic incision is an easy and efficient method of relieving the obstruction; however, many patients require further surgery to correct iatrogenically induced VUR as a result of the endoscopic incision. The prognosis is excellent in most cases after surgical correction of UPJ obstruction, UVJ obstruction, ectopic ureter, and ureterocele. Patients with severe PUV can have long-term sequelae such as renal insufficiency, renal failure, bladder instability, urinary incontinence, and hypertension. Consequently, these patients need long-term follow-up and coordinated care with a pediatric nephrologist.

Consultation and Admission Criteria

• Very early consultation with a pediatric urologist is appropriate in nearly all cases of obstruction.
• Infants with obstruction and sepsis require immediate surgical intervention.

VESICOURETERAL REFLUX

VUR is a common condition that occurs in healthy children. It is secondary to an abnormally positioned ureter within the bladder (detrusor) muscle that results in an

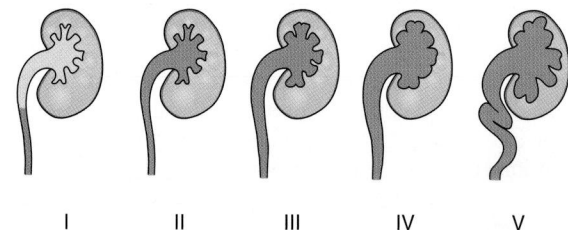

Figure 148-3   Grading of vesicoureteral reflux: grade 1—ureter only; grade II—ureter, renal pelvis, calyces without dilation; grade III—dilation or tortuosity of the ureter and/or dilated pelvis; grade IV—shape of the calyces maintained but dilated; grade V—gross dilation of the collecting system.

incompetent UVJ that allows urine to freely reflux from the bladder into the ureter during filling or emptying of the bladder. In fact, 15% to 35% of girls with UTI have VUR.[6] Although UTI is less common in boys, VUR is found in up to 50% when these boys are investigated for infection. In infants there is an almost equal incidence of reflux in males and females. VUR should never be considered a normal phenomenon because reflux with infection could have a devastating effect on renal function. Children with signs of hydronephrosis, UTIs, and known syndromes associated with VUR should be evaluated.

Grading of Vesicoureteral Reflux

VUR is graded on a scale of I to V by an internationally agreed upon classification (Fig. 148-3).[7] Grade I is the least and grade V is the most severe. Grading of VUR allows health care providers to estimate the probability of spontaneous resolution. Grades I and II reflux have an 80% to 90% chance of spontaneous resolution. Grade III has a 50% spontaneous resolution rate. Grade IV has a relatively low spontaneous resolution rate, in the range of 10% to 20%. Grade V is considered a surgical problem. The observation period is generally 3 to 5 years.

Consequences of Vesicoureteral Reflux

VUR alone is not generally considered harmful to the kidney. It is the combination of VUR and infection that can produce renal parenchymal damage. Bacterial colonization of the renal parenchyma results in an inflammatory response that leads to pyelonephritic scarring, papillary damage, and cortical loss. Prophylactic antibiotics should be used to prevent infection while reflux is present.

Diagnosis

VUR is diagnosed by VCUG (see Fig. 148-3) or radionuclide cystography (RNC). Often, reflux will not occur during filling of the bladder but may be seen only during voiding, thus illustrating the importance of the voiding phase of the cystogram. It is preferable that all boys and infant girls undergo VCUG as their initial study, whereas in older girls with their first UTI, RNC may be used. RNC is used for serial studies. VCUG provides more anatomic detail than RNC does. RNC is being used with increasing frequency, particularly in females with infection, in siblings as screening for reflux, and in children with VUR as annual follow-up. RNC is not good at delineating anatomic abnormalities such as bladder diverticula or PUV. Ultrasound and IVP are poor

screening tests for VUR. Patients with known VUR will have normal IVP and renal ultrasound findings in more than 50% of cases.

Treatment

Grades I to III VUR are best managed with low-dose antibiotic therapy and yearly follow-up. Many parents are concerned about long-term antibiotic use, but low-dose prophylaxis has proved to be safe and effective. Prophylactic antibiotic therapy in the management of VUR is defined as 20% to 25% of the normal antibiotic dose. Higher doses result in higher serum levels and can potentially lead to antibiotic resistance in the intestinal bacteria that ultimately colonize the perineum; such resistance can result in ascending infection. Urinary antibiotic concentrations are much higher because these antibiotics are excreted in urine, and the concentrations are sufficient to prevent bacterial colonization of the urinary tract. If free of recurrent UTI, yearly follow-up includes renal/bladder ultrasonography and RNC. Children with grades IV and V are usually surgical candidates. Children with nonfebrile UTIs (cystitis) may be screened by renal/bladder ultrasound alone. In voiding individuals, infrequent voiding behavior is the most likely reason for recurrent cystitis, and thus a careful voiding history is essential.

Controversy exists regarding surveillance by periodic urine culture. Although some advocate urine cultures every 3 months, others recommend urine cultures only when there are signs or symptoms of UTI. Either method is acceptable and should be individualized according to the circumstances of the patient and the philosophy of the health care providers. Bag specimens are notoriously inaccurate, particularly in females and non–toilet-trained children. A catheterized urine specimen is the only way to accurately detect an infection in babies and pre–toilet-trained infants. Indications for antireflux surgery include breakthrough infections despite prophylactic antibiotics, reflux with an anatomic abnormality at the UVJ (i.e., diverticulum), development or progression of renal parenchymal scarring, poor compliance in taking antibiotics, and persistent reflux.

Surgery

Ureteroneocystostomy (antireflux surgery or ureteral reimplantation) involves repositioning of the affected ureter or ureters within the bladder in such a way that a longer tunnel is created through the bladder wall to prevent reflux. Various open operations have been devised to achieve this result. Surgical success rates exceed 95% with these open procedures. In recent years, some surgeons have advocated cystoscopic injection therapy for the ureteral orifice to "bulk up" the intramural tunnel and prevent reflux. Cystoscopic injection therapy is a brief outpatient procedure. Dextranomer/hyaluronic acid (Deflux) is now approved by the Food and Drug Administration for the treatment of VUR. It has a 60% to 80% success rate, but its long-term efficacy remains to be determined.

Postoperatively, all children are maintained on antibiotics for approximately 3 to 4 months. Renal and bladder ultrasonography is performed 4 weeks after surgery to assess for hydronephrosis. RNC is performed 4 months after surgery to document resolution of the reflux. Antibiotics are discontinued at this point if the operation has been successful, and patients are reminded to void regularly (every 3 hours). Postoperative UTIs develop in some children (approximately 15% of girls and 1% of boys), but pyelonephritis is unusual. In most instances, postsurgical nonfebrile UTIs are the result of infrequent daytime voiding or voiding dysfunction, or both. Postoperatively, it is important to continue to assess the child's voiding habits to identify this condition and suggest corrective behavioral management.

Consultation

- Pediatric urology for initial management, evaluation, and follow-up.

Admission Criteria

- Febrile UTI in neonates
- Febrile UTI in infants and toddlers with poor oral intake

In a Nutshell

- VUR is common.
- All febrile UTIs warrant evaluation with renal/bladder ultrasound and VCUG.
- Medical management with prophylactic antibiotics is the initial treatment in most cases.
- Surgical treatment is recommended for nonresolving or breakthrough UTIs.
  Surgical success rates exceed 95%.

On the Horizon

- The genetic locus will probably be determined soon.
- Look for endoscopic management to continue and accelerate.
- Look for the launching of large clinic studies to determine the best management regimen.

NEPHROLITHIASIS

The prevalence of nephrolithiasis in American children ranges from 1 in 1000 to 1 in 7600. Some of the variability is due to geographic differences, with stone disease being more common in the Southeast and southern California. In general, there is an equal prevalence with regard to gender. Race is a risk factor. Whites have the greatest incidence, whereas African Americans have low risk. The presentation, evaluation, and management of children with stone disease are unique because of the variability in symptoms and normative values. These parameters vary according to the stage of development and age of the child.

Clinical Presentation

The characteristic renal colic that occurs in adults is present in only half the children with urolithiasis; therefore, establishing the diagnosis can be a challenge. Presenting symptoms may include UTIs, hematuria both microscopic and macroscopic, sterile pyuria, dysuria, or generalized irritability. The combination of stones and UTIs is most common in preschool children. The incidence of hematuria

varies widely (30% to 90%), and it can be either microscopic or macroscopic. Sterile pyuria should always trigger further evaluation for urolithiasis. Dysuria or urinary frequency (or both) may be due to bladder stones and the resultant local irritation to the bladder wall. Patients with congenital urinary tract anomalies or urinary diversions are also at increased risk for urolithiasis.

Stone Formation

Stone formation is a complex process. Simplistically stated, it represents a delicate chemical balance between substances that induce and substances that inhibit stone formation. A full discussion of physiochemical properties, such as the free ion concentration, activity product, and equilibrium solubility product, is beyond the scope of this chapter. Interested readers are referred to more comprehensive sources listed at the end of this chapter. Clinically speaking, the most important factors include urinary volume, solute excretion (i.e., calcium, oxalate, uric acid), urinary pH, and inhibitors (citrate, magnesium).

For example, urinary pH can have a dramatic effect on the solubility of stone-forming ions. Acidic urine favors uric acid and cystine stones. Alkaline urine (pH >6.5) favors calcium phosphate stones. Struvite stones occur in alkaline urine because bacterial action on urea produces ammonia and thus results in alkaline urine.

Free ions such as magnesium and citrate bind calcium and reduce the free ion concentration of calcium, which reduces the chance of crystal formation.

Causative factors for pediatric urolithiasis vary widely in the literature. The most common factor is hypercalciuria, but other factors include infection, genitourinary abnormalities, and congenital enzymatic deficiencies.

Evaluation

The initial evaluation includes a complete history and physical examination. A thorough family history is essential, particularly in regard to urolithiasis and inheritable metabolic abnormalities. A dietary history should be obtained with notation of dietary excesses and fluid intake. Urinalysis and urine culture should be performed. Findings on urinalysis should be assessed, particularly for pH, hematuria, and sedimentary crystals. Further urinary studies include a 24-hour urine collection for calcium, cystine, citrate, oxalate, and uric acid. Serum studies include calcium, potassium, creatinine, bicarbonate, blood urea nitrogen, phosphorus, magnesium, and uric acid. In children with hypercalcemia or hypercalciuria, a serum intact parathyroid hormone level should be obtained. The least invasive and oftentimes most expeditious method to evaluate the upper urinary tracts is renal and bladder ultrasonography. Current ultrasound technology has greatly improved the ability to image small stones in the kidney and ureter (Fig. 148-4). The degree of hydronephrosis is also easily assessed. The most sensitive test is a non–contrast-enhanced computed tomography scan. Its disadvantages include ionizing radiation exposure and the occasional need for sedation in pediatric patients.

Common Stone Compositions

Calcium stones are the most common type of stones seen. The two major causes of calcium stone formation are hypercalciuria and hyperoxaluria, with hypercalciuria being more

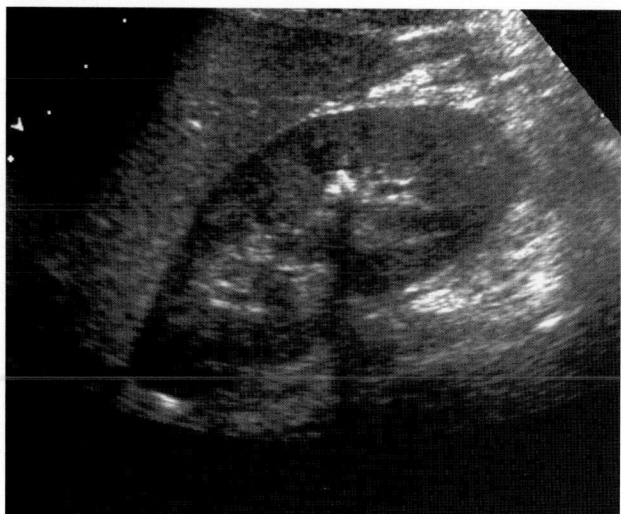

Figure 148–4 This sagittal image of the right kidney demonstrates two abutting small renal stones in the midportion of the kidney. The stones are characteristically echogenic with posterior acoustic shadowing.

common than hyperoxaluria. There are many causes of increased urinary excretion of calcium. Idiopathic hypercalciuria accounts for the largest percentage of children with this diagnosis. Other causes include distal renal tubular acidosis, furosemide therapy, and prednisone therapy. Normal urinary calcium excretion should be less than 4 mg/kg body weight per day. Spot urinary assessment of the ratio of calcium to creatinine correlates well with 24-hour assessment of calcium excretion. In infants younger than 6 months, the ratio should be less than 0.6; in children 7 to 12 months of age, the ratio should also be less than 0.6; and in children 2 years or older, it should be less than 0.2. Calcium excretion is affected by dietary intake of milk and various formulas. Intake of soy-based formulas is associated with the lowest calcium excretion. Treatment of hypercalciuria consists of hydration and restriction of dietary sodium. Hydrochlorothiazide (1 to 2 mg/kg/day) can also be used to treat hypercalciuria when necessary.

Oxalic acid is an end product of metabolism. Of the daily oxalate excretion, 90% is derived from metabolism and 10% from dietary sources. Normal children excrete less than 50 mg/1.73 m²/day of oxalate. Oxalate excretion in infants can be four times higher. Causes of increased oxalate excretion include increased dietary intake, inborn errors of metabolism, and enteric hyperabsorption.

Uric acid stones account for 4% of pediatric stones. These stones can be the result of overproduction of uric acid or volume contraction, or they can be idiopathic. The disorders associated with overproduction are many, and interested readers are referred to sources presented at the end of the chapter. Uric acid is an end product of metabolism, and the kidney removes two thirds of the amount produced. Excretion varies by age, and age-related normative values need to be used to assess excretion status. Medical therapy includes alkalinization of urine (pH >6.0) to facilitate dissolution of the stone and adequate hydration. Sodium citrate, sodium bicarbonate, and potassium citrate are all used to help alkalinize the urine.

Struvite stones result from specific bacterial action on the urea contained in urine. The bacterial enzyme urease hydrolyzes urea into ammonium and carbon dioxide, which results in an alkaline urine. This process favors the formation of magnesium-ammonium-phosphate stones (struvite). Organisms known to contain urease are *Pseudomonas, Klebsiella, Proteus, Staphylococcus, Serratia, Candida,* and *Mycoplasma.* If left untreated or undiagnosed, these stones become large and form staghorn calculi that fill the entire renal collecting system. Renal damage, pyelonephritis, sepsis, and obstruction can occur.

For other stones such as cystine, xanthine, adenine, and orotic acid stones, please refer to the references at the end of the chapter.

Surgical Therapy

Extracorporeal shock wave lithotripsy (ESWL) has rapidly replaced open and endoscopic surgery as the primary treatment of upper urinary tract stones. Most of the initial reluctance to use this technologic advancement in children has dissipated as experience has shown there to be no long-term consequences on renal growth or development. Nevertheless, further long-term studies need to be done to confirm these initial findings. The ESWL machine generates a shock wave that is focused by a hemielliptical reflector. The shock wave is generated within a liquid medium that is similar in density to human tissue and therefore transitions from the machine to the patient with little attenuation. The hemielliptical reflector allows the surgeon to focus the shock wave on the renal stone with the aid of ultrasound or fluoroscopy. The stone is fragmented into small pieces that are spontaneously passed. In adults, current ESWL technology allows these procedures to be performed under intravenous sedation; however, general anesthesia is needed in infants and children, primarily to manage pain and anxiety. Modifications are often required when using this therapy in children, including changes in positioning, shielding of the lung, and reduced power settings. Some contraindications to ESWL in children include a bleeding disorder, severe anatomic anomalies, or hypertension. The overall results are similar to the adult experience, with success rates ranging from 50% to 100%. Factors that affect success rates include the type of machine used, in addition to stone size, location, and composition.

Endoscopic surgery involves fiberoptic instrumentation such as a ureteroscope or nephroscope. The nephroscope is used percutaneously after establishing a percutaneous working port from the flank skin to the renal pelvis. In this fashion, a stone can be directly visualized with the nephroscope. Once visualized and depending on its size, the stone can be grasped and removed in toto or fragmented and removed in pieces. Complications include loss of access, bleeding or hemorrhage, electrolyte and fluid disturbances, and perforation of the collecting system. Ureteroscopy involves the use of a flexible fiberoptic scope that is passed up the urethra and into the bladder and ureter. It is most commonly used for ureteral stones but can also be used to access stones within the renal pelvis. Once visualized, the stone can be grasped or ensnared by small flexible instruments passed through the working port of the ureteroscope. The trapped stone and ureteroscope are then removed. This therapy is highly effective in adults and also successful in children. In infants and some children, technical limitations because of the small-caliber ureter and larger ureteroscope diameter may limit access. Complications can include perforation of the ureter, bleeding, and ureteral or urethral stricture formation.

Open Surgery

Open surgery for stone removal is an uncommon occurrence in infants and children. When needed, it is a well-established and effective method of removal. A detailed discussion of the various open surgical procedures is not the subject of this chapter. Interested readers are referred to any standard urologic textbook.

Consultation and Admission Criteria

- Patients with UTIs and urinary tract stones require urologic consultation and admission.
- Patients with a solitary kidney and urinary tract stones require urologic consultation.
- Patients with any suggestion of obstruction require admission and immediate urologic consultation.

In a Nutshell

- Stones are relatively uncommon in children and infants: 1 in 1000.
- The presentation can vary in infants and children. Stones rarely require open surgery.

On the Horizon

- Look for the genetics of stone formation to continue to develop.
- Look for new genetically based treatments for prevention of recurrent stone formation.
- Look for continued improvements in endoscopic equipment.

SUGGESTED READING

Diagnostic maneuvers to differentiate obstructive from nonobstructive ureteral dilation. In Gonzales ET, Bauer SB (eds): Pediatric Urologic Practice. Philadelphia, Lippincott Williams & Wilkins, 1999.

Megaureter. In Gonzales ET, Bauer SB (eds): Pediatric Urologic Practice. Philadelphia, Lippincott Williams & Wilkins, 1999.

Posterior urethral valves. In Gonzales ET, Bauer SB (eds): Pediatric Urologic Practice. Philadelphia, Lippincott Williams & Wilkins, 1999.

Testicular torsion. In King LR (ed): Urologic Surgery in Infants and Children. Philadelphia, WB Saunders, 1998.

UPJ obstruction. In King LR (ed): Urologic Surgery in Infants and Children. Philadelphia, WB Saunders, 1998.

Urolithiasis in children. In Gonzales ET, Bauer SB (eds): Pediatric Urologic Practice. Philadelphia, Lippincott Williams & Wilkins, 1999.

Vesicoureteral reflux. In Gonzales ET, Bauer SB (eds): Pediatric Urologic Practice. Philadelphia, Lippincott Williams & Wilkins, 1999.

REFERENCES

1. Deeg KH, Wild F: Colour Doppler imaging—a new method to differentiate torsion of the spermatic cord and epididymo-orchitis. Eur J Pediatr 1990;149:253-255.
2. Brandt MT, Sheldon CA, Wacksman J, Matthews P: Prenatal testicular torsion: Principles of management. J Urol 1992;147:670-672.
3. Nussbaum Blask AR, Bulas D, Shalaby-Rana E, et al: Color Doppler sonography and scintigraphy of the testis: A prospective, comparative analysis in children with acute scrotal pain. Pediatr Emerg Care 2002;18(2):67-71.
4. Kass EJ, Lundak B: The acute scrotum. Pediatr Clin North Am 1997;44:1251-1266.
5. Woodward M, Frank D: Postnatal management of antenatal hydronephrosis. BJU Int 2002;89:149-156.
6. Smellie JM, Normand IC, Katz G: Children with urinary infection: A comparison of those with and without vesicoureteric reflux. Kidney Int 1981;20:717-722.
7. Medical versus surgical treatment of primary vesicoureteral reflux: Report of the International Reflux Study Committee. Pediatrics 1981;67:392-400.

CHAPTER 149

Lumps and Bumps: Benign and Malignant Tumors

Brandie J. Roberts and Bari B. Cunningham

The spectrum of cutaneous tumors, or lumps and bumps, in children is broad. A range of tumors, from benign, self-limited lesions to malignant and life-threatening conditions, is reviewed in this chapter. The signs of a benign versus a malignant tumor are covered, followed by a discussion of some of the most commonly encountered skin tumors seen by pediatricians in an inpatient hospital environment. Appropriate imaging and subspecialty consultation (dermatology, surgery, oncology) are important in the diagnosis and management of these tumors.

BENIGN VERSUS MALIGNANT

There are specific tumor features that should increase the index of suspicion for malignancy. Although this generalization is not entirely foolproof, when all of the following features are present in a skin tumor, the possibility of malignancy should be strongly considered[1]:

1. Neonatal onset
2. History of rapid growth
3. Firm mass greater than 3 cm in diameter
4. Skin ulceration
5. Fixation to deep tissues or location below the fascia

EPIDERMAL TUMORS

Epidermal Inclusion Cyst

An epidermal cyst (epidermoid cyst, epidermal inclusion cyst) is a dermal or subcutaneous nodule composed of an epithelium-lined cavity filled with keratin. Epidermoid cysts are rare in early childhood and occur most frequently in adolescence and adulthood. There is no racial or gender predilection. The presence of multiple epidermal inclusion cysts, particularly early in life, should lead to a consideration of Gardner syndrome, an autosomal dominant genodermatosis characterized by multiple epidermal cysts, intestinal polyps, desmoid tumors, lipomas, and osteomas, often in the mandible.

Physical examination of an epidermal cyst reveals a firm spherical nodule that varies in size but usually measures 1 to 2 cm. There is often a central 1-mm depression (punctum), a feature that helps distinguish it from other cystic masses

(Fig. 149-1). An inflamed cyst may be red and tender and, rarely, accompanied by fever.

The differential diagnosis of an epidermal inclusion cyst includes pilomatricoma, superficial lymph node, lipoma, and dermoid cyst. Epidermal inclusion cysts must be differentiated from developmental cysts, such as thyroglossal, bronchogenic, branchial cleft, and preauricular cysts, owing to their varying therapy. Thyroglossal cysts occur on the midline of the neck and may move upward with swallowing and protrusion of the tongue. Bronchogenic cysts are found most commonly on the suprasternal notch, and branchial cleft cysts occur on the lateral neck overlying the edge of the sternocleidomastoid muscle. Preauricular cysts occur in front of the ear and may overlie complex anatomy; they may occur alone or in conjunction with hearing loss. All these developmental cysts are prone to infection and may present with erythema, edema, abscess, or purulent drainage. Patients who fail outpatient oral antibiotic therapy or have systemic illness may warrant hospitalization. Consultation with an otorhinolaryngologist or plastic surgeon should be considered, especially if repeated infections have occurred. Incision and drainage are not routinely required. Definitive exploration and excision are rarely performed at the time of an acute infection.

A solitary, asymptomatic epidermoid cyst does not require any intervention. If the lesion is cosmetically disfiguring, tender, or inflamed, therapy is indicated. Surgical excision is a simple, rapid outpatient procedure that leaves minimal scarring. Care must be taken to ensure that the entire sac or epithelial lining is removed; otherwise, recurrence of the cyst is likely. For inflamed or infected lesions, surgery should be delayed, and antibiotics, warm compresses, and intralesional corticosteroids may be indicated.

Dermoid Cyst

Dermoid cysts are congenital nodules that occur along predictable embryonic fusion lines. These should not be confused with benign cystic teratomas, which are sometimes referred to as "dermoids." All dermoid cysts are congenital, although only 40% of these lesions are recognized at birth.[2] Lesions present as hard, oval to round subcutaneous tumors that do not move with the overlying skin. Dermoid cysts are

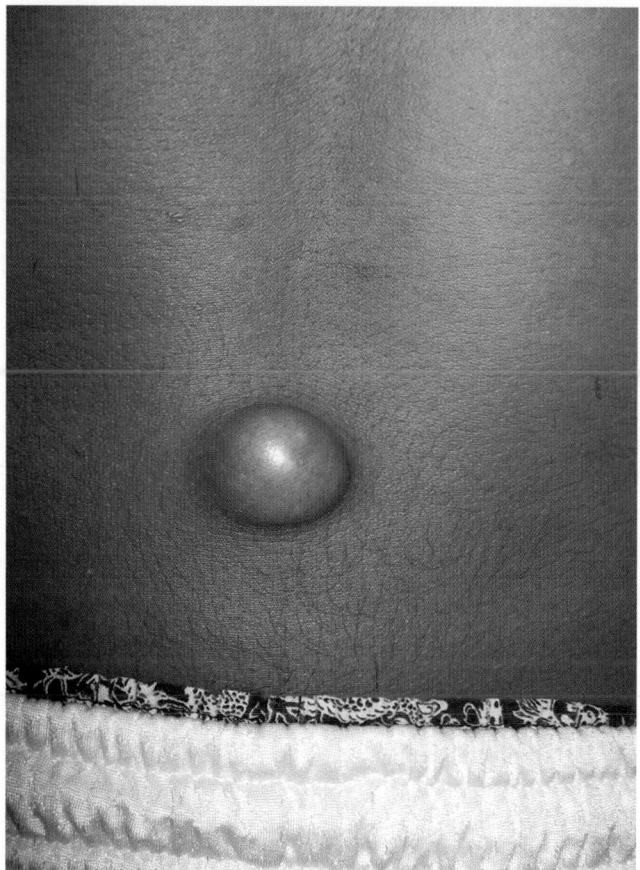

Figure 149-1   Epidermal cyst with central punctum on the back of an adolescent.

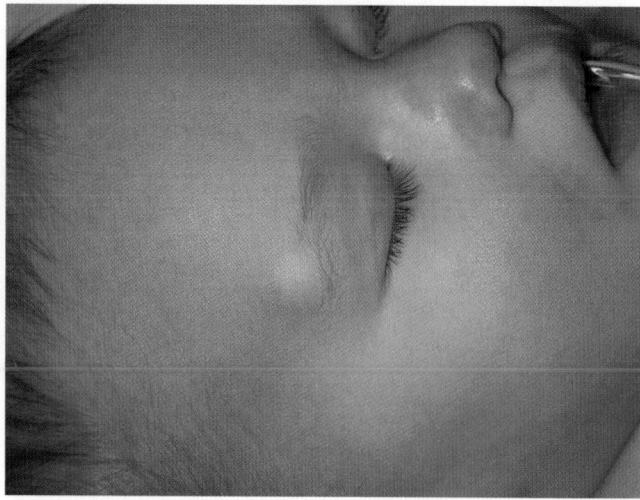

Figure 149-2   Dermoid cyst located on the lateral third of the eyebrow, the most common location.

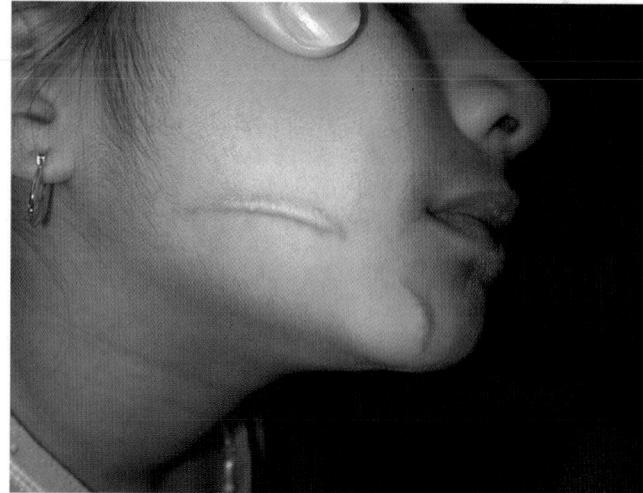

Figure 149-3   In a hypertrophic scar, the fibrous tissue is limited to the original site of skin injury.

usually 1 to 4 cm in diameter and fixed posteriorly to the underlying periosteum. These lesions do not compress with manipulation and do not enlarge with Valsalva maneuvers.

Dermoid cysts are most commonly located on the lateral third of the eyebrow (Fig. 149-2); other common locations include midline nasal bridge, overlying the anterior fontanelle, and the submental crease, but they may be found anywhere on the scalp, face, or spinal axis. A sinus opening from which hairs project may be present; this increases the likelihood of an intracranial connection (cranial dysraphism).[3] Most dermoid cysts are superficial, located in the submuscular layer and adherent to the periosteum. However, up to 45% of dermoid cysts have an associated intracranial connection.[4] Although dermoid cysts are usually asymptomatic, they can be complicated by cellulitis, abscess, osteomyelitis, meningitis, or pressure erosion of the underlying bone. Surgical excision is the treatment of choice.

Basal Cell Carcinoma

Basal cell carcinoma usually presents as a single pearly, translucent papule or plaque on the head or neck. It is exceedingly rare in children and accounts for only 0.24% of all tumors in childhood and 13% of pediatric malignancies of the skin.[5] Often the diagnosis is delayed in children because the index of suspicion is so low. Basal cell carcinoma may be locally aggressive and destroy surrounding tissue; it typically does not metastasize. A diagnosis of basal cell carcinoma in childhood should prompt an investigation to rule

out an underlying syndrome predisposing to cutaneous malignancy. These syndromes include xeroderma pigmentosum, basal cell nevus syndrome, and Rombo, Bazex, and Oley syndromes. Excision is the treatment of choice, although other less invasive therapies may be considered, including imiquimod cream, 5-fluorouracil cream, cryotherapy, and electrodesiccation and curettage.

FIBROUS TUMORS

Keloid and Hypertrophic Scarring

A scar is termed *hypertrophic* if it remains confined to the original site of skin injury (Fig. 149-3). If it extends beyond the injured skin and invades the once normal, uninvolved skin, it is termed a *keloid* (Fig. 149-4). Hypertrophic scars are common in childhood and typically resolve spontaneously within a year after the original injury. Keloids are thick bands of fibrous tissue elevated above the skin. They can occur at any age but are most often seen in patients between 10 and

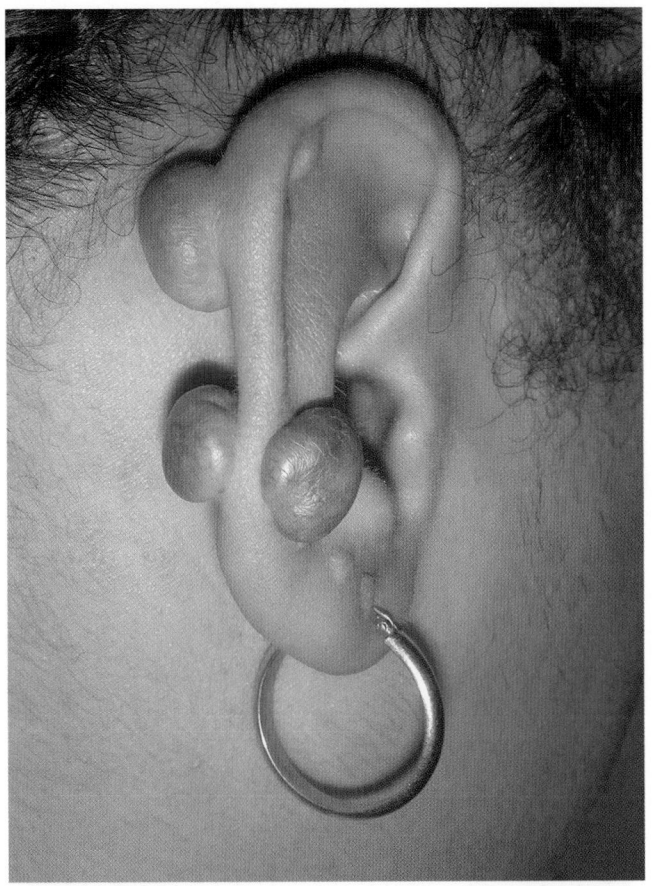

Figure 149-4 In a keloid, the scar tissue extends beyond the injured skin to form large nodules.

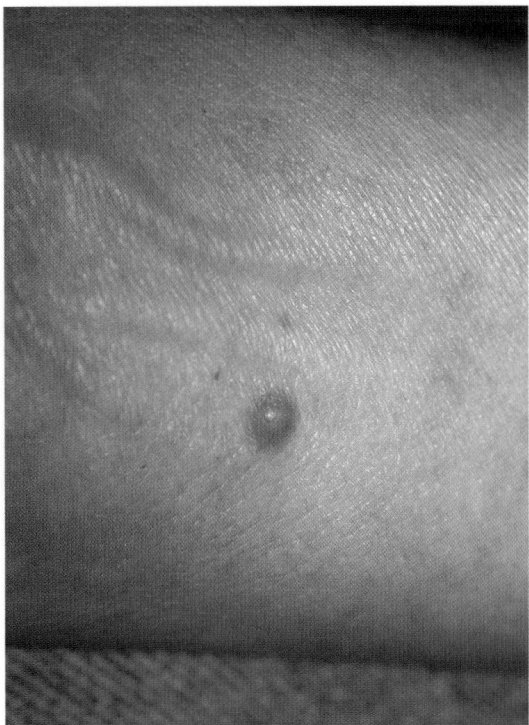

Figure 149-5 Dermatofibroma on the wrist. (Courtesy of Eric Parlette, MD.)

30 years old. They are most common on the chest, earlobes, and proximal upper extremities. There is no gender predilection.[6]

The clinical appearance of a keloid is usually so distinctive that a diagnosis is readily made. At times, a keloid may be confused with dermatofibrosarcoma protuberans (DFSP), an indolent, slow-growing, slowing invasive malignant plaque. In cases in which the diagnosis is in question, a biopsy should be performed to differentiate these biologically distinct neoplasms. Extensive, spontaneous keloid formation can be seen in Rubinstein-Taybi syndrome, which should be considered in a dysmorphic child with keloids and hypertrichosis.[7]

Treatment of keloids is challenging. Smaller lesions are usually managed with intralesional corticosteroid injections in concentrations from 10 to 40 mg/mL every 2 to 4 weeks. Corticosteroids lead to collagen breakdown and softening of the keloid. Other treatment options include silicon gel sheeting, imiquimod cream, carbon dioxide laser ablation, intralesional methotrexate or 5-fluorouracil, and surgical excision. In general, keloids recur after simple excision. Therefore, surgery is usually combined with other modalities, such as postoperative radiation, intralesional steroid injections, or imiquimod cream, to minimize the risk of recurrence. Even with a multimodal approach, keloids frequently recur, and treatments are often palliative rather than curative.

Dermatofibroma

Dermatofibroma (fibrous histiocytoma, histiocytoma cutis, sclerosing hemangioma) is a small, firm, benign papule limited to the skin (Fig. 149-5). This lesion usually occurs in early adulthood and is commonly located on the lower extremities of women. Dermatofibroma is not common in young children and is almost never seen in infancy. Most lesions are 3 to 4 mm in diameter, but giant variants do exist. Lateral pressure on a dermatofibroma leads to dimpling of its surface, known as the dimple sign. The cause of dermatofibroma has not been clearly established,[8] but it is believed to be a benign, reactive proliferation of skin that occurs as a result of minor trauma, such as an insect bite. In adults, the presence of multiple dermatofibromas has been associated with connective tissue diseases such as lupus erythematosus. Treatment for dermatofibroma is generally not indicated unless the lesion is symptomatic. If the diagnosis is in question, an excisional biopsy should be performed.

Dermatofibrosarcoma Protuberans and Giant Cell Fibroblastoma

DFSP is a slowly growing, indolent, malignant fibrous tumor. It can occur anywhere on the body but is most commonly seen on the chest and in the shoulder region. Most cases occur in adults, but occasional pediatric and even congenital cases have been reported.[9] Typically, lesions are nodular, lumpy, ill-defined plaques referred to by the patient as "scar" despite the fact that no antecedent trauma occurred. Tissue diagnosis is essential; DFSP has characteristic histologic features, making differentiation from other fibrous tumors relatively easy. Surgical excision and Mohs micrographic surgery are the treatments of choice.[10] Recurrences

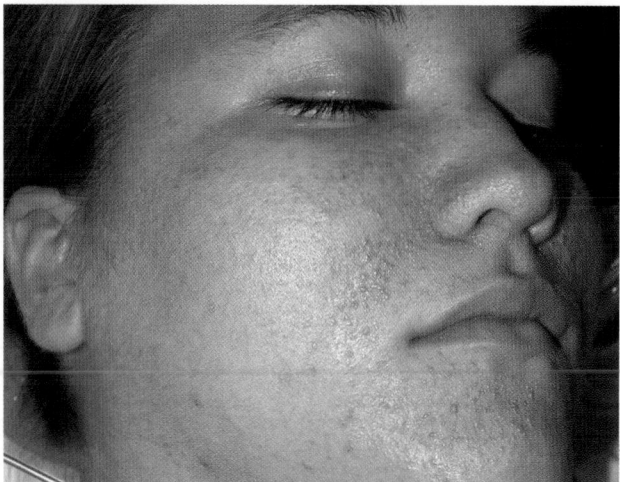

Figure 149-6   Angiofibromas, small pink papules over the nasal bridge and cheeks, in a patient with tuberous sclerosis.

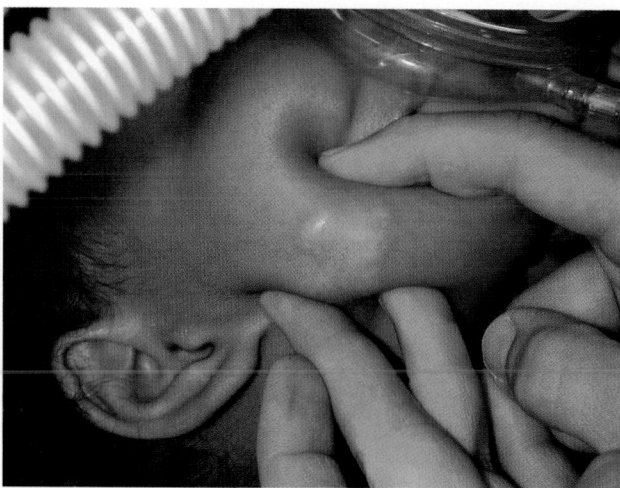

Figure 149-7   Pilomatricoma. Rock-hard subcutaneous nodule with a bluish hue on the cheek.

after standard excision are common, but metastases are uncommon.

Giant cell fibroblastoma is a DFSP variant usually seen in young children and infants. It presents as a single dermal nodule on the lower abdomen, thigh, or trunk. Histologically, this tumor looks like DFSP, but with sinusoidal spaces lined with characteristic giant cells and atypical spindle cells in a myxoid stroma. Recurrences are common, but, like DFSP, metastases are unusual.

Angiofibroma

Angiofibroma is a pink, firm, 1- to 2-mm dome-shaped papule most commonly located over the nasal bridge and cheeks (Fig. 149-6). Histologically, angiofibromas are characterized by fibrosis of the dermis and blood vessels. A number of childhood conditions are characterized by angiofibromas, but the most common is tuberous sclerosis. The term *adenoma sebaceum,* which is used to describe the lesions of tuberous sclerosis, is a misnomer; angiofibromas are not sebaceous in origin. Multiple angiofibromas may also be seen in patients with multiple endocrine neoplasia type I (MEN I) or in isolation in patients with no stigmata of MEN I. When a solitary angiofibroma occurs on the nose or face of a child, it is referred to as a *fibrous papule;* this is a benign process and requires no treatment.

ADNEXAL TUMORS

Pilomatricoma

Pilomatricoma (calcifying epithelioma) is by far the most common adnexal tumor in childhood. It is a benign tumor derived from hair matrix cells with a predilection for the head and neck. It commonly appears in the first or second decade of life and has a slight female preponderance.[11] Most are solitary nodules, but multiple lesions are present in approximately 5% to 8% of patients.[12] Although it is usually an isolated finding, the occurrence of multiple pilomatricomas can be seen with sarcoidosis, myotonic dystrophy,[13] Gardner syndrome,[14] and Rubinstein-Taybi syndrome.[15]

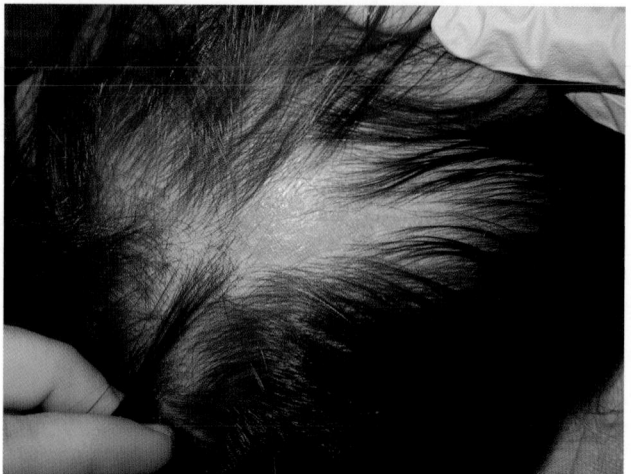

Figure 149-8   Nevus sebaceus. Hairless, waxy, yellow-orange plaque on the scalp.

Pilomatricomas are slowly growing, rock-hard nodules of varying size, usually 0.5 to 5 cm, that are fixed within the epidermis but freely mobile over underlying structures. The overlying skin is typically a normal color but may show a bluish discoloration (Fig. 149-7). These lesions frequently display the "teeter-totter" sign: one side of the lesion elevates when the other side is pushed down. The differential diagnosis includes epidermal inclusion cyst and other adnexal tumors. A pilomatricoma can discharge a chalky material and will continue to grow slowly if left untreated; it may also become inflamed and tender. Therefore, surgical excision is the treatment of choice.

Nevus Sebaceus

Nevus sebaceus, which was first described by Jadassohn in 1895, is a hamartoma composed of an excess of epidermal and glandular skin structures. This congenital hamartoma of the skin is usually seen on the head and neck. Lesions are typically round or oval, hairless, waxy, yellow-orange plaques on the scalp or linear plaques on the face (Fig. 149-8).

Because these lesions are stimulated by androgenic hormones, they may grow in early infancy due to maternal hormones and then become more verrucous at puberty. Histologically, these lesions contain sebaceous glands, abortive hair follicles, and apocrine sweat glands.

In addition to their cosmetic significance, these lesions may undergo benign or malignant transformation following puberty. In the past, this was believed to occur in 15% to 30% of lesions, and they were routinely excised to prevent deterioration into basal cell carcinoma and other cutaneous malignancies. It is now accepted that most of the basaloid tumors arising within nevus sebaceus are trichoblastomas, benign tumors that are histologically similar to basal cell carcinoma. There is increasing recognition that the rate of malignant transformation may be much lower than was previously thought—as low as 1%—and occurs predominantly after the fourth decade of life.[16]

The approach to nevus sebaceus is generally surgical excision in preadolescence under local anesthesia. Some large, cosmetically disfiguring lesions may be excised under general anesthesia in infants or toddlers. In addition, biopsy or excision is indicated if suspicious tumors develop within the nevus.

MALIGNANT TUMORS

Rhabdomyosarcoma

Rhabdomyosarcoma is the most common childhood sarcoma. It is also the most common malignant cutaneous sarcoma in childhood, although less than 1% of rhabdomyosarcomas involve the skin.[17] Approximately 50% of cases occur in children younger than 5 years, with 2% present at birth.[18] A cutaneous origin of rhabdomyosarcoma is rare. Most commonly, extension from the soft tissue into the dermis results in a papule, plaque, or nodule (Fig. 149-9). Given their vascular appearance, these lesions can be

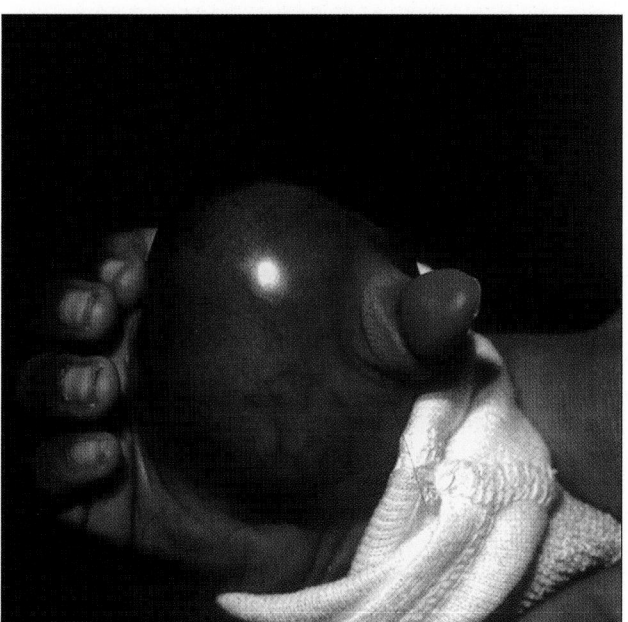

Figure 149-9 Rhabdomysarcoma. Given their vascular appearance, both clinically and on magnetic resonance imaging, these lesions may be misdiagnosed as hemangioma.

misdiagnosed as hemangiomas, cysts, or other malignancies (neuroblastoma, lymphoma). The radiographic interpretation of magnetic resonance imaging (MRI) findings is notoriously challenging. The diagnosis of rhabdomyosarcoma is therefore made by tissue biopsy.

Treatment is based on the extent of local, regional, and distant disease and consists of combinations of surgery, radiation, and chemotherapy.[19]

Fibrosarcoma

Although rare, fibrosarcoma is the second most common childhood sarcoma involving the skin. Lesions can present congenitally or during infancy, and almost all appear before 5 years of age. The tumors most frequently occur on the extremities and grow rapidly. The overlying skin may be tense, shiny, and erythematous, and ulceration may occur.[20] MRI may be useful in delineating the extent of the lesion, but diagnosis is based on histology.

Because the risk of metastasis is considerably lower in infants than in adults, surgery is the treatment of choice, with radiation and chemotherapy reserved for recurrences and metastases.

Neuroblastoma

Neuroblastoma arises from the primitive neurocrest cells that form the adrenal medulla and the sympathetic nervous system. This malignancy usually appears in newborns or young children, with 50% diagnosed in the first 2 years of life. Primary cutaneous neuroblastoma is a tumor of adulthood and is exceedingly rare. Although metastasis to the skin is rare, it is more common in newborns; 32% of newborns with neuroblastoma have cutaneous lesions.

The cutaneous metastases of neuroblastoma in children present as multiple blue to purple dermal papules or nodules. Manual rubbing of a neuroblastoma may lead to a ring of pallor known as an "icy blanch" due to local catecholamine release.[21] Serum and urine catecholamines are elevated in the majority of patients. Periorbital ecchymoses, due to orbital metastases, may also occur. Metastatic disease, characterized by fever, hepatomegaly, and failure to thrive, is often present at the time of diagnosis. The primary lesion is usually located in the upper abdomen, arising within the adrenal gland. The most common presentation is a hard abdominal mass, palpable in the flank.

The clinical differential diagnosis includes other cutaneous metastases, mastocytoma, angiolipoma, adnexal tumor, and cutaneous lymphoma. Clinically and histologically, the lesions of neuroblastoma must be differentiated from lymphoma and leukemia. In addition, the "blueberry muffin" appearance of some lesions may mimic congenital infections such as rubella or cytomegalovirus (see Chapter 164).

Important prognostic factors include age of the patient, clinical stage (based on tumor size and presence of metastasis), and type of tumor suppressor gene expression.[22] Treatment involves various combinations of surgery, radiation therapy, and chemotherapy, depending on staging. Children younger than 1 year at the time of diagnosis generally do well, with a 90% survival rate at 2 years.

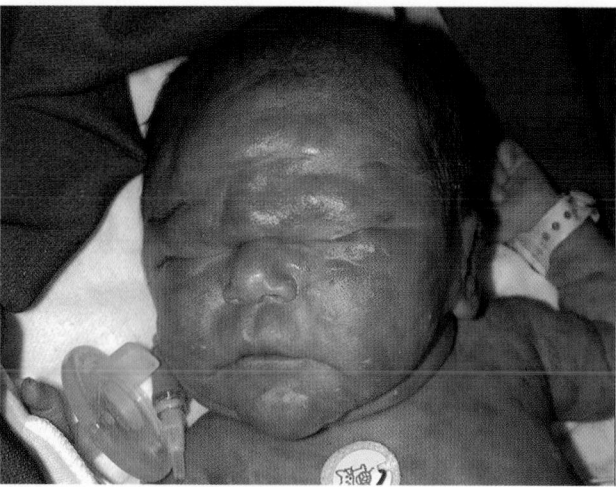

Figure 149-10 Leukemic infiltrates can cause thickening of the eyebrows and cheeks, producing a leonine facies.

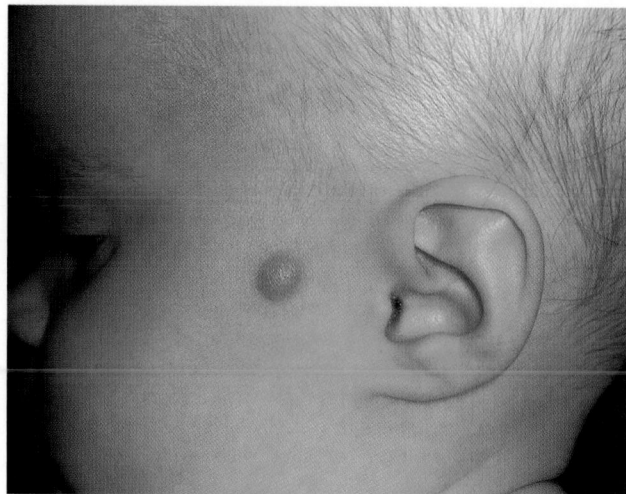

Figure 149-11 Juvenile xanthogranuloma. A yellow papule, most commonly located on the head or neck of a young child.

Leukemia Cutis

Cutaneous findings in leukemia include both leukemic infiltrates (occurring in approximately 1% of children with leukemia) and a host of secondary lesions such as petechiae, hemorrhage, Sweet syndrome, and erythema nodosum.[23] Leukemic infiltrates, known as leukemia cutis, appear as multiple discrete red-brown to violaceous papules and nodules. Leukemic infiltrates can also cause plaquelike thickening of the scalp, eyebrows, and cheeks, producing a typical leonine facies (Fig. 149-10). A biopsy of one of these lesions may show leukemic cells around blood vessels and between collagen bundles, although the type of leukemia cannot be determined from skin biopsy specimens. For diagnosis, the physical findings must be correlated with the interpretation of peripheral blood smears and bone marrow. Chemotherapy is the mainstay of treatment and varies with the type of leukemia.

Lymphoma Cutis

The lymphomas are a heterogeneous group of malignant neoplasms derived from B or T lymphocytes. They include Hodgkin's disease, non-Hodgkin's lymphoma, and mycosis fungoides (cutaneous T-cell lymphoma).

Hodgkin's disease is limited to the lymph nodes in 90% of cases, with cutaneous manifestations found in 13% to 40% of patients. Similarly, cutaneous manifestations occur in up to 26% of patients with non-Hodgkin's lymphoma; in about 5% of patients, they are the initial manifestation of the disease. As in patients with leukemia, the skin lesions may be specific (with histologic features of the disease) or nonspecific. Nonspecific skin signs include pruritus, purpura, hyperpigmentation, acquired ichthyosis, erythema nodosum, erythema multiforme, and urticaria.[24] Specific cutaneous lesions with histologic features of Hodgkin's disease are rare, occurring in 0.5% to 7.5% of patients, and are generally late manifestations. Such lesions are pink, reddish brown, or violaceous papules or nodules that may coalesce to form large tumors or plaques.[25] The lesions of non-Hodgkin's lymphoma are typically red, brown, or plum-colored and are often found in groups.

The treatment of this variable group of diseases includes combinations of surgery, chemotherapy, and radiation.

OTHER LESIONS

Juvenile Xanthogranuloma

Juvenile xanthogranuloma (JXG) is a fairly common disorder characterized by one or a few yellow, dome-shaped papules or nodules 1 to 2 cm in diameter, usually occurring in infancy or early childhood (Fig. 149-11). Almost 75% of lesions appear within the first year of life. No treatment is indicated in patients with disease limited to the skin, because the course is self-limited and benign. Cutaneous lesions usually regress spontaneously within 3 to 6 years.

Extracutaneous JXG has been reported in many organs, with the eye being the most commonly affected. Ocular JXG occurs in patients younger than 2 years and develops in less than 0.5% of patients with cutaneous lesions. However, approximately 40% of patients with ocular JXG have cutaneous lesions (always multiple) at the time of diagnosis. Because ocular JXG can lead to blindness, referral for slit-lamp examination to rule out ocular involvement is recommended in patients younger than 2 years with multiple cutaneous lesions.[26]

The association of JXG, neurofibromatosis 1 (NF1), and juvenile chronic myelogenous leukemia is well recognized. Patients with NF1 and JXG have at least a 20 times greater risk of developing juvenile chronic myelogenous leukemia, so patients with this conjunction should be followed closely for hematologic dyscrasias.[27]

SUGGESTED READING

Burgdorf WH, Ruiz-Maldonado R: Benign and malignant tumors. In Schachner LA, Hansen RC (eds): Pediatric Dermatology. Edinburgh, Mosby, 2003, p 881.

Knight PJ, Raimer SB: Superficial bumps in children: What, when and why? Pediatrics 1983;72:147-153.

REFERENCES

1. Knight PJ, Raimer SB: Superficial bumps in children: What, when and why? Pediatrics 1983;72:147-153.
2. Brownstein MH, Helwig EB: Subcutaneous dermoid cysts. Arch Dermatol 1973;107:237.
3. Paller AS, Pensler J, Tomita T: Nasal midline masses in infants and children: Dermoids, encephaloceles, and nasal gliomas. Arch Dermatol 1991;127:362-366.
4. Wardinsky TD, Poagon RA, Kropp RJ, et al: Nasal dermoid cysts: Association with intracranial extension and multiple malformations. Cleft Palate Craniofac J 1991;28:87.
5. Burgdorf WH, Ruiz-Maldonado R: Benign and malignant tumors. In Schachner LA, Hansen RC (eds): Pediatric Dermatology. Edinburgh, Mosby, 2003, p 881.
6. Muray JC, Pollack SV, Pinnell SR: Keloids: A review. J Am Acad Dermatol 1981;4:461.
7. Selmanowitz VJ, Stiller MJ: Rubinstein-Taybi syndrome: Cutaneous manifestations and colossal keloids. Arch Dermatol 1981;117:504.
8. Sanchez RL: The elusive dermatofibromas. Arch Dermatol 1990;126:522-523.
9. Checketts SR, Hamilton RK, Baughman RD: Congenital and childhood dermatofibrosarcoma protuberans: A case report and review of the literature. J Am Acad Dermatol 2000;42:907-913.
10. Snow SN, Gordon EM, Larson PO, et al: Dermatofibrosarcoma protuberans: A report of 29 patients treated by Mohs micrographic surgery with long-term follow-up and review of the literature. Cancer 2004;101:28-38.
11. Moehlenbeck FW: Pilomatricoma (calcifying epithelioma): A statistical study. Arch Dermatol 1973;109:532-534.
12. Agarwal RP, Handler SD, Matthews MR, Carpentieri D: Pilomatrixoma of the head and neck in children. Otolaryngol Head Neck Surg 2001;125:510-515.
13. Geh JL, Moss AI: Multiple pilomatrixomata and myotonic dystrophy: A familial association. Br J Dermatol 1999;52:143-146.
14. Pujol RM, Cassanova JM, Egido R, et al: Multiple familial pilomatricomas: A cutaneous marker for Gardner syndrome? Pediatr Dermatol 1995;12:331-335.
15. Cambiaghi S, Ermacora E, Brusasco A, et al: Multiple pilomatricomas in Rubinstein-Taybi syndrome: A case report. Pediatr Dermatol 1994;11:21-25.
16. Cribier B, Scrivener Y, Grosshans E: Tumors arising in nevus sebaceus: A study of 596 cases. J Am Acad Dermatol 2000;42:263-268.
17. Schmidt D, Fletcher CD, Harris D: Rhabdomyosarcomas with primary presentation in the skin. Pathol Res Pract 1993;189:422-427.
18. Ahmed OA, Hussain A, King DJ, et al: Congenital rhabdomyosarcoma. Br J Plast Surg 1999;52:304-307.
19. Maurer HM, Gehan EA, Beltangady M, et al: The Intergroup Rhabdomyosarcoma Study-II. Cancer 1993;71:1904-1922.
20. Balsaver AM, Butler JJ, Martin RG: Congenital fibrosarcoma. Cancer 1967;20:1607-1616.
21. Lucky AW, McGuire J, Komp DM: Infantile neuroblastoma presenting with cutaneous blanching nodules. J Am Acad Dermatol 1982;6:389-391.
22. Enzinger FM, Weiss SW: Benign tumors of peripheral nerves. In Soft Tissue Tumors, 4th ed. St Louis, Mosby, 2001, pp 1111-1207.
23. Su WP, Buechner SA, Li CY: Clinicopathologic correlations in leukemia cutis. J Am Acad Dermatol 1984;11:121-128.
24. Simon S, Azevedo SJ, Byrnes LL: Erythema nodosum heralding recurrent Hodgkin's disease. Cancer 1985;56:1470-1472.
25. White RM, Patterson JW: Cutaneous involvement in Hodgkin's disease. Cancer 1985;55:1136-1145.
26. Chang MW, Frieden IJ, Good W: The risk of intraocular juvenile xanthogranuloma: Survey of current practices and assessment of risk. J Am Acad Dermatol 1996;34:445-449.
27. Zvulunov A, Barak Y, Metzker A: Juvenile xanthogranuloma, neurofibromatosis, and juvenile chronic myelogenous leukemia: World statistical analysis. Arch Dermatol 1995;131:904-908.

CHAPTER 150

Purpura

Bernard A. Cohen

Purpura, or bleeding into the skin, may be an innocent finding in minor trauma or the first sign of a life-threatening disease. Pinpoint areas of hemorrhage are called petechiae; large, confluent patches are referred to as ecchymoses. Purpura may result from extravascular, intravascular, or vascular processes. Nonpalpable purpuric lesions develop from extravascular and intravascular phenomena, whereas those that are palpable result from a vascular process. Conditions associated with each type are listed in Table 150-1.

PATHOPHYSIOLOGY

Extravascular Purpura

Trauma is the most common cause of extravascular purpura in children. Nonblanching, nonpalpable purple patches following accidental trauma vary from a few millimeters to many centimeters in diameter and are usually located over bony prominences such as the knees, elbows, extensor surfaces of the lower legs, forehead, nose, and chin. In otherwise healthy children, petechiae occur occasionally on the face and chest after vigorous coughing or vomiting and in dependent areas after standing in place or engaging in vigorous physical activity for long periods.

The presence of purpura on protected or unexposed sites, such as the buttocks, spine, genitalia, upper thighs, and upper inner arms, suggests the possibility of nonaccidental trauma (Fig. 150-1). In some cases, the shape of the bruise provides a clue as to the object used to inflict the injury (see Chapter 175).[1]

Scars, nutritional deficiencies (e.g., vitamin C, protein), hereditary defects in collagen synthesis (e.g., Ehlers-Danlos syndrome), and other factors that increase skin fragility and decrease the tensile strength of the tissue surrounding vessels in the dermis and fat increase the risk of extravascular purpura after trauma.

Intravascular Purpura

Intravascular purpura results from disorders that interfere with normal coagulation. Nonpalpable petechiae and large ecchymoses may be present, and mucosal bleeding may be evident; in severe cases, bleeding may occur in the joints, deep soft tissues, kidneys, gastrointestinal tract, central nervous system, and other viscera. Disorders associated with intravascular purpura may result from abnormalities in platelet number or function or from deficiencies in coagulation factors. These disorders include autoimmune thrombocytopenic purpura, acute leukemia with thrombocytopenia, aplastic anemia, sepsis with disseminated intravascular coagulation (DIC), and various coagulation factor deficiencies.

Autoimmune thrombocytopenic purpura (ATP) is the most common type of intravascular purpura in previously healthy children. This condition was previously termed idiopathic or immune thrombocytopenic purpura. Patients typically present 2 to 4 weeks after a viral illness with petechiae and ecchymoses after minimal or no apparent trauma (Fig. 150-2). The incidence peaks in the later winter and early spring. Occult blood can often be detected in the stool and urine, but clinically significant hemorrhage is unusual. ATP is associated with the development of immunoglobulin (Ig) G antibodies that bind to platelets and trigger increased destruction by the reticuloendothelial system. Platelet counts may dip below 10,000/mm^3 for several weeks but usually return to normal within 4 to 6 weeks. Other cell lines are unaffected. Antiplatelet antibodies and thrombocytopenia can also develop in other less common disorders, including systemic lupus erythematosus, leukemia, lymphoma, and drug reactions.

Purpura can be an early manifestation of leukemia or aplastic anemia. These disorders may also be associated with anorexia, weight loss, fatigue, joint pain, and a persistent flulike illness. Hepatosplenomegaly, lymphadenopathy, and bone tenderness may be prominent. Bone marrow dysfunction from both leukemia and aplastic anemia may affect all cell lines, and patients may present with serious cutaneous infections or sepsis.

Purpura fulminans presents with rapidly progressive ecchymoses that may cover large areas of skin (Fig. 150-3). It represents the cutaneous manifestation of sepsis and DIC. Hemorrhage into multiple organs may also occur in this life-threatening process. Purpura is usually associated with ischemia, and in patients who survive, large areas of necrosis can develop. In normal children, meningococcal infections, Rocky Mountain spotted fever, and streptococcal infections are the most common cause of purpura fulminans, but a number of other bacterial, viral, and fungal organisms have been implicated in immunocompromised patients.[2,3]

Hereditary coagulation defects can also cause nonpalpable purpura. Children with hereditary deficiency or dysfunction of coagulation factors, most commonly factor VIII or IX, bruise easily but are less likely to develop petechiae. Patients with less than 1% of normal factor activity develop spontaneous hemorrhage and are usually diagnosed in early infancy; those with 1% to 5% of normal factor activity develop exaggerated bleeding at sites of trauma. Individuals with moderate reductions in factor function may not demonstrate cutaneous bleeding, and diagnosis may be delayed until they bleed excessively after major trauma or surgery.

Vascular Purpura

Vascular purpura develops when an inflammatory process involves the vessel wall, resulting in vasculitis. Leukocytoclastic vasculitis (LCV) is mediated by immune complex

Table 150-1 Pathophysiology of Purpura

Extravascular
Trauma
Accidental
Nonaccidental (iatrogenic, self-induced, abuse)
Defective collagen synthesis
Nutritional deficiency (vitamin C, protein, calorie)
Hereditary disorders (Ehlers-Danlos syndrome)

Intravascular
Thrombocytopenia
Autoimmune thrombocytopenic purpura
Systemic lupus erythematosus
Marrow failure (leukemia, lymphoma, aplastic anemia)
Drug induced
Infection and disseminated intravascular coagulation
Hereditary coagulation defects
Factor VIII or IX deficiency or dysfunction

Vascular
Small-vessel leukocytoclastic vasculitis
Henoch-Schönlein purpura
Drug induced
Collagen vascular disease (systemic lupus erythematosus)
Medium-sized arteritis
Polyarteritis nodosa
Lymphocytic vasculitis
Progressive pigmented purpuric dermatosis
Autoimmune? (Sjögren syndrome, drug reaction)

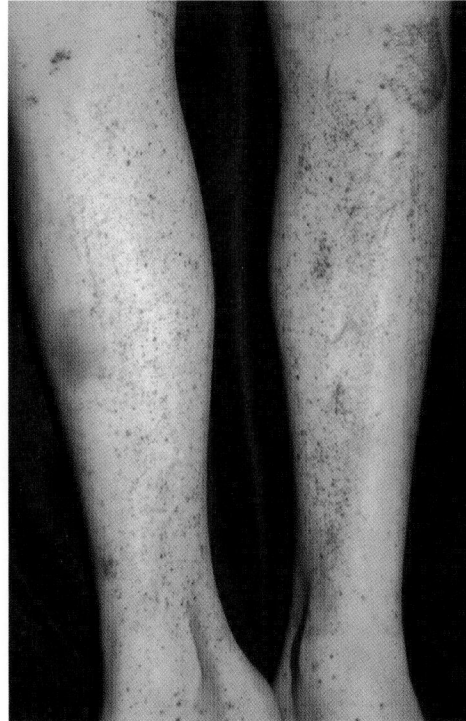

Figure 150-2 Autoimmune thrombocytopenic purpura, petechiae, and bruises in a 10-year-old boy.

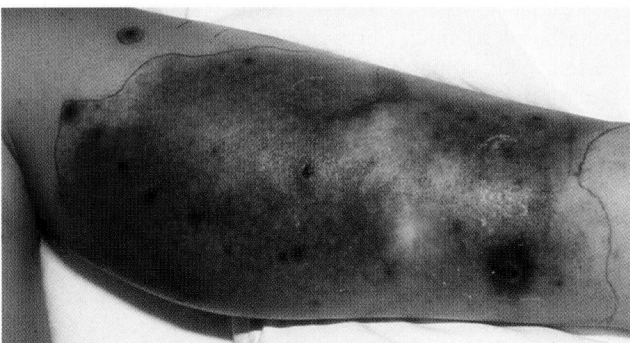

Figure 150-3 Purpura fulminans. Widespread purpura in a 9-year-old girl with disseminated intravascular coagulation following group A β-hemolytic streptococcal infection secondary to varicella.

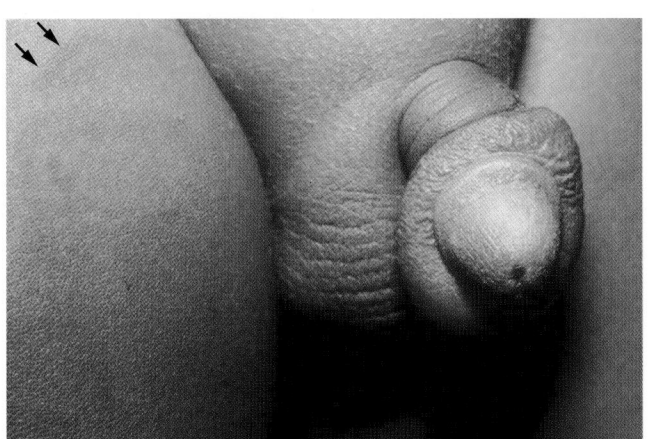

Figure 150-1 Belt-buckle imprint from a beating (*arrow*).

formation and deposition in the vascular basement membrane zone, with subsequent activation of complement and influx of neutrophils. The inflammatory process and subsequent destruction of vessels result in hemorrhagic papules and nodules referred to as palpable purpura. Lesions tend to produce angulated and starburst patterns conforming to the area of distribution of the involved vessels.[4]

Infectious agents, medications, autoimmune disorders, and malignancies can trigger LCV. Infectious agents (e.g., Rocky Mountain spotted fever, meningococcemia) can also invade and damage the vascular endothelium directly,

followed by leukocyte invasion. Therefore, the purpura associated with these infectious agents may be nonpalpable (related to DIC and sepsis), palpable (infectious vasculitis), or both.

In Henoch-Schönlein purpura (HSP), the most common vascular purpuric process in children, a small-vessel LCV typically results in palpable purpuric lesions less than 1 cm in diameter on the extensor surfaces of the arms, legs, buttocks, cheeks, and ears. Although early lesions may appear urticarial, as they evolve, confluent lesions may produce larger areas of purpura, bullae, necrosis, and ulceration (Fig. 150-4). HSP is also characteristically associated with crampy abdominal pain and periarticular swelling, but patients often appear well and are usually afebrile. Recurrences are seen in about half of patients for up to several months, but these

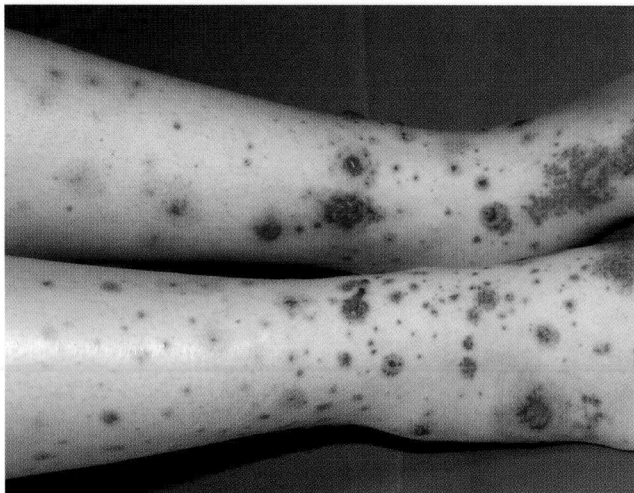

Figure 150-4 Leukocytoclastic vasculitis in 10-year-old boy with Henoch-Schönlein purpura.

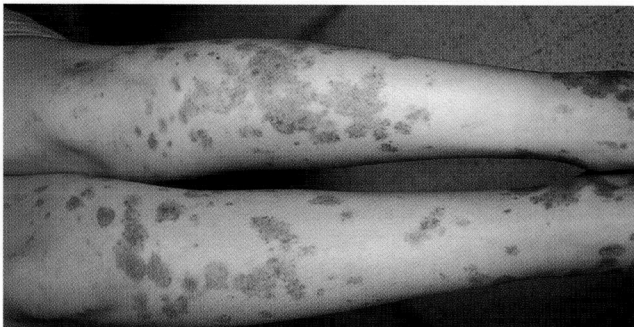

Figure 150-5 Progressive pigmented purpura in a 14-year-old with chronic bronze-red macules on the extremities for more than 1 year.

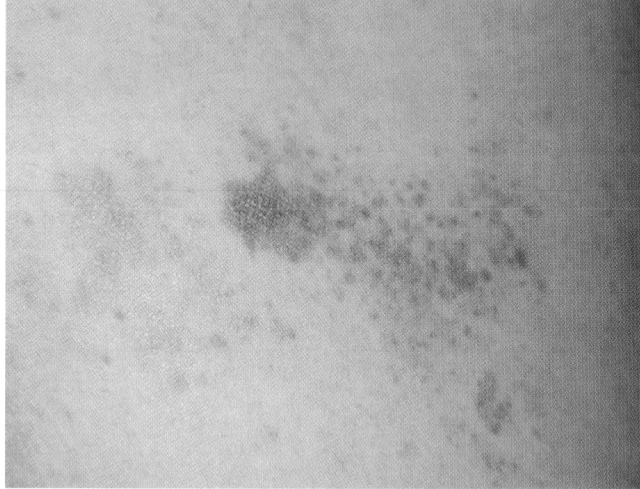

Figure 150-6 Pigmented purpura.

episodes are usually mild. In most cases, visceral disease is self-limited. However, renal involvement, consisting of nephritis or nephrosis, may precede, accompany, or follow the cutaneous manifestations. Patients with prolonged or serious cutaneous lesions may be at greater risk for the development of chronic renal disease.[5] HSP is discussed in greater detail in Chapter 103.

LCV in HSP involves small dermal blood vessels, usually postcapillary venules. Classic histologic findings include endothelial swelling, fibrin deposition within and around vessels, neutrophilic infiltrate within the vessel walls, and nuclear dust (scattered nuclear fragments from neutrophils). Direct immunofluorescence from biopsies of fresh skin lesions demonstrates IgA and C3 deposition around dermal blood vessels. A normal blood count, platelet count, and coagulation studies help differentiate HSP from disorders causing intravascular purpura. Typical clinical findings and clinical course, histopathology, and other screening laboratory studies exclude lupus and other connective tissue disorders.

Medication-induced LCV can produce a similar clinical and histologic picture, but immunofluorescence findings are negative. Although many drugs have been implicated as triggers of LCV, the most commonly reported medications include allopurinol, antibiotics, nonsteroidal anti-inflammatory drugs, diphenylhydantoin (phenytoin), and thiazide diuretics.

Polyarteritis nodosa (PAN) is an LCV involving small and medium-sized arteries but is rare in children. A systemic form presents acutely with high fever, weakness, abdominal pain, and cardiac failure. Despite aggressive treatment with anti-inflammatory and immunosuppressive medications, death may ensue quickly from renal failure, gastrointestinal bleeding, and bowel perforation. Nonspecific cutaneous findings include livedo reticularis, erythema, and purpura on the extremities. Livedo reticularis appears as a red to purple fishnet-like blanching or marbling of the skin. Cutaneous PAN is a distinct variant in which skin findings predominate and systemic disease is minimal. Crops of painful purpuric nodules and annular plaques erupt on the hands and feet and, less commonly, on the trunk, face, and neck.

Urticaria, livedo reticularis, and ulcerations may develop. Although life-threatening visceral disease does not occur in this form of PAN, fever, arthralgias, myalgias, and periarticular swelling may accompany flares of cutaneous lesions. PAN is diagnosed by skin biopsy, and patients require long-term monitoring to exclude progression to systemic disease.[6,7]

Lymphocytic vasculitis refers to a reaction pattern in the skin that is associated with a number of disorders in which lymphocytic inflammation predominates in the walls and around superficial dermal capillaries. Lymphocytic vasculitis has been described in cutaneous drug reactions, Sjögren syndrome, and the late phase of LCV. Progressive pigmented purpuric dermatosis (PPPD) is the only disorder in which lymphocytic vasculitis occurs consistently (Fig. 150-5). The development of asymptomatic patches of petechiae and confluent purpura, particularly on the lower extremities, characterizes PPPD. Hemosiderin deposition and postinflammatory hyperpigmentation in the chronic lesions lead to shades of brown, gold, and bronze as the lesions evolve (Fig. 150-6). Although the lesions are usually macular, subtle eczematous and lichenoid papules may develop. Eruptions may persist for years, but systemic symptoms do not occur, and laboratory studies are normal.[8]

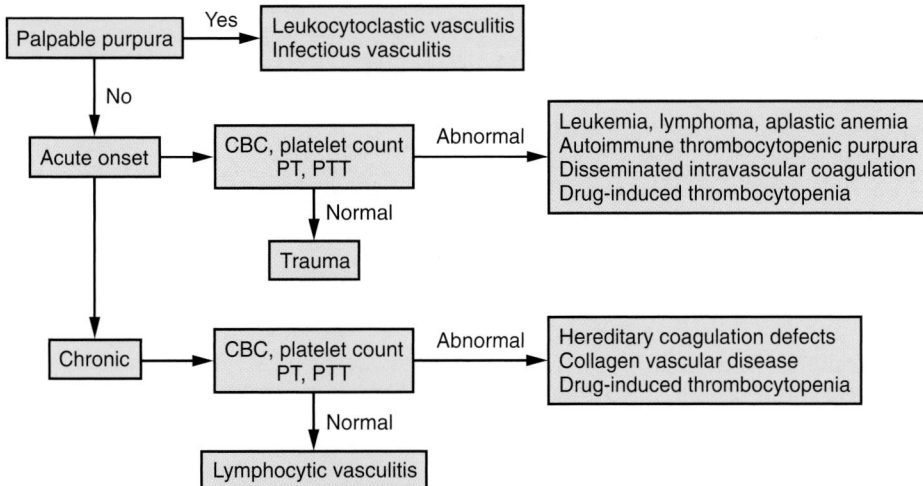

Figure 150-7 Algorithm for the diagnosis of purpura. CBC, complete blood count; PT, prothrombin time; PTT, partial thromboplastin time.

CLINICAL PRESENTATION

Any child who presents with purpura requires a complete history, review of systems, family history, and physical examination with an emphasis on cutaneous and systemic findings that may provide diagnostic clues (Fig. 150-7).

Purpura may resemble hyperemia that results from increased blood flow through dilated vessels. Diascopy is used to differentiate hyperemia from the cutaneous hemorrhage of purpura. Diascopy involves applying pressure to the skin either by pressing it apart between the thumb and index finger or by applying a glass or plastic slide over the involved skin surface. Hyperemic areas blanch with diascopy, but purpuric lesions do not.

During the first few minutes of the visit, the clinician should determine whether the child is acutely ill. A toxic-appearing patient with fever, headache, hypotension, or diffuse purpura requires an immediate evaluation for septicemia and DIC. Transfer to a facility that can provide rapid clinical and laboratory assessment, cardiovascular and respiratory support, and prompt initiation of therapy (e.g., empirical antibiotics) is required.

In a well-appearing child, a thorough history and physical examination can be completed. Aside from a description of the rash and its evolution and the events surrounding its appearance, questions regarding recent illnesses or medication use should be asked. Exploration of the child's past medical history should include previously diagnosed coagulation disorders or collagen vascular diseases, unusual diet, weight loss, bone pain, anemia, joint laxity, poor wound healing, abnormal scarring, or easy bruising. A surgical history is important to determine whether abnormal bleeding was detected.

Children with suspected nonaccidental trauma, as well as healthy children with no history of trauma or unusually shaped skin lesions, warrant laboratory evaluation. Consultation with a child protective agency may be indicated. A family history of skin fragility, poor skin healing, wide disfiguring scars, increased bruising, anemia, hemophilia, or collagen vascular disease should prompt an evaluation for hereditary disorders that predispose to bleeding and cutaneous purpura.

In a well-appearing child with unexplained petechiae or purpura, the entire skin surface and the mucous membranes should be examined, and all findings should be carefully documented. Bruises in unusual shapes suggesting nonaccidental trauma should prompt an evaluation for other signs of occult physical trauma and child abuse, and cutaneous findings should be photographed.

LABORATORY EVALUATION

When the cause of cutaneous bleeding is not apparent, a complete blood count and coagulation studies can help exclude intravascular purpura. When indicated, specific quantitative and functional coagulation factor studies should be performed.

In children with doughy or hyperextensible skin and wide disfiguring scars, particularly if there is a family history of similar findings, a skin biopsy for routine pathology or electron microscopy may confirm the suspicion of Ehlers-Danlos syndrome or other genodermatoses associated with increased bruisability.

The evaluation of palpable purpura should include a biopsy with direct immunofluorescence. When septicemia is suspected, tissue should also be submitted for bacterial or fungal culture. Tissue may also be subjected to marker studies (polymerase chain reaction, immunoperoxidase, double fluorescent antibody) for specific organisms, if available. PPPD can be confirmed by characteristic histologic findings.

TREATMENT

Treatment should be tailored to the specific disorder when a cause is identified, such as coagulopathy (see Chapter 120), malignancy, autoimmune disorder, or infection (see Chapter 62).[2] Patients with hyperextensibility syndrome and Ehlers-Danlos syndrome should take precautions to protect the skin from trauma. There is no uniformly effective therapy for PPPD. However, treatment with topical steroids, topical nonsteroidal anti-inflammatory agents, and yellow pulsed dye laser has been successful in some patients.

IN A NUTSHELL

- Nonblanching red eruptions in the skin should prompt an evaluation for purpura.
- The initial evaluation should promptly determine whether a life-threatening infectious process is present.
- Purpura can arise from intravascular, extravascular, and vascular causes. Intravascular and extravascular purpura cause nonpalpable lesions; a vascular process leads to palpable lesions.
- Trauma is the most common cause of purpura, but nonaccidental injury should be considered when the distribution is not typical of accidental injury or the history is not consistent with a plausible mechanism of injury.

ON THE HORIZON

- In patients with a family history of coagulation defects, genetic markers may allow early detection and prophylactic therapy. Specific mutational analysis is increasingly available for disorders that predispose to coagulopathy, LCV, and genodermatoses associated with platelet dysfunction and easy bruisability.

SUGGESTED READING

Ballinger S: Henoch-Schönlein purpura. Curr Opin Rheumatol 2003;15:591-594.

Bauzo A, Espana A, Idoate M: Cutaneous polyarteritis nodosa. Br J Dermatol 2002;146:694-699.

Darmstadt GL: Acute infectious purpura fulminans: Pathogenesis and medical management. Pediatr Dermatol 1998;15:169-183.

Siberry GK, Cohen BA, Johnson B: Cutaneous polyarteritis nodosa: Report of cases in children and review of the literature. Arch Dermatol 1994;130:884-889.

Tristani-Firouzi P, Meadous KP, Vanderhooft S: Pigmented purpuric eruption of childhood. Pediatr Dermatol 2001;18:299-304.

Warren PM, Kagan RJ, Yakaboff KP, et al: Current management of purpura fulminans: A multicenter study. J Burn Care Rehabil 2003;24:119-126.

Yalcindag A, Sundel R: Vasculitis in childhood. Curr Opin Rheumatol 2001;13:422-427.

REFERENCES

1. Mudd SS, Findlay JS: The cutaneous manifestations and common mimickers of physical child abuse. J Pediatr Health Care 2004;18:123-129.
2. Warren PM, Kagan RJ, Yakaboff KP, et al: Current management of purpura fulminans: A multicenter study. J Burn Care Rehabil 2003;24:119-126.
3. Darmstadt GL: Acute infectious purpura fulminans: Pathogenesis and medical management. Pediatr Dermatol 1998;15:169-183.
4. Yalcindag A, Sundel R: Vasculitis in childhood. Curr Opin Rheumatol 2001;13:422-427.
5. Ballinger S: Henöch-Schonlein purpura. Curr Opin Rheumatol 2003;15:591-594.
6. Bauzo A, Espana A, Idoate M: Cutaneous polyarteritis nodosa. Br J Dermatol 2002;146:694-699.
7. Siberry GK, Cohen BA, Johnson B: Cutaneous polyarteritis nodosa: Report of cases in children and review of the literature. Arch Dermatol 1994;130:884-889.
8. Tristani-Firouzi P, Meadous KP, Vanderhooft S: Pigmented purpuric eruption of childhood. Pediatr Dermatol 2001;18:299-304.

CHAPTER 151

Vesicles and Bullae

Andrea L. Zaenglein

The diagnosis of vesicular and bullous diseases in childhood can be a difficult task. To better understand the defining characteristics of vesiculobullous disorders, a general knowledge of skin anatomy is helpful. Figure 151-1 illustrates normal skin histology. The numerous causative entities can be divided into those with neonatal and childhood onsets. Secondary characteristics, such as distribution and morphology, further limit the differential diagnosis.

It is important to have a clear understanding of the terminology used to describe vesicular or bullous lesions and their associated physical features. A *vesicle* is a fluid-filled, dome-shaped lesion of 0.5 cm or less; if such a lesion is greater than 0.5 cm, it is termed a *bulla*. The fluid inside may be clear or hemorrhagic in nature. If the material is purulent, the lesion is called a *pustule*. Secondary lesions, including crusting, excoriation, scaling, milia, and scarring, may also be noted. An *erosion* is a superficially denuded vesicle with damage confined to the epidermis. *Ulceration* is a deeper lesion, with loss of the entire depth of the epidermis. Secondary scarring does not usually result from erosion but is common with ulceration, given the depth of the injury, or it may result from a secondary infectious process (Table 151-1; Fig. 151-2).

Whether the vesicle or bulla is flaccid or tense is another defining characteristic. A tense bulla suggests a deeper process in which the split in the epidermis lies below the level of the lamina lucida located in the basement membrane zone. This gives the lesion enough support to hold the fluid tense under pressure. In contrast, a flaccid bulla is a more superficial process that generally occurs higher in the epidermis, where skin tension may easily disrupt the lesion's integrity (Fig. 151-3). Helpful in differentiating a tense from a flaccid bulla are the Nikolsky and Asboe-Hansen signs. A positive Nikolsky sign occurs when a blister is induced by rubbing normal-appearing skin with the eraser of a pencil. The Asboe-Hansen sign is elicited by applying lateral pressure to the edge of a bulla away from the center. If the lesion extends, the spilt is higher up in the epidermis, and the lesion is classified as flaccid. If the lesion does not extend, a deeper split is suggested, and the lesion is defined as tense.

CLINICAL PRESENTATION

The clinical presentation of the numerous vesiculobullous conditions varies tremendously, depending on whether the lesion is a primary process or a manifestation of an underlying illness. A complete history should include the duration of disease, previous or current infection, other family members affected, recent travel, environmental or household exposures, and associated symptoms. A thorough review of systems can help ascertain the severity of the illness, and systemic complaints such as fever, arthralgias, lethargy, and weight loss may help define a cause. Special care must be taken in the evaluation of neonates, because associated symptoms are not always well defined in this age group, and occult infection can easily be missed. If an adverse drug reaction is suspected, a detailed drug history is essential. Even regularly used over-the-counter medications, such as nonsteroidal anti-inflammatory drugs, can cause blistering reactions, including bullous fixed drug reactions, pseudoporphyria, or even toxic epidermal necrolysis. A detailed family history is vital to the diagnosis of many genetic vesiculobullous disorders, including various forms of epidermolysis bullosa simplex and Hailey-Hailey disease. A positive family history of autoimmune diseases may also assist in making a diagnosis.

Aside from identifying the nondermatologic features on physical examination, a clear description of the skin lesions is necessary, using the terms defined earlier. Delineating the nature of the lesions, the pattern of eruption, and its arrangement and distribution can be invaluable in differentiating among vesiculobullous diseases. Note whether the lesions are grouped or scattered, localized to a specific area or generalized, or linear or annular in configuration; note whether they follow the lines of Blaschko or occur in a dermatomal distribution. It is also important to identify the duration and timing of the lesions. The history should reveal whether the lesions are acute, subacute, or chronic in duration. Lesions may appear at the same time, in crops, or follow a cyclical pattern, with periods of activity followed by resolution. The lesions may appear to be recently erupted, resolving, or a mixed pattern. Attention to the mucosal surfaces is important, because many systemic blistering disorders involve the oral, genital, or ocular mucosal surfaces.

DIFFERENTIAL DIAGNOSIS

As previously stated, the age of onset of a disorder is an important clue in the diagnosis of vesiculobullous disorders. The differential diagnoses of neonatal and childhood vesiculobullous disorders are described in Tables 151-2 and 151-3, respectively.[1-6] Lesions that appear in the neonatal period may be genetic, infectious, or even iatrogenic. Infectious causes should always be considered in a newborn with vesiculobullous findings. If the lesions are congenital, a genetic blistering disorder should be considered. Some autoimmune disorders can be transferred through the presence of maternal antibodies, up to about 6 months of age. Disorders in this category include neonatal lupus, neonatal pemphigus, and pemphigus foliaceus.

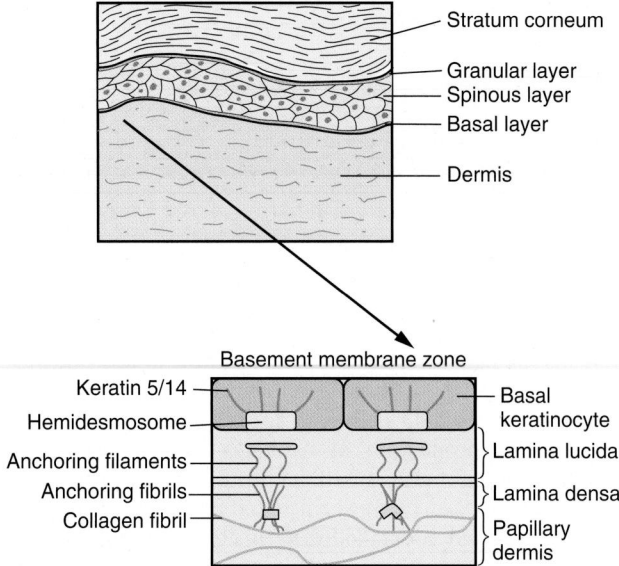

Keratin 5/14
Hemidesmosome
Anchoring filaments
Anchoring fibrils
Collagen fibril

Stratum corneum
Granular layer
Spinous layer
Basal layer
Dermis

Basement membrane zone

Basal keratinocyte
Lamina lucida
Lamina densa
Papillary dermis

Figure 151–1   Normal skin histology.

Table 151–1   Definition of Vesiculobullous Lesions: Primary and Secondary Findings

Lesion	Definition
Primary	
Vesicle	Fluid-filled lesion ≤0.5 cm
Bulla	Fluid-filled lesion >0.5 cm
Pustule	Blistering lesion filled with purulent exudate
Secondary	
Erosion	Partial loss of epidermis
Ulceration	Complete loss of epidermis with extension into dermis
Excoriation	Scratched primary lesions; may be linear or crusted
Scaling	Dry, superficial accumulations of keratin
Crusting	Dried serous, hemorrhagic, or purulent exudate (i.e., scabbing)
Milia	Small 1-2 mm epidermal cysts

EVALUATION

Although in many cases the clinical picture is sufficient to determine the diagnosis, laboratory testing is indicated in certain situations. The laboratory workup of a patient with a vesiculobullous disorder should include investigations to rule out plausible causes and those that may place the patient at risk for significant morbidity or mortality, whether benign, infectious, acquired, or genetic. If a viral cause is suspected, a Tzanck smear, rapid fluorescent antibody stain, polymerase chain reaction assay, or viral culture should be considered to rule out herpes and varicella infections. If a bacterial cause is suspected, a Gram stain and appropriate cultures can aid in the diagnosis of gram-positive and gram-negative bacterial infections. A Wright stain can help elucidate the predominant inflammatory cell type (e.g., neutrophils, eosinophils, or mixed infiltrates). For suspected fungal infections, Giemsa stain or a potassium hydroxide preparation can help identify hyphal and yeast forms. A particularly thorough workup should be done in neonates and in immunocompromised children of all ages. Infectious diseases can present atypically in these special patients, and without timely diagnosis and treatment, the outcome can be devastating. The workup of a neonate with a blistering disorder of unknown cause is outlined in Table 151-4.

TREATMENT

Aside from treatment of the underlying cause or condition, there are some general principles regarding the management of vesicles and bullae. As a rule, vesicles and small bullae should not be disturbed. Open lesions should kept clean by gentle washing with a soapless cleanser, coating with bland petrolatum (Aquaphor is typically used in the neonatal population), and covering with a sterile bandage if needed. If a large bulla is intact and in an area that causes pain, or if it keeps expanding due to pressure, the fluid can be drained using a sterile large-bore needle or number 11

blade. A linear incision should be made near the base of the bulla to allow drainage of the fluid contents. The incision should be large enough to ensure that the bulla will not reform after drainage but small enough to keep the blister roof in place, because unroofed lesions are more painful. With extensive denudation, fluid and electrolyte management may be challenging owing to the increased insensible losses. Temperature control may be disrupted, especially in neonates. Pain may be significant and requires special attention. Pain control may be needed around the clock or during certain activities such as dressing changes and physical therapy.

CONSULTATION

- Dermatology for assistance with diagnosis, inpatient management, and, if the condition is ongoing, outpatient follow-up.
- Infectious diseases for recommended testing and interpretation of results, empirical antibiotic therapy, and adjustment of therapy.
- Critical care or burn center when cardiorespiratory support is needed, the extent of bedside interventions exceeds the capacity of a noncritical care setting, or resources and expertise are unavailable at the existing institution.
- Physical or occupational therapy for maintaining or reestablishing mobility, reconditioning, or implementing medical equipment (e.g., splints).
- Plastic surgery for the management of skin lesions that may require grafting or the revision of scars.

ADMISSION CRITERIA

- Because neonates with blistering conditions are at high risk for serious infectious or other life-threatening conditions, they require hospitalization to conduct an appropriate evaluation, initiate therapy, and manage potential complications.

Text continued on p. 966.

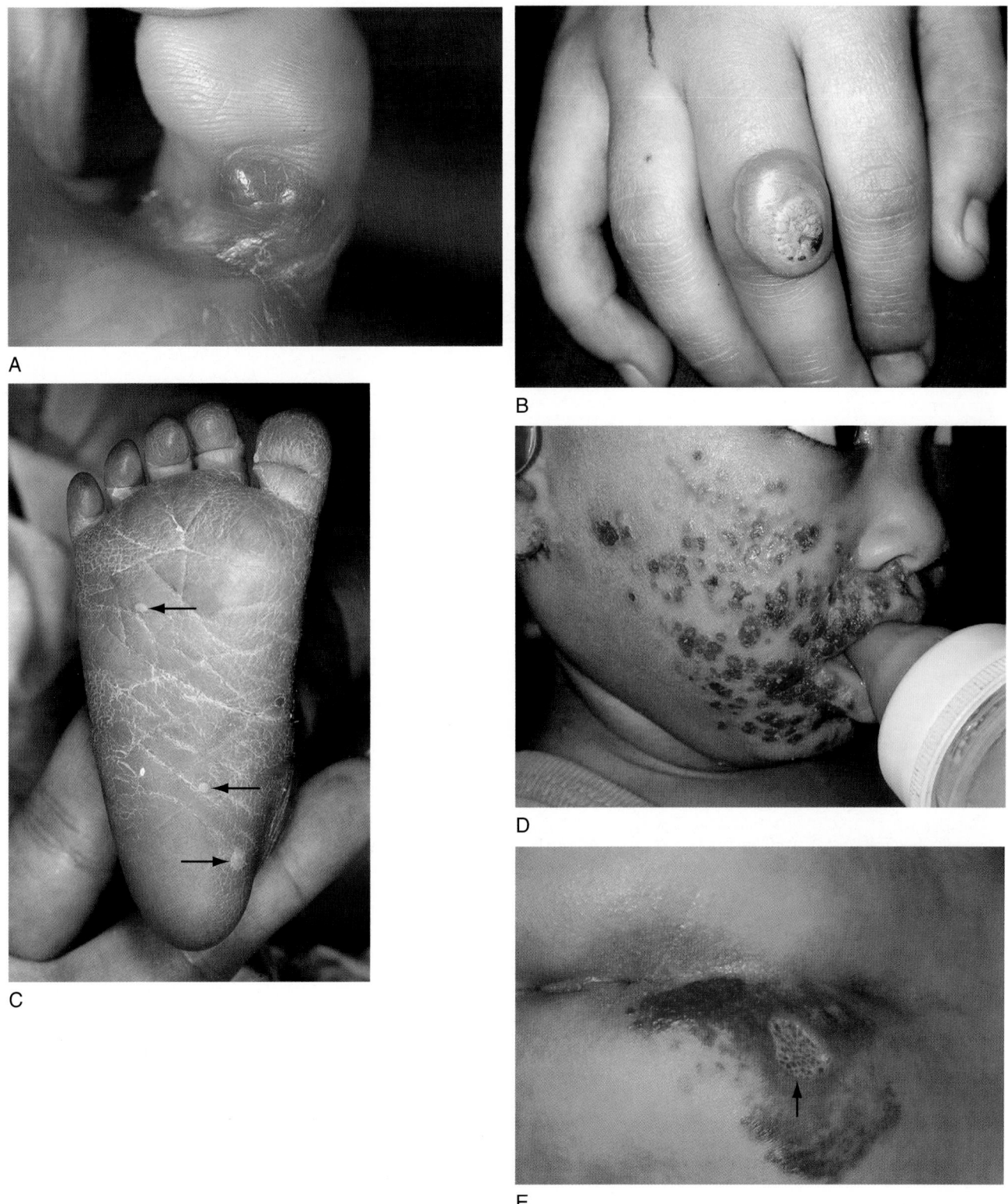

Figure 151-2 Clinical examples. A, Vesicle (scabies). B, Bulla (adverse reaction to topical cantharidin). C, Pustules (transient neonatal pustular melanosis). D, Erosion (eczema herpeticum). E, Ulcer (ulcerated infantile hemangioma).

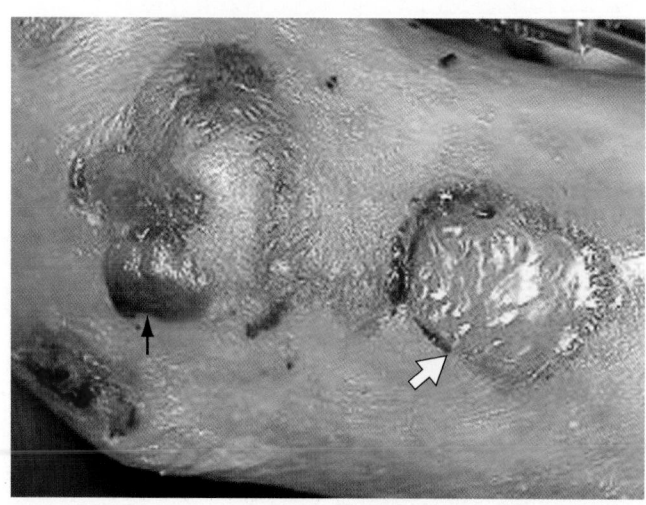

Figure 151-3 Flaccid (*open arrow*) and tense (*solid arrow*) bullae in a patient with recessive dystrophic epidermolysis bullosa.

Table 151-2 Neonatal Vesiculobullous Disorders

Disorder	Onset and Duration	Clinical Characteristics	Diagnosis
Benign, transient			
Erythema toxicum neonatorum	24-72 hr after birth; lasts 1 wk	Blotchy erythema with small central pustule; generalized, except palms and soles; full-term, healthy infants	Clinical; Gram stain: eosinophils
Neonatal acne	Weeks to months	Erythematous papules and pustules on face and chest; healthy neonates	Clinical; stains mostly negative, but may see yeast forms
Transient neonatal pustular melanosis	Birth; hyperpigmentation lasts months	Pustules without erythema; collarette when wiped away; heals, but hyperpigmentation lasts months; generalized, palms, and soles; healthy neonates; more common in darker pigmented skin types	Clinical; Gram stain: neutrophils
Miliaria (rubra or crystallina)	Days to months; lasts hours to days	Small erythematous papules (rubra) to clear vesicles (crystallina) on forehead, upper chest, and back; history of fever, overheating	Clinical; all stains negative
Infantile acropustulosis	Days to months; may last 2-3 yr	Extremely pruritic vesicles and pustules occurring in crops on hands and feet	Clinical; biopsy
Eosinophilic pustular folliculitis	Birth to 1 yr; may last years	Pruritic follicular-based papules and pustules on scalp and face; very rare	Biopsy
Congenital Langerhans cell histiocytosis	Birth to days	Vesicles to crusted papules, petechiae; solitary to numerous; scalp, groin, flexures most common	Biopsy; electron microscopy
Sucking blister	Birth or later	Noninflamed blister; usually solitary; most often on hands or wrists	Clinical; all stains negative
Inflammatory			
Mastocytosis	Birth to several months	Mastocytoma: solitary pink, tan, or brown macule to indurated plaque with overlying bullae	Clinical; all stains negative; biopsy showing mast cells
		Urticaria pigmentosa: multiple lesions as described for mastocytoma	
		Diffuse cutaneous mastocytosis: peau d'orange (indurated yellowish orange skin) with vesicles and bullae at sites of trauma	
Infectious			
Syphilis	Birth	Vesicles and bullae, often eroded; perioralo (snuffles), hands, and feet; may be localized or generalized; associated with hepatosplenomegaly and pseudoparalysis	Serology; DFA; darkfield examination
Candidiasis, congenital	Birth to 24 hr; lasts 2 wk	Generalized erythema and pustules or vesicles	KOH: pseudohyphae

Table 151-2 Neonatal Vesiculobullous Disorders—cont'd

Disorder	Onset and Duration	Clinical Characteristics	Diagnosis
Candidiasis, neonatal	Past 1 wk of age	Erythematous macules or papules with satellite pustules; diaper area and flexures most commonly affected	KOH: pseudohyphae
Herpes simplex	Birth to weeks	Vesicles or pustules; erosions to scarring; localized to generalized	Tzanck, DFA, PCR, culture, or serology
Varicella	Birth	Linear scarring, erosions; often affects extremities; fetal anomalies occur with first- or second-trimester infection	Tzanck, DFA, PCR, culture, or serology
Scabies	Weeks	Vesicles to crusted papules, nodules with burrows; hands, feet, axilla, scalp	Mineral oil preparation
Genetic			
Incontinentia pigmenti	Birth	Linear and whorled vesicles along lines of Blaschko; progresses to verrucous lesions; localized to limb or generalized; may be associated with seizures, retinopathy, and eosinophilia	Biopsy; genetic testing (*NEMO* gene)
Epidermolysis bullosa	Birth to teens (for certain forms such as Weber-Cockayne)	Noninflammmatory vesicles, bullae; often eroded; milia with dystrophic forms; extremities most often affected; severity depends on type; some forms associated with pyloric atresia, GI involvement, failure to thrive	Biopsy; electron microscopy; genetic testing (keratins 5/14, plectin, laminin 5, collagen XVII, α6β4 integrin, collagen VII)
Transient bullous dermolysis of the newborn	Birth; resolves within months	Extensive blistering due to transient defect in collagen VII	Biopsy; electron microscopy
Epidermolytic hyperkeratosis (bullous congenital ichthyosiform erythroderma)	Birth	Generalized erythema and scaling with bullae and erosions; evolves to generalized ichthyosis with flexural predominance	Biopsy; genetic testing (keratins 1/10)
Ichthyosis bullosa of Siemens	Birth	Milder blisters and erosions than epidermolytic hyperkeratosis; episodic superficial peeling	Clinical; biopsy; genetic testing (keratin 2e)
AEC syndrome (Hay-Wells)	Birth	Associated with erosive scalp dermatitis	Clinical; genetic testing (*p63* gene)
Ectodermal dysplasia; skin fragility syndrome	Birth	Generalized erythema with superimposed bullae, erosions; perioral redness and desquamation; sparse hair and dystrophic nails; abnormal sweating	Biopsy; genetic testing (plakophilin)
Congenital erosive and vesicular dermatosis	Birth; heals in weeks to months	Premature infants; diffuse vesicles, erosions, and crusting; palms, soles, face relatively spared; heals with reticulated scarring	Biopsy
Kindler syndrome	Birth to months	Acral blistering that later develops poikiloderma	Biopsy; electron microscopy
Metabolic			
Acrodermatitis enteropathica	Birth to 6 mo	Copper-colored patches and plaques; perioral region, groin, hands, and feet; overlying vesicles and bullae	Low serum zinc level; low alkaline phosphatase
Autoimmune			
Herpes gestationis	Birth; resolves in weeks	Very pruritic, urticarial plaques with overlying tense vesicles, bullae; results from transfer of maternal antibodies; self-limited	Biopsy; direct and indirect immunofluorescence
Neonatal pemphigus	Birth; resolves in a few weeks	Pruritic, urticarial plaques with flaccid bullae, erosions; occurs in infants of mothers with active pemphigus vulgaris or foliaceus due to transfer of maternal antibodies	Maternal history; biopsy; direct and indirect immunofluorescence

AEC, ankyloblepharon–ectodermal dysplasia–clefting; DFA, direct fluorescent antibody; GI, gastrointestinal; KOH, potassium hydroxide; NEMO, NF-kappa B essential modulator; PCR, polymerase chain reaction.

Table 151-3 Infantile and Childhood Vesiculobullous Disorders

Disorder	Clinical Characteristics	Diagnosis
Acquired		
Psoriasis (pustular)	Widespread erythematous, well-defined papules with overlying pustules; may be exacerbated by systemic corticosteroid use	Biopsy; Giemsa stain shows sterile neutrophils
Allergic contact dermatitis	Very pruritic; may be localized or generalized; erythematous papulovesicles to bullae; linear distribution with poison ivy	Clinical; biopsy
Dyshidrotic eczema	Erythematous papulovesicles to bullae on hands and feet; may have generalized reaction	Clinical; biopsy
Erythema multiforme	Targetoid to bullous erythematous macules or maculopapules; palms, soles, mucous membranes frequently affected; HSV most common trigger	Clinical; biopsy
Stevens-Johnson syndrome; toxic epidermal necrolysis	Generalized erythematous macules to morbilliform eruption, with frequent progression to flaccid bulla formation and widespread desquamation; mucosal involvement common; drugs, infections, vaccinations may trigger	Clinical; biopsy
Phototoxic; drug	Erythematous macules or papulovesicles with vesicle or bulla formation in photodistribution	Clinical; biopsy
Acute generalized exanthematous pustulosis	Generalized erythematous small papules or erythroderma studded with numerous small pustules; associated with sudden fever; drug, viral, mercury, immunization triggers possible	Clinical; biopsy
Burn	Well-defined to figured erythema with overlying vesicle or bulla formation; may be sign of abuse	Clinical
Friction blister	Noninflamed vesicle to bulla at site of friction	Clinical
Coma blister	Noninflamed bulla occurring in comatose patient; possible associated bruising; generally occurs 24 hr after onset of coma	Clinical
Hydroa vacciniforme	Crusted erosions with varioliform scarring; photodistribution	Clinical
Autoimmune		
Pemphigus vulgaris	Generalized flaccid, easily eroded, crusted bullae; Nikolsky sign positive; may be drug induced	Biopsy with direct and indirect immunofluorescence
Pemphigus foliaceus	Erythematous, very superficially crusted, eroded, polycyclic plaques; most common on the head and neck	Biopsy with direct and indirect immunofluorescence
Paraneoplastic pemphigus	Generalized pemphigus lesions with severe mucosal lesions common; often refractory to treatment; may be associated with lymphoma or Castleman tumor	Biopsy with direct and indirect immunofluorescence
Epidermolysis bullosa acquista	Skin fragility to tense bulla formation; healing with scarring and milia; mucous membranes may be involved	Biopsy with immunofluorescence
Bullous pemphigoid	Urticarial plaques with overlying tense bullae; may be annular or polycyclic; facial and palmar or plantar involvement more common in children	Biopsy with direct and indirect immunofluorescence
Bullous lupus erythematosus	Generalized, pruritic, tense bullae; predominantly photodistributed; very rare in childhood	Biopsy with immunofluorescence; antinuclear antibodies
Dermatitis herpetiformis	Intensely pruritic papulovesicles to vesicles; symmetrical over extensor surfaces; often associated with gluten-sensitive enteropathy	Biopsy with immunofluorescence
Linear IgA disease (chronic bullous disease of childhood)	Abrupt onset of tense vesicles or bullae, often in string-of-pearls configuration; groin and perioral region favored; mucous membrane involvement common	Biopsy with immunofluorescence
Genetic		
Hailey-Hailey disease	Moist, erythemtous, eroded plaques in flexures; may have vesicles or pustules; presents in second to fourth decades	Biopsy; family history; genetic testing (*ATP2C1* gene)
Epidermolysis bullosa	Noninflammatory bullae appearing at sites of trauma; may present from birth to teen years	Biopsy; family history; genetic testing
Pachyonychia congenita	Hypertrophic nails, hyperkeratotic palms and soles, leukokeratosis beginning in infancy to childhood; bullae may form at sites of friction usually in late childhood	Clinical; genetic testing (keratins 6/16 or 17)

Table 151-3 Infantile and Childhood Vesiculobullous Disorders—cont'd

Disorder	Clinical Characteristics	Diagnosis
Porphyrias (congenital erythropoietic porphyria, porphyria cutanea tarda, variegate porphyria)	All may have varying degrees of photosensitivity with blistering; severe types present early, porphyria cutanea tarda in childhood	Biopsy; porphyrin testing
Infectious		
Impetigo	Honey-colored, crusted, oozing vesicles with erythema; may be primary infection (common in perioral, perinasal regions) or secondary infection (atopic dermatitis, varicella); caused by *Staphylococcus, Streptococcus,* or both	Clinical; Gram stain; culture
Blistering distal dactylitis	Erythema with bullae on distal fingers; caused by β-hemolytic streptococci	Clinical; Gram stain; culture
Staphylococcal scalded skin syndrome	Painful erythema with localized flaccid bullae; may generalize to erythroderma; patient is ill appearing, with malaise, fever; Nikolsky sign positive; neonates most susceptible; caused by staphylococcal exfoliative toxins	Clinical; cultures from mucosal surfaces and blood
Scabies	Vesicles to crusted papules or nodules with burrows; hands, feet, axilla, scalp (in infants)	Mineral oil preparation
Bullous arthropod reaction	Pruritic vesicles, bullae, pustules on exposed areas; causes include fleas, red ants	Clinical; biopsy
Herpes simplex	Grouped vesicles on erythematous base; erosions may heal with scarring; painful oral ulcerations in primary outbreaks; localized (perioral, genital) to generalized (eczema herpeticum)	Tzanck, DFA, PCR, culture, or serology
Varicella (chickenpox)	Crops of pruritic vesicles that are pustular and crusted; can heal with scarring; caused by varicella-zoster virus	Clinical, DFA, PCR, culture
Zoster	Dermatomal distribution of urticarial papules or plaques to vesicles; pain may be associated, but less than in adults	Clinical, DFA, PCR, culture
Dermatophytosis	Annular, pink, scaling pruritic plaques; often bullous on the feet or hands	KOH
Hand-foot-and-mouth disease	Oval vesicles and bullae on hands and feet; painful erosions in mouth; caused by coxsackievirus A16	Clinical

DFA, direct fluorescent antibody; HSV, herpes simplex virus; KOH, potassium hydroxide; PCR, polymerase chain reaction.

Table 151-4 Workup for Unidentified Vesicular or Pustular Rash in Neonates

Study	Cause
Direct preparations	
Tzanck	Herpesviruses
Gram	Bacteria
Potassium hydroxide	Fungal elements
Mineral oil	Scabies
Giemsa or Wright	Inflammatory cell type
Darkfield	Syphilis
Fluorescent antibody testing	Herpes simplex virus, varicella-zoster virus, syphilis, immunobullous disorders
Histology	
Biopsy	If cause cannot otherwise be ascertained
Electron microscopy	Epidermolysis bullosa, Langerhans cell histiocytosis
Laboratory	
Complete blood count with differential	Infectious and parasitic causes, incontinentia pigmenti (eosinophils)
Zinc, alkaline phosphatase	Acrodermatitis enteropathica
Polymerase chain reaction	Herpes simplex virus, varicella-zoster virus, enterovirus
Porphyrins	Porphyria
Antinuclear antibody	Lupus erythematosus

- Infants and children with vesiculobullous eruptions warrant admission when a serious condition is suspected that requires prompt diagnosis or therapy.
- Patients demonstrating rapid progression or extensive skin involvement merit hospitalization.
- Patients unable to tolerate sufficient oral intake or manage skin care in the outpatient setting should be admitted.

DISCHARGE CRITERIA

- Stabilization of the patient and control of the underlying condition.
- Ability to complete necessary therapy in the outpatient setting.
- Adequate follow-up in place.

IN A NUTSHELL

- Vesiculobullous disorders constitute a wide variety of conditions, including some that are benign and self-limited, acute or chronic, disfiguring, debilitating, or even life-threatening.
- The clinical presentation often provides sufficient diagnostic information, but when a serious causative or underlying condition is suspected, appropriate infectious, immunologic, genetic, or autoimmune testing is indicated.
- Many vesiculobullous conditions are self-limited, but complications of the skin lesions can include scarring, deformities, recurrence, superinfection, fluid and electrolyte imbalance, and pain.
- In general, skin care involves gentle cleansing and application of bland petroleum jelly to all open areas. Any infectious causes should be treated concomitantly.

ON THE HORIZON

- Rapid techniques to identify herpes simplex virus and varicella-zoster virus are becoming more widespread. Real-time detection methods using polymerase chain reaction technology allow the earlier identification of herpesviruses.[7]
- Gene therapy for genetic blistering disorders such as epidermolysis bullosa is currently being explored.[8]

SUGGESTED READING

Eichenfield LF, Larralde MM: Neonatal skin and skin disorders. In Schachner LA, Hansen RC (eds): Pediatric Dermatology, 3rd ed. London, Mosby, 2003, pp 205-262.

Frieden IJ, Howard R: Vesicle, pustules, bullae, erosions and ulceration. In Eichenfield LF, Frieden IJ, Esterly NB (eds): Textbook of Neonatal Dermatology. Philadelphia, WB Saunders, 2001, pp 137-178.

Lucky AW: Transient benign cutaneous lesions in the newborn. In Eichenfield LF, Frieden IJ, Esterly NB (eds): Textbook of Neonatal Dermatology. Philadelphia, WB Saunders, 2001, pp 88-102.

Pauporte MC, Frieden IJ: Vesiculobullous and erosive diseases in the newborn. In Bolognia JL, Jorizzo JL, Rapini RP (eds): Dermatology. London, Mosby, 2003, pp 509-524.

Van Praag MCG, Van Rooij RWG, Folkers E, et al: Diagnosis and treatment of pustular disorders in the neonate. Pediatr Dermatol 1997;14:131-143.

REFERENCES

1. Eichenfield LF, Larralde MM: Neonatal skin and skin disorders. In Schachner LA, Hansen RC (eds): Pediatric Dermatology, 3rd ed. London, Mosby, 2003, pp 205-262.
2. Pauporte MC, Frieden IJ: Vesiculobullous and erosive diseases in the newborn. In Bolognia JL, Jorizzo JL, Rapini RP (eds): Dermatology. London, Mosby, 2003, pp 509-524.
3. Lucky AW: Transient benign cutaneous lesions in the newborn. In Eichenfield LF, Frieden IJ, Esterly NB (eds): Textbook of Neonatal Dermatology. Philadelphia, WB Saunders, 2001, pp 88-102.
4. Frieden IJ, Howard R: Vesicle, pustules, bullae, erosions and ulceration. In Eichenfield LF, Frieden IJ, Esterly NB (eds): Textbook of Neonatal Dermatology. Philadelphia, WB Saunders, 2001, pp 137-178.
5. Van Praag MCG, Van Rooij RWG, Folkers E, et al: Diagnosis and treatment of pustular disorders in the neonate. Pediatr Dermatol 1997;14:131-143.
6. Meadows KP, Egan CA, Vanderhooft S: Acute generalized exanthematous pustulosis, an uncommon condition in children: Case report and review of the literature. Pediatr Dermatol 2000;17:399-402.
7. van Doornum GJ, Guldemeester J, Osterhaus AD, Niesters HG: Diagnosing herpesvirus infections by real-time amplification and rapid culture. J Clin Microbiol 2003;41:576-580.
8. Ferrari S, Pellegrini G, Mavilio F, De Luca M: Gene therapy approaches for epidermolysis bullosa. Clin Dermatol 2005;23:430-436.

CHAPTER 152

Psoriasis

James G. H. Dinulos

Psoriasis is a papulosquamous skin condition characterized by red, scaly papules and plaques. It accounts for approximately 4% of all scaly rashes seen in children younger than 16 years.[1] The incidence is higher in the United States (4.6%) than in Europe (1.5%), with a peak incidence between age 20 to 30 years and 50 to 60 years. Genetic factors are important in the underlying cause of psoriasis. Thirty percent to 90% of patients have a family history of psoriasis.[2] When both parents have psoriasis, the risk of a child developing psoriasis is 41%; when one parent has psoriasis, the risk is 14%; and if one sibling has psoriasis, the risk is 6%.[3] Environmental influences can unmask a genetic susceptibility for psoriasis. Group A streptococcal pharyngitis commonly precedes guttate psoriasis, suggesting that superantigens or other bacterial influences are important underlying causes of this form of psoriasis. Often, human immunodeficiency virus (HIV) unmasks an underlying genetic susceptibility, causing patients to develop psoriasis or exacerbating preexisting psoriasis. Psychological stress and medications such as beta-blockers, antimalarial drugs, and lithium have long been known to exacerbate psoriasis. Intense social stigmatization and emotional disability can be brought on by even a few psoriatic plaques; thus, children with psoriasis must be approached with compassion and followed closely. The pediatric hospitalist must be able to recognize the various clinical presentations, identify environmental factors that exacerbate psoriasis, assist dermatologists in developing appropriate inpatient treatment regimens, and arrange for close outpatient follow-up care. Although hospitalization is rare for this condition, some complications of the disease, such as cellulitis or sepsis, may warrant admission.

PATHOPHYSIOLOGY

Psoriatic plaques develop thick scales in large part because of the increased number of keratinocytes recruited to proliferate and differentiate, although the cell cycle in psoriasis is thought to be normal.[3] The reasons for this increased keratinocyte recruitment are unknown but are thought to be driven by the inflammatory infiltrate seen in psoriatic lesions. T lymphocytes account for the majority of inflammatory cells seen in psoriatic plaques, and activated T lymphocytes ($CD4^+$ and $CD8^+$) are present in psoriatic lesions. It is currently thought that these T lymphocytes produce cytokines capable of interacting with keratinocytes to produce altered cellular differentiation and proliferation. T lymphocytes produce a number of cytokines, such as interleukin-10, tumor necrosis factor-α, and interleukin-8, that are thought to be relevant to the altered cellular proliferation and differentiation.

CLINICAL PRESENTATION

Psoriasis is a highly heterogeneous skin condition with varying degrees of severity and many possible clinical presentations (Table 152-1). The most common type of psoriasis is psoriasis vulgaris, or plaque psoriasis (Fig. 152-1). Classically, the lesions are described as having a mica-like scale that is adherent peripherally to the plaque. Removal of this scale can result in bleeding at the site of detachment (Auspitz sign). Commonly, psoriatic plaques are distributed on the scalp, elbows, knees, torso, and buttocks. Psoriasis may occur at sites of skin trauma. This isomorphic or Koebner phenomenon can assist in the diagnosis of psoriasis, and patients should be warned to avoid cuts and abrasions. Usually, plaque psoriasis begins subtly with one or two isolated lesions. Some children continue to have minimal skin findings; however, many go on to develop more widespread, recalcitrant plaque psoriasis.

Guttate psoriasis is characterized by widespread round to oval plaques. Frequently, there is a preceding streptococcal pharyngitis. Guttate psoriasis can disappear as quickly as it appears and has a better prognosis than does plaque psoriasis (Fig. 152-2).

In addition to lesions that have thick, white (micaceous) scales, psoriatic lesions can form pustules, especially at the edges of the plaques. This form of psoriasis, called pustular psoriasis, is more difficult to treat, often requiring systemic therapy. Pustular psoriasis seen on the palms and soles can be exacerbated by smoking. Fortunately, pustular psoriasis is less common in children.

Psoriasis can also manifest as acute, widespread plaques coalescing into diffuse whole-body redness (erythroderma) (Fig. 152-3). Patients are often acutely ill with fever and malaise. When the skin barrier is compromised with erosions, patients are at risk for sepsis.

Arthritis can occur in 5% to 30% of patients with psoriasis,[4] but this is less common in children than in adults. Psoriatic arthritis can be associated with minimal psoriasis, and the extent of the skin lesions does not appear to correlate with the severity of the arthritis. The most common presentation of psoriatic arthritis is involvement of the proximal and distal interphalangeal joints of the hands and feet (asymmetrical oligoarthritis). Rarely, psoriatic arthritis is progressive and results in extensive joint destruction (arthritis mutilans).

Psoriasis is a condition that can be localized to specific sites, such as the scalp, palms and soles (palmar-plantar psoriasis), nails, and tongue (geographic tongue). Characteristic nail changes include nail pitting and onycholysis (separation of the nail plate from the nail bed). Patients with psoriasis can develop yellow spots within the nail that look like oil droplets.

Table 152-1 Variants of Psoriasis

Variant	Clinical Features	Treatment	Special Considerations
Plaque psoriasis	Sharply demarcated plaques, most commonly on scalp and extensor surfaces but can be isolated, especially in children	Low-strength corticosteroids for face and folds; medium- to high-strength for torso, extremities, and scalp	Can start with one isolated plaque; usually chronic
Guttate psoriasis	Generalized small, oval plaques with abrupt onset; often associated with streptococcal disease (pharyngitis > perianal > impetigo)	Topical medium-potency corticosteroids with sauna suit; consider phototherapy and oral antibiotic (penicillin)	Prognosis is better than for plaque psoriasis; many children have spontaneous remission in weeks to months
Pustular psoriasis	Pustules may be subtle, occurring at edges of a plaque, or widespread, with formation of "lakes of pus"; may be localized to palms and soles	Systemic therapy with cyclosporine and acitretin indicated for widespread pustular psoriasis or debilitating localized palmar or plantar pustular psoriasis	Rare in children
Erythrodermic psoriasis	Generalized redness with scaling and skin barrier breakdown	Wet dressings or sauna suit with medium-potency corticosteroids; consider systemic therapy with cyclosporine	Often seen with taper of systemic corticosteroids

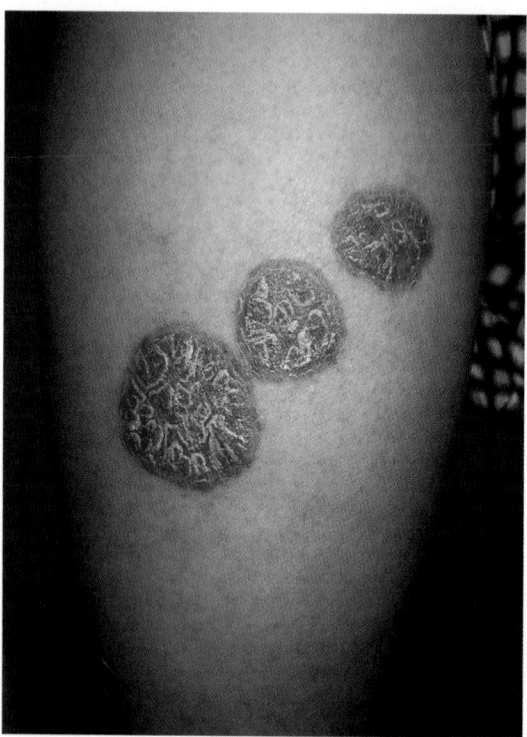

Figure 152-1 Plaque psoriasis. (Courtesy of Albert C. Yan, MD.)

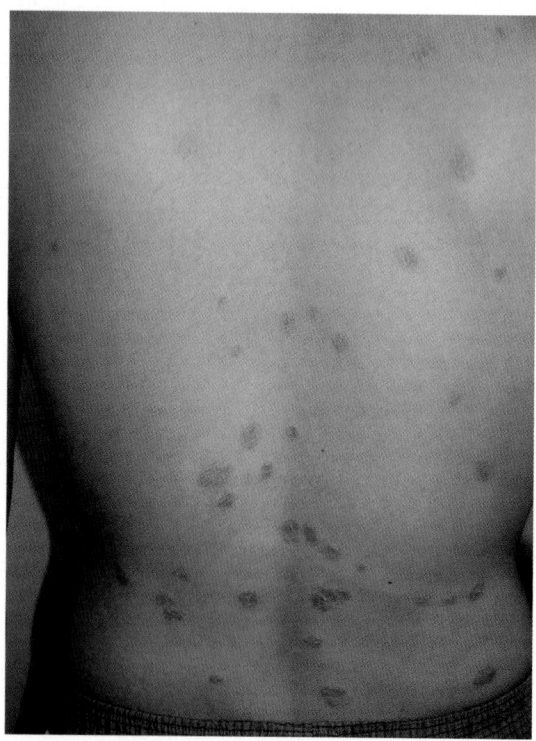

Figure 152-2 Guttate psoriasis. (Courtesy of Albert C. Yan, MD.)

When psoriasis involves primarily the intertriginous regions, it is referred to as inverse psoriasis. Pink, weepy plaques in the gluteal cleft and characteristic nail changes may be helpful in diagnosing more localized, subtle cases.

DIFFERENTIAL DIAGNOSIS

Many other skin disorders manifest with scaly "psoriasiform" plaques, including pityriasis rosea; tinea corporis, capitis, or cruris (dermatophytosis); seborrheic dermatitis; syphilis; ichthyosis; tinea versicolor; nummular eczema; discoid lupus erythematosus; lichen planus; T-cell lymphoma; and pityriasis lichenoides.[5]

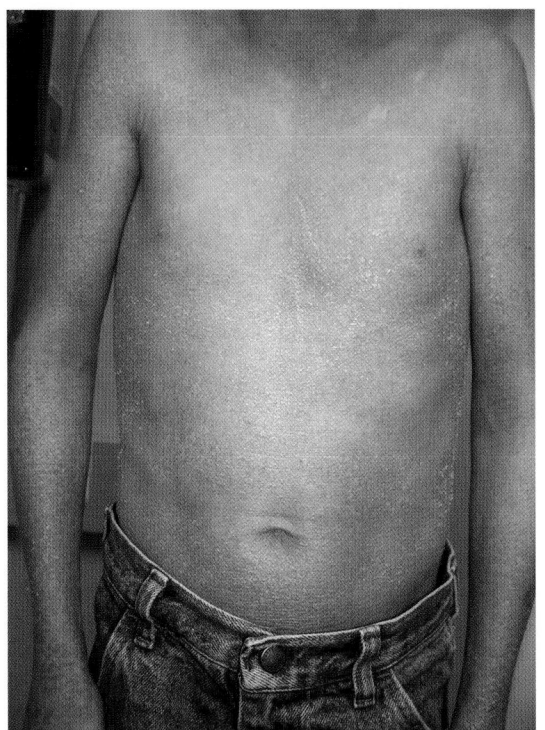

Figure 152-3 Erythrodermic psoriasis. (Courtesy of Albert C. Yan, MD.)

Table 152-2 Topical Medications for Childhood Psoriasis

Corticosteroids
    Low potency: hydrocortisone acetonide 1%, desonide 0.05%,
        fluocinolone acetonide 0.01%
    Medium potency: triamcinolone acetonide 0.1%,
        mometasone furoate 0.1%, hydrocortisone valerate 0.2%
    High potency: clobetasol propionate, betamethasone
        dipropionate 0.05%, halobetasol propionate 0.05%

Calcipotriene
Coal tar
Anthralin
Tazarotene
Tacrolimus
Pimecrolimus

DIAGNOSIS

Diagnosis is based on the complete clinical picture. No specific laboratory testing can confirm the diagnosis; however, some tests may help eliminate alternative diagnoses under consideration. Patients presenting with infectious complications such as cellulitis or sepsis warrant wound and blood cultures and a complete blood count. Evidence of the involvement of other organs with septic shock is evaluated as appropriate.

TREATMENT

Most childhood psoriasis is managed with topical medications applied directly to the skin. For more widespread skin lesions, phototherapy (ultraviolet B; psoralen plus ultraviolet A) and systemic medications are helpful. The type and severity of psoriasis determine treatment regimens. The impact of psoriasis on psychosocial development and long-term safety issues must be addressed when treating children. For example, there are critical junctures in psychosocial development (e.g., adolescence) when tight control of psoriasis is essential. In addition, because psoriasis is a chronic condition that usually requires many years of therapy, long-term medication toxicity must be considered.

Psoriasis may be the primary reason for hospital admission, or it may be a secondary issue unrelated to the reason for admission. Topical corticosteroids are the mainstay of therapy for mild to moderate plaque psoriasis (Table 152-2). Medium- to high-strength corticosteroids are useful for plaque psoriasis on the extremities and body, and low-strength corticosteroids should be applied to plaques on the face and intertriginous areas. Wet dressings are useful to decrease cutaneous inflammation and augment the penetration of topical corticosteroids. One method of applying wet dressings in children is to have them wear wet pajamas, covered with dry pajamas. Topical medications are applied after the pajamas are removed and the skin dried. Occlusion with plastic wraps or sauna suits can be helpful for recalcitrant lesions. Care must be taken when applying corticosteroids under the diaper, because the occlusion increases the corticosteroid's potency. Topical medications are generally applied twice daily. In the inpatient setting, they can be applied three times a day for more widespread skin involvement. In most cases, ointments are preferable to creams; however, some children do not like the greasiness of ointments.

Corticosteroids used over large surface areas or on small infants can cause suppression of the hypothalamic-pituitary axis. Skin thinning, acneiform eruptions, and telangiectasia are potential side effects of corticosteroids. For this reason, corticosteroids are combined with another topical medications to limit corticosteroid exposure. These "steroid-sparing" agents often improve the efficacy of the corticosteroid and prevent tachyphylaxis, which is sometimes seen with long-term corticosteroid use. Triamcinolone acetonide 0.1% is commonly compounded with tar (5% to 10%). Topical vitamin D_3 (calcipotriene), tacrolimus, pimecrolimus, and anthralin may be helpful adjuncts to topical corticosteroids.

Scalp psoriasis can be difficult to treat because the scale is typically thick and the hair impedes application of the medication. Massaging olive oil into the whole scalp and then covering the head with a moist, warm towel (olive oil turban) for 30 minutes, followed by gentle combing, is an effective method of removing excess scale. Over-the-counter tar shampoos with or without salicylic acid are effective to decrease inflammation and remove thick scale. Fluocinolone shampoo (for mild scalp psoriasis) and clobetasol shampoo (for more severe cases) are effective treatments. Corticosteroid solutions and foams are also available to treat scalp psoriasis.

Inverse psoriasis and facial psoriasis can be effectively controlled with low-strength corticosteroids, tacrolimus, and pimecrolimus. Tacrolimus and pimecrolimus do not thin

Table 152-3	Systemic Medications for Childhood Psoriasis		
Medication	Mechanism of Action	Oral Dose	Short-Term Side Effects
Methotrexate	Binds dihydrofolate reductase—decreases folates and inhibits DNA synthesis	0.3-0.5 mg/kg (max 25 mg), given weekly	Nausea, vomiting, malaise
Cyclosporine	Binds cyclophilin—decreases T-lymphocyte production	2-5 mg/kg, given daily in divided doses, 1.0 mg/kg-2.5 mg/kg per dose	Hypertension
Acitretin	Binds retinoid receptors (RXRα/RARγ)—inhibits epidermal proliferation	0.25-1 mg/kg, given daily (maximum 50 mg/day)	Cheilitis, dry skin

the skin, but they can cause a mild degree of burning when first applied. This side effect improves over time.

Rarely, medications such as cyclosporine, methotrexate, and acitretin are administered to abate an acute flare of psoriasis (Table 152-3). Pediatric patients with more severe forms of psoriasis—pustular flares or erythroderma—may require both topical and systemic therapy. Consultation with a specialist is strongly recommended in these cases. Subsequent maintenance therapy with topical and systemic medications, or transition to newer targeted biologic agents, can then be considered.

Systemic corticosteroids such as prednisone should not be used to treat severe psoriasis, because rebound erythroderma or a diffuse flare of pustules can occur with steroid withdrawal. Children with psoriasis who are placed on systemic corticosteroids for other comorbid conditions, such as asthma, should be monitored closely for psoriasis flares after discontinuing the corticosteroids.

CONSULTATION

A dermatologist can provide a definitive diagnosis of psoriasis, help with inpatient management, and establish a relationship with the patient for ongoing outpatient therapy.

Infectious disease specialists can offer guidance with empirical therapy or ongoing management of infectious complications.

Critical care services may be necessary if sepsis with cardiovascular instability develops.

ADMISSION CRITERIA

Widespread psoriasis with erythroderma is associated with systemic illness (fever, malaise) that may necessitate hospital admission for hydration. Prompt evaluation is needed, because these patients are at risk for sepsis or extensive cellulitis due to skin erosions.

DISCHARGE CRITERIA

Patients admitted for infectious complications can be discharged to complete therapy as outpatients when they are cardiovascularly stable, afebrile, and tolerating oral hydration, and when appropriate outpatient follow-up is in place.

IN A NUTSHELL

- Psoriasis, although an uncommon reason for hospitalization, may be a concomitant condition in hospitalized patients.
- Four variants of psoriasis are recognized: plaque, guttate, pustular, and erythrodermic.
- Infectious complications of psoriasis, such as cellulitis or sepsis, are conditions that warrant admission.
- Topical treatments may include topical steroids or topical steroid-sparing agents (e.g., tar). Thick scaling, especially of the scalp, may improve with applications of olive oil or over-the-counter tar shampoos.
- Phototherapy with ultraviolet light is effective for moderate to severe psoriasis.
- Severe or recalcitrant psoriasis may require systemic therapy and is best managed in conjunction with a specialist in dermatology.

ON THE HORIZON

- Targeted medical therapy, using molecules capable of blocking key steps in T-lymphocyte activation and cytokine production, are being developed for the treatment of psoriasis.

SUGGESTED READING

Lebwohl M: Psoriasis. Lancet 2003;361:1197-1204.

van de Kerkhof P: Psoriasis. In Bolognia GL, Jorizzo JL, Rapini RP (eds): Dermatology. London, Mosby, 2003, pp 125-149.

REFERENCES

1. Watson W, Cann HM, Farber EM, et al: The genetics of psoriasis. Arch Dermatol 1972;105:197-207.
2. Farber EM, Bright RD, Nall ML: Psoriasis: A questionnaire survey of 2144 patients. Arch Dermatol 1968;98:248-259.
3. van de Kerkhof P: Psoriasis. In Bolognia GL, Jorizzo JL, Rapini RP (eds): Dermatology. London, Mosby, 2003, pp 125-149.
4. Espinoza LR, Cuellar ML, Silveira LH: Psoriatic arthritis. Curr Opin Rheumatol 1992;4:470-478.
5. In Habif: Clinical Dermatology, 4th ed. Mosby, 2004, pp 2-12.

CHAPTER 153

Vascular Anomalies

Caroline C. Kim, Marilyn G. Liang, and John B. Mulliken

Vascular anomalies are relatively common in the pediatric age group. Approximately a third of infants are born with a vascular birthmark. Although most lesions are uncomplicated and benign, some require treatment and inpatient care. The pediatric hospitalist should be able to recognize the major kinds of vascular anomalies and appreciate which lesions require referral or immediate medical care in collaboration with vascular anomalies specialists in the fields of dermatology, surgery, hematology/oncology, pathology, and radiology.

CLASSIFICATION

In 1996, vascular anomalies were reclassified into malformations and tumors.[1,2] Vascular malformations are composed of structurally abnormal vessels with normal endothelial turnover and can consist of capillary, venous, lymphatic, arterial, or arteriovenous vessels alone or in combination. Vascular malformations are subcategorized by channel architecture and rheology as slow flow or fast flow. These anomalies can be stable or progressive; they never regress. In contrast, vascular tumors arise by endothelial hyperplasia; they can be benign, borderline, or sometimes malignant. Each of these two categories is addressed separately in this chapter.

Malformations
    Capillary
    Venous
    Arterial
    Lymphatic
    Combined
Tumors
    Infantile hemangioma
    Congenital hemangioma
    Kaposiform hemangioendothelioma
    Tufted angioma

VASCULAR MALFORMATIONS

Capillary malformations are usually slow flow, localized, and well circumscribed, but they can also be regional, diffuse, or part of a syndrome. The 19th century term for capillary malformation is "port-wine" stain. Capillary malformations are pink to red homogeneous patches at birth and are permanent. They must be differentiated from the common fading macular stains of infancy, commonly called angel's kiss, stork bite, or salmon patch. These evanescent vascular marks typically present at or shortly after birth as a pink to red, nonblanching patch on the forehead or nape of the neck and can also be seen on the upper eyelids, nose, and lips. Most of these lesions disappear after 1 or 2 years; however, some, such as those on the nape of the neck, may

persist for life and are therefore recategorized as capillary malformations. A variant, the butterfly-shaped mark, which has been described as occurring in the midline sacral area, also tends to persist. As with other congenital lesions in the midline of the spine such as an asymmetric gluteal cleft, hair, or dimpling, stains in this location warrant further evaluation for occult spinal dysraphism. Capillary malformations may occur anywhere, but those occurring in the ophthalmic branch of the fifth cranial nerve, alone or in combination with other sites, can be signs of Sturge-Weber syndrome.[3] Capillary malformations evolve with time and become thicker, nodular, and darker purple. In addition, soft tissue and bony overgrowth may be associated with more extensive lesions.

Venous malformations are composed of irregular, ectatic slow-flow channels that present at birth or appear later as localized bluish compressible lesions. They typically swell in a dependent position or when the child cries. Blue rubber bleb nevus syndrome is a rare disorder of discrete venous malformations on the skin, in the gastrointestinal tract, and less often in other organ systems and is discussed in further detail later.

Lymphatic malformations are composed of irregular, ectatic lymph channels and are classified as macrocystic or microcystic according to the size of the cystic spaces. Microcystic lesions can also form clear or hemorrhagic vesicles at the surface of the skin, formerly called lymphangioma circumscriptum. Macrocystic lesions (formerly called "cystic hygroma") commonly occur on the neck and axilla and are visible at birth as large subcutaneous compressible masses.

Arteriovenous malformations (AVMs) present as pink or red, flat or slightly raised lesions with localized warmth, commonly on the head or neck. They are fast-flow lesions; therefore, a thrill or bruit may be felt on palpation or documented by Doppler ultrasonography. Only 40% are manifested at birth. An AVM may mimic a capillary malformation or infantile hemangioma initially, but they progressively grow and often worsen at puberty. AVMs may also expand after trauma, infection, or radiologic or surgical intervention.

Combined malformations present in association with soft tissue and bony abnormalities. Klippel-Trenaunay syndrome encompasses capillary, lymphatic, and venous malformations with overgrowth of soft tissue and bone on the affected limb. Parkes Weber syndrome is a microfistulous AVM of the skin and muscle of an extremity with overgrowth.

Evaluation and Treatment

Assessment and management of vascular malformations depends on the type, location, and extent of the lesion. An infant with a capillary malformation should be sent to dermatology or plastic surgery within the first few months of

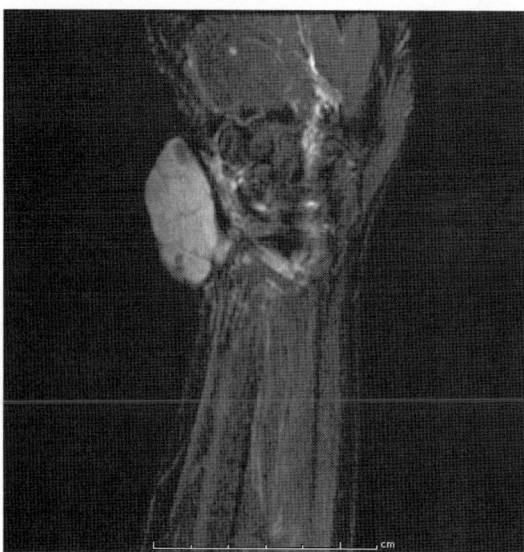

Figure 153-1 Coronal fat-saturated T2-weighted MRI of the right wrist area demonstrating a large hyperintense exophytic venous malformation in the radial aspect of the wrist with surrounding prominent veins. Two phleboliths are seen within the malformation.

life for consideration of treatment with the pulsed dye laser. If a capillary malformation involves the ophthalmic branch of the fifth cranial nerve distribution, further workup should be considered to evaluate for Sturge-Weber syndrome, which affects 10% of these cases. Neurologic workup should include magnetic resonance imaging (MRI) with gadolinium contrast for possible leptomeningeal enhancement and an ophthalmologic examination for choroidal vascular lesions and glaucoma. Venous malformations and lymphatic malformations can be diagnosed clinically or with the aid of MRI with gadolinium (Fig. 153-1). AVMs can be diagnosed by ultrasonography or MRI.

Pulsed dye laser therapy is usually warranted for capillary malformations. Larger capillary malformations on the trunk and extremity should be referred to appropriate surgical specialists, particularly if there is associated soft or bony tissue overgrowth. Treatment of venous malformations and lymphatic malformations is considered for functional impairment, disfigurement, pain, or bleeding. Treatment options are elective sclerotherapy or surgical excision.

Admission Criteria

A few rare clinical scenarios require immediate attention and possible inpatient admission for complications of vascular malformations:

- A patient with Sturge-Weber syndrome and extensive brain involvement may need to be hospitalized for management of seizures.
- Extensive venous malformations can cause intravascular consumption coagulopathy, particularly after intervention by sclerotherapy or surgical procedures; prompt attention is required.

- Blue rubber bleb nevus syndrome causes chronic gastrointestinal bleeding, in addition to abdominal pain, intussusception, volvulus, infarction, or internal hemorrhage, and requires inpatient stabilization and possible surgical intervention.
- Patients with lymphatic malformations are frequently hospitalized for cellulitis, which can be difficult to treat and requires intravenous antibiotic therapy.
- Large AVMs can lead to ulceration, pain, bleeding, or very rarely, high-output heart failure and warrant inpatient management with endovascular embolization.
- Combined vascular lesions of an extremity can also be complicated by ulceration, pain, bleeding, and clotting, which may require admission.

Discharge Criteria

- Patients are discharged after thorough evaluation has been completed, after the acute problem is treated or controlled, and when appropriate outpatient follow-up has been arranged.

VASCULAR TUMORS

Hemangiomas

Infantile hemangioma is the most common vascular tumor in infancy and affects 1% to 2.6% of healthy newborns[4] and up to 10% of white children by 1 year of age. It is more common in females in a ratio of 3:1 to 5:1, and it is more prevalent in premature infants. These benign tumors are made up of proliferating endothelial cells. They are described as superficial if the lesion is in the uppermost layer of skin, deep if the lesion is in the deeper portion of skin, or combined if it has elements of both superficial and deep lesions. Older terms such as "strawberry" or "cavernous" should be avoided. Superficial lesions are bright red, flat or raised, whereas deep lesions are bluish, soft, and compressible. About 40% of infantile hemangiomas are present at birth as a nascent mark: either an erythematous patch or pale area with or without telangiectases. Rarely, infantile hemangioma presents as a nonhealing ulcer on the lip or perineal area. They grow rapidly in the first year of life and regress slowly over a period of years: 50% of lesions involute by 5 years of age, 70% by 7 years, and the remainder by 10 to 12 years of age. There is an uncommon variant called congenital hemangioma that arises in utero and presents as a fully developed lesion at birth. These congenital lesions are divided into two categories: rapidly involuting congenital hemangioma (RICH) and noninvoluting congenital hemangioma (NICH). RICH involutes by 6 to 10 months of age, whereas NICH never involutes. Repeated examinations are required to make a definitive diagnosis.

Other Vascular Tumors

Kaposiform hemangioendothelioma (KHE) is an uncommon vascular tumor associated with Kasabach-Merritt phenomenon, a severe type of thrombocytopenic coagulopathy (see later).[5,6] KHE may present at birth and partially regresses over a period of years. Tufted angioma tends to occur in early childhood and presents as large warm, firm inhomogeneous red or violaceous nodules or plaques. The tumor may regress completely or partially or persist. Infantile tufted angioma is believed to be on a spectrum of KHE but is less likely to be associated with Kasabach-Merritt phenomenon.

Evaluation and Treatment

The type of vascular tumor can be correctly diagnosed by history and physical examination in more than 90% of patients and by radiologic confirmation in more than 95% of patients. Whenever there is any question of diagnosis, biopsy is mandated. Other tumors such as sarcoma and rhabdomyosarcoma can mimic infantile hemangioma and KHE.

Hemangiomas

Hemangiomas are diagnosed clinically, and because of spontaneous involution, most lesions are simply observed. Complications arise in about 10% of infantile hemangiomas and require treatment. Complications include ulceration, obstruction, deformation, bleeding, hypothyroidism, and rarely, high-output cardiac failure.

Ulceration (Fig. 153-2) can occur with rapid growth, particularly in the lip or perineal area. An ulcer can become infected and is often painful. In these instances, referral should be made to a vascular anomalies specialist. Treatment options include liberal lubrication with a moisturizer or barrier cream, topical or oral antibiotic, pain control, intralesional or oral corticosteroid, or laser therapy.[7,8] Surgical excision may also be considered if easily accomplished.

Obstruction or structural anomalies caused by infantile hemangioma that impair an infant's normal function require prompt treatment. Periorbital hemangiomas should be assessed and monitored by a pediatric ophthalmologist to evaluate for signs of obstruction of vision and astigmatic amblyopia caused by deformation of the cornea. Prompt treatment is important in these children because other long-term visual sequelae such as ptosis, proptosis, and strabismus can occur. Lumbosacral hemangioma, as with all congenital lesions in the midline sacral distribution, should be further evaluated in the outpatient setting to rule out underlying spinal dysraphism, a tethered spinal cord, or lipoma.

A large hemangioma may be associated with hypothyroidism from increased type 3 iodothyronine deiodinase activity in the tumor[9] and rarely with high-output cardiac failure, especially in patients with multifocal intrahepatic hemangioma. Multiple neonatal hemangiomas are often associated with visceral hemangiomas, most commonly found in the liver. For this reason, an infant presenting with five or more hemangiomas when younger than a few months of age should undergo hepatic ultrasonography. Other less common complications associated with multiple hemangiomas include involvement of the gastrointestinal tract, lungs, and central nervous system.

Several structural abnormalities are associated with large facial hemangiomas,[10] as denoted by the acronym PHACES:

Posterior brain fossa abnormalities (Dandy-Walker most commonly)
Hemangioma

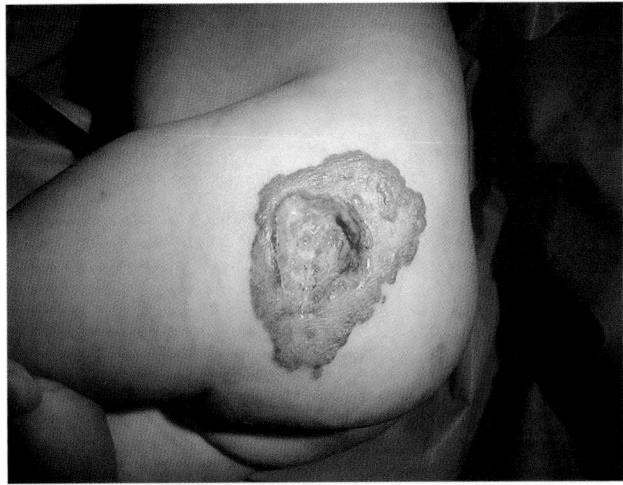

Figure 153-2 Ulcerated hemangioma.

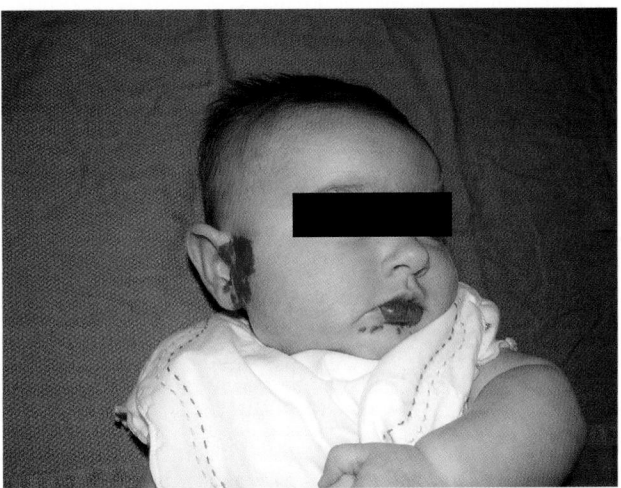

Figure 153-3 Hemangioma in a beard distribution.

Arterial anomalies (cervical and intracranial)
Coarctation of the aorta and other cardiac defects
Eye abnormalities
Sternal clefting

Evaluation for this association includes MRI of the brain and an echocardiogram.

A hemangioma in a partial or full beard distribution (the preauricular areas, chin, anterior neck, and lower lip) (Fig. 153-3) has been shown to be associated with upper airway or subglottic hemangiomas.[11] Therefore, an infant who has a hemangioma in this distribution with any signs of stridor, cough, cyanosis, or hoarseness needs to be immediately evaluated by endoscopic examination for airway involvement. Often, the symptoms in these patients are initially misdiagnosed as croup.

First-line treatment of problematic hemangiomas is systemic corticosteroids, usually initiated at 2 to 3 mg/kg/day for 4 weeks and then a slow taper over months. Corticosteroids have been shown to stabilize or reduce the size of a growing hemangioma in 85% of cases.[12] An alternative treatment of a tumor unresponsive to corticosteroid is interferon alfa-2a or alfa-2b,[13] usually started in the inpatient setting at 1 million U/m²/day and increased to a treatment dose of 3 million U/m²/day. However, interferon therapy has been controversial given the rare side effect of spastic diplegia.[14] Vincristine is now considered second-line therapy if there is failure to respond to corticosteroids.[15] Surgical excision may be considered if feasible, and tracheostomy may be necessary in some cases of upper airway or subglottic hemangiomas.

Kasabach-Merritt Phenomenon

Kasabach-Merritt phenomenon is manifested as severe thrombocytopenia secondary to platelet trapping by the tumor. It does not occur with infantile hemangioma, but rather with other vascular tumors such as KHE, tufted angioma, and congenital hemangiopericytoma. The presentation is an enlarging vascular lesion that becomes violaceous, indurated, and ecchymotic. Inpatient admission and consultation by vascular anomalies specialists is warranted because patients are at high risk for hemorrhage and infection. Laboratory workup is significant for thrombocytopenia as low as 5000/mm³, decreased fibrinogen levels, and increased fibrin split products and D-dimers. MRI is often needed to confirm and document the extension of KHE. Treatment should be initiated promptly. High-dose oral prednisone (2 to 4 mg/kg/day) has been shown to be effective in only about 10% of patients.[16] Interferon alfa-2a at 3 million U/m²/day and vincristine are other treatment options. Platelet transfusions should be avoided because platelets are trapped in the tumor and release growth factors that stimulate the tumor. Heparin should also be avoided. Once stabilized, patients may be slowly tapered from their medication with close outpatient follow-up.

Admission Criteria

A few rare clinical scenarios require immediate attention and possible inpatient admission for complications of vascular tumors of infancy:

* Ulcerated hemangioma can be an indication for admission for pain control, antibiotics, dressings, and if appropriate, pharmacologic treatment or excision.
* Rapid growth may result in impairment of vital functions, most commonly breathing and vision and, less commonly, for gastrointestinal involvement.
* Infants with large hemangiomas may also need to be admitted for intravenous thyroid hormone replacement therapy, abdominal compartment syndrome, or rarely, management of congestive cardiac failure, which can be seen with large or multiple intrahepatic hemangiomas.

IN A NUTSHELL

* Vascular malformations are composed of structurally abnormal vessels with normal endothelial turnover and can be composed of capillary, venous, lymphatic, arterial, or arteriovenous vessels alone or in combination.
* Congenital malformations are large pink to red homogeneous patches at birth; it is important to differentiate them from common fading macular stains of infancy because congenital malformations require referral to a vascular specialist.
* Treatment of vascular malformations is dictated by degree of functional impairment, disfigurement, pain, bleeding, or problems related to associated syndromes.
* Complications of vascular malformations that may warrant admission include management of airway involvement, coagulopathy, bleeding, cellulitis, or rarely, high-output cardiac failure.
* Infantile hemangioma is the most common vascular tumor of infancy; it grows rapidly in the first year of life and regresses slowly over a period of years, with 50% of lesions involuting by age 5, 70% by age 7, and most by 10 to 12 years of age.
* About 10% of infantile hemangiomas are associated with complications that require treatment. Such complications include ulceration, obstruction, bleeding, hypothyroidism, and rarely, high-output cardiac failure.
* Treatment options for infantile hemangioma include systemic corticosteroid, interferon alfa-2a or alfa-2b, vincristine, and sometimes surgical excision.
* Kasabach-Merritt phenomenon is severe thrombocytopenia secondary to platelet trapping by KHE or tufted angioma—it does not occur with infantile hemangioma.

ON THE HORIZON

* The recently discovered mutations responsible for vascular malformations permit study of these anomalies in genetically engineered mice and in vitro systems. Thus, in the future it might be possible to test new therapies in murine models. Endovascular therapy is playing an increasing role in the management of these anomalies. As the pathogenesis is better understood, targeted agents could be injected. Vessel proliferation may be the cause of expansion in some types of vascular malformation, and thus antiangiogenic therapy is a possibility.
* A search for the molecular basis of the genesis of hemangioma is actively being pursued by several laboratories. There is evidence that hemangiomas are clonal and that endothelial stem cells play an important role in their rapid growth.[17,18] Genetics studies in families with hemangiomas are also being performed to look for causative mutations. Animal models of hemangioma are also under investigation. Once the molecular defect or defects are known, targeted pharmacologic therapy will be possible.

SUGGESTED READING

Drolet BA, Esterly NB, Frieden IJ: Hemangiomas in children. N Engl J Med 1999;341:173-181.

Fishman SF, Mulliken JB: Vascular anomalies. A primer for pediatricians. Pediatr Clin North Am 1998;45:1455-1477.

Mulliken JB, Fishman SF, Burrows PE: Vascular anomalies. Curr Probl Surg 2000;37:517-584.

Mulliken JB, Young A: Vascular Birthmarks: Hemangiomas and Malformations. Philadelphia, WB Saunders, 1988.

REFERENCES

1. Mulliken JB, Glowacki J: Hemangiomas and vascular malformations in infants and children: A classification based on endothelial characteristics. Plast Reconstr Surg 1982;69:412-420.
2. Enjolras O, Mulliken JB: Vascular tumors and vascular malformations (new issues). Adv Dermatol 1998;13:375-422.
3. Enjolras O, Riche MC, Merland JJ: Facial port-wine stains and Sturge-Weber syndrome. Pediatrics 1985;76:48-51.
4. Jacobs AH, Walton R: The incidence of birthmarks in neonate. Pediatrics 1976;58:218-222.
5. Sarkar M, Mulliken JB, Kozakewich HPW, et al: Thrombocytopenic coagulopathy (Kasabach-Merritt phenomenon) is associated with kaposiform hemangioendothelioma and not with common infantile hemangioma. Plast Reconstr Surg 1997;100:1377-1386.
6. Enjolras O, Wassef M, Mazoyer E, et al: Infants with Kasabach-Merritt syndrome do not have "true" hemangiomas. J Pediatr 1997;130:631-640.
7. Kim HJ, Colombo M, Frieden IJ: Ulcerated hemangiomas: Clinical characteristics and response to therapy. J Am Acad Dermatol 2001;44:962-972.
8. Frieden IJ, Eichenfield LF, Esterly NB: Guidelines of care for hemangiomas of infancy. American Academy of Dermatology Guidelines/Outcomes Committee. J Am Acad Dermatol 1997;37:631-637.
9. Huang SA, Tu HM, Harney JW, et al: Severe hypothyroidism caused by type 3 iodothyronine deiodinase in infantile hemangiomas. N Engl J Med 2000;343:185-189.
10. Metry DW, Dowd CF, Barkovich AJ, Frieden IJ: The many faces of PHACE syndrome. J Pediatr 2001;139:117-123.
11. Orlow SJ, Isakoff MS, Blei F: Increased risk of symptomatic hemangiomas of the airway in association with cutaneous hemangiomas in a "beard" distribution. J Pediatr 1997;131:643-646.
12. Bennett ML, Fleisher AB Jr, Chamlin SL, Frieden IJ: Oral corticosteroid use is effective for cutaneous hemangiomas: An evidence-based evaluation. Arch Dermatol 2001;137:1208-1213.
13. Ezekowitz RAB, Mulliken JB, Folkman J: Interferon alfa-2a for life-threatening hemangiomas of infancy. N Engl J Med 1992;326:1456-1463.
14. Barlow CF, Priebe CJ, Mulliken JB, et al: Spastic diplegia as a complication of interferon alfa-2a treatment of hemangiomas of infancy. J Pediatr 1998;132:527-530.
15. Haisley-Royster C, Enjolras O, Frieden IJ, et al: Kasabach-Merritt phenomenon: A retrospective study of treatment with vincristine. J Pediatr Hematol Oncol 2002;24:459-462.
16. Mulliken JB, Anupindi S, Ezekowitz RA, Mihm MC: Case 13-2004: A newborn girl with a large cutaneous lesion, thrombocytopenia, and anemia. N Engl J Med 2004;350:1764-1775.
17. Boye E, Yu Y, Paranya G, et al: Clonality and altered behavior of endothelial cells from hemangiomas. J Clin Invest 2001;107:745-752.
18. Walter JW, North PE, Waner M, et al: Somatic mutation of vascular endothelial growth factor receptors in juvenile hemangioma. Genes Chromosomes Cancer 2002;33:295-303.

CHAPTER 154

Head Lice and Scabies

Jessica L. Hills and Albert C. Yan

HEAD LICE

Pediculosis capitis is caused by infestation of the scalp with the head louse, *Pediculus humanus capitis*. Transmission occurs by direct contact with the hair of infested patients and, less commonly, by contact with fomites such as hats, brushes, or linens.[1] Infestation is endemic worldwide, affecting people of all ages, socioeconomic levels, and race,[2] but it is less common in African Americans.[3] There is a predominance in children, particularly in girls aged 3 to 12 years. Head lice are not a sign of poor hygiene, and infestation is not significantly influenced by hair length or frequent brushing and shampooing.[1]

The head louse is a wingless insect measuring 3 to 4 mm long with three pairs of clawed legs that are adapted to grasp hairs (Fig. 154-1).[4] The life cycle of the head louse consists of three stages: egg, nymph, and adult. Head lice lay ova within a case referred to as a nit. The ova or nits are translucent, measure less than 1 mm, and firmly attach to the hair shaft with a gluelike substance.[5,6] The nits hatch after about a week of incubation, giving rise to nymphs that leave behind white casings that remain tightly adherent to the hair shaft. Nymphs mature into adults over a period of 9 to12 days.[2] Mating occurs, and if treatment is not instituted, the cycle repeats. Head lice are obligate parasites of humans. They are blood-sucking insects and temperature sensitive. Typically, head lice cannot survive for more than a day or two away from the scalp.[1] Head lice do not commonly transmit any other diseases.

Clinical Presentation

Nits attach themselves to hair shafts approximately 1 to 3 mm from the scalp, particularly in the occipital and retroauricular regions.[4] Pruritus is the principal symptom of head lice infestation, and children may be seen scratching the posterior scalp (Fig. 154-2); however, many children are asymptomatic.[7] With the first exposure to lice, itching may not develop for 4 to 6 weeks until sensitization occurs.[4] Scratching may result in excoriation, eczematous changes, or secondary bacterial infection. Other findings include bite reactions and cervical lymphadenopathy.

Differential Diagnosis

The differential diagnosis of pediculosis capitis includes hair casts; hair debris; flakes of seborrheic dermatitis, scalp psoriasis, scalp atopic dermatitis, and tinea capitis; trichodystrophies such as monilethrix and trichorrhexis nodosa; and black and white piedra.[7] Nits are firmly attached to the hair shafts and difficult to remove, distinguishing them from scales or hair casts, which can slide along the hair shaft. In addition, microscopic examination allows the easy identification of nits.[4]

Diagnosis and Evaluation

A definitive diagnosis can be made when crawling lice are seen in the hair or are combed from the scalp. This may be difficult to do, because the lice move quickly and prefer to avoid light. An average host carries fewer than 20 adult lice.[6] Louse combs are a useful screening tool and can aid in finding live lice. Nits alone are not diagnostic of active infection, but if they are found within $1/4$ inch from the scalp, active infestation is more likely.[4] Nits found more than 1 cm from the scalp are not likely to be viable.[2] The duration of infestation can be approximated by measuring the distance from the nit to the surface of the scalp, assuming hair growth of about 1 cm per month.[7]

Treatment

Treatment requires the killing of both adult lice and eggs. The safety of pediculicides is emphasized because the infestation itself usually does not present a risk to the host.[1] However, some children who scratch intensely may become secondarily infected and develop a frank pyoderma. Most therapeutic shampoos or cream rinses recommend application to dry hair for maximum effectiveness.[2] Wet hair leads to dilution and poor penetration of the active ingredients into the lice. All topical pediculicides should be rinsed from the hair over a sink rather than in a bath to limit exposure, and cool water should be used to minimize absorption secondary to vasodilation.[3] Because cream rinses and conditioning shampoos coat the hair and protect the lice from the pediculicide, these products should not be used for 2 weeks after treatment.[6]

Permethrin 1% is the recommended first-line treatment for head lice owing to its safety and efficacy. Initial studies showed a clinical efficacy greater than 95%, and it is available without a prescription.[6] The product is a cream rinse applied for 10 minutes to hair that has first been shampooed and towel dried. Permethrin leaves a residue on the hair that kills nymphs hatched from the 20% to 30% of eggs that are not killed with the first application.[3] However, retreatment after 1 week is still widely recommended.[4] Significant resistance to permethrin 1% has begun to emerge in the United States, and alternative therapies may be necessary.

Pyrethrin is a natural extract from chrysanthemum flowers combined with piperonyl butoxide to provide stability and synergy. Pyrethrin-based products are neurotoxic to lice but have extremely low mammalian toxicity. These products are applied to dry hair, lathered with small amounts of water, and then rinsed off after 10 minutes. Because ovicidal activity is low, a second treatment 7 to 10 days later is necessary to kill newly hatched lice.[3] Products containing pyrethrins should be avoided in patients allergic to chrysanthemums. Resistance to these products has been reported in the United States as well as in other countries.

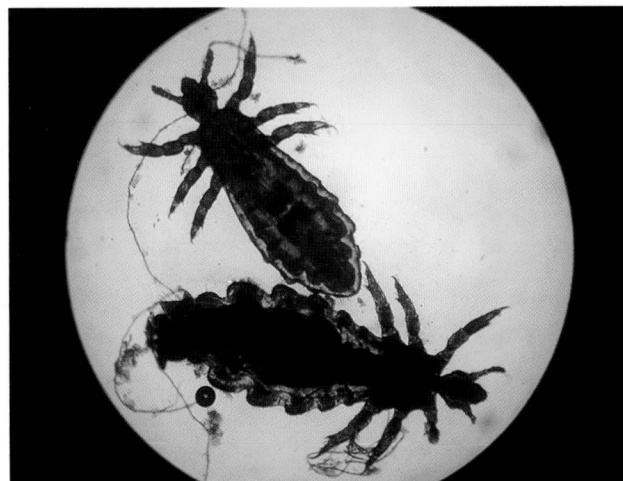

Figure 154-1 Head lice under light microscopy.

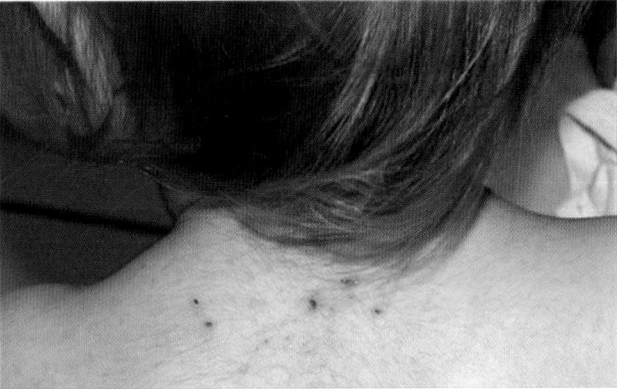

Figure 154-2 Head lice dermatitis involving the posterior scalp of this school-aged girl.

Second-line pediculicides include lindane 1% and malathion 0.5%. Lindane 1% is available only by prescription and is no longer widely used because of its toxicity profile. It may be used as a shampoo, with a repeat application in 7 to 10 days to eradicate any newly hatched lice. It has low ovicidal activity, and resistance has been reported worldwide for years.[3] Adverse side effects, which usually occur as a result of exposure to high doses from overuse or ingestion, include neurotoxicity. Lindane 1% is contraindicated in preterm infants, pregnant or nursing women, and patients with seizure disorders.[1]

Malathion 0.5% is an organophosphate recently reintroduced to the U.S. market. It requires a prescription and is available as a lotion applied to the hair, left to air dry, and then washed off after 8 to 12 hours. It has high ovicidal activity but should be reapplied if live lice are seen in 7 to 10 days. Major concerns are the high alcohol content, which makes it flammable, and the risk of severe respiratory distress if it is accidentally ingested.[3] Malathion 0.5% is contraindicated in neonates and infants because their increased scalp permeability leads to higher levels of absorption.[1]

In vitro studies have shown Ovide lotion (0.5% malathion) to be the fastest killing pediculicide and the most effective agent when compared with lindane, pyrethrin-based products such as RID and A-200, and 1% permethrin. This study found that although RID and A-200 have the same active ingredients (synthetic pyrethrins and piperonyl butoxide), A-200 is significantly more effective, owing to differences in vehicle composition.[8]

A fine-toothed comb should be used a day or two after the final application of a pediculicide to confirm that treatment has been successful. Regular weekly combing is recommended for several weeks after cure.[2] After treatment, nits remain in the scalp. Removal is not necessary to prevent the spread of infection but may be done for aesthetic reasons. Inflammation of the skin in response to topical agents may result in itching or mild burning of the scalp that can persist for many days. Topical corticosteroids or oral antihistamines may be beneficial for symptomatic relief.[3]

Causes of treatment failure include improper dilution or duration of application, noncompliance, reinfestation from untreated contacts, and drug resistance. After proper application of an appropriate pediculicide, reinfestation from an untreated infested contact is more common than treatment failure. If true treatment failure occurs, immediate retreatment with a different pediculicide, followed by a second application 7 days later, is recommended.[1] Resistance patterns vary in different geographic areas, and treatment should be tailored to local resistance patterns and the availability of agents.[4]

Other treatments that are not currently approved by the Food and Drug Administration for use as pediculicides include permethrin 5% (Elimite), which is a cream available by prescription only. It is typically used to treat scabies but has been recommended for the treatment of head lice that are resistant to other treatments. It should be applied to the scalp, left on for several hours or overnight, and then rinsed off.[3] Oral trimethoprim-sulfamethoxazole (TMP-SMZ) given at typical otitis media doses for 5 to 10 days or ivermectin 200 µg/kg given as a single oral dose have also been cited as effective against head lice.[1] Oral TMP-SMZ is presumably ingested during the louse's blood meal and kills the symbiotic parasite residing in the louse's gut. Ivermectin is neurotoxic to the louse and kills the organism as it is ingested during blood meals. Alternative treatments such as petrolatum, mayonnaise, kerosene, and electrocution by battery-powered combs have not been assessed with regard to efficacy or safety in published trials.[2] Use of a new physical suffocant has been reported in a preliminary case series, and utilizes an over-the-counter product (Cetaphil Cleanser) applied to the scalp and hair, combed out, and then blow-dried with a standard hair dryer. The material is washed out the next morning. Three weekly treatments reportedly clear head lice with a greater than 90% efficacy. This product, however, is not commercially available.[9]

Mechanical removal is another treatment method that entails combing the wet hair with a specially designed comb. The rationale behind wet combing is that because lice do not move to another host within 7 days of hatching, they do not reproduce for 10 days, and all eggs hatch in about a week.[2] If all young lice are combed out within a few days after hatching, the infestation can be eradicated. The combing procedure should be done on wet hair and continued until no lice are found. It may be aided by soaking the hair in a vinegar solution, which helps loosen the glue that holds the nits to the hair, or by using a formic acid rinse.[7] Combing is repeated every 3 to 4 days for several weeks and should continue for 2 weeks after any session in which an adult louse is found.[2] However, this method is quite time-consuming, it can be painful for the patient, and its efficacy is dependent on the skill of the comber.

Admission Criteria

Head lice infestation is not typically an indication for hospitalization, and most complications that arise—such as bacterial superinfection—can be treated on an outpatient basis.

Prevention

A hospitalized patient with pediculosis capitis should be isolated, and contact precautions are recommended until the patient has completed appropriate treament.[1] Because this problem can be spread among pediatric inpatients who have close contact, we recommend the following:

- Close examination of household and other close contacts, including hospital staff, bedmates, and inpatient roommates.
- Treatment of infested patients and contacts.
- Cleaning of hair-care items and bedding, as well as clothing, furniture, and carpeting that was in close contact with the patient.
- Education for staff, patients, and visitors regarding the diagnosis, treatment, and prevention of head lice.

Because lice cannot survive off the scalp beyond 48 hours, only clothing, furniture, and carpeting that were in contact with the head of the infested patient in the 24 to 48 hours before treatment require cleaning.[3] Washing, soaking, or drying items at temperatures greater than 130°F will kill stray lice or nits.[7] Furniture, carpeting, and other fabrics can be vacuumed. Items that cannot be washed can be placed in sealed bags for 2 weeks, by which time any nits that may have survived would have hatched, and hymphs would die without a feeding source.[3]

Data are lacking to assess whether disinfection of personal or household items influences the likelihood of cure or recurrence.[2] Children should be taught not to share personal items such as hats, combs, or brushes.

In a Nutshell

- Head lice are obligate human parasites that feed on human blood.
- Head lice cannot live for more than 48 hours off the human body.
- Pruritus is the most common presenting symptom, especially when it occurs on the occipital scalp.
- Bacterial superinfection, lymphadenopathy, and bite reactions are the most likely secondary complications of head lice infestation.
- Diagnosis is typically made by inspection and microscopy, if needed.
- Treatment involves the use of physical agents that suffocate the lice or chemical agents that are neurotoxic to them.
- Resistance to chemical pediculicides is an emerging problem.

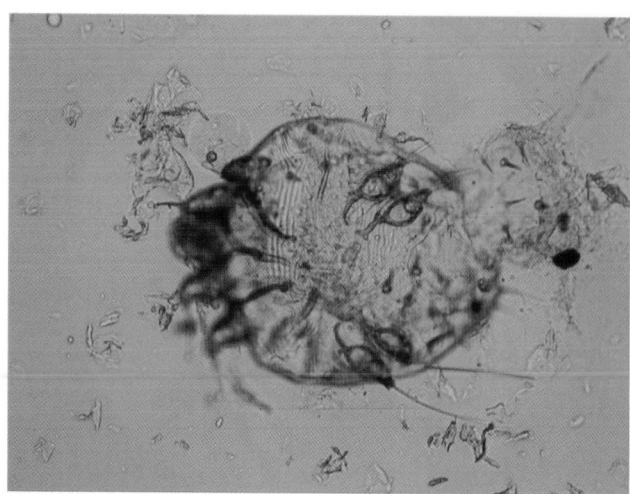

Figure 154-3 Scabies mite under light microscopy.

On the Horizon

- Better understanding of the mechanisms associated with resistance to pediculicides is emerging.
- Newer, less toxic pediculicidal formulations are under investigation.

SCABIES

Scabies is a highly contagious infestation caused by the itch mite *Sarcoptes scabiei* (Fig. 154-3). Transmission occurs through prolonged, close personal contact. Infestation is common, occurs worldwide, and affects people of all ages, socioeconomic levels, and standards of personal hygiene.[10] Scabies spreads rapidly under crowded conditions where people have frequent skin-to-skin contact. Therefore, hospitals, child-care facilities, and nursing homes may all experience widespread scabies epidemics that are difficult to control. Epidemics of scabies seem to occur in 30-year cycles, with each one lasting about 15 years.[10]

The adult female mite is oval, has four pairs of legs, and measures about 0.4 mm long. Infestation begins as a female exudes a keratolytic substance on the skin surface and burrows into the stratum corneum. She gradually extends this tract while depositing two or three eggs daily.[11] In 4 to 5 weeks, egg laying is complete, and the female dies in the burrow. Eggs hatch in 3 to 4 days; the larvae leave the burrow to molt into nymphs, and they achieve maturity in 2 to 3 weeks.[12] Mating takes place, and the gravid female tunnels into the skin, completing the life cycle.

Clinical Presentation

Patients without prior exposure to scabies often do not exhibit symptoms for 4 to 6 weeks, during which time sensitization to the mite occurs.[13] For patients who were previously infested, symptoms develop 1 to 3 days after repeated exposure to the mite.[5] The eruption consists of intensely pruritic papules, vesicles, pustules, and linear burrows. Itching peaks at night and is thought to be secondary to a hypersensitivity reaction to the mites.

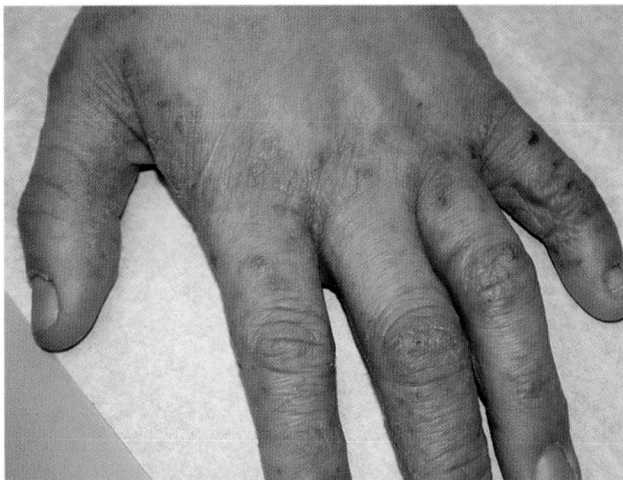

Figure 154-4 Scabietic vesicle involving the web space between the thumb and forefinger.

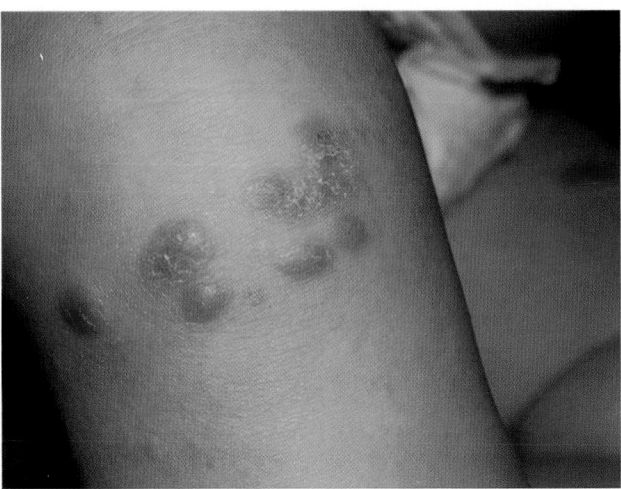

Figure 154-5 Nodular scabies involving the limb of this infant.

In older children and adults, the mites have a predilection for the finger and toe webs, axillae, flexor surfaces of the wrist and elbows, around the nipples and waistline, and over the inguinal areas and buttocks (Fig. 154-4). In infants and toddlers, the characteristic distribution of lesions differs, with involvement of the head, neck, trunk, palms, and soles. In addition, patients may develop reddish brown nodules (nodular scabies) that are most prominent in covered areas of the body such as the axillae, inguinal areas, and buttocks (Fig. 154-5). These lesions often persist for weeks to months even after effective treatment.[14]

Norwegian scabies is a variant characterized by extensive crusted skin lesions with thick hyperkeratosis.[5] It is highly contagious, and even casual contact can lead to transmission. Norwegian scabies is most commonly found in patients who are immunosuppressed, physically debilitated, or developmentally disabled.[10] Localized outbreaks of scabies are often traced to someone infested with Norwegian scabies, particularly in institutionalized settings.[13]

Differential Diagnosis

The differential diagnosis includes atopic or contact dermatitis, seborrheic dermatitis, infantile acropustulosis, insect bites, papular urticaria, dyshidrotic eczema, and Langerhans cell histiocytosis.

Diagnosis and Evaluation

The burrow is pathognomonic for scabies, which can frequently be diagnosed clinically. However, the appearance of primary lesions—papules, vesicles, and pustules—is often altered as a result of excoriation, secondary bacterial infection, or an eczematous eruption due to scratching. Burrows are present in less than 25% of infants.[14] Therefore, scabies can be misdiagnosed. A definitive diagnosis can be made by microscopic examination of scrapings of suspicious lesions and identification of the adult mites, ova, or fecal matter.[11] The best lesions to examine are fresh papules or intact burrows from the terminal portion, most commonly identified on the wrists, finger webs, elbows, or feet. Mineral oil, microscope oil, or water applied to the skin aids in the collection of scrapings with a scalpel, which are then examined microscopically under low power. However, there are usually fewer than a dozen mites present on an infested patient's skin, so a negative result does not rule out the disorder.[5]

Treatment

Successful treatment requires a careful explanation of the nature of the infestation to the patient and parent, appropriate administration of antiscabietic therapy, and thorough inquiry into the infested patient's close contacts. For children and adults, treatment consists of applying a scabicide-containing cream or lotion over the entire body below the head. In infants and toddlers, treatment of the entire head and neck is also required because these areas can be involved in this age group.[14] The first-line treatment—except for neonates and pregnant women—is 5% permethrin cream (Elimite). Permethrin should be removed by bathing after 8 to 14 hours. Studies have shown a cure rate of 89% and minimal side effects.[15] Second-line therapies include 1% lindane cream or lotion, crotamiton (Eurax), and 6% to 10% sulfur precipitate in petrolatum.

Lindane lotion (as stated earlier, no longer widely used because of potential toxicity) is applied to the body and then removed by bathing after 8 to 12 hours; the treatment is repeated in 4 to 7 days. There is a risk of neurotoxicity from absorption through the skin, so the frequency of application should not exceed that recommended by the manufacturer. Lindane should not be used immediately after a bath to limit its transcutaneous permeability.[10] The risk of side effects is maximal in young children secondary to an increased risk of accidental ingestion and their larger body surface area and consequent greater percutaneous absorption. This treatment is contraindicated in patients with crusted scabies or an extensive dermatitis, those with known seizure disorders, young infants, and women who are pregnant or breastfeeding.

Crotamiton is applied once or twice daily for 3 to 5 days. Crotamiton is safe in young infants, but studies show only a 60% cure rate.[15] In addition, it can be irritating on raw or denuded skin.

Sulfur precipitate 5% in petrolatum—considered a safer option for neonates and pregnant women—can be applied for 3 consecutive nights, but the treatment is malodorous as well as messy. Ivermectin is emerging as a treatment choice for severe or Norwegian scabies and for patients whose infestation is refractory to topical treatment. The drug acts as a neurotoxin on the scabies mite but is well tolerated in humans. A single oral dose of 200 µg/kg has been shown to be effective for uncomplicated scabies in both immunocompetent and immunosuppressed patients.[16] However, ivermectin is not licensed for this indication by the Food and Drug Administration, nor is it approved for use in children younger than 5 years old. It should not be used in children weighing less than 15 kg, in pregnant women, or in patients with other contraindications.

After treatment, pruritus can persist for days to weeks until mites, eggs, and feces are shed from the stratum corneum. Symptomatic relief can be achieved with oral antihistamines and topical corticosteroids. Topical or systemic antimicrobial therapy is indicated for secondary bacterial infections of excoriated lesions.

Admission Criteria

Scabies infestation is not typically an indication for hospitalization, and most complications that arise—such as bacterial superinfection—can be treated on an outpatient basis. This condition may be encountered incidentally among inpatients admitted for other indications.

Prevention

Scabies can be transmitted via clothing and bedding to household contacts, but direct skin contact is the predominant means of transmission in the hospital setting. A hospitalized patient should be isolated, and contact precautions are recommended until the patient has completed appropriate therapy, because scabies can be transmitted as long as the patient remains infested and untreated.

Clinical symptoms of scabies infestation can appear up to 2 months after exposure. Therefore, all household members should be treated simultaneously, regardless of the presence of symptoms, to prevent reinfestation. The mites can survive on clothing for 3 to 4 days without skin contact. Thus, all clothing, towels, and bedding used by the infested patient during the 4 days before the initiation of therapy should be washed with hot water at least 120°F and dried using a hot cycle, or dry-cleaned.[10] Alternatively, items can be placed in a sealed bag for a week to prevent reinfestation.[14]

Patients, staff members, and visitors who have prolonged skin-to-skin contact with infested patients should also be considered for treatment.[13] Visitors should be notified that the hospital has recently experienced a scabies infestation and should be advised to contact their physicians if they have any symptoms. Staff should be educated to ensure compliance with therapy and to reassure them that patients and staff are receiving appropriate treatment.[13]

In a Nutshell

- Scabies mites are transmitted through prolonged, close contact. They cannot survive off the human body for more than 4 days.

- Intense pruritus is a characteristic finding. Lesions—papules, vesicles, and burrows—are commonly found in intertriginous zones, including web spaces between fingers.
- Infested patients may remain asymptomatic for up to 4 to 6 weeks.
- The diagnosis may be suspected on clinical grounds—based on characteristic skin lesions—and confirmed by taking scrapings of burrows or lesions to identify the mites or eggs.
- Treatment typically involves the use of topical antiscabietic medications.

On the Horizon

- Topical antiscabietic medications continue to be quite effective, and so far, there is little evidence of resistance. Because of their ease of use and high efficacy, oral antiscabietic medications are a useful option, especially for recalcitrant or severe scabies infestations.

REFERENCES

1. American Academy of Pediatrics: Pediculosis capitis. In Pickering LK (ed): Red Book: 2003 Report of the Committee on Infectious Diseases, 26th ed. Elk Grove Village, Ill, American Academy of Pediatrics, 2003, pp 547-549.
2. Roberts RJ: Head lice. N Engl J Med 2002;346:1645-1650.
3. Frankowski BL, Weiner LB: American Academy of Pediatrics, Committee on School Health and Committee on Infectious Diseases: Head lice. Pediatrics 2002;110:638-643.
4. Ko CJ, Elston DM: Pediculosis. J Am Acad Dermatol 2004;50:1-12.
5. Chosidow O: Scabies and pediculosis. Lancet 2000;355:819-826.
6. Burkhart CN, Burkhart CG, Burkhart KM: An assessment of topical and oral prescription and over-the-counter treatments for head lice. J Am Acad Dermatol 1998;38:979-982.
7. Elgart ML: Pediculosis. Dermatol Clin 1990;8:219-228.
8. Meinking TL, Entzel P, Villar ME, et al: Comparative efficacy of treatments for pediculosis capitis infestations. Arch Dermatol 2001;137:287-292.
9. Pearlman DL: A simple treatment for head lice: Dry-on, suffocation-based pediculicide. Pediatrics 2004;114:e275-e279.
10. American Academy of Pediatrics: Scabies. In Pickering LK (ed): Red Book: 2003 Report of the Committee on Infectious Diseases, 26th ed. Elk Grove Village, Ill, American Academy of Pediatrics, 2003, pp 547-549.
11. Elgart ML: Scabies. Dermatol Clin 1990;8:253-263.
12. Angel TA, Nigro J, Levy ML: Infestations in the pediatric patient. Pediatr Clin North Am 2000;47:921-935.
13. Estes SA, Estes J: Therapy of scabies: Nursing homes, hospital, and the homeless. Semin Dermatol 1993;12:26-33.
14. Paller AS: Scabies in infants and small children. Semin Dermatol 1993;12:3-8.
15. Taplin D, Meinking TL, Chen JA, et al: Comparison of crotamiton 10% cream (Eurax) and permethrin 5% cream (Elimite) for the treatment of scabies in children. Pediatr Dermatol 1990;7:67-73.
16. Meinking TL, Taplin D, Hermida JL, et al: The treatment of scabies with ivermectin. N Engl J Med 1995;333:26-30.

CHAPTER 155

Atopic Dermatitis

Albert C. Yan, Christine Lauren, Paul J. Honig, and Jonathan M. Spergel

Atopic dermatitis (AD), or atopic eczema, is a common inflammatory skin disorder characterized by pruritus, a chronic and recurrent course, and a distinctive anatomic distribution and morphology. It is often accompanied by a personal or family history of other allergic disorders. Epidemiologic data indicate that AD has been increasing in prevalence, with rates as high as 17% in the United States.[1] Socioeconomic studies estimate that the annual financial impact of AD may be as high as $4400 per patient in the United States.[2] Although most patients are treated in the outpatient setting, one third to one half of the yearly expenditures for AD are directly related to the costs of hospitalization.

Patients may require hospitalization because of the severity of their primary skin disease or as a result of secondary complications, predominantly bacterial or viral superinfections. Some patients presenting with an eczematous dermatitis along with other comorbidities may require inpatient evaluation for potential underlying causes, such as Wiskott-Aldrich syndrome, hyper-IgE syndrome, or a variety of metabolic disorders.

PATHOPHYSIOLOGY

AD appears to be a multifactorial disease that involves dysregulation of the immune response, with resulting alterations in skin barrier integrity and associated cutaneous hyperreactivity. Studies suggest that T cells, particularly those expressing markers for the Th2-response, are upregulated in acute AD. The elaboration of Th2-related cytokines such as interleukin (IL)-4, IL-5, and IL-13 indirectly results in increased immunoglobulin E (IgE) production and eosinophilia. In the chronic phase of AD, there is a switch to the Th1-related cytokines IL-12 and interferon-γ. Other pathobiologic abnormalities noted in patients with AD include a genetic background of atopy, disturbed essential fatty acid metabolism, increased leukocyte phosphodiesterase activity, autonomic nervous system dysregulation, pruritus,[3-5] and a predisposition to infection.[6]

The specific genetic basis of the disease has yet to be elucidated. Studies of twins and families clearly indicate a familial predisposition in approximately two thirds of patients. Twin studies suggest an 85% concordance among monozygotic twins, but only a 21% concordance among dizygotic twins and nontwin siblings.[7] If one parent has AD, 59% of offspring will develop AD; if both parents have AD, 81% of offspring will develop the disease. It now appears unlikely that AD is the result of a single gene; rather, it appears to be the result of multiple genes interacting to produce the disorder. Recent research does, however, suggest that filaggrin mutations may play a central role in some subsets of patients with atopic dermatitis and indicates that defects in

barrier function are important in the pathogenesis of atopic dermatitis.

Patients with AD have an increased propensity for other atopic diseases such as asthma and allergic rhinitis. Based on clinical observations, patients sometimes progress sequentially from AD to the development of asthma and allergic rhinitis in what has been referred to as the "atopic march."[8]

The threefold increase in the prevalence of AD over the past three decades has been attributed to the hygiene hypothesis, which suggests that reduced childhood exposure to microbial antigens that are thought to be mediated by Th1-related immune responses leads to an increased propensity for Th2-related diseases.[4,9,10]

CLINICAL PRESENTATION

The diagnosis of AD involves the identification of characteristic clinical criteria. Although a broad spectrum of history and physical examination findings has been associated with AD, certain features have greater sensitivity and specificity. Diagnostic criteria described for the purposes of AD research have been difficult to apply in the clinical setting (Table 155-1).[11,12] A recent consensus conference on AD proposed a set of practical working guidelines for its diagnosis.[13] These guidelines characterize AD on the basis of essential and supporting criteria. The presence of pruritus and a chronic and relapsing skin rash with a typical morphology and distribution are considered essential to the diagnosis of AD. Most cases are also associated with an early age of onset (typically younger than 2 years) and a personal or family history of atopy (e.g., asthma, allergic rhinitis, IgE reactivity). Supportive, but not entirely specific, findings can help confirm the diagnosis (Table 155-2). These guidelines emphasize that AD is principally a clinical diagnosis that generally does not require confirmatory laboratory testing or histopathologic analysis.

Pruritus is a hallmark feature of AD, and patients often complain of nighttime exacerbations. Exposed skin surfaces not covered by clothing are especially predisposed to itch, although certain rough fabrics, such as wool, may aggravate pruritus in atopic patients.

The skin in early atopic eczema may itch without obvious cutaneous findings. With continued scratching, the skin becomes erythematous, scaly, and excoriated. The term *eczema* has its origins in a Greek word meaning "boiling over," and this accurately describes the morphology of an acute lesion of atopic eczema, with its exuberant oozing and crusting. Chronic excoriation may lead to thickening and altered pigmentation of the skin. Patients with significant involvement of the hands may also manifest nail pitting.

The distribution of AD lesions evolves with age. Infants generally show more widespread disease, with generalized

Table 155-1   Criteria for the Diagnosis of Atopic Dermatitis*

Major Criteria	Minor Criteria

Typical morphology and distribution
    Children: facial and extensor involvement
    Adults: flexural lichenification or linearity
Chronic or relapsing dermatitis
Personal or family history
Pruritus
	Xerosis
	Ichthyosis, keratosis pilaris, palmar hyperlinearity
	Immediate (type I) skin test reactivity
	Elevated serum immunoglobulin E
	Early age of onset
	Tendency for skin infection (*Staphylococcus aureus*, herpes), impaired cellular immunity
	Hand or foot dermatitis
	Nipple eczema
	Conjunctivitis
	Dennie-Morgan fold
	Keratoconus
	Anterior subcapsular cataracts
	Orbital darkening
	Facial pallor, erythema
	Pityriasis alba
	Anterior neck folds
	Itch when sweating
	Intolerance to wool or lipid solvents
	Perifollicular accentuation
	Food intolerance
	Course influenced by environmental or emotional factors
	White dermatographic, delayed blanch

*Patients must have three of four major criteria and three minor criteria.
From Hanifin JM, Rajka G: Diagnostic features of atopic dermatitis. Acta Derm Venereol 1980;92(Suppl):44-47.

Table 155-2   Clinical Features of Atopic Dermatitis

Essential Features
Pruritus
Eczema (acute, subacute, chronic)—typical morphology and
    age-specific patterns with chronic or relapsing history

Important Features
Early age of onset
Atopy—manifested by personal or family history or
    immunoglobulin E reactivity

Associated Features
Atypical vascular responses—dermatographism, delayed blanch
    response, facial pallor
Keratosis pilaris, hyperlinear palms, ichthyosis
Ocular or periorbital changes
Other areas of change (e.g., periorbital, periauricular)
Perifollicular accentuation, lichenification, prurigo lesions

From Eichenfield LF, Hanifin JM, Luger TA, et al: Consensus conference on pediatric atopic dermatitis. J Am Acad Dermatol 2003;49:1088-1095.

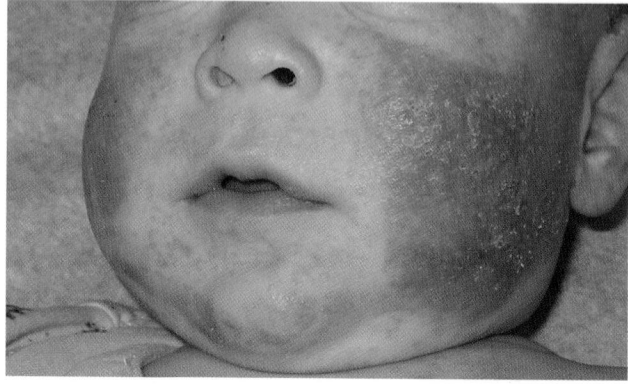

Figure 155-1   Atopic dermatitis of the face. Note the characteristic sparing of the perinasal areas.

involvement of the face, neck, extremities, and torso. Sparing of the nose, perinasal area, and diaper area is characteristic; this helps distinguish AD from seborrheic dermatitis and other skin disorders (Fig. 155-1). Accentuation within the flexural creases—the wrist, antecubital, proximal posterior thigh, popliteal (Fig. 155-2), and ankle (Fig. 155-3) areas—may be evident in infancy but is more frequently observed in toddlers and older children. Children may also suffer from scalp pruritus, scaling, and lymphadenopathy, which may make it difficult to distinguish AD from other scalp dermatoses such as tinea capitis. The majority of affected adolescents and adults demonstrate only limited disease on the hands or face, including the eyelids. When the hands are affected, the eczema is often more pronounced on the dorsal aspect.

The majority of patients with AD manifest features of the disease within the first 2 years of life, and 80% show signs of AD by age 5 years. Fortunately, most children who develop AD improve with age. Remission rates as high as 92% by age 10 years have been reported; 10-year clearance rates appear to be closer to 50% to 70% for those who develop signs of AD during childhood. Approximately 84% of children diagnosed with AD have mild to moderate disease, and 16% have

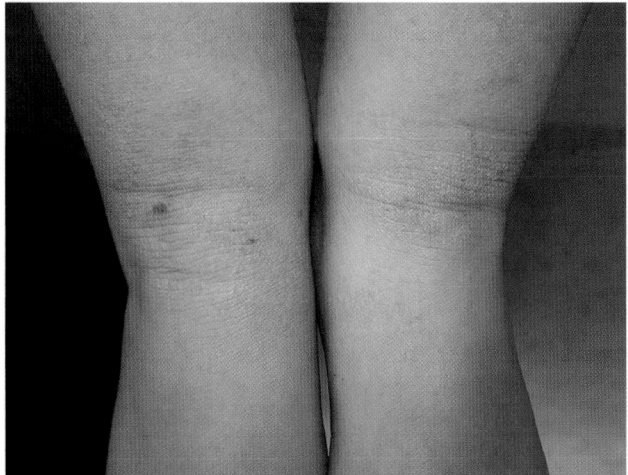

Figure 155-2 Atopic dermatitis involving the popliteal spaces.

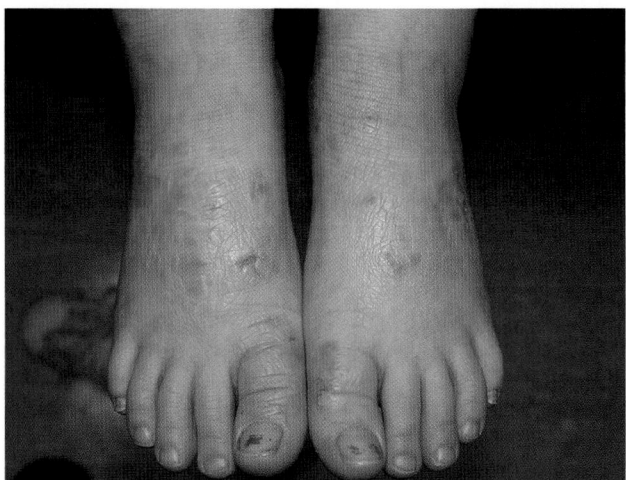

Figure 155-3 Atopic dermatitis involving the ankles.

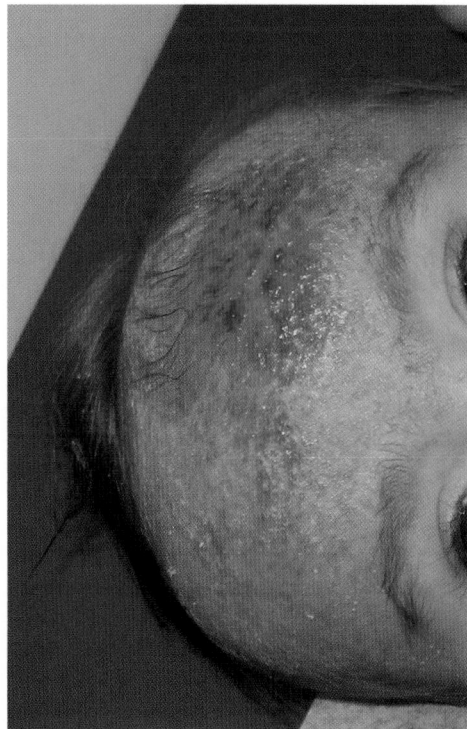

Figure 155-4 Atopic dermatitis associated with staphylococcal superinfection.

more severe disease.[14] Those suffering from severe disease also have a lower rate of spontaneous remission than do those with milder disease.

The findings of xerosis, ichthyosis, keratosis pilaris, pityriasis alba, pruritus with sweating, perifollicular accentuation, orbital darkening, hand and foot dermatitis, conjunctivitis, white dermatographism, and nipple eczema are all associated with AD.[11] Although these findings have low individual sensitivity and specificity, the presence of multiple corroborating features can be helpful in confirming the diagnosis of AD when the presentation is atypical.

The signs and symptoms of AD can be a major burden for patients and their families. Children may suffer bouts of itching and scratching that are hard to control, and sleep may be disturbed for both the child and the family. Children may have difficulty in school because they are distracted by their disease or fatigued due to poor sleep at night, or they may have secondary complications necessitating hospitalization. The treatments for AD are often both time and labor intensive. The psychosocial and socioeconomic costs of this disease are significant and should not be underestimated.

SUPERINFECTION

Patients with AD have a predilection for colonization and infection by both bacterial and viral organisms, especially *Staphylococcus aureus*, herpes simplex virus (HSV), and molluscum contagiosum virus. The propensity for microbial colonization in AD patients is likely multifactorial—a combination of impaired skin integrity permitting a favorable environment for adherence of the organism and a disease-associated decrease in antimicrobial skin properties. Naturally occurring peptides known as cathelicidins and defensins possess antimicrobial activity against organisms such as *Staphylococcus* species as well as viruses and fungi, and recent data suggest that patients with AD produce less of these peptides on the skin compared with controls.[6] These factors predispose AD patients to staphylococcal superinfection, Kaposi varicelliform eruption (or, more specifically, eczema herpeticum), and extensive outbreaks of molluscum contagiosum. This has led to speculation that because certain bacterial superantigens are known to bind glucocorticoid receptors, patients with significant bacterial colonization may show apparent steroid resistance[15] or apparent tachyphylaxis.

Bacterial Superinfection

Although patients with AD are nearly universally colonized by *S. aureus*, approximately half go on to develop frank signs and symptoms of infection at some point in their disease (Fig. 155-4). Patients who show evidence of fever with cellulitis may require hospitalization for intravenous antibiotic therapy and appropriate skin care. Severe AD flares with impetiginization may require hospitalization for

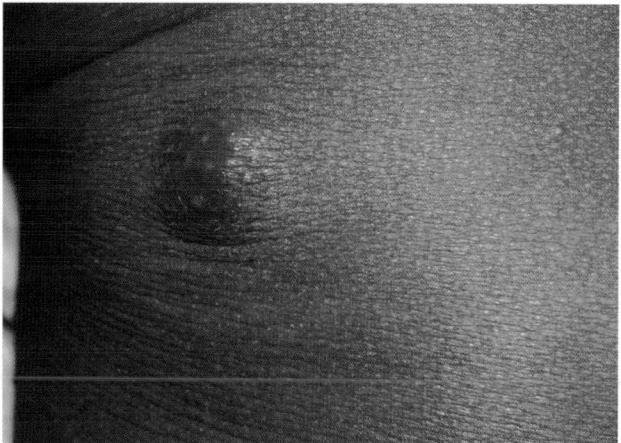

Figure 155-5 Atopic dermatitis complicated by methicillin-resistant staphylococcal furunculosis.

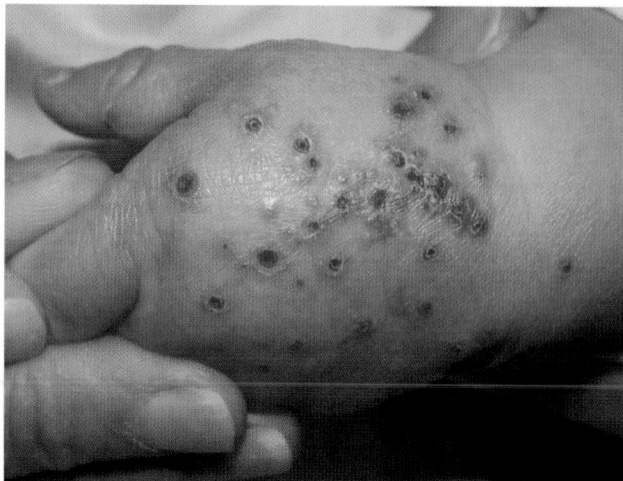

Figure 155-6 Note the "punched out" erosions characteristic of eczema herpeticum.

more potent topical therapy as well as antibiotic therapy to reduce cutaneous bacterial populations. Studies suggest that patients with AD clear faster with oral antistaphylococcal antibiotic therapy, so judicious use of these drugs is reasonable. Superinfection limited to small areas may be treated with topical mupirocin. Larger areas may require systemic antibiotics. However, this approach needs to be balanced against the increased potential for the development of antibiotic resistance. Community-acquired *S. aureus* has become a significant problem in several major urban areas. Surveys at the Children's Hospital of Philadelphia indicate that approximately 50% of all invasive *S. aureus* infections presenting to the hospital were methicillin-resistant species, indicating the need to reconsider appropriate first-line therapy for such infections.[16] At present, it is unclear whether the high prevalence of methicillin resistance among hospitalized patients affects those with AD to the same degree, but preliminary surveys of AD outpatients suggest that the rate of methicillin-resistant *S. aureus* is approximately 15% in our institution.

When AD patients present with invasive infections such as cellulitis or furuncles (Fig. 155-5), treatment with penicillinase-resistant penicillins or first-generation cephalosporins is indicated, but due consideration should be given to the potential for antibiotic resistance. With severe infections such as bacteremia or sepsis, empirical therapy with clindamycin, trimethoprim-sulfamethoxazole, or vancomycin should be considered. It should be noted that with increased use of these antibiotics, resistance to them may emerge as well.

Patients who have staphylococcal carriage in reservoir areas such as the nares, fingertips, or perianal area may benefit from treatment with mupirocin applied to these reservoir areas to reduce the carrier state.

Kaposi Varicelliform Eruption

Patients with AD may suffer acute superimposed eruptions of umbilicated vesicular or pustular lesions due to superinfection by HSV, coxsackievirus, vaccinia virus, and variola virus. The phenomenon has been referred to as Kaposi varicelliform eruption because of its resemblance to severe varicella infection. When the causative agent is HSV, the condition is specifically called eczema herpeticum; when

it is vaccinia, the term eczema vaccinatum is used. The risk of eczema vaccinatum is one of the primary reasons that smallpox vaccination is contraindicated in patients with AD. As individual lesions evolve, they become hemorrhagic and then develop a more typical "punched-out" appearance (Fig. 155-6). Often, clusters of vesicles and pustules localize to facial or flexural areas and may be superimposed on areas of existing AD. Children may have fever, lymphadenopathy, and poor oral intake, especially if there is an associated gingivostomatitis.

Diagnostic workup of Kaposi varicelliform eruption includes swabs of the affected area for fluorescent antibody testing (HSV) and polymerase chain reaction (HSV, coxsackie, vaccinia); for more atypical cases, skin biopsy for histology and electron microscopy (variola) may be warranted. All patients require close follow-up of hydration status and nutrition, as well as management of any primary viral and secondary bacterial infections with appropriate antivirals (e.g., acyclovir) and antibiotics. Tap-water soaks of affected skin areas two to four times daily may help reduce crusting.

Ophthalmic complications of eczema herpeticum require consultation with an ophthalmologist, aggressive therapy, and probably hospitalization. Patients with severe gingivostomatitis may benefit from soothing mouth rinses commonly known as "Magic Mouthwash"; these are typically a mixture of diphenhydramine liquid mixed with agents such as aluminum and magnesium hydroxide (Maalox or Mylanta) or bismuth subsalicylate (Kaopectate). During the acute phase, discontinuation of topical immunosuppressive agents such as corticosteroids or calcineurin inhibitors may be advisable. As the patient improves, reintroduction of low-potency topical steroid agents and later calcineurin inhibitors is reasonable. It is important to realize that patients with eczema herpeticum have a one in four chance of developing a reactivation of HSV on the skin within 6 months of the primary episode.

DIFFERENTIAL DIAGNOSIS

Pityriasis alba is characterized by patches of indistinct hypopigmentation and scaling, often on the face or extremities. This may represent a forme fruste of AD, a feature

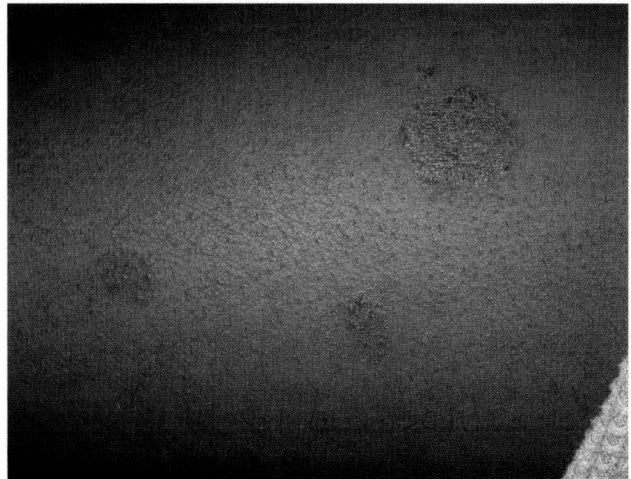

Figure 155-7 Coin-shaped lesions of nummular dermatitis.

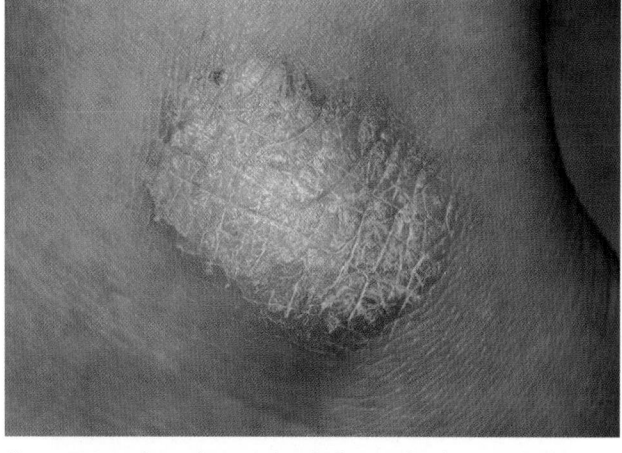

Figure 155-8 Areas that are chronically excoriated can evolve into lichen simplex chronicus.

supportive of a diagnosis of AD, or an independent phenomenon. It is often aggravated by the use of harsh soaps or cleansers.

Nummular dermatitis (nummular eczema) consists of discrete, coin-shaped areas of erythema, lichenification, and scaling (Fig. 155-7). It may occur on extensor surfaces. This disease is often less responsive to low-potency topical agents and may require higher-potency agents. Although nummular dermatitis may represent a form of AD, others argue that it is a distinct entity.

Keratosis pilaris is identified by perifollicular keratotic papules on the face, upper arms, or legs. Although keratosis pilaris is a minor manifestation associated with AD, it is a distinct clinical disorder that is frequently mistaken for AD. The condition tends not to respond significantly to topical therapies, although the use of moisturizers, especially keratolytic moisturizers (those containing urea or lactate), can be helpful in moderating the appearance of the lesions.

Prurigo lesions are often lichenified or even keratotic papules and nodules, whereas lichen simplex chronicus manifests as lichenified plaques (Fig. 155-8). Both result from chronic excoriation of an area of skin. These dermatoses may occur as a result of AD or may be initiated by some other pruritic process. These diseases are often less responsive to low-potency topical agents and may require higher-potency agents.

Seborrheic dermatitis (seborrheic eczema) is a salmon-colored erythema and scaling of the scalp, perinasal area (Fig. 155-9), eyebrows, ears, axillae, or diaper area; often, little pruritus is observed.

Contact dermatitis (contact eczema) consists of patterned areas of erythema, scaling, oozing, or frank vesiculation. Linear or geometric areas may be noted in response to an allergen (e.g., poison ivy, nickel, fragrances).

Scabies infestation may resemble AD due to involvement of the hands, feet, wrists, ankles, and other flexural creases. In addition, scratching may cause secondary eczematous changes. However, involvement of atypical areas such as the axillae, inguinal creases, scrotum, and inframammary areas suggests scabies rather than AD (Fig. 155-10). Also, an initial onset outside of the typical age range favors scabies over AD.

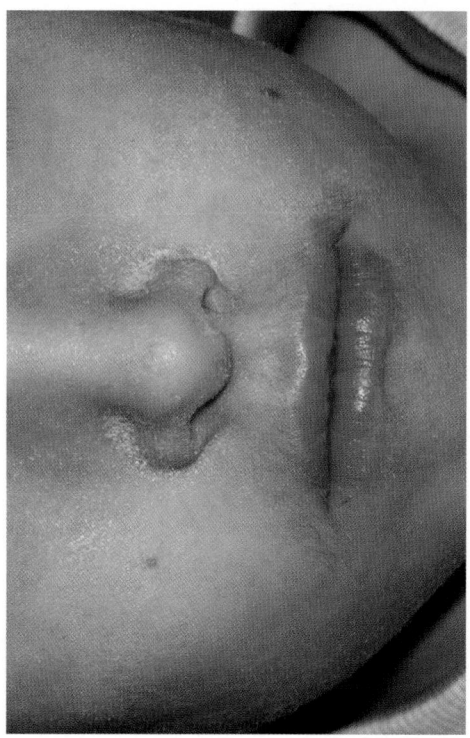

Figure 155-9 Note the contrasting perinasal involvement observed in a patient with seborrheic dermatitis.

Although there may be some similarities between the skin lesions of AD and psoriasis, several distinguishing features can be observed on clinical examination. Psoriatic lesions typically consist of well-demarcated plaques with beefy erythema and superficial white scale (Fig. 155-11). Lesions are classically located on extensor surfaces, as opposed to flexural creases. The scalp, palms, soles, and intertriginous (axillae, inguinal, genital, intergluteal) areas may also be involved. Nail pitting may be seen in both AD and psoriasis.

The differential diagnosis for scalp scaling includes scalp AD as well as psoriasis, seborrheic dermatitis, tinea capitis, and Langerhans cell histiocytosis. In areas endemic for tinea

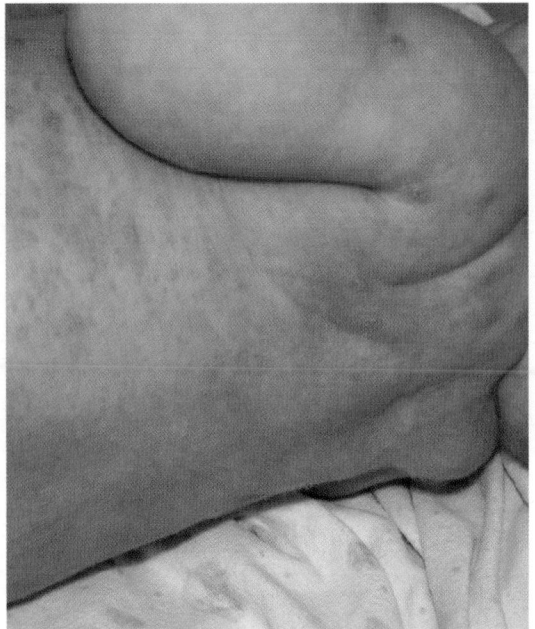

Figure 155-10 Scabies in an infant may manifest with vesicles and papules associated with excoriations.

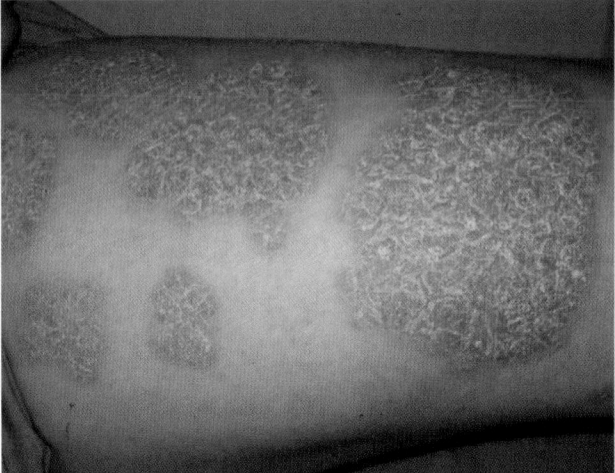

Figure 155-11 Plaque-type psoriasis. Note the well-demarcated plaques on extensor surfaces.

capitis, patients with scalp scaling should be screened for dermatophytosis.

The facial (often U-shaped around the mouth) and acrally located dermatitis of acrodermatitis enteropathica (Fig. 155-12) may resemble AD. However, there is typically chronic diaper-area involvement, as well as symptoms of diarrhea, hair loss, and irritability.

Wiskott-Aldrich syndrome and hyper-IgE syndrome are associated with chronic severe AD. A number of other diseases result in an eczematous dermatitis that resembles AD. They include ataxia-telangiectasia, cutaneous T-cell lymphoma, dermatophytosis, Dubowitz syndrome, gluten-sensitive enteropathy, Hartnup syndrome, histidinemia, Hurler syndrome, hypervitaminosis A, ichthyosis, kwashior-

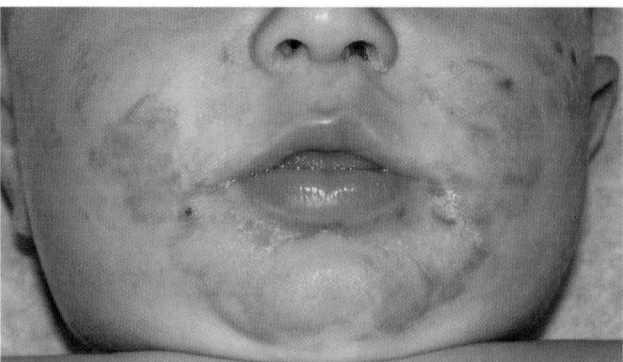

Figure 155-12 Acrodermatitis enteropathica. Note the U-shaped distribution of the facial dermatitis that is typical of patients with this condition.

kor, Langerhans cell histiocytosis, necrolytic erythema, Netherton syndrome, phenylketonuria, selective IgA deficiency, severe combined immunodeficiency, secondary syphilis, and X-linked agammaglobulinemia.

DIAGNOSIS AND EVALUATION

Diagnosis is most often made on clinical grounds (see Tables 155-1 and 155-2) using the features of pruritus, eczematous eruption (erythema, scaling, oozing, crusting), and a typical distribution and age of onset. A personal or family history of atopic disease, associated physical examination findings, and a chronic and recurrent course strengthen the diagnosis. Laboratory screening is used on occasion to assess complications or to differentiate AD from other disorders (Table 155-3).

TREATMENT

Most patients with AD are successfully managed in the outpatient setting. Children with AD may, however, require hospitalization for severe flares of the primary skin condition or as a result of significant secondary infection.

The goals of AD management include (1) optimizing skin care; (2) reducing pruritus and cutaneous inflammation; (3) avoiding potential aggravating factors, including environmental and food allergens; and (4) treating secondary infection.

Atopic Skin Care

Bathing

Controversy exists regarding bathing. Some practitioners advocate an increased frequency and duration of baths to reduce exposure to environmental allergens and hydrate the skin (the "wet school"). Others argue that bathing alters normal skin pH and reduces normal skin proteins that help maintain skin hydration status and that frequent bathing is more laborious for the family (the "dry school"). The choice of a wet versus a dry approach depends on the clinician's expertise and experience, as well as the individual patient. A mild soap with a neutral or acidic pH, such as Dove, Oil of Olay, or Cetaphil, is recommended.

Table 155-3 Laboratory Assessment for Atopic Dermatitis

Laboratory Test	Rationale
Complete blood count with differential; blood culture	Eosinophilia may be present; leukocytosis may be compatible with superinfection
Immunoglobulin E (IgE) levels	May be very elevated; may be associated with hyper-IgE syndrome
Serum zinc levels	Increased skin turnover may result in low serum zinc levels; patients with irritability and chronic facial and acral dermatitis may have acquired zinc deficiency, which may resemble atopic dermatitis
Skin culture	Bacterial culture may help determine the antibiotic-resistance profile of resident *Staphylococcus* species and may be useful in superinfected patients to determine optimal antibiotic therapy
Direct fluorescent antibody testing, polymerase chain reaction, or viral culture of skin lesions	May be helpful in identifying viral agents causing secondary infection or Kaposi varicelliform eruption (e.g., herpes simplex virus, coxsackievirus, vaccinia virus)
Skin biopsy	May be helpful in differentiating atopic dermatitis from other scaly skin disorders (e.g., psoriasis, ichthyosis, nutritional deficiency syndromes)
Skin testing or RAST	Food allergy may occur in up to 30% of severe cases of atopic dermatitis

RAST, radioallergosorbent test.

Emollients

Frequent use of emollients can improve skin barrier integrity and reduce reliance on other pharmacologic agents. Because lotions have a high alcohol content, children may complain of burning or stinging when they are applied; therefore, creams and ointments are the preferred vehicles for emollients. These include petrolatum-based moisturizers and various hydrophilic ointments such as petroleum jelly, Aquaphor, Eucerin, Absorbase, Acid Mantle cream, Cetaphil cream, and Vanicream.

Pruritus and Inflammation

Children with AD often require topical anti-inflammatory agents to reduce pruritus and inflammation. When selecting topical agents, the choice of vehicle is important in terms of both efficacy and compliance. Ointments are more occlusive and tend to contain fewer ingredients and less alcohol and therefore cause less stinging and burning; however, they may leave the patient feeling greasy. Ointments are best tolerated by infants and young children. Creams are less occlusive, have a greater propensity to cause stinging and burning, but may be better tolerated by older children and adults. Lotions and solutions are generally less effective emollients and contain higher concentrations of alcohol, but these may be better tolerated in hair-bearing areas such as the scalp.

Topical Corticosteroids

There is extensive experience in the use of topical corticosteroids, and these agents are safe when used under appropriate medical supervision. They act by binding to cytoplasmic receptors and translocating to the nucleus, where they decrease the transcription of a variety of proinflammatory cytokines, thereby reducing inflammation. The choice of topical corticosteroid should be based on the patient's age, the anatomic site being treated, and the disease severity. Although high-potency topical steroids are more effective than low-potency agents, they are also associated with a greater risk of side effects, including cutaneous atrophy and striae, Cushing syndrome, and hypothalamic-pituitary-adrenal axis suppression.

Low-potency topical corticosteroids (e.g., hydrocortisone acetonide 1% or 2.5%, desonide 0.05%, alclometasone 0.05%) can be used safely on all areas of the body, including the face or intertriginous areas for short periods. Medium-potency agents (e.g., fluocinolone 0.025%, hydrocortisone valerate 0.2%, triamcinolone 0.1%, fluticasone 0.05%) may be necessary for patients with more active disease. These agents should be avoided on the face and intertriginous areas and warrant closer medical supervision. High-potency corticosteroids (e.g., fluocinonide 0.05%, desoximetasone 0.25%, betamethasone dipropionate 0.05%) may be considered for short-term, supervised use for recalcitrant disease on the hands and feet.

Topical Calcineurin Inhibitors

Topical calcineurin inhibitors have been approved by the Food and Drug Administration (FDA) for the treatment of AD. Tacrolimus (Protopic) 0.03% and 0.1% ointment and pimecrolimus (Elidel) 1% cream are macrolide immunosuppressive agents that act by binding to cytoplasmic macrophilin receptors; they reduce inflammation by decreasing the production of proinflammatory cytokines through actions on the NF-κB pathway. Because these agents are nonsteroidal, they do not have the side effects of the topical corticosteroids. As a result, both agents can be used on any affected cutaneous surface, including the face, eyelids, and perineal area. Both carry an indication for the treatment of acute flares of AD as well as for long-term, intermittent therapy.

Pimecrolimus is available as a 1% cream and is indicated for the treatment of mild to moderate AD. Topical tacrolimus is available as an ointment in both 0.03% and 0.1% concentrations; these are indicated for the treatment of moderate to severe AD. For both agents, application twice daily is recommended for optimal effect. Topical tacrolimus appears to have greater efficacy but is also somewhat more irritating than pimecrolimus.

In February 2005 the FDA issued a public health advisory regarding the use of topical calcineurin inhibitors, citing the increased risk of lymphoma and skin cancers observed in animal studies in which very high doses of the drugs were ingested or applied to the skin.[17] It is unclear whether clinically useful doses of topical calcineurin inhibitors pose any significant risk to humans. Population-based studies, as well as most laboratory and theoretical models, have not found an increased incidence of cancer among pediatric and adult patients using either medication.[18] At this time, the FDA recommends that both tacrolimus and pimecrolimus continue to be considered as second-line agents in the treatment of AD. Manufacturers of both agents have established long-term patient registries in an effort to gather safety information. Both drugs continue to represent useful additions to the pharmacopeia for AD.

Antihistamines

Studies have reached conflicting conclusions regarding the efficacy of antihistamines for the pruritus of AD. If patients complain of nighttime itching, it may be helpful to try using a sedating antihistamine at night. If the child has a beneficial response, the medication can be continued. Sedating antihistamines such as hydroxyzine, cetirizine, diphenhydramine, and doxepin appear to be more effective than less sedating antihistamines.

Systemic Corticosteroids

Prednisone, prednisolone, methylprednisolone, and dexamethasone are more commonly prescribed for patients with asthma than for those with AD. Many patients who suffer from both disorders note that although their asthma may improve following systemic therapy, they experience flares of AD following steroid withdrawal. Some clinicians have anecdotally observed that patients receiving multiple courses of systemic steroids subsequently suffer from more brittle AD; however, it is also possible that patients with more severe AD are treated with systemic steroids more often than are those with less severe disease. In general, in patients who suffer from AD alone, the use of systemic steroids should be avoided. If steroids are necessary for the management of other comorbid conditions such as asthma, they should be tapered gradually over 7 to 14 days, and topical steroids should be instituted as part of the regimen to minimize the potential for AD flare with steroid withdrawal.

Wet Wraps

An effective method that may obviate the need for systemic corticosteroids involves the use of wet wraps. This technique can be initiated while the child is an inpatient and continued on an outpatient basis if necessary. After the patient is bathed in lukewarm water, a low-potency topical steroid is applied to all affected areas of skin. Soft, moist, water-soaked dressing material (e.g., Tubifast)—with excess water removed by squeezing—is applied to the skin, followed by a layer of similar dry dressing. This can be continued for 1 to 2 weeks. Application of the topical steroid under occlusion promotes penetration as well as hydration of the skin. At home, the child can substitute moist cotton pajamas for the water-soaked dressing.

Alternative Agents

Patients who suffer from severe AD may be prescribed other medications or therapeutic options.[19] Ultraviolet (UV) light has a number of effects on the skin; in patients with AD, it reduces the presence of cutaneous inflammatory T cells. Patients on UV treatment may have tanned skin and run the risk of ultraviolet light burns, especially those receiving photosensitizing agents as part of their therapy.

Cyclosporine, a potent, broad-spectrum, systemic immunosuppressive, has been used successfully in patients with severe, recalcitrant AD. Its use is limited, however, by the potential side effects, ranging from nausea, fatigue, and hirsutism to hypertension, renal insufficiency, immune suppression, and increased risk for malignancy.

Methotrexate, a well-known antimetabolite anti-inflammatory agent, improves the clinical findings in some patients with severe AD. Its use is limited by potential mucositis, marrow suppression, hepatotoxicity, and, less commonly, pulmonary complications.

The cytokine interferon-γ exerts its effects on patients with AD through the inhibition of IgE synthesis, the depletion of activated EG2-reactive eosinophils, and the decrease in circulating CD25$^+$-activated T cells, thereby reducing IL-4 and IL-5. This medication is typically administered subcutaneously three times a week for 4 to 12 weeks. Fever, myalgia, respiratory symptoms, and hepatic dysfunction (elevated lactate dehydrogenase or transaminitis) are the principal adverse effects.

A few case reports have documented the use of the potent broad-spectrum immunosuppressives azathioprine and mycophenolate mofetil, but they carry the side effects of immune suppression and an increased risk for malignancy. Of note, patients who are deficient in the enzyme thiopurine *S*-methyltransferase may suffer severe marrow suppression when azathioprine or its derivatives are administered.

Aggravating Factors

Although patients may be unable to identify specific triggers for their AD flares, several environmental factors have been associated with the aggravation of AD. Wool or other abrasive fabrics, pets, dust mites, and specific foods may trigger flares in certain patients. Food allergens are associated with AD in a minority of patients (5% to 30%); the likelihood of a food allergy tends to increase with the severity of AD. The most common foods implicated in AD exacerbations include milk, eggs, wheat, soy, and nuts. Because it is difficult to eliminate all these foods in a growing child, consultation with an allergist may be helpful when environmental or specific food allergens are suspected.

Secondary Infection

Patients with AD are frequently colonized by *S. aureus*, and a subset of patients develops secondary infection. Use of a diluted formulation of chlorine bleach may help reduce bacterial skin colonization. Typically, one capful per gallon of water, or approximately $1/4$ to $1/2$ cup of bleach per bathtub of water, is used once or twice a week for 5 minutes. It should be noted that patients may feel stinging or burning if there is fissured skin. Children should be patted dry with a white towel.

Studies indicate that AD patients with secondary infection improve more rapidly when treated with antistaphylococcal antibiotics such as clindamycin or dicloxacillin. Given that only a minority of patients are infected with bacteria that are methicillin resistant, first-line therapy typically includes a penicillinase-resistant penicillin such as dicloxacillin or a first-generation cephalosporin such as cephalexin.

For more severe infections, and especially in communities where methicillin resistance is high, clindamycin, trimethoprim-sulfamethoxazole, or vancomycin should be considered. Although routine first-line use of clindamycin or trimethoprim-sulfamethoxazole on an outpatient basis is not recommended, owing to their propensity for adverse effects, these drugs or linezolid, the quinolones, and vancomycin may be appropriate for the management of superinfected AD. Superinfected patients who do not respond to first-generation cephalosporins or penicillinase-resistant antibiotics may benefit from treatment with clindamycin or trimethoprim-sulfamethoxazole. The possibility of inducible clindamycin resistance should be considered in patients who do not respond as expected to antibiotic treatment. If clindamycin resistance is suspected, a D-test can be ordered on a positive staphylococcal bacterial culture to determine whether inducible resistance is present. In these instances, trimethoprim-sulfamethoxazole or inpatient therapy should be considered.

Acyclovir is indicated for the treatment of eczema herpeticum.

CONSULTATION

- Dermatology: for severe cases of atopic dermatitis unresponsive to typical outpatient therapy.
- Allergy: for evaluation of food or environmental allergies.
- Ophthalmology: for evaluation and management of ophthalmic complications of Kaposi varicelliform eruption.
- Infectious disease: for severe complications due to secondary infections.

ADMISSION CRITERIA

- Severe flare of AD unresponsive to outpatient therapy.
- Secondary infection unresponsive to outpatient therapy.
- Severe secondary infection—for example, bacterial superinfection necessitating intravenous antibiotic therapy or severe Kaposi varicelliform eruption.
- Persistent eczematous dermatitis unresponsive to outpatient therapy, necessitating further evaluation for other underlying causes.

DISCHARGE CRITERIA

- Clinical improvement of AD flare.
- Signs of resolving infection: for bacterial infection, resolution of fever, absence of bacteremia, and clinical improvement; for viral infection, resolution of vesicular lesions and crusting over of initial lesions.

- Adequate oral intake and hydration status.
- Education of caretakers regarding appropriate atopic skin care and use of pharmacologic agents such as topical corticosteroids, calcineurin inhibitors, antihistamines, emollients, and other adjuncts to therapy.
- Appropriate follow-up established.

IN A NUTSHELL

- AD is an increasingly common, pruritic, inflammatory skin disorder characterized by a chronic course of intermittent, recurrent flares.
- Patients with AD may suffer from associated atopic disorders, including asthma and allergic rhinitis, and demonstrate an increased predisposition to secondary skin infection.
- It is important to realize that not all eczematous dermatitides are AD. Some forms of eczema may resemble AD but are associated with other systemic metabolic disorders.
- AD patients may require hospitalization for a severe flare or superinfection by bacterial or viral pathogens.
- Treatment should optimize the impaired skin barrier, minimize exposure to environmental allergens, reduce pruritus and inflammation, and eliminate secondary infection.
- With appropriate intervention, patients and their clinicians can hope to achieve stable and adequate control of the signs and symptoms of AD.

ON THE HORIZON

- As a more sophisticated understanding of AD pathophysiology emerges, a number of potential therapeutic options may become available. Some agents are already being implemented as adjuncts to conventional treatment, including the use of probiotics such as *Lactobacillus* and new nonsteroidal anti-inflammatory products containing glycyrrhetinic acid (Atopiclair) and palmitimide MEA (Mimyx).
- The use of biologic agents that target specific immunologic pathways has revolutionized the treatment of psoriasis. Because of their effects on T-cell function, some of these same agents—efalizumab, infliximab, etanercept, alefacept—have been evaluated in small series for the treatment of AD, with variable responses. Similarly, omalizumab, a humanized monoclonal anti-IgE antibody currently indicated for the treatment of asthma, has shown mixed results in patients with AD.
- Investigations into the commercial development of antimicrobial peptides may also provide AD patients with an alternative to currently available antibiotics and antimicrobial products.

SUGGESTED READING

Eichenfield LF, Hanifin JM, Luger TA, et al: Consensus conference on pediatric atopic dermatitis. J Am Acad Dermatol 2003,49:1088-1095.

Paller AS, Mancini AJ: Atopic dermatitis. In Hurwitz Clinical Pediatric Dermatology. Philadelphia, Elsevier Saunders, 2006, pp 49-64.

Sturgill S, Bernard LA: Atopic dermatitis update. Curr Opin Pediatr 2004;16:396-401.

REFERENCES

1. Laughter D, Istvan JA, Tofte SJ, et al: The prevalence of atopic dermatitis in Oregon schoolchildren. J Am Acad Dermatol 2000;43:649-655.
2. Ellis CN, Drake LA, Prendergast MM, et al: Cost of atopic dermatitis and eczema in the United States. J Am Acad Dermatol 2002;46:361-370.
3. Paller AS, Mancini AJ: Atopic dermatitis. In Hurwitz Clinical Pediatric Dermatology. Philadelphia, Elsevier Saunders, 2006, pp 49-64.
4. Leung DYM, Boguniewicz M, Howell MD, et al: New insights into atopic dermatitis. J Clin Invest 2004;113:651-657.
5. Bos JD, Kapsenberg ML, Smitt JH: Pathogenesis of atopic eczema. Lancet 1994;343:1338-1341.
6. Ong PY, Ohtake T, Brandt C, et al: Endogenous antimicrobial peptides and skin infections in atopic dermatitis. N Engl J Med 2002;347:1151-1160.
7. Schultz-Larsen F: Atopic dermatitis: A genetic-epidemiological study in a population-based twin sample. J Am Acad Dermatol 1993;28:719-723.
8. Spergel JM, Paller A: Atopic dermatitis and atopic march. J Allergy Clin Immunol 2003;112(6 Suppl):S118-S127.
9. Strachan DP: Hay fever, hygiene, and household size. BMJ 1989;299:1259-1260.
10. Bach J-F: The effect of infections on susceptibility to autoimmune and allergic diseases. N Engl J Med 2002;347:911-920.
11. Hanifin JM, Rajka G: Diagnostic features of atopic dermatitis. Acta Derm Venereol 1980;92(Suppl):44-47.
12. Williams HC, Burney PGL, Hay RJ, et al: The UK Working Party's diagnostic criteria for atopic dermatitis. I. Derivation of a minimum set of discriminators for atopic dermatitis. Br J Dermatol 1994;31:386-396.
13. Eichenfield LF, Hanifin JM, Luger TA, et al: Consensus conference on pediatric atopic dermatitis. J Am Acad Dermatol 2003;49:1088-1095.
14. International Study of Asthma and Allergies in Childhood (ISAAC) Steering Committee: Worldwide variation in prevalence of symptoms of asthma, allergic rhinoconjunctivitis, and atopic eczema. Lancet 1998;351:1225-1232.
15. Sturgill S, Bernard LA: Atopic dermatitis update. Curr Opin Pediatr 2004;16:396-401.
16. Coffin SE, Zaoutis T: Rising incidence of community-onset MRSA infection. Children's Hospital of Philadelphia memorandum, Nov 24, 2003.
17. US Food and Drug Administration: FDA public health advisory: Elidel (pimecrolimus) cream and Protopic (tacrolimus) ointment. Feb 15, 2005. *http://www.fda.gov/cder/drug/advisory/elidel_protopic.htm.*
18. Fonacier L, Spergel JM, Charlesworth EN, et al: Report of the Topical Calcineurin Inhibitor Task Force of the ACAAI and AAAAI. J Allergy Clin Immunol 2005;115:1249-1253.
19. Meagher LJ, Wines NY, Cooper AJ: Atopic dermatitis: Review of immunopathogenesis and advances in immunosuppressive therapy. Australas J Dermatol 2002;43:247-254.

CHAPTER 156

Cellulitis and Erysipelas

Howard B. Pride

Cellulitis is an acute, noncontagious infection of the skin and subcutaneous tissue. It most commonly involves an extremity and is often associated with an underlying wound, ulcer, or chronic limb edema. Erysipelas is a superficial form of cellulitis with prominent lymphatic involvement; the bright red color and sharp line of demarcation from normal skin help differentiate erysipelas from cellulitis. Both conditions require prompt diagnosis and antibiotic therapy to prevent complications. The majority of children can be managed safely and effectively in the outpatient setting, but hospital admission may be prudent in some cases. In addition, cellulitis or erysipelas may develop in a patient hospitalized for a related or unrelated condition.

CLINICAL PRESENTATION

Cellulitis presents as ill-defined erythema, warmth, edema, and pain in a child who may have systemic symptoms of fever, chills, and malaise. Although a leading edge of the erythema can be determined, this edge is not raised or sharply demarcated from the adjacent normal skin. Bullae and petechiae may be noted in dependent limbs (Fig. 156-1). Portals of entry for the infection include an abrasion, ulcer, body piercing, toe web fissure, insect or animal bite, or surgical site. Venous and lymphatic damage from past surgeries, trauma, thromboses, or congenital vascular malformations may result in chronic limb edema and serve as predisposing factors for cellulitis.

The most common causative organisms are *Streptococcus pyogenes* (group A β-hemolytic streptococcus) and *Staphylococcus aureus*, but other gram-positive bacteria such as *Streptococcus pneumoniae* and group C or G streptococci may be involved.[1] Although not reliable distinguishing features, infection with *S. aureus* tends to be more localized and may suppurate, whereas *S. pyogenes* tends to spread more rapidly, with associated lymphangitis.

Erysipelas is characterized by the abrupt onset of fever, chills, and malaise, followed by the development of a warm, shiny, bright red, confluent, indurated, tender plaque with elevated, sharply defined margins (Fig. 156-2). The lower extremity is the most common location, but the face and, less commonly, other areas can be affected. *S. pyogenes* is by far the most common causative organism, although group B, C, D, and G streptococci and, uncommonly, *S. aureus*, *Klebsiella pneumoniae*, and *Yersinia enterocolitica* may be involved.[2]

Since the mid-1980s, there has been an increase in the incidence and severity of skin and soft tissue infections caused by group A β-hemolytic streptococcus (GABHS). This correlates with the increased prevalence of GABHS serotypes that produce a virulent exotoxin[3,4]; however, an increase in antibiotic resistance has not been associated with these serotypes.

Distinct clinical settings or presentations suggest different infectious agents. In neonates, group B streptococcus should be suspected and a full septic workup instituted. Buccal cellulitis, a purplish red swelling of the cheek, suggests infection with *Haemophilus influenzae* type B, but this is rarely seen since the advent of routine immunization. Hematogenous seeding of the skin may be a mechanism of infection for these organisms. Invasive GABHS causing cellulitis, lymphangitis, and necrotizing fasciitis is a recognized complication of varicella infection. It has been estimated that 15% of invasive GABHS infections in children are varicella related, and a decline in these infections has been temporally associated with use of the varicella vaccine.[5,6] Infection after contact with fresh or salt water should raise the possibility of *Aeromonas hydrophila* or *Vibrio vulnificus,* respectively. Crepitation suggests infection with clostridia or nonspore-forming anaerobes such as *Bacteroides* species, peptostreptococci, and peptococci. Circumstances such as the subcutaneous injection of medications (e.g., insulin) or illicit drugs ("skin popping") or iatrogenic or congenital immunosuppression open the door to a large array of bacterial, fungal, and mycobacterial organisms, necessitating greater scrutiny in terms of diagnosis and management.[7]

Complications of cellulitis include abscess formation, bacteremia, osteomyelitis, septic arthritis, necrotizing fasciitis (see Chapter 70), and streptococcus-associated nephritis. Recurrent bouts of cellulitis may occur after successful treatment, possibly due to lymphatic damage.

DIFFERENTIAL DIAGNOSIS

There are several noninfectious causes of swollen, warm, red skin that must be considered in the differential diagnosis of cellulitis and erysipelas. Most can be distinguished by the history and the lack of systemic symptoms, but in some cases, a skin biopsy may be needed to make the correct diagnosis. With insect bite hypersensitivity reaction or allergic contact dermatitis, itch is usually the dominant symptom, and the history may provide a clue to the cause. Familial Mediterranean fever and other periodic fever syndromes sometimes have a cellulitis-like presentation. The history of recurrent episodes resolving with and without antibiotics and the family history are helpful, but differentiating this condition from bacterial cellulitis can be extremely challenging. Wells syndrome is a rare condition characterized by urticarial plaques with central clearing that persist for weeks and may be associated with a peripheral eosinophilia. This condition responds well to systemic corticosteroids but not to antibiotics.

Fixed drug eruption remains fairly stable, without the progression seen in cellulitis, and is usually associated with the use of a medication. The tender lower extremity nodules

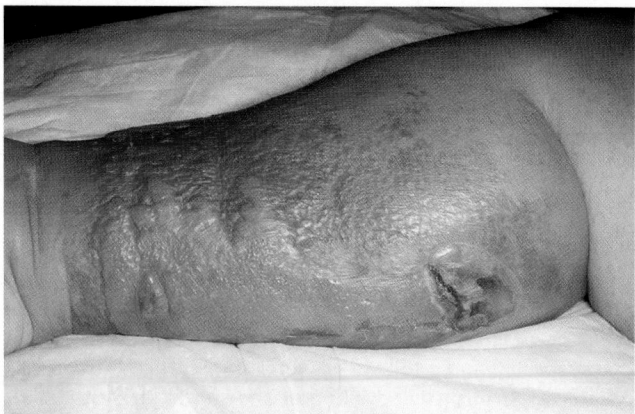

Figure 156-1 Ill-defined erythema and edema with bullae formation, characteristic of lower extremity cellulitis.

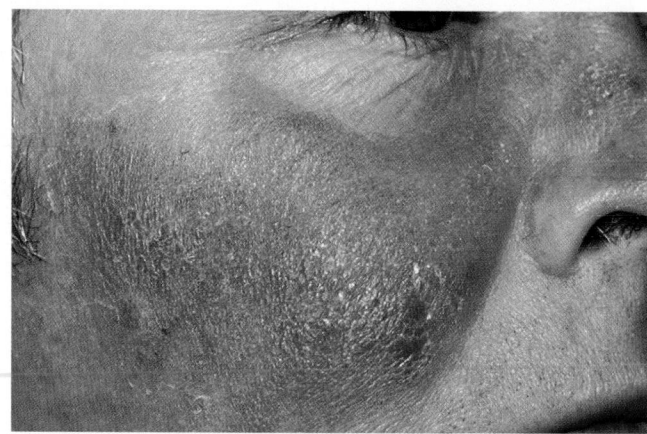

Figure 156-2 Sharply defined erythema and edema, characteristic of erysipelas.

Table 156-1 Empirical Antibiotic Therapy for Cellulitis

Clinical Presentation	Antibiotic
Typical Group A β-hemolytic streptococcus *Staphylococcus aureus** Group B streptococcus† Group C, D, or G streptococcus *Streptococcus pneumoniae*	Penicillinase-resistant penicillin (e.g., oxacillin) or first-generation cephalosporin (e.g., cephalexin)
Exposure to fresh or salt water *Aeromonas hydrophila* *Vibrio vulnificus*	In addition to coverage for typical presentation, add TMP-SMX, a quinolone (e.g., ciprofloxacin), or a third-generation cephalosporin
Presence of crepitance or gangrene *Clostridium* spp. *Bacteroides* Peptococci or streptopeptococci	In addition to coverage for typical presentation, add metronidazole

*Add vancomycin if methicillin-resistant *Staphylococcus aureus* is a concern.
†A consideration in neonates.
TMP-SMX, trimethoprim-sulfamethoxazole.

of erythema nodosum or early pyoderma gangrenosum may be mistaken for cellulitis. Reflex sympathetic dystrophy, a syndrome of unknown cause, may present with pain, hyperesthesia, swelling, and erythema of a limb, generally following some traumatic injury.

DIAGNOSIS AND EVALUATION

Cellulitis can usually be diagnosed by its typical clinical presentation, and diagnostic studies are not routinely needed. Wound aspirates are positive in only about 25% of cases, although the yield can be increased slightly by aspirating at the point of maximal inflammation rather than at the leading edge.[8] Two 3-mm punch biopsies afford enough tissue for multiple cultures as well as histologic evaluation; this is particularly helpful when the diagnosis is in question, the response to therapy has been poor, or more unusual organisms are suspected (e.g., in an immunocompromised patient).[9] Blood cultures are usually negative in routine cases of cellulitis, but they should be obtained in very ill children.

Radiologic studies are not helpful in managing cellulitis but should be obtained if symptoms suggest an associated osteomyelitis. Magnetic resonance imaging may help distinguish cellulitis from necrotizing fasciitis, but immediate surgical exploration is indicated if necrotizing fasciitis is suspected.

TREATMENT

Uncomplicated cellulitis in an immunocompetent host can be treated with oral β-lactam antibiotics with activity against GABHS and penicillinase-producing *S. aureus*. Dicloxacillin, a first-generation cephalosporin (e.g., cephalexin), and amoxicillin-sulbactam are good choices for most patients. Oral clindamycin, quinolones, or macrolide antibiotics can be substituted for uncomplicated infections in patients allergic to β-lactam antibiotics.[9]

For those who require hospitalization, antibiotics are administered intravenously. As for outpatient therapy, β-lactams with antistaphylococcal activity are recommended for empirical therapy in uncomplicated cases (Table 156-1). An increasing percentage of North American communities has seen the emergence of community-acquired methicillin-resistant *S. aureus*, and the possibility that this pathogen could be causing cellulitis must be weighed, based on the antibiotic resistance profile in the practitioner's geographic area. In extremely ill children, intravenous vancomycin or linezolid (either intravenous or oral) should be used as initial therapy and then adjusted as cultures become available or as the patient's clinical condition allows. The total duration of antibiotic therapy should be 7 to 14 days and must be gauged by the health of the patient and the response to therapy.

When the presentation or clinical setting increases the concern for uncommon pathogens, antibiotic coverage should be broadened appropriately. Empirical therapy is initiated based on the presentation, particular exposures, and the appearance of the involved skin (see Table 156-1). If the pathogen is identified and antibiotic susceptibilities are available, coverage can be adjusted.

Abscesses must be surgically drained or aspirated.

ADMISSION CRITERIA

- Ill appearance.
- Rapid progression of skin findings.
- Worsening clinical picture despite appropriate outpatient therapy.
- Inability to tolerate oral medications.
- Inability to ensure compliance with treatment or adequate follow-up.

DISCHARGE CRITERIA

- Ability to take adequate oral fluids.
- Ability to take oral medications or the capacity to perform home intravenous therapy.
- Lack of fever or systemic symptoms for 12 to 24 hours.
- Clinical improvement.

IN A NUTSHELL

- Fever, chills, and malaise are accompanied by ill-defined soft tissue erythema, warmth, and edema, indicating cellulitis; raised, sharply defined margins suggest erysipelas.
- Despite modest help from tissue aspiration or biopsy, cellulitis remains a clinical diagnosis.
- Oral or intravenous antibiotics effective against *S. aureus* and *S. pyogenes* are needed for 7 to 14 days.

ON THE HORIZON

- Reports of vancomycin-resistant *S. aureus* are surfacing in adults, and this pathogen will eventually be seen in childhood infections.
- The decoding of the genomic sequences of many bacterial pathogens has facilitated vaccine development, including for those organisms responsible for cellulitis.
- Bacterial agents compete for areas of colonization, such as the nares, and it has been found that *S. aureus* carriage decreases with nasal carriage of the vaccine strain of *S. pneumoniae*, offering the possibility of a new preventive strategy.

SUGGESTED READING

Morris A: Cellulitis and erysipelas. Clin Evid 2002;7:1483-1487.
Swartz MN: Cellulitis. N Engl J Med 2004;350:904-912.

REFERENCES

1. Sigurdsson AF, Gudmundsson S: The etiology of bacterial cellulitis as determined by fine-needle aspiration. Scand J Infect Dis 1989;21:537-542.
2. Jorup-Ronstrom C: Epidemiological, bacteriological and complication features of erysipelas. Scand J Infect Dis 1986;18:519-524.
3. Schwartz B, Facklam RR, Breiman F: Changing epidemiology of group A streptococcal infection in the USA. Lancet 1990;336:1167-1171.
4. Belani K, Schlievert PM, Kaplan EL, Ferrieri P: Association of exotoxin-producing group A streptococci and severe disease in children. Pediatr Infect Dis J 1991;10:351-354.
5. Laupland KB, Davies HD, Low DE, et al: Invasive group A streptococcal disease in children and association with varicella-zoster virus infection. Pediatrics 2000;105:60.
6. Patel RA, Binns HJ, Shulman ST: Reduction in pediatric hospitalizations for varicella-related invasive group A streptococcal infections in the varicella vaccine era. J Pedatr 2004;144:68-74.
7. Swartz MN: Cellulitis. N Engl J Med 2004;350:904-912.
8. Howe PM, Eduardo-Fajardo J, Orcutt MA: Etiologic diagnosis of cellulitis: Comparison of aspirates obtained from the leading edge and the point of maximal inflammation. Pediatr Infect Dis J 1987;6:685-686.
9. Duvanel T, Auckenthaler R, Rohner P, et al: Quantitative cultures of biopsy specimens from cutaneous cellulitis. Arch Intern Med 1989;149:293-296.

CHAPTER 157

Staphylococcal Scalded Skin Syndrome

Kimberly D. Morel

Staphylococcal scalded skin syndrome (SSSS) is a toxin-mediated systemic illness that is manifested as an epidermal blistering disorder. Certain strains of *Staphylococcus aureus* elaborate an exfoliative toxin that is responsible for the cutaneous manifestations of the condition. In neonates, SSSS has previously been called Ritter syndrome, named after the first person to describe the condition in 1878.[1] The disorder occurs most commonly in children younger than 5 years. Neonates are especially susceptible to the toxin, probably because of their renal immaturity and inability to clear the toxin from their bloodstream.

PATHOPHYSIOLOGY

Certain strains of *S. aureus* elaborate exfoliative toxins A and B. Phage groups I, II, and III may elaborate exotoxin, with phage group II strains 71 and 55 being the most common. An understanding of the pathogenesis of SSSS involves recognizing that bullous impetigo is essentially a localized form of SSSS. The toxin may act locally to cause bullous impetigo and can also spread hematogenously from an infected site and act by cleaving the superficial layer of the epidermis, the stratum granulosum, just below the stratum corneum (Fig. 157-1). The exfoliative toxin produced by pathogenic strains of *S. aureus* cleaves the same superficial level of the epidermis in SSSS as in bullous impetigo.[2] The target antigen of the exfoliative toxin is desmoglein 1, a desmosomal protein involved in intercellular adhesion. Unlike the toxin produced in staphylococcal toxic shock syndrome, the exfoliative toxin of SSSS is not thought to induce hemodynamic compromise (see Chapter 62).

As mentioned, neonates are at higher risk for this condition, probably because of their renal immaturity and decreased ability to clear the toxins from their bloodstream. In this same regard, adults with renal insufficiency also have increased susceptibility to the toxin-mediated effects of *S. aureus* infections.

CLINICAL PRESENTATION

Neonates may present initially with fever or temperature instability and irritability. In young children, the syndrome often begins with a prodrome of fever, irritability, and coryza. The initial symptoms are followed by the abrupt onset of tender cutaneous erythema. An important clinical clue is the Nikolsky sign, in which gentle lateral pressure on the skin causes separation of the superficial layer of the epidermis. Bullae and diffuse erosions then develop over the next 1 to 2 days. Conjunctivitis may be present, but other mucous membranes are spared. Perioral radial scaling can occur (Figs. 157-2 and 157-3).

The most common timing of neonatal presentations of SSSS is 3 to 16 days after birth.[3] Congenital cases and presentations in the first 24 hours after birth are uncommon but can occur.[4,5] A case of intrauterine SSSS with positive amniotic fluid cultures has also been reported.[6] Nursery outbreaks, as well as neonatal intensive care unit outbreaks involving premature babies, have also been well described.[7] Very low birth weight premature infants also have increased susceptibility to the toxin-mediated effects of the condition.[8,9]

DIAGNOSIS AND EVALUATION

Cultures should be performed before initiation of antibiotics to search for an infectious source, as well as to check sites of bacterial colonization. With the emergence of methicillin-resistant *S. aureus* (MRSA), bacterial cultures are imperative to help in choosing antibiotic coverage for the patient. Cultures should include blood, urine, nasal swab, throat, wound (if present), umbilicus, and any other potentially contaminated body fluid. Cerebrospinal fluid should be examined in neonates. A conjunctiva swab should also be considered.

The most common site of colonization is the nasopharynx, especially the anterior nares (vestibulum). Other typical sites include the umbilicus, axillary skin folds, and perineum. The cleaved skin or bulla fluid itself is expected to be sterile because it is the toxin, not the bacterium, that produces the cutaneous manifestations.

Histopathologic evaluation of SSSS reveals a separation of the stratum granulosum, the most superficial layer of the epidermis, from the underlying epidermis. Minimal to no inflammation is seen. A skin biopsy is useful to help differentiate SSSS from other disorders such as toxic epidermal necrolysis, which involves full-thickness necrosis of the epidermis.

DIFFERENTIAL DIAGNOSIS

The differential diagnosis of SSSS includes burn injury, generalized bullous impetigo, scarlet fever, toxic epidermal necrolysis, graft-versus-host disease, and boric acid poisoning. In neonates, the differential diagnosis should also include other rare conditions such as epidermolysis bullosa, epidermolytic hyperkeratosis, diffuse cutaneous mastocyto-

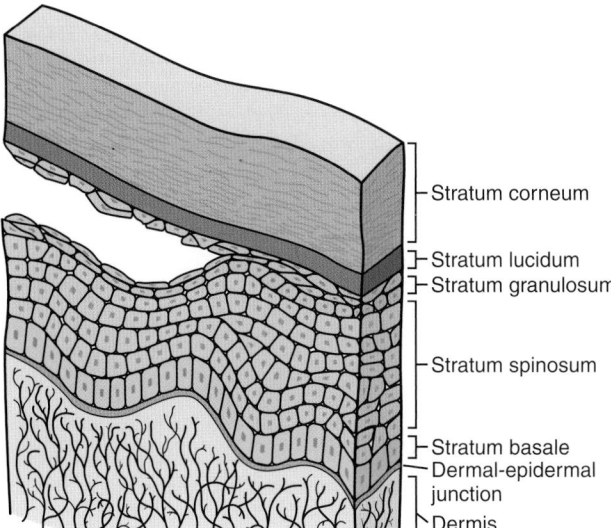

Figure 157-1   Level of cleavage in staphylococcal scalded skin syndrome.

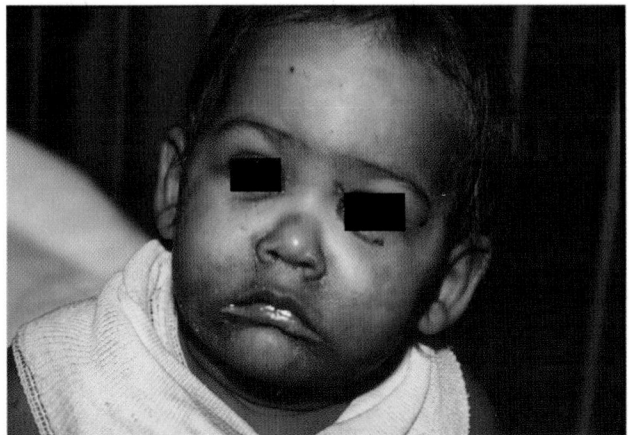

Figure 157-2   Facial erythema, crusted erosions, and perioral scaling in a child who presented with a prodrome of fever, irritability, and coryza. Truncal dressings overlie superficially eroded skin.

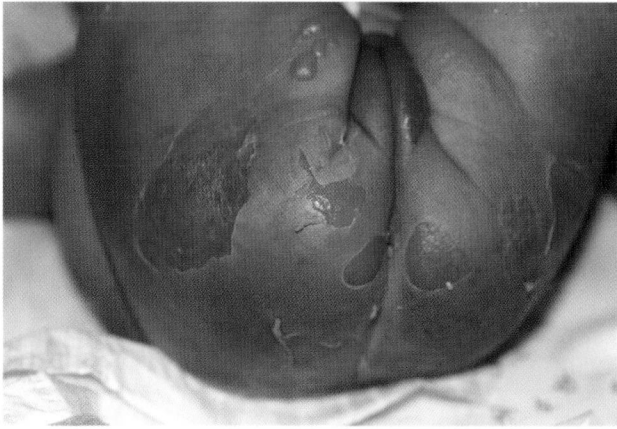

Figure 157-3   This neonate presented with fever, superficial erosions of the perineum, and bullae on the thighs. The Nikolsky sign was positive.

sis, other infectious processes such as syphilis, metabolic disorders such as methylmalonic acidemia, and familial peeling skin syndrome.

TREATMENT AND PROGNOSIS

Essential treatment includes prompt initiation of intravenous antibiotics with activity against *S. aureus.* Early treatment against MRSA should also be considered in consultation with an infectious disease specialist based on the epidemiology of local *S. aureus* sensitivity patterns. Coverage can then be narrowed after culture sensitivity results return. The addition of clindamycin can also be considered because its mechanism of action, inhibition of 30S ribosomal synthesis, may inhibit further bacterial exfoliative toxin production. However, it is not generally appropriate as single-agent therapy. Inducible clindamycin resistance may develop rapidly in certain strains of *S. aureus.*[10] Topical care

includes bland emollients (such as petrolatum) and semiocclusive, nonadherent dressings applied and changed once or twice a day. The patient should be placed on strict contact isolation with minimal handling. Applying tape in direct contact with the skin should be avoided whenever possible. Fluids and electrolytes must be monitored closely because of the increased insensible losses related to the denuded skin. Topical antibiotics should be avoided, especially in neonates, given the high risk for systemic absorption. For example, topical application of neomycin to neonatal skin has been associated with ototoxicity and deafness.

Hand hygiene is crucial for helping prevent nursery outbreaks of SSSS. Hospital epidemiologists should be involved to investigate and control nursery outbreaks of SSSS.[7]

The mortality rate has been reported to be 4% in infants and as high as 60% or more in adults and may depend on the baseline health status of the affected individual. Prompt recognition of the condition plus initiation of antibiotic treatment is imperative to decrease morbidity and mortality. With extensive loss of skin, temperature regulation and maintenance of fluid and electrolyte balance become important issues. Risk factors for increased mortality include younger age, whereas immunosuppression is an important risk factor for increased mortality in adults.[11] Given the superficial nature of the skin blistering and desquamation, permanent scarring is unusual. Morbidity and mortality are related to complications such as superinfection of the skin, bacteremia, and sepsis.

In most children, this syndrome does not recur because of the development of neutralizing antibodies. However, recurrence may develop in children and adults in the context of immunosuppression or renal insufficiency (resulting in an inability to clear the toxin).

CONSULTATION

- Dermatology can assist with diagnosis and ongoing management.
- Infectious disease consultation can guide empirical therapy and ongoing antimicrobial choices.
- Hospital epidemiology or infection control services (or both) should be involved with outbreaks.

- Critical care may be needed if intensive care services are required.

ADMISSION CRITERIA

Admission is generally required for prompt initiation of intravenous antibiotics and local wound care. Transfer to an intensive care setting may be necessary if hemodynamic instability develops, fluid and electrolyte management becomes difficult, or bedside care of the skin exceeds the staffing capabilities in a non–intensive care setting.

DISCHARGE CRITERIA

- Completion of an appropriate course of intravenous antibiotics. Consider the age of the patient and the source of infection because neonates or those with bacteremia may require a full course of intravenous antibiotics before discharge.
- Hemodynamic stabilization with the patient able to maintain adequate hydration and nutrition orally.
- Ability of caregivers to provide necessary wound and skin care. Home nursing services are useful to assist families and monitor for signs of deterioration.

IN A NUTSHELL

- SSSS is a toxin-mediated illness.
- Fever, irritability, rhinitis, and tender cutaneous erythema are often the initial presenting features.
- The Nikolsky sign is positive in SSSS.
- Bullae and superficial desquamation follow soon after the appearance of tender cutaneous erythema.
- Common sources of bacterial infection and colonization should be cultured before the initiation of antibiotics.
- Neonates are more susceptible to this toxin-mediated illness because of their immature renal function.
- Treatment involves prompt initiation of intravenous antibiotics effective against known resistance patterns of *S. aureus*. Coverage can then be narrowed as sensitivity results become available.
- The increasing incidence of MRSA necessitates vigilance for MRSA-associated SSSS.

ON THE HORIZON

- Community-acquired, as well as hospital-acquired, strains of MRSA are on the rise.[12] Of notable concern, young age has been identified as a risk factor for MRSA in some population-based studies.[13] MRSA-associated SSSS has been reported to occur.[14-16] A nursery outbreak of MRSA has also been described.[17] Therefore, consideration should be given to starting empirical treatment of MRSA in consultation with an infectious disease specialist based on *S. aureus* resistance patterns in the area. MRSA should also be considered in children who do not demonstrate a response to treatment or worsen despite treatment.

- Inducible clindamycin resistance is another factor that has limited the spectrum of appropriate antibiotic choices for treating infections caused by *S. aureus*. The "D zone reaction" may be performed to analyze whether inducible clindamycin resistance, caused by the *erm* gene, is present.[10]
- Research into neutralizing antitoxin antibody for the treatment and prevention of SSSS is being performed but is not clinically available at the present time.[18]

SUGGESTED READING

Ladhani S, Evans RW: Staphylococcal scalded skin syndrome. Arch Dis Child 1998;78:85-88.
Prevost G, Couppie P, Monteil H: Staphylococcal epidermolysins. Curr Opin Infect Dis 2003;16:71-76.

REFERENCES

1. Ritter von Rittershain G: Die exfoliative Dermatitis jungerer Sauglinge. Zentralzeit Kinderheilkd 1878;2:3-23.
2. Dancer SJ, Simmons NA, Poston SM, Noble WC: Outbreak of staphylococcal scalded skin syndrome among neonates. J Infect 1988;16:87-103.
3. Haveman LM, Fleer A, de Vries LS, Gerards LJ: Congenital staphylococcal scalded skin syndrome in a premature infant. Acta Paediatr 2004;93:1661-1662.
4. Loughead JL: Congenital staphylococcal scalded skin syndrome: Report of a case. Pediatr Infect Dis J 1992;11:413-414.
5. Lo WT, Wang CC, Chu ML: Intrauterine staphylococcal scalded skin syndrome: Report of a case. Pediatr Infect Dis J 2000;19:481-482.
6. Saiman L, Jakob K, Holmes KW, et al: Molecular epidemiology of staphylococcal scalded skin syndrome in premature infants. Pediatr Infect Dis 1998;17:329-334.
7. Haveman LM, Fleer A, Gerards LJ: Staphylococcal scalded skin syndrome in two very low birth weight infants. J Perinat Med 2003;31:515-519.
8. Makhoul IR, Kassis I, Hashman N, Sujov P: Staphylococcal scalded-skin syndrome in a very low birth weight premature infant. Pediatrics 2001;108(1):E16.
9. Amagai M, Matsuyoshi N, Wang ZH, et al: Toxin in bullous impetigo and staphylococcal scalded skin syndrome targets desmoglein 1. Nat Med 2000;6:1213-1214.
10. Lewis JS 2nd, Jorgensen JH: Inducible clindamycin resistance in staphylococci: Should clinicians and microbiologists be concerned? Clin Infect Dis 2005;40:280-285.
11. Mockenhaupt M, Idzko M, Grosber M, et al: Epidemiology of staphylococcal scalded skin syndrome in Germany. J Invest Dermatol 2005;124:700-703.
12. Zetola N, Francis JS, Nuermberger EL, Bishai WR: Community-acquired methicillin-resistant Staphylococcus aureus: An emerging threat. Lancet Infect Dis 2005;5:275-286.
13. Fridkin SK, Hageman JC, Morrison M, et al: Methicillin-resistant Staphylococcus aureus disease in three communities. N Engl J Med 2005;352:1436-1444.
14. Acland KM, Darvey A, Griffin C, et al: Staphylococcal scalded skin syndrome in an adult associated with methicillin-resistant Staphylococcus aureus. Br J Dermatol 1999;140:518-520.
15. Yamaguchi T, Yokota Y, Terajima J, et al: Clonal association of Staphylococcus aureus causing bullous impetigo and the emergence of new methicillin-resistant clonal groups in Kansai district in Japan. J Infect Dis 2002;185:1511-1516.

16. Yokota S, Imagawa T, Katakura S, et al: Staphylococcal scalded skin syndrome caused by exfoliative toxin B–producing methicillin-resistant *Staphylococcus aureus.* Eur J Pediatr 1996;155:722.

17. Richardson JF, Quoraishi AH, Francis BJ, Marples RR: Beta-lactamase–negative, methicillin-resistant *Staphylococcus aureus* in a newborn nursery: Report of an outbreak and laboratory investigations. J Hosp Infect 1990;16:109-121.

18. Ladhani S: Understanding the mechanism of action of the exfoliative toxins of *Staphylococcus aureus.* FEMS Immunol Med Microbiol 2003;39:181-189.

CHAPTER 158

Ecthyma Gangrenosum

Julie V. Schaffer and Mary Wu Chang

In 1897 Barker first described skin lesions evolving from erythematous macules to vesicles to necrotic ulcers in the setting of septicemia secondary to *Pseudomonas aeruginosa*.[1] In the same year, Hitschmann and Kreibich coined the term *ecthyma gangrenosum* (EG) for this characteristic cutaneous manifestation of pseudomonal septicemia.[2] Although *P. aeruginosa* is the classic pathogen in EG, over the past several decades, other infectious causes have been reported for clinically identical lesions (Box 158-1).[3] Regardless of the causative organism, EG tends to occur in immunocompromised hosts, particularly individuals with neutropenia and hematologic malignancies.[4] EG represents a morphologic pattern of cutaneous necrosis that results from vascular occlusion by organisms proliferating within the adventitia and media of subcutaneous blood vessels.

EPIDEMIOLOGY

Conditions that have been associated with EG in children are listed in Table 158-1. Almost half of pediatric patients with EG have leukemia or aplastic anemia, and the occurrence of EG usually coincides with neutropenia related to the administration of chemotherapy or myeloablative regimens for peripheral blood stem cell transplantation. However, EG occasionally heralds the onset of leukemia in a previously healthy child.[5] Additional predisposing factors for the development of EG in cancer patients and other immunocompromised hosts include prior antibiotic therapy, treatment with systemic corticosteroids or other immunosuppressive medications, diabetes mellitus, hypocomplementemia, occlusion or maceration of the skin, and, particularly in premature neonates, a high-humidity environment.[6-8] Intravenous catheters and invasive procedures represent additional iatrogenic risk factors.[9] Finally, bacterial contamination (e.g., with *P. aeruginosa*) of "moist" hospital equipment and supplies, ranging from nebulizers to antiseptic solutions to bath toys, can be a source of nosocomial infections manifesting as EG in immunocompromised patients.[10,11]

Approximately one third of reported pediatric cases of EG occurred in previously healthy children (see Table 158-1). The median age of these patients was younger than 1 year, compared with approximately 4 years for children known to have an underlying medical disorder. Most cases developed in the setting of an acute gastrointestinal illness, and more than half the children were subsequently found to have X-linked recessive agammaglobulinemia or another immunodeficiency syndrome.

Regardless of the underlying medical condition, EG is observed in approximately 20% to 50% of children with pseudomonal septicemia.[8] Cutaneous lesions that may be clinically identical to pseudomonal EG can also be seen in the setting of disseminated candidiasis (10% to 15% of cases) or aspergillosis (<5% of cases), which represent the most common systemic mycoses in neutropenic patients. Of note, EG-like skin lesions occur in 70% to 90% of disseminated infections with *Fusarium*, the mold second most likely to cause systemic disease in immunocompromised hosts.[12]

PATHOGENESIS

There are two major routes to the development of EG: (1) a classic bacteremic (or fungemic) form, caused by hematogenous dissemination of the organism to the skin; and (2) a nonbacteremic form in which the skin lesions are located at a cutaneous site of inoculation of the organism.[10,13,14] Although blood cultures are initially negative in the latter scenario, secondary bacteremia and clinical decompensation may occur if treatment is delayed.

The most recognized pathogen of EG, *P. aeruginosa* is a gram-negative bacillus that is a component of the normal intestinal flora in 10% to 15% of healthy individuals and in more than 33% of hospitalized patients.[15] Although it cannot survive on intact, dry skin, *P. aeruginosa* colonizes moist intertriginous areas, such as the groin and axillae, in approximately 2% of the population. Based on the frequent localization of pseudomonal EG to these intertriginous areas, as well as documentation of EG in association with blood cultures that are initially negative but later positive, some authors have postulated that the source of *P. aeruginosa* infection manifesting with EG in immunologically impaired hosts is often the skin itself.[8]

Abnormal neutrophil function (resulting from quantitative or qualitative defects) represents the most important risk factor for both disseminated *P. aeruginosa* infection and opportunistic mycoses. The vascular destruction that leads to EG lesions in septicemia due to *P. aeruginosa* is thought to be related to dissolution of the elastic lamina by pseudomonal elastase. Not unexpectedly, other bacteria (e.g., *Aeromonas maltophilia*) that have been implicated in the development of EG also produce elastase and various proteases.[16] Likewise, several of the opportunistic mycoses that can cause lesions resembling EG (e.g., aspergillosis, fusariosis, zygomycosis) have a propensity to invade blood vessel walls, resulting in thrombosis and tissue necrosis.

CLINICAL PRESENTATION

EG typically begins as a painless, erythematous macule, often with a relatively blanched or grayish center. Over a 12- to 24-hour period, the lesion becomes indurated, and a hemorrhagic vesicle or pustule develops centrally (Fig. 158-1). Rupture then leads to the formation of a necrotic ulcer with a gray-black eschar and a red to violaceous border (Fig. 158-2).[17] One or multiple lesions may be present, either

Box 158-1   Organisms That Have Been Reported to Cause Ecthyma Gangrenosum-Like Lesions

BACTERIA

Gram-negative rods
  Pseudomonas aeruginosa
  Pseudomonas stutzeri
  Burkholderia (Pseudomonas) cepacia
  Methylobacterium (Pseudomonas) mesophilica
  Stenotrophomonas (Xanthomonas) maltophilia
  Aeromonas hydrophila
  Klebsiella pneumoniae
  Serratia marcescens
  Citrobacter freundii
  Morganella morganii
  Escherichia coli
  Vibrio vulnificus
  Yersinia pestis
Gram-negative cocci
  Moraxella (Branhamella) catarrhalis
  Neisseria gonorrhoeae
Gram-positive rods
  Corynebacterium diphtheriae
Gram-positive cocci
  Staphylococcus aureus
  *Streptococcus pyogenes**

FUNGI

Candida spp.
  C. albicans
  C. tropicalis
Aspergillus spp.[†]
  A. fumigatus
  A. niger
Zygomycetes[†]
  Mucor
  Rhizopus
  Absidia
Other organisms causing hyalohyphomycosis[†,‡]
  Fusarium solani
  Pseudoallescheria boydii
  Metarrhizium anisopliae
Organisms causing phaeohyphomycosis[†,§]
  Curvularia
  Exserohilum
  Drechslera
  Scytalidium dimidiatum

VIRUSES

Herpes simplex virus

*Local infection can result in ecthyma, a condition distinct from ecthyma gangrenosum (see Table 158-2).
[†]Primarily soil saprophytes found in decaying vegetation.
[‡]Representing molds with hyaline (nonpigmented) hyphae.
[§]Representing molds with dematiaceous (brown-black) hyphae.

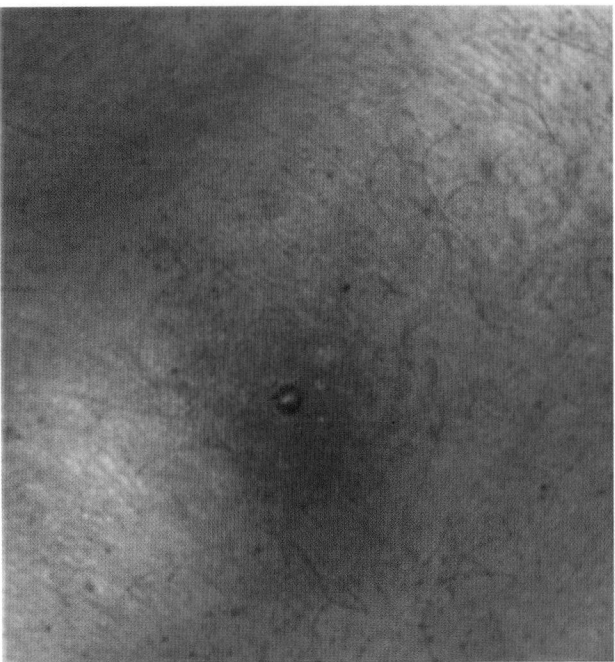

Figure 158-1   Hemorrhagic pustule with surrounding erythema in a patient with *Staphylococcus aureus* septicemia. (Courtesy of Yale Dermatology Residents' Slide Collection.)

grouped or in a scattered distribution, with sizes ranging from a few millimeters to several centimeters in diameter.

EG due to *P. aeruginosa* has a predilection for the groin, buttocks, and anogenital area; in children, more than 50% of all cases and more than 90% of nonbacteremic cases involve these sites.[7] Bacteremic pseudomonal EG also favors the extremities, as does nonpseudomonal EG. However, EG can develop anywhere on the cutaneous surface and occasionally affects the oral, nasal, and conjunctival mucosa. Widespread EG lesions represent "septic emboli" resulting from bacteremia or fungemia; EG localized to moist, occluded sites (e.g., the diaper area or the skin underlying adhesive tape securing an intravenous catheter) may be due to primary inoculation of the skin.

The spectrum of cutaneous lesions that can develop in association with septicemia (due to *P. aeruginosa* as well as other bacterial and fungal organisms) also includes purpuric macules or papules (especially in thrombocytopenic patients), subcutaneous nodules, and necrotic cellulitis.[18,19] Pseudomonal infections in immunocompromised hosts may have atypical presentations, such as edematous follicular papulopustules in the groin (resembling "hot tub" folliculitis) that subsequently evolve into classic EG.[10] Of note, the gangrenous orofacial and anogenital lesions of noma neonatorum are thought to represent a neonatal form of EG secondary to *P. aeruginosa* infection in debilitated premature infants.[20] Infections with some pathogens that can cause EG-like lesions may have other characteristic manifestations in immunocompromised patients (Table 158-2).

In the classic bacteremic form of EG that occurs in immunocompromised individuals, patients are critically ill and typically present with fever, hypotension, tachycardia, and altered mental status. In contrast, *P. aeruginosa* gastrointestinal infections, which represent the most common

Table 158-1 Underlying Conditions in 114 Children with Ecthyma Gangrenosum

Underlying Condition*	% of Total Cases	Median Age at Presentation with EG (yr)	Bacteremia or Fungemia (% of Cases)	Neutropenia (% of Cases)
Acute leukemia[†]	33	4	60	100
Solid tumors[†,‡]	4	2	75	100
Aplastic anemia[†]	4	15	100	100
Hypogammaglobulinemia[§]	15	1	95	90
Neutropenia or abnormal neutrophil function[§]	6	0.7	30	70
HIV/AIDS	4	1	100	50
Severe burns	11	5	100	NA
Nutritional deficiency[¶]	4	0.5	100	NA
Extreme prematurity	2	0	50	0
Recent major surgery or trauma	2	3	100	NA
None identified[§]	15	0.5	95	50

*Single cases of EG have also been reported in children with Wiskott-Aldrich syndrome, harlequin ichthyosis, and Hirschsprung disease.
[†]Most occurred after receiving chemotherapy or after a bone marrow or peripheral blood stem cell transplant.
[‡]Included cases of neuroblastoma, osteosarcoma, and rhabdomyosarcoma.
[§]The vast majority of patients were previously healthy, and most presented with fever and diarrhea in the setting of a gastrointestinal infection with *Pseudomonas aeruginosa.*
[¶]One patient also had underlying methylmalonicacidemia.
EG, ecthyma gangrenosum; HIV/AIDS, human immunodeficiency virus/acquired immunodeficiency syndrome; NA, not applicable.

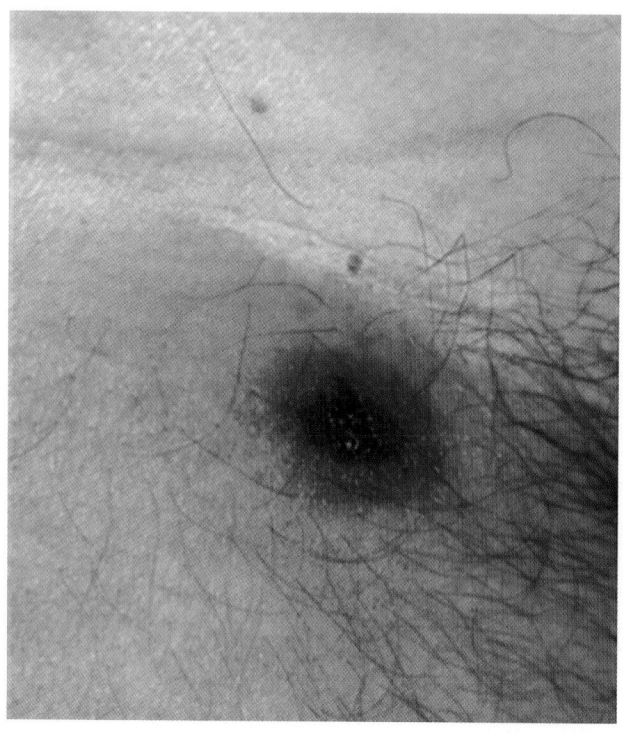

A

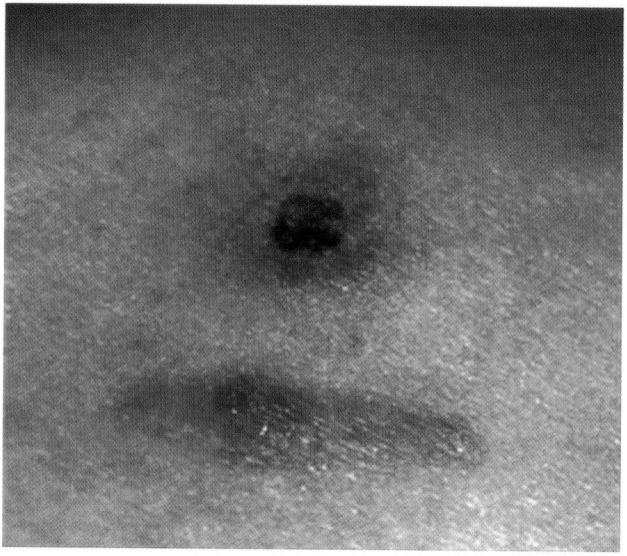

B

Figure 158-2 *A,* Necrotic ulcer with a red halo in the inguinal area of an adolescent with *Pseudomonas aeruginosa* septicemia. *B,* Similar necrotic ulcer on the chest (superior to a surgical scar), representing a septic embolus due to *Aspergillus.* (Courtesy of Yale Dermatology Residents' Slide Collection.)

Table 158-2 Differential Diagnosis of Ecthyma Gangrenosum

Disorder	Distinctive Clinical Features	Distinctive Microscopic Features
Disseminated Infections Causing EG-Like Lesions in Immunocompromised Hosts		
Pseudomonas	EG favors the groin, buttocks, and anogenital area	Presence of gram-negative rods
Staphylococcus aureus	Disseminated pustular purpura	Presence of gram-positive cocci
Candida	In addition to EG, often presents with pustules (may be misdiagnosed as folliculitis) or multiple firm, pink papules with central pallor	Budding yeast and pseudohyphae in dermis*
Aspergillus	EG lesions are relatively large (≥2–3 cm) and few in number; propensity for primary infections at sites of intravenous catheters	45-degree dichotomous branching of septate, medium-width, uniform hyphae in an "oriented" array in dermis
Mucor, Rhizopus, and *Absidia*	Cutaneous extension of an underlying fungal sinus infection can initially present as subtle, unilateral facial swelling and erythema that, without therapy, leads to extensive necrosis†; poorly controlled diabetes mellitus is a risk factor	90-degree branching of broad, nonseptate, ribbon-like hyphae in dermis
Fusarium	Widespread, painful EG lesions with high fever and severe myalgias; primary site of infection is often paronychia or insect bite	45- or 90-degree branching of septate hyphae in dermis (less uniformity and orientation than *Aspergillus*)
Herpes simplex virus	Chronic ulcers with scalloped borders in perioral, perinasal, and perianal areas (preceded by vesicles); disseminated vesicles and crusted erosions†	Tzanck preparation reveals multinucleated giant cells (representing virally infected keratinocytes)
Other Infections§		
Ecthyma (deep form of impetigo, most often caused by *Streptococcus pyogenes*)	Round, punched-out, shallow ulcers on legs, with thick crust covering purulent base; setting of poor hygiene and minor trauma	Presence of gram-positive cocci
Necrotizing fasciitis	Rapidly spreading, dusky grayish purple erythema and tense edema, with development of bullae, malodorous watery discharge, and deep necrotic ulcers; favors extremities and perineum	Presence of gram-positive cocci or mixed flora
Bacillus cereus infection	Single necrotic bulla on extremity of neutropenic patient	Presence of gram-positive rods
Cutaneous diphtheria	Punched-out ulcer with rolled borders and grayish membrane-like eschar on acral site	Presence of gram-positive rods
Cutaneous anthrax	Painless eschar with surrounding edema and vesiculation	Presence of gram-positive rods
Atypical mycobacterial infections	Protean manifestations in immunocompromised hosts, including necrotic ulcers	Presence of acid-fast bacilli
Dimorphic fungal infections (e.g., histoplasmosis, blastomycosis, coccidioidomycosis)	Protean manifestations in immunocompromised hosts, including mucocutaneous ulcers	Characteristic yeast forms (or, in coccidioidomycosis, spherules with endospores) within neutrophilic and granulomatous infiltrates
Noninfectious Disorders		
Sweet syndrome	Painful, edematous, erythematous plaques; may be pseudovesicular or pustular; favors the face and dorsal hands; particular association with AML	Dense neutrophilic infiltrate¶
Pyoderma gangrenosum	Inflammatory pustule progressing to painful, necrotic ulcer with irregular, purple, undermined borders and purulent base; favors the legs	Neutrophilic infiltrate in active lesions¶
Primary vasculitides	Manifestations include purpuric papules and nodules, hemorrhagic bullae, and necrotic ulcers; favors the lower legs and dependent sites	Neutrophilic infiltrate or dust and fibrin deposition within vessel walls¶
Vaso-occlusive disorders (e.g., monoclonal cryoglobulinemia)	Retiform (branching, netlike) purpura progressing to necrotic ulcers with angular shape; favor acral sites	Intravascular thrombi and erythrocyte extravasation with minimal inflammation¶

Table 158-2   Differential Diagnosis of Ecthyma Gangrenosum—cont'd

Disorder	Distinctive Clinical Features	Distinctive Microscopic Features
Spider bite	Single painful, edematous, inflammatory plaque progressing to necrotic ulcer	Neutrophilic infiltrate and cutaneous necrosis¶
Erythema multiforme (see Chapter 160)	Target lesions with a dusky or bullous center, pale edematous ring, and peripheral erythema; oral erosions	Vacuolar interface dermatitis with lymphocytic infiltrate¶

*Rather than in the stratum corneum, as in mucocutaneous candidiasis.
†*Aspergillus* and *Fusarium* infections may also originate from the sinuses.
‡Similar lesions may be seen in disseminated zoster.
§Additional considerations may include leprosy (Lucio phenomenon) and parasitic infections such as leishmaniasis or amebiasis.
¶Negative cultures and special stains for organisms.
AML, acute myelogenous leukemia; EG, ecthyma gangrenosum.

setting of EG in previously healthy children, often manifest with fever and diarrhea alone. Such infections can occur in conjunction with enteroviral gastroenteritis or ruptured appendicitis. The development of EG in a child with a clinical presentation that otherwise suggests viral gastroenteritis represents an important diagnostic clue, allowing early recognition and appropriate treatment of a potentially life-threatening bacterial infection. Last, the presence of EG-like lesions in the context of persistent fever, prolonged neutropenia, and broad-spectrum antibiotic therapy should raise the suspicion of a fungal infection, especially in patients who are also being treated with systemic corticosteroids.

DIFFERENTIAL DIAGNOSIS

Infectious and noninfectious entities in the differential diagnosis of EG-like skin lesions are presented in Table 158-2. Although early EG lesions can mimic insect bites, the latter differ in their prominent pruritus and inflammatory (rather than necrotic) evolution. In infants, the differential diagnosis of EG localized to the diaper area may also include subcutaneous fat necrosis, Jacquet erosive diaper dermatitis, and ulcerating hemangioma.

DIAGNOSIS AND EVALUATION

When skin lesions resembling EG are seen, particularly in immunocompromised or acutely ill patients, the evaluation (preferably before the initiation of antimicrobial therapy) should include the following:

- A sterile skin biopsy specimen for culture (bacterial, mycobacterial, fungal, and viral).
- A skin biopsy specimen for histologic examination, including special stains for bacteria (e.g., a tissue Gram stain), mycobacteria (e.g., a Fite stain), and fungi (e.g., a periodic acid–Schiff stain or Gomori methenamine silver stain).
- Examination of a Gram stain of the vesicular contents or a touch preparation from the biopsy specimen (looking for the presence of bacteria).
- Examination of a potassium hydroxide preparation of dermal scrapings (looking for the presence of hyphae or pseudohyphae).
- Examination of a Tzanck smear or viral direct fluorescent antibody testing of scrapings from the base of a vesicle or edge of an ulcer (looking for evidence of herpes simplex or varicella-zoster viral infection of keratinocytes). In some institutions, polymerase chain reaction studies may be available if direct fluorescent antibody testing is inconclusive.
- Blood, urine, and (if indicated clinically) stool or cerebrospinal fluid cultures.

A complete blood count with differential, serum electrolyte panel, serum creatinine level, blood urea nitrogen level, prothrombin time, partial thromboplastin time, hepatic function panel, serum complement levels or CH50 assay, and urinalysis should also be obtained. If clinically indicated, additional laboratory tests and imaging studies may be needed to rule out systemic involvement. When EG develops in previously healthy infants and children, the evaluation should include serum immunoglobulin levels, analysis of lymphocyte subsets, assays of neutrophil function (including a nitroblue tetrazolium reduction), and human immunodeficiency virus testing. In addition, it is important to exclude the possibility of an underlying leukemia. Because initial neutropenia may be due to toxic effects of the infecting organism, the complete blood count and differential should be followed longitudinally; this also enables the detection of cyclic neutropenia.

The typical histologic findings of EG include cutaneous necrosis, extravasated erythrocytes, and extensive collections of organisms within the media, adventitia, and surrounding regions of dermal and subcutaneous vessels. The intima and lumina are characteristically spared, and inflammation is often minimal (particularly in neutropenic patients).[7] Obtaining a deep tissue biopsy specimen for culture is particularly important in the diagnosis of invasive fungal infections, because cultures obtained by swabbing the surface of necrotic ulcerations will likely reveal only bacterial colonization.

COURSE OF ILLNESS

Factors associated with increased mortality in pseudomonal EG include multiple lesions, a delay in the institution of appropriate antimicrobial therapy, and persistent neutropenia.[7] Nonbacteremic pseudomonal EG has a better prognosis than the bacteremic form, with mortality rates of 5% to 15% and 25% to 50%, respectively.[8,14] EG due to opportunistic mycoses is a particularly ominous sign, with the presence of disseminated skin lesions portending mortality rates of 70% to 90%. In any situation, recovery of neutrophil-mediated immunity is imperative for survival of the patient and eventual healing of the necrotic ulcerations.[7]

TREATMENT

Patients with EG require hospitalization and aggressive systemic therapy. If pseudomonal EG is suspected, intravenous administration of a combination of an antipseudomonal β-lactam antibiotic and an aminoglycoside should be initiated immediately after obtaining blood, urine, and skin samples for culture. The decision to begin treatment with a systemic antifungal or antiviral agent should be based on clinical suspicion and the findings of the aforementioned bedside evaluations. Adjustment of the antimicrobial regimen may be necessary when culture and sensitivity results are available, or sooner if the patient's clinical condition deteriorates. For neutropenic patients, administration of granulolyte colony-stimulating factor to expedite neutrophil recovery can accelerate the healing of EG lesions.[21] Granulocyte infusions represent another therapeutic option for patients with profound, refractory neutropenia.

In most cases of EG due to *P. aeruginosa* or other bacterial pathogens, surgical débridement is not required. However, wide surgical débridement represents an important component of therapy for EG secondary to infections with opportunistic molds, and surgical excision may be an option for localized fungal lesions.[22] Nonetheless, persistent infection and extremely poor wound healing are commonly seen until the patient's neutropenia resolves.

CONSULTATION

Consultations by a dermatologist (to evaluate the cutaneous lesions) and infectious disease specialist (to evaluate for systemic infection and institute appropriate antimicrobial coverage) are recommended for all patients suspected of having EG. Depending on the clinical situation, the input of hematology-oncology or immunology teams might be helpful in the diagnosis and treatment of underlying medical conditions. The assistance of additional pediatric subspecialists may be useful for patients in whom other organ systems are involved.

PREVENTION

Although pseudomonal septicemia accounted for one quarter of life-threatening infections in cancer patients during the 1950s,[7] it is seen less frequently today because of shorter durations of neutropenia (due to the use of granulocyte colony-stimulating factors and peripheral blood stem cell rather than bone marrow transplantation), as well as the prophylactic administration of antibiotics (e.g., fluoroquinolones). Likewise, the incidence of disseminated candidiasis has decreased significantly with the use of prophylactic fluconazole. As a result, the spectrum of pathogens that cause septicemia and EG-like lesions in oncology patients has changed and now includes a wider variety of bacterial and fungal organisms (see Box 158-1).

Meticulous skin care, especially in the diaper area, for pediatric patients with hematologic malignancies may help prevent EG arising from a cutaneous portal of entry. Patients should receive a thorough skin examination and treatment of preexisting dermatoses before commencing myelosuppressive regimens. During periods of profound neutropenia, exposure to potential environmental sources of *Pseudomonas* and opportunistic molds should be avoided (e.g., cut flowers in vases).

CONCLUSION

EG represents an important cutaneous sign of systemic disease. Recognition of these skin lesions can enable prompt diagnosis and treatment of life-threatening infections not only with *P. aeruginosa* but also with an expanding list of other bacterial and fungal pathogens in immunocompromised hosts. Moreover, in previously healthy children, the development of EG can serve as a valuable clue to the presence of an underlying immunodeficiency.

IN A NUTSHELL

- The skin lesions of EG evolve from an erythematous macule to a hemorrhagic vesicle to a necrotic eschar in neutropenic patients, often with an underlying hematologic malignancy or immunodeficiency.
- Diagnosis is based on histologic examination and culture of a skin biopsy specimen.
- Hospitalization is required, with immediate initiation of intravenous antimicrobial therapy.

ON THE HORIZON

- With the introduction of new antimicrobial agents and prophylactic regimens, the spectrum of organisms responsible for EG-like lesions in immunocompromised patients will continue to evolve. As the frequency of disseminated infections with established pathogens susceptible to modern regimens decreases, both resistant organisms and novel opportunistic pathogens will inevitably emerge. For example, the prophylactic administration of voriconazole to hematopoietic stem cell transplant recipients may have decreased the incidence of aspergillosis, but an increase in the frequency of invasive zygomycosis (caused by fungi with intrinsic resistance to this agent) has been reported.
- In the future, polymerase chain reaction and other molecular diagnostic techniques will enable earlier identification of the causative organisms in disseminated bacterial and fungal infections than is possible with culture alone.[23] The timely institution of effective antimicrobial regimens, together with improved supportive care for neutropenic patients, will lead to a reduction in the incidence of EG as well as its morbidity and mortality.

REFERENCES

1. Barker LF: The clinical symptoms, bacteriologic findings and postmortem appearances in cases of infection of human beings with the *Bacillus pyocyaneus*. JAMA 1897;29:213-216.

2. Hitschmann F, Kreibich K: Zur Pathogenese des *Bacillus pyocyaneus* und zur Aetiologie des Ekthyma gangraenosum. Wien Klin Wochenschr 1897;10:1093-1101.

3. Reich HL, Fadeyi DW, Naik NS, et al: Nonpseudomonal ecthyma gangrenosum. J Am Acad Dermatol 2004;50:S114-S117.

4. Wolfson JS, Sober AJ, Rubin RH: Dermatologic manifestations of infections in immunocompromised patients. Medicine 1985;64:113-133.

5. Pouryousefi A, Foland J, Michie CA, Cummuns M: Ecthyma gangrenosum as a very early herald of acute lymphoblastic leukaemia. J Paediatr Child Health 1999;35:505-506.

6. Hoffman MA, Finberg L: *Pseudomonas* infections in infants associated with high-humidity environments. J Pediatr 1955;46:626-630.

7. Greene SL, Su WP, Muller SA: Ecthyma gangrenosum: Report of clinical, histopathologic, and bacteriologic aspects of eight cases. J Am Acad Dermatol 1984;11:781-787.

8. El Baze P, Thyss A, Vinti H, et al: A study of nineteen immunocompromised patients with extensive skin lesions caused by *Pseudomonas aeruginosa* with and without bacteremia. Acta Derm Venereol 1991;71:411-415.

9. Murphy O, Marsh PJ, Gray J, et al: Ecthyma gangrenosum occurring at sites of iatrogenic trauma in pediatric oncology patients. Med Pediatr Oncol 1996;27:62-63.

10. El Baze P, Thyss A, Caldani C, et al: *Pseudomonas aeruginosa* O-11 folliculitis: Development into ecthyma gangrenosum in immunosuppressed patients. Arch Dermatol 1985;121:873-876.

11. Buttery JP, Alabaster SJ, Heine RG, et al: Multiresistant *Pseudomonas aeruginosa* outbreak in a pediatric oncology ward related to bath toys. Pediatr Infect Dis J 1998;17:509-513.

12. Bodey GP, Boktour M, Mays S, et al: Skin lesions associated with *Fusarium* infection. J Am Acad Dermatol 2002;47:659-666.

13. Huminer D, Siegman-Igra Y, Morduchowicz G, Pitlik SD: Ecthyma gangrenosum without bacteremia: Report of six cases and review of the literature. Arch Intern Med 1987;147:299-301.

14. Fergie JE, Patrick CC, Lott L: *Pseudomonas aeruginosa* cellulitis and ecthyma gangrenosum in immunocompromised children. Pediatr Infect Dis J 1991;10:496-500.

15. Silvestre JF, Betloch MI: Cutaneous manifestations due to *Pseudomonas* infection. Int J Dermatol 1999;38:419-431.

16. Bottone EJ, Reitano M, Janda M, et al: *Pseudomonas maltophilia* exoenzyme activity as correlate in pathogenesis of ecthyma gangrenosum. J Clin Microbiol 1986;24:995-997.

17. Dorff GJ, Geimer NF, Rosenthal DR, Rytel MW: *Pseudomonas* septicemia: Illustrated evolution of its skin lesion. Arch Intern Med 1971;128:591-595.

18. Schlossberg D: Multiple erythematous nodules as a manifestation of *Pseudomonas aeruginosa* septicemia. Arch Dermatol 1980;116:446-447.

19. Hurwitz RM, Leaming RD, Horine RK: Necrotic cellulitis: A localized form of septic vasculitis. Arch Dermatol 1984;120:87-92.

20. Freeman A, Mancina A, Yogev R: Is noma neonatorum a presentation of ecthyma gangrenosum in the newborn? Pediatr Infect Dis J 2002;21:83-85.

21. Becherel PA, Chosidow O, Berger E, et al: Granulocyte-macrophage colony-stimulating factor in the management of severe ecthyma gangrenosum related to myelodysplastic syndrome. Arch Dermatol 1995;131:892-894.

22. Radhakrishnan R, Donato ML, Prieto VG, et al: Invasive cutaneous fungal infections requiring radical resection in cancer patients undergoing chemotherapy. J Surg Oncol 2004;88:21-26.

23. Xu J, Moore JE, Millar BC, et al: Improved laboratory diagnosis of bacterial and fungal infection in patients with hematological malignancies using PCR and ribosomal RNA sequence analysis. Leuk Lymphoma 2004;45:1637-1641.

CHAPTER 159

Drug-Associated Rashes

Laurie A. Bernard and Lawrence F. Eichenfield

Drug-associated rashes are very common in hospitalized patients and, uncommonly, can be associated with conditions that prompt admission. Approximately 4% of pediatric hospital admissions are related to adverse drug reactions.[1] Additionally, the Boston Drug Surveillance Project published data in 1986 estimating that approximately 30% of hospitalized patients experience adverse drug events,[2] and in 1991 the Harvard Medical Practice Study II published data showing that drug events were the most common type of adverse event in the hospital.[3] A study in the 1980s in New York State estimated that as many as 20% of serious drug reactions involve the skin. Certain categories of common pediatric medications, including antibiotics and anticonvulsants, are associated with rates of drug eruption ranging from as high as 1% to 5%.[4] Many unique cutaneous reaction patterns have been described, and the same medication may cause different reaction patterns in different patients, thus making accurate diagnosis challenging. A subset of drug eruptions are serious and may even be life threatening and require rapid diagnosis and intervention. Therefore, it is important in the inpatient setting to be able to recognize the common patterns of cutaneous drug reaction, identify the probable causative agent, and institute appropriate therapy when indicated.

PATHOGENESIS

Drug reactions result from both immunologic and non-immunologic mechanisms. Nonimmunologic adverse reactions account for the majority of drug reactions and include those related to factors such as overdose, cumulative toxicity, metabolic alterations, drug-drug interactions, and idiosyncrasy. Alternatively, many drug eruptions are mediated by immunologic mechanisms. Generally, these eruptions are hypersensitivity reactions and are classified by the Gell and Coombs classification of hypersensitivity: types I to IV. They are described in Chapter 135.

DIAGNOSIS

The diagnosis of a drug-induced eruption begins with a careful history and physical examination. The clinician should evaluate the timeline of initiation of the medication as it relates to development of the rash. Frequently, chronology is the most helpful factor in correctly diagnosing a drug reaction. Most reactions occur within 1 to 3 weeks of starting a new medication and resolve when the medication is fully excreted or metabolized. An accurate description of the eruption is extremely important, including the morphology and distribution of the rash. Additionally, the patient's current medication list, including over-the-counter drugs, should be carefully reviewed for possible offending agents. In general, diagnostic tests are of limited value in the evalu-

ation of drug eruptions, although skin biopsy, radioallergosorbent testing (RAST), and patch testing may be helpful in selected cases. Additionally, for a subset of patients with nonserious reactions (e.g., fixed drug eruptions), rechallenge with the medication may be appropriate.[5]

Exanthematous Drug Eruptions

An exanthem is the most common type of cutaneous drug eruption. The terms *maculopapular* and *morbilliform* ("measles-like") are also often used to describe this class of drug rash. The eruption is characterized by pruritic, red to salmon-colored macules or papules that at times coalesce into plaques (Fig. 159-1). The lesions tend to be bilateral and symmetrical; they generally appear on the trunk initially and then spread peripherally to the extremities. They may spare the face, palms, and soles, but this is inconsistent. A long list of drugs may cause exanthematous eruptions (Table 159-1), but penicillin antibiotics are among the most frequently implicated agents. The eruption classically appears 7 to 14 days after the start of a new medication, although it may appear sooner or later. The presence of a viral infection is thought to increase the likelihood of an exanthematous drug eruption. The most well recognized example occurs in patients with mononucleosis who experience a morbilliform eruption when exposed to aminopenicillin agents (e.g., amoxicillin).

The most common differential diagnosis of an exanthematous drug eruption is primary viral exanthems, although other conditions to be considered include eczematous dermatitis and graft-versus-host disease, among others. Viruses often cause rashes identical to those of drug eruptions. If histopathology is available, the presence of an eosinophilic infiltrate supports a drug etiology, but the findings are generally nonspecific. Drug hypersensitivity syndrome (see discussion later in this chapter) can also initially present with an exanthematous rash, although these patients typically have high fever, characteristic facial edema, eosinophilia, and other evidence of organ system involvement.

The mechanism behind the development of exanthematous drug eruptions is unclear, even though a T-cell–mediated process seems likely based on the time delay between exposure and the development of symptoms. It appears, however, that this is not a classic Gell and Coombs type IV reaction because it does not consistently occur on rechallenge.

Exanthematous eruptions typically last days to weeks but almost universally resolve after removal of the offending agent. Time to resolution is dependent on a variety of factors, including the half-life of the involved drug. Specific therapeutic interventions are not required, but topical corticosteroids may be useful in providing symptomatic relief, and antihistamines may be helpful for relief of itching. An

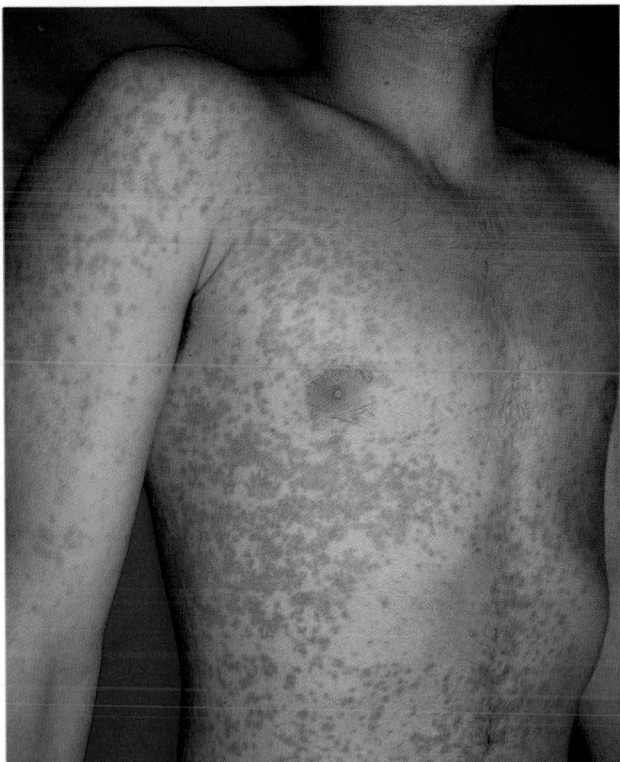

Figure 159-1 Morbilliform drug eruption.

Table 159-1 Drugs Commonly Causing Exanthematous Eruptions In Pediatric Patients

Penicillin derivatives
Sulfonamides
Phenytoin
Carbamazepine
Barbiturates
Amphotericin B
Oral hypoglycemic agents
Thiazides
Benzodiazepines
Phenothiazines
Allopurinol
Antimalarials
Captopril
Nonsteroidal anti-inflammatory drugs
Gentamicin
Lithium

exanthematous reaction is not necessarily an absolute contraindication to future use of the drug, although many patients will experience recurrence of the rash with rechallenge. Therefore, in the majority of cases, the patient should be considered "allergic" to the medication.

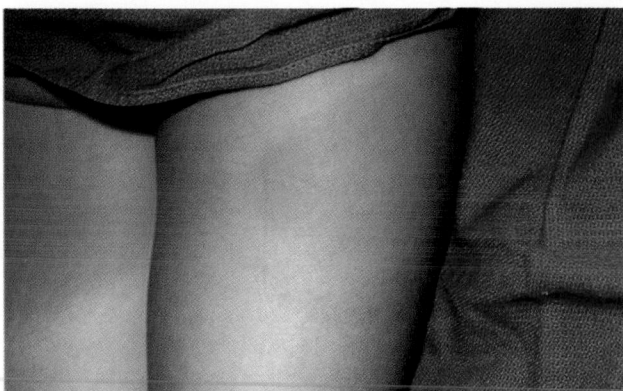

Figure 159-2 Fixed drug eruption secondary to acetaminophen.

Fixed Drug Eruption

A fixed drug eruption presents as a distinct lesion or lesions after systemic drug exposure. It is often underdiagnosed, which leads to recurrences when and if the drug is readministered. This eruption generally appears as sharply circumscribed, round to oval patches or plaques that may be single or multiple (Fig. 159-2). The lesions are usually asymptomatic or only mildly pruritic. The eruption typically develops within 1 to 2 weeks of starting a new medication. The lesions may be red, gray, violaceous, or brown, and a central vesicle or bullae may be present. They tend to progress from erythematous to hyperpigmented. The rash may occur anywhere on the body, but the most common locations are the face, lips, hands, feet, and genitalia. A classic characteristic of a fixed drug eruption is that when patients are rechallenged with the offending medication, the lesion reappears in the same anatomic location and tends to appear much more rapidly, even within hours of taking the medication.[6] The most common agents implicated in fixed drug eruptions include sulfonamides, tetracyclines, nonsteroidal anti-inflammatory drugs (NSAIDs), barbiturates, and carbamazepine, although a large number of other medications have been reported (Table 159-2).[7-9] Cross-reactivity may occur within a class of similar drugs. Biopsy of an early lesion of a fixed drug eruption reveals a lichenoid infiltrate, hydropic degeneration of the basal cell layer, and dyskeratotic keratinocytes. A later-stage biopsy will reveal large amount of melanin within macrophages in the upper dermis.[10]

The differential diagnosis includes an insect bite when the lesion is solitary and urticaria and erythema multiforme when multiple lesions are present. Diagnosis may be aided by biopsy. If the diagnosis is unclear, the physician may choose to rechallenge the patient with the medication.

Treatment involves removal of the offending agent. The eruption generally resolves after discontinuation of the medication, but hyperpigmentation in the area may persist for months to years. The cause of the disorder is unknown, although familial cases have been described, as well as an association with HLA-B22.[11]

Urticarial Drug Eruptions

Urticaria is among the most frequent of the drug eruptions. It may be IgE induced, such as with antibiotics, or non–IgE induced, such as a pseudoallergic reaction seen with

Table 159-2   Drugs Commonly Associated with Fixed Drug Eruptions in Pediatric Patients

Sulfonamides
Trimethoprim
Tetracyclines
Penicillin derivatives
Clindamycin
Erythromycin
Antifungal agents
Dapsone
Antimalarials
Metronidazole
Barbiturates
Opiates
Benzodiazepines
Anticonvulsants
Nonsteroidal anti-inflammatory drugs (acetaminophen, ibuprofen, paracetamol)
Dextromethorphan
Allopurinol
Sympathomimetics (pseudoephedrine)

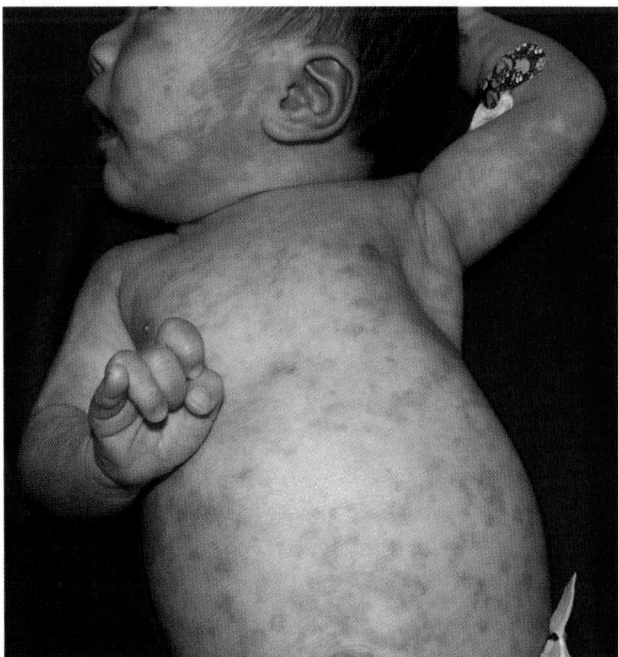

Figure 159-3   Diffuse urticarial drug eruption.

NSAIDs or opiates. Intensely pruritic erythematous, edematous papules and plaques characterize an urticarial rash (Fig. 159-3). Lesions occur anywhere on the body, including the palms and soles, and occasionally have a "dusky" appearance or central pallor. The rash may appear within minutes of exposure to the offending agent or as long as several days later. Each individual hive usually persists for a period of hours but less than 24 hours. If lesions remain fixed for longer than 24 hours, other diagnoses should be entertained, such as urticarial vasculitis, erythema multiforme, or acute hemorrhagic edema of infancy.

A number of inflammatory mediators are thought to be involved in the pathogenesis of urticaria. Release of histamine from mast cells plays an important role. Additional mediators that may be involved include prostaglandins, leukotrienes, neutrophil and eosinophil chemotactic factors, platelet-activating factor, interleukin-1, and kinins. Urticarial lesions occur when these inflammatory mediators cause a local increase in the permeability of capillaries in the skin with subsequent dermal edema.

Urticaria may be acute or chronic and is classified as the latter when persistent beyond 6 weeks. Many drugs can induce acute urticaria. Antibiotics are commonly implicated, with penicillin being the most frequent. Other important agents include cephalosporins, sulfonamides, and tetracyclines. The urticaria caused by factors other than drug exposure is morphologically identical. Such factors include infection, autoimmune disease, temperature changes, pressure, sunlight, and exercise, among others.[12]

The first line of therapy is removal of the offending agent. Oral antihistamines are the recommended therapy for uncomplicated acute urticaria and are generally sufficient to control symptoms. Depending on the individual situation, both sedating and nonsedating H_1 blockers may be appropriate. There is also evidence to support adjunctive use of H_2 blockers. Patients with very severe acute urticaria may occasional require systemic corticosteroids, although the vast majority can be managed with antihistamines alone. Allergy to the medication should be documented in the medical record.[13]

The hospitalist should be aware that acute urticaria may progress to angioedema or anaphylaxis, or both. Angioedema refers to transient edema of subcutaneous or submucosal tissue. Common areas of involvement include the lips, eyelids, oropharynx, and tongue. If deeper airway structures such as the larynx become involved, stridor and airway obstruction can result. Patients may also experience nausea, emesis, and diarrhea. Anaphylaxis is defined as a hypersensitivity reaction to a substance that results in severe systemic symptoms. Anaphylaxis represents an emergency, and acute management can be lifesaving and is discussed in Chapter 134.

Drug Hypersensitivity Syndrome

Drug hypersensitivity syndrome, or drug rash with eosinophilia and systemic symptoms (DRESS), refers to a subset of severe drug reactions characterized by the triad of cutaneous eruption, fever, and internal organ dysfunction caused by exposure to a drug. This entity was previously known as anticonvulsant hypersensitivity syndrome but is now reported in association with several other categories of drugs. DRESS is the most recently proposed nomenclature for the syndrome and is significantly more descriptive and clinically precise.[14] A number of medications that can cause drug hypersensitivity are commonly used in pediatric hospitals, including anticonvulsants (phenytoin, phenobarbital, carbamazepine, and lamotrigine), sulfonamides, trimethoprim, minocycline, dapsone, azathioprine, and allopurinol.[15] Anticonvulsant hypersensitivity is the most studied of the hypersensitivity syndromes, and genetics probably plays a role in development of the disease. The implicated anticonvulsants have in common an aromatic benzene ring that is metabolized by cytochrome P-450 enzymes to an arene oxide metabolite. These metabolites are highly unstable and can cause cytotoxicity, as well as form neoantigens leading to an immune response. In a normal host, arene oxides are detoxified by a number of enzymatic pathways, the most significant being the pathway involving the enzyme epoxide hydrolase. It is theorized that patients in whom anticonvulsant hypersensitivity develops may have a genetically determined deficiency of this enzyme that leads to buildup of toxic metabolites and finally cell death, thereby resulting in the clinical manifestations of the syndrome.[16]

The syndrome usually occurs from 1 to 6 weeks into therapy with the drug but may occur as late as a few months after initiation. The majority of patients with DRESS experience a prodrome consisting of fever, malaise, and upper respiratory symptoms often mimicking a viral illness. Lymphadenopathy and a generalized rash of varying severity develop in most patients. The rash is generally a morbilliform exanthem, but erythroderma and exfoliative dermatitis can occur, as can eruptions seen in Stevens-Johnson syndrome or toxic epidermal necrolysis (Fig. 159-4). Mucous membrane lesions may or may not be present. The rash usually involves the upper part of the trunk, face, and extremities. Dramatic facial swelling is often seen, and patients are generally quite ill.

Recognition of the temporal association between initiation of the drug and onset of the syndrome is key to establishing the diagnosis. If the diagnosis is in question, skin biopsy may be contributory in establishing the rash as a drug reaction by revealing a dense infiltrate of eosinophils or lymphocytes in the papillary dermis. Unfortunately, no specific test exists for definitively establishing the diagnosis.

The hallmark of the disease is multisystem internal organ involvement; the most frequently seen findings include hepatitis, pneumonitis, hematologic abnormalities, nephritis, and hypothyroidism. Hematologic findings are variable in severity; the most common findings are eosinophilia and atypical lymphocytosis, although agranulocytosis, thrombocytopenia, hemolytic anemia, and aplastic anemia have been described. Hepatic involvement ranges from mild elevation of transaminases to frank hepatic necrosis. The disorder carries a 10% mortality rate, and the prognosis depends on the extent and severity of organ involvement. Fulminant hepatic failure is the most common cause of death.

Treatment begins with recognition of the diagnosis and removal of the offending agent. A delay in diagnosis may increase morbidity and mortality. The use of multiple medications can make assessment difficult; if it is unclear which agent is causative, the usual practice is to stop administering all possible offending drugs that are not lifesaving, especially in patients with severe reactions. Because drugs with long half-lives may be difficult to remove, dialysis may be indicated. Compromised organ function (e.g., liver dysfunction)

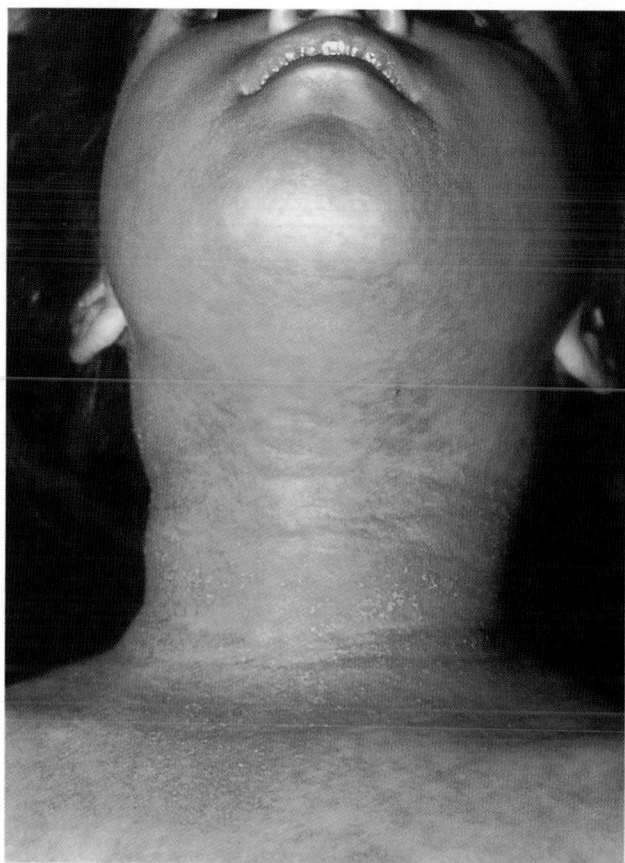

Figure 159-4 Exanthem and fine scaling associated with drug rash with eosinophilia and systemic symptoms (DRESS) from carbamazepine.

may have an impact on drug clearance, and monitoring of serum drug levels is appropriate when available. Cross-reactivity is common among the implicated anticonvulsants (phenobarbital, phenytoin, carbamazepine, and lamotrigine), so alternative antiseizure therapy must be chosen carefully. Benzodiazepines, valproate, and gabapentin are among the commonly suggested alternatives, although they should be used with caution in patients with hepatic dysfunction.[17,18]

Many experts recommend that patients with DRESS be hospitalized and closely monitored for signs of severe organ involvement, which may develop even after cessation of the offending drug. Intensive supportive care, including aggressive nutritional support, fluid/electrolyte replacement, and meticulous skin care, is critical in managing the disorder. Many experts recommend that patients with DRESS and severe organ involvement be treated with corticosteroids. A number of case reports have described dramatic improvement in visceral organ dysfunction after the administration of steroids.[19] Prolonged, tapering courses of medication may be required, and the disease often relapses after cessation of therapy. It is not uncommon for the disease to fluctuate for many months before finally resolving. There is some evidence to support adjuvant use of intravenous immunoglobulin (IVIG), although IVIG has been studied predominantly in patients with toxic epidermal necrolysis.[20]

Drug-Induced Vasculitis

Cutaneous vasculitis is a physical finding seen in association with a number of disorders, as well as with the systemic administration of certain drugs. It is associated with immune complex deposition in the skin, but the precise mechanism is poorly understood. Clinically, lesion morphology is quite variable, although urticaria-like plaques and palpable purpura concentrated on the lower extremities develop in most patients (Fig. 159-5). The plaques may blister or ulcerate. Progression to systemic disease is rare but has been reported; the liver, kidney, joints, and brain may be involved. A definitive diagnosis is made by histopathologic detection of characteristic inflammation of small vessels within the dermis. A perivascular disintegrating neutrophilic infiltrate accompanied by fibrin deposition and hemorrhage is seen. Tissue eosinophilia may also be present. Immunofluorescence studies characteristically reveal deposition of immunoglobulin and complement.

The drugs most commonly implicated in cutaneous vasculitis are β-lactam antibiotics, sulfonamides, NSAIDs, diuretics, and the thiouracils, although any drug is a potential cause. Henoch-Schönlein purpura is a cutaneous vasculitis that may occasionally be associated with administration of a medication.

Once a diagnosis of cutaneous vasculitis is established, attempts should be made to identify an underlying cause. The differential diagnosis is broad and includes medication reaction, connective tissue disease, primary systemic vasculitis, infection, and malignancy. A diagnosis of idiopathic vasculitis can be made only after all other possibilities have been fully evaluated. A careful history and physical examination will often reveal clues to the specific systemic process, although most patients will also require laboratory tests to fully exclude disorders such as systemic lupus erythematosus (SLE), primary vasculitides, and infection.

Treatment of cutaneous vasculitis is directed toward the underlying cause. If the rash is suspected to be drug induced, removal of the offending agent generally results in rapid improvement over a period of 1 to 3 weeks. Occasionally, patients will require more aggressive therapy with systemic corticosteroids or other immunosuppressive agents, although this is usually necessary only in patients with an underlying systemic process such as a connective tissue

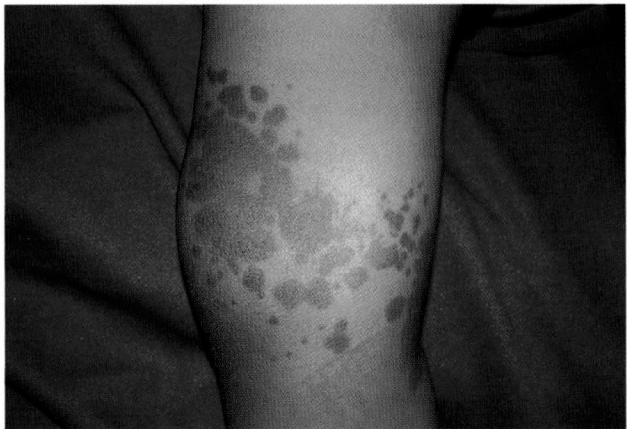

Figure 159-5   Drug-induced vasculitis with palpable purpura

disease. Two excellent reviews of drug-induced vasculitis are available for further reference.[21,22]

Drug-Induced Lupus

Drug-induced lupus is a disorder characterized by a constellation of symptoms mimicking those of SLE. The most frequently implicated drugs are procainamide, hydralazine, isoniazid, lithium, phenytoin, and oral contraceptives. Clinically, patients present with fever, malaise, myalgias, polyarthritis, pleuritis, cutaneous vasculitis, or any combination of these findings. Systemic symptoms are more common than skin manifestations. Laboratory analysis will reveal antinuclear antibodies in the majority of patients, and many will also have an elevated erythrocyte sedimentation rate, hypocomplementemia, and additional SLE-associated antibodies such as anti–double-stranded DNA.

The most important initial intervention for patients with drug-induced lupus is discontinuation of the offending drug. The majority of patients will improve, albeit slowly, with this intervention alone, although occasionally, persistence of symptoms necessitates therapy with immunosuppressive agents. NSAIDs can provide symptomatic relief during the resolution phase. Rheumatology consultation may be helpful in the diagnosis and management of this disorder in hospitalized patients.

Serum Sickness

Serum sickness is an illness caused by circulating immune complexes. The syndrome was initially described in the early 1900s when it was seen in association with the use of horse serum containing diphtheria antitoxin. Approximately 8 to 13 days after injection of the serum, a syndrome consisting of fever, malaise, lymphadenopathy, rash, proteinuria, and arthralgias developed. The syndrome was termed *serum sickness* and a half-century later was reported to be linked to the creation and deposition of circulating immune complexes in tissues and activation of complement. This was demonstrated in patients receiving antithymocyte globulin before bone marrow transplantation.

Serum sickness is now most commonly seen after the administration of animal-derived immunoglobulins such as snake antivenin. The illness usually begins 2 to 21 days after the offending medication is given. The most frequent clinical findings are fever, malaise, rash, arthralgias, gastrointestinal symptoms, and lymphadenopathy. Demonstration of low C3 and C4 and abnormal findings on urinalysis can be helpful in establishing the diagnosis. Treatment is supportive because the illness is self-limited. NSAIDs and corticosteroids may be helpful if symptoms are severe or bothersome.

A serum sickness–like reaction is also well described. Patients have similar symptoms (fever, rash, and arthralgias); however, immune complex deposition is not seen. Medications most commonly associated with serum sickness–like reactions include penicillins, cephalosporins (particularly cefaclor), sulfonamides, phenytoin, and salicylates. The mechanism of the syndrome is poorly understood, but it has been proposed to be due to a cytotoxic effect on cells. Treatment is primarily supportive because the illness is self-resolving, although NSAIDs may help control the symptoms. An excellent published review of serum sickness is available for further reference.[23]

CONSULTATION

Dermatology should be involved when there is diagnostic uncertainty, especially if skin biopsy is being considered, such as in the case of drug-induced vasculitis. These specialists can obtain specimens for histopathology and assist in the management of complex or recalcitrant cases. Their input is especially useful for exfoliative conditions, where management of skin care is particularly challenging.

Involving rheumatology consultants can be helpful in drug-induced vasculitides and serum sickness, especially if the symptoms are severe, progressive, recurrent, or recalcitrant to initial therapy.

ADMISSION CRITERIA

Hospitalization is not necessary for many patients with one of the common drug eruptions, such as exanthematous or fixed drug reactions, because they are not typically associated with severe or progressive symptoms. Patients with localized urticarial reactions without evidence of progression and without airway involvement often do not require admission, especially if the symptoms are stable or improving during a period of observation. Hospitalization should be considered in the following cases:

- There is concern for systemic conditions such as anaphylaxis or DRESS.
- Discontinuation of a drug may lead to instability of an underlying condition, such as discontinuation of an anticonvulsant in a patients with severe epilepsy.
- Stabilization of the reaction requires inpatient support (e.g., intravenous fluids) or therapy (e.g., IVIG).

DISCHARGE CRITERIA

Patients may be discharged after the following conditions have been met:

- Symptoms have stabilized, are improving, or are well controlled by therapy that is able to be continued after discharge.
- The underlying condition is well controlled despite discontinuation of medication.
- Adequate follow-up has been arranged with the primary care physician or, if needed, with subspecialists.

IN A NUTSHELL

- Drug eruptions are common in hospitalized pediatric patients, and the majority are benign and self-limited.
- A subset of drug-associated rashes can be serious and even life threatening.
- Drug reactions result from both immunologic (e.g., IgE or T cell mediated) and nonimmunologic (e.g., cumulative toxicity, drug-drug interactions, or idiosyncrasy) mechanisms.
- The drug hypersensitivity syndrome (DRESS) refers to a subset of severe drug reactions characterized by the triad of cutaneous eruption, fever, and internal organ dysfunction associated with exposure to a drug. Dramatic facial swelling is often seen, and patients are

generally quite ill. There is a 10% mortality rate, with fulminant hepatic failure being the most common cause of death.
- Drug-induced vasculitis, drug-induced lupus, and serum sickness may present as rheumatologic conditions, but identification and discontinuation of the inciting agent are key to treatment.

ON THE HORIZON

- The evolution of biotechnology and the development of new medications bring the possibility of new cutaneous and systemic drug reactions, as well as drug interactions.
- Increasing knowledge of the genetic influences on pharmacology, known as pharmacogenetics, may allow prospective assessment of individual differences in drug metabolism, efficacy, tolerance, and interactions with other drugs, infections, and disease states. This may have a significant impact on avoidance, prediction, and diagnosis of drug reactions.

SUGGESTED READING

Baker H: Drug reactions. In Rook A, Wilkinson DS, Ebling FG, et al (eds): Textbook of Dermatology, 4th ed. Oxford, Blackwell Scientific, 1986.

Beltrani VS: Cutaneous manifestations of adverse drug reactions. Immunol Allergy Clin North Am 1998;18(4):867-895.

McKenna JK, Leiferman KM: Dermatologic drug eruptions. Immunol Allergy Clin North Am 2004;24:399-423, vi.

Nigen S, Knowles SR, Shear NH: Drug eruptions: Approaching the diagnosis of drug-induced skin diseases. J Drugs Dermatol 2003;2:278-299.

Revuz J: New advances in severe adverse drug reactions. Dermatol Clin 2001;19:679-709, ix.

Volchek GW: Clinical evaluation and management of drug hypersensitivity. Immunol Allergy Clin North Am 2004;24:357-371, v.

REFERENCES

1. Martinez-Mir I, Garcia-Lopez M, Palop V, et al: A prospective study of adverse drug reactions as a cause of admission to a pediatric hospital. Br J Clin Pharmacol 1996;42:319-324.
2. Bigby M, Jick S, Jick H, et al: Drug-induced cutaneous reactions: A report from the Boston Collaborative Drug Surveillance Program on 15,438 consecutive inpatients, 1975-1982. JAMA 1986;256:3358-3365.
3. Leape LL, Brennan TA, Laird N, et al: The nature of adverse events in hospitalized patients: Results of the Harvard Medical Practice Study. N Engl J Med 1991;324:377-384.
4. Bigby M: Rates of cutaneous reactions to drugs. Arch Dermatol 2001;137:765-770.
5. Drake LA, Dinehart SM, Farmer ER, et al: Guidelines of care for cutaneous adverse drug reactions. Guideline/Outcome Committee of the American Academy of Dermatology. J Am Acad Dermatol 1996 35(3 pt 1):458-461.
6. Ozkaya-Bayazit E: Specific site involvement in fixed drug eruption. J Am Acad Dermatol 2003;49:1003-1007.
7. Mahboob A, Haroon TS: Drugs causing fixed eruptions: A study of 450 cases. Int J Dermatol 1998;37:833-838.
8. Crowson AN, Magro CM: Recent advances in the pathology of cutaneous drug eruptions. Dermatol Clin 1999;17:537-560, viii.
9. Morelli JG, Yong-Kwang T, Rogers M, et al: Fixed drug eruptions in children: Clinical and laboratory observations. J Pediatr 1999;134:365-367.

10. Crowson AN, Magro CM: Drug eruptions. In Barnhill R, Crowson AN, Busam K, et al (eds): Textbook of Dermatopathology. New York, McGraw-Hill, 1998, pp 257-270.

11. Pellicano R, Ciavarella G, Lomuto M, Di Giorgio G: Genetic susceptibility to FDE: Evidence for a link with HLA B22. J Am Acad Dermatol 1994;30:52-54.

12. Greaves MW: Chronic idiopathic urticaria. Curr Opin Allergy Clin Immunol 2003;3:363-368.

13. Zuberbier T, Greaves MW, Juhlin L, et al: Management of urticaria: A consensus report. J Invest Dermatol Symp Proc 2001;6:128-131.

14. Bocquet H, Bagot M, Roujeau J: Drug-induced pseudolymphoma and drug hypersensitivity syndrome (drug rash with eosinophilia and systemic symptoms—DRESS). Semin Cutan Med Surg 1996;15:250-257.

15. Kaur S, Sarkar R, Thami GP, Kanwar AJ: Anticonvulsant hypersensitivity syndrome. Pediatr Dermatol 2002;19:142-145.

16. Lowitt M, Shear N: Pharmacogenomics and dermatologic therapeutics. Arch Dermatol 2001;137:1512-1514.

17. Tas S, Simonart T: Management of drug rash with eosinophilia and systemic symptoms (DRESS): An update. Dermatology 2003;206:353-356.

18. Volchek GW: Clinical evaluation and management of drug hypersensitivity. Immunol Allergy Clin North Am 2004;24:357-371, v.

19. Chopra S, Levell NJ, Cowley G, Gilkes JH: Systemic corticosteroids in the phenytoin hypersensitivity syndrome. Br J Dermatol 1996;134:1109-1112.

20. Scheuerman O, Nofech-Moses Y, Rachmel A, Ashkenazi S: Successful treatment of antiepileptic drug hypersensitivity syndrome with IVIG. Pediatrics 2001;107(1):E14.

21. Doyle MK, Cuellar ML: Drug-Induced vasculitis. Exp Opin Drug Saf 2003;2:401-409.

22. Calabrese LH, Duna GF: Drug-induced vasculitis. Curr Opin Rheumatol 1996;8:34-40.

23. Lawley TJ, Bielory L, Gascon P, et al: A prospective clinical and immunologic analysis of patients with serum sickness. N Engl J Med 1984;311:1407-1413.

CHAPTER *160*

Erythema Multiforme

Douglas E. Moses

Erythema multiforme (EM) is thought to be an acute hypersensitivity reaction to a variety of inciting agents. The cutaneous lesions of EM have been described for centuries, with the current name having been adopted in the 1860s.[1] Stevens and Johnson described a more severe form with significant mucosal changes in the 1920s.[2]

The spectrum of associated illness can be separated into two forms: EM minor and EM major.[3,4] About 20% of cases of EM minor occur in children and adolescents,[3] with a small male preponderance.[2] EM major is less common than its EM minor counterpart, but it has a higher predilection for the pediatric population, especially adolescents. Stevens-Johnson syndrome is a severe form of EM major associated with significant mucosal sloughing.[3] The most severe presentation of this spectrum is called toxic epidermal necrolysis, thought by some to be a form of EM major with abundant sloughing of the skin and increased mortality. These two entities are discussed in Chapter 161.

In both EM minor and Stevens-Johnson syndrome, a local cell-mediated response to an inciting antigen occurs at the site of lesion eruption and leads to local tissue damage.[2,4] Skin cells demonstrate a change in the histocompatibility antigens displayed that is thought to be induced by infiltration of T cells into dermal tissues.[2,4]

CLINICAL PRESENTATION

Many patients with EM minor do not have prodromal symptoms; however, in those suffering from recurrent EM minor, a relationship with previous herpes simplex virus (HSV) eruption is well established.[1,2,4,5] Those with EM major often have a prodrome of symptoms such as headache, fever, and malaise that may occur from a few days to 2 weeks before onset of the eruption. The EM spectrum can be seen anytime throughout the year; however, there is an increase in incidence during the spring and fall.

The classic skin finding in EM is a fixed target or iris lesion. This finding is manifested as an area of central duskiness surrounded by a circular plaque of pallor and a peripheral rim of erythema yielding a ringlike shape.[2-5] There may be varying intensity of the red rings leading to the target appearance (Figs. 160-1 and 160-2). Once lesions appear, they remain fixed in the affected areas for at least a week or longer.

The rash is symmetrical and may develop anywhere on the body but often presents on the extensor surfaces of the extremities. The palms and soles may be involved. Erythematous macules may be the first sign of the rash, but progression to the classic target lesion is often rapid. These lesions may be pruritic or painful, or both. The lesions may uncommonly become vesicular or bullous but frequently retain the target shape. EM minor often involves a single mucous membrane, which is most commonly seen as localized mouth lesions (see Fig. 160-1).[2] The mucous membrane lesions are similar to those seen in HSV, with some appearing vesicular and others appearing ulcerated and even blood crusted, but they generally avoid the gingiva. Arthralgia may also be a symptom in patients with EM minor. Systemic symptoms are rare; however, mild fever and malaise may be present. Table 160-1 lists the commonly encountered potential triggers of EM in children.

In EM major, the nonspecific prodromal symptoms are followed by an abrupt and rapid onset of cutaneous and mucosal lesions.[3] The skin may become red and tender and then rapidly progress to vesicles and ulcerations, with bullous lesions being much more common in EM major than EM minor. Large areas of skin may be left with tender ulcers exposed as the illness progresses. Unlike EM minor, EM major often has systemic symptoms, as well as involvement of other organ systems.[1,3] By definition, mucous membrane involvement in this circumstance is present in at least two sites.[3] The eyes may present with signs and symptoms of injection, ulceration, and discharge. Dysuria may result from inflammation of the genitourinary mucosa and dyschezia from involvement of the gastrointestinal tract. Rarely, pulmonary mucosal involvement may also be encountered. Most cases of EM major result from exposure to medications, although a subset of cases have been linked to infection with *Mycoplasma pneumoniae* or coxsackievirus.[1,3,5]

DIFFERENTIAL DIAGNOSIS

The classic target lesion of EM is nearly diagnostic; however, forms of annular urticaria must be entertained.[2,4,5] In contrast to EM, lesions of annular urticaria are evanescent, with lesions resolving and appearing elsewhere within 24 hours.[5] In addition, lesions of annular urticaria show central clearing and are often pruritic, whereas lesions of EM show central duskiness and may be tender or painful but are less likely to be pruritic. The combination of rash and arthralgia may be seen early in the course of serum sickness–like reaction, Henoch-Schönlein purpura, juvenile rheumatoid arthritis, and systemic lupus erythematosus, before the appearance of definitive arthritis. Kawasaki syndrome may present with target-like lesions and should be strongly considered when evaluating for EM major because both conditions are accompanied by fever, eye involvement, oral mucosal changes, and occasionally, inflammatory urethritis. However, patients with Kawasaki syndrome may have a polymorphous eruption with nonexudative conjunctival injection, strawberry tongue, and red lips, as opposed to the targetoid lesions of EM major, which may also be associated with erosive mucosal involvement of the eyes and oral mucous membranes. Finally, an individual lesion of a fixed

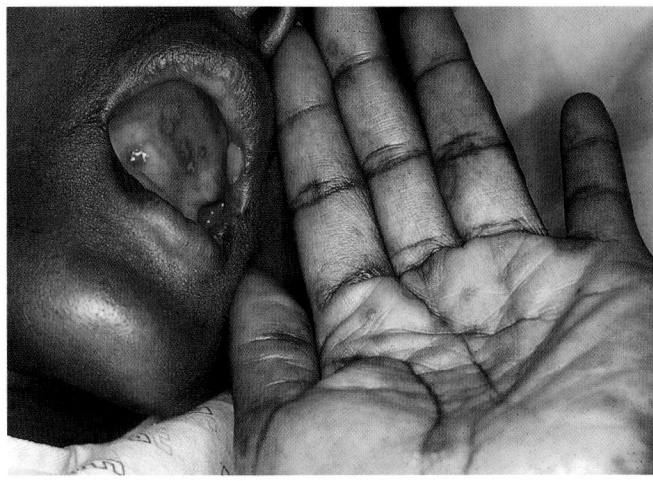

Figure 160-1 Classic appearance of erythema multiforme minor with target (iris) lesions on the palm and fingers and single mucous membrane involvement. (Courtesy of Robert Brodell, M.D.)

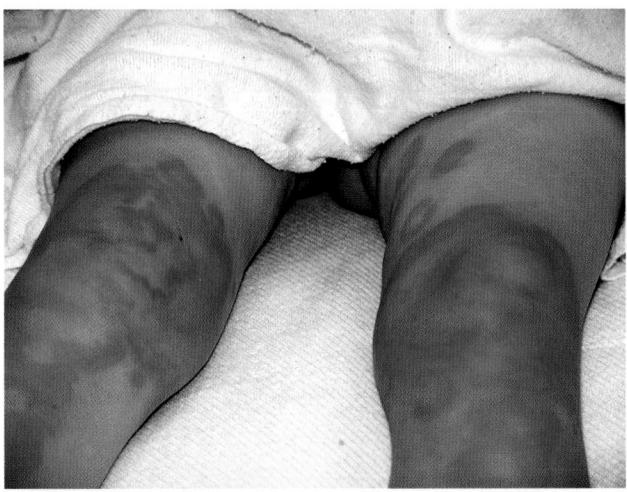

Figure 160-2 Multiple annular, polycyclic and arcuate lesions representative of annular urticaria. Note the areas of central clearing and the incomplete circles that differentiate this form of urticaria from erythema multiforme, which presents with targetoid lesions with dusky centers.

drug eruption may mimic that of EM both clinically and histologically, but in EM, the lesions are more numerous and more widely distributed.

DIAGNOSIS AND EVALUATION

The diagnosis of EM minor or EM major is principally a clinical diagnosis. Determining that at least some of the lesions present conform to the target shape is the hallmark of the diagnosis.[3] Finding associated mucous membrane lesions may aid in the diagnosis and also differentiation of EM minor from EM major based on the degree of involvement of these tissues.

Laboratory tests are not specifically indicated in EM minor because there are no consistent abnormalities, although they may be helpful in pointing toward another diagnosis if the results are significantly abnormal. Elevated indices of acute inflammation (i.e., erythrocyte sedimentation rate, C-reactive protein, ferritin), as well as elevated

Table 160-1 Potential Triggers of Erythema Multiforme in Children
Idiopathic
Viral
Herpes simplex virus (often implicated in recurrent bouts)
Enterovirus (e.g., coxsackievirus)
Epstein-Barr virus
Bacterial
Streptococcus (e.g., group A streptococcus, pneumococcus)
Mycoplasma pneumoniae (generally erythema multiforme major)
Drug induced
Nonsteroidal anti-inflammatory drugs
Antiepileptic medications
Antibiotics (e.g., sulfonamides, penicillins)

white blood cell counts and, if dehydrated, related electrolyte changes, may be seen in EM major. Biopsy demonstrates characteristic findings for the EM spectrum and may help differentiate the condition from other dermatologic diagnoses, especially in patients with vesiculobullous eruptions.[2]

COURSE OF ILLNESS

EM minor is generally a self-limited illness that typically lasts about 4 weeks. The lesions develop over the first week and the symptoms often resolve over the next 1 to 2 weeks.[3] Recurrent lesions may erupt as the first batch of lesions resolves; however, the total course still lasts about 4 weeks.

EM major, in contrast, tends to last somewhat longer,[1] and resolution often takes up to 6 weeks. Long-term sequelae are related to unresolved organ system involvement in EM major. If all organ systems recover without incident, there are no long-term associated risks. Mortality is very low in EM minor and estimated to be about 10% in EM major.[3]

TREATMENT

For all forms of EM, removal or treatment of the causative factor, if identified, is crucial.[3]

The vast majority of patients with EM minor can be managed outside the hospital, with the exception generally being younger children, who may refuse to drink adequately because of malaise and oral mucositis and may require hospitalization for intravenous rehydration.[3]

In mild forms of EM minor, treatment is essentially symptomatic.[2] The use of antihistamines to control itch[2-4] and oral solutions combining diphenhydramine elixir with aluminum/magnesium hydroxide suspension (Maalox) and at times viscous lidocaine (the so-called magic mouthwash) may reduce oral symptoms and improve liquid intake.[2,3] Nonsteroidal anti-inflammatory medications may be used with caution for the arthralgia. Attention to open skin lesions with good hygiene and oatmeal baths may help control symptoms.

EM major, in contrast, often warrants admission to manage the localized, organ-specific or systemic complications. Prompt discontinuation of any etiologic drug triggers and identification of any underlying infections (such as

Mycoplasma) are essential.[3] In more advanced forms of EM the potential use of corticosteroids must be considered. This issue is controversial, with support for and against the use of these medications.[1-4] If diagnosed promptly, the early use of systemic corticosteroids may be helpful if initiated within the first 24 to 72 hours of the eruption and if not contraindicated by an underlying infectious trigger for the EM (e.g., a herpesvirus infection[2]). If it is thought that a child's condition warrants a course of corticosteroids, short courses of 3 to 5 days are generally used with monitoring for improvement. If no improvement is seen, the medications should be discontinued.[3]

Several case reports have suggested a possible role for administration of intravenous immunoglobulin, particularly when ocular integrity is at risk or the EM major is particularly severe.

Intravenous crystalloid solution with electrolyte replacement may be needed to maintain hydration in severely affected children because of both less intake and increased loss through the damaged skin. It is rare that colloid solutions would be needed.

CONSULTATION

- Dermatology: Uncertain diagnosis, severe skin sloughing
- Ophthalmology: Ocular involvement
- Infectious disease: Concern for alternative infectious processes, such as recurrent HSV as a cause of repeated episodes of EM minor and *M. pneumoniae* as a cause of EM major
- Rheumatology: Progressive arthralgia, concern for other causes of arthralgia
- Plastic surgery: Extensive skin sloughing or ulcerations
- Critical care: Severe skin sloughing, significant electrolyte abnormalities, pulmonary involvement
- Urology: Treatment of urethral strictures when present

ADMISSION CRITERIA

Hospitalization is indicated if there is a need for any of the following:

- Clarification of a definitive diagnosis, including evaluation for other diagnostic considerations (e.g., Kawasaki disease)
- Maintenance of adequate hydration
- Correction of electrolyte abnormalities
- Wound management of large areas of denuded skin to decrease the risk for infection or dehydration (or both) or for management of infections
- Involvement of other organs requiring subspecialty involvement, ongoing observation, stabilization, or treatment

DISCHARGE CRITERIA

The following will be needed before discharge:

- Ability to maintain adequate oral/enteral hydration
- Resolution of symptoms to the point that the family can manage them at home
- Arrangement of follow-up appropriate to the organ system involvement

PREVENTION

Prevention of EM is a difficult task because there are several suspected causes. Most commonly in EM minor, viral infections are implicated, especially those caused by herpesviruses. Because recurrent symptoms may be seen after outbreaks of HSV in an individual, controlling these outbreaks may theoretically lessen or eliminate symptoms of EM minor.

Avoidance of medications that are more commonly associated with EM is difficult because the reaction is uncommon and, if it is the first episode, unpredictable. If there is a history of EM after a specific medication, other drugs in that class should be avoided.

IN A NUTSHELL

Presentation
- EM minor: Symmetrically distributed, erythematous papules evolving into classic target lesions with involvement of the extremities, as well as the palms and soles. A single mucous membrane may be involved.
- EM major: Atypical target lesions that may show blistering. At least two mucous membranes are involved by definition. Other organ systems may also be involved.

Diagnosis
- EM is clinically diagnosed by the appearance of at least a few target lesions.
- Occasionally, skin biopsy may be necessary to confirm the diagnosis

Treatment
- Discontinuation of etiologic drug triggers or treatment of inciting infections is key for both the minor and major forms.
- EM minor is typically managed on an outpatient basis, but hospitalization may be required if there is concern for dehydration or electrolyte disturbances or for management of extensive severe skin involvement. Symptomatic relief with nonsteroidal anti-inflammatory drugs and pain-relieving mouthwashes is the mainstay of treatment.
- EM major is often managed in the inpatient setting for timely definitive diagnosis, supportive care, subspecialty involvement as needed, or consideration of corticosteroid or immunoglobulin therapy.

ON THE HORIZON

- Look for improved understanding of the pathophysiology of EM, which may help delineate better prevention measures.
- The benefit of corticosteroids in cases of EM should become better understood.
- The use of intravenous immunoglobulin in severe cases will continue to be studied as a potential method of controlling the disease.

REFERENCES

1. Stiehm ER (ed): Immunologic Disorders in Infants and Children, 4th ed. Philadelphia, Saunders, 1996, pp 649-651.
2. Brice SL, Huff JC, Weston WL: Erythema multiforme in children. Pediatrician 1991;18:188-194.
3. Hurwitz S: Erythema multiforme: A review of characteristics, diagnostic criteria, and management. Pediatr Rev 1990;11:217-222.
4. Salman SM, Kibbi AG: Vascular reactions in children. Clin Dermatol 2002;20:11-15.
5. Weston WL: What is erythema multiforme? Pediatr Ann 1996;25:106-109.

CHAPTER 161

Stevens-Johnson Syndrome and Toxic Epidermal Necrolysis

Denise W. Metry

Stevens-Johnson syndrome (SJS) and toxic epidermal necrolysis (TEN) are severe cutaneous reactions that are best considered part of the same disease process. In the past, erythema multiforme (see Chapter 160) was classified into minor and major forms, the major form being synonymous with SJS. However, it is now recognized that despite histologic similarities, SJS and erythema multiforme are best regarded as separate entities with distinct clinical presentations and causes.[1]

SJS was first described by Stevens and Johnson in 1922 as a symptom complex in children involving "an eruptive fever associated with stomatitis and ophthalmia."[2] In 1956, Lyell described a cutaneous process in adults as "an eruption resembling scalding of the skin" that he called *toxic epidermal necrolysis* (although this original report included at least one patient with what is now recognized as staphylococcal scalded skin syndrome [SSSS]).[3] SJS and TEN are rare; however, these illnesses often present in the hospital, are certainly managed within the inpatient setting, and are diagnostic considerations in many circumstances and therefore important entities to hospitalists.

ETIOPATHOGENESIS

SJS and TEN are most commonly triggered by drugs. Other causes such as infections (particularly *Mycoplasma pneumoniae*) and immunizations are much less common. Although more than 100 drugs have been associated with SJS/TEN, the most frequently implicated are nonsteroidal anti-inflammatory drugs (especially ibuprofen and naproxen), anticonvulsants (especially hydantoins such as phenytoin and barbiturates), and antibiotics (especially sulfonamides, penicillins, tetracycline, and doxycycline).[1] There is compelling evidence to suggest that a genetic susceptibility to SJS/TEN exists; those afflicted have an impaired capacity to detoxify reactive intermediate drug metabolites.[4] Immunocompromised patients, especially those who are human immunodeficiency virus positive, are known to be at particular risk for the development of SJS/TEN.

The histologic features of SJS include extensive epidermal necrosis with sparse inflammatory cells. The severe epidermal necrosis is accompanied by incontinence of melanin pigment, colloid bodies, and subepidermal blister formation.

TEN includes full-thickness necrosis of the epidermal layer with cleavage at the level of the upper dermis.[5]

CLINICAL PRESENTATION

SJS/TEN most commonly develops 2 to 8 weeks after drug exposure and is heralded by a prodrome of nonspecific constitutional symptoms that generally occur 1 to 14 days before the onset of mucosal or skin lesions. Children with SJS/TEN appear acutely ill. Fever and malaise are universal and often accompanied by upper respiratory or gastrointestinal symptoms, or both. Mucosal involvement, most commonly intraoral, ocular, and genital, may occur with or without cutaneous lesions. Classically, hemorrhagic crusts develop on the lips (Fig. 161-1), and painful stomatitis leads to decreased oral intake. A purulent conjunctivitis, with the lids often adherent to one another, is also characteristic, along with photophobia. Genital mucosal involvement is complicated by pain and bleeding. Respiratory or gastrointestinal involvement may also occur in more severe cases.[5,6]

Skin lesions, which may begin simultaneously or after the onset of mucosal lesions, consist of tender, red to dusky macules that are often targetoid. Lesions generally appear first on the trunk; spread to the face, neck, proximal ends of the extremities, and palms and soles; and rapidly coalesce (see Fig. 161-1). Blistering, often heralded by the development of central graying within the skin lesions, may develop within hours or after several days and may be limited or consist of widespread epidermal detachment. In the latter case, large areas of raw, bleeding dermis may be seen. Both SJS and TEN are characterized by epidermal detachment in addition to mucosal involvement, although the development of large sheets of epidermal detachment in the absence of mucosal involvement is more characteristic of TEN.[6] The frequent presence of overlapping clinical features in a given patient often makes definitive classification difficult. According to a consensus definition for the classification of SJS and TEN, epidermal detachment of 10% or less of total body surface area is classified as SJS, greater than 30% as TEN, and between 10% and 30% as SJS-TEN overlap.[5]

Other potential systemic complications of SJS/TEN include generalized lymphadenopathy, hepatosplenomegaly, hepatitis, arthritis, and arthralgias. Less common are

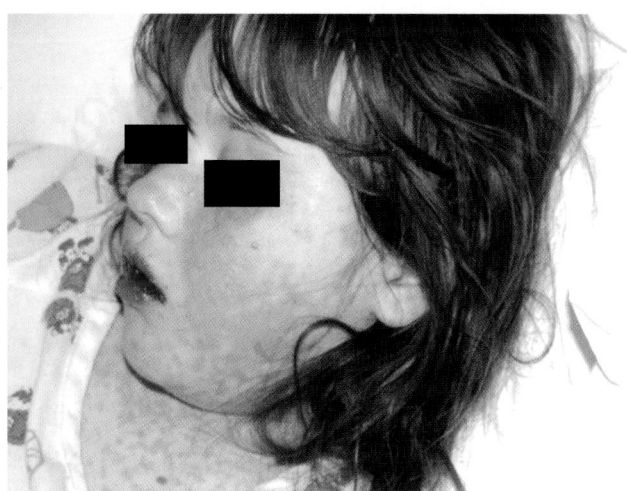

Figure 161-1 Oxcarbazepine-induced Stevens–Johnson syndrome. On the day of admission, hemorrhagic crusting of the lips and coalescing erythematous macules on the face and upper part of the trunk were apparent, along with early blister formation.

myocarditis, pancreatitis, pulmonary complications (especially pneumonia and pneumothorax), and nephritis.[7]

DIFFERENTIAL DIAGNOSIS

The two most common entities in children confused with SJS/TEN are Kawasaki disease (KD) and SSSS. In KD, mucosal involvement consists of chapped, red lips, without the erosions and hemorrhagic crusts typical of SJS. In addition, the conjunctival injection associated with KD lacks the purulent exudate of SJS. The skin lesions of KD are polymorphous and generally transient, without targetoid lesions or blistering, although superficial peeling of the fingertips and perineum is a characteristic finding seen later in the course of KD (see Chapter 102). SSSS, which usually occurs in infants and children younger than 2 years, is characterized by the onset of widespread, tender erythema (see Chapter 157). Crusting and superficial fissuring of the perioral and periocular skin is common, although mucous membrane involvement is absent. Very superficial erosions, which most commonly occur in flexural areas, are a feature of SSSS, but they are clinically and histologically distinct from the blistering and deeper skin separation seen in SJS/TEN.

Although rare, paraneoplastic pemphigus can present with mucosal findings identical to those of SJS. The malignancy most commonly associated with paraneoplastic pemphigus in children is Castleman disease, followed by lymphoma. Paraneoplastic pemphigus can be diagnosed with a skin biopsy, which shows features distinct from SJS on routine histology, and positive direct and indirect immunofluorescence studies. Grade IV acute graft-versus-host disease and burns can also mimic TEN and should be considered in the appropriate clinical setting.

TREATMENT

As soon as the diagnosis of SJS/TEN is suspected, any potential drug trigger should be immediately discontinued. Early withdrawal of the causative drug may reduce mortal-

ity.[8] Supportive therapy is the standard of care for SJS/TEN and includes close monitoring of fluid and electrolyte status, hydration, nutritional support, ophthalmologic care, wound care, and control of pain and infection.

Oral intake is often limited because of intraoral mucositis, and insensible losses are increased as a result of fever and open skin lesions. Administration of parenteral fluids with careful monitoring of urine output and electrolytes is needed. Nutritional support may become necessary when oral intake is inadequate for a prolonged period.

Attempts to limit ongoing skin loss should be instituted. Even minor manipulation of intact skin can cause sloughing. Maneuvers to protect fragile skin may include assistance with repositioning, devices to protect against friction and pressure, and assistance with activities of daily living. Use of a controlled-pressure, thermoregulated bed can also be beneficial.

Meticulous wound care is of utmost importance. Detached areas are handled similarly to burns. They can be covered with petroleum gauze or biologic dressings. Periorificial erosions and hemorrhagic crusts should be gently cleansed daily and protected with petrolatum or a similar ointment. The mouth should be rinsed several times daily with a solution such as sterile isotonic saline.

Because sepsis is the principal cause of death, patients should be closely monitored for signs of secondary infection. A complete blood cell count, liver enzyme analysis, urinalysis, and chest radiography should be performed to evaluate for associated visceral complications.

The importance of early ophthalmologic consultation cannot be overemphasized because ocular complications, including blindness, are an important potential source of morbidity.

There is currently no evidence-based, specific therapy accepted as the standard of care for SJS/TEN. Because of the rarity of such disorders and the frequent delay in diagnosis, no large, controlled studies have been undertaken. The literature consists mainly of scattered case reports, in which several treatments, including cyclosporine, cyclophosphamide, plasmapheresis, and N-acetylcysteine, have been reported to be beneficial. Of these, only plasmapheresis for TEN has been reported in children. In contrast, the use of systemic corticosteroids in patients with SJS/TEN has been widely debated and remains controversial. Although some advocate early, short-term use in drug-induced cases, a number of retrospective studies have suggested that systemic corticosteroids not only fail to improve prognosis but also adversely affect outcome by increasing patient susceptibility to sepsis and gastrointestinal tract hemorrhage. Despite decades of controversy, the efficacy of systemic corticosteroids in patients with SJS/TEN has yet to be demonstrated by any controlled clinical trial.[7,9]

Intravenous immunoglobulin (IVIG) has emerged as a potential immunomodulatory therapy for SJS/TEN. Recent studies have demonstrated arrest in the progression of skin blistering and associated rapid recovery after IVIG infusion (Fig. 161-2; also see Fig. 161-1).[7] As with other therapeutic modalities reported for SJS/TEN, treatment is most effective when initiated as early as possible in the disease course. IVIG appears to be a useful and safe therapy for children with SJS/TEN, although well-controlled, prospective, multicentered clinical trials are needed to determine optimal dosing

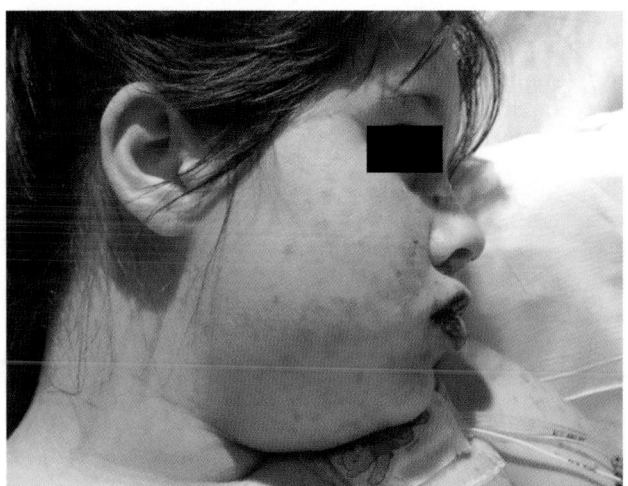

Figure 161-2   Clinical improvement (hospital day 5) of the patient in Figure 161-1 after four consecutive daily doses of intravenous immunoglobulin.

guidelines and to compare the efficacy and safety of IVIG with other potentially effective modalities.

PROGNOSIS

As expected, cases of TEN with the most extensive skin detachment are associated with the highest mortality rates, with large case series pointing to a mortality rate of approximately 30% in such instances. Cases of SJS/TEN triggered by drugs with a long half-life are more likely to result in a fatal outcome. However, with appropriate medical management the prognosis in children is good, with lower mortality than in adults.

Late cutaneous complications of SJS/TEN include scarring, dyspigmentation, and fingernail loss and deformity. Large areas of scarring over joints may cause contractures, so physical therapy is an important prophylactic measure for patients at risk. As previously mentioned, ocular sequelae are the most common serious cause of morbidity from SJS/TEN. Potential complications include psuedomembrane formation with immobility of the eyelids, symblepharon, entropion, trichiasis, corneal scarring, and permanent visual impairment. Lacrimal scarring with subsequent excessive tearing, anterior uveitis, and panophthalmitis may also occur. Although mouth and lip lesions usually heal without sequelae, mucous membrane involvement at other sites may result in esophageal and anal strictures, vaginal stenosis, urethral meatal stenosis, and phimosis.[9]

CONSULTATION

- Dermatology: Can assist with diagnosis and wound management
- Ophthalmology: Can help monitor for and prevent ocular complications
- Plastic surgery: For wound management, acutely and long-term if needed
- Critical care: When an intensive level of care is required

ADMISSION CRITERIA

Patients are managed in the hospital setting because progression of the illness can be swift. Inpatient care centers on

- Fluid and electrolyte management and nutritional support
- Meticulous care of areas of denuded skin and monitoring for secondary infection
- Close observation for multiorgan involvement, including respiratory compromise as a result of mucosal injury
- Coordination of subspecialty services

Transfer to a critical care setting is warranted in patients with cardiorespiratory instability or sepsis or if the level of bedside care needed exceeds the capacity of non–intensive care unit staffing. Care in a burn center is often optimal for patients with extensive skin loss.

DISCHARGE CRITERIA

Care can be transitioned to the outpatient setting when

- Progression of the illness has ceased and the patient has stabilized.
- Hydration and nutrition can be maintained.
- Wound care can be managed.
- Appropriate outpatient follow-up is in place.

IN A NUTSHELL

- SJS and TEN are severe cutaneous reactions that carry a significant risk for morbidity in affected children.
- Drugs are by far the most common cause of SJS/TEN, with infectious precipitants being much less common.
- Presentation: Nonspecific febrile illness followed by mucosal involvement and skin lesions. Hemorrhagic crusting of the lips, stomatitis, and purulent conjunctivitis are salient features of the mucositis. Skin findings progress from tender, red to dusky macules or targetoid lesions to blistering or sheets of epidermal skin loss.
- Treatment includes prompt discontinuation of any potential inciting drug. Supportive care is the mainstay of therapy.
- Sepsis is the principal cause of death. Ocular injury and skin/joint contractures are responsible for serious morbidity.

ON THE HORIZON

- Investigation is ongoing regarding potentially effective immunomodulatory agents for the treatment of SJS/TEN. In addition, advances in genetics research may help identify patients at higher risk for SJS/TEN.

SUGGESTED READING

Prendiville J: Stevens-Johnson syndrome and toxic epidermal necrolysis. Adv Dermatol 2002;18:151-173.

Ringheanu M, Laude TA: Toxic epidermal necrolysis in children—an update. Clin Pediatr (Phila) 2000;39:687-694.

REFERENCES

1. Assier H, Bastuji-Garin S, Revuz J, Roujeau JC: Erythema multiforme with mucous membrane involvement and Stevens-Johnson syndrome are clinically different disorders with distinct causes. Arch Dermatol 1995;131:539-543.
2. Stevens AM, Johnson FC: A new eruptive fever associated with stomatitis and ophthalmia: Report of two cases in children. Am J Dis Child 1922;24:526-533.
3. Lyell A: Toxic epidermal necrolysis: An eruption resembling scalding of the skin. Br J Dermatol 1956;68:355-361.
4. Sullivan JR, Shear NH: The drug hypersensitivity syndrome. What is the pathogenesis? Arch Dermatol 2001;137:357-364.
5. Bastuji-Garin S, Rzany B, Stern RS, et al: Clinical classification of cases of toxic epidermal necrolysis, Stevens-Johnson syndrome, and erythema multiforme. Arch Dermatol 1993;129:92-96.
6. Roujeau JC: The spectrum of Stevens-Johnson syndrome and toxic epidermal necrolysis: A clinical classification. J Invest Dermatol 1994;102:28S-30S.
7. Metry DW, Jung P, Levy ML: Use of intravenous immunoglobulin (IVIG) in children with Stevens-Johnson syndrome and toxic epidermal necrolysis: 7 cases and review of the literature. Pediatrics 2003;112:1430-1436.
8. Garcia-Doval I, LeCleach L, Bocquet H, et al: Toxic epidermal necrolysis and Stevens-Johnson syndrome: Does early withdrawal of causative drugs decrease the risk of death? Arch Dermatol 2000;136:323-327.
9. Chave TA, Mortimer NJ, Sladden MJ, et al: Toxic epidermal necrolysis: Current evidence, practical management and future directions. Br J Dermatol 2005;153:241-253.

CHAPTER 162

Skin Disease in Immunosuppressed Hosts

Maria C. Garzon

A wide variety of cutaneous disorders may affect pediatric patients who have undergone immunosuppressive therapy for a wide range of reasons, including solid organ transplantation, bone marrow transplantation, and various chronic rheumatologic conditions. Skin lesions are most frequently a consequence of drug side effects or infection caused by immunosuppression.[1,2]

The cutaneous disorders associated with immunosuppression range in severity. Some disorders typically occur in the early post-transplant period or during periods of acute rejection and are associated with high levels of immunosuppression. Others are a consequence of prolonged exposure to medications (Table 162-1).

Graft-versus-host disease, an important disorder with cutaneous manifestations, is discussed in Chapter 125.

INFECTIOUS COMPLICATIONS

Infections with common and unusual organisms are a complication of immunosuppression. Extensive involvement caused by relatively minor, but still problematic, skin infections such as tinea corporis, pityriasis (tinea) versicolor, or viral warts is a consequence of long-term immunosuppression.[1-3] The most worrisome complication of chronic immunosuppression is the increased risk of significant morbidity or life-threatening infection.

Bacterial infections such as impetigo, folliculitis, and cellulitis may arise in transplant recipients. Moreover, skin infection may herald or coincide with systemic infection with a variety of pathogens. Common pathogens such as *Staphylococcus aureus* and group A streptococci may be causative agents, but less common pathogens, including gram-negative organisms, may also cause skin disease (Fig. 162-1). Ecthyma gangrenosum is a manifestation of *Pseudomonas* sepsis that can occur in debilitated and immunocompromised hosts. It begins as an erythematous to purpuric patch that evolves into a hemorrhagic bulla, which progresses to a necrotic ulcer or eschar. This life-threatening infection must be recognized early and treated promptly (see Chapter 158). Disseminated nocardiosis from a pulmonary source may occur in severely immunocompromised individuals presenting with nonspecific skin lesions (papules and nodules).[4,5]

Infections caused by yeasts and molds typically occur when immunosuppression is greatest. This is often during the first few months after transplantation or when increased immunosuppression is instituted to treat a later rejection.[6,7] Systemic disease caused by a variety of pathogens, including *Aspergillus, Rhizomucor fusarium, Alternaria,* and *Paecilomyces,* may present as an erythematous patch or nodule that in some cases evolves into an ulcerated, necrotic lesion

(Fig. 162-2).[8-11] Skin lesions of aspergillosis often present at sites of intravenous catheterization.[12] These skin lesions may represent primary infection with the potential for dissemination to other organs or "metastatic" disease from preexisting systemic organ involvement. *Candida* species may cause localized skin disease such as intertrigo and folliculitis or *Candida* sepsis. *Candida* sepsis may present as erythematous papules, often on the trunk and extremities. Disseminated cryptococcosis presents as nonspecific papules or areas of cellulitis.[6,13] Dermatophyte fungus (*Trichophyton* species) may cause widespread superficial skin infections, including tinea capitis, tinea pedis, and tinea corporis. These common infections are usually not life threatening but may serve as a portal of entry for other pathogens that cause systemic disease.

Nontuberculous mycobacteria (*Mycobacterium kansasii, Mycobacterium avium-intracellulare, Mycobacterium fortuitum, Mycobacterium marinum, Mycobacterium abscessus,* and others) may present as subcutaneous nodules and abscesses.[14,15] In addition to these pathogens, parasites such as *Leishmania* are reported to cause visceral disease and subsequent cutaneous infection in young adults following organ transplantation.[16]

Cutaneous viral infections caused by herpes simplex virus 1 and 2 may be more extensive in transplant recipients and cause lesions that mimic pressure ulcers. Reactivation of varicella-zoster virus, a common cutaneous complication in immunocompromised hosts, leads to herpes zoster in transplant recipients. The presentation may not be limited to a strictly dermatomal distribution. Cytomegalovirus, a common cause of systemic infection in solid organ transplant recipients, may also cause a wide variety of skin lesions, including periorificial ulcers, nodules, and plaques and a diffuse exanthem.[17] Skin biopsy of suspicious lesions for histologic evaluation, including special stains and culture, is essential, because superficial skin cultures are often not sufficient to establish a diagnosis, and the clinical presentation of skin diseases caused by a variety of different pathogens is often similar. Prompt evaluation and treatment of these life-threatening infections can reduce morbidity and mortality.

Viral warts caused by human papillomavirus (HPV) are common and troublesome to transplant recipients. They are often numerous, painful, and unsightly (Fig. 162-3). Moreover, the association of HPV with squamous cell carcinoma in transplant recipients is troubling. Verruca vulgaris is very common and is reported to occur in 13% to 54% of organ transplant recipients.[1,2] Warts can occur anywhere on the skin or mucosal surfaces. There is often a history of common viral warts before transplantation, and the prevalence increases over time. Spontaneous regression is uncommon, and treatment is often challenging. Destructive treatments

Table 162-1 Skin Diseases in Pediatric Organ Transplant Recipients

Immunosuppression

Infection
  Bacterial
  Viral
  Fungal, yeast
  Other
Neoplasia
  Malignant
    Skin cancer
    Post-transplant lymphoproliferative disorder
  Benign
    Melanocytic nevi
    Pyogenic granuloma

Medication Side Effects

Calcineurin inhibitors
  Hypertrichosis
  Gingival hyperplasia
  Acne vulgaris
Corticosteroids
  Acne vulgaris
  Striae distensae
  Cushingoid facies

Other

Atopic dermatitis
Dry skin
Hyperpigmentation

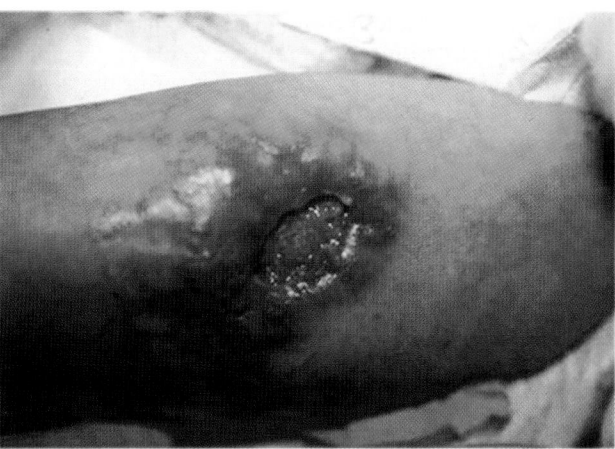

Figure 162-2 Skin ulcer caused by mucormycosis in a cardiac transplant patient.

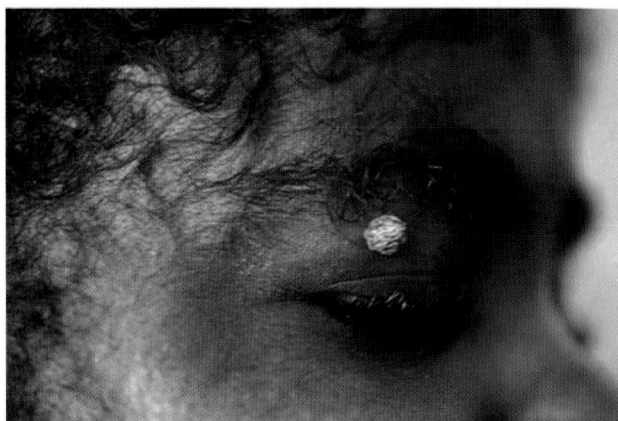

Figure 162-3 Cyclosporine-induced hypertrichosis and verruca vulgaris.

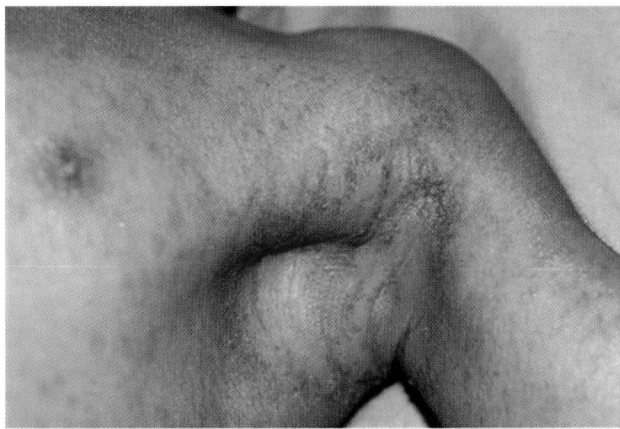

Figure 162-1 Superficial skin infection caused by *Staphylococcus aureus* in a pediatric solid organ transplant recipient.

are often used, but these are painful and may be complicated by poor wound healing or infection. Imiquimod, a topical immunomodulator, has been used in adult transplant recipients[18,19]; however, its safety and efficacy remain to be determined in pediatric organ transplant recipients. Molluscum contagiosum occurs in 7% of pediatric organ transplant recipients. These lesions arise in typical locations on the face, trunk, and extremities but are often multiple and resistant to conventional treatment.[1]

NEOPLASIA

An increased risk of malignant neoplasms is one of the most concerning consequences of immunosuppression. Chronic immunosuppression causing reduced immune-mediated tumor surveillance is believed to lead to the increased incidence of cancer. An overall three- to fourfold increase in cancer risk is reported.[20] Cutaneous cancers (squamous cell, basal cell, and melanoma), post-transplant lymphoproliferative disorder, Kaposi sarcoma, and other sarcomas are commonly reported malignancies.[20] Factors increasing the skin cancer incidence in organ transplant recipients include older patient age, longer immunosuppression, intensity of immunosuppression, ultraviolet light exposure, infection with HPV, and fair skin. Lymphomas, skin and lip carcinomas, sarcomas, and anal and vulvar carcinomas are the most frequently reported malignant neoplasms in pediatric transplant recipients.[21,22] Post-transplant lymphoproliferative disorder may present in the skin as subcutaneous nodules.[23] Squamous cell carcinoma is the most common skin cancer in solid organ transplant recipients; there is a 65-fold increase in the overall incidence of squamous cell carcinoma, a 20-fold increase in squamous cell carcinoma of the lip, a 10-fold increase in basal cell carcinoma, and 3- to 4-fold increase in melanoma.[20] Squamous cell carcinomas arising in transplant recipients are often multiple, have a younger age of onset than in the general population, and are more aggressive. Pediatric transplant recipients also show increased rates of metastases from skin tumors and increased mortality.

Owing to this significant increase in skin cancer risk, which may take years to develop, protective strategies should be implemented in all transplant recipients. Parents and organ recipients need to be counseled about the importance of sun protection, including the use of protective clothing, broad-spectrum sunscreens and lip balms, and behavioral strategies (e.g., avoidance of sun exposure during peak hours). Education should be undertaken before the transplant and reinforced by transplant physicians and primary care providers in the post-transplant period. Annual skin examinations are suggested; these should occur more often if suspicious lesions develop. Examining physicians should have a very low threshold for performing skin biopsies of suspicious lesions.

MEDICATION SIDE EFFECTS

Acne vulgaris, gingival hyperplasia, striae distensae, and hypertrichosis arise after the immediate transplant period and are cutaneous side effects of immunosuppressive medications. Although these conditions are medically benign, they are disfiguring and adversely affect the patient's quality of life.[1,3] Acne vulgaris is a very common disorder in adolescent transplant recipients and may appear rapidly after transplantation, when immunosuppression is at its peak (Fig. 162-4). Several immunosuppressive medications contribute to the development of acne, including corticosteroids, cyclosporine, and sirolimus. Because combination immunosuppressive therapy is common, it may be difficult to determine the exacerbating drug. Systemic corticosteroids may worsen typical adolescent acne as well as cause "steroid acne." Steroid acne is characterized by the abrupt onset of monomorphous pink papules on the face and trunk.[1] Further evaluation to differentiate this condition from infectious causes of skin lesions may be warranted. Steroid acne improves as corticosteroid doses are reduced. Topical retinoids such as tretinoin cream or gel may be beneficial if active treatment is desired.

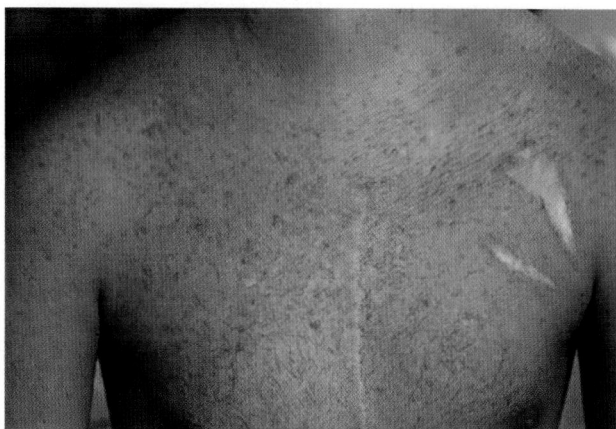

Figure 162-4 Acne vulgaris in an adolescent transplant recipient.

Nodulocystic acne has been described in individuals taking cyclosporine.[24] It is less frequently associated with tacrolimus treatment. Tender, draining nodules and cysts characterize this form of acne. Lesions may be very disfiguring, and the course may be complicated by bacterial superinfection.[24] The differential diagnosis for this condition includes other infectious causes, but the distribution of lesions on the skin surface and the lack of systemic symptoms are useful to differentiate it from more serious conditions. Nodulocystic acne is difficult to treat in this setting. Patients can be managed with traditional acne therapy, including topical retinoids and antibiotics and systemic antibiotics; however, individuals need to be monitored for medication interactions. There are a few reports of the successful use of the systemic retinoid isotretinoin in young adults who have undergone organ transplantation.[24-26] Specific guidelines for the use of isotretinoin in this population do not exist. The potential for systemic toxicities, including pancreatitis and hyperlipidemia, and early experimental evidence that vitamin A derivatives may increase the likelihood of allograft rejection need to be carefully considered.[24-27] It is essential that the dermatologist caring for these individuals work closely with the transplantation team and patient to determine the best course of therapy.

Gingival hyperplasia is commonly seen in individuals receiving cyclosporine and infrequently with tacrolimus administration. It is characterized by thickening of the gingiva and may be widespread or limited to intradental papillae. It often improves as cyclosporine is reduced or replaced with another immunosuppressive agent.[28] Surgical intervention is required in rare cases.[1] Cushingoid facies is a common side effect of steroid administration and improves as corticosteroid doses are reduced. Striae distensae may be very pronounced, and the severity is not directly proportional to steroid doses. Treatment is unsatisfactory.

Cyclosporine-induced hypertrichosis is a common complication, occurring in as many as 69% of children receiving this agent after transplantation (see Fig. 162-3).[3] It is a dose-dependent effect and improves with the reduction of cyclosporine doses. Parents and patients are very troubled by this complication and may go to great lengths to remove hair. Many modalities are used to treat hypertrichosis, but most are uncomfortable and expensive and do not result in permanent hair removal. Waxing and shaving may be complicated by folliculitis or local irritation. Electrolysis and laser hair removal are costly and may be painful, making them difficult for younger patients to tolerate. Wendelin and colleagues reported the successful treatment of cyclosporine-induced hypertrichosis using a low-strength depilatory followed by the application of hydrocortisone to a limited body surface area.[29] Patients and their families should be reassured that their appearance will improve, but if treatment is desired, it should be limited to visible areas and a small body surface area.

CONCLUSION

Organ transplantation and immunosuppressive therapy have increased in the general population. Skin disease is extremely common in these individuals and encompasses a wide spectrum of disorders ranging from minor conditions that may nevertheless be life altering to those that are truly life threatening. Involvement of dermatologists in the care of these children throughout their lifetimes is important.

SUGGESTED READING

Euvrard S, Kanitakis J, Cochat P, et al: Skin diseases in children with organ transplants. J Am Acad Dermatol 2001;44:932-939.

Hibberd PL, Rubin RH: Clinical aspects of fungal infection in organ transplant recipients. Clin Infect Dis 1994;19:S33-S40.

REFERENCES

1. Euvrard S, Kanitakis J, Cochat P, et al: Skin diseases in children with organ transplants. J Am Acad Dermatol 2001;44:932-939.

2. Menni S, Beretta D, Piccinno R, Ghio L: Cutaneous and oral lesions in 32 children after renal transplantation. Pediatr Dermatol 1991;8:194-198.

3. Halpert E, Tunnessen WW, Fivush B, Case B: Cutaneous lesions associated with cyclosporine therapy in pediatric renal transplant recipients. J Pediatr 1991;119:489-491.

4. Kibbler CC: Infections in solid organ transplant recipients. Skin Pharmacol Appl Skin Physiol 2001;14:332-343.

5. Tsambaos D, Badavanis G: Skin manifestations in solid organ transplant recipients. Skin Pharmacol Appl Skin Physiol 2001;14:332-343.

6. Hibberd PL, Rubin RH: Clinical aspects of fungal infection in organ transplant recipients. Clin Infect Dis 1994;19:S33-S40.

7. Hadley S, Karchmer AW: Fungal infections in solid organ transplant recipients. Infect Dis Clin North Am 1995;9:1045-1074.

8. Pfundstein J: *Aspergillus* infections among solid organ transplant recipients: A case study. J Transpl Coord 1997;7:187-189.

9. Boyd AS, Wiser B, Sams HH, King LE: Gangrenous cutaneous mucormycosis in a child with a solid organ transplant: A case report and review of the literature. Pediatr Dermatol 2003;20:411-415.

10. Singh N: Fungal infections in the recipients of solid organ transplantation. Infect Dis Clin North Am 2003;17:113-134.

11. Benedict LM, Kusne S, Torre-Cisneros J, Hunt SJ: Primary cutaneous fungal infection after solid-organ transplantation: Report of five cases and review. Clin Infect Dis 1992;15:17-21.

12. Grossman ME, Fithian EC, Behrens C, et al: Primary cutaneous aspergillosis in six leukemic children. J Am Acad Dermatol 1985;12:313-318.

13. Singh N, Rihs JD, Gayowski T, Yu VL: Cutaneous cryptococcosis mimicking bacterial cellulitis in a liver transplant recipient: Case report and review in solid organ transplant recipients. Clin Transplant 1994;8:365-368.

14. Patel R, Roberts GD, Keating MR, Paya CV: Infections due to nontuberculous mycobacteria in kidney, heart, and liver transplant recipients. Clin Infect Dis 1994;19:263-273.

15. Farooqui MA, Berenson C, Lohr JW: *Mycobacterium marinum* infection in a renal transplant recipient. Transplantation 1999;67:1495-1496.

16. Hernandez-Perez J, Yebra-Bango M, Jimenez-Martinez E, et al: Visceral leishmaniasis (kala-azar) in solid organ transplantation: Report of five cases and review. Clin Infect Dis 1999;29:218-221.

17. Wong J, McCracken G, Ronan S, Aronson I: Coexistent cutaneous *Aspergillus* and cytomegalovirus infection in a liver transplant recipient. J Am Acad Dermatol 2001;44:370-372.

18. Schmook T, Nindl I, Ulrich C, et al: Viral warts in organ transplant recipients: New aspects in therapy. Br J Dermatol 2003;149:20-24.

19. Dupin N, Soubrane O, Escande JP: Eficacite partielle de l'imiquimod sur des verrues plantaires de l'immunodeprime. Ann Dermatol Venereol 2003;130:210-213.

20. Berg D, Otley CC: Skin cancer in organ transplant recipients: Epidemiology, pathogenesis, and management. J Am Acad Dermatol 2002;47:1-17.

21. Penn I: Posttransplant malignancies in pediatric organ transplant recipients. Transplant Proc 1994;26:2763-2765.

22. Penn I: De novo malignancies in pediatric organ transplant recipients. Pediatr Transplant 1998;2:56-63.

23. Schumann KW, Oriba HA, Begfeld WF, et al: Cutaneous presentation of posttransplant lymphoproliferative disorder. J Am Acad Dermatol 2000;42:923-926.

24. El-Shahaway MA, Gadallah MF, Massry SG: Acne: A potential side effect of cyclosporine A therapy. Nephron 1996;72:679-682.

25. Bunker CB, Rustin MHA, Dowd PM: Isotretinoin treatment of severe acne in posttransplant patients taking cyclosporine. J Am Acad Dermatol 1990;22:693-694.

26. Abel EA: Isotretinoin treatment of severe cystic acne in a heart transplant patient receiving cyclosporine: Consideration of drug interactions. J Am Acad Dermatol 1991;24:511.

27. Floersheim GL, Bollag W: Accelerated rejection of skin homografts by vitamin A acid. Transplantation 1972;14:564-567.

28. Thorp M, DeMattos A, Bennett W, et al: The effect of conversion from cyclosporine to tacrolimus on gingival hyperplasia, hirsutism and cholesterol. Transplantation 2000;69:1218-1224.

29. Wendelin DS, Mallory GB, Mallory SB: Depilation in a 6-month-old with hypertrichosis: A case report. Pediatr Dermatol 1999;16:311-313.

CHAPTER 163

Epidermolysis Bullosa

Kara N. Shah, Paul J. Honig, and Albert C. Yan

Epidermolysis bullosa (EB) refers to a family of rare genodermatoses characterized by an inherited tendency toward recurrent cutaneous and sometimes mucosal blistering at sites of mechanical trauma. According to the National Epidermolysis Bullosa Registry, EB affects approximately 12,500 individuals in the United States, with an incidence of 50 new EB cases per 1 million live births annually. More than 3200 individuals are listed on the registry.

Depending on the particular genotype, the clinical manifestations of EB may range from minimal blistering of the hands and feet to severe, widespread, mutilating blistering that can involve the epithelial mucosa of other organ systems. Historically, EB has been classified into a variety of subtypes based on clinical findings, and a growing number of eponyms and otherwise distinctive EB variants have been described in the literature. The current classification system divides EB into three main types based on the ultrastructural level of blister formation: EB simplex, junctional EB, and dystrophic EB (Fig. 163-1). In general, patients with EB simplex have a milder phenotype, and patients with junctional and dystrophic EB have a more severe phenotype; however, there are particularly severe variants of EB simplex, as well as milder forms of junctional and dystrophic EB (Table 163-1).

Although all patients with EB are at risk for complications such as pain, infection, and scarring, those with more severe variants are also at risk for a multitude of chronic morbidities, including nutritional deficiencies and failure to thrive, severe scarring and contractures, cutaneous squamous cell carcinomas, esophageal strictures, and ocular complications that may lead to blindness. All patients with chronic skin disease are at an increased risk of infection as a result of immunologic suppression. The care of a patient with EB involves a multidisciplinary approach and must incorporate a variety of lifestyle modifications and specialized skin care to minimize disease severity and complications. Some of the acute complications associated with EB lead to hospitalization for inpatient management. In addition, hospitalists may be involved with the initial presentation of EB.

CLINICAL PRESENTATION

In general, blistering in EB simplex is limited to the skin, without significant involvement of the mucosal epithelia, and blisters usually heal without scarring (Fig. 163-2).[1] Milia, though classically associated with dystrophic forms of EB, are also encountered in EB simplex, but with less frequency. Other abnormalities may include dystrophic nails, focal keratoderma of the palms and soles, and dental enamel hypoplasia. Patients with EB simplex may not present with blistering until later childhood (Fig. 163-3).

Junctional EB, a result of defective adhesion proteins within the dermal-epidermal junction, presents at birth with generalized blistering. Perhaps even more concerning is the significant risk of extracutaneous involvement of the ocular, gastrointestinal, genitourinary, and respiratory systems, which may result in blistering and stricture formation.[2] Affected patients are therefore at increased risk for nutritional compromise, anemia, respiratory complications, and infection and sepsis. Associated findings include atrophic scarring, exuberant granulation tissue, dystrophic or absent nails, milia formation, significant dental enamel hypoplasia with dental caries, and scalp abnormalities. Patients with the more severe subtype, junctional EB Herlitz, usually do not survive infancy, whereas those with the non-Herlitz subtype display clinical improvement with age.

Dystrophic EB typically presents at birth with generalized blistering that heals with significant scarring. Milia formation, dystrophic or absent nails, and scalp abnormalities are also commonly seen. (Fig. 163-4). Recessive dystrophic EB results in significant, severe scarring that leads to pseudosyndactyly and flexion contractures (Fig. 163-5).[3] Significant systemic involvement can occur, with esophageal stricture formation, dysphagia, and urethral stenosis, leading to malabsorption, anemia, and failure to thrive. Patients with recessive dystrophic EB also have a significant risk of developing squamous cell carcinoma of the skin, corneal ulcerations and scarring, and dental caries. Dominant dystrophic EB generally has a milder phenotype, with less significant systemic involvement and a tendency toward reduced blistering with advancing age. Pseudosyndactyly, ocular complications, squamous cell skin cancers, and respiratory tract involvement are not seen with dominant dystrophic EB.

Chronic skin blistering and ulceration, as well as immunologic suppression as a result of chronic disease and poor nutrition, predisposes EB patients to infection. Although *Staphylococcus aureus* and *Streptococcus pyogenes* are the most commonly isolated organisms, gram-negative, anaerobic, and mixed infections can also occur. Superinfection with *Candida* species is also common in chronic wounds.

Systemic manifestations of mucosal blistering can affect the gastrointestinal, genitourinary, and respiratory tracts, as well as the eyes (Table 163-2). Because of potential injury to the respiratory tract, great care should be taken if children with EB require endotracheal intubation.

DIFFERENTIAL DIAGNOSIS

The differential diagnosis of blistering disorders in neonates and infants is extensive and includes other inherited diseases characterized by skin blistering or erosions, infectious diseases, and immunobullous disorders (Table 163-3). Common disorders to be considered include herpes simplex virus infection, staphylococcal scalded skin syndrome, bullous impetigo, traumatic blisters, and child abuse.

Table 163-1 Classification and Features of Selected Forms of Epidermolysis Bullosa (EB)

EB Type	Level of Defect on Skin Biopsy	Age of Onset	Extracutaneous Involvement	Mortality
EB simplex Weber-Cockayne Koebner Dowling-Meara Muscular dystrophy	Epidermis (basal layer)	Birth or later childhood	Less common	Low
Junctional EB Herlitz Non-Herlitz Pyloric stenosis	Basement membrane zone	Birth	Common	Herlitz and pyloric stenosis: death during early childhood Non-Herlitz: low
Dystrophic EB (recessive)	Dermis	Birth	Common	High; death during adolescence or adulthood from skin cancer
Dystrophic EB (dominant)	Dermis	Birth or later childhood	Less common	Low
Dystrophic EB (transient bullous dermolysis of the newborn)	Dermis	Birth	Less common	Low

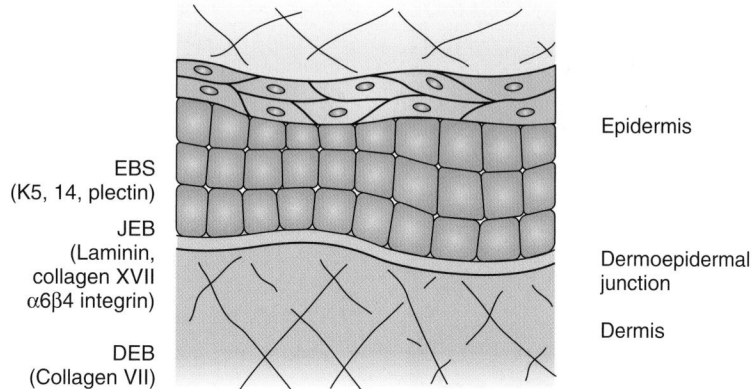

EBS
(K5, 14, plectin)

JEB
(Laminin,
collagen XVII
α6β4 integrin)

DEB
(Collagen VII)

Epidermis

Dermoepidermal
junction

Dermis

Figure 163-1 Location of pathology in epidermolysis bullosa. EB, epidermolysis bullosa—S (simplex); J, junctional; D, dystrophic.

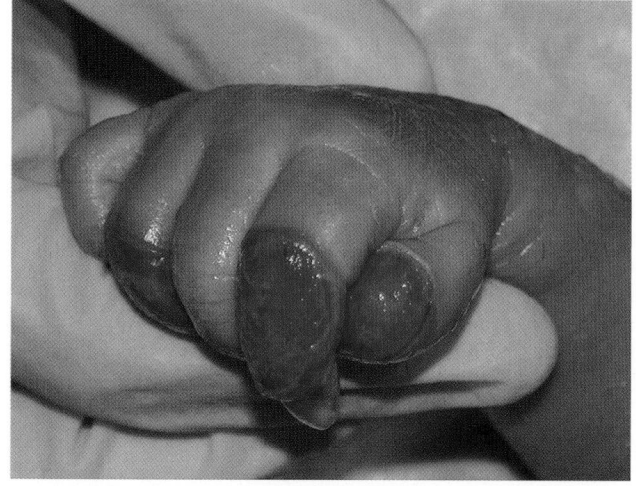

Figure 163-2 Erosions of epidermolysis bullosa simplex on the hand of an infant.

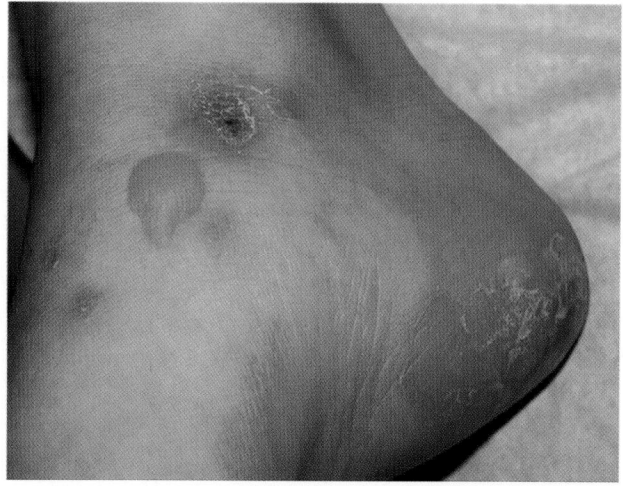

Figure 163-3 Blisters of epidermolysis bullosa simplex located on areas prone to friction.

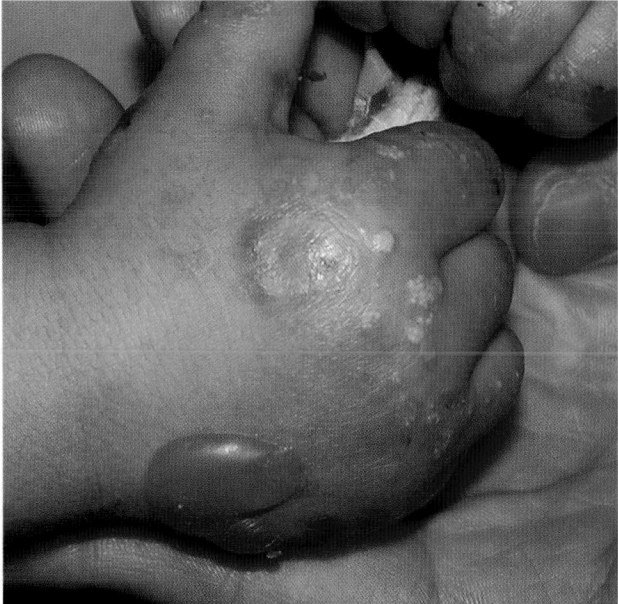

Figure 163-4 Bullae and milia on the hand of a patient with dystrophic epidermolysis bullosa.

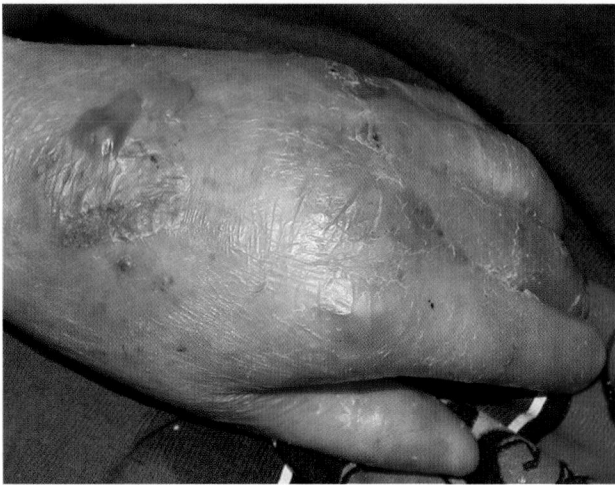

Figure 163-5 Pseudosyndactyly on the hand of a patient with recessive dystrophic epidermolysis bullosa.

Table 163-2 Complications Associated with Epidermolysis Bullosa

System	Complications
Skin	Infection, scarring, milia formation, excessive granulation tissue
Musculoskeletal	Pseudosyndactyly, contractures
Gastrointestinal	Esophageal strictures, dysphagia, anal stenosis, constipation, malnutrition, iron-deficiency anemia, failure to thrive
Ocular	Blepharitis, keratitis, conjunctivitis, corneal scarring, ectropion
Genitourinary	Urethral strictures, phimosis
Respiratory	Laryngeal and tracheal strictures, tracheal stenosis, stridor, hoarseness

Table 163-3 Differential Diagnosis of Epidermolysis Bullosa in Neonate and Infants

Congenital Disorders
Epidermolytic hyperkeratosis
Ichthyosis bullosa of Siemens
Pachyonychia congenita
Incontinentia pigmenti
Ankyloblepharon–ectodermal dysplasia–cleft lip syndrome
Aplasia cutis congenita

Immunobullous Disorders
Bullous pemphigoid
Pemphigus vulgaris (includes transplacentally transferred antibodies)
Chronic bullous dermatosis of childhood (linear IgA disease of childhood)
Epidermolysis acquisita

Infectious Diseases
Staphylococcal scalded skin syndrome
Bullous impetigo
Herpes simplex
Congenital syphilis (congenital blisters on palms and soles)

Other
Bullous mastocytosis
Traumatic blisters
Thermal or chemical burns

DIAGNOSIS AND EVALUATION

Proper diagnosis of EB depends on identifying the site of blister formation in the skin and excluding other causes of blistering disease.[4] An initial skin biopsy for routine histology may help exclude other blistering diseases. When EB is suspected, a freshly induced blister can be created by using a pencil eraser held against the skin with moderate pressure and rotated several times with a twisting motion, thus creating a shear force that results in separation of the dermal-epidermal junction and blister formation. The skin biopsy should be performed at the edge of the blister and processed for examination under both light microscopy and transmission electron microscopy, the findings of which can be diagnostic for each specific form of EB. Immunoepitope mapping of the basement membrane zone can also be performed using a panel of antibodies to basement membrane components that allows the level of the split to be determined precisely. Specific molecular diagnostic mutation analysis is available only in specialized research laboratories but can be helpful in differentiating EB subtypes.

COURSE OF ILLNESS

Although some subtypes of EB may improve with age, it is generally a chronic disease punctuated by recurrent exacerbations. In those with the more severe forms of EB, life

Table 163-4 General Care for Infants and Children with Epidermolysis Bullosa

Type of Care	Recommendations
General skin care	Lift infants by supporting buttocks and head; avoid lifting from under the arms Provide a cool, air-conditioned environment Avoid taking rectal temperatures Take blood pressure readings only when necessary; use soft gauze beneath the blood pressure cuff Use petrolatum gauze under pulse oximetry probes and a hydrogel dressing such as Duoderm under electrocardiogram electrodes Do not use tape to secure dressings or intravenous lines; use gauze or tubular dressings When tape is necessary, use the "tape-to-tape" method: (1) apply a strip of petrolatum gauze against skin, (2) apply a layer of tape to gauze, (3) fasten equipment to tape, (4) apply tape to underlying tape to anchor equipment Monitor for signs of skin infection
Bath care	Avoid rubbing the skin vigorously; pat the skin instead Cleanse skin gently with a mild nonsoap cleanser such as Dove or Cetaphil Apply an emollient such as petrolatum twice daily to decrease friction Give weekly baths using dilute bleach or dilute chlorhexidine to help reduce bacterial skin colonization

Diet, nutrition, and oral care	For infants: use soft nipples on bottles and avoid pacifiers
	For older infants and children:
	    Provide soft, cool foods and teething gels
	    Clean the mouth gently using a soft toothbrush and toothpaste
	    Avoid suctioning the oropharynx
	    Give multivitamins, stool softeners

Bedding and clothing	Use loose-fitting clothing and cloth diapers; avoid elastic Use protective foam or fleece padding on seatbelts and shoes and over elbows and knees Pad mattresses and cribs with foam or fleece For poorly mobile inpatients, use air-cushioned mattresses to help reduce blisters
Wound care and dressings	Clean erosions with saline-soaked gauze Decompress blisters by puncturing with a sterile needle; leave blister roof intact where possible as a natural sterile dressing Apply bacitracin or silver sulfadiazine to erosions Apply petrolatum gauze or nonadherent dressing (e.g., Telfa, Mepilex Transfer, Mepitel) Use self-adhering gauze or tubular dressings; avoid tape and adhesive bandages Soak old dressings before removal if there is crusting or if the dressing sticks to the skin

expectancy can be significantly reduced as a result of failure to thrive, recurrent infections, and sepsis during infancy. Mortality in early adulthood is usually the result of aggressive squamous cell carcinoma. Patients with milder forms of EB may have a normal life expectancy (see Table 163-1).

TREATMENT

Management of patients with EB focuses on the prevention and treatment of skin blistering and infections, as well as on careful monitoring for EB-related complications (see Table 163-2).[5-7] General guidelines are designed to reduce frictional forces on the skin and are summarized in Table 163-4.

Caretakers should avoid adhesive tape and Band-Aids on the skin. If tape is necessary, a layer of gauze can be placed first, followed by an overlying layer of tape. Equipment can then be anchored by taping devices down to the already placed tape (Fig. 163-6). G-tube sites may cause local erosions, and placement of a layer of petrolatum gauze or a silicone-based dressing such as Mepilex Transfer may prevent further blistering at these sites (Fig. 163-7). Intravenous lines

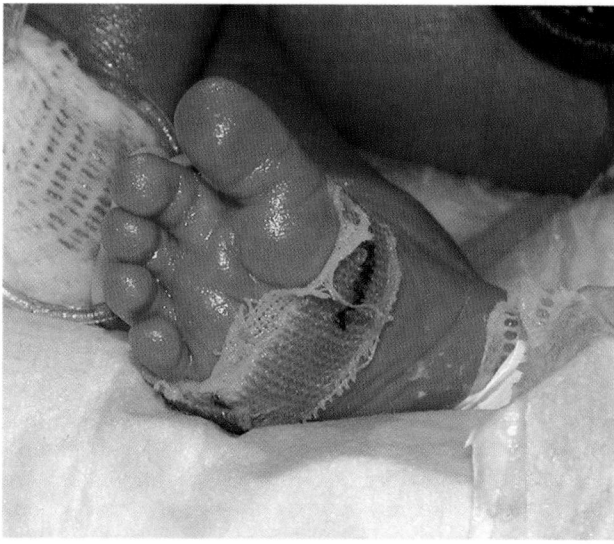

Figure 163-6 Petrolatum gauze is used to protect the skin underneath oximeter tape.

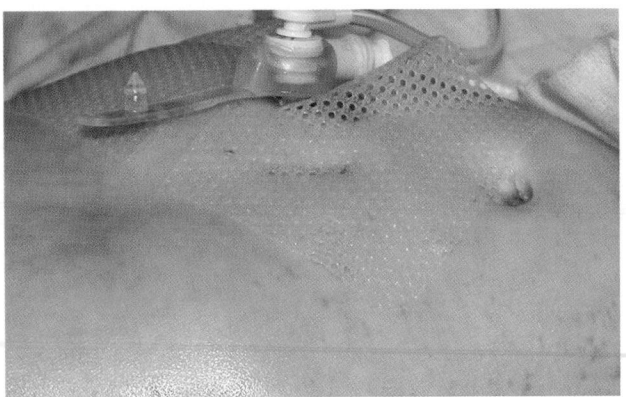

Figure 163-7 Mepilex Transfer is used to protect the skin around a gastrostomy tube.

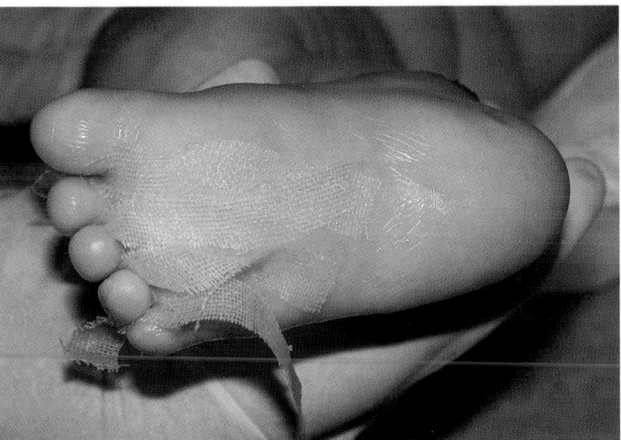

Figure 163-8 Strips of petrolatum gauze are placed between the toes to prevent pseudosyndactyly.

can be addressed similarly, or they may need to be sutured in place. Infants should not be picked up by grasping under the arms but should be lifted by the buttocks with one hand while the other hand supports the head. Soft leather shoes and loose clothing without elastic are recommended. Soft fleece coverings on mattresses and car seats can help reduce skin friction. Cribs should be padded with foam or sheepskin, and foam crib bumpers should be placed inside.

Use of emollients such as petrolatum to reduce skin friction and avoidance of vigorous rubbing of the skin are essential. A cool environment also helps minimize blistering. Gentle skin care is recommended with a mild nonsoap cleanser such as Dove or Cetaphil. In patients prone to recurrent skin infections, the use of additives in the bath water may help reduce bacterial overgrowth. Weekly baths in diluted bleach (1 capful of common household bleach per gallon of water; $\frac{1}{8}$ to $\frac{1}{4}$ cup per bathtub of water) or diluted chlorhexidine (10 mL per tubful) may help reduce bacterial skin colonization and thus reduce the risk of infection; dilute formulations of acetic acid (0.25%) may help reduce the presence of gram-negative organisms in particular.

Infants benefit from teething gels, and soft nipples are preferred for feeding. Frequent small-volume feedings are tolerated best. Use of pacifiers may lead to intraoral blistering and should be avoided. Older children may prefer soft, pureed, cool food; harder foods such as potato chips should be avoided. Good oral hygiene consists of frequent saline rinses and use of a soft toothbrush or gentle water massage device, with avoidance of both harsh mouthwashes and vigorous brushing of the teeth. Routine dental care with an experienced dentist is recommended. Regular use of ocular lubricants is important in the prevention of ocular complications.

In addition, patients with EB require an adequate nutritional intake to aid in wound healing and general immune system function.[8] Multivitamin supplementation, including iron, should be provided. Stool softeners, a high-fiber diet, and adequate fluid intake can help prevent constipation. Pruritus can be managed with oral antihistamines, and patients with significant pain may require analgesics.

There are no therapies that consistently reduce blister formation in patients with EB. Inpatients with poor mobility may require airbeds to reduce pressure on the skin. Blisters

should be punctured and drained using sterile technique to reduce pressure inside the blister cavity, thereby preventing extension. The blister roof, however, should be left intact to provide a natural sterile dressing. Eroded wounds should be covered with petrolatum gauze and a nonadherent gauze bandage or a tubular dressing such as Kling. Interdigitating the fingers and toes using petrolatum gauze may help minimize adhesions or pseudosyndactyly (Fig. 163-8). Areas that require extra padding, such as the diaper area and bony prominences, should be covered with thicker gauze dressings. An elastic net dressing such as Spandage can be used to secure gauze dressings. Other types of dressings, including hydrogel (Aquasorb, Duoderm), fenestrated silicone (Mepitel), or absorbent foam silicone (Mepilex), are also appropriate but are significantly more expensive. New techniques, including the use of nanocrystalline silver dressings, which have antibacterial properties, may reduce the risk of infection.

Although children with EB may be hospitalized for a variety of EB-related complications, they may also be admitted for non-EB indications. The inpatient team should be aware of the myriad complications and issues that may arise with EB patients. Because these children and their families are often well educated about this chronic condition, they can often describe the optimal skin care regimen that has worked well at home, and the hospital team can continue this regimen while the child is hospitalized.

General guidelines for all patients with EB admitted to the hospital include avoidance of friction or iatrogenic skin trauma (see Table 163-4). For patients admitted with significant cutaneous blistering, whirlpool therapy can help clean and débride wounds, and application of semiocclusive nonadherent dressings, such as petrolatum gauze covered with self-adhering gauze or tubular dressings, protects denuded areas and aids in re-epithelialization. Dressings should be changed once daily after gentle bathing in warm water with a gentle nonsoap cleanser. Dressings should never be forcibly removed but should be soaked off in a warm bath.

Careful monitoring of fluid status is important, because patients with skin erosions and subsequent loss of skin barrier function can have significant transepidermal water loss and quickly become dehydrated, especially if they are febrile or unable to take in sufficient oral fluids.

Routine use of topical antibiotics such as mupirocin is not recommended owing to the potential for the development of drug-resistant organisms. Bacitracin or silver sulfadiazine (Silvadene) is an acceptable alternative. Acute skin infections as well as chronic, poorly healing wounds should be evaluated for infection with appropriate wound cultures and Gram stain evaluation. Patients in whom atypical or unusual infections are suspected may need a skin biopsy for aerobic and anaerobic bacterial cultures as well as fungal and mycobacterial cultures. Systemic antibiotics are indicated for the treatment of cellulitis or extensive wound infections. Prolonged use of topical steroids is contraindicated in patients with EB owing to impairment of wound healing.

Patients with significant blistering and skin erosions have an impaired skin barrier; therefore, medications applied topically may be absorbed to a significant degree. In particular, emollients and medicaments containing salicylic acid, prilocaine or lidocaine, or lactic acid should not be applied to patients with EB. Patients with severe skin and mucosal erosions experience a significant degree of pain that should be identified and treated. In general, the use of narcotic analgesics is reserved for the short-term control of acute, severe pain.

A complete nutritional assessment should be performed in all patients with EB who are admitted to the hospital. A complete blood count and iron studies are useful in monitoring for anemia. Other screening serum laboratory studies, including albumin, prealbumin, electrolytes, blood urea nitrogen, liver transaminases, triglycerides, calcium, magnesium, and phosphate, should be evaluated. Serum levels of specific vitamins and minerals may also be evaluated as indicated. Careful monitoring of growth parameters, in conjunction with dietary assessments to ensure adequate calorie and protein intake, is essential for the maintenance of proper growth and nutrition.

Patients with dysphagia or odynophagia and infants who feed poorly should be evaluated for gastrointestinal dysfunction, including esophageal stricture formation. An upper gastrointestinal radiographic series is indicated to evaluate the anatomy and function of the esophagus. Neonates in whom pyloric atresia is suspected should be evaluated and managed appropriately (see Chapter 138).

Patients with ocular manifestations, including pain, discharge, and blepharitis, should undergo a full ocular examination. Patients with urinary symptoms, including dysuria, hematuria, or recurrent urinary tract infections, may have urethral strictures and should be seen by a urologist for a full evaluation of the genitourinary system; this may include imaging studies such as renal ultrasonography or a voiding cystourethrogram.

Musculoskeletal complications are a major cause of morbidity in patients with EB. Therefore, physical and occupational therapy evaluation is essential in all patients with significant pain and blistering to maintain adequate function and range of motion.

CONSULTATION

Dermatologists' expertise may be required to identify the specific EB subtype, determine the patient's prognosis, and perform a diagnostic skin biopsy. In addition, they can educate the patient and family on proper wound care and general skin care to maintain skin integrity.

Pediatric surgeons or gastroenterologists can perform esophageal dilation for symptomatic esophageal strictures; colonic interposition may be required for severe cases.[9,10] Pyloric atresia requires urgent surgical correction in the neonatal period. Patients with significant oropharyngeal erosions and failure to thrive may require gastrostomy tube placement for nutrition.

Nutritionists who have experience treating patients with chronic skin diseases can help maximize nutritional intake, which aids in wound healing.[11]

Plastic surgeons can perform surgical correction of pseudosyndactyly and contractures, although the recurrence rate is high.[12] In addition, wide resection of aggressive squamous cell carcinoma is indicated and requires careful planning to provide an appropriate closure. Plastic surgeons also have training in the use of skin grafting and bioengineered skin equivalents, which may be helpful in patients with chronic nonhealing wounds.[13,14]

Urologists should be consulted for further evaluation and treatment if phimosis or urethral strictures are suspected.[15]

Ophthalmologists can perform detailed examinations of the eyes and adnexa and identify and treat potential complications, including chronic blepharitis, conjunctivitis, keratitis, corneal scarring, and ectropion. Ocular antibiotics, analgesics, and cycloplegics may be required to treat corneal erosions.[16]

Anesthesiologists or otolaryngologists experienced in treating patients with EB may be required if endotracheal intubation is indicated. Their expertise is invaluable in preventing trauma to the upper airway that may result in blistering and scarring.[17]

Physical and occupational therapists are an integral part of the team of specialists who care for patients with EB. Regular exercises and conditioning can help maintain function, and splinting may be helpful in preventing contracture formation. In patients with pseudosyndactyly and contractures, therapy is important to maintain quality of life.

Geneticists can provide counseling on inheritance patterns and prenatal counseling and testing for families considering additional children. Prenatal diagnosis with the use of chorionic villus sampling or amniocentesis is available for families in which the proband has a known genetic mutation.

ADMISSION CRITERIA

- Severe or extensive skin blistering not responsive to outpatient management.
  Admission to optimize wound care and educate caretakers.
- Secondary infection, such as cellulitis.
  Admission for systemic antibiotics and skin care.
- Management of squamous cell carcinoma.
  Although patients may be managed in the outpatient setting, metastatic or large tumors may require inpatient care.
- Severe malnutrition and failure to thrive.
  Admission for evaluation and management of nutritional issues and consultation with appropriate services (e.g., nutrition, gastroenterology, surgery), depending on the active problems.
- Esophageal strictures that prevent adequate oral intake.

Admission for evaluation and management by a surgeon or gastroenterologist.

- Respiratory compromise in more severe forms of EB (junctional or dystrophic).

  Admission for evaluation and management by appropriate services; severely affected patients may require airway support or tracheostomy due to development of tracheobronchial strictures.

- Pseudosyndactyly with mitten-hand deformities or contractures.

  Admission for surgical correction, including skin grafting or specialized postoperative wound care and physical and occupational therapy.

DISCHARGE CRITERIA

- Presence of a significant degree of skin re-epithelialization, no signs or symptoms of persistent infection, and ability to receive adequate nutritional support either enterally or parenterally.
- Pain is adequately controlled, and there is a postdischarge plan for physical and occupational therapy.
- Parents and caregivers demonstrate the appropriate skills required for general skin and wound care and are able to recognize the signs of local or systemic infection.

PREVENTION

EB is an inherited blistering disorder that has no cure. Preventive care includes general strategies to minimize skin blistering and prevent infection. Use of phenytoin and tetracyclines has shown some benefit in reducing the frequency and severity of blistering in some patients, but these drugs are not used routinely.

IN A NUTSHELL

- EB is a diverse group of inherited blistering diseases that can result in severe, generalized blistering with mucosal involvement and significant morbidity and mortality.
- Three types of EB have been established—EB simplex, junctional EB, and dystrophic EB—based on their clinical presentation and an ultrastructural evaluation of the level at which the skin blister occurs.
- Junctional and dystrophic forms of EB are more severe and may result in significant morbidity and mortality.
- Preventive care in patients with EB focuses on general skin care and prevention of blistering. Extensive blistering, wound infections, and systemic complications may require hospitalization for supportive care and subspecialty consultation.
- Malnutrition with failure to thrive, esophageal strictures, ocular complications, and significant scarring with contractures and pseudosyndactyly are common complications.
- Caring for patients with EB requires a multidisciplinary approach involving general pediatrics, dermatology, ophthalmology, general surgery, plastic surgery, and nutrition experts.

ON THE HORIZON

- Current investigations include the refinement of wound healing strategies and the development of gene transfer therapies to provide a potential cure for this devastating disease. New bioengineered skin substitutes that provide long-term re-epithelialization are under development. One strategy uses bioengineered tissues that contain recombinant proteins—either cytokines or extracellular matrix proteins—that are missing or dysfunctional in certain EB subtypes, such as laminin 5 and type VII collagen. Exogenous production of these proteins may enhance wound healing. Gene therapy for EB is still in its infancy, but pilot studies are under way to evaluate the use of keratinocyte stem cells in the treatment of the Herlitz subtype of junctional EB and the Hallopeau-Siemens subtype of recessive dystrophic EB.
- The Dystrophic Epidermolysis Bullosa Research Association of America (*http://www.debra.org*) is a national organization that provides support to families of children with EB. It also supports EB-related research and educational initiatives.

SUGGESTED READING

Bello YM, Falabella AF, Schachner LA: Management of epidermolysis bullosa in infants and children. Clin Dermatol 2003;21:278-282.

Gannon BA: Epidermolysis bullosa: Pathophysiology and nursing care. Neonatal Netw 2004;23:25-32.

Herod J, Denyer J, Goldman A, et al: Epidermolysis bullosa in children: Pathophysiology, anaesthesia and pain management. Paediatr Anaesth 2002;12:388-397.

REFERENCES

1. Horn HM, Tidman MJ: The clinical spectrum of epidermolysis bullosa simplex. Br J Dermatol 2000;142:468-472.
2. Goldstein AM, Davenport T, Sheridan RL: Junctional epidermolysis bullosa: Diagnosis and management of a patient with the Herlitz variant. J Pediatr Surg 1998;33:756-758.
3. Horn HM, Tidman MJ: The clinical spectrum of dystrophic epidermolysis bullosa. Br J Dermatol 2002;146:267-274.
4. Fine JD, Eady RA, Bauer EA, et al: Revised classification system for inherited epidermolysis bullosa: Report of the second international consensus meeting on diagnosis and classification of epidermolysis bullosa. J Am Acad Dermatol 2000;42:1051-1066.
5. Bello YM, Falabella AF, Schachner LA: Management of epidermolysis bullosa in infants and children. Clin Dermatol 2003;21:278-282.
6. Gannon BA: Epidermolysis bullosa: Pathophysiology and nursing care. Neonatal Netw 2004;23:25-32.
7. Schachner L, Feiner A, Camisulli S: Epidermolysis bullosa: Management principles for the neonate, infant, and young child. Dermatol Nurs 2005;17:56-59.
8. Gruskay DM: Nutritional management in the child with epidermolysis bullosa. Arch Dermatol 1988;124:760-761.
9. Castillo RO, Davies YK, Lin YC, et al: Management of esophageal strictures in children with recessive dystrophic epidermolysis bullosa. J Pediatr Gastroenterol Nutr 2002;34:535-541.
10. Demirogullari B, Sonmez K, Turkyilmaz Z, et al: Colon interposition for esophageal stenosis in a patient with epidermolysis bullosa. J Pediatr Surg 2001;36:1861-1863.
11. Allman S, Haynes L, MacKinnon P, et al: Nutrition in dystrophic epidermolysis bullosa. Pediatr Dermatol 1992;9:231-238.
12. Fine JD, Johnson LB, Weiner M, et al: Pseudosyndactyly and musculoskeletal contractures in inherited epidermolysis bullosa: Experience of

the National Epidermolysis Bullosa Registry, 1986-2002. J Hand Surg [Br] 2005;30:14-22.

13. Fivenson DP, Scherschun L, Choucair M, et al: Graftskin therapy in epidermolysis bullosa. J Am Acad Dermatol 2003;48:886-892.

14. Glicenstein J, Mariani D, Haddad R: The hand in recessive dystrophic epidermolysis bullosa. Hand Clin 2000;16:637-645.

15. Fine JD, Johnson LB, Weiner M, et al: Genitourinary complications of inherited epidermolysis bullosa: Experience of the National Epi-

dermylosis Bullosa Registry and review of the literature. J Urol 2004;172:2040-2044.

16. Lin AN, Murphy F, Brodie SE, et al: Review of ophthalmic findings in 204 patients with epidermolysis bullosa. Am J Ophthalmol 1994;118:384-390.

17. Herod J, Denyer J, Goldman A, et al: Epidermolysis bullosa in children: Pathophysiology, anaesthesia and pain management. Paediatr Anaesth 2002;12:388-397.

CHAPTER 164

Transplacentally Acquired Dermatoses of the Newborn

Amy E. Gilliam and Ilona J. Frieden

Transplacentally acquired dermatoses of the newborn are cutaneous diseases transmitted from mother to fetus in utero through the placental circulation. These dermatoses can be subdivided into those due to infectious agents and neoplastic cells and those that are immunologically mediated.

INFECTIOUS TRANSPLACENTAL DERMATOSES

Transplacental transfer of infectious agents can result in the TORCH syndrome, which describes the clinical findings seen in children who have contracted a congenital infection with toxoplasmosis, other (syphilis, listeriosis), rubella, cytomegalovirus, and herpesvirus. Transplacental infection with these organisms can cause clinically similar dermatologic findings, and distinguishing the causative agent is often based on serologic or microbiologic tests.[1,2] Extracutaneous features of the TORCH syndrome often include neurologic, ophthalmic, and hematologic, among other systemic abnormalities. Most TORCH infections result in more profound fetal anomalies when acquired during the first and second trimesters, which are the critical periods for organogenesis. However, infections with organisms such as *Listeria* can cause severe neonatal illness when acquired late in pregnancy as well, because the immunologically immature infant is susceptible to disseminated infection. Cutaneous manifestations of these infections are summarized in Table 164-1. A more complete discussion of perinatal infections appears in Chapter 53.

The most common cutaneous features associated with TORCH infections include jaundice, petechiae, purpura, ecchymoses, and "blueberry muffin" lesions, which are infiltrative, blue-red plaques or nodules that represent dermal erythropoiesis (Fig. 164-1).[1,2] This extramedullary hematopoiesis is secondary to either bone marrow suppression from infection or hematologic dyscrasias such as Rh hemolytic disease, maternal-fetal ABO incompatibility, twin-twin transfusion syndrome, and hereditary spherocytosis. The differential diagnosis for blueberry muffin skin lesions in a neonate should also include neoplastic infiltration of the dermis due to a malignancy such as congenital leukemia, neuroblastoma, Langerhans cell histiocytosis, and rhabdomyosarcoma. However, blueberry muffin lesions are not seen exclusively in the setting of TORCH intrauterine infection. Other viral infections described in association with blueberry muffin lesions include parvovirus B19 and coxsackievirus B2.[3]

NEOPLASTIC TRANSPLACENTAL DERMATOSES

Transplacental passage of neoplastic agents in the setting of maternal metastatic cancer is extremely rare. Melanoma is the most common neoplasm reported to affect both the placenta and the fetus, despite the fact that cervical and breast cancer account for more than 50% of the malignancies in pregnant women. This suggests that hormonal or immunologic mechanisms may affect the fetus's susceptibility to certain types of cancer.

In the few reported cases of transplacental transmission of malignant melanoma, cutaneous pigmented papules and nodules as well as multiorgan metastases have been described. Liver involvement is usually significant, and death occurs in the first year of life in many cases.[4]

IMMUNOLOGICALLY MEDIATED TRANSPLACENTAL DERMATOSES

Immunologically mediated transplacentally acquired dermatoses occur as a result of both antibody-mediated and cell-mediated mechanisms. The skin disorders seen in the newborn period that are caused by transplacental autoantibody transfer include neonatal lupus erythematosus (NLE), neonatal pemphigus, and herpes gestationis.

NLE is an acquired autoimmune disorder characterized by maternal autoantibodies against RNA protein complexes that cross the placenta and lead to the clinical manifestations of NLE, which include cutaneous, cardiac, hematologic, and hepatic disorders. Mothers of affected infants may have systemic lupus erythematosus (see Chapter 107) or Sjögren syndrome, or they may be asymptomatic.

Cutaneous lesions occur in approximately half of infants with NLE and are characterized by erythematous, scaling, annular plaques on sun-exposed areas such as the head and neck, particularly on the scalp and malar and periorbital regions (Fig. 164-2).[5] The eruption can occur at birth but more commonly appears within the first 8 weeks of life, after exposure to ultraviolet light, including phototherapy for hyperbilirubinema. After 3 to 5 months, the lesions resolve, with residual hyperpigmentation, telangiectases, or mild atrophy. The resolution of the skin rash parallels the disappearance of the maternal autoantibodies from the infant's serum by 6 months of age. Additionally, neonates with NLE may have petechiae or purpura secondary to thrombocytopenia, as well as jaundice due to hepatic involvement.[6] Recommended treatment for the skin lesions of NLE includes sun avoidance and low-potency topical corticosteroids.

Neonatal pemphigus and herpes gestationis are extremely rare mucocutaneous blistering disorders seen in the early neonatal period. They are caused by passive transplacental transfer of pathogenic immunoglobulin G autoantibodies to specific epithelial surface peptides. Infants with these disorders are born to mothers with autoimmune blistering disorders, including pemphigus vulgaris, pemphigus foliaceus, and herpes gestationis (also called pemphigoid gestationis).

Table 164-1 Clinical Features, Diagnosis, and Treatment of TORCH Syndrome Infections

Disease: Causative Organism	Cutaneous Signs	Systemic Signs	Laboratory Diagnosis	Treatment
Congenital toxoplasmosis: *Toxoplasma gondii*	Jaundice, petechiae, ecchymoses, purpura, "blueberry muffin" lesions	General: hepatosplenomegaly, lymphadenopathy, intrauterine growth retardation Eye: chorioretinitis > 50%, iridocyclitis, microphthalmia Neurologic: hydrocephalus, microcephaly, seizures, mental retardation, encephalomyelitis, intracranial calcifications Hematologic: anemia, thrombocytopenia	Detection of *Toxoplasma*-specific IgM (however, absent in 25% of infected infants) or PCR for *T. gondii* DNA from CSF, blood, or urine	Sulfadiazine, pyrimethamine, and folinic acid for up to 1 yr to prevent late sequelae
Congenital cytomegalovirus: cytomegalovirus (CMV)	Jaundice, petechiae, purpura, "blueberry muffin" lesions	General: nontender hepatosplenomegaly, intrauterine growth retardation Eye: chorioretinitis Neurologic: sensorineural hearing loss, microcephaly, seizures, intracranial calcifications Pulmonary: pneumonitis, respiratory distress	Viral culture of infant's saliva, urine, or tissue by shell vial assay in first 3 wk of life Detection of CMV-specific IgM or persistent or increasing titer of IgG during first 4-6 mo of life	Clinical trials ongoing using ganciclovir; no approved treatment
Congenital rubella: rubella virus	Petechiae, purpura, "blueberry muffin" lesions; generalized maculopapular eruption; reticulated erythema and signs of vasomotor instability (e.g., mottling, dependent cyanosis, temperature-dependent flushing)	Classic triad of cataracts, sensorineural deafness, and cardiac malformations (e.g., patent ductus arteriosus, valvular stenosis, septal defect) General: prematurity, intrauterine growth retardation, hepatosplenomegaly Eye: cataracts, chorioretinitis Neurologic: sensorineural hearing loss, microcephaly, psychomotor retardation Pulmonary: pneumonitis	Viral culture of pharynx or Demonstration of rubella-specific IgM antibodies in infant's serum	No treatment; universal immunization is designed for prevention
Congenital syphilis: *Treponema pallidum*	Early: petechiae; hemorrhagic vesicles and bullae; erythematous papular, papulosquamous, annular, or polymorphous eruption; "snuffles"; condyloma latum; rhagades Late: rare skin findings	Early: hepatosplenomegaly, lymphadenopathy, pneumonia, anemia, thrombocytopenia, nephrotic syndrome, chorioretinitis, meningitis, seizures Late: Hutchinson teeth, mulberry molars, saber shins, Clutton joints, interstitial keratitis, optic atrophy, sensorineural hearing loss, frontal bossing, concave central face	Demonstration of spirochetes in exudates or tissues using darkfield or direct immunofluorescence microscopy or Demonstration of reactive CSF VDRL or serum quantitative treponemal tests 4 × higher than mother's	IV penicillin over 10 days

Table 164-1   Clinical Features, Diagnosis, and Treatment of TORCH Syndrome Infections—cont'd

Disease: Causative Organism	Cutaneous Signs	Systemic Signs	Laboratory Diagnosis	Treatment
Intrauterine herpes simplex: herpes simplex virus types 1, 2	Single or grouped vesicles, vesicopustules, erosions, scarring, or areas of absent skin	Low birth weight, microcephaly, chorioretinitis, microphthalmia	Detection of virus using DFA or cell culture or PCR from skin lesions or body fluids	IV acyclovir
Congenital varicella syndrome: varicella-zoster virus	Denuded areas of skin with stellate or angular scarring in a dermatomal distribution; may be associated with hypoplasia of underlying tissues	General: low birth weight, colonic atresia Skeletal: limb hypoplasia Eye: chorioretinitis, microphthalmia, cataracts, nystagmus Neurologic: microcephaly, hydrocephalus, mental retardation, seizures, limb paresis	Serology demonstrating varicella-specific IgM or Persistence of varicella-specific IgG beyond 1 yr of life	Supportive only; prevention of maternal infection
Listeriosis: *Listeria monocytogenes*	Generalized erythematous papules, petechiae, and pustules; also mucopurulent conjunctivitis	Acute neonatal sepsis, meningitis, pneumonia, premature birth	Gram + coccobacilli in stains or cultures of infant's blood, urine, CSF, skin lesions, meconium, and gastric aspirates	Ampicillin + aminoglycoside such as gentamicin for synergy

CSF, cerebrospinal fluid; DFA, direct fluorescent antibody; Ig, immunoglobulin; PCR, polymerase chain reaction; TORCH, toxoplasmosis, other agents, rubella, cytomegalovirus, herpes simplex.

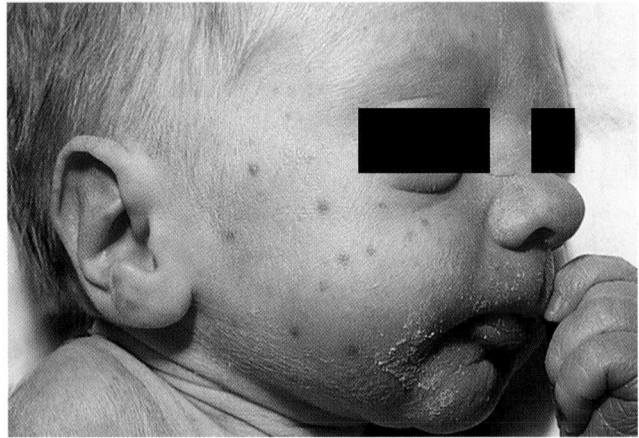

Figure 164-1   "Blueberry muffin" lesions associated with congenital cytomegalovirus infection. (From Eichenfield LF, Frieden IJ, Esterly NB: Textbook of Neonatal Dermatology. Philadelphia, WB Saunders, 2001, p 313.)

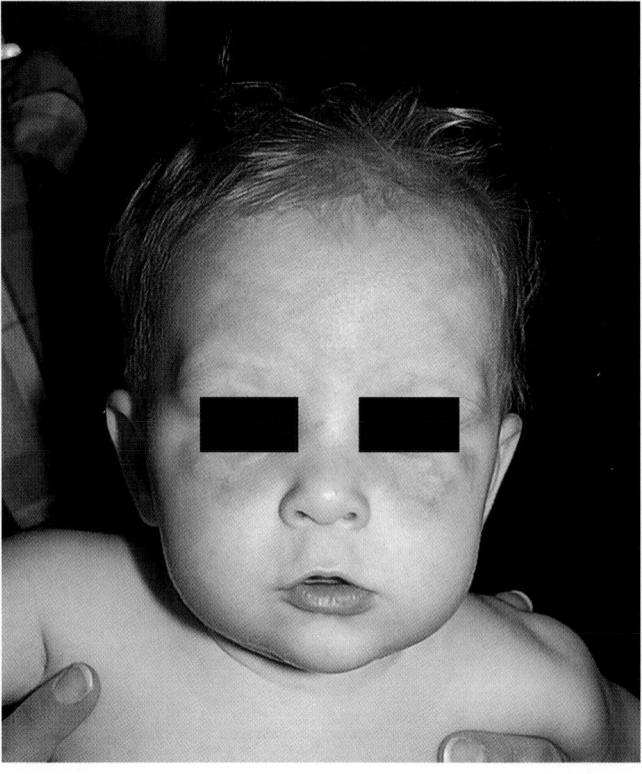

Figure 164-2   "Raccoon eyes" eruption of neonatal lupus erythematosus. (From Eichenfield LF, Frieden IJ, Esterly NB: Textbook of Neonatal Dermatology. Philadelphia, WB Saunders, 2001, p 297.)

These neonates present at birth or within the first few days of life with mucosal and skin blistering or erosions, often located on the trunk, arms, and legs. Healing of the skin lesions usually occurs within several weeks, coincident with waning maternal autoantibodies, much like the process in NLE. Treatment is not required but may consist of topical corticosteroids or topical antibacterials if there are signs of secondary infection.

Neonatal Behçet disease has been described in infants born to mothers with oral and genital Behçet ulcerations during pregnancy.[7] Cutaneous findings in neonatal Behçet disease are transient, suggesting the placental transfer of maternal immunoglobulin; they include ulcerations on the oral and genital mucosa, as well as vesicular and vasculitic skin lesions.

Cell-mediated transplacentally acquired dermatoses occur when maternal lymphocytes traverse the placenta into the fetal circulation of an immunocompromised fetus, resulting in maternal engraftment. This is seen in the setting of severe combined immunodeficiency (SCID) as the transplacentally derived maternal T lymphocytes cause graft-versus-host disease (GVHD) in affected infants. This phenomenon has been described in approximately 25% of all patients with SCID, and the cutaneous manifestations of GVHD due to maternal engraftment can be striking.[8] Fortunately, systemic or multiorgan involvement is rare, although associated hepatic, renal, and hematologic abnormalities have been reported. Maternal engraftment can also be asymptomatic. Interestingly, engraftment is often incomplete, and maternally engrafted T cells fail to protect infants with SCID from opportunistic infections.

The dermatologic manifestations of GVHD due to maternal engraftment resemble those seen in patients with GVHD after bone marrow transplantation. The cutaneous eruptions usually present as either a chronic eczematous skin rash that develops insidiously during the second or third month of life or as a severe exfoliative erythroderma that develops 2 to 6 weeks after birth.[9] Patients with the latter presentation may have associated lymphadenopathy, hepatosplenomegaly, and alopecia. The skin findings often appear first on the face,

neck, palms, and soles before generalizing. In severe cases, bullae or toxic epidermal necrolysis can occur. GVHD due to maternal engraftment should be considered in the differential diagnosis for any neonate with erythroderma, which includes immunodeficiency disorders without maternal engraftment, viral exanthems, drug eruptions, seborrheic dermatitis, Langerhans cell histiocytosis, ichthyosis, erythrodermic psoriasis, and staphylococcal scalded skin syndrome, as well as other infections.

SUGGESTED READING

Boh EE: Neonatal lupus erythematosus. Clin Dermatol 2004;22:125-128.
Eichenfield LF, Frieden IJ, Esterly NB: Textbook of Neonatal Dermatology. Philadelphia, WB Saunders, 2001.
Krusinski PA, Saurat JH: Transplacentally transferred dermatoses. Pediatr Dermatol 1989;6:166-177.

REFERENCES

1. Krusinski PA, Saurat JH: Transplacentally transferred dermatoses. Pediatr Dermatol 1989;6:166-177.
2. Fine JD, Arndt KA: The TORCH syndrome: A clinical review. J Am Acad Dermatol 1985;12:697-706.
3. Bowden JB, Hebert AA, Rapini RP: Dermal hematopoiesis in neonates: Report of five cases. J Am Acad Dermatol 1989;29:1104-1110.
4. Richardson SK, Tannous ZS, Mihm MC: Congenital and infantile melanoma: Review of the literature and report of an uncommon variant, pigment-synthesizing melanoma. J Am Acad Dermatol 2002;47:77-90.
5. Eichenfield LF, Frieden IJ, Esterly NB: Textbook of Neonatal Dermatology. Philadelphia, WB Saunders, 2001.
6. Boh EE: Neonatal lupus erythematosus. Clin Dermatol 2004;22:125-128.
7. Stark AC, Bhakta B, Chamberlain MA, et al: Life-threatening transient neonatal Behcet's disease. Br J Rheumatol 1997;36:700-702.
8. Müller SM, Ege M, Pottharst A, et al: Transplacentally acquired maternal T lymphocytes in severe combined immunodeficiency: A study of 121 patients. Blood 2001;98:1847-1851.
9. Denianke KS, Frieden IJ, Cowan MJ, et al: Severe combined immunodeficiency: Cutaneous manifestations of maternal engraftment in patient with severe combined immunodeficiency: A clinicopathologic study. Bone Marrow Transplant 2001;28:227-233.

Psychiatry

CHAPTER 165

Depression and Physical Illness

Pamela J. Beasley and Harsh K. Trivedi

Children and adolescents hospitalized for the treatment of physical illness often have feelings of sadness, frustration, or irritability that represent a normal response to their experience. These feelings may result from many factors, including disruption of routine, separation from family and peers, uncertainty and anxiety regarding diagnosis and prognosis, pain related to the illness or its treatment, and fear of the illness or its sequelae. When the sadness becomes pervasive and is associated with cognitive or physiologic symptoms, however, a depressive disorder must be considered.

Because of the association between physical illness and depression, it is incumbent on the hospitalist to distinguish normal feelings of sadness from a depressive disorder and to implement treatment when necessary. Chronically ill children are at increased risk for developing depressive, anxiety, and eating disorders.[1-5] Clinical depression has been reported to increase the risk of poor physical health in the future[6] and has been associated with poor adherence to treatment regimens,[7] reduced immune function,[8] increased disease severity, and death due to nonadherence.[9] Emerging data suggest that depression in patients with human immunodeficiency virus (HIV) and acquired immunodeficiency syndrome (AIDS) is associated with declining CD4 counts, accelerated disease progression, and increased mortality.[10] In addition, suicidal ideation and suicide attempts are tragic consequences of depression that increase with the onset of puberty.[11] Depressive disorders cause significant suffering on the part of the child and family and are generally highly treatable once they are recognized. The purpose of this chapter is to provide the pediatric hospitalist with a framework for understanding the diagnosis and treatment of depressive disorders in children and adolescents with physical illness.

BACKGROUND

Making the diagnosis of a depressive disorder in physically ill youngsters may be complicated for several reasons. First, the term *depression* is ambiguous and has many connotations. It may be used to describe a transient mood state or one of several clinical syndromes of varying severity. Second, because symptoms of depressive disorders are subject to developmental variation, they may present differently depending on the child's stage of development.[11]

Third, because medical and nursing staff often view depression as a normal and understandable response to a chronic, terminal, or disfiguring illness, psychiatric evaluation and treatment may not be pursued.[12] Fourth, patients and families may be resistant to exploring the possibility of a depressive disorder because of the perceived stigma of a psychiatric diagnosis. Last, the diagnosis of depression is made on the basis of a constellation of psychological and somatic symptoms. Because somatic symptoms are commonly seen in physical illness, it is often difficult to determine whether the symptoms are related to the physical illness or to a depressive disorder.

CLINICAL PRESENTATION

The symptoms of depressive disorders can be divided into two general realms: psychological and somatic. Psychological symptoms include dysphoric mood, anhedonia (loss of interest in usual, pleasurable activities), feelings of helplessness or hopelessness, feelings of guilt or worthlessness, loss of self-esteem, decreased ability to concentrate, and thoughts of suicide. Somatic symptoms of depression include fatigue, sleep disturbance (insomnia or hypersomnia), appetite changes (decrease or increase), and motor restlessness or retardation (see Chapter 167 for a discussion of somatoform disorders). The hospitalist should focus on the psychological symptoms because of the frequent overlap between somatic symptoms of depression and symptoms of the physical illness.

The presentation of depression depends on the child's stage of development, and depression in children may manifest differently from depression in adolescents. Signs of depression in children (or in older children with developmental delay) may include feelings of sadness, a depressed appearance, somatic complaints (most commonly stomachaches and headaches), separation anxiety, low self-esteem, social withdrawal, decline in academic performance, sleep or appetite disturbances, decreased concentration, and suicidal thoughts.[11,13]

In adolescents, depression frequently presents with an irritable rather than a depressed mood. Additional symptoms commonly associated with depression in adolescents include behavioral disturbances, motor hyperactivity, feelings of being unloved, self-deprecation, tearfulness, hopelessness, low self-esteem, hypersomnia, lethargy, anhedonia, weight gain, decreased concentration, declining school performance, psychomotor retardation, feelings of being misunderstood, and suicidal ideation. Adolescents frequently do not recognize their symptoms as being part of a depressive disorder and may not report them unless specifically asked.[11]

The hospitalist should consider the diagnosis of depression in patients who report feelings of sadness or who appear sad or withdrawn, in patients who exhibit oppositional behavior (e.g., refusal to participate in self-care or nonadherence to a treatment plan), or in patients with a history of other psychiatric disorders (e.g., anxiety, bipolar disorder, substance abuse). Studies have estimated that 40% to 70% of adolescents with depressive disorders also meet the criteria for at least one other psychiatric disorder.[11]

EVALUATION

When the hospitalist suspects depression, psychiatric consultation should be obtained if available. If unavailable, the hospitalist should complete the assessment as follows. The first step is to meet with the patient and his or her parents or guardians to obtain the following information: past individual and family psychiatric histories, description of academic performance and peer relations, and drug or alcohol use. In addition, the hospitalist should inquire about current and past psychosocial stressors, perform a mental status examination (see Chapter 166), and screen for the psychological and somatic symptoms of depression. These symptoms can be remembered using the mnemonic SIGECAPS, which refers to a prescription one might write for a depressed person (sig.: energy capsules). Each letter refers to one of the diagnostic criteria for a major or clinical depressive episode (Table 165-1).[14,15]

Elements of the psychiatric history that should be elicited from both the patient and the family include current and past histories of psychiatric disorders, treatments, and medications. A personal or family history of depression predisposes children and adolescents to develop a primary depressive disorder in the face of the stress of illness and hospitalization.[15,16] The mental status examination should focus on evidence of the presence of mood dysphoria, suicidal ideation, and thought disorder (e.g., hallucinations, delusions).

It is important for the hospitalist to meet with the patient and parents separately for part of the evaluation to encourage full reporting of symptoms and concerns. If they are interviewed together, the patient or parents may not feel comfortable speaking freely and may withhold valuable diagnostic information. The evaluation should include the following:

- Onset, severity, and duration of symptoms.
- Functioning in various domains (e.g., family, school, peers).
- Burden of suffering imposed by the symptoms (e.g., depth of distress, difficulty coping).
- Presence or absence of suicidal ideation.

Together, these factors help determine the type and level of depression.[11]

The hospitalist should obtain collateral information from as many sources as possible. Teachers, guidance counselors,

Table 165-1   SIGECAPS: A Mnemonic for Symptoms of Depressive Disorders

S	Sleep	Insomnia or hypersomnia*
I	Interests	Loss of interest or pleasure in activities (anhedonia)
G	Guilt	Excessive guilt, worthlessness*, hopelessness*
E	Energy	Loss of energy or fatigue*
C	Concentration	Decreased ability to concentrate*
A	Appetite	Appetite disturbance (decreased or increased)*
P	Psychomotor	Psychomotor retardation or agitation
S	Suicidality	Suicidal thoughts or plans; feeling that life is not worth living

SIG: E CAPS (prescribe energy capsules).
To meet the criteria for a major depressive episode, a patient must have four of the above symptoms, in addition to depressed mood or anhedonia, for at least 2 weeks. To meet the criteria for dysthymic disorder, a patient must have two of the six symptoms marked with an asterisk, in addition to a depressed or irritable mood for at least 1 year (2 years in adults).
Adapted from Wise MG, Rundell JR: Concise Guide to Consultation Psychiatry. Washington, DC, American Psychiatric Press, 1998; and Carlat DJ: The psychiatric review of symptoms: A screening tool for family physicians. Am Fam Physician 1998;58:1617-1624.

and therapists may provide helpful information about the patient's mood and level of functioning outside the hospital. Within the hospital, nurses and child life specialists may provide valuable information about the patient's symptoms and level of functioning throughout the course of each day. Assessments of the patient's mood at different points during the day may also assist in making the diagnosis. For example, a patient who presents with a depressed mood and withdrawn behavior during morning rounds but who appears cheerful and engaged when observed in the playroom later in the day is less likely to be suffering from clinical depression than is a patient whose depressive symptoms persist without change over the course of several days.

It is important to recognize that suicidal ideation and suicide attempts may be tragic consequences of depression in children and adolescents. If there is any concern about suicide, a risk assessment should be conducted to determine the history of previous suicide attempts, family history of suicide, exposure to family violence or abuse, level of impulsivity, accessibility to lethal agents, and presence of comorbid psychiatric disorders. For those patients deemed to be at risk for suicide, constant observation in the form of a one-to-one sitter should be implemented to monitor the patient around the clock until the patient is no longer a suicide risk or is transferred to a psychiatric hospital (see Chapter 166).

DIFFERENTIAL DIAGNOSIS

The next step is to determine into which diagnostic category the patient's symptoms best fit. Depressive symptoms in hospitalized children and adolescents typically fall into

Table 165-2 DSM-IV-TR Criteria for Major Depressive Episode

A. Five (or more) of the following symptoms have been present during the same 2-week period and represent a change from previous functioning; at least one of the symptoms is either depressed mood or loss of interest or pleasure. Do not include symptoms that are clearly due to a general medical condition or mood-incongruent delusions or hallucinations.
   1. Depressed mood (or irritable mood in children and adolescents) most of the day, nearly every day, as indicated by either subjective report (e.g., feels sad or empty) or observation by others (e.g., appears tearful).
   2. Markedly diminished interest or pleasure in all, or almost all, activities most of the day, nearly every day (as indicated by either subjective account or observation by others).
   3. Significant weight loss when not dieting or weight gain (e.g., change of >5% of body weight in a month), or decrease or increase in appetite nearly every day. In children, consider failure to make expected weight gains.
   4. Insomnia or hypersomnia nearly every day.
   5. Psychomotor agitation or retardation nearly every day (observable by others, not merely subjective feelings of restlessness or being slowed down).
   6. Fatigue or loss of energy nearly every day.
   7. Feelings of worthlessness or excessive or inappropriate guilt (which may be delusional) nearly every day (not merely self-reproach or guilt about being sick).
   8. Diminished ability to think or concentrate, or indecisiveness, nearly every day (either by subjective account or as observed by others).
   9. Recurrent thoughts of death (not just fear of dying), recurrent suicidal ideation without a specific plan, or a suicide attempt or a specific plan for committing suicide.

B. The symptoms cause clinically significant distress or impairment in social, occupational, or other important areas of functioning.

C. The symptoms are not due to the direct physiologic effects of a substance (e.g., drug of abuse, medication) or a general medical condition (e.g., hypothyroidism).

D. The symptoms are not better accounted for by bereavement (i.e., after the loss of a loved one), and the symptoms persist for longer than 2 months or are characterized by marked functional impairment, morbid preoccupation with worthlessness, suicidal ideation, psychotic symptoms, or psychomotor retardation.

Adapted from American Psychiatric Association: Diagnostic and Statistical Manual of Mental Disorders, 4th ed, text revision. Washington, DC, American Psychiatric Association, 2000.

one of three categories, although overlap is common: adjustment disorder with depressed mood (situational depression), depressive disorder related to a general medical condition or substance, and primary psychiatric disorders, such as major depressive episode or dysthymia (chronic depression). Tables 165-2 through 165-5 provide diagnostic criteria, and Table 165-6 provides a comparison of the three types of depression.

Adjustment disorder with depressed mood (situational depression) involves symptoms such as depressed mood, tearfulness, or feelings of hopelessness that arise in response to an identifiable stressor. Illness, hospitalization, and medical or surgical procedures are the stressors typically identified in hospitalized children. Patients frequently appear sad and tearful and may not be motivated to participate in their treatment regimens. They may describe feeling overwhelmed by their illness or its treatments and may report feeling hopelessness or fear that they will never leave the hospital. Depressive symptoms typically resolve when the stressor is removed and the patient is able to resume his or her usual routine following discharge from the hospital.

Certain medical conditions, medications, and drugs of abuse may be associated with depressive symptoms and should be considered in the differential diagnosis of depression (Table 165-7). A mood disorder due to a general medical condition refers to a significant and persistent disturbance in mood that is the direct physiologic effect of a medical condition. A substance-induced mood disorder is

the direct effect of a medication or drug of abuse. In both disorders, symptoms may range from depressed mood or anhedonia to multiple psychological and somatic symptoms of depression. A clue to the diagnosis is a temporal relationship between the onset, exacerbation, or remission of the mood disturbance and the medical disorder, medication, or drug of abuse.[16,17]

Primary psychiatric disorders such as major depressive episode and dysthymic disorder should also be considered in the differential diagnosis of depressive symptoms. A major depressive episode is an acute episode (at least 2 weeks) of pervasive sadness or anhedonia in conjunction with four or more other symptoms of depression (see Table 165-2). The patient must experience significant distress or functional impairment (e.g., decline in social or academic performance), and the symptoms cannot be the direct physiologic effects of a medical condition or substance (e.g., medication, drug of abuse).[17] Dysthymic disorder refers to a chronically depressed or irritable mood for at least 1 year (2 years in adults) in conjunction with two or more of the following symptoms: insomnia or hypersomnia, poor or excessive appetite, decreased energy, poor concentration, low self-esteem, and feelings of helplessness. The symptoms must cause significant distress or functional impairment and cannot be the direct physiologic effects of a medical condition or substance.[17] Primary psychiatric disorders are more common in patients with a history of previous depressive episodes or a family history of depression.

Table 165-3   **DSM–IV–TR Criteria for Dysthymic Disorder**

A. Depressed mood for most of the day, for more days than not, as indicated by either subjective account or observation by others, for at least 2 years (in children and adolescents, mood can be irritable, and duration must be at least 1 year).

B. Presence, while depressed, of two (or more) of the following:
   1. Poor appetite or overeating.
   2. Insomnia or hypersomnia.
   3. Low energy or fatigue.
   4. Low self-esteem.
   5. Poor concentration or difficulty making decisions.
   6. Feelings of hopelessness.

C. During the 2-year period (1 year for children and adolescents) of the disturbance, the person has never been without the symptoms in criteria A and B for more than 2 months at a time.

D. No major depressive episode has been present during the first 2 years of the disturbance (1 year for children and adolescents); that is, the disturbance is not better accounted for by chronic major depressive disorder or major depressive disorder in partial remission.*

E. There has never been a manic episode, a mixed episode, or a hypomanic episode, and criteria have never been met for cyclothymic disorder.

F. The disturbance does not occur exclusively during the course of a chronic psychotic disorder, such as schizophrenia or delusional disorder.

G. The symptoms are not due to the direct physiologic effects of a substance (e.g., drug of abuse, medication) or a general medical condition (e.g., hypothyroidism).

H. The symptoms cause clinically significant distress or impairment in social, occupational, or other important areas of functioning.

*There may have been a previous major depressive episode, provided there was full remission (no significant signs or symptoms for 2 months) before development of the dysthymic disorder. In addition, after the initial 2 years (1 year in children and adolescents) of dysthymic disorder, there may be superimposed episodes of major depressive disorder, in which case both diagnoses may apply when the criteria are met for a major depressive episode.
Adapted from American Psychiatric Association: Diagnostic and Statistical Manual of Mental Disorders, 4th ed, text revision. Washington, DC, American Psychiatric Association, 2000.

Table 165-4   **DSM–IV–TR Criteria for Mood Disorder Due to a General Medical Condition**

A. A prominent and persistent disturbance in mood predominates in the clinical picture and is characterized by either (or both) of the following:
   1. Depressed mood or markedly diminished interest or pleasure in all, or almost all, activities.
   2. Elevated, expansive, or irritable mood.

B. Evidence from the history, physical examination, or laboratory findings that the disturbance is the direct physiologic consequence of a general medical condition.

C. The disturbance is not better accounted for by another mental disorder (e.g., adjustment disorder with depressed mood in response to the stress of being ill).

D. The disturbance does not occur exclusively during the course of delirium.

E. The symptoms cause clinically significant distress or impairment in social, occupational, or other important areas of functioning.
Specify type:
   With depressive features: if the predominant mood is depressed, but the full criteria for a major depressive episode are not met.
   With major depressive-like episode: if the full criteria are met (except criterion D) for a major depressive episode.
   With manic features: if the predominant mood is elevated, euphoric, or irritable.
   With mixed features: if the symptoms of both mania and depression are present, but neither predominates.

Adapted from American Psychiatric Association: Diagnostic and Statistical Manual of Mental Disorders, 4th ed, text revision. Washington, DC, American Psychiatric Association, 2000.

TREATMENT

The treatment of depression in hospitalized children and adolescents varies, depending on the cause. It requires both an acute intervention in the hospital and a plan for follow-up after discharge, if necessary. If available, a psychiatric consultant can be helpful in guiding the initial evaluation and diagnosis and creating a treatment plan appropriate to the child's developmental level that incorporates the patient and his or her family, medical and nursing staff, social workers, and child life specialists. The symptoms of depression in patients with situational depression (adjustment

Table 165-5	DSM-IV-TR Criteria for Adjustment Disorder with Depressed Mood

A. Emotional or behavioral symptoms develop in response to an identifiable stressor or stressors within 3 months of the onset of the stressors.

B. The predominant manifestations are symptoms such as depressed mood, tearfulness, or feelings of hopelessness.

C. These symptoms or behaviors are clinically significant, as evidenced by either of the following:
   1. Marked distress in excess of what would be expected from exposure to the stressor.
   2. Significant impairment in social or occupational (or academic) functioning.

D. The stress-related disturbance does not meet the criteria for another specific axis I disorder and is not merely an exacerbation of a preexisting axis I or axis II disorder.

E. The symptoms do not represent bereavement.

F. Once the stressor (or its consequences) has terminated, the symptoms do not persist for more than an additional 6 months.
Specify whether the disorder is:
   Acute: if the disturbance lasts less than 6 months.
   Chronic: if the disturbance lasts for 6 months or longer. By definition, symptoms cannot persist for more than 6 months after the termination of the stressor or its consequences. The chronic specifier therefore applies when the duration of the disturbance is longer than 6 months in response to a chronic stressor or to a stressor that has enduring consequences.

Adapted from American Psychiatric Association: Diagnostic and Statistical Manual of Mental Disorders, 4th ed, text revision. Washington, DC, American Psychiatric Association, 2000.

Table 165-6	Working Model for Distinguishing the Three Types of Depression		
Criterion	Primary Psychiatric Disorder (Major Depression or Dysthymia)	Mood Disorder Due to Medical Condition or Substance	Adjustment Disorder with Depressed Mood (Situational Depression)
DSM-IV criteria for major depressive episode	++	+	±
Preoccupied with worthlessness	++	+	−
Mood or affect flat, with malaise quality	+	++	−
Positive family history of depression	++	−	±
Previous depressive episodes	+	±	±
Greater than expected reaction to being sick	+	+	−
Weight loss of >25%	+	++	−
Temporal relationship to physical condition	−	++	+
Positive neurologic signs or laboratory findings (e.g., abnormal EEG)	−	++	−
Taking medications that can cause depression	−	+	−
Environmental stresses evident	±	±	++
Mood improves with distraction	±	±	++
Expect antidepressants to help	++	−	−
Expect supportive psychotherapy to help	±	±	++
Behavioral interventions may be helpful	±	±	++

DSM-IV, *Diagnostic and Statistical Manual of Mental Disorders*, 4th ed; EEG, electroencephalogram.
Adapted from Waller DA, Rush AJ: Differentiating primary affective disease, organic affective syndromes, and situational depression on a pediatric service. J Am Acad Child Psychiatry 1983;22:52-58.

disorder with depressed mood) are frequently related to unexpressed anxiety or fears about the illness and its treatment, feeling "out of control," and disruption of routine. In these cases, patients typically respond well to a combination of psychosocial and behavioral interventions, and antidepressant therapy is usually not necessary.[18]

Psychosocial interventions are designed to help the patient and family better understand the medical condition and its treatment and to facilitate coping with the illness and hospitalization. For example, the psychiatric consultant can help explain medical issues and treatments to children in a developmentally appropriate manner to encourage feelings

Table 165-7   Common Medical and Pharmacologic Causes of Depression

Endocrine	Infectious	Neurologic	Medications	Other
Diabetes mellitus	Encephalitis	Epilepsy	Benzodiazepines	Drug abuse and
Cushing disease	Hepatitis	Multiple sclerosis	Corticosteroids	withdrawal (cocaine,
Hypothyroidism	Pneumonia	Trauma	Oral contraceptives	amphetamines,
Addison disease	Mononucleosis	Sleep apnea	Anticonvulsants	opiates)
Hypopituitarism	AIDS	Cerebrovascular	Antihypertensives	Alcohol abuse
Parathyroid disorders	Chronic fatigue	accident	Aminophylline	Electrolyte
(hyper- and hypo-)	syndrome	Huntington disease	Clonidine	abnormalities
		Hydrocephalus	Ibuprofen	Anemia
		Migraine	Ampicillin	Failure to thrive
		Neoplasm	Tetracycline	Lupus erythematosus
			Sulfonamides	Wilson disease
			C-Asparaginase	Uremia
			Azathioprine	Porphyria
			Bleomycin	
			Vincristine	
			Cimetidine	
			Stimulants	

Adapted from Wise MG, Rundell JR: Concise Guide to Consultation Psychiatry. Washington, DC, American Psychiatric Press, 1998.

of mastery and control. Supportive therapy may include engaging younger children in therapeutic play with medical toys and dolls or having older patients create a scrapbook or a mood journal to cope with their feelings related to the illness and hospitalization.[18] Adolescents may benefit from a trial of cognitive behavioral therapy to help them cope.[13] Validating a child's experience of sadness, fear, or anxiety may be an important component of supportive therapy. Family members may benefit from meeting with the psychiatric consultant or social worker to address their feelings related to the child's illness and to receive ongoing support.

Parents should be encouraged to bring special items from home (e.g., favorite blanket, toys, pictures) to help the child feel more comfortable in the hospital. If possible, the child's teacher should be informed of the hospitalization to help facilitate contact between the patient and friends at school. Contact with other patients can provide peer support and help the child understand that he or she is not alone.

Behavioral interventions can be helpful in creating a routine and allowing the child to feel more in control. If available, a child life specialist can help the patient develop a daily schedule to add structure and predictability to his or her day. This can be written on poster board and hung in the hospital room. The psychiatric consultant or child life specialist can also develop a reward system (e.g., sticker chart) to encourage the patient to participate in his or her treatment. Mobilizing the child as much as possible—getting the child out of bed and into a chair or into the activity room for a certain number of times per day—can also be helpful in providing structure and routine.[18] Distraction, in the form of movies, visitors, and crafts projects, may also be helpful in alleviating depressive symptoms.

Ongoing pain may be another source of depression. The importance of adequately treating pain cannot be overstated. Behavioral therapies such as hypnosis, relaxation, and guided imagery can be helpful adjuncts in the management of both acute and chronic pain.

Children and adolescents with mood disorder due to a general medical condition or substance generally improve with treatment of the underlying medical condition or removal of the substance causing the depressive symptoms (medication or drug of abuse). These patients may also benefit from the psychosocial and behavioral interventions previously described.

If psychosocial and behavioral interventions fail, or if the patient's symptoms are severe (e.g., major depressive disorder), a trial of an antidepressant medication should be considered. It is important to note that there are no controlled studies addressing the use of antidepressants in children or adolescents with physical illnesses. Because most antidepressants take weeks to reach maximal efficacy, the formation of a treatment alliance with the patient and parents is crucial. Before treatment begins, a meeting should occur at which the specific target symptoms are defined and the risks, benefits, and goals of treatment are delineated. It is imperative to inform the patient and parents about side effects, dosage schedule, lag in therapeutic efficacy, and danger of overdose for each agent prescribed.[18] Following discharge from the hospital, the parents should be responsible for storing and administering these medications to minimize the risk of overdose.

The choice of medication depends on several variables, including the patient's concomitant medical or psychiatric condition, potential drug interactions with other medications, and medication side effects.[19] For example, an antidepressant such as mirtazapine, with the primary side effects of appetite stimulation and weight gain, would not be the first choice for a patient with diabetes. It is important to keep in mind that certain antidepressants (e.g., tricyclic antidepressants, selective serotonin reuptake inhibitors) are metabolized by the cytochrome P-450 enzyme system and may interfere with the metabolism of other medications.[17]

Selective serotonin reuptake inhibitors (SSRIs) are the first line of treatment for depressive disorders. Fluoxetine

Table 165-8 Selective Serotonin Reuptake Inhibitors

Medication	Dosage Range	Available Forms	Cytochrome P-450 System Isoenzyme Involved	Selected Drug Interactions*
Citalopram (Celexa)	10-40 mg qd	10-, 20-, 40-mg tablets 10 mg/5 mL solution	3A4 2C19	MAOIs, ketoconazole, itraconazole, macrolides, omeprazole
Escitalopram (Lexapro)	5-20 mg qd	5-, 10-, 20-mg tablets 1 mg/mL solution	3A4 2C19	MAOIs, sumatriptan, cimetidine; minimal clinically significant effects on pharmacokinetic properties of other medications
Fluoxetine (Prozac)†	5-60 mg qd	10-, 20-mg capsules 20 mg/5 mL solution 90-mg time-release capsule	2D6 2C19	MAOIs, ketoconazole, phenytoin, carbamazepine, omeprazole, digoxin, lithium, warfarin, ritonavir, tramadol, clozapine
Fluvoxamine (Luvox)	25-300 mg qd	25-, 50-, 100-mg coated tablets	1A2 2C19 3A4	MAOIs, ketoconazole, carbamazepine, omeprazole, ciprofloxacin, methadone, lithium, theophylline, warfarin, clozapine
Paroxetine (Paxil)	5-30 mg qd	10-, 20-, 30-, 40-mg tablets 10 mg/5 mL suspension 12.5-, 25-, 37.5-mg controlled-release tablets	2D6 3A4	MAOIs, warfarin, cimetidine, phenobarbital, phenytoin, digoxin, theophylline, tramadol
Sertraline (Zoloft)	25-200 mg qd	25-, 50-, 100-mg tablets 20 mg/mL concentrated solution	2D6 3A4	MAOIs, warfarin, cimetidine, phenobarbital, phenytoin, digoxin, theophylline, tramadol

*Check for specific drug-drug interactions before initiating treatment with an SSRI.
†Fluoxetine (Prozac) is currently the only antidepressant that has received FDA approval for the treatment of depression in children and adolescents.
MAOI, monoamine oxidase inhibitor.
Adapted from Physician's Desk Reference, 59th ed. Montvale, New Jersey, Thomson PDR, 2005.

(Prozac) is currently the only antidepressant that has received Food and Drug Administration (FDA) approval for the treatment of depression in children and adolescents.[18]

Citalopram (Celexa) and escitalopram (Lexapro) have very little cytochrome P-450 activity and therefore less potential for drug-drug interactions. Although baseline laboratory testing is not required, it is prudent to obtain liver function tests and a complete blood count with differential and platelets before initiating therapy.[19] Initial adverse effects of SSRIs may include nausea, dizziness, drowsiness, insomnia, nervousness, behavioral activation, and memory problems. These symptoms typically abate within the first few weeks of treatment and may be minimized by starting with a low dose and slowly increasing the dosage as tolerated.

Longer-term adverse effects of SSRIs may include weight gain or loss, sexual dysfunction, and an amotivational syndrome characterized by the development of apathy, indifference, amotivation, or disinhibition.[18] In addition, the hospitalist should be aware of a potentially lethal condition of serotonergic hyperstimulation known as the serotonin syndrome, which can be produced by the concurrent use of drugs that enhance central nervous system serotonin (e.g., linezolid [Zyvox], voriconazole [Vfend]). Common clinical features include altered mental status, diaphoresis, myoclonus, diarrhea, tremors, shivering, restlessness, and hyperreflexia.

The FDA recently issued a public health advisory requiring that antidepressant labels carry a "black box warning" informing patients of an increased risk of suicidal thoughts and behaviors among children and adolescents taking these medications. These potential risks should be discussed with patients and their families and balanced against clinical need. Patients who are started on antidepressant therapy should be observed closely for clinical worsening, suicidality, or unusual changes in behavior. Families and caregivers should be advised of the need for close observation and communication with the prescriber.[20] Table 165-8 provides a list of SSRIs and dosage guidelines. Currently, recommendations for weight-based dosing are not available.

Stimulants have been used with success in the treatment of depression in adults with physical illnesses and should be considered in children and adolescents. Although these agents are approved for use in youngsters with attention-deficit hyperactivity disorder, there have been no controlled studies addressing their use in the treatment of depression in the pediatric population. Studies in medically ill adults have demonstrated improvement in depressive symptoms, including mood, appetite, and energy level. Stimulants generally have a rapid onset of action (often within days) and are relatively safe, with a short half-life. Side effects may include insomnia, agitation, anxiety, confusion, and paranoia. Stimulants should be used with caution in patients with tic disorders and Tourette disorder, because they may exacerbate tics.[3,21,22]

A comprehensive follow-up treatment plan should be developed for the patient and family before discharge. This may include referrals to mental health providers for outpatient psychotherapy, pharmacotherapy, family therapy, or group therapy. For children and adolescents with severe depression or suicidal ideation, transfer to an inpatient psychiatric unit or enrollment in a partial hospital program may be warranted.[18]

CONSULTATION

Mental health services should be incorporated into the patient's care when depressive symptoms are recognized. Psychiatrists can provide guidance for diagnosis and treatment and help organize the multidisciplinary mental health team. Input from these specialists also assists the medical team members. The mental health team may provide guidance for proper interactions with the patient and family and insights into the interactions between depression and medical illness. They are also helpful in establishing continued mental health support after discharge from the hospital.

IN A NUTSHELL

- Feelings of sadness, frustration, and irritability are common in hospitalized children and adolescents. However, when these symptoms persist and are associated with certain cognitive and somatic symptoms, the clinician should consider the diagnosis of a depressive disorder.
- The major categories of depressive disorders in physically ill children and adolescents include adjustment disorder with depressed mood (situational depression), depressive disorder related to a general medical condition or substance, and primary psychiatric disorders such as major depressive episode or dysthymic disorder (chronic depression).
- Depending on the severity of the depressive disorder, treatment may consist of psychosocial and behavioral interventions and pharmacotherapy, including SSRIs and stimulants.

ON THE HORIZON

- Recent studies have identified high rates of clinically significant depression among children and adolescents with inflammatory bowel disease. In addition, a strong relationship has been found between steroid usage and depressive symptoms. These results highlight the importance of screening for depression in children and adolescents with inflammatory bowel disease. Future studies examining rates of depression in children and adolescents with other medical illnesses will enable us to develop more effective preventive and treatments strategies for this population.[23]
- Recent pilot study data suggest that manual-based cognitive-behavioral therapy is a safe and effective nonpharmacologic intervention in children and adolescents with inflammatory bowel disease. This approach is associated with a significant reduction in depressive symptoms as well as improvement in adolescents' perceptions of their general health and physical functioning. Future studies examining the efficacy of manual-based therapy in patients with other physical illnesses will have important treatment implications.[24]
- Researchers at Children's Hospital Boston have developed the Experience Journal, a web-based intervention designed to promote healthy coping among children and families facing various physical and emotional illnesses. Experience journals currently exist for patients and families coping with heart disease, depression, organ transplantation, inflammatory bowel disease, and obesity. Access the Experience Journal at *www.experiencejournal.com*.[25,26]

SUGGESTED READING

American Academy of Child and Adolescent Psychiatry: Practice parameters for the assessment and treatment of children and adolescents with depressive disorders. J Am Acad Child Adolesc Psychiatry 1998;37(Suppl 10):63S–83S.

Beasley PJ, Beardslee WR: Depression in the adolescent patient. Adolesc Med State Art Rev 1998;9:351–362.

Sutor B, Rummans TA, Jowsey SG, et al: Major depression in medically ill patients. Mayo Clin Proc 1998;73:329–337.

REFERENCES

1. Burke P: Depression in pediatric illness. Behav Modif 1991;15:486–500.
2. Canning EH, Kelleher K: Performance of screening tools for mental health problems in chronically ill children. Arch Pediatr Adolesc Med 1994;148:272–277.
3. Katon WJ: Clinical and health services relationships between major depression, depressive symptoms, and general medical illness. Soc Biol Psychiatry 2003;54:216–226.
4. Vitulano LA: Psychosocial issues for children and adolescents with chronic illness: Self-esteem, school functioning and sports participation. Child Adolesc Psychiatr Clin North Am 2003;12:585–592.
5. Kashani JH, Venzke R, Milar EA: Depression in children admitted to hospital for orthopaedic procedures. Br J Psychiatry 1981;138:21–25.
6. Cohen P, Pine DS, Must A, et al: Prospective associations between somatic illness and mental illness from childhood to adulthood. Am J Epidemiol 1998;147:232–239.
7. Ciechanowski PS, Katon WJ, Russo JE: Depression and diabetes: Impact of depressive symptoms on adherence, function, and costs. Arch Intern Med 2000;160:3278–3284.
8. Leonard B: Stress, depression and the activation of the immune system. World J Biol Psychiatry 2000;1:17–25.
9. Shemesh E, Bartell A, Newcorn J: Assessment and treatment of depression in medically ill children. Curr Psychiatry Rep 2002;4:88–92.
10. Evans DL, Charney DS: Mood disorders and medical illness: A major public health problem. Biol Psychiatry 2003;54:177–180.
11. Beasley PJ, Beardslee WR: Depression in the adolescent patient. Adolesc Med State Art Rev 1998;9:351–362.

12. Neese JB: Depression in the general hospital. Nurs Clin North Am 1991; 26:613-622.
13. Weller EB, Weller RA, Svadjian H: Mood disorders. In Lewis M (ed): Child and Adolescent Psychiatry. Baltimore, Williams & Wilkins, 1991, p 657.
14. Carlat DJ: The psychiatric review of symptoms: A screening tool for family physicians. Am Fam Physician 1998;58:1617-1624.
15. Wise MJ, Rundell JR: Effective psychiatric consultation. In Hales RE (ed): Concise Guide to Consultation Psychiatry. Washington, DC, American Psychiatric Press, 1994, pp 1-10.
16. Sutor B, Rummans TA, Jowsey SG, et al: Major depression in medically ill patients. Mayo Clin Proc 1998;73:329-337.
17. Rush JA, Keller MB, Bauer MS, et al: Mood disorders. In American Psychiatric Association: Diagnostic and Statistical Manual of Mental Disorders, 4th ed. Washington, DC, American Psychiatric Association, 1994, pp 317-393.
18. American Academy of Child and Adolescent Psychiatry: Practice parameters for the assessment and treatment of children and adolescents with depressive disorders. J Am Acad Child Adolesc Psychiatry 1998;37(Suppl 10):63S-83S.
19. Birmaher B, Brent D: Depressive disorders. In Martin A, Scahill L, Charney DS, Leckman J (eds): Pediatric Psychopharmacology: Principles and Practice. New York, Oxford University Press, 2003, pp 466-483.
20. Pappadopulos EA, Tate Guelzow B, Wong C, et al: A review of the growing evidence base for pediatric psychopharmacology. Child Adolesc Psychiatr Clin North Am 2004;13:817-855.
21. Masand P, Pickett P, Murray G: Psychostimulants for secondary depression in medical illness. Psychosomatics 1991;32:203-208.
22. Beliles K, Stoudemire A: Psychopharmacologic treatment of depression in the medically ill. Psychosomatics 1998;39:S2-S19.
23. Szigethy E, Levy-Warren A, Whitton S, et al: Depressive symptoms and inflammatory bowel disease in children and adolescents: A cross-sectional study. J Pediatr Gastroenterol Nutr 2004;39:395-403.
24. Szigethy E, Whitton SW, Levy-Warren A, et al: Cognitive-behavioral therapy for depression in adolescents with inflammatory bowel disease: A pilot study. J Am Acad Child Adolesc Psychiatry 2004;43:1469-1477.
25. DeMaso DR, Gonzalez-Heydrich J, Dahlmeier Erickson J, et al: The experience journal: A computer-based intervention for families facing congenital heart disease. J Am Acad Child Adolesc Psychiatry 2000;39:727-734.
26. DeMaso DR, Marcus NE, Kinnamon C, Gonzalez-Heydrich J: The depression experience journal: A computer-based intervention for families facing childhood depression. J Am Acad Child Adolesc Psychiatry 2006;45(2):158-165.

Assessment and Management of Suicidal Patients

Elizabeth A. Wharff and Katherine B. Ginnis

Among adolescents, suicide is the third leading cause of death, exceeded only by unintentional injury and homicide. More teenagers die as a result of suicide than from cancer, heart disease, AIDS, birth defects, stroke, pneumonia, influenza, and chronic lung disease combined.[1] In 2000 the incidence of suicide was 10.4 per 100,000 for 15- to 24-year olds and 1.5 per 100,000 for 10- to 14-year-olds. The suicide rate for 15- to 19-year-olds was 8.2 deaths per 100,000. Five times as many males as females killed themselves.[2]

Suicide has become a problem of national importance. In 1999 Surgeon General David Satcher published *Call to Action to Prevent Suicide*,[1] declaring suicide a public health problem that must be addressed on a national level. That was followed in 2000 by the development of a national strategy for suicide prevention, a collaborative effort among several governmental and private agencies designed to reduce the rate of suicide and its sequelae.[3] *Healthy People 2010* declared that significant reductions in both suicide and suicide attempts among adolescents were important goals for national health.[4]

There has been extensive research into the factors that may be predictive of completed adolescent suicide. Male gender, current psychiatric disorder, substance abuse, and sexual orientation issues place youths at higher risk for completed suicide.[5,6]

Suicidal children and adolescents can be worrisome and difficult to work with, even in the context of a psychiatric setting. In a hospital setting, these issues are complicated by the medical comorbidity that may accompany a patient's psychiatric presentation. Consideration must be given to the environment where a patient receives inpatient medical care, which is not designed to provide the level of safety and containment of an inpatient psychiatric facility. The duty of the hospitalist is to provide medical care while also assessing and attending to the psychiatric needs of patients. Medical and nursing staff members who are not trained to work with suicidal patients are often frightened and frustrated by them. The following guidelines are intended to assist the hospitalist in the assessment and treatment of suicidal patients.

EVALUATION

Any patient admitted to the hospital who has a history of suicidal ideation or suicide attempt or who has a potential psychiatric disorder should receive a careful psychiatric assessment. This assessment should occur immediately upon the patient's arrival to determine whether special precautions are needed (e.g., one-to-one observation). In situations in which a patient is unresponsive following a serious suicide attempt, the mental status should be assessed as soon as the child or adolescent is alert enough to allow an examination.

To fully understand the patient's mental status, his or her medical condition must be carefully assessed. For instance, racing thoughts and rapid speech might be symptomatic of mania caused by bipolar disorder, but they also might be caused by stimulant abuse. Hospitalists are often called on to provide "medical clearance" for inpatients with suicidal concerns or to act as consultants for such patients in the emergency department. The hospitalist may also be asked to "medically clear" a patient who is going to be transferred from the medical service to a psychiatric facility. In either case, certain guidelines should be followed.

Generally, the minimal laboratory studies include a urine toxicology screen for drugs of abuse, a serum toxicology screen if there is a suspected or known ingestion, and a urine pregnancy test for postmenarchal females. For patients who are being treated with lithium or valproate acid, a serum level is suggested to inform any changes to those medications once the patient is admitted to a psychiatric facility. In most cases, patients who are being transferred to a psychiatric facility must be as medically stable as if they were being discharged home. Although some psychiatric facilities have the capacity to treat patients' medical conditions, patients must generally be stable enough to function in a psychiatric milieu where there is little or no medical staff on site.

The following guidelines are intended to provide the hospitalist with a framework for the direct assessment of each patient. If psychiatric consultation is available, these guidelines will facilitate communication of the hospitalist's findings to the consulting psychiatrist and will assist the hospitalist in understanding the findings and recommendations of the psychiatric consultant.

Interview Process

A thorough assessment begins with a careful interview of both the patient and the parents or guardians. Unlike medical interviews, where the patient and parents may be interviewed together, a psychiatric interview must include some time alone with each party, especially when assessing the patient's potential dangerousness, to obtain a complete picture of the problem. Many suicidal children or adolescents will not be completely truthful in front of their parents, and many parents will not be frank and open in front of their children. Complex family interactions often contribute to the patient's presentation and should be explored in a nonthreatening manner with both the patient and his or her caregivers.

History and Physical Examination

Acquiring a psychiatric history follows the same format as any medical history, with particular emphasis on developmental and social factors. It must also include the patient's past mental health history, including treatment and medications, and a history of family psychiatric disorders and treatment. Besides gathering information about the patient's suicidality and other symptoms, it is important to gather information about the patient's and family's strengths and resources. Knowing their strengths can often help galvanize the patient and his or her family in the struggle toward recovery. This information about positive aspects of the patient's life may also help counter his or her depression and suicidality. The interviewer must determine whether the patient has been suicidal in the past, what the precipitants were, and how the patient and family dealt with that incident. This can provide a sense of the current situation and clues to management. Inquiries about the family's previous experiences with mental health care are relevant and may also provide insight into the patient's and family's attitudes about mental illness and mental health care.

Mental Status Examination

In addition to a thorough physical examination, a complete mental status examination is essential to assess overall psychiatric functioning (Table 166-1).

Suicidal Ideation

Contrary to popular myth, children and adolescents do not become suicidal when asked about suicidal thoughts. It is extremely important that the physician ask about suicidal ideation, plans, or attempts openly and frankly: "Have you been having thoughts about hurting or killing yourself either now or in the past?" "Do you ever feel that life isn't worth living?" "Have you ever wished you could just go to sleep and not wake up?" A patient with a known history of either suicidal ideation or attempt who answers no to these questions is probably not telling the full story. Be sure to gather information from *both* the patient and the family whenever possible. Family members may have good insight into current or ongoing stressors, even if the patient is not forthcoming. If a patient answers yes to any of these questions, ask all the interrogatories: who, what, when, where, why, and how. For example, ask the patient the following:

- Who knows about this?
- Who are the supports in your life?
- What could help you not hurt or kill yourself?
- What are you thinking about doing?
- When do you think you might do it?
- Where might you hurt or kill yourself?
- Why do you want to hurt or kill yourself?
- How might you hurt or kill yourself?

Assessment of Risk and Dangerousness

When assessing the patient's suicide risk and degree of dangerousness to him- or herself, the following issues should be considered (Table 166-2):

- Is the patient engaged in risk-taking behaviors? A patient who is a mountain biker or bungee jumper is more likely to kill himself or herself than is someone whose recreational activities are less risky.
- Has there been recent exposure to suicide, either personally or in the media? Recent exposure to suicide increases the likelihood of a completed suicide, and teenagers often do not make a distinction between people they know in real life and the movie or rock stars they idolize.

- Is there a family history of violence or suicide? Even though the family may report, "Jimmy doesn't know that Uncle Bob killed himself," Jimmy probably does know. Knowing that someone in the family committed suicide and that the family survived this horror removes some of the "guilt barrier" that might otherwise prevent a serious attempt.
- Does the patient have access to a weapon? Access to firearms increases the likelihood of completed suicide.
- Does the patient have a problem that impairs thinking or judgment? If thinking or judgment is impaired by substance abuse, mental retardation, or psychosis, the interviewer cannot rely on a child's claim that he or she is not planning to commit suicide.
- What are the stressors in the child's life? What were the precipitating events for the suicidal ideation or the suicide plan or attempt? Are they acute or chronic? If the stressors in a child's life are chronic and serious, the child is much more likely to be hopeless, and there is a greater likelihood of suicide. For example, a child who is moving from foster home to foster home or one who suffers from chronic neglect is at greater risk than a child with an acute stressor that can be remedied.
- What was the patient's intent? It is not safe to assume that a previous nonlethal attempt lacked serious intent. Many patients do not know what will kill them, and they may intend to die even if the attempt seems feeble. Others who make apparently serious attempts have no intent to kill themselves. Important questions include the following: Did the child want to die? Is he or she sorry to still be living?
- Was the attempt planned? Was there a suicide note? Both these factors are correlated with completed suicide.
- Did the patient engage in help-seeking behavior? If so, how soon after the attempt did he or she seek help? Was the patient remorseful, guilty, or sorry about making the attempt or that it failed? Does the patient seem hopeful about the future? If the child was able to reach out to family and friends, he or she is more likely to accept help from professionals.
- Does the patient acknowledge his or her behavior and have insight into the problem? The presence of these features offers a more positive prognosis.
- What are the patient's supports? What was the family's reaction to the suicidal ideation, plan, or attempt? The family's reaction is the most important element in the management and treatment plan. Parents who can acknowledge the seriousness of the problem and problem-solve about how to support their child can make the difference between a child who continues to be suicidal and one who uses parental support to move toward mental health. Research has shown that family "connectedness" is a protective factor against suicide.[7]

TREATMENT

At the end of the assessment, the goal is to have a biopsychosocial understanding of the patient's suicidal thinking or suicide attempt and to reduce his or her risk factors for suicide. The hospitalist together with the psychiatric consultant uses clinical considerations (e.g., current psychiatric disorder, substance abuse, psychosis, precipitants) and the

Table 166-1	Components of Mental Status Examination

Physical Appearance
Note child's size for age, grooming, dress, nutritional state, and mannerisms.

Parent-Child Interaction
Observe interactions between caretakers and child.

Attitude toward Examiner
Judge level of cooperation, hostility, guardedness, and attentiveness.

Motor Activity
Observe level of activity, ability to attend, and motor coordination, as well as any involuntary movements.

Cognitive Functioning
Assess orientation to person, place, and date.
Assess memory.
  Immediate retention and recall:
    Ask child to repeat 3 objects immediately, and again after 5 minutes.
    Test digit span (ability to repeat a series of numbers forward and backward).
    School-age children should be able to remember 3 objects after 5 minutes, and repeat 5 digits forward and 3 digits backward.
  Recent memory: ask what the patient did yesterday.
  Remote memory: ask about events earlier in the patient's life.
Assess general intellectual level, as measured by impression of age-appropriate knowledge, vocabulary, and comprehension.

Speech and Language
Note whether speech and language acquisition are appropriate for the child's age, as well as the rate and rhythm of speech, articulation of words, and spontaneity of speech.

Mood and Affect Disturbances
Mood describes pervasive and sustained emotion that colors one's perception of the world. Mood is evidenced by sad expression, tearfulness, anxiety, or anger.
  Adolescents can report their own mood and may report more sadness than has been recognized by parents.
  Children younger than 13 years can describe the mood state of the moment but cannot reliably report on mood over time.
  Children younger than 10 years are generally unable to provide an accurate report of their mood, so parental input is required.
Affect describes the child's current range of emotional expression and its appropriateness to his or her thought content. It is described as follows:
  Within normal range (normal variation in facial expression, tone of voice, body movements)
  Constricted (reduction in range and intensity of expression)
  Blunted (greater reduction in emotional expression)
  Flat (no signs of emotional expression, monotonous voice, immobile face)

Thought Disturbances
Thought process describes the capacity for developmentally appropriate goal-directed thinking. Note any disturbances, including loosening of associations (unrelated ideas connected idiosyncratically), inability to distinguish fantasy from reality, or inability to reason logically.
Thought content describes the following disturbances:
  Suicidal or homicidal thoughts
  Delusions (fixed false beliefs not consistent with cultural background)
  Obsessions (intrusive and repetitive thoughts)
  Compulsions (repetitive acts patient feels driven to do)
  Phobias (irrational fears of heights, crowds, etc.)
Perceptual disturbances describe the following problems:
  Illusions: misperception of a real sensory experience
  Hallucinations: sensory perception in the absence of an external stimulus
    Auditory: "Have you ever heard voices or sounds that no one else can hear?"
    Visual: "Have you ever had visions or seen things that no one else can see?"
  Depersonalization or derealization (i.e., extreme feelings of detachment from oneself or the environment)

Adapted from Kaplan H, Sadock B, Grebb J: Kaplan and Sadock's Synopsis of Psychiatry: Behavioral Sciences and Clinical Psychiatry, 7th ed. New York, Williams & Wilkins, 1994.

Table 166-2 Risk and Protective Factors for Childhood Suicide

Risk	Protection
Risk-taking activities	Peer social support
Friend or family member with prior attempt or completed suicide	Help-seeking behavior
	Future-oriented thinking
	Insight into problem
Impaired thinking or judgment	Family support and adaptability
Current social stressors and family conflict	Well-developed coping strategies
Substance abuse	
Access to firearms	Female gender
Male gender	Religion or spirituality
Peer victimization	Hopefulness
Sexual orientation conflicts	
Current psychiatric illness (especially depressive disorders)	

assessment of risk and dangerousness queries to estimate a "risk-rescue ratio." This ratio contrasts the relative strength of the suicidal intent (risk) versus the wish for help (rescue). For example, a patient who, without prior warning, makes a suicide attempt when the family is away clearly has fewer wishes for rescue than one who makes a noisy and dramatic attempt. Thus, the assessment notes the interaction among the psychiatric disorder (e.g., depression), the trigger factors (e.g., stress events, altered state of mind), and the social milieu (e.g., isolation versus support).

Prompt consultation with psychiatry is appropriate for risk-rescue determinations. Collaboration with social workers can provide critical additional psychosocial assessment and ongoing support and treatment interventions for the patient and family.

If psychiatry or social work consultation is unavailable, the hospitalist must complete the assessment and provide initial interventions. The clinician should strive to galvanize the family's support of the child, which can significantly reduce suicidality. Consideration should also be given to contacting preexisting supports available to the child, including psychotherapist, clergy, school counselor, and other family members.

The nursing staff needs to be aware of the assessment and the specific concerns of the clinicians and the family. The hospital's established protocol for suicide precautions should be implemented. This generally involves one-to-one observation by having a staff member (a "sitter") present with the patient at all times. Because relationships appear to be protective in terms of preventing a suicide attempt, an individually assigned nurse or sitter is important. In some circumstances, a family member may serve as the sitter. The sitter must be given clear instructions as to the extent of observation needed (e.g., including bathroom visits) and should be made aware of the means by which the patient might attempt to harm him- or herself. This may include sharing specific information about the patient's lethality and the specific methods he or she might use for self-injury.

All objects that could be used by the patient to harm him- or herself must be removed from the room. This includes

personal items as well as all intravenous lines or other medical instruments, such as insulin pumps. If this is not possible, the sitter should be alerted to these dangers.

The family should be engaged in managing the patient. When a child attempts or plans suicide, parents are often in a state of disbelief, denial, or emotional shock, especially if this is the first evidence of psychiatric illness. Frank conversations with the family must take place, and family members should be encouraged to think of ways that they might support the child and thus decrease his or her suicidality.

Most states and hospitals have guidelines mandating the use of restraints as a last resort; however, chemical or mechanical restraints may be necessary if the patient continues to attempt to harm him- or herself despite psychosocial interventions (see Chapter 168).

ADMISSION CRITERIA

- If, after assessment, the hospitalist believes that a child or adolescent is in imminent danger of harming him- or herself or others, or that the child's judgment is impaired to a degree that he or she cannot maintain his or her own safety, the patient should be admitted to an acute psychiatric setting as soon as medically stable.
- If the patient is stabilized medically and deemed not to be at imminent risk for harming him- or herself or others, the patient should be discharged with a plan for close outpatient follow-up by the primary pediatrician, in conjunction with a referral for outpatient mental health follow-up. If available, mental health consultants within the hospital may be a source of referrals. Otherwise, the patient's pediatrician may be able to facilitate a referral for outpatient mental health services.

DISCHARGE CRITERIA

- The patient, family, and clinical team are in agreement that the patient is not at imminent risk of harming him- or herself.
- Aftercare services are in place, which may include outpatient therapy, psychopharmacology, day treatment, or home-based services. Keep in mind that the patient may not have follow-up appointments for up to several weeks after discharge.
- The patient and family must be engaged in safety planning, which may consist of any or all of the following:
  - Increasing the family's supervision of the patient.
  - Removing all medications, sharp objects, or other means of self-harm from the patient's access.
  - Identifying additional supports for the patient, including family, friends, school counselors, and clergy, and ensuring that the patient is willing to access them and knows how to do so.
  - Identifying positive coping strategies that the patient can use instead of hurting him- or herself, such as writing, music, exercise, and other positive activities.
- Discharge home is contraindicated if, despite attempts to stabilize the patient's mental status and provide additional support, he or she remains unable to engage in treatment and safety planning. In this case, the patient should be transferred to an inpatient psychiatric facility.

IN A NUTSHELL

- Patients admitted with suicidal ideation or for a suicide attempt may be at imminent risk of killing themselves. Hospitalists should take every precaution until these patients can be thoroughly assessed and the level of danger determined.
- If possible, psychiatrists and social workers should be involved in the assessment and management of the patient.
- If mental health consultation is unavailable, the hospitalist should use the guidelines described to complete a medical and mental health assessment and initiate appropriate management.
- Although the hospital stay for an acutely suicidal patient is a key part of the initial assessment and management, it represents only a small period of the overall illness. Family involvement and appropriate referrals are essential elements for safe discharge or transfer of care.

ON THE HORIZON

- Novel approaches are being developed for the treatment of suicidal adolescents using family-based crisis intervention in emergency departments. The aim is to help stabilize children in crisis and thus decrease the need for inpatient hospitalization.
- Data demonstrating that such family-based crisis interventions decrease suicidal ideation and behavior would enable families to maintain some children at home with outpatient support.

SUGGESTED READING

Borowsky I, Ireland M, Resnick M: Adolescent suicide attempts: Risks and protectors. Pediatrics 2001;107:485-493.

Shaffer D, Pfeffer C: Summary of the practice parameters for the assessment and treatment of children and adolescents with suicidal behavior. J Am Acad Child Adolesc Psychiatry 2001;40:495-499.

REFERENCES

1. US Public Health Service: The Surgeon General's Call to Action to Prevent Suicide. Washington, DC, US Public Health Service, 1999.
2. National Institutes of Mental Health: In Harm's Way: Suicide in America. National Institutes of Mental Health, 2003.
3. US Department of Health and Human Services: National Strategy for Suicide Prevention: Goals and Objectives for Action. Washington, DC, US Government Printing Office, 2001.
4. US Department of Health and Human Services: Healthy People 2010, 2nd ed. Washington, DC, US Government Printing Office, 2000.
5. Shaffer D, Pfeffer C: Summary of the practice parameters for the assessment and treatment of children and adolescents with suicidal behavior. J Am Acad Child Adolesc Psychiatry 2001;40:495-499.
6. Garafolo R, Wolf RC, Wissow LS, et al: Sexual orientation and risk of suicide attempts among a representative sample of youth. Arch Pediatr Adolesc Med 1999;153:487-493.
7. Borowsky I, Ireland M, Resnick M: Adolescent suicide attempts: Risks and protectors. Pediatrics 2001;107:485-493.
8. Kaplan H, Sadock B, Grebb J: Kaplan and Sadock's Synopsis of Psychiatry: Behavioral Sciences and Clinical Psychiatry, 7th ed. New York, Williams & Wilkins, 1994.

CHAPTER 167

Conversion and Pain Disorders

Pamela J. Beasley and David Ray DeMaso

The assessment and management of children and adolescents who are exhibiting physical or pain symptoms that are unsupported by medical findings and the physical examination or that are grossly in excess of what would be expected given the medical findings can be daunting. These symptoms are considered part of a psychosomatic disorder, or, in the terminology of the fourth edition of the *Diagnostic and Statistical Manual of Mental Disorders* (DSM-IV), a somatoform disorder.[1]

Conversion and pain syndromes are the most common somatoform disorders seen in the pediatric hospital setting. These problems are not mutually exclusive, and in fact, conversion disorders are often accompanied by pain symptoms. The complex interactions between mind and body are apparent in these two emotional disorders. The psychological and economic costs of somatization are great in terms of patient disability, decreased patient and family productivity, and negative impact on health care costs and delivery of service. In this chapter, the assessment of conversion and pain disorders is outlined, followed by recommendations for an integrated medical and psychiatric management approach to these disorders.

CONVERSION DISORDERS

Conversion disorders are characterized by symptoms affecting voluntary motor or sensory function that suggest a neurologic or other physical condition (Table 167-1).[1] A list of symptoms seen in conversion disorders is provided in Table 167-2. Pseudoseizures, unexplained falls, and episodes of fainting are the most common abnormalities. These symptoms are not intentionally produced or feigned. They cannot be fully explained by a physical illness, by the direct effects of a substance, or as a culturally sanctioned behavior.[1] They typically occur suddenly and temporarily but can be chronic. These disorders cause clinically significant distress or impairment in social or academic functioning.

A temporal relationship between significant emotional stressors and the development of symptoms is important.[2,3] A prior history of conversion symptoms or recurrent somatic complaints is helpful in making the diagnosis. Psychiatric disorders occur at a high frequency in these patients or in family members. The presence of a symptom model, such as a family member with similar deficits, is common. *La belle indifference* (a patient seemingly indifferent to what appears to be a major impairment) and histrionic personality traits have not proved to be reliable diagnostic criteria.[2,3]

On physical examination, the symptoms do not conform to known anatomic pathways and physiologic mechanisms. If physical findings are present, they may be related to either muscle atrophy from disuse or sequelae of medical procedures.

There are no specific laboratory studies that can rule out a conversion disorder. The lack of brain wave abnormalities on video-electroencephalographic monitoring in association with seizure-like behavior makes pseudoseizures a likely diagnosis.[4] Psychological testing cannot confirm the diagnosis and generally is not performed during a medical hospitalization.[4]

Hospitalists typically see these patients in the context of symptoms that have become ingrained and disabling. Persistent stress, significant psychopathology, or symptoms that provide for significant secondary gain are usually evident. Although early studies found that a significant percentage of patients with an initial diagnosis of conversion disorder was subsequently diagnosed with a medical illness,[5] recent samples have revealed a more modest risk (<10%) of faulty diagnosis.[6]

Cause

In psychodynamic theory, the symptoms are thought to be the direct symbolic expression of an underlying unconscious emotional conflict that is "converted" into somatic symptoms.[7] "Primary gain" is obtained by keeping the conflict from consciousness and thus minimizing anxiety. The symptoms can also provide "secondary gain" by allowing for an escape from unwanted responsibilities or consequences.[1]

Increased parental attention and avoidance of unpleasant peer or school pressures may reinforce the symptoms. High-achieving children who cannot admit that they are under too much pressure may present with symptoms related to the avoidance of academic stress. Physical symptoms have been viewed as a form of body language in children who have difficulty expressing their emotions verbally. Social learning theory suggests that some symptoms are a result of "modeling" or "observational learning" within the family.[8] A central focus on the symptoms may allow the avoidance of conflict within a family, which can reinforce the illness behavior.[9]

There is some evidence that conversion symptoms may be precipitated by excessive central nervous system arousal. This triggers reactive inhibition signals at synapses in peripheral sensorimotor pathways by way of negative feedback relationships between the cerebral cortex and the brainstem reticular formation.[10] This may help explain the consistent relationship among stressors, the appearance of symptoms, and the subsequent reduction of anxiety.

Differential Diagnosis

It is critical to exclude neurologic or medical conditions. Migraine syndromes, temporal lobe epilepsy, and central nervous system tumors can present particularly difficult diagnostic dilemmas. Hospitalists should be alert to the

Table 167-1   DSM-IV Criteria for Conversion Disorders
A. One or more symptoms or deficits affecting voluntary motor or sensory function that suggest a neurologic or other general medical condition.
B. Psychological factors are judged to be associated with the symptom or deficit because its initiation or exacerbation is preceded by conflicts or stressors.
C. The symptom or deficit is not intentionally produced or feigned (as in factitious disorder or malingering).
D. The symptom or deficit cannot, after appropriate investigation, be fully explained by a general medical condition, by the direct effects of a substance, or as a culturally sanctioned behavior or experience.
E. The symptom or deficit causes clinically significant distress or impairment in social, occupational, or other important areas of functioning or warrants medical evaluation.
F. The symptom or deficit is not limited to pain or sexual dysfunction, does not occur exclusively during the course of somatization disorder, and is not better accounted for by another mental disorder.

Adapted from American Psychiatric Association: Diagnostic and Statistical Manual of Mental Disorders, 4th ed. Washington, DC, American Psychiatric Association, 1994.

Table 167-2   Motor and Sensory Symptoms in Conversion Disorders
Motor Symptoms
Paralysis
Ataxia
Aphonia
Dysphagia
Urinary retention
Seizures
Syncope
Sensory Symptoms
Blindness
Deafness
Paresthesia
Diplopia

possibility of the dual existence of a medical condition and conversion symptoms in the same patient.

Psychological factors affecting medical conditions are characterized by the presence of emotional reactions that adversely impact a physical illness.[1] Premorbid emotional disorders, personality traits, coping styles, or maladaptive health behaviors are some emotional factors that can directly impact a patient's coping responses to a physical illness.

Depressive and anxiety disorders can all present with somatic symptoms (see Chapter 165).[2,3] A conversion disorder should not be diagnosed if the symptoms are better accounted for by one or more of these disorders.[1]

Conversion symptoms can occur in undifferentiated somatization disorders.[1-3] These disorders extend over several years and are characterized by combinations of pain, gastrointestinal, sexual, and pseudoneurologic symptoms. The multiple symptom patterns of somatization disorders distinguish them from the frequently monosymptomatic and time-limited conversion disorders. Somatization disorders are usually diagnosed in adulthood, although the medical history generally reveals that the symptom pattern began in adolescence.

Neurasthenia is historically similar to chronic fatigue syndrome.[11] Both are characterized by persistent, relapsing, or debilitating fatigue that impairs daily activity. The fatigue cannot be explained by either medical or psychiatric illness. Additional symptoms may include weakness, headaches, fever, painful adenopathy, and migratory arthralgia. Depression and anxiety-related symptoms are common. Viral infections, immune dysfunction, and neuropsychological problems are thought to be inciting or perpetuating factors.[11] These syndromes are most likely a result of multiple causes, one of which is an undifferentiated somatoform disorder.

Malingering involves the intentional production or feigning of symptoms.[1] The motivation for the behavior is the conscious goal of gaining or avoiding something, such as avoiding criminal prosecution. This diagnosis is rarely seen in pediatrics, although occasionally an oppositional or antisocial adolescent may present with somatic symptoms.

Factitious disorder by proxy (or Munchausen syndrome by proxy) refers to the production of symptoms in a person (e.g., a child) who is under the care of another individual (e.g., a parent).[12] This syndrome most often presents in the preschool-age population (see Chapter 176).

Pain disorders with psychological factors are diagnosed if the symptoms are limited to pain.[1] Physical changes resembling conversion symptoms are common aspects of certain culturally sanctioned religious and healing rituals, such as syncopal episodes or seizure-like activity associated with certain religious rituals or ceremonies.[1]

PAIN DISORDERS ASSOCIATED WITH PSYCHOLOGICAL FACTORS

Pain disorders associated with psychological factors are divided into two DSM-IV subtypes: (1) pain disorders associated with psychological factors in which emotional factors alone play a major role, and (2) pain disorders associated with both psychological factors and a general medical condition, both of which have important roles in the onset, severity, exacerbation, or maintenance of pain.[1] The pain is not intentionally produced or feigned and is of sufficient severity to cause significant distress or impairment in functioning (Table 167-3).[1]

As with conversion disorders, hospitalists are generally asked to assess patients with a history of debilitating and disabling chronic pain that necessitates hospitalization. Pain that is entirely related to a general medical condition is not considered a psychiatric disorder.

Cause

Analogous to conversion disorders, psychodynamic theory holds that the defense mechanism of conversion underlies medically unexplained pain. Somatic preoccupa-

Table 167-3 DSM-IV Criteria for Pain Disorders

A. Pain in one or more anatomic sites is the predominant focus of the clinical presentation and is of sufficient severity to warrant clinical attention.

B. The pain causes clinically significant distress or impairment in social, occupational, or other important areas of functioning.

C. Psychological factors are judged to have an important role in the onset, severity, exacerbation, or maintenance of the pain.

D. The symptom or deficit is not intentionally produced or feigned (as in factitious disorder or malingering).

E. The pain is not better accounted for by a mood, anxiety, or psychotic disorder and does not meet the criteria for dyspareunia.

F. Code as follows:
  1. Pain disorder associated with psychological factors.
  2. Pain disorder associated with both psychological factors and a general medical condition.
  3. Pain disorder associated with a general medical condition.*

*This is not considered a mental disorder and is included to facilitate the differential diagnosis.
Adapted from American Psychiatric Association: Diagnostic and Statistical Manual of Mental Disorders, 4th ed. Washington, DC, American Psychiatric Association, 1994.

tion, recurrent pain complaints, alcohol abuse, and psychiatric disorders are family factors that have been associated with pain disorders.[8,13] Family models may result in a pain didsorder.[8] The focus on the child's illness allows the avoidance of conflict within the family and may reinforce the child's illness behavior.

Classic conditioning results from the repeated pairing of a neutral stimulus and an unconditioned stimulus that evokes a response, such that the neutral stimulus eventually evokes the response. For example, when a physician wearing a white coat (neutral stimulus) repeatedly performs a medical procedure (unconditioned stimulus) that causes pain (unconditioned response), a white coat alone may induce a pain-related behavior (conditioned response).

Operant conditioning holds that behaviors that are rewarded will increase in strength or frequency, while behaviors that are inhibited or punished will decrease. Attention and sympathy from others, euphoric effects of pain medications, or a decrease in responsibilities may reinforce pain behaviors. If the pain behaviors are reinforced early on, these behaviors will likely continue even after removal of the original painful stimulus.[10,14]

There are no unifying biologic explanations for pain disorders.[10,15] The neurobiologic components of pain involve complex interactions between ascending and descending pain pathways within the central and peripheral nervous systems. Endorphins and biogenic amine neurotransmitters such as serotonin and norepinephrine play important modulating roles in descending analgesic tracts. Drugs such as antidepressants that potentiate the central effects of biogenic

amines have been useful in producing analgesia by increasing their concentrations in these descending pathways.

Chronic pain often causes decreased mobility and poor posture that may result in the development of secondary pathologic changes such as osteoporosis, contractures, myofibrositis, and circulatory and respiratory disturbances. These conditions often lead to the stimulation of peripheral afferent fibers, which creates a cycle of progressive deterioration.[10]

Evaluation

The presence of psychiatric disorders and situation-dependent or temporally related stressors is critical.[1] It is important to determine whether these problems exist simultaneously with a pain syndrome secondary to a physical illness or exist independently and are the cause of the pain syndrome.[16] A history of prior pain episodes as well as pain syndromes in other family members should be obtained.[16,17]

In pain disorders associated with psychological factors, the pain is neuroanatomically inconsistent with known pathways or is grossly in excess of what would be expected based on the physical findings. If physical findings are present, they are secondary to pathologic changes associated with immobilization. The diagnosis of a pain disorder with psychological factors is made when the patient's response is out of proportion to the physical condition and when deficits or impairment in psychosocial functioning occur.

There are no specific laboratory abnormalities associated with pain disorders. Infrared thermography may be helpful in identifying changes in temperature and vascular flow associated with certain disorders that can cause chronic pain.[10]

Differential Diagnosis

It is critical to assess all potential neurologic or medical conditions that may be contributing to the patient's pain symptoms. Complex regional pain syndrome (or reflex sympathetic dystrophy), headache syndromes, myofascial pain, post-traumatic syndromes, neuropathies, and tumors are important considerations. Hospitalists need to be aware of the potential existence of both a physical condition and a pain disorder with psychological factors.

Depressive disorders and pain frequently occur together. The term *masked depression* has been used to refer to presentations in which pain is the primary complaint. Demoralization and learned helplessness associated with pain may lead to depressive symptoms.[2,3] Pain disorders should be diagnosed only if the symptoms cannot be better accounted for by depressive disorders or if the symptoms exceed those associated with depression.

Psychological factors affecting medical conditions, undifferentiated somatization disorder, malingering, and factitious disorders may have significant pain symptoms.[1-3] These disorders were previously described in the discussion of conversion disorders.

TREATMENT

An integrated medical and psychiatric management approach is warranted when somatoform conditions are being considered. The biologic, psychological, and social realms need to be evaluated both separately and in relation to one another in patients with conversion and pain disorders.[18] Given the common diagnostic uncertainty in these disorders and the frequency of dual physical and emotional diagnoses, an integrated medical and psychiatric treatment approach is strongly recommended. This combined approach sidesteps the organic versus psychiatric dilemma that is often faced by hospitalists.[19]

When a child and his or her family present to the hospitalist, they are usually certain that there is a medical cause for the symptoms. The hospitalist should begin the assessment with an exploration of both medical and psychiatric factors that may be contributing to the presenting symptoms. Given the expected complexity of cases requiring hospitalization, psychiatric consultation is generally indicated. This consultation can proceed simultaneously with the medical examinations. The hospitalist can tell the patient and family that the psychiatric consultation is part of a comprehensive biopsychosocial evaluation that includes all aspects of the child's life. The hospitalist should also communicate to the family that the findings of all consultants will be integrated into a comprehensive understanding of the child's symptoms.

The hospitalist should expect the psychiatric consultant to take a full history and perform a mental status examination that focuses on the areas highlighted in the previous sections. These somatoform disorders are not diagnoses of exclusion. If the psychiatric consultant is unable to elicit any of the diagnostic criteria except for motor or sensory symptoms, the possibility of an underlying medical diagnosis should be reconsidered. In addition to the presence or absence of specific psychiatric diagnoses, the hospitalist should expect to gain a logical and thoughtful understanding of the family's experience and the words they use to describe it. It is often helpful for the hospitalist to incorporate the family's words into his or her formulation of the problem during discussions with the family.

Once the medical and psychiatric assessments have been completed, it is crucial for the hospitalist to present the findings to the patient and his or her family. Families are often convinced that the symptoms are due solely to a medical condition. This view of the problem needs to be reframed into a broader biopsychosocial understanding. An "informing conference" is the best way to convey the findings to the family. The goal of this meeting is for the hospitalist to convey a comprehensive biopsychosocial formulation of the child's problem.

This meeting generally begins with a review of the medical findings. The family should be told that many important things have been discovered, such as, "We have good news. We have ruled out a number of serious illnesses, such as. . . ." Statements such as "We couldn't find anything," "It's in your mind," and "The symptoms are not real" should be avoided. It is then critical for the hospitalist to outline his or her understanding of the significant emotional aspects of the case in a supportive and nonjudgmental manner. Although the psychiatric consultant may also attend this meeting, it is important for the family to hear directly from the hospitalist that the symptoms are not solely due to a medical condition, thereby facilitating family acceptance.

Following the family's acceptance of the findings, the hospitalist and the psychiatric consultant should create an integrated medical and psychiatric treatment team. This team arranges for ongoing medical follow-up of any symptoms or physical illness and initiates further psychiatric evaluation and treatment. This approach should begin in the hospital, coupled with a planned transition to either outpatient care or more intensive psychiatric treatment (e.g., inpatient, day program).

Psychiatric treatment is directed toward understanding the child and the family dynamics and the reasons for the child's assumption of the sick role. Individual, behavioral, cognitive, family, and pharmacologic therapies are potential interventions that the psychiatric consultant may initiate during the hospitalization or make arrangements for following discharge.

During the hospitalization, it is useful for the hospitalist to work closely with the psychiatric consultant to implement a treatment plan aimed at decreasing reinforcement of the sick role, as well as encouraging mobilization of the patient. Physical therapy consisting of a gradual return to the child's usual activities before the symptoms began is helpful for many patients.

It is not uncommon for families to remain resistant to psychiatric intervention. In these situations, the psychiatric consultant can advise whether social services intervention to investigate possible parental neglect or abuse is indicated (e.g., parents seeking multiple unnecessary medical procedures).

IN A NUTSHELL

- Conversion disorders and pain syndromes are the most common somatoform disorders seen in the pediatric hospital setting.
- Voluntary motor or sensory symptoms that suggest a neurologic or physical condition are characteristic of conversion disorders.
- Pain disorders are associated with psychological factors and are differentiated by the presence or absence of general medical conditions.
- In somatoform disorders, biologic, psychological, and social realms need to be evaluated both separately and in relation to one another; therefore, an integrated medical and psychiatric evaluation and treatment approach are best.

ON THE HORIZON

- Citalopram (Celexa) has recently been identified as a promising treatment for functional recurrent abdominal pain in pediatric patients.[20]
- Researchers are focusing on the role of serotonin dysregulation in the pathophysiology of both functional gastrointestinal disorders and emotional disorders such as anxiety and depression. Recent studies have suggested an important link between the two that may be mediated by the serotonergic neurotransmitter system.[21] Further studies of this comorbidity will be important in the development of more effective treatment strategies.

SUGGESTED READING

Campo JV, Fritsch SL: Somatization in children and adolescents. J Am Acad Child Adolesc Psychiatry 1994;33:1223-1235.

DeMaso DR, Beasley PJ: The somatoform disorders. In Klykylo WM, Kay JL (eds): Clinical Child Psychiatry. Philadelphia, Wiley, 2005, pp 471-486.

Jamison RN, Walker LS: Illness behavior in children of chronic pain patients. Int J Psychiatry Med 1992;22:329-342.

Minuchin S, Baker L, Rosman BL, et al: A conceptual model of psychosomatic illness in children. Arch Gen Psychiatry 1975;32:1031-1038.

REFERENCES

1. American Psychiatric Association: Diagnostic and Statistical Manual of Mental Disorders, 4th ed. Washington, DC, American Psychiatric Association, 1994.

2. Beasley PJ, DeMaso DR: Conversion and somatoform disorders. In Steiner H (ed): Treating School Age Children. San Francisco, Jossey Bass, 1997, pp 123-151.

3. DeMaso DR, Beasley PJ: The somatoform disorders. In Klykylo WM, Kay JL (eds): Clinical Child Psychiatry. Philadelphia, Wiley, 2005, pp 471-486.

4. Nemzer ED: Somatoform disorders. In Lewis M (ed): Child and Adolescent Psychiatry: A Comprehensive Textbook. Baltimore, Williams & Wilkins, 1991, p 697.

5. Ramsay AR: The relationship of pathogenetic mechanisms to treatment in patients with pain. Psychother Psychosom 1984;42:69-79.

6. Campo JV, Fritsch SL: Somatization in children and adolescents. J Am Acad Child Adolesc Psychiatry 1994;33:1223-1235.

7. Stinnett JL: The functional somatic symptom. Psychiatr Clin North Am 1987;10:19-33.

8. Jamison RN, Walker LS: Illness behavior in children of chronic pain patients. Int J Psychiatry Med 1992;22:329-342.

9. Minuchin S, Baker L, Rosman BL, et al: A conceptual model of psychosomatic illness in children. Arch Gen Psychiatry 1975;32:1031-1038.

10. Cloninger CR: Somatoform and dissociative disorders. In Winokur G, Clayton PJ (eds): The Medical Basis of Psychiatry, 2nd ed. Philadelphia, WB Saunders, 1994, p 169.

11. Dale JK, Straus SE: The chronic fatigue syndrome: Considerations relevant to children and adolescents. Adv Pediatr Infect Dis 1992;7:63-83.

12. Schreier HA, Libow JA: Hurting for Love: Munchausen by Proxy Syndrome. New York, Guilford Press, 1993.

13. Mohamad SN, Weisz GM, Waring EM: The relationship of chronic pain to depression, marital adjustment, and family dynamics. Pain 1978;5:285-292.

14. Fordyce WE, Fowler RS, Lehmann JF, et al: Operant conditioning in the treatment of chronic pain. Arch Phys Med Rehab 1973;54:399-408.

15. Kaufman DM: Clinical Neurology for Psychiatrists, 3rd ed. Philadelphia, WB Saunders, 1990, p 286.

16. Mufson MJ: Chronic pain syndrome: Integrating the medical and psychiatric evaluation and treatment. In Branch WT (ed): Office Practice of Medicine, 3rd ed. Philadelphia, WB Saunders, 1994, pp 1019-1027.

17. McGrath PJ: Annotation: Aspects of pain in children and adolescents. J Child Psychol Psychiatry 1995;36:717-730.

18. Richtesmeier AJ, Aschkenasy JR: Psychological consultation and psychosomatic diagnosis. Psychosomatics 1988;29:338-341.

19. Woodbury MM, DeMaso DR, Goldman SJ: An integrated medical and psychiatric approach to conversion symptoms in a four-year-old. J Am Acad Child Adolesc Psychiatry 1992;31:1095-1097.

20. Campo JV, Dahl RE, Williamson DE, et al: Gastrointestinal distress to serotonergic challenge: A risk marker for emotional disorder? J Am Acad Child Adolesc Psychiatry 2003;42:1221-1226.

21. Campo JV, Perel J, Lucas A: Citalopram treatment of pediatric recurrent abdominal pain and comorbid internalizing disorders: An exploratory study. J Am Acad Child Adolesc Psychiatry 2004;43:1234-1242.

CHAPTER 168

Agitation

Lourival Baptista-Neto and Pamela J. Beasley

Although a violent, aggressive pediatric patient is rare, the presence of such a patient in a medical inpatient unit poses a significant risk to other patients and staff and constitutes an emergency.[1] Attempts have been made to standardize the approach to managing agitation in children and adolescents in psychiatric settings,[2] but there are few data regarding its management in a pediatric medical unit. The recognition of risk factors for agitation and aggressive behavior can be of great value in terms of early intervention and can prevent escalation of the behavior to a more dangerous level (Table 168-1). This chapter describes the causes of out-of-control behavior, the agitation continuum, the assessment of imminent risk, and strategies for managing disruptive behavior in the pediatric hospital setting.

CAUSE

Out-of-control, agitated behavior in the hospital setting is a nonspecific symptom that may be seen in a variety of disorders; however, they typically fall into three interrelated realms: medical conditions, primary psychiatric illnesses, and developmental disorders.

Medical Conditions

Many general medical conditions may be accompanied by agitation and aggressive behavior. These include metabolic disturbances, infections, hyperthyroidism, and neurologic disorders (e.g., epilepsy, central nervous system tumors, traumatic brain injury). Agitation can be a behavioral side effect of certain medications, including corticosteroids, antihistamines, and benzodiazepines, or it may develop as a result of drug or alcohol intoxication or withdrawal syndromes.[3-5] Pain and physical discomfort can also precipitate agitation in vulnerable children.

Delirium is a transient and usually reversible dysfunction in cerebral metabolism that is largely underdiagnosed in the pediatric population. The hallmark symptom is an alteration in the level of consciousness with cognitive changes affecting orientation, memory, and attention span.[6] The onset is often acute or subacute, characterized by a fluctuating level of consciousness and periods of agitation and lethargy. Psychotic symptoms (e.g., illusions, hallucinations, delusions), aggressive behavior, and sleep disturbances are frequent components. The differential diagnosis is extensive (e.g., metabolic disturbances, central nervous system hypoperfusion, high fever, infections, medications, drug intoxication and withdrawal).[3] On the electroencephalogram, the usual pattern observed is generalized slowing.[6] Delirium may be preceded for several days by prodromal symptoms such as insomnia, anxiety, mood lability, and mild to moderate agitation.

In severe cases of delirium, agitation and violence may be extreme. When mechanical restraint is required, rapid sedation with medications that can be given parenterally (e.g., haloperidol, lorazepam) is often critical. Haloperidol has the advantage of keeping the patient calm without causing a major clouding of consciousness or respiratory depression, thus allowing for better monitoring of the patient's mental status and medical condition. The use of newer atypical antipsychotics (e.g., risperidone) for the treatment of delirium requires more study in the pediatric hospital setting. However, clinical experience to date has shown behavioral improvements similar to those seen with haloperidol. The hospitalist's goal is to control the disruptive behavior while simultaneously treating the underlying medical condition.

Primary Psychiatric Illnesses

Children and adolescents with disruptive behavior disorders as identified by the *Diagnostic and Statistical Manual of Mental Disorders,* 4th edition, text revision (DSM-IV-TR), including conduct, oppositional defiant, and attention-deficit hyperactivity disorders, are vulnerable to the development of agitated or aggressive behavior in the hospital setting, particularly with longer stays.[4] Patients with psychotic disorders (e.g., major depression, schizophrenia, bipolar disorder) may misperceive the hospital environment as hostile and overreact with out-of-control behavior. Acute psychosis is discussed in Chapter 169. Patients with histories of substance abuse or childhood trauma (physical or sexual abuse) and those with a family history of violence or criminal arrest are also at greater risk for developing aggressive behavior in the hospital setting.[3-5] Family psychopathology may play a major role in precipitating, exacerbating, or maintaining agitation; disruptive, highly anxious, or hostile family members can have a significant negative effect on a patient's adjustment to the hospital setting and on interactions with medical and nursing staff.

Developmental Disorders

Children and adolescents with developmental disorders or mental retardation are at higher risk for behavioral disturbances owing to their limited cognitive capacity to mediate conflicts verbally and understand events. Because of their central nervous system vulnerabilities, they are also more susceptible to the side effects of medications, including idiosyncratic reactions. DSM-IV-TR diagnoses within this category include autism, pervasive developmental disorder not otherwise specified, and mental retardation of various etiologies.[4] Children and adolescents with dementia have similar vulnerabilities. These patients are at higher risk of developing delirium and behavioral changes induced by

Table 168-1 Risk Factors for Out-of-Control Behaviors

Primary psychiatric illness
  Attention-deficit hyperactivity disorder
  Oppositional defiant disorder
  Conduct disorder
  Psychotic disorder
  Bipolar disorder
  Pervasive developmental disorder

Delirium and dementia

Substance dependence and abuse

History of physical abuse

Family history of violence and criminal arrest

Low verbal IQ

Highly anxious or angry caretakers

medications, and they have a limited capacity to negotiate conflicts and adapt to adverse situations.

CLINICAL PRESENTATION

Agitation refers to behaviors that fall along a continuum ranging from verbal threats and motor restlessness to harmful aggressive and destructive behaviors. Mild agitation includes symptoms such as irritability, oppositional behavior, inappropriate language, and pacing. These patients do not pose an immediate risk of harming themselves or others. Moderate agitation includes escalating verbal threats and increased motor restlessness. Although these patients are not an immediate risk to themselves or others, rapid escalation to an emergency situation may occur at any time. Severely agitated patients are at immediate risk of harming themselves or others through assaultive or self-injurious behavior, and they are capable of causing property damage.

The critical first step is to evaluate the patient's symptoms of agitation and their severity to assess the risk of imminent violence. Acutely combative, agitated, or violent patients constitute an emergency situation in which immediate chemical or mechanical restraint (or both) is required to prevent patients from harming themselves or others. In these circumstances, the hospitalist must focus on rapidly getting the patient's behavior under control. Only then can the hospitalist perform the necessary medical and psychiatric assessments to determine the cause of the behavioral disturbance and develop a specific treatment plan.

TREATMENT

For patients with behavioral disturbances caused by a medical condition or delirium, it is critical that the underlying disorder be aggressively pursued and treated. Children and adolescents manifesting out-of-control behavior such as agitation or aggression require both preventive interventions and rapid, well-thought-out responses to the acute behavioral disruption. Hospitalists must be aware of the stresses associated with a hospital admission and be prepared to use both preventive and responsive management strategies. An algorithm to help direct management in a hospital setting is provided in Figure 168-1.

Behavioral Interventions

The hospitalist's goal is to reduce aggressive or out-of-control behavior to a level where no one is endangered. At all times, the hospitalist must strive to provide the least restrictive environment that protects the safety of the patient, family members, other patients, and medical staff.

Mild agitation may respond to psychosocial and environmental interventions that diminish stimulation and help the patient regain control. These include providing a quiet environment, speaking in soothing tones, offering food or drink, praising appropriate behavior, ignoring bad behavior, and setting limits.[4] It may also be helpful to set limits for family members whose behaviors are adversely affecting the patient. Supportive and reassuring family members are often helpful in calming a patient and can be permitted to remain at the bedside; those whose presence only escalates the child's behavior should be asked to leave.

Despite these interventions, the situation may escalate and require more intensive management. The patient should be monitored closely for behavioral symptoms and risk of violence. It may be necessary to implement a series of pharmacologic and behavioral strategies to protect the patient and others. The hospitalist can have a one-to-one sitter at the patient's bedside or security staff at the door to provide constant monitoring and ensure patient and staff safety. In some situations, this close level of monitoring may be better accomplished in an intensive care setting.

Psychopharmacologic Intervention

Medications ("chemical restraints") should be offered whenever attempts to de-escalate or contain behavior fail. As with behavioral interventions, medications should ideally be given in the early stages of agitation to prevent escalation to violence. The class, dose, and method of administration depend on the child's age, weight, level of agitation, concurrent medical and psychiatric conditions, concomitant medications, and previous responses to treatment. Antihistamines, benzodiazepines, and antipsychotics are among the most frequently used medications for the acute treatment of agitation. Table 168-2 provides dosing guidelines for antihistamines and benzodiazepines. Antipsychotic medications are used for severe agitation or agitation with psychosis (see Chapter 169).

Antihistamines

Diphenhydramine, the most commonly used antihistamine, is generally well tolerated, and its sedating properties are helpful in decreasing agitation. Behavioral disinhibition may be a rare side effect. Antihistamines are generally used in the treatment of mild to moderate levels of agitation. They may also be used in conjunction with antipsychotics to prevent or treat extrapyramidal side effects. Diphenhydramine can be administered orally, intravenously, or intramuscularly.

Benzodiazepines

Lorazepam is the benzodiazepine most commonly used for rapid sedation owing to its quick onset of action, relatively short half-life, lack of active metabolites, and avail-

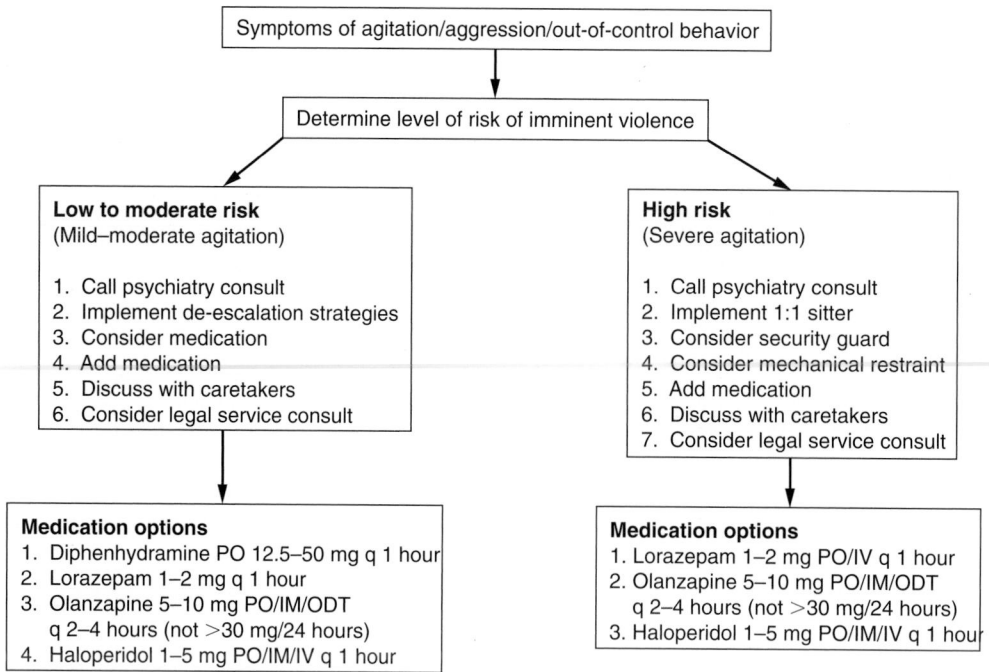

Figure 168-1   Algorithm for the management of agitation in the pediatric hospital setting.

Table 168-2   Dosing Guidelines for Emergency Use of Antihistamines or Benzodiazepines in Patients with Mild to Moderate Agitation

Diphenhydramine*

Children: 5 mg/kg/24 hr PO, IV, or IM, divided every 6 hr as needed for sedation, up to a maximum of 300 mg/day

Adults: 12.5-50 mg/dose PO, IV, or IM every 4-6 hr as needed for sedation, up to a maximum of 300 mg/day

Lorazepam†

Children: 0.05 mg/kg/dose PO or IV as needed for sedation, up to a maximum of 2 mg/dose

Adults: 0.5-2 mg/dose PO, IM, or IV every 1-6 hr as needed for sedation, up to a maximum of 10 mg/day

*Occasionally causes behavioral disinhibition.

†Occasionally causes behavioral disinhibition; helpful in agitation secondary to drug or alcohol intoxication or withdrawal; may cause respiratory depression.

ability in preparations for oral, intramuscular, intravenous, and sublingual administration.[1] Lorazepam is highly effective in the treatment of agitation related to drug or alcohol intoxication or withdrawal states. In addition, it may potentiate the effects of an antipsychotic medication when the two are used together. Studies in adults suggest that the combination of lorazepam and haloperidol is superior to lorazepam alone in the management of agitation.[7] Possible side effects of lorazepam include sedation, ataxia, and confusion. Because of its respiratory depressant properties, lorazepam should be used with caution in patients with pulmonary disease or in those taking other medications with potential respiratory depressant properties.[5] Paradoxical behavioral disinhibition may occur, especially in children with central nervous system vulnerability (e.g., developmental delay, organic brain syndrome).[1] Midazolam, a benzodiazepine with a rapid onset and short half-life, is used for the acute sedation of agitated patients. It has a rapid effect, but this drug may be less desirable when more prolonged control is needed. As the medication effect wears off, other interventions should be in place. Respiratory depression is a known side effect, even with oral dosing, so appropriate monitoring should be considered.

Psychopharmacologic interventions should occur in conjunction with ongoing efforts to de-escalate the patient's agitation with behavioral interventions. If safety remains a concern despite the use of behavioral and pharmacologic interventions, the use of mechanical restraints should be considered.

Mechanical Restraints

The only indication for the use of mechanical restraints is to prevent the patient from harming him- or herself or others when all other interventions have failed. Restraints should never be used as a punishment and should never be instituted by untrained staff.[2] Unique to general medical units is the concept of "medically necessary restraints." This refers to a situation in which the patient is not self-injurious or threatening others but is exhibiting symptoms of agitation that may pose serious risks to his or her medical condition. The hospitalist, unit staff, and hospital security staff need to be aware of both institutional and state guidelines regarding the application and use of physical restraint. There should be someone in charge who can direct the restraint process. Security staff may be quick to arrive, but they must often wait for instructions. Staff should be familiar with regulations about the use of restraints, including documentation, such as the following sample note: "The patient became agitated and combative; attempts to de-escalate his behavior were not successful. The patient attempted to pull his IV line and threatened to punch staff if not allowed to leave. The patient refused to take medications offered to help him calm down. Security was called; patient was placed in four-point restraints for protection of self and others. Patient also received Haldol 2 mg IM and Ativan 1mg IM."

Restraint orders are time-limited, and patients must be observed constantly while in restraints. Restraints must be removed as soon as the patient has achieved behavioral control and is no longer at risk for harming him- or herself or others.[4] During and after the period of mechanical restraint, patients and families should be given the opportunity to process and understand the event.

CONSULTATION

The psychiatric consultant should be involved early in the process. This consultant can assist in emergency management, diagnosis of underlying or contributing processes, assembly of a multidisciplinary team (e.g., pediatrics, nursing, psychiatry, social work, child life specialist), and transition to an appropriate outpatient or inpatient program.

DISCHARGE CRITERIA

Once the patient is medically stable and behavior is under control, the psychiatric consultant can assist in developing a discharge plan. This usually consists of follow-up psychiatric care, which might include outpatient psychotherapy, pharmacotherapy, family therapy, or group therapy. If aggressive behaviors have not resolved, transfer to a more intensive level of treatment (e.g., inpatient psychiatric unit, partial hospital program) may be indicated.

PREVENTION

Ideally, the best strategy is one of prevention.[2,8] It is helpful to inquire about a history of aggressive or out-of-control behavior during the admission process, keeping in mind the previously outlined risk factors (see Table 168-1). The hospitalist should be alert to any feelings of fear or worry during interactions with patients and their families. These feelings may be early-warning signals that there will be problems with behavioral control. Determining the cause of the symptoms is required to create a treatment plan that specifically targets the individual patient and his or her family. Psychiatric consultation is most effective when it occurs in response to suspected or potential concerns rather than after a patient is already displaying out-of-control behavior.

Anger management and stress reduction techniques are important tools in the prevention of higher levels of agitation.[2,8] Medical and nursing staff who are familiar with basic stress reduction strategies can promote a child's self-control and reduce behavioral disruption. It is also helpful to structure the patient's day by creating a schedule and mobilizing the patient as much as possible within the constraints of his or her medical illness. Nursing staff and child life specialists (when available) can develop daily schedules that can be posted at the bedside.

IN A NUTSHELL

- Agitated and aggressive behaviors are nonspecific symptoms that may be seen in a variety of disorders that typically fall into three realms: general medical conditions, primary psychiatric illnesses, and developmental disorders.
- These behaviors may constitute an emergency requiring rapid intervention to maintain a safe environment and prevent patients from harming themselves or others.
- Interventions may require any or all of the following: behavioral and environmental strategies, psychopharmacologic agents, and mechanical restraints. At all times, the least restrictive environment that maintains the safety of the patient, caregivers, other patients, and medical staff should be pursued.
- Antihistamines, benzodiazepines, and antipsychotics may be helpful when used judiciously in the treatment of a medically ill child who is agitated.
- Physical restraints may be required in cases of severe agitation to maintain safety. Documentation should clearly indicate all efforts made to control the patient's behavior before the restraints were used.
- Once safety has been ensured, treatment of the underlying disorder can be pursued or resumed.

ON THE HORIZON

- Clinical practice guidelines addressing aggression and agitation in the inpatient setting are needed, including recognition of risk factors and prevention.

- Alternative routes of administration of atypical antipsychotic medications are being explored, including intramuscular administration of olanzapine and ziprasidone and orally disintegrating forms of risperidone and olanzapine.[9]

SUGGESTED READING

Cummings MR, Miller BD: Pharmacologic management of behavioral instability in medically pediatric patients. Curr Opin Pediatr 2004;16:516-522.

Heyneman EK: The aggressive child. Child Adolesc Psychiatr Clin North Am 2003;12:667-677.

REFERENCES

1. Pappadopulos E, Macintyre JC, Crismon ML, et al: Treatment recommendations for the use of antipsychotics for aggressive youth (TRAYY). Part II. J Am Acad Child Adolesc Psychiatry 2003;42:2.

2. Barnett SR, Dosreis S, Riddle MA: Improving the management of acute aggression in state residential and inpatient psychiatric facilities for youths. J Am Acad Child Adolesc Psychiatry 2002;41:8.

3. Wise MJ, Rundell JR: Effective psychiatric consultation. In Hales RE (ed): Concise Guide to Consultation Psychiatry. Washington, DC, American Psychiatric Press, 1994, pp 1-10.

4. Heyneman EK: The aggressive child. Child Adolesc Psychiatr Clin North Am 2003;12:667-677.

5. Sorrentino A: Chemical restraints for the agitated, violent, or psychotic pediatric patient in the emergency department: Controversies and recommendations. Curr Opin Pediatr 2004;16:2.

6. Bieniek SA, Ownby RL, Penalver A, et al: A double-blind study of lorazepam versus the combination of haloperidol and lorazepam in managing agitation. Pharmacotherapy 1998;18:57-62.

7. Green WH: Antipsychotics. In Mitchell CW, Kairis LR (eds): Child and Adolescent Clinical Psychopharmacology. Philadelphia, Lippincott Williams & Wilkins, 2001, pp 89-149.

8. Masters KJ, Bellonci C, Bernet W, et al: Summary of the practice parameter for the prevention and management of aggressive behavior in child and adolescent psychiatric institutions with special reference to seclusion and restraint. J Am Acad Child Adolesc Psychiatry 2001;40:11.

9. Citrome L: Atypical antipsychotics for acute agitation: New intramuscular options offer advantages. Postgrad Med 2002;112:85-96.

CHAPTER 169

New-Onset Psychosis

Brigid L. Vaughan and Pamela J. Beasley

Psychosis is not a diagnosis but a symptom cluster that may play a role in many psychiatric illnesses. Psychotic symptoms include hallucinations, or delusions, with variable manifestations. Children and adolescents exhibiting psychotic symptoms may be suffering from bipolar, major depressive, post-traumatic stress, substance abuse, or schizophrenia spectrum disorders. Psychosis may also be caused by physical illnesses or their treatments.

There are no definitive data regarding the prevalence of psychosis in childhood. Schizophrenia has a prevalence of 0.5% to 1.5% in adults,[1] with a peak onset during the late adolescent and young adult years. Depressive disorders, seen in 2% of children and 4% to 8% of adolescents,[2] can include psychosis, but the prevalence of this symptom complex in depressed youth is not known. A review of 2031 consecutive referrals to a pediatric mood and anxiety disorders clinic found that 4.5% of the patients had psychotic symptoms, typically auditory hallucinations.[3] Information primarily from adult studies of schizophrenia suggests that the frontal and temporal lobes are involved in the pathophysiology of psychosis.[4]

CLINICAL PRESENTATION

Psychosis can present in a number of ways, based in part on the underlying cause. Psychosis in children and adolescents may be heralded by premorbid difficulties with speech and language and peer relationships or by social withdrawal or disruptive behaviors.[5] When the premorbid history involves primarily social isolation and problematic peer relations, early-onset schizophrenia is more likely than bipolar disorder.[6]

The acute presentation of psychosis may be quite dramatic, with prominent thought disturbances such as hallucinations, delusions, illogical thinking, and loose associations. Patients may be frightened, confused, agitated, or even suicidal.[3] Hallucinations can be auditory, visual, olfactory, or tactile; auditory presentations account for more than 74% of hallucinations in children and adolescents.[3,7-10] Of note, hallucinations of any type are extremely rare in patients younger than 7 years.[4]

Delusions are fixed false beliefs that cannot be corrected by reasoning. There are many categories of delusions. The content of a mood-congruent delusion is mood-appropriate, involving themes of guilt, worthlessness, and failure (e.g., a depressed patient who believes that she will develop cancer as a punishment for misdeeds), whereas the content of a mood-incongruent delusion has no association to mood or is mood-inappropriate (e.g., a depressed patient who believes that his food is being poisoned). Bizarre delusions are implausible or strange false beliefs (e.g., the belief that

space invaders have implanted electrodes in the patient's brain), somatic delusions are false beliefs regarding bodily functions (e.g., the belief that one's brain is melting), delusions of reference are false beliefs that the behavior of others refers to oneself (e.g., a television actor's words are actually a special message directed toward the patient), and systematized delusions are false beliefs united by a single theme (e.g., a patient being persecuted by the Mafia or the FBI). Delusions tend to become more complex and systematized with increasing age.[10,11] Additionally, patients presenting with psychosis typically exhibit disordered thought processes, including loose associations, tangentiality, and incoherence.

The patient's stage of development is an important factor to consider when a child presents with psychosis. For example, illogical thinking and loose associations, common in schizophrenia, are normal for children younger than 7 years and may also be seen in older children and adolescents who are developmentally delayed.[4]

DIFFERENTIAL DIAGNOSIS

The critical first step in establishing a diagnosis is to rule out a medical cause. In children and adolescents, physical illnesses that may present with psychosis include seizures, delirium, central nervous system injuries or lesions (e.g., cranial malformations, brain tumors), metabolic diseases (e.g., Wilson disease), neurodegenerative disorders (e.g., Huntington disease), developmental disorders, infectious diseases (e.g., meningitis, encephalitis, human immunodeficiency virus-related syndromes), and toxic encephalopathies (e.g., substance abuse, anticholinergic medications, stimulants, corticosteroids, other toxins).[5]

Delirium, which can closely mimic acute psychosis, is an acute confusional state. Overlapping symptoms may include hallucinations and sensory misperceptions. Some distinguishing characteristics include the waxing and waning presentation seen with delirium. Additionally, patients with psychosis are usually not disoriented, as is frequently seen with delirium. Further discussion of delirium is provided in Chapter 168.

As noted earlier, many psychiatric conditions can present with psychosis. These include mood disorders (e.g., major depressive and bipolar disorders) and certain nonpsychotic psychiatric disorders (e.g., personality and post-traumatic stress disorders), as well as substance abuse, pervasive developmental disorders, developmental language disorders, obsessive-compulsive disorders, and schizophrenia spectrum disorders.[5] In an examination of psychosis in a pediatric mood and anxiety disorders program, 41% of the patients with psychosis met the *Diagnostic and Statistical*

Table 169-1   DSM-IV-TR Criteria for Major Depressive Episode

A. Five (or more) of the following symptoms have been present during the same 2-week period and represent a change from previous functioning; at least one of the symptoms is either depressed mood or loss of interest or pleasure. Do not include symptoms that are clearly due to a general medical condition or mood-incongruent delusions or hallucinations.
  1. Depressed mood (or irritable mood in children and adolescents) most of the day, nearly every day, as indicated by either subjective report (e.g., feels sad or empty) or observation by others (e.g., appears tearful).
  2. Markedly diminished interest or pleasure in all, or almost all, activities most of the day, nearly every day (as indicated by either subjective account or observation by others).
  3. Significant weight loss when not dieting or weight gain (e.g., change of >5% of body weight in a month), or decrease or increase in appetite nearly every day. In children, consider failure to make expected weight gains.
  4. Insomnia or hypersomnia nearly every day.
  5. Psychomotor agitation or retardation nearly every day (observable by others, not merely subjective feelings of restlessness or being slowed down).
  6. Fatigue or loss of energy nearly every day.
  7. Feelings of worthlessness or excessive or inappropriate guilt (which may be delusional) nearly every day (not merely self-reproach or guilt about being sick).
  8. Diminished ability to think or concentrate, or indecisiveness, nearly every day (either by subjective account or as observed by others).
  9. Recurrent thoughts of death (not just fear of dying), recurrent suicidal ideation without a specific plan, or a suicide attempt or a specific plan for committing suicide.

B. The symptoms cause clinically significant distress or impairment in social, occupational, or other important areas of functioning.

C. The symptoms are not due to the direct physiologic effects of a substance (e.g., drug of abuse, medication) or a general medical condition (e.g., hypothyroidism).

D. The symptoms are not better accounted for by bereavement (i.e., after the loss of a loved one), and the symptoms persist for longer than 2 months or are characterized by marked functional impairment, morbid preoccupation with worthlessness, suicidal ideation, psychotic symptoms, or psychomotor retardation.

Adapted from American Psychiatric Association: Diagnostic and Statistical Manual of Mental Disorders, 4th ed, text revision. Washington, DC, American Psychiatric Association, 2000.

Manual of Mental Disorders, 4th edition, text revision (DSM-IV-TR), criteria for a major depressive disorder, 21% exhibited subthreshold depressive disorder symptoms, 25% met DSM-IV-TR criteria for a bipolar disorder, and 14% had a schizophrenia spectrum disorder.[3]

Major depressive episode refers to at least 2 weeks of depressed or irritable mood that is associated with neurovegetative symptoms of depression (Table 169-1). A disabling depression may occur with or without psychotic features. A major depressive disorder with psychotic features (psychotic depression) typically presents with hallucinations or delusions that are not bizarre.

Patients who experience manic episodes (Table 169-2) with or without depressive episodes qualify for the diagnosis of bipolar disorder. The manic and depressive phases of the illness may present with or without psychotic symptoms. A manic episode with psychotic features may present with delusions that are grandiose and paranoid, along with either a congruent or incongruent mood.[4,12] The depressed phase of bipolar disorder with psychotic features presents similarly to major depressive disorder with psychotic features.

Patients with schizophrenia spectrum disorders (Table 169-3) typically present with hallucinations and delusions in association with a flat or inappropriate affect. The hallucinations are commonly auditory, often with one or more voices of a threatening, insulting, or obscene nature. The delusions tend to be bizarre, paranoid, referential, or somatic.[4]

Patients with obsessive-compulsive disorder may rarely exhibit psychotic behavior, such as believing that the world will end unless certain counting rituals are performed many times a day. Patients with post-traumatic stress disorder may present with hallucinations related to the trauma experienced. Patients who abuse psychoactive substances may present with hallucinations or delusions related to intoxication or withdrawal syndromes.

DIAGNOSIS AND EVALUATION

It is important for the hospitalist to evaluate the patient for a general medical condition that might cause psychotic symptoms. A thorough history and physical examination, including neurologic assessment, may help identify organic causes of psychosis.[5,13,14] The performance of laboratory and imaging studies should be determined by the results of the history and physical examination. Given that drug and alcohol intoxication may present with psychotic symptoms, it is important to obtain a toxicology screen as soon as possible after the initial presentation. The routine use of endocrinologic and radiologic tests for new-onset psychosis is not supported in the literature and does not have much yield.[13,15] However, some researchers have suggested an electroencephalogram; comprehensive laboratory testing, including thyroid function tests, ceruloplasmin, erythrocyte sedimentation rate, complete blood count, renal and liver function tests, pregnancy test, and antinuclear factor; and

Table 169-2 DSM-IV-TR Criteria for Manic Episode

A. A distinct period of abnormally and persistently elevated, expansive, or irritable mood lasting at least 1 week (or any duration if hospitalization is necessary).

B. During the period of mood disturbance, three (or more) of the following symptoms have persisted (four if the mood is only irritable) and have been present to a significant degree:
   1. Inflated self-esteem or grandiosity.
   2. Decreased need for sleep (e.g., feels rested after only 3 hours of sleep).
   3. More talkative than usual or feels pressure to keep talking.
   4. Flight of ideas or subjective experience that thoughts are racing.
   5. Distractibility (i.e., attention too easily drawn to unimportant or irrelevant external stimuli).
   6. Increase in goal-directed activity (socially, at work or school, or sexually) or psychomotor agitation.
   7. Excessive involvement in pleasurable activities that have a high potential for painful consequences (e.g., unrestrained buying sprees, sexual indiscretions, foolish business investments).

C. The mood disturbance is sufficiently severe to cause marked impairment in occupational functioning or in usual social activities or relationships with others, or to necessitate hospitalization to prevent harm to self or others, or there are psychotic features.

D. The symptoms are not due to the direct physiologic effects of a substance (e.g., drug of abuse, medication) or a general medical condition (e.g., hypothyroidism).

Adapted from American Psychiatric Association: Diagnostic and Statistical Manual of Mental Disorders, 4th ed, text revision. Washington, DC, American Psychiatric Association, 2000.

Table 169-3 DSM-IV-TR Criteria for Schizophrenia

A. Characteristic symptoms: Two (or more) of the following, each present for a significant portion of time during a 1-month period (or less if successfully treated)*:
   1. Delusions.
   2. Hallucinations.
   3. Disorganized speech (e.g., frequent derailment or incoherence).
   4. Grossly disorganized or catatonic behavior.
   5. Negative symptoms (e.g., affective flattening, alogia, avolition).

B. Social or occupational dysfunction: For a significant portion of the time since the onset of the disturbance, one or more areas of functioning such as work, interpersonal relations, or self-care are markedly below the level achieved before the onset (or, when the onset is in childhood or adolescence, failure to achieve expected level of interpersonal, academic, or occupational achievement).

C. Duration: Continuous signs of the disturbance persist for at least 6 months. This 6-month period must include at least 1 month of symptoms (or less if successfully treated) that meet criterion A (i.e., active-phase symptoms) and may include periods of prodromal or residual symptoms. During these prodromal or residual periods, the signs of the disturbance may be manifested by only negative symptoms or two or more symptoms listed in criterion A present in an attenuated form (e.g., odd beliefs, unusual perceptual experiences).

D. Schizoaffective and mood disorder exclusion: Schizoaffective disorder and mood disorder with psychotic features have been ruled out because either (1) no major depressive, manic, or mixed episodes have occurred concurrently with the active-phase symptoms or (2) if mood episodes have occurred during active-phase symptoms, their total duration has been brief relative to the duration of the active and residual periods.

E. Substance and general medical condition exclusion: The disturbance is not due to the direct physiologic effects of a substance (e.g., drug of abuse, medication) or a general medical condition.

F. Relationship to a pervasive developmental disorder: If there is a history of autistic disorder or another pervasive developmental disorder, the additional diagnosis of schizophrenia is made only if prominent delusions or hallucinations are also present for at least a month (or less if successfully treated).

*Only one criterion A symptom is required if delusions are bizarre or hallucinations consist of a voice keeping up a running commentary on the person's behavior or thoughts or two or more voices conversing with each other.
Adapted from American Psychiatric Association: Diagnostic and Statistical Manual of Mental Disorders, 4th ed, text revision. Washington, DC, American Psychiatric Association, 2000.

neuroimaging tests. These are especially useful in patients with an uncertain or poor medical history, atypical symptoms, poor response to antipsychotic medication, recurring illness, or a strong familial history of medical illness that may be associated with psychotic symptoms.[14,15]

When a medical cause cannot be identified, a psychiatric evaluation should be performed to determine the underlying psychiatric illness responsible for the psychosis. The focus of the psychiatric evaluation is to identify and organize the features detailed in Tables 169-1, 169-2, and 169-3 to determine a unifying diagnosis.

COURSE OF ILLNESS

The course of psychosis depends on the underlying cause. Psychotic symptoms due to a general medical condition generally resolve with treatment of the underlying disorder.

In schizophrenia, the onset of psychotic symptoms may be acute or insidious, with a prodromal phase characterized by social withdrawal and a gradual decline in functioning.[1] It is generally considered to be a phasic disorder with variability in the expression of phases.[5]

Bipolar disorder by definition has a cyclical course and can present with manic or depressive symptoms.[1] Pediatric patients with bipolar disorder may be more likely than adults to have a rapidly cycling mood (i.e., at least four episodes of mood disturbance in the previous 12 months).[1,12] Additionally, some researchers have found adolescents with bipolar illnesses to be more resistant to treatment than adults are.[16,17]

The typical duration of a major depressive episode is 7 to 9 months for clinically referred pediatric patients and 1 to 2 months in community samples. Greater severity, associated in part with psychotic features, predicts a longer duration for a depressive episode.[2]

The long-term outcome for children and adolescents with new-onset psychosis is dependent on the diagnosis. In a study examining the adult outcome for patients hospitalized with adolescent-onset psychosis, 79% of those diagnosed with schizophrenia spectrum illnesses had a poor outcome, compared with 26% of those hospitalized with mood disorders.[18]

TREATMENT

When a child or adolescent presents with new-onset psychosis, both the patient and the family are in dire need of assistance. The patient is generally functioning quite poorly and may be unable to participate in the initial assessment. Family members are likely to be frightened, worried, and confused by what has happened to their child.

Ideally, the assessment and treatment of new-onset psychosis in children and adolescents should be provided in an intensive psychiatric treatment setting.[14] If this is not possible, it is critical that a multidisciplinary team (e.g., pediatrics, nursing, psychiatry, psychology, social work) be available to assess and treat the youngster and provide education and support for the family. One-to-one observation is necessary whenever there is the possibility of harmful behavior.

Initial Agitation

Particularly for agitated or combative patients, ensuring the safety of the patient, family, and health care providers is the primary objective. *Agitation* refers to behaviors that fall

Table 169-4   Levels of Agitation

Level	Features
Mild	Irritability, oppositional behavior, inappropriate language, pacing
Moderate	Escalating verbal threats, increased motor restlessness
Severe	Aggressive, destructive, or self-injurious behavior

on a continuum ranging from verbal threats and motor restlessness to aggressive and destructive behaviors that may cause physical harm to the patient or staff. The appropriate interventions depend on the hospitalist's assessment of the level of agitation (Table 169-4), keeping in mind that patients may escalate or drop from one level to another very quickly. At all times, the hospitalist should strive to provide the least restrictive environment that preserves the safety of the patient, family, and medical staff.

In an emergency situation, the purpose of medications is to decrease the behavioral symptoms associated with agitation. Choice of medication and route of administration depend on several factors, including the patient's level of agitation, any concomitant medical problems, and the side effect profile of the agent. Table 169-5 provides dosage guidelines for the emergency use of antipsychotic medications for patients with severe agitation or agitation with psychosis.

For ongoing treatment, the medications to consider include antihistamines, benzodiazepines, and antipsychotics. Typically, mild and moderate levels of agitation are not treated with antipsychotic medications (see Chapter 168). Severe agitation or agitation with psychosis often requires the use of all three classes of medications. It may take several weeks of treatment with antipsychotic medications to alleviate the symptoms of psychosis. Antipsychotic medications consist of the older, typical antipsychotics (e.g., haloperidol, chlorpromazine) and the newer, atypical antipsychotics (e.g., risperidone, olanzapine, quetiapine, ziprasidone).[13] Olanzapine, risperidone, and ziprasidone are more widely used because of their availability in both oral and intramuscular forms. The recent introduction of an orally disintegrating form of olanzapine may provide an easier and less painful route of administration.

Although both classes of antipsychotics are used in the treatment of acutely agitated patients, the newer-generation antipsychotic medications are preferred owing to their lower risk of extrapyramidal side effects (e.g., muscle rigidity, dyskinesia, akathisia, tremors), tardive dyskinesia, neuroleptic malignant syndrome, and acute dystonic reaction. Of these, neuroleptic malignant syndrome is the rarest but most serious complication of antipsychotic medications. It can result in hyperthermia, rigidity, autonomic dysregulation, mental status changes, and rhabdomyolysis. Treatment of this medical emergency includes aggressive supportive care with ventilatory and circulatory support, cooling blanket and antipyretics, and fluid administration to prevent renal injury from myoglobinemia. The value of other interventions, such as dantrolene, amantadine, bromocriptine, and electroconvulsive therapy, is uncertain.

Table 169-5 Guidelines for Emergency Use of Antipsychotic Medications in Patients with Severe Agitation or Agitation with Psychosis

Drug	Oral Dosage	Intramuscular Dosage	Q-T Interval	Comments
New-Generation ("Atypical") Antipsychotics*				
Risperidone	0.5-1 mg, up to 4-6 mg/day	0.5-1 mg, up to 4-6 mg/day	Minimal increase	Higher dosage (>4 mg/day) may be associated with greater risk of extrapyramidal symptoms
Olanzapine	2.5-5 mg, up to 20 mg/day	2.5-5 mg, up to 20 mg/day	Minimal increase	Available in orally disintegrating tablet; use same dosage as oral and IM forms
Ziprasidone	10 mg, up to 20 mg/day	10 mg, up to 20 mg/day	Minimal to moderate increase	Do not use with drugs or in conditions associated with prolonged Q-T interval
Typical Antipsychotics				
Haloperidol	Children: 0.05-0.15 mg/kg/day in 2-3 divided doses; starting dose 0.025-0.05 mg/kg/day; not to exceed 0.15 mg/kg/day Adolescents: 0.5-5 mg bid-tid; starting dose 0.5-2 mg bid-tid; not to exceed 100 mg/day	Children: 1-3 mg tid-qid; not to exceed 0.15 mg/kg/day[†] Adolescents: 2-5 mg; not to exceed 100 mg/day[†]	Rare increase	Higher incidence of extrapyramidal symptoms, neuroleptic malignant syndrome, and hypotension compared with atypicals; to reduce risk of extrapyramidal symptoms, administer with either diphenhydramine 25-50 mg PO or IM or benztropine 1 mg PO or IM, especially with IM dosing of haloperidol
Chlorpromazine	Children: 0.5-1 mg/kg, 4-6 doses/day[†] Adults: 200-800 mg/day in 3-4 divided doses; starting dose 10-25 mg in 2-4 divided doses; not to exceed total dose of 1 g/day	Children: 0.5-1 mg/kg, 3-4 doses/day; not to exceed 40 mg/day for children <5 yr and 75 mg/day for those 5-12 yr Adults: 200-800 mg/day in 3-4 divided doses; starting dose 25-50 mg q4-6 hr; not to exceed total dose of 1 g/day	Rare increase	Same as haloperidol

*Although they are routinely used in clinical practice, the atypical antipsychotics are not approved by the Food and Drug Administration for emergency use in agitation; dosages are extrapolated from those used in the treatment of psychiatric disorders.
[†]Switch to oral dosing as soon as possible.
[‡]Not recommended as a standing medication.

Symptoms of acute dystonic reaction include torticollis, oculogyric crisis, dysarthria secondary to buccal-lingual crisis, and difficulty ambulating secondary to spasm of the abdominal and pelvic musculature. Mental status is not affected. Although usually not life threatening (with the exception of laryngospasm), these reactions can be very painful and frightening. Younger males are at higher risk for developing an acute dystonic reaction. Fortunately, this complication responds promptly to the administration of anticholinergics such as diphenhydramine or benztropine (Cogentin), which can be administered orally, intramuscularly, or intravenously (Table 169-6). Because antipsychotic medications may have long half-lives, dosing with anticholinergics may need to be continued to avoid a recurrence of the dystonic reaction.

Table 169-6 Medications for Acute Dystonic Reactions

Diphenhydramine*
Children: 5 mg/kg/day in 3-4 divided doses, not to exceed 300 mg/day
Adults: 10-50 mg in a single dose every 4 hr, not to exceed 400 mg/day

Benztropine (Cogentin)*
Children >3 yr: 0.02-0.05 mg/kg/dose administered 1-2 times/day
Adults: 1-4 mg/dose administered 1-2 times/day

*Dosing is the same for the oral, intramuscular, and intravenous routes of administration, all of which are acceptable.

Tardive dyskinesia is manifested by involuntary movements of the tongue, lips, jaw, facial musculature, and trunk. Although this late-onset movement disorder may be reversible with early recognition, many features may be permanent. Control of this complication rarely requires acute intervention by a general hospitalist.

Other side effects of the atypical antipsychotics include sedation, postural hypotension, dizziness, tachycardia, anticholinergic effects, and prolongation of the Q-T interval.[5] Note that although atypical antipsychotics are commonly used in clinical practice, their safety and efficacy in the pediatric population have not been established.

Common side effects of the typical antipsychotics include sedation, anticholinergic effects, orthostatic hypotension, and extrapyramidal symptoms. Haloperidol is widely used in the management of acute agitation related to delirium in medically compromised patients. It has virtually no hypotensive or anticholinergic properties and therefore minimal effects on cardiovascular and respiratory systems. Haloperidol has a lower incidence of side effects when given parenterally. Although intravenous administration is widely used, the Food and Drug Administration has not officially approved this route.[5]

If one of the older antipsychotic medications (e.g., haloperidol, chlorpromazine) is used, concomitant administration of benztropine or diphenhydramine is recommended to decrease the risk of extrapyramidal symptoms. An uncomfortable or frightening adverse reaction to medication can have deleterious and long-lasting effects on a patient's adherence to the treatment regimen. If the patient is cooperative, oral medications should be first-line therapy; however, if the patient is agitated or noncompliant, intramuscular administration may be necessary.

Ongoing Treatment after Stabilization

After initial stabilization, the assessment should lead to provisional diagnostic impressions, which dictate the next steps in treatment, such as the choice of psychotropic medications to be used for ongoing psychiatric care. Accurate diagnosis and selection of optimal pharmacologic therapy are best accomplished in conjunction with a pediatric psychiatrist. A detailed discussion of the use of antipsychotic medications is beyond the scope of this chapter; however, general guidelines regarding their use in children and adolescents are provided. Readers can refer to other sources for additional information.[5,19,20]

Psychotic illnesses in the pediatric population are believed to be similar to adult-onset forms.[5,21] In the absence of a substantial body of research on the pharmacologic treatment of pediatric psychosis, the use of antipsychotic medications in children is extrapolated largely from the extensive adult literature.[20] Although there are limited data regarding the use of new-generation antipsychotic medications in children and adolescents,[5,14] they are used as first-line treatment for adults because of their desirable side effect profiles and should be similarly considered in the pediatric population.

Before initiating ongoing antipsychotic treatment, baseline assessment and laboratory studies should be obtained, including complete blood count; electrolytes; renal, liver, and thyroid function tests; hyperprolactinemia screening; fasting lipid panel; fasting glucose; pregnancy test; electrocardiogram; and weight, height, and body mass index. Patients should receive baseline and then ongoing monitoring for the development of extrapyramidal side effects.[5,20] This monitoring may be facilitated by the use of a validated instrument such as the Abnormal Involuntary Movement Scale (AIMS).[22]

The treatment of a depressive disorder with psychotic features generally includes both an antipsychotic and an antidepressant medication (e.g., selective serotonin reuptake inhibitor). The treatment of bipolar disorder with psychosis generally includes an antipsychotic and a mood stabilizer (e.g., lithium, divalproex sodium, carbamazepine). Pharmacologic management of schizophrenia includes an antipsychotic medication (e.g., risperidone, olanzapine).

Informed consent addressing the potential risks, benefits, and alternatives to treatment should be obtained from the guardian and the patient. The patient's age or developmental level may prevent his or her participation in the informed consent process; each state may have its own regulations regarding how to proceed in this situation.[5]

CONSULTATION

Mental health clinicians can provide important assistance in diagnosing and treating the patient's illness, educating the family, and obtaining referrals for inpatient hospitalization, day treatment programs, or outpatient treatment.

ADMISSION CRITERIA

Hospitalization on a medical service may be warranted in the following situations:

- The patient is medically unstable. This could be related to a variety of conditions, such as an inability to care for him- or herself by maintaining adequate hydration or nutrition or the need for detoxification.
- Observation during imposed abstinence from substances of abuse is needed to clarify the cause of psychotic symptoms.
- Based on physical findings, the patient requires medical investigation to exclude medical causes of the psychotic symptoms.
- Lack of adequate outpatient support or treatment.
- The patient is awaiting placement in an appropriate psychiatric facility. Reasons for psychiatric admission could include psychomotor agitation, suicidal or homicidal ideation or behavior, need for close medical monitoring during medication initiation (e.g., in the presence of comorbid physical illness), or marked disorganization requiring constant supervision for the patient's safety.

DISCHARGE CRITERIA

- The patient is medically stable, and appropriate arrangements have been made for follow-up psychiatric care, including psychiatric evaluation and treatment for the patient and family, as well as psychopharmacologic care when indicated.
- If psychotic symptoms have resolved sufficiently that the family can adequately supervise the patient at home, a day

treatment program or outpatient psychiatric follow-up is indicated.

- If psychotic symptoms have not resolved, transfer to an inpatient psychiatric unit is indicated.

PREVENTION

There are no known strategies for preventing psychosis in children and adolescents. A possible exception may be the prevention of substance abuse among adolescents because of the increased risk of schizophrenia in teens with history of chronic cannabis use[23]; however, this has not been studied.

IN A NUTSHELL

- Acute psychosis may have an insidious or acute onset, but hallmarks include illogical thinking, loose associations, hallucinations, or delusions.
- New-onset psychosis has multiple potential causes, both medical and psychiatric. The need for an extensive organic workup is determined by the outcome of a thorough history and physical examination.
- Acute management of agitation is required to prevent injury to the patient, the family, and the medical staff.
- Regardless of the cause, nonorganic psychosis requires multidisciplinary treatment and usually the administration of antipsychotic medications. Close outpatient care and monitoring are imperative.

ON THE HORIZON

- The results of studies of the efficacy of new-generation antipsychotic medications in the pediatric population will be published.
- Look for additional clarification of appropriate baseline and monitoring studies as more specific information regarding antipsychotic medication side effects in children and adolescents is uncovered.
- Guidelines for the early diagnosis of specific psychiatric causes of psychosis will be delineated.

SUGGESTED READING

American Academy of Child and Adolescent Psychiatry: Practice parameters for the assessment and treatment of children and adolescents with depressive disorders. J Am Acad Child Adolesc Psychiatry 1998;37(10 Suppl):63S-83S.

American Academy of Child and Adolescent Psychiatry: Practice parameter for the assessment and treatment of children and adolescents with schizophrenia. J Am Acad Child Adolesc Psychiatry 2001;4S-23S.

American Academy of Child and Adolescent Psychiatry: Practice parameter for the prevention and management of aggressive behavior in child and adolescent psychiatric institutions, with special reference to seclusion and restraint. J Am Acad Child Adolesc Psychiatry 2002;41:4S-25S.

Semper T, McClellan J: The psychotic child. Child Adolesc Psychiatr Clin North Am 2003;12:679-691.

REFERENCES

1. American Psychiatric Association: Diagnostic and Statistical Manual of Mental Disorders, 4th ed, text revision. Washington, DC, American Psychiatric Association, 2000.
2. American Academy of Child and Adolescent Psychiatry: Practice parameters for the assessment and treatment of children and adolescents with depressive disorders. J Am Acad Child Adolesc Psychiatry 1998; 7(10 Suppl):63S-83S.
3. Ulloa RE, Birmaher B, Axelson D, et al: Psychosis in a pediatric mood and anxiety disorders clinic: Phenomenology and correlates. J Am Acad Child Adolesc Psychiatry 2000;39:337-345.
4. Caplan R, Tanguay PE: Development of psychotic thinking in children. In Lewis M (ed): Child and Adolescent Psychiatry: A Comprehensive Textbook. Philadelphia, Lippincott Williams & Wilkins, 2002, pp 359-366.
5. American Academy of Child and Adolescent Psychiatry: Practice parameter for the assessment and treatment of children and adolescents with schizophrenia. J Am Acad Child Adolesc Psychiatry 2001;4S-23S.
6. McClellan J, McCurry C: Neurocognitive pathways in the development of schizophrenia. Semin Clin Neuropsychiatry 1998;3:320-332.
7. Gordon CT, Frazier JA, McKenna K, et al: Childhood-onset schizophrenia: An NIMH study in progress. Schizophr Bull 1994;20:697-712.
8. Kolvin I, Ounsted C, Humphrey M, et al: Studies in the childhood psychoses. I. The phenomenology of childhood psychoses. Br J Psychiatry 1971;118:385-395.
9. McKenna K, Gordon CT, Lenane M, et al: Looking for childhood-onset schizophrenia: The first 71 cases screened. J Am Acad Child Adolesc Psychiatry 1994;33:636-644.
10. Russell AT, Bott L, Sammons C: The phenomenology of schizophrenia occurring in childhood. J Am Acad Child Adolesc Psychiatry 1989;28:399-407.
11. Apter A, Spivak B, Weizman A, et al: Paranoid schizophrenia in adolescence. J Clin Psychiatry 1991;52:365-368.
12. American Academy of Child and Adolescent Psychiatry: Practice parameters for the assessment and treatment of children and adolescents with bipolar disorder. J Am Acad Child Adolesc Psychiatry 1997;36:157S-176S.
13. Semper T, McClellan J: The psychotic child. Child Adolesc Psychiatr Clin North Am 2003;12:679-691.
14. Kumra S: The diagnosis and treatment of children and adolescents with schizophrenia. Child Adolesc Psychiatr Clin North Am 2000;9:183-199.
15. Adams M, Kutcher S, Antoniw E, Bird D: Diagnostic utility of endocrine and neuroimaging screening tests in first-onset adolescent psychosis. J Am Acad Child Adolesc Psychiatry 1996;35:67-73.
16. McGlashan TH: Adolescent versus adult onset of mania. Am J Psychiatry 1988;145:221-223.
17. Strober M, Schmidt-Lackner S, Freeman R, et al: Recovery and relapse in adolescents with bipolar affective illness: A five-year naturalistic, prospective follow-up. J Am Acad Child Adolesc Psychiatry 1995;34:724-731.
18. Jarbin H, Ott Y, Von Knorring AL: Adult outcome of social function in adolescent-onset schizophrenia and affective psychosis. J Am Acad Child Adolesc Psychiatry 2003;42:176-183.
19. Kutcher S (ed): Practical Child and Adolescent Psychopharmacology. Cambridge, Cambridge University Press, 2002.
20. American Psychiatric Association: Practice guidelines for the treatment of patients with schizophrenia, 2nd ed. Am J Psychiatry 2004;161(2 Suppl):1-56.
21. McClellan J, McCurry C, Snell J, DuBose A: Early-onset psychotic disorders: Course and outcome over a 2-year period. J Am Acad Child Adolesc Psychiatry 1999;38:1380-1388.
22. Rating scales and assessment instruments for use in pediatric psychopharmacology research. Psychopharmacol Bull 1985;21:1077-1080.
23. Arseneault L, Cannon M, Witton J, Murray RM: Causal association between cannabis and psychosis: Examination of the evidence. Br J Psychiatry 2004;184:110-117.

CHAPTER 170

Eating Disorders

Daniel H. Reirden and Donald F. Schwarz

Eating disorders are complex conditions that require the coordinated effort of a team of individuals—consisting of a physician (either the patient's primary care physician, if he or she is comfortable in that role, or a physician specializing in eating disorders), a nutritionist, and a mental health provider—for optimal management.[1] The course of treatment may extend for many years after the initial diagnosis.[2] Although most patients with eating disorders are managed in an outpatient setting, this chapter provides a framework for the general pediatric hospitalist to begin the initial management and stabilization of a patient with an eating disorder.

EPIDEMIOLOGY

Eating disorders are affecting adolescents with increasing frequency.[3] The three major subgroups of eating disorders are anorexia nervosa, bulimia nervosa, and eating disorder not otherwise specified (EDNOS).[3] Anorexia is further subdivided into a purely restrictive type and a binge-eating and purging type.[4] Anorexia is estimated to affect 1% of adolescents and young adults. Bulimia has a much higher prevalence, ranging from 1% to 19%. The prevalence of EDNOS has been estimated to be as high as 67% among college athletes.[5] Females account for the overwhelming majority of cases of anorexia nervosa and bulimia nervosa, but the disorders are also found in males. Males make up only a fraction of the cases of anorexia but may account for 15% of bulimia cases[6] and as many as 40% of cases of binge eating that do not meet the criteria for bulimia.[7] In the United States, most patients with eating disorders are from white families of middle to upper socioeconomic status; however, eating disorders occur in all races and socioeconomic strata.[7,8] These disorders appear to be the manifestation of a complex combination of developmental events.[9] Studies have suggested the contribution of genetic, neurochemical, psychodevelopmental, and sociocultural factors.[7]

CLINICAL PRESENTATION

A patient presenting with a refusal to maintain a minimally normal body weight should prompt a consideration of the diagnosis of anorexia nervosa. Bulimia nervosa classically presents as recurrent episodes of binge eating followed by unhealthy behaviors to avoid weight gain, such as induced vomiting or laxative use.[10] The consequences of the weight loss or purging activity are usually the entry point for hospitalization.

Anorexia Nervosa

For a patient with anorexia nervosa, failure to maintain a minimally acceptable body weight or recent rapid weight loss is the core of the clinical picture. There is an intense fear of weight gain and a relentless pursuit of thinness. There is often a history of overactivity or excessive exercise. Many patients also exhibit elaborate rituals pertaining to food or an intense interest in para-eating behaviors, such as collecting recipes or watching food-related television programs. Patients often have an unrealistic perception of their body image and display little concern over their weight loss, and they are often described as being excellent students or overachievers. Postmenarchal females with anorexia nervosa are amenorrheic. Patients may have some of the following physical complaints: early satiety; abdominal bloating, discomfort, or pain; nausea or vomiting; constipation; dizziness or fainting; cold intolerance; dry or yellow skin; fatigue, weakness, or muscle cramps.[4]

Bulimia Nervosa

The key distinguishing feature of bulimia nervosa is repeated episodes of binge eating. These episodes are characterized by (1) the consumption of an amount of food in a fixed period that is larger than what most people would eat and (2) a sense of loss of control over the eating episode. In response to an episode of bingeing, the individual often displays maladaptive behaviors to prevent weight gain. These behaviors take one of two forms:

1. Purging: the patient engages in self-induced vomiting or the use of laxatives, enemas, or diuretics.
2. Nonpurging: the patient engages in fasting or excessive exercise as compensatory methods.

An individual with bulimia is usually aware that his or her eating pattern is abnormal. The profound emaciation exhibited in anorexia is not found in the bulimic patient, and this

Table 170-1 Differential Diagnosis of Eating Disorders
Malignancy: central nervous system tumor
Gastrointestinal: inflammatory bowel disease, malabsorption, celiac disease
Endocrine: diabetes, thyroid disease, Addison disease, hypopituitarism
Psychiatric: depression, obsessive-compulsive disorder, other psychiatric diagnoses
Infectious: tuberculosis, HIV
Rheumatologic: collagen vascular disease

Adapted from American Academy of Pediatrics, Committee on Adolescence: Identifying and treating eating disorders. Pediatrics 2003;111:204-211.

Table 170-2 DSM-IV Criteria for Anorexia Nervosa
A. Refusal to maintain body weight at or above a minimally normal weight for age and height (e.g., weight loss leading to maintenance of body weight <85% of that expected or failure to make expected weight gain during period of growth, leading to body weight <85% of that expected).
B. Intense fear of gaining weight or becoming fat, even though underweight.
C. Disturbance in the way one's body weight or shape is experienced, undue influence of body weight or shape on self-evaluation, or denial of the seriousness of the current low body weight.
D. In postmenarchal females, amenorrhea (i.e., absence of at least three consecutive menstrual cycles). (A woman is considered to have amenorrhea if her periods occur only following hormone [e.g., estrogen] administration.)
Restricting type: During the current episode of anorexia nervosa, the person has not regularly engaged in binge-eating or purging behavior (i.e., self-induced vomiting or the misuse of laxatives, diuretics, or enemas).
Binge-eating–purging type: During the current episode of anorexia nervosa, the person has regularly engaged in binge-eating or purging behavior (i.e., self-induced vomiting or the misuse of laxatives, diuretics, or enemas).

Adapted from American Psychiatric Association: Diagnostic and Statistical Manual of Mental Disorders, 4th ed. Washington, DC, American Psychiatric Association, 1994.

can help distinguish an anorexic who purges from a bulimic individual.[4]

DIFFERENTIAL DIAGNOSIS

The initial assessment of a patient with a suspected eating disorder should be sufficiently complete to ensure that another cause of weight loss is not present. Table 170-1 provides a list of conditions that may present as an eating disorder.[11]

DIAGNOSIS AND EVALUATION

The starting point for the diagnosis of an eating disorder is generally found in the psychiatric literature. The diagnostic criteria for eating disorders are published in the fourth edition of the *Diagnostic and Statistical Manual of Mental Disorders* (DSM-IV; Tables 170-2 and 170-3).[12] In assessing an individual with a suspected eating disorder, the provider must first determine the patient's current weight, the history of weight loss (peak weight and rate of loss), and how the current weight compares with an ideal body weight.

There are several methods for determining how a patient's weight compares with an ideal body weight. One method is to use the patient's height as a starting point; then, using the growth charts published by the Centers for Disease Control and Prevention, determine the percentile value for the patient's height and compare his or her weight to the ideal weight for that percentile value. For example, a 16-year-old girl is 5 feet 6 inches (167 cm) tall and her weight is 100 pounds (45.5 kg). Her height corresponds to approximately the 25th percentile, and the value for weight that represents the 25th percentile for her age is 120 pounds (approximately 55 kg). Thus, the patient's actual weight of 45.5 kg is 83% of her ideal weight of 55 kg. For older adolescents who have presumably completed their growth, the body mass index may be a useful tool for assessing weight. Anorexia nervosa has been defined as a body mass index less than 17.5.[7]

It is important to note that formal weight criteria should be used only as guidelines when assessing pediatric patients. An eating disorder may initially appear when a child fails to make expected gains in growth parameters. The diagnosis should also be considered within the context of normal pubertal growth and adolescent development.[3]

The evaluation of a patient with a suspected eating disorder includes a complete history and physical examination. In addition to standard history questions, special attention should be paid to questions regarding dieting, body image, weight-control measures, and associated psychiatric conditions. Table 170-4 suggests pertinent questions for a patient with a suspected eating disorder,[11] and Table 170-5 lists the potential physical findings in a patient with an eating disorder.

The diagnosis of an eating disorder is a clinical diagnosis; one cannot perform a confirmatory laboratory test. However, some laboratory and ancillary testing may be indicated in the evaluation of a patient with an eating disorder (Table 170-6). The purpose of such testing is to exclude other disease processes, detect complications of purging or vomiting, and monitor the effects of nutritional rehabilitation. An erythrocyte sedimentation rate can be helpful in screening for chronic inflammatory diseases as the cause of weight loss. The erythrocyte sedimentation rate is characteristically low (usually <5) in patients with eating disorders. A higher value, even if within the normal range, should prompt a search for another diagnosis.[13] Laboratory values are often in the normal range, even in the presence of severe malnutrition. Hyponatremia may be present if the patient is practicing water loading (often accompanied by a low urine specific gravity). A patient who is vomiting frequently may have hypokalemia with elevated serum bicarbonate. A clue to laxative abuse may be a metabolic acidosis without an anion gap.[4] Electrocardiographic findings may include bradycardia

Table 170-3 DSM-IV Criteria for Bulimia Nervosa

A. Recurrent episodes of binge eating. An episode of binge eating is characterized by both of the following:
  1. Eating, in a discrete period (e.g., within any 2-hour period), an amount of food that is definitely larger than most people would eat in a similar period and under similar circumstances.
  2. A sense of lack of control over eating during the episode (e.g., a feeling that one cannot stop eating or control what or how much one is eating).

B. Recurrent inappropriate compensatory behavior to prevent weight gain, such as self-induced vomiting; misuse of laxatives, diuretics, enemas, or other medications; fasting; or excessive exercise.

C. The binge eating and inappropriate compensatory behaviors both occur, on average, at least twice a week for 3 months.

D. Self-evaluation is unduly influenced by body shape and weight.

E. The disturbance does not occur exclusively during episodes of anorexia nervosa.

Purging type: During the current episode of bulimia nervosa, the person has regularly engaged in self-induced vomiting or the misuse of laxatives, diuretics, or enemas.

Nonpurging type: During the current episode of bulimia nervosa, the person has used other inappropriate compensatory behaviors, such as fasting or excessive exercise, but has not regularly engaged in self-induced vomiting or the misuse of laxatives, diuretics, or enemas.

Adapted from American Psychiatric Association: Diagnostic and Statistical Manual of Mental Disorders, 4th ed. Washington, DC, American Psychiatric Association, 1994.

Table 170-4 Screening Questions for Patients with Suspected Eating Disorders

What is the most and least you have ever weighed, and when was that?

What do you think you ought to weigh?

How much do you exercise? Are you stressed if you miss a workout?

What is your self-image (thin or fat)? Are there any particular areas of your body that bother you?

What are your current dietary practices?
  24-hour diet history
  Taboo foods
  Binge eating—frequency and triggers
  Purging—frequency and triggers
  Use of diet pills, laxatives, or diuretics
  Vomiting
  Rituals around food preparation or eating

What is your past medical history?

Is there a family history of eating disorders, obesity, or mental illness?

What is your menstrual history—menarche, regularity, date of last menstrual period?

Do you have any social support systems?

Do you use cigarettes, drugs, or alcohol?

What is your sexual history?

Have you ever been abused physically or sexually?

Have you experienced any of the following (review of symptoms)?
  Dizziness, syncope, weakness, or fatigue
  Cold intolerance
  Fevers
  Vomiting, diarrhea, or constipation
  Abdominal or epigastric pain, bloating or fullness
  Hair loss, lanugo, or dry skin
  Pallor, bleeding, or bruising
  Chest pain or palpitations
  Muscle cramps or joint pain
  Menstrual irregularities

Adapted from Rome ES, Ammerman S, Rosen DS, et al: Children and adolescents with eating disorders: The state of the art. Pediatrics 2003;111:e98-e108.

or a prolonged Q-T interval in an anorexic or low-weight bulimic patient. These findings may exist even in the absence of abnormal serum electrolytes. Additional testing, such as computed tomography or magnetic resonance imaging of the head and a gastrointestinal or endocrine workup, should be performed if clinical suspicion warrants it.

TREATMENT

Eating disorders are complex and are ideally treated by a team of medical, nursing, nutrition, and mental health professionals. Clearly defining the role of each team member and the expectations of the patient can help avoid frustration for everyone involved. Many facilities that treat patients with eating disorders are using specific protocols. For example, clinicians from the Lucile Salter Packard Children's Hospital have published the first clinical pathway for treating anorexia nervosa in adolescents.[14] Table 170-7 provides treatment guidelines for a severe eating disorder that warrants inpatient admission.

MEDICAL COMPLICATIONS

Various organ systems can be adversely affected by eating disorders as a result of starvation, purging, or bingeing (Table 170-8).[5] Two important considerations for clinicians

in the inpatient setting are cardiac complications and refeeding syndrome.

Cardiac Complications

Both starvation and the electrolyte abnormalities induced by purging can lead to cardiac complications. Starvation can lead to decreased cardiac muscle, systolic dysfunction, and blood pressure changes. One third of patients with anorexia may have mitral valve prolapse secondary to wasted cardiac muscle.[5] Many of the cardiac vital sign changes are believed to be secondary to the decrease in basal metabolic rate

Table 170–5 Potential Physical Findings in Patients with Eating Disorders

Anorexia Nervosa	Bulimia Nervosa
Bradycardia	Bradycardia
Orthostasis	Orthostasis
Hypothermia	Hypothermia
Thinning scalp hair	Parotitis
Cardiac murmur (one third have mitral valve prolapse)	Russell sign*
Lanugo	Mouth sores
Sunken cheeks; sallow, yellowish skin	Dry skin
Pitting edema of extremities	Palatal or tonsillar pillar scratches
Flat affect	Dental enamel erosion
Cold extremities, acrocyanosis	

*Callused knuckles from inducing gagging or vomiting by pushing fingers down throat.
Adapted from American Academy of Pediatrics, Committee on Adolescence: Identifying and treating eating disorders. Pediatrics 2003;111:204-211.

Table 170–6 Laboratory Evaluation in Patients with Eating Disorders

Complete blood cell count
Erythrocyte sedimentation rate
Serum electrolytes with glucose
Blood urea nitrogen and creatinine
Serum calcium, magnesium, phosphorus concentrations
Liver tests: transaminases, albumin, prealbumin
Urinalysis with specific gravity

Table 170–7 Guidelines for Inpatient Treatment of Eating Disorders

Nursing staff is essential. Their approach should be firm yet supportive, and there should be no bargaining with the patient.
Nutrition is restored through food trays planned by a nutritionist, and the patient is expected to finish each meal.
Calories are provided through 3 meals and 3 snacks over the course of the day. In general, start at 1200-1500 calories/day and increase by 200 calories/day until the patient is gaining 0.2 kg/day; then increase by 200 calories every 2-3 days until the goal calorie level is achieved.
The patient must wear a hospital gown during meals, and all meals are supervised by a team member. Family members or friends are not allowed in the room during mealtimes, and distractions such as television or music are avoided.
The medical team monitors electrolytes and fluid shifts, cardiac status, and other potential medical complications.
The patient must rest for 1 hour after each meal; observation is maintained during this time.
The patient is allowed 30 minutes to finish each meal. If the patient is unable to do so, a nutritional supplement such as Boost may be used to attain the allotted calories. If patient is unable to comply with the nutritional supplement, a nasogastric tube is inserted, the nutritional supplement is provided by that means, and the tube is removed.
The patient is weighed daily in a hospital gown, and a urine specific gravity is obtained around that time.
During the initial phase of hospitalization, the patient must be closely monitored to avoid excess exercise or purging.
A member of the mental health team should be involved in the initial assessment to screen for comorbid psychiatric diagnoses and to provide ongoing care. Cognition is often limited in cases of severe malnutrition, and therapy may not begin until the patient's nutritional status improves.
Hospitalization should continue long enough for the patient to stop losing weight, establish a weight-gaining trend, normalize vital signs and laboratory studies, and be able to eat adequately.
Social workers and case managers should be available to help arrange for care outside the hospital, whether in an inpatient eating disorder facility, a partial hospitalization program, or outpatient treatment with adequate mental health, nutrition, and medical follow-up.

Adapted from Rome ES, Ammerman S, Rosen DS, et al: Children and adolescents with eating disorders: The state of the art. Pediatrics 2003;111:e98-e108.

brought on by reduced energy consumption.[5] A prolonged Q-Tc interval can be a harbinger of cardiac arrhythmias, and a baseline electrocardiogram is warranted to screen for this abnormality. Unlike earlier studies in adults, a study in adolescents did not find an association between prolonged Q-Tc and anorexia nervosa. The authors speculate that disease duration may be a factor, but they caution that the finding of a normal Q-Tc interval does not indicate less severe disease.[15]

Refeeding Syndrome

When an anorexic patient is provided with sufficient energy intake, the body shifts from the catabolic state of starvation to an anabolic state. It is during this time that the patient is at risk for refeeding syndrome, which is characterized by cardiovascular collapse and possible death; the condition may also be marked by fluid and electrolyte shifts and delirium.[16] Prolonged starvation results in a decreased level of total body phosphorus. When calories are added to the patient's diet, particularly glucose calories, there is a shift of extracellular phosphate to intracellular sites for incorporation into cell products. This may result in severely decreased

Table 170-8 Medical Complications of Eating Disorders

Starvation-Related Effects
Amenorrhea
Arrested growth
Atrophic vaginitis
Breast atrophy
Cardiac muscle wasting
Constipation
Cortical atrophy
Decreased antidiuretic hormone secretion
Delayed puberty
Hypercholesterolemia
Hypercortisolemia
Hypophosphatemia
Infertility
Osteopenia
Pancytopenia
Peripheral neuropathy
Vital sign abnormalities
  Bradycardia: pulse <50 beats/min daytime or <45 beats/min overnight
  Hypotension: systolic blood pressure <90 mm Hg or diastolic blood pressure <45 mm Hg
  Orthostatic blood pressure
  Hypothermia: temperature <36.3°C daytime or <36.0°C overnight

Purging-Related Effects
Cardiac arrhythmias
Chronic hypovolemia
Dental enamel erosion
Electrolyte abnormalities
Esophagitis
Mallory-Weiss tears
Parotid gland swelling
Pneumothorax or pneumomediastinum
Pseudo-Bartter syndrome
Renal calculi
Russell sign (callused knuckles from using fingers to induce vomiting)
Vital sign abnormalities

Bingeing-Related Effects
Esophageal rupture
Gastric rupture

Adapted from Rome ES, Ammerman S: Medical complications of eating disorders: An update. J Adolesc Health 2003;33:418-426; and Becker AD, Grinspoon SK, Klibanksi A, Herzog DB: Eating disorders. N Engl J Med 1999;340:1092-1098.

Table 170-9 Indications for Inpatient Admission

Severe malnutrition: body weight <75% of ideal weight

Significant hypovolemia or hypotension

Bradycardia (heart rate <45 beats/min)

Cardiac dysfunction or arrhythmia (e.g., prolonged Q-Tc interval)

Significant laboratory abnormalities
  Potassium <2 mmol/L
  Blood glucose <50 mg/dL

Intractable multiple bingeing or purging episodes per day

Failure of outpatient management (e.g., no weight gain, no reduction in bingeing or purging episodes, failure to keep appointments)

Suicidal thoughts or gestures

Adapted from The American Psychiatric Association Practice Guideline for the Treatment of Patients with Eating Disorders, 2nd ed. Washington, DC, American Psychiatric Association, 2000.

total body phosphorus stores, leading to cardiovascular collapse. A case series published in 1998 described the clinical manifestations of refeeding syndrome in three adolescent women.[17] Those affected were severely malnourished (<70% of ideal body weight), and the cardiac complications occurred in the first week. Delirium occurred later in the refeeding process, and interestingly, the repletion of serum phosphorus had less of an effect on correcting the delirium.

In general, refeeding syndrome can be prevented by slowly initiating caloric intake, ideally with the assistance of a registered dietitian to calculate the proper amounts. A patient can safely be started on 1500 calories/day, and this amount can be increased by 100 to 250 calories/day for each day that the patient does not gain 0.2 kg.[5] Serum electrolytes, including calcium, magnesium, and phosphorus, should be monitored on a daily basis. Oral phosphorus supplementation can be initiated during the first week of refeeding to help prevent complications.[5]

ADMISSION CRITERIA

Hospital admission of a patient with an eating disorder is occasionally necessary for initial diagnosis or if the patient fails an outpatient program. The goal of admission to a general pediatric service is stabilization of the patient's acute medical or nutritional needs. Treatment is directed at correcting and preventing the complications associated with abnormal weight loss; thus, admission is more often required for patients with anorexia nervosa.[7] Psychiatric risk factors may also precipitate admission, and mental health professionals should determine the most appropriate setting for this care. See Table 170-9 for indications for inpatient admission.

DISCHARGE CRITERIA

There is no established optimal length of hospitalization. Some data suggest that patients discharged closer to their ideal weight have a more favorable outcome.[18] When a patient with an eating disorder is discharged from an acute care hospital, it is essential to address his or her ongoing medical, nutritional, and mental health needs. This may require transfer directly to an inpatient facility that can provide the necessary expertise for a multidisciplinary approach. Another option is for patients to participate in intensive day programs coordinated through a single source. Alternatively, outpatient follow-up can be arranged with the experts on the team. This requires the identification of a coordinator who can ensure compliance, orchestrate communication among the specialists, and help the patient and family navigate the complex process.

IN A NUTSHELL

- The three major categories of eating disorders are anorexia nervosa, bulimia nervosa, and eating disorder not otherwise specified. The diagnostic criteria are published in DSM-IV.
- The role of inpatient clinicians is stabilization of the patient and establishment of the medical, nutritional, and mental health support needed during hospitalization and after discharge.
- Although there are many complications related to eating disorders, cardiac dysfunction and refeeding syndrome are the major considerations in the acute inpatient setting.

ON THE HORIZON

- Improved access to outpatient or inpatient eating disorder programs is needed after the acute hospitalization.
- With the increased recognition of early manifestations of eating disorders among younger children, age-appropriate treatment is required.
- Research into the societal influences that contribute to the growing prevalence of eating disorders is needed, as well as investigation of interventions that can prevent these disorders.

SUGGESTED READING

American Academy of Pediatrics, Committee on Adolescence: Identifying and treating eating disorders. Pediatrics 2003;111:204-211.

Becker AD, Grinspoon SK, Klibanski A, Herzog DB: Eating disorders. N Engl J Med 1999;340:1092-1098.

Golden NH, Katzman DK, Kreipe RE, et al: Eating disorders in adolescents: Position paper of the Society for Adolescent Medicine. J Adolesc Health 2003;33:496-503.

Rome ES, Ammerman S, Rosen DS, et al: Children and adolescents with eating disorders: The state of the art. Pediatrics 2003;111:e98-e108.

REFERENCES

1. Fisher M, Golden NH, Katzman DK, et al: Eating disorders in adolescents: A background paper. J Adolesc Health 1995;16:420-437.
2. Strober M, Freeman R, Morrell W: The long-term course of severe anorexia nervosa in adolescents: Survival analysis of recovery, relapse, and outcome predictors over 10-15 years in a prospective study. Int J Eat Disord 1997;22:339-360.
3. Golden NH, Katzman DK, Kreipe RE, et al: Eating disorders in adolescents: Position paper of the Society for Adolescent Medicine. J Adolesc Health 2003;33:496-503.
4. Neinstein LS, MacKenzie RG: Anorexia nervosa and bulimia nervosa. In Neinstein LS (ed): Adolescent Health Care: A Practical Guide, 4th ed. Philadelphia, Lippincott Williams & Wilkins, 2002, pp 700-726.
5. Rome ES, Ammerman S: Medical complications of eating disorders: An update. J Adolesc Health 2003;33:418-426.
6. Muise AM, Stein DG, Arbess G: Eating disorders in adolescent boys: A review of the adolescent and young adult literature. J Adolesc Health 2003;33:427-435.
7. Becker AD, Grinspoon SK, Klibanksi A, Herzog DB: Eating disorders. N Engl J Med 1999;340:1092-1098.
8. Kreipe RE, Dukarm CP: Eating disorders in adolescents and older children. Pediatr Rev 1999;20:410-421.
9. Rome ES, Ammerman S, Rosen DS, et al: Children and adolescents with eating disorders: The state of the art. Pediatrics 2003;111:e98-e108.
10. Klein DA, Walsh BT: Eating disorders: Clinical features and pathophysiology. Physiol Behav 2004;81:359-374.
11. American Academy of Pediatrics, Committee on Adolescence: Identifying and treating eating disorders. Pediatrics 2003;111:204-211.
12. American Psychiatric Association: Diagnostic and Statistical Manual of Mental Disorders, 4th ed. Washington, DC, American Psychiatric Association, 1994, pp 539-550, 729-731.
13. Seidenfeld MK, Sosin E, Rickert VI: Nutrition and eating disorders in adolescents. Mt Sinai J Med 2004;71:155-161.
14. Lock J: How clinical pathways can be useful: An example of a clinical pathway for the treatment of anorexia nervosa in adolescents. Clin Child Psychol Psychiatry 1999;4:331-340.
15. Panagiotopoulos C, McCrindle BW, Hick K, Katzman DK: Electrocardiographic findings in adolescents with eating disorders. Pediatrics 2000; 105:1100-1105.
16. Solomon SM, Kirby DF: The refeeding syndrome: A review. JPEN J Parenter Enteral Nutr 2000;14:90-97.
17. Kohn MR, Golden NH, Shenker IR: Cardiac arrest and delirium: Presentations of the refeeding syndrome in severely malnourished adolescents with anorexia nervosa. J Adolesc Health 1998;22:239-243.
18. Baran SA, Weltzin TE, Kaye WH: Low discharge weight and outcome in anorexia nervosa. Am J Psychiatry 1995;152:1070-1072.

CHAPTER 171

Sexually Transmitted Diseases

Stephanie B. Dewar

Sexually transmitted diseases (STDs) in adolescents encompass a wide variety of clinical conditions. Although diagnosis and management are handled predominantly in the outpatient setting, some illnesses warrant hospitalization. In addition, STDs may coexist with or are included in the differential diagnoses of other medical or surgical conditions of hospitalized patients.

A large number of sexually transmitted organisms can result in localized, regional, or systemic illness. This chapter focuses on the genitourinary or regional diseases that are transmitted sexually. A list of the organisms that cause primarily genitourinary disease is provided in Table 171-1. Human immunodeficiency virus (HIV) (Chapter 72) and hepatitis A, B, and C viruses (Chapter 68) are sexually transmitted organisms that result in systemic illness; they are not addressed in this chapter. There are approximately 15 million new cases of STDs in the United States each year, with the majority of these infections occurring among people younger than 25 years. The most common sexually transmitted infection in the United States is anogenital human papillomavirus, with up to 40% of sexually active teenage girls affected. Chlamydia is the most common bacterial STD, with an estimated 3 million new cases each year; infection rates are especially high in teenagers. The STD infection rate in sexually active girls between the ages of 15 and 19 is up to 10 times the rate among women aged 30 to 34. Adolescent populations that are at particularly high risk for STDs include youth in detention facilities, STD clinic patients, male homosexuals, and injection-drug users.

Sexually active adolescents are especially prone to infection with gonorrhea and chlamydia. The smaller introitus of the adolescent female makes it more susceptible to trauma and the exchange of body fluids during intercourse. The cervix is relatively immature, with mucosal tissue (columnar epithelium) lining the canal instead of the squamous epithelium seen in older women, further predisposing young women to infection. Adolescents who have been sexually active for only a short time are less likely to have partial protective immunity from prior infections. Adolescents are also less likely to plan ahead for consistent and responsible condom use and are less likely to schedule routine visits for asymptomatic screening.

The diagnosis of one STD in an adolescent makes infection with other STDs more likely. Any diagnosis of an STD in a child should prompt an evaluation for possible sexual abuse.

CLINICAL PRESENTATION

Although most sexually transmitted diseases in adolescents are asymptomatic, some specific disease entities present with the following signs and symptoms.

Women

Vaginitis may present with a vaginal odor, vaginal discharge, or vulval itching and irritation. The most common infectious agent is *Trichomonas vaginalis*. Bacterial vaginosis and candidiasis are seen in sexually active females but are not thought to be sexually transmitted. Clinical features of the most common infections are listed in Table 171-2.

Mucopurulent cervicitis is characterized by a purulent or mucopurulent endocervical exudate that is visible in the endocervical canal or on an endocervical swab specimen. Easily induced cervical bleeding is evident. Patients may also report vaginal discharge and bleeding, especially after intercourse. Gonococcal (*Neisseria gonorrhoeae*) and chlamydial infections are the most common causes. Trichomoniasis is associated with a classic "strawberry cervix," with pinpoint hemorrhagic lesions and friabilitiy, often accompanied by a foamy, grayish yellow discharge with a musty odor.

Pelvic inflammatory disease (PID) is an infection of the upper genital tract in females; included entities are endometritis, salpingitis, tubo-ovarian abscess, peritonitis, and perihepatitis (Fitz-Hugh–Curtis syndrome). PID is most often caused by untreated chlamydial and gonococcal infections, although uncommonly, vaginal flora may cause this infection. PID can be difficult to diagnose owing to the wide range of symptoms, which may be absent, vague, or nonspecific. An "acute" or "surgical" abdomen with peritoneal signs may be present, along with McBurney point tenderness when the infection involves predominantly right-sided structures. A thorough history, physical examination, and routine laboratory studies cannot reliably detect PID or exclude the diagnosis. The diagnostic criteria for suspected, likely, and definite PID are provided in Table 171-3. Empirical treatment is recommended for sexually active young women with suspected PID, even those who meet the minimum criteria.[1]

Both Genders

Urethritis is characterized by urethral discharge of mucopurulent or purulent material and sometimes by dysuria or urethral pruritus. Gonococcus and chlamydia are the principal bacterial pathogens responsible. *T. vaginalis* and herpes simplex virus (HSV) can also cause urethritis, either in isolation or as part of a more proximal genitourinary infection. Reiter syndrome (arthritis, urethritis, and bilateral conjunctivitis) is thought to be a reactive inflammatory condition that may follow chlamydial infection.

Pharyngitis may result from primary gonococcal or chlamydial infection. Although patients are usually asymptomatic, both infections may present with throat pain, dysphagia, erythema of the posterior pharynx, or cervical adenopathy. Gonococcal infection can cause an exudative tonsillopharyingitis.[2,3] It is very uncommon for the pharynx to be the sole locus of infection, so it is prudent to evaluate for anourogenital disease as well.

Ulcers or vesicles of the genital organs or perineum in sexually active teenagers are most commonly caused by HSV, with HSV 2 infections outnumbering HSV 1 by approximately 2:1. The lesions are painful, and with primary infection, there is often systemic illness with fever, myalgias, and malaise. Other important ulcer-forming infections include syphilis, chancroid, lymphogranuloma venereum, and granuloma inguinale. The clinical features are detailed in Table 171-4.

Anogenital warts (condylomata acuminata) may present as skin-colored flat or papillary lesions with a cauliflower or frondlike appearance. They range in size from a few millimeters to several centimeters and may be found on the penis, scrotum, anal area, perianal area, vulva, vagina, or cervix. Patients are usually asymptomatic, but the lesions are easily visualized, which often prompts patients to seek medical attention. If the warts become irritated, they may cause itching, burning, local pain, or bleeding.

Anorectal infections may be seen in patients who engage in receptive anal intercourse. These infections manifest as proctitis, which is limited to the rectum and is associated with anorectal pain, tenesmus, or rectal discharge; proctocolitis, which has the additional symptoms of diarrhea and abdominal cramps; or enteritis, which manifests as abdominal cramping and diarrhea without evidence of proctitis or proctocolitis. The most common causative organisms in proctitis are gonococci, *Chlamydia trachomatis*, *Treponema pallidum*, and HSV. *Campylobacter* species, *Shigella* species, and *Entamoeba histolytica* cause proctocolitis, and *Giardia lamblia* is the most common cause of enteritis.[1]

Disseminated (systemic) gonococcal infection is also known as acute arthritis and dermatitis syndrome. The nongenital sites of infection are seeded hematogenously from a preceding gonococcal bacteremia. The most common findings include arthritis, tenosynovitis, dermatitis, and, uncommonly, endocarditis, meningitis, and hepatitis. The classic skin findings are pustules on an erythematous base that are

Table 171-1 Sexually Transmitted Diseases by Organism

Organism	Clinical Illness
Chlamydia trachomatis	Urethritis, epididymitis, proctitis, cervicitis, pharyngitis, pelvic inflammatory disease, lymphogranuloma venereum
Neisseria gonorrhoeae	Urethritis, epididymitis, proctitis, cervicitis, pharyngitis, pelvic inflammatory disease, disseminated infection, septic or reactive arthritis
Trichomonas vaginalis	Vaginitis, urethritis
Treponema pallidum	Syphilis: primary chancre or ulcer, secondary, tertiary, and neurosyphilis
Haemophilus ducreyi	Chancroid
Calymmatobacterium granulomatis	Granuloma inguinale
Herpes simplex viruses	Genital, oral, rectoanal ulcerations and vesicles; "flulike" illness with primary infection
Human papillomavirus	Condyloma acuminatum

Table 171-2 Features of Vaginitis

Organism	Appearance of Discharge	pH of Vaginal Fluid	Microscopic Findings
Trichomoniasis	Frothy, purulent, yellow-green, profuse	>4.5	Flagellated organisms, WBCs
Bacterial vaginosis	Thin, homogeneous, gray-white	>4.5	"Clue" cells; positive whiff test with addition of KOH
Vulvovaginal candidiasis	Thick, "cottage cheesy," adherent, white	4-4.5	Budding yeast and hyphae on KOH preparation

KOH, 10% potassium hydroxide solution; WBCs, white blood cells.

Table 171-3 Criteria for the Diagnosis of Pelvic Inflammatory Disease (PID)

Suspected PID	Likely PID	Definite PID
Lower abdominal tenderness Adnexal tenderness Cervical motion tenderness	Those listed under "Suspected" plus: Fever (>38.3°C) Abnormal vaginal or cervical discharge Elevated ESR or CRP Laboratory evidence of gonococcal or *Chlamydia trachomatis* cervicitis	Those listed under "Suspected" and "Likely" plus: Histopathologic evidence of endometritis on endometrial biopsy Pelvic imaging that demonstrates thickened, fluid-filled fallopian tubes or tubo-ovarian abscess Laparoscopic abnormalities consistent with PID

CRP, C-reactive protein; ESR, erythrocyte sedimentation rate.
Adapted from Centers for Disease Control and Prevention: 1998 Guidelines for treatment of sexually transmitted diseases. MMWR Recomm Rep 1997;47(RR-1):80.

Table 171-4 Clinical Features of Genital Ulcerative Syndromes

| Illness (Pathogen) | FEATURES OF ULCERS | | | |
	Site	*No. of Lesions*	*Pain*	*Inguinal Adenopathy*
Herpes simplex virus (HSV 1 and 2)	Male: penile glans, prepuce Female: cervix (primary); vulva, perineum, buttocks (recurrent); anus, rectum (either)	Multiple; can coalesce	Common	Firm, tender, often bilateral
Syphilis (*Treponema pallidum*)	Site of inoculation	Usually single	Not usual	Firm, nontender, bilateral
Chancroid (*Haemophilus ducreyi*)	Site of inoculation	Often multiple; can coalesce	Usually very tender	Tender, can suppurate; unilateral; superinfection
Lymphogranuloma venereum (*Chlamydia trachomatis*)	Site of inoculation	Usually single	Variable	Tender, can suppurate; unilateral
Granuloma inguinale (*Calymmatobacterium granulomatis*)	Site of inoculation	Single or multiple	Not usual	Pseudobuboes; regional lymphadenopathy with superinfection

Adapted from McDonald NE, Patrick DM: Sexually transmitted disease syndromes. In Long SS, Pickering LK, Prober CG (eds): Principles and Practices of Pediatric Infectious Diseases, 2nd ed. New York, Churchill Livingstone, 2003, p 340.

Table 171-5 Signs and Symptoms of Syphilis by Stage of Infection

Primary	Secondary	Tertiary
Incubation period: 1-4 wk Painless ulcer or chancre at inoculation site Lesion resolves in 3-6 wk*	Begins after 6-12 wk Rash: salmon-pink macules progress to copper-colored papules; evolves centrifugally, eventually involving palms and soles Adenopathy: generalized, painless Mucosa: grayish patches Condyloma latum: broad, flat macules, especially on vulva, scrotum, anus, axilla Constitutional: fever, malaise, myalgias, sore throat Other: patchy alopecia, arthritis, osteitis, gastritis, hepatitis, splenomegaly, nephrotic syndrome Resolution in 1-3 mo*	Cardiac Occurs 10-40 yr after infection Aneurysm of ascending aorta ± aortic insufficiency Neurologic Can occur 3 mo to 30 yr after infection Meningeal: cranial nerve palsies, sensorineural deafness, hydrocephalus Meningovascular: endarteritis leading to stroke Tabes dorsalis: demyelination of posterior columns, roots of spinal cord leading to large joint destruction (Charcot joint), incontinence, ataxia, hyporeflexia General paresis: progressive loss of cognitive functions Asymptomatic: cerebrospinal fluid abnormalities without signs or symptoms Late benign Destructive gummas (granulomas) form after 1-10 yr May involve skin, respiratory tract, gastrointestinal tract, bones Nocturnal pain is characteristic

*Even without treatment.

tender and show evidence of necrosis. The distribution favors the distal upper extremities.

Syphilis can present in any of the three symptomatic phases of the illness (primary, secondary, and tertiary) or may be detected during the asymptomatic latent phase. The clinical findings in the different stages of syphilis are provided in Table 171-5. The asymptomatic latent phase is considered "early" if the infection was acquired within the preceding year; otherwise, it is classified as "late" latent

(acquired >1 year previously) or syphilis of unknown duration. During the latent phase, patients are noninfectious except for transplacental transmission from mother to fetus.

Men

Epididymitis presents with unilateral testicular pain and tenderness, hydrocele, and palpable swelling of the epididymis. Symptoms of urethritis often accompany or precede the epididymal infection.[4] As with urethritis, the most common pathogens are *C. trachomatis* and gonococci, with *Ureaplasma urealyticum* the next most likely.[5]

DIFFERENTIAL DIAGNOSIS

In patients presenting with vaginitis, one might also consider candidiasis, bacterial vaginosis, foreign body, or accidental trauma.

When considering the diagnosis of PID, the following are considered: appendicitis, vaginal foreign body, trauma, pyelonephritis, enteritis, cholecystitis, mesenteric lymphadenitis, pelvic thrombophlebitis, pregnancy (intrauterine or ectopic), ovarian cyst or torsion, endometriosis, teratoma or other mass, and chronic pelvic pain secondary to adhesions from previous infection or prior surgery.

Epididymitis might be confused with testicular torsion, testicular infarction, or abscess.

The differential diagnosis for disseminated gonococcal infection includes hematogenously seeded infections from other bacteria, including *Neisseria meningitidis, Staphylococcus aureus, Streptococcus pneumoniae, Salmonella* species, and *Stretpococcus pyogenes.*

Syphilis is included in the differential diagnosis of a host of disorders. Primary syphilis is a consideration in all patients with ulcerative genital lesions. The rash of secondary syphilis may resemble pityriasis rosea, drug eruptions, viral exanthems (e.g., hand-foot-and-mouth disease secondary to coxsackievirus), and many other papulosquamous cutaneous disorders. Condyloma latum may be confused with condyloma acuminatum, and the mucosal patches may resemble thrush. Tertiary syphilis is a consideration in a wide range of cardiovascular, cerebrovascular, encephalopathic, and progressive spinal cord processes.

EVALUATION

Most STDs are diagnosed and treated as a result of routine screening of asymptomatic sexually active patients in the outpatient setting. All symptomatic adolescents require a full genital examination, and screening for other STDs is a warranted.

The measurement of pH and microscopic examination of vaginal discharge with saline and 10% potassium hydroxide solution (KOH) can identify the cause of most cases of vaginitis (see Table 171-2). The presence of "clue" cells is particularly helpful in the diagnosis of bacterial vaginosis; they represent the epithelial cells that are studded with bacteria on their surface. With vaginosis, the "whiff" test may be positive; this is an amine odor from the vaginal fluid on the KOH preparation. With trichomoniasis, the whipping of the flagella and motility of the trichomonad are diagnostic; therefore, culture or immunofluorescence for *Trichomonas* is generally not required.

Definitive diagnosis of gonococcal and chlamydial infection can be made by isolation of the organism in culture. Swabs for gonococcal culture must be plated on nonselective chocolate agar with incubation in 5% to 10% carbon dioxide. Gram stain of urethral or cervical discharge may reveal the gram-negative intracellular diplococci of gonorrhea. An increased number of polymorphonuclear leukocytes may be evident on Gram stain of cervical or urethral discharge. Tests detecting chlamydial antigen (enzyme immunoassays, direct fluorescent antibody, DNA probe tests, and nucleic acid amplification tests) are useful for the evaluation of urethral swab specimens from males and endocervical swab specimens from females but are not approved for use on pharyngeal or anal samples. Nucleic acid amplification tests such as polymerase chain reaction, ligase chain reaction, and others are more sensitive than cell culture, DNA probe, direct fluorescent antibody, and enzyme immunoassays for the detection of chlamydia; they can be used to screen urine samples from either sex to diagnose chlamydia and gonorrhea. Some authorities recommend obtaining at least two bacteriologic tests involving different principles to confirm a diagnosis of gonococcus or chlamydia if a positive culture is not available.

The diagnosis of disseminated gonococcal infection is suggested by the clinical picture and is confirmed by isolation of the organism, most reliably from urethral or anogenital mucosa. Less than 50% of patients have positive culture from blood, skin lesions, or other sterile sites.[5]

A diagnosis of PID is based largely on the clinical presentation as described earlier. Definitive diagnosis requires biopsy, imaging, or laparoscopic testing (see Table 171-3). Negative endocervical culture does not preclude upper reproductive tract infection.

All patients presenting with genital ulcers should be tested for syphilis and herpes, and if chancroid is prevalent, a culture for *Haemophilus ducreyi* should be performed. A definitive diagnosis of syphilis can be made with a darkfield examination or direct immunofluorescent antibody testing of lesion exudate. Screening for syphilis is done with a nontreponemal test, either rapid plasma reagin (RPR) or VDRL (Venereal Disease Research Laboratory). A presumptive diagnosis can be established with a treponemal test such as fluorescent treponemal antibody absorption (FTA-ABS) or *T. pallidum* particle agglutination (TP-PA). False positives may occur with FTA-ABS and TP-PA in patients infected with other spirochetal diseases such as yaws, pinta, leptospirosis, rat-bite fever, relapsing fever, and Lyme disease. The VDRL is negative in Lyme disease. Isolation of HSV in culture from infected lesions is the preferred method of diagnosis and is much more reliable when obtained from vesicular lesions compared with crusted lesions. Direct immunofluorescent staining is a rapid test that is preferred over a Tzanck test. The high specificity and sensitivity and increasing availability of polymerase chain reaction techniques make detection by this method possible in many cases. Type-specific serologic tests may be helpful in diagnosing unrecognized infection.

Most anogenital warts are diagnosed through clinical inspection. Specific identification may be made through Papanicolaou smear or biopsy of lesions, but this is generally not necessary.

TREATMENT

Treatment should be guided by the results of diagnostic testing and the clinical syndrome. All sexual partners of persons diagnosed with gonorrhea, chlamydia, trichomoniasis, and PID within the past 60 days, or the most recent partner if it has been longer than 60 days, should be notified and offered treatment. Patients should abstain from sexual

Table 171-6 Treatment of Uncomplicated and Complicated Gonococcal Infections

Uncomplicated: Cervicitis, Urethritis, Proctitis, Conjunctivitis, Pharyngitis
Ceftriaxone 125 mg IM × 1
or
Ciprofloxacin 500 mg PO × 1
or
Ofloxacin 400 mg PO × 1
plus (to treat undiagnosed *Chlamydia*)
Azithromycin 1 g PO × 1
or
Doxycycline 100 mg PO bid × 7 days

Complicated*: Disseminated Gonococcal Infection
Ceftriaxone 1 g IV daily
or
Spectinomycin 2 g IV bid
Continue for at least 24-48 hr after evidence of clinical improvement, then switch to one of the following to complete a 7-day course:
Cefixime 400 mg PO bid
or
Ciprofloxacin 500 mg PO bid

*See Table 171-7 for the treatment of pelvic inflammatory disease.

Table 171-7 Treatment of Pelvic Inflammatory Disease

Inpatient	Ambulatory
Regimen A	**Regimen A**
Cefotetan 2 g IV q12h	Ofloxacin 400 mg PO bid × 14 days
or	with or without
Cefoxitin 2 g IV q6h until improvement	Metronidazole 500 mg PO bid × 14 days
plus	
Doxycycline 100 mg PO or IV q12h × 14 days	
Regimen B	**Regimen B**
Clindamycin 900 mg IV q8h	Ceftriaxone 250 mg IM once
plus	or
Gentamicin IV or IM 2 mg/kg loading dose, then 1.5 mg/kg q8h	Cefoxitin 2 g IM plus probenecid 1 g PO in a single dose
	or
	Other IV third-generation cephalosporin
	plus
	Doxycycline 100 mg PO bid × 14 days with or without
	Metronidazole 500 mg PO bid × 14 days

intercourse for at least 7 days, until treatment is complete and they are asymptomatic. Patients generally do not need follow-up evaluations if the recommended regimen has been followed, unless they are persistently symptomatic or symptoms recur.

Metronidazole is an effective treatment for both trichomoniasis and bacterial vaginosis.

The treatment of gonorrhea is evolving as a result of the increasing resistance to β-lactams and the emerging resistance to fluoroquinolones (especially in Hawaii, California, Asia, and the Pacific). Parenteral ceftriaxone remains the drug of choice for uncomplicated gonococcal infections. An oral third-generation cephalosporin is an alternative when available. Azithromycin as a single oral dose is effective but has not been recommended because of its cost and the frequency of gastrointestinal intolerance. Complicated gonococcal infections such as arthritis, meningitis, or endocarditis require longer therapy at higher doses (Table 171-6). Treatment of PID is detailed in Table 171-7. Either doxycycline or azithromycin can be used for uncomplicated chlamydial infections of the genital tract. Longer treatment is required for lymphogranuloma venereum. Patients who present with mucopurulent cervicitis or urethritis should be treated for both gonococcus and chlamydia because of the high rates of coinfection.

Most patients with primary genital herpes eruption should receive antiviral therapy. Acyclovir decreases the duration of symptoms and viral shedding and should be initiated within 6 days of the eruption of lesions. Topical therapy is not recommended. For patients with recurrent lesions, acyclovir can be administered either episodically (within 2 days of the onset of symptoms) or, for suppressive therapy, continuously (if the patient is experiencing six or more recurrences a year).

Parenteral penicillin G is the mainstay of therapy for *T. pallidum* infections. Recommendations for dosage and duration of therapy vary, depending on the stage of disease and the clinical manifestations (Table 171-8).

Topical regimens are available for the treatment of human papillomavirus, including podofilox 0.5% solution or gel or imiquimod 5% cream applied by the patient. Provider-administered therapy includes cryotherapy, topical podophyllum resin 10% to 25%, trichloroacetic acid, dichloroacetic acid 80% to 90%, and surgical removal.

ADMISSION CRITERIA

Most patients with STDs do not require hospitalization; however, those with a toxic appearance and those unlikely to comply with therapy should be admitted. If urgent or emergent surgical intervention is a consideration (e.g., acute abdomen, testicular torsion), evaluation and observation should be performed as an inpatient.

Patients with disseminated gonococcal infection warrant admission for intravenous therapy until clinical improvement is demonstrated. Disseminated HSV infections such as pneumonitis, hepatitis, or complications of the central nervous system also require inpatient admission and therapy.

Hospitalization is recommended by the Centers for Disease Control and Prevention for women with PID who meet the following criteria:

● May have a condition requiring emergent surgery, such as appendicitis.
● Do not respond clinically to oral antimicrobial therapy.
● Are unable to follow or tolerate an oral outpatient regimen.

Table 171–8   Specific Therapy by Organism

Pathogen	Treatment*
Chlamydia trachomatis	Children <8 yr: <45 kg: erythromycin base 50 mg/kg/day PO divided qid × 10-14 days ≥45 kg: azithromycin 1 g PO × 1 Children ≥8 yr: Azithromycin 1 g PO × 1 or Doxycycline 100 mg PO bid × 7 days (21 days for LGV)
Trichomonas vaginalis	Metronidazole 2 g PO in a single dose or Metronidazole 500 mg PO bid × 7 days
Mixed organisms of bacterial vaginosis (including anaerobes, *Gardnerella vaginalis,* mycoplasmas)	Metronidazole 500 mg PO bid × 7 days or Metronidazole 2 g PO × 1 or 0.75% Metronidazole gel 5 g (1 applicator full) intravaginally bid × 5 days or 2% Clindamycin cream 5 g (1 applicator full) intravaginally at bedtime × 7 days or Clindamycin 300 mg PO bid × 7 days
Calymmatobacterium granulomatis	Trimethoprim-sulfamethoxazole 1 double-strength tablet PO bid × at least 3 wk or Doxycycline 100 mg PO bid × at least 3 wk or Ciprofloxacin 750 mg PO bid × at least 3 wk or Erythromycin base 500 mg PO qid × at least 3 wk
Haemophilus ducreyi	Azithromycin 1 g PO × 1 or Ceftriaxone 250 mg IM × 1 or Ciprofloxacin 500 mg PO bid × 3 days or Erythromycin base 500 mg PO qid × 7 days
Herpes simplex virus	Primary: Acyclovir 400 mg PO tid × 7-10 days or Acyclovir 200 mg PO 5 times/day × 7-10 days or Famciclovir 250 mg PO tid × 7-10 days or Valacyclovir 1 g PO bid × 7-10 days Recurrence: Acyclovir 400 mg PO tid × 5 days or Acyclovir 200 mg PO 5 times/day × 5 days or Acyclovir 800 mg PO bid × 5 days or Famciclovir 125 mg PO bid × 5 days or Valacyclovir 500 mg PO bid × 5 days Suppressive: Acyclovir 400 mg PO bid daily continuously or Famciclovir 250 mg PO bid daily continuously

Table 171-8 Specific Therapy by Organism—cont'd	
Pathogen	Treatment*
	or
	Valacyclovir 500-1000 mg PO daily
	Severe disease (disseminated, pneumonitis, hepatitis, central nervous system):
	Acyclovir 5-10 mg/kg IV q8h × 5-7 days
Treponema pallidum	Primary, secondary, early latent syphilis:
	Penicillin G benzathine 50,000 units/kg (max 2.4 million units) IM × 1
	or
	Doxycycline 100 mg PO bid × 14 days
	Late latent, disease of unknown duration, tertiary syphilis:
	Penicillin G benzathine 50,000 units/kg (max 2.4 million units) IM weekly × 3
	or
	Doxycycline 100 mg PO bid × 4 wk
	Neurosyphilis:
	Aqueous crystalline penicillin G 200,000-400,000 units/kg/day IM divided q4h × 10-14 days (max 18-24 million units/day divided q4h)
	or
	Procaine penicillin 2.4 million units IM daily and probenecid 500 mg PO qid, both × 10-14 days

*See Table 171-6 for the treatment of uncomplicated and dissmeminated gonococcal infections and Table 171-7 for the treatment of pelvic inflammatory disease.

LGV, lymphogranuloma venereum.

Dosing information from Centers for Disease Control and Prevention: 1998 Guidelines for treatment of sexually transmitted diseases. MMWR Recomm Rep 1997;47(RR-1).

- Have severe illness, nausea, vomiting, or high fever.
- Have a tubo-ovarian abscess.
- Are pregnant.

DISCHARGE CRITERIA

Patients may be discharged when they are able to tolerate and comply with an oral regimen or are clinically improved from a systemic infection.

PREVENTION

The most reliable way to avoid transmission of STDs is to abstain from sexual intercourse (oral, anal, or vaginal) or to be in a long-term, mutually monogamous relationship with an uninfected partner. Consistent use of condoms may decrease the transmission of STDs. Currently, only hepatitis B infection can be avoided through the use of routine immunization. The spread of infection may be reduced through the routine screening of asymptomatic sexually active teens.

IN A NUTSHELL

- Most STDs are managed in the outpatient setting, but hospitalization may be warranted for systemic illness, toxic appearance, potential need for urgent surgical intervention, or poor compliance.
- The presentation of STDs in adolescents is highly variable, from asymptomatic to specific clinical syndromes.

- Diagnosis is organism and symptom specific. Culture is the gold standard for most infections, but more rapid tests such as DNA probes, enzyme immunoassays, and nuclei acid amplification tests are available.
- Treatment is specific to the infecting organism or clinical syndrome.

ON THE HORIZON

- Improved, more affordable, less invasive diagnostic tests such as polymerase chain reaction, strand-displacement amplification, or transcription-mediated amplification will become available for the detection of chlamydia, gonococcal infection, HIV, and hepatitis, among others.
- New vaccines are being developed to prevent hepatitis C and HIV.
- Expect expanding resistance of gonococci against fluoroquinolones.

SUGGESTED READING

American Academy of Pediatrics: *Chlamydia trachomatis,* gonococcal infections, herpes simplex. In Pickering LD (ed): Red Book: 2003 Report of the Committee on Infectious Diseases, 26th ed. Elk Grove Village, Ill, American Academy of Pediatrics, 2003, pp 238-243, 285-291, 344-353.

Centers for Disease Control and Prevention: Oral alternatives to cefixime for the treatment of uncomplicated *Neisseria gonorrhoeae* urogenital infections. MMWR 2002. http://www.cdc.gov/std/treatment/Cefixime/htm.

Centers for Disease Control and Prevention: Sexually transmitted disease treatment guidelines 2002. MMWR Recomm Rep 2002;51(RR-6):1-73.

REFERENCES

1. Centers for Disease Control and Prevention: 1998 Guidelines for treatment of sexually transmitted diseases. MMWR Recomm Rep 1997;47(RR-1).

2. Weisner PJ, Tronca E, Bonin P, et al: Clinical spectrum of pharyngeal gonococcal infections. N Engl J Med 1973;288:181.

3. Tice AW, Rodriguez VL: Pharygeal gonorrhea. JAMA 1981;246:2717.

4. Martin DH, Bowie WR: Urethritis in males. In Holmes KK, Sparling PF, Mardh P-E, et al (eds): Sexually Transmitted Diseases, 3rd ed. New York, McGraw-Hill, 1999, pp 833-845.

5. Woodin KA: *Neisseria gonorrhoeae.* In Long SS, Pickering LK, Prober CG (eds): Principles and Practices of Pediatric Infectious Diseases. New York, Churchill Livingstone, 1997, pp 847-848.

CHAPTER 172

Dysfunctional Uterine Bleeding

Leonard J. Levine and Donald F. Schwarz

Dysfunctional uterine bleeding (DUB) is defined as bleeding from the uterine endometrium that is not related to an anatomic lesion of the uterus.[1,2] Abnormal uterine bleeding includes menstrual cycles that occur less than 21 or more than 45 days apart, bleeding that lasts more than 8 days, or blood loss greater than 80 mL.[1,3-8] DUB can present as heavy and prolonged bleeding with associated periods of amenorrhea or frequent and excessive bleeding that occurs every 1 to 2 weeks.[9]

Immaturity of the hypothalamic-pituitary-ovarian (HPO) axis, resulting in anovulatory cycles, is the most common cause of DUB in adolescents. Until this axis is fully mature, ovulation may not occur each month. In fact, ovulation is associated with only 50% of menstrual cycles 1 year after menarche and 80% at 2 years.[3,5,7] Without ovulation, there is no corpus luteum or associated progesterone secretion to provide stromal support to an endometrium continuously stimulated by estrogen. As a result, proliferation of the vascular and glandular endometrial elements is unopposed. Menstrual cycles can appear normal because increased estrogen levels provide feedback to the hypothalamic-pituitary axis to inhibit the release of gonadotropins; this decreases estrogen levels, causing cyclic, controlled bleeding. When there are problems with this negative feedback system, the estrogen levels cannot suppress gonadotropin release or the continued production of estrogen, leading to irregular or heavy bleeding. The endometrium, which continues to grow and thicken under the influence of unopposed estrogen, eventually breaks down in an irregular and often prolonged manner. As the endometrium outgrows its blood supply, there is variable shedding, necrosis, and withdrawal bleeding, with inadequate hemostasis and menorrhagia.[3,7]

Although pubertal immaturity of the HPO axis is the most common cause of DUB, other organic causes should be considered when confronted with an adolescent with vaginal bleeding.[3,7]

CLINICAL PRESENTATION

An adolescent with menstrual irregularities secondary to anovulatory cycles may have a normal clinical presentation if her hemoglobin has not been dramatically affected. However, blood loss leading to anemia can cause pallor, dizziness, lightheadedness, fatigue, and even hemodynamic instability. Heavy, irregular bleeding can also cause psychological distress in a young adolescent, limiting her activity and perhaps even interfering with school attendance. Vaginal bleeding due to organic causes other than anovulatory cycles usually presents with signs and symptoms consistent with the underlying disorder (see subsequent sections).

DIFFERENTIAL DIAGNOSIS

Although 75% to 80% of abnormal menses in adolescent females can be attributed to anovulatory cycles,[1,5] it is important to rule out other organic causes for irregular or heavy vaginal bleeding. The source of bleeding can be the lower reproductive tract (vagina) or upper reproductive tract organs (uterus, fallopian tubes). The most important diagnosis to consider in an adolescent with vaginal bleeding is pregnancy. Other possibilities include infectious,[5,10,11] hematologic,[12,13] or endocrinologic[14-19] causes, as well as trauma, retained foreign body, systemic or chronic disease,[20,21] medication effects, structural pathology, and endometriosis (Box 172-1). These disorders can lead to bleeding via inflammation of the vaginal or uterine lining, interference with hemostasis, direct trauma, or disruption of the HPO axis.

EVALUATION

The evaluation of an adolescent who presents with abnormal or heavy vaginal bleeding should focus on assessing the patient's hemodynamic stability and degree of anemia and ruling out underlying causes other than anovulatory cycles. A menstrual history should include age of menarche, interval between menses, duration and amount of menstrual flow, and presence or absence of cramping. Uterine cramping, caused by progesterone secreted from the corpus luteum, can serve as a marker of ovulatory cycles. It can be helpful to determine whether cyclic intervals are normal with increased bleeding during each cycle (e.g., bleeding disorder), normal with bleeding between cycles (e.g., trauma, foreign body), or abnormal with no cycle regularity (e.g., anovulatory cycles, endocrinopathy, hormonal contraception). Other key elements of the history include the amount of bleeding (best estimated by how often tampons or pads need to be changed), recent sexual activity, abdominal pain, trauma, masturbation with a foreign object, history of abuse, dizziness or lightheadedness (suggestive of anemia), and history of easy bruising or bleeding. The review of systems should also include recent weight changes, headaches, visual disturbances, nipple discharge, hirsutism, and symptoms associated with thyroid disorders (e.g., diarrhea or constipation, palpitations, heat or cold intolerance) or other chronic diseases. The patient's sexual history and medication use (including hormonal contraception), as well as any family history of irregular menses, polycystic ovary syndrome, or bleeding disorders, are important.

The physical examination should start with an assessment of the patient's vital signs. Tachycardia, orthostatic blood pressure changes, and decreased capillary refill, suggesting significant blood loss and anemia, should be addressed immediately. The degree of pallor should be assessed, as well as the presence of any ecchymoses or petechiae. The patient's sexual maturity rating can help determine whether bleeding is truly menstrual in nature, because menarche usually does not occur prior to Tanner stage 3. Special attention should also be given to nutritional status, visual fields (e.g., pituitary lesion), thyroid size, breast examination (galactorrhea), and any evidence of androgen excess (e.g., hirsutism, acne). All adolescents with abnormal bleeding should have a pelvic examination if they have ever been sexually active. If the history points strongly to anovulatory cycles and the patient has never been sexually active, bimanual or digital examination can be performed instead of a speculum examination

to rule out foreign body or structural abnormality. Alternatively, patients can have pelvic ultrasonography to rule out structural abnormalities.

A pregnancy test must be obtained on every adolescent female presenting with vaginal bleeding, regardless of the sexual history she provides. A complete blood count should also be obtained for evaluation of all three cell lines. The hemoglobin level indicates the degree of blood loss. However, it is important to remember that a patient presenting with severe hemorrhage may have a normal hemoglobin level initially. Ongoing or chronic blood loss may present as a normocytic anemia, but more commonly it presents as a microcytic anemia with reduced reticulocyte response due to iron deficiency from blood loss. An elevated white blood cell (WBC) count may indicate infection or inflammation. A markedly elevated WBC count or depression of more than one cell line suggests a leukemic process, especially if immature forms (e.g., blasts) are present. The platelet count can identify thrombocytopenia, although it does not reflect platelet function. The presence of thrombocytosis may be a marker for inflammation.

If a speculum examination is performed, a wet mount can be obtained to look for *Trichomonas*, and cervical specimens can be obtained for *Chlamydia* and gonorrhea. Alternatively, urine can be collected for nuclear DNA testing (e.g., polymerase chain reaction, ligase chain reaction) for *Chlamydia* and gonorrhea. If a bleeding disorder is suspected, evaluation of the prothrombin time, partial thromboplastin time, and von Willebrand factor is indicated. For a patient with a prolonged history of abnormal vaginal bleeding, laboratory studies such as an erythrocyte sedimentation rate, thyroid-stimulating hormone, and prolactin levels can screen for inflammatory and pituitary disturbances. If hyperandrogenism or polycystic ovary syndrome is a concern, luteinizing hormone and follicle-stimulating hormone levels are obtained, along with serum androgen levels (e.g., testosterone, dehydroepiandrosterone). Imaging with pelvic ultrasonography is appropriate to evaluate any masses palpated on the bimanual examination or if there are concerns about structural abnormalities.

TREATMENT

In hemodynamically stable patients, the initial management of abnormal uterine bleeding depends on the severity of the bleeding and the degree of anemia. In the immediate treatment period, the main goals are control of excess bleeding and prevention of future episodes.[1,4-6] Any underlying pathology, such as infection or coagulopathy, must be identified and addressed. Menstrual diaries, iron supplementation, and close follow-up are important adjuncts in the care of these patients.

Medical management consists largely of hormonal therapy with estrogen and progesterone to provide hemostasis and stabilize the endometrium (Box 172-2). If DUB is largely due to unopposed estrogen, it may seem counterintuitive to give estrogen as treatment. However, its role is twofold. First, estrogen promotes better hemostasis through its procoagulation effects, which include increasing platelet aggregation and raising the levels of fibrinogen and clotting factors (factors V and IX).[1] Second, prolonged bleeding may leave patches of the endometrium either too thin for pro-

Box 172-2 Treatment of Dysfunctional Uterine Bleeding

MILD DUB* WITHOUT ACTIVE BLEEDING

Reassurance
Menstrual calendar
Iron supplementation
Observation

MODERATE DUB† WITHOUT ACTIVE BLEEDING

Combined OCP: 30 to 35 μg ethinyl estradiol + progestin (e.g., norgestrel); one pill daily × 6 months, then reevaluate
or
Oral progestin only: medroxyprogesterone acetate 10 mg × 10 days; repeat regimen monthly × 6 months (start dosing on day 14 of the cycle), then reevaluate
Iron supplementation

MODERATE DUB† WITH ACTIVE BLEEDING

Combined OCP
  One pill qid until bleeding stops, followed by pill taper
  Taper: 1 pill qid × 4 days, then tid × 3 days, then bid × 2 days, then daily
  After taper, continue daily OCP × at least 6 months or cyclic oral medroxyprogesterone acetate (as above) × 6 months, then reevaluate
Antiemetics with high-dose estrogen
Iron supplementation

SEVERE DUB† WITH ACTIVE BLEEDING

Outpatient
  Combined OCP with high-dose estrogen
    50 μg ethinyl estradiol + progestin (e.g., norgestrel)
    One pill qid until bleeding stops, followed by pill taper
    Taper: 1 pill qid × 4 days, then tid × 3 days, then bid × 2 days, then daily
    After taper, continue daily OCP × at least 6 months, then reevaluate
    Skip placebo pills for one to three cycles if necessary for recovery of hemoglobin level
  Antiemetics with high-dose estrogen
  Iron supplementation
Inpatient
  Combined OCP with high-dose estrogen
    50 μg ethinyl estradiol + progestin (e.g., norgestrel)
    One pill every 4 to 6 hours until bleeding stops, then taper
  If unable to take oral regimen as above:
    IV conjugated estrogen every 4 hours until bleeding stops
    Antiemetics with high-dose estrogen
    Add OCP when able to tolerate oral intake
    Taper schedule as above
    Continue pills at least 6 months, then reevaluate
  Iron supplementation

*Hemoglobin >12 g/dL.
†Hemoglobin 10-12 g/dL.
‡Hemoglobin <10 g/dL.
DUB, dysfunctional uterine bleeding; OCP, oral contraceptive pill.

gesterone to act on or bare enough to expose bleeding vessels in the wall that are difficult to control. Therefore, estrogen promotes a more uniform growth of the lining, with endometrial tissue distributed more evenly throughout the uterus. Progesterone can then act to decidualize the lining, and a controlled withdrawal of both of these hormones can lead to more synchronized and milder menstrual bleeding.

Mild Dysfunctional Uterine Bleeding

If an adolescent with a history of prolonged menses or shortened cycles presents with a normal hemoglobin level (>12 g/dL) and no active bleeding, she can be managed with reassurance and observation. Teaching the patient how to use a menstrual calendar can be helpful not only to track her bleeding patterns but also to give her a sense of involvement and control over her irregular or heavy periods. Iron supplementation can also be useful at this stage. Hormonal therapy is not necessary.

Moderate Dysfunctional Uterine Bleeding

If a patient with more prolonged menses or shortened cycles has evidence of moderate blood loss (hemoglobin 10 to 12 g/dL), hormonal therapy can be introduced after any necessary laboratory evaluation. A combined oral contraceptive pill (OCP), usually with 30 to 35 μg of ethinyl estradiol and a potent progestin such as norgestrel, continued for at least 6 months is a common regimen. A good alternative is a progestin-only regimen; this is especially useful for patients who are unable to take estrogen. Cyclic oral medroxyprogesterone (Provera) is used to stabilize the endometrial stroma in anticipation of a withdrawal bleed. This regimen is then repeated monthly for three to six cycles.[10] Details of dosing are provided in Box 172-2. Iron supplementation should accompany both these regimens.

If the patient is actively bleeding, multiple daily doses of a monophasic OCP containing at least 35 μg of ethinyl estradiol should be used. The patient takes one pill every 6 hours until the bleeding stops, which usually takes 24 to 48 hours. Because high doses of estrogen can cause extreme nausea, concomitant use of antiemetics is important. The dose is then tapered to one pill daily.[10] After a pill-free week to allow a withdrawal bleed and a recheck of the hemoglobin level, a new pack of pills is started, continuing the once-daily regimen. This can be continued for 6 months, after which the patient can discontinue the OCPs to see whether her cycles have normalized (unless she is sexually active and desires contraception, in which case the OCPs can be continued). If the initial taper of a combined OCP is completed but the patient still has a moderate degree of anemia, it may be appropriate to avoid the monthly withdrawal bleeds, thus allowing the hemoglobin level to recover.[4] This is accomplished by skipping the last 7 days of placebo pills and starting a fresh pill pack on day 22 of the cycle. Iron supplementation is an important adjunct to therapy. Again, cyclic oral medroxyprogesterone is an alternative if estrogen must be avoided.

Severe Dysfunctional Uterine Bleeding

Excessively heavy or prolonged bleeding with significant anemia (hemoglobin <10 g/dL) requires treatment with a higher dose of estrogen. This can be done with an OCP containing 50 µg of ethinyl estradiol and a potent progestin, again given every 6 hours until bleeding stops. Severe anemia (hemoglobin <7 g/dL) or evidence of hemodynamic instability merits hospital admission for this treatment regimen. If the patient cannot tolerate oral medication or is acutely unstable, high-dose conjugated estrogen (Premarin) can be given intravenously every 4 hours for up to 24 hours to control bleeding.[22] Because of the heavy estrogen withdrawal bleed that follows this therapy, oral progesterone, usually in the form of a combined OCP, should be added to this regimen as soon as possible to help stabilize the endometrium. Again, with these doses of estrogen, antiemetics are often necessary. A tapering schedule should be followed, and skipping the withdrawal bleed for a few cycles may be required to allow the hemoglobin level to normalize. Iron supplementation should be part of the regimen. If a high dose of estrogen is used initially, it should be reduced to a 30- or 35-µg pill after the first withdrawal bleed.

If high-dose estrogen does not stop the acute bleeding, other organic pathology (e.g., coagulopathy) should be more thoroughly investigated. It is rare for an adolescent to fail medical management and require surgical intervention with dilation and curettage, although this remains an option.[1,3,6] The patient's clinical status and response to therapy should guide decisions regarding the need for blood transfusions.

ADMISSION CRITERIA

Mild to moderate DUB can be managed in the outpatient setting with close follow-up. However, hospital admission may be necessary to stop the bleeding in the following situations:

- Hemodynamic instability.
- Inability to tolerate oral intake and oral medications.
- Severe anemia (hemoglobin <7 g/dL).
- Extremely heavy flow and hemoglobin less than 9 g/dL.
- Psychological stress associated with heavy bleeding.
- Inadequate follow-up.

DISCHARGE CRITERIA

- Hemodynamically stable, with control of excessive bleeding.
- Ability to tolerate oral hormonal therapy.
- Reliable outpatient follow-up.

IN A NUTSHELL

- Anovulatory cycles are a common cause of DUB in adolescent females.
- Anovulatory cycles remain a diagnosis of exclusion in the workup of DUB.
- Treatment for DUB is determined by the underlying pathology, extent of bleeding, and degree of anemia.
- Hormonal therapy is the mainstay of treatment for DUB.
- Antiemetics are important with high-dose estrogen therapy.

SUGGESTED READING

Bravender T, Emans SJ: Menstrual disorders: Dysfunctional uterine bleeding. Pediatr Clin North Am 1999;46:545-553.

Emans SJ, Laufer MR, Goldstein DP: Pediatric and Adolescent Gynecology, 4th ed. Philadelphia, Lippincott-Raven, 1998.

Mitan LA, Slap GB: Dysfunctional uterine bleeding. In Neinstein LS (ed): Adolescent Health Care: A Practical Guide, 4th ed. Philadelphia, Lippincott Williams & Wilkins 2002, pp 966-972.

Rimsza ME: Dysfunctional uterine bleeding. Pediatr Rev 2002;23:227-232.

REFERENCES

1. Hertweck SP: Dysfunctional uterine bleeding. Pediatr Adolesc Gynecol 1992;19:129-149.
2. Dysfunctional Uterine Bleeding. ACOG Technical Bulletin No. 134, 1989.
3. Rimsza ME: Dysfunctional uterine bleeding. Pediatric Rev 2002;23:227-232.
4. Bravender T, Emans SJ: Menstrual disorders: Dysfunctional uterine bleeding. Pediatr Clin North Am 1999;46:545-553.
5. Lavin C: Dysfunctional uterine bleeding in adolescents. Curr Opin Pediatr 1996;8:328-332.
6. Bayer SR, DeCherney AH: Clinical manifestations and treatment of dysfunctional uterine bleeding. JAMA 1993;269:1823-1828.
7. Mitan LA, Slap GB: Adolescent menstrual disorders: Update. Med Clin North Am 2000;84:851-868.
8. Shwayder JM: Pathophysiology of abnormal uterine bleeding. Obstet Gynecol Clin North Am 2000;27:219-234.
9. Polaneczky MM, Slap GB: Menstrual disorders in the adolescent: Dysmenorrhea and dysfunctional uterine bleeding. Pediatr Rev 1992;13:83-87.
10. Emans SJ, Laufer MR, Goldstein DP: Pediatric and Adolescent Gynecology, 4th ed. Philadelphia, Lippincott-Raven, 1998.
11. Neinstein LS (ed): Adolescent Health Care: A Practical Guide, 4th ed. Philadelphia, Lippincott Williams & Wilkins 2002.
12. Claessens EA, Cowell CA: Acute adolescent menorrhagia. Am J Obstet Gynecol 1981;139:277-280.
13. Falcone T, Desjardins C, Bourque J, et al: Dysfunctional uterine bleeding in adolescents. J Reprod Med 1994;39:761-764.
14. Krassas GE, Pontikides N, Kaltsas T, et al: Disturbances of menstruation in hypothyroidism. Clin Endocrinol 1999;50:653-659.
15. Krassas GE: Thyroid disease and female reproduction. Fertil Steril 2000;74:1063-1070.
16. Koutras DA: Disturbances of menstruation in thyroid disease. Ann N Y Acad Sci 1997;816:280-284.
17. Wilansky DL, Greisman B: Early hypothyroidism in patients with menorrhagia. Am J Obstet Gynecol 1989;160:673-677.
18. Vaitukaitis JL, Melby JC: Menstrual disorders associated with adrenal dysfunction. Clin Obstet Gynecol 1969;12:771-785.
19. Gordon CM: Menstrual disorders in adolescents: Excess androgens and the polycystic ovary syndrome. Pediatr Clin North Am 1999;46:519-543.
20. Lim VS, Henriquez C, Sievertsen G, Frohman LA: Ovarian function in chronic renal failure: Evidence suggesting hypothalamic anovulation. Ann Intern Med 1980;93:21-27.
21. Steinkampf MP: Systemic illness and menstrual dysfunction. Obstet Gynecol Clin North Am 1990;17:311-319.
22. DeVore GR, Owens O, Kase N: Use of intravenous Premarin in the treatment of dysfunctional uterine bleeding—a double-blind randomized control study. Obstet Gynecol 1982;59:285-291.

Child Abuse and Neglect

CHAPTER 173

Inflicted Traumatic Brain Injury

Alice W. Newton

The term inflicted traumatic brain injury (ITBI) is used to describe a constellation of inflicted injuries resulting from the violent shaking of a child. Although a child of any age can be a victim of ITBI, typically infants and young children are at greatest risk. The classic triad of injuries consists of subdural hemorrhage, brain injury, and retinal hemorrhage. Other injuries such as spinal cord trauma, skull fracture, rib or long bone fractures, and external bruising are sometimes associated with ITBI but do not occur in every case.[1]

Evidence about the mechanism of injury in ITBI has been gathered from confessions and witnessed shaking events. In general, accurate information is difficult to obtain because perpetrator confessions are completely lacking or only partially describe the events leading to the child's injuries. The injuries seen in ITBI are caused by vigorous shaking of the child while grasping him or her by the chest, neck, or extremities. In some cases, there may also be blunt force impact if the child is thrown down after the shaking event. Perpetrators often shake children in response to inconsolable crying.[2] It is not uncommon for perpetrators to shake their victims on multiple occasions rather than just in response to a one-time episode of frustration.[3]

The brain injuries seen in ITBI are caused by repetitive acceleration-deceleration trauma to the brain, combined with rotational forces generated as the head rotates about its axis. The movement of the brain within the skull leads to tearing of bridging vessels, resulting in subdural hemorrhage. This subdural bleeding serves as a marker of ITBI but may not contribute significantly to symptoms. The shaking episode can cause direct injury to the brain parenchyma, resulting in contusions, shearing injuries, and diffuse axonal injury.[4] Additionally, there may be significant brain edema related to hypoxia. Children who are shaken often have a period of apnea immediately after sustaining the injury. They may have seizures and sustain damage to the spinal cord and brainstem, all of which contributes to apnea and decreased brain perfusion.

CLINICAL PRESENTATION

Children with ITBI present with a spectrum of injuries ranging from mild to severe. Victims with mild injury often present with poor feeding, vomiting, or irritability, which can be misdiagnosed as colic or gastroenteritis. Many times, there are no external signs of trauma. Often, caretakers do not seek medical attention for days or weeks, and symptoms may resolve without the true cause being identified. Because presenting symptoms in mild cases can be nonspecific, it is important to have a high index of suspicion when treating any young child with unexplained symptoms of vomiting, irritability, or lethargy.

More severe injury results in clear and immediate symptoms of lethargy, apnea, seizures, and cardiopulmonary instability. These injured children suffer from progressive worsening of symptoms as central nervous system dysfunction ensues. As brain edema increases over 24 to 48 hours, many of these children become unstable and experience an evolution of symptoms, including coma or even death.

Further medical evaluation may reveal fractures. Rib fractures are sustained from forceful compression of the chest, and metaphyseal fractures of the long bones occur as the child's arms and legs flail about during the shaking event. However, many victims of ITBI have no evidence of skeletal trauma.

Retinal hemorrhage is present in 75% to 90% of cases. The hemorrhage is usually diffuse and widespread, extending to the periphery of the retina and occurring in multiple layers. Retinal hemorrhages may be unilateral or bilateral, the latter often presenting with asymmetry. Vitreous hemorrhage, retinal folds, and traumatic retinoschisis (splitting of the layers of the retina) may also be present.[5]

The timing of injury can be difficult to determine in children who do not sustain severe injuries; however, interviews with confessed perpetrators indicate that the onset of symptoms is immediate after shaking. An accurate history of when the child was last seen behaving normally is often the most helpful clue to determine when the injury may have occurred.

DIFFERENTIAL DIAGNOSIS

Because some of the isolated findings such as subdural hemorrhage or retinal hemorrhage can be caused by other conditions, it is important to consider and rule out other underlying medical causes. Although each of these injuries in isolation can result from other mechanisms, there are few, if any, clinical scenarios in which these findings occur together. Clarification can usually be accomplished by obtaining a thorough history, physical examination, and simple laboratory evaluation.

Accidental head trauma can result in intracranial hemorrhage. Falls from significant heights and accidents that involve a parent, a car seat, or a walker that falls with the child have a greater momentum and may include not only angular but also rotational forces. Such falls can therefore result in more severe head injuries. However, falls from modest heights (e.g., bed or changing table) rarely result in significant brain injury and do not cause diffuse retinal hemorrhage. Also, children with large extra-axial fluid collections (e.g., hydrocephalus) may be at increased risk of sustaining intracranial hemorrhage with minor trauma; however, severe brain injury and retinal hemorrhage are generally not seen in these cases.[6]

Birth trauma can also lead to intracranial hemorrhage. Most commonly, subdural hemorrhage is seen along the tentorium; it is usually small and clinically insignificant and resolves within the first few weeks of life. More significant intracranial injury generally results in symptoms that occur within the first 36 hours of life and is therefore detected before or shortly after newborns are discharged home.

Retinal hemorrhage can also result from birth. It is most commonly associated with vaginal delivery (20% to 30%), although it can occur with cesarean sections as well (1% to 12%). These retinal hemorrhages are usually not associated with intracranial injury. The hemorrhage can be widespread but usually resolves within 1 to 6 weeks. In general, the extensive, diffuse retinal hemorrhages seen in ITBI do not result from chest compression with resuscitation, minor head trauma, or elevated intracranial pressure.[5]

The differential diagnosis also includes meningitis, bleeding disorders (e.g., vitamin K deficiency), and glutaric-aciduria type I. All these conditions have other classic findings associated with them, and further testing can rule out the presence of underlying infectious, metabolic, or hematologic abnormalities.[6]

DIAGNOSIS AND EVALUATION

The diagnosis of ITBI is based on a constellation of findings, including intracranial hemorrhage, brain injury, and retinal hemorrhage. The initial history given by caretakers is crucial to establishing the diagnosis because it usually includes a history of minor trauma that could not result in such severe injuries or a complete lack of witnessed trauma. The history should be taken as soon as possible, focusing on a detailed description of the events leading up to the child's presentation to medical personnel, as well as the child's appearance and activities before developing symptoms. When obtaining the past medical history, it is crucial to include the birth history, prior minor falls or injuries, developmental abilities, and family history, including specific questions about bleeding disorders or relatives with multiple fractures. Discussion with the child's primary care physician is an integral part of this history-gathering process.

Social work staff can often be extraordinarily helpful in obtaining a detailed social history, including information about substance abuse, mental health issues, and other psychosocial stressors. Ideally, parents should be interviewed

separately to screen for domestic violence and to obtain their individual accounts of the events leading up to the child's hospitalization.

In any case in which an infant presents with signs that might be related to abuse, a thorough evaluation, including radiologic and hematologic studies, should be performed. In most cases, computed tomography (CT) is the initial method to assess for intracranial hemorrhage or brain injury. CT is very helpful in detecting an acute bleed and screening for injuries that may need urgent surgical intervention. However, the initial CT scan does not always detect small amounts of intracranial hemorrhage, especially if located along the vertex or parietal convexities. Magnetic resonance imaging (MRI), with its high resolution, can help differentiate subdural from subarachnoid collections and should be performed 2 to 3 days after the initial presentation. Also, MRI can be helpful in identifying intraparenchymal injury and defining the nature of fluid collections that have mixed signal intensities.[7] However, care should be taken when describing fluid collections as "subdural hemorrhage of differing ages," because subdural fluid collections with mixed signal intensities can also be seen in "hyperacute" bleeds or as a result of arachnoid tears that lead to leakage of cerebrospinal fluid into the subdural space.

A dilated eye examination by an ophthalmologist should be performed as soon as possible in cases of suspected traumatic brain injury. The purpose of this examination is to document the number, size, and distribution of any retinal hemorrhages present, as well as to detect any accompanying ocular injury (e.g., retinal detachment, retinal folds, retinoschisis).

Serology studies may include a complete blood count with differential, prothrombin time, partial thromboplastin time, liver function tests, and possibly a toxicology screen. Any young infant with possible abusive injuries should also have a skeletal survey to assess for occult skeletal injuries. A bone scan can supplement the skeletal survey and may be desirable in some cases. A repeat skeletal survey should be performed in 2 weeks to detect healing fractures that were not visible on the initial skeletal examination, differentiate normal variants, and assess for new injuries.

TREATMENT

The treatment of ITBI entails a combination of supportive medical therapy and psychosocial intervention. The repercussions of the traumatic brain injury dictate the medical management. In rare cases, there may be a significant subdural hemorrhage that requires surgical evacuation. More commonly, the child's symptoms are related to brain edema; consequently, there is minimal need for operative management. Children who are severely injured may deteriorate in the first 24 to 48 hours as brain swelling increases and may require transfer to the intensive care unit for respiratory support and close monitoring. Seizures may require the use of anticonvulsant therapy. Severely injured children often develop coagulopathies and may require blood products such as platelets and fresh frozen plasma.

Children who survive ITBI often require ongoing medical management. They may have visual loss from damage to the occipital cortex. They may be unable to feed due to a poorly functioning gag reflex and may require placement of a feeding tube. Physical and occupational therapy services are often involved long term, and these patients may require a prolonged stay in a rehabilitation facility owing to permanent neurologic damage.[8]

CONSULTATION

Cases of abusive head trauma are often best managed by a multidisciplinary team. If a child protection team is available, it should be consulted as soon as possible. Additionally, social work staff should be involved, as well as specialists in neurosurgery, ophthalmology, orthopedics, hematology, and genetics, if indicated.

Any case in which there is a strong suspicion of child abuse requires a mandatory report to the state child protective services agency. This agency will determine whether there are other children exposed to the offending caretaker who may be at risk. Staff should be prepared to interface with outside agencies, including representatives of child protective services and law enforcement. Accurate diagnosis and documentation are essential. Throughout the hospital admission, parents and guardians of the patient should be treated with respect and kept apprised of both medical management issues and necessary social work interventions.

ADMISSION CRITERIA

Any child who is thought to have a diagnosis of SBS should be admitted for further medical evaluation, social work assessment, and child protective services involvement.

DISCHARGE CRITERIA

Once medically stable, the child may be discharged home or to a rehabilitation facility. Often, the timeline for discharge planning is dictated by the ability of child protective services to locate a safe environment for the child, either with relatives or by placing the child in foster care.

PREVENTION

Prevention programs are being started throughout the United States, and preliminary data suggest a reduction in the rate of ITBI. These programs focus not only on educating caretakers about the dangers of shaking infants but also on teaching parents how to cope with crying infants.[9]

IN A NUTSHELL

- ITBI presents with a variety of symptoms, ranging from mild to severe. In any young child with unexplained vomiting, lethargy, or irritability, the possibility of inflicted head trauma should be considered, and further medical evaluation should be conducted.

- ITBI cases are best managed by a multidisciplinary team, including multiple medical specialties, social work, and child protection professionals.
- Although there are often contributing psychosocial stressors such as substance abuse, mental illness, domestic violence, or poverty, ITBI occurs in all types of families from every socioeconomic background.

ON THE HORIZON

- As physicians develop a greater understanding of the widely varying presentations of head trauma, differentiating abusive and accidental injury becomes more challenging and requires greater expertise. "Child abuse pediatrics" has become a board-certified specialty, and it is likely that many more pediatric hospitals will provide access to a child protection team to assist in these difficult cases.

SUGGESTED READING

Duhame AC, Christian CW, Rorke LB, et al: Nonaccidental head injury in infants—the "shaken-baby syndrome." N Engl J Med 1998;338: 1822.

REFERENCES

1. American Academy of Pediatrics Committee on Child Abuse and Neglect: Shaken baby syndrome: Rotational cranial injuries. Technical report. Pediatrics 2001;108:206.
2. Starling SP, Patal S, Burke BL, et al: Analysis of perpetrator admissions to inflicted traumatic brain injury in children. Arch Pediatr Adolesc Med 2004;158:454.
3. Jenny C, Hymel KP, Ritzen A, et al: Analysis of missed cases of abusive head trauma. JAMA 1999;281:621.
4. Duhame AC, Christian CW, Rorke LB, et al: Nonaccidental head injury in infants—the "shaken-baby syndrome." N Engl J Med 1998;338: 1822.
5. Levin AV: The ocular findings in child abuse. Focal Points—Clinical Modules for Ophthalmologists 1998;16(7).
6. Reece RM, Ludwig S (eds): Child Abuse: Medical Diagnosis and Management, 2nd ed. Philadelphia, Lippincott Williams & Wilkins, 2001.
7. Kleinman PK (ed): Diagnostic Imaging of Child Abuse, 2nd ed. St Louis, Mosby, 1998.
8. Libby AM, Sills MR, Thurston NK, et al: Costs of childhood physical abuse: Comparing inflicted and unintentional traumatic brain injuries. Pediatrics 2003;112:58.
9. Dias MS, Smith K, DeGuehery K, et al: Preventing abusive head trauma among infants and young children: A hospital-based, parent education program. Pediatrics 2005;115:e470-e477.

CHAPTER 174

Imaging of Child Abuse

Jeannette M. Perez-Rossello and Paul K. Kleinman

In 1946 Caffey described the association of subdural hematomas and fractures in infants and raised the possibility of maltreatment to explain these injuries.[1] Later, in a landmark article, Kempe and colleagues described the characteristic radiologic features seen in abused children and coined the term *battered child syndrome*.[2] Modern diagnostic imaging is crucial in the evaluation of child abuse and its imitators.

SKELETAL TRAUMA

Skeletal injuries can be classified with regard to their relative specificity for abuse based on their imaging pattern and location (Table 174-1).[3] Highly specific fractures are usually identified in infants and are typically clinically occult.[3] Most of these injuries occur from indirect forces rather than direct blows, explaining the usual absence of bruising overlying the fracture sites. Rib fractures near the costovertebral articulations occur with anteroposterior compression of the thorax, which may be associated with violent shaking (Fig. 174-1). The classic metaphyseal lesion results from torsional and tractional forces applied to the extremities (Fig. 174-2); it may also occur with acceleration forces associated with infant shaking. Highly specific injuries are not caused by simple falls[3-6] or by cardiopulmonary resuscitation efforts in normal infants.[7,8]

Skull fractures have been noted in 10% of abused children. Although the fractures are usually linear, they may be multiple, diastatic, complex, bilateral, and depressed.[9-11] Skull fractures can occur with short falls to firm surfaces in young infants; therefore, simple linear skull fractures carry a low specificity for abuse. Although long bone shaft fractures have a strong association with abuse in infancy, they can occur with household and playground accidents in toddlers and older children. Thus, any long bone shaft fracture, including those with oblique and spiral patterns, must be viewed in conjunction with the clinical history.

Adequate imaging is critical for the detection of subtle fractures specific for abuse. Failure to perform an adequate skeletal survey may result in returning a child to a potentially dangerous environment. The detection of skeletal injuries depends on the technical quality and thoroughness of the skeletal survey. Traditional film-based surveys should be performed with a high-detail screen-film imaging system. Digital imaging should be optimized to a high-resolution technique.[12-14] The skeletal survey protocol is shown in Table 174-2. The study should be reviewed before completion by a radiologist, and positive sites should be imaged in at least two projections.[13,14]

Skeletal surveys are recommended in all infants and toddlers younger than 2 years when there is suspicion of abuse.

Clinically occult trauma in children older than 2 years is less common than in infants[9]; therefore, in older children, skeletal surveys should be reserved for situations in which there is a strong suspicion of physical abuse. There is little value in global screening for inflicted skeletal injury beyond age 5 years.[14]

Additional imaging studies may complement the skeletal survey in problematic cases. High-quality skeletal scintigraphy may be performed when a skeletal survey is negative or equivocal in infants or as an alternative to radiography in toddlers and young children. Scintigraphy can identify acute rib fractures not apparent on plain films, but it is less sensitive than radiography in the detection of classic metaphyseal lesions and skull fractures.[15,16] A follow-up skeletal survey at 2 weeks can identify fractures that were subtle initially but have become more evident with healing. This approach can increase the degree of certainty of fracture, assist in dating, and differentiate fractures from developmental variants that may simulate abuse.[17] Magnetic resonance imaging (MRI) and ultrasonography are useful in the evaluation of epiphyseal separations and may have a role in the evaluation of soft tissue injuries.

Patterns of fracture healing vary, depending on the patient's age, injury site, and fracture displacement and motion. Infants heal faster than older children. Subperiosteal new bone formation usually occurs between 7 and 10 days, soft callus is seen at about 10 to 14 days, and hard callus forms between 14 and 21 days. Serial examinations are useful in assigning ages to specific fractures such as classic metaphyseal lesions.

VISCERAL TRAUMA

Abdominal and thoracic trauma is more common in toddlers and young children than in infants. The mechanisms of injury include direct blows and decelerational impacts. Children may present with nonspecific complaints. Intraabdominal injuries include small intestinal perforation, duodenal or jejunal hematoma, adrenal hemorrhage, pancreatic laceration and pseudocyst formation, and liver laceration. Gastric, renal, splenic, and bladder injuries are uncommon. Neck and chest injuries include pharyngeal or esophageal perforation, pulmonary contusion, pneumothorax, and hemothorax. Many visceral injuries are not associated with bruising, and the clinical picture may suggest a naturally occurring illness. Failure to diagnose visceral injury can result in up to 50% mortality.[3,18] Multidetector helical computed tomography (CT) with intravenous contrast is sensitive in the detection of significant thoracoabdominal injuries and can be performed in seconds without sedation.

HEAD TRAUMA

Intracranial injury is a major cause of morbidity and mortality in abused children. Subdural hematomas (SDHs) are common in severely abused infants and children. A SDH without a skull fracture or in the presence of retinal hemor-rhages raises the suspicion of shaking. In addition, infants who are shaken may have signs of blunt force trauma resulting from impact, including skull fractures and subgaleal hematomas. CT is highly sensitive in the detection of inter-hemispheric SDHs but may miss small convexity collections. MRI is more sensitive in the detection of subacute SDHs but may miss significant acute SDHs as well as subarachnoid hemorrhage. Other common findings in abused infants are

Table 174-1   Specificity of Fractures for Abuse*

High specificity
  Metaphyseal lesions
  Posterior rib fractures
  Scapular fractures
  Spinous process fractures
  Sternal fractures

Moderate specificity
  Multiple fractures, especially bilateral
  Fractures of different ages
  Epiphyseal separations
  Vertebral body fractures and subluxations
  Digital fractures
  Complex skull fractures
  Pelvic fractures

Common but low specificity
  Subperiosteal new bone formation
  Clavicular fractures
  Long bone shaft fractures
  Linear skull fractures

*Fractures carry the highest specificity in infants.

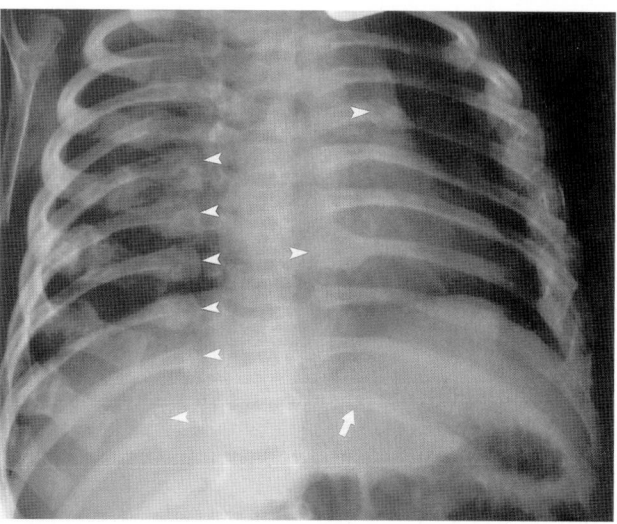

Figure 174-1   Two-month-old abused infant. The chest film shows multiple healing rib fractures *(arrowheads)* and a single acute rib fracture *(arrow)* near the costovertebral articulations. Also note the multiple lateral and anterior rib fractures.

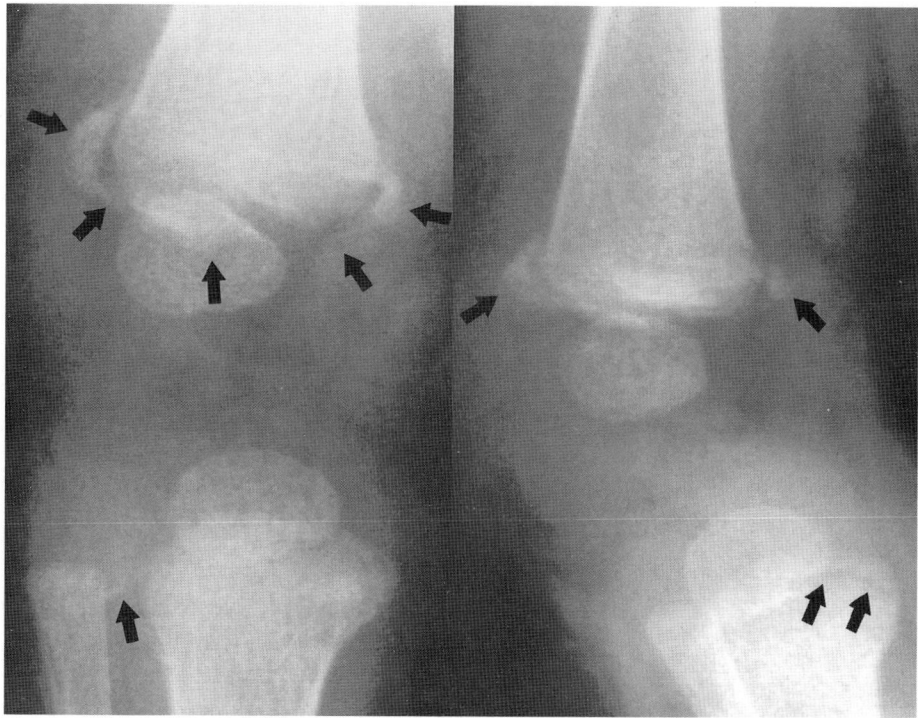

Figure 174-2   The same patient as in Figure 174-1 manifests classic multiple metaphyseal lesions in a variety of patterns. The anteroposterior and lateral views of the knee show a bucket-handle fracture of the distal femur, metaphyseal irregularity of the proximal tibia, and a corner fracture of the proximal fibula.

Table 174-2 The Skeletal Survey: Children's Hospital Boston

Axial Skeleton	Views Acquired*	Appendicular Skeleton	Views Acquired*
Skull	AP, lateral (opposite lateral and Towne view if head trauma)	Humerus	AP
Cervical spine	Lateral	Radius, ulna	AP
Chest	AP, lateral, oblique	Hand	Oblique PA
Pelvis	AP to include lower lumbar spine	Femur	AP
Lumbar spine	Lateral	Tibia, fibula	AP
		Foot	AP

*All views done with high-detail technique.
AP, anteroposterior; PA, posteroanterior.

hypoxic-ischemic injury, focal or diffuse cerebral edema, nonhemorrhagic contusions, gross white matter tears, and diffuse axonal injury. In general, these patterns of injury are better displayed with MRI.[3,19] Diffusion-weighted MRI may show hypoxic-ischemic injury earlier than is possible with conventional pulse sequences.[20,21] MRI can also provide valuable information with respect to the age and multiplicity of injury events. Ultrasonography is useful to differentiate convexity SDHs from large extra-axial cerebrospinal fluid spaces and in the detection of subcortical white matter tears.[22-24]

Suspected acute inflicted head trauma should be evaluated with CT to exclude life-threatening injuries.[25] Abnormal findings on CT should be further assessed with MRI. It may be useful to perform MRI 5 to 7 days after the initial CT scan to assess the evolution of the injuries and to identify additional findings that may have become more evident with time. MRI is indicated in suspicious cases even when the initial CT scan is negative, when high-specificity skeletal injuries are present in infants, or when there is evidence of chronic neurologic injury.[26]

DIFFERENTIAL DIAGNOSIS

Diagnostic imaging can identify a variety of conditions that can be confused with child abuse. Multiple fractures or metaphyseal irregularities simulating classic metaphyseal lesions can be seen in osteogenesis imperfecta, rickets, syphilis, certain bone dysplasias, and as a result of traumatic delivery. Subperiosteal new bone formation can be seen with Caffey disease, sickle cell anemia, leukemia, and osteomyelitis. A variety of developmental variants, such as physiologic subperiosteal new bone formation, can easily be confused with skeletal injury. These entities can generally be distinguished from abuse by the history, physical examination, laboratory data, and careful imaging in consultation with a pediatric radiologist.

IN A NUTSHELL

- The diagnosis of child abuse requires a multidisciplinary approach. The pediatric radiologist plays a crucial role in the evaluation and documentation of inflicted injuries. Rigorous imaging technique and analysis, in conjunction with clinical history and laboratory data, are all critical to accurately diagnose child abuse.

ON THE HORIZON

- The diagnostic imaging of suspected child abuse has been revolutionized with advances in digital technologies. Multidetector helical CT technologies are rapidly evolving and currently permit cranial and body examinations in seconds. Multiplanar reformations can be generated that are comparable in quality to the original direct axial acquisitions. However, these benefits generally come at the cost of increased radiation exposure. MRI continues to be at the forefront of technical innovations, and new pulse sequences such as diffusion-weighted imaging will provide useful tools in the assessment of inflicted central nervous system injuries. New magnetic resonance coil technologies, electronics, and image processing will permit improved temporal and spatial resolution, which may promote the use of total-body MRI for suspected abuse.[27]

- Plain radiography is still the mainstay of imaging in cases of suspected abuse. Images are now easily retrieved, viewed by clinicians, and transported to consultants around the world. The process of displaying images in court during civil and criminal child abuse proceedings has been simplified and vastly improved in the digital environment. Unfortunately, most digital radiographic systems perform at a level well below that of the high-detail screen-film systems currently recommended for skeletal surveys by the American College of Radiology and the American Academy of Pediatrics.[12] These guidelines were developed to ensure the identification of the subtle and highly specific fractures seen in child abuse. High-detail digital imaging systems that offer relatively high resolution and contrast are being developed and evaluated. It is clear that these advances will provide a satisfactory alternative to high-detail screen-film imaging in the future. Until these systems are fully deployed, however, specialists should be cautious and adequately informed regarding the advantages and limitations of this new and exciting technology when applied in cases of suspected child abuse.

SUGGESTED READING

ACR practice guideline for skeletal surveys in children. In American College of Radiology: ACR Standards. Reston, Va, American College of Radiology, 2001, p 107.

American Academy of Pediatrics: Diagnostic imaging of child abuse. Pediatrics 2000;105:1345.

Kleinman PK: Diagnostic Imaging of Child Abuse, 2nd ed. St Louis, Mosby, 1998.

REFERENCES

1. Caffey J: Multiple fractures in the long bones of infants suffering from chronic subdural hematoma. AJR Am J Roentgenol 1946;56:163.
2. Kempe CH, Silverman FN, Steele BF, et al: The battered-child syndrome. JAMA 1962;181:105.
3. Kleinman PK: Diagnostic Imaging of Child Abuse, 2nd ed. St Louis, Mosby, 1998.
4. Helfer RE, Slovis TL, Black M: Injuries resulting when small children fall out of bed. Pediatrics 1977;60:533.
5. Lyons TJ, Oates RK: Falling out of bed: A relatively benign occurrence. Pediatrics 1993;92:125.
6. Williams RA: Injuries in infants and small children resulting from witnessed and corroborated free falls. J Trauma 1991;31:1350.
7. Spevak MR, Kleinman PK, Belanger PL, et al: Cardiopulmonary resuscitation and rib fractures in infants: A postmortem radiologic-pathologic study. JAMA 1994;272:617.
8. Feldman KW, Brewer DK: Child abuse, cardiopulmonary resuscitation, and rib fractures. Pediatrics 1984;73:339.
9. Merten DF, Radkowski MA, Leonidas JC: The abused child: A radiological reappraisal. Radiology 1983;146:377.
10. Rao P, Carty H: Non-accidental injury: Review of the radiology. Clin Radiol 1999;54:11.
11. Meservy CJ, Towbin R, McLaurin RL, et al: Radiographic characteristics of skull fractures resulting from child abuse. AJNR Am J Neuroradiol 1987;8:455.
12. Kleinman PL, Kleinman PK, Savageau JA: Suspected infant abuse: Radiographic skeletal survey practices in pediatric health care facilities. Radiology 2004;233:477.
13. ACR practice guideline for skeletal surveys in children. In American College of Radiology: ACR Standards. Reston, Va, American College of Radiology, 2001, p 107.
14. American Academy of Pediatrics: Diagnostic imaging of child abuse. Pediatrics 2000;105:1345.
15. Mandelstam SA, Cook D, Fitzgerald M, et al: Complementary use of radiological skeletal survey and bone scintigraphy in detection of bony injuries in suspected child abuse. Arch Dis Child 2003;88:387.
16. Cadzow SP, Armstrong KL: Rib fractures in infants: Red alert! The clinical features, investigations and child protection outcomes. J Paediatr Child Health 2000;36:322.
17. Kleinman PK, Nimkin K, Spevak MR, et al: Follow-up skeletal surveys in suspected child abuse. AJR Am J Roentgenol 1996;167:893.
18. Ledbetter DJ, Hatch EI Jr, Feldman KW, et al: Diagnostic and surgical implications of child abuse. Arch Surg 1988;123:1101.
19. Alexander RC, Schor DP, Smith WL Jr: Magnetic resonance imaging of intracranial injuries from child abuse. J Pediatr 1986;109:975.
20. Biousse V, Suh DY, Newman NJ, et al: Diffusion-weighted magnetic resonance imaging in shaken baby syndrome. Am J Ophthalmol 2002;133:249.
21. Suh DY, Davis PC, Hopkins KL, et al: Nonaccidental pediatric head injury: Diffusion-weighted imaging findings. Neurosurgery 2001;49:309.
22. Chen CY, Chou TY, Zimmerman RA, et al: Pericerebral fluid collection: Differentiation of enlarged subarachnoid spaces from subdural collections with color Doppler US. Radiology 1996;201:389.
23. Veyrac C, Couture A, Baud C: Pericerebral fluid collections and ultrasound. Pediatr Radiol 1990;20:236.
24. Jaspan T, Narborough G, Punt JA, et al: Cerebral contusional tears as a marker of child abuse—detection by cranial sonography. Pediatr Radiol 1992;22:237.
25. Schutzman SA, Barnes P, Duhaime AC, et al: Evaluation and management of children younger than two years old with apparently minor head trauma: Proposed guidelines. Pediatrics 2001;107:983.
26. Rubin DM, Christian CW, Bilaniuk LT, et al: Occult head injury in high-risk abused children. Pediatrics 2003;111:1382.
27. Eustace S, Walker RE, Blake M, Yucel EK: Whole body MR imaging, practical issues, clinical applications and future directions. Magn Reson Imaging Clin North Am 1999;9:209.

CHAPTER 175

Injuries: Signs and Symptoms of Concern for Nonaccidental Trauma

Amy Goldberg

Injury may be the primary reason for a child's hospital admission, as in the case of anterior rib fractures sustained in a motor vehicle accident. Or a child may be hospitalized with an injury secondary to a medical condition, such as pathologic rib fractures in a child diagnosed with rickets. Finally, injury may be an incidental finding noted during the workup for an unrelated diagnosis, such as posteromedial rib fractures noted on the chest radiograph of an infant admitted with bronchiolitis.

CLINICAL PRESENTATION

History

Although certain injuries are considered pathognomonic for physical abuse, obtaining a thorough history is critical for determining whether an injury is accidental or nonaccidental. Even if there is suspicion that a child has been abused, the clinician must maintain a nonjudgmental demeanor when obtaining the history. The physician's responsibility is not to determine who inflicted an injury but rather to recognize when the explanation or mechanism is inconsistent with the injury (Table 175-1). When there is suspicion of abuse, it is the physician's responsibility to make a report to the state child protective agency.

Certain social risk factors may put a child at increased risk for injury and abuse, but they do not by themselves constitute the basis for a diagnosis of nonaccidental trauma. Clinicians must be careful not to exclude the possibility of abuse because certain characteristics of the child's caretakers (e.g., age, sex, socioeconomic status, education) make them appear to be unlikely perpetrators. One study found that the diagnosis of abusive head trauma was most likely to be missed in younger white infants with two parents living in the home. This suggests that a physician's personal bias can impede a coherent approach to a child with signs and symptoms that are potentially consistent with inflicted injury.[1]

Physical Examination

Cutaneous injuries, including bruises, abrasions, lacerations, and burns, are commonly found in both abused and nonabused children. However, certain factors, including age, developmental stage, and location and pattern of injury, can aid the clinician in distinguishing accidental from nonaccidental trauma. When abuse is suspected, all cutaneous injuries should be measured and documented photographically, if possible, or using a body chart.

Bruises

A normative study of bruising patterns in children 0 to 36 months old found that as children age and their developmental level increases, so do the number of bruises they sustain.[2] Bruising over bony prominences (forehead, knee, anterior tibia) is common in a child who is learning to walk. As the child gains greater stability and learns to run, climb, and jump, the number and site of bruises expand. Several sites, however, including the ears, face, neck, chest, buttocks, and genitals, are less common locations for bruises in all age groups and should raise the index of suspicion for inflicted injury. Bruising is extremely uncommon in infants younger than 6 months regardless of the location, and in the absence of a plausible mechanism, the physician should initiate a complete workup for physical abuse (head computed tomography, ophthalmologic examination, and skeletal survey). Certain patterns should be readily recognized as pathognomonic for inflicted injuries. For example, when injuries are inflicted with an object, the silhouette or outline of that object may be left behind (Fig. 175-1). Human bite marks should be measured and swabbed with sterile water to collect genetic markers from residual saliva. When abuse is suspected, a forensic dentist can be consulted to imprint the bitten skin and possibly identify the assailant or at least determine whether the injury was inflicted by an adult or a child.

Depth, location, and skin complexion all affect the timing of the appearance of a bruise, as well as its color. Thus, the age of a bruise cannot be estimated solely by color. Timing injuries in this way is not supported in the literature and is not recommended.

Thermal Injury

The temperature of a burning agent, the length of time it had contact with the skin, and the thickness of the skin determine the severity of a thermal injury and can help the physician determine whether the caretaker's history is consistent with the injury. Scald burns are the most common inflicted burns and can be divided into splash-spill and immersion types. Splash-spill burns occur when a hot liquid falls from a height onto a child. The natural tendency of liquid is to flow downward and to cool, producing an arrowhead pattern of nonuniform depth. These burns usually occur on the face, upper extremities, and chest and are not circumferential or symmetrical. Splash-spill burns are most frequently accidental and occur when a developmentally able child pulls down a vessel filled with hot liquid.

Immersion burns are characterized by a clear demarcation between burned and normal skin. Inflicted immersion burns have a paucity of splash marks, reflecting the child's suppressed attempt to escape from the injury. Typically, abusive immersion burn patterns are uniformly deep and bilateral, involving the hands or feet in a stocking or glove distribution or localized to the perineum and buttocks. Inflicted immersion burns are often associated with "discipline" surrounding toilet training or the soiling of clothing.

Table 175-1   Examples of a History Suspicious for Nonaccidental Injury

Suspicious History	Example
Reported mechanism of injury is not consistent with findings	24-month-old with clearly demarcated deep partial-thickness burns to buttocks, sparing hands and feet, and paucity of splash-mark burns, with a history of climbing into bathtub and turning on hot water
History provided by caretakers changes over time	Multiple versions of events are provided, and explanations are modified throughout evaluation process
Delay in seeking medical attention after injury is noted	Periorbital ecchymosis noted by caretaker 3 days before medical evaluation
Developmental stage of child is incompatible with activity reported to cause injury	1-month-old infant has subdural hemorrhage, with a history of rolling off a bed

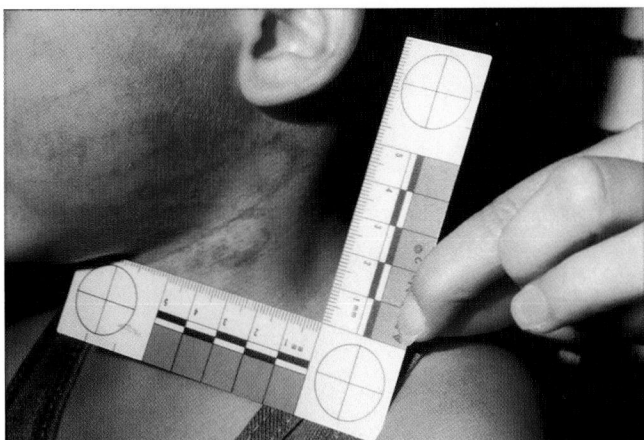

Figure 175-1   Slap marks can leave a negative imprint of the abuser's hand on the skin.

The child's body is held in flexion at the waist under hot water, resulting in sparing of the buttocks, soles of the feet, and flexor creases when the child's body is pushed down against the cooler tub or sink.

Inflicted contact burns with cigarettes, hot irons, radiators, or other objects are uniformly deep, with well-defined borders. They typically result in a characteristic pattern, enabling the examining physician to identify the object. Conversely, accidental contact burns are usually less clearly demarcated, and the skin lesion may appear as a "brush" against the hot object.

Clear documentation of the workup, including the complete history, physical examination, and radiographic imaging, that led the physician to a diagnosis of physical abuse or caused him or her to initiate an investigation by the state's child protective agency is critical. The medical record should clearly reflect the physician's opinion (e.g., "this injury is inconsistent with the history provided and with the child's developmental level") and what evaluations have been done to secure or exclude the diagnosis.

DIFFERENTIAL DIAGNOSIS

Accidental mechanisms as well as organic causes of the patient's injury must be fully explored and excluded with the appropriate tests before making the diagnosis of nonaccidental injury. For example, when a child presents with bruising, laboratory studies are recommended to screen for a bleeding disorder that might make the child more likely to bruise from minor accidental trauma. A child with a bleeding disorder might still be abused, however; the history and location and pattern of the injury will ultimately determine whether it is suggestive of abuse. Infectious diseases (e.g., staphylococcal bullous impetigo) and other skin conditions (e.g., phytophotodermatitis) must be excluded before diagnosing inflicted thermal injury. Cultural practices such as coining (Cao gio) or cupping leave a characteristic pattern and must also be considered in the differential diagnosis.

CONSULTATION

Suspected nonaccidental trauma is best evaluated by a multidisciplinary team with experience in such cases. Social work staff should be involved, as well as other specialists as indicated, including neurosurgery, ophthalmology, orthopedics, hematology, and genetics. Finally, in any case in which there is a strong suspicion of nonaccidental trauma, a report to the state child protective services agency is mandatory.

ADMISSION CRITERIA

Any child who is thought to be at risk for nonaccidental trauma should be admitted for further medical evaluation, social work assessment, and child protective services involvement.

DISCHARGE CRITERIA

Discharge of a patient admitted for known or suspected nonaccidental trauma depends on two major factors. First, the patient must be medically ready to be discharged. Second, the patient must be discharged to a safe environment. Depending on the findings of the state child protective services agency, this may involve having the child remain in the home of origin or placing the child in substitute care with a relative or nonrelative. This may be home, with relatives, or in foster care, depending on the findings of the state child protective services agency.

PREVENTION

Prevention of nonaccidental trauma mainly involves education for caretakers, especially with regard to the dangers of shaking infants (see Chapter 173).

IN A NUTSHELL

- Injuries from nonaccidental trauma may be the primary reason for a child's hospital admission. Although certain injuries are pathognomonic for physical abuse, a thorough history and physical examination are critical to determine whether an injury is accidental or nonaccidental.

ON THE HORIZON

- There is growing recognition that expertise is required to manage cases of suspected nonaccidental trauma. "Child abuse pediatrics" has been approved by the American Board of Pediatrics as a distinct subspecialty.
- With advances in radiographic technologies, imaging may assist in identifying nonaccidental trauma (see Chapter 174).

SUGGESTED READING

Kleinman P: Diagnostic Imaging of Child Abuse, 2nd ed. St Louis, Mosby, 1998.

Myers J, Berliner L, et al: The APSAC Handbook on Child Maltreatment, 2nd ed. Thousand Oaks, Calif, Sage Publications, 2002.

Reece R, Ludwig S: Child Abuse Medical Diagnosis and Management, 2nd ed. Philadelphia, Lippincott Williams & Wilkins, 2001.

REFERENCES

1. Jenny C, Hymel KP, Ritzen A, et al: Analysis of missed cases of abusive head trauma. JAMA 1999;281:621-626.
2. Sugar NF, Taylor JA, Feldman KW: Bruises in infants and toddlers: Those who don't cruise rarely bruise. Arch Pediatr Adolesc Med 1999;153:399-403.

CHAPTER 176

Munchausen by Proxy

Andrea M. Vandeven

Munchausen by proxy (MBP), a type of child abuse first described by Meadow in the 1970s, is characterized by the deliberate falsification of symptoms in a child by an adult caretaker so that the child is rendered ill or impaired.[1] Symptoms and signs of illness are intentionally exaggerated, fabricated, or induced, and as a result, the child is subjected to medical testing, treatment, and even surgery, none of which is warranted. MBP is seen in situations in which the child would be considered healthy but for the maneuvers of the caretaker, as well as in situations in which the child has a mild or treatable medical condition that is dramatically and intentionally worsened by the actions of the caretaker. Within the maltreatment and psychiatry community, there is controversy over the precise definition of the parental behaviors and motivations in MBP.[2] The complicated psychological factors that cause caretakers (who are almost always mothers) to abuse their children in this way are the subject of active study; there is no diagnostic "profile" of the MBP mother. Because it is problematic for the pediatrician to accurately identify the caretaker's motivation or underlying mental state, this chapter addresses the diagnosis of factitious illness in the child victim. *Factitious illness* is the general term for cases in which the caretaker exaggerates or invents a child's medical symptoms.

Owing to definitional controversies and the inherent problem of underreporting of child maltreatment, the true incidence of MBP is unknown, although it is thought to be much less common than other forms of child abuse. A large prospective series of cases in Ireland and the United Kingdom reported that the incidence of MBP was 0.5 per 100,000 children younger than 16 years, with a higher incidence in early childhood.[3]

CLINICAL PRESENTATION

Although a child with MBP may present in myriad ways, certain symptoms are commonly seen, including unexplained bleeding, apnea, seizures, vomiting, skin rashes and bruising, and metabolic derangements such as hypoglycemia (Table 176-1). Often the symptoms are reported as occurring only in the presence of the caregiver and have never been objectively documented by medical personnel. The initial presentation of illness may be completely straightforward, leading to an appropriate medical investigation. However, suspicions arise when no underlying medical condition is identified, a reasonable course of treatment is ineffective, bizarre laboratory results are obtained, or symptoms recur inexplicably—in other words, when the pattern of disease just does not make sense. At this point, the child may have already received the "million-dollar workup" and seen multiple subspecialists in an attempt to find a unifying diagnosis. Adding to the diagnostic complexity is the possibility that the child is quite disabled as a result of iatrogenic complications of medical treatment and may be legitimately unable to attend school or perform other age-appropriate activities.

Much has been made of the "profile" of the MBP mother, but this is a complex and controversial topic. It is generally inappropriate for pediatricians who are not trained in forensics to attempt to analyze the motivation or psychological state of the child's caregiver.[4]

DIFFERENTIAL DIAGNOSIS

Factitious illness and MBP exist on a spectrum ranging from situations of caretaker underinvolvement (i.e., child neglect) to excessive involvement, the extreme of which is MBP.[5] The MBP caretaker has a pattern of repeatedly seeking medical evaluation for "unexplained" episodes. In contrast, in cases of non-MBP abuse or neglect, although the caregiver may attempt to obscure the real story, he or she is typically not trying to elicit a prolonged evaluation of the child.

One can also differentiate factitious illness from the more extreme MBP. In cases of factitious illness, the caretaker may "overreport" or "pathologize" symptoms that are in fact unremarkable, leading to inappropriate testing or treatment. The crucial difference is that the non-MBP caretaker does not intend to deceive. Factitious disorders that are not MBP can also be seen when the caregiver is psychotic and in children with somatoform disorder and some eating and feeding disorders.[2] Regardless of the terminology, such caretaker behavior places the child's overall health and well-being at risk.

DIAGNOSIS AND EVALUATION

A multidisciplinary approach is invaluable when making the diagnosis of MBP. The hospitalist is in the unique position of being able to convene a meeting of the entire inpatient and outpatient care team for the purpose of comparing observations and impressions. Commonly, multiple subspecialists are involved in the child's care, and they are not communicating directly with one another. Additionally, there may be miscommunication among these professionals, resulting from the caretaker's relaying of information back and forth with either intentional or unintentional distortions. Because no one has the complete picture, a team meeting is extremely helpful to clarify contradictory information and review the original data that resulted in the preliminary diagnosis and the subsequent course of treatment.

If MBP or factitious illness is being considered, it is also essential to obtain original laboratory and other test results

Table 176-1   Presentations in Munchausen by Proxy

System	Symptom, Sign, Disease	Cause
Neurologic	Seizures, collapse and loss of consciousness, ataxia, drowsiness, developmental delay, deafness	Drugs, poisons, suffocation, pressure on carotid sinus
Cardiorespiratory	Apneic and cyanotic episodes, cardiac arrest, "near-miss SIDS"	Suffocation
	Cystic fibrosis	Altering laboratory investigations and stealing sputum from other patients
	Asthma	Deliberate under- or overtreatment
Gastrointestinal	Recurring vomiting and diarrhea	Drugs, poisons, mechanically induced
	Failure to thrive	Restricting intake, altering IV infusion, aspirating nasogastric tube
Renal	Polyuria, polydipsia	Drugs
	Hematuria, renal stone	Adding stone, parental blood, coloring substances to urine
	Bacteriuria	Swapping urine specimens with parent or other patients
Hematologic	Purpura	Injecting blood under skin, rubbing skin
	Hematemesis, hemoptysis, rectal bleeding	Adding parental blood to specimens, clothing, diapers
Immunologic	Recurrent fever, sepsis	Heating thermometer, injecting bacteriologically contaminated material, interfering with IV sites
	Allergy	Applying excessive environmental and dietary measures to avoid "allergen"
Dermatologic	Rashes	Applying irritants, scratching or injecting skin
Metabolic	Hypoglycemia, glycosuria	Abuse of insulin and sugar solution, drugs
	Hypernatremia	Adding salt to formula

SIDS, sudden infant death syndrome.
Adapted from Plunkett MCB, Southall DP: The presentation and natural history of Munchausen syndrome by proxy. In Adshead G, Brooke D (eds): Munchausen's Syndrome by Proxy: Current Issues in Assessment, Treatment and Research. London, Imperial College Press, 2001, pp 77-87.

rather than relying on the caretaker's report or summaries that do not include objective information. If the medical evaluation is not complete, the requisite consultations or testing should be arranged. Information about the child's social and intellectual development should be obtained from outside individuals such as teachers and visiting nurses. Nurses and child life specialists may be able to provide observations about the child's behavior when the caretaker is not at the bedside. A social work assessment is important in evaluating the family's life stresses and general functioning. If the family is willing, a psychiatric consultation is often very helpful. Child protective and legal consultants can offer insight into reporting obligations to the state child protective services agency, issues surrounding the use of covert video monitoring, and the appropriateness of separating mother and child.

Ultimately, for the child to be diagnosed as a victim of MBP, it must be found that the child's illness was *intentionally* feigned or induced. If that strict standard is not met, it is not MBP. However, if the child has no real organic disease process but is treated as though ill by caregivers, the diagnosis of factitious illness can be made. Finally, if the child has an underlying medical condition that could be appropriately managed by the family with proper support but is not, consideration should be given to the diagnosis of child neglect or abuse.

COURSE OF ILLNESS

Untreated MBP can result in death or severe and permanent disability. Long-term physical and psychological morbidity is high if intervention does not occur expeditiously. Because of MBP, children may be deprived of a normal childhood and may develop into adults with severely compromised mental and physical health.

TREATMENT

If there is evidence of intentionally fabricated or induced illness (MBP), a child abuse report must be filed with the state child protective services agency. It is not necessary to complete a full assessment of the caretaker; that will be done by a qualified forensic clinician. When the diagnosis is factitious illness (not MBP), consultation with legal and child protective professionals can help determine whether the threshold for filing a report with the state has been reached.

In cases of factitious illness or situations in which the caretaker perceives the child as ill despite evidence to the contrary, the emphasis of management is to provide unambiguous information to the family and devise a plan to wean the child off unneeded medications and treatments. To achieve these goals, it is recommended that one physician be designated to manage and monitor the child's care in an effort to minimize miscommunication and misunderstanding of the treatment plan. With regard to communication, careful, objective, precise documentation is absolutely necessary, particularly when recording comments or behaviors by the caretaker that may be concerning for MBP.

Once the diagnosis of factitious illness or MBP is made, it is helpful to create a treatment contract with the family that defines objective goals and measures. An outpatient clinician (usually the primary care clinician) manages all aspects of care, including communication with subspecialists. Typically, mental health counseling for the caretaker is indicated. If the family is unable to comply with the contract despite maximal support, the state child protective services agency should be notified. The ultimate aim is to help the child achieve a normal or near-normal level of age-appropriate functioning, including participation in social activities and school.

ADMISSION CRITERIA

Hospitalization is indicated for the following reasons:

- To protect the child when it is believed that the child will be unsafe at home and the state child protective services agency has not yet intervened.
- To complete an appropriate medical workup under the supervision of all subspecialists involved and to jointly evaluate medical data.
- To observe interactions between the child and caretaker and to monitor for events that have been witnessed only by the caretaker. Consideration should be given to separating the caretaker and child to see whether symptoms improve in the caretaker's absence.
- To observe the effects of medical interventions, especially the effect of removing treatments and medications that are thought to be unwarranted.

DISCHARGE CRITERIA

- Discharge to home is allowed if a safe environment can be ensured and close medical follow-up has been arranged.
- In some cases, discharge to a psychiatric or rehabilitation facility is warranted.

PREVENTION

No interventions are known to prevent MBP.

IN A NUTSHELL

- The child presents with signs and symptoms of illness that are exaggerated, fabricated, or intentionally induced by a caregiver for the purpose of obtaining medical attention and treatment for the child.
- Alternative medical conditions must be excluded.
- Management goals are to eliminate unnecessary medical treatments and return the child to healthy, age-appropriate activities. Involvement of the state child protective services agency may be required.

ON THE HORIZON

- Within the child maltreatment field, efforts are being directed at defining the characteristics of perpetrators of MBP. Additionally, the effects of social services intervention and psychiatric treatment are being evaluated to define best treatment practices.

SUGGESTED READING

Eminson DM, Postlethwaite RJ: Factitious illness: Recognition and management. Arch Dis Child 1992;67:1510-1516.

Meadow R: Munchausen syndrome by proxy: The hinterland of child abuse. Lancet 1977;2:343-345.

REFERENCES

1. Meadow R: Munchausen syndrome by proxy: The hinterland of child abuse. Lancet 1977;2:343-345.
2. Schreier H: Munchausen by proxy. Curr Probl Pediatr Adolesc Health Care 2004;34:126-143.
3. McClure RJ, Davis PM, Meadow SR, Sibert JR: Epidemiology of Munchausen syndrome by proxy, non-accidental poisoning, and non-accidental suffocation. Arch Dis Child 1996;75:57-61.
4. Sanders MJ, Bursch B: Forensic assessment of illness falsification, Munchausen by proxy, and factitious disorder, NOS. Child Maltreat 2002;7:112-124.
5. Eminson DM, Postlethwaite RJ: Factitious illness: Recognition and management. Arch Dis Child 1992;67:1510-1516.

CHAPTER 177

Legal Issues

Lisa Santos Kresnicka

Physicians do not learn much about the law during their training, yet in pediatric practice, there is an increasing need for legal knowledge, especially in the area of child maltreatment. Medical professionals often have questions regarding the process of mandated reporting of child abuse to state agencies, as well as the civil and criminal court actions that may result from those reports, which may require physicians to provide factual and expert testimony.

REPORTING

All 50 states have statutes requiring certain professionals to report incidents of suspected child abuse and neglect to the state child protective services agency. *Abuse* includes physical, emotional, and sexual injury or exploitation. *Neglect* includes physical harm, emotional deprivation, failure to monitor, and medical or emotional neglect.[1] Common mandated reporters are physicians, nurses, teachers, psychologists, social workers, and law enforcement personnel.[2,3] Only a reasonable suspicion or belief of abuse is needed to make a report to state authorities; a person does not need to know that abuse or neglect exists.

All states have immunity provisions for mandated reporters, so that the reporter is protected from any civil or criminal liability if a report is later deemed to be erroneous or unsubstantiated.[1] In contrast, failure of a mandated reporter to report suspected child abuse may result in a fine, malpractice suit, or criminal sanctions. Therefore, it is best to make a report any time there is "reasonable cause" to believe that abuse or neglect exits.

As an inpatient pediatrician, it is essential to confirm that a report has been made in all cases in which doing so is necessary. It is important to note that if another person or institution has filed a report about the same episode of abuse, no other professionals are required to duplicate that report.[1] However, if a new indicator of abuse is observed, a new report must be filed. For example, a report is filed for a non-ambulatory child with an unexplained femur fracture. He is subsequently transferred to another hospital for further treatment, where he is found to have suspicious rib fractures as well. The accepting physician must make a supplementary report about the rib fractures.

CHILD PROTECTIVE SERVICES

Child protective services (CPS) is a governmental agency responsible for investigating reports of child maltreatment, determining whether child abuse or neglect has occurred, and intervening to ensure a safe environment for the child. In most cases, CPS agencies assist families in finding appropriate support services to protect and improve the well-being of their children. When it is deemed necessary, these agencies also secure alternative placements for children or pursue

the termination of parental rights. Although CPS agencies vary by state and county, professional standards of practice have been widely accepted and implemented.

When a report is made to CPS, it is important to provide as much information as possible regarding the child and the incident or circumstances that led to the suspicion of maltreatment. State laws protect the identity of reporters if they choose to remain anonymous. However, especially in the inpatient setting, it is recommended that parents or guardians be notified when a medical professional is going to make a report to preserve (to the extent possible) an open, honest relationship with the child's caretakers. The most effective means of notifying parents or guardians is to express concern that someone may be harming their child, not to accuse them of maltreatment. When providing this information, the physician can ask whether the parents know of anyone who might be hurting their child. Although the physician-parent relationship may become strained, parents generally respond better to honesty and directness than to secretiveness. This should facilitate a more comfortable working relationship while the child remains in the hospital and encourage appropriate follow-up care.

Once a report is made, the CPS agency has an obligation to investigate the allegation of abuse. Rules vary by state whether the CPS agency must thoroughly investigate every report.[4] This remains a controversial issue as states attempt to balance their mandates for child protection with limited financial resources.

The CPS investigation begins by gathering all the relevant information about the case. Many state laws and regulations outline the investigative procedure in great detail. Most require contact with the child and family within 24 hours of the most serious reports of abuse and within 72 hours for other reports.[4] Interviews are conducted with the child, the parents, other family members, and other individuals who might have knowledge about the specific allegations or about the family's treatment of the child in general.

Many jurisdictions have children's advocacy centers in place to assist and guide the child interview process. Children's advocacy centers provide a multidisciplinary team approach to investigations of child abuse, including forensic interviews, therapeutic interventions, victim support and advocacy, and case management. Such facilities provide a safe, child-friendly environment to conduct forensic interviews of a neutral, fact-finding nature. Often these agencies work in collaboration with law enforcement and CPS to minimize the number of times the child victim is interviewed.

If the alleged maltreatment constitutes criminal behavior, law enforcement personnel should be brought into the investigation to ensure that the criminal aspect of suspected maltreatment is thoroughly investigated and that the evidence necessary for criminal prosecution is adequately safeguarded.[3,4] The reporter may contact the police directly, or this may be done through an established mechanism within CPS. Many jurisdictions have guidelines to ensure cooperation between law enforcement and CPS.

One of the most important aspects of the child protection system is the ability to take a child into protective custody on an emergency basis if his or her safety is believed to be in jeopardy. Once this is done, the CPS agency must obtain a court order granting it temporary legal custody of the child within 24 hours from the time the child was placed in protective custody. Then, within 72 hours, the matter must be brought before the court to determine whether there is enough evidence that the child would be at risk if he or she were returned to the family environment. If so, further legal procedures must be initiated and followed.

State laws and regulations require that the CPS agency conclude the investigative process by arriving at a disposition, or a formal finding of whether child abuse or neglect has occurred, within a given time frame.[4] A number of terms, including *indicated, supported, confirmed,* or *substantiated,* are used when CPS believes that the child was a victim of maltreatment; words such as *unfounded* or *unsubstantiated* indicate that there was insufficient evidence to conclude that child maltreatment occurred. It is important to keep in mind that these CPS conclusions are not the result of a hearing.

Although an unsubstantiated report seldom involves additional action on the part of CPS, a finding that abuse or neglect has been substantiated frequently requires further action by the child welfare agency and the family, unless the perpetrator no longer has access to the child and the child is not at any additional risk. The next step often involves the formulation of a case plan by CPS, with the main goals of ensuring the child's safety and stabilizing the family system. The case plan reflects the expectations and responsibilities of family members, as well as the role and contributions of the CPS agency, which often involves the provision of assistance through other community agencies. CPS staff then follows the progress of the family in accomplishing the changes set forth in the case plan. If the family does not follow the plan and the child continues to be at risk, CPS can take further steps.

A minority of substantiated cases of child maltreatment result in some type of court proceeding. This occurs when the child is thought to be in imminent danger of repeated maltreatment or when it is perceived that social services will not be sufficient to effect the desired family changes. A small percentage of the cases filed in court result in the child's removal from the home and placement with a third party. Federal law requires the juvenile court to (1) conclude affirmatively that the CPS agency has made reasonable efforts to avoid removing a child from his or her family home before authorizing an out-of-home placement for the child, and (2) review the actions of CPS periodically to ensure that reasonable efforts are being made to return the child to his or her birth family.[4]

Cases investigated by CPS become "closed" for a variety of reasons, ranging from the conclusion that the child is safe insofar as can be determined to the termination of parental rights and placement of the child in a permanent substitute family.[4] Infrequently, under certain circumstances, cases may be closed for less legitimate reasons.

LEGAL PROCEEDINGS

Medical testimony may be used in a variety of legal proceedings in civil and criminal courts, including child custody disputes, criminal prosecution of alleged perpetrators of child maltreatment, and civil actions for damages from injuries. Most child abuse and neglect cases are heard in state courts. Civil cases usually involve the juvenile court, with the CPS agency initiating the action. In juvenile court, ideally, the focus is on the child—whether he or she has been subjected to abuse or neglect and, if so, what intervention is needed not only to protect the child but also, unless contraindicated, to strengthen the child's family.[5] It is not always necessary to prove that a specific parent or guardian injured a child.

Civil court cases are begun with the filing of a complaint or petition. In criminal court, cases are begun with the filing of an indictment or other charge. In civil actions, the standard of proof is less than that required in criminal court. The moving party usually has the burden of persuading the factfinder by a "preponderance of the evidence" or by "clear and convincing evidence," meaning the state must prove that it is more likely than not that the allegations are true.[6] In contrast, criminal cases require a higher degree of certainty—"beyond a reasonable doubt"—to prove guilt. Therefore, even if there is insufficient evidence to convict a perpetrator in a criminal trial, it may be sufficient to give the juvenile court protective jurisdiction over the child.[5]

Criminal cases involve the prosecution of individuals by the state or federal government to establish their guilt or innocence of particular charges and to determine appropriate sentences for those found guilty.[6] All sexual abuse and unlawful sexual conduct or contact with a child (as defined by state law) as well as severe physical abuse are criminal acts.[7] In the event the government believes that it cannot prove the suspect guilty beyond a reasonable doubt, the government may instead seek a court order adjudicating the child a dependent, which is a civil proceeding.

Once the legal process has begun, there is frequently a period of "discovery" whereby both sides exchange information regarding the case. Physicians may be involved in the discovery process by means of a subpoena. A subpoena ad testificandum is a court order requiring an individual to appear at a designated time and place to provide sworn testimony.[6] A subpoena duces tecum requires the production of records or documents relevant to the matter being litigated.[8]

It is very important for physicians to be complete, accurate, and legible when documenting events in a patient's medical records. In the event those records will be used as evidence in court, it is even more vital that they be comprehensive. Correct, thorough, decipherable medical records can help the treating physician recall his or her findings when preparing for a hearing or a trial, which may occur several months after the physician's initial involvement with the patient, and they can help the lawyer have a better understanding of the medical findings. If the medical records become evidence, they will help the fact-finder understand the case and render the proper resolution.

A deposition is part of the discovery process whereby the parties learn about and evaluate the other's case through the testimony of witnesses before the trial.[6] In a civil case, it is possible that the opposing attorney will depose the treating physician. It is an informal setting, without a presiding judge or jury. It is important for the physician to be well prepared and to confer with the patient's attorney before the deposition. The testimony is given under oath and is recorded by a stenographer. After the deposition, a transcript is printed and signed by the witness, with amendments limited to corrections and clarifications.[6]

Providing Expert and Nonexpert Testimony

The rules of evidence provide the statutory and case-law framework by which information is deemed by a judge to be relevant, material, and therefore ordinarily admissible for consideration by the fact-finder (judge or jury) at a hearing or trial.[6] Although the rules of evidence may vary between federal and state proceedings and from state to state, most jurisdictions have evidentiary rules consistent with the federal rules of evidence as provided in Title 28 of the U.S. Code.

Evidence can be testimonial or "real," in the form of documents, pictures, or things (e.g., weapons). There are two types of witnesses. A fact witness provides factual testimony based on personal knowledge and is not allowed to express an opinion based on that knowledge.[6] An expert witness can formulate a professional opinion on the matter at hand, assist the fact-finder in understanding the evidence, or answer a hypothetical question. The judge decides whether a professional possesses sufficient knowledge, skill, experience, training, or education to qualify as an expert witness.[9]

Preparing to Testify

Testifying in a court hearing can be stressful, even for the most experienced professionals. It is crucial to be well prepared to ease anxiety, decrease the risk of surprises, and ensure that the court is provided with the most helpful information possible.[6] This involves reviewing all the medical records related to the case and any subsequent letters or documents generated.

It is crucial for the physician to confer with the attorney who subpoenaed him or her before the court date. This allows the physician to share knowledge or concerns that may be of interest to the lawyer, as well as any fears or past experiences.[6] The attorney should provide the physician with the theories of the case and a list of questions he or she intends to ask. The attorney may also discuss the opposing counsel's theories and anticipated questions. The physician should inquire whether documents will be admitted partially or entirely into evidence and whether he or she will be asked to use them as part of the testimony.[6] It is critical that the attorney be aware of the physician's opinion and understand the reasoning behind that opinion. The physician must be firm about the limits or scope of both his or her factual testimony and opinions. If the attorney presses for answers or opinions that the physician is uncomfortable giving, this must be expressed.[6]

Testifying in Court

On the day of the trial, the physician should dress professionally, arrive early, and notify the attorney of his or her presence. This allows time to clarify any new issues that may have arisen since the last contact. Of note, witnesses often

are sequestered, meaning that they are allowed in the courtroom only during their own testimony. In some cases, the court may permit the physician to be in the courtroom during the opposing side's expert testimony.

While on the witness stand, it is imperative that the physician listen to and understand each question. If the question is not fully heard or comprehended, the physician must ask the attorney to repeat the question. Questions should be answered with truthfulness, precision, and clarity. It may be necessary to define unfamiliar terms and explain difficult concepts. Always attempt to answer questions in language that is understandable to laypeople. In the event the physician does not know the answer to a question or cannot remember, he or she must say so.[6]

The initial part of expert testimony involves qualifying the physician as an expert. The attorney begins by asking a series of identifying and qualifying questions regarding the physician's professional education and experience.[6] In some instances, the physician's curriculum vitae will be admitted as an exhibit. The opposing counsel then has an opportunity to ask further questions to refute this qualification.

Once the physician is qualified as an expert, testimony can take one of three forms: an opinion, an answer to a hypothetical question, or a lecture that provides background information for the judge or jury.[8] Most often the expert is asked to render an opinion based on the facts of the case. Sometimes the expert's testimony is in the form of an answer to a hypothetical question that includes significant facts relevant to the case at hand. On occasion, an expert may testify in the form of a lecture that provides the fact-finder (judge or jury) with background information on technical, clinical, or scientific issues.[8]

Whatever the form of question and answer, it is important that the answer be well thought out, accurate, and clearly articulated. The physician should explain all conclusions and analyses in terms that are understood by the fact-finder and ensure that he or she does not exceed the bounds of his or her expertise or exaggerate in any manner. In formulating an opinion, an expert may rely on information that the prosecutor would not be permitted to offer in evidence to prove abuse, as long as it is based on information relied on by other experts.[9] This includes all relevant clinical, scientific, historical, and factual information. Experts are not allowed to express an opinion on legal issues such as the guilt or innocence of a defendant.

During cross-examination, the opposing counsel will attempt to show the fact-finder that the expert's testimony is flawed in some way. This may involve trying to discredit the expert's knowledge of the relevant evidence or posing other theories to explain the child's condition. An expert who has thoroughly reviewed all medical documents and relies on up-to-date knowledge in the field will be well equipped for cross-examination. The expert should also be prepared to explain the nature of possible differential diagnoses, their manifestations, and why they are not a plausible explanation for the matter on which the expert has given his or her opinion.[6]

Once again, it is imperative that the physician be attentive and understands each question asked by the opposing counsel. Although attorneys are not allowed to ask "leading" questions during direct examination, such questions are allowed and are often used during cross-examination.

Usually these take the form of yes or no questions, which the opposing counsel uses to control the witness and the testimony. If a question cannot be answered truthfully yes or no, the expert should say so and qualify the answer. The expert is also entitled to request to clarify a previous answer if it appears that he or she misspoke or misunderstood the question.[6]

If the expert was not allowed to fully answer a question or the expert's testimony was undercut during cross-examination, the direct examiner will attempt to clarify the expert's testimony during the redirect examination. This portion is usually limited to areas of inquiry pursued in or raised by cross-examination.[6]

IN A NUTSHELL

- As a physician, being involved in a case of suspected child abuse or neglect can be difficult both mentally and emotionally. It can be easier if the physician has a good knowledge base of the legal system and its intricacies. Physicians should know their state laws, hospital practice procedures, and venues for support services.
- If there is "reasonable cause" to suspect that a child has been maltreated, the physician must file a report with the state CPS agency or a law enforcement agency. In questionable cases, one can always call CPS to inquire whether a certain incident or circumstance should be reported.
- Ensure complete, accurate, legible documentation in patients' medical records, especially when dealing with cases of suspected child maltreatment. Those records may be subpoenaed by a court of law.
- Physicians should be well prepared before testifying in court, whether as a factual witness or an expert witness. This includes reviewing all medical records and conferring with the attorney who subpoenaed the physician.
- While testifying, if a question is not fully heard or comprehended, the physician should ask the attorney to repeat it. During testimony, the physician should explain all conclusions and analyses in terms understandable by the fact-finder and should not exceed the limits of his or her expertise or knowledge. If a question posed by the attorney cannot be answered yes or no, the physician should feel free to qualify the answer.

SUGGESTED READING

Myers JEB: Medicolegal aspects of child abuse. In Reece RM, Ludwig S (eds): Child Abuse Medical Diagnosis and Management, 2nd ed. Philadelphia, Lippincott Williams & Wilkins, 2001, pp 545-562.

Weber MW: The assessment of child abuse: A primary function of child protective services. In Helfer ME, Kempe RS, Krugman RD (eds): The Battered Child, 5th ed. Chicago, University of Chicago Press, 1997, pp 120-149.

REFERENCES

1. Bourne R: Child abuse and the law I: General Issues for the radiologist. In Kleinman PK (ed): Diagnostic Imaging of Child Abuse, 2nd ed. St Louis, Mosby, 1998, pp 371-374.
2. Melton GB, Limber S: Psychologist's involvement in cases of child maltreatment. Am Psychol 1989;44:1225-1233.
3. Shepherd JR: The role of law enforcement in the investigation of child abuse and neglect. In Helfer ME, Kempe RS, Krugman RD (eds): The Battered Child, 5th ed. Chicago, University of Chicago Press, 1997, pp 451-459.
4. Weber MW: The assessment of child abuse: A primary function of child protective services. In Helfer ME, Kempe RS, Krugman RD (eds): The Battered Child, 5th ed. Chicago, University of Chicago Press, 1997, pp 120-149.
5. Davidson HA: The courts and child maltreatment. In Helfer ME, Kempe RS, Krugman RD (eds): The Battered Child, 5th ed. Chicago, University of Chicago Press, 1997, pp 482-499.
6. Coakley M: Child abuse and the law II: The radiologist in court. In Kleinman PK (ed): Diagnostic Imaging of Child Abuse, 2nd ed. St Louis, Mosby, 1998, pp 375-382.
7. Trost T, Bulkley J: Child Maltreatment: A Summary and Analysis of Criminal Statutes. Washington, DC, ABA Center on Children and the Law, 1993.
8. Myers JEB: Medicolegal aspects of child abuse. In Reece RM, Ludwig S (eds): Child Abuse Medical Diagnosis and Management, 2nd ed. Philadelphia, Lippincott Williams & Wilkins, 2001, pp 545-562.
9. Myers JEB: Expert testimony regarding child sexual abuse. Child Abuse Negl 1993;17:175-185.

Toxins, Substance Abuse, and Environmental Exposures

CHAPTER 178

Stabilization and Hospitalization of the Poisoned Child

Kevin C. Osterhoudt

Approximately 2.4 million poisoning exposures are reported to the American Association of Poison Control Centers' Toxic Exposure Surveillance System each year.[1] More than half of all reported exposures involve children aged 5 years or younger, and two thirds can be considered "pediatric" exposures. Seventy-four percent of poisoning exposures reported to poison centers are managed at home, with less than 10% of exposures leading to hospitalization. The federally commissioned Institute of Medicine has determined that poisoning is the second leading cause of injury-related death in the United States, with costs exceeding $12.6 billion each year.[2]

The epidemiology of pediatric poisoning is bimodal: young, curiosity-driven children encounter toxicants through normal exploration of their environment, whereas adolescents become poisoned through substance abuse, experimentation, and intentional self-harm. Hospitalization rates, morbidity, and mortality are higher among the older group. Both groups are appropriate targets for preventive education in the hospital setting.

Poisoned children are frequently encountered by pediatric hospitalists. Typically, the poisoning scenario has been identified before inpatient hospitalization; however, pediatric poisoning may occasionally present as a diagnostic dilemma. The families of all children admitted to the hospital should be queried with regard to medication use; use of vitamins, herbs, or ethnic remedies; recreational drug abuse; occupational drug and chemical exposure; and environmental drug and chemical exposure. Several features of childhood illnesses that should raise the suspicion for poisoning are detailed in Table 178-1.

INITIAL STABILIZATION

Respiratory arrest, shock, cardiac arrhythmia, and neurologic injury are the most acute threats to life from poisoning. A standardized approach to initial life support is recommended (Table 178-2). Central nervous system depression due to poisoning may be most effectively assessed and communicated using the "AVPU" system (A, alert; V, opens eyes to verbal stimuli; P, opens eyes to painful stimuli; U, unresponsive). The Glasgow Coma Scale was developed for trauma evaluation, and its prognostic properties do not apply to acute poisoning. It is important to identify hypoglycemia or hypoxia as a cause of altered mentation early in the resuscitative process.

With critical life functions stabilized, attention should be given to decontamination of the patient from offending poisons. Topical contamination of the eyes can be flushed with warmed normal saline, and skin can be washed with soap and copious water. Based on the recommendations of the American Academy of Pediatrics, inducing emesis with syrup of ipecac has largely been abandoned as a means of decontaminating ingested poisons.[3] Gastric lavage, once a mainstay of gastric decontamination, has also fallen out of favor and should be considered only in rare circumstances (Table 178-3). Activated charcoal administration is the decontamination strategy of choice for most potentially toxic pediatric ingestions (Tables 178-4 and 178-5).[4] Activated charcoal is typically administered as a slurry at a dose of 1 g/kg, up to a maximum of 75 g. Charcoal should be regarded as a drug, and vomiting, constipation, pulmonary aspiration, and death have complicated its clinical use.[5] Naso- or orogastric tube administration of charcoal appears to be more commonly associated with severe adverse events. Whole-bowel irrigation with a polyethylene glycol–balanced electrolyte solution can be used as a cathartic to prevent the absorption of ingested toxic substances (Table 178-6). It is typically administered via nasogastric tube at rates titrated to 500 mL/hour in young children and 2 L/hour in adolescents. It is continued until the rectal effluent is clear but should be discontinued for refractory vomiting, abdominal pain, or abdominal distention.

Table 178-1   Features That Suggest a Diagnosis of Poisoning

Acute onset of illness
Age range 1 to 5 yr
Suspected exploratory or intentional ingestion of drug or chemical
Evidence of interpersonal conflict or chronic illness in the home
History of depression
Significant alteration in level of consciousness
Involvement of multiple organ systems
Puzzling clinical picture

Adapted from Osterhoudt KC, Burns Ewald M, Shannon M, Henretig FM: Toxicologic emergencies. In Fleisher G, Ludwig S (eds): Textbook of Pediatric Emergency Medicine, 5th ed. Philadelphia, Lippincott Williams & Wilkins, 2006, pp 951-1007.

Table 178-2   Initial Resuscitation of a Poisoned Patient

A: Airway—maintain adequate airway
B: Breathing—ensure adequate oxygenation and ventilation
C: Circulation—support circulation and perfusion
D: Disability—altered consciousness merits resuscitation Oxygen Dextrose (0.2-0.5 g/kg) Naloxone (0.4-2 mg initially, up to 10 mg) Treat hyperthermia if present

Table 178-3   Indications for Gastric Lavage*

Suspected life-threatening toxic ingestion
Procedure can be performed early after ingestion, when significant amount of drug remains in stomach
Symptoms of poisoning not yet floridly apparent
Airway patency can be maintained
General supportive care, or antidotal therapy, expected to be ineffectual
Procedure can be performed with proper technique, including large-bore orogastric tube, body positioned on left side with head lower than feet

*All must apply.

CLINICAL PRESENTATION

Clinical signs can be categorized into characteristic poisoning syndromes known as toxidromes.[6] During a thorough physical examination, careful attention should be paid

Table 178-4   Indications for Single-Dose Activated Charcoal*

Potentially injurious toxic ingestion
Toxicant can be adsorbed by activated charcoal (see Table 178-5)
Charcoal can be given early after ingestion, when significant amount of drug remains in stomach
Charcoal can be administered safely, with attention to the prevention of pulmonary aspiration

*All must apply.

Table 178-5   Poisons for Which Activated Charcoal Is Not Helpful

Ineffective Alcohols Iron Lithium
Poorly Effective Hydrocarbons Metals

Table 178-6   Poisons for Which Whole-Bowel Irrigation Might Be Considered

Ingested packages of drugs of abuse
Iron pills
Lithium pills
Sustained-release drugs
Medicinal patches
Pill concretions

to suspected poisoning patients' mentation, vital signs, pupil size and reactivity, bowel and bladder function, and skin moisture and color (Table 178-7).

LABORATORY EVALUATION

Many drugs become concentrated upon elimination in the urine, and urine is the preferred specimen for toxicology screening. Blood or serum testing is typically reserved for quantification of specific drug or chemical levels such as acetaminophen, aspirin, toxic alcohols, anticonvulsants, lithium, iron, or lead. Most hospitals offer a urine immunoassay for drugs of abuse, including amphetamines, barbiturates, benzodiazepines, cocaine, and opiates. Toxidrome analysis, as described earlier, is typically faster, cheaper, and more clinically useful than urine screening.

Table 178-7 Common Toxidromes

Physical Findings	Sympathomimetics (Cocaine, Amphetamine)	Anticholinergics	Organophosphates	Opiates, Clonidine	Barbiturates, Sedative-Hypnotics	Salicylates
Mental status	A, D, P, S	C, D, P, S	C, D, F	C	C	C, S
Heart rate	↑	↑	↓ (↑)	↑	–	– (↑)
Blood pressure	↑	↑	– (↑)	↓	↓	–
Temperature	↑	↑	–	↓	↓	↑
Respirations	–	–	↑	↓	↓	↑
Pupil size	↑ (reactive)	↑ (sluggish)	↓	↓↓	–	–
Bowel sounds	–	↓	↑	↓	–	–
Skin	Sweaty	Flushed, dry	Sweaty	–	Bullae (IV use)	Sweaty

A, agitation; C, somnolence/coma; D, delirium; F, fasciculations; P, psychosis; S, seizure.
From Osterhoudt KC, Wiley J: Poisonings. In Selbst SM, Cronan K (eds): Pediatric Emergency Medicine Secrets, 2nd ed. Philadelphia, Elsevier, 2006.

Whenever the urine of a young child is analyzed for drugs of abuse, it must be considered that a positive result is likely to have medicolegal implications. Therefore, a sufficient sample should be provided to the laboratory in a timely and organized fashion. Because urine drug immunoassays can have both false-positive and false-negative results, they should always be confirmed by another method. Some reference laboratories offer more comprehensive testing of urine for drugs, chemicals, or elemental metals. Hair testing is sometimes used to determine the chronology of poison exposure.

When the poisoning exposure is well defined, as is common with exploratory ingestions in young children, laboratory analysis and diagnostic studies may be goal directed. When the exposure history is unreliable, as is often the case with adolescents' polypharmacy attempts at suicide, some empirical testing may be warranted. Acetaminophen poisoning may be asymptomatic until hepatic failure ensues, so an acetaminophen level should be strongly considered. Heart blocks or conduction delays on electrocardiography may foretell cardiac complications. Tests for metabolic acidosis, serum electrolytes, serum ammonia, osmolar gap calculation, rhabdomyolysis, hepatic and renal function, and hemoglobin co-oximetry are sometimes indicated.

TREATMENT

The physiologic derangements caused by acute poisoning are typically of finite duration, until the drug or chemical is eliminated from the body, and good supportive care suffices for the majority of patients. Some poisons have specific or nonspecific antidotes (Table 178-8), and some poisons are amenable to methods that speed their elimination from the body. Urinary alkalization leads to "ion trapping" in the kidney and enhanced elimination of salicylates. Hemodialysis assists in the clearance of lithium, methanol and ethylene glycol, and salicylates; charcoal hemoperfusion enhances the elimination of theophylline and paraquat. Multiple doses of activated charcoal, given every 4 to 6 hours, may disrupt enterohepatic circulation and hasten the elimination of carbamazepine, dapsone, phenobarbital, quinine, and theophylline.[7]

DISPOSITION

In the United States, regional poison control centers can be contacted by telephone at 1-800-222-1222. Poison control centers play an important public health role by triaging nontoxic exposures away from hospitals and assisting health care providers with hospitalization decisions. A modest list of pharmaceutical agents is thought to be potentially life threatening to curiosity-driven children ingesting only one or two dosage forms (Table 178-9).[8] Children exposed to arrhythmogenic poisons such as chloroquine, cyclic antidepressants, and selected psychotropic medications merit telemetry monitoring when available. Children with impending or existing failure of the respiratory, cardiovascular, or neurologic systems or those with special needs (e.g., hemodialysis) are good candidates for intensive care. Although the advice of medical toxicologists is frequently available through the regional poison control center network, selected poisoned patients may benefit from transfer to a specialized center for poisoning treatment (Table 178-10; more information is available from the American College of Medical Toxicology website at *http://www.acmt. net/main/resources_guidelines.asp#anchor265036*). Most patients who will become ill following a poisoning exposure develop symptoms or signs within 6 hours. However, several "toxic time bombs" are notorious for causing relatively late clinical deterioration (Table 178-11), and due caution should be exercised when discharging patients with these exposures from medical care.

Table 178-8   Common Antidotes Used to Treat Poisoning and Envenomation

Antidote*	Indications
N-Acetylcysteine	Acetaminophen
Antivenin	Snake, spider, scorpion envenomation
Atropine	Organophosphates, carbamates
Bicarbonate (sodium)	Cyclic antidepressant cardiotoxicity
Bromocriptine	Neuroleptic malignant syndrome
Calcium	Calcium channel blockers, hydrogen fluoride
Dantrolene	Malignant hyperthermia
Deferoxamine	Iron
Digoxin-specific Fab	Digoxin, digitalis
Dimercaprol (BAL)	Lead, other metals
Diphenhydramine	Neuroleptic dystonia
Edetate calcium disodium	Lead, other metals
Ethanol	Ethylene glycol, methanol
Flumazenil	Benzodiazepines
Folic acid	Methanol
Folinic acid (leucovorin)	Methotrexate
Glucagon	Beta-blocker-induced bradycardia and hypotension
Hyperbaric oxygen	Carbon monoxide
Methylene blue	Methemoglobinemia
Naloxone, nalmefene	Opioids
Nitrite (amyl, sodium)	Cyanide
Penicillamine	Lead, other metals
Physostigmine	Anticholinergic agents
Pralidoxime (2-PAM)	Organophosphates, carbamates
Protamine	Heparin
Pyridoxine	Isoniazid, ethylene glycol
Sodium thiosulfate	Cyanide
Succimer (DMSA)	Lead, other metals
Thiamine	Wernicke encephalopathy, ethylene glycol
Thiosulfate	Cyanide
Vitamin K_1	Warfarins

*Does not include gastrointestinal decontamination agents, routine supportive pressor agents, sedatives, and anticonvulsants.

Table 178-9   Pharmaceuticals Highly Dangerous to Young Children*

Benzocaine

Calcium channel blockers

Camphor

Chloroquine

Clonidine

Cyclic antidepressants

Diphenoxylate, atropine (Lomotil)

Lindane

Methadone (and other opioids)

Methyl salicylate (oil of wintergreen)

Oral hypoglycemics

Propranolol

Quinidine

Theophylline

Thioridazine

*Poisoning can occur with one or two pills or swallows.
Adapted from Osterhoudt KC: The toxic toddler: Drugs that can kill in small doses. Contemp Pediatr 2000;17:73-88.

Table 178-10   Indications for Transfer to a Poisoning Treatment Center

Lack of familiarity with an unusual poison

Unavailability of, or unfamiliarity with, an unusual antidote

Need for enhanced toxicology laboratory services

Need for unavailable medical technology or services

Table 178-11   Drugs That Can Cause Toxicity after a Prolonged Asymptomatic Period

Acetaminophen

Oral hypoglycemic agents

Toxic alcohols, glycols

Warfarin products

Thyroid hormones

Monoamine oxidase inhibitors

Sustained-release preparations

Drugs causing acute withdrawal syndromes

SUGGESTED READING

Osterhoudt KC, Burns Ewald M, Shannon M, Henretig FM: Toxicologic emergencies. In Fleisher G, Ludwig S (eds): Textbook of Pediatric Emergency Medicine, 5th ed. Philadelphia, Lippincott Williams & Wilkins, 2006, pp 951-1007.

Osterhoudt KC, Perrone J, De Roos F, Henretig FM (eds): Toxicology Pearls. Philadelphia, Elsevier Mosby, 2004.

Shannon MW: Ingestion of toxic substances by children. N Engl J Med 2000;342:186-191.

REFERENCES

1. Watson WA, Litovitz TL, Rodgers GC Jr, et al: 2004 Annual report of the American Association of Poison Control Centers Toxic Exposure Surveillance System. Am J Emerg Med 2005;23:589-666.

2. Institute of Medicine: Forging a Poison Prevention and Control System. Washington, DC, National Academies Press, 2004.

3. American Academy of Pediatrics, Committee on Injury, Violence, and Poison Prevention: Poison treatment in the home. Pediatrics 2003;112:1182-1185.

4. Bond GR: The role of activated charcoal and gastric emptying in gastrointestinal decontamination: A state-of-the-art review. Ann Emerg Med 2002;39:273-286.

5. Osterhoudt KC, Durbin D, Alpern ER, et al: Activated charcoal administration in a pediatric emergency department. Pediatr Emerg Care 2004;20:493-498.

6. Osterhoudt KC: No sympathy for a boy with obtundation. Pediatr Emerg Care 2004;20:403-406.

7. American Academy of Clinical Toxicology, European Association of Poisons Centres and Clinical Toxicologists: Position statement and practice guideline on the use of multi-dose activated charcoal in the treatment of acute poisoning. Clin Toxicol 1999;37:731-751.

8. Osterhoudt KC: The toxic toddler: Drugs that can kill in small doses. Contemp Pediatr 2000;17:73-88.

CHAPTER 179

Toxicity of Over-the-Counter and Oral Hypoglycemic Agents

Rebekah Mannix and Michele Burns Ewald

The household medicine cabinet is filled with products that are potentially toxic, many of which have been obtained over the counter. According to the 2004 American Association of Poison Control Centers' Toxic Exposure Surveillance System (TESS), analgesics, vitamins, antihistamines, and cough and cold preparations account for approximately 20% of all exposures in children younger than 6 years.[1] Oral hypoglycemics, which are also ubiquitous, are another common household danger that cause significant morbidity and mortality in children.

IRON

Historically, iron preparations have been a leading cause of pediatric mortality from exploratory drug overdose. In 1997, the Food and Drug Administration issued a regulation requiring warning labels and childproof packaging for iron-containing products with 30 mg or more of iron per dosage unit.[2] Since the implementation of childproof packaging and warning labels, the trend in TESS data suggests that iron poisoning and fatalities are decreasing.[3] In 2004, the iron-packaging regulations were repealed, and ferrous sulfate tablets and prenatal vitamins remain a toxic threat.

Clinical Presentation

Different formulations of iron contain disparate amounts of elemental iron (Table 179-1). Mild toxicity, expressed in terms of milligrams of elemental iron per kilogram body weight, is seen with doses as low as 20 mg/kg elemental iron, whereas systemic illness generally occurs with doses in the range of 40 to 60 mg/kg. The pharmacokinetics of iron in an overdose remains somewhat of a mystery.[4] Peak iron levels are thought to occur between 2 and 6 hours after ingestion. Serum iron levels generally correlate with clinical severity: mild symptomatology (vomiting, diarrhea) is seen with levels less than 300 μg/dL, moderate symptoms with levels of 300 to 500 μg/dL, and severe manifestations (shock, acidosis, seizures, coma) with levels exceeding 500 μg/dL.[5]

Iron toxicity is described in phases. Early toxicity is caused by local irritant effects, whereas later findings are thought to be due to mitochondrial damage, particularly in the liver (Table 179-2).

Diagnosis and Evaluation

An abdominal radiograph is indicated to look for the presence and location of iron tablets. Completely dissolved iron tablets/capsules/liquid preparations may not be radiopaque; consequently, a negative radiograph does not rule out the possibility of toxic iron ingestion.[6] However, patients with negative abdominal radiographs may be discharged after a 6-hour period of observation if they remain asymptomatic.[7] Baseline laboratory studies, including serum iron levels (if available), hepatic studies (serum transaminases, albumin, and coagulation studies), and electrolytes, including the serum bicarbonate concentration, should be obtained 4 to 6 hours after ingestion for any patient with symptoms of toxicity or a significant history of ingestion. Leukocytosis (>15,000/mm³) and hyperglycemia (>150 mg/dL) are sometimes seen after iron poisoning, but these laboratory findings are neither sensitive nor specific. Metabolic acidosis should be regarded with concern.

Treatment

Whole-bowel irrigation with a polyethylene glycol balanced electrolyte solution may be considered as a means of gastrointestinal decontamination. Iron is not adsorbed by activated charcoal. Further therapeutic guidelines, including deferoxamine chelation, are presented in Table 179-3.

Intravenous deferoxamine remains the mainstay of treatment after gut decontamination. Oral deferoxamine is not recommended. Deferoxamine may be administered intramuscularly, but the injections are painful and may cause local tissue inflammation. Although previously advocated, the intramuscular deferoxamine challenge test is no longer recommended. In patients with serious systemic toxicity, a deferoxamine infusion should be started and gradually increased to a rate of 15 mg/kg/hr.

Once therapy with deferoxamine is instituted, clinical monitoring should include serial measurements of blood pressure, serum iron concentration (if available), hepatic transaminases, electrolytes, and the prothrombin time. Of note, serum iron levels may be falsely lowered by the presence of deferoxamine. Therapeutic end points for deferoxamine therapy include resolution of clinical symptoms and metabolic acidosis, as well as narrowing of the anion gap. In the presence of deferoxamine, iron levels may not be accurate, but persistently elevated levels should raise concern. Recurrent symptomatology may warrant reinstitution of deferoxamine, which should be undertaken carefully and at a lower dose.

The most dreaded complications of therapy with deferoxamine are *Yersinia enterocolitica* septicemia and mucormycosis. The mechanism of this complication is unclear, but deferoxamine may provide the iron siderophore complex growth factor needed by the bacteria to induce overgrowth.[8,9] Pulmonary toxicity, which is manifested as tachypnea, hypoxemia, fever, eosinophilia, preceding urticaria, and pulmonary infiltrates, may be seen in patients receiving both prolonged (>24 hours) and high (>15 mg/kg/hr) doses of intravenous deferoxamine.[10-12] Hypotension, too, appears to be a dose-related effect. Ocular and otic toxicity has also been reported.

Admission Criteria

Patients in whom signs of mild poisoning (vomiting, diarrhea) develop should be admitted for inpatient management. Patients who demonstrate serious systemic signs of toxicity (shock, central nervous system depression) should be considered candidates for an intensive care setting.

Discharge Criteria

Discharge from inpatient medical care may occur when symptoms and laboratory abnormalities have resolved and no clinical deterioration is noted after cessation of deferoxamine therapy.

ANTIHISTAMINES

Over-the-counter antihistamines are ubiquitous and used for cold and allergy symptoms. Most of the toxicity associated with an overdose of antihistamines is due to their anticholinergic effects. Recently, two of the nonsedating antihistamines, terfenadine (Seldane) and astemizole (Hismanal), were discontinued because of reports of significant cardiac toxicity when combined with drugs that impair their

Table 179-1 Iron Formulations

Formulation	Elemental Iron (%)
Ferrous sulfate	20
Ferrous sulfate (anhydrous)	30
Ferrous gluconate	12
Ferrous fumarate	33
Ferrous lactate	19
Ferrous chloride	28

Table 179-2 Phases of Iron Toxicity

Phase	Time from Ingestion	Symptoms	Pathophysiology
1	0-6 hr	Emesis, diarrhea, abdominal pain Can progress to hypovolemic shock	Direct local irritant effect on gastrointestinal mucosa
2	6-12 hr	Improvement of phase 1 symptoms	Iron entering cells
3	12-24 hr	Gastrointestinal fluid losses lead to hypovolemic shock. Wide anion gap acidosis. Depressed myocardial function. Increased pulmonary vascular resistance. Liver failure with hypoglycemia and coagulopathy	Iron concentrates intracellularly in mitochondria and disrupts oxidative phosphorylation, thereby resulting in free radical formation and lipid peroxidation Free iron may exhibit a direct inhibitory effect on the formation of thrombin and thrombin's effect on fibrinogen in vitro
4	2-6 wk and beyond	Emesis Liver failure	Emesis secondary to pyloric stricture, liver failure secondary to hepatic cirrhosis

Table 179-3 Treatment of Iron Toxicity (Ingestion >20 mg/kg Elemental Iron)

Symptom	Laboratory Finding	Treatment
Asymptomatic	Negative KUB	Observe for 6 hr—discharge home if no symptoms develop
Asymptomatic	Radiopaque pills on KUB	WBI and repeat KUB Determine electrolytes and SI 4-6 hr after ingestion Start deferoxamine if peak SI >500 µg/dL or metabolic acidosis
Symptomatic	Radiopaque pills on KUB or Peak SI >350-500 µg/dL or Patient is symptomatic and SI cannot readily be obtained	As above Start deferoxamine by continuous infusion at a rate of up to 15 mg/kg/hr
Symptomatic	Anion gap acidosis	Aggressive fluid resuscitation
Hypotension, shock		Watch for cardiogenic pulmonary edema. Dopamine and/or norepinephrine may be needed for refractory hypotension
Symptomatic	Hypoglycemia	Watch for hypoglycemia and correct as needed
Acute liver failure	Coagulopathy	FFP, cryoprecipitate as needed

FFP, fresh frozen plasma; KUB, abdominal radiograph; SI, serum iron concentration; WBI, whole-bowel irrigation.

Table 179-4   Common Histamine Receptor Antagonists

Azelastine (Astelin)
Brompheniramine (Dimetane)*
Cetirizine (Zyrtec)
Chlorpheniramine (Chlor-Trimeton)*
Cyclizine (Marezine)*
Dimenhydrinate (Dramamine)*
Diphenhydramine (Benadryl)*
Doxylamine*
Fexofenadine (Allegra)
Hydroxyzine (Atarax, Vistaril)*
Loratadine (Claritin)
Meclizine (Antivert)*
Promethazine (Phenergan)*

*Prominent anticholinergic symptoms.

metabolism through cytochrome 3A4, such as ketoconazole or erythromycin.[13] Cardiotoxicity has not been reported with the use of fexofenadine (Allegra), cetirizine (Zyrtec), loratadine (Claritin), or azelastine (Astelin), all of which have limited anticholinergic side effects.[14] A list of some common antihistamines is provided in Table 179-4.

Clinical Presentation

Absorption of antihistamines from the gastrointestinal tract is rapid, with the peak drug effect usually seen in 1 hour. However, after large ingestions, symptoms may not occur for several hours and may last for days. Patients who have taken an overdose of antihistamines may present with the classic anticholinergic toxidrome (Chapter 178). In addition, seizures are common after large overdoses of antihistamines. Some antihistamines, especially diphenhydramine, can cause wide-QRS tachyarrhythmias from sodium channel blockade. Antihistamines are often combined with other drugs in commercial products, so concomitant toxicity from sympathomimetic agents or dextromethorphan may be encountered.

Diagnosis and Evaluation

The toxic effects of antihistamines are due mostly to anticholinergic phenomena through inhibition of both central and peripheral muscarinic cholinergic receptors. The diagnostic course for patients with a suspected overdose of antihistamines depends somewhat on the symptomatology and dose ingested. The mean dose in symptomatic children was 17.3 mg/kg in a study of 184 cases; deaths have been reported with doses as low as 33 mg/kg.[15] The delirium associated with anticholinergic poisoning may lead to evaluation for central nervous system infection. Acetaminophen levels are of particular importance because many cold products contain both antihistamines and acetaminophen. Diphenhydramine may result in a false-positive urine immunoassay for phencyclidine. Electrocardiographic evaluation, specifi-

cally checking for widening of the QRS, is warranted to look for signs of impending arrhythmia, as well as the possibility of co-ingestants.

Treatment

Activated charcoal may reduce the absorption of antihistamine drugs if administered soon after ingestion. Inpatient care should be directed at symptoms (Table 179-5). Physostigmine should be considered for both diagnosis and symptom management.[16] The benefits of physostigmine, which include restoration of gastrointestinal motility and improvement in mental status, must outweigh the potential risks (worsening of cardiac conduction delays). Physostigmine may be used safely when the patient has a narrow QRS complex on electrocardiography and no evidence of ingestion of other agents (e.g., class IA or IC antiarrhythmics) that may cause intraventricular conduction delays. Intravenous access and cardiovascular monitoring must be established before the use of physostigmine. The initial dose of physostigmine, 0.02 mg/kg in children or 1 to 2 mg in adults, may be administered by slow intravenous push every 5 minutes until the anticholinergic symptoms are reversed. Additional physostigmine should not be administered if significant cholinergic symptoms develop, particularly bradycardia or excessive salivation. A dose of atropine, approximately half the dose of physostigmine, should be readily available. Redosing of physostigmine may be needed every 30 to 60 minutes. Patients considered at high risk for the development of seizures may be coadministered a prophylactic dose of benzodiazepine.

Admission Criteria

Patients displaying persistent changes in mental status, abnormalities in vital signs, electrocardiographic changes, or seizures should be admitted to the hospital. The severity of symptomatology may warrant admission to an intensive care setting.

Discharge Criteria

Discharge from inpatient medical care may occur when the patient has become asymptomatic and no further drug absorption is anticipated.

ACETAMINOPHEN

Acetaminophen, also known as paracetamol, is responsible for a large number of toxic ingestions in children each year.[1] Hepatic injury is the most frequent cause of morbidity and mortality after an overdose of acetaminophen. Extensive clinical research and experience have allowed clinicians to better predict and prevent the development of hepatotoxicity.[17,18]

Most forms of acetaminophen are rapidly absorbed after ingestion. The newer extended-release acetaminophen preparations have similar pharmacokinetics as the regular-release formulations, with peak levels occurring less than 4 hours after ingestion.[19]

Acetaminophen is metabolized almost exclusively in the liver; approximately 90% is glucuronidated or sulfated, 5% is excreted unchanged in urine, and the remaining 5% is oxidized by liver cytochrome enzymes, specifically CYP2E1,

Table 179-5   Treatment of Antihistamine Overdose

Symptom	Treatment	Comments
Agitation/delirium	Physostigmine IV over 5-min period (adults, 1-2 mg; pediatric, 0.02 mg/kg) Benzodiazepines IV	Electrocardiographic conduction delay (wide PR, QRS) is relative contraindication for physostigmine
Seizures	Benzodiazepines IV Physostigmine IV over 5-min period (adults, 1-2 mg; pediatric, 0.02 mg/kg)	In the setting of tricyclic antidepressant overdose, use of physostigmine has been associated with seizures and intractable cardiac arrest
Hyperthermia	Cool bath, fans, sedation	
Ventricular arrhythmia	Sodium bicarbonate bolus (1-2 mEq/kg), then drip (in D5W) Lidocaine bolus (1 mg/kg), then drip as needed (20-50 µg/kg/min)	Monitor electrocardiogram continuously; monitor serum electrolytes and arterial blood gases Goal serum pH, 7.45-7.55. Continue 24 hr past end points of cessation of dysrhythmias, normalization of QRS complexes
Other tachyarrhythmia	Supportive treatment if hemodynamically stable May consider beta-blocker (propranolol) May consider physostigmine if refractory	See above
Torsades de pointes	Cardioversion Magnesium sulfate IV (adults, 2-6 g; pediatric, 25-50 mg/kg) Overdrive pacing	
Rhabdomyolysis	Fluid resuscitation, urinary alkalinization, and maintenance of urine output at 1-2 mL/kg/hr	

D5W, 5% dextrose in water.

CYP1A2, and CYP3A4. Oxidation produces the reactive electrophile *N*-acetyl-*p*-benzoquinone imine (NAPQI). In conditions of therapeutic dosing, NAPQI is detoxified by glutathione, whereas in conditions of decreased glutathione stores, large doses of acetaminophen, or induction of cytochrome enzymes, NAPQI overwhelms the capacity of glutathione. Free NAPQI binds instead to hepatocytes and causes hepatocellular damage.

The risk for hepatocellular injury can be assessed by the dose ingested, the acetaminophen level, or both. In acute ingestion, patients who take more than 150 to 200 mg/kg (children) or 7.5 g (adults) are at risk for acetaminophen toxicity. Some patients who chronically exceed the recommended doses of acetaminophen appear to be particularly at risk for hepatotoxicity; such patients include those with pre-existing liver disease, children with acute febrile illnesses, and patients who chronically ingest inducers of CYP2E1.[20-22]

Clinical Presentation

Patients who have been exposed to toxic doses of acetaminophen may have a paucity of findings on physical examination. Acetaminophen toxicity is divided into four clinical stages, and the findings of each phase are presented in Table 179-6.[23]

Diagnosis and Evaluation

Initial laboratory analysis for a patient with a known acetaminophen overdose should begin with a serum acetaminophen level. Acetaminophen levels should be obtained in all cases of intentional overdose because acetaminophen is a

Table 179-6   Stages of Acetaminophen Toxicity

Stage	Time after Ingestion	Clinical Findings
I	0.5 to 24 hr	Anorexia, nausea, vomiting, malaise, pallor, diaphoresis
II	24 to 48 hr	Resolution of early symptoms; right upper quadrant abdominal pain and tenderness; elevated bilirubin, prothrombin time, hepatic transaminases, oliguria
III	72 to 96 hr	Peak of liver function abnormalities Reappearance of anorexia, nausea, vomiting Onset of fulminant hepatic failure with metabolic acidosis, coagulopathy, and renal dysfunction
IV	4 days to 2 wk	Resolution of hepatic dysfunction or progression to oliguric renal failure and death

frequent co-ingestant. Levels obtained before 4 hours after ingestion are difficult to interpret. The standard acetaminophen nomogram may be used to predict the risk for acetaminophen toxicity in patients in whom levels were obtained 4 hours or longer after ingestion (Fig. 179-1).

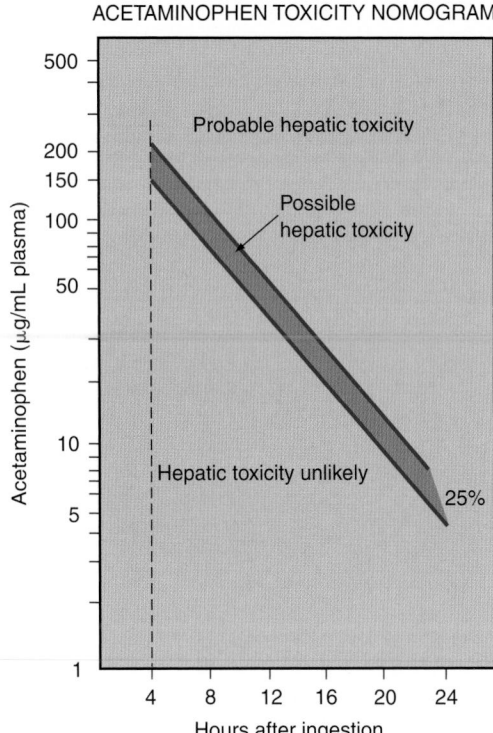

ACETAMINOPHEN TOXICITY NOMOGRAM

Figure 179-1 The Rumack-Matthew nomogram relating expected severity of liver toxicity to serum acetaminophen concentrations. (From Smilkstein MJ, Bronstein AC, Linden C, et al: Acetaminophen overdose: A 48-hour intravenous *N*-acetylcysteine treatment protocol. Ann Emerg Med 1991;20:1058.)

Table 179-7 Criteria for Referral to a Transplant Center and Criteria for Transplantation	
Referral to a Transplant Center	Transplantation
INR >5 *or*	Arterial pH <7.3 any time after FHF that fails to correct
Serum creatinine >2.3 mg/dL *or*	with colloid *or* Prothrombin time >100 seconds *and*
Arterial pH <7.35 *or* Serum HCO₃ <18 mEq/L *or*	Creatinine >3.4 mg/dL *and* Grade III or grade IV hepatic encephalopathy
Hypotension *or*	
Hepatic encephalopathy *or*	
Hypoglycemia	

FHF, fulminant hepatic failure; INR, international normalized ratio.
Adapted from Makin AJ, Williams R: Acetaminophen-induced hepatotoxicity: Predisposing factors and treatments. Adv Intern Med 1997;42:453–483.

Levels obtained after the ingestion of extended-release products may also be plotted on the nomogram.[24] In the United States, the lower line of the nomogram is used as the clinical indicator to begin treatment. Additional laboratory evaluation should consist of measurement of hepatic transaminases and determination of liver synthetic function (coagulation studies and albumin) and renal function. Repeated supratherapeutic overdoses of acetaminophen are difficult to plot on the nomogram, although some will conservatively extrapolate as though the total ingested dose was taken at the time of the first ingestion.

Treatment

N-acetylcysteine (NAC) is effective when administered by both the oral and intravenous routes. A 72-hour oral regimen has historically been used in the United States; the intravenous preparation has recently become more available after U.S. Food and Drug Administration approval, and this 21-hour regimen is as efficacious as the oral regimen. No deaths from hepatic injury have been reported in patients treated with NAC within 8 hours of overdose. No serious complications have been reported after the use of oral NAC.[25] In contrast, intravenous NAC has been shown to cause urticaria, anaphylactoid reactions, and rarely, death.[26,27] The risk seems to be highest in asthmatic patients. Intravenous NAC is preferred in patients with intractable vomiting despite the use of antiemetics, fulminant hepatic failure (FHF), or pregnancy.

The treatment regimen for oral NAC is a loading dose of 140 mg/kg, followed by 70 mg/kg every 4 hours for a total of 17 doses (not including the loading dose). Shorter courses have been proposed. Patients with persistent laboratory abnormalities may benefit from NAC past the standard 72-hour regimen. NAC may be given intravenously as a 3% solution (in 5% dextrose) as follows: 150-mg/kg loading dose over a 1-hour period, then 50 mg/kg over a 4-hour period, and then 100 mg/kg over a 16-hour period. The last infusion may be continued beyond 16 hours if hepatitis occurs.

Transaminases, liver synthetic function (coagulation studies and albumin), and renal function should be checked initially and daily during therapy in any patient with a serum acetaminophen concentration above the treatment nomogram line. Worsening hepatic function may necessitate more frequent laboratory studies. Patients who demonstrate hepatotoxicity despite treatment with NAC will need further clinical and laboratory monitoring, including the prothrombin time, international normalized ratio (INR) clotting measure, arterial pH, and serum creatinine. Patients with an INR greater than 2 at 24 hours, 4 at 48 hours, or 6 at 72 hours are at high risk for the development of FHF. Any patient in whom FHF develops should be referred for possible liver transplantation. Criteria for referral and transplantation are found in Table 179-7.

Admission Criteria

Treatment with NAC is the mainstay of acetaminophen poisoning and necessitates admission to the hospital. For a single acute overdose taken at a known time, NAC should be administered to all patients with an acetaminophen level in the "possible and probable hepatotoxicity" range. When the time of ingestion is unknown or in cases of repeated supratherapeutic overdoses, NAC may be administered while the acetaminophen is eliminated and hepatic transaminases are monitored.

Discharge Criteria

Demonstration of a normal serum aspartate transaminase (AST) level 36 hours after acetaminophen ingestion essentially eliminates the possibility of liver toxicity.[28] In the face of hepatic toxicity, a decline in the serum AST level may indicate clinical recovery or complete hepatocellular death and must be interpreted in the context of liver function. Patients suffering hepatic toxicity may be discharged once hepatic recovery is clearly in progress.

SALICYLATES

From its introduction 100 years ago, aspirin (acetylsalicylic acid) has remained a mainstay of clinical medicine. Despite the development of newer and more specific nonsteroidal anti-inflammatory drugs (NSAIDs), aspirin continues to be widely used because of its multiple applications and benefits. Although reported cases of aspirin toxicity have declined in the last 2 decades, aspirin still accounts for tens of thousand of cases reported to poison control centers and approximately 30 deaths each year. Moreover, aspirin has a significantly higher fatality ratio than acetaminophen or ibuprofen does.[1]

In addition to aspirin, other salicylate-containing products are commonly used, including liniments for arthritis, acne creams, sunscreens, antidiarrheals, and Chinese proprietary medications. There are also numerous combination preparations of aspirin.

Clinical Presentation

Salicylates produce analgesic, antipyretic, and anti-inflammatory effects, mostly through inhibition of cyclo-oxygenase and a subsequent decrease in the production of prostaglandins. Therapeutic doses of acetylsalicylic acid, 10 to 20 mg/kg for children and 650 to 1000 mg every 4 to 6 hours for adults, produce a serum salicylate level of 3 to 6 mg/dL. Of note, there are several circumstances, including Kawasaki disease and rheumatoid arthritis, in which high-dose therapy is used, with dosing in the range of 80 to 100 mg/kg.

Evidence of toxicity usually appears around serum levels of 30 mg/dL. The potentially toxic acute dose is greater than 150 mg/kg, whereas chronic toxicity may occur with doses that exceed 100 mg/kg/day.[29] Toxic doses for other salicylate formulations may be calculated by using known aspirin equivalencies.

Salicylates are absorbed in the stomach and proximal part of the intestine. Peak serum levels in therapeutic doses occur at 1 to 2 hours (4 to 6 hours for enteric-coated tablets) but may be delayed to 10 to 60 hours in cases of overdose.[30,31] The most notorious reason for delayed absorption is an aspirin bezoar, but other causes include enteric-coated products, contraction of the pylorus, and delayed gastric emptying from other ingestants. The elimination half-life of salicylate in therapeutic doses is 4 hours, but it increases to 15 to 29 hours with toxic plasma levels.[30]

The pathophysiology of salicylate toxicity is complex. Salicylates directly stimulate the respiratory center of the medulla and result in hyperventilation and hyperpnea. In an attempt to compensate for the respiratory alkalosis, the kidney excretes bicarbonate, thereby producing metabolic acidosis. This metabolic acidosis is exacerbated by the salicylate-driven uncoupling of mitochondrial oxidative phosphorylation, which causes an increase in oxygen consumption and carbon dioxide production, as well as accumulation of lactic and pyruvic acids.[32] Disruption of Krebs cycle metabolism leads to gluconeogenesis, lipolysis, and increased ketone formation. The salicylate ion itself contributes very little to the metabolic acidosis. The differential diagnosis of anion gap acidosis should be considered. The pathophysiology of the most common presenting symptoms in salicylate toxicity is found in Table 179-8.

Diagnosis and Evaluation

Evaluation of salicylate toxicity should begin with assessment of the chronicity of the toxicity. Patients with chronic toxicity can be identified by historical clues such as extremes of age, chronic medical problems, mental status changes out of proportion to the serum salicylate level, late presentation, and severe dehydration. Laboratory studies should include a serum salicylate level, serum chemistry panels, coagulation profile, and blood gas analysis. Evaluation for other co-ingestants is warranted. A chest radiograph may be indicated to evaluate for noncardiogenic pulmonary edema or aspiration pneumonitis.

Treatment

As stated earlier, peak salicylate levels may be significantly delayed. Serial salicylate levels should be obtained at least every 2 to 4 hours until they are clearly decreasing, then every 4 to 6 hours until less than 30 mg/dL. Units (mg/dL versus mg/L) should be confirmed before declaration of toxic levels because there is some variability among hospitals in units of measure that are used. The Done nomogram is no longer recommended for prediction of the severity of salicylate toxicity. Serum levels that have wide vacillations or seem to be rising despite treatment may indicate the presence of a bezoar.

Treatment of salicylate toxicity centers around gastrointestinal decontamination and correction of fluid, electrolyte, and acid-base disturbances. Strict measurement of urine output is necessary. The various modalities for treatment of salicylate toxicity can be found in Table 179-9. Special note should be made to clinicians regarding the dangers of assistance with ventilation. Patients with salicylate-induced hyperpnea may easily be misdiagnosed as being in imminent respiratory failure. However, endotracheal intubation in these patients is a particular risk and may contribute to mortality. Mechanical ventilation rarely achieves the degree of respiratory alkalosis attained by unassisted ventilation, and the worsening acidosis associated with sedation and paralysis increases entry of salicylate into the brain. Moreover, mechanical ventilation should never be considered an adequate substitute for intravenous bicarbonate therapy and, if necessary, hemodialysis.

Admission Criteria

Patients who have a history of significant exposure (>150 mg/kg) should be admitted to the hospital. Other criteria for admission include rising salicylate levels, acidosis,

Table 179-8 Pathophysiology of Symptoms in Salicylate Toxicity

Symptom	Pathophysiology/Etiology
Nausea, vomiting, and epigastric discomfort	Gastrointestinal irritation Stimulation of the medullary chemoreceptor trigger zone
Tinnitus and deafness	Vasoconstriction of the auditory microvasculature
Sweating, hyperpyrexia, and dehydration	Uncoupling of mitochondrial oxidative phosphorylation and increased metabolism of skeletal muscle
Dehydration	Decreased oral intake, vomiting, tachypnea, diaphoresis, and obligatory early diuresis
Hyperpnea and tachypnea	Direct stimulation of the medullary respiratory center
Disorientation, hallucinations, lethargy, agitation, coma, and seizures	Acidosis, cerebral edema
Noncardiogenic pulmonary edema	Leukotriene-induced increased permeability of the microvasculature
Renal failure	
Acid-base disorders (e.g., respiratory alkalosis, mixed respiratory alkalosis, and anion gap metabolic acidosis)	Combination of direct stimulation of the medullary respiratory center (respiratory alkalosis) with renal compensation (metabolic acidosis) and uncoupling mitochondrial respiration (metabolic acid acidosis)
Hypokalemia and hyponatremia or hypernatremia	Increased renal excretion of potassium/sodium because of the anion drag of bicarbonate Hypernatremia may ensue if free H_2O is lost in excess of salt in the kidneys and sweat
Hypoglycemia/hyperglycemia	Salicylates enhance insulin secretion from pancreatic islet cells (hypoglycemia); also decrease peripheral glucose utilization (hyperglycemia)
Hypoprothrombinemia	

Table 179-9 Treatment of Salicylate Toxicity

Treatment	Method	Comments
Activated charcoal	1 g/kg PO initially. Repeat doses of 25 g or 0.5 g/kg at 2-4 hr	MDAC useful in cases of prolonged absorption Uncertain whether MDAC adds benefit once urinary alkalinzation is achieved
Urinary alkalinization	1-2 mEq/kg of $NaHCO_3$ by IV bolus, then D5W with 100-150 mEq/L $NaHCO_3$ at 1-2 times maintenance requirements	Traps ionized salicylate in proximal tubule Start when salicylate levels >30 mg/dL Goal is urine pH of 7.5-8.0 (should be monitored hourly). Also monitor serum pH (should be 7.45-7.55). Watch carefully and correct for hypokalemia or other electrolyte imbalances Watch for fluid overload
Indications for hemodialysis		Serum levels >100 mg/dL with acute ingestion Serum levels >60 mg/dL with chronic intoxication Pulmonary edema Renal failure Congestive heart failure No response to standard therapies Altered mental status and acidemia

D5W, 5% dextrose in water; MDAC, multiple-dose activated charcoal.

coagulopathy, mental status changes, or persistent abnormalities in vital signs. Admission to an intensive care setting may be warranted for patients with abnormal mental status, severe acidosis, renal failure, or coagulation abnormalities.

Discharge Criteria

Discharge from inpatient medical care may occur when the patient has been asymptomatic and has serial falling salicylate levels below 30 mg/dL after cessation of bicarbonate therapy.

ORAL HYPOGLYCEMICS

Non-insulin-dependent diabetes mellitus (NIDDM) affects 2% to 3% of adults in industrialized countries, with approximately 15 million affected individuals in the United States alone.[33] NIDDM is a growing entity in the pediatric population as well. Oral hypoglycemics are the mainstay of treatment of NIDDM. A brief review of glycemic control is necessary to better understand the mechanism of toxicity after an overdose of oral hypoglycemics.

Glycemic control is achieved through the careful balance of hormonal, neural, and substrate mechanisms. Plasma glucose is maintained within a narrow range of 72 to 144 mg/dL. In conditions of hyperglycemia, pancreatic beta cells secrete insulin. Insulin binds to the insulin receptor, which unleashes a signaling cascade. The biologic activity of insulin results in a decrease in plasma glucose that occurs by inhibition of hepatic glucose production, increased glucose uptake, and increased glycogen stores in insulin-sensitive tissues.

Hypoglycemia is corrected by the counterregulatory hormones glucagon, epinephrine, norepinephrine, cortisol, growth hormone, and adrenocorticotropic hormone. The initial response to hypoglycemia is release of glucagon, secreted from pancreatic alpha cells. Glucagon acts on the liver to increase glycogenolysis and gluconeogenesis.[34] Epinephrine, synthesized in the adrenal medulla, constitutes the bulk of circulating catecholamines released in response to hypoglycemia.[34] Epinephrine works primarily through β_2-adrenergic receptors to increase plasma glucose by indirect stimulation of lipolysis. Cortisol is necessary for the liver to respond appropriately to glucagon and epinephrine. Long-standing hypoglycemia raises plasma cortisol levels, thereby reducing the autonomic adrenomedullary response to subsequent hypoglycemia. The combination of hypoglycemia-induced autonomic failure and glucagon depletion that occurs in patients with NIDDM increases the risk and decreases the awareness of severe hypoglycemia.[35]

The oral hypoglycemics work by either increasing insulin production, increasing insulin receptor sensitivity, or decreasing serum glucose levels. Table 179-10 lists the most common oral hypoglycemics and their mechanism of action.

Clinical Presentation

Although the sulfonylureas and thiazolidinediones can cause hypoglycemia in overdose, the other oral hypoglycemics can only potentiate these effects. The clinical symptoms of hypoglycemia are protean and can include unstable vital signs, fixed and dilated pupils, dysrhythmias, diaphoresis, and altered mental status. Neurologic symptoms are often most prominent: mild neurologic symptoms of hypoglycemia include weakness, fatigue, and behavioral and cognitive dysfunction, whereas severe hypoglycemia can result in hemiplegia, decerebrate posturing, ataxia, choreoathetosis, and seizures.[35] The cerebral cortex and hippocampus are the most sensitive to neuroglycopenia, and the brainstem and spinal cord are the most resistant.

Diagnosis and Evaluation

The onset and duration of symptoms can be predicted if the type of oral hypoglycemic agent and the time of ingestion are known. Although hypoglycemia can occur early after the ingestion of oral hypoglycemic agents, hypoglycemia may be delayed up to 48 hours after ingestion. Recurrent hypoglycemia has been reported as long as 94 hours after ingestion. A combination of a history of ingestion or rapid bedside testing (or both) may be needed to confirm the diagnosis of exposure to oral hypoglycemic agents. Lactic acidosis from biguanide use should be suspected in patients presenting with lethargy, vomiting, diarrhea, and an elevated anion gap metabolic acidosis.[36] In patients presenting with nausea, vomiting, fatigue, dark urine, or jaundice, hepatic failure secondary to troglitazone should be considered.

Treatment

The possibility of hypoglycemia must be considered in any patient with an onset of central nervous system dysfunction. Intravenous dextrose can be administered empirically if bedside testing is unavailable. Delay in treatment may result in profound sequelae, including death. The most common sequelae are neurologic, and the risk increases with prolonged hypoglycemia. Recurrent, severe hypoglycemia is associated with electroencephalographic changes and cognitive impairment, particularly in children, with reported IQ deficiencies of 6 points.[37,38] Treatment of hypoglycemia is presented in Table 179-11. Octreotide is considered the first-line agent, and subcutaneous preparations are used more commonly than intravenous ones. The dose of octreotide is 4 to 5 µg/kg/day divided every 6 hours. Other metabolic abnormalities such as lactic acidosis may also need to be corrected. Sodium bicarbonate should be administered if serum pH falls below 7.1. Hemodialysis, which removes ketones, lactate, and metformin, may be necessary if the acidosis is refractory. Thiamine, 100 mg, should be administered to adults receiving glucose to prevent Wernicke encephalopathy.

Admission Criteria

Ingestion of just one tablet of chlorpropamide, glipizide, or glyburide can produce hypoglycemia. Because of the long half-life and duration of action of these drugs, clinicians should have a low threshold for admitting a patient with a suspected exposure. A patient who ingests an oral hypoglycemic agent should be admitted if (1) hypoglycemia develops, (2) it is a deliberate overdose, or (3) the patient is a child, even in the absence of hypoglycemia. The absence of hypoglycemia within the first 8 hours of ingestion may be predictive of a benign outcome after exploratory pediatric sulfonylurea ingestion, although one study of sulfonylurea ingestion in children showed that hypoglycemia can occur as late as 16 hours after ingestion.[39,40] Even though the nonsulfonylurea oral agents do not generally cause hypoglycemia,

Table 179-10   Oral Hypoglycemics

Class	Examples	Mechanism of Action	Comments
Sulfonylureas (first generation)	Acetohexamide Chlorpropamide Tolazamide Tolbutamide	Increased insulin release Bind to the sulfonylurea receptor and inhibit the pore-forming unit of the adenosine triphosphate-sensitive potassium channel, which ultimately causes insulin secretion from the beta cell	High risk for hypoglycemia. Many drug interactions. Exhibit ionic protein binding and are displaced by various drugs, including phenylbutazone, salicylates, sulfonamides, and warfarin
Sulfonylureas (second generation)	Glipizide Glyburide Glimepiride		100 times more potent than 1st generation, although better safety profile. Increased risk for hypoglycemia in patients with renal insufficiency. Should be avoided in patients with severe liver disease
Biguanides	Metformin Phenformin (not available in the U.S.)	No increase in insulin release Inhibit lipolysis, which causes increased glucose uptake, decreased hepatic glucose production, decreased intestinal absorption of glucose, and increased insulin receptor binding	Lactic acidosis: metformin > phenformin Does not cause hypoglycemia when taken alone Should not be used in patients with congestive heart failure, metabolic acidosis, drug hypersensitivity, and renal impairment Use of iodinated radiographic contrast dyes can also precipitate metformin-associated lactic acidosis
			Avoid using with other drugs that affect creatinine clearance or compete with renal tubular secretion, including vancomycin, trimethoprim, triamterene, quinidine, quinine, morphine, digoxin, amiloride, ranitidine, cimetidine, nifedipine, furosemide, nonsteroidal anti-inflammatory drugs, and loop diuretics
α-Glucosidase inhibitors	Acarbose Miglitol	No increase in insulin release Reversible competitive inhibition of α-glucosidase on the brush border of the small bowel, delayed carbohydrate absorption, and lower postprandial glucose and insulin concentrations	Does not cause hypoglycemia when taken alone Effects by concomitant administration of intestinal absorbing agents (charcoal) or carbohydrate-splitting enzymes (amylase, pancreatin) Flatulence, borborygmi, abdominal pain, and diarrhea the most common side effects. Transaminitis and decreased serum iron also reported
Thiazolidinediones	Troglitazone* Rosiglitazone Pioglitazone Meglitinide Repaglinide	Increase sensitivity to insulin Bind to nuclear peroxisome proliferator–activated receptors involved in the transcription of insulin-responsive genes and in the regulation of adipocyte differentiation and lipid metabolism	Hepatotoxicity with troglitazone Hypoglycemia can occur with repaglinide, although less frequently than with sulfonylureas. No significant drug interactions have been reported. However, concomitant use of other agents that affect the CYP3A4 system should be done with caution

*Withdrawn from the U.S. market because of severe hepatotoxicity.

even after an overdose, patients in whom hypoglycemia develops from these agents should be admitted. Patients who present with lactic acidosis secondary to biguanide use should also be admitted.

If euglycemia is achieved in the emergency department and the patient is asymptomatic, the patient can be admitted to a general medical unit with the capability of frequent glucose monitoring. Patients with metabolic acidosis, continued neurologic symptoms/signs, and continued episodes of hypoglycemia despite treatment should be admitted to an intensive care setting.

Discharge Criteria

Patients with suspected or evident sulfonylurea poisoning may be considered safe for discharge if they can tolerate a normal overnight fast without hypoglycemia developing. Children with biguanide-induced acidosis may be discharged once the acidosis has resolved.

Table 179-11 Treatment of Hypoglycemia

Treatment	Mechanism of Action	Dose
Dextrose	Raises serum glucose	*Neonate*: 200 mg/kg (2 mL/kg of D10 by IV bolus) *Child*: 0.5 g/kg (2 mL/kg of D25 by IV bolus) *Adult*: 25 g (50 mL of D50 by IV bolus) Then continuous infusion of D5, D10, or D20 while monitoring serum glucose
Octreotide*	Inhibits insulin release from pancreatic beta cells	*Adult*: 50-100 µg q12h SC *Child*: 4-5 µg/kg/day divided q6h
Glucagon	Acts on the liver to increase glycogenolysis and gluconeogenesis. Requires adequate glycogen stores	*Neonate*: 0.3 mg/kg IV, SC (concentration ≤1.0 mg/mL). Can repeat in 4 hr *Child*: 0.03-0.1 mg/kg IV, SC (concentration ≤1.0 mg/mL). Can repeat in 20 min or use drip 0.05-0.1 mg/kg/hour *Adult*: 0.5-2.0 mg IM, SC, IV. May repeat twice or use drip 1-5 mg/hour
Diazoxide	Inhibits insulin secretion by opening K⁺ channels, increases hepatic glucose production, and decreases cellular glucose utilization	*Newborn/infant*: 8-15 mg/kg/day PO divided into 2-3 doses given q8-12h *Child*: 3-8 mg/kg/day PO divided into 2-3 doses given q8-12h *Adult*: 200 mg PO q4h

*Octreotide preferred over diazoxide.
D10, 10% dextrose.

IN A NUTSHELL

- Over-the-counter medications account for at least 20% of all toxic exposures in children younger than 6 years.
- Childproof packaging has significantly reduced the incidence of childhood iron poisoning, although recent repeal of iron-packaging laws may result in a rise in such exposures, which can lead to gastritis, acidosis, and death.
- Physostigmine should be considered both for diagnosis and for symptom management of an antihistamine overdose, but the benefits must outweigh the potential risks, which include worsening of cardiac conduction delays.
- Use of NAC for the treatment of acetaminophen toxicity is based on the clinical scenario and serum acetaminophen levels as guided by the Rumack nomogram.
- Treatment of salicylate toxicity focuses on gastrointestinal decontamination and correction of fluid, electrolyte, and acid-base disturbances. Activated charcoal, urinary alkalinization, and hemodialysis are adjunctive therapies that can be used.
- Children may have a prolonged risk for hypoglycemia after exposure to oral hypoglycemics, even after the ingestion of a single tablet or capsule, so hospitalization and close monitoring of blood glucose are usually warranted.

ON THE HORIZON

- With the repeal of iron-packaging laws, clinicians may face iron poisoning more frequently.
- Intravenous NAC is increasingly available, and its use is rising in comparison to the oral form for the treatment of acetaminophen toxicity.
- Therapies targeted at inhibition of CYP2E1 may further reduce the hepatotoxicity associated with acetaminophen overdose.
- Increased use of oral hypoglycemics in the American population will make this class of medications a more frequent toxic exposure faced by clinicians.

SUGGESTED READINGS

Burns MJ, Linden CH, Graudins A, et al: A comparison of physostigmine and benzodiazepines for the treatment of anticholinergic poisoning. Ann Emerg Med 2001;37:374-381.
Krause DS, Wolf BA, Shaw LM: Acute aspirin overdose: Mechanisms of toxicity. Ther Drug Monit 1992;14:441-451.
Mcguigan MA: Acute iron poisoning. Pediatr Ann 1996;25:33-38.
Quadrani DA, Spiller HA, Widder P: Five year retrospective evaluation of sulfonylurea ingestion in children. J Toxicol Clin Toxicol 1996;34:267-270.
Rumack BH: Acetaminophen overdose in children and adolescents. Pediatr Clin North Am 1986;33:691-701.

REFERENCES

1. Watson WA, Litovitz TL, Rodgers GC Jr, et al: 2004 Annual report of the American Association of Poison Control Centers Toxic Exposure Surveillance System. Am J Emerg Med 2005;23:589-666.
2. Nightingale SL: From the Food and Drug Administration. JAMA 1997;277:1343.

3. Tenenbein M: Unit-dose packaging of iron supplements and reduction of iron poisoning in young children. Arch Pediatr Adolesc Med 2005;159:557-560.

4. Mcguigan MA: Acute iron poisoning. Pediatr Ann 1996;25:33-38.

5. Chyka PA, Butler AY, Holley JE: Serum iron concentrations and symptoms of acute iron poisoning in children. Pharmacotherapy 1996;16:1053-1058.

6. Jaeger RW, Decastro FJ, Barry RC, et al: Radiopacity of drugs and plants in vivo—limited usefulness. Vet Hum Toxicol 1981;23(Suppl 1):2-4.

7. Lacouture PG, Wason S, Temple AR, et al: Emergency assessment of severity in iron overdose by clinical and laboratory methods. J Pediatr 1981;99:89-91.

8. Mofenson HC, Caraccio TR, Sharieff N: Iron sepsis: *Yersinia enterocolitica* septicemia possibly caused by an overdose of iron. N Engl J Med 1987;316:1092-1093.

9. Howland MA: Risks of parenteral deferoxamine for acute iron poisoning. J Toxicol Clin Toxicol 1996;34:491-497.

10. Macarol V, Yawalkar SJ: Desferrioxamine in acute iron poisoning. Lancet 1992;339:1601.

11. Tenenbein M, Adamson IY: Desferrioxamine and pulmonary injury. Lancet 1992;340:428-429.

12. Tenenbein M, Kowalski S, Sienko A, et al: Pulmonary toxic effects of continuous desferrioxamine administration in acute iron poisoning. Lancet 1992;339:699-701.

13. Rao KA, Adlakha A, Verma-Ansil B, et al: Torsades de pointes ventricular tachycardia associated with overdose of astemizole. Mayo Clin Proc 1994;69:589-593.

14. Brannan MD, Reidenberg P, Radwanski E, et al: Loratadine administered concomitantly with erythromycin: Pharmacokinetic and electrocardiographic evaluations. Clin Pharmacol Ther 1995;58:269-278.

15. Goetz CM, Lopez G, Dean BS, Krenzelok EP: Accidental childhood death from diphenhydramine overdosage. Am J Emerg Med 1990;8:321-322.

16. Burns MJ, Linden CH, Graudins A, et al: A comparison of physostigmine and benzodiazepines for the treatment of anticholinergic poisoning. Ann Emerg Med 2001;37:374-381.

17. Prescott LF: Paracetamol poisoning. Prevention of liver damage. Med Chir Dig 1979;8:391-393.

18. Rumack BH: Acetaminophen overdose in children and adolescents. Pediatr Clin North Am 1986;33:691-701.

19. Temple AR, Mrazik TJ: More on extended-release acetaminophen. N Engl J Med 1995;333:1508-1509.

20. Henretig FM, Selbst SM, Forrest C, et al: Repeated acetaminophen overdosing causing hepatotoxicity in children. Clinical reports and literature review. Clin Pediatr (Phila) 1989;28:525-528.

21. Cytochrome P-450 web page on the Internet (last updated Aug 19, 2006). Available at *http://medicine.iupui.edu/flockhart/table.htm*.

22. Schiodt FV, Rochling FA, Casey DL, Lee WM: Acetaminophen toxicity in an urban county hospital. N Engl J Med 1997;337:1112-1117.

23. Linden CH, Rumack BH: Acetaminophen overdose. Emerg Med Clin North Am 1984;2:103-119.

24. Douglas DR, Sholar JB, Smilkstein MJ: A pharmacokinetic comparison of acetaminophen products (Tylenol Extended Relief vs regular Tylenol). Acad Emerg Med 1996;3:740-744.

25. Miller LF, Rumack BH: Clinical safety of high oral doses of acetylcysteine. Semin Oncol 1983;10:76-85.

26. Mant TG, Tempowski JH, Volans GN, Talbot JC: Adverse reactions to acetylcysteine and effects of overdose. Br Med J (Clin Res Ed) 1984;289:217-219.

27. Smilkstein MJ, Bronstein AC, Linden C, et al: Acetaminophen overdose: A 48-hour intravenous *N*-acetylcysteine treatment protocol. Ann Emerg Med 1991;20:1058-1063.

28. Anker AL, Smilkstein MJ: Acetaminophen. Concepts and controversies. Emerg Med Clin North Am 1994;12:335-349.

29. Temple AR: Acute and chronic effects of aspirin toxicity and their treatment. Arch Intern Med 1981;141:364-369.

30. Krause DS, Wolf BA, Shaw LM: Acute aspirin overdose: Mechanisms of toxicity. Ther Drug Monit 1992;14:441-451.

31. Wortzman DJ, Grunfeld A: Delayed absorption following enteric-coated aspirin overdose. Ann Emerg Med 1987;16:434-436.

32. Yip L, Dart RC, Gabow PA: Concepts and controversies in salicylate toxicity. Emerg Med Clin North Am 1994;12:351-364.

33. Martin AE, Montgomery PA: Acarbose: An alpha-glucosidase inhibitor. Am J Health Syst Pharm 1996;53:2277-2290.

34. Maggs DG, Jacob R, Rife R, et al: Counterregulation in peripheral tissues: Effect of systemic hypoglycemia on levels of substrates and catecholamines in human skeletal muscle and adipose tissue. Diabetes 1997;46:70-76.

35. Cryer PE: Hierarchy of physiological responses to hypoglycemia: Relevance to clinical hypoglycemia in type I (insulin dependent) diabetes mellitus. Horm Metab Res 1997;29:92-96.

36. Lu HC, Parikh PP, Lorber DL: Phenformin-associated lactic acidosis due to imported phenformin. Diabetes Care 1996;19:1449-1450.

37. Tribl G, Howorka K, Heger G, et al: EEG topography during insulin-induced hypoglycemia in patients with insulin-dependent diabetes mellitus. Eur Neurol 1996;36:303-309.

38. Perros P, Frier BM: The long-term sequelae of severe hypoglycemia on the brain in insulin-dependent diabetes mellitus. Horm Metab Res 1997;29:197-202.

39. Quadrani DA, Spiller HA, Widder P: Five year retrospective evaluation of sulfonylurea ingestion in children. J Toxicol Clin Toxicol 1996;34:267-270.

40. Spiller HA, Villalobos D, Krenselok EP, et al: Prospective multicenter study of sulfonylurea ingestion in children. J Pediatr 1997;131:141-146.

Hazardous Household Chemicals: Hydrocarbons, Alcohols, and Caustics

Diane P. Calello

Young children are typically poisoned by agents that are attractive and readily available to them. The combination of curiosity, desire to mimic parental behavior (such as drinking from a bottle or can), newly acquired developmental milestones, and ready availability of household products makes children younger than 6 years particularly vulnerable to hazardous chemicals. In fact, these substances represent the second most common poisoning exposure in young children each year.[1]

Most concerning household chemicals fall into three categories: hydrocarbons, alcohols, and caustics. Table 180-1 lists some common products and their potentially toxic components. Among children for whom medical attention is sought for poisoning from such agents, ingestion is by far a much more common route of exposure than topical or inhalational exposure is.

HYDROCARBONS

Hydrocarbon compounds include petroleum distillates (lighter fluid, kerosene, mineral oil, naphtha, gasoline, butane), plant extract oils, also referred to as terpenes (turpentine, lamp oil, menthol, eucalyptus oil), camphor, inhalants (toluene, chlorofluorocarbons), and organic solvents (toluene, xylene, benzene).

Pathophysiology

After ingestion, hydrocarbon compounds not only enter the esophagus but also spread into the tracheobronchial tree, with the lungs becoming the primary target of injury. The potential for a given substance to cause direct lung injury is influenced by its (1) viscosity, (2) surface tension, and (3) volatility. Low-viscosity liquids with high volatility and low surface tension have the highest potential for pulmonary injury. Highly viscous hydrocarbons (motor oil, paraffin) very seldom cause lung injury, whereas low-viscosity substances (gasoline, kerosene) easily enter the lungs. The chemical can cause alveolar collapse and destroy surfactant, which can lead to pneumonitis and in some cases can progress to respiratory failure.

In addition, lipid-soluble hydrocarbons such as terpenes and aromatics easily cross the blood-brain barrier and cause central nervous system (CNS) depression. Other organ damage may result from a particular compound's inherent toxicity. Table 180-2 offers a mnemonic listing of hydrocarbons with specific systemic toxicity. Inhalant abuse of organic solvents is associated with a sudden death syndrome via sensitization of the myocardium to catecholamines and can also cause a chronic encephalopathy. Because petroleum distillates and terpenes account for the majority of pediatric hydrocarbon exposures, the remainder of this discussion will focus on pulmonary toxicity.

Clinical Presentation

Children may be brought to medical attention for a witnessed or suspected ingestion, even if asymptomatic. Patients with severe ingestion may have signs of lung injury promptly after ingestion, including tachypnea, hypoxia, cough, wheezing, or evidence of increased work of breathing. A child in whom respiratory distress develops within the first hours is very concerning and may progress quickly to respiratory failure. Fever is present in 50% of patients with chemical pneumonitis and reflects the inflammatory response to the noninfectious lung injury.

An aroma of the hydrocarbon may remain on the skin, clothing, or breath and suggest ingestion or exposure. Some hydrocarbon compounds may produce mild mucosal irritation as well.

Evaluation

Evaluation of a child after hydrocarbon ingestion or exposure should focus on the patient's respiratory status. Careful physical examination with measurement of the respiratory rate and work of breathing, as well as pulse oximetry, should be performed immediately and repeated frequently. A chest radiograph should be performed on initial assessment and repeated with clinical deterioration or as part of clinical reassessment (e.g., consideration for admission or discharge). One large review of 950 children found that all patients who were both asymptomatic and had normal chest radiographs at 6 hours after exposure were suitable for discharge and did not deteriorate. In contrast, patients who have initial symptoms and infiltrates on chest radiographs usually worsen and require hospitalization.[2]

An elevation of the white blood count and neutrophil count may be seen in patients with significant chemical pneumonitis. Such leukocytosis early after ingestion reflects the noninfectious inflammation associated with the lung injury.

Further evaluation may be indicated, depending on the toxicities of the particular substance involved (see Table 180-2). For example, serum transaminase studies should be considered for patients exposed to halogenated compounds.

Treatment

The mainstay of treatment for these patients involves supportive care with careful monitoring of respiratory status, as well as respiratory support and treatment of other concomitant organ dysfunction as necessary. Endotracheal

Table 180-1   Contents of Common Household Products

Product	Contents	Category
Toilet bowl, porcelain cleaners	Sulfuric, hydrochloric acid	Caustic/corrosive, acid
Drain/pipe openers	Sodium, potassium hydroxide	Caustic/corrosive, alkali
Lighter fluid (naphtha), gasoline, kerosene, butane	Petroleum distillates	Hydrocarbons
Pine oil, lamp oil, potpourri oil	Terpenes (plant extracts)	Hydrocarbons
Mouthwash	Ethanol	Alcohols
Sterno fuel, windshield wiper fluid	Methanol	Alcohols
Antifreeze	Ethylene glycol	Alcohols
Rubbing alcohol	Isopropyl alcohol	Alcohols
Airplane glue, inhalants	Toluene, xylene	Aromatic/halogenated hydrocarbons
Hair relaxer crème	Sodium hydroxide	Caustic/corrosive, alkali
"No-lye" hair relaxer crème	Calcium hydroxide	Caustic/corrosive, alkali
Mothballs	Camphor	Aromatic hydrocarbons

Table 180-2   "CHAMP" Mnemonic for Hydrocarbons with Systemic Toxicity

C: *Camphor*	Seizures, CNS depression
H: *Halogenated* compounds (carbon tetrachloride, chloral hydrate)	Hepatic necrosis, arrhythmias
A: *Aromatic* compounds (benzene, toluene)	CNS depression, arrhythmias, white matter degeneration
M: Hydrocarbons that contain heavy *metals*	Heavy metal poisoning (multisystem)
P: Hydrocarbons as vehicles for *pesticides*, other toxic compounds	Organophosphate, other compound poisoning

intubation and ventilation or extracorporeal support may be needed with profound lung injury.

Corticosteroids do not improve the course of hydrocarbon pneumonitis and have caused increased bacterial superinfection in animal studies.[3] Antibiotics have also failed to show benefit, may increase infection with resistant organisms, and are therefore indicated only for patients in whom fever and leukocytosis persist and bacterial infection seems likely.

Consultation

- Involvement of critical care specialists may be warranted in patients whose clinical condition is deteriorating and when there is an anticipated need for increasing respiratory support or level of monitoring.
- Social work or social services consultation may be indicated if the circumstances surrounding the ingestion raise suspicion of abuse or neglect.

- Consultation with a regional poison control center is appropriate, especially for children with severe or atypical symptoms or when the compound involved is highly toxic.

Admission Criteria

- Any patient in whom respiratory symptoms develop should be admitted for monitoring and support. Patients who remain asymptomatic for 6 hours after exposure may be candidates for outpatient follow-up with parental surveillance.

Discharge Criteria

- Patients whose respiratory symptoms have resolved sufficiently to be discharged have no further risk from hydrocarbon pneumonitis and can be sent home.

ALCOHOLS

The major compounds involved in pediatric alcohol exposure include ethylene glycol, methanol, isopropanol, and most commonly, ethanol. Ethanol is readily available for adult consumption in most households and may also be found in toiletries such as mouthwash and antibacterial soap. Isopropanol is the active ingredient in rubbing alcohol. Ethylene glycol is found in antifreeze, and methanol can be found in windshield wiper fluid and Sterno fuel.

Pathophysiology

All these alcohols act to some degree on the CNS to cause intoxication, CNS depression, and hypothermia, and all are metabolized by the enzyme alcohol dehydrogenase (Fig. 180-1). The mechanism of hypothermia is complex and not entirely understood; however, it stems from the depth of CNS depression and resultant loss of behavioral responses to cold. In young children, ethanol metabolism suppresses

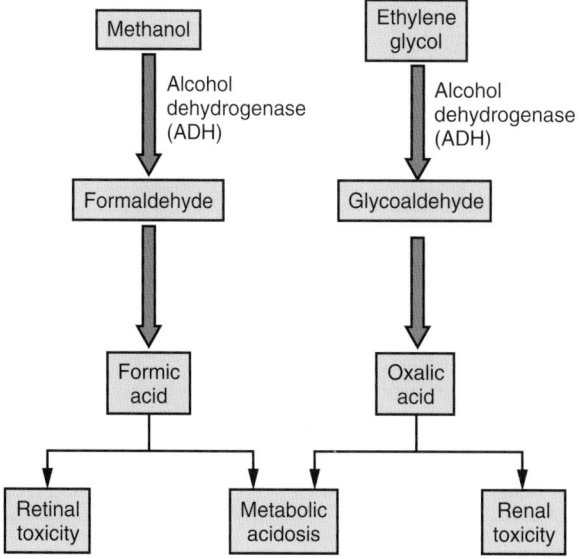

Figure 180-1 Toxic alcohol metabolism. Both methanol and ethylene glycol undergo transformation to toxic metabolites via the enzyme alcohol dehydrogenase (ADH). ADH is inhibited by ethanol and fomepizole therapy.

gluconeogenesis and may cause hypoglycemia hours after exposure. Isopropanol is metabolized to acetone, which causes ketonemia and ketonuria without acidosis; in addition, isopropanol is a gastrointestinal irritant that often causes bleeding, although it is not usually life threatening.

Ethylene glycol and methanol are referred to as "toxic alcohols" because of their conversion through alcohol dehydrogenase to highly toxic metabolites (see Fig. 180-1). Ethylene glycol is metabolized to glycolic and oxalic acid, which cause profound acidosis and renal failure, partially as a result of oxalate crystalluria. In addition, oxalate forms complexes with calcium, which can lead to systemic hypocalcemia and its attendant complications (e.g., seizures, tetany, dysrhythmia). Methanol is metabolized to formic acid, which also causes severe metabolic acidosis, as well as retinal toxicity.

Clinical Presentation

After any of these ingestions patients will be intoxicated and may have profound CNS depression and hypothermia in extreme cases. Young children and malnourished adults may become hypoglycemic between 2 and 8 hours after alcohol ingestion and present with jitters, combativeness, obtundation, or other symptoms of low blood glucose. Ingestion of isopropanol can cause intoxication along with hematemesis, ketonuria, and a strong acetone odor.

Patients with ethylene glycol or methanol poisoning may initially appear intoxicated, with severe metabolic acidosis and organ failure developing within the next 24 hours. These toxic alcohols are osmotically active and can lead to dehydration because of the osmotic diuresis that ensues after ingestion. Retinal toxicity secondary to the toxic metabolite of methanol can cause a number of visual abnormalities, including blurred vision, spots, and scotomas, a condition collectively described as "snowstorm" vision; it can progress

to complete irreversible blindness. Patients poisoned with ethylene glycol are at risk for anuria and renal failure. Fatalities result from profound acidosis and metabolic perturbation.

Evaluation

Serum levels of ethanol, isopropanol, methanol, and ethylene glycol may be obtained and correspond well with toxicity. However, these tests are not rapidly available in all hospitals. Indirect evidence of their presence may be revealed through measurements of serum electrolytes and osmolality and blood gas analysis. Within an hour after ingestion, the presence of alcohols in serum may be detected by an elevated osmolar gap (the difference between calculated serum osmolarity and measured serum osmolality). As metabolism of ethylene glycol and methanol progresses, metabolic acidosis with an elevated anion gap develops; this is uncommon with ethanol or isopropanol metabolism.

Additional testing should include urinalysis, serum creatinine, and ophthalmologic examination, depending on the toxicities associated with the suspected alcohol ingested. After ethylene glycol ingestion, oxalate crystals may be visible in urine; ketonuria occurs with isopropanol metabolism. Because fluorescein is often used as an additive to antifreeze, demonstration of fluorescence by Wood lamp examination of urine may be a sign of ingestion of this material. However, not all preparations of antifreeze contain fluorescein, and therefore such examination cannot reliably eliminate the concern for ingestion.

Treatment

For ethanol and isopropanol ingestion, close observation and supportive care are required, along with careful attention to blood glucose monitoring in young children. Although ethanol and isopropanol ingestions are associated with few complications, the clinician should be particularly observant of the patient's potentially depressed mental status and respiratory rate.

In ethylene glycol or methanol poisoning, the mainstay of therapy is reducing the formation of toxic metabolites by inhibiting the action of alcohol dehydrogenase on the toxic alcohols. Substances such as ethanol or fomepizole (4-methylpyrazole [4-MP]) can be administered to compete with the toxic alcohols in binding to alcohol dehydrogenase. Fomepizole is preferable to ethanol if available because ethanol infusions are intoxicating and warrant frequent monitoring of blood glucose and ethanol levels (desired level, 100 mg/dL). Fomepizole has been shown to be safe and effective in children as well as adults.[4-6] See Table 180-3 for more details of ethanol and fomepizole therapy.

It is important to remember that the use of ethanol or fomepizole prevents the ongoing production of toxic metabolites but does not treat the toxic effects of metabolites already present. A number of treatments may help prevent end-organ damage and reverse acidosis. Sodium bicarbonate therapy can treat acidosis and reduce further entry of toxic metabolites into target tissues. Pyridoxine (1 mg/kg intravenously, maximum of 100 mg, every 6 hours) and thiamine (50 mg intravenously every 8 hours) may help

Table 180-3 Antidotes for Toxic Alcohol Ingestion

Agent	Dosage/Administration	Comment
Ethanol	10% solution for IV use Loading dose: 0.8 g/kg Maintenance: 80-130 mg/kg/hr Target level: 100 mg/dL	Side effects: obtundation, hyperosmolarity, hypothermia, hypoglycemia Frequent monitoring of levels May necessitate central venous access
Fomepizole (4-methylpyrazole)	Loading dose: 15 mg/kg IV over 15-min period Maintenance: 10 mg/kg q12h Increase to 15 mg/kg after 4 doses	Fewer side effects than ethanol Less availability Administer of 4h during dialysis

detoxify the acid metabolites of ethylene glycol, and folic acid (1 mg/kg intravenously, maximum of 50 mg, every 4 hours) may help detoxify the metabolites of methanol.

Hemodialysis is very effective in removing both ethylene glycol and methanol and their toxic metabolites. Hemodialysis should be considered when the serum ethylene glycol or methanol level is higher than 50 mg/dL or in the context of refractory acidosis. Many experts recommend that ethanol or 4-MP infusion accompany hemodialysis because the dialysis process is not instantaneous and residual toxic alcohol may still be metabolized. However, others eschew hemodialysis in favor of prolonged alcohol dehydrogenase blockade with ethanol or 4-MP, and this option might be considered by those with considerable expertise in the treatment of toxic alcohol ingestion.

Consultation

- Social work or social services should be considered if circumstances surrounding the ingestion raise suspicion of abuse or neglect.
- Ophthalmology should be consulted in cases of methanol poisoning.
- Nephrology should be consulted if there is a credible history of ingestion of a toxic alcohol, especially when hemodialysis is being considered.

Admission Criteria

- Any patient in whom ingestion of a toxic alcohol is suspected should be admitted unless negative serum levels are obtained or the anion and osmolar gaps remain normal on serial measurement. Abnormalities in the osmolar and anion gap should appear within 12 hours after ingestion, so a patient in whom abnormalities do not develop within this time is reassuring. It is important to note that a normal osmolar gap should be interpreted in the context of the anion gap and vice versa; as the toxic alcohol compound is metabolized, the osmolar gap will decrease and the anion gap will rise. However, patients who exhibit the CNS depression of alcohol ingestion should be admitted regardless of acid-base status.
- All intoxicated children should be admitted or observed until the intoxication resolves.

Discharge Criteria

- Patients may be discharged once the intoxication resolves, levels of toxic alcohols are undetectable, and end-organ toxicity is either resolved or stable.

CAUSTICS

Caustic substances are found in a number of readily available household products (see Table 180-1), including drain and oven cleaners, porcelain cleaners, and some detergents. Of note, ammonia and bleach packaged for household use are significantly less concentrated than many commercial preparations and are therefore associated with a much lower risk of injury.

The Federal Poisoning Prevention Act of 1970 mandates that alkaline caustics greater than 2% in concentration and other caustics greater than 10% in concentration be sold in childproof containers. As a result, the number of serious pediatric caustic injuries has vastly decreased. However, severe injuries still occur, often with industrial-strength chemicals or products inappropriately transferred to non-childproof containers.

Pathophysiology

The degree of caustic injury depends on the properties of the substance (e.g., pH, viscosity), the nature of the exposure (e.g., splash, ingestion), and the timeliness of initiating appropriate therapy. Severe caustic injuries are more likely to occur with a strong acid or base and in the context of large-volume or suicidal ingestion. Aside from injury as a result of direct contact with the caustic agent, some compounds cause additional toxicity through systemic absorption of components. For example, acids may be absorbed and cause metabolic acidosis, and zinc and mercuric chloride ($ZnCl_2$, $HgCl_2$) can be associated with heavy metal toxicity.

The most common targets of caustic injury are the airway, esophagus, and gastrointestinal tract. Although acid and alkali substances produce different histopathologic patterns of injury, the clinical picture appears similar. On ingestion, the liquid traveling down the gastrointestinal tract comes in contact with esophageal epithelium and causes damage ranging from edema and erythema to necrosis and perforation. Fluid reaching the stomach may also cause burns of varying degrees to the gastric mucosa, including perforation.

Clinical Presentation

Because the tissue damage from caustic ingestion begins immediately, patients generally become symptomatic quickly. Signs and symptoms of esophageal injury predominate, including vomiting, dysphagia, refusal to drink, hematemesis, drooling, and associated oral and oropharyngeal burns. In addition, airway injury or impending collapse

Table 180-4   Indications for Endoscopy after Caustic Ingestion

History of large-volume, intentional or suicidal ingestion, especially highly caustic products (e.g., drain cleaner)

Any *symptoms*, including vomiting, dysphagia, hematemesis, chest or abdominal pain, drooling, refusal to drink

Any *signs*, including stridor, respiratory distress, oropharyngeal burns, abdominal tenderness, peritoneal signs

Further evaluation reveals acidosis, anemia, coagulopathy, or radiographs suggestive of perforation or mediastinitis

Table 180-5   Endoscopic Classification of Esophageal Injury

Class	Characteristics	Prognosis
I	Edema, hyperemia	Excellent; no strictures
IIa	Ulcerated, discrete	Up to 75% chance of stricture
IIb	Ulcerated, circumferential	75% chance of stricture
III	Necrosis	100% stricture formation

may cause stridor, respiratory distress, cough, and wheezing. A patient with overwhelming tissue destruction may be hemodynamically unstable with metabolic acidosis. Life-threatening complications can ensue, many of which may not occur until 72 hours after the ingestion. Severe chest pain and shortness of breath may be a sign of esophageal perforation and mediastinitis. Perforation of the stomach with resultant caustic peritonitis usually causes severe abdominal pain, a rigid abdomen, acidosis, and hemodynamic instability. Gastrointestinal hemorrhage from direct vessel injury can present with hematemesis, melena, or shock.

After the acute phase of injury, the healing process may cause gastrointestinal strictures to form, most commonly in the esophagus. Strictures should be suspected in a patient in whom dysphagia or failure to thrive develops.

Evaluation

Endoscopy of the upper gastrointestinal tract can delineate the location and degree of injury to the hypopharynx, esophagus, and stomach. To reduce the risk of perforation, the procedure is performed within the first 48 hours after injury. Table 180-4 provides a list of indications for this diagnostic procedure, and Table 180-5 describes the endoscopic classification system most commonly used to grade esophageal injuries.

Radiographs of the chest may be useful if there is concern for aspiration with chemical pneumonitis, esophageal perforation, or mediastinitis. An abdominal obstruction series may reveal intraperitoneal free air in patients with distal esophageal or gastric perforation. Lateral neck films may be useful to evaluate the upper airway in cases in which stridor or respiratory distress is present and may demonstrate airway narrowing or epiglottic swelling.

Laboratory studies may be warranted in some situations. For patients at risk for systemic absorption of caustic agents or with concern for severe injury, a complete blood count, coagulation studies, electrolyte determinations, and blood gas analysis should be performed. A blood type and cross-match should be obtained for patients with hemorrhage or peritonitis or for those in need of surgical intervention.

Surgical exploration is reserved for patients with abdominal pain, tachycardia and worsening acidosis, or radiographic evidence of catastrophic visceral perforation or mediastinitis.

Management of an asymptomatic toddler who has ingested an unknown quantity of a caustic substance presents a particular challenge. A number of prospective studies in the last 20 years have demonstrated that children without symptoms or signs after 6 hours of observation will have no significant endoscopic injury and therefore do not warrant endoscopy.[7,8] In addition, young children who ingest thick crème hair relaxer products may have isolated oral burns, but episodes of more extensive injury are exceedingly rare.

Treatment

In the emergency department, patients may require resuscitation, including endotracheal intubation if airway collapse is imminent. Gastrointestinal decontamination is not generally indicated. Tissue injury will have already occurred on arrival, so the introduction of either activated charcoal or a lavage tube into a potentially damaged esophagus incurs futile risk. Dilution, a process by which patients drink milk or water to decrease the concentration of the caustic substance, also has little benefit beyond the first 1 to 2 minutes of ingestion.

On admission, corticosteroid therapy to prevent stricture formation is controversial but often used. Theoretically, corticosteroids prevent the collagen cross-linking that takes place during healing and stricture formation. Whereas patients with type I burns uniformly do well and patients with type III injury nearly always form strictures, patients with type II burns may be good candidates for this therapy. A number of studies have attempted to evaluate the efficacy of this treatment, but the data are insufficient to make definitive recommendations.[9] Most clinicians use either methylprednisolone, 2 mg/kg/day, or dexamethasone, 1 mg/kg/day, for patients with circumferential second-degree esophageal burns. Antibiotics are often given concurrently.

Consultation with a specialist, usually a gastroenterologist or a general surgeon, is recommended to aid in decisions such as when to institute oral feeding and whether nasogastric tube placement is needed. In general, patients with mild (type I, IIa) burns can be started slowly on a liquid diet as soon as tolerated, but in patients with more advanced disease, longer periods of restricted oral intake may be advised because of the risk for perforation.

Swallowing difficulty, gastric outlet obstruction, or dysmotility may develop in patients with strictures, most often in the weeks to months after the ingestion. Alternative enteral feeding regimens may be needed and might include nasogastric, gastrostomy, or transpyloric feeding. Revision of strictures may be required for severely narrowed or obstructing segments, and therapy can include dilation or surgical resection. Patients with significant esophageal injury require lifelong surveillance for esophageal carcinoma because they are at greatly increased risk after caustic ingestion.[10]

Consultation

- Gastroenterologists are often involved in the assessment of symptomatic children. Ongoing involvement is appropriate for children with evidence of mucosal injury, feeding difficulties, or gastrointestinal bleeding.
- Surgical involvement should be sought early in children at risk for perforation, mediastinitis, or peritonitis. Further along the course of management, surgical services may be needed for placement of gastrostomy feeding tubes or for evaluation of strictures that may need resection.
- Critical care should be consulted for patients with hemodynamic instability and those in need of airway management.
- Patients with injury to the upper or lower airways may warrant input from otolaryngology or pulmonology.
- Social services should be contacted if circumstances surrounding the ingestion raise suspicion of abuse or neglect.

Admission Criteria

- Any patient with symptoms or abnormal physical examination findings after caustic ingestion.
- Any patient with a large-volume or intentional ingestion.
- Observation and discharge may be considered for a completely asymptomatic toddler in whom significant ingestion is in doubt or for a patient with crème hair relaxer exposure and oral burns only. However, such management is advisable only with close follow-up and a reliable situation in the home.

Discharge Criteria

- Patients may be discharged when asymptomatic and able to tolerate oral feeding. For patients unable to feed orally, alternative enteral nutritional therapy must be established.
- Appropriate outpatient follow-up is needed for ongoing evaluation of known complications, most commonly stricture formation.

PREVENTION

The great advances in preventive legislation have already made a significant impact on household poisonings in the United States; however, exposures still occur and are largely preventable. Careful education on the part of health care providers regarding the safe storage of household chemicals, both out of reach and out of attractive non-childproof containers, is still needed. Awareness of the national poison control center system can be lifesaving, so each household should have contact information readily available.

IN A NUTSHELL

- The risk for injury secondary to hydrocarbon ingestion is related to the nature of the substance (e.g., volatility), as well as the toxicants dissolved in the product (e.g., organophosphates).

- Hydrocarbons with high volatility, low viscosity, and low surface tension (e.g., gasoline, kerosene) can cause aspiration and pneumonitis.
- After hydrocarbon ingestion, symptomatic patients should be monitored closely.
- Ethanol and isopropanol can cause hypoglycemia in young children.
- Ethylene glycol and methanol ingestion can be life threatening, and treatment may include hemodialysis and inhibition of alcohol dehydrogenase.
- Caustic ingestion can cause acute life-threatening injuries, including airway damage, gastrointestinal hemorrhage, and esophageal or gastric perforation with mediastinitis or peritonitis.
- Endoscopy within 48 hours of caustic ingestion can delineate the severity and location of the caustic injury.
- Children who remain asymptomatic for at least 6 hours after caustic ingestion are at low risk for injury and may be discharged if close observation can be maintained.

ON THE HORIZON

- Future research directions currently include investigation of the use of fomepizole for toxic alcohol poisoning as not only an adjunct for but also in lieu of hemodialysis, as well as evaluation of the use of extracorporeal membrane oxygenation in patients with severe hydrocarbon pneumonitis. Both these experimental methods of treatment have thus far shown favorable results.

REFERENCES

1. Watson WA, Litovitz TL, Rodgers GC Jr, et al: 2004 Annual Report of the American Association of Poison Control Centers Toxic Exposure Surveillance System. Am J Emerg Med 2005;23:589-666.
2. Anas N, Namasonthi V, Ginsburg CM: Criteria for hospitalizing children who have ingested products containing hydrocarbon. JAMA 1981;246: 840-843.
3. Marks MI, Chicoine L, Legere G, Hillman E: Adrenocorticosteroid treatment of hydrocarbon pneumonia in children—a cooperative study. J Pediatr 1972;81:366-369.
4. Brent J, McMartin K, Phillips S, et al: Fomepizole for the treatment of ethylene glycol poisoning. N Engl J Med 1999;340:832-838.
5. Brent J, McMartin K, Phillips S, et al: Fomepizole for the treatment of methanol poisoning. N Engl J Med 2001;344:424-429.
6. Borron SW, Megarbane B, Baud FJ: Fomepizole in treatment of uncomplicated ethylene glycol poisoning. Lancet 1999;354:831.
7. Crain E, Gershel J, Mezey A: Caustic ingestions: Symptoms as predictors of esophageal injury. Am J Dis Child 1984;138:863-865.
8. Gaudreault P, Parent M, McGuigan M, et al: Predictability of esophageal injury from signs and symptoms: A study of caustic ingestion in 378 children. Pediatrics 1983;71:7676-7770.
9. Anderson KD, Rouse TM, Randolph JG: A controlled trial of corticosteroids in children with corrosive injury of the esophagus. N Engl J Med 1990;323:637-640.
10. Appelqvist P, Salmo S: Lye corrosion carcinoma of the esophagus: A review of 63 cases. Cancer 1980;45:2655-2658.

CHAPTER 181

Lead, Other Metals, and Chelation Therapy

April A. Harper and Michael W. Shannon

LEAD

Lead is a highly toxic metal, and exposure to it can produce a wide range of adverse health effects. The most common cause of childhood lead poisoning is ingestion of lead-containing paint chips or lead-contaminated dust as a result of normal hand-to-mouth activity. Until 1978, lead was commonly used in paints to provide pigment and color stability. According to the U.S. Department of Housing and Urban Development, about 25% of the nation's current housing stock—some 24 million homes—still contains significant lead-based paint hazards. Although lead paint that is in intact does not pose an immediate concern, lead paint that is deteriorating or is disturbed during repair or renovation activities creates a hazard. There is new evidence that lead poisoning is harmful at blood levels that were once thought safe. The effects of sustained exposure, such as learning disabilities, shortened attention span, and lowered IQ, have been observed in children with lead levels as low as 10 μg/dL. Lead poisoning was once a disease of poor or minority children living in older housing in the inner cities. Unfortunately, the number of at-risk groups has expanded as families from all strata inadvertently expose their children through home renovation activities.

Toxicokinetics

Lead ingestion is the primary route of exposure for children, whose gut absorbs 45% to 50% of a lead dose, compared with 10% to 15% in adults. After absorption occurs, the amount of lead entering the bloodstream is dependent on several factors: the amount or concentration of lead in the specific medium; the physicochemical characteristics of the lead compound; and specific host factors such as age, nutritional status, and fasting conditions. Once absorbed, 99% of lead binds to erythrocytes, and the remaining 1% is free to diffuse into soft tissues and bone, where it equilibrates with blood lead. In the body, the total lead burden can be divided into four compartments: blood (half-life 35 days), soft tissue (half-life 40 days), and the trabecular (half-life 3 to 4 years) and cortical components (half-life 16 to 20 years) of bone.

In terms of lead's toxicity, the most notable effect is seen in the heme synthetic pathway. Lead inhibits δ-aminolevulinic acid dehydrase and ferrochelatase (heme synthetase). As a result, δ-aminolevulinic acid cannot be converted into porphobilinogen, nor can iron be incorporated into the protoporphyrin ring. The heme precursor erythrocyte protoporphyrin (EP), commonly assayed as zinc protoporphyrin (ZPP; zinc substitutes for iron in the porphyrin moiety), increases, and heme synthesis is subsequently reduced. The biologic dysfunction produced by lead appears to be associated with the metal's ability not only to bind sulfhydryl ligands but also to mimic or inhibit the action of calcium. At low concentrations, lead increases the basal release of neurotransmitters from a presynaptic nerve ending in both the peripheral and central nervous systems. Lead also has the ability to block the release of neurotransmitters during the normal action potential. This twofold effect has significant consequences on the developing nervous system and may be one of the underlying causes of the cognitive and behavioral problems seen in lead-poisoned children.

Clinical Presentation

The clinical presentation of lead poisoning varies widely, depending on blood lead level (BLL), age at exposure, and amount and duration of exposure. Children presenting with possible lead poisoning should be assessed for correlates of exposure and recognizable sequelae. These sequelae can include gastrointestinal (GI) complaints such as colicky pain, constipation, anorexia, and intermittent vomiting. Signs and symptoms suggestive of central nervous system involvement include irritability, lethargy, alterations in sleep pattern, decreased attention span, and developmental delay. Acute encephalopathy may be seen in children with BLLs greater than 70 μg/dL. These children can develop persistent vomiting and become drowsy and possibly ataxic. As the encephalopathy worsens, the level of consciousness deteriorates further, and seizures or even coma can occur.

The decision to admit a child for the treatment of lead poisoning is multifaceted and is never based solely on the BLL. Besides the BLL, the medical evaluation, environmental history, social history, and laboratory facilities available at the admitting hospital are all important factors. It is important that the hospital laboratory have the capacity to run a BLL with a relatively prompt turnaround of results. Asymptomatic patients with BLLs greater than 45 to 50 μg/dL are generally managed as inpatients. Involvement by a medical toxicologist or pediatric environmental health subspecialist is not essential but may be valuable. Symptomatic children, regardless of BLL, should receive immediate subspecialty consultation. All children with signs or symptoms suggesting lead encephalopathy should be evaluated for admission to the pediatric intensive care unit or transfer to a tertiary center where critical care can be provided if necessary.

Diagnosis

The evaluation of lead poisoning includes a venous BLL, detailed environmental and social histories, and systematic physical examination.

Laboratory Studies

The following laboratory data should be obtained to aid in making the diagnosis:

- Repeat BLL—confirmatory test must be a venous BLL, because specimens obtained by finger stick are less reliable.
- ZPP or EP level.
- Complete blood count with differential.
- Serum iron studies: iron, ferritin, total iron binding capacity, or, if available, reticulolyte hemoglobin content.

Radiographic Studies

An abdominal radiograph is recommended for any child admitted with newly diagnosed lead poisoning or a child with known lead poisoning who has an abrupt increase in BLL. Radiopaque specks in the GI tract, particularly the stomach and small intestine, may represent lead-containing particles, leading to consideration of gut decontamination. Radiographs of the long bones (distal radius or proximal tibia-fibula) may be indicated in growing children with BLLs in excess of 40 µg/dL over a protracted period. Characteristic lead lines are radiodensities in metaphyseal plates of the long bones; these represent periods of bone growth arrest.

Developmental Evaluation

Children with BLLs greater than 20 µg/dL should have thorough neurologic evaluations, including developmental screening tests to identify possible developmental delay. Speech and language screening is recommended on admission, because speech delay is very common in lead-poisoned children. Children with abnormal screening tests should be referred for formal neuropsychological testing.

Social and Environmental Assessment

All families warrant a complete social work assessment. The local health department's childhood lead poisoning prevention program should be notified of the child's admission and can advise pediatric care providers and families how to obtain environmental assessments. Local public health nurses may be able to identify lead hazards when they make home visits. They can also provide risk-reduction education and make recommendations to the family about how to diminish the hazard.

Treatment

The treatment of childhood lead poisoning involves the elimination of additional exposure and adequate nutrition. When these measures fail, chelation therapy should be considered.

Gut Decontamination

When there is radiographic evidence of lead densities in the stomach or small intestine of children with BLLs greater than 45 µg/dL, the GI tract must be evacuated to eliminate further absorption. Gut decontamination should occur before chelation. For small radiodensities, a cathartic such as magnesium citrate can be administered once orally at a dose of 4 mL/kg. An effect is usually seen in 30 minutes to 3 hours. Magnesium citrate may cause hypovolemia and electrolyte imbalance and should not be used repeatedly or in patients with renal impairment. Adequate hydration should be established before initiating this therapy.

For larger or multiple radiodensities, whole-bowel irrigation is preferable. This can be accomplished with a polyethylene glycol solution (GoLYTELY, CoLyte). Polyethylene glycol solution is given orally or instilled by nasogastric tube at a dose of 20 to 40 mL/kg per hour, up to a maximum of 1000 mL/hr for a minimum of 4 hours, or until the rectal effluent is clear. Effect of action is usually 30 to 60 minutes. Contraindications to polyethylene glycol solution include bowel perforation, adynamic ileus, significant GI hemorrhage, intestinal obstruction, and inability to protect the airway. A follow-up radiograph may be indicated to document removal or transit of the density after GI decontamination.

Nutrition

Nutrition can play a pivotal role in the prevention and treatment of lead poisoning, especially in young children. To decrease their susceptibility to lead intoxication, children should be provided with balanced nutrition, including adequate amounts of foods rich in calcium (e.g., milk, cheese, yogurt), iron (e.g., beef, ham, beans, green leafy vegetables), and ascorbic acid (e.g., citrus fruit, tomatoes, broccoli). Lead-poisoned children should be assessed for iron deficiency, because lead is more readily absorbed when iron stores are depleted. Lead-poisoned children who are iron deficient should receive oral iron supplementation at a dose of 4 to 6 mg/kg per day.

Chelation Therapy

Table 181-1 provides a quick guide to chelation therapy.

Asymptomatic Patients with Blood Lead Levels 45 to 70 µg/dL

Asymptomatic children with BLLs of 45 to 70 µg/dL can be treated with either oral succimer or parenteral calcium disodium edetate ($CaNa_2EDTA$). Succimer and $CaNa_2EDTA$ are similar in terms of safety and efficacy. The advantages of oral succimer include ease of administration and the potential for outpatient treatment (although this is generally not advised for children with BLLs in this range). Its adverse effects include nausea, rash, and liver function abnormalities. Also, because it is formulated as a capsule, succimer may be difficult to administer in young children. $CaNa_2EDTA$ can be administered only intravenously or intramuscularly, necessitating greater resource utilization; because of the pain of intramuscular administration, it should be given intravenously when possible, which may require hospitalization. The half-life of $CaNa_2EDTA$ is 20 to 60 minutes with intravenous administration and 60 to 90 minutes with intramuscular administration. If given intramuscularly, $CaNa_2EDTA$ should be mixed with procaine to decrease injection site pain. $CaNa_2EDTA$ should not be confused with disodium edetate (sodium EDTA); use of the latter may result in severe hypocalcemia and possible death.

The baseline laboratory studies listed in Table 181-2 should be done before administering $CaNa_2EDTA$. After ensuring adequate urine output, chelation can be initiated with an intravenous infusion of $CaNa_2EDTA$ for 3 to 5 consecutive days. The dosage of $CaNa_2EDTA$ is 35 to 50 mg/kg per day and must be diluted to 2 to 4 mg/mL in either 5% dextrose or 0.9% saline solution. It is incompatible with high-concentration dextrose solution or lactated Ringer's solution. The rate of infusion is calculated to deliver the total

Table 181–1 Chelation Therapy Based on Clinical Presentation and Blood Lead Level

Clinical Presentation	Chelating Agent and Dose	Route	Duration
Asymptomatic patients with BLL <25 µg/dL	Not routinely indicated	N/A	N/A
Asymptomatic patients with BLL 25–45 µg/dL	Typically not indicated but may have a role in select patients; consult lead poisoning treatment program or medical toxicologist	N/A	N/A
Asymptomatic patients with BLL 46–69 µg/dL	Succimer (Chemet) 10 mg/kg/dose 3 times/day for 5 days, then twice/day for remaining 14 days or CaNa$_2$EDTA 35–50 mg/kg/day	PO or nasogastric tube; 100-mg capsules of medicated beads can be opened and sprinkled on food or dissolved in juice IM (with procaine) IV (24-hr infusion)	19 days; may repeat course, with a minimum of 2 wk between courses 3–5 days; may repeat course, with 2–5 days between courses
Asymptomatic patients with BLL ≥70 µg/dL and all symptomatic patients without encephalopathy	BAL 3–5 mg/kg/dose every 4–6 hr and CaNa$_2$EDTA 50 mg/kg/day	IM IV (24-hr continuous infusion)	Up to a total of 12 doses Begin 4–5 hr after first dose of BAL and continue for 5 days
All patients with BLL ≥100 µg/dL and acute encephalopathy	BAL 3–5 mg/kg/dose every 4–6 hr and CaNa$_2$EDTA 50 mg/kg/day	IM IV (24-hr continuous infusion)	Total of 12 doses Begin 4–5 hr after first dose of BAL and continue for 5 days

BAL, British antilewisite (dimercaprol); BLL, blood lead level; CaNa$_2$EDTA, calcium disodium edetate; N/A, not applicable.

Table 181–2 Monitoring Laboratory Studies for Patients Receiving CaNa$_2$EDTA and BAL

Baseline (Before Infusion)	Daily	Day 3	Day 5
Venous BLL, G6PD level[†] Serum electrolytes (Na, K, Cl, CO$_2$, BUN, Cr, glucose, Ca, Mg, phosphate) Liver enzymes (AST, ALT, alkaline phosphatase) ZPP or EP (reference level ≤35 µg/dL whole blood) CBC with indices Iron studies: iron, ferritin, TIBC, if available Chr Urinalysis with urine specific gravity	Urinalysis with urine specific gravity every day plus Urine dip and urine specific gravity every 8 hr	Venous BLL* Serum electrolytes (Na, K, Cl, CO$_2$, BUN, Cr, glucose, Ca, Mg, phosphate) Liver enzymes (AST, ALT, alkaline phosphatase) ZPP or EP CBC with indices Iron studies: iron, ferritin, TIBC, if available Chr	Venous BLL* Serum electrolytes (Na, K, Cl, CO$_2$, BUN, Cr, glucose, Ca, Mg, phosphate) Liver enzymes (AST, ALT, alkaline phosphatase) ZPP or EP CBC with indices Iron studies: iron, ferritin, TIBC, if available Chr

*Stop infusion for 1 hour before drawing blood to avoid falsely elevated lead level.
[†]Consider in patients before receiving BAL.
ALT, alanine transaminase; AST, aspartate transaminase; BAL, British antilewisite (dimercaprol); BLL, blood lead level; BUN, blood urea nitrogen; CaNa$_2$EDTA, calcium disodium edetate; CBC, complete blood count; Chr, reticulocyte hemoglobin content; EP, erythrocyte protoporphyrin; G6PD, glucose-6-phosphate dehydrogenase; TIBC, total iron binding capacity; ZPP, zinc protoporphyrin.

dose over a 24-hour continuous infusion. If administered intramuscularly, the total daily dose is divided into two doses given 12 hours apart (with procaine added). Regardless of the route of administration of CaNa$_2$EDTA, vigorous hydration (intravenous or oral) should be provided to reduce the risk of nephrotoxicity; urine specific gravity should be maintained at less than 1.020 at all times. Total fluid intake should

be 1.5 times the maintenance fluid requirements. The patient should receive strict input and output monitoring, with vital signs checked every 4 hours. Electrocardiogram monitoring is also recommended. The suggested schedule of laboratory monitoring studies is given in Table 181-2.

CaNa$_2$EDTA is excreted renally; as a result, the major adverse effects include acute necrosis of proximal tubules (exhibited by glycosuria, proteinuria, microscopic hematuria) and large epithelial cells in urinary sediment. Hypotension and cardiac rhythm irregularities have been documented. Mild increases in serum transaminases are common, with a return to normal within 48 hours after cessation of therapy. Elevation of serum transaminases also occurs with plumbism, so it may precede CaNa₂EDTA chelation and is not a contraindication. CaNa₂EDTA also increases the urinary excretion of zinc, but this is clinically insignificant unless therapy is continued for more than 5 days.

Alternatively, asymptomatic patients with BLLs of 45 to 70 μg/dL can be chelated with oral succimer (Chemet). Succimer is rapidly absorbed from the GI tract, with a peak concentration at 3 hours and an elimination half-life in children of 3 ± 0.2 hours. Succimer has a small volume of distribution, with 95% binding in blood, and the succimer-lead complex is excreted renally. Baseline laboratory studies that should be obtained before treatment with succimer include confirmation venous BLL, ZPP or EP level, complete blood count (with differential and platelets), and liver function tests (alanine transaminase, aspartate transaminase, alkaline phosphatase). Succimer is given orally at 10 mg/kg per dose (rounded to the nearest 100 mg) three times a day for 5 days, then twice a day for 14 days. Initial laboratory studies should be repeated on days 6 and 20 of treatment to monitor for adverse effects.

The foul smell and taste of succimer make oral administration a challenge in young children. Administration via a nasogastric tube is an alternative. The most common adverse effects in children are nausea, vomiting, diarrhea, appetite loss, and loose stools. Hypersensitivity reactions have been reported, including chills, fever, urticaria, and rashes, which occur in approximately 4% of patients. Some skin rashes may necessitate the discontinuation of therapy; however, if a rash occurs, other causes should be considered before ascribing it to a drug reaction. Mild, transient elevations of serum transaminases have been observed in 6% to 10% of patients. Mild to moderate reversible neutropenia has also been noted. Therapy should be withheld or discontinued if the absolute neutrophil count falls below 1200/μL.

Asymptomatic Patients with Blood Lead Levels Greater Than 70 μg/dL and Symptomatic Patients without Encephalopathy

Asymptomatic patients with BLLs greater than 70 μg/dL and symptomatic patients without encephalopathy require combination therapy with CaNa₂EDTA and dimercaprol. Dimercaprol, or British antilewisite (BAL), is used for a wide variety of heavy metal poisonings because of its ability to form stable complexes with many metals, facilitating solubility and elimination. Peak BAL concentrations are obtained in 30 to 60 minutes, with a duration of action of 4 hours. As a result, frequent doses at 3- to 4-hour intervals are necessary to maintain the therapeutic effect. The BAL-metal complex is eliminated via the renal and biliary tracts. Table 181-2 lists the baseline laboratory studies that should be performed before chelation with BAL and during therapy. In addition, before beginning therapy, one must identify any allergy to peanuts, because BAL is suspended in peanut oil. BAL may also induce hemolysis in those with glucose-6-

phosphate dehydrogenase (G6PD) deficiency; therefore, a G6PD assay should be obtained if the patient's G6PD status is not known. Withhold oral iron supplementation during BAL treatment to avoid potential toxic interactions.

BAL is given by deep intramuscular injection in a dose of 3 to 5 mg/kg every 4 to 6 hours. CaNa₂EDTA (50 mg/kg per day) is started 4 to 5 hours after the first dose of BAL and given as a continuous intravenous infusion (over 24 hours). The hemodynamic stability of severely lead-poisoned children, as well as changes in neurologic status that may indicate encephalopathy, should be closely monitored. Just as when administering CaNa₂EDTA alone, intravenous fluids are given to ensure adequate hydration and urine output and to facilitate renal excretion. Dual therapy should be continued for a minimum of 72 hours, and a BLL should be repeated. If the BLL is greater than 50 μg/dL, BAL is continued for an additional 48 hours in conjunction with CaNa₂EDTA, for up to a total of 12 doses. If the BLL is less than 50 μg/dL, CaNa₂EDTA alone is continued for a total of 5 days.

Between 30% and 50% of patients who receive BAL experience side effects. Mild febrile reactions and transient elevations in serum transaminases may be observed. Hypertension and tachycardia can also occur. Other minor adverse effects include, in order of frequency, nausea, vomiting, headache, lacrimation, rhinorrhea, and salivation. These side effects are transient and usually disappear with cessation of the drug.

Patients with Clinical Signs and Symptoms of Acute Encephalopathy

Children with signs and symptoms of acute encephalopathy (usually seen with a BLL >70 μg/dL) should be evaluated for admission to an intensive care setting; the poison control center, toxicology consulting service, or pediatric environmental health service should be consulted immediately. Lead encephalopathy is a life-threatening emergency that should be treated using contemporary standards for the intensive care treatment of increased intracranial pressure, including appropriate pressure monitoring, osmotic therapy, and drug therapy in addition to chelation therapy. If the admitting hospital does not have intensive care services, toxicology or the local poison control center should be asked for advice on stabilizing the patient for transfer. A lumbar puncture should *not* be performed on any child suspected of having lead encephalopathy.

Children with signs and symptoms of encephalopathy or a venous BLL greater than 100 μg/dL should receive nothing by mouth (usually for the first 24 hours), and parenteral fluid therapy should begin immediately; total volume is restricted to basal requirements plus ongoing losses to avoid excessive intravenous fluid administration. Although it is desirable to evacuate residual lead from the gut, this should not delay the start of chelation therapy in severely lead-poisoned children. For acute encephalopathy or a BLL greater than 100 μg/dL, BAL and CaNa₂EDTA are coadministered for a total of 5 consecutive days, as detailed earlier. The use of CaNa₂EDTA alone is avoided in children with lead levels greater than 70 μg/dL because it may precipitate encephalopathy by causing a redistribution of lead to the brain, resulting in a lethal increase in intracranial pressure.

Consultation

Consider consultation with toxicology or a poison control center for guidance in treatment and acute and long-term management. If encephalopathy is present, the inclusion of critical care specialists and neurology services is warranted. Contact local authorities for lead abatement programs and referral for early intervention.

Admission Criteria

- All children with elevated BLLs and symptoms of toxicity, particularly encephalopathy (e.g., headache, ataxia, sleepiness) or evidence of raised intracranial pressure.
- Children with venous BLLs of 45 to 69 μg/dL who are not candidates for oral therapy with succimer (e.g., no lead-free housing available, unable to tolerate enteral therapy, concern about noncompliance, inadequate follow-up).
- Children with venous BLLs greater than 70 μg/dL.

Discharge Criteria

- A repeat BLL obtained at the end of chelation determines the need for reinstitution of chelation therapy:

  Children with BLLs less than 45 μg/dL can be discharged home, with the understanding that outpatient chelation will most likely be required. As a general rule, children whose admission BLL is less than 70 μg/dL will have an end-of-chelation BLL of less than 45 μg/dL, making them candidates for discharge after a single course of chelation.

  If the BLL is 45 to 69 μg/dL at the end of the first course, a second course of chelation therapy is necessary, which is best done as an inpatient.

  If, at the end of the first course of chelation, the BLL is 70 μg/dL or greater, dual therapy with BAL and CaNa$_2$EDTA should be reinitiated. A minimum of 2 days must elapse before restarting intravenous CaNa$_2$EDTA (a chelation "honeymoon") to minimize the risk of nephrotoxicity and permit at least partial recovery from the urinary losses of zinc produced by CaNa$_2$EDTA.
- Referral to an early intervention program is advised for lead-poisoned children suspected of having a developmental handicap (e.g., speech delay).
- Availability of lead-safe housing at the time of discharge (e.g., with friends or relatives or in designated transitional housing) if the child's residence remains contaminated.
- Institution of plans for lead abatement in the home where the exposure occurred.

Follow-up Care

The first follow-up visit should be scheduled for 7 to 14 days after chelation to allow for a period of reequilibration. At this visit, a BLL and ZPP or EP level are repeated to determine whether subsequent outpatient chelation is needed. Many children require more than one round of outpatient chelation therapy. The time interval of follow-up care is detailed in the Centers for Disease Control and Prevention lead screening guidelines. During follow-up visits, pediatric care providers can assess the patient's and family's compli-

ance with recommended risk-reduction practices and the abatement or reduction of lead hazards, as well as address dietary factors to ensure an adequate intake of calcium, ascorbic acid, and iron. All children with significant lead exposure, and especially those who have undergone chelation, need routine screening for lead-induced developmental injuries such as speech or language impairments, learning disabilities, and behavioral disturbances. If at any time during follow-up a possible developmental delay is identified, the child should immediately be referred for a complete developmental evaluation and for neuropsychological testing if older than 4 years.

In a Nutshell

- Lead poisoning remains a common problem, affecting an estimated 300,000 children in the United States.
- Severe lead poisoning, defined as a BLL greater than 45 μg/dL, requires immediate intervention. Hospitalization is recommended for these children, with the goals of providing immediate environmental protection and the rapid institution of chelation therapy. In rare circumstances, children with BLLs of 45 to 55 μg/dL can be considered for outpatient therapy if a safe environment and 100% compliance with the outpatient chelation regimen can be assured.
- The chelation agents of choice for asymptomatic hospitalized children with BLLs of 45 to 70 μg/dL are succimer and CaNa$_2$EDTA. Children with BLLs greater than 70 μg/dL should receive dual chelation therapy with CaNa$_2$EDTA and BAL. BAL, which should be initiated before CaNa$_2$EDTA, is given until the BLL has fallen below 70 μg/dL, at which time CaNa$_2$EDTA alone can be given.

On the Horizon

- Clinical and laboratory investigations of childhood lead poisoning, the molecular and genetic basis of its toxicity, and the clinical consequences continue to advance our understanding of this environmental illness. For example, recent clinical investigations have disclosed that during pregnancy, lead is mobilized along with calcium, initiating lead exposure in utero. Early data suggest that this mobilization can be diminished through prenatal calcium supplementation.
- Investigations by Lanphear, Canfield, Bellinger, and others have shown that lead is a no-threshold toxin; that is, even BLLs less than 10 μg/dL—the current definition of lead poisoning—can produce demonstrable toxicity.
- A growing body of literature suggests that school-aged children (i.e., those older than 6 years) may demonstrate neurodevelopmental deficits that correlate more closely to their BLLs at the time of testing than their BLLs in early childhood. Even children with BLLs as low as 5 to 8 μg/dL perform worse than their peers with lower BLLs. This finding may force a reexamination of the value of chelation therapy, because the most common cause of

elevated BLLs in school-aged children can be presumed to result from lead poisoning in infancy.

- Chelation therapy with the agent succimer, when provided to children with BLLs of 25 to 44 µg/dL, does not appear to improve neurodevelopmental outcome (although other studies have suggested long-term improvement after chelation with other agents). This finding—the result of a rigorous, randomized clinical trial—has called into question the value of chelating any child with a BLL less than 45 µg/dL. Although this will remain an area of controversy until additional investigation is done, the prevailing practice among lead poisoning treatment programs is to treat select children with BLLs of 20 to 44 µg/dL.

ARSENIC

Arsenic is the 20th most abundant element in the earth's crust. It is released into the environment by volcanoes, through the weathering and smelting of arsenic-containing minerals and ores, and by commercial and industrial processes. It is also found in some folk and naturopathic remedies. Children are commonly exposed to arsenic by the ingestion of contaminated well water or by contact with arsenate wood preservatives, such as copper chromium arsenate found in pressure-treated wood. Arsenic exists in organic and inorganic forms. Trivalent arsenic (As^{+3}) is considered the most toxic form, followed by pentavalent arsenic (As^{+5}). Organic arsenic is the nontoxic form that is commonly found in seafood, particularly shellfish. Arsenic is well absorbed by all routes. Once absorbed, arsenicals disrupt cellular metabolism by interacting with sulfhydryl groups and by inhibiting enzymatic pathways required for the production of adenosine triphosphate. Arsenic is rapidly cleared from the blood (1-hour half-life), and excretion is almost exclusively renal.

Clinical Presentation

The clinical presentation of arsenic poisoning depends on the route, dose, timing, and duration of exposure. The characteristic presentation of acute arsenic poisoning is described as dysphagia associated with a metallic taste. Within hours of exposure, diffuse capillary and endothelial cell damage results in vasodilation and leakage of plasma, which precipitates a hemorrhagic gastroenteritis. In severe cases, extensive third spacing of fluids combined with fluid loss may lead to cardiovascular collapse consisting of hypotension, shock, and even death. Electrocardiogram findings may include nonspecific T-wave changes and a prolonged Q-Tc interval that may occur promptly or after a delay of several days. Acute tubular necrosis may also occur after a large ingestion. Acute poisoning can cause delirium, encephalopathy, seizures, and coma. A delayed sensorimotor peripheral neuropathy may appear within 3 weeks after acute ingestion.

Chronic arsenic poisoning develops insidiously and includes peripheral neuropathy and dermal changes. "Raindrop" lesions of the skin can take years to manifest and are characteristically described as hypo- and hyperpigmentation with hyperkeratosis. Skin, bladder, and lung malignancies have been observed in adults. General manifestations of chronic arsenic toxicity can include malaise, weakness, anorexia, alopecia, headache, diarrhea, nausea, vomiting, leukopenia, and anemia.

Diagnosis and Treatment

The diagnosis of arsenic poisoning is based on a history of exposure combined with a characteristic presentation. Arsenic levels can be obtained from urine, blood, hair, and nail samples. Urine is the preferred biomarker for arsenic exposure and must be obtained as a timed (8- to 24-hour) urine collection. A "spot" urine sample is not accurate but may be helpful in acute poisoning. There are two methods of measuring arsenic in urine samples: fractionated (speciated) measurement for inorganic plus organic arsenic, or total arsenic level (this must be done 1 week after seafood abstinence to avoid false-positive results). Urine arsenic has a reference value of less than 25 µg/L. Blood arsenic levels are rarely useful because of the short half-life. Normal blood levels vary based on background exposures but are typically less than 3 µg/dL. Hair and nail levels are of limited value owing to external contamination.

Because arsenic is readily excreted in urine, elimination of exposure is the most effective treatment. In symptomatic patients, BAL at a dose of 3 to 5 mg/kg intramuscularly every 4 to 6 hours can be administered and should continue until the urinary arsenic level is less than 50 µg/L per 24 hours. Chelation is rarely needed outside the setting of symptomatic acute poisoning; however, if chelation is prescribed, succimer is the preferred agent at a dose of 10 mg/kg orally three times a day for 5 days, then twice a day for 14 days.

Consultation

Chelation should be undertaken only after consultation with a medical toxicologist.

Admission Criteria

- Symptomatic arsenic poisoning requiring parenteral chelation therapy.

Discharge Criteria

- Completion of parenteral therapy, with resolution of symptoms.
- Identification and elimination of source of arsenic exposure.

In a Nutshell

- Arsenic is a heavy metal with a short half-life.
- Exposure commonly occurs from ingestion of contaminated well water or by contact with arsenate wood preservatives (e.g., pressure-treated wood).
- Acute toxicity presents initially with dysphagia associated with a metallic taste. Endothelial damage ensues, with vasodilation and leakage of plasma, which can lead to hemorrhagic gastroenteritis and progress to cardiovascular collapse. Neurotoxic effects can progress to coma.
- Evidence of chronic poisoning develops over years with peripheral neuropathy, dermal changes, and hair loss.
- Chelation therapy is indicated for symptomatic patients with acute poisoning.

Table 181-3 Mercury Absorption and Target Organs

Mercury Form	EXPOSURE		Target Organ
	Inhalation	*Oral*	
Elemental (metallic) mercury Hg^0 liquid, Hg^0 vapor	Major	Minor	Acute: lungs Chronic: CNS/PNS, erethism Other: kidney, acrodynia
Inorganic mercury salts Hg^{+1} (mercurous), Hg^{+2} (mercuric)	Minor	Major	Acute: GI (caustic injury) Chronic: CNS/PNS, erethism, triad (tremor, neuropsychiatric disturbances, gingivostomatitis) Other: kidney, acrodynia
Organic (alkyl) mercury methylmercury, ethylmercury, dimethylmercury	Minor	Major	Acute and chronic: CNS/PNS, teratogen Other: kidney, liver

CNS/PNS, central nervous system/peripheral nervous system; erethism, irritability, excitability, decreased concentration; GI, gastrointestinal.

MERCURY

Mercury is a naturally occurring metal that is present throughout the environment. It has been used in medications, disinfectants, thermometers, dental amalgams, and ethnic remedies. In the United States, coal-fired power plants are the biggest source of mercury emissions in the air. Mercury exists in three primary forms, each with a different toxicity: elemental or metallic mercury (Hg^0), inorganic mercury salts (Hg^{+1} [mercurous], Hg^{+2} [mercuric]), and organic or alkyl mercury (e.g., methylmercury). Inorganic mercury is readily converted to methylmercury by aquatic microorganisms and can bioaccumulate in the tissues of large carnivorous fish. The toxicokinetics of mercury vary, depending on the route of absorption and chemical form. Elemental, inorganic, and organic mercury can all be absorbed after inhalation. Elemental mercury is poorly absorbed orally; conversely; organic mercury is well absorbed (Table 181-3). Dermal absorption is limited for all forms of mercury. Elemental and inorganic mercury have a half-life of 40 to 60 days and are excreted via urine. Organic mercury has a half-life of 70 to 90 days and is eliminated via bile and feces.

Clinical Presentation

Acute inhalation of elemental mercury vapor is the main cause of toxicity. Symptoms may develop within a few hours and include nausea, vomiting, chills, metallic taste, tachypnea, dyspnea, abdominal pain, and diarrhea. These symptoms may subside in a few days or progress to interstitial pulmonary fibrosis, noncardiogenic pulmonary edema, interstitial chemical pneumonitis, and hemoptysis. Elemental liquid mercury can irritate the skin and cause allergic reactions. Chronic inhalation of elemental mercury vapor produces the classic triad of tremor, neuropsychiatric disturbances, and gingivostomatitis. Acrodynia (painful extremities) is a rare disease that affects primarily young children with chronic exposure. Symptoms include irritability, photophobia, pink discoloration of the hands and feet, and polyneuritis.

Acute ingestion of inorganic mercury salts is caustic to the GI tract and can produce a sudden onset of corrosive stomatitis, hemorrhagic gastroenteritis, and abdominal pain.

Acute oliguric renal failure from acute tubular necrosis may also occur within days of exposure. Chronic manifestations of inorganic mercury toxicity are similar to those of elemental mercury.

Organic mercury affects primarily the central nervous system, causing paresthesias, ataxia, dysarthria, spasticity, hearing impairment, and progressive visual field constriction. Perinatal exposure to methylmercury, a known potent teratogen, can produce severe congenital abnormalities such as neuroencephalopathy and micrognathia.

Diagnosis and Treatment

The diagnosis of mercury poisoning depends on the integration of characteristic findings with a history of known or potential exposure and the presence of a positive biomarker. Whole blood or, preferably, urine can be used to determine metallic and inorganic mercury levels. Whole blood samples are preferred for organic mercury levels, because that form is excreted in feces. Hair samples have limited value.

Removing the mercury source and preventing additional exposure are the best treatments. Elemental and inorganic mercury poisoning can be treated with oral succimer at a dose of 10 mg/kg orally three times a day for 5 days, then twice a day for 14 days. Alternatively, intramuscular BAL can be given initially at a dose of 3 to 5 mg/kg every 4 hours for 2 days, then 2.5 to 3 mg/kg every 6 hours for 2 days, then 2.5 to 3 mg/kg every 12 hours for 1 to 3 days. Organic mercury has been treated with oral succimer; however, data on its effectiveness are limited. Chelation therapy is rarely indicated and should be initiated only after consultation with a medical toxicologist.

SUGGESTED READING

Agency for Toxic Substances and Disease Registry: Toxicological Profile for Arsenic. Atlanta, US Department of Health and Human Services, 2000.

Agency for Toxic Substances and Disease Registry: Toxicological Profile for Mercury. Atlanta, US Public Health Service, 1999.

American Academy of Pediatrics, Committee on Drugs: Treatment guidelines for lead exposure in children. Pediatrics 1995;96:155-160.

American Academy of Pediatrics, Committee on Environmental Health: Technical report: Mercury in the environment: Implications for pediatricians. Pediatrics 2001;108:1505-1510.

Baum CR: Treatment of mercury intoxication. Curr Opin Pediatr 1999;11: 2675-2684.

Canfield RL, Henderson CR Jr, Cory-Slechta DA, et al: Intellectual impairment in children with blood lead concentrations below 10 µg per deciliter. N Engl J Med 2003;348:1517-1526.

Centers for Disease Control and Prevention: Managing Elevated Blood Lead Levels among Young Children: Recommendations from the Advisory Committee on Childhood Lead Poisoning Prevention. Atlanta, CDC, 2002.

Centers for Disease Control and Prevention: Screening Young Children for Lead Poisoning: Guidance for State and Local Public Health Officials. Atlanta, CDC, 1997.

Cullen NM, Wolf LR, St Clair D: Pediatric arsenic ingestion. Am J Emerg Med 1995;13:432-435.

Hall AH: Chronic arsenic poisoning. Toxicol Lett 2002;128:69-72.

Ozuah PO: Mercury poisoning. Curr Probl Pediatr 2000;30:91-99.

Piomelli S, Rosen JF, Chisolm JJ Jr, Graef JW: Management of childhood lead poisoning. J Pediatr 1984;105:523-532.

REFERENCES

1. Angle CR: Childhood lead poisoning and its treatment. Annu Rev Pharmacol Toxicol 1993;33:409-434.
2. Kosnett MJ: Lead. In Ford MD, Delaney KA, Ling LJ, Erickson T (eds): Clinical Toxicology. Philadelphia, WB Saunders, 2001, pp 723-735.
3. Weitzman M, Glotzer D: Lead poisoning. Pediatr Rev 1992;13:461-468.
4. Yip L: Heavy metal poisoning. In Irwin RS, Rippe JM (eds): Irwin & Rippe's Intensive Care Medicine, 4th ed. Philadelphia, Lippincott-Raven, 1999, pp 1637-1653.
5. Jacobs DE, Clickner RP, Zhou JY, et al: The prevalence of lead-based paint hazards in US housing. Environ Health Perspect 2002;110:A599-A606.
6. Lanphear BP, Roghmann KJ: Pathways of lead exposure in urban children. Environ Res 1997;74:67-73.
7. Taketomo CK: Pediatric Dosage Handbook, 11th ed. Hudson, Ohio, Lexi-Comp, 2004, p 445.
8. Dart RC, Bond GR: Gastrointestinal decontamination. In Dart RC (ed): Medical Toxicology, 3rd ed. Philadelphia, Lippincott-Williams & Wilkins, 2001, pp 32-39.
9. Agency for Toxic Substances and Disease Registry: Toxicological Profile for Lead. Atlanta, US Department of Health and Human Services, 2003.
10. Dart RC: Succimer. In Dart RC (ed): Medical Toxicology, 3rd ed. Philadelphia, Lippincott-Williams & Wilkins, 2001, pp 266-268.
11. Centers for Disease Control and Prevention: Screening Young Children for Lead Poisoning: Guidance for State and Local Public Health Officials. Atlanta, CDC, 1997.
12. Jones AL, Flanagan RJ: Dimercaprol. In Dart RC (ed): Medical Toxicology, 3rd ed. Philadelphia, Lippincott-Williams & Wilkins, 2001, pp 185-186.
13. Canfield RL, Henderson CR Jr, Cory-Slechta DA, et al: Intellectual impairment in children with blood lead concentrations below 10 µg per deciliter. N Engl J Med 2003;348:1517-1526.
14. Pirkle JL, Brody DJ, Gunter EW, et al: The decline in blood lead levels in the United States: The National Health and Nutrition Examination Surveys (NHANES). JAMA 1994;272:284-329.
15. Shannon MW: Etiology of lead poisoning. In Pueschel SM, Linakis JG, Anderson AC (eds): Lead Poisoning in Childhood. Baltimore, Paul H. Brookes, 1996, pp 37-57.
16. Yip L: Calcium disodium ethylenediaminetetraacetic acid (CaNa$_2$EDTA). In Dart RC (ed): Medical Toxicology, 3rd ed. Philadelphia, Lippincott-Williams & Wilkins, 2001, pp 169-172.
17. American Academy of Pediatrics, Committee on Drugs: Treatment guidelines for lead exposure in children. Pediatrics 1995;96:155-160.
18. Piomelli S, Rosen JF, Chisolm JJ Jr, Graef JW: Management of childhood lead poisoning. J Pediatr 1984;105:523-532.
19. Shannon MW, Graef JW: Lead intoxication in infancy. Pediatrics 1992;89:87-90.
20. Ziegler EE, Edwards BB, Jensen RL, et al: Absorption and retention of lead by infants. Pediatr Res 1978;12:29-34.
21. Rabinowitz MB, Wetherill GW, Kopple JD: Kinetic analysis of lead metabolism in healthy humans. J Clin Invest 1976;58:260-270.
22. Bellinger D, Sloman J, Leviton A, et al: Low-level lead exposure and children's cognitive function in the preschool years. Pediatrics 1991;87:219-227.
23. Bellinger DC, Stiles KM, Needleman HL: Low-level lead exposure, intelligence and academic achievement: A long-term follow-up study. Pediatrics 1992;90:855-861.
24. Liebelt EL, Shannon MW: Oral chelators for childhood lead poisoning. Pediatr Annu 1994;23:616-619.
25. Hryhorczuk D, Eng J: Arsenic. In Ford MD, Delaney KA, Ling LJ, Erickson T (eds): Clinical Toxicology. Philadelphia, WB Saunders, 2001, pp 716-721.
26. Concha G, Nermell B, Vahter M: Metabolism of inorganic arsenic in children with chronic high arsenic exposure in northern Argentina. Environ Health Perspect 1998;106:355-359.
27. Agency for Toxic Substances and Disease Registry: Toxicological Profile for Arsenic. Atlanta, US Department of Health and Human Services, 2000.
28. Cullen NM, Wolf LR, St Clair D: Pediatric arsenic ingestion. Am J Emerg Med 1995;13:432-435.
29. Hall AH: Chronic arsenic poisoning. Toxicol Lett 2002;128:69-72.
30. Agency for Toxic Substances and Disease Registry: Toxicological Profile for Mercury. Atlanta, US Public Health Service, 1999.
31. Myers G, Davidson P, et al: Effects of prenatal methylmercury exposure from a high fish diet on developmental milestones in the Seychelles Child Development Study. Neurotoxicology 1997;18:819-830.
32. Chiang WK: Mercury. In Dart RC (ed): Medical Toxicology, 3rd ed. Philadelphia, WB Saunders, 2001, pp 737-1153.
33. American Academy of Pediatrics, Committee on Environmental Health: Technical report: Mercury in the environment: Implications for pediatricians. Pediatrics 2001;108:1505-1510.
34. Baum CR: Treatment of mercury intoxication. Curr Opin Pediatr 1999;11:265-268.
35. Ozuah PO: Mercury poisoning. Curr Probl Pediatr 2000;30:91-99.

CHAPTER 182

Drugs of Abuse

Carl R. Baum

Drugs of abuse continue to have a significant impact on health care utilization in the pediatric population. The pediatric hospitalist should consider drugs of abuse in the differential diagnosis of any patient who presents with altered mental status (hallucinations, stupor, coma), abnormal motor activity (tremor, seizure), or behavioral disturbance (agitation, outburst, withdrawal, depression, suicidal or homicidal ideation).

Each fall, the American Association of Poison Control Centers publishes its annual summary of poisoning exposures reported to its member centers. In 2003, there were a total of 2.4 million exposures reported, 1106 of which led to a fatality.[1] Of these fatalities, 34 (3.1%) involved a child (<20 years of age) who intentionally abused (alone or in combination with other substances) cannabis, hallucinogens, inhalants, narcotics, or stimulants (Table 182-1).

Another annual resource is the National Institute on Drug Abuse's Monitoring the Future surveys of 8th-, 10th-, and 12th-grade students conducted to gauge trends in drug use, as well as levels of perceived risk and disapproval among these children. First performed in 1975, the most recent of these extensive studies is in the public domain and posted on the organization's website.[2] The 2005 survey of nearly 50,000 students in 402 secondary schools revealed that although several drugs showed declines in use, the declines were in general not statistically significant. There were increases in the use of three types of drugs: inhalants, controlled-release oxycodone (OxyContin), and sedatives.

CLINICAL PRESENTATION

Initial assessment of a patient who may have been exposed to any drugs of abuse follows the principles outlined in Chapter 178. Reassessment should occur periodically, even in patients who appear to be stable on initial evaluation; if drug absorption and distribution are not complete at the time of presentation, the clinical condition may worsen with the passage of time.

After the initial assessment, the hospitalist should attempt to elicit a complete history from the patient, if lucid and cooperative, or from a parent, guardian, or other companion who may be able to provide details of the exposure. Prehospital personnel may be able to shed additional light, particularly if pill containers or other items are available at the scene.

A thorough history often elicits clues about specific drugs of abuse. A number of surveys around the world have documented the use of illicit drugs in various populations and social settings. For example, a survey in the United Kingdom identified risk taking, male gender, higher educational level, single marital status, unemployment, age younger than 25 years, smoking, and heavy alcohol consumption among the social factors associated with the use of these drugs.[3] In another survey conducted at the University of Michigan, 3% of students who responded reported illicit use of methylphenidate, often abused as a study aid, in the previous year.[4] A decade-long series of surveys of psychotropic drug use among 10- to 18-year-old Brazilian students revealed significant increases over the study period in the use of many drugs, including amphetamines, anxiolytics, cocaine, and marijuana.[5] Another survey of French school athletes[6] documented their use of illicit substances, including those that the International Olympic Committee (IOC) lists as banned "doping agents": stimulants, narcotics, anabolic agents, peptide hormones, corticosteroids, and diuretics. First published in 1963 under the leadership of the IOC, the "prohibited list" of banned agents now falls under the aegis of the World Anti-Doping Agency.[7]

Injuries may be associated with drugs of abuse because risk seeking is a closely linked behavior and judgment is often impaired while under the influence of drugs. An individual who attempts to operate a motor vehicle while under the influence of drugs or alcohol (or both) is at increased risk for collisions and resultant trauma. Researchers in the Netherlands conducted a prospective observational case-control study in which drivers hospitalized after collisions were compared with those randomly recruited on the roads. In this study population, no increased risk for road trauma was found in those who used cannabis; risk was increased (but did not achieve statistical significance) in those who used amphetamines, cocaine, or opiates. The highest relative risks occurred in drivers who used a combination of drugs and alcohol.[8] Alcohol (ethanol) presents an interesting problem because it is so broadly tolerated in a social context yet can be considered a drug of abuse that accounts for significant morbidity/mortality. For example, ethanol has an effect on slow eye movements, the basis for horizontal gaze nystagmus that law enforcement officials may observe in field sobriety tests. Recent work suggests that this effect leads to impaired "motion parallax" and depth perception.[9] The epidemic of methamphetamine abuse deserves special note; this highly addictive drug causes significant morbidity and mortality, but it also creates a significant environmental hazard to children exposed to its clandestine production.[10,11]

Exposure to drugs of abuse often occurs at bars, parties, or rave dances, and in such cases "club" drugs such as methylenedioxymethamphetamine (MDMA) or "date rape" drugs (see discussion in Diagnosis and Evaluation) should be suspected.

DIFFERENTIAL DIAGNOSIS

Patients suspected of intentional or unintentional exposure to drugs of abuse may present with symptom/sign complexes or toxic syndromes (toxidromes) that suggest a

Table 182–1 Drugs of Abuse (Intentional) in Pediatric Fatalities Reported to U.S. Poison Centers, 2003

Class	Substances	Fatalities	Age Range (yr)
Cannabinoids	Cannabis + unknown	1	16
Hallucinogens	Dextromethorphan + others Cough/cold preparation	2	17–18
Inhalants	Air freshener (aerosol) Butane Chlorofluorocarbon Gasoline Helium	6	11–18
Narcotics	Fentanyl patch Heroin Hydrocodone Methadone Morphine (RA, LA) Oxycodone (RA, LA)	12	13–19
Narcotics plus stimulants	Methadone + cocaine Morphine (LA) + amphetamine Oxycodone (LA) + cocaine	3	15–19
Stimulants	Amphetamine Amphetamine/dextroamphetamine Caffeine Cocaine Ma huang MDMA ("ecstasy") Methamphetamine Methylphenidate (Ritalin)	10	17–19

LA, long-acting; MDMA, methylenedioxymethamphetamine; RA, regular-acting.
Adapted from Watson WA, Litovitz TL, Klein-Schwartz W, et al: 2003 Annual report of the American Association of Poison Control Centers Toxic Exposure Surveillance System. Am J Emerg Med 2004;22:335-404.

specific drug class. Commonly abused drugs and related symptoms and signs are listed in Table 182-2.

Although considerable symptom/sign overlap exists among the drugs listed, a presenting toxidrome may refine the search to some degree. A broad range of neurologic, infectious, or metabolic conditions, including seizures and postictal states, encephalitis, encephalopathy, cerebrovascular accidents, hypoglycemia, and hyperammonemia, can present with features of altered mental status (see Chapter 28) similar to those of drug abuse. Primary cardiovascular dysfunction, including myocarditis, severe hypertension, and conduction abnormalities, can mimic some of the cardiac features. Acute psychiatric disorders can have overlapping signs and symptoms or may coexist with drug ingestions.

DIAGNOSIS AND EVALUATION

Often initiated in the emergency department, the diagnostic evaluation may include a number of tests, including the electrocardiogram and various chemistry panels and toxicology screens.

The cardiac rhythm strip may provide the first clues of a drug-induced arrhythmia, and a 12-lead electrocardiogram should be obtained for diagnostic purposes. Urinalysis may reveal rhabdomyolysis or pregnancy. Alterations in blood chemistry, including serum glucose, electrolytes, renal and liver function tests, and cardiac enzymes, may provide additional if indirect evidence of drug toxicity, such as metabolic acidosis, hepatic failure, or cardiac ischemia.

The hospitalist should avoid viewing the toxicology screen as a "black box" that provides a simple list of ingested or inhaled substances, because hospital laboratories may offer a number of screens with varying capability. Drugs of abuse may be detected in serum/plasma, gastric aspirates, and urine, although most hospital laboratories offer a drugs-of-abuse panel to screen urine samples. A number of techniques may be used: thin-layer chromatography, high-pressure/performance liquid chromatography, immunoassay, and gas chromatography/mass spectrometry. Some laboratories may not be able to perform all these techniques and must instead send samples to reference laboratories. In general, immunoassays offer high sensitivity, rapid turnaround time, low cost, and relatively simple technical protocols, and are therefore often used to screen for drugs of abuse. Typical drugs-of-abuse panels may include amphetamines, barbiturates, benzodiazepines, cannabinoids, cocaine metabolites, methadone, opiates, and phencyclidine.[12]

The hospitalist should consider the possibility of both false-negative and false-positive screening tests. False-negative results may arise because many of these immunoas-

Table 182–2 Symptoms/Signs of Common Drugs of Abuse

Class	Symptoms/Signs
Cannabinoids	Conjunctival injection, slowed reflexes, tachycardia, xerostomia
GHB and precursors	Amnesia, apnea, arrhythmias, coma, respiratory depression
Hallucinogens Dextromethorphan (e.g., Coricidin)	Ataxia, coma, drowsiness, dystonia, fevers, hallucinations, miosis, respiratory depression, tachycardia, tremors
Ketamine	Emergence reactions, hallucinations, hypersalivation, hypertension, nystagmus, seizures, tachycardia, vivid dreams
Inhalants	Arrhythmias, coma, drowsiness, encephalopathy, frostbite, paint stains, respiratory depression
Narcotics	Bradycardia, coma, constipation, dizziness, histamine release, hypotension, miosis, respiratory depression
Stimulants	General: arrhythmias, euphoria, hallucinations, insomnia, mydriasis, nervousness, restlessness, seizures
Methamphetamine	"Meth mouth" (dental decay)
Cocaine	Chest pain, nasal congestion, rhinitis
MDMA (ecstasy)	Empathy, talkativeness

GHB, γ-hydroxybutyrate; MDMA, methylenedioxymethamphetamine.
Adapted from Leikin JB, Paloucek FP (eds): Poisoning & Toxicology [electronic book for the PDA]. Hudson, OH, Lexi-Comp, 2004.

say panels do not detect a number of common substances, including anabolic steroids, the benzodiazepines alprazolam and flunitrazepam (Rohypnol), ethanol, γ-hydroxybutyrate (GHB), ketamine, lysergic acid diethylamide (LSD), and synthetic opioids such as fentanyl. The screen for phencyclidine will not usually detect the structurally similar ketamine. Thus, a "negative tox screen" may falsely reassure a hospitalist who is not familiar with the limitations of a particular laboratory's immunoassay.[12] The presence of amnesia or coma, for example, should raise the possibility of Rohypnol, GHB, or ketamine, common "date rape" drugs. Furthermore, a negative test may occur when the concentration of the metabolite falls below the federally mandated threshold or cutoff value established by the Substance Abuse and Mental Health Services Administration for that particular substance.[13]

In contrast, false-positive results may arise because immunoassays are intended to maximize sensitivity, so confirmatory testing with a highly specific technique should follow any positive result. Fluoroquinolones, for example, may cause a screen to be positive for opiates,[14] whereas high concentrations of dextromethorphan may screen positive for phencyclidine. Screens may remain positive for days to weeks, depending on the drug and the pattern of use. Cocaine metabolites such as benzoylecgonine and ecgonine methylester typically persist for up to 72 hours, whereas cannabinoids may yield a positive test in the urine of a heavy marijuana user for weeks after the last use.[15]

Plasma toxicology screens for coingestants, such as acetaminophen, acetylsalicylic acid (aspirin), alcohols (ethanol, isopropyl, methanol), barbiturates, ethylene glycol, and tricyclic antidepressants, are generally available and should be considered. For example, children may abuse easily available over-the-counter products, particularly dextromethorphan-containing cough and cold preparations, for their euphoric effects, but some combination products also contain aceta-

minophen, the toxicity of which may not be apparent on presentation.[16]

Parents or guardians who inquire about home kits that test breath, hair, saliva, or urine for drugs of abuse should be advised of the significant limitations of these products. It is important to emphasize that asymptomatic children should not be tested without their consent or assent.[17]

TREATMENT

Stabilization and ongoing support of the respiratory, circulatory, and neurologic systems are fundamental management principles. An ABCDEF mnemonic, introducing *d*econtamination, *e*nhancement, and *f*ollow-up, helps guide further care of a drug-of-abuse patient (Table 182–3).

Enhancement is a reference to the use of drugs that serve as antidotes, including those that correct physiologic abnormalities, or to methods for enhancing elimination of the absorbed toxicant. Examples of these drugs are dextrose and specific antidotes such as naloxone (Narcan), fomepizole (Antizol), and *N*-acetylcysteine (Mucomyst, Acetadote). Enhanced elimination methods include hemodialysis, multidose activated charcoal (although indications are limited), urinary alkalinization, and whole-bowel irrigation. The latter technique uses nonabsorbable polyethylene glycol in a balanced electrolyte solution, administered by mouth or via nasogastric tube, to clear the gastrointestinal tract of ingested substances. Whole-bowel irrigation may be particularly useful when the hospitalist encounters a body stuffer (drug packets hastily ingested to avoid police detection) or packer (drug packets sealed and ingested, often for transport across international borders). Specific treatment strategies are summarized in Table 182–4.

Follow-up refers to the importance of reviewing all consultations and laboratory investigations and ensuring

Table 182-3 Priorities in the General Approach to a Poisoned Patient

	Priority	Examples of Interventions
A	Airway	Endotracheal intubation
B	Breathing	Supplemental oxygen, ventilatory support
C	Circulation	Antiarrhythmics, pressor support
D	Decontamination	Activated charcoal Whole-bowel irrigation
E	Enhancement	Dextrose Antidotes Enhanced elimination Hemodialysis Multidose activated charcoal Urinary alkalinization Whole-bowel irrigation
F	Follow-up	Social work/psychiatric consultations Laboratory and toxicology screen results Inpatient detox(ification) Outpatient follow-up Primary care provider Toxicology clinic

Table 182-4 Management Strategies for Drugs of Abuse

Class	Monitor for	Treatment
GHB and congeners	Apnea	Respiratory support
Hallucinogens		
Dextromethorphan	Respiratory depression	Naloxone
Ketamine	Dystonia Hypersalivation Hypertension/ emergence reactions/ seizures	Diphenhydramine Atropine Benzodiazepines
Inhalants	Apnea Arrhythmias	Respiratory support Avoid catecholamine stimulation of sensitized myocardium
Narcotics	Apnea	Naloxone, respiratory support
Stimulants	Arrhythmias Seizures	Lidocaine (caution if cocaine exposed) Sodium bicarbonate Benzodiazepines

GHB, γ-hydroxybutyrate.
Adapted from Leikin JB, Paloucek FP (eds): Poisoning & Toxicology [electronic book for the PDA]. Hudson, OH, Lexi-Comp, 2004.

appropriate disposition for a patient who has been exposed to drugs of abuse. Social workers and psychiatrists may have been consulted as part of the evaluation, and the results of some laboratory investigations, particularly "send-out" tests, may not be available immediately on admission to the hospital. Appropriate disposition may require inpatient detoxification services; patients discharged home may require follow-up with a primary care provider or toxicology clinic. Preventive strategies should always be considered to prevent the morbidity and mortality associated with drug abuse.

Observation and cardiorespiratory monitoring may suffice as the drug of abuse is being metabolized. Specific treatment strategies are summarized in Table 182-4.

CONSULTATION

The hospitalist should consider regional poison control center (1-800-222-1222) and medical toxicology consultation, which may provide clinically relevant guidance about management and disposition of the patient and may be aware of local trends in the use or abuse of certain substances. Calls to the regional poison control center also help document exposures that will contribute to the annual statistics reported to the American Association of Poison Control Centers.

ADMISSION CRITERIA

Hospitalization is indicated for either of the following reasons:

- Altered mental status or vital signs that do not return to baseline within 4 to 6 hours of presentation

- Exposures that require prolonged monitoring or therapy (e.g., acetaminophen coingestion, which presents a risk for hepatotoxicity and requires a course of *N*-acetylcysteine)

DISCHARGE CRITERIA

- Mental status and vital signs returned to baseline
- All pending laboratory investigations reviewed
- Social work/psychiatric consultations completed (if appropriate) and discussion and resolution of the need for an inpatient detoxification program
- Primary care provider contacted and outpatient follow-up arranged

PREVENTION

Many reliable online resources are available (see Table 182-5) to provide accurate information about drugs of abuse and the risks associated with them. However, information consumers should be aware that Internet search engines may direct children to websites, such as the Vaults of Erowid, that contain misinformation about drugs of abuse.[18]

IN A NUTSHELL

- Suspicion of exposure to drugs of abuse should be prompted by signs and symptoms, as well as by associated risk factors such as age (<25 years), smoking,

Table 182-5 Online Information and Prevention Resources (Accessed July 2006)

Organization	Internet Address (URL)
Al-Anon	*alateen.org*
American Academy of Pediatrics	*aap.org/healthtopics/subabuse.cfm*
American Association of Poison Control Centers	*aapcc.org*
Monitoring the Future	*monitoringthefuture.org*
National Institute on Drug Abuse	*nida.nih.gov*
Substance Abuse and Mental Health Services Administration	*health.org/kidsarea*
U.S. Drug Enforcement Administration	*www.dea.gov*
World Anti-Doping Agency	*www.wada-ama.org/en*

social setting (dance clubs, bars), and alcohol ingestion.
- Toxicology screens should be ordered judiciously and interpreted cautiously because false-positive and false-negative results are important considerations and vary by the method of testing performed.
- Drugs of abuse are often ingested or inhaled along with other medications. Common coingestants include acetaminophen, aspirin, and alcohols.
- Consultation with a regional poison control center or medical toxicologist provides clinically relevant guidance about management and disposition of the patient; in addition, such resources may be aware of local trends in the use or abuse of certain substances.

ON THE HORIZON

- Although some drugs of abuse seem to be omnipresent standards, others may appear on the scene in specific regions or populations. The hospitalist should be cognizant of this shifting landscape, particularly when novel synthetic analogues or combinations of drugs present unusual patterns of morbidity and mortality. Local police and health departments, as well as emergency departments, medical toxicologists, and poison control centers, may be the first to identify new trends of abuse.

SUGGESTED READINGS

Babu K, Boyer EW, Hernon C, et al: Emerging drugs of abuse. Clin Pediatr Emerg Med 2005;6:81-84.
Haroz R, Greenberg M: Emerging drugs of abuse. Med Clin North Am 2005;89:1256-1259.
Henretig F: Inhalant abuse in children and adolescents. Pediatr Ann 1996;25:47-52.
Osterhoudt KC: Experiencing ecstasy: Is it all the rave? Pediatr Case Rev 2002;2:126-129.
Osterhoudt KC, Henretig FM: Comatose teenagers at a party: What a tangled "web" we weave. Pediatr Case Rev 2003;3:171-173.

REFERENCES

1. Watson WA, Litovitz TL, Klein-Schwartz W, et al: 2003 Annual report of the American Association of Poison Control Centers Toxic Exposure Surveillance System. Am J Emerg Med 2004;22:335-404.
2. Johnston LD, O'Malley PM, Bachman JG, Schulenberg JE: Monitoring the Future national results on adolescent drug use: Overview of key findings, 2005 (NIH Publication No. 06-5882). Bethesda, MD, National Institute on Drug Abuse, 2006.
3. Wadsworth EJK, Moss SC, Simpson SA, Smith AP: Factors associated with recreational drug use. J Psychopharmacol 2004;18:238-248.
4. Teter CJ, McCabe SE, Boyd CJ, Guthrie SK: Illicit methylphenidate use in an undergraduate student sample: Prevalence and risk factors. Pharmacotherapy 2003;23:609-617.
5. Galduroz JCF, Noto AR, Nappo SA, Carlini EA: Trends in drug use among students in Brazil: Analysis of four surveys in 1987, 1989, 1993 and 1997. Braz J Med Biol Res 2004;37:523-531.
6. Laure P, Lecerf T, Friser A, Binsinger C: Drugs, recreational drug use and attitudes toward doping of high school athletes. Int J Sports Med 2004;25:133-138.
7. Prohibited List. World Anti-Doping Agency. Available at http://www.wada-ama.org/en/prohibitedlist.ch2. Accessed July 26, 2006.
8. Movig KLL, Mathijssen MPM, Nagel PHA, et al: Psychoactive substance abuse and the risk of motor vehicle accidents. Accid Anal Prev 2004;36:631-636.
9. Nawrot M, Nordenstrom B, Olson A: Disruption of eye movements by ethanol intoxication affects perception of depth from motion parallax. Psychol Sci 2004;15:858-865.
10. Porter CJ, Armstrong JR: Burns from illegal drug manufacture: Case series and management. J Burn Care Rehabil 2004;25:314-318.
11. Marris E: Police urge speedy action to clean up home drug factories. Nature 2005;434:129.
12. Cox MN, Baum CR: Toxicology reviews: Immunoassay in detecting drugs of abuse. Pediatr Emerg Care 1998;14:372-375.
13. Luzzi VI, Saunders AN, Koenig JW, et al: Analytic performance of immunoassays for drugs of abuse below established cutoff values. Clin Chem 2004;50:717-722.
14. Zacher JL, Givone DM: False-positive urine opiate screening associated with fluoroquinolone use. Ann Pharmacother 2004;38:1525-1528.
15. Leikin JB, Paloucek FP (eds): Poisoning & Toxicology [electronic book for the PDA]. Hudson, OH, Lexi-Comp, 2004.
16. Kirages TJ, Sule HP, Mycyk MB: Severe manifestations of Coricidin intoxication. Am J Emerg Med 2003;21:473-475.
17. Levy S, Van Hook S, Knight J: A review of Internet-based home drug-testing products for parents. Pediatrics 2004;113:720-726.
18. Boyer EW, Shannon M, Hibberd PL: Web sites with misinformation about illicit drugs [letter]. N Engl J Med 2001;345:469-471.

CHAPTER 183

Withdrawal Syndromes

Robert J. Hoffman and Adhi N. Sharma

Drug withdrawal is a physiologic response to an effectively lowered drug concentration in a patient tolerant to the drug in question. Withdrawal results in a predictable constellation of symptoms that are reversible if the drug is reintroduced. Withdrawal is a phenomenon of altered neurochemistry, and the central nervous system (CNS) is the most consequential target. Under normal conditions, the CNS maintains a balance between excitation and inhibition. Although such balance can be achieved by several means, excitation is constant and actions occur through removal of inhibitory tone.[1]

Clinicians may encounter withdrawal symptoms as the primary reason for hospitalization or as a consequence of hospitalization when interruption of drug use occurs, either intentionally or unintentionally. This chapter focuses on syndromes associated with withdrawal from the following classes of agents: ethanol, sedative-hypnotics, opioids, and selective serotonin reuptake inhibitors (SSRIs).

CLINICAL PRESENTATION

The onset, progression, duration, and severity of withdrawal symptoms depend on both the patient's degree of tolerance and the half-life of the drug involved. In general, drugs with shorter half-lives produce withdrawal symptoms sooner after discontinuation, and the symptoms tend to be more severe (Table 183-1).

Ethanol Withdrawal

Ethanol withdrawal is one of the most common withdrawal syndromes, behind those of nicotine and caffeine. The alcohol withdrawal syndrome is multifaceted and should be considered a spectrum. The discrete aspects of alcohol withdrawal can follow a progression or occur independently. These aspects include alcoholic tremulousness, hypertension, tachycardia, diaphoresis, agitation, and seizures. Alcohol withdrawal rarely if ever occurs in children other than neonates.

Sedative–Hypnotic Withdrawal

Sedative-hypnotic agents include benzodiazepines, barbiturates, γ-hydroxybutyric acid (GHB), and γ-butyrolactone (GBL), and withdrawal from these drugs may be indistinguishable from alcohol withdrawal because the presenting symptoms are nearly identical. However, the chronology may offer a clue to the cause of the withdrawal. Because of rapid metabolism and the lack of active metabolites, withdrawal from GHB or GBL generally occurs within 2 to 3 hours of cessation of drug use.[2] In contrast, diazepam has active metabolites, and thus withdrawal symptoms may not be manifested for a week. Seizures may result from any sedative-hypnotic withdrawal. Different sedative-hypnotic agents often share enough common receptor or metabolic activity that one drug can be substituted for the other to treat withdrawal—a phenomenon known as cross-tolerance.

Opioid Withdrawal

Opioid withdrawal can be divided into physical signs and symptoms and psychological symptoms. Piloerection, yawning, and lacrimation are some of the physical signs, whereas nausea, vomiting, and diarrhea are common symptoms. Withdrawing patients also have intense opioid craving associated with the feeling of being unwell. In contrast to sedative-hypnotic withdrawal, opioid withdrawal is associated with minimal autonomic instability. Patients may be tachycardic and have a slight elevation in blood pressure, but this is partly in response to their physical and emotional symptoms. Furthermore, other than agitation, opioid withdrawal is associated with normal mental status.

Selective Serotonin Reuptake Inhibitor Withdrawal

The most recently described withdrawal syndrome is that of SSRIs, probably related to temporary and self-limited serotonin dysregulation.[3,4] Signs and symptoms include dizziness, gastrointestinal disturbances, headaches, lethargy, anxiety or agitation (or both), paresthesias, tremors, sweating, insomnia, and irritability. The onset is usually within 1 week of abrupt cessation of treatment, and symptoms generally resolve within 3 weeks. Most reports describe symptoms associated with withdrawal from venlafaxine, but the syndrome, which occurs in both neonates and children, has also been reported with citalopram, fluoxetine, fluvoxamine, paroxetine, and sertraline.[5]

Neonatal Withdrawal Syndromes

Maternal addiction can lead to neonatal withdrawal. The time to symptom presentation after birth varies with the agent in question. Neonatal alcohol withdrawal typically begins within 3 days of parturition. Symptoms most typically include agitation, irritability, crying, tremors, tachycardia, hypertension, insomnia, and diaphoresis.[6] Opisthotonos, nystagmus, clonus, seizures, hypertonia, hyperactive or asymmetric reflexes, excessive rooting, diarrhea, vomiting, and inability to thermoregulate may also occur.[7] Opisthotonos and abdominal distention rarely occur in opioid withdrawal and can help differentiate the two when the mother has abused multiple substances. Although initially thought to occur only as a complication of fetal alcohol syndrome (FAS), neonatal alcohol withdrawal can occur independently of FAS. The presentation of neonates withdrawing from sedative-hypnotics would be indistinguishable.

Table 183-1 Expected Onset and Duration of Withdrawal Symptoms by Agent in Children

	Symptom Onset	Duration
Alcohol	Hours	5-7 days
Alprazolam	24-48 hours	4-5 days
Diazepam	5-7 days	Weeks
Lorazepam	2-4 days	Weeks
Heroin/morphine	Hours	3-5 days
Methadone	1-2 days	5-7 days
Phenobarbital	7-10 days	3-5 days
GHB/GBL	Hours	3-5 days

GBL, γ-butyrolactone; GHB, γ-hydroxybutyric acid.

Table 183-2 Vital Signs and Mental Status Changes in Withdrawal

	Opioids	Sedative/Hypnotics	Alcohol
Heart rate	↑	↑↑	↑↑
Blood pressure	↑	↑↑	↑↑
Respiratory rate	↑	↑↑	↑↑
Hyperthermia	−	+	+
Altered mental status	−	+/−	+/−

Table 183-3 Nontoxic Differential Diagnosis of Sedative-Hypnotic Withdrawal

Hypoglycemia
Encephalitis
Hypomagnesemia
Meningitis
Neuroleptic malignant syndrome
Pneumonia
Serotonin syndrome
Thyrotoxicosis

Table 183-4 Poisoning Syndromes That May Mimic Withdrawal Syndromes

Amphetamines
Carbamates
Cocaine
Lithium
Organophosphates
Salicylates
Theophylline

Withdrawal from caffeine, inhalants, and SSRIs has been reported in neonates, and it is estimated that 20% to 30% of newborns exposed in the third trimester are affected. Symptoms include jitteriness, agitation, crying, shivering, increased muscle tone, breathing and sucking problems, and seizures.[8]

Neonatal opioid withdrawal (abstinence) syndrome is discussed in Chapter 56.

DIFFERENTIAL DIAGNOSIS

The withdrawal symptoms described have some distinguishing and overlapping features (see Table 183-2), and a number of nontoxic disorders may be mistaken for withdrawal (Table 183-3). In addition, certain toxic agents can mimic withdrawal symptoms. Organophosphate poisoning can result in constricted pupils, diaphoresis, vomiting, agitation, seizures, and altered mental status. A combination of these symptoms could easily be confused for either opioid or sedative-hypnotic withdrawal. Sympathomimetic intoxication can present in a manner similar to sedative-hypnotic withdrawal and create the same diagnostic dilemma. Additionally, a patient with anticholinergic toxicity may present with hallucinations, tachycardia, and hyperthermia. Other drugs that may mimic substance withdrawal in overdose are listed in Table 183-4.

Symptoms associated with SSRI withdrawal may be difficult to distinguish from features of the underlying anxiety or depressive disorder or side effects of the therapy, especially in patients with unreliable compliance in taking medication. When the timing of discontinuation of SSRI therapy is known, it is easier to distinguish withdrawal symptoms (usually within 1 week) from relapse of depression (more commonly after 2 or more weeks). Withdrawal symptoms are uncommon in patients who have been taking SSRIs for less than 7 weeks.[9]

TREATMENT

Ethanol and Sedative-Hypnotic

Mild to moderate ethanol or sedative-hypnotic withdrawal usually responds well to low-dose oral benzodiazepines. Current practice guidelines for the treatment of ethanol withdrawal recommend benzodiazepines as first-line therapy.[10] Benzodiazepines are also preferred to treat benzodiazepine withdrawal, and barbiturates are used for barbiturate withdrawal. Various treatment regimens exist and fixed-schedule treatments are common. However, studies demonstrate that "front-loading" benzodiazepines by giving diazepam in repeated doses on an hourly basis until the patient is asymptomatic relieves withdrawal symptoms more promptly than fixed-schedule treatment alone does.[11] Additionally, symptom-triggered therapy has been demon-

Table 183-5 Pharmacologic Therapy for Withdrawal

Drug Causing Withdrawal	Therapeutic Agent Used	Dose
Alcohol Sedative-hypnotic drugs Benzodiazepines	Diazepam	0.1 mg/kg IV q30min. Double dose every 3rd administration until sedate Once sedate, continue last dose administered q1h as needed for agitation. Taper dose by 10% daily
Barbiturates	Phenobarbital	Loading dose of 20 mg/kg IV, followed by maintenance dosing of 2-8 mg/kg/day Taper dose by 10% daily
Baclofen	Baclofen Benzodiazepine	Same dose and route used before withdrawal Administer high-dose benzodiazepine until baclofen can be administered
Caffeine	Children—caffeine Neonates—no treatment	Caffeine as a soft drink or tea taken to treat headache or agitation
Opioid—neonatal	Paregoric	0.1 mL/kg of a 0.4-mg/mL solution q4h with feeding Dose may be doubled to control symptoms. After 3-5 days, taper by decreasing the dose without altering the frequency of administration
	Tincture of opium	Diluted solution (1:25) at 0.1 mL/kg orally with feeding q4h. Dosing may be doubled to control symptoms. After 3-5 days, taper by decreasing the dose without altering the frequency of administration
	Methadone	0.05 to 0.1 mg/kg PO (max 20 mg) given q6h until symptoms are controlled Then dose daily, weaning dose to 0.05 mg/kg/day. Discontinue drug at that point and self-taper will occur
	Morphine	Orally administered to deliver the same morphine-equivalent dose as paregoric Dosing may be doubled to control symptoms. After 3-5 days, taper by decreasing the dose without altering the frequency of administration
Selective serotonin reuptake inhibitor (SSRI)		Children: Administer the same agent in the same dose used before withdrawal. Taper by 10% daily Neonates: No consensus on treatment of neonates. Diazepam may be used

strated to be superior to fixed-dose regimens. Patients who experience benzodiazepine or barbiturate withdrawal in the setting of chronic or intensive care may be treated by reinstituting the infusion or dosing of the drug that they were taking before withdrawal symptoms and then tapering the dose of the drug, typically by 10% daily.[12]

Baclofen withdrawal is unique because of the fact that cross-tolerance between baclofen and benzodiazepines or barbiturates is much less than that of other sedative-hypnotics. Baclofen withdrawal, which is more frequently severe and life threatening than benzodiazepine withdrawal, should be treated with the same dosing of baclofen used before withdrawal symptoms.[13] If baclofen cannot be administered immediately, such as in circumstances of a failed intrathecal pump, high-dose benzodiazepines should be used until baclofen can be administered.

Specific dosing recommendations are provided in Table 183-5.

Opioid

Heroin withdrawal (as well as withdrawal from other opioids) is best treated with an opioid of similar potency and equal or longer duration of action. Methadone is a preferred

treatment of withdrawal in children, adolescents, and adults. In neonates, a neonatal opiate solution containing an aqueous solution of morphine sulfate is often used (see Chapter 56). Patients who experience opioid withdrawal in the setting of chronic or intensive care may be treated by reinstituting the infusion or dosing of the drug that they were taking before withdrawal symptoms and then tapering the dose, typically by 10% daily. A number of oral opioid agents are available and can be dosed similarly by using morphine equivalents. Adolescents for whom an opioid-tapering plan is judged undesirable may be symptomatically supported through the withdrawal process; clonidine (oral or transcutaneous patch), which decreases sympathetic outflow, and antinausea drugs have proved useful in this regard.

Selective Serotonin Reuptake Inhibitor

Primary prevention of withdrawal symptoms can often be accomplished by slowly tapering the SSRI. Recommended strategies for managing withdrawal symptoms include reassurance, especially when the symptoms are mild. Patients may be relieved to understand that the symptoms are not related to relapse or reactions to coincident life events and that resolution is likely within days. If withdrawal symptoms are not well tolerated, reinitiation of therapeutic doses followed by a more slowly tapered dosing regimen may be appropriate. In some cases, substitution of a longer-acting SSRI (e.g., fluoxetine) may be needed to complete a slow discontinuation program.

ADMISSION CRITERIA

- Withdrawal symptoms in a neonate
- Initial presentation of withdrawal from a sedative-hypnotic agent, including benzodiazepines, baclofen, barbiturates, ethanol, GHB, or any similar drug
- Withdrawal associated with derangement of vital signs beyond acceptable limits that are not corrected with outpatient-congruent therapy, such as oral medication or patch treatment

DISCHARGE CRITERIA

- Stability of vital signs and neurologic symptoms that can be maintained with outpatient-congruent therapy, such as oral medication or patch treatment.

IN A NUTSHELL

- Withdrawal from substances that have γ-aminobutyric acid activity, including benzodiazepines, baclofen, barbiturates, alcohol, GHB, and similar drugs, can produce life-threatening withdrawal symptoms.
- Drugs with shorter half-lives produce withdrawal symptoms that tend to be more severe with onset sooner after discontinuation.
- Withdrawal from sedative-hypnotic drugs may progress rapidly from mild symptoms to severe or life-threatening withdrawal. Failure to estimate the potential severity of withdrawal because of initially mild symptoms could be catastrophic.
- Withdrawal from opioids should not result in alteration of cognition, although changes in mood and behavior typically occur.
- A number of drug overdose syndromes may cause poisoning that mimics sedative-hypnotic withdrawal.

ON THE HORIZON

- Ultrarapid detoxification techniques are being investigated to help addicts recover from drugs without suffering prolonged withdrawal symptoms. These treatments remain experimental.
- Investigation of biologic mechanisms and genetic markers is continuing, especially in the area of SSRI withdrawal.[14]

- The social impact of programs pertaining to legalization of narcotics, monitored drug provision sites, and other nonjudgmental addiction programs continues to be debated.

SUGGESTED READING

Cunliffe M, McArthur L, Dooley F: Managing sedation withdrawal in children who undergo prolonged PICU admission after discharge to the ward. Paediatr Anaesth 2004;4:293-298.

Hamilton RJ: Substance withdrawal. In Flomenbaum NE, Goldfrank LR, Hoffman RS, et al (eds): Goldfrank's Toxicologic Emergencies, 8th ed. New York, McGraw-Hill, 2006.

Kosten TR, O'Connor PG: Management of drug and alcohol withdrawal. N Engl J Med 2003;348:1786-1795.

REFERENCES

1. Glue P, Nutt D: Overexcitement and disinhibition. Dynamic neurotransmitter interactions in alcohol withdrawal. Br J Psychiatry 1990;157:491-499.
2. Dyer JE, Roth B, Hyma BA: Gamma-hydroxybutyrate withdrawal syndrome. Ann Emerg Med 2001;37:147-153.
3. Zajecka J, Tracey KA, Mitchell S: Discontinuation symptoms after treatment with serotonin reuptake inhibitors: A literature review. J Clin Psychiatry 1997;58:291-297.
4. Haddad P: The SSRI discontinuation syndrome. J Psychopharmacol 1998;12:305-313.
5. Sanz EJ, De-las-Cuevas C, Kiuru A, et al: Selective serotonin reuptake inhibitors in pregnant women and neonatal withdrawal syndrome: A database analysis. Lancet 2005;365:482-487.
6. Scott CS, Decker JL, Edwards ML, Freid EB: Withdrawal after narcotic therapy: A survey of neonatal and pediatric clinicians. Pharmacotherapy 1998;28:1308-1312.
7. Coles CD, Smith IE, Fernhoff PM, et al: Neonatal ethanol withdrawal: Characteristics in clinically normal, nondysmorphic neonates. J Pediatr 1984;105:445-451.
8. Nordeng H, Lindeman R, Perminov KV, Reikvam A: Neonatal withdrawal syndrome after in utero exposure to selective serotonin reuptake inhibitors. Acta Paediatr 2001;90:288-291.
9. Rosenbaum JF, Zajecka J: Clinical management of antidepressant discontinuation. J Clin Psychiatry 1997;58(Suppl 7):37-40.
10. Mayo-Smith MF: Pharmacological management of alcohol withdrawal. A meta-analysis and evidence-based practice guideline. American Society of Addiction Medicine Working Group on Pharmacological Management of Alcohol Withdrawal. JAMA 1997;278:144-151.
11. Manikant S, Tripathi BM, Chavan BS: Loading dose diazepam therapy for alcohol withdrawal state. Indian J Med Res 1993;98:170-173.
12. Tobias JD: Tolerance, withdrawal, and physical dependency after long-term sedation and analgesia of children in the pediatric intensive care unit. Crit Care Med 2000;28:2122-2132.
13. Coffey RJ, Edgar TS, Francisco GE, et al: Abrupt withdrawal from intrathecal baclofen: Recognition and management of a potentially life-threatening syndrome. Arch Phys Med Rehabil 2002;83:735-741.
14. Schatzberg AF, Haddad P, Kaplan EM, et al: Possible biological mechanisms of the serotonin reuptake inhibitor discontinuation syndrome. J Psychiatry 1997;58(Suppl 7):23-27.

CHAPTER 184

Fire-Related Inhalation Injury

Karen J. O'Connell and Paul E. Manicone

Fire-related injuries constitute a major health hazard to the children of the United States. In 2004, burn-related injuries were the fifth leading cause of accidental injury–related death in children 14 years and younger and accounted for approximately 10% of childhood deaths.[1,2] The injury to the skin can be just one facet of the potentially multisystem insults that occur. Smoke inhalation is the leading cause of death in house fires, with mortality rates of approximately 5% to 8%.[3] The focus of this chapter is inhalation injury associated with fires and incomplete combustion, specifically, thermal airway injuries, smoke inhalation, and carbon monoxide (CO) poisoning. Dermal burns are discussed in Chapter 146.

PATHOPHYSIOLOGY

Inhalation of superheated air can cause thermal injury to the airway, but injury is often limited to structures above the carina.[4] Swelling of these structures ensues in the hours following the injury and can result in critical upper airway obstruction.

A child who has a history of exposure to fire in an enclosed space is at risk for lower airway injury from inhaled toxicants. Even without skin burns, significant lower airway involvement can occur in a child who inhales toxic particles in smoke. The injury from smoke inhalation is a combination of systemic toxicity and direct pulmonary injury. A material's toxicity is dependent on its chemical composition, the dose inhaled, and the duration of exposure.[5] The high minute ventilation characteristic of children puts them at increased risk for toxic exposure as compared with adults.[5] Certain inhaled toxicants act as systemic asphyxiants, such as CO and cyanide. Others act as chemical irritants and cause direct mucosal injury, inflammation, edema, interference with surfactant production, and loss of normal protective ciliary action. The resultant ventilation-perfusion mismatch exacerbates hypoxemia.

CO is a colorless, odorless gas produced from the incomplete combustion of carbon-containing substances. Exposure to combustion or smoke in a closed or partially closed space puts the patient at high risk for CO poisoning. Other important sources of CO exposure include car exhaust fumes, furnaces, and wood-burning stoves. Epidemics tend to occur in winter months, especially during winter storms associated with power outages. Alternative methods of heating and cooking and snow-obstructed motor vehicle exhaust systems are more common under these conditions.[6-8]

CO is a tissue asphyxiant that disrupts hemoglobin's oxygen-carrying capacity and cellular metabolism. CO binds to hemoglobin with an affinity 200 to 300 times greater than that of oxygen. The resultant carboxyhemoglobin (COHb) shifts the oxyhemoglobin dissociation curve to the left, thereby resulting in impaired oxygen delivery at the tissue level. CO also affects cellular metabolism and oxidative energy production and can cause inflammatory vasculitis within the brain.

INITIAL ASSESSMENT AND STABILIZATION

The initial evaluation plus stabilization of a child with suspected airway or inhalation injury most often occurs in the field or in an emergency department. Basic principles of resuscitation with concentration on the overall physiologic state of the child should be applied. Evaluation and management of life-threatening injuries are the first priorities. Immediate decompensation usually results from hypoxemia, airway obstruction, and CO or cyanide poisoning.[9] In accordance with the "ABCs" (airway, breathing, circulation) of trauma resuscitation, airway patency and the risk for upper airway injury should be evaluated. All patients should receive maximum oxygenation with a 100% concentration of inspired oxygen and assisted ventilation when necessary. The airway should be protected and early intubation considered in burn patients with signs of upper airway involvement, significant smoke inhalation, or altered mental status. The cervical spine should be immobilized in all burn patients who have a history of a traumatic injury mechanism or if the mechanism is unknown. Hypotonic pharyngeal structures can obstruct the upper airway in unconscious patients, thus making a chin lift maneuver critical in the preservation of airway patency. After adequate control of the airway and ventilation, assessment of the circulation can proceed with appropriate interventions as needed.

After initial stabilization, further assessment should concentrate on identifying potential inhalational injury and CO poisoning.

CLINICAL PRESENTATION AND EVALUATION

Airway and Lung Injury

Symptoms of acute lung injury (cough, respiratory distress, tachypnea, wheezing, rales, rhonchi) may have developed by the time of patient presentation but are most often delayed up to 24 hours after the initial insult.[10,11] The peak in mucosal changes with sloughing and mucopurulent membrane production may be delayed up to 72 hours. Clinical findings on lung auscultation often precede abnormalities seen on chest radiograph, such as atelectasis, edema, or interstitial infiltrates, by 12 to 24 hours.[11]

Children who have suffered burns by flame or have a history of smoke inhalation or smoke exposure in a closed space are at increased risk for airway compromise. Even without the classic signs of facial burns, singed nasal or facial hairs, hoarseness, stridor, and carbonaceous sputum,

Table 184-1	Symptoms of Acute Carbon Monoxide Poisoning Based on Carboxyhemoglobin Levels*
COHb%	Symptoms
10	Asymptomatic or headache
20	Dizziness, nausea, dyspnea
30	Visual disturbances
40	Confusion, syncope
50	Seizures, coma
≥60	Cardiopulmonary dysfunction, death

*Note: COHb levels often do not closely correlate with symptoms, especially if there has been a delay in determining levels after exposure or if the patient has been pretreated with supplemental oxygen.
COHb%, carboxyhemoglobin percentage from CO-oximetry.
From Varon J, Marik PE, Fromm RE, Gueler A: Carbon monoxide poisoning: A review for clinicians. J Emerg Med 1999;17:87-93.

Table 184-2	Indications for Early Endotracheal Intubation
Signs of upper airway obstruction	
Altered level of consciousness associated with loss of cough or gag reflex	
Persistent hypoxia (PaO_2, 60 mm Hg on >60% inspired oxygen)	
Need for aggressive pulmonary toilet	

significant airway inflammation and edema can ensue. Mucosal injury threatens airway patency as a consequence of increased capillary permeability, tissue swelling, and plugging of distal airways with sloughed, injured tissue. Progressive upper airway edema and bronchospasm are often responsible for deterioration within the first 12 hours.[9] Vigilant airway surveillance is critical when monitoring for early mucosal edema. Serial observation by fiberoptic laryngoscopy and bronchoscopy can be used in an intensive care setting to assess the degree and extent of injury.

Carbon Monoxide Poisoning

Acute symptoms of CO toxicity range from headache, nausea, and ataxia in mild cases to severe neurologic impairment with loss of consciousness and seizures, pulmonary edema, respiratory failure, myocardial ischemia, and cardiac arrest.

Any child who underwent cardiopulmonary resuscitation at the scene or had loss of consciousness or an altered level of consciousness should be considered to have potentially significant CO exposure. In classic teaching, the lips and nail beds have a "cherry red" appearance, but unfortunately, these findings are uncommon.

Diagnosis of CO poisoning is made through the history and detection of COHb. CO-oximetry, a spectrophotometric laboratory test, can directly measure abnormal COHb saturation. Peak levels less than 20% are often associated with mild toxicity, and those above 60% are associated with coma and death (Table 184-1). However, the COHb level does not accurately correlate with the severity of poisoning, especially in children, and should not be used alone in the diagnosis of CO toxicity. Symptomatic patients receiving supplemental oxygen during prolonged transport to an emergency department may have nearly normal COHb levels on arrival. Arterial blood gas (ABG) measurement is not useful in the detection of CO toxicity, but it may be used to assess for metabolic acidosis. The partial pressure of oxygen (PaO_2) measured on ABG analysis is a measurement of the amount of oxygen dissolved in blood (not bound to hemoglobin). Because CO does not affect the amount of dissolved oxygen, PaO_2 may be normal in patients with CO poisoning. Because PaO_2 is normal, the calculated oxygen saturation level on ABG analysis (SaO_2) will also be "normal," even in the setting of substantial CO toxicity. Pulse oximetry also fails to detect CO poisoning and does not accurately measure oxygen saturation (SpO_2) in this condition. Pulse oximetry uses only two wavelengths of light to determine hemoglobin saturation and divides the molecules into oxyhemoglobin and deoxyhemoglobin. COHb is misread as oxyhemoglobin, thus giving a CO-poisoned patient a falsely elevated and often normal reading of oxygen saturation.

TREATMENT

Airway and Lung Injury

Any signs of airway compromise indicate the need for direct laryngoscopy and should prompt the medical provider to consider early, elective endotracheal intubation to avoid a potential critical airway. Indications for early endotracheal intubation and mechanical ventilation are provided in Table 184-2. In the setting of acute mucosal inflammation, intubation with smaller endotracheal tubes than expected for age may be necessary. Cuffed endotracheal tubes provide better cushioning and control in the effort to prevent pressure necrosis.

Treatment of smoke inhalation and parenchymal lung damage focuses on supportive care to maximize respiratory function. All patients should initially receive the maximum concentration of inspired oxygen. Weaning of the oxygen concentration should begin only after there is confirmation of a normal COHb level (by CO-oximetry) and correction of ventilation-perfusion mismatch. Oxygen saturation and serial ABG measurement can help guide treatment options. ABG analysis is a valuable tool for monitoring acid-base status (pH), oxygenation (as measured by the arterial partial pressure of dissolved oxygen [PaO_2] and the calculated arterial saturation level [SaO_2]), ventilation (measured by the arterial partial pressure of dissolved carbon dioxide [PaCO_2]), and gas exchange at the alveolar level (assessed by the alveolar-arterial gradient).

In the setting of pulmonary edema from increased capillary leak, delivery of peak end-expiratory pressure support by endotracheal tube will maintain small-airway patency and improve oxygenation. Because airway obstruction is usually mechanical, adequate humidification and pulmonary toilet are the mainstays of supportive care. Particulate matter may cause hypersensitivity and bronchoconstriction, especially in children with a previous reactive airway history. Bronchodilators such as nebulized albuterol may help alleviate lower airway obstruction. The use of steroids and prophylactic antibiotics is not indicated in the setting of acute lung injury from smoke inhalation. Corticosteroids have been associated with a significant increase in the risk for death and infectious complications and should not be used in the treatment of burn patients.[3,12] Antibiotic use should be reserved for clinical signs of infectious pneumonia, which rarely occur during the first 24 hours.[3] Prophylactic antibiotics may select for more resistant organisms and are not recommended.[3] The use of certain exogenous surfactants has been shown to effectively restore endogenous surfactant function after inhalational injury by wood smoke.[13,14]

Carbon Monoxide Poisoning

Patients suspected of suffering CO poisoning should have 100% oxygen therapy initiated with the intention of decreasing the blood half-life of COHb. Delivery of 100% inspired oxygen should be continued until COHb has fallen below 5%, and some clinicians prefer to continue oxygen therapy for several hours longer. The half-life of COHb is decreased from approximately 4 to 6 hours in patients breathing room air at sea level (normobaric, 1 atm) to 60 to 90 minutes with 100% inspired oxygen. Treatment with 100% oxygen at hyperbaric treatment pressures (usually 3 atm) increases the oxygen concentration in blood and further shortens the half-life of COHb to 20 to 30 minutes. By increasing the competition for hemoglobin binding sites, elimination of CO occurs more quickly.[15] Patients with significant CO poisoning are at risk for delayed neurologic sequelae, including cognitive and memory difficulties, personality changes, peripheral neuropathies, and neurologic deficits. The role of hyperbaric oxygen (HBO) therapy in the prevention of delayed neurologic sequelae is still unclear, and its use in the acute management of CO poisoning is controversial. HBO therapy can inhibit the leukocyte adherence that initiates the cerebral vasculitis from severe CO poisoning. However, several randomized controlled trials in adults have failed to establish whether HBO therapy in patients with acute CO poisoning reduces the incidence of adverse neurologic sequelae.[16,17] Some patients with moderate to severe CO poisoning may benefit from HBO therapy, and this decision should be made individually based on the history, clinical presentation, and degree of neurologic impairment. Certain criteria that have been used include any history of loss of consciousness, focal or persistent neurologic symptoms, ischemic changes on electrocardiography, pregnant patients with COHb levels higher than 15%, and significantly elevated COHb levels (>25%).[18,19] Measured COHb levels do not correlate with the severity of CO poisoning and should not be used alone when deciding on appropriate therapy. HBO therapy can be safely administered to patients who are hemodynamically stable and those without pulmonary air trapping.

Concurrent poisoning with hydrogen cyanide has been reported and should be considered in patients who are victims of a closed-space fire. Cyanide toxicity should be suspected in those who have altered levels of consciousness and persistent or worsening lactic acidosis (blood lactate level >10 mmol/L) not responsive to maximal oxygenation and fluid resuscitation. A cyanide antidote kit is available and consists of three components. The first steps of the kit, amyl nitrite and sodium nitrite, induce methemoglobinemia, which reduces oxygen delivery to tissues, and should not be

given. The third step of the kit involves using sodium thiosulfate to safely scavenge cyanide. The intravenous dose of sodium thiosulfate is 12.5 g for adults and 1.65 mL/kg of 25% sodium thiosulfate for children.

CONSULTATION

- Critical care: For patients with a severe cardiopulmonary insult or instability
- Otolaryngology/pulmonology: For patients with evidence of airway injury
- Toxicology: For patients with significant CO poisoning or exposure to other inhaled toxins

ADMISSION CRITERIA

Hospitalization is indicated for patients with

- Hemodynamic instability (intensive care setting)
- The need or potential need for endotracheal intubation and mechanical ventilation (consider the intensive care setting)
- Evidence of airway compromise that has yet to demonstrate steady improvement
- High risk for airway injury despite being asymptomatic during the initial period of observation (e.g., signs of airway erythema or edema, prolonged or severe exposure to smoke, other victims with similar exposure who have demonstrated clinical deterioration)
- Evidence of significant CO poisoning, especially if symptoms persist after normalization of COHb levels
- Need or potential need for HBO therapy

DISCHARGE CRITERIA

- Stabilization of all airway and pulmonary issues
- Normalization of COHb levels, including rebound levels
- Resolution of all toxin-associated symptoms

IN A NUTSHELL

- Immediate decompensation usually results from hypoxemia, asphyxia, and airway obstruction in patients with airway burns and smoke inhalation.
- Exposure to smoke in a closed space puts the patient at high risk for CO and cyanide poisoning.
- CO poisoning is not detected by pulse oximetry or by the pressure of oxygen (PaO_2) from ABG analysis. These tests can give falsely normal readings in the setting of significant CO poisoning.
- CO-oximetry can measure the CO bound to hemoglobin, although delays in obtaining the specimen and pretreatment with oxygen may result in levels that have diminished since the time of exposure.
- Treatment of CO poisoning is 100% oxygen therapy, which decreases the blood half-life of the CO bound to hemoglobin (COHb). The administration of 100% oxygen at hyperbaric treatment pressures further shortens the half-life of COHb. It remains unclear whether this therapy diminishes the risk for delayed neurologic sequelae.

ON THE HORIZON

• Investigations continue in the development of exogenous surfactants for the acute management of inhalational injury. Further studies will help define the role of HBO therapy in the prevention of delayed neurologic sequelae in the pediatric population.
• Hydroxocobalamin is being investigated as an antidote for cyanide poisoning due to smoke inhalation.

SUGGESTED READING

Assessment and management: Burn service manual. In Eichelberger M, et al (eds): Trauma Resource Manual. Washington, DC, Children's National Medical Center.
Martin JD, Osterhoudt KC, Thom SR: Recognition and management of carbon monoxide poisoning in children. Clin Pediatr Emerg Med 2000;1:244-250.
McCall JE, Cahill TJ: Respiratory care of the burn patient. J Burn Care Rehabil 2005;26:200-206.
Reed JL, Pomerantz WJ: Emergency management of pediatric burns. Pediatr Emerg Care 2005;21:118-129.
Varon J, Marik PE, Fromm RE, Gueler A: Carbon monoxide poisoning: A review for clinicians. J Emerg Med 1999;17:87-93.

REFERENCES

1. Burn incidence and treatment in the US: 2005 Fact Sheet. American Burn Association, 2005. Available at *www.ameriburn.org*.
2. Facts about childhood burns. Safe Kids Worldwide Fact Sheet, 2005. Available at *www.safekids.org*.
3. Miller K, Chang A: Acute inhalation injury. Emerg Med Clin North Am 2003;21:533-557.
4. Pruitt BA, Flemma RJ, DiVincenti FC, et al: Pulmonary complications in burn patients. A comparative study of 697 patients. J Thorac Cardiovasc Surg 1970;59:7-20.
5. Ciorciari AJ: Environmental emergencies. In Crain EF, Gershel JC (eds): Clinical Manual of Emergency Pediatrics, 3rd ed. New York, McGraw-Hill, 1997, pp 163-189.
6. From the Centers for Disease Control and Prevention: Deaths from motor-vehicle–related unintentional carbon monoxide poisoning—Colorado, 1996, New Mexico, 1980-1995, and United States, 1979-1992. JAMA 1996;276:1942-1943.
7. Geehr EC, Saluzzo R, Bosco S, et al: Emergency health impact of a severe storm. Am J Emerg Med 1989;7:598-604.
8. Varon J, Marik PE, Fromm RE, Gueler A: Carbon monoxide poisoning: A review for clinicians. J Emerg Med 1999;17:87-93.
9. Carvajal HF, Griffith JA: Burn and inhalation injuries. In Fuhrman BP, Zimmerman JJ (eds): Pediatric Critical Care, 3rd ed. Philadelphia, CV Mosby, 2006, pp 1565-1576.
10. Duffy BJ, McLaughlin PM, Eichelberger MR: Assessment, triage, and early management of burns in children. Clin Pediatr Emerg Med 2006;7:82-93.
11. Joffe MD: Burns. In Fleisher GR, Ludwig S, Henretig FM (eds): Textbook of Pediatric Emergency Medicine. Philadelphia, Lippincott Williams & Wilkins, 2005, pp 1517-1524.
12. Rabinowitz PM, Siegel MD: Acute inhalation injury. Clin Chest Med 2002;23:707-715.
13. Jeng M, Kou YR, Sheu C, Hwang B: Effects of exogenous surfactant supplementation and partial liquid ventilation on acute lung injury induced by wood smoke inhalation in newborn piglets. Crit Care Med 2003;31:1166-1174.
14. Nieman GF, Paskanik AM, Fluck RR, Clark WR: Comparison of exogenous surfactants in the treatment of wood smoke inhalation. Am J Respir Crit Care Med 1995;152:597-602.
15. Martin JD, Osterhoudt KC, Thom SR: Recognition and management of carbon monoxide poisoning in children. Clin Pediatr Emerg Med 2000;1:244-250.
16. Judge BS, Brown MD: To dive or not to dive? Use of hyperbaric oxygen therapy to prevent neurologic sequelae in patients acutely poisoned with carbon monoxide. Ann Emerg Med 2005;46:462-466.
17. Juurlink DN, Buckley NA, Stanbrook MB, et al: Hyperbaric oxygen for carbon monoxide poisoning. Cochrane Database Syst Rev 2005;1:CD002041.
18. Kao LW, Nanagas KA: Carbon monoxide poisoning. Med Clin North Am 2005;89:1161-1194.
19. Wratney AT, Cheifetz IM: Gases and drugs used in support of the respiratory system. In Slonim AD, Pollack MM (eds): Pediatric Critical Care Medicine. Philadelphia, Lippincott Williams & Wilkins, 2006, pp 717-729.

CHAPTER 185

Heat Disorders

Lise E. Nigrovic and Michele Burns Ewald

Heat disorders such as heat exhaustion and heatstroke result from a failure of the body's regulatory mechanisms to maintain a constant body temperature. Individuals at the extremes of age and those with chronic diseases are the most vulnerable. Approximately 400 people die annually in the United States from heat-related illness.[1] In distinction to hyperthermia, fever is an elevation in body temperature secondary to mediators of inflammation and involves an adjustment in the physiologic setpoint (see Chapter 33). Malignant hyperthermia, another thermoregulatory disorder, results from a triggering exposure in a genetically susceptible individual.

Heat disorders occur most commonly in the summer months or in tropical regions. Although elderly patients are most severely affected, healthy children are also susceptible. Young children have suboptimally developed thermoregulatory controls and are dependent on others to provide them with fluids and to keep them from unsafe environments. Four percent of the heat-related deaths in the United States occur in children younger than 14 years.[1] Comorbid conditions such as obesity, physical disabilities that limit rapid egress from a warm environment, or cystic fibrosis increase a child's susceptibility to heat stress.

PHYSIOLOGY

The human body maintains a relatively constant body temperature despite wide swings in environmental temperature. Heat is acquired both endogenously (from basal metabolism, muscle activity, hormonal effects, and sympathetic stimulation) and exogenously (when environmental temperature exceeds body temperature). Heat is lost to the environment by radiation (up to 60% of losses), evaporation of sweat (22% to 25%), conduction (3%), and convection (12% to 15%).

The hypothalamus, the body's primary thermoregulator, maintains the core body temperature within a narrow range. Increases in body temperature result in sympathetically mediated peripheral blood vessel dilation (increased radiation losses), increased sweat gland activity (higher evaporative losses), and reduced endogenous heat production. Hyperthermia occurs when the body cannot adequately dissipate excess exogenous or endogenous heat.

Malignant hyperthermia is a group of genetic myopathies associated with a defect in the calcium channels of skeletal muscles.[2] Most patients are asymptomatic until exposed to the triggering agent. A muscle biopsy is needed to confirm the diagnosis. Implicated triggers include medications such as inhaled anesthetics and neuromuscular blockers, as well as physical stressors (Table 185-1).

CLINICAL PRESENTATION

Table 185-2 describes the symptoms, clinical and laboratory findings, treatment, and prognosis of the three major types of heat-related illnesses: heat cramps, heat exhaustion, and heatstroke.

Heat Cramps

Heat cramps are painful muscle spasms that typically occur several hours after vigorous exertion. They are thought to be due to repletion of water without adequate salt intake. The voluntary muscles of the calves, thighs, and shoulders are most commonly affected. Symptoms typically last only a few minutes but may recur. The affected muscles feel hard to palpation. Laboratory abnormalities include hyponatremia with very low or undetectable urine sodium.

Heat Exhaustion

Heat exhaustion occurs secondary to water or salt depletion, or both. Affected patients experience systemic complaints, including fatigue, weakness, nausea, vomiting, diarrhea, and headache. Irritability may be a prominent sign in infants and nonverbal children. The core temperature is mildly elevated (<39°C), and the patient often experiences tachycardia, orthostatic hypotension, profuse sweating, and flushed skin. Laboratory abnormalities include hyponatremia or hypernatremia and hemo- and urinary concentration.

Heatstroke

Without adequate recognition and initiation of effective therapies, heat exhaustion can progress to life-threatening heatstroke. Classic heatstroke, also referred to as nonexertional heatstroke, typically occurs in children with predisposing factors that put them at increased risk. These factors include children's limited ability to increase their fluid intake (e.g., young infancy, nonverbal status), remove themselves from a hot environment (e.g., immobility), or dissipate heat (e.g., overdressing, obesity, underlying medical condition). Exertional heatstroke usually occurs in otherwise healthy individuals who participate in vigorous activities when it is hot and humid, often with inadequate efforts to maintain hydration.

Patients present with a significantly elevated core body temperature (>40°C) associated with central nervous system dysfunction. Anhidrosis is frequently but not universally observed. Neurologic symptoms include progressive lethargy, confusion, headache, delirium, seizures, and coma. On physical examination, patients are tachycardic, hypotensive, and tachypneic (hyperventilation causes a respiratory alkalosis). Laboratory abnormalities include hyponatremia or hypernatremia, hypokalemia, hemo- and urinary concentration, acute renal failure, and elevated liver function tests.

The extent and severity of the central effects depend on the extent of the hyperpyrexia. Rhabdomyolysis may occur as a result of thermal injury to myocytes. Circulating myoglobin as well as thermal and ischemic insults can result in acute renal compromise.

Malignant Hyperthermia

When a susceptible individual is exposed to a triggering agent, the uncontrolled influx of calcium into the muscle cell results in muscle contraction, accelerated metabolism, and resultant hyperthermia. Initially, end-tidal carbon dioxide increases and arterial oxygen decreases, with muscle rigidity and a rapid rise in body temperature.[2,3]

Laboratory evaluation reveals acidosis as well as hyperkalemia, hyperphosphatemia, hypocalcemia, and myoglobinuria from muscle breakdown. Although serum creatinine

starts to rise almost immediately due to the rhabdomyolysis, peak levels are not seen until several days after the exposure.

DIFFERENTIAL DIAGNOSIS

Other causes of myositis or tonic muscle contractions can present with features similar to heat cramps, including viral or drug-induced myositis and electrolyte imbalances leading to tetany. Increased body temperature can occur secondary to a wide range of causes (Table 185-3). Encephalitis or other causes of encephalopathy, especially when accompanied by fever, can mimic heatstroke.

Many drug-induced hyperthermia syndromes exist. These include the serotonin syndrome, neuroleptic malignant

Table 185-1 Drugs That Can Cause Malignant Hyperthermia

Type of Agent	Causative Drugs
Inhalation anesthetic	Halothane Isoflurane Enflurane Desflurane Sevoflurane
Depolarizing muscle relaxant	Succinylcholine
Other	Phenothiazines

Table 185-3 Causes of Hyperthermia

Sepsis
Central nervous system infection
Environmental exposure
Tetanus
Typhoid fever
Thyroid storm
Pheochromocytoma
Catatonia
Hypothalamic stroke
Status epilepticus
Cerebral hemorrhage
Dystonic reaction

Adapted from Lanken PN, Manaker S, Hanson CW III (eds): The Intensive Care Unit Manual. Philadelphia, Saunders (in press).

Table 185-2 Descriptions of Heat Illnesses

	Heat Cramps	Heat Exhaustion	Heatstroke
Core body temperature	Normal	Elevated (≤39°C)	Very elevated (≥40°C)
Symptoms	Painful muscle spasms	Weakness Thirst Headache Nausea, vomiting Diarrhea	Confusion Delirium Seizures Coma
Physical examination	Hard knot in muscle belly	Tachycardia Orthostatic hypotension Diffuse sweating	Tachycardia Circulatory collapse Anhidrosis Central nervous system dysfunction
Laboratory studies	Hyponatremia Low urine sodium	Hypo- or hypernatremia Hemoconcentration Urinary concentration	Hypo- or hypernatremia Hemoconcentration Acute renal failure Rhabdomyolysis
Therapy	Oral rehydration Electrolyte solutions	Passive cooling IV rehydration	Active cooling Cardiorespiratory support (dobutamine)
Prognosis	Excellent	Excellent	High mortality

Table 185-4   Laboratory Studies for the Evaluation of Heat Disorders

Study	Common Abnormalities
Complete blood count	Leukocytosis, hemoconcentration, and, if DIC is present, thrombocytopenia
Serum electrolytes: sodium, potassium, chloride, bicarbonate, calcium, phosphate, magnesium	Variable derangements indicative of dehydration
Blood urea nitrogen, serum creatinine	Elevations consistent with dehydration or renal injury
Hepatic enzymes	Elevated if there is hepatic injury
Creatine kinase	Elevated with rhabdomyolysis
PT, INR, PTT, D dimer	Elevated with DIC
Urinalysis	Elevated specific gravity, proteinuria, ketonuria, dipstick-positive for blood without red blood cells on microscopic examination

DIC, disseminated intravascular coagulation; INR, international normalized ratio; PT, prothrombin time; PTT, partial thromboplastin time.

syndrome, acute drug withdrawal, and poisoning with sympathomimetic drugs, salicylates, lithium, or anticholinergics.

DIAGNOSIS AND EVALUATION

Obtaining a history that identifies heat exposure, inadequate hydration, and predisposing factors for problems with heat dissipation is key for the diagnosis of heat-related disorders. The physical examination should focus on identifying the signs of heat illness, the severity of the condition, and any underlying conditions. Laboratory assessments that may aid in the evaluation are listed in Table 185-4, along with typical derangements. Depending on the other diagnostic concerns, additional studies such as imaging of the head; urine toxicology screen; cultures of blood, urine, or cerebrospinal fluid; and chest radiograph may be indicated.

TREATMENT

Heatstroke victims should have careful cardiovascular monitoring. Airway protection may be required to prevent aspiration. Patients with elevated core body temperatures should be aggressively cooled. Core body temperature should always be checked with a rectal or esophageal thermometer and monitored frequently. Active cooling should be initiated to bring core body temperature down to 38.5°C to 39.0°C.[4] Victims should be first removed from the hot environment and their clothing removed. Rapid cooling can begin either by emersion in cold water with ice or by evaporative cooling. Gastric or peritoneal lavage can be considered as a supplemental cooling method in severe cases. Cooled intravenous fluids are not used because of the risk of an arrhythmia with an already stressed myocardium. Benzodiazepines may be useful to help control shivering.

Fluid and electrolyte replacement is extremely important in the effective therapy of heat illnesses. Heat cramps can be effectively treated with rest as well as oral salt and water replacement. Heat exhaustion requires intravenous rehydration with unrestricted dietary sodium. Electrolyte imbalances should be corrected slowly over 12 to 24 hours. Heatstroke victims require aggressive fluid resuscitation to maintain central perfusion. If urine output cannot be maintained at greater than 1 mL/kg per hour by aggressive fluid repletion, the addition of diuretics (e.g., furosemide, mannitol) should be considered.[4]

Hypotension refractory to intravenous fluids warrants vasopressor therapy. Dobutamine (5 to 20 µg/kg per minute), a β_1-adrenergic agent, should be selected because it increases cardiac contractility, thus raising blood pressure, and the peripheral vasodilation allows ongoing heat loss. Agents with α-adrenergic activity, such as dopamine, epinephrine, and norepinephrine, should be avoided because the resulting peripheral vasoconstriction minimizes heat dissipation. Isoproterenol, a β-adrenergic agent, may increase myocardial oxygen consumption beyond oxygen delivery capacity.

The initial management of malignant hyperthermia involves discontinuing the offending agent. Hyperventilation with 100% oxygen and volume replacement should begin immediately. As soon as the diagnosis of malignant hyperthermia has been made, dantrolene should be given (2.5 mg/kg body weight up to every 5 minutes until muscle relaxation is achieved; only rarely is a total dose of 10 mg/kg needed to control rigidity and tachycardia).[5] Dantrolene causes muscle relaxation directly by blocking the release of calcium from the sarcoplasmic reticulum. Each 20-mg vial of dantrolene contains 3 g of mannitol, which should be taken into account if further diuretic therapy is being considered. External cooling measures should be initiated to treat hyperthermia. Benzodiazepines or paralysis should be considered for patients with persistent shivering. Cardiac arrhythmias resulting from malignant hyperthermia should be treated with procainamide and calcium chloride.

Rhabdomyolysis may develop as a complication of heatstroke or malignant hyperthermia. Creatine kinase levels typically peak several days after the heat or drug exposure. Monitoring for electrolyte imbalances and renal injury (evidenced by urine myoglobin) is required. Ample hydration should be maintained, and some experts recommend alkalization (target urine pH >6.5).

Disseminated intravascular coagulation, seizure, renal failure, hepatic dysfunction, and acute respiratory distress syndrome can complicate heatstroke and should be managed appropriately, often in an intensive care setting.

CONSULTATION

Involvement of critical care specialists is indicated for patients who require or are anticipated to need intensive care support. Nephrologists may be helpful for patients at risk for or with evidence of renal injury, especially those with severe rhabdomyolysis.

Emergency consultation for a patient thought to have malignant hyperthermia can be obtained by calling the emergency hotline (800-MH-HYPER or 800-644-9737) or reviewing the website (*www.mhaus.org/hotline.html*).

ADMISSION CRITERIA

The majority of otherwise healthy patients with heat cramps and heat exhaustion can be treated with cooling and rehydration in the office or emergency room setting without hospital admission. Patients with heatstroke or other evidence of end-organ injury (e.g., rhabdomyolysis), drug-induced hyperthermia syndromes, coexisting chronic medical conditions, or malignant hyperthermia generally warrant inpatient stabilization.

DISCHARGE CRITERIA

- Hemodynamic stability.
- Return to baseline mental status.
- Ability to maintain adequate hydration.
- Resolution of rhabdomyolysis with decreasing levels of creatine kinase and clearance of myoglobinuria.

PREVENTION

Avoidance of situations that put patients at risk for heat illness is the most important preventive measure. The National Weather Service and the Centers for Disease Control and Prevention issue heat advisories through local broadcasting systems that can alert individuals and communities to dangerous conditions. Prevention tips are provided in Table 185-5.

Early recognition of malignant hyperthermia and prevention of exposure to triggering agents are the most effective therapies for this life-threatening condition. Preoperative assessments should include careful questioning about reactions to anesthesia in the patient or family members. To prevent recurrences, patients should carry malignant hyperthermia medical identification bands at all times.

IN A NUTSHELL

- Heat-related conditions are usually a result of heat exposure and inadequate hydration.
- Heat cramps typically involve the calves, thighs, and shoulders and are usually managed with rest and hydration.
- Features of heat exhaustion include weakness, irritability, vomiting, diarrhea, diaphoresis, elevated body temperature, and orthostasis.
- Heatstroke is a life-threatening condition that presents with a significant elevation in core body temperature, changes in mental status, and often cardiovascular instability. Sweating may be absent.
- Malignant hyperthermia represents a group of genetic myopathies that result in muscle rigidity and severe elevations in core body temperature upon exposure to triggers (e.g., anesthetic agents).
- Rapid cooling and appropriate management of fluid and electrolyte derangements are the mainstays of therapy for heat disorders.
- Dantrolene is used in the treatment of malignant hyperthermia.

ON THE HORIZON

- New treatments are being studied to improve the outcome in heatstroke, including the use of glutamine[6] and dantrolene.[7] Optimal hydration regimens for the prevention of heatstroke are also being explored for individuals involved in prolonged endurance activities.[8]

Table 185-5 Recommendations for the Prevention of Heat Illness

Drink plenty of nonalcoholic fluids
Replace salts and minerals (e.g., salt-containing foods, sports drinks)
Dress in lightweight, light-colored, loosely fitted clothing
Avoid or limit sun exposure
Avoid outdoor activity, especially during midday and afternoon
Seek out air-conditioned environments (e.g., shopping mall, public library, heat-relief shelter)
Check on individuals at increased risk for heat injury

Adapted from the Centers for Disease Control and Prevention website: Extreme Heat: A Prevention Guide to Promote Your Personal Health and Safety.

SUGGESTED READING

Denborough M: Malignant hyperthermia. Lancet 1998;352:1131-1136.

Halloran LL, Bernard DW: Management of drug-induced hyperthermia. Curr Opin Pediatr 2004;16:211-215.

Hoffman JL: Heat-related illness in children. Clin Pediatr Emerg Med 2001; 2:203-210.

Lugo-Amador NM, Rothenhaus T, Moyer P: Heat-related illness. Emerg Med Clin North Am 2004;22:315-327.

REFERENCES

1. Hoffman JL: Heat-related illness in children. Clin Pediatr Emerg Med 2001;2:203-210.
2. Denborough M: Malignant hyperthermia. Lancet 1998;352:1131-1136.
3. Litman RS, Rosenberg H: Malignant hyperthermia: Update on susceptibility testing. JAMA 2005;293:2918-2924.
4. Lugo-Amador NM, Rothenhaus T, Moyer P: Heat-related illness. Emerg Med Clin North Am 2004;22:315-327.

5. Halloran LL, Bernard DW: Management of drug-induced hyperthermia. Curr Opin Pediatr 2004;16:211-215.

6. Singleton KD, Wischmeyer PE: Oral glutamine enhances heat shock protein expression and improves survival following hyperthermia. Shock 2006;25:295-299.

7. Hadad E, Cohen-Sivan Y, Heled Y, Epstein Y: Clinical review: Treatment of heat stroke: Should dantrolene be considered? Crit Care 2005;9:86-91.

8. Von Duvillard SP, Braun WA, Markofski M, et al: Fluids and hydration in prolonged endurance performance. Nutrition 2004;20:651-656.

CHAPTER 186

Hypothermia and Cold-Related Injuries

Jeffrey P. Louie

Hypothermia should be a preventable disease, yet in 2001, 599 people died of cold exposure in the United States.[1] The majority of reported mortality cases involve victims older than 19 years, and two thirds of all victims are male. Predisposing factors that increase the risk for hypothermia are listed in Table 186-1.

Maintaining the body's core temperature is essential for human life. It is dependent on basal metabolism and physical activity. The human body can lose heat by four mechanisms: (1) radiation, or transfer of heat through infrared energy, accounts for 55% to 65% of heat loss; (2) evaporation, which includes respiration, accounts for 20% to 30% of heat energy loss; (3) convection, or transfer of heat by the movement of air currents; and (4) conduction, or heat loss through direct contact with another object. When conduction and convection are combined, heat loss may be as high as 10% to 15%, which is why removing cold and wet clothes is essential in the initial management of these patients.

Hypothermic patients are traditionally classified into three categories according to core temperature: mild (32° C to 35° C), moderate (30° C to 31.9° C), and severe (less than 30° C). The lower the core temperature, the more organ systems involved and the greater the potential for morbidity and mortality.

Another form of morbidity that is not solely related to hypothermia is frostbite. Frostbite represents a continuum from tissue injury to irreversible tissue damage. Two mechanisms are responsible.[2] The first is cellular death at the time of cold exposure and involves ice crystal formation in the extracellular space, which induces an osmotic shift; the end result is intracellular dehydration and cell death. As the tissue is continually exposed to cooler temperatures, intracellular ice crystals are formed and cause more cellular destruction. The body's response to this localized trauma is to alternate vasoconstriction and vasodilation. As a whole, this thawing and refreezing causes most of the cellular damage. The second mechanism of injury is very similar to thermal burns and is a result of prolonged, progressive dermal ischemia. Once the exposure occurs, inflammatory mediators are produced: thromboxanes, prostaglandins, histamine, and bradykinins. These mediators promote edema, which results in the formation of blisters.

CLINICAL PRESENTATION

The signs and symptoms of a hypothermic patient are inherently associated with the person's core temperature. Table 186-2 outlines the core temperatures associated with clinical findings.

Central Nervous System

Hypothermia results in decreased metabolism and blood flow to the brain. Brain function, thought processes, and motor skills decline as the body's core temperature drops below 35° C. Fine motor skills decline, which leads to frank clumsiness. Dysarthria and ataxia follow. As the hypothermia worsens, a phenomenon known as "paradoxical undressing" may occur whereby the victims undress themselves. It is thought that this phenomenon signifies impending thermoregulatory collapse. By 32° C, confusion and drowsiness become evident. Below 32° C, the person becomes unconscious.

Cardiovascular System

The early cardiovascular response to hypothermia is tachycardia. However, as the body cools below 35° C, the heart rate slows and cardiac output decreases. Hypotension may occur secondary to decreased cardiac output, cardiac contractility, and intravascular volume. Electrocardiographic findings are nonspecific and include prolongation of the PR, QRS, and QTc intervals, as well as ST-segment and T-wave changes. As the core temperature drops to 32° C, roughly 30% of hypothermic victims will demonstrate the J wave, or Osborn wave, on electrocardiograms.[3] The Osborn wave is an upward deflection after the QRS complex (Fig. 186-1). There are no arrhythmias specific to hypothermia, but atrial and ventricular fibrillation has been documented.

Respiratory System

Tachypnea is initially seen in mild hypothermia, but as the core temperature continues to decline, hypopnea will follow. Hypoxia and hypercapnia ensue and produce both metabolic and respiratory acidosis. Ciliary function ceases as hypothermia intensifies, thus predisposing the victim to pneumonia.

Muscular and Peripheral Vascular System

Shivering produces heat as a means to maintain core temperature. This mechanism of heat production stops when the core temperature drops below 32° C. Cessation of shivering signifies the body's inability to combat hypothermia.

Arteriolar vasoconstriction decreases blood flow to the skin. A slight increase in blood pressure may be noted. However, as the body's temperature drops, blood pressure also declines as a result of loss of sympathetic tone. Conversely, intense peripheral vasoconstriction leads to pallor. Facial puffiness may ensue secondary to increased capillary permeability with subcutaneous edema.

Table 186-1   Risk Factors Predisposing to Hypothermia

General conditions
  Malnutrition
  Hypothyroidism
  Hypoglycemia

Immobility
  Extreme ages: neonates and geriatrics
  Intoxications/ingestions
  Trauma
  Neuromuscular disorders

Infection   Sepsis

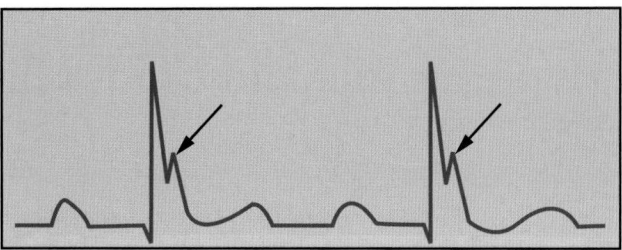

Figure 186-1   Example of a J or Osborn waves (*arrows*) from an individual with a core temperature below 32° C.

Table 186-2 Core Temperature Associated with Clinical Findings	
35° C	Confusion, dysarthria, shivering, cold diuresis
34° C	Impaired judgment
33° C	Apathy
32° C	Decreased level of consciousness, hallucinations, appearance of J wave
31° C	Stupor, loss of shivering
30° C	Onset of arrhythmias
28° C	Coma, loss of reflexes, decreases in blood pressure and heart rate
24° C	Apnea and asystole
19° C	Flat electroencephalogram

Skin

Blisters may be found with any prolonged, cold exposure. They are typically superficial or deep dermal injuries. Superficial injuries portend a good prognosis and on examination include normal-colored skin and blisters filled with clear fluid. In addition, the skin will have the ability to deform with palpation. The physical findings after deep dermal injury suggest long-term morbidity and include dark, hemorrhagic blisters, and hard, non-deforming skin on palpation.[2]

Frostbite is classified into four categories—first to fourth degree—based on severity. First-degree frostbite is characterized by an anesthetic central white area with peripheral erythema. Second-degree injury represents blisters filled with either clear or milky fluid, surrounded by erythema or edema, and appears in the first 24 hours. Third-degree frostbite is associated with hemorrhagic blisters that progress over a course of 2 to 4 weeks, with the end result being a thick, black eschar. Fourth-degree frostbite produces complete tissue necrosis and autoamputation.

Renal System

Peripheral vasoconstriction increases blood flow to the kidneys, which induces diuresis. In addition, there is a decrease in circulating antidiuretic hormone. These two factors, along with insensible water loss (sweating and respiration) and tissue third spacing, lead to a decrease in intravascular volume. Renal failure may occur secondary to rhabdomyolysis or acute tubular necrosis.[4]

DIFFERENTIAL DIAGNOSIS

The clinical presentation, along with a clear history from first responders, witnesses, or family members, makes the diagnosis of hypothermia or frostbite straightforward. Underlying medical conditions that may predispose the patient to hypothermia (e.g., malnutrition), as well as intercurrent processes (e.g., trauma, overdose), are important to consider. Signs and symptoms of these coexistent conditions may overlap with those of hypothermia.

DIAGNOSIS AND EVALUATION

Hypothermia is a clinical diagnosis based on the patient's core body temperature. Patients presenting in extremis should have their core temperatures obtained by thermometer probe inserted into the esophagus. Rectal temperatures are useful for initial assessment, but after rewarming has begun, they may be falsely low secondary to unintentional insertion of the thermometer probe into stool. Handheld, digital thermometers may or may not be capable of registering temperatures below 34° C and thus may be useful and accurate only in mildly hypothermic patients. Cardiac and respiratory monitoring leads must be placed, but because the victim's skin is usually very slick, even after drying, proper placement may be difficult.

The initial evaluation of hypothermic patients focuses on cervical spine immobilization (if trauma is suspected); support of airway, breathing, and circulation; and removal of wet clothes. A secondary survey should also be performed, much like the secondary survey during trauma resuscitation. The skin should be thoroughly inspected and documented for sensation to light touch and noxious stimuli. Blister formation secondary to frostbite may be found and should be categorized as either superficial or deep. Lacerations, fractures, and bruises should all be noted and addressed appropriately. Laboratory data to be considered include serum electrolytes, complete blood cell count, coagulopathy studies (prothrombin time, partial thromboplastin time, fibrinogen), blood gas analysis, blood type and screen, and hepatic and pancreatic enzymes. Urine and serum toxicology testing may be indicated in some scenarios. A bedside blood sugar quantification should also be obtained. Blood gas interpretation does not need to be adjusted for the victim's core temperature. It is now believed that the metabolic and respiratory acidosis will resolve as core temperature rises and that management of acidosis is more successful with uncorrected gases.[5]

Imaging studies should be performed if indicated. A chest radiograph is useful if pulmonary edema or aspiration pneumonia is suspected or to verify endotracheal tube placement. Head or abdominal computed tomography is indicated if trauma or abuse is suspected.

An electrocardiogram should be performed if any arrhythmia is suspected. Likewise, it may be useful to document cardiac electrical activity, J waves, and cardiac ischemia or infarcts.

COURSE OF ILLNESS

Mild hypothermic patients will recover fully without any complications. The mental confusion or dysarthria will resolve once normal core temperature returns. Moderate to severe hypothermic patients tend to do well if successfully rewarmed. Survival rates have ranged from 47% to 71%.[2,4] Patients with chronic medical conditions tend to have a worse prognosis. Frostbite injuries may take as long as 4 weeks for definitive care. Decisions for débridement are rarely necessary in the acute phase of treatment because delineation of viable versus nonviable tissue is difficult to determine in the early phases.

TREATMENT

Rewarming any hypothermic patient, which typically begins in an emergency department setting, is divided into two methods: passive and active rewarming. Active rewarming is further differentiated into active external and active core rewarming. Passive rewarming is noninvasive and involves removing wet clothes, drying and wrapping the patient in a blanket. This is suitable for mild hypothermic patients who are stable. Their temperature can be expected to rise by 0.5° C to 2° C per hour.[2] Warmed blankets or heating blankets (which can raise the body's temperature by up to 0.8° C per hour) and heat lamps or forced heated air are examples of active external rewarming.[2] These modalities are typically for moderate hypothermia victims who are not in shock. "Afterdrop" of body temperature has been described in some case reports with active external rewarming. This rare phenomenon is hypothesized to occur when the rewarming process has begun and resulted in vasodilation in the cooler extremities. The cooler, acidotic venous blood then returns to the body's core, thereby decreasing core temperature. The clinical significance of "afterdrop" remains a controversy.[6]

Active core rewarming techniques are the most efficient and rapid methods of warming patients. Intravenous administration of warmed crystalloid is the initial step in the treatment of a profoundly hypothermic patient. Intravenous warmers are now available and are used at the bedside. These portable devices can warm any intravenous fluids to 43° C.

If the patient is endotracheally intubated, humidified, warmed oxygen is essential. Bladder irrigation, peritoneal dialysis, and even thoracostomy tube placement for saline lavage are all effective. If the patient is pulseless, cardiopulmonary bypass is the method of choice. Bypass can raise a patient's core temperature by 1° C to 2° C every 5 minutes.[7] Indications for bypass are (1) cardiac arrest or instability with a temperature lower than 32° C, (2) suboptimal response to other warming measures, (3) frozen extremities, or (4) severe hyperkalemia secondary to rhabdomyolyisis.[4,6,7]

During resuscitation, if pulses are noted in the face of profound bradycardia, most researchers argue to forgo any chest compressions because of the possibility that external cardiac massage might induce arrhythmias. In addition, given the depressed metabolic demands of the brain and body, a slow pulsatile rate may be sufficient to sustain survival.[8] The only true indication for chest compressions is asystole. Electrical defibrillation is warranted with ventricular fibrillation but may not be effective until core temperature rises. Likewise, resuscitation medications are also rarely effective. It should be noted that once the body is sufficiently rewarmed, J waves will disappear and the heart rate, blood pressure, and hypopnea or apnea will slowly resolve. Supportive care is the rule.

Patients who are rewarmed and resuscitated but continue to be pulseless should be declared dead only after core temperature rises above 35° C.[8] Defibrillation and resuscitation medications are thought to be more effective at core temperatures higher than 30° C. Patients with severe hypothermia may experience renal failure, coagulopathies, hyperglycemia or hypoglycemia, electrolyte disturbances, pulmonary edema, or aspiration pneumonia. Dialysis may be required for renal failure. Coagulopathies should be corrected with fresh frozen plasma (10 mL/kg). Electrolyte disturbances, hyperkalemia in particular, will often resolve with rewarming. Patients who are hypothermic secondary to cold water submersion may also present with seizures related to a cerebral hypoxic-ischemic event.

Treatment of frostbite is a three-phase approach. The initial phase is the prethaw care, typically started by prehospital care providers. This phase involves using soft padding to protect the affected area. No other treatment should be initiated. No rubbing or rewarming of tissues is indicated because this may potentially do more damage. The second phase, emergency department treatment, is the rewarming process. Rewarming should be done for 15 to 30 minutes or until thawing is complete by immersing the involved area in circulating water at a temperature between 40° C and 42° C.[2] Tissue that has been adequately rewarmed will become supple and demonstrate capillary refill. Intravenous analgesics may be necessary during the rewarming phase because it can be severely painful. Blisters should be left intact and a topical antibiotic ointment applied every 6 hours. Tetanus prophylaxis is indicated for potentially contaminated wounds. The post-thaw, or third, phase requires gentle handling of injured tissue. Areas of injury should be covered with dry, sterile dressings; the dressings should be loosely secured, noncompressive, and nonadhesive. If the hands or feet are involved, they should be splinted and placed in an elevated position. Digits must be separated with cotton gauze.[7]

Patients successfully rewarmed in the emergency department may warrant observation. Patients with frostbite typically require inpatient wound care, pain control, and rehabilitation. Most deep frostbite wounds may take 3 to 4 weeks for the skin or digits to clearly demarcate areas of necrosis or autoamputate.

CONSULTATION

For Hypothermia

- Critical care: For patients with cardiovascular instability or for patients requiring bedside services and monitoring that exceed the capacity of general inpatient unit
- Nephrology: For patients with renal failure or at risk for it (e.g., rhabdomyolysis)
- Cardiology/cardiothoracic surgery: For patients who have suffered a cardiac infarct or demonstrate persistent conduction abnormalities or patients in need of cardiopulmonary bypass

For Frostbite

- Pain team: To provide adequate short- and long-term analgesics
- General, plastic, or otolaryngologic surgery: For débridement of open blisters and amputation of necrotic, dead tissue, digits, limbs, nose, and ears.
- Nutrition: For the caloric adjustment needed for recovery from severe frostbite
- Rehabilitation: For the daily physical and occupational therapy required
- Psychological services: For ongoing support, especially if extremities and digits are expected to be amputated.

Criteria for Transfer to a Burn Center

- Severe frostbite
- Inability to provide adequate care with appropriate services: surgical, physical, and occupational care

ADMISSION CRITERIA

Hospitalization is indicated for any of the following criteria:

- Moderate to severe hypothermia
- Hypothermia associated with physical findings of frostbite
- Altered mental status despite adequate rewarming
- Inadequate social situation
- Questions of abuse or neglect
- Suicidal attempt

DISCHARGE CRITERIA

- Normal physical and mental examination
- Normal laboratory data
- Acceptable social environment
- Frostbite injuries suitable for outpatient follow-up

IN A NUTSHELL

- Clinical presentation: The spectrum of physical signs and symptoms is dependent on the victim's temperature and can be as simple as dysarthria and shivering to frank coma or shock. Early frostbite injuries are typically apparent at presentation.
- Initial management of hypothermia includes removal of all wet clothes, rewarming, supportive care, and cardiopulmonary resuscitation (until the body is at least 35° C).
- Frostbite treatment starts with prethaw care, which involves the use of soft padding to protect the affected area. The second phase is the rewarming process, usually involving immersion in warm water, pain control, and tetanus prophylaxis. The post-thaw, or third, phase includes the application of dry, sterile, noncompressive, and nonadhesive dressings.

ON THE HORIZON

- Advances are being made in rewarming technology, including cardiopulmonary bypass, extracorporeal membrane oxygenation,[9] and continuous arteriovenous blood rewarming.[10]
- New treatment modalities being investigated in the management of frostbite include hyperbaric oxygen[11] and tissue plasminogen activator,[12] as well as new topical agents. Triple-phase bone scanning is increasingly being used to help define the extent of fatally damaged deep tissue and guide earlier débridement for improved limb salvage.[13]

SUGGESTED READING

Epstein E, Anna K: Accidental hypothermia. BMJ 2006;332:706-709.

Urlich SA, Rathlev NK: Hypothermia and localized cold injuries. Emerg Med Clin North Am 2004;22:281-298.

REFERENCES

1. Centers for Disease Control and Prevention (CDC): Hypothermia-related deaths: United States, 2003. MMWR Morb Mortal Wkly Rep 2003;58(8):172-173.
2. Urlich SA, Rathlev NK: Hypothermia and localized cold injuries. Emerg Med Clin North Am 2004;22:281-298.
3. Aslam AF, Aslam AK, Vasavada BC, et al: Hypothermia: Evaluation, electrocardiographic manifestations, and management. Am J Med 2006;119:297-301.
4. Mccullough L, Arora S: Diagnosis and management of hypothermia. Am Fam Physician 2004;70:2325-2332.
5. Kempainen RR, Brunette DD: The evaluation and management of accidental hypothermia. Respir Care 2004;49:192-205.
6. Epstein E, Anna K: Accidental hypothermia. BMJ 2006;332:706-709.
7. Biem J, Koehncke N, Classen D, Dogman J: Out of the cold: Management of hypothermia and frostbite. CMAJ 2003;168:305-311.
8. Guidelines for cardiopulmonary resuscitation and emergency cardiac care. Emergency Cardiac Care Committee and Subcommittees, American Heart Asssociation. Part IV. Special resuscitation situations. JAMA 1992;268:2242-2250.

9. Tiruvoipati R, Balasubramanian SK, Koshbin E, et al: Successful use of venovenous extracorporeal membrane oxygenation in accidental hypothermic cardiac arrest. ASAIO J 2005;51:474-476.
10. Kirkpatrick AW, Garraway N, Brown DR, et al: Use of a centrifugal vortex blood pump and heparin-bound circuit for extracorporeal rewarming of severe hypothermia in acutely injured and coagulopathic patients. J Trauma 2003;55:407-412.
11. von Heimburg D, Noah EM, Sieckmann UP, Pallua N: Hyperbaric oxygen treatment in deep frostbite of both hands in a boy. Burns 2001;27:404-408.
12. Twomey JA, Peltier GL, Zera RT: An open-label study to evaluate the safety and efficacy of tissue plasminogen activator in treatment of severe frostbite. J Trauma 2005;59:1350-1355.
13. Greenwald D, Cooper B, Gottlieb L: An algorithm for early aggressive treatment of frostbite with limb salvage directed by triple-phase scanning. Plast Reconstr Surg 1998;102:1069-1074.

CHAPTER 187

Near Drowning

Frances M. Nadel

Submersion events have been described in various ways in the medical literature. The international panel of resuscitation experts convened to devise the Guidelines 2000 for Cardiopulmonary Resuscitation and Emergency Cardiovascular Care proposed the standardization of definitions, so that *submersion* is an event in which a person experiences swimming-related distress that requires emergency medical care; *drowning* refers to death within 24 hours of a submersion event; and *near drowning* refers to a submersion or immersion event that is significant enough to require medical attention but the victim survives longer than 24 hours.

EPIDEMIOLOGY

Near drowning is a significant pediatric problem.[1] In the United States, drowning is the second leading cause of traumatic death in children 1 to 14 years of age. Toddlers and teenagers are particularly at risk, and males are two to four times more likely to drown than females. African American males aged 5 to 14 years have a 4- to 15-fold higher drowning rate compared with their white counterparts. Morbidity and mortality are high; 15% of admitted patients die, and 20% of survivors have permanent severe neurologic sequelae. Although most submersion events occur in open water sites, bathtubs, toilets, and buckets of water can be dangerous for infants and toddlers.

PATHOPHYSIOLOGY

Hypoxemia is the final common pathway of injury in submersion events, with the pulmonary and neurologic systems being primary sites of damage. During the initial phases of submersion, victims hold their breath and struggle until they reflexively breathe, causing the aspiration of fluid. This aspiration results in laryngospasm, and if it is sustained, the victims do not aspirate any more fluid. This is often referred to as a "dry drowning." In most cases, however, the laryngospasm resolves and the victims aspirate more fluid. Because of progressive neurologic failure and the swallowing of fluid, victims often vomit and may aspirate gastric contents as well. Although the mechanisms of injury are different with freshwater versus seawater aspiration, there is no clinical significance unless submersion occurs in a hypertonic fluid, such as the Dead Sea. Acute impaired lung function results from loss of surfactant, caustic injury from aspirated contents, and pulmonary edema, all contributing to worsening hypoxemia. Atelectasis, ventilation-perfusion mismatch, and acute respiratory distress syndrome (ARDS) may result. Pneumonia may develop later in the course, especially in intubated patients. Neurologic sequelae are often the most devastating for submersion victims. Hypoxic-ischemic injury causes cerebral edema and increased intracranial pressure. Submersion in very cold water may provide cerebral protection by slowing down cerebral metabolism, especially in children (hypothermia is covered in Chapter 186). The effects of hypoxemia on cardiovascular function include decreased cardiac output and increased systemic and pulmonary resistance. Arrhythmias occur because of hypoxemia, hypothermia, and other metabolic derangements. Common arrhythmias include sinus bradycardia, pulseless electrical activity, and asystole, but ventricular fibrillation is rare. Hypoxic injury may occur in all end organs. Less common complications include renal insufficiency or failure, acute tubular necrosis, and disseminated intravascular coagulopathy.

CLINICAL PRESENTATION

The initial presentation of a submersion victim varies from asymptomatic to critically ill. This presentation often reflects the severity of injury. Children who present alert and without respiratory distress usually continue to stay well, with no deterioration in their clinical status. Critically ill patients often appear dead; they are cold, poorly perfused, and an ashen color. Body temperature rapidly decreases in submersion victims. Lung sounds may be coarse, clear, or absent. Pulses may be diminished or absent, and perfusion is decreased due to peripheral vasoconstriction.

The history focuses on identifying the life-threatening injury or insult, determining the details of the submersion and rescue, and obtaining the pertinent medical history (Table 187-1). Basic life support by laypersons appears to be critical in patient survival. The physical examination consists of an assessment of the airway, breathing, and circulation (ABCs), followed by a full head-to-toe examination.

DIFFERENTIAL DIAGNOSIS

For older children, the diagnosis of submersion is obvious. However, it is important to consider comorbidities that may have placed the patient at higher risk, such as long QT syndrome, alcohol or drug intoxication, or a poorly controlled seizure disorder.[2] Although cervical spine injuries are rare, they should be considered, especially if the patient was diving into the water.[3] Inflicted submersion should be suspected when the reported history is not consistent with the child's developmental stage or physical examination. Inflicted submersions are seen predominantly in children younger than 2 years, and they are often reported to occur in the bathtub.[4]

EVALUATION AND TREATMENT

The initial evaluation and treatment proceed in tandem, so they are discussed together.

Table 187-1   Focused History for the Near-Drowning Patient

Scene Events

When was the victim last seen alive? How long was he or she underwater?

Where did the event occur? Was the water excessively contaminated or stagnant?

What is the estimated water temperature?

Was diving involved? Is head trauma suspected?

Did the patient vomit?

Is alcohol or drug use suspected, especially in teenagers?

Rescue Events

Was the patient responsive and breathing when rescued? Did he or she have a pulse?

Was the patient removed with cervical spine precautions (if necessary)?

What initial rescue maneuvers were done? Who performed these maneuvers? How long did it take emergency technicians to arrive, and what steps did they take? What response did the patient have to these maneuvers?

Past Medical History

Underlying seizure disorder

History of syncope, long QT syndrome

Other History

Allergies

Last meal

Initial Stabilization

To date, no set of prognostic factors has been found to reliably predict survival or neurologic outcome for patients in the emergency department. Additionally, there are many case reports of survival after prolonged down times and significantly abnormal physiologic parameters. Therefore, in the emergency department, all patients should undergo initial resuscitation unless there are signs of irreversible death.

The initial stabilization of a submersion victim depends on the patient's severity of injury at the time of presentation. Those who are critically ill are treated like any other critically ill or injured patient, focusing primarily on the immediate identification and treatment of life-threatening conditions. A stepwise approach begins with an assessment of the patient's ABCs.

For asystolic patients, intubation with positive-pressure ventilation, initiation of chest compressions, and parenteral administration of epinephrine should occur immediately. For other patients, airway attention remains important because the airway may be obstructed from secretions or because of an altered sensorium. Clear the airway with suctioning, positioning, and the use of adjunctive airways. Consider cervical spine immobilization if there is suspicion of a cervical spine injury. Provide 100% oxygen, because hypoxemia is the final common pathway of injury. If there is still ineffective ventilation or oxygenation after these airway maneuvers, endotracheal intubation may be necessary. Other indications for intubation include apnea or significant neurologic injury. Except for asystolic patients, use of rapid-sequence intubation medications can facilitate mechanical airway control. If pulmonary edema is suspected because of pink, frothy pulmonary secretions or an inability to adequately oxygenate, the peak inspiratory pressures should be increased to a maximum of 15 mm Hg, and administration of a diuretic (e.g., furosemide) should be considered.

Circulatory assessment should focus on the patient's pulse, perfusion, and pressure. Bradycardic patients may require only simple airway maneuvers to relieve upper airway obstruction. If the patient remains bradycardic despite these maneuvers, pediatric advanced life support guidelines should be instituted, including administration of epinephrine and initiation of chest compressions. Fluid resuscitation may be required if there is evidence of inadequate perfusion (e.g., 20 mL/kg of crystalloid or colloid). The patient should be remain on a cardiorespiratory monitor and pulse oximetry.

The ABCs should be expanded to include an assessment of disability and exposure ("D" and "E"). A quick assessment of disability includes the patient's pupillary response and assignment of a mental status: alert, responds to verbal stimuli, responds to painful stimuli, or unresponsive (AVPU). The Glasgow Coma Scale provides a baseline measure of neurologic status. The head-to-toe examination should be done to identify signs of coexisting trauma (whether intentional or nonintentional), toxidromes, and signs of death, such as dependent lividity or rigor mortis. The patient should be undressed completely to allow a full assessment for other injuries and to remove wet clothing to minimize further heat loss. The patient should then be covered with warm blankets, and body temperature should be monitored.

Further Management

In the emergency department, patients should be triaged into one of two groups: those who have moderate to severe perturbations in their cardiorespiratory or central nervous systems, and those who have minimal or no changes. For the first group, the primary focus is the immediate identification and treatment of life-threatening conditions. Following the ABCs described in the previous section, an arterial blood gas measurement, pulse oximetry, and a chest radiograph provide important information. Consider serial arterial blood gas levels in patients who are hypoxemic, acidotic, deteriorating, or not responding to interventions. Chest radiographs are often normal initially but later reveal evidence of pulmonary injury or aspiration (Fig. 187-1). Increasing hypoxia as shown by continuous pulse oximetry can identify children who are developing pulmonary edema or ARDS. Consider bedside glucose measurement to identify hypoglycemia in infants and young children, whose limited glycogen stores may be depleted by the increased demands associated with the event. Laboratory studies may be normal initially or may reflect derangements from initial fluid shifts (e.g., hypo- or hypernatremia) or secondary to cardiovascular and respiratory compromise. A complete blood cell count may reveal elevations in the neutrophil count secondary to demargination from the intravascular endothelium. Serum liver transaminases or creatinine may be elevated due to end-organ hypoperfusion. Serum bicarbonate levels are often reduced when lactic acidosis develops secondary to shock.

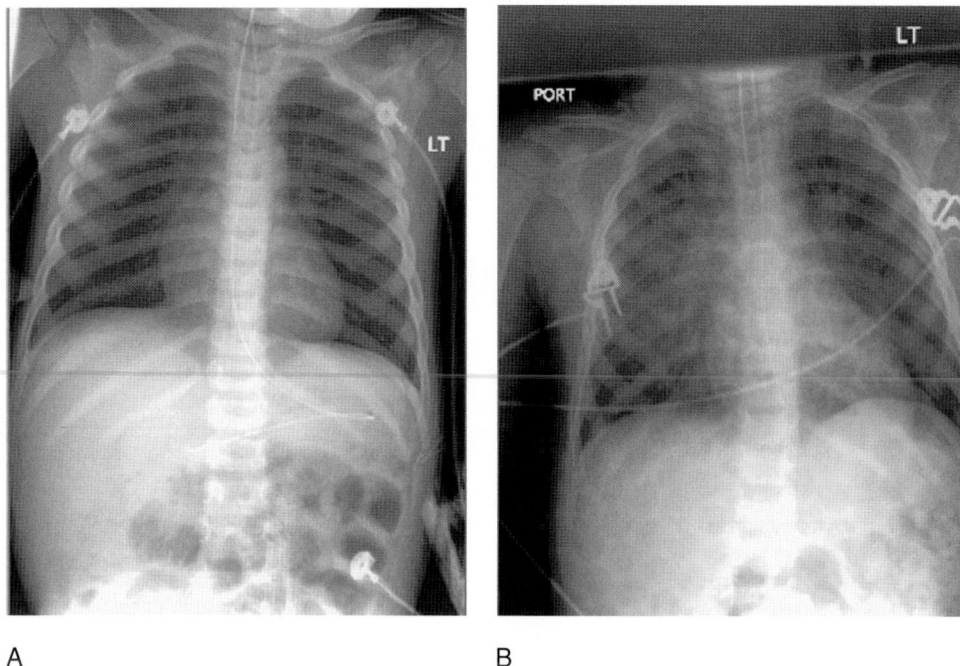

A

B

Figure 187-1   Initial chest radiograph *(A)* and radiograph taken 2 days later *(B)* in a 4-year-old boy who was found submerged in a bathtub after being left unattended for a few minutes. Note the initially clear lungs and the subsequent development of pulmonary edema, as evidenced by increased interstitial markings.

A urine toxicology screen or serum alcohol level is indicated in the appropriate clinical setting. Computed tomography of the head is useful in neurologically compromised patients. If there is a suspicion of syncope or a family history of syncope or early unexplained death, consider an electrocardiogram to determine the Q-Tc interval (decreased in short QT syndrome) and the P-R interval (shortened with an accessory atrioventricular pathway).

Well-appearing patients with little or no disturbance in their respiratory and neurologic status can be evaluated with a careful history and physical examination, along with an initial and discharge pulse oximetry and a chest radiograph. Careful observation for 6 to 12 hours after the event should be sufficient to identify the small proportion of children who become progressively worse despite their reassuring appearance on initial presentation. It is unlikely that an arterial blood gas measurement will provide relevant data to assist in this evaluation.

After the initial stabilization, treatment is directed toward limiting further injury and identifying disease progression. When hypoxemia persists despite adequate ventilation, pulmonary edema should be suspected. In this setting, diuresis with furosemide may be beneficial, although hypovolemia should be corrected before this treatment is initiated. Fluid restriction to two thirds of maintenance may be warranted if the patient is hemodynamically stable.

Extracorporeal membrane oxygenation may be necessary in patients who progress to ARDS or when there is profound hypothermia requiring rewarming. Pressors are used when adequate perfusion cannot be established despite fluid resuscitation. Prophylactic antibiotics do not prevent the development of pneumonia, even in the setting of suspected aspiration of orogastric fluid, and are not recommended.

Steroids do not improve outcome and should not be used routinely.

Moderately affected patients should be observed closely for progression of disease, particularly respiratory status, because signs and symptoms may be subtle and delayed. Incremental decreases in the amount of supplemental oxygen delivered can proceed if oxygen saturation levels, as measured by pulse oximetry, remain greater than 94% without evidence of cardiac arrhythmia or hemodynamic decompensation. Wheezing may develop due to airway edema, increased airway debris or secretions, or bronchospasm. The inhalation of albuterol or some other β-agonist may help reduce the bronchospastic component. Some believe that chest physiotherapy helps mobilize secretions.

Complications

Complications from near drowning are common among critically ill patients and result from the initial hypoxic-ischemic insult or the primary lung injury. Pulmonary edema, ventilation-perfusion mismatch, pneumothorax, and ARDS are often encountered, especially among patients requiring mechanical ventilation. Although it may be difficult to determine which of these conditions coexist, the need for increased supplemental oxygen or ventilatory support may suggest pneumonia, especially if the chest radiography shows a new infiltrate. Common pathogens are those aspirated from the body of water or the human oropharyngeal tract. Although antibiotics are not indicated for prophylaxis, patients with a clinical picture consistent with bacterial pneumonia warrant empirical antibiotic therapy, such as an extended-spectrum penicillin–β-lactamase inhibitor combination.[5]

Cerebral edema and resultant permanent neurologic injury are the most feared complications. Rhabdomyolysis, renal failure, and multiorgan system failure have also been described in critically ill victims of near drowning.

CONSULTATION

- Critical care when cardiorespiratory support is needed.
- Subspecialty medical consultation based on organ system involvement.
- Child protective services when there is suspicion of nonaccidental events or negligence.

ADMISSION CRITERIA

- Critically ill patients or those with a deteriorating status should be transferred to an intensive care setting.
- Patients with mild to moderate symptoms should be admitted for close observation, including continuous pulse oximetry and cardiorespiratory monitoring. Observe mildly symptomatic patients until they have returned to baseline.
- The management of asymptomatic children is somewhat controversial because of rare reports of late respiratory decompensation.[6] However, for the vast majority of well-appearing children, observation for at least 6 to 12 hours after the event is warranted. If they remain well and there is a reliable guardian who can return them to the hospital if needed, these patients can be discharged after the period of observation.

DISCHARGE CRITERIA

- Patients should demonstrate normal heart and respiratory rates and oxygen saturation greater than 94% on room air.
- Patients should have no increase in the work of breathing, and breath sounds should be clear on auscultation.
- Caretakers should be available who are able to detect signs and symptoms of clinical deterioration and return the child to the hospital if necessary.
- For children with long-term sequelae, institution of appropriate home care and follow-up is needed.
- If an accidental near drowning occurred, the caretakers should receive counseling for injury prevention.
- If nonaccidental injury is suspected, child protective services should be notified, and discharge to a safe environment must be assured.

PREVENTION

Toddlers and teenage boys are especially at risk of drowning and near drowning. For young children, many events occur while under the supervision of a guardian who looks away for just a moment. Safe bathing as well as safe swimming practices should be emphasized to all parents. Swimming lessons at a young age, adequate supervision of events that occur near bodies of water, protective swimwear, and restrictive barriers around pools can all help decrease this common but unfortunate occurrence.[7]

IN A NUTSHELL

- Drowning and near drowning are predominantly events of childhood and adolescence.
- Rapid response and delivery of basic life support at the scene are critical for survival.
- The initial presentation can be an inaccurate measure of outcome or disease progression.
- Children who present in extremis, even with cessation of cardiopulmonary function, have survived with minimal neurologic injury.
- Victims who are asymptomatic on presentation or who have minimal signs of respiratory compromise warrant a period of observation because their condition can deteriorate.
- Consider comorbidities, such as child abuse in a toddler who nearly drowned in the bathtub or alcohol or drug use in a teenager.

ON THE HORIZON

- For the critically ill, many novel therapies are being explored, including surfactant replacement, prone positioning during artificial ventilation, and extracorporeal membrane oxygenation. Prone positioning is also being considered for unintubated, moderately symptomatic victims.
- New methods of assessing cerebral injury are being studied, which may be helpful in predicting prognosis. To date, pharmacologic therapies to prevent or reverse cerebral injury have not shown any benefit in near-drowning victims. However, there is ongoing interest in the role of controlled hypothermia in cerebral protection after hypoxemic insult.

SUGGESTED READING

Bierens JJ, Knape JT, Gelissen HP: Drowning. Curr Opin Crit Care 2002;8:578-586.

Christensen DW, Jansen P, Perkin RM: Outcome and acute care hospital costs after warm water near drowning in children. Pediatrics 1997;99:715-721.

European Resuscitation Council: Part 8: Advanced challenges in resuscitation. Section 3: Special challenges in ECC. 3B: Submersion or near-drowning. Resuscitation 2000;46:273-277.

Ibsen LM, Koch T: Submersion and asphyxial injury. Crit Care Med 2002;30:S402-S408.

National SAFE KIDS Campaign (NSKC): Drowning Fact Sheet. Washington, DC, NSKC, 2004.

Weinstein MD, Krieger BP: Near-drowning: Epidemiology, pathophysiology, and initial treatment. J Emerg Med 1996;14:461-467.

REFERENCES

1. Zuckerman GB, Conway EE Jr: Drowning and near drowning: A pediatric epidemic. Pediatr Ann 2000;29:360-366.
2. Yoshinaga M, Kamimura J, Fukushige T, et al: Face immersion in cold water induces prolongation of the QT interval and T-wave changes in children with nonfamilial long QT syndrome. Am J Cardiol 1999;83:1494-1497.

3. Hwang V, Shofer FS, Durbin DR, Baren JM: Prevalence of traumatic injuries in drowning and near drowning in children and adolescents. Arch Pediatr Adolesc Med 2003;157:50-53.

4. Gillenwater JM, Quan L, Feldman KW: Inflicted submersion in childhood. Arch Pediatr Adolesc Med 1996;150:298-303.

5. Encler PT, Dolan MJ: Pneumonia associated with near-drowning. Clin Infect Dis 1997;25:899-907.

6. Causey AL, Tilelli JA, Swanson ME: Predicting discharge in uncomplicated near-drowning. Am J Emerg Med 2000;18:9-11.

7. Thompson DC, Rivara FP: Pool fencing for preventing drowning in children. Cochrane Database Syst Rev 2000;2:CD001047.

CHAPTER 188

Human and Animal Bites

Rebecca G. Carlisle and Phyllis Lewis

In the United States, it is estimated that annually there are 4.5 million dog bites, 400,000 cat bites, and 250,000 human bites. As many as 1% of all pediatric visits to emergency departments during the summer months are for the treatment of human or animal bite wounds, and an estimated 1% to 2% of all bite wounds require hospitalization.[1] Each type of bite carries a risk of morbidity and sometimes mortality. Physical trauma certainly plays a role, but infection is the most common complication. The rate of infection can be higher than 50% after cat bites, 15% after dog bites, and 20% after human bites.[2]

In general, bite wounds that most often require medical attention are those to the extremities, especially the dominant hand. Facial bites, most commonly from dogs, are more frequent in children younger than 10 years and lead to 5 to 10 deaths per year, often because of exsanguination. Of 12,777 mammalian bites reported from 1990 through 1992, 25% occurred in children younger than 6 years, and 34% were in children 6 to 17 years old.

The time of presentation of the patient to medical care can be telling. Patients who present for medical care within 8 to 12 hours after injury are usually concerned with crush injury, care of disfiguring wounds, or the need for rabies or tetanus therapy. These wounds are frequently contaminated with multiple strains of aerobic and anaerobic bacteria. An estimated 2% to 30% of "treated" wounds will still become infected and may require hospitalization. Patients presenting longer than 12 hours after injury usually have established infection.

In this chapter, both mechanical injury and infection as a result of dog, cat, and human bites are discussed. Included are topics that warrant special consideration, such as clenched-fist injuries, bites to the face, bites to the hand, immunocompromised hosts, and rabies. Although other mammalian bites are not discussed, it is of note that monkey and simian bites are becoming more common, and other types that may be seen include those by horses, pigs, aquatic animals, ferrets, and bird pecking and bites. Rodent bites carry a low risk of secondary infection. Rat-bite fever is a rare infection manifested by fever, chills, headache, malaise, and rash 1 to 3 weeks after the bite. Rabbit bites can cause tularemia, most frequently of the ulceroglandular type.

PATHOPHYSIOLOGY

Bite wounds result in morbidity and mortality through both physical trauma and infection. Dog bites can cause a spectrum of injuries from lacerations to avulsions and crush injuries. A dog's teeth are not sharp but can exert a pressure of 200 to 450 psi.[3] This pressure is strong enough to perforate sheet metal and result in a crush injury with much devital-ized tissue. Such bites can result in physical trauma, as well as infection-prone devitalized tissue. The scalp, face, and neck are sites of injury in more than 80% of dog bites in the United States each year. The thin and immature calvaria of a young child has little resistance to the pressure that can be exerted by a dog bite, and a small, apparently minor cranial puncture can be associated with a breach in dural integrity, which carries with it a high risk of intracranial infection.

Dog bites can also result in vascular injuries. Injuries to the brachial artery are regularly encountered and have an attendant risk of significant blood loss. Cat bites have the highest infection rates, probably because they are usually puncture wounds that inoculate the bacteria deeply, thus making wound care more difficult. In addition, there is a high prevalence of *Pasturella multocida*. Human bites commonly involve injury to the hand after fist-to-mouth contact in teens, although in younger children, a bite to the face or trunk is more common. Child abuse needs to be considered when human bites are involved.

Infection generally results from mouth organisms of the biting mammal. The type of infection depends on the nature of the injury and the proximity/involvement of bones or joints. Infections can be manifested as cellulitis, septic arthritis, osteomyelitis, tenosynovitis, or local abscesses in any potential anatomic space. Regional lymphadenopathy or lymphangitis may be seen. Penetrating skull wounds may result in meningitis or a brain abscess. Septicemia occurs primarily in immunocompromised patients, particularly those who are asplenic and therefore more susceptible to infection with encapsulated organisms. Endocarditis is likewise a rare complication. More severe infections are also likely to occur in women who have undergone radical or modified radical mastectomy, patients with edema of an extremity of any cause, and patients with lupus erythematosus, especially if taking steroids. Important prognostic factors for the development of infection include the extent of tissue damage, the depth of the wound and which compartments are entered, the pathogenicity of the inoculated oral bacteria, and the immunocompetence of the host.

The infectious organism varies with the source of the bite. Bites should be considered polymicrobial infections, including both aerobes and anaerobes. The organism most commonly found in both dog and cat bites is *Pasteurella*, with *P. canis* being the most common from dogs and *P. multocida* the most common from cats. Other species commonly isolated from these bites include streptococci, staphylococci, *Moraxella* species, *Neisseria* species, enterococcus, and *Corynebacterium* species. Common anaerobic isolates include *Fusobacterium, Bacteroides, Porphyromonas, Prevotella, Propionibacterium,* and *Peptostreptococcus. Capnocytophaga* species (formerly the DF-2 bacillus) have been implicated in endocarditis, septicemia, and other more severe infections, primarily in immunocompromised hosts.

In human bites, the most common aerobic organisms isolated are streptococci and *Staphylococcus aureus*, and the most common anaerobic organisms are *Bacteroides, Peptostreptococcus* species, and *Fusobacterium* species. More serious morbidity of human bites correlates with *S. aureus* and *Eikenella corrodens* infection. Human bite injuries also represent a potential means of transmitting human immunodeficiency virus (HIV), hepatitis B, and hepatitis C infections. HIV transmission by this route has been reported rarely.[4,5] Transmission could theoretically occur either through biting or receiving a bite from an HIV-infected person. Biting an HIV-infected person, with a break in the skin, exposes the oral mucous membranes to infected blood; being bitten by an HIV-infected person exposes nonintact skin to saliva. Saliva that is contaminated with infected blood poses a more substantial exposure risk. Saliva that is not contaminated with blood contains HIV in much lower titer and constitutes a negligible exposure risk.[6] There are also case reports documenting transmission of hepatitis C virus (HCV) through human bites, although numbers defining absolute risk are not available.

Death can occur from massive trauma to vessels in the neck.[7] Sepsis with *Capnocytophaga canimorsus* or *Eubacterium plautii* has been described in immunocompromised hosts.[8] Endocarditis from *Pasteurella* species other than *multocida, C. canimorsus,* and *S. aureus* has occurred after minor bites.[9,10] Patients with crush injuries to the limbs are at risk for compartment syndrome. Joint and bone infections; meningitis or brain abscess; facial, neck, or limb deformities; or limb loss can occur after bites.

EVALUATION

Certain features of a routine complete history and physical examination warrant particular attention. The focus may vary by type of bite and time of presentation after the bite (Tables 188-1 and 188-2).

Further evaluation focuses on determining the extent of injury or the extent or type of complicating infection (or both). Plain radiographs are helpful if a fracture, foreign body (teeth or teeth fragments), or bone penetration is suspected. Radiographic evaluation of dog bite injuries to the scalp, face, and neck in children helps identify occult cranial puncture wounds, which can result in the introduction of microbes into the intracranial space. Skull films in both the anteroposterior and lateral projections need to be obtained and scrutinized carefully for evidence of fracture. For deep puncture wounds to the extremities, multiple views may reveal small cortical defects. Such findings can serve as baseline information if concerns of osteomyelitis arise in the future.

Because of the polymicrobial nature of bite wounds, aerobic cultures and Gram stain are paramount in the evaluation of wounds suspected of infection. Anaerobic cultures should be performed if there is abscess formation, sepsis, serious cellulitis, devitalized tissue, or a foul odor of any exudate. Culture and Gram stain of fresh uninfected wounds are not recommended. Blood cultures should be considered if fever or other systemic signs of sepsis are present, especially in immunocompromised children.

Table 188-1   History
Description of the Event and Injury
Date and time of injury
Mechanism of injury
Circumstances and environment in which the bite occurred
History of discharge, redness, or increasing pain at the site of injury
For animal bites
Type of animal
Provoked versus unprovoked attack
Assess risk for rabies—immunization status of the animal, ability to observe the animal
For human bites
Recognize clenched-fist injuries as possible bites
Recognize human bites as possible abuse
Assess possible risk of transmission of viruses, such as HIV, hepatitis B, and hepatitis C
Past Medical History
Drug allergies
Current medications
Immunization status
History of splenectomy, mastectomy, liver disease, diabetes mellitus, immunosuppression, or immunocompromise, any of which would put the person at increased risk for systemic infection after a bite

Table 188-2   Physical Examination
Systemic Signs
Fever
Tachycardia
Tachypnea
Hypotension or widened pulse pressure
Other signs of injury or infection
Local Findings
Diagram or photograph the wound
Note the location, type, and depth of injury
Note joint or bone penetration
Note edema or crush injuries, including distal pulses, nerve and tendon function, and range of motion
Assess pain
Note erythema, including lymphatic streaking
Note regional adenopathy
Note the type and odor of any exudates

TREATMENT

Initial Stabilization

Patients presenting for care secondary to a bite wound should first be assessed for adequate airway, breathing, and circulation (ABCs), especially if the wound involves the head and neck. After stabilization of the ABCs, the secondary survey should be attentive to large areas of devitalized tissue, possible neurovascular injuries, or penetrating injuries to any bone or organ. Once life-threatening or catastrophic injuries have been stabilized or excluded from consideration, attention can be directed toward local wound assessment and care.

Initial management of bite wounds involves irrigation, débridement, wound closure if indicated, and protection from infection. These management steps are usually carried out before hospitalization but are discussed here briefly.

Bite wounds should be meticulously cleansed. High-pressure irrigation is accomplished with large volumes (at least 200 mL) of sterile normal saline delivered via a 20-mL syringe and 18-gauge catheter.[11] Irrigation of puncture wounds is controversial because irrigation of this type of wound may merely infiltrate the surrounding tissue.[12] Surgical débridement is necessary to remove any devitalized or necrotic tissue, as well as any debris or foreign bodies not removed with irrigation. Operative exploration and débridement may be necessary if there is extensive tissue damage, involvement of the metacarpophalangeal (MCP) joint from a clenched-fist injury, or cranial injury from the bite of a large animal.

Wound closure may be necessary for selected, fresh uninfected wounds, especially on the face because of the risk of scarring and disfigurement without primary closure. However, primary wound closure is not indicated for wounds at high risk for infection, including puncture wounds, human or cat bites, bites on the hand or foot, bites more than 8 to 12 hours old, or bites in immunocompromised hosts. Other bite wounds can be closed with delayed primary closure techniques. Recent small wounds, not at high risk for infection, can be treated by approximating the wound edges with adhesive strips.[13]

Elevation of edematous wounds or wounds in dependent areas is an important aspect of successful treatment. Immobilization of extremity injuries, especially hand injuries, is essential to prevent spread of infection along tendon sheaths (Fig. 188-1). They should be splinted in a position of function.

Only limited data are available to support the use of prophylactic antibiotics. There is some evidence that the use of prophylactic antibiotics reduces the risk of infection after human bites and bites to the hand.[13] Presently, there is little evidence that the use of prophylactic antibiotics reduces the risk for infection after dog or cat bites. Because the evidence is still insufficient to draw a firm conclusion, prophylaxis is generally recommended for moderate to severe injuries less than 8 hours old; for puncture wounds; if bone or joint penetration is suspected; for wounds of the face, hand, foot, or genitals; for cat bites; and for bites in immunocompromised patients. The drug of choice is amoxicillin–clavulanic acid for 2 to 3 days.

Empirical treatment of infected wounds should be aimed at the following potential pathogens: *Pasteurella* sp. (*multocida* and *canis*), *S. aureus*, streptococci, *Moraxella* sp., *Neisseria* sp., enterococcus, *Corynebacterium* sp., and anaerobes in animal bites; and streptococci, *S. aureus*, *E. corrodens*, and anaerobes in human bites. Amoxicillin–clavulanic acid will cover most animal and human bite pathogens. Alternatives in penicillin-allergic patients are not well established, but the American Academy of Pediatrics Red Book recommends an extended-spectrum cephalosporin or trimethoprim-sulfamethoxazole plus clindamycin. Preferred parenteral antibiotic coverage is ampicillin-sulbactam for both animal and human bites. The duration of therapy is not well defined and should be individualized on the basis of the infection site, culture results, and response to therapy.

Tetanus immunization status should be ascertained and appropriate dosing provided as detailed in Table 188-3. Baseline HIV testing should be performed on all persons seeking evaluation for potential HIV exposure. When the HIV status of the source is unknown, it should be determined whether the source is available for HIV testing. Based on assessment of the risk, postexposure prophylaxis should be initiated according to current recommendations from the U.S. Department of Health and Human Services Working Group on Nonoccupational Postexposure Prophylaxis (nPEP).[14] For exposure to blood that contains (or might contain) hepatitis B surface antigen, the decision to give hepatitis B immune globulin prophylaxis and hepatitis B vaccine is based on the infectious status of the source of the exposure and the immunization status (including response to immunization) of the exposed person.[15] Immunization is recommended for any person who was exposed but does not have evidence of immunity. No vaccine for hepatitis C is available, and prophylaxis with immune globulin is not effective in preventing HCV infection after exposure. If possible, the HCV status of the source and the exposed person should be determined.[16]

Special Considerations
Clenched-Fist Hand Injuries

Clenched-fist injuries are caused by a blow to the teeth from a clenched fist during a fight, with the blow resulting in a bite, usually to the dorsum of the hand or over an MCP joint. The penetrating tooth may cause injury to the extensor tendon or the MCP joint capsule or fracture a metacarpal or phalangeal bone (or both). It is often not recognized as a bite, and patients may not seek medical care until the hand has become infected.

Injuries to the extensor tendon and joint capsule can be overlooked, especially if the MCP joint is examined in extension when the injury occurred with the joint in flexion. In one study, as many as 75% of clenched-fist injuries resulted in an injury to tendon, bone, joint, or cartilage.[17] Examina-

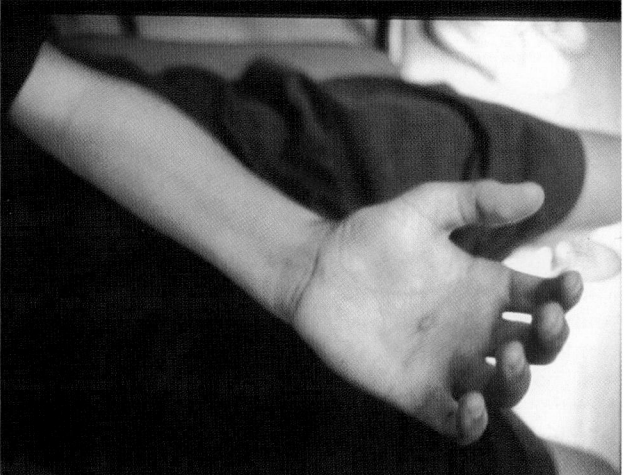

Figure 188-1 Infected cat bite. Note the streak of erythema extending proximally along the anterior forearm.

Table 188-3 Guide to Tetanus Prophylaxis in Wound Management

History of Absorbed Tetanus Toxoid (No. Doses)	CLEAN, MINOR WOUNDS		ALL OTHER WOUNDS*	
	Td or Tdap[†]	TIG[‡]	Td or Tdap[†]	TIG[‡]
<3 or unknown	Yes	No	Yes	Yes
≥3[§]	No	No	No[¶]	No[¶¶]

*Such as, but not limited to, wounds contaminated with dirt, feces, soil, and saliva; puncture wounds; avulsions; and wounds resulting from missiles, crushing, burns, and frostbite.

[†]Tdap is preferred to Td for adolescents who never received Tdap. Td is preferred to tetanus toxoid (TT) for adolescents who received Tdap previously or when Tdap is not available.

[‡]Intravenous immune globulin should be used when TIG is not available.

[§]If only three doses of fluid toxoid have been received, a fourth dose of toxoid, preferably an adsorbed toxoid, should be given. Although licensed, fluid tetanus toxoid is rarely used.

[¶¶]Yes, if 10 or more years since the last tetanus-containing vaccine dose.

[¶]Yes, if 5 or more years since the last tetanus-containing vaccine dose. More frequent boosters are not needed and can accentuate adverse effects.

Td, adult-type diphtheria and tetanus toxoid vaccine; Tdap, booster tetanus toxoid, reduced diphtheria toxoid, and acellular pertussis; TIG, tetanus immune globulin (human).

Taken from American Academy of Pediatrics: Tetanus. In Pickering LK (ed): 2006 Red Book: Report of the Committee on Infectious Diseases, 27th ed. Elk Grove Village, Ill, American Academy of Pediatrics, 2006, p 650.

tion of the hand should include a musculoskeletal and neurovascular examination, with documentation of extensor tendon function. Radiography should be performed to exclude fractures, foreign bodies, gas, or osteomyelitis. As with other bite wounds, copious irrigation and surgical débridement are recommended. Wounds should not be sutured. The hand should be splinted in a position of function and elevated. If the wound is fresh, antibiotic prophylaxis is recommended.[18] If infected, antibiotics should be instituted after tissue for aerobic and anaerobic culture and Gram stain is obtained.

Rabies

Rabies virus is a neurotropic RNA virus in the Rhabdoviridae family that causes an acute encephalitis with atypical focal neurologic signs or paralysis, or both. It is almost always fatal. Rabies is transmitted by the bite or saliva of an infected animal. Between 1990 and 2001 there were 35 human deaths from rabies in the United States.[19] Any mammal can carry and potentially transmit rabies, but carnivorous species and bats are usually the agents of transmission. Transmission is by bite, aerosolization of virus in laboratories, and corneal transplantation from infected donors. It is still unclear how bat-variant rabies is transmitted; 92% of human cases of bat-variant rabies since 1990 do not have a record of a definitive bite. It is hypothesized that the bites may be minimized or unrecognized or that aerosol transmission may have taken place. Therefore, postexposure prophylaxis should be considered for any direct contact between a human and a bat, regardless of bite history.[20]

The incubation period is 5 days to 7 years but averages 4 to 6 weeks. Diagnosis is by virus-specific fluorescent antigen testing of brain tissue, fluorescent microscopy of a skin biopsy specimen from the nape of the neck, isolation of virus in saliva, detection of antibody in unimmunized people in cerebrospinal fluid or serum, or detection of viral nucleic acid in infected tissues. Treatment is supportive.

Recommendations for rabies postexposure prophylaxis can be found in Table 188-4.

Human rabies immune globulin (RIG) is used concomitantly with the first dose of vaccine to provide passive immunity until the vaccine induces active immunity. The recommended dose is 20 IU/kg. As much of the dose as possible should be infiltrated into the wound or wounds, with the rest given intramuscularly. If more volume is needed for infiltration, the dose should not be increased, but RIG may be diluted twofold or threefold to provide more volume for large wounds. RIG should not be used in individuals previously immunized for rabies.

Presently, three rabies vaccines are approved for use in the United States. The dose of vaccine is 1 mL intramuscularly (deltoid or anterolateral aspect of the thigh) on days 0, 3, 7, 14, and 28. If possible, the brand of vaccine should not be changed during the series. The dose is the same for infants and children.

Those at high risk for rabies exposure should undergo pre-exposure vaccination. This category would include veterinarians, animal handlers, laboratory workers, spelunkers, and travelers to areas of the world where canine rabies is common. The dose for pre-exposure immunization is 1 mL intramuscularly on days 0, 7, and 21 or 28. Booster doses may be needed in high-risk groups.

CONSULTATION

Plastic surgery consultation is recommended for disfiguring injuries, especially those involving the face. Ophthalmologic consultation is indicated for the treatment of wounds involving the eye or orbit, or both. Surgical (vascular, general, hand, orthopedic) consultation is needed for wounds with involvement of major blood vessels, a risk for compartment syndrome, abscesses or deep tissue infections, or a potential for loss of hand function (clenched-fist wounds). Depending on the community and the specifics of the injury, the appropriate surgical consultant or consultants may be general, vascular, hand, or orthopedic. An infectious disease specialist can provide advice regarding antibiotic choices, especially if the infection is not responding to initial

Table 188-4 Rabies Postexposure Prophylaxis

Animal Type	Evaluation and Disposition of Animal	Postexposure Prophylaxis Recommendations
Dogs, cats, and ferrets	Healthy and available for 10 days of observation	Prophylaxis only if signs of rabies develop in the animal[†]
	Rabid or suspected of being rabid*	Immediate immunization and human RIG
	Unknown (escaped)	Consult public health officials for advice
Bats, skunks, raccoons, foxes, and most other carnivores; woodchucks (groundhogs)	Regarded as rabid unless the geographic area is known to be free of rabies or until the animal is proved negative by laboratory tests*	Immediate immunization and human RIG
Livestock, rodents, and lagomorphs (rabbits and hares)	Consider individually	Consult public health officials. Bites of squirrels, hamsters, guinea pigs, gerbils, chipmunks, rats, mice, other rodents, rabbits, and hares almost never require antirabies treatment.

*The animal should be euthanized and tested as soon as possible. Holding for observation is not recommended. Immunization can be discontinued if testing of the animal is negative for rabies.
[†]During the 10-day holding period, at the first signs of rabies in the biting animal, treatment with human RIG and vaccine should be initiated. The animal should immediately be euthanized and tested.
RIG, rabies immune globulin.
Adapted from American Academy of Pediatrics: Rabies. In Pickering LK (ed): 2006 Red Book: Report of the Committee on Infectious Diseases, 27th ed. Elk Grove Village, Ill, American Academy of Pediatrics, 2006, p 555.

antibiotic therapy. Neurosurgery should be consulted for penetrating wounds to the skull.

Involvement of physical and occupational therapy may be helpful, especially with immobilization or when activities are limited. Psychology services should be solicited as appropriate, especially when the event was particularly frightening or when there is concern for disfigurement.

ADMISSION CRITERIA

Hospitalization is indicated for the treatment of infected wounds complicated by fever, sepsis, or spreading cellulitis. Wounds with significant edema or crush injury causing loss of function, at high risk for cosmetic morbidity, at risk for joint infection or osteomyelitis, or occurring in an immunocompromised host or a noncompliant patient are best managed in the hospital setting. Some recommend hospitalization, surgical consultation, and surgical wound exploration for all clenched-fist injuries to the hand.[21]

DISCHARGE CRITERIA

- Completion of the necessary surgical débridement and repair
- Clear improvement in signs of infection with either completion of antibiotic therapy or arrangements for completion of therapy after discharge
- Close outpatient follow-up with the primary care physician and surgical specialists, if involved

PREVENTION

Parents and children should be educated regarding behavior around animals, especially those that are unfamiliar to the child. Teasing animals and approaching them when sleeping, eating, or caring for their young are especially risky.

Dogs that are spayed or neutered are less likely to bite, as are trained and socialized dogs. Encourage local leash laws and reporting of bites, and educate the public about responsible dog selection, ownership, and training.

Prevention of human rabies involves vaccinating animals, limiting exposure to potentially rabid animals, and immunoprophylaxis for exposure. An estimated 20,000 to 30,000 people per year receive treatment for potential rabies exposure.[22]

IN A NUTSHELL

- More than 5 million animal and human bites occur each year in the United States, and approximately 1% to 2% require hospitalization.
- Dog bites are often associated with crush injury at the site because of the powerful jaws of the animal. Such injury can lead to devascularized tissue and an increased risk for infection.
- Cat bites are associated with the highest rate of infection related to the nature of the bite. The puncture wound inoculates mouth flora deep into soft tissues, thus making decontamination of the wound difficult.
- Clenched-fist hand injuries from a punch to the mouth are often associated with delay in seeking treatment. Injuries from the penetrating tooth can cause laceration of the extensor tendon and result in infection of the skin, tendon, bones, or joints of the hand. These injuries are often managed with the assistance of surgical specialists.
- Primary wound closure is generally deferred unless the risk for infection is low. In selected situations, especially those associated with a high risk for disfigurement, early wound closure may be considered.

- Although not routinely administered, prophylactic antibiotics may be appropriate for moderate to severe injuries less than 8 hours old; puncture wounds; suspected bone or joint penetration; wounds to the face, hand, foot, or genitals; cat bites; and immunocompromised patients.
- Empirical therapy for infected bites is amoxicillin-clavulanate or ampicillin-sulbactam or, for penicillin-allergic patients, an extended-spectrum cephalosporin or trimethoprim-sulfamethoxazole plus clindamycin.
- Tetanus immunization should be administered to unimmunized or underimmunized patients.

ON THE HORIZON

- Rabies has been considered a nearly uniformly fatal disease if untreated. Immunoprophylaxis before the onset of symptoms has led to survival in a few patients.[23,24] A report of a 15-year-old girl who survived rabies was published in 2005.[25] The patient did not receive immune prophylaxis but was treated by induction of coma, intense antiviral therapy, and full critical care level of support. She survived, although with some neurologic impairment, but is sufficiently functional to attend high school on a part-time basis. The intervention provided this patient might lead to greater survival and improved neurologic outcome in the future.

SUGGESTED READING

Animal bites: *http://www.emedicine.com/ped/topic107.htm.*
Goldstein EJ: Bites. In Mandell G, Bennett J, Dolin R (eds): Principles and Practice of Infectious Diseases, 5th ed. Philadelphia, Churchill Livingstone, 2000.
Lieberman JM: Infection following bites. In Long S, Pickering L, Prober C (eds): Principles and Practice of Pediatric Infectious Diseases, 2nd ed. New York, Churchill Livingstone, 2003.
Rabies: *http://www.emedicine.com/ped/topic1974.htm.*

REFERENCES

1. Brook I: Microbiology and management of human and animal bite wound infections. Prim Care 2003;30:25-39.
2. American Academy of Pediatrics: Bite wounds. In Pickering LK (ed): 2003 Red Book: Report of the Committee on Infectious Diseases, 26th ed. Elk Grove Village, IL, American Academy of Pediatrics, 2003, pp 182-186.
3. Chambers G, Payne J: Treatment of dog bite wounds. Minn Med 1969;52:427-430.
4. Vidmar L, Poljak M, Tomazic J, et al: Transmission of HIV-1 by a human bite. Lancet 1996;347:1762.
5. Abel S, Cesaire R, Cales-Quist D, et al: Occupational transmission of human immunodeficiency virus and hepatitis C virus after a punch. Clin Infect Dis 2000;31:1494-1495.
6. Richman KM, Rickman LS: The potential for transmission of human immunodeficiency virus through human bites. J Acquir Immune Defic Syndr 1993;6:402-406.
7. Centers for Disease Control and Prevention (CDC): Dog-bite-related fatalities—United States, 1995-1996. MMWR Morb Mortal Wkly Rep 1997;46(21):463-467.
8. Carpenter PD, Heppner BT, Gnann JW Jr: DF-2 bacteremia following cat bites. Report of two cases. Am J Med 1987;82(3 Spec No):621-623.
9. Sandoe JA: *Capnocytophaga canimorsus* endocarditis. J Med Microbiol 2004;53:245-248.
10. Bradshaw SE: Endocarditis due to *Staph aureus* after minor dog bite. South Med J 2003;96:407-409.
11. Bravo A, Paidas C: Trauma and burns. In Siberry G, Iannone R (eds): Johns Hopkins: The Harriet Lane Handbook: A Manual for Pediatric House Officers, 16th ed. Baltimore, CV Mosby, 2002, pp 82-84.
12. Capellan O, Hollander JE: Management of lacerations in the emergency department. Emerg Med Clin North Am 2003;21:205-231.
13. Broder J, Jerrard D, Olshaker J, Witting M: Low risk of infection in selected human bites treated without antibiotics. Am J Emerg Med 2004;22(1):10-13.
14. Smith DK, Grohskopf LA, Black RJ, et al: Antiretroviral postexposure prophylaxis after sexual, injection-drug use, or other nonoccupational exposure to HIV in the United States: Recommendations from the U.S. Department of Health and Human Services. MMWR Recomm Rep 2005;54(RR-2):1-20.
15. American Academy of Pediatrics: Hepatitis B. In Pickering LK (ed): 2003 Red Book: Report of the Committee on Infectious Diseases, 26th ed. Elk Grove Village, IL, American Academy of Pediatrics, 2003, pp 334-335.
16. Sexually transmitted diseases guidelines, 2002. Centers for Disease Control and Prevention. MMWR Recomm Rep 2002;51(RR-6):1-78.
17. Patzakis MJ, Wilkins J, Bassett RL: Surgical findings in clenched-fist injuries. Clin Orthop 1987;220:114-117.
18. Zubowicz VN, Gravier M: Management of early human bites of the hand: A prospective randomized study. Plast Reconstr Surg 1991;188:111-114.
19. American Academy of Pediatrics: Rabies. In Pickering LK (ed): 2003 Red Book: Report of the Committee on Infectious Diseases, 26th ed. Elk Grove Village, IL, American Academy of Pediatrics, 2003, pp 514-521.
20. Gibbons RV: Cryptogenic rabies, bats, and the question of aerosol transmission. Ann Emerg Med 2002;39(5):528-536.
21. Clark D: Common acute hand infections. Am Fam Physician 2003;68(11):2167-2176.
22. Human rabies prevention—United States, 1999. Recommendations of the Advisory Committee on Immunization Practices (ACIP). MMWR Recomm Rep 48(RR-1):1-21.
23. Jackson AC, Warrell MJ, Ruprecht CE, et al: Management of rabies in humans. Clin Infect Dis 2003;36:60-63.
24. Centers for Disease Control and Prevention (CDC): Recovery of a patient from clinical rabies—Wisconsin, 2004. MMWR Morb Mortal Wkly Rep 2005;53(50):1171-1173.
25. Willoughby RE, Tieves KS, Hoffman GM, et al: Survival after treatment of rabies with induction of coma. N Engl J Med 2005;352:2508-2514.

CHAPTER 189

Envenomation

Christine S. Cho and Kevin C. Osterhoudt

Bites and envenomations account for 4% of phone calls to poison control centers (approximately 50,000 calls a year).[1] In North America, venomous animals vary by specific region and include varied terrestrial vertebrates and invertebrates. Venomous bites are of particular concern in the pediatric population, with the highest morbidity and mortality occurring in smaller patients. Diagnosis and management strategies for envenomation vary according to the type of animal, specific toxic properties of the venom, location of the bite, time elapsed since exposure, appearance of the wound, systemic symptoms, size of the child, and history and physical examination findings (Table 189-1). It is important to keep in mind that unwitnessed bites can occur in younger children. This chapter specifically addresses the presentation and management of common snake bites, as well as black widow and brown recluse spider bites.

SNAKE BITES

In North America, the most common venomous snakes belong to the Viperidae family (Crotalinae subfamily) and are commonly referred to as pit vipers.

Common features of their general appearance that differentiate them from nonpoisonous snakes include a triangular head, vertically positioned elliptical pupils, heat-sensing nostril pits, and a single row of scales at the tail. In North America, common crotaline snakes include (1) eastern and western diamondbacks and other multiple species of rattlesnakes, (2) copperheads, and (3) water moccasins (also called cottonmouths); envenomation by rattlesnakes is usually more severe. In addition to pit vipers, coral snakes (Elapidae family) can be found in the southeastern and southwestern United States. Coral snake envenomation is less common than pit viper bites but can cause serious neurologic dysfunction.

Clinical Presentation

About 75% of snake bites occur with envenomation. It is important to remember that a snake bite deposits the same amount of venom regardless of the size of the victim. Therefore, a smaller patient will have a more significant venom load per kilogram and will be at higher risk for morbidity and mortality than larger children and adults. Crotaline venom contains a mixture of multiple enzymes and toxic substances. It is usually deposited subcutaneously, but rarely there can be subfascial or intravascular deposition. Local effects start approximately 15 to 30 minutes after the bite and include pain, paresthesias, numbness, edema, ecchymosis, necrosis, bleeding, and hemorrhagic blisters and blebs. Swelling can be extensive and is of particular concern if respiratory obstruction occurs from bites to the mouth, face, or neck. Although the appearance of a swollen bite site may mimic compartment syndrome, the subcutaneous location of envenomation makes compartment syndrome unlikely.

Systemic symptoms can include diaphoresis, lightheadedness, chills, nausea, and vomiting. Rhabdomyolysis is a rare complication. With crotaline snakes, systemic effects primarily involve the hematologic system, with laboratory abnormalities typical of disseminated intravascular coagulation: decreased fibrinogen and platelets and increased prothrombin and partial thromboplastin times, fibrin split products, and D-dimer. Certain crotaline snakes (Mojave rattlesnakes) have neurotoxic venom. Coral snake envenomation also has neurologic sequelae as its primary feature and minimal local effects. Neurologic symptoms of Mojave and coral snake envenomation can include fasciculations, paresthesias, cranial nerve deficits, and muscular weakness that could involve the respiratory muscles (Table 189-2).

Treatment

For every envenomation, initial management includes stabilization of respiratory and cardiovascular status and local wound care. Local wound care with irrigation is important. Venom should never be removed by oral suction because it has not been proved to be effective and may increase the risk for infection. Use of tourniquets is not recommended, but the affected location should be immobilized and not elevated to minimize mobilization of toxins. Tetanus immunization status should be confirmed and toxoid administered if indicated. Prophylactic antibiotics have not been shown to be helpful. Laboratory markers that should be monitored for suspected crotaline envenomation include complete blood count, prothrombin and partial thromboplastin times, fibrinogen, fibrin split products, D-dimer, electrolytes, blood urea nitrogen, creatinine, creatine kinase, urinalysis, and type and screen.

Crotaline antivenom is indicated for swelling that compromises local structures, in particular, airway-compromising obstruction at the neck or face, and for neurologic and hematologic abnormalities. Crotalidae polyvalent immune Fab—ovine (CroFab) is an ovine antibody preparation that has become the preferred antivenom for the treatment of evenomation by North American crotaline snakes and is safe for use in the pediatric population.[2,3] It is less immunogenic and better tolerated than the older horse serum–derived antivenoms, which have a high incidence of anaphylaxis and serum sickness. Crotaline polyvalent immune Fab is administered at a dose sufficient to neutralize the injected venom, and therefore the recommended dose is identical for patients of all sizes and ages. Four to six vials should be administered initially, with additional vials given to achieve clinical control of the envenomation syndrome. The Fab antivenom has a short pharmacodynamic half-life, and the manufacturer recommends maintenance dosing at 6-hour intervals. Antivenom administration is a complicated procedure that is best performed by clinicians with experience in caring for snake envenomation and should be done in consultation with a toxicologist or regional poison control center. If Crotalidae polyvalent immune Fab is not available, patients may be treated with Crotalidae antivenom-equine.

Fasciotomy is not indicated except for the rare situation of subfascial envenomation with resultant compartment syndrome.

Table 189-1 Important Details to Elicit on History and Physical Examination

History
Description of animal (identification may not always be possible)
Time of exposure
Location of wound on the body
Changes in appearance of wounds before presentation
Pain
Local symptoms (paresthesia, weakness, swelling)
Systemic symptoms (dizziness, diaphoresis, respiratory compromise, seizures, muscle cramping, bleeding)

Physical Examination
Patient's weight
Wound characteristics (erythema, edema, target lesion, bleeding, necrosis, hemorrhagic blebs)
Local compromise (airway compromise, perfusion, neurovascular status)
Systemic compromise (vital signs and end-organ perfusion)

Admission Criteria

A patient may be discharged home with close follow-up after a 6- to 8-hour period of observation that reveals no worsening local effects, laboratory abnormalities, or systemic symptoms. Any patient with moderate or severe symptoms (see Table 189-2) should be admitted for neurovascular assessment of the wound and its extension or for hematologic and neurologic monitoring by serial physical examination and laboratory evaluation.

Discharge Criteria

Children may be discharged when the progression of local injury has halted, any coagulation abnormalities have subsided, and no further antivenom administration is warranted. Physical therapy may be indicated for functional disability. Children treated with antivenom warrant outpatient observation for serum sickness.

SPIDER BITES

Black Widow Spider

Widow spiders (genus *Latrodectus*) are indigenous throughout North America. Black widow spider (*Latrodectus mactans*) envenomation occurs with bites by females, identifiable by the red hourglass-shaped mark on the abdomen. Symptoms of black widow spider bites arise from the activation of nerve cells when toxins cause release of neurotransmitters via calcium channel modulation.

Clinical Presentation

Initially after a black widow spider bite, pain may develop at the site and at times becomes severe (Table 189-3). The wound may develop a characteristic target appearance with

Table 189-2 Severity of Snake Bite Envenomation

	Mild	Moderate	Severe
Wound (all bites)	Pain, erythema, mild swelling	Increased pain, mild bleeding, moderate swelling	Hemorrhagic blisters and blebs, extensive swelling (at risk for compromising local structures)
Hematologic (most pit vipers)	Limited local bleeding, normal laboratory values	Mild abnormalities in laboratory values	Disseminated intravascular coagulation
Neurologic (Mojave rattlesnake, coral snakes, other neurotoxic envenomation)	Local paresthesias	Local extension of paresthesias and weakness	Systemic weakness

Table 189-3 Severity of Spider Bite Envenomation

	Mild	Moderate	Severe
Black widow	Local pain, target lesion, erythema, normal vital signs	Muscular cramps at local bite and proximal muscles, normal vital signs	Generalized muscle cramps (abdomen, back, thighs), diaphoresis, tachycardia, hypertension
Brown recluse	Local pain, erythema	Extension of wound and blistering	Large necrosis and ulceration

blanching immediately surrounding the bite and an outer erythematous ring. Systemic symptoms develop between 1 and 8 hours after the bite, with most occurring by 2 to 3 hours. Stimulation of the neurologic and autonomic nervous systems causes muscle cramping and rigidity at the site of the bite or in large muscle groups such as the abdomen, thighs, and back. Other symptoms can include facial spasm, diaphoresis, vomiting, tachycardia, hypertension, and rarely, priapism. Systemic toxicity can occur in varying degrees, with mild bites having only local effects and severe envenomation causing marked abnormalities (see Table 189-3).

Treatment

Local wound care, as well as attention to support of the cardiorespiratory systems, is important in the initial management. Pain control and relief from systemic symptoms can often be achieved with the use of benzodiazepines and opioids. Despite calcium channel pathology, intravenous calcium does not mitigate the symptoms.[4] A horse serum immunoglobulin antivenom is available for black widow spider envenomation; administered intravenously, it reduces both the duration and severity of symptoms.[5] It should be administered in consultation with a toxicologist for severe envenomation or inability to control symptoms with supportive care, or both. The preparation is associated with a high incidence of immediate and delayed hypersensitivity reactions. Serum sickness is common and should be treated with antihistamines and corticosteroids.

Admission/Discharge Criteria

Patients with moderate or severe toxicity should be hospitalized for symptom control and monitoring. Discharge is safe when symptoms have resolved.

Brown Recluse Spider

Recluse spiders (genus *Loxosceles*) are distributed throughout temperate regions of the United States, with the most common one in America being the brown recluse spider (*Loxosceles reclusa*). Many spiders are misidentified as brown recluse spiders by the public despite the characteristic brown violin-shaped marking on their dorsal surface.

Clinical Presentation

Initial bites are often not detected, but severe pain can develop over the ensuing 8 hours. The cytotoxic properties of the venom cause erythema and edema with mild envenomation. Moderate to severe bites can lead to the formation of blisters that develop into a necrotic ulcer over the next 3 to 4 days. In smaller children, systemic symptoms such as weakness, emesis, and hematologic abnormalities can also occur (see Table 189-3).

Evaluation

Accurate diagnosis of brown recluse spider bites is a challenge, and overdiagnosis remains a problem with dermonecrotic wounds. Especially in nonendemic areas, a wide

Table 189-4 Differential Diagnosis of Necrotic Arachnidism
Envenomation from *Loxosceles* species
Bites from other spiders/arthropods
Impetigo/cellulitis
Contact/chemical dermatitis
Soft tissue trauma
Lyme disease
Anthrax
Herpes simplex or varicella-zoster
Toxic epidermal necrolysis
Ecthyma gangrenosum
Pyoderma gangrenosum
Pyogenic granuloma
Sporotrichosis
Focal vasculitis
Bedsore
Diabetic ulcer
Erythema nodosum
Dermatitis of gonococcal arthritis
Barbiturate blisters
Warfarin-induced skin necrosis
Periarteritis nodosum
Lymphomatoid papulosis
Tularemia
Chagas disease

From Osterhoudt KC, Zaoutis T, Zorc JJ: Lyme disease masquerading as brown recluse spider bite. Ann Emerg Med 2002;39:558-561.

variety of illnesses can mimic necrotic arachnidism (Table 189-4).[6-8] Although rare, if systemic symptoms are present, laboratory evaluation for disseminated intravascular coagulation and renal function should be performed, including a complete blood count, prothrombin and partial thromboplastin times, fibrinogen, D-dimer, fibrin split products, serum electrolytes, blood urea nitrogen and creatinine, and urinalysis.

Treatment

In managing brown recluse spider bites, local wound care is the priority. Large wounds with extension of necrosis may eventually require skin grafting. Tetanus immunization should be addressed. Prophylactic antibiotics do not prevent infection; however, wound infection can often occur, and appropriate antibiotic therapy should be initiated if secondary infection is suspected. Typical pathogens, such as *Staphylococcus aureus* and group A streptococcus, are the common pathogens that lead to skin infection in this setting.

Admission and Discharge Criteria

Patients with systemic symptoms should be admitted for observation and supportive treatment and may be discharged when symptoms resolve. In a randomized controlled trial of brown recluse spider envenomation in an animal model, neither diphenhydramine, colchicine, dapsone, nor triamcinolone was efficacious in improving wound healing.[9]

IN A NUTSHELL

- Crotaline, or "pit viper," snake envenomation causes soft tissue destruction and coagulopathy and may be treated with antivenom.
- Elapid snake envenomation may cause neurorespiratory failure.
- Black widow (*Latrodectus* sp.) spider bites may cause painful muscle cramping and hyperautonomicity; they are best treated with sedatives, analgesics, and antivenom (when necessary).
- Brown recluse spiders (*Loxosceles* sp.) may cause necrotic skin lesions, but clinicians are encouraged to consider a broad differential diagnosis for focal necrosis.

ON THE HORIZON

- Because of the difficulty of diagnosing envenomation by history and physical examination alone, novel methods of venom detection are being developed. In particular, given the large differential diagnosis for dermonecrotic wounds, assays for brown recluse spider venom[10] and studies exploring which specimens are best used to detect venom[11] are among the current literature topics. Active research in enzyme immunoassays for snake venom is also prominent in regions with a high incidence of snake bites.[12]

SUGGESTED READING

Gold BS, Dart RC, Barish RA: Bites of venomous snakes. N Engl J Med 2002;347:347-356.
Isbister GK, White J: Clinical consequences of spider bites: Recent advances in our understanding. Toxicon 2004;43:477-492.
Swanson DL, Vetter RS: Loxoscelism. Clin Dermatol 2006;24:213-221.

REFERENCES

1. Watson WA, Litovitz TL, Rodgers GC, et al: 2004 Annual Report of the American Association of Poison Control Centers Toxic Exposure Surveillance System. Am J Emerg Med 2005;23:589-666.
2. Schmidt JM: Antivenom therapy for snakebites in children: Is there evidence? Curr Opin Pediatr 2005;17:234-238.
3. Offerman SR, Bush SP, Moynihan JA, et al: Crotaline Fab antivenom for the treatment of children with rattlesnake envenomation. Pediatrics 2002;110:968-971.
4. Clark RF, Wethern-Kestner S, Vance MV, et al: Clinical presentation and treatment of black widow spider envenomation: A review of 163 cases. Ann Emerg Med 1992;21:782-787.
5. Isbister GK, Graudins A, White J, et al: Antivenom treatment in arachnidism. J Toxicol Clin Toxicol 2003;41:291-300.
6. Osterhoudt KC: Diagnosis of brown recluse spider bites in absence of spiders [letter]. Clin Pediatr 2004;43:407.
7. Vetter RS, Bush SP: The diagnosis of brown recluse spider bite is overused for dermonecrotic wounds of uncertain etiology. Ann Emerg Med 2002;39:544-546.
8. Osterhoudt KC, Zaoutis T, Zorc JJ: Lyme disease masquerading as brown recluse spider bite. Ann Emerg Med 2002;39:558-561.
9. Elston DM, Miller MS, Young RJ, et al: Comparison of colchicine, dapsone, triamcinolone, and diphenhydramine therapy for the treatment of brown recluse spider envenomation. Arch Dermatol 2005;141:595-597.
10. Gomez HF, Krywko DM, Stoecker WV: A new assay for the detection of *Loxosceles* species (brown recluse) spider venom. Ann Emerg Med 2002;39:469-474.
11. Krywko DM, Gomez FH: Detection of *Loxosceles* species venom in dermal lesions: A comparison of 4 venom recovery methods. Ann Emerg Med 2002;39:475-480.
12. O'Leary MA, Isbister GK, Schneider JJ, et al: Enzyme immunoassays in brown snake (*Pseudonaja* spp.) envenoming: Detecting venom, antivenom and venom-antivenom complexes. Toxicon 2006;48:4-11.

CHAPTER 190

Infant Botulism

Michael DelVecchio

Infant botulism, the most common form seen in the United States, has a unique pathogenesis. Unlike food-borne botulism, which occurs from the ingestion of preformed toxin, infant botulism occurs following the ingestion of *Clostridium botulinum* spores that germinate and colonize the infant gut. Botulinum neurotoxin is produced in vivo and absorbed, producing clinical disease. This form of botulism occurs almost exclusively in children younger than 1 year.[1] The first clear association of in vivo production of botulinum neurotoxin and a syndrome of weakness in infants was described in 1976.[2] Subsequently, the pathophysiology, epidemiology, clinical manifestations, and specific therapy have been elucidated.

PATHOPHYSIOLOGY

C. botulinum is a gram-positive, spore-forming, obligate anaerobe that is found worldwide in soil and dust. The spores can be found on fresh fruits and vegetables and in honey. The infant intestinal microflora plays a critical role in the pathophysiology of infant botulism. Experiments in mice show that adult mouse microflora completely inhibits gut colonization with *C. botulinum* or that significantly higher numbers of spores are required for successful colonization than in infant mice.[3] Diet is also a critical factor because it determines the intestinal microflora. Although it is unclear whether breastfeeding is a risk factor for infant botulism, the introduction of nonhuman milk or other foods perturbs the microflora of exclusively breast-fed infants and may increase the susceptibility of the gut to colonization with *C. botulinum*. Honey is the only food that has been unequivocally linked to specific cases of infant botulism.[4] Corn syrup was implicated as a source of infection in the past, but recent changes in the production process have largely eliminated the risk of infection with corn syrup.[5] After botulinum toxin is produced in the gut, it is absorbed into the bloodstream and carried to peripheral cholinergic synapses, where it blocks the release of acetylcholine. Autonomic effects occur, as well as the classic somatic muscle weakness or paralysis. Botulinum toxin does not enter the central nervous system.[1]

EPIDEMIOLOGY

Although *C. botulinum* spores are ubiquitous, there is a clear geographic clustering of cases. The majority of reported cases are from California and the eastern Pennsylvania, New Jersey, and Delaware region, apparently mirroring the geographic distribution of spores. Toxin serotype also varies geographically. Type B toxin causes about 90% of cases in Pennsylvania, whereas the majority of California cases are due to type A toxin.[4] All but four reported cases have been caused by toxin A or B. All reported cases of infant botulism have occurred in patients between 6 and 351 days of age, and 95% of cases occurred in the first 6 months of life. Arnon and colleagues showed that the age distribution of infant botulism is almost identical to that of sudden infant death syndrome.[6] No sex, race, or seasonal risk factors have been identified.

CLINICAL PRESENTATION

The clinical severity of infant botulism varies widely. The onset of symptoms may be gradual (days) or abrupt (hours). Some infants, regardless of treatment, never require airway intervention, whereas others need prolonged endotracheal intubation.[1] In California as many as 5% of cases of sudden infant death syndrome have been attributed to fulminant infant botulism.[6] If the patient is evaluated early in the course of disease or has a slowly progressive course, the initial abnormal physical findings may be limited to weakness of the muscles innervated by the cranial nerves. Clinical assessment should include careful and repeated examination of pupillary constriction, extraocular movement, and gag, suck, and swallow reflexes. Repeated stimulation of a muscle is the most sensitive way to induce a clinically evident palsy.[7] The paralysis of infant botulism is symmetrical, flaccid, and descending. Weakness is detectable in all affected infants on presentation. Initial deep tendon reflexes may be normal, only to diminish later. The majority of patients are afebrile on presentation. Constipation, present in approximately 95% of patients at the time of presentation, is frequently overlooked.[1]

DIFFERENTIAL DIAGNOSIS

Other diagnostic considerations such as myasthenia gravis, Guillain-Barré syndrome, and spinal muscular atrophy can usually be eliminated by history and physical examination. Constipation and abnormal cranial nerve function are key features in distinguishing infant botulism from these other entities.[1] Sepsis is the most common clinical diagnosis at the time of hospital admission in patients later found to have infant botulism.

EVALUATION

Laboratory confirmation of the diagnosis requires the isolation of *C. botulinum* or the demonstration of botulinum toxin from the patient's stool. The mouse neutralization test is preferred for confirmation and is available from state health laboratories or from the Centers for Disease Control and Prevention in Atlanta. Because of severe constipation, an enema with sterile, nonbacteriostatic water is often required to obtain a sample. The stool sample must be kept at 4°C during transport.[4] Polymerase chain reaction testing has not been clinically useful.[4,8] Other laboratory examinations are typically normal. Electromyography demonstrates brief, small, abundant motor unit potentials, and repetitive stimulation of peripheral nerves shows facilitation of neuromuscular transmission. This testing is uncomfortable and technically challenging and is rarely needed for the initial diagnosis.[4]

TREATMENT

Intravenous botulism immune globulin (BabyBIG), a human-derived antitoxin, has been developed by the California Department of Health Services (CDHS). A single dose of BabyBIG was found to be safe and effective in a 5-year placebo-controlled trial. Mean hospital stay and costs were significantly reduced. Subsequently, a 6-year nationwide open-label study confirmed the safety and efficacy of the drug and led to the approval of BabyBIG for the treatment of infant botulism, both type A and type B. The earlier that BabyBIG is administered, the sooner specific intervention can begin; treatment should not be delayed for laboratory confirmation. The half-life of the immune globulin preparation is approximately 28 days. A single infusion is sufficient to neutralize any ongoing toxin production or absorption for at least 6 months.[9] The CDHS Infant Botulism Treatment and Prevention Program is accessible at telephone number 510-231-7600.

Even with specific therapy, meticulous supportive care is essential. Because botulinum toxin has a prolonged duration of action following its binding to receptors in the presynaptic membrane and internalization, symptoms may persist for days to weeks, even with the administration of BabyBIG. Nutritional, airway, and respiratory support are the most important measures. Nutritional support can be effectively accomplished by enteral tube feeding, including nasogastric feeding. Enteral feeding can be initiated immediately on presentation, beginning with a low rate of continuous ("drip") feedings to reduce the risk of aspiration.[10] Constipation usually continues but should not interrupt enteral feedings. Other than the initial removal of an inspissated fecal plug, constipation can be managed with routine measures.[1]

Loss of protective airway reflexes is the primary indication for placement of an artificial airway.[10] However, meticulous attention to positioning can reduce the need for one (the CDHS Infant Botulism Treatment and Prevention Program website describes the optimal positioning).[7] Frequent assessment of airway status and respiratory effort is required and should include continuous pulse oximetry, continuous measurement of carbon dioxide, maximum inspiratory pressure, and crying vital capacity.[10]

Urinary retention can occur, but catheter placement should be avoided. Gentle manual pressure over the suprapubic region (the Credé method) is usually sufficient to empty the bladder.[1]

Antibiotics are not effective for the primary treatment of infant botulism but may be indicated for complications. Previously, there were concerns about administering antibiotics, which could lyse *C. botulinum,* lead to additional intraintestinal toxin release, and potentially result in increased absorption of the toxin. When BabyBIG is used, however, this is not a concern because the antitoxin has the capacity to bind any additional toxin released. Thus, any suitable antibiotic can be prescribed to treat an infectious complication. However, aminoglycosides are contraindicated because they can potentiate the action of the toxin at the neuromuscular junction.

CLINICAL COURSE AND PROGNOSIS

With the use of BabyBIG, the average hospital stay has been lowered to 2.2 weeks. Treatment within 3 days of hospitalization decreases the length of stay by an additional week, compared with infants treated 4 to 7 days after admission.[9]

Patients reach a peak of paralysis, followed by a period of stability and then gradual recovery. The clinical time course shows considerable individual variation, so careful anticipatory guidance must be given to the child's parents or primary caregivers. Recovery from infant botulism requires regeneration of nerve endings and subsequent induction of new motor end plates, because antitoxin does not remove any toxin already bound to nerve synapses. The entire process of regeneration takes several weeks.[11]

In the absence of secondary complications, complete recovery can be expected. Relapses are rare, if they occur at all. Deterioration after initial clinical improvement suggests a complication.[1] The most common complications are pneumonia, otitis media, and urinary tract infection; others are listed in Table 190-1. There are no reports of reinfection with *C. botulinum.* Profound hyponatremia has been reported and appears to be secondary to increased secretion of antidiuretic hormone as a result of venous pooling in paralyzed patients.[12]

CONSULTATION

Neurologists can provide guidance in terms of clinical evaluation and diagnostic testing. Infants with incomplete recovery at the time of discharge may benefit from their ongoing involvement. Input from critical care physicians can assist in the assessment of clinical status, including signs of deterioration that warrant transfer to an intensive care setting. Pulmonologists can offer management expertise if respiratory insufficiency develops.

ADMISSION CRITERIA

Infants suffering from botulism are often hospitalized before consideration or confirmation of the diagnosis owing to their worrisome clinical presentation. All infants with suspected or confirmed botulism require hospitalization. The course of the illness is not predictable at the time of presentation; therefore, close observation is required. The hospital should have the capacity to provide full cardiopulmonary support, if needed. Prompt therapy is provided in the inpatient setting.

DISCHARGE CRITERIA

The infant must demonstrate unequivocal and sustained improvement in symptoms. Adequate ventilation must be demonstrated, and ability to protect the airway is essential. Safe and sufficient means for hydration and nutrition must be in place. Most patients can tolerate oral feedings at discharge, but some may go home on a combination of oral and gastric tube feedings. Physical, speech, and occupational therapy may be warranted after discharge to speed recovery, maintain developmental skills, and avoid complications. Standard infection control measures are usually adequate, but ongoing excretion of spores from the stools can continue for months.

Table 190-1 Complications of Infant Botulism

Acute respiratory distress syndrome
Anemia
Aspiration
Bacteremia
Clostridium difficile colitis, including toxic megacolon
Fracture of the femur (nosocomial)
Inappropriate secretion of antidiuretic hormone
Misplaced or plugged endotracheal tube
Otitis media
Pneumonia
Recurrent atelectasis
Seizures secondary to hyponatremia
Sepsis
Pneumothorax, including tension pneumothorax
Tracheal granuloma
Tracheal stenosis
Tracheitis
Tracheomalacia
Transfusion reaction
Urinary tract infection

From *http://www.infantbotulism.org.*

IN A NUTSHELL

- Infant botulism is the most common form of botulism in the United States.
- Infant botulism has a unique pathogenesis. It is caused by colonization of the infant gut with *Clostridium botulinum*, whereas in adults, the disease is caused by ingestion of the preformed toxin.
- Diagnosis is based on the history and physical examination. Although rarely necessary, distinctive findings on the electromyogram can help confirm the diagnosis.
- A specific treatment is now available: BabyBIG. Call the California Department of Health Services at 510-231-7600.
- Management consists of meticulous airway and nutritional support.
- Long-term prognosis is excellent.

ON THE HORIZON

- Bioterrorism is an ongoing threat around the globe. Botulinum toxin is considered a category A (maximum threat) bioweapon.[13] Therefore, a much larger supply of antitoxin is needed, and a recombinant product is under development.[14]

SUGGESTED READING

Arnon SS: Infant botulism. In Feigin RD, Cherry JD, Demmler GJ, Kaplan SL (eds): Textbook of Pediatric Infectious Diseases, 5th ed. Philadelphia, WB Saunders, 2004, pp 1758-1766.

Arnon SS, Schechter R, Maslanka S, et al: Human botulism immune globulin for the treatment of infant botulism. N Engl J Med 2006;354:462-471.

Infant Botulism Treatment and Prevention Program, California Department of Health Services. *http://www.infantbotulism.org.*

REFERENCES

1. Arnon SS: Infant botulism. In Feigin RD, Cherry JD, Demmler GJ, Kaplan SL (eds): Textbook of Pediatric Infectious Diseases, 5th ed. Philadelphia, WB Saunders, 2004, pp 1758-1766.
2. Pickett J, Berg B, Chaplin E, et al: Syndrome of botulism in infancy: Clinical and electrophysiologic study. N Engl J Med 1976;295:770-772.
3. Sugiyama H, Mills D: Intraintestinal toxin in infant mice challenged intragastrically with *Clostridium botulinum* spores. Infect Immun 1978;21:59-63.
4. Long SS: Infant botulism. Pediatr Infect Dis J 2001;20:707-709.
5. Lilly T, Rhodehamel E, Kautter D, Solomon H: *Clostridium botulinum* spores in corn syrup and other syrups. J Food Prot 1991;54:585-587.
6. Arnon S, Damus K, Chin J: Infant botulism: Epidemiology and relation to sudden infant death syndrome. Epidemiol Rev 1981;3:45-66.
7. Infant Botulism Treatment and Prevention Program, California Department of Health Services. *http://www.infantbotulism.org.*
8. Franciosa G, Ferreira J, Hatheway C: Detection of type A, B and E botulism neurotoxin genes in *Clostridium botulinum* and other *Clostridium* species by PCR: Evidence of unexpressed type B toxin genes in type A toxigenic organisms. J Clin Microbiol 1994;32:1911-1916.
9. Arnon SS, Schechter R, Maslanka S, et al: Human botulism immune globulin for the treatment of infant botulism. N Engl J Med 2006;354:462-471.
10. Schreiner M, Field E, Ruddy R: Infant botulism: A review of 12 years' experience at the Children's Hospital of Philadelphia. Pediatrics 1991;87:159-165.
11. Duchen L: Motor nerve growth induced by botulinum toxin as a regenerative phenomenon. Proc R Soc Med 1972;65:196-197.
12. Kurland G, Seltzer J: Antidiuretic hormone excess in infant with botulism. Am J Dis Child 1987;141:1227-1229.
13. Arnon SS: Botulinum toxin as a biological weapon: Medical and public health management. JAMA 2001;285:1059-1070.
14. Nowakowski A: Potent neutralization of botulinum neurotoxin by recombinant oligoclonal antibody. Proc Natl Acad Sci U S A 2002;99:11346-11350.

CHAPTER 191

Biologic, Chemical, and Radiologic Terrorism

Michele R. McKee

The terrorist use of weapons of mass effect predates the catastrophic events of September 11, 2001. Almost a decade earlier another assault on the World Trade Center (the bombing of 1993) included sodium cyanide. Fortunately, the sodium cyanide burned instead of being vaporized. In another bombing event, dissemination of an anticoagulant (rat poison) on a bus in Jerusalem caused a 14-year-old girl to have a refractory bleeding diathesis. The Aum Shinrikyo cult in Japan used anthrax (1993) and sarin (1994 and 1995)—a nerve agent—in three separate attacks on civilians. The 1995 subway attack caused 11 deaths with more than 5500 casualties, including the "worried well." Clearly, such a volume of patients is overwhelming to even the most sophisticated all-hazards response system.

All systems, from hospitals to mobile search and rescue, have implemented enhanced planned responses when dealing with weapons of mass effect. Facility disaster management encompasses a myriad of issues ranging from medical staffing and antidotes to bed surge and alternative facilities. A heightened awareness of mass casualty, including radiation, biologic and chemical exposure, promotes the need for all health care providers to be well versed in rapid identification and management of these cases. Hospitalists are routinely tasked with the acute and chronic care of patients, a unique and important skill set to be used for such an adverse event. Integration of the hospitalist into ongoing education, drills, and facility planning is important for a cohesive, powerful response.

The following overview emphasizes the most commonly cited threats, key parameters helpful in narrowing a differential diagnosis, and mainstays for therapy. There are other more in-depth review articles and consensus guidelines,[1-6] as well as online references.[7-9] These references, in tandem with up-to-date internet sources, can provide a more exhaustive reserve of information.

EPIDEMIOLOGY OF RADIOLOGIC, BIOLOGIC, OR CHEMICAL TERRORISM

The most probable mode of dispersal for a biologic or chemical agent is via an aerosol route. Radiologic exposures might include nuclear reactor site explosions, a conventional bomb to disperse radioactive material (a "dirty bomb"), or nuclear weapons. Traditional mass casualty disaster and hazardous material incident elements would be combined when considering a chemical or radiologic attack. Preparation for such an event goes beyond entity or syndromic recognition. Preparedness now extends to the knowledge and availability of specific antidotes, decontamination, and appropriate personal protective equipment and postevent surveillance for health care providers.

A biologic event has an inherent delay in presentation because of variable incubation times. The point of source and time of exposure will not be as clearly delineated as in chemical or radiologic events. Clues to purposeful biologic exposure include diseases not ordinarily prevalent for a given geographic location and an abrupt increase in the incidence of disease and high degrees of morbidity and mortality. On the surface, a biologic event might not appear to deserve the same acuity of response as a chemical or radiologic event. However, because of potential person-to-person transmission, early, appropriate medications to lessen mortality are of supreme value.

PEDIATRIC VULNERABILITIES

Children have a higher degree of vulnerability because of physiologic, developmental, and psychological differences from the adult population. Pediatric patients have higher minute ventilation and comparably shorter stature, both of which would potentially enhance exposure to airborne culprits such as aerosols or radioactive fallout. Emotional and analytical maturity could thwart a toddler from fleeing danger, or an older child could suffer an increased rate of posttraumatic stress disorder. Children of all ages could be further stressed by issues such as the appearance of hospital providers in personal protective equipment, water decontamination in inclement weather, and medical care taking them away from their parent or caretaker.

CLINICAL PRESENTATIONS, DIAGNOSIS, EVALUATION, AND MANAGEMENT

Biologic Agents

The Centers for Disease Control and Prevention has highlighted six biologic diseases/agents posing the greatest threat: anthrax, smallpox, plague, botulinum toxin, tularemia, and viral hemorrhagic fevers.[10]

These agents possess variable incubation times and pathogenicity. Of considerable note are the few illnesses that can be transmitted from person to person and those requiring early, appropriate medication to lessen morbidity and mortality. In the early stages these illnesses can all appear to mimic nonspecific viral illness—a typical prodrome of fever, fatigue, malaise, and headache—which complicates early recognition. Table 191-1 is an overview of the biologic diseases/agents, clinical and laboratory diagnostics, precautions, and treatments.[11]

Anthrax is caused by *Bacillus anthracis*, a gram-positive sporulating rod that can be manifested as cutaneous, gastrointestinal, or inhalational illness, depending on the vector.

Table 191–1 Biologic Agents of Terrorism

Disease	Etiology	Clinical Findings*	Incubation Period	Diagnostic Samples	Diagnostic Assay	Isolation Precautions	Initial Treatment†	Prophylaxis
Anthrax	*Bacillus anthracis*	Inhalational: febrile prodrome with rapid progression to mediastinal lymphadenitis, mediastinitis (chest radiograph: ± infiltrates, widened mediastinum, pleural effusions), sepsis, shock, meningitis	1–5 days (up to 6 wk?)	Blood CSF Pleural fluid	Culture Gram stain ELISA PCR	Standard	Ciprofloxacin, 10–15 mg/kg (max 400 mg) IV q12h, or Doxycycline, 2.2 mg/kg (max 100 mg) IV q12h†	Ciprofloxacin, 10–15 mg/kg (max 500 mg) PO q12h × 60 days, *or* Doxycycline, 2.5 mg/kg (max 100 mg) PO q12h × 60 days†
		Cutaneous: papule progressing to vesicle, to ulcer, then to depressed black eschar, with marked edema		Skin biopsy	Immunohistochemical assay			
Plague	*Yersinia pestis*	Febrile prodrome with rapid progression to fulminant pneumonia with bloody sputum, sepsis, DIC	2–3 days	Blood Sputum Lymph node aspirate	Culture Gram or Wright-Giemsa stain ELISA IFA Ag-ELISA	Pneumonic: droplet until patient treated for 3 days	Gentamicin, 2.5 mg/kg IV q8h,§ or Doxycycline, 2.2 mg/kg IV (max 100 mg) IV q12h, or Ciprofloxacin, 15 mg/kg (max 500 mg) IV q12h, or Chloramphenicol, 25 mg/kg (max 1 g) q6h	Doxycycline, 2.2 mg/kg (max 100 mg) PO q12h × 7 days, or Ciprofloxacin, 20 mg/kg (max 500 mg) PO q12h × 7days, or Chloramphenicol, 25 mg/kg (max 1 g) PO q6h × 7 days
Smallpox	Variola virus	Febrile prodrome Synchronous vesicopustular eruption, predominantly on the face and extremities	7–17 days	Pharyngeal swab Scab material	ELISA PCR Virus isolation	Airborne, droplet, contact	Supportive care	Vaccination within 4 days (consider vaccinia immunoglobulin, 0.6 mL/kg IM within 3 days of exposure for vaccine complications, immunocompromised persons)

Continued

Table 191–1 Biologic Agents of Terrorism—cont'd

Disease	Etiology	Clinical Findings*	Incubation Period	Diagnostic Samples	Diagnostic Assay	Isolation Precautions	Initial Treatment†	Prophylaxis
Tularemia	*Francisella tularensis*	Pneumonic: abrupt onset of fever, fulminant pneumonia (chest radiograph: prominent hilar adenopathy) Typhoidal: fever, malaise, abdominal pain	2–10 days	Blood Sputum Serum Tissue	Culture Serology: agglutination EM	Standard	Gentamicin, 2.5 mg/kg IV q8h,¶ or Doxycycline, 2.2 mg/kg (max 100 mg) IV q12h, or Ciprofloxacin, 15 mg/kg (max 500 mg) IV q12h, or Chloramphenicol, 15 mg/kg (max 1 g) IV q6h	Doxycycline, 2.2 mg/kg (max 100 mg) PO q12h, or Ciprofloxacin, 15 mg/kg (max 500 mg) PO q12h
Botulism	*Clostridium botulinum* toxin	Afebrile Descending flaccid paralysis Cranial nerve palsies Sensation and mentation intact	1–5 days	Nasal swab?	Mouse bioassay Ag-ELISA	Standard	CDC trivalent antitoxin (serotypes A, B, E), 1 vial (10 mL) IV DOD heptavalent antitoxin (serotypes A–G) (IND) California Dept of Health immunoglobulin (IND)	None
Viral hemorrhagic fevers	Arenaviridae (e.g., Lassa fever) Filoviridae (Ebola, Marburg)	Febrile prodrome; rapid progression to shock, purpura, bleeding diathesis	4–21 days	Serum Blood	Viral isolation Ag-ELISA RT-PCR Serology: Ab-ELISA	Contact, droplet; consider airborne if massive hemorrhage	Supportive care Ribavirin (arenaviruses): 30 mg/kg IV initially, 15 mg/kg IV q6h × 4 days, 7.5 mg/kg IV q8h × 6 days	None

*Syndrome expected after aerosol exposure.
†The Centers for Disease Control and Prevention (CDC) recommended one or two additional antibiotics for inhalational anthrax in the fall 2001 outbreak: rifampin, vancomycin, penicillin or ampicillin, clindamycin, imipenem, or clarithromycin. Recommendations in future outbreaks may evolve rapidly, and frequent consultation with local health departments and the CDC (1-770-488-7100; *www.bt.cdc.gov*) is encouraged.
‡Amoxicillin, 80 mg/kg/day divided every 8 hours, can be substituted if the strain proves susceptible.
§Streptomycin, 15 mg/kg intramuscularly every 12 hours, may be substituted if available.
¶The laboratory must be notified that tularemia is suspected.
CSF, cerebrospinal fluid; DIC, disseminated intravascular coagulation; DOD, Department of Defense; ELISA, enzyme-linked immunosorbent assay; EM, electron microscopy; IFA, immunofluorescent assay; IND, investigational new drug; PCR, polymerase chain reaction; RT-PCR, reverse transcriptase PCR.
Reproduced with permission from Henretig FM, Cieslak TJ, Madsen JM, et al: Emergency department awareness and response to incidents of biological and chemical terrorism. In Fleisher G, Ludwig S, Henretig F (eds): Textbook of Pediatric Emergency Medicine, 5th ed. Philadelphia, Lippincott Williams & Wilkins, 2005, pp 135–162.

Naturally occurring vectors include infected animals or animal products such as unprocessed wool or animal hides. The cutaneous form begins as a papular lesion and rapidly progresses to a vesicle, an ulcer, and then a deep, black eschar with surrounding edema and little associated pain. Inhalational anthrax is similar to flu symptoms in that afflicted patients have fever, malaise, and arthralgias, but with a paucity of upper respiratory symptoms during the prodromal phase. The subsequent phase shows an abrupt onset of severe respiratory symptoms, shock, and necrotizing mediastinitis. A widened mediastinum, infiltrates, and pleural effusions may be evident on chest radiographs. There may be progression to sepsis and meningitis. It is crucial to implement appropriate antibiotic therapy before the onset of fulminant symptoms to lessen mortality.

Smallpox presents with a febrile prodrome followed by a synchronous, centripetally located vesiculopustular exanthem. This disease differs from varicella (chickenpox) in that the rash is synchronous and centripetal and the fever tends to be more pronounced than in uncomplicated varicella. Hypotension and immune complex–associated toxemia contribute to a historical mortality rate near 30%. There is the potential for person-to-person transmission of this highly contagious disease. Postexposure vaccination within 3 to 4 days may prevent or mitigate infection.

Plague is caused by *Yersinia pestis*, a gram-negative coccobacillus that has caused several cases per year in the endemic southwestern United States. Plague may present as a pneumonic or bubonic illness, with potential spread to septicemia. Pneumonic plague presents early with severe respiratory symptoms and complications such as hemoptysis and toxemia and is almost always fatal if not treated within 24 hours of the onset of symptoms. This form of plague can be transmitted from person to person.

Botulism toxin may be used as a terrorist weapon. Natural cases of infant botulism occur throughout the United States, but the majority of cases are clustered in California and a region of eastern Pennsylvania (see Chapter 190). Natural vectors for adult illness include contaminated foods containing preformed toxin or, less frequently, wound contamination. Botulinum toxin blocks neurotransmission by inhibiting the release of presynaptic acetylcholine. Hallmarks of botulism include an afebrile patient with a symmetrical, descending flaccid bulbar and skeletal paralysis. There are no sensory or cognitive changes. Treatment is largely supportive, and a human-derived antitoxin is available.

Tularemia, also known as rabbit fever and deer fly fever, is caused by *Francisella tularensis*, an intracellular gram-negative coccobacillus. The ulceroglandular form presents with a local ulcer and regional lymphadenopathy, fever, chills, headache, and malaise. The typhoidal form includes cough and substernal discomfort. Chest radiographs may show mediastinal lymphadenopathy or pleural effusion. The greatest risk for spread to health care workers is to laboratory staff isolating the prolific bacterium.

Viral hemorrhagic fevers are highly lethal and very contagious. They include Ebola, Marburg, and Lassa fevers. As with many of the other entities, there is a febrile prodrome, but hallmarks of hemorrhagic fever include flushing, conjunctival injection, and petechiae with generalized signs of vascular permeability. Supportive treatment is the mainstay, with the addition of ribavirin for Lassa fever.

Chemical Agents

Chemical weapons include nerve agents, cyanide, vesicants, pulmonary agents, and riot agents. The nerve agents and cyanide can contaminate and affect health care providers and require specific antidotes. The other agents require termination of exposure and supportive therapy. Table 191-2 outlines the primary chemical threats, clinical findings, and treatment.[11]

Nerve agents are organophosphate compounds that inhibit acetylcholinesterase and butyrylcholinesterase (i.e., inhibit acetylcholine degradation). Decontamination (soap and water shower) and removal of contaminated clothing are essential to prevent further exposure to patients and secondary exposure ("off-gassing") to health care providers. Symptoms include miosis, rhinorrhea and sialorrhea (copious secretions), seizures, incontinence, and paralysis. In addition to airway and circulatory support, specific antidote therapy is warranted: atropine to counter the muscarinic effects (end point: drying of secretions), pralidoxime to reverse the agent-acetylcholinesterase bond if irreversible enzyme changes have not occurred (expect prolonged infusions, on the order of days to weeks for severe exposures), and benzodiazepines for seizure control.

Vesicants include mustard and lewisite. Mustard is an alkylating agent that forms cross-links between the double strands of DNA. It has an asymptomatic period for up to hours, although irreversible bonding occurs within minutes. It causes blistering, conjunctivitis, lacrimation, and respiratory irritation ranging from mild upper airway signs to hemorrhagic pulmonary edema. Large exposures can produce gastrointestinal, bone, and central nervous system involvement. The risk of cross-contamination of caregivers warrants decontamination and precautions similar to those for nerve agents. Lewisite causes blisters with more tissue necrosis or sloughing than seen with mustard, conjunctival and lid edema, respiratory irritation, diarrhea, and cardiovascular effects. Treatment includes immediate decontamination, supportive treatment, and use of the antidote dimercaprol (British antilewisite) to promote excretion of the heavy metal by chelation.

Cyanide poisons the electron transport chain and inhibits mitochondrial oxygen utilization. The physical findings are few and nonspecific; seizures develop and patients become apneic with little other symptomatology, including a lack of cyanosis because of poor tissue extraction of oxygen. Therapy includes oxygen, cardiopulmonary resuscitation, and antidotes (sodium nitrite and sodium thiosulfate) to facilitate the formation of methemoglobin and thiocyanate, which is cleared renally. Sodium nitrite dosing is best based on the patient's hemoglobin status; care must be taken to prevent excess formation of methemoglobin. Consequently, mild cases of toxicity may be managed by oxygen and sodium thiosulfate alone.

Radiologic Exposures

Radiation exposure may come from nonexplosive dispersal, a "dirty bomb," conventional attacks on nuclear power plants, or detonation of a nuclear weapon. In general, the radiation exposure to health care workers from patients classified as "walking wounded" carries minimal risk. True nuclear detonation is the exception, with the blast and

Table 191-2   Chemical Agents of Terrorism

Agent	Toxicity	Clinical Findings	Onset	Decontamination*	Management

Nerve agents
  Tabun
  Sarin
  Soman
  VX
	Anticholinesterase: muscarinic, nicotinic, and CNS effects	Vapor: miosis, rhinorrhea, dyspnea
		Liquid: diaphoresis, vomiting
		Both: coma, paralysis, seizures, apnea
			Seconds: vapor
			Minutes-hours: liquid
				Vapor: fresh air, remove clothes, wash hair
				Liquid: remove clothes, copious washing of skin and hair with soap and water, ocular irrigation
					ABCs
					Atropine, 0.05 mg/kg IV,[†] IM[†] (min 0.1 mg, max for a child (0.5 mg, max for an adolescent 1 mg) repeat q2-5min prn for marked secretions, bronchospasm
					
					Pralidoxime, 25 mg/kg IV, IM[§] (max 1 g IV; 2 g IM), may repeat within 30-60 min prn, then again q1h for 1 or 2 doses prn for persistent weakness, high atropine requirement
					Diazepam, 0.3 mg/kg IV (max 10 mg)
					Lorazepam, 0.1 mg/kg IV, IM (max 4 mg)
					Midazolam, 0.2 mg/kg IM (max 10 mg) prn for seizures or severe exposure

Vesicants
  Mustard
 	
  Lewisite
	Alkylation
	
	Arsenical
		Skin: erythema, vesicles
		Eye: inflammation
		Respiratory tract: inflammation
			Hours
			
			Immediate pain with lewisite
				Skin: soap and water
				Eyes: water
				Both: major impact only if done within minutes of exposure
					Symptomatic care
					
					Possibly BAL, 3 mg/kg IM q4-6h, for systemic effects of lewisite in severe cases

Pulmonary agents
  Chlorine
 	
  Phosgene
	Liberate HCl, alkylation	Eyes, nose, throat irritation (especially chlorine)
		Respiratory: bronchospasm, pulmonary edema (especially phosgene)
			Minutes: eyes, nose, throat irritation, bronchospasm
			Hours: pulmonary edema
				Fresh air
				Skin: water
					Symptomatic care

Cyanide	Cytochrome oxidase inhibition: cellular anoxia, lactic acidosis	Tachypnea, coma, seizures, apnea	Seconds	Fresh air Skin: soap and water	ABCs, 100% oxygen Na bicarbonate prn for metabolic acidosis Na nitrite (3%): **Dose (mL/kg) Estimated Hgb (g/dL)** 0.27 10 0.33 12 (est. for average child) 0.39 (max 14 10 mL) Na thiosulfate (25%), 1.65 mL/kg (max 50 mL)

Table 191-2 Chemical Agents of Terrorism—cont'd

Agent	Toxicity	Clinical Findings	Onset	Decontamination*	Management
Riot control agents CS CN (Mace) Capsaicin (pepper spray)	Neuropeptide substance P release, alkylation	Eye: tearing, pain, blepharospasm Nose and throat irritation Pulmonary failure (rare)	Seconds	Fresh air Eyes: lavage	Ophthalmic agents topically, symptomatic care

*Decontamination, especially for patients with significant nerve agent or vesicant exposure, should be performed by health care providers garbed in adequate personal protective equipment. For emergency department staff, this consists of a nonencapsulated, chemically resistant body suit, boots, and gloves with a full-face air purifier mask/hood.

†The intraosseous route is probably equivalent to the intravenous route.

‡Atropine might have some benefit via endotracheal tube or inhalation, as might aerosolized ipratropium. As of July 2004, the Food and Drug Administration has approved pediatric autoinjectors of atropine in 0.25-, 0.5-, and 1-mg sizes. Recommendations are as follows:

Approx Age	Approx Weight	Auoinjector Size
<6 mo	<15 lb	0.25 mg (not available as of this writing, but in development)
6 mo-4 yr	15-40 lb	0.5 mg
5-10 yr	41-90 lb	1 mg
>10 yr	>90 lb	2 mg (adult-sized)

§Pralidoxime is reconstituted to 50 mg/mL (1 g in 20 mL water) for intravenous administration, and the total dose is infused over a 30-minute period or may be given by continuous infusion (loading dose, 25 mg/kg over a 30-minute period, then 10 mg/kg/hr). For intramuscular use, it might be diluted to a concentration of 300 mg/mL (1 g added to 3 mL water—by analogy to the U.S. Army's Mark 1 autoinjector concentration) to achieve a reasonable volume for injection. Pediatric autoinjectors of pralidoxime are not approved by the Food and Drug Administration or available at this time. The Mark 1 autoinjector kits contain 2 mg (0.7 mL) atropine and 600 mg (2 mL) pralidoxime, delivered into two separate intramuscular sites; although not approved for pediatric use, the pralidoxime autoinjector might be considered as initial treatment in dire (especially prehospital) circumstances, for children with severe, life-threatening nerve agent toxicity who lack intravenous access, and for children for whom more precise, mg/kg intramuscular dosing would be logistically impossible. Suggested dosing guidelines are offered; note the potential excess of the initial pralidoxime dose for age/weight, although it is within general guidelines for the recommended total over the first 60 to 90 minutes of therapy for severe exposure:

Approx Age	Approx Weight	Number of Autoinjectors	Pralidoxime Dose Range (mg/kg)
3 –7 yr	13-25 kg	1	24-46
8-14 yr	26-50 kg	2	24-46
>14 yr	>51 kg	3	35 or less

ABCs, airway, breathing, and circulatory support; BAL, British antilewisite; CNS, central nervous system; Hgb, hemoglobin concentration; est., estimated; max, maximum; min, minimum; prn, as needed.

Reproduced with permission from Henretig FM, Cieslak TJ, Madsen JM, et al: Emergency department awareness and response to incidents of biological and chemical terrorism. In Fleisher G, Ludwig S, Henretig F (eds): Textbook of Pediatric Emergency Medicine, 5th ed. Philadelphia, Lippincott Williams & Wilkins, 2005, pp 135-162.

thermal effects and subsequent radiation fallout causing widespread death and morbidity.

Radiation contamination can be local or involve the whole body and is caused by cutaneous contact, inhalation, ingestion, or absorption through the skin. The rapidly dividing cells of the body are those most affected (i.e., bone marrow and intestinal mucosa). High doses also cause injury to the microvasculature, with marked fluid and electrolyte loss contributing to hypovolemic shock and neurologic effects secondary to cerebral vascular leak and edema.

Localized radiation injury, or burns, are associated with direct handling of radioactive sources. Areas of the body most often affected include the hands and buttocks or upper part of the thigh (consider a source in a pants pocket). Radiation burns are similar to thermal burns, but less painful with a latent period. Erythema precedes blistering and subsequent ulceration or tissue necrosis (or both). Treatment is primarily supportive, and overly aggressive débridement should be avoided.

Acute radiation syndrome (Table 191-3)[12] results from penetrating or internal radiation exposure. Symptoms vary with individual radiation sensitivity, the type of radiation, and the dose absorbed. A prodromal phase of nausea, vomiting, diarrhea, fatigue, weakness, fever, and headache begins within 6 to 12 hours after significant exposure. The gastrointestinal manifestations last 24 to 48 hours; however, the fatigue and weakness can persist indefinitely. A latent, relatively asymptomatic phase follows and lasts up to 2 or more weeks, although this latent phase may be absent after severe exposure. Subsequent dose-dependent manifestations include effects on the hematopoietic, gastrointestinal, and neurovascular systems. Treatment is again primarily supportive. Most medical challenges will not occur for days to weeks after the initial presentation.

Hematopoietic Syndrome

Bone marrow injury is seen at doses exceeding 2 Gy. Lymphopenia within 48 hours of exposure serves as a marker of this syndrome. The absolute lymphocyte count obtained soon after exposure can be used to specify the relative degree of exposure; a count less than 1000/mm³ is moderate, whereas a count less than 500/mm³ is severe. Maximal neutropenia and thrombocytopenia usually occur 3 to 4 weeks after exposure, with resultant opportunistic infection and hemorrhage.

Table 191-3 Acute Radiation Syndrome

Phase of Syndrome	Feature	Whole-Body Radiation from External Radiation or Internal Absorption					
		Subclinical Range		Sublethal Range		Lethal Range	
		0-100 cGy (rad)	100-200 cGy (rad)	200-600 cGy (rad)	600-800 cGy (rad)	800-3000 cGy (rad)	>3000 cGy (rad)
Initial or prodromal	Nausea, vomiting	None	5%-50%	50%-100%	75%-100%	90%-100%	100%
	Time of onset		3-6 hr	2-4 hr	1-2 hr	<1 hr	<1 hr
	Duration		<24 hr	<24 hr	<48 hr	<48 hr	<48 hr
	Lymphocyte count			<1000 at 24 hr	<500 at 24 hr		
	Central nervous system function	No impairment	No impairment	Routine task performance Cognitive impairment for 6-20 hr	Simple and routine task performance Cognitive impairment for >24 hr	Progressive incapacitation	
Latent	Duration	>2 wk	7-15 days	0-7 days	0-2 days	None	
"Manifest illness" (obvious illness)	Signs and symptoms	None	Moderate leukopenia	Severe leukopenia, purpura, hemorrhage Pneumonia Hair loss after 300 cGy	Diarrhea Fever Electrolyte disturbance	Convulsions Ataxia Tremor Lethargy	
	Time of onset	>2 wk	>2 wk	2 days-2 wk	2-3 days	1-48 hr	
	Critical period	None	None	4-6 wk	5-14 days		
	Organ system	None		Hematopoietic and respiratory (mucosal) systems	GI tract Mucosal systems	CNS	
Hospitalization	Percent	0%	<5%	90%	100%	100%	
	Duration	0%	45-60 days	60-90 days	90+ days	2 wk	2 days
Fatality	Percent	0%	0%	0%-80%	90%-100%	90%-100%	100%
	Time to death			3 wk-3 mo	1-2 wk	1-2 days	

Available at: *http://www.homelandsecurityweekly.com/7.05.04.html.*

Table 191-4   Potassium Iodide Therapy after Radioactive Iodide Exposure

Patient Age	Predicted Thyroid Exposure (cGy)	KI dose (mg)	No. 130-mg Tablets	No. 65-mg Tablets
>40 yr*	≥500	130	1	2
>18-40 yr	≥10	130	1	2
Pregnant or lactating	≥5	130	1	2
>12-18 yr[†]	≥5	65	$^1/_2$	1
>3-12 yr	≥5	65	$^1/_2$	1
>1 mo-3 yr[†]	≥5	32	$^1/_4$	$^1/_2$
Birth-1 mo[†§]	≥5	16	$^1/_8$	$^1/_4$

Side effects may also include gastrointestinal distress, rash, and sialadenitis.

*Older patients are more likely to suffer side effects from KI, including iodine-induced thyrotoxicosis, goiter, and hypothyroidism in iodide-deficient areas.

[†]Adolescents approaching 70 kg or more should be given the full adult dose (130 mg).

[†]Infants may be given KI as a fresh saturated solution diluted in milk, formula, or water.

[§]Neonates should have thyroid-stimulating hormone and free levothyroxine (T$_4$) monitored, with free T$_4$ replacement therapy as needed.

From U.S. FDA Center for Drug Evaluation and Research Guidance: Potassium Iodide as a Thyroid Blocking Agent in Radiation Emergencies Rockville, MD, November 2001.

Gastrointestinal Syndrome

A recurrence of nausea, vomiting, and diarrhea at about 1 week or less after the prodromal phase is seen in exposures of 6 to 30 Gy. Sepsis quickly follows, along with metabolic disturbances and a very high incidence of mortality.

Neurovascular Syndrome

Seen with doses in excess of 30 Gy, neurovascular syndrome is characterized by the nearly immediate development of nausea, vomiting, and prostration, quickly followed by shock, ataxia, and seizures. Diffuse vascular injury leads to hypotension and cerebral edema. Death generally occurs within several days.

External, inhaled, ingested, or absorbed radioactive contamination is the only form of radiation exposure that presents a risk to health care workers; the danger is minimal in treating patients during transport to local facilities. External contamination is rarely a significant risk, even to the patient directly. However, when possible, decontamination along with disrobement is recommended before further medical care. Providers should be garbed in attire that adheres to traditional universal precautions for treating life-threatening conditions. Wrapping patients in cloth sheets can aid in minimizing contamination of the facility. The treatment area should have controlled access. Radiation counters can aid in assessing both the degree and effectiveness of decontamination. Decontamination via clothing removal is about 80% to 90% effective in and of itself and is augmented by washing with soap and water. Gentle washing is recommended to avoid abrading the skin, and extra attention should be given to the hair, face, hands, skin folds, and area under nails. Open wounds should be covered to avoid internal contamination, and wounds that are already contaminated should be irrigated and treated conventionally. Skin closure should be performed as soon as possible with exposures exceeding 1 Gy to mitigate opportunistic infection when bone narrow suppression occurs.

Decontamination from internal exposure involves the use of several generic principles: reduction of absorption, enhancement of elimination, chelation, and blockage or displacement by nonradioactive materials. Potassium iodide (KI) is used to prevent the accumulation of radioactive iodine in the thyroid. Treatment with KI as soon as possible within 24 hours after exposure is indicated as an adjunct to evacuation, sheltering, and containment of contaminated food. The protective effects of KI last approximately 24 hours, and it can be redosed daily in most individuals until a significant risk of exposure no longer exists. Careful monitoring for hypothyroidism is indicated, especially in newborns or infants. Pregnant or lactating females also deserve special consideration in that redosing of KI may be contraindicated for this population. It should be used only at the suggestion of local authorities while carefully weighing radiation exposure against newborn or unborn hypothyroidism and mental retardation (Table 191-4).[13] Readers are encouraged to also seek current recommendations because a more uniform dose, regardless of patient age, may be quoted as an aid to rapid mass administration.

PREVENTION

Education on the "exotic" entities of radiation, biologic, or chemical exposure coupled with keen public awareness of the terrorist threat could lead to early recognition and treatment by health care workers. Hospitalists may be asked to perform roles ranging from decontamination outside the emergency department doors in personal protective equipment to management of prolonged pralidoxime infusions. Ongoing education and participation in facility disaster drills will enable the hospitalist to be prepared for such all-hazards threats.

IN A NUTSHELL

- The most probable mode of dispersal for a biologic or chemical agent is via an aerosol route.
- In unwitnessed or unsuspected terrorist exposures, providers may be well poised to recognize atypical patterns and unusual distribution of illness that could be manifestations of an event.

- Beyond recognition of exposure, preparedness includes knowledge and availability of specific antidotes, decontamination, appropriate personal protective equipment, and postevent surveillance for health care providers.
- The six biologic diseases/agents that are considered to pose the greatest terrorist threat are anthrax, smallpox, plague, botulinum toxin, tularemia, and viral hemorrhagic fevers.
- Exposure to chemical and radiation agents often requires decontamination to arrest primary and secondary spread.

ON THE HORIZON

- Updates to antimicrobial therapies to counter engineered or natural resistance
- Availability of autoinjectors beyond atropine to aid in rapid, mass treatment
- Additional "standardized" radiation treatments as we extend our concerns beyond radioactive iodine

SUGGESTED READING

Henretig FM, Cieslak TJ, Madsen JM, et al: Emergency department awareness and response to incidents of biological and chemical terrorism. In Fleisher G, Ludwig S, Henretig F (eds): Textbook of Pediatric Emergency Medicine, 5th ed. Philadelphia, Lippincott Williams & Wilkins, 2005, pp 135-162.

Henretig FM, McKee MR: Preparedness for acts of nuclear, biological and chemical terrorism. In Gausche-Hill M, Fuchs S, Yamamoto L (eds): APLS The Pediatric Emergency Medicine Resource, 4th ed. Sudbury, MA, AAP and ACEP, Jones & Bartlett, 2003, pp 568-591.

REFERENCES

1. Inglesby TV, Henderson DA, Bartlett JG, et al: Anthrax as a biological weapon: Medical and public health management [consensus statement]. JAMA 1999;281:1735-1745.
2. Henderson DA, Inglesby TV, Bartlett JG, et al: Smallpox as a biological weapon: Medical and public health management [consensus statement]. JAMA 1999;281:2127-2137.
3. Inglesby TV, Dennis DT, Henderson DA, et al: Plague as a biological weapon: Medical and public health management [consensus statement]. JAMA 2000;283:2281-2290.
4. Arnon SS, Schechter R, Inglesby TV, et al: Botulinum toxin as a biological weapon: Medical and public health management [consensus statement]. JAMA 2001;285:1059-1070.
5. Dennis DT, Inglesby TV, Henderson DA, et al: Tularemia as a biological weapon: Medical and public health management [consensus statement]. JAMA 2001;285:2763-2773.
6. Inglesby TV, O'Toole T, Henderson DA, et al: Anthrax as a biological weapon, 2002: Updated recommendations for management. JAMA 2002;287:2236-2252.
7. U.S. Army Medical Research Institute of Infectious Diseases (USAMRIID). Available at http:/www.usamriid.army.mil.
8. U.S. Army Medical Research Institute of Chemical Defense (USAMRICD). Available at http:/ccc.apgea.army.mil.
9. Armed Forces Radiobiology Research Institute (AFRRI). Available at http:/www.afrri.usuhs.mil.
10. Centers for Disease Control and Prevention (CDC). Available at http://www.bt.cdc.gov/agent/agentlist-category.asp#adef.
11. Henretig FM, Cieslak TJ, Madsen JM, et al: Emergency department awareness and response to incidents of biological and chemical terrorism. In Fleisher G, Ludwig S, Henretig F (eds): Textbook of Pediatric Emergency Medicine, 5th ed. Philadelphia, Lippincott Williams & Wilkins, 2005, pp 135-162.
12. Terrorism with Ionizing Radiation General Guidance Pocket Guide. Bethesda, MD, USAFRRI, 2001. Available at http://www.afrri.usuhs.mil/www/outreach/pdf/pcktcard.pdf.
13. U.S. FDA Center for Drug Evaluation and Research Guidance: Potassium Iodide as a Thyroid Blocking Agent in Radiation Emergencies. Rockville, MD, November 2001. Available at http://www.fda.gov/cder/guidance/index.htm.

Care of the Medically Complex Child

CHAPTER 192

Introduction to the Medically Complex Child

Sherri L. Adams and Sanjay Mahant

A recent survey in the United States demonstrated a growing number of children with special health care needs (CSHCN).[1] These children require special, comprehensive medical care and resources that traditional medical systems may be ill equipped to provide. The pediatric hospitalist is often central to the care of medically complex children who require frequent hospitalization. This chapter provides an overview of various definitions that apply to medically complex children, discusses the principles of caring for this population, and examines the role of the pediatric hospitalist in managing these children.

DEFINITIONS AND DEMOGRAPHICS

There is no formally accepted definition of *medically complex children*. Accepted definitions exist for *technologically dependent children* and *children with special health care needs,* with CSHCN being one of the most commonly used terms. Other terms include *children with multiple impairments* and *medically fragile children*. Children with multiple impairments are those with significant physical disabilities combined with sensory or cognitive deficits.[2] Medically fragile children are complex, fragile, technology-dependent CSHCN; however, children who do not require technology can be medically fragile as well. Technologically dependent children are those who require both medical devices to compensate for the loss of a vital body function and significant and sustained care to avert death or further disability.[3]

The Maternal and Child Health Bureau (MCHB) and the American Academy of Pediatrics (AAP) define CSHCN as "those who have or are at increased risk for chronic physical, developmental, behavioral, or emotional conditions and who require health and related services of a type or amount beyond that required by children generally."[4] According to a national survey, CSHCN account for 12.8% of the pediatric population in the United States.[1] In addition, the survival rate of chronically ill children is increasing. On average, 90% of children with chronic illnesses will reach their 20th birthdays.[5] This poses an enormous challenge to health care providers and the health care system. Children with chronic health conditions have annual health care costs that are more than five times that of healthy children.[6]

CARE COORDINATION AND THE MEDICAL HOME

Care coordination is defined by the MCHB and the AAP as "a process that links CSHCN and their families to services and resources in a coordinated effort to maximize the potential of the children and provide them with optimal health care."[7] It is a proactive process that should be implemented in various settings in conjunction with the family and the child's care providers.[8] Care coordination is best exemplified when a patient's care plan is understood and followed by all care providers and programs. Care coordination involves many settings, including the health care system, the educational system, the social services and public health system, and the home setting.

The concept of a medical home embodies the ideal situation for the provision of comprehensive care. The medical home should be accessible, continuous, comprehensive, family centered, coordinated, compassionate, and culturally effective.[9] It should be centered around the child and located in the most suitable environment. Key to the medical home is the partnership of trust and responsibility between the child and his or her family and the physician and the health care team. All aspects of care can be managed or facilitated through this partnership. Ensuring that all CSHCN have a primary care physician on discharge is just one way to promote the medical home and prevent the inappropriate use of emergency rooms and walk-in clinics and subsequent unnecessary treatment.

The AAP refers to care coordination and the medical home in the context of the primary care pediatrician; however, these concepts can be implemented by any care provider who is familiar with the system and the child's and family's needs. Because medically complex children often have multiple entry points into the health care system, care coordination is often best facilitated by the care provider with whom they have the most contact. Other care providers, such as pediatric nurse practitioners, may also be good choices to coordinate the care of CSHCN.

Table 192-1 Components of the Standard Care Plan

Patient's name, nickname

Date of birth

Hospital number

Allergies

Wishes about cardiopulmonary resuscitation (if applicable)

Primary diagnosis
   Common presenting problems
   Suggested management
   Relevant physical examination findings

Secondary diagnoses
   Related information (e.g., gastrostomy tube feeding,
    ventilator setting, physiotherapy needs)
   Relevant physical examination findings

Medication list

Hospital and community contacts (e.g., pediatric hospitalist,
  pediatrician, pediatric nurse practitioner, interdisciplinary
  team members, specialists)

Family contact information

Home-care providers' contact information (e.g., nurses,
  therapists)

CARE PLANNING AND EMERGENCY PREPAREDNESS

Medically complex children have frequent admissions to the hospital. Therefore, care coordination and emergency preparedness are preventive strategies that can improve the quality and efficiency of patient care. Emergency preparedness is the concept of preparing a patient and family for potential life-threatening events that require emergency intervention.[10] One of the most useful ways to assist families is to create a care plan that includes emergency and general care information. For such information to continue to be useful once the child has entered the health care system, it must be revised on a regular basis. Table 192-1 lists the components of a standard care plan. Other items, such as a detailed medical history, relevant social information, and information regarding inpatient care, may facilitate care during repeat admissions to the hospital.

THE PEDIATRIC HOSPITALIST AND THE INPATIENT TEAM

The pediatric hospitalist can play an integral role in the care of medically complex children. To ensure continuity and consistency of care, such children benefit from one inpatient care provider who is familiar with all their issues and can oversee their care. These children often have multisystem disease, require frequent inpatient admissions, have chronic illnesses, are technologically dependent, and require significant nursing care and services at home. For example, a child with cerebral palsy and severe neurologic impairment typically has multisystem medical problems that require hospitalization. Such a child often has admissions for seizures, gastroesophageal reflux and nutritional manage-

ment, aspiration pneumonia, and intercurrent illnesses. On one level, these children are diverse, with different underlying disease processes, age of onset of illness, need for technologic assistance, and types of disability. However, these diverse disease processes have common themes that lead to similar life experiences for these children and their families. The pediatric hospitalist and multidisciplinary team must appreciate these common themes to provide comprehensive and family-centered care.

Caring for this population of children is often difficult. There may be a lack of continuity in care, both within the hospital and in the outpatient setting. A number of subspecialists may be involved, each one focusing on a specific system or problem. However, there may be no cohesive team that manages the child and the family from the generalist perspective. There is often a lack of coordination in terms of appointments and investigations, as well as a lack of communication among the various health care providers. This can lead to duplication and inappropriate use of resources. Families often require help navigating the health care system and gaining access to resources. These families are often socially isolated and have stressed support systems.[11]

The pediatric hospitalist and a multidisciplinary team can play an important role in overseeing the care of these children and their families. In the inpatient setting, the pediatric hospitalist is ideally positioned to direct the care of a medically complex child. As a generalist, the hospitalist can assess all aspects of the patient's care rather than just one specific system. The hospitalist should direct and provide the framework for care, especially when multiple specialists are involved. The hospitalist should evaluate recommendations and help the family make decisions about tests and treatment. The hospitalist is also the one who sees the patient on a daily basis and communicates with the patient and the family. However, the hospitalist cannot do this alone. An ideal model of care includes not only the medical specialties but also other professional services, such as advance practice nurses, social workers, dietitians, therapists, and others.

IN A NUTSHELL

- Medically complicated children are an important and growing subset of children with special health care needs, especially within the field of inpatient pediatrics.
- Care coordination, medical home, and emergency preparedness are important principles for these children.
- The hospitalist is ideally positioned to provide care coordination and deal with multiple specialists in the context of a medical home.

ON THE HORIZON

- Topics for future research in this area include (1) tools for the prospective identification of medically complex children, (2) interaction between patients and the health care system and communication during transitions of care (e.g., outpatient to inpatient settings, intensive care unit to ward), (3) the quality of inpatient care, and (4) opportunities to improve care.

SUGGESTED READING

American Academy of Pediatrics, Committee on Children with Disabilities: Care coordination: Integrating health and related systems of care for children with special health care needs. Pediatrics 1999;104:978-981.

Lindeke LL, Leonard BJ, Presler B, Garwick A: Family centered care coordination for children with special needs across multiple settings. J Pediatr Health Care 2002;16:290-297.

REFERENCES

1. Centers for Disease Control and Prevention, National Center for Health Statistics: National Survey of Children with Special Health Care Needs (state and local area integrated telephone survey), 2001.

2. International Classification of Impairments, Disabilities and Handicaps: A Manual of Classification Relating to the Consequences of Diseases. Geneva, World Health Organization, 1980.

3. Wegner J, Power E, Fox H: Technology Dependent Children: Hospital versus Home Care. Office of Technology Assessment Task Force. Philadelphia, Lippincott, 1988.

4. McPherson M, Arango P, Fox H, et al: A new definition of children with special health care needs. Pediatrics 1998;102:137-140.

5. Blum R: Transitioning to adult health care: Setting the stage. J Adolesc Health 1995;17:3-5.

6. Hoffman C, Rice D, Sung HY: Persons with chronic conditions: Their prevalence and costs. JAMA 1996;276:1473-1479.

7. American Academy of Pediatrics, Committee on Children with Disabilities: Care coordination: Integrating health and related systems of care for children with special health care needs. Pediatrics 1999;104:978-981.

8. Jackson PL, Vessey JA: Primary Care and the Child with a Chronic Condition, 4th ed. St Louis, Mosby, 2004.

9. American Academy of Pediatrics, Medical Home Initiatives for Children with Special Needs Project Advisory Committee: The medical home. Pediatrics 2004;113:1545-1547.

10. Committee on Pediatric Emergency Medicine: Emergency preparedness for children with special health needs. Pediatrics 1999;104:1-6.

11. Ratliffe CE, Harrigan RC, Haley J, et al: Stress in families with medically fragile children. Issues Comprehens Pediatr Nurs 2002;25;167-188.

CHAPTER 193

Acute Care of the Medically Complex Child

Nancy Murphy and Lisa Samson-Fang

In the United States, there are 12.6 million children with special health care needs (CSHCN).[1] Because of the dynamic and fragile nature of their medical conditions, acute or chronic hospitalization is not uncommon. This population's inpatient needs are complex and different from those of children without underlying chronic conditions. This chapter presents a general, family-centered approach to the care of medically complex children and discusses the role of the multidisciplinary team, unique aspects of the history and physical examination, and the multifaceted nature of the medical assessment and treatment planning for CSHCN, including pharmacologic, nutritional, developmental, and familial needs.

FAMILY-CENTERED APPROACH

Children with complex health conditions and their families are experienced consumers of in-hospital care. Optimally, these children are cared for with a family-centered approach. Although many institutions strive to provide all children with this type of care, it is believed to be crucial for children whose medical issues have far-reaching implications for the family. The concept of family-centered care as described by the American Academy of Pediatrics includes physician recognition of key family members and their values and shared decision making between medical providers and families[2] (Table 193-1). Family-centered care begins when the hospitalist discusses the child's medical history and establishes rapport with the parents, who should be regarded as the experts in their child's condition. Parents can provide meaningful and unique information, such as tips on successful feeding approaches, optimal positions to promote sleep or inhibit involuntary movements, and how to interpret the communications of children with dysarthria.

SPECIFIC COMPLEXITIES

Multidisciplinary Care Coordination

Multidisciplinary care is the delivery of coordinated and goal-directed interventions by a team of skilled clinicians with myriad skills. CSHCN often require the expertise of multiple consultants, including medical, nursing, rehabilitation, and nutrition specialists. A key responsibility of the pediatric hospitalist is care coordination, including the facilitation of medical team and family meetings when appropriate. The hospitalist serves as the primary communicator of the child's diagnoses, acuity, plans for ongoing hospitalization, and discharge planning with the child, family, and primary care physician.[3]

Children with special medical needs or dependence on medical technology have higher rates of hospital-reported medical errors.[4] A hospitalist who carefully coordinates family-centered and multidisciplinary care can minimize such events.

Multiple Organ System Involvement

CSHCN frequently present with the involvement of multiple systems. For example, a child with cystic fibrosis may present with pulmonary, gastrointestinal, endocrinologic, and nutritional issues. Optimal management requires a systematic approach and an awareness of the interplay of these systems. Although numerous specialists may be involved, each views the child's illness from his or her unique perspective. Hospitalists, in collaboration with families, understand these interactions, set priorities, and manage from the standpoint of the global perspective.

Multiple Medications

The avoidance of drug interactions, the early recognition of adverse drug effects, and the prevention and early detection of secondary complications are critical roles for the hospitalist. On admission, each child's medications should be reviewed. When many medications have been prescribed, the potential for error increases, and careful attention to doses and dosing schedules is imperative. It is important to record the indication for each medication. For example, valproic acid may be prescribed for aggressive outbursts and gabapentin for neuropathic pain syndromes. The assumption that either of these medications is administered to treat a seizure disorder could be an error. During the usual review of food and drug allergies, the hospitalist should explore each child's history of latex reactions, especially among those who have had multiple reactions. A review of the home medication schedule can reveal meaningful information, such as administration of phenytoin with meals rather than nonadherence to explain subtherapeutic blood levels.[5] Providing medications in liquid or tablet form according to the preference of the child and family promotes comfort and confidence in the health care team. It is wise not to interrupt medications that have been given on a long-term basis to avoid the risk of withdrawal syndromes. For example, abrupt cessation of baclofen can lead to rebound spasticity, acute agitation, and seizures. Use of complementary and alternative medicines and over-the-counter medications should also be discussed.

Complicated Physical Examination

CSHCN are more likely to have abnormalities on the baseline physical examination, making assessment difficult if the hospitalist has not met the child previously. Children with neurodevelopmental disabilities who are particularly stressed by unfamiliar settings and medical providers can be especially hard to assess. Parental input can be invaluable in

Table 193-1 Principles of Family-Centered Care

Be respectful
Honor racial, ethnic, cultural, and socioeconomic diversity
Recognize and build on the family's strengths
Support and facilitate choice
Ensure flexibility in organizational policies, procedures, and provider practices to accommodate the family's needs and cultural values
Share honest and unbiased information that is ongoing, useful, and affirming
Provide or ensure formal and informal support (e.g., family-to-family support)
Collaborate at all levels of health care, including professional education, policy making, and program development
Empower the family to discover its own strengths, build confidence, and make choices and health care decisions

providing information regarding the child's baseline and any change from that baseline. Engaging in a few minutes of reassurance and play before the examination allows the hospitalist to observe developmental and functional skills while providing the child time to acclimate to a new situation.

A systematic and detailed approach to each child with a complex condition and a careful documentation of findings and medical plans require an investment of the hospitalist's time on admission, but this can expedite the hospital stay by streamlining communications among consultants and various team members. During lengthy hospitalizations, the admitting document also provides a basis to detect changes in status.

Nutritional Issues

CSHCN often have special dietary needs and an underlying vulnerability to nutritional compromise. On admission, historical information should include details of the child's feeding program, including route (e.g., oral, tube feedings), modifications to diet (e.g., altered texture), specialized supplements (e.g., formulas, vitamins, herbs), and feeding schedule. If a child has significant dysphagia, it is important to determine whether and how the child is fed orally. Parents may be using special cups, spoons, nipples, oral stimulation techniques, or positioning strategies to facilitate feeding. These procedures need to be replicated throughout the hospitalization, or the child might not eat for staff.

Hospitalized CSHCN should have baseline nutritional assessments and periodic reassessments during prolonged stays. In addition to plotting height and weight on a standard growth curve, for certain populations (e.g., those with Down syndrome), growth parameters should be plotted on specialized growth curves, and data points should be obtained from prior evaluations. For some children, detailed assessments by nutritional specialists are indicated, including measurements of skinfold thickness, serum nutritional markers such as albumin and prealbumin, segmental measures (e.g., in patients with contractures or scoliosis, in whom

height is not a reliable measure), and vitamin levels. The child's usual feeding program or typical diet may need to be modified based on current nutritional status or to accommodate periods when the child is not allowed intake because of scheduled procedures. The intake of calories and fluids should be monitored regularly, and the hospitalist should intervene with enteral feedings or hyperalimentation when nutritional intake or status is deemed inadequate.

Technology Needs

CSHCN frequently use technology and specialized adaptive equipment in their everyday lives (see Chapter 195). Other equipment may be required to allow the child mobility, minimize the development of musculoskeletal complications, or promote independence in activities of daily living and environmental control. Whenever possible, children with functional limitations who use adaptive equipment at home and in the community should be encouraged to do so while hospitalized to maximize their sense of control, independence, and participation. The family should be encouraged to bring the child's assistive devices, such as walkers or wheelchairs, to the hospital. If the child's usual equipment cannot be obtained, loaner equipment should be sought through physical and occupational therapy consultation. If ankle-foot orthoses or other braces are worn on a nightly basis at home to prevent deformity, they should be used on the same schedule during hospitalization to prevent secondary complications of the acute condition.

Ancillary Staff Support

A wide variety of hospital professionals is available for consultative support, and in the case of CSHCN, their input is critical (Table 193-2). The hospitalist should be aware of the various skills of the team members, how they can help in the care of medically complex children, and when to consult them.

Developmental and Behavioral Concerns

For CSHCN, repeated or prolonged hospitalization can impact psychological development. During infancy, prolonged hospitalization places children at risk for attachment disorders. Toddlers may experience behavioral regression. Adolescents, whose major psychological developmental task is separation and individuation, experience increased dependence. The medical team can support and promote the psychological development of children with complex needs as they confront these challenges during hospitalization.

Education is another aspect of development that is impacted by repeated and prolonged hospitalization. Efforts are necessary to prevent the child from losing educational ground. When the child's clinical status permits, schoolwork should continue at the bedside. For children with recurrent hospitalizations (e.g., those with cystic fibrosis), preemptive educational plans should be in place. For children experiencing acute changes in function (e.g., after a head or spinal cord injury), a plan should be in place before discharge to determine how and when the child will return to school. Parents need information about how to deal with school systems to obtain the services needed to meet their child's unique needs. This might include special educational programming through an individualized educational plan (IEP)

Table 193-2   Roles of Ancillary Staff

Health Care Professional	Risks for Medically Complex Children	Reasons to Consult
Physical therapist	Children limited to bed rest are at increased risk for complications of immobility, including muscle atrophy, joint contractures, decubitus ulcers, deep venous thrombosis, constipation, atelectasis	Provide wheelchairs, ambulation aids, transfer equipment, or mobility training Facilitate transitions from hospital to home by coordinating home equipment needs (e.g., hospital bed, rented or purchased wheelchair) Educate families in individualized programs of home exercise, provide strategies to overcome architectural barriers in the home and community, oversee adequacy of car seats and transportation systems Identify physical therapy needs after discharge
Occupational therapist	Prolonged hospitalization may impact self-care skills	Address feeding issues, positioning, and environmental control during the hospital stay Evaluate and treat children who lack age-appropriate skills and attitudes for independent feeding, self-care, play, and school performance
Speech-language pathologist	Condition-specific needs (e.g., failure to thrive, risk of aspiration, tracheostomy)	Facilitate the child's expression and staff's interpretation of basic needs, including hunger, pain, toileting, fatigue, stress Enhance communication with use of augmentative devices, gestures, signing Provide multidisciplinary treatment, along with respiratory therapists and physicians, in promoting communication and feeding skills in children with tracheostomies In some institutions, speech pathologists investigate the safety of oral intake and optimal feeding interfaces, especially for infants
Respiratory therapist	Children with generalized muscular weakness or incoordination are at risk for hospital-acquired and aspiration pneumonia Condition-specific needs (e.g., cystic fibrosis)	Decrease the occurrence and limit the severity of respiratory complications through chest physical therapy, assisted coughing techniques, postural drainage interventions
Child life specialist, psychologist	Chronically or repeatedly hospitalized children are at risk for psychological and developmental problems	Work one-on-one with children and their families to explain the child's perspective, provide normalization activities, teach coping strategies Aid the staff in creating bedside behavioral or developmental programs to minimize the impact of hospitalization Help children cope during specific procedures
Social work	Chronic or recurrent health care needs affect families emotionally, physically, and economically	Assess stressors and identify available supports and resources Assist families in applying for financial resources such as Medicaid and Social Security Provide emotional support at the bedside as families confront grief and loss, and educate families on how to emotionally support siblings and spouses during hospitalization Serve as a family advocate when conflict or confusion arises, and help families solve problems during periods of crisis
Discharge planner, case manager, home-care coordinator	Children may need many services and equipment for home care Admissions may be prolonged if proper resources are not in place at home	Organize funding (with social worker) for services and equipment Explain issues related to funding, and facilitate home-care or long-term care placements

Table 193-2   Roles of Ancillary Staff—cont'd

Health Care Professional	Risks for Medically Complex Children	Reasons to Consult
Dietitian	Specialized feeding regimens include enteral or parenteral nutrition	Lead nutritional aspects of inpatient care (total parenteral nutrition, enteral feeding) Provide education to care providers and family regarding nutritional aspects of care
Pharmacist	Multiple medications result in increased potential interactions and side effects	Monitor drugs at admission and discharge to minimize errors due to transitions in care settings Provide hospitalist and family with information on medication options, dosing, potential side effects, contraindications, cost, interactions, administration
Teacher	School year or semester often jeopardized due to frequent admissions	Provide education to hospitalized child, in conjunction with current education outside of hospital

or physical accommodations through a health or 504 plan. For children unable to return to school in the short term (e.g., a child with cardiomyopathy on strict bed rest), the hospitalist has the important duty of prescribing homebound education and determining the appropriate time for community-based school reentry.

Children with underlying cognitive or behavioral impairments may endanger their own safety when removed from familiar routines and environments. The treatment team has the responsibility of ensuring the safety of each child in the hospital. This may require environmental modifications such as direct observation, physical restraint devices such as enclosed beds, pharmacologic restraints, or behavioral programs.

Unmet Needs

CSHCN have more unmet medical needs than do typically developing children.[6] Because hospitalists and specialists provide most of their care, primary care issues may be overlooked. It is therefore particularly important to review the immunization records of medically complex children. The hospitalist can provide immunizations against influenza or pneumococcal infections or prophylaxis against severe infections with respiratory syncytial virus during winter months. For a child with unaddressed developmental delays, the hospital admission may present a critical opportunity to obtain early intervention, discuss eligibility for Social Security, or explore community-based services for recreation and socialization.

Advance Planning

Given the complexity of their conditions, advance planning is vital in the optimal management of hospitalized CSHCN. Hospitalists often engage in discussions about advance directives with medically complex patients and their families (see also Chapters 12 and 196).

IN A NUTSHELL

* Hospitalists who care for medically complex children should render family-centered, coordinated, and multidisciplinary care.
* Hospitalists should be aware of the unique aspects of the history, physical examination, medications, and nutritional, technologic, and developmental needs of these children.
* Hospitalists need an increased awareness of the value of all potential team members involved in the care of these children.

SUGGESTED READING

AAP policy statement: Family centered care and the pediatrician's role. Pediatrics 2003;112:691-696.
Percelay JM, Committee on Hospital Care: Physician's role in coordinating care of hospitalized children. Pediatrics 2003;111:707-709.

REFERENCES

1. Newacheck P, Strickland B, Shonkoff JP, et al: An epidemiologic profile of children with special health care needs. Pediatrics 1998;102:117-123.
2. AAP policy statement: Family centered care and the pediatrician's role. Pediatrics 2003;112:691-696.
3. Percelay JM, Committee on Hospital Care: Physician's role in coordinating care of hospitalized children. Pediatrics 2003;111:707-709.
4. Slonim AD, LaFleur BJ, Ahmed W, Joseph JG: Hospital reported medical errors in children. Pediatrics 2003;111:617-621.
5. Sacchetti A, Sacchetti C, Carraccio C, Gerardi M: The potential errors in children with special health care needs. Acad Emerg Med 2000;7:1330-1333.
6. Mayer ML, Skinner AC, Slifkin RT: Unmet need for routine and specialty care: Data from the National Survey of Children with Special Health Care Needs. Pediatrics 2004;113:109-115.

CHAPTER 194

Common Reasons for Admission

Raj Srivastava, Sherri Adams, and Nancy Murphy

With increasing pressure from managed care to decrease length of stay, the advent of observation units in emergency departments, and a change in the mind-set of clinicians regarding what can be treated on an outpatient basis (e.g., home oxygen use for bronchiolitis, home intravenous therapy), the nature of inpatient pediatrics has changed. Recently, there has been a shift in the relative proportion of children who present with common versus uncommon conditions, and more complex children with a variety of acute and chronic medical problems are being hospitalized. These children may need technologic support and may have multisystem diseases and varying degrees of functional, social, or communication impairments. They are frequently cared for by an array of specialists in both the inpatient and the outpatient setting.

When children with complex medical conditions present to the emergency department, they are often admitted to the hospital. Because their care is so complex and many of their chief complaints cannot be easily addressed, further inpatient evaluation and management may be warranted. Also, the emergency physician may not know the child and his or her baseline functional or general health status, increasing the complexity of medical decision making.

A comprehensive approach to the inpatient care of children with complex medical needs is essential to deliver effective, efficient, and family-centered care that best meets the multifaceted needs of this special population. Families of children with special health care needs are typically frequent users of the health care system and benefit from the involvement of pediatric hospitalists who can skillfully communicate and coordinate care throughout the entire hospital stay.

POPULATION

It is difficult to precisely define children with complex medical needs. They are often placed into categories such as technology-dependent children, children with multisystem disease processes, children with neurologic impairments, and children with special health care needs (see Chapter 192). Although research into the prospective identification of such children is limited, the astute hospitalist should be aware of which children meet the criteria for medical complexity. The pediatric hospitalist also needs to recognize the special concerns that are pertinent to children with medically complex conditions and meet the needs of this population in the following ways:

- Understand the child's baseline functional status by interviewing the child, family members, outpatient physicians, specialists, therapists, educators, and others.
- Recognize that a child may have multiple reasons for admission.
- Employ an evidence-based approach to care.

- Prioritize goals for admission, knowing that not all issues need to be resolved during the hospitalization.
- Ensure timely transitions to community-based care and consistent communication with outpatient health care providers.

The largest single group of medically complex patients the hospitalist is likely to encounter consists of children with neurologic impairments due to congenital or acquired conditions (e.g., disorders of neuronal migration, intraventricular hemorrhage associated with prematurity, trauma). These children often have developmental delays, cerebral palsy, gastrointestinal motility disorders, dysphagia with recurrent aspiration events, failure to thrive, seizures, and many functional limitations. Table 194-1 outlines some common reasons for the hospitalization of children with neurologic impairments.

IN-HOSPITAL CARE

The care of medically complex children in the hospital can be especially challenging and time-consuming.[1] The multisystem nature of their illnesses requires a comprehensive assessment to prevent or minimize readmissions. Applying a consistent, systematic approach ensures that their care is not only thorough but also organized and efficient (see Chapter 193).

Care of the medically complex child must be family centered.[2] Coordination of care and the medical home are mainstays of caring for this population (see Chapter 192).[3,4] In most instances, the parents should lead the care coordination process; they play a critical role on the treatment team and should be included in all decision making, particularly when it comes to admission and discharge planning. If the parents believe that their child's needs are not being addressed, this may result in repeat visits to the hospital or an increased length of stay. Understanding the family's rationale for bringing the child to the hospital is important, and it may be very different from the medical interpretation. Forming a trusting and communicative relationship with the family can decrease frustrations and allow for mutual goal setting.

To ensure that all aspects of care are addressed comprehensively during hospitalization and that discharge is timely, a multidisciplinary approach is essential.[5] Each member of the inpatient team contributes unique aspects of care and plays an integral role in the management of these children (see Chapter 193). Allowing each team member to practice to his or her full capacity not only distributes the workload but also provides the team with multiple insights into the family's functioning and coping. Each professional has different strengths, and combining them effectively maximizes the outcome.[5]

Table 194-1 Reasons for the Hospitalization of Children with Neurologic Impairments

Fever

Unexplained irritability

Seizures

Respiratory distress, pneumonia (viral, bacterial, aspiration), asthma

Poor feeding and enterostomy tube–related complications

Failure to thrive

Gastroesophageal reflux disease

Planned and unplanned surgeries (fundoplication, orthopedic, ventricular shunts)

Table 194-2 Complications in Children with Neurologic Impairments

Signs and Symptoms	Possible Causes
Exacerbation of well-controlled epilepsy	Fever, food-drug interactions, change in drug formulation or route of delivery, sleep deprivation
Acute respiratory distress	Silent aspiration, atelectasis secondary to prolonged immobility, deep venous thrombosis with pulmonary embolism, inadvertent latex exposure
Nausea, vomiting, abdominal distention	Superior mesenteric artery syndrome, obstipation, malposition of enteral feeding devices, adverse drug reactions, dietary changes, gastroesophageal reflux disease
Increased spasticity	Pain, sleep deprivation, stress, abrupt cessation of spasmolytic medications, constipation, urinary retention, ventricular shunt malfunction, occult neurologic event

In addition to a multidisciplinary approach, care must be coordinated within the hospital. The hospitalist or another team member, such as a pediatric nurse practitioner, can do this. In the inpatient setting, a care coordinator is a person who works with the family and the treatment team members to facilitate the provision of care that is both holistic and comprehensive.[6]

The hospitalist must be familiar with all aspects of the child's care; the entire past medical history, the specialists involved and their suggestions, any previous tests performed and treatments given, and the outcomes of these must all be carefully considered. Team meetings, in which the parents are central participants, ensure that everyone shares a common understanding of the medical plan and is working toward the same treatment goals. Maintaining open communication among all medical specialists promotes a unified medical approach while preventing the duplication of tests and treatments.

Creating care plans for complex patients (see Chapter 192) is useful not only in emergency situations but also during inpatient stays.[7] Care plans outline all medical problems, relevant medical history, and therapeutic interventions. Copies of the care plan should be given to the family and kept in a central location in the medical record for all team members to see.[8] These plans should be updated by the care coordinator and family as often as necessary.

COMPLICATIONS THAT PROLONG HOSPITALIZATION

Children with chronic illnesses not only have an acute primary diagnosis that triggers the hospitalization but also may have multiple secondary conditions. Although the pediatric hospitalist focuses on diagnostic and therapeutic interventions, it is important to ensure that secondary conditions remain stable during the course of hospitalization. The interdependent nature of organ systems and the inherent medical fragility of children with medically complex conditions means that the health care team must remain vigilant to avoid secondary complications that may prolong hospitalization and add to the stress of these children and their families.

Consider, for example, a child with spastic quadriplegic cerebral palsy who is hospitalized for interstitial viral pneu-

monia. With a focus on good respiratory care, the child begins to improve clinically over 1 to 2 days. The child then experiences a generalized tonic-clonic seizure, associated with vomiting and significant aspiration pneumonitis. Could this scenario have been prevented? On careful review, it is noted that when gastrostomy tube feedings were resumed, the formula was delivered via continuous infusion rather than periodic boluses. This child's previously diagnosed seizure disorder had been managed successfully on stable doses of phenytoin, but the serum drug concentration was found to be markedly subtherapeutic. Phenytoin absorption is impeded in the presence of food or formula and therefore must be given at least 1 hour before or 2 hours after meals.[9,10] As this example shows, the physician must remain alert for potential food and drug interactions in children receiving multiple medications.

Children with complex medical conditions often have secondary diagnoses of gastroesophageal reflux, delayed gastric emptying, and slow colonic transit times, all as a manifestation of gastrointestinal dysmotility. When such children are hospitalized for unrelated acute conditions or elective surgical procedures, the frequency and volume of stool output must be monitored. Immobility associated with bed rest, as well as analgesics, anesthetics, anxiolytics, and other medications, can further reduce gut motility. Constipation can present as anorexia, abdominal pain, sleep disturbance, irritability, urinary retention, nausea, and vomiting. These nonspecific symptoms can be related to a multitude of other factors, and a comprehensive approach to children with complex medical conditions is the primary strategy for the prevention and early recognition of complications associated with hospitalization (Table 194-2). Although less common than in the adult population, pediatric patients are not immune to deep venous thrombosis, pulmonary emboli, and decubitus ulcers.[11]

When a child with a chronic condition is hospitalized for an acute illness, a family-centered approach to care is most effective. In the process of obtaining a complete history, details of the child's daily schedule, medications, dietary intake, sleep patterns, typical stool output, and usual behaviors and activities can establish a baseline picture of the child's abilities. Without such insights, it is difficult for health care providers who are unfamiliar with the patient to promptly identify and address any changes in status. However, with careful attention to the details provided by parents, secondary complications can often be avoided or dealt with quickly.

DISCHARGE PLANNING

Discharge planning should begin at admission to minimize the time the child spends in the hospital.[1] Many children with complex conditions are technology dependent, and securing the appropriate equipment for home care and ensuring that caregivers are competent in its use can be time-consuming and costly. Further, the coordination of home care can be difficult, depending on the child's needs. One must ensure that home-care providers are adequately trained, that homes are equipped with proper medical equipment and accessible (e.g., to wheelchairs), and that support systems and safety nets (e.g., electricity, telephone, transportation) are in place.[12] When a discharge date is planned, the care coordinator and the parents should collaborate to establish and maintain a calendar for medical scheduling. These children often have numerous follow-up appointments and treatments, and the care coordinator may be able to consolidate them. It is often useful to establish a specific discharge date to ensure goal-directed care, keeping in mind the needs of individual families and that flexibility may be required. Communication with the primary care physician promotes an effective transition to the outpatient arena and minimizes the loss of critical information that could lead to poor outcomes. When discharge home is not possible, options such as a long-term care facility or short-term placement in a rehabilitation facility should be considered. These placements may be difficult to arrange, however, resulting in long waiting periods in the hospital. Addressing these options with families from the start allows the team to begin the planning process immediately.

IN A NUTSHELL

- The inpatient care of children with complex medical conditions must be comprehensive, encompassing both the acute reason for admission and all comorbidities.
- Building a trusting relationship with the family and having a solid understanding of the child's social situ-

ation and medical history are essential. Family-centered and coordinated care facilitates the process and promotes the best interests of the child and family throughout the hospitalization.
- A multidisciplinary team approach is indispensable, providing an abundance of clinical expertise in an efficient model of care delivery.
- Discharge planning can be complicated and should begin at admission. A care plan is an excellent way to summarize important medical and nonmedical issues, involve the family in the child's care, and provide comprehensive, seamless care in a goal-directed manner.

SUGGESTED READING

American Academy of Pediatrics, Committee on Hospital Care: Physician's role in coordinating care of hospitalized children. Pediatrics 1996;98:509-510.

Lindeke LL, Leonard BJ, Presler B, Garwick A: Family centered care coordination for children with special needs across multiple settings. J Pediatr Health Care 2002;16:290-297.

REFERENCES

1. Oleske JM, Boland M: When a child with a chronic condition needs hospitalization. Hosp Pract 1997;32:167-181.
2. Lindeke LL, Leonard BJ, Presler B, Garwick A: Family centered care coordination for children with special needs across multiple settings. J Pediatr Health Care 2002;16:290-297.
3. American Academy of Pediatrics, Committee on Children with Disabilities: Care coordination: Integrating health and related systems of care for children with special health care needs. Pediatrics 1999;104:978-981.
4. American Academy of Pediatrics, Medical Home Initiatives for Children with Special Needs Project Advisory Committee: The medical home. Pediatrics 2004;113:1545-1547.
5. Capen CL, Dedlow ER: Discharging ventilator-dependant children: A continuing challenge. J Pediatr Nurs 1998;13:175-184.
6. American Academy of Pediatrics, Committee on Hospital Care: Physician's role in coordinating care of hospitalized children. Pediatrics 1996;98:509-510.
7. Committee on Pediatric Emergency Medicine: Emergency preparedness for children with special health needs. Pediatrics 1999;104:1-6.
8. Emergency Medical Services for Children, National Task Force on Children with Special Health Care Needs: EMS for children: Recommendations for coordinating care for children with special health care needs. Ann Emerg Med 1997;30:274-280.
9. Au Yeung SC, Ensom MH: Phenytoin and enteral feedings: Does evidence support an interaction? Ann Pharmacother 2000;34:896-905.
10. Faraji B, Yu PP: Serum phenytoin levels of patients on gastrostomy tube feeding. J Neurosci Nurs 1998;30:55-59.
11. Curley MA, Quigley SM, Lin M: Pressure ulcers in pediatric intensive care: Incidence and associated factors. Pediatr Crit Care Med 2003;4:284-290.
12. Bakwell-Sachs S, Carlino H, Ash L, et al: Home care considerations for chronic and vulnerable populations. Nurse Pract Forum 2000;11:65-72.

CHAPTER 195

Technologic Devices in the Medically Complex Child

Jeremy Friedman

Medically complex children have an array of technologic devices to allow preservation of some of the basic life functions, including vascular and enteral access for nutrition and medications. Hospitalists who care for these children need to be familiar with the devices that they may encounter. This chapter focuses on vascular and enterostomy access and provides an overview of various types of devices, indications, and complications. Other common forms of technologic support are discussed elsewhere (noninvasive respiratory support is discussed in Chapter 209 and cerebrospinal fluid shunts are discussed in Chapters 143, 213, and 214).

VASCULAR ACCESS

Most medically complex patients require vascular access when admitted to the hospital. If the anticipated need for access is short, a peripheral intravenous (PIV) catheter may be adequate. Central venous catheters (CVCs) are usually required if therapy is long term, if it involves hypertonic or vasoactive medications or includes parenteral nutrition, or if peripheral access is impossible to obtain or maintain. Use of central catheters has also allowed patients to receive their intravenous therapy at home. Although these intravascular catheters facilitate management, they do put the patient at risk for many complications, including local and systemic infections, thrombosis, and mechanical problems. This section describes the various vascular access options available and their indications and specific characteristics, as well as gives a broad overview of the management and complications encountered with the different intravascular catheter options.

Vascular Access Devices

Short Term

PIV catheters are the devices most frequently used for vascular access and are generally placed in the veins of the arm, the dorsum of the foot, or the scalp (in neonates). These devices are the least invasive with the lowest risk of causing systemic infection. If the duration of intravenous therapy is likely to exceed 6 days, a midline catheter or central line may be considered. Removal of the PIV catheter is required if there is evidence of phlebitis, infection, or extravasation. The rate of PIV catheter–related bacteremia is 0.2%, or 0.6 per 1000 catheter days.[1] Infiltration of hypotonic or isotonic solution into tissues is generally treated by removal of the catheter and elevation of the limb. In the case of extravasation of a hypertonic solution (e.g., parenteral nutrition, calcium chloride, bicarbonate), subcutaneous or intradermal injection of dilute hyaluronidase into the leading edge can be used to help avert tissue necrosis. Full parenteral nutrition and certain medications cannot be given through a PIV catheter, and repeated blood sampling cannot be performed through this catheter.

Midline catheters are peripherally inserted catheters placed around the antecubital fossa into the proximal basilic or cephalic veins, with optimal tip placement in the proximal portion of the upper part of the arm. They are not used at all institutions. Midline catheters may be inserted with topical anesthesia, as well as oral sedation if necessary. They are ideal for children older than 3 years and can be left in place for up to 6 weeks, although they may not last that long because of phlebitis or extravasation. Medications and infusates requiring central access cannot be administered, and only a single lumen is available. There are no blood sampling capabilities.

Percutaneous CVCs are placed directly into the jugular, subclavian, or femoral veins. They are commonly used in critical care areas for short-term, acute central access or during resuscitative efforts. They can be single or double lumen, and all medications and infusates can be administered. Blood sampling is possible through these catheters. They do, however, have the highest risk of all CVCs for catheter-related infections, as well as the development of deep vein thrombosis (DVT). The recommended dwell time is therefore as short as possible and not longer than 2 weeks.

Long Term

Peripherally inserted central catheters (PICCs) are placed peripherally, usually around the antecubital fossa with the tip in the superior vena cava (SVC)/right atrial junction. PICCs are ideal for patients requiring therapy for a few weeks to 6 months and are the CVCs most commonly used in routine inpatient pediatrics. As with other CVCs, they can be single or double lumen, and infusion of all medications and infusates, as well as blood sampling, is possible. In some patients, insertion may be performed under local anesthesia. The most common complications include accidental displacement, occlusion, venous thrombosis, and infection.

External tunneled CVCs are tunneled through subcutaneous tissue and commonly inserted into the right internal jugular vein with tip placement in the SVC/right atrial junction. Less commonly, they can also be placed in the femoral veins. These catheters are generally used in patients requiring therapy longer than 6 months and are usually the catheter of choice in patients requiring hemodialysis, plasma exchange, chemotherapy, and bone marrow transplantation. The "tunneling" adds increased stability, but general anesthesia is frequently required for placement and sometimes for removal. These catheters are associated with a greater risk for intraoperative bleeding and pneumothorax than PICCs are.

Totally implanted intravascular devices (ports) are placed in a pocket in subcutaneous tissue and tunneled upward, usually into the right internal jugular vein, with tip placement in the SVC/right atrial junction. Ports are ideal for patients requiring long-term intermittent therapy (e.g.,

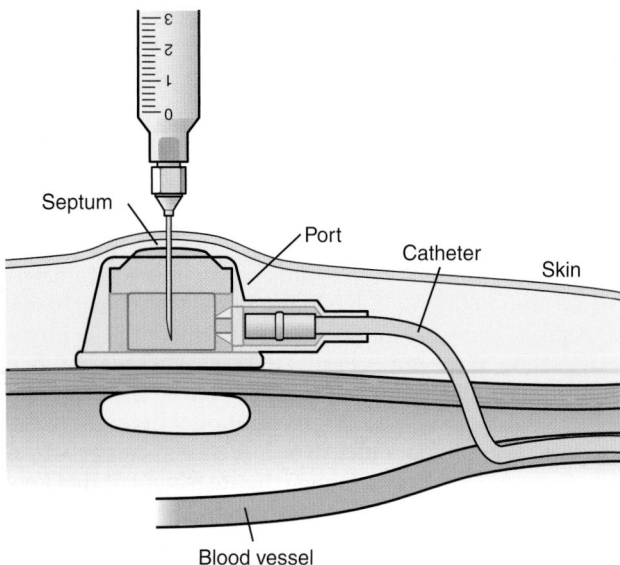

Figure 195-1   Schematic of a needle entering ("accessing") a port.

chemotherapy) and are less obtrusive and require fewer restrictions on activity. They have the lowest risk of catheter-related infections of the CVCs, 0.3 to 1.8 per 1000 catheter days versus 2.2 per 1000 catheter days for external tunneled lines.[2] They do require needle access to use (Fig. 195-1).

Complications

Acute

There are always risks associated with CVCs, although they differ somewhat depending on the technique and type of CVC used. Attempts to cannulate the internal jugular or subclavian vein can result in inadvertent needle puncture of the lung (leading to pneumothorax) or a large vein or artery (resulting in bleeding). Any mechanical damage to the thoracic duct can lead to chylothorax. On occasion, intravascular loss of the guidewire, bleeding, apnea, and oversedation may be seen during insertion. If the catheter is open to the atmosphere and the patient creates negative intrathoracic pressure by taking a breath, it is possible for an air embolus to develop, which can also occur during removal of the CVC. Mechanical breakage of part of the catheter and aberrant catheter localization can occur. When the tip of the line is in the heart adjacent to the sinoatrial node, arrhythmias may occur. Cardiac tamponade is a rare, but very serious complication caused by cardiac perforation. Immediately after insertion of a CVC, a plain film is indicated to confirm the location of the catheter and to detect complications.

Chronic

Long-term complications can include infection, occlusion (fibrin sheath, thrombosis), and venous obstruction. Over time, the catheter can migrate and cause perforation of the vessel wall with extravasation of the infusion.

Infections

Infections are the most common and can be a life-threatening complication of CVCs. For a complete discussion of infectious issues related to CVCs, please see Chapter 71.

Thrombosis and Occlusion

There is evidence that DVT develops in as many as 50% of children with catheters.[3] Thrombosis of the line can act as a nidus for infection, occlude the vessel, or result in fracture and pulmonary embolism. For a full discussion of these issues, please see Chapter 120 on disorders of coagulation.

In addition to DVT, CVCs can also result in a thin peri-catheter thrombus (fibrin sheath) that gradually encroaches on the catheter tip and can create a ball-valve effect leading to difficulty with aspiration from the catheter or initiation of large-vessel thrombosis. Blockage of the catheter can also be caused by a small intraluminal thrombus at the tip.

Clues to the presence of thrombosis may include a sudden decrease in the platelet count, difficulty aspirating from or flushing the catheter, and facial or extremity edema. Sometimes an increase in prominent blood vessels over the chest wall may be noted. However, most patients with CVC-related thrombosis are clinically asymptomatic. Nevertheless, there are potential serious complications, including recurrent thrombosis, pulmonary embolism, thrombi in the heart, loss of potential sites for future venous access, postthrombotic syndrome, and even death. The long-term outcome of the vascular damage and occlusion from CVCs is not clear in children.

In the case of occlusion of a CVC, chest radiography and a contrast study of the catheter are helpful in ruling out migration or breakage of the line. Use of intraluminal thrombolytics (e.g., urokinase, alteplase) is often successful in restoring patency. If attempts at unblocking the line are unsuccessful or if occlusion recurs, further investigation for thrombosis is essential. It is important to note that a contrast study through the CVC may not rule out the presence of clot in a large vessel (within which the CVC is located).

Many imaging options are available to assist in the diagnosis of DVT. Most imaging tests are helpful with diagnosis of thrombosis in the lower venous system. Consistent data suggest that contrast venography (with ultrasound of the jugular veins) is the most reliable means of detecting DVT in the upper venous system.

Decreased thrombosis in adult cancer patients is noted with the prophylactic use of low-dose warfarin or low-molecular-weight heparin, but there is minimal evidence for such a decrease in children. Prophylactic flushes with heparinized saline have been used for catheter maintenance, but the best agent, timing, volume, and so forth have yet to be established.

ENTEROSTOMY ACCESS (GASTROSTOMY, JEJUNOSTOMY, AND GASTROJEJUNOSTOMY TUBES)

If the gastrointestinal tract is functioning adequately, enteral nutrition is preferable to parenteral nutrition in a medically complex child. When compared with parenteral nutrition, enterostomy tubes are easier to handle and less expensive, and several randomized trials have shown that complications (e.g., sepsis, thrombosis, liver dysfunction) are less common. Enteral feeding prevents mucosal atrophy, maintains gut flora, and plays an important role in preserving the enteral immune system. In recent times, gastrostomy (G), jejunostomy (J), and gastrojejunostomy (GJ) tubes have replaced nasogastric (NG) and nasojejunal (NJ) tubes when the anticipated length of enteral feeding exceeds 4 to 8 weeks.

Tubes through the nose, although simple to place, are not well tolerated in the long term and are cosmetically unappealing. They may lead to sinusitis and nasal ulceration and could predispose to gastroesophageal reflux, esophagitis, and strictures. They are easily displaced and may result in aspiration, especially in neurologically impaired children. This section outlines the indications for enterostomy tube placement, the different techniques available to place tubes, and the outcomes reported and complications encountered.

Indications

There are a number of reasons to consider placement of an enteral tube:

- Oral motor feeding problems, which can result in an inability to maintain hydration or aspiration of orally ingested food into the lungs
- Failure to thrive as a result of oral motor feeding problems, malabsorption, or a specific disease process (e.g., congenital heart disease, cystic fibrosis, chronic renal failure, cancer)
- Need for an unpalatable elemental diet (e.g., inflammatory bowel disease, various metabolic diseases)
- Feeding aversion that is resistant to other therapy
- Administration of medications (e.g., for human immunodeficiency virus infection)
- Decompression ("venting") for functional or mechanical bowel obstruction
- As part of palliative care

On occasion, a J or GJ tube may be more appropriate, for example, in the management of severe gastroesophageal reflux disease (GERD) resistant to maximal medical therapy and still symptomatic with NG or G tube feeding. Anatomic or mechanical issues, such as superior mesenteric artery syndrome, would be another indication for a GJ or J tube (where the tip of the feeding tube is passed distal to the obstruction).

Method of Placement

There are three well-accepted techniques for placement of enterostomy tubes in children:

- Surgical
- Percutaneous endoscopic gastrostomy (PEG)
- Percutaneous radiologic gastrostomy (PRG)

Surgical gastrostomy is technically simple and has been performed since the late 1800s. Since the 1990s, an increasing number of these procedures are being performed laparoscopically. PEG, first performed in 1980, is a quick and low-cost method of placing a tube percutaneously under endoscopic guidance by the "pull" or "push" technique, according to the preference of the endoscopist. Percutaneous nonendoscopic or radiologic gastrostomy done under fluoroscopic guidance was first performed in 1981 and has the advantage of being able to be performed in children without general anesthesia if necessary. The nonsurgical techniques of PEG (most commonly performed) and PRG have largely replaced surgery for enterostomy tube placement. Surgical gastrostomy is still indicated for patients requiring laparotomy/laparoscopy for related or unrelated abdominal problems.

No study has compared the three techniques in a pediatric population, but a meta-analysis of all patients in the literature who underwent enterostomy over a 15-year period, largely an adult population, was performed to evaluate the effectiveness and safety of the different techniques. Rates of successful tube placement varied from 100% for surgical G tubes, 99.2% for PRG, and 95.7% for PEG. Major complications were most common after surgical G tube placement at 19.9%, lower at 9.4% in PEG, and least common after PRG at 5.9%.[4]

The technique used will probably depend on what is most readily available in the particular institution. However, certain conditions may be important to consider. In a medically complex patient, avoidance of general anesthesia may be of significant benefit, thus arguing against a surgically placed tube. However, patients requiring another surgical procedure, such as fundoplication, are better served through surgical tube placement at the same time. In patients with portal hypertension and gastric varices, simultaneous endoscopy may be helpful to avoid puncturing a varix and causing bleeding. Unfavorable anatomy, such as previous gastric surgery or interposition of the liver resulting in absence of a safe access route, is also a relative contraindication to the PEG or PRG technique.

Many different types of G tubes are available, and no single catheter is appropriate for all patients. Most are secured by a pigtail, balloon, or bulb in the stomach, which helps prevent accidental dislodgement (Fig. 195-2). After 6 to 12 weeks the tube can be changed to a low-profile device (e.g., MIC-KEY, Bard button) (Fig. 195-3), although low-profile tubes tend to not be available in smaller sizes. They are more cosmetically appealing, tend to move less, and are more difficult to remove accidentally.

Outcomes

It is generally assumed that enterostomy feeding is a necessary, safe, and effective intervention in the group of complex medical patients with oral motor feeding problems. The finding in some earlier cohort studies of a higher death rate and an increase in GERD in children with cerebral palsy

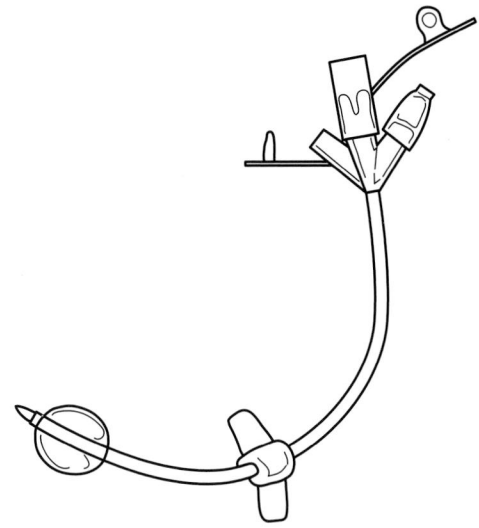

Figure 195-2 Typical gastrostomy tube. Note the inflated balloon at the tip, which helps prevent the tube from becoming dislodged.

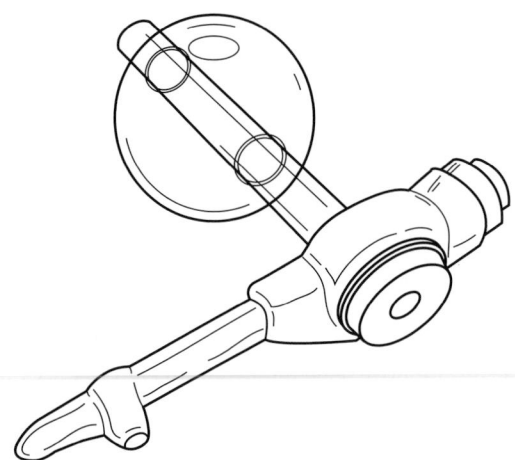

Figure 195-3   Typical low-profile gastrostomy tube device.

(CP) who were fed by gastrostomy is cause for concern. It has been hypothesized that the increased mortality may be due to an increase in pulmonary disease secondary to overly vigorous nutritional maintenance and subsequent aspiration. Unfortunately, no randomized controlled trials of enterostomy tube feeding have been conducted in neurologically impaired children, which raises the question of whether the control group was really equally severely disabled before the intervention. This is supported by noting that the association between feeding and death was substantially reduced when other confounding factors were controlled for. Most studies investigating the risks and benefits of tube feeding in neurologically impaired children are limited by methodologic weaknesses, thus making it difficult to draw any firm conclusions in this regard.

Based on the literature to date, it appears that children generally show improved weight gain after initiation of G tube feeding. Change in the rate of growth in height is less predictable in the population of children with CP. Although weight gain is generally a good thing, it can have some disadvantages in the severely disabled, neurologically impaired population, for example, making the child more difficult to lift and carry.

Caregivers of children with CP generally report an increase in the ease and a decrease in the time taken up by feeding after enterostomy tube placement. They usually see an improvement in the child's disposition and nutrition and often report that they are pleased with the G tube and enhancement of the child's comfort and abilities. There are also caregivers who report on the difficulty of getting respite care because of the tube feeding, as well as the restricted mobility if pump feeding is required. Furthermore, some have commented on a "changed" relationship with their child, in addition to their child missing the taste of food.

Although G tubes are often placed because of concern about the risk for direct aspiration with oral feeding, it is also possible to aspirate saliva as well as refluxed gastric contents. It is therefore important to know whether G tube placement will cause reflux or worsen preexisting GERD. Unless the child's GERD symptoms are very severe despite maximal medical therapy, fundoplication at the time of G tube inser-

tion is not usually recommended. If severe GERD is present, another option would be to feed via a GJ tube. Reflux can, of course, be clinically silent, and investigations for GERD are far from perfect. This makes it very difficult to decide what effect tube placement has on the child's reflux, and studies thus far remain inconclusive.

Given all the uncertainties regarding the outcomes of G tube placement, specifically in neurologically impaired children, a prospective randomized controlled trial in this group of patients would be very helpful in providing more definitive answers to the questions that have been raised.

Complications

Complications can be classified as early (within 30 days of the procedure) or late (after 30 days). They may also be divided into major and minor complications, which is less consistently defined in the literature. One clinically useful definition would be that major complications require a significant medical or surgical intervention. For example, tube dislodgement occurring in the first week before the tract has matured would be considered "major" because it may need to be replaced in a new site; displacement after the first few weeks would be "minor" because the tube could easily be replaced through the same stoma. Some authors include tube "maintenance" problems as minor complications, such as unscheduled tube changes caused by blockage or dislodgement. Complication rates vary depending on the technique used, with one large meta-analysis quoting major complications with surgical gastrostomy (19.9%), PEG (9.4%), and PRG (5.9%).[4] Minor complication rates can vary greatly, depending on differences in definition, but the same study calculated figures for surgical gastrostomy (9%), PEG (5.9%), and PRG (7.8%). The 30-day mortality rate from the procedure was 2.5% for surgical gastrostomy, 0.53% for PEG, and 0.3% for PRG.[4]

Some of the more commonly reported *major complications* include

- Aspiration (as a direct result of the procedure)
- Peritonitis
- Premature removal of the G tube
- Gastrointestinal bleeding
- Severe wound and abdominal wall infection
- Sepsis
- Death

Peritonitis may result from leakage into the peritoneal cavity from around the G tube site or from a dislodged or misplaced tube. Children in whom peritonitis develops after G tube insertion may present with vomiting, fever, irritability, tachycardia, and progressive peritoneal signs, with progression to sepsis and death if not recognized. Early recognition is especially difficult in younger infants and those with neurologic impairment. If peritonitis is suspected, feeding should be withheld and an urgent contrast study performed through the tube to rule out leakage and confirm tube position. Pneumoperitoneum can be a normal finding after G tube placement, but late-onset or increasing pneumoperitoneum may represent unrecognized perforation of the gastrointestinal tract or ongoing leakage around the tube site. Peritonitis can usually be managed with bowel rest, total parenteral nutrition, empirical antibiotic therapy, and close observation, but surgical intervention is occasionally required.

Minor complications, including the tube maintenance problems most commonly encountered, may consist of

- Tube dislodgement
- Tube leakage
- Tube migration
- Tube blockage
- G tube site infection
- Intussusception

Dislodged tubes should be replaced as promptly as possible. Caregivers can be taught to place a Foley catheter to keep the stoma open once the tract has matured. If this is achieved without difficulty and gastric contents can be aspirated, patients can resume feeding through the Foley catheter.

Pericatheter leakage can sometimes become a problem. If the leakage is the result of excessive external tube motion, external fasteners may successfully stabilize the tube. If the stomal site enlargement is due to skin breakdown as a result of infection, antibiotic therapy and replacement with a GJ tube (to minimize fluid contact at the stomal site) may be helpful.

Tubes can migrate into the duodenum or the esophagus (and in the case of GJ tubes, retrogradely into the stomach) and result in obstruction and vomiting. Migration is generally diagnosed by means of a contrast study through the tube.

Tube blockage usually results from failing to flush the tube after feeding or administration of medications or from certain medications that are notorious for their ability to clog up G and GJ tubes. Flushing the tube with warm water or a carbonated beverage may unblock the tube. Alternatively, blockage can sometimes be corrected with a guidewire, or else the tube will need to be changed. Tubes should be flushed with a minimum of 5 to 20 mL of water after feeding or medications, and medications should be given in liquid format or, if not feasible, then finely crushed and completely dissolved in water before administration through the tube.

Infections around the G tube site can lead to cellulitis and occasionally a subcutaneous abscess. Infection can result in redness, swelling, tenderness, and increased discharge that may be foul smelling. Children rarely have constitutional symptoms, and the infection usually resolves rapidly with local wound care and topical or oral antibiotics. G tube site infections are often polymicrobial, but *Staphylococcus aureus* and β-hemolytic streptococci are commonly involved, as is fungal superinfection. It is important to distinguish infection from skin redness and irritation caused by sensitivity to acidic gastric contents. The latter may respond to a non-medicated barrier cream or benefit from acid-suppressing agents. The skin can also become reddened because of a reaction to the tape used to hold the tube in place. Granulation tissue around the stoma is caused by an overgrowth of dark pink "cauliflower-like" tissue, which bleeds easily but generally responds to repeated applications of silver nitrate.

Intussusception of the small bowel is not uncommonly seen with GJ tubes, especially in young infants and in the presence of a tube with a distal pigtail. This complication should be suspected in patients with a GJ tube presenting with bilious vomiting and feed intolerance. The diagnosis of intussusception can be made by ultrasonography or fluoroscopy, and it is usually managed by changing the tube and replacing with a shorter GJ tube or removing the distal pigtail, or both.

ON THE HORIZON

- Prevention of bloodstream infections is an area of tremendous research, and it is hoped that new techniques and technology will bear fruit in the next several years.
- Research is under way to prospectively look at the risks and benefits of J tubes versus fundoplication in the management of GERD.

SUGGESTED READING

Campos ACL, Marchesini JB: Recent advances in the placement of tubes for enteral nutrition. Curr Opin Clin Nutr Metab Care 1999;2:265-269.

Friedman JN: Enterostomy tube feeding: The ins and outs. Paediatr Child Health 2004;9:695-699.

Friedman JN, Ahmed S, Connolly B, et al: Complications associated with image guided gastrostomy and gastrojejunostomy tubes in children. Pediatrics 2004;114:458-461.

Journeycake JM, Buchanan GR: Thrombotic complications of central venous catheters in children. Curr Opin Hematol 2003;10:369-374.

McGee DC, Gould MK: Preventing complications of central venous catheterization. N Engl J Med 2003;348:1123-1133.

Sleigh G, Brocklehurst P: Gastrostomy feeding in cerebral palsy: A systematic review. Arch Dis Child 2004;89:534-539.

Stovroff M, Teague WG: Intravenous access in infants and children. Pediatr Clin North Am 1998;45:1373-1393.

REFERENCES

1. Robinson J: Practical approach to catheter-related bloodstream infections in paediatrics. Paediatr Child Health 2005;10:465-470.
2. Salzman MB, Rubin LG: Intravenous catheter–related infections. Adv Pediatr Infect Dis 1995;10:337-368.
3. Journeycake JM, Buchanan GR: Thrombotic complications of central venous catheters in children. Curr Opin Hematol 2003;10:369-374.
4. Wollman BS, Horacio BD, Walus-Wigle J, et al: Radiologic, endoscopic and surgical gastrostomy: An institutional evaluation and meta-analysis of the literature. Radiology 1995;197:699-704.

CHAPTER 196

Do-Not-Resuscitate Orders

Armand H. Matheny Antommaria

With medicine's increasing capabilities, situations arise in which possible interventions will not serve the patient's or the family's goals of care. Under such circumstances, the decision to forgo treatment, even potentially lifesaving treatment, may be appropriate. This chapter discusses one means of limiting treatment: the do-not-resuscitate (DNR) order. It describes the historical development of DNR orders, outlines the process of writing such orders, and explains why they should not be written unilaterally. The related issues of family presence during resuscitation and DNR orders in the operating room and outside the hospital are also reviewed.

CARDIOPULMONARY RESUSCITATION AND DO-NOT-RESUSCITATE ORDERS

DNR or do-not-attempt-resuscitation (DNAR) orders developed out of the recognition that cardiopulmonary resuscitation (CPR) lacks efficacy in certain patient populations and that a formal process of advance planning was needed. Some authors prefer the language of DNAR, believing that it reflects the fact that not all resuscitation attempts are effective.[1] Although modern CPR was initially developed for patients suffering anesthesia-induced cardiac arrest, it became the standard of care for cardiac arrest in hospitalized patients regardless of their underlying diagnosis. Experience, however, demonstrated that the effects of CPR were often transient. In some institutions, covert decision-making processes evolved to withhold or limit resuscitation efforts. Hospitals developed DNR policies in the 1970s to address the need for both a decision-making process and a means to communicate these decisions.[2]

There are limited data in the pediatric literature regarding the efficacy of CPR in hospitalized patients. A nonconcurrent cohort study of consecutive pediatric intensive care unit admissions found that 13.7% of patients (28 of 205) requiring cardiac massage for at least 2 minutes survived to hospital discharge.[3] Another study, a retrospective medical records review combined with a prospective telephone follow-up, reported that 36% of patients who received CPR survived 24 hours, but only 10% (9 of 92) survived 1 year. The majority of survivors were moderately to severely disabled, but this represented little to no change from their pre-arrest level of functioning.[4] Information regarding the efficacy of CPR within specific diagnostic categories is even more limited. These studies identified different indicators of a low likelihood of survival: trauma and "other etiologies" versus sepsis syndrome.

Even if CPR might be effective, there may be situations in which it is ethical to withhold it. For example, in terminally ill patients, it may only prolong the dying process. More controversially, the patient's quality of life may be so diminished that it need not be maintained.

The Patient Self-Determination Act, which became effective in 1991, requires most health care institutions to ask adult patients on admission whether they have advance directives; however, there are few mechanisms for parents or guardians to express their wishes for their children or for adolescents to express their wishes should they become incompetent.[5,6] Hospitalists should review the goals of treatment—curative, uncertain, or primarily comfort—with the families of children with special health care needs (Box 196-1). The patient's primary care provider may be a valuable resource, especially if he or she has a long-standing or close relationship with the patient and family and has discussed treatment goals with them. Discussing the goals of treatment is particularly important when significant changes occur in the child's clinical condition. If there is a possibility of cardiorespiratory arrest, especially if there is a low likelihood of survival or survival would not be in the child's best interest, the hospitalist should discuss the risks and benefits of CPR, and a DNR order should be considered. This difficult topic can be broached by asking, "What is your hope for your child?"

The hospitalist should carefully document conversations with the patient and the patient's family in the medical record. This is particularly important because of the limited continuity within some hospitalist systems. DNR orders generally prohibit CPR regardless of the cause of the arrest. If the DNR order is based on a low likelihood of survival and if different causes of arrest have different survival rates, this should be discussed.[7] For example, a family might desire intubation and mechanical ventilation for respiratory depression that is a side effect of anticonvulsants. The hospitalist should also write a formal order, ensuring that it is internally consistent. DNR orders should be reviewed periodically and any time there is a significant change in the patient's medical condition. Hospitalists should communicate the substance of their discussions to primary care providers and complete out-of-hospital DNR orders (see later), if appropriate, at the time of discharge.

DNR orders should not be interpreted to represent a broad decrease in the intensity of care, especially when such limitations have not been discussed and agreed on.[8] DNR orders should be implemented in the context of palliative care (see Chapter 12), including managing pain and symptoms and addressing emotional and spiritual needs (see Chapter 11).[9]

Hospitalists should be familiar with the policies of the hospitals and the laws of the states where they practice. Hospitals may require the attending physician to write the initial DNR order, prohibit verbal or telephone orders, and specify how frequently the order must be renewed. States may restrict the circumstances in which a DNR order can be entered, such as only if the patient is terminally ill. These statutes are controversial; some consider them unconstitutional or unethical.[10]

Evidence of low survival rates after CPR in specific patient populations has led some authors to argue that it is futile and that physicians can unilaterally withhold it.[11] Definitions of futility are problematic, however, because they incorporate values that the patient may not share. The disputed procedure generally has a physiologic effect, but parties disagree on what likelihood of success justifies the procedure or the value of the outcome to the patient. Permitting physicians to unilaterally withhold treatment violates patients' autonomy. Such decisions are particularly problematic because physicians tend to undervalue the quality of life of individuals with disabilities.[12,13] Disagreements between patients or other decision makers and the medical staff have led to the implementation of specific procedural steps to mediate such disagreements or to facilitate the transfer of care to a physician willing to carry out the family's wishes.[14]

FAMILY PRESENCE

There is a growing move to permit families to be present during resuscitation attempts. For example, the American Heart Association's *PALS Provider Manual* states, "Healthcare providers should offer the opportunity [for family members to be present during the attempted resuscitation of a loved one] whenever possible."[15] It should be noted that family presence protocols are structured and include an assessment of the patient and the family, preparation of the family for the event, and support of the family by a trained facilitator during and after the experience.[16] Proponents contend that this practice benefits family members in terms of knowing that everything possible was done, feeling that they supported the patient, and easing their bereavement, without disrupting the provision of care.[17] Much of the research has focused on family members, and studies are needed on the effects of family presence, both medical and psychological, on the children themselves.

OTHER CONTEXTS

Anesthesia and Surgery

DNR orders during anesthesia and surgery may be problematic because anesthesia promotes some degree of cardiovascular instability, and it can be difficult and artificial to separate anesthesia from resuscitation. Additionally, procedure-specific DNR orders may restrict anesthesiologists' and surgeons' discretion in cases of unexpected but easily reversible events. Professional organizations contend that DNR orders should not be automatically rescinded in the operating room but should be reevaluated. Hospitalists should review the DNR order and treatment goals with the patient and his or her parents, as well as the anesthesiologists and surgeons, before sedation or surgery. If the DNR order is suspended, a temporal end point should be established.[18,19]

Outside the Hospital

Children with special health care needs live in many contexts: they may live at home or in an extended-care facility, they may attend school, and they may be hospitalized intermittently. Sometimes the families of children with DNR orders may legitimately need to activate the emergency medical services (EMS) system. For example, the child could be in status epilepticus or suddenly develop distressing symptoms. Performing CPR is, however, the default for first responders and EMS personnel. Many states authorize "portable" or out-of-hospital DNR orders that EMS personnel are required to comply with and that protect them from liability for doing so. Some programs are applicable to minors. Hospitalists should be aware of state regulations and complete such documents if available (Fig. 196-1).[20,21] Otherwise, they should discuss the risks and benefits of calling 911 with the family. Code status should also be part of the child's emergency care plan, which includes a concise summary of his or her medical conditions, precautions needed, and special management plans.[22,23] Out-of-hospital DNR orders and emergency care plans may also facilitate patients' readmission to the hospital.

Children with chronic or terminal conditions who are at risk of dying may also attend school. The American Academy of Pediatrics recommends that pediatricians and parents meet with school officials to reach an agreement about the goals of in-school medical interventions and the best means to implement those goals.[24] Hospitalists must continue to define their role in such conversations, particularly when patients do not have a functional medical home.

IN A NUTSHELL

- Given their responsibilities for patient care, education, administration, and research, hospitalists have many opportunities to improve the treatment of children with special health care needs, especially at the end of life.[25] In terms of direct patient care, they can participate in discussions about the patient's prognosis and help clarify the goals of treatment. They coordinate care with other disciplines, such as anesthesia and surgery, and facilitate transitions home or to extended-care facilities. Additionally, given their teaching roles, hospitalists can educate students and residents about these important issues.[26,27] Many hospitalists also have administrative responsibilities and may be involved in formulating, revising, or updating hospital policies on DNR orders and related matters.

HIPAA PERMITS DISCLOSURE OF POLST TO OTHER HEALTH CARE PROFESSIONALS AS NECESSARY

Physician Orders
for Life-Sustaining Treatment (POLST)

First follow these orders, then contact physician or NP. This is a Physician Order Sheet based on the person's medical condition and wishes.
Any section not completed implies full treatment for that section.
Everyone shall be treated with dignity and respect.

Last Name
First Name/Middle Initial
Date of Birth

A	**CARDIOPULMONARY RESUSCITATION (CPR):** **Person has no pulse and is not breathing.**
Check one	☐ Resuscitate/CPR ☐ Do Not Attempt Resuscitation (DNR/no CPR)
	When not in cardiopulmonary arrest, follow orders in **B**, **C** and **D**.

B	**MEDICAL INTERVENTIONS:** **Person has pulse and/or is breathing.**
Check one	☐ **Comfort Measures Only** Use medication by any route, positioning, wound care and other measures to relieve pain and suffering. Use oxygen, suction and manual treatment of airway obstruction as needed for comfort. ***Do not transfer*** to hospital for life-sustaining treatment. ***Transfer*** *if comfort needs cannot be met in current location.*
	☐ **Limited Additional Interventions** Includes care described above. Use medical treatment, IV fluids and cardiac monitor as indicated. Do not use intubation, advanced airway interventions, or mechanical ventilation. ***Transfer*** *to hospital if indicated.* *Avoid intensive care.*
	☐ **Full Treatment** Includes care described above. Use intubation, advanced airway interventions, mechanical ventilation, and cardioversion as indicated. ***Transfer*** *to hospital if indicated. Includes intensive care.*
	Additional Orders: _____

C	**ANTIBIOTICS**
Check one	☐ No antibiotics. Use other measures to relieve symptoms.
	☐ Determine use or limitation of antibiotics when infection occurs.
	☐ Use antibiotics if life can be prolonged.
	Additional Orders: _____

D	**ARTIFICIALLY ADMINISTERED NUTRITION:** **Always offer food by mouth if feasible.**
Check one	☐ No artificial nutrition by tube.
	☐ Defined trial period of artificial nutrition by tube.
	☐ Long-term artificial nutrition by tube.
	Additional Orders: _____

E	**SUMMARY OF MEDICAL CONDITION AND SIGNATURES**	
	Discussed with: ☐ Patient ☐ Parent of Minor ☐ Health Care Representative ☐ Court-Appointed Guardian ☐ Other: _____	**Summary of Medical Condition**
	Print Physician / Nurse Practitioner Name	MD/DO/NP Phone Number	Office Use Only
	Physician / NP Signature (mandatory)	Date	

SEND FORM WITH PERSON WHENEVER TRANSFERRED OR DISCHARGED

© CENTER FOR ETHICS IN HEALTH CARE, Oregon Health & Science University, 3181 Sam Jackson Park Rd, UHN-86, Portland, OR 97239-3098 (503) 494-3965

Figure 196–1   Sample physician order for life–sustaining treatment.

HIPAA PERMITS DISCLOSURE OF POLST TO OTHER HEALTH CARE PROFESSIONALS AS NECESSARY

Signature of Person, Parent of Minor, or Guardian/Health Care Representative

Significant thought has been given to life-sustaining treatment. Preferences have been expressed to a physician and/or health care professional(s). This document reflects those treatment preferences.

(If signed by surrogate, preferences expressed must reflect patient's wishes as best understood by surrogate.)

Signature (optional)	Name (print)	Relationship (write "self" if patient)

Contact Information

Surrogate (optional)	Relationship	Phone Number	
Health Care Professional Preparing Form (optional)	Preparer Title	Phone Number	Date Prepared

Directions for Health Care Professionals

Completing POLST

Must be completed by a health care professional based on patient preferences and medical indications.

POLST must be signed by a physician or nurse practitioner to be valid. Verbal orders are acceptable with follow-up signature by physician or nurse practitioner in accordance with facility/community policy.

Use of original form is strongly encouraged. Photocopies and FAXes of signed POLST forms are legal and valid.

Using POLST

Any incomplete section of POLST implies full treatment for that section.

No defibrillator (including AEDs) should be used on a person who has chosen "Do Not Attempt Resuscitation."

Oral fluids and nutrition must always be offered if medically feasible.

When comfort cannot be achieved in the current setting, the person, including someone with "Comfort Measures Only," should be transferred to a setting able to provide comfort (e.g., treatment of a hip fracture).

IV medication to enhance comfort may be appropriate for a person who has chosen "Comfort Measures Only."

Treatment of dehydration is a measure which prolongs life. A person who desires IV fluids should indicate "Limited Interventions" or "Full Treatment."

A person with capacity, or the surrogate of a person without capacity, can request alternative treatment.

Reviewing POLST

This POLST should be reviewed periodically and if:

(1) The person is transferred from one care setting or care level to another, or

(2) There is a substantial change in the person's health status, or

(3) The person's treatment preferences change.

Draw line through sections A through E and write "VOID" in large letters if POLST is replaced or becomes invalid.

The Oregon POLST Task Force

The POLST program was developed by the Oregon POLST Task Force. The POLST program is administratively housed at Oregon Health & Science University's Center for Ethics in Health Care. Research about the safety and effectiveness of the POLST program is available online at <**www.polst.org**> or by contacting the Task Force at <**polst@ohsu.edu**>.

SEND FORM WITH PERSON WHENEVER TRANSFERRED OR DISCHARGED

© CENTER FOR ETHICS IN HEALTH CARE, Oregon Health & Science University, 3181 Sam Jackson Park Rd, UHN-86, Portland, OR 97239-3098 (503) 494-3965

Figure 196-1, cont'd

ON THE HORIZON

- Research is needed into the efficacy of CPR in specific patient population to inform decision making.
- Training programs are being developed to help health care providers become more comfortable discussing resuscitation status.
- Systems must be implemented to help patients and their families achieve their goals for end-of-life care in all of the contexts in which they live.

SUGGESTED READING

Burns JP, Edwards J, Johnson J, et al: Do-not-resuscitate order after 25 years. Crit Care Med 2003;31:1543-1550.

Schmidt TA, Hickman SE, Toole SW: Honoring treatment preferences near the end of life: The Oregon physician orders for life-sustaining treatment (POLST) program. Adv Exp Med Biol 2004;550:255-262.

REFERENCES

1. Hadorn DG: DNAR: Do not attempt resuscitation. N Engl J Med 1989;320:673.
2. Burns J: DNR (do not resuscitate). In Post SG (ed): Encyclopedia of Bioethics, vol 2, 3rd ed. New York, Macmillan Reference, 2003, pp 683-685.
3. Slonim AD, Patel KM, Ruttimann UE, Pollack MM: Cardiopulmonary resuscitation in pediatric intensive care units. Crit Care Med 1997;25:1951-1955.
4. Torres A Jr, Pickert CB, Firestone J, et al: Long-term functional outcome of inpatient pediatric cardiopulmonary resuscitation. Pediatr Emerg Care 1997;13:369-373.
5. Sahler OJ, Greenlaw J: Pediatrics and the Patient Self-Determination Act. Pediatrics 1992;90:999-1001.
6. Weir RF, Peters C: Affirming the decisions adolescents make about life and death. Hastings Cent Rep 1997;27(6):29-40.
7. Choudhry NK, Choudhry S, Singer PA: CPR for patients labeled DNR: The role of the limited aggressive therapy order. Ann Intern Med 2003;138:65-68.
8. Henneman EA, Baird B, Bellamy PE, et al: Effect of do-not-resuscitate orders on the nursing care of critically ill patients. Am J Crit Care 1994;3:467-472.
9. Himelstein BP, Hilden JM, Boldt AM, Weissman D: Pediatric palliative care. N Engl J Med 2004;350:1752-1762.
10. Burns JP, Edwards J, Johnson J, et al: Do-not-resuscitate order after 25 years. Crit Care Med 2003;31:1543-1550.
11. Blackhall LJ: Must we always use CPR? N Engl J Med 1987;317:1281-1285.
12. Blaymore Bier JA, Liebling JA, Morales Y, Carlucci M: Parents' and pediatricians' views of individuals with meningomyelocele. Clin Pediatr (Phila) 1996;35:113-117.
13. Wolraich ML, Siperstein GN, O'Keefe P: Pediatricians' perceptions of mentally retarded individuals. Pediatrics 1987;80:643-649.
14. Medical futility in end-of-life care: Report of the Council on Ethical and Judicial Affairs. JAMA 1999;281:937-941.
15. PALS Provider Manual. American Heart Association, 2002.
16. Eckle NJ (ed): Presenting the Option for Family Presence, 2nd ed. Des Plaines, Ill, Emergency Nurses Association, 2001.
17. Meyers TA, Eichhorn DJ, Guzzetta CE, et al: Family presence during invasive procedures and resuscitation. Am J Nurs 2000;100:32-42.
18. Waisel DB, Burns JP, Johnson JA, et al: Guidelines for perioperative do-not-resuscitate policies. J Clin Anesth 2002;14:467-473.
19. Fallat ME, Deshpande JK: Do-not-resuscitate orders for pediatric patients who require anesthesia and surgery. Pediatrics 2004;114:1686-1692.
20. Sabatino CP: Survey of state EMS-DNR laws and protocols. J Law Med Ethics 1999;27:297-315.
21. Schmidt TA, Hickman SE, Tolle SW: Honoring treatment preferences near the end of life: The Oregon physician orders for life-sustaining treatment (POLST) program. Adv Exp Med Biol 2004;550:255-262.
22. American Academy of Pediatrics, Committee on Pediatric Emergency Medicine: Emergency preparedness for children with special health care needs. Pediatrics 1999;104:e53.
23. Emergency Information Form for Children with Special Needs. http://www.acep.org/library/pdf/EIF.pdf.
24. American Academy of Pediatrics, Committee on School Health and Committee on Bioethics: Do not resuscitate orders in schools. Pediatrics 2000;105:878-879.
25. Srivastava R, Landrigan C, Gidwani P, et al: Pediatric hospitalists in Canada and the United States: A survey of pediatric academic department chairs. Ambul Pediatr 2001;1:338-339.
26. Khaneja S, Milrod B: Educational needs among pediatricians regarding caring for terminally ill children. Arch Pediatr Adolesc Med 1998;152:909-914.
27. Sahler OJ, Frager G, Levetown M, et al: Medical education about end-of-life care in the pediatric setting: Principles, challenges, and opportunities. Pediatrics 2000;105:575-584.

PART IV

Procedures

CHAPTER 197

Procedural Sedation

Douglas W. Carlson

SEDATION AND ANALGESIA

The goals of sedation and analgesia are to relieve pain and suffering and to allow diagnostic and therapeutic procedures to proceed with comfort, safety, efficacy, and efficiency. The needs of the patient and the specific goals of sedation must be considered on an individual basis, with attention to patient safety and minimization of anxiety, pain, and memory. Attainment of these goals requires careful preparation and monitoring of the patient during the procedure and while he or she is recovering from sedation. Adherence to the guidelines for the monitoring of sedated patients developed by the American Academy of Pediatrics (AAP), American Society of Anesthesiologists (ASA), and Joint Commission on Accreditation of Healthcare Organizations (JCAHO) is essential.[1-3] Please note that the information provided in this chapter is not sufficient guidance for the safe administration of procedural sedation. Each institution should have its own training and certification requirement, as well as a procedure for maintaining competence in providing procedural sedation.

The following definitions for the level of sedation have been adopted by the AAP, ASA, and JCAHO.[1-3]

Minimal sedation (anxiolysis): A drug-induced state during which patients respond normally to verbal commands. Although cognitive function and coordination may be impaired, ventilatory and cardiovascular functions are usually maintained.

Moderate sedation or analgesia: A drug-induced depression of consciousness during which patients respond purposefully to verbal commands, either alone or accompanied by light to moderate tactile stimulation. No interventions are required to maintain a patent airway, and spontaneous ventilation is adequate. Cardiovascular function is usually maintained.

Deep sedation or analgesia: A drug-induced depression of consciousness during which patients cannot be easily aroused but respond purposefully following repeated or painful stimulation. The ability to maintain independent ventilatory function may be impaired. Patients may require assistance in maintaining a patent airway, and spontaneous ventilation may be inadequate. Cardiovascular function is usually maintained.

General anesthesia: A drug-induced loss of consciousness during which patients cannot be aroused, even by painful stimulation. The ability to maintain independent ventilatory function is often impaired. Patients often require assistance in maintaining a patent airway, and positive-pressure ventilation may be required because of depressed spontaneous ventilation or depression of neuromuscular function.

It is important to note that patients' responses to medications and doses can vary tremendously. Thus, health care providers intending to achieve moderate sedation should be prepared to manage unintended deep sedation, and during attempts to achieve deep sedation, the provider should be capable of managing a brief period of general anesthesia, including maintaining a patent airway, effective ventilation, and cardiovascular function.

PRESEDATION EVALUATION

History and Physical Examination

All children scheduled to undergo sedation should be screened for potential adverse events during sedation and recovery. A presedation evaluation includes a focused history and physical examination, with attention to the airway and cardiorespiratory status. A focused history can be guided by the mnemonic AMPLE (Table 197-1).

The evaluation of a potentially difficult airway includes a history of previous problems with sedation or anesthesia, stridor, snoring, sleep apnea, and any recent respiratory illness. Patients with significant obesity, short neck, small mandible, dysmorphic facial features, small mouth opening, large tongue or tonsils, or nonvisible uvula are at increased risk of airway obstruction even with moderate sedation.

The patient's physical status, as classified by the ASA, can be useful in assessing sedation risk (Table 197-2).[2] ASA class I and II children are at low risk for adverse events during sedation when they are carefully monitored. Anesthesiology consultation should be considered when planning the sedation of an ASA class III to V patient.

Presedation Fasting

There is no proven relationship between the duration of fasting before sedation and the risk of aspiration in humans. However, the general consensus is that fasting likely reduces the risk of aspiration. For elective procedures, the ASA consensus recommendations should be followed (Table 197-3).[4] For nonelective procedures, the patient should be fasted as soon as the potential need for sedation is identified. Although the risk of clinically significant aspiration is low, it should be weighed carefully against the need to perform a diagnostic or therapeutic procedure quickly. The lightest effective sedation should be used.

SEDATION PLANNING

Selection of an Agent

The selection of medications is guided by the desired effect: analgesia, anxiolysis, amnesia, or some combination. Desired depth of sedation must be considered carefully. The

Table 197–1	AMPLE History
A	Allergies to medications, latex, food
M	Medications—current
P	Past medical history, including sedation history
L	Last meal, fluid intake
E	Events leading to procedure

Table 197–2 American Society of Anesthesiologists Physical Status Classification

Class	Disease State
I	No organic, physiologic, biochemical, or psychiatric disturbance
II	Mild to moderate systemic disturbance
III	Severe systemic disturbance
IV	Severe systemic disturbance that is life-threatening
V	Moribund patient with little chance of survival

Table 197–3 Fasting Guidelines for Elective Sedation

Type of Food of Liquid	Age	Time (hr)
Clear liquids	All ages	2
Breast milk	Newborn-6 mo	4
Infant formula	All ages	6
Solids	>6 mo	6

lightest effective sedation is preferred, but because of the wide variety of individual responses, clinicians should be trained and prepared to administer increasingly deeper sedation, guided by the patient's response. The clinician should consider using effective nonpharmacologic techniques, such as distraction, imagery, and parental involvement, whenever possible.

Personnel

For minimal and moderate sedation, one person with the appropriate training and experience is responsible for the procedural sedation and analgesia. This person may be the same individual who will be performing the procedure. A second person who is knowledgeable in basic pediatric life support is also required. That person is responsible for monitoring the patient's cardiopulmonary status and for recording these data on a sedation record; he or she may also assist in brief, interruptible tasks once the level of sedation is stabilized.

For deep sedation, a provider with training in advanced pediatric life support must be in the room. The person administering deep sedation should perform direct monitoring of the patient and should not be the person primarily

responsible for the procedure. The sedation provider can offer brief assistance with the procedure, as long as attention is still being paid to the patient's physiologic status. Problems with ventilation and oxygenation are easily managed when they are recognized quickly. Because deeper than intended sedation may occur in any patient, it is generally recommended that the sedation provider be prepared to manage deep sedation even when only moderate sedation is intended.

Monitoring

For minimal and moderate sedation, a minimum of pulse oximetry is strongly recommended.[1-3] In addition, continuous monitoring of the heart rate and respiratory rate and intermittent noninvasive blood pressure measurements are recommended by most. If intravenous access is not otherwise established, it is not required but should be carefully considered.

For deep sedation, continuous electrocardiographic heart rate and respiratory rate, as well as pulse oximetry and noninvasive blood pressure monitoring, are strongly recommended.[1-3] If available, end-tidal carbon dioxide monitoring is also recommended throughout the sedation and recovery. Intravenous access is also recommended. In addition to electrophysiologic monitoring, the child's color, airway patency, and rate and depth of respiration should be monitored by direct observation. This is especially important when giving additional medicine and immediately after the procedure. Completion of the painful parts of the procedure may cause children to experience deepening of the sedated state.

MEDICATIONS

There are many reasonable choices for safe sedation and analgesia. It is probably best for clinicians to become familiar with a limited number of agents or combinations of agents to meet sedation goals. This allows health care providers to become more experienced with each drug's indications, dosing, responses, and adverse effects and develop a more thorough understanding of its use. It is also important to use agents that best meet the needs of the individual patient and the procedure, based on whether the goal is simple anxiolysis, prolonged decreased motion, pain control, or some combination.

Chloral Hydrate

Choral hydrate is a halogenated hydrocarbon with sedative-hypnotic effects, but it provides no analgesia.

Route: Oral (PO) or rectal (PR).
Dose: 25 to 100 mg/kg PO or PR (common dose is 75 mg/kg); maximum 2 g total dose.
Pharmacokinetics: The drug has a half-life of 4 to 9 hours; it generally produces sedation within 30 to 60 minutes, with recovery by 60 to 120 minutes.
Side effects: Respiratory depression and hypotension.[5]
Reversal agent: None.
Uses: Its effects can be variable, but the drug is most successful when motionless sedation is needed for children younger than 12 months for nonpainful procedures (e.g., computed tomography scan, echocardiogram).

Pentobarbital

Pentobarbital is a short-acting barbiturate with sedative-hypnotic effects without analgesia.

Route: Intravenous (IV) is preferred, but intramuscular (IM) administration is also possible.
Dose: 4 to 6 mg/kg IM; 2 to 6 mg/kg IV (typically given in 1 to 2 mg/kg increments to achieve desired effect); maximum dose 150 mg.
Pharmacokinetics: The onset of action is less than 60 seconds when given intravenously and 10 to 30 minutes when given intramuscularly. Recovery time is dependent on the drug's redistribution, based on lipid solubility and protein binding. This typically occurs in 50 to 75 minutes, even though the half-life is 15 to 20 hours.
Side effects: Respiratory depression associated with pentobarbital is dose dependent.[6]
Reversal agent: None.
Uses: Pentobarbital is used primarily for nonpainful radiologic procedures.

Midazolam

Midazolam is a water-soluble benzodiazepine that has more potent amnestic effects and a quicker onset than diazepam.

Route: IV, PO.
Dose: IV: 0.05 mg/kg for anxiolysis, 0.1 mg/kg for sedation; subsequent doses of 0.05 mg/kg may be given every 2 to 5 minutes to reach desired effect; maximum single dose 2.5 to 5 mg. PO: 0.5 to 1 mg/kg; maximum dose 20 mg.
Pharmacokinetics: With IV administration, onset is usually within 1 minute, with a peak at 2 to 6 minutes and recovery within 30 to 60 minutes. With PO administration, onset is 15 to 20 minutes, with recovery in 60 to 90 minutes.
Side effects: Respiratory depression, which is much more common when administered with opioids.
Reversal agent: IV flumazenil 0.02 mg/kg repeated at 60-second intervals as needed.
Uses: As an amnestic, midazolam is used alone to provide anxiolysis. It may also be combined with an analgesic (e.g., fentanyl) for painful procedures.

Ketamine

Ketamine is a dissociative agent that rapidly induces profound sedation and analgesia.

Route: IV, IM.
Dose: IV: 1 to 2 mg/kg (given over 1 to 2 minutes); 0.5- to 1-mg injections can be given to maintain a dissociative state. IM: 2 to 6 mg/kg.
Pharmacokinetics: IV: The dissociative state usually occurs within 1 minute of administration, and coherence begins to return in approximately 15 minutes. IM: The dissociative state usually occurs within 5 minutes, and coherence begins to return in 15 to 30 minutes.
Side effects: Respiratory depression can occur, especially if an IV dose is given too quickly. However, effective spontaneous respirations are generally preserved, and airway reflexes remain intact.[7] Laryngospasm is a rare but potentially serious adverse reaction. Ketamine is contraindi-

cated in patients who have increased intracranial pressure or increased intraocular pressure. Because ketamine can cause increased salivation and bronchorrhea, glycopyrrolate (5 µg/kg) or atropine (0.01 to 0.02 mg/kg) is often given in conjunction. Coadministration with midazolam is also a common practice, because it may both decrease the incidence of dysphoria and other unpleasant emergence phenomena and treat patients who are experiencing these reactions. This, however, increases the risk of respiratory depression.
Reversal agent: None.
Uses: The relative lack of respiratory depression and sparing of airway reflexes make ketamine a popular choice for short, painful procedures.

Propofol

Propofol is a nonbarbiturate sedative-hypnotic agent that has no analgesic effect.

Route: IV.
Dose: Doses of 1 to 2 mg/kg can provide sedation for short procedures. For prolonged painless sedation, propofol is maintained at a constant infusion rate of 150 to 200 µg/kg per minute.
Pharmacokinetics: The plasma concentration of propofol rapidly equilibrates with brain concentrations, and its onset of action is usually less than 1 minute. Plasma levels fall quickly because of metabolic clearance and rapid redistribution, so a continuous infusion is needed to maintain sedation longer than a few minutes.
Side effects: Propofol can cause both apnea and hypotension.[8,9] Owing to its extremely short half-life, it can be difficult to titrate its effect. Thus, propofol should be administered only by experienced providers with advanced airway skills. (When using propofol, the sedation provider must be dedicated to monitoring the patient and should not be involved in the procedure being performed.)
Reversal agent: None.
Uses: The quick onset of action and short duration make propofol an attractive drug for brief, nonpainful procedures.

Fentanyl

Fentanyl is a high-potency opioid that has minimal adverse hemodynamic effects.

Route: IV.
Dose: 1-2 µg/kg, usually given as 0.5 µg/kg infused over 30 to 60 seconds and repeated to effect.
Pharmacokinetics: The onset of action is 30 to 60 seconds, and the duration of action is 5 to 10 minutes.[10]
Side effects: The major side effect of fentanyl is respiratory depression, which is clearly dose related but can occasionally occur with low doses. The risk of respiratory depression is significantly increased when fentanyl is given with benzodiazepines or barbiturates. Hypotension and chest wall rigidity are rare adverse events that can occur with rapid infusion of large doses.
Reversal agent: Naloxone 0.001 to 0.01 mg/kg, given every 60 seconds until the patient awakens.

Uses: As an analgesic, fentanyl is used for painful procedures. It is frequently combined with a sedative-hypnotic for procedural sedation.

SUGGESTED READING

American Academy of Pediatrics, Committee on Drugs: Guidelines for monitoring and management of pediatric patients during and after sedation for diagnostic and therapeutic procedures. Pediatrics 1992;89:1110-1115.

Joint Commission on Accreditation of Healthcare Organizations: Standards and intents for sedation and anesthesia care. In Revisions to Anesthesia Care Standards, Comprehensive Accreditation Manual for Hospitals. Oakbrook Terrace, Ill, Joint Commission on Accreditation of Healthcare Organizations, 2001. *http://www.jcaho.org/standard/aneshap.html.*

REFERENCES

1. American Academy of Pediatrics, Committee on Drugs: Guidelines for monitoring and management of pediatric patients during and after sedation for diagnostic and therapeutic procedures. Pediatrics 1992;89:1110-1115.

2. American Society of Anesthesiologists: Practice guidelines for sedation and analgesia by non-anesthesiologists. Anesthesiology 2002;96:1004-1017.

3. Joint Commission on Accreditation of Healthcare Organizations: Standards and intents for sedation and anesthesia care. In Revisions to Anesthesia Care Standards, Comprehensive Accreditation Manual for Hospitals. Oakbrook Terrace, Ill, Joint Commission on Accreditation of Healthcare Organizations, 2001. *http://www.jcaho.org/standard/aneshap.html.*

4. American Society of Anesthesiologists: Practice guidelines for preoperative fasting and the use of pharmacologic agents to reduce the risk of pulmonary aspirations: Application to healthy patients undergoing elective procedures. Anesthesiology 1999;90:896-905.

5. Lacouture PG: Chloral hydrate. Clin Toxicol Rev 1983;5:6.

6. Strain JD, Harvey LA, Foley LC, et al: Intravenously administered pentobarbital sodium for sedation in pediatric CT. Radiology 1986;161:105-108.

7. White PF, Way WL, Trevor AJ: Ketamine—its pharmacology and therapeutic uses. Anesthesiology 1982;56:119-136.

8. Bryson HM, Fulton BR, Faulds D: Propofol: An update on its clinical use. Drugs 1995;50:513-559.

9. Green SM: Propofol for emergency department procedural sedation—not yet ready for prime time. Acad Emerg Med 1999;6:975-978.

10. McCain DA, Hug CC: Intravenous fentanyl kinetics. Clin Pharmacol Ther 1980;28:106-114.

CHAPTER 198

Radiology for the Pediatric Hospitalist

Jeanne S. Chow, Anna M. Golja, and Horacio M. Padua

The purpose of this chapter is to familiarize hospitalists with common pediatric imaging examinations so that they can order the most appropriate test for the patient, as well as be able to properly inform and prepare the patient and family before the study. This chapter describes the techniques, indications, and patient preparation for common pediatric imaging examinations.

After a discussion of radiation safety and sedation techniques, the chapter is divided into imaging studies that require ionizing radiation and those that do not. Studies that use ionizing radiation include conventional radiographs, fluoroscopy, computed tomography (CT), and nuclear medicine examinations. Studies that do not use ionizing radiation include ultrasound (US) and magnetic resonance imaging (MRI). Vascular and nonvascular interventional procedures are described at the end of the chapter.

RADIATION SAFETY

Whenever considering a radiographic examination for any patient, one must be cognizant of the amount of radiation that the patient will receive, especially if the patient has a chronic condition. The guiding principle behind radiation protection is that radiation exposures should be kept "as low as reasonably achievable (ALARA)." This principle must be especially adhered to in children because it is well known that for the same dose, children are more susceptible to radiation effects than adults are. The 1-year-old "lifetime" cancer mortality from radiation is higher than in adults by an entire order of magnitude.[1] Children incur a far greater effective dose of radiation when undergoing CT than plain radiography or fluoroscopy. It is estimated that if 600,000 pediatric CT procedures are performed per year, approximately 500 of these patients will eventually die of radiation-induced cancer.[1] Appropriate indications for evaluation of a pediatric patient with CT cannot be stressed enough. Other imaging modalities such as ultrasound or MRI should be considered whenever possible.

BASIC RADIATION PHYSICS

Plain radiographs are produced when a beam of photons penetrates through an object and strikes a film. Electrons pass from a tungsten cathode filament to a surrounding rotating anode, where the electronic energy is converted to x-rays. The cathode and anode are collectively known as the x-ray tube. Only about 1% of the electron energy is converted to radiation, and the remainder is converted to heat energy. An even smaller number of photons actually pass completely through the patient to strike the film. The remainder of these photons scatter throughout the air.[2]

Fluoroscopy uses continuous x-rays to evaluate a real-time dynamic process in the patient. The radiologist watches a monitor, which resembles a TV, during this real-time evaluation. To decrease the radiation dose, pulsed fluoroscopy has been developed, which emits a beam of photons only a fraction of the time as opposed to a continuous beam.[3]

Images acquired with CT are based on the same principles; however, to obtain cross-sectional images, the x-ray tube in CT rotates, and a ring of detectors replaces the film.[4] With the advent of multidetector CT scanners, the number of rings or rows of detectors continues to increase, which has decreased scan time considerably but potentially increases the radiation dose. Multidetector CT scanners, however, have made it possible to scan pediatric patients without the need for sedation, thereby reducing risks related to the sedating agents.

Parents may remain with their child when any of these radiologic examinations are performed, unless the mother is pregnant; ionizing radiation exposure in the fetus is known to cause miscarriages and malformations and carries a small, but real risk for the development of childhood cancers.[5] Parents and other personnel who remain in the same room where the x-ray tube is located must wear lead shielding for protection. Special shields are provided to protect the thyroid gland, which is especially susceptible to radiation-induced malignancy.

CONTRAST MATERIALS

The different contrasts one sees on radiologic images are based on differences in tissue density or water composition. Contrast agents are often used to enhance these differences. These agents aid in visualizing certain organ systems, such as the gastrointestinal (GI) tract or the genitourinary system, but they can also more accurately assess certain disease processes, for example, the spread of tumor along the craniospinal axis.

Barium and Gastrografin (a combination of sodium amidotrizoate and meglumine amidotrizoate) are often used for evaluation of the GI tract along with other contrast agents. Many different iodinated contrast agents are available that can be used to evaluate the GI tract, but they may also be administered intravenously for the evaluation of certain organ systems, such as the genitourinary tract or central nervous system (CNS). Similarly, other contrast agents are available for specific indications in imaging modalities such as US or MRI. Although US contrast agents are more widely used in adult patients, their use is still experimental in the pediatric population in the United States. The MRI contrast agent gadolinium is frequently used in the pediatric population. This contrast agent is administered intravenously. Some MRI contrast agents may also be administered parenterally.

As with any medication, administration of contrast agents is generally safe but may cause adverse reactions ranging from benign urticaria to death from fulminant anaphylaxis. An in-depth discussion of these contrast agents and treatment of the adverse events follows in this chapter.

SEDATION/GENERAL ANESTHESIA

For most imaging examinations performed in children, sedation or general anesthesia is not necessary. As described previously, with the advent of multidetector CT scanners increasing the speed with which information is obtained, far fewer patients need to be sedated to obtain diagnostic images. However, a small number of patients undergoing CT and a larger number undergoing MRI need to be sedated or even placed under general anesthesia. In our hospital, strict practice guidelines have been established by the Radiology Sedation Committee, which in turn comply with policies established by the Children's Hospital Boston Sedation Task Force. Quality assurance indicators for this sedation program are reviewed monthly.

Each patient receives a presedation evaluation, which is usually performed by telephone contact with the parent before arrival at the department, as well as by history and physical examination before sedation. If sedation is deemed appropriate, informed written consent is obtained and the appropriate sedative is ordered. The child is generally fasted for approximately 4 hours. Eight hours of fasting is usually the requirement before general anesthesia. Generally, pentobarbital is used as the first-line sedative agent and may be administered orally, intramuscularly, or intravenously, depending on the age of the patient and state of intravenous access. If the child has received the maximum dose of pentobarbital and is not motionless, midazolam and fentanyl citrate may be additionally administered. If during the presedation evaluation sedation is not deemed appropriate, general anesthesia or alternative sedative drugs may be ordered. When ordering any CT or MRI examination, careful consideration must be given to these issues. The benefit of information obtained from these studies must outweigh the risk of possible adverse events from sedation or general anesthesia.

As an alternative to sedation and general anesthesia, distraction methods practiced by our child life experts are used to get some patients through the examination with the least amount of motion and stress. Child life experts may, for example, use play or diversional talk with preschool- or school-aged children and guided imagery with school-aged children or adolescents. All children are unique, and how they function while undergoing a radiologic examination depends on family dynamics and the child's individual personality and coping ability.

IMAGING IN CHILD ABUSE

In 2002, approximately 896,000 children were abused or neglected, with close to 20% being physically abused, and an estimated 1400 child fatalities occurred in 2002 because of neglect or abuse.[6] It has been shown that radiologic examinations may aid in investigation and prosecution of cases of fatal infant abuse.[7] Even more important is the evidence that radiologic examinations can provide help to protect a still living infant or child. Although skeletal surveys play a major role in the evaluation of suspected abuse, US, nuclear

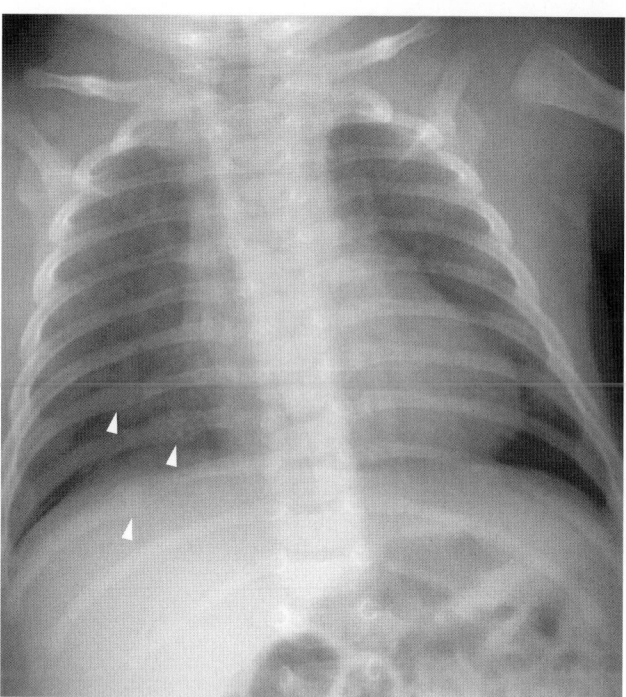

Figure 198-1 Multiple posterior rib fractures involving the right 8th, 9th, and 10th ribs (*arrowheads*) in an 8-week-old who concomitantly sustained a femur fracture. The infant was reportedly sleeping on the edge of the bed next to his father when he fell on the floor. The radiographic findings along with the given clinical history are consistent with trauma.

medicine, CT, and MRI examinations provide important information as well.

Certain abnormal skeletal findings have high specificity for diagnosing inflicted trauma, including the classic metaphyseal fracture; rib fractures, especially posterior ones (Fig. 198-1); and scapular, spinous process, and sternal fractures.[8] The skeletal survey plays a key role in evaluating a suspected abused infant or child because a subtle skeletal abnormality may be very specific for this diagnosis. Although techniques for skeletal survey imaging vary widely across the United States,[9] we recommend high-detail screen-film imaging of the appendicular skeleton in the anteroposterior (AP) projection and the axial skeleton in the AP and lateral projections. Any area of abnormality should be imaged in two views. If rib fractures are suspected, oblique views are recommended (Fig. 198-2). Likewise, additional images of the calvaria should be obtained if there is suspicion of a fracture in this region. If a skull fracture is present, a head CT scan should be obtained. There should be a low threshold for performing head CT or even brain MRI in cases of suspected abuse.[10,11] A subdural hematoma is an important feature in the diagnosis of infant abuse (Fig. 198-3).

Prominent subarachnoid spaces are most commonly seen from 2 months to 2 years of age,[12] yet this same age group is especially vulnerable to abuse; the greatest number of fatalities occurs in children 3 years and younger,[6] and therefore it is imperative to evaluate the extra-axial spaces carefully for any difference in density that may represent a concomitant subdural or even epidural hematoma. In the event of any concern, US or MRI, or both, may aid in distinguishing a

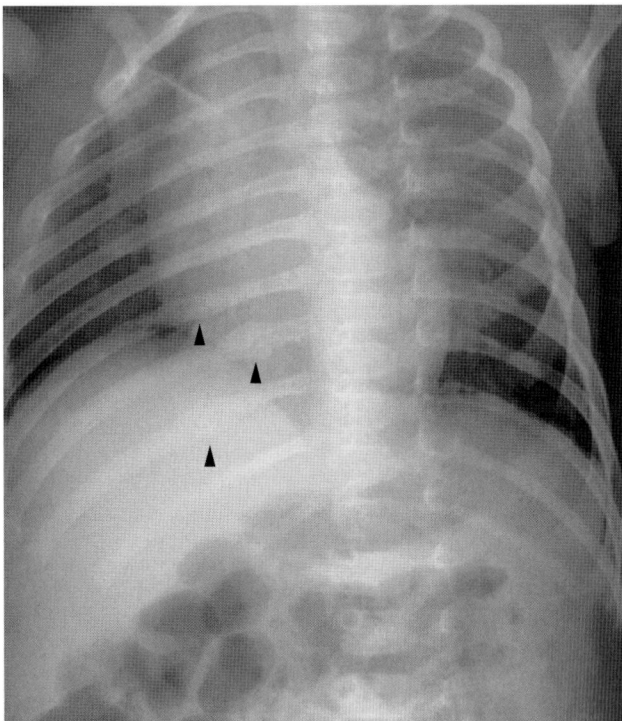

Figure 198-2 Oblique chest radiograph, which is very helpful to obtain in skeletal surveys because it may better depict posterior or lateral rib fractures. Callus formation can be appreciated surrounding the posterior aspect of the right 9th and 10th ribs and to a lesser degree surrounding the posterior of the right 8th rib (*arrowheads*) of the same infant shown in Figure 198-1.

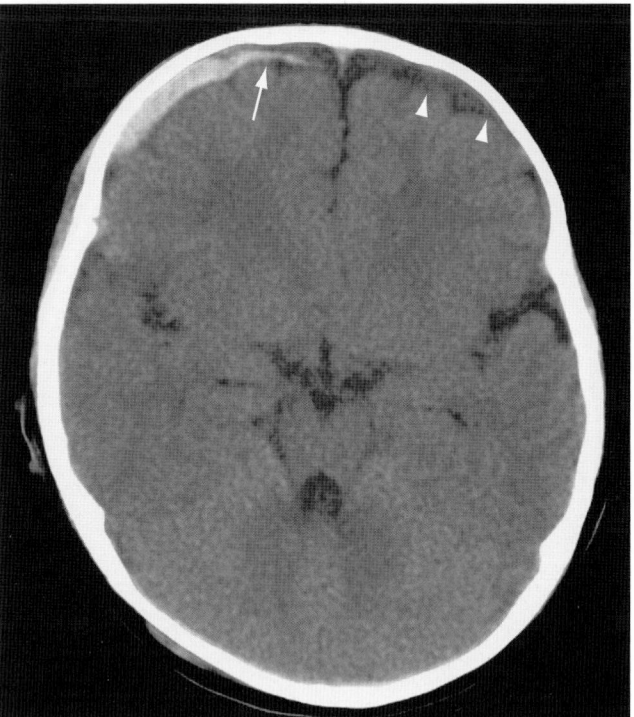

Figure 198-3 Right frontal subdural hematoma (*arrowhead*) that extends minimally into the interhemispheric region (*arrow*) in a 10-month-old who presented to the emergency department (ED) limp and unresponsive. During an ED visit only 9 days earlier for a nonfebrile seizure, an unremarkable head computed tomography scan was demonstrated. The extra-axial spaces overall are minimally prominent, which can be a normal variant in this age group, thus making the diagnosis of an isointense subdural hematoma challenging.
From Egelhoff JC, Caré MM: Pediatric Head Trauma. In Slovis TL: Caffey's Pediatric Diagnostic Imaging, 11th ed. Philadelphia: Elsevier Mosby, in press.

prominent subarachnoid space from a subdural collection (Fig. 198-4).

Although it is important to recognize radiographic abnormalities caused by inflicted trauma, it is also of utmost importance to recognize normal variants and other disease entities that can simulate the appearance of child abuse, such as Caffey disease, osteogenesis imperfecta, Menkes kinky hair syndrome, congenital insensitivity to pain, bone dysplasias, and others. Diagnostic imaging is essential in recognizing physical abuse and supporting this diagnosis in suspected cases; however, it is also essential in excluding the diagnosis when true accidental injury, normal variants, and other mimics exist. It is because of these variations that communication with the radiologist regarding the historical and clinical information is crucial.

CONVENTIONAL RADIOGRAPHS

Although far more sophisticated imaging modalities exist, the conventional radiograph remains an invaluable means by which to evaluate certain organ systems. An area of interest can be evaluated in many ways with the plain film. In the chest, for example, posteroanterior and lateral views are the standard projections obtained when a chest radiograph is ordered. Beyond these two, there are many other projections with differing obliquities that the radiologist may use to further evaluate a specific area. Some of these additional views include inspiratory/expiratory, lordotic, or decubitus projections.

Skull radiographs remain an especially invaluable means by which to evaluate any infant or child suspected of having a calvarial fracture. Although CT and MRI are far better for evaluation of the brain and even bone in some cases, a fracture can very easily be overlooked with these imaging modalities, especially if the orientation of the fracture is in the axial plane. Additionally, skull radiographs are useful for evaluation of the sutures in suspected cases of craniosynostosis. AP, bilateral lateral (with each side of the head close to the film cassette), and the Towne's view (the x-ray tube is angled inferiorly to better visualize the occipital bone) projections are routinely obtained in the skull series (Fig. 198-5A-C).[13]

In radiographic evaluation of the spine, the number of views obtained depends on which part of the spine is studied (i.e., cervical, thoracic, or lumbar) and the indication. For example, in the setting of trauma, additional views are obtained to visualize the dens and the C7-T1 junction. If the dens or the C7-T1 junction is not clearly visualized, the radiologist cannot "clear" the cervical spine. For further evaluation of these focal areas, CT is sometimes needed. Alternatively, bilateral oblique or "swimmer's" views may be obtained to visualize the C7-T1 junction. Because the incidence of spinal fractures is relatively low in the pediatric population and to keep the radiation dose as low as reason-

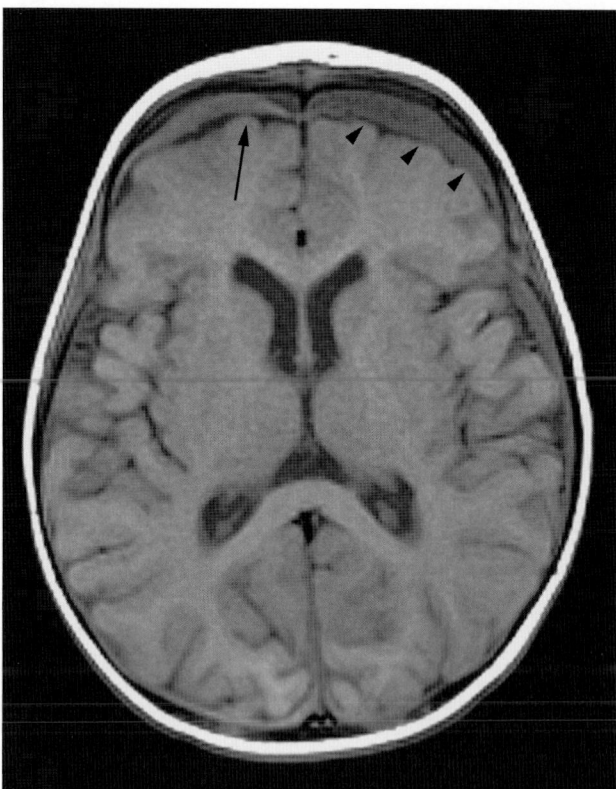

Figure 198-4 Importance of obtaining a brain magnetic resonance image in patients suspected of sustaining inflicted trauma. A T1-weighted image of the same patient as in Figure 198-3 at a comparable level shows that the prominent extra-axial space on the left is consistent with a subdural collection (*arrowheads*) and not a prominent subarachnoid space; this information is crucial for medicolegal purposes. Again shown is the right-sided subdural hematoma (*arrow*).

ably achievable, full cervical spine CT evaluation is not performed at our institution. CT is reserved for further investigation of any focal area of tenderness that the patient may have or for more thorough evaluation of any region of abnormality seen on plain films. For the evaluation of lower back pain in an adolescent, bilateral oblique views are obtained in addition to the standard AP and lateral views to better evaluate the pars interarticularis. If a fracture or spondylolysis is noted on plain films and grading of the pars defect is necessary, obtaining a focused CT scan limited to the region of abnormality is recommended to decrease the amount of radiation that the pelvis receives. This practice is especially important in females because the ovaries may be in the radiation field.

AP and lateral radiographs are the typical projections obtained when evaluating the soft tissues of the neck for epiglottitis, croup, and other conditions. In a case of suspected epiglottitis, a health care provider should accompany the patient to the radiology department in case the airway becomes obstructed. To prevent airway obstruction, placing the patient in a supine position to obtain radiographs is contraindicated.

As described earlier, radiologists have many projections available in their armamentarium to evaluate the chest. In a child suspected of aspirating a foreign body, inspiratory/

expiratory or bilateral decubitus films are very helpful. A chest radiograph is perhaps most commonly ordered for the evaluation of pneumonia in the pediatric population, and although the lungs do occupy the majority of the chest, the mediastinum, heart, pulmonary vasculature, diaphragm, pleura, and bones can be initially evaluated on the chest radiograph. For example, a chest radiograph may be the only vehicle with which posterior rib fractures are identified in an infant who is being abused, something that may be initially unsuspected during evaluation of an unrelated condition such as pneumonia.

No description of a chest radiograph would be complete without some mention of the thymus in a pediatric patient. One must be familiar with the normally large thymus seen in infants and not mistake this normal structure for mediastinal pathology.

Both chest and abdominal radiographs are frequently evaluated for the placement of various lines and tubes. This is especially important in a neonate, in whom tube malpositioning can have deleterious complications. The tip of the endotracheal tube should be located between the level of the thoracic inlet and the carina. If well secured in this anatomically "safe" location, the tube should not be displaced very far inferiorly into one of the bronchi and should not fall out of the trachea. In neonates, the tip of the endotracheal tube is especially sensitive to flexion and extension of the neck, and radiographs should be interpreted with this in mind.

The tip of an umbilical arterial catheter should be below the ductus arteriosus, approximately below the T6 vertebral body. The tip should not approximate the celiac, superior mesenteric, inferior mesenteric, or renal artery branches and should therefore be above the level of T11 or below the level of the L2 vertebral artery. Similarly, the tip of an umbilical venous catheter should not approximate any tributary veins and should therefore be positioned in the lower portion of the right atrium near the inferior vena cava junction.[14]

Aside from evaluation of line and tube positioning, perhaps the most important indication for obtaining an abdominal radiograph is to assess the bowel gas pattern. Supine and upright views are obtained in any radiographic evaluation of the abdomen. If the patient is too young or sick to stand, in place of the upright view, a left lateral decubitus film is obtained. If intussusception is suspected, a prone view is additionally obtained to aid in filling the cecum with air, which would then exclude the more common ileocolic intussusception. For the evaluation of renal calculi, a single "KUB" view suffices; this radiograph includes the *k*idneys, *u*reters, and *b*ladder. The superimposition of many densities within the abdomen may simulate the appearance of calculus. Oblique views are frequently obtained when this occurs to confirm or dismiss the finding. One may further evaluate the suspicion of calculus with US or even CT. Finally, although abdominal radiographs are more commonly ordered to assess the bowel gas pattern, the bony structures need to be carefully examined, especially in a very young patient, who has difficulty expressing precisely where the pain is coming from. Vertebral body and disk space heights, spinal alignment, and pedicle size are only a few of the things to check in regard to the skeleton on the abdominal film.

When the area of abnormality can be localized to a particular joint or location, such as the forearm, a dedicated

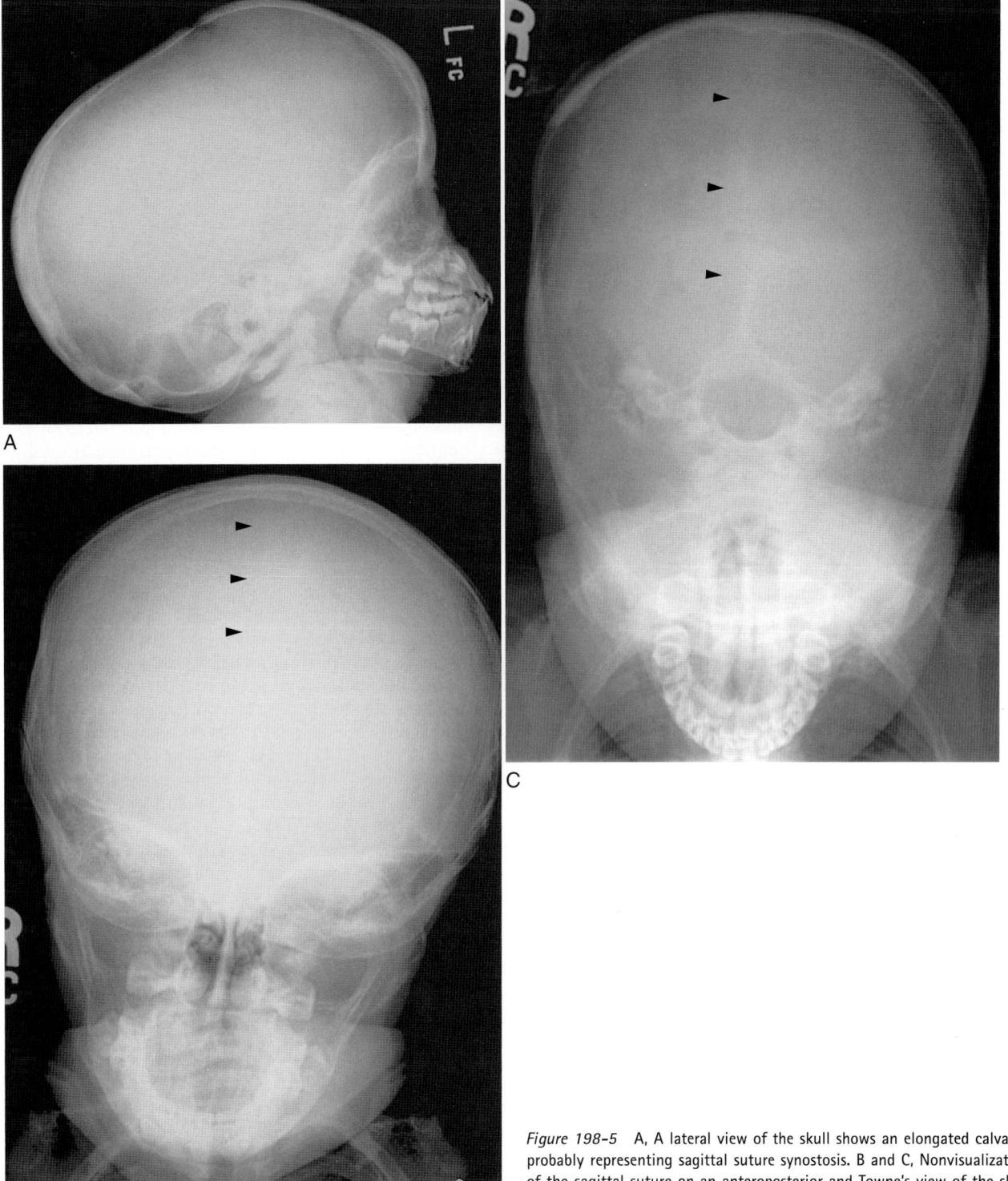

Figure 198-5 A, A lateral view of the skull shows an elongated calvaria, probably representing sagittal suture synostosis. B and C, Nonvisualization of the sagittal suture on an anteroposterior and Towne's view of the skull (*arrowheads*) confirms the diagnosis.

radiographic series coned down to that anatomic location is performed. AP and lateral views are the basic radiographs obtained when evaluating the musculoskeletal system. These projections are frequently supplemented with an oblique view, sometimes even bilateral oblique views when evaluating particular regions, such as the elbow. More specialized projections such as the "sunrise" or "tunnel" views of the knee or the "Harris" view of the calcaneus may be obtained, depending on the clinical indication. Although CT and MRI may evaluate the musculoskeletal system in greater detail, one can obtain important diagnostic information from the standard radiograph. In certain cases, radiography alone can be diagnostic without the aid of additional imaging. Therefore, radiography remains extremely important and should not be dismissed in the evaluation of any bone pathology.

The radiographic series just described are typically performed within the radiology department; however, sometimes the patient is too sick to leave the intensive care unit or emergency room, and thus portable radiographs may be obtained. Portable series should be truly reserved for critically ill patients. When interpreting portable radiographs, one must take into account suboptimal patient positioning and external conditions that may limit the evaluation.

FLUOROSCOPY

Fluoroscopy uses radiation to dynamically observe the form and function of the body. The information obtained from a fluoroscopic examination can be stored as a video or as a series of individual images that represent the most important information from the examination. Most fluoroscopy studies also use a contrast material to better demarcate the anatomic area of interest.

Digital pulsed fluoroscopy units are recommended for use in children. Unlike conventional fluoroscopy, pulsed fluoroscopy creates high-quality diagnostic images[15,16] while substantially reducing the radiation dose associated with older standard fluoroscopic units and conventional film-screen combinations.[3,17,18] Gonadal shielding and careful image coning also significantly decrease patient radiation exposure.

Chest/Neck/Airway Imaging

Fluoroscopy is very useful in the dynamic evaluation of the airway, glottis, and diaphragm. CT and MRI are gradually replacing fluoroscopy in evaluation of the tracheobronchial tree and soft tissues of the neck. Fluoroscopy of these anatomic locations requires no patient preparation or sedation. The natural difference between the density of gas in the airways and lungs and the adjacent soft tissues provides the contrast for these studies; no additional contrast is necessary.

Fluoroscopy is a simple noninvasive test to evaluate children who are suspected of having aspirated a foreign body. When plain radiographs are equivocal or further confirmation is necessary, fluoroscopy can show persistent air trapping in the area blocked by the foreign body.

In addition, fluoroscopy is frequently used for further evaluation after plain radiographs suggest a prevertebral soft tissue mass. With this imaging modality, redundant yet normal prevertebral soft tissues flatten during inspiration, whereas prominence secondary to an abscess or mass will persist throughout the respiratory cycle. Similarly, fluoroscopy can be used to evaluate movement of the vocal cords and diaphragm. Asymmetric movement of these structures can point to the site of injury.

Gastrointestinal Imaging

Several fluoroscopic examinations are available to evaluate the GI system: swallowing studies, esophagograms, upper gastrointestinal (UGI) series, small bowel series, enemas, and stomagrams. These studies all require that the patient receive contrast either orally, per rectum, or into the stoma. The contrast is necessary to visualize the bowel. All studies except the swallowing studies require a "scout" film of the area of interest before administering contrast.

Table 198-1   Hours a Patient Is Restricted from Oral Intake before an Upper Gastrointestinal Series

Newborn-6 months old	2 hours before the procedure
6 months-2 years old	3 hours before the procedure
2-4 years old	4 hours before the procedure
4 years or older	6 hours before the procedure

Patients and their families should be informed of their scheduled examination and how the test is performed. Before a UGI study or small bowel series, the patient is restricted from food or drink for a number of hours, depending on the patient's age (Table 198-1).

In our institution, we do not require bowel cleansing before most gastrointestinal contrast studies. Bowel preparation is, however, required before any double-contrast (air and barium) lower intestinal study. Performance of a double-contrast study is dependent on the institution and age of the child. Sedation is contraindicated because the patient should be alert and cooperative during these examinations. If a patient cannot drink the barium or the water-soluble contrast from a cup, barium can be fed by bottle, syringe, or straw or administered via nasogastric tube.

Barium, water-soluble low-osmolar nonionic contrast, and air are the three most widely used contrast agents for the GI system. Barium sulfate suspension is an inert white liquid that attenuates the passage of x-rays. It comes in different consistencies, depending on its required use. Barium has a chalk-like taste, but its palatability is improved with mild flavoring.

Double-contrast barium studies involve the use of barium and gas. These studies introduce gas into the intestines to distend the bowel and create a thin coat of barium on the bowel mucosal surfaces to assess mucosal detail. Patients undergoing double-contrast esophagography and UGI studies quickly swallow effervescent granules, which produce carbon dioxide and distend the stomach and intestines. During double-contrast enemas, gas is insufflated into the colon per rectum. Because double-contrast studies require strict patient cooperation and are most useful for mucosal detail, they are not routinely performed in the pediatric population; more typically, single-contrast studies are performed.

The use of barium for GI studies is contraindicated in patients in whom aspiration, a tracheoesophageal fistula, bowel perforation or obstruction, or constipation is suspected. Barium clears very slowly from the lungs, contaminates the peritoneal cavity, and can cause constipation. Water-soluble low-osmolar nonionic contrast is used in neonates in cases in which barium use is contraindicated. Water-soluble high-osmolar contrast agents are used for therapeutic enemas, for example, in a cystic fibrosis patient with meconium ileus equivalent or in a neonate with meconium ileus. Gas or barium is used to reduce ileocolic intussusception.

A swallowing study evaluates the oral and pharyngeal phases of swallowing and can detect the presence of aspiration with different food textures; the swallowing phases are observed during fluoroscopy with different consistencies

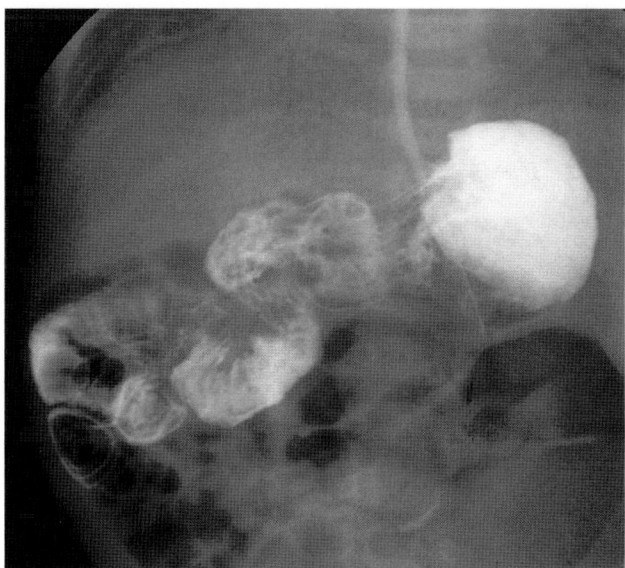

Figure 198-6 A single image from an upper gastrointestinal series in a patient with bilious vomiting demonstrates malrotation; the fourth portion of the duodenum does not reach the expected location of the ligament of Treitz to the left of the spine at the level of the pylorus.

of barium preparations, including solids, purees, and thick and thin liquids. At our institution, this examination is performed in conjunction with the speech pathologist.

Esophagograms evaluate the patient's ability to swallow and the appearance and motility of the esophagus. Indications depend on the patient's age; newborns are most commonly evaluated for symptoms of choking or wheezing to look for a vascular ring or sling, esophageal stricture, or tracheoesophageal fistula. Older children with symptoms of dysphagia or a feeling that something is "stuck" in the throat may have esophageal narrowing or a foreign body obstructing the esophagus.

A UGI examination studies the digestive system from the mouth to the duodenojejunal junction. This study is preformed on an emergency basis in a child suspected of having malrotation with symptoms of obstruction (Fig. 198-6), but it is more commonly ordered for evaluation of unexplained vomiting and detection of gastroesophageal reflux. It is useful for evaluating the esophagus, stomach, and duodenum and the location of the ligament of Treitz. Because the column of contrast is followed dynamically, peristalsis, as well as the appearance of the intestine, is evaluated.

The duodenojejunal junction on a UGI study is normally to the left of the spine and at the same level as the pyloric bulb. The radiographic definition of malrotation is any deviation from the normal definition of the duodenojejunal junction on a UGI examination. For patients suspected of having an obstruction at the level of the second portion of the duodenum (i.e., secondary to duodenal atresia, an annular pancreas, or a duodenal web), UGI examination is not necessary; a plain film of the abdomen is usually diagnostic because gas within the distended stomach and proximal duodenum serves as a good contrast agent to delineate the level of obstruction.

A small bowel series is used to evaluate the small intestine from the ligament of Treitz to the ileocecal valve. It is usually

performed with a UGI series but can be performed separately. It is useful in evaluating the site of small bowel obstruction, focal abdominal pain, small bowel masses, and inflammatory bowel disease. The examination is performed almost exclusively with barium because water-soluble contrast tends to become diluted and lose its opacity before reaching the ileum. This examination requires a cooperative child because a large volume of barium is required to opacify the entire small bowel. After the patient finishes drinking the contrast agent, movement of the contrast column is monitored by a series of radiographs. Fluoroscopy is used to evaluate peristalsis and pliability of the small bowel. The duration of this examination depends on the time needed for the contrast to pass through the small intestine, which can take up to several hours in some cases. This is particularly important because many small bowel diseases arise in the distal part of the small bowel. Patients should be informed of this possibility before the examination.

Although other imaging modalities are being explored for evaluation of the colon, a contrast enema is most commonly used in the pediatric population for studying the large bowel. Contrast is instilled into the rectum by gravity technique via a soft catheter. The patient is often rotated during the examination to allow visualization of the various curves and flexures of the colon. This examination is frequently used for the evaluation of distal obstruction in a newborn infant secondary to Hirschsprung's disease, ileal atresia, or meconium ileus. Older patients with a suspected mass, inflammatory bowel disease, or a stricture can likewise be evaluated with a contrast enema. A scout film of the abdomen before the examination is necessary to assess whether there is any evidence of pneumoperitoneum, but this film is also useful in assessing whether there has been any change in the bowel gas pattern in an obstructed patient.

Contrast can also be injected into ostomy sites to evaluate the internal anatomy. Fluoroscopic examination of an ostomy site is frequently requested in the setting of a suspected stricture. Water-soluble contrast is preferred over barium for this evaluation. The location and complications of gastric and gastrojejunal tubes can also be assessed with an injection of contrast into the tube under fluoroscopic visualization.

An important diagnostic and therapeutic use for GI fluoroscopy is diagnosis and reduction of ileocolic intussusception. Institutions vary greatly in the workup of suspected intussusception. We recommend an abdominal radiograph as the screening examination. When the cecum is clearly identified or other causes of abdominal pain are revealed, further imaging may not be necessary. Alternatively, an abdominal radiograph may show definite evidence of intussusception. If plain films are unrevealing and additional imaging is needed, abdominal US is recommended. US can reliably demonstrate intussusception with high specificity and sensitivity. It can also evaluate for other causes of the patient's symptoms. Rather than obtaining a US examination, some pediatric radiologists prefer to proceed directly to an enema, which may both diagnose and reduce the intussusception (Fig. 198-7).

Before enema reduction, the surgical staff should be notified of the impending procedure, and the patient should receive prophylactic antibiotics. As previously described, a scout film of the abdomen is obtained to evaluate for pneu-

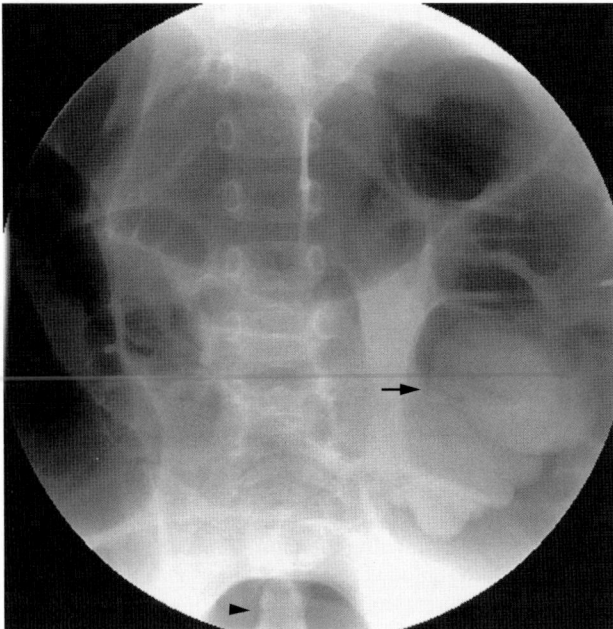

Figure 198-7 A single image from an air enema reduction of intussusception demonstrates the intussusceptum as a soft tissue density within the colon (*arrow*). Air is being insufflated into the rectum via a soft catheter (*arrowhead*). This 2-year-old presented with intermittent abdominal pain and bloody stools.

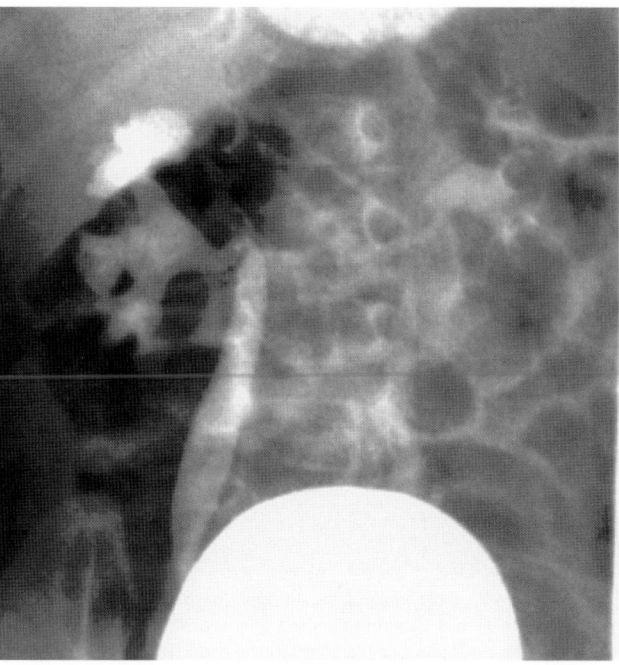

Figure 198-8 A voiding cystourethrogram demonstrates bilateral vesicoureteral reflux, grade 3 on the right and grade 2 on the left. This child presented with a febrile urinary tract infection diagnosed by catheter specimen.

moperitoneum, but this film is especially important to obtain before enema reduction. During the enema, a surgeon should be in attendance in the event of bowel perforation and the need for emergency surgery. The risks and benefits of the procedure are explained to the parents in detail before the examination and informed consent is obtained. The patient should not be sedated because, as the patient's colon is filled with gas or contrast, the patient usually performs a Valsalva maneuver as a natural protective mechanism to prevent bowel perforation, as well as to provide a higher-pressure gradient to aid in reduction of the intussusception. Gas or barium is instilled per rectum under fluoroscopic guidance. The pressure of the contrast or gas reduces the intussusception. After the procedure, radiographs are obtained to assess for successful reduction and any complications. Contraindications to enema reduction are bowel perforation or signs of peritonitis.

Genitourinary Imaging

Common fluoroscopic evaluations of the genitourinary system include voiding cystourethrography (VCUG), retrograde urethrography, and intravenous pyelography (IVP). During VCUG, the urethra is catheterized and contrast is instilled into the bladder. High-osmolar ionic contrast material is generally safe for these studies. High- or low-osmolar contrast material can be injected intravenously for IVP. Low-osmolar contrast is 10 to 20 times the price of high-osmolar contrast but has definite advantages and is recommended by the American College of Radiology[19] for the following indications:

1. Patients with a history of a previous adverse reaction to contrast material, with the exception of a sensation

of heat, flushing, or a single episode of nausea or vomiting
2. Patients with a history of asthma or allergy
3. Patients with known cardiac dysfunction, including recent or potentially imminent cardiac decompensation, severe arrhythmias, unstable angina, recent myocardial infarction, and pulmonary hypertension
4. Patients with generalized severe debilitation
5. Any other circumstances in which after due consideration, the radiologist believes that there is a specific indication for the use of low-osmolar contrast material

Most hospitals now primarily use low-osmolar contrast. If there has been a previous contrast reaction, premedication with steroids is mandatory or an alternative examination should be sought. At our institution, we recommend an H_1 blocker, diphenhydramine, 1 mg/kg orally or intravenously 1 hour before intravenous contrast injection (maximum of 50 mg), and the following:

Older patients: Prednisone, 1 mg/kg orally (maximum of 20 mg per dose and 60 mg/day) at 13 hours, 7 hours, and 1 hour before contrast injection
Younger patients: Prednisolone, 15 mg/5 mL; 1 mg/kg orally (maximum of 20 mg per dose and 60 mg/day) at 13 hours, 7 hours, and 1 hour before contrast injection
Those who can take medication only intravenously: Methylprednisolone, 1 mg/kg intravenously 12 hours and 2 hours before contrast injection

VCUG evaluates for the presence/absence of vesicoureteral reflux (Fig. 198-8) and the function and appearance of the bladder and urethra. This study is indicated in patients with a history of well-documented pyelonephritis, abnormal prenatal or postnatal US findings, and a family history of reflux. This study can also show abnormalities of the bladder such as diverticula or bladder wall thickening. VCUG can demonstrate abnormalities of the urethra, such as posterior urethral valves. It can also be used to evaluate complex congenital anomalies such as ambiguous genitalia and anorectal malformations.

During VCUG, dilute water-soluble contrast is instilled into the bladder through a sterile urethral catheter via gravity under fluoroscopic guidance. Fluoroscopy is performed during bladder filling and voiding. A cyclic study, when the bladder is refilled after voiding, is performed in infants. For older children, the bladder is typically filled one time only to its predicted capacity based on age.

When the study is performed in an environment comfortable for the patient, family, and physician and the parents and children are well informed and reassured, no sedation is necessary. Sedation can prolong and complicate this otherwise simple examination, as well as elevate the risk incurred by the patient. If sedation is used, midazolam can be administered without any negative outcome on the results of the examination.[20,21]

Patients at moderate to high risk for endocarditis need prophylactic antibiotics before VCUG, as recommended by the American Heart Association. High-risk patients include those with complex cyanotic congenital heart disease and surgically constructed systemic-pulmonary shunts or conduits. Moderate-risk patients include those with congenital cardiac malformations, hypertrophic cardiomyopathy and mitral valve prolapse with regurgitation or thickened leaflets (or both).[22] Many patients who are suspected of having reflux because of prenatal hydronephrosis or who have pyelonephritis are already taking antibiotics. Radionuclide cystography (RNC) is an alternative to VCUG for evaluating reflux and is discussed in the Nuclear Medicine section.

A retrograde urethrogram is used to examine the urethra. The most common indication for this examination is evaluation for urethral trauma (Fig. 198-9) or stricture. A catheter is gently placed in the very tip of the urethra, and contrast is then slowly introduced under fluoroscopic visualization.

IVP examines the form and function of the kidneys, ureters, and bladder. After a scout film of the abdomen is obtained, intravenous contrast is injected. Radiographs taken at 3 and 15 minutes after injection show the ability of the kidneys to concentrate and excrete contrast, respectively. Anatomic variants or abnormalities of the kidneys may be evaluated at this stage of the examination. IVP is commonly used for the evaluation of complex anatomy and obstruction, whether due to a congenital abnormality, stones, or any other cause. CT, MRI, and nuclear medicine studies are slowly replacing IVP; however, IVP does not require sedation, and the radiation incurred by the patient is far less than that from a CT scan.

NUCLEAR MEDICINE

Nuclear medicine studies generate diagnostic information by recording the distribution of the radiopharmaceuticals administered. Radiopharmaceuticals are chemicals that are bound to radionuclides. Radiopharmaceuticals have a typical distribution pattern in the body, and therefore an atypical distribution can be a marker for disease or functional abnormality. Gamma scintillation cameras record the radioactivity emitted by radionuclides in the body. Unlike many other imaging studies, nuclear medicine examinations provide both anatomic and functional information. However, the anatomic resolution is not generally as clear as with other imaging studies. New image fusion techniques combine the functional information from positron-emission tomography (PET) and single photon emission computed tomography (SPECT), for example, with the clearer anatomic images of CT and MRI. Many nuclear medicine studies, especially for brain imaging, require sedation for young and uncooperative patients.

Genitourinary Imaging

A variety of nuclear medicine studies demonstrate the form and function of the kidneys. Dynamic renal scintigraphy and diuresis renography evaluate the renal cortex and collecting system over time without and with diuretic challenge, respectively. Renal cortical scintigraphy is a static imaging study that quantifies the functional tissue of each kidney. RNC assesses for vesicoureteral reflux. A nonimaging nuclear medicine study measures the glomerular filtration rate. These examinations may require venous access or bladder catheterization (or both) and hydration before the examination.

During dynamic renal scintigraphy, the activity of intravenously injected technetium Tc 99m mercaptoacetyltriglycine (MAG3) is imaged and measured to assess the form and function of each kidney and collecting system. MAG3 is excreted by active renal tubular transport. The time-activity curve, or the time needed for uptake and excretion of the radiotracer, is measured and compared with normal values. Technetium Tc 99m stannous diethylenetriamine pentaacetic acid (DTPA) is a less commonly used alternative to MAG3. This study is commonly used to assess patients with hydronephrosis or hydroureteronephrosis, reflux nephropathy, surgery on the kidneys, transplanted kidneys, acute renal failure, and hypertension. Diuresis renography is performed to help distinguish urinary obstruction from a dilated nonobstructed renal collecting system.[23] After initial imaging during a dynamic renal scan, a diuretic, typically furosemide, is injected intravenously. The kidneys' ability to drain the radiopharmaceutical over

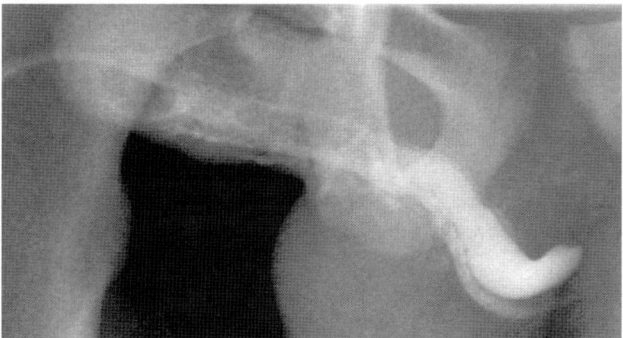

Figure 198-9 An oblique view of the urethra during a retrograde urethrogram demonstrates extravasation of contrast along the course of the urethra as a result of a tear in the bulbar urethra. This boy suffered a skateboard injury.

WHOLE KIDNEY (–bkg)

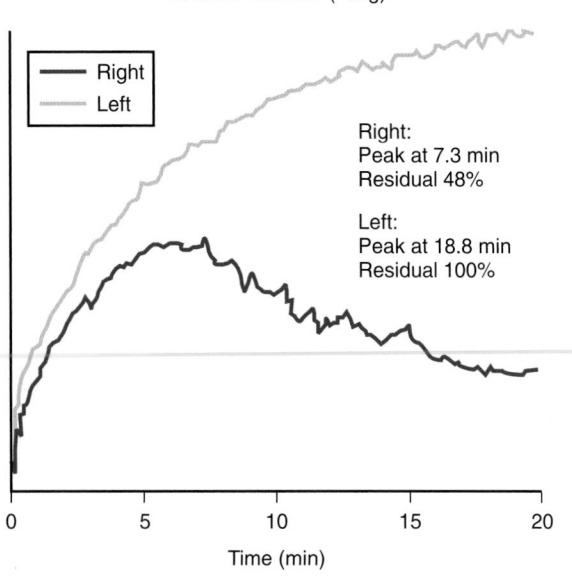

Right:
Peak at 7.3 min
Residual 48%

Left:
Peak at 18.8 min
Residual 100%

Time (min)

CORTEX (–bkg)

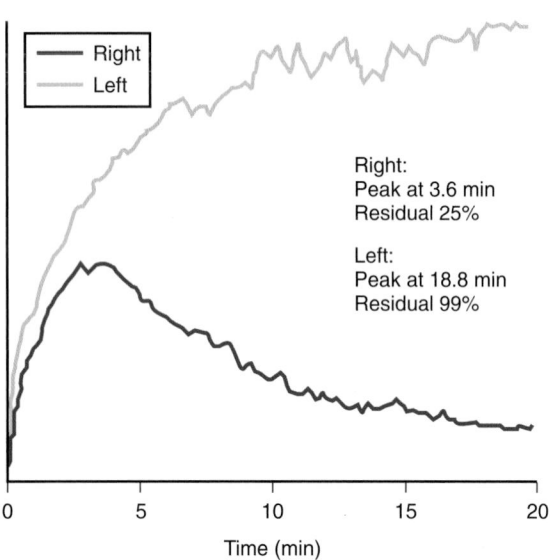

Right:
Peak at 3.6 min
Residual 25%

Left:
Peak at 18.8 min
Residual 99%

Time (min)

A

Figure 198-10   A and B, Images from a Tc 99m mercaptoacetyltriglycine (MAG3) study demonstrate left-sided obstruction with a time–activity curve showing that the half time of radiotracer excretion is greater than 20 minutes, or in the obstruction range. The curve for the right kidney is normal. It was known prenatally that the patient had left-sided pelvic dilation.

time is measured. In significantly obstructed kidneys, radiotracer fails to be excreted normally (Fig. 198-10A and B).

Several patient factors can confound interpretation of the studies. Infants, especially those younger than 1 month, have functionally immature kidneys and do not concentrate the radiopharmaceutical into urine well.[24,25] Studies performed in the first month of life should be interpreted with this in mind. Similarly, kidneys with impaired function may not respond to diuresis as well as kidneys with normal function. Intravenous urography, renal angiography, and other tests

using contrast agents eliminated by the kidneys may reduce renal uptake and prolong the examination.

During renal cortical scintigraphy, the radiopharmaceutical technetium Tc 99m dimercaptosuccinic acid (DMSA) is injected intravenously and concentrates in the renal parenchyma. Four hours after injection, images are obtained. The main indication for cortical scintigraphy is evaluation of pyelonephritis, renal scarring, renal ectopia, renal dysplasia, and the functional contribution of each kidney.

RNC is performed to diagnose vesicoureteral reflux. For RNC, preparation and bladder catheterization of the patient are identical to that for VCUG, described earlier in this chapter. The activity of technetium Tc 99m pertechnetate instilled into the bladder is recorded by a gamma camera. The radiation dose of RNC is approximately $\frac{1}{100}$ that of traditional VCUG and $\frac{1}{30}$ that of low-dose pulse fluoroscopy VCUG.[17,26]

The indications for whether to perform RNC or VCUG to evaluate reflux vary from institution to institution and from physician to physician. RNC is a very sensitive examination for determining the presence of reflux (Fig. 198-11) and exposes the patient to a low dose of radiation. However, VCUG provides more detailed anatomic information about the bladder, sites of ureteral insertion, the male urethra, and the possibility of duplex collecting systems. The risks and benefits of each examination should be considered and tailored to each patient.

Angiotensin-converting enzyme (ACE) inhibition scintigraphy is performed to evaluate patients suspected of having hypertension secondary to renal artery stenosis.[27,28] If renal artery stenosis is causing decreased perfusion of the kidney, angiotensin II, a potent vasoconstrictor, is released to restore perfusion pressure to the kidneys. During ACE inhibition scintigraphy, excretion of the kidneys is evaluated after the administration of an ACE inhibitor, typically oral captopril. In significant renal artery stenosis, excretion of the radiotracer is slowed. Patients allergic to ACE inhibitors should not undergo this examination.

Renal scintigraphy complements the use of US and renal biopsy in the evaluation of renal transplant complications.[29,30] Vascular compromise, either from renal artery stenosis or from renal vein thrombosis, can be evaluated with dynamic renal imaging. Fluid collections such as hematomas, urinomas, or lymphoceles can be demonstrated.

Tc 99m DTPA is used to estimate the glomerular filtration rate. The patient is well hydrated before the examination. Blood samples are obtained 2, 3, and 4 hours after radiopharmaceutical injection. No imaging is performed.

Skeletal Imaging

Bone scans are one of the most frequently performed nuclear medicine examinations. The radiopharmaceutical technetium Tc 99m methylene diphosphonate (MDP) is taken up in areas of increased osteogenic activity and hyperemia. It is intravenously administered, and scanning can be performed at various times up to 3 hours after injection, depending on the indication. Common clinical indications for skeletal scintigraphy are osteomyelitis, low back pain, bone pain, fractures or suspected stress fractures, avascular necrosis, osteoid osteoma, sacroiliitis, osteochondritis, reflex sympathetic dystrophy, and primary and secondary bone tumors. Bone scans also have high sensitivity in the

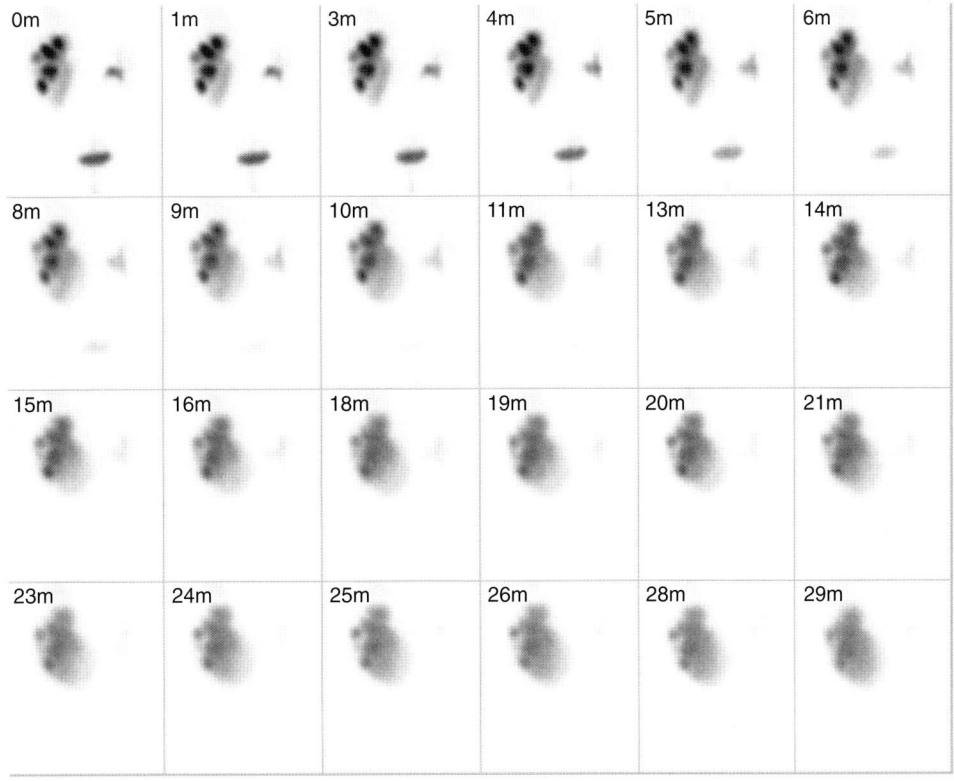

B

Figure 198-10, cont'd

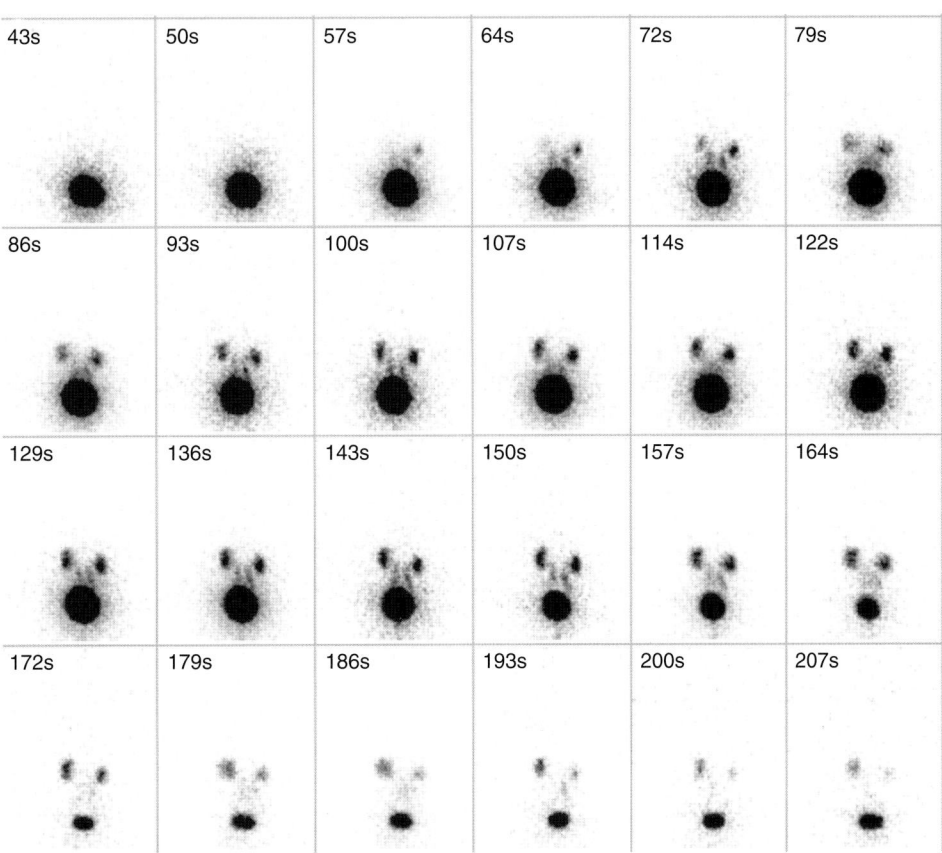

Figure 198-11   Selected images from a radionuclide cystogram demonstrate bilateral grade 2 vesicoureteral reflux in a child whose sibling has reflux. The refluxed material drains promptly.

evaluation of skeletal trauma in children suspected of being abused. Despite the examination's high sensitivity, bone scans are not highly specific because fractures, infections, acute infarctions, and tumors can all increase osteogenesis. The distribution of radiotracer depends on blood flow. In children, the growth plates have increased blood flow, and high activity in the region of the physes is normal. Areas of decreased activity represent sites of decreased osteogenesis or decreased perfusion and can be caused by tumors, infections, or infarctions. It is helpful to correlate findings on bone scan with the patient's age, clinical history, symptoms, and radiographs or other imaging studies. Patients should refrain from having barium studies performed 24 to 48 hours before the examination because the barium attenuates the radioactivity of the technetium.

When findings need to be clarified on a bone scan, adjunct nuclear medicine studies may be helpful. For example, when osteomyelitis is suspected but the bone scan is normal, an abnormal gallium 67 scan, indium 111 scan, or technetium 99m white blood cell scan can help in the diagnosis of osteomyelitis.[31] Gallium citrate Ga 67 binds to transferrin and localizes at sites of infection. *m*-Iodobenzylguanidine (iobenguane, MIBG; see later discussion) can be used to detect cortical, medullary, and soft tissue metastases from neuroblastoma when a bone scan may appear normal.

Additionally, the sensitivity and specificity of conventional radiographs can be increased with the addition of information from a bone scan. Abnormal activity on a bone scan can lead to a targeted search on the conventional radiograph.

Tumor Imaging

Different radiopharmaceuticals are used for the evaluation of tumors based on the agent's avidity for the tumor.

MIBG labeled with iodine 131 or iodine 123 and octreotide labeled with indium 111 are three radiopharmaceutical agents specific to tumors of neuroectodermal origin.[32] MIBG is much more commonly used than octreotide. The main indication is to diagnose or evaluate children with neuroblastoma (Fig. 198-12A and B). MIBG is more specific than CT or MRI for preoperative and postoperative evaluation of neuroblastoma.[33] Many medications interfere with the activity of iodine I 123 MIBG, and therefore the patient's medications must be checked carefully before the examination. If MIBG is unavailable, octreotide is an alternative for the evaluation of neuroendocrine tumors.

Tc 99m MDP (see Skeletal Imaging) is used for the evaluation of primary bone tumors, especially osteosarcomas and metastatic bone tumors. Tumors with increased osteogenic activity cause areas of increased radiotracer uptake on bone scans. Tumors that cause pure osteolysis demonstrate decreased uptake, but this is rarely encountered by bone scan.

Gallium 67 scintigraphy is useful for the evaluation of Hodgkin's and non-Hodgkin's lymphoma, rhabdomyosarcoma, soft tissue sarcoma, and infection.[34,35] Unlike US, CT, or MRI, gallium scans are able to distinguish inactive disease or scars from active disease. The patient is injected with the radiopharmaceutical 3 days before imaging, and delayed imaging may be performed up to 72 hours after the initial imaging.

PET is another method to evaluate tumors. The most commonly used radiopharmaceutical, fluorine F 18 fluo-

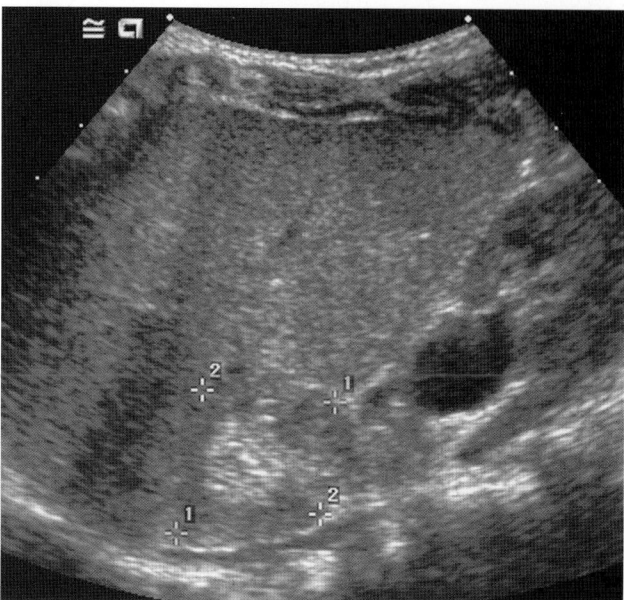

A

B

Figure 198-12 This 6-month-old underwent renal ultrasound (US) for follow-up of prenatal renal pelvic dilation. A, US demonstrates an echogenic mass cephalad to the right kidney (marked). B, An *m*-iodobenzylguanidine (MIBG) study demonstrates abnormal radiotracer uptake in the area seen on US (*arrowhead*) and in the left humerus (*arrow*). This patient had metastatic neuroblastoma.

rodeoxyglucose (FDG), accumulates within cells with increased glycolysis, such as malignant cells. PET scans have been more thoroughly researched and applied to the evaluation of tumors in adults than in children. We currently use PET for the evaluation of tumors such as lymphoma, osteosarcoma, Ewing sarcoma, brain tumors, and neuroblastoma. PET has a variety of other indications as well, which will be discussed later in this section.

Brain tumors can be evaluated with a variety of agents, including FDG, thallium 201, and technetium Tc 99m sestamibi. Sestamibi has been used to assess the viability of brain tumors in children.[36] It is common for children undergoing evaluation of the brain to require sedation.

Lymphoscintigraphy assesses areas of lymphatic drainage and is useful in evaluating patients with lymphedema and chylothorax.

Hepatobiliary and Spleen Imaging

Biliary scanning using technetium Tc 99m disofenin (diisopropyl iminodiacetic acid; DISIDA) evaluates the function of hepatocytes. This intravenously injected radiopharmaceutical shares the same hepatocyte uptake, transport, and excretion pathways as bilirubin. In infants, this test is most commonly used to differentiate neonatal hepatitis from congenital biliary atresia.[37] DISIDA is also useful for the evaluation of choledochal cysts, acute and chronic cholecystitis, biliary obstruction, and potential biliary leakage after gallbladder surgery. Perfusion and excretion of the liver after transplantation can also be assessed.[38]

In patients in whom biliary atresia is being distinguished from neonatal hepatitis, the patient does not need to be restricted from oral intake. Pretreatment with phenobarbital 3 to 5 days before the examination, 5 mg/kg/day in two equal doses, is highly recommended. Phenobarbital enhances biliary excretion of the radiotracer and the specificity of the examination. In patients with biliary atresia, no excretion of contrast into the bowel is seen (Fig. 198-13A and B).

All other patients need to fast for 4 hours before the examination and should not undergo barium studies for 48 hours before the examination. The scintigraphic findings in children with cholecystitis are often different from those in adults. For example, in a teenage girl presenting with symptoms of cholecystitis, the study may show the gallbladder filling with radiotracer and very slow excretion, consistent with acalculous cholecystitis. In children with cholecystitis secondary to obstructing calculi, findings may be similar to those of adults, with nonvisualization of the gallbladder. For patients who have been fasting longer than 24 hours, a fatty meal is preferred to the intravenous injection of a cholecystokinin analogue to decrease the possibility of a false-positive examination.

The nuclear medicine study of choice for the evaluation of asplenia and polysplenia is a spleen scan using denatured red blood cells (technetium Tc 99m denatured RBCs).

Gastrointestinal Imaging

A variety of imaging studies can be used to evaluate the GI system. Studies that evaluate for active GI bleeding, Meckel's diverticulum, gastroesophageal reflux, esophageal emptying, gastric emptying, and aspiration are discussed here. For many studies the patient must fast for 4 hours before the examination. No barium must be present in the GI system.

Active GI bleeding is best evaluated with Tc 99m–labeled RBCs. The radiopharmaceutical is injected intravenously and the abdomen is imaged for 60 minutes, with additional spot views if necessary. Only areas of active bleeding during the time of imaging are revealed, which is the main limita-

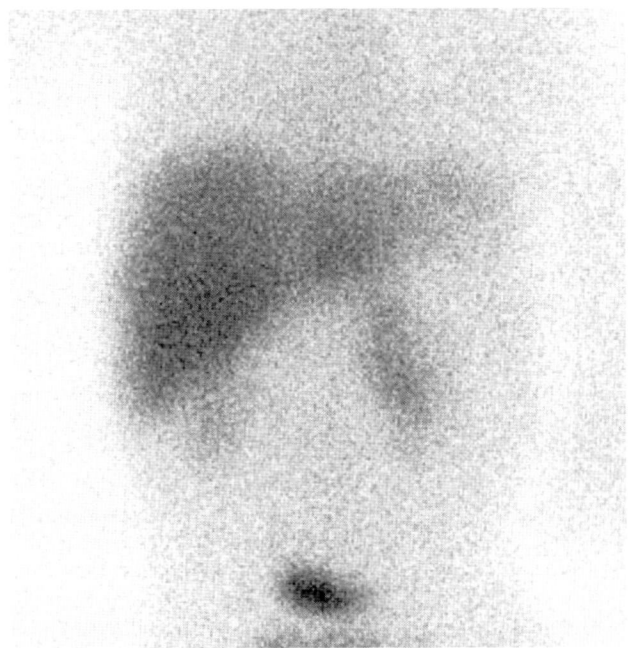

A

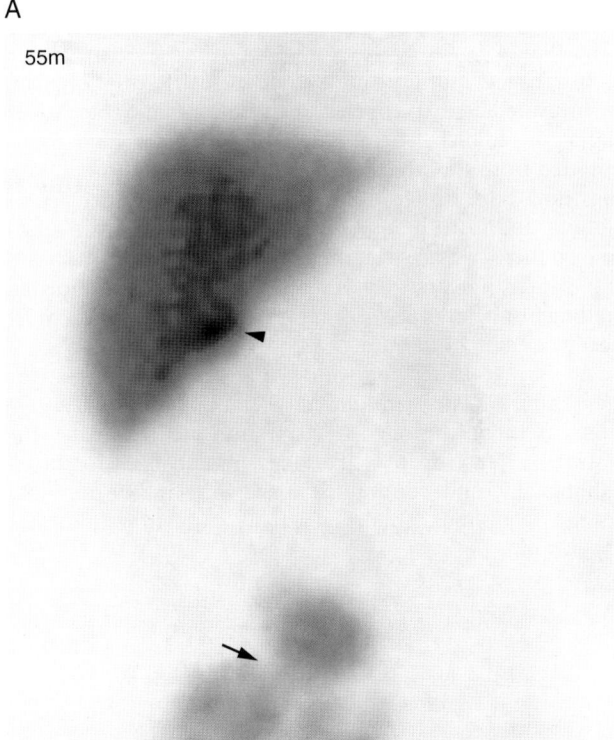

55m

B

Figure 198-13 A, A Tc 99m disofenin (diisopropyl iminodiacetic acid; DISIDA) scan of a 5-week-old with elevated direct bilirubin and nonvisualization of the gallbladder on ultrasound demonstrates no radiotracer uptake in the gallbladder or bowel after 4.5 hours. The patient was pretreated with phenobarbital before the examination. Exploratory laparotomy demonstrated biliary atresia, and the patient underwent a Kasai portoenterostomy. B, In an example of a normal DISIDA scan, radiotracer is seen in the gallbladder (*arrowhead*) and within the bowel (*arrow*).

tion of the examination. Delayed imaging, however, as long as 24 hours after injection, may help in resolving subtle bleeding. No patient preparation is necessary.

Symptomatic Meckel's diverticula contain gastric mucosa in 60% of children. In the presence of GI bleeding, the frequency increases to greater than 95%. A Meckel scan demonstrates whether intravenously injected Tc 99m pertechnetate, a radiopharmaceutical that targets gastric mucosa, is present in the region of the small intestine. During the examination, the patient should have an empty bladder for better conspicuity of the diverticulum. If Meckel's diverticulum is actively bleeding, a bleeding scan may also show the diverticulum.

In evaluation of gastroesophageal reflux, the gold standard is 24-hour monitoring with an intraesophageal pH probe.[39] Barium esophagograms can demonstrate reflux but have a high rate of false-negative results because of their intermittent nature.[40] Radionuclide studies are more sensitive than esophagograms and less invasive than pH probe monitoring. The patient must fast before the examination. Technetium Tc 99m sulfur colloid mixed with food or drink is ingested and its radioactivity imaged over time. If there is abnormal activity within the esophagus after the radiotracer has passed into the stomach, reflux is diagnosed (Fig. 198-14).

Esophageal motility and the rate of gastric emptying can be measured easily by nuclear medicine studies. The patient ingests a radiolabeled meal, and the time for food to be emptied from the stomach or esophagus is monitored with a gamma camera. Because meal composition, patient positioning, and instrumentation vary from laboratory to laboratory, there are no generally applicable standard values.[41] The patient must fast for at least 4 hours or miss a normal feeding just before a gastric emptying study. The bowel must also be cleared of barium.

A salivagram is the study of choice to assess for aspiration. Patients with difficulty handling their oral secretions or those suspected of aspiration are candidates for testing. A small drop of Tc 99m sulfur colloid is placed sublingually, and continuous images are taken every 30 seconds for 1 hour. Abnormal activity in the lungs indicates aspiration.

Cardiac Imaging

Pediatric cardiovascular nuclear medicine studies detect and quantify abnormal cardiac shunts, measure myocardial perfusion, determine cardiac output and ejection fraction, and demonstrate cardiac function and wall motion. Echocardiography and MRI are also used cooperatively in these indications.

Myocardial perfusion is assessed with technetium Tc 99m methoxyisobutyl isonitrile (sestamibi; MIBI). Fluorine F 18 FDG–labeled PET scans have also been useful in the evaluation of viable myocardium.[42] The most common indications for myocardial perfusion imaging at our institution are for cardiac transplantation, Kawasaki disease, anomalous coronary arteries, trauma, and chest pain. Before this examination, patients fast for 3 to 4 hours to decrease blood flow to the splanchnic bed.

Radionuclide ventriculography assesses global and regional ventricular function. Autologous RBCs labeled with technetium 99m in vitro are reinjected into the patient. Data acquisition is synchronized with the electrocardiographic signal. Cardiac output, right and left ventricular ejection fractions, stroke volume, and end-diastolic and end-systolic volumes can be determined.

Pulmonary Imaging

Pulmonary nuclear medicine studies assess regional pulmonary blood flow and ventilation and are useful for a variety of clinical indications.

Regional ventilation is assessed when the distribution of inhaled radioactive gases such as xenon 133 is imaged over time. Asymmetric ventilation may be detected in a variety of diseases, including cystic fibrosis, lobar emphysema, congenital diaphragmatic hernia, asthma, and pulmonary hypoplasia. Ventilation studies are useful both before and after pulmonary transplantation and in the evaluation of congenital and acquired anomalies of the heart and great vessels.[43]

A ventilation-perfusion ($\dot{V}/\dot{Q}$) scan of the lungs evaluates differences in lung ventilation and vascular perfusion. A common indication for this examination is assessment of pulmonary perfusion before and after cardiac surgery or

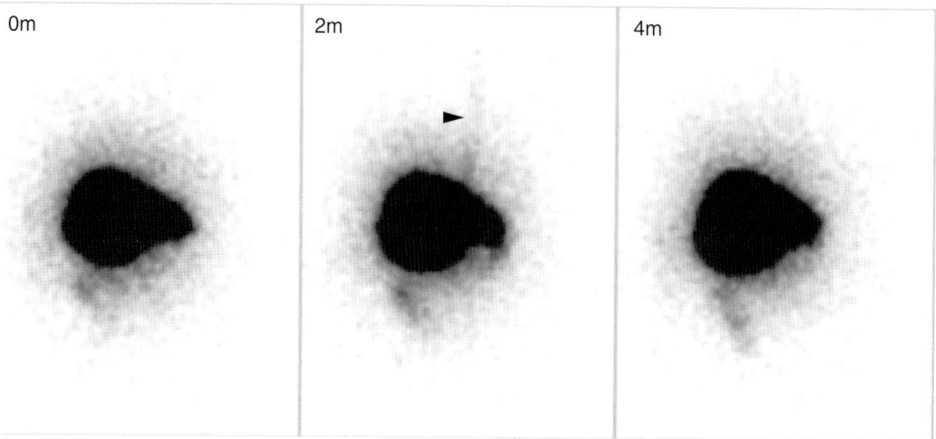

Figure 198-14 Selected images from a gastric emptying study demonstrate intermittent gastroesophageal reflux (*arrowhead*) in a patient with persistent vomiting after feeding.

cardiopulmonary interventional procedures. This study is much less commonly used to diagnose pulmonary emboli in children at our institution.

A V̇/Q̇ scan requires that a patient first inhale xenon 133 with subsequent lung imaging. Then technetium Tc 99m microaggregated albumin (MAA) is injected intravenously. The intravenous particles are trapped in the pulmonary vascular bed. When there is decreased or absent perfusion, fewer particles are trapped, thereby resulting in an area of decreased radioactivity. The V̇/Q̇ studies are compared, and mismatches may represent areas of infarction. Correlation with chest radiography is essential.

Thyroid Imaging

Scintigraphy can provide anatomic and physiologic information about the thyroid gland. Common indications are evaluation of hypothyroidism, hyperthyroidism, and neck masses.[44] Iodine I 123 and technetium Tc 99m pertechnetate are the most common radiopharmaceuticals used for thyroid scintigraphy. The only patient preparation for patients undergoing iodine 123 studies is to discontinue any medications that interfere with thyroid uptake of radioiodine. Iodine 131 has limited application in pediatric thyroid scintigraphy because of its high radiation absorbed dose. It may be used to detect and treat recurrent or metastatic thyroid carcinoma and treat hyperthyroidism.[45]

Brain Imaging

Nuclear medicine studies are most useful in the evaluation of seizure disorders, but they are also indicated for cerebral vascular disorders, trauma, and brain tumors.

SPECT is used to assess regional brain perfusion. The radiopharmaceutical technetium Tc 99m hexamethylpropyleneamine oxime (HMPAO) remains within the brain for several hours after intravenous administration, and therefore the patient can be imaged at a later time. This is a major advantage over contrast agents used for CT and MRI, for which imaging must occur within seconds to minutes after contrast injection. This difference is especially useful in the evaluation of seizures. The radiotracer can be injected during ictal or interictal activity; differences in brain perfusion are studied in regard to the brain's activity at the point of injection (Fig. 198-15).

These agents are also useful in assessing brain perfusion in patients with cerebrovascular conditions such as moyamoya disease or decreased brain perfusion from hypotension after extracorporeal membrane oxygenation or repair of complex congenital heart disease. Perfusion brain SPECT and cerebral radionuclide angiography are used to help in the assessment of brain death.

PET is also used to evaluate children with refractory epilepsy who are being considered for surgical cure. Functional alterations related to ictal or interictal states can be detected with FDG-PET.[46]

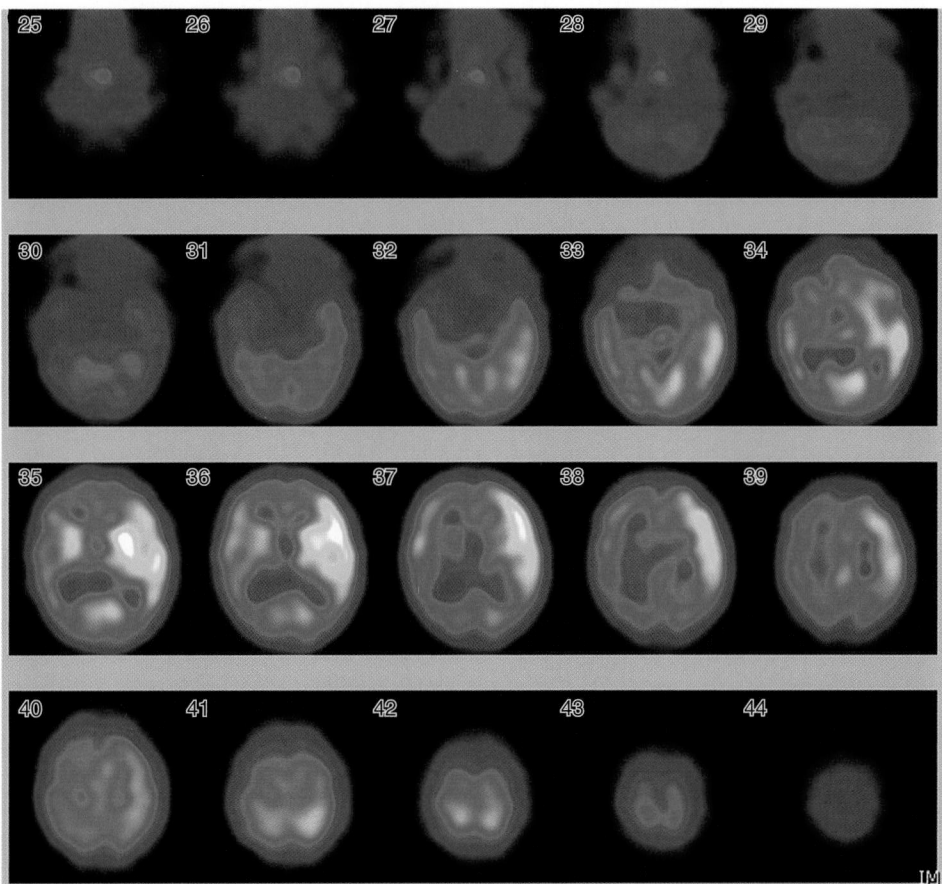

Figure 198-15 Single photon emission computed tomography images from a brain scan obtained in the interictal state in a child with seizures demonstrates marked asymmetric uptake in the left temporal lobe.

Normal and abnormal flow of cerebrospinal fluid (CSF) can be assessed by radionuclide cisternography. MRI is also very useful in the evaluation of CSF flow. Indications for radionuclide cisternography include communicating hydrocephalus and CSF liquorrhea (CSF dripping from the nose or ear). The patency of CSF shunts can also be assessed with a similar method.

COMPUTED TOMOGRAPHY/COMPUTED AXIAL TOMOGRAPHY

CT or computed axial tomography (CAT) scans, like conventional radiographs and fluoroscopy, create images based on the variable absorption of x-rays by different body tissues. Differences in tissue density and composition affect the ability of x-rays to pass through the body and ultimately create images.

Early CT scans acquired one "slice" or axial cross section of information at a time. With spiral scanners, x-rays are emitted and detected as the patient moves continuously through the scanner, thereby creating a volume of information. Multislice or multidetector CT scanners have multiple cameras and detectors rotating simultaneously around the patient with the effect of increasing spatial resolution and decreasing the time to perform a study over standard spiral scanners.

CT scans have excellent spatial resolution, and large areas of the body may be rapidly imaged. With the volume-spatial data acquired, images can be reconstructed in many planes and formatted to enhance the conspicuity of soft tissues, bones, or vascular structures. Viewing these reformatted images can be very helpful, especially with regard to preoperative planning (Fig. 198-16A and B). The ease and speed of obtaining this type of information need to be weighed against the patient's potential radiation risk and cost of the examination. Based on measurements in our department, the average absorbed radiation dose of a chest CT scan is 100 times that of a chest radiograph, and an abdominal CT scan is 8 times that of an abdominal radiograph.

The diagnostic quality of CT scans is improved with contrast agents. The appearance of bowel without contrast may mimic abdominal masses, lymph nodes, or fluid collections. Bowel contrast agents include radiodense materials such as dilute barium sulfate or Gastrografin. Contrast can be given by mouth or via stomas, nasogastric or gastric tubes, or rectum according to the indication. The quantity depends on the patient's age. Patients may also receive intravenous low-osmolar contrast to enhance the conspicuity of vascular and soft tissue structures. Because many times these agents are machine injected at a high flow rate and can be painful, most institutions now use low-osmolar contrast agents because they are better tolerated than high-osmolar contrast agents. Patients with previous contrast allergies need to be premedicated, or other tests should be considered.

During a CT examination, the patient must hold still, which can be accomplished with minimal or no sedation. Multidetector CT scan times are now often less than 30 seconds, but any motion during the scan can degrade the imaging. Additionally, once intravenous contrast is administered, it generally cannot be readministered for 24 hours after the first injection. Therefore, careful assessment of a

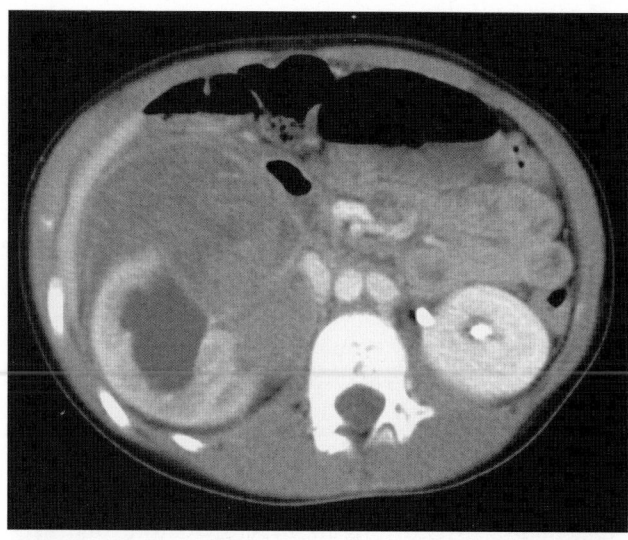

A

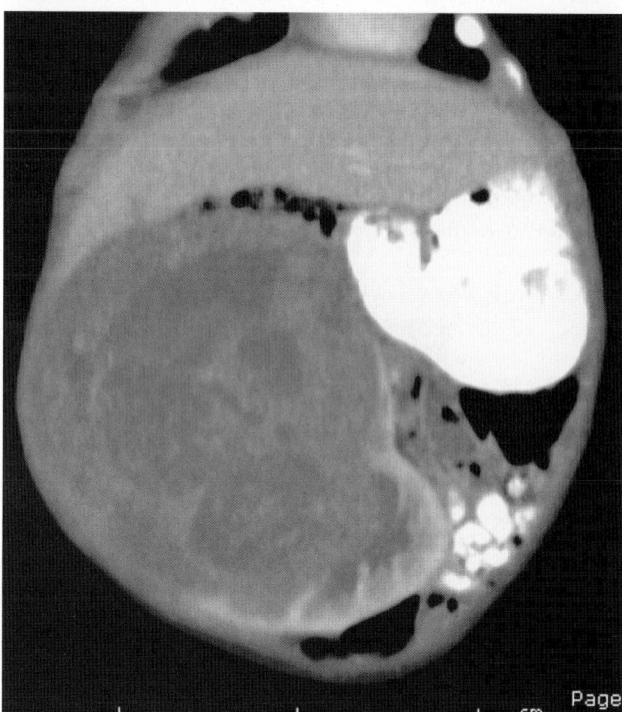

B

Figure 198-16 A, An axial image of a large mass, probably renal in nature, is seen here. B, With a reformatted image in the coronal plane, the tumor can be seen in its craniocaudal extent, with a rim of renal parenchyma visualized at the inferior aspect of the mass, thus confirming its renal origin, consistent with a Wilms tumor in this young child.

child's ability to hold still before examination is recommended.

Brain Imaging

Head CT is often requested in the pediatric population for the evaluation of acute change in neurologic status secondary to trauma, infarction, or a seizure, for example. CT is widely available, and image acquisition is rapid. In a critically ill patient, all life support systems are compatible

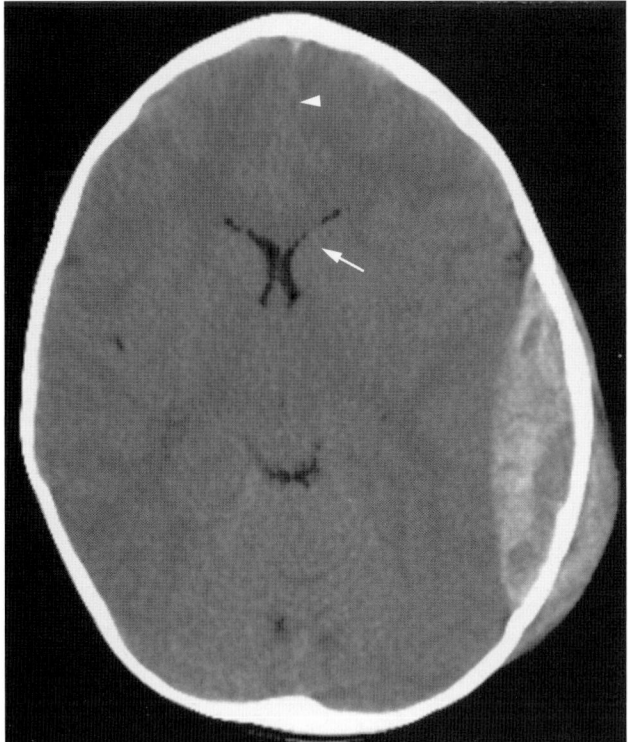

Figure 198-17 A large epidural hematoma is causing a mass effect with minimal splaying of the falx to the contralateral side (*arrowhead*) and mild effacement of the left frontal horn (*arrow*). This hematoma was associated with a skull fracture. The patient was brought to the operating room on an emergency basis after the computed tomography scan.

with the CT scanner, unlike MRI, which has restrictions regarding metallic objects in the scanner area. With CT, beam-hardening artifact can limit assessment of the posterior fossa and temporal lobe regions. MRI offers superior brain parenchymal and other soft tissue evaluation without the effects of ionizing radiation. One must take these factors into consideration when imaging of the brain is indicated.

For the evaluation of trauma, both accidental and nonaccidental, head CT is the imaging modality of choice. CT is excellent for the evaluation of intracranial hemorrhage, which may be epidural, subdural, subarachnoid, or intraparenchymal in location. Head CT is ideal for the evaluation of a suspected epidural hematoma, for which emergency surgical decompression may be necessary (Fig. 198-17). Once the initial CT scan is obtained and the patient is stable, further evaluation of the brain parenchyma for prognostication in the setting of trauma may be performed, but it is advisable to wait 5 to 7 days after the initial incident because such delay will allow greater conspicuity of traumatic brain injury. In cases of nonaccidental trauma, we recommend that brain MRI be obtained when clinically feasible to acquire additional evidence of injury, which may be important for legal proceedings in the future.

CT is also the preferred imaging modality for the evaluation of intracranial calcifications. When a mass lesion is suspected, CT's ability to demonstrate tiny calcifications can aid in narrowing the differential diagnosis. The typical pattern

of calcifications associated with certain syndromes, as seen in the subependymal lesions in tuberous sclerosis or along the gyri in Sturge-Weber syndrome, is also well evaluated with CT.

In children with shunted hydrocephalus, head CT is the quickest imaging modality with which to assess ventricular size if shunt malfunction is suspected. In the evaluation of these patients, it is imperative to compare the current examination with the most recent neuroimaging available, whether it is previous head US or brain MRI. Although the imaging modalities are different, comparison of ventricular size is possible, and the information gleaned from such comparison may make a vast difference in patient care. Comparisons of multiple studies over a long period may also reveal a slowly progressive shunt malfunction that may be overlooked if only a single recent comparison is used.

Head CT may be performed without or with the administration of an intravenous contrast agent. Depending on the urgency of the examination, our practice is to administer contrast in cases in which treatment may be altered immediately based on the findings, for example, in the evaluation of an extra-axial abscess. In cases in which a lesion is suspected on CT and contrast would aid in further evaluation but the information is not going to change the immediate course of management, administering contrast is deferred and instead brain MRI is obtained. An exception to this practice is CT venography. Because CT is not susceptible to as many artifacts related to intravascular flow as MRI is, we would recommend CT venography over MR venography for the evaluation of suspected venous thrombosis.

Head and Neck Imaging

For the evaluation of infection involving the head and neck, contrast is administered in most cases unless the patient is going to be further evaluated with MRI for better soft tissue evaluation, and then the CT technique is optimized for studying the adjacent bony structures for osteomyelitis. Although exposing the orbits to ionizing radiation should be avoided as much as possible, contrast-enhanced CT of the orbits is necessary in cases of suspected deeper extension of orbital cellulitis, where there is a potential risk for loss of vision (Fig. 198-18A and B). Reviewing images in both the axial and coronal planes is imperative when evaluating any of the facial structures. Obtaining the images in the axial plane with a spiral technique allows the imaging data to be reconstructed in multiple anatomic planes or even three-dimensional models. Whereas a patient was scanned twice to obtain axial and coronal images, new technology with the capability of obtaining reformatted images after scanning only in the axial plane allows a significant reduction in the radiation dose to the patient. Reviewing images in the orthogonal planes is especially important for the evaluation of any facial fracture. From our experience, we believe that facial CT is far more sensitive for the evaluation of fractures than plain radiographs of the face are. Regarding whether the potential risks of receiving a greater dose of ionizing radiation outweigh the benefits, the additional information that CT provides over plain radiographs has not yet been evaluated.

Evaluation of the temporal bone is typically performed by spiral technique in the axial plane with coronal reformatted

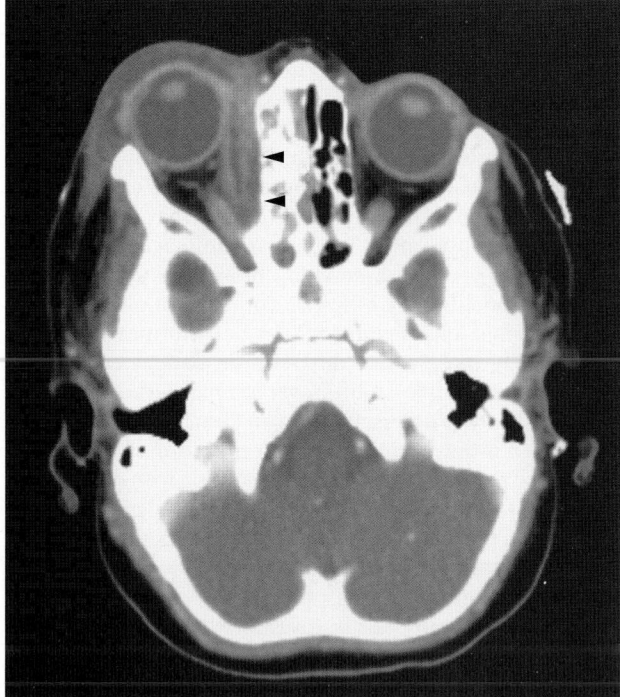

A

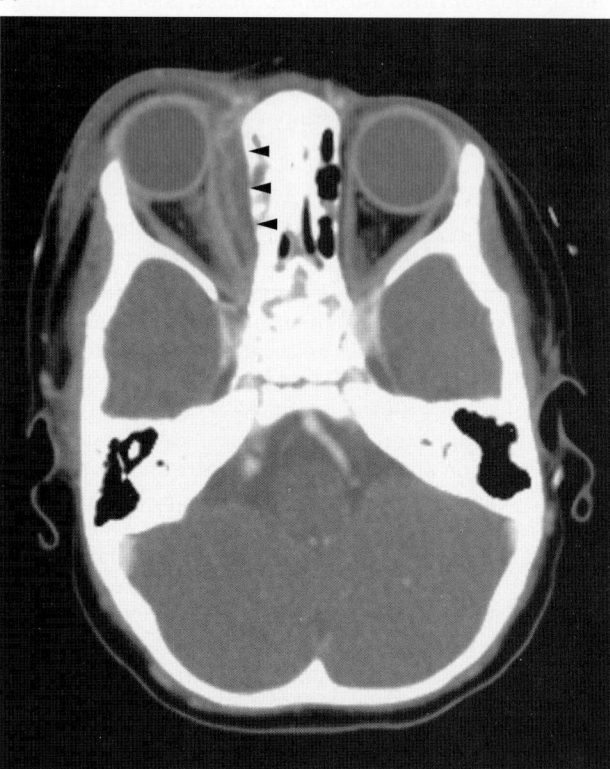

B

Figure 198–18   A and B, Contrast-enhanced axial images through the orbits demonstrate right-sided preseptal soft tissue inflammatory changes, proptosis, and a mass effect on the globe from the adjacent subperiosteal abscess (*arrowheads*). These findings are secondary to spread of infection from adjacent sinusitis; note the opacification of the right-sided paranasal sinuses.

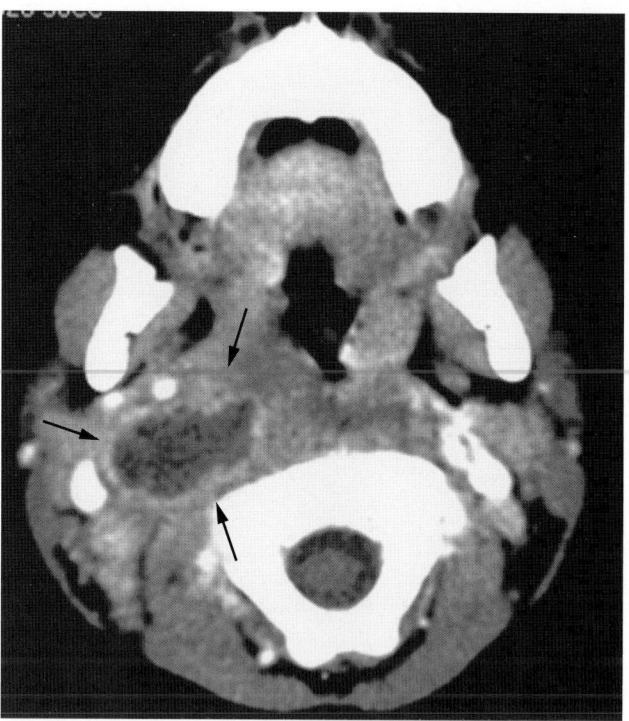

Figure 198–19   A contrast-enhanced axial image through the neck demonstrates a low-density lesion in the right lateral retropharynx with scalloping wall enhancement, consistent with an abscess.

images from the axial data. Temporal bone CT is frequently part of the workup in cases of sensorineural or conductive hearing loss. In patients with suspected branchial cleft cysts about this region, contrast-enhanced temporal bone CT is performed. If there is no sign of infection and a cutaneous defect may be appreciated on physical examination, the radiologist sometimes injects iodinated contrast into this defect in the hope of better delineating a sinus tract, which may aid in preoperative planning.

To provide better surgical guidance, evaluation of the paranasal sinuses with CT is also performed in an axial plane with coronal reformatted images. The raw data obtained from the axial images is used intraoperatively to guide the surgeon during functional endoscopic sinus surgery.

Although many abnormalities of the neck may be evaluated with US, neck CT may be preferred by some surgeons because it allows easier assessment of the surrounding anatomic structures. Contrast-enhanced neck CT is recommended for the evaluation of any neck mass and is very useful in distinguishing the many reactive lymph nodes located in this region in a pediatric patient versus a mass lesion of another cause. To better differentiate suppurative lymphadenitis from an organized abscess, additional delayed axial images through the area of interest are obtained. A persistent lobulated rim or scalloping wall enhancement surrounding a low-density center has been shown to correlate highly with the presence of an abscess (Fig. 198-19).[47] Neck CT at our institution is performed with a nonspiral technique, which renders better soft tissue detail, unlike cervical spine CT, which is performed with a spiral technique. It is important for the clinician to understand the differences in technique between neck CT, which optimizes soft tissue evaluation, and cervical spine CT, which optimizes bony evaluation. Cervical spine CT is performed with a spiral technique so that reformatted images may be obtained, especially in the sagittal plane, which aids in the diagnosis of compression fractures and subluxation.

Spine Imaging

In general, spine CT performed with a spiral technique allows one to reconstruct the images in the sagittal and coronal planes and construct a three-dimensional model if necessary. To keep the radiation dose as low as reasonably acceptable, only the area of clinical concern should be scanned. In the setting of trauma, images of the cervical spine obtained at our institution are limited to the area of concern. This same concept holds true for imaging the lumbar spine in cases of suspected trauma or spondylolysis. Sometimes patients have previous plain radiographs or bone scans that can aid the radiologist in scanning a limited area of interest; at other times, relying on the referring clinician's assessment of the level of concern is necessary. Larger portions of the spine are sometimes imaged for preoperative planning in patients with severe scoliosis, where the formation of a three-dimensional model is very helpful to the surgeon. For evaluation of the intervertebral disks or paraspinal soft tissues, MRI should be performed (discussed later in this chapter).

Chest and Cardiovascular Imaging

Indications for chest CT are evaluation of the lung parenchyma, mediastinum, pleural spaces, soft tissues, bones, and cardiovascular structures (Fig. 198-20A and B). Because of the natural density difference between normal lung parenchyma and abnormal soft tissues within the lung, studies to evaluate the lungs may not require intravenous contrast. High-resolution images are useful to assess for interstitial lung disease. Evaluation of the mediastinum, great vessels, pulmonary masses, and pleural disease typically requires intravenous contrast administration. The use of CT to assess heart disease is controversial in children because of the high radiation dose.

Abdomen/Pelvis Imaging

Indications for abdominal and pelvic CT are numerous. However, because US is nonradiating and does not require sedation, it is the study of choice for the initial investigation of most abdominal and pelvic abnormalities in children. US and MRI are superior to CT in evaluation of the uterus and ovaries. Administration of bowel and intravenous contrast is typically required for imaging the abdomen and pelvis, with the exception of evaluating renal stone disease.

Extremity Imaging

The ability to create multiplanar reconstructions makes CT ideal for the evaluation of complex fractures, especially before surgery, as well as congenital anomalies. After surgery, metallic hardware artifact may obscure bony and soft tissue detail. CT and MRI better characterize bone lesions, which are not obviously diagnosed by plain film. Masses within the soft tissues of the extremities are usually better characterized by US or MRI than by CT.

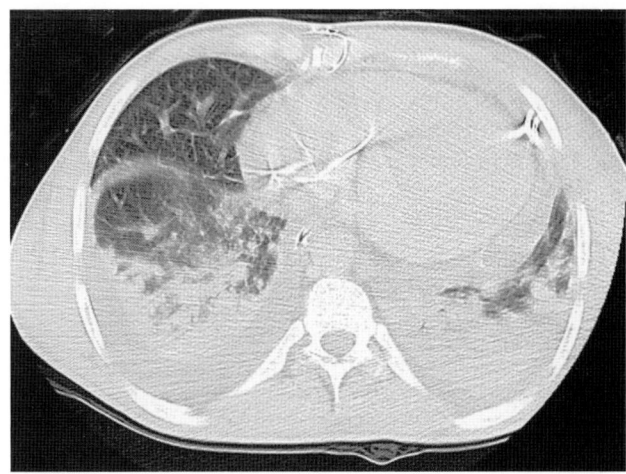

A

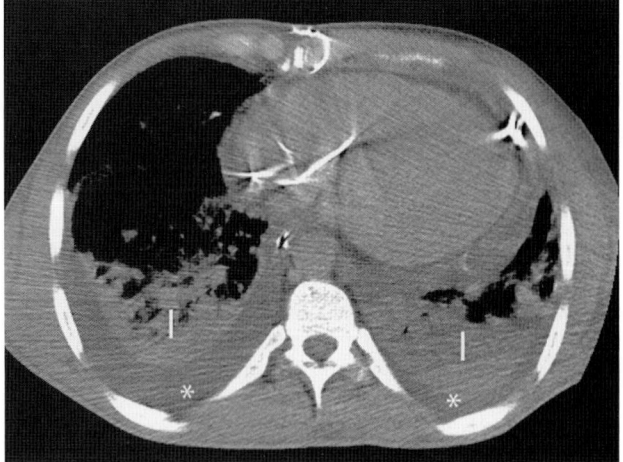

B

Figure 198-20 Computed tomography scan of the chest. These axial images of the lower part of the chest demonstrate the difference in lung and soft tissue windows. This patient had a history of congenital heart disease and presented with sepsis from bilateral pneumonia. A, Lung windows emphasize the lung parenchyma. B, Soft tissue windows help distinguish the different soft tissues, including the consolidated lung (l) and pleural effusions (*asterisk*) bilaterally.

ULTRASOUND

US produces images based on the different reflectivity of sound waves that each tissue inherently possesses. Because this study is nonradiating, provides images in real time, and rarely requires sedation, it is often the first cross-sectional imaging examination of choice for the abdomen and pelvis, gonads, infant hips, neonatal brain, and neonatal spine. US can be used to assess blood flow and is an excellent noninvasive test to evaluate the patency of arteries and veins throughout the body. US also provides images in real time, which is extremely useful in evaluation of the bowel and heart. Cardiac US or echocardiography will not be discussed in this section. Most US examinations do not require patient preparation, with the exception of abdominal and pelvic US, which will be discussed later in this section.

Head, Neck, and Spine Imaging

US plays a major role in evaluation of the brain, particularly in a premature or near-term infant who is critically ill and cannot be transported to radiology or cannot undergo a lengthy examination such as MRI. US may be performed at the bedside, is quick, and provides crucial information needed to manage some of these patients. The American College of Radiology and the American Institute of Ultrasound Medicine have proposed guidelines regarding which standard images must be obtained when evaluating the head.[48] However, evaluation with US is a dynamic process, and the images captured during the evaluation are but a fraction of the sonographer's examination. The real-time capability of US examination has some advantages over other imaging modalities. Not only is a gray-scale index used to evaluate the brain parenchyma, but color Doppler imaging capabilities also make evaluation of intracranial arteries and veins possible. Color Doppler imaging plus real-time examination capability makes it possible to evaluate change in intracranial arterial resistive indices in response to increased intracranial pressure.

Head US is mostly used to evaluate for the presence of intracranial hemorrhage at the germinal matrix (Fig. 198-21A and B) and periventricular leukomalacia in preterm infants. More definitive characterization of periventricular leukomalacia suspected on US may be made with MRI when the patient is stable. Serial US examination in a patient known to have an intracranial hemorrhage is a means with which to monitor ventricular size and spare the patient the considerable amount of ionizing radiation that would be incurred if head CT were used. Ventricular size in a young child may be monitored until the anterior fontanelle is too small to image through; the age at which this occurs is variable, and although the fontanelle may not completely close until 18 to 24 months, one must take into account the size of the transducer used to obtain images. The smallest transducer used in our department for head US has an interface measuring up to 2.5 cm. Imaging via the anterior fontanelle is used first and foremost because it is the largest nonossified membranous junction of the parietal bone. For better evaluation of intracranial abnormality, such as hemorrhage involving the posterior cerebral hemispheres or posterior fossa, the sonographer may examine the brain in a young child through the posterior fontanelle or posterolateral (mastoid) fontanelle if these nonossified membranous junctions of the parietal bone are patent.[49] Head US may also be used for the evaluation of parenchymal calcifications or septations in a cyst, both of which may be too small to be seen with CT or MRI. US is useful in the evaluation of midline congenital anomalies, vascular malformations, and extra-axial collections. The sonographer may "sweep" the transducer laterally for the evaluation of extra-axial collections. Using this technique along with color Doppler is helpful in distinguishing subarachnoid from subdural collections, especially in cases of suspected inflicted trauma.

US evaluation of neck masses is commonly used to distinguish lymphadenitis from other neck masses such as a second branchial cleft cyst or a lymphatic malformation. Evaluation of midline neck masses such as a thyroglossal duct cyst or a dermoid is also possible with US. With color Doppler, increased or decreased vascularity of a neck mass

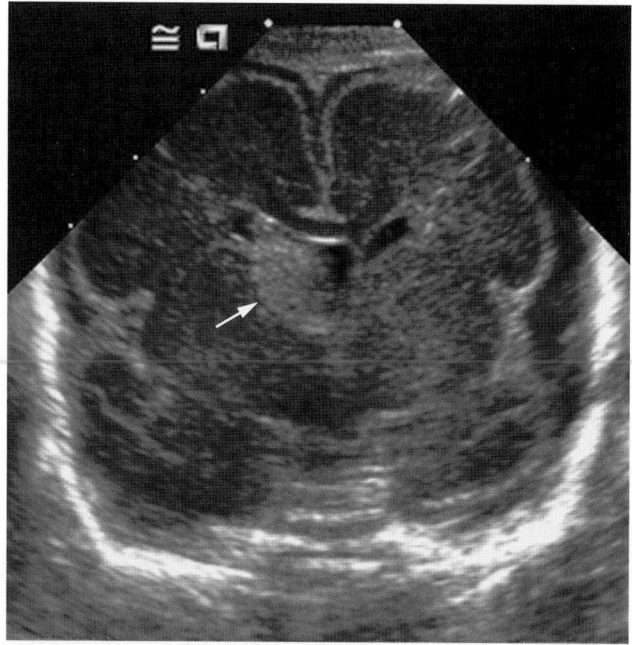

A

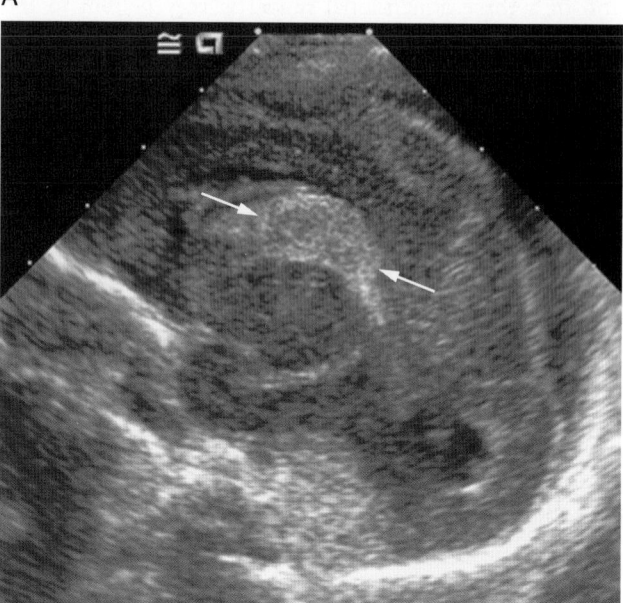

B

Figure 198-21 Coronal (A) and sagittal (B) views from head ultrasonography show relatively large bleeding (*white arrow*) at the caudothalamic groove.

may be demonstrated and can aid in determining the cause of the mass. The advantages of US over CT in the evaluation of neck masses are that the patient is neither exposed to ionizing radiation nor incurs the risk of an allergic reaction secondary to the intravenous contrast needed for CT. Administration of drugs for sedation can be avoided by using neck US over other imaging modalities such as CT or MRI, where it is imperative that the patient remain perfectly still to acquire diagnostic images; with US, the examination is usually possible even if the child is crying and moving.

Sedation is also avoided in US evaluation of the neonatal spine. Evaluation of a suspected tethered cord, fatty filum, or distal thecal sac mass is possible until the posterior elements ossify, between 2 and 3 months of age. Although US examination of the lumbar spine is frequently requested because a sacral dimple or pit or a hairy patch is found on neonatal physical examination,[50] a recent study demonstrated that all spinal US findings for the indication of simple sacral dimples, pits, or sinuses were normal.[51] This study recommends that patients with an abnormal antenatal scan, a cutaneous lesion other than a simple dimple or pit, and any congenital abnormality or any neurologic signs or symptoms associated with occult spinal dysraphism be evaluated with lumbar spine US.

Abdomen and Pelvis Imaging

Patients undergoing abdominal or pelvic US typically need to be prepared before the examination. Before abdominal US, patients need to fast for 2 to 6 hours, depending on the age and indication. Before pelvic US in females, a full urinary bladder is necessary to best view the pelvic organs. A full urinary bladder is also useful to evaluate the bladder itself. The main deterrents to obtaining diagnostic-quality images are bowel gas, large body habitus, and difficulty positioning the patient.

US is excellent for evaluation of the intra-abdominal and pelvic solid organs, the bowel, and blood flow. The liver, spleen, kidneys, pancreas, and gallbladder are easily assessed with US; the size and configuration, as well as blood flow, of these organs is examined in real time, and masses can be excluded with this imaging modality. The uterus and ovaries can be evaluated by transabdominal scanning, with a full urinary bladder used as the acoustic window as previously discussed, or by transvaginal scanning in sexually active females. US is the best imaging modality for the evaluation of ovarian torsion and is useful in the initial evaluation of pelvic pain, any pelvic mass, amenorrhea or dysmenorrhea, and müllerian duct anomalies. MRI is also useful in evaluation of the female pelvic organs and will be discussed later. US is useful in evaluation of the bowel, especially in the evaluation of pyloric stenosis (Fig. 198-22), intussusception, appendicitis, and bowel wall thickening.

Extremity and Superficial Organ Imaging

US is useful in the evaluation of palpable soft tissue masses anywhere in the body, including the extremities, to determine whether they are solid, cystic, or vascular (or any combination) in nature.

US is also very useful to evaluate superficial organs such as the thyroid gland or testes. The combination of high-resolution imaging and no ionizing radiation makes US especially ideal in examining the testes. US is the best imaging modality for the evaluation of a painful scrotum and easily distinguishes testicular torsion (Fig. 198-23) from other causes of pain.

MAGNETIC RESONANCE IMAGING

Brain Imaging

Another imaging modality with which to examine the CNS is MRI. Depending on the age of the patient, sedation or even general anesthesia may need to be administered to obtain images of diagnostic quality. For a newborn, we use

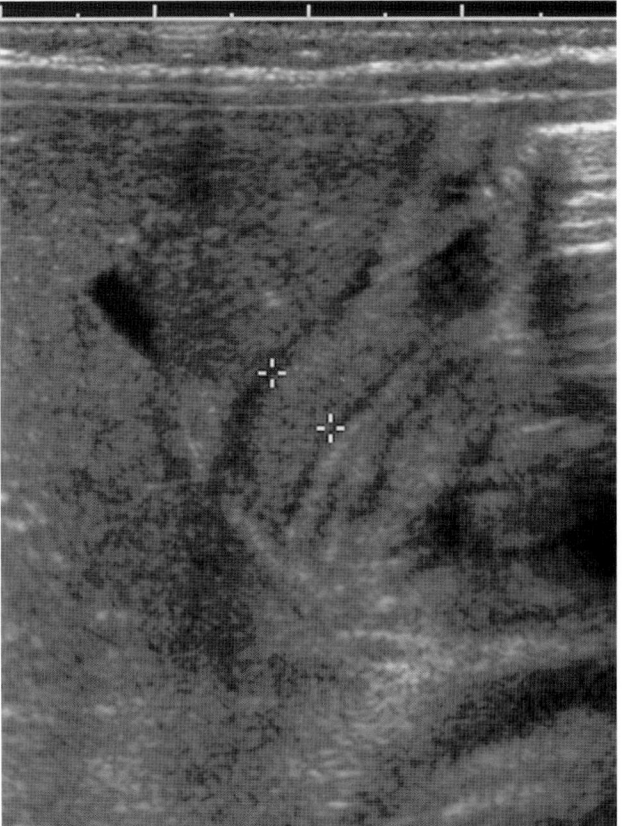

Figure 198-22 An ultrasound image of the right upper quadrant in a 4-week-old boy with projectile vomiting demonstrates pyloric stenosis. The thickened muscularis of the pylorus (marked) measures greater than 3 mm.

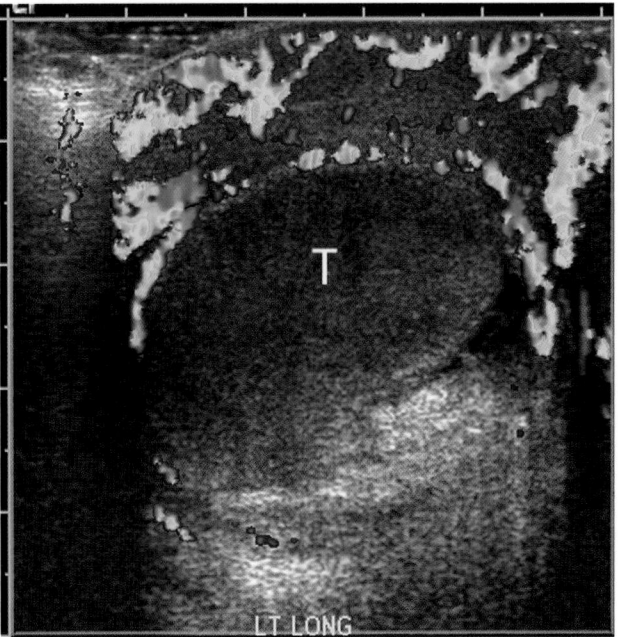

Figure 198-23 Ultrasound of the left scrotum in a boy who presented with acute left scrotal pain demonstrates skin thickening and hypervascularity surrounding the testicle (T), which shows no internal flow by color Doppler. At surgery the patient was found to have testicular torsion.

the "feed and wrap" method as an alternative to sedation. Every patient and any family member wishing to accompany the patient into the room for the examination must be cleared before entering the magnetic field, where potential complications may arise if there has been any recent surgery or if the individual possesses any noncompatible metallic objects.

Brain MRI is the most frequently requested examination of the CNS using this modality. The superb brain parenchymal depiction by MRI makes it possible to diagnose subtle lesions, particularly in regions where one is limited with CT because of beam-hardening artifact, specifically, the temporal lobe or posterior fossa. MRI is also superior when evaluation of small structures is needed, such as in the sellar and suprasellar regions. Gray-white differentiation may be thoroughly evaluated with brain MRI, thus making the diagnosis of infarction straightforward. MRI offers diffusion-weighted imaging, which in turn has made earlier and easier diagnosis of an acute ischemic event possible. For example, diffuse hypoxic ischemic encephalopathy in a newborn, which is difficult to diagnose because the normal high water content of the white matter may mask the presence of underlying edema, can be better assessed with diffusion-weighted imaging. Because of MRI's ability to demonstrate myelination patterns, MRI exceeds any imaging modality for the evaluation of developmental delay. Almost any white matter abnormality, whether a focal or diffuse process such as acute disseminated encephalomyelitis or a systemic metabolic disorder, is best evaluated with MRI because CT lacks the conspicuity to differentiate lesions from normal brain in many instances. Although CT is useful in the acute setting, brain MRI is the gold standard for evaluation of the brain parenchyma when imaging is indicated in the workup of a patient with seizures (Fig. 198-24A and B). Similarly, although CT is useful in the acute management of any patient with new signs or symptoms that suggest the possibility of an intracranial lesion or mass, brain MRI is often necessary to better distinguish not only the lesion but also the lesion's effects on adjacent parenchymal structures.

Face/Neck Imaging

Face or neck lesions, or both, in the pediatric population are frequently examined with MRI because of its excellent soft tissue differentiation, especially when intracranial extension is suspected, for example, with skull base, nasal, or orbital lesions. In addition, if cross-sectional imaging of an isolated neck mass is needed and the patient has a contraindication to the administration of iodinated contrast for CT, MRI or US should be performed instead.

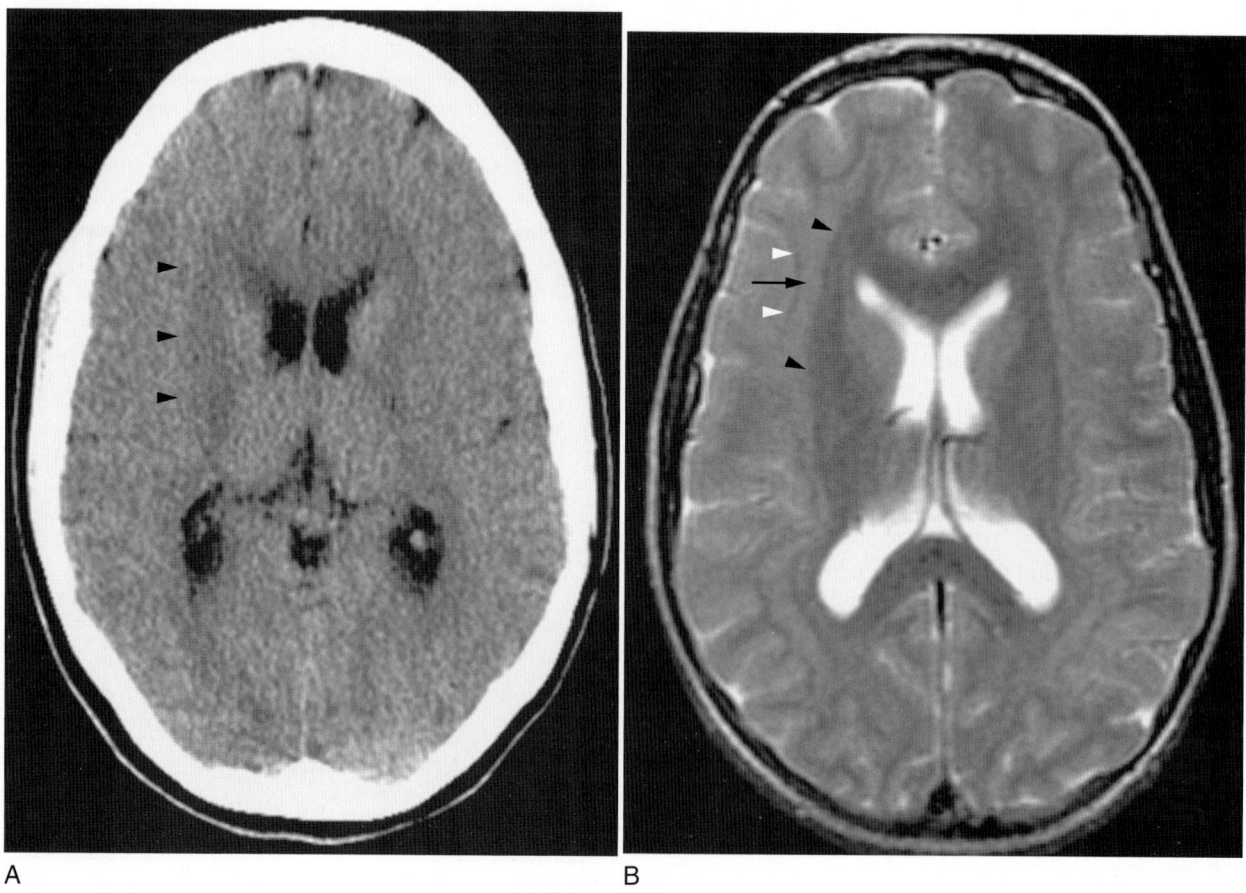

A   B

Figure 198-24   A, Head computed tomography in this child with seizures does not show the white matter to extend well into the periphery, as it should, but rather shows the low density of the white matter located more centrally (*arrowheads*). This patient has band heterotopia, also known as double cortex, better depicted on brain magnetic resonance imaging. B, White matter (*black arrowheads*) followed by a "band" of cortex (*black arrow*), followed by a thin layer of white matter (*white arrowheads*), followed by cortical gray matter as one proceeds peripherally.

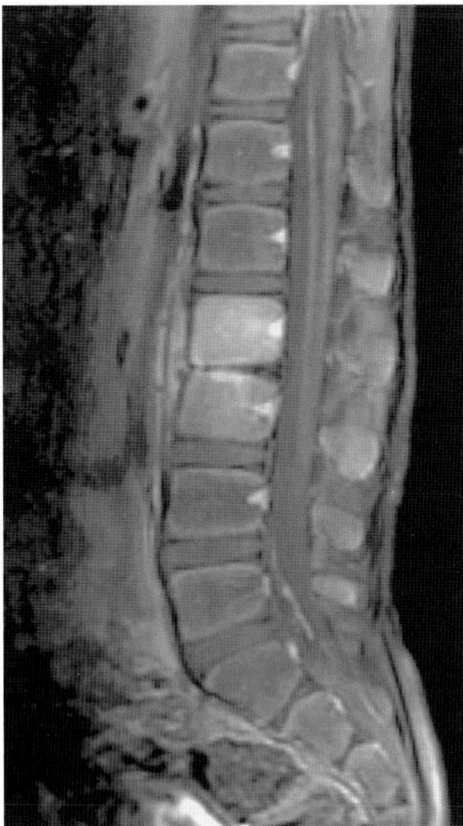

Figure 198-25 This sagittal T1-weighted contrast-enhanced image of the lumbosacral spine shows abnormal enhancement involving the L2 and L3 vertebrae, abnormal enhancement involving the prevertebral soft tissues, and a marked decrease in disk height at this level. These findings are consistent with vertebral osteomyelitis/diskitis. There is no evidence of epidural extent of the infection, but the disk minimally bulges posteriorly.

Spine Imaging

The indications for spine MRI are vast and include evaluation of developmental abnormalities such as diastematomyelia, lipomyelomeningocele, or a Chiari type I malformation. Increasingly, spine MRI is being used at our institution for the evaluation of scoliosis. An abnormality of the CNS is present in approximately 10% of patients with presumed adolescent idiopathic scoliosis in whom only subtle abnormalities are identified on the basis of the clinical history or physical or radiographic examination.[52] Knowledge of these indicators can help the clinician more effectively determine when advanced imaging of the CNS should be performed. Spine MRI is also used for the evaluation of any inflammatory process, whether it involves the vertebrae or is located deeper in the central canal (i.e., osteomyelitis or transverse myelitis, respectively) (Fig. 198-25). In the evaluation of spinal ligamentous injury after trauma, MRI is also superior to CT despite the latter's superior ability to detect fractures. Certain sequelae of spine trauma such as nerve root avulsion can be depicted with MRI as well. Finally, for any pediatric patient with back pain, MRI may be indicated in the search for an intraspinal or paraspinal mass.

Cardiac/Chest/Vascular Imaging

MRI is useful for the evaluation of cardiac, vascular, and soft tissue structures of the chest. CT currently remains superior to MRI in evaluating parenchymal lung disease.

Cardiovascular anatomy, cardiac function, perfusion and blood flow, and pulmonary vascular anatomy can be assessed with cardiac MRI, an examination that complements echocardiography. Cardiovascular imaging is performed with cardiac gating, which means that images are timed to the cardiac cycle. Because patient cooperation is crucial and breath holding is often required, young or uncooperative patients typically undergo general anesthesia for cardiovascular imaging.

Although CT scans are generally the initial cross-sectional imaging modality for evaluating noncardiac anatomy of the chest, MRI is particularly useful for evaluating the mediastinum and soft tissues of the chest wall. Chest MRI is excellent in the evaluation of congenital abnormalities of this region such as bronchopulmonary foregut malformations.

Vascular imaging throughout the body can be achieved with or without the use of gadolinium intravenous contrast. MR angiograms and MR venograms are excellent noninvasive studies for assessing vascular anatomy and patency.

Extremity Imaging

One of the most common indications for MRI is evaluation of the extremities. MRI is used to evaluate the joints for bony, ligamentous, tendinous, and cartilaginous injury. It is very useful in evaluating the composition and extent of soft tissue and bony masses and infections.

Abdomen and Pelvis Imaging

Like CT, MRI offers multiplanar evaluation of the abdominal and pelvic solid organs, the bowel, the peritoneal cavity, surrounding soft tissues, and bones. CT and US are often preferred over MRI because MRI is more time consuming and thus more often requires sedation, is more costly, and is less available. MRI is superior to CT for evaluation of the female pelvic organs and is a useful adjunct to US.

INTERVENTIONAL RADIOLOGY

Interventional radiology has grown significantly in the last 15 years.[53,54] Many procedures previously relegated to surgeons can now be performed with minimally invasive techniques by interventional radiologists. Image-guided therapy and interventions, which are minimally invasive, have a low risk for complications and morbidity. On an outpatient basis, interventional radiologists now perform many procedures previously done surgically and requiring a lengthier hospital admission. With new advances in this field, the radiologist can not only provide diagnostic information but also deliver primary therapy in many instances and frequently during the same visit. The possibility of diagnosis and treatment in one setting is important to consider, especially if the patient will need sedation under general anesthesia. Consultation with the interventional radiologist is important for comprehensive patient care. In the workup of complex cases, multiple subspecialty consultation along with the interventional radiologist may be needed.

There are important differences that arise when interventional radiology procedures are performed on pediatric versus adult patients. The first involves sedation and anesthesia. Many procedures, although minimally invasive, are painful. Certain procedures also stand a greater chance for success with a quiet, still patient. With this in mind, procedural sedation and anesthesia are far more frequently administered to pediatric patients. Not only does one need to administer the appropriate sedative in these cases so that the patient remains motionless as for other diagnostic imaging studies, but administration of an analgesic is also usually necessary.[53] In general, the level of sedation is usually deeper for interventional radiology procedures, and general anesthesia is frequently administered, thereby increasing the overall risk associated with the procedure. In addition, patients in a hospital setting requiring an interventional radiology procedure have a far more complex medical history and usually have an acute abnormality, which in turn further increases the overall risk associated with the procedure when combined with the need for sedation. The overall risk should always be weighed against the benefits gained by performing the particular interventional procedure. Consulting the anesthesiologist and interventional radiologist during complex clinical scenarios cannot be stressed enough. At our institution, there is an anesthesiologist dedicated to the interventional division. This person is familiar with the various procedures performed and tailors the sedation to the particular case being performed.

In addition to differences in sedation between pediatric and adult patients, there are differences related to iodinated contrast administration, technique, and equipment needed to perform a given procedure, not to mention the overall difference in pathophysiology between pediatric and adult disease. Nonetheless, many of the interventional techniques are directly transferable from adult patients to children, particularly nonvascular interventions. It is, however, not unusual for interventional radiologists and surgeons trained and experienced with adults to refer pediatric patients to our institution for image-guided procedures because of the aforementioned issues. Conversely, pediatric interventional radiologists may not be facile in all interventional radiology techniques, and collaboration with their adult counterparts is common. It should be noted that there are very few dedicated training programs in pediatric interventional radiology, and these specialists primarily practice at tertiary pediatric referral centers.

Another issue regarding pediatric interventional procedures relates to radiation exposure. Many adult interventional radiologists use fluoroscopy and CT as image guidance modalities for the sake of speed and ease of use; they tend to use US guidance less frequently. Typical radiation doses for an adult interventional procedure can sometimes be unacceptable for a pediatric patient. To avoid ionizing radiation, most pediatric interventional radiologists use US whenever possible. Altering the fluoroscopy and CT parameters during interventional procedures also helps in decreasing the overall radiation dose to the patient.

Vascular Procedures

Diagnostic Angiography

Diagnostic angiography is not performed as routinely in the pediatric population because of the availability of less invasive modalities such as CT or MR angiography. Still, this procedure remains the gold standard for the diagnosis of vascular diseases. Some of the indications for conventional angiography in children include localization of hemorrhage, renal vascular hypertension, complications of organ transplantation, and the workup of vascular malformations.[55-66] Important precautionary measures need to be taken during this procedure for a pediatric patient because the risk for complications, particularly those related to the puncture site (i.e., vasospasm with the potential for arterial thrombosis), is higher than in an adult patient. This procedure is contraindicated in a patient who is medically unstable. Relative contraindications include substantial electrolyte imbalance, cardiac arrhythmia, a documented serious reaction to contrast administration, impaired renal status, coagulopathy, inability to lie flat on the table, residual barium in the abdomen, and pregnancy.[67] A comprehensive clinical history and physical examination, with special attention to the common femoral and more distal arterial pulses, should be obtained. Screening laboratory studies may include a complete blood count (CBC), Chem-7, prothrombin time (PT), partial thromboplastin time (PTT), and international normalized ratio (INR). All patients require some form of sedation. Previous imaging studies, when necessary, should be available. Informed consent for the procedure is necessary. The interventional radiologist performing the procedure should obtain this consent so that the procedure itself, its benefits and risks, and any questions can be fully discussed. Preprocedural medications such as antibiotics are not routinely used.

Angiography is performed in a dedicated angiography suite with sterile technique. Arterial access is typically gained via puncture of the right common femoral artery. A vascular sheath is placed to lessen trauma to the vessel during catheter exchanges. Catheters and guidewires are placed under fluoroscopic guidance to access the desired vessels. Intravascular contrast is administered via a mechanical injector at a high flow rate through the catheter as serial radiographic images are obtained. Digital techniques are used to subtract background information, such as bony structures, so that only images of the blood vessels remain (Fig. 198-26). It is essential that no motion be present during this process to avoid blurring of images. Typically, images are obtained during a breath hold. During abdominal imaging, glucagon is routinely given to slow bowel motility, which can also interfere with optimal imaging.

As mentioned previously, vessels in children are particularly prone to vasospasm and thrombosis. The presence of a catheter and guidewire in the vessel may be enough to induce spasm. It is not unusual to heparinize a patient during this procedure, particularly infants. Induced hypercapnia during anesthesia is another strategy used to reduce the propensity for vasospasm.

After completion of the procedure, pressure on the arterial puncture site is typically held for 5 to 10 minutes, depending on the patient's coagulation status. It is suggested that patients attempt to limit activity for approximately 24 hours after arterial puncture, after which they may resume normal activity. Lower extremity pulses, particularly on the puncture side, are monitored for possible spasm or impending thrombosis. Hydration at one to two times maintenance is recommended to promote renal clearance of contrast.

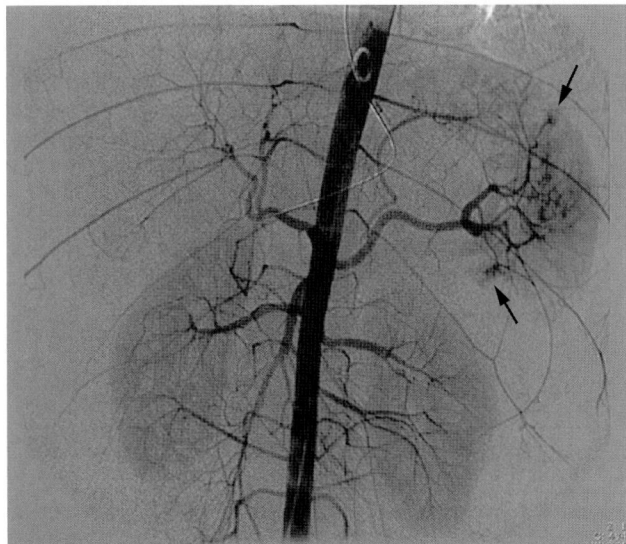

Figure 198-26 Abdominal aortogram performed with digital subtraction. This 13-year-old girl was under general anesthesia, and breath hold and glucagon were used to reduce motion artifact. The patient was involved in a fall and suffered a splenic laceration shown by computed tomography. Multiple areas of contrast extravasation consistent with bleeding are noted (*arrows*).

There are maximum limits on the amount of contrast that can be administered to a patient because of nephrotoxicity. At our institution, this limit is 7 mL/kg in 24 hours, including any other contrast administration on the same day that may have been used for diagnostic imaging (CT, IVP, etc.). Monitoring of renal function by serum creatinine levels is not an absolute requirement after the procedure except in high-risk patients.

Primary Vascular Interventions

Many new techniques are being developed with regard to image-guided minimally invasive treatment of the vascular system. In the vascular arena, primary interventions can be divided into opening up blood vessels (angioplasty, stenting) and blocking them off (embolization, sclerotherapy). One of the more common uses of angioplasty is for evaluation of patients with renovascular hypertension secondary to either fibromuscular dysplasia or renal artery stenosis. On the other end of the spectrum, one of the typical scenarios for occluding vessels via particle embolization is a patient with cystic fibrosis and massive hemoptysis. Recent reports continue to support the usefulness of this technique.[68] Embolization and sclerotherapy are used for the treatment of congenital vascular malformations (arteriovenous, venous, or lymphatic malformations).[69-74] In general, preprocedural preparation is similar to that for diagnostic angiography. For certain procedures, corticosteroids may be administered to reduce the inflammatory response. Prophylactic antibiotics may also be administered during certain vascular interventions. Because treatment of vascular malformations may be complicated and require staged interventions, consultation with the interventional radiologist is essential before discussing these procedures and treatment options with the parents.

Vascular Access Procedures

Image-guided venous access, which includes peripherally inserted central catheter (PICC) and central venous line placement, is generally reserved for patients in whom multiple attempts at gaining venous access without image guidance have proved futile. Success rates for placement of PICCs and central venous catheters under US and fluoroscopic guidance are excellent.[75] Preprocedural preparation usually involves fasting for sedation or anesthesia and is generally reserved for younger patients. Review of the patient's previous imaging examinations and history of previous line placement is essential before the procedure to assess whether there is any known venous obstruction, thrombosis, or stricture. Under US guidance, PICC placement is usually performed in the upper part of the arm with a basilic vein puncture. US guidance is also used for placement of central venous lines and is typically performed via an internal jugular vein approach. Preservation of venous access, particularly in a pediatric patient with chronic disease, is important, so the smallest, least invasive catheters are used to reduce repetitive trauma to the veins. Most catheters placed under image guidance can be used immediately after the procedure.

Nonvascular Interventions

Percutaneous Drainage of Fluid Collections and Abscesses

Minimally invasive image-guided drainage of fluid collections and abscesses is becoming the first-line approach to treatment of these abnormalities at our institution. Collections or abscesses, or both, that arise as a result of complications of appendicitis are commonly treated with this approach.[76-78] Indications for the procedure include (1) reduction in size of collections causing symptoms (such as bowel or urinary obstruction), (2) characterization of fluid (both chemical and microbiologic), and (3) prevention of sepsis in patients with infected collections not responding to antibiotic treatment alone. Contraindications include a percutaneously inaccessible area, surrounding normal bowel being the most common cause of an inaccessible area, and coagulopathy. Review of previous imaging studies and laboratory values and consultation with the pediatric surgeon are needed before performing this procedure. Sedation or general anesthesia is needed in all age groups. The procedure can usually be performed under US guidance. CT guidance is occasionally used for more difficult collections. In most cases, after aspiration a drainage catheter is left within the cavity for several days. Fluid output from these catheters is monitored daily. The catheters may become obstructed, which would require tube flushing, repositioning, or even tube replacement in certain cases. Drainage catheters are removed at the bedside without sedation in most instances.

Image-guided thoracentesis and paracentesis can be performed with similar techniques and preprocedural preparation as for the procedures described earlier. With regard to thoracentesis, consultation with a pediatric surgeon is recommended, particularly for complex effusions or empyemas because the patient may be a more suitable candidate for video-assisted thoracoscopic surgery (VATS) or large-bore chest tube drainage (or both). Use of tissue plasminogen

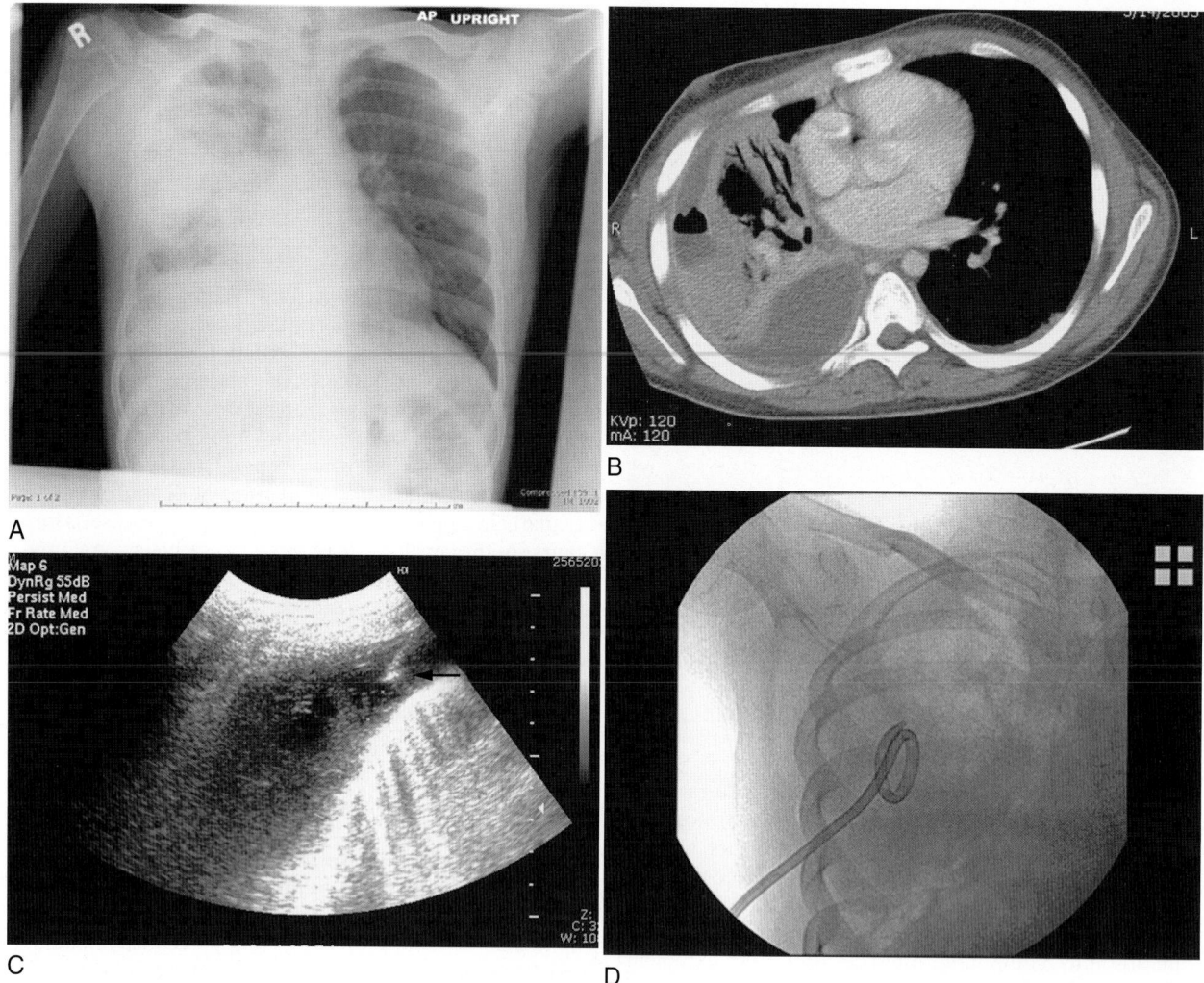

Figure 198-27 Ultrasound-guided thoracentesis and chest tube placement. Right lower lobe pneumonia with complex pleural effusion developed in this 18-year-old male with developmental delay. A and B, Preprocedure appearance by chest radiography and computed tomography, respectively. C, Ultrasound appearance of the collection with a catheter needle in position. D, Placement of a pigtail catheter in the collection under fluoroscopy.

activator through small-bore pigtail catheters has been very successful in draining complex collections that may be loculated.[79,80] Given this, image-guided chest tube placement tends to be the first line of therapy at our institution in these situations (Fig. 198-27A-D).

Percutaneous Image-Guided Biopsy

Minimally invasive biopsy of tumors and other lesions is gaining more acceptance as histologic techniques become more sophisticated. Imaging guidance not only increases the safety of the procedure but also affords the ability to be very precise in targeting specific abnormalities, particularly if they are small. The vast majority of these biopsies can be performed on an outpatient basis under conscious sedation or with a short-lasting general anesthetic. Fine-needle aspirates, as well as small core biopsies, can be obtained by the interventional radiologist. Preprocedural preparation is similar to that for other percutaneous techniques described earlier: fasting status for the patient before sedation/anesthesia, evaluation of the patient's history, imaging examinations, laboratory analysis (CBC, PT/PTT, INR), and

cessation of anticoagulant medications for at least 10 days before biopsy. Open surgical biopsy is necessary in certain cases, such as a large tumor that is partially necrotic, because fine-needle aspiration or even a small core biopsy may not yield adequate specimens. Similarly, in certain cases the patient may need to proceed to immediate surgical excision because of a deleterious mass effect on adjacent structures. Seeding of the biopsy tract is another complication that one must keep in mind for certain tumors. It is best to consult with the oncologist and oncology surgeon when contemplating ordering a minimally invasive biopsy of a presumed tumor.

Percutaneous Gastrostomy/Gastrojejunostomy Placement

At our institution, primary gastrostomy placement is generally performed endoscopically. However, percutaneous image-guided gastrostomy placement is gaining more acceptance because it is less costly and quicker to perform and may be associated with fewer complications. In the pediatric population, gastrostomy placement is essential if nutritional requirements for growth and development are not being met. In patients with severe reflux, who are at increased risk for aspiration, transgastric jejunal feeding tubes can be placed. The techniques and results of percutaneous placement have been reviewed.[81] Both fluoroscopy and US may be used for image guidance to place this feeding tube. The procedure can be performed on an outpatient basis. The stoma is allowed to mature for about 8 to 12 weeks before attempting to place a transgastric jejunal tube. These tubes are placed under fluoroscopic guidance to ensure placement in the proximal jejunum. Getting the feeding tube to the proximal jejunum can be challenging in many instances, and it is not uncommon that radiation exposure is prolonged in both the patient and operator. These feeding tubes frequently need to be replaced because they can become obstructed or the patient inadvertently pulls the tube out, which in turn increases the cumulative radiation exposure. Consideration for this increased radiation dose must be balanced against the potential benefits/risks of surgical fundoplication for treating the reflux.

Percutaneous Cecostomy

Many patients with chronic neurologic, developmental, or metabolic diseases are plagued with chronic constipation. In this group of patients, placement of a catheter within the cecum with the administration of regular antegrade enemas can be life changing.[82] Placement of a cecostomy tube is similar to placement of a gastrostomy tube, again performed under US and fluoroscopic guidance. Preprocedural preparation is similar.

Hepatic and Biliary Interventions

In the pediatric population, interventions involving the liver are common. Image-guided liver biopsy is now the preferred standard of care at our institution and has replaced blind biopsies. Several papers have shown a decrease in bleeding complications with image-guided biopsy.[83] At our institution, many children with metabolic or infectious diseases involving the liver, most commonly viral hepatitis, require liver biopsy for diagnosis, as well as monitoring of therapy. Many of our patients are taking hepatotoxic medications, which also require monitoring. As an institution that performs liver transplantation, biopsy is routinely performed to monitor for organ rejection. Thalassemia patients, who require multiple transfusions, are often evaluated for iron overload. Percutaneous liver biopsy is performed with the same techniques as described earlier for image-guided biopsy, with careful attention to avoiding adjacent vessels or transgressing the liver capsule and inadvertently puncturing nearby structures. Performance of the procedure can be challenging in that many of these patients may be coagulopathic. Performance of a coagulation profile, as well as preparing blood products for administration to correct the coagulopathy or resuscitate the patient in case of bleeding, is standard protocol at our institution. The procedure is performed with sedation or anesthesia. A hematocrit level is obtained 4 hours after the procedure. A significant decrease in hematocrit or the presence of pain after the procedure warrants further workup and possible blood transfusion.

In patients with severe uncorrectable coagulopathy, liver biopsy can alternatively be performed with a transvenous approach via the right internal jugular vein and the liver parenchymal specimen obtained by puncturing through the right or middle hepatic vein with specialized technology.

Biliary interventions are not common in the pediatric population. Most biliary procedures in this population are performed through endoscopic or surgical methods. Noninvasive methods for evaluation of the biliary system, such as magnetic resonance cholangiopancreatography (MRCP), are becoming more available, thus precluding the need for endoscopy and cholangiopancreatography. Interventional biliary procedures are sometimes performed in liver transplantation patients with complications involving the biliary-enteric anastomosis. Balloon cholangioplasty of strictures at these anastomoses is performed at our institution with mixed results. Other biliary interventions that are common in the adult population, such as biliary stone removal or common bile duct stenting, are performed rarely in children. Preprocedure preparation for biliary interventions includes the administration of prophylactic antibiotics to cover gram-negative organisms.

Urologic Interventions

Percutaneous nephrostomy is performed primarily for relief of urinary tract obstruction. In the pediatric population, this is usually in the setting of congenital obstruction of the ureteropelvic junction. The next most common indication in our practice is in the setting of postoperative edema of the ureterovesical junction after ureteral reimplantation surgery for vesicoureteral reflux. Relief of obstruction secondary to nephrolithiasis, the most frequent indication in the adult population, is not as common in children. Techniques are similar to that for drainage of fluid collections, with the same preprocedure preparation of the patient. Prophylactic antibiotics are usually administered. Whereas in adult institutions the procedure is performed under fluoroscopic guidance, US guidance is almost exclusively used in our practice. Using US reduces the radiation dose to the patient, and having Doppler affords one the ability to locate an avascular plane to access the collecting system. A small pigtail catheter is placed within the renal pelvis after aspiration of urine. This catheter can form a mature tract, thus making the renal pelvis easier to access so that future interventions can be performed, such as balloon dilation or stent placement for a stricture. The catheter can remain within the renal pelvis for several weeks with proper care on an outpatient basis.

Musculoskeletal Interventions

Musculoskeletal interventions account for a major portion of the nonvascular pediatric interventional radiology practice. Percutaneous bone biopsy under either fluoroscopic or CT guidance is gaining more acceptance in the diagnosis of both neoplastic and infectious disease. Therapeutic interventions are also becoming more commonplace as technology advances. Biopsy plus treatment of osteoid osteomas with radiofrequency ablation under imaging guidance is well documented and highly effective.[84] Percutaneous biopsy of presumed histiocytosis lesions can be followed by direct injection of a steroid into the lesion with good results.[85] Preoperative embolization of aneurysmal bone cysts and tumors has significantly reduced the morbidity associated with these operations. Primary sclerotherapy for aneurysmal bone cysts is also being performed.[86] Because most of these procedures can be quite painful, general anesthesia is usually required with the same preprocedural preparation as for image-guided biopsy. Most of these procedures can be performed on a day surgery basis. Again, consultation with the orthopedic surgeon, oncologist, and interventional radiologist is essential.

ACKNOWLEDGMENT

We would like to give thanks for the efforts, support, and expertise of Dr. Ted Treves and Rhonda Johnson in making this chapter come to fruition. We would like to give a special thank you to Max, who gave us the motivation to finish this chapter.

REFERENCES

1. Brenner D, Elliston C, Hall E, et al: Estimated risks of radiation-induced fatal cancer from pediatric CT. AJR Am J Roentgenol 2001;176:289-296.
2. Bushberg J, Seibert J, Leidholdt E Jr: Projection radiography. In Bushberg JT, Seibert JA, Leidholdt EM Jr, Boone JM (eds): The Essential Physics of Medical Imaging. Baltimore, Williams & Wilkins, 1994, pp 139-168.
3. Hernandez RJ, Goodsitt MM: Reduction of radiation dose in pediatric patients using pulsed fluoroscopy. AJR Am J Roentgenol 1996;167:1247-1253.
4. Bushberg J, Seibert J, Leidholdt E Jr: X-ray computed tomography. In Bushberg JT, Seibert JA, Leidholdt EM Jr, Boone JM (eds): The Essential Physics of Medical Imaging. Baltimore, Williams & Wilkins, 1994, pp 239-289.
5. Lowe SA: Diagnostic radiography in pregnancy: Risks and reality. Aust N Z J Obstet Gynaecol 2004;44:191-196.
6. US Department of Health and Human Services: Child Maltreatment 2002: Summary of Key Findings. Washington, DC, US Government Printing Office, 2004.
7. Kleinman PK, Blackbourne BD, Marks SC, et al: Radiologic contributions to the investigation and prosecution of cases of fatal infant abuse. N Engl J Med 1989;320:507-511.
8. Nimkin K, Kleinman PK: Imaging of child abuse. Radiol Clin North Am 2001;39:843-864.
9. Kleinman PL, Kleinman PK, Savageau JA: Suspected infant abuse: Radiographic skeletal survey practices in pediatric health care facilities. Radiology 2004;233:477-485.
10. Rubin DM, Christian CW, Bilaniuk LT, et al: Occult head injury in high-risk abused children. Pediatrics 2003;111:1382-1386.
11. Jaspan T, Griffiths PD, McConachie NS, et al: Neuroimaging for non-accidental head injury in childhood: A proposed protocol. Clin Radiol 2003;58:44-53.
12. Barkovich A: Hydrocephalus: In Barkovich AJ (ed): Pediatric Neuroimaging. New York, Lippincott Williams & Wilkins, 2000, pp 606-607.
13. Novelline R: The central nervous system. In Novelline RA (ed): Squire's Fundamentals of Radiology. Cambridge, MA, Harvard University Press, 1997, pp 506-511.
14. Donnelly L: Chest. In Donnelly LF (ed): Fundamentals of Pediatric Radiology. Philadelphia, WB Saunders, 2001, pp 27-29.
15. Boland GW, Murphy B, Arellano R, et al: Dose reduction in gastrointestinal and genitourinary fluoroscopy: Use of grid-controlled pulsed fluoroscopy. AJR Am J Roentgenol 2000;175:1453-1457.
16. Ward L, Barnewolt C, Strauss K, et al: Radiation exposure and image quality: Preliminary results of a comparison of variable-rate pulsed fluoroscopy with continuous fluoroscopy in a swine model of pediatric genitourinary abnormalities [Scientific Presentation 08-54]. Paper presented at the annual meeting of the Association of University Radiologists, 2003, Miami.
17. Diamond DA, Kleinman PK, Spevak M, et al: The tailored low dose fluoroscopic voiding cystogram for familial reflux screening. J Urol 1996;155:681-682.
18. Persliden J, Helmrot E, Hjort P, et al: Dose and image quality in the comparison of analogue and digital techniques in paediatric urology examinations. Eur Radiol 2004;14:638-644.
19. American College of Radiology: Current criteria of the use of water soluble contrast agents for intravenous injections. ACR Bulletin, Reston, VA, 1990.
20. Elder JS, Longenecker R: Premedication with oral midazolam for voiding cystourethrography in children: Safety and efficacy. AJR Am J Roentgenol 1995;164:1229-1232.
21. Stokland E, Andreasson S, Jacobsson B, et al: Sedation with midazolam for voiding cystourethrography in children: A randomised double-blind study. Pediatr Radiol 2003;33:247-249.
22. Dajani AS, Taubert KA, Wilson W, et al: Prevention of bacterial endocarditis. Recommendations by the American Heart Association. JAMA 1997;277:1794-1801.
23. Conway JJ, Maizels M: The "well tempered" diuretic renogram: A standard method to examine the asymptomatic neonate with hydronephrosis or hydroureteronephrosis. A report from combined meetings of The Society for Fetal Urology and members of The Pediatric Nuclear Medicine Council—The Society of Nuclear Medicine. J Nucl Med 1992;33:2047-2051.
24. Treves S, Majd M, Kuruc A, et al: Kidneys. In Treves ST (ed): Pediatric Nuclear Medicine, 2nd ed. New York, Springer-Verlag, 1995, pp 339-399.
25. Schofer O, Konig G, Bartels U, et al: Technetium-99m mercaptoacetyltriglycine clearance: Reference values for infants and children. Eur J Nucl Med 1995;22:1278-1281.
26. Kleinman PK, Diamond DA, Karellas A, et al: Tailored low-dose fluoroscopic voiding cystourethrography for the reevaluation of vesicoureteral reflux in girls. AJR Am J Roentgenol 1994;162:1151-1154; discussion 1155-1156.
27. Taylor A, Nally J, Aurell M, et al: Consensus report on ACE inhibitor renography for detecting renovascular hypertension. Radionuclides in Nephrourology Group. Consensus Group on ACEI Renography. J Nucl Med 1996;37:1876-1882.
28. Lagomarsino E, Orellana P, Munoz J, et al: Captopril scintigraphy in the study of arterial hypertension in pediatrics. Pediatr Nephrol 2004;19:66-70.
29. Brown ED, Chen MY, Wolfman NT, et al: Complications of renal transplantation: Evaluation with US and radionuclide imaging. Radiographics 2000;20:607-622.
30. Dubovsky EV, Russell CD, Bischof-Delaloye A, et al: Report of the Radionuclides in Nephrourology Committee for evaluation of transplanted kidney (review of techniques). Semin Nucl Med 1999;29:175-188.
31. Palestro CJ, Torres MA: Radionuclide imaging in orthopedic infections. Semin Nucl Med 1997;27:334-345.
32. Bombardieri E, Maccauro M, De Deckere E, et al: Nuclear medicine imaging of neuroendocrine tumours. Ann Oncol 2001;12(Suppl 2):S51-S61.
33. Maurea S, Cuocolo A, Reynolds JC, et al: Iodine-131-metaiodobenzylguanidine scintigraphy in preoperative and postoperative evaluation of paragangliomas: Comparison with CT and MRI. J Nucl Med 1993;34:173-179.
34. van Amsterdam JA, Kluin-Nelemans JC, van Eck-Smit BL, et al: Role of ^{67}Ga scintigraphy in localization of lymphoma. Ann Hematol 1996;72:202-207.
35. Bekerman C, Hoffer PB, Bitran JD: The role of gallium-67 in the clinical evaluation of cancer. Semin Nucl Med 1984;14:296-323.
36. Nadel H, Rossleigh M: Tumor imaging. In Treves ST (ed): Pediatric Nuclear Medicine, 2nd ed. New York, Springer-Verlag, 1995, pp 496-527.
37. Kirks DR, Coleman RE, Filston HC, et al: An imaging approach to persistent neonatal jaundice. AJR Am J Roentgenol 1984;142:461-465.
38. Treves S, Jones A, Markisz J: Liver and spleen. In Treves ST (ed): Pediatric Nuclear Medicine, 2nd ed. New York, Springer-Verlag, 1995, pp 466-495.

39. Tappin DM, King C, Paton JY: Lower oesophageal pH monitoring—a useful clinical tool. Arch Dis Child 1992;67:146-148.

40. Al-Khawari HA, Sinan TS, Seymour H: Diagnosis of gastro-oesophageal reflux in children. Comparison between oesophageal pH and barium examinations. Pediatr Radiol 2002;32:765-770.

41. Heyman S: Gastric emptying in children. J Nucl Med 1998;39:865-869.

42. Gropler RJ, Soto P: Recent advances in cardiac positron emission tomography in the clinical management of the cardiac patient. Curr Cardiol Rep 2004;6:20-26.

43. Treves S, Packard A: Lungs. In Treves ST (ed): Pediatric Nuclear Medicine, 2nd ed. New York, Springer-Verlag, 1995, pp 159-197.

44. Paltiel HJ, Summerville DA, Treves ST: Iodine-123 scintigraphy in the evaluation of pediatric thyroid disorders: A ten year experience. Pediatr Radiol 1992;22:251-256.

45. Paltiel H, Larsen R, Treves S: Thyroid. In Treves ST (ed): Pediatric Nuclear Medicine, 2nd ed. New York, Springer-Verlag, 1995, pp 135-148.

46. Juhasz C, Chugani HT: Imaging the epileptic brain with positron emission tomography. Neuroimaging Clin N Am 2003;13:705-716, viii.

47. Kirse DJ, Roberson DW: Surgical management of retropharyngeal space infections in children. Laryngoscope 2001;111:1413-1422.

48. American College of Radiology: ACR practice guidelines for the performance of neurosonography in neonates and young children. In American College of Radiology (ed): Practice Guidelines and Technical Standards 2004. Reston, VA, ACR, 2004, pp 645-648.

49. Slovis T: Cranial ultrasound. In Khun JP, Slovis TL, Haller JO (eds): Caffey's Pediatric Diagnostic Imaging, 10th ed. Philadelphia, CV Mosby, 2004, pp 277-310.

50. Slovis T: Ultrasound of the neonatal spinal canal. In Kuhn JP, Slovis TL, Haller JO (eds): Caffey's Pediatric Diagnostic Imaging, 10th ed. Philadelphia, CV Mosby, 2004, pp 311-316.

51. Robinson AJ, Russell S, Rimmer S: The value of ultrasonic examination of the lumbar spine in infants with specific reference to cutaneous markers of occult spinal dysraphism. Clin Radiol 2005;60:72-77.

52. Davids JR, Chamberlin E, Blackhurst DW: Indications for magnetic resonance imaging in presumed adolescent idiopathic scoliosis. J Bone Joint Surg Am 2004;86:2187-2195.

53. Kaye RD, Sane SS, Towbin RB: Pediatric intervention: An update—part I. J Vasc Interv Radiol 2000;11:683-697.

54. Kaye R, Sane SS, Towbin RB: Pediatric intervention: An update—part II. J Vasc Interv Radiol 2000;11:807-822.

55. Burrows PF, Robertson RL, Barnes PD: Angiography and the evaluation of cerebrovascular disease in childhood. Neuroimaging Clin N Am 1996;6:561-588.

56. Burrows PE, Laor T, Paltiel H, et al: Diagnostic imaging in the evaluation of vascular birthmarks. Dermatol Clin 1998;16:455-488.

57. Christensen R: Invasive radiology for pediatric trauma. Semin Pediatr Surg 2001;10:7-11.

58. D'Souza SJ, Tsai WS, Silver MM, et al: Diagnosis and management of stenotic aorto-arteriopathy in childhood. J Pediatr 1998;132:1016-1022.

59. Jain S, Sharma N, Singh S, et al: Takayasu arteritis in children and young Indians. Int J Cardiol 2000;75(Suppl 1):S153-S157.

60. Johnson JW, Gracias VH, Gupta R, et al: Hepatic angiography in patients undergoing damage control laparotomy. J Trauma 2002;52:1102-1106.

61. Kassarjian A, Dubois J, Burrows PE: Angiographic classification of hepatic hemangiomas in infants. Radiology 2002;222:693-698.

62. Ng CS, de Bruyn R, Gordon I: The investigation of renovascular hypertension in children: The accuracy of radio-isotopes in detecting renovascular disease. Nucl Med Commun 1997;18:1017-1028.

63. Opatowsky MJ, Browne JD, McGuirt WF Jr, et al: Endovascular treatment of hemorrhage after tonsillectomy in children. AJNR Am J Neuroradiol 2001;22:713-716.

64. Rozycki GS, Tremblay L, Feliciano DV, et al: A prospective study for the detection of vascular injury in adult and pediatric patients with cervicothoracic seat belt signs. J Trauma 2002;52:618-623; discussion 623-624.

65. Yamada I, Himeno Y, Matsushima Y, et al: Renal artery lesions in patients with moyamoya disease: Angiographic findings. Stroke 2000;31:733-737.

66. Yalcindag A, Sundel R: Vasculitis in childhood. Curr Opin Rheumatol 2001;13:422-427.

67. Kandarpa K, Gardiner G: Peripheral arteriography. In Kandarpa K, Aruny J (eds): Handbook of Interventional Radiologic Procedures, 3rd ed. Philadelphia, Lippincott Williams & Wilkins, 2002, pp 3-7.

68. Barben J, Robertson D, Olinsky A, et al: Bronchial artery embolization for hemoptysis in young patients with cystic fibrosis. Radiology 2002;224:124-130.

69. Mason KP, Michna E, Zurakowski D, et al: Serum ethanol levels in children and adults after ethanol embolization or sclerotherapy for vascular anomalies. Radiology 2000;217:127-132.

70. Yakes WF, Rossi P, Odink H: How I do it. Arteriovenous malformation management. Cardiovasc Intervent Radiol 1996;19:65-71.

71. Behnia R: Systemic effects of absolute alcohol embolization in a patient with a congenital arteriovenous malformation of the lower extremity. Anesth Analg 1995;80:415-417.

72. Berenguer B, Burrows PE, Zurakowski D, et al: Sclerotherapy of craniofacial venous malformations: Complications and results. Plast Reconstr Surg 1999;104:1-11; discussion 12-15.

73. Cabrera J, Cabrera J Jr, Garcia-Olmedo MA: Sclerosants in microfoam. A new approach in angiology. Int Angiol 2001;20:322-329.

74. Choi YH, Han MH, O-Ki K, et al: Craniofacial cavernous venous malformations: Percutaneous sclerotherapy with use of ethanolamine oleate. J Vasc Interv Radiol 2002;13:475-482.

75. Chait PG, Ingram J, Phillips-Gordon C, et al: Peripherally inserted central catheters in children. Radiology 1995;197:775-778.

76. Jamieson DH, Chait PG, Filler R: Interventional drainage of appendiceal abscesses in children. AJR Am J Roentgenol 1997;169:1619-1622.

77. Gervais DA, Hahn PF, O'Neill MJ, et al: CT-guided transgluteal drainage of deep pelvic abscesses in children: Selective use as an alternative to transrectal drainage. AJR Am J Roentgenol 2000;175:1393-1396.

78. Pereira JK, Chait PG, Miller SF: Deep pelvic abscesses in children: Transrectal drainage under radiologic guidance. Radiology 1996;198:393-396.

79. Mitri RK, Brown SD, Zurakowski D, et al: Outcomes of primary image-guided drainage of parapneumonic effusions in children. Pediatrics 2002;110:e37.

80. Ray TL, Berkenbosch JW, Russo P, et al: Tissue plasminogen activator as an adjuvant therapy for pleural empyema in pediatric patients. J Intensive Care Med 2004;19:44-50.

81. Kaye RD, Towbin RB: Imaging and intervention in the gastrointestinal tract in children. Gastroenterol Clin North Am 2002;31:897-923, viii.

82. Chait PG, Shandling B, Richards HM, et al: Fecal incontinence in children: Treatment with percutaneous cecostomy tube placement—a prospective study. Radiology 1997;203:621-624.

83. Nobili V, Comparcola D, Sartorelli MR, et al: Blind and ultrasound-guided percutaneous liver biopsy in children. Pediatr Radiol 2003;33:772-775.

84. Torriani M, Rosenthal DI: Percutaneous radiofrequency treatment of osteoid osteoma. Pediatr Radiol 2002;32:615-618.

85. Yasko AW, Fanning CV, Ayala AG, et al: Percutaneous techniques for the diagnosis and treatment of localized Langerhans-cell histiocytosis (eosinophilic granuloma of bone). J Bone Joint Surg Am 1998;80:219-228.

86. Falappa P, Fassari FM, Fanelli A, et al: Aneurysmal bone cysts: Treatment with direct percutaneous Ethibloc injection: Long-term results. Cardiovasc Intervent Radiol 2002;25:282-290.

CHAPTER 199

Lumbar Puncture

Timothy Gibson

Lumbar puncture (LP) is a frequently performed procedure by hospital-based physicians. Although its description may sound frightening to parents or other laypersons, in actuality, it is a fairly simple and straightforward procedure in most patients.

INDICATIONS

LP is performed whenever cerebrospinal fluid (CSF) is needed for evaluation. The most typical scenario for a pediatric hospitalist is a febrile patient in whom meningitis is a concern, and a majority of such patients are neonates or infants with nonspecific signs and symptoms of meningitis. Other indications include evaluation of suspected central nervous system (CNS) bleeding, measurement of intracranial pressure (ICP) as in pseudotumor cerebri, and investigation of suspected inflammatory conditions of the CNS.

CONTRAINDICATIONS

The practitioner should always consider whether it is safe to perform LP. If a patient has increased ICP, such as from a cerebral mass, release of pressure during LP may potentially precipitate shifting of intracranial contents from an area of high pressure to one of low pressure (i.e., cerebral herniation). If this is at all a possibility, the patient should have CNS imaging performed before a spinal tap is done. The risk is significantly less in infants who have an open fontanelle. The same is true for significant intracranial bleeding. In general, if the patient does not have focal neurologic findings on physical examination or demonstrate signs or symptoms of increased ICP by history or on physical examination, it is safe to perform LP before imaging. LP is relatively contraindicated in patients with underlying bleeding diatheses to avoid the formation of a hematoma around the spinal column or within the surrounding soft tissues. If this problem is suspected, blood studies such as a complete blood count and coagulation studies should be performed before LP is attempted.

EQUIPMENT

Virtually all hospitals will have a commercially made LP tray that contains most of the equipment needed to perform LP (Table 199-1). Although these kits all contain local anesthetic, most do not contain topical anesthetic (e.g., EMLA, ELA-Max). One will also need to obtain an appropriately sized spinal needle based on the age or size of the patient (Table 199-2). It should also be noted that some pediatric LP kits have no manometer, so to measure opening pressure, a manometer must be obtained from an adult LP kit.

ANATOMY

CSF is produced in the choroid plexuses of the lateral ventricles. It circulates between the lateral ventricles and around the spinal cord and cerebrum in the subarachnoid space. The goal of LP is to obtain a sample of CSF in the safest possible manner, which is achieved by puncturing the dura mater in the lumbar region, below the termination of the spinal cord itself, where only the cauda equina is found. In young children, the inferior termination of the spinal cord is at the level of L3, and in older children, it is even higher. Thus, LP can nearly always be performed safely, barring any anatomic anomaly, which is usually obvious, by inserting the spinal needle between the L4 and L5 vertebrae. To locate this interspace, palpate the posterior superior iliac crests; the L4-L5 interspace is located at that level. On the patient's back you will feel the spinous processes of the vertebrae. When the needle is inserted, it will penetrate the skin and then the supraspinous ligament, the interspinous ligament, and the ligamentum flavum before puncturing the dura mater to enter the subarachnoid space, where CSF is found (Fig. 199-1).

PREPARATION

Before beginning, the practitioner should consider issues of analgesia. If LP is anticipated, the patient should have a topical anesthetic applied widely to the lower lumbar area in the midline. Topical anesthetics take approximately 35 to 50 minutes to take effect, so some foresight is needed. For positioning, the two options are to have the patient either sitting up or lying on the side. In either case, the goal is to get the patient to flex the neck and back while drawing up the legs to maximize the size of the intervertebral space between L4 and L5. Older patients often prefer to be sitting, but infants are more often positioned on their side. The latter will be discussed because an infant requiring LP will be encountered much more frequently.

PROCEDURE

As a right-handed person, I prefer to have the patient lying in the right lateral decubitus position with the head on my right and the feet to my left. An important factor in determining the eventual success of LP is the skill of the person who restrains the patient. The holder should flex the neck and pull the knees to the chest while keeping the patient as still as possible. It is also important that the holder keep the back vertical, with an imaginary line between the posterior superior iliac crests lying perpendicular to the table. Open the LP tray in sterile fashion and place it close by so that you can reach the tray with one hand during the procedure. The kit also has only one spinal needle. Not only should one make sure that it is an appropriate size, but it is also a good idea to have one or two extra needles on the tray to open in case they are needed. Once the patient is positioned, put on sterile gloves and use gauze or a swab stick soaked with povidone-iodine (Betadine) to sterilize the site of entry in a circular fashion. Place a fenestrated drape over the patient such that only the lumbosacral spine is visible. The drape is large enough in an infant to cover the posterior superior iliac spines and will be sterile; thus, one is able to palpate the spines and locate the L4-L5 interspace simultaneously. The L3-L4 interspace is also acceptable. When the space is located, draw up 1 to 2 mL of lidocaine included in

Table 199–1 Equipment Needed for Lumbar Puncture

Lumbar puncture tray
  Spinal needle (see Table 199-2)
  Sterile collecting tubes
  Sterile drapes
  Povidone-iodine (Betadine) swabs or sterile sponges and tray
    to pour Betadine
  Gauze
  Manometer (may need to be added)
  Syringe and local anesthetic (1% lidocaine)

Sterile gloves

Betadine solution

Bandage

Table 199–2 Spinal Needle Size Based on Age

Neonate-2 years	22-gauge, 1½-inch needle
2-12 years	22-gauge, 2½-inch needle
Older than 12 years	20- or 22-gauge, 3½-inch needle

the kit. With the use of topical anesthetics, the skin in the area should be blanched and anesthetized. Create a wheal with lidocaine just below the skin, and proceed as deep into the intervertebral space as the ⅝-inch needle will allow. Pull the needle out slowly while injecting the lidocaine as you go. Once the lidocaine is administered, you are ready to insert the spinal needle, again making sure that it is the appropriate size. It should be noted that the larger the gauge of the needle, the more likely the patient will have a "spinal headache" because of CSF leakage after the procedure (see Complications). Place your left thumb over the lower of the spinous processes that you have chosen (i.e., L5 for the L4-L5 interspace). With your thumb on the spinous process, the rest of your left hand can still be on the left posterior superior iliac crest. While holding the spinal needle with your right thumb and first finger close to its end, insert it, bevel up, through the skin pointing toward the umbilicus (slightly cephalad). Use the left thumb as a fulcrum to steady the needle as you insert it. If there is immediate bony resistance, you are probably in contact with the spinous process, so pull the needle back and redirect it, most commonly more cephalad. Once you are past the superficial bony structures, insert the needle slowly. If you think that you may be in the subarachnoid space, remove the stylet and watch for CSF flow. Experienced practitioners may feel a "pop" as they penetrate the dura mater to enter the subarachnoid space. If there is no flow of CSF, it may help to rotate the needle 90 degrees. If there is still no flow of CSF, reinsert the stylet and advance the needle a few millimeters further. This process is performed repeatedly until flow of CSF is obtained. If blood flows from the needle, the venous plexus just outside the epidural space (see Fig. 199-1) may have been punctured, a so-called traumatic tap. Blood from a traumatic tap will clot, as opposed to bloody CSF, which will not. In addition, blood from a traumatic tap will gradually lessen as flow occurs, whereas bloody CSF will be homogeneous. If a traumatic tap occurs, remove the needle completely and start in a different interspace.

Once CSF flow has begun, opening pressure can be measured by attaching a manometer. This apparatus is a bit

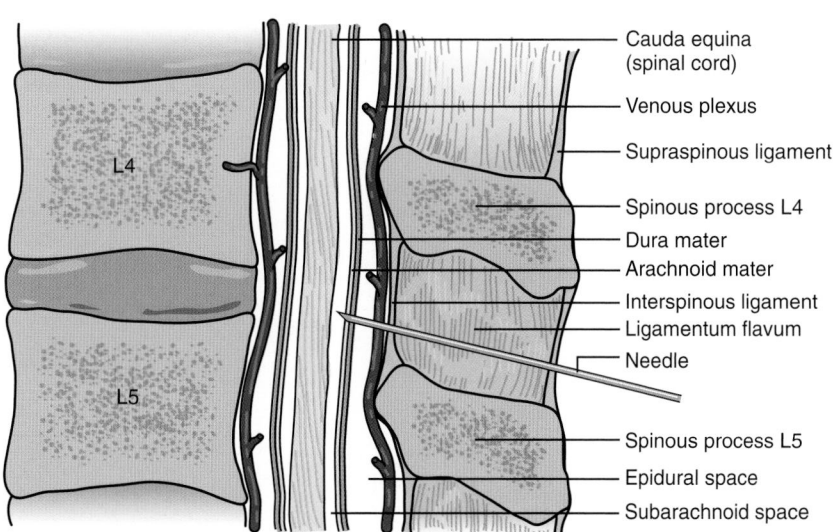

Figure 199–1 The spinal needle is inserted between the L4 and L5 vertebrae.

clumsy, and attaching it often requires the help of an assistant. The patient must be still and not struggling to obtain an accurate reading, which is often impossible in infants. Either way, once flow begins, collect specimens in the sterile tubes included in the kit, 1 mL per tube. Tube 1 is sent for culture, Gram stain, and bacterial antigen detection; tube 2 is sent for protein and glucose; and tube 3 is sent for cell counts. It is often good practice to draw off a fourth tube and have the laboratory store it in case other studies are desired later. Once the desired amount of CSF is removed, reinsert the stylet and remove the needle in one quick movement. Apply a bandage and make sure that any excess Betadine is wiped off the patient.

COMPLICATIONS

There is always the risk of bleeding or infection when performing an LP, and this possibility should be discussed with the family in advance. The risk of herniation was discussed earlier. In small infants, respiratory compromise can occur, but more as a result of positioning and restraint than the LP itself. In general, young patients should be on a monitor while being tightly held. In the adult or older adolescent population, headaches are relatively common after LP. This is thought to be due to a small leak of CSF through the puncture in the dura. These headaches usually respond to analgesics and fluids. Caffeine may also be effective. For a prolonged headache, an epidural blood patch can be applied to stop the leak, but this is not generally necessary. Hematomas in the subdural or epidural space are reported but are not common. If the patient has neurologic deficits after LP, traumatic bleeding must be ruled out. Finally, there is a risk of pushing superficial dermal material into the subarachnoid space during LP. This can generally be avoided by having the stylet in the needle whenever it is advanced.

SUGGESTED READING

Cronan K, Wiley J: Lumbar puncture. In Henretig F, King C (eds): Textbook of Pediatric Emergency Procedures. Baltimore, Williams & Wilkins, 1997, pp 541-552.

Janssens E, Aerssens P, Alliet P, et al: Post–dural puncture headache in children. A literature review. Eur J Pediatr 2003;162:117-121.

CHAPTER 200

Bladder Catheterization

Sandra Schwab

Urinary bladder catheterization in children can serve as both a diagnostic and a therapeutic intervention. Catheterization is a simple, sterile procedure that can be performed at the bedside in most circumstances. Children usually tolerate the procedure well when it is done carefully, requiring only a topical anesthetic, if any.[1,2]

INDICATIONS

The most common indication for urinary bladder catheterization is collection of urine for analysis and culture. A catheter specimen is recommended to rule out urinary tract infection in those children who are not yet toilet trained or who are unable to cooperate with a midstream clean-catch specimen.[3] Catheterization is also indicated to relieve urinary retention or obstruction. This may be due to anatomic abnormalities such as posterior urethral valves or prolapsing ureterocele, inflammation of the urethra, or mechanical obstruction related to blood clots or debris in the bladder. Neurogenic bladder may also cause retention requiring catheterization. In critically ill patients, urinary catheterization is used to monitor urine output and assess fluid status.

CONTRAINDICATIONS

There are few contraindications for urinary catheterization. A general practitioner should not catheterize patients with known urethral trauma or acute pelvic fracture, and careful consideration should be given to catheterization in patients with recent genitourinary surgery. Consultation with a urologist is recommended before placing a catheter in any of these patients.

EQUIPMENT

Catheters come in many shapes and sizes; common sizes are listed in Table 200-1. The two most common catheters used in children are a straight catheter and a self-retaining Foley catheter. A straight catheter is used for one-time or intermittent catheterization. If long-term catheterization is anticipated, a Foley catheter is appropriate. Choose the smallest lumen possible to pass the catheter easily and accomplish the goals of catheterization. In a newborn or infant, a 5-French feeding tube can be used if an 8-French catheter is too large. Table 200-2 lists the other supplies needed to perform a bladder catheterization.

PROCEDURE

Position the patient supine, and restrain as necessary for age. Sterile technique should be maintained throughout the procedure. If using a Foley catheter, test the balloon for competency by filling it with sterile water; then empty it. Place sterile drapes around the penis or perineum. Using the non-dominant hand, retract the foreskin and grasp the penis or spread the labia to expose the urethral meatus (Fig. 200-1). Cleanse the urethral opening and surrounding tissue with antiseptic solution. If desired, slowly inject viscous lidocaine into the urethral opening. Extend the penile shaft so that it is perpendicular to the abdomen in order to straighten the urethra in males (Fig. 200-2). After lubricating the tip, slowly advance the catheter into the bladder. Resistance in males is frequently the result of volitional constriction of the external sphincter and can usually be overcome with firm, steady pressure. Advance a Foley catheter its entire length into the bladder. Stop advancing a straight catheter once urine is obtained. Urine should flow easily into the collection container. If no urine is obtained, consider irrigating the catheter with sterile water to confirm urine return. In females, absence of urine return may indicate misplacement into the vagina. Once the Foley catheter is advanced its entire length, inflate the balloon with sterile water, and pull the catheter back until resistance is met, indicating that the balloon is at the bladder neck. If using a straight catheter, remove the catheter after the bladder is emptied. If the patient is an uncircumcised male, be sure to replace the foreskin to its original position. Secure the catheter by taping it to the child's leg.

COMPLICATIONS

If continued resistance is met while attempting catheterization, stop. Potential complications of catheterization include localized trauma or creation of a false passage, with future stricture formation.[3-8] An exceedingly rare complication is bladder perforation. Introduction of bacteria with resultant infection may occur following catheterization. Another rare but possible complication is knotting of the catheter while in the bladder. Finally, some patients may experience urinary retention on removal of the catheter, especially after prolonged catheter placement.

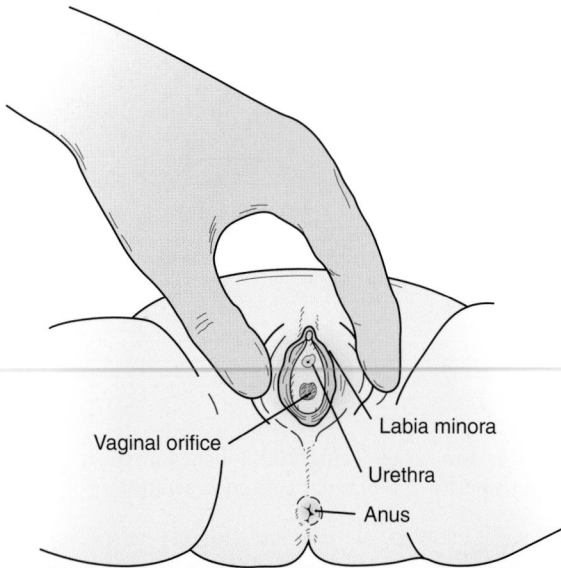

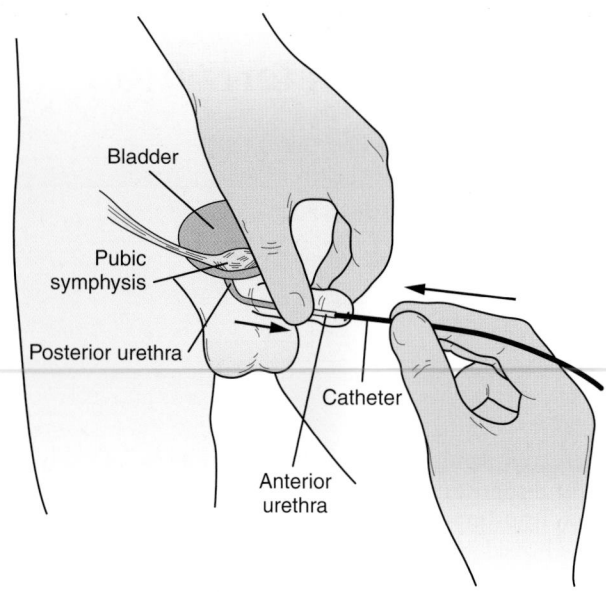

Figure 200-2   Transurethral bladder catheterization; position in the male. (From Dieckmann RA, Fiser DH, Selbst SM [eds]: Illustrated Textbook of Pediatric Emergency and Critical Care Procedures. St Louis, Mosby, 1997, p 415.)

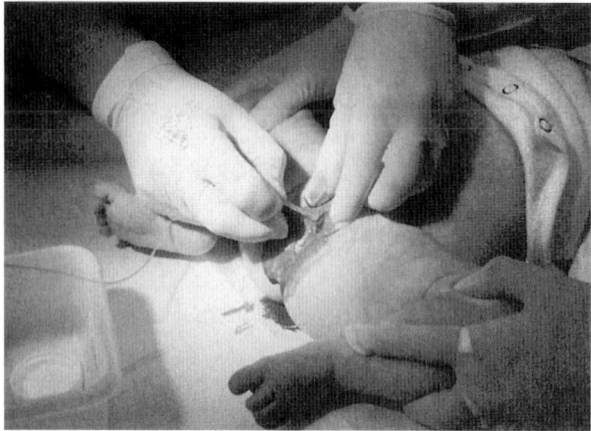

Figure 200-1   Transurethral bladder catheterization; position in the female. (From Dieckmann RA, Fiser DH, Selbst SM [eds]: Illustrated Textbook of Pediatric Emergency and Critical Care Procedures. St Louis, Mosby, 1997, p 415.)

Table 200-2   Catheterization Supplies
Antiseptic solution (iodine, povidone-iodine [Betadine])
Sterile drapes
Sterile gloves
Lubricant
Catheter
Syringe
Sterile water
Collection device
2% Lidocaine hydrochloride jelly (optional)

Table 200-1 Catheter Sizes	
Age	Size (French)
Newborn	8
Young child	10
Adolescent	12
Adult	16

SUGGESTED READING

Boenning DA, Henretig FM: Bladder catheterization. In Henretig F, King C (eds): Textbook of Pediatric Emergency Procedures. Baltimore, Williams & Wilkins, 1997, pp 991-998.

Carlson DW, Digiulio GA, Gewitz MH, et al: Catheterization of the bladder. In Fleisher GR, Ludwig S (eds): Textbook of Pediatric Emergency Medicine. Philadelphia, Lippincott Williams & Wilkins, 2000, p 1857.

REFERENCES

1. Gerard LL, Cooper CS, Duethman KS, et al: Effectiveness of lidocaine lubricant for discomfort during pediatric urethral catheterization. J Urol 2003;170:564-567.
2. Tanabe P, Steinmann R, Anderson J, et al: Factors affecting pain scores during female urethral catheterization. Acad Emerg Med 2004;11:699-702.
3. Basha M, Subhani M, Mersal A, et al: Urinary bladder perforation in a premature infant with Down syndrome. Pediatr Nephrol 2003;18:1189-1190.
4. Campbell JB, Moore KN, Voaklander DC, et al: Complications associated with clean intermittent catheterization in children with spina bifida. J Urol 2004;171:2420-2422.
5. Lindehall B, Abrahamsson K, Hjalmas K, et al: Complications of clean intermittent catheterization in boys and young males with neurogenic bladder dysfunction. J Urol 2004;172:1686-1688.
6. Matlow AG, Wray RD, Cox PN: Nosocomial urinary tract infections in children in a pediatric intensive care unit: A follow-up after 10 years. Pediatr Crit Care Med 2003;4:74-77.
7. Peniakov M, Antonelli J, Naor O, et al: Reduction in contamination of urine samples obtained by in-out catheterization by culturing the later urine stream. Pediatr Emerg Care 2004;20:418-419.
8. Turner TWS: Intravesical catheter knotting: An uncommon complication of urinary catheterization. Pediatr Emerg Care 2004;20:115-117.

Arterial Blood Gas

Esther Maria Sampayo and Mirna M. Farah

Arterial puncture or arterial blood gas sampling is a necessary procedure in the evaluation of any critically ill patient, especially those with significant respiratory distress or compromise. The ability to measure (and interpret) pH, P_{CO_2}, and P_{O_2} in these patients is an essential skill for the pediatric hospitalist. Although the procedure itself is similar to venipuncture or phlebotomy, there are significant potential complications that all people who perform the procedure must be aware of.

INDICATIONS

Arterial puncture is performed for limited sampling and is a routine procedure in the management of critically ill and injured children.[1] Arterial blood gas sampling provides information about lung ventilation through the interpretation of P_{CO_2} and information about tissue oxygenation through the interpretation of P_{O_2} for patients with respiratory distress or compromise. Acid-base problems are associated with a number of diseases, such as diabetic ketoacidosis, shock, severe dehydration, metabolic diseases, and certain toxic ingestions. These conditions are often diagnosed by, or treatment decisions are based on, the interpretation of arterial pH, P_{CO_2}, and bicarbonate (HCO_3) levels.

CONTRAINDICATIONS

Collateral circulation of the hand must be assessed when attempting radial artery puncture or catheterization. The Allen test is a simple procedure that has demonstrated consistent and valid results in the assessment of collateral blood flow to the hand.[2,3] It is performed by placing pressure to occlude the radial and ulnar arteries simultaneously for 20 seconds at the wrist. During that time, the patient's hand is elevated above the level of the heart while making a tight fist. The clenched fist is released, and one observes the hand become pale from decreased circulation. After the hand blanches white, one releases pressure over the ulnar artery while retaining pressure over the radial artery. If the patient has adequate collateral circulation, the hand should flush or become pink again as a sign of restored circulation within 5 to 7 seconds. Arterial puncture should not be attempted at that site if return of perfusion takes longer, indicating inadequate collateral circulation. In a young, difficult, or unconscious patient, a modified Allen test can be performed (Fig. 201-1).

Extra precautions should be taken when performing arterial blood sampling on patients receiving anticoagulants or those with bleeding disorders. Arterial access should be avoided when the patient has an infection or burn of the overlying skin puncture site.

EQUIPMENT

Although prepackaged arterial puncture kits are commercially available, only minimal equipment is needed:

- Butterfly or regular needle (25 gauge for newborns, 23 gauge for older infants or young children)
- Heparinized syringe that can be sealed air-tight
- Alcohol or other antiseptic solution to prepare the puncture site
- Gauze
- Gloves
- Arm board and tape
- Local or topical anesthetic (in an awake or conscious patient)

One should place an arterial catheter if it is determined that frequent arterial blood gas sampling will be required during the patient's care.[4]

ANATOMY

Arterial blood gas samples can be obtained from a number of sites, including the following:

- Radial artery at the wrist—the most popular site for arterial blood sampling because of its easy accessibility, superficial location, and availability of collateral circulation.
- Brachial artery at the antecubital fossa, right above the crease and just medial to the biceps tendon.
- Dorsalis pedis artery on the dorsal aspect of the midfoot between the extensor hallucis and extensor digitorum longus while the foot is in plantar flexion.
- Posterior tibial artery at the foot between the medial malleolus and the calcaneal tendon while the foot is in dorsiflexion.
- Femoral artery below the midpoint of the inguinal ligament. This site should be used only as a last resort in emergent situations because of the increased risk of side effects.

PROCEDURE

Hold the wrist in extension 30 to 45 degrees, or affix the extended joint to an arm board with tape. Do not overextend the wrist, because this may occlude the pulse. The point of maximal impulse of the radial artery can be palpated on

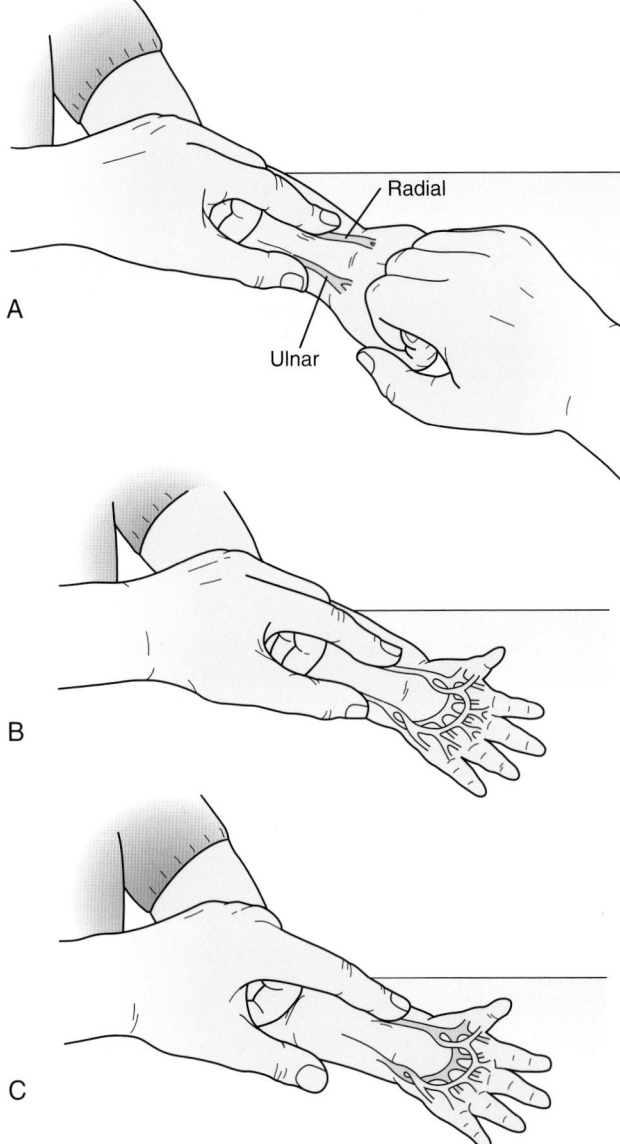

Table 201-1	Blood Gas Sampling Errors
Air or air bubbles in the syringe: equilibration between blood and air causes PO_2 to be altered, PCO_2 to decrease, and pH to increase	
Delay in icing or analyzing blood gas sample: allows for metabolism, causing a decrease in PO_2 and pH and an increase in PCO_2	
Venous or venous admixture sample: correlates with clinical presentation and oxygen saturation as measured by pulse oximetry (SpO_2)	
Alterations in temperature (< or > 37°C): Fever: PO_2 and PCO_2 are increased and pH decreased Hypothermia: PO_2 and PCO_2 are decreased and pH increased	
Excess heparin in syringe: dilutional effect causes alterations in PO_2, PCO_2, and pH	
Leukocytosis and thrombocytosis may elevate PCO_2 and lower pH	

Figure 201-1 Modified Allen test. A, Close the child's hand with firm pressure while simultaneously occluding the ipsilateral radial and ulnar arteries with the index finger and thumb of the opposite hand. B, After a few seconds to allow an adequate reduction of blood volume in the hand, release the hand while maintaining point pressure on the radial and ulnar arteries. When this maneuver is performed properly, this hand should appear paler than the other one. C, Release the pressure applied to the ulnar artery while maintaining point pressure on the radial artery. Reperfusion of the entire hand should occur within a few seconds if sufficient collateral circulation is present. (From Dieckmann RA, Fiser DH, Selbst SM [eds]: Illustrated Textbook of Pediatric Emergency and Critical Care Procedures. St Louis, Mosby, 1997, p 166.)

the vessel. Hold the 23- to 25-gauge butterfly needle or prepackaged heparinized syringe with the dominant hand like a pencil or a dart, with the bevel of the needle upward. Holding the needle at about a 30- to 45-degree angle, puncture the skin just distal to where the index finger is palpating the radial pulsation, aiming away from the hand. Slowly advance the needle until there is a pulsating flash of blood in the hub of the needle, indicating arterial rather than venous access. Hold the needle and syringe in that position, allowing the syringe to fill with blood to the amount desired. If no blood return occurs before meeting bony resistance, the needle should be slowly withdrawn in order to reenter the arterial lumen. When finished, remove the needle and immediately apply firm pressure at the puncture site for at least 5 minutes. Place an alcohol gauze over the needle, and expel any air bubbles in the upright syringe by tapping the bubbles to the top. Seal the syringe with the cap provided. Deposit the syringe in a bag of ice, and send it to the laboratory immediately.

COMPLICATIONS

The most significant potential complication of arterial puncture is permanent damage to the artery that interferes with the arterial supply to the distal aspect of the extremity. This is especially serious in patients who have absent or reduced collateral circulation. Also, this is more commonly seen as a result of catheter placement or repetitive punctures. Hematoma formation can also be quite significant after arterial puncture and can be reduced with the proper application of direct pressure. To reduce infection, one should always employ sterile technique and avoid using sites with overlying cellulitis.

There are also a number of potential errors that can occur owing to the transport or timing of the blood gas sample or to the patient's underlying condition (Table 201-1).[5]

the palmar aspect of the wrist at the second transverse wrist crease proximal to the hand. Perform the Allen test for collateral flow. Prepare the area in a sterile fashion. Slightly anchor the artery with the index and middle fingers of the nondominant hand to prevent rolling. Local anesthesia is optional and can be achieved with topical cream anesthetic or local infiltration of 1% lidocaine, avoiding infusion into

REFERENCES

1. Saladino R, Bachman D, Fleisher G: Arterial access in the pediatric emergency department. Ann Emerg Med 1990;19:382-385.
2. Hosokawa K, Hata Y, Yano K, et al: Results of Allen test on 2940 arms. Ann Plast Surg 1990;24:149-151.
3. Cable DG, Mullany CJ, Schaff HV: The Allen test. Ann Thoracic Surg 1999;67:876-877.
4. Henretig FM, King C: Arterial puncture and catheterization. In Henretig FM, King C (eds): Textbook of Pediatric Emergency Procedures. Baltimore, Williams & Wilkins, 1997, pp 783-795.
5. Bageant RA: Variations in arterial blood gas measurements due to sampling techniques. Respir Care 1975;20:565.

CHAPTER 202

Peripheral Intravenous Access

Philip R. Spandorfer

Of all the procedures that a pediatric hospitalist performs, placement of an intravenous (IV) catheter is among the most common and the most difficult.

INDICATIONS

Peripheral IV access is obtained to administer medications, fluids, or blood products intravenously. It may also be used for frequent phlebotomy draws.

CONTRAINDICATIONS

The contraindications of IV access are related primarily to location. Specifically, placement of an IV line should be avoided in a fractured or burned extremity (unless a Bier block will be performed for fracture reduction). Dermatologic conditions that preclude proper securing of the IV line (e.g., epidermolysis bullosa syndrome) are relative contraindications. Additionally, if alternative treatment techniques are available, such as oral rehydration therapy for a patient who is dehydrated, the decision to place an IV line should be reconsidered.

EQUIPMENT

Table 202-1 lists the equipment needed to place an IV line. "Over-the-needle" catheters come in different models (e.g., intracaths, angiocaths) and are sized by gauge. Typically, 22- or 24-gauge catheters are used for infants; 20 or 22 gauge in children; and 18, 20, or 22 gauge in adolescents and adults. Larger-bore catheters (e.g., 14 or 16 gauge) are typically reserved for resuscitation. It should also be noted that many of the newer catheters have self-retracting needles to avoid accidental needlesticks.

PROCEDURE

Setup and Preparation

Although children typically rate the pain of IV line insertion as only a 3 on a 10-point scale, the procedure can cause apprehension, making pain management and anxiety reduction crucial. If family members choose to stay for the procedure, they should be given specific instructions, such as to sing the child's favorite song, stroke the child's forehead, tell the child that it will be all right, and the like. Involvement of a child life specialist is helpful to provide distraction during the procedure. An additional person may be needed to help restrain the patient.

Assess several potential sites for the IV catheter. Attempt access distally first, in case additional attempts are required in the proximal extremities. If the upper extremity is being used, the nondominant hand is preferable. Figure 202-1 shows common sites for placement of an IV catheter in the upper extremity. In infants, the lower extremities (i.e., feet) or the scalp can be considered as sites for IV placement.

Technique

Universal precautions should be used during the entire procedure. Connect the needleless access port to the extension tubing and flush saline through both the port and the tubing (unless phlebotomy is to be performed at the time of IV line insertion). Remove any topical anesthetic (if applicable), and apply a tourniquet proximal to the desired location. Clean the site with appropriate skin cleanser, and spray topical anesthetic (if applicable). Using the catheter with the bevel side up, enter the skin at approximately a 30- to 45-degree angle, just distal to the desired entry point into the vein (Fig. 202-2). Because the needle enters the vein before the catheter does (Fig. 202-3), continue to insert the needle and catheter just slightly once there is a flash of blood in the hub of the catheter to ensure that the catheter is in the vein (Fig. 202-4). Slide the catheter over the needle into the vessel (Fig. 202-5). Apply pressure proximal to the IV catheter to prevent blood from flowing out of it. Remove the needle, leaving the catheter in place, by pressing the button to autoretract the needle or simply by removing it (depending on the type used). Connect the extension tubing and needleless access port to the IV line. Apply tape or a transparent occlusive dressing on top to hold the catheter in place. Remove the tourniquet, and flush the catheter (or obtain a phlebotomy specimen). If the catheter does not flush easily, it may not be placed intravenously. If there is swelling at the site, the IV line should be removed. Secure the catheter to the patient, applying a board and cover as needed.

Follow-up

The IV line should be checked by medical personnel to ensure the adequacy of the site (no signs of infection, no erythema) and that it is infusing without any problem (e.g., pain, high pressure on the pump).

COMPLICATIONS

The most common complication is IV infiltrate when the catheter becomes dislodged and a substance is infused into the subcutaneous tissues. The substance that is extravasated

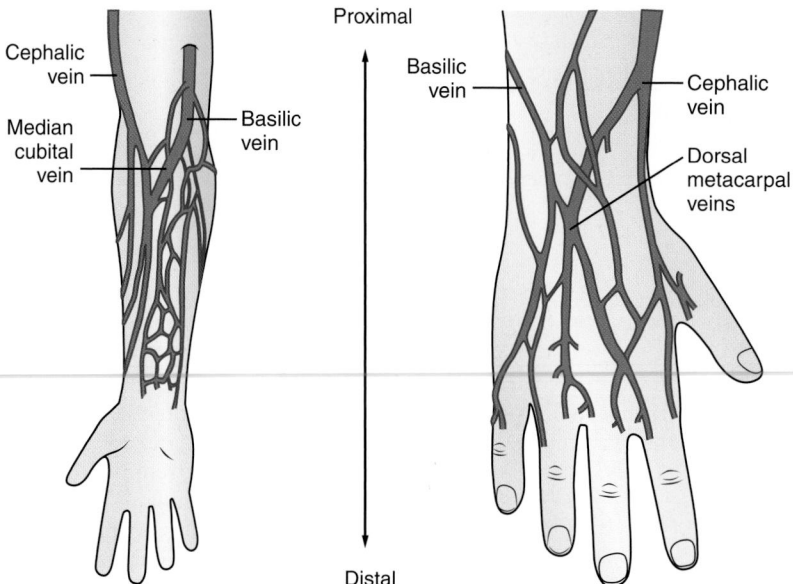

Figure 202-1   Venous anatomy of the upper extremity.

Table 202-1   Equipment Needed for Placement of an Intravenous Line
Catheter
Skin cleanser (e.g., 70% ethyl alcohol, povidone-iodine)
Tourniquet (or rubber bands if placing a scalp IV line)
T-connectors and needleless port
Normal saline flush
Tape, transparent dressing, arm board, and other devices to secure the catheter in place
3- or 5-mL syringes if blood is being drawn simultaneously
Gauze
Gloves
Topical anesthetic—cream or spray (optional)

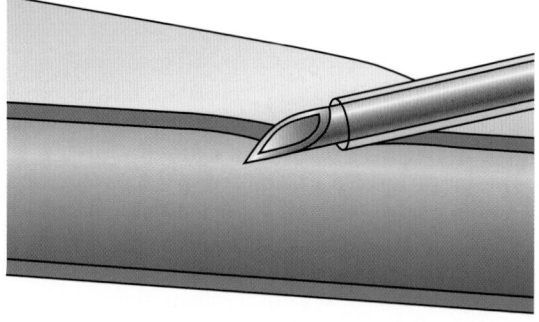

Figure 202-3   The needle punctures the vein before the catheter does.

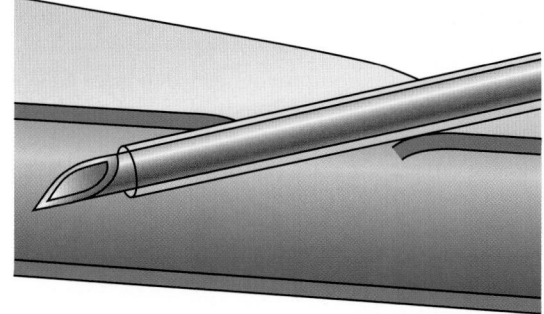

Figure 202-4   Advance the needle and catheter into the vein.

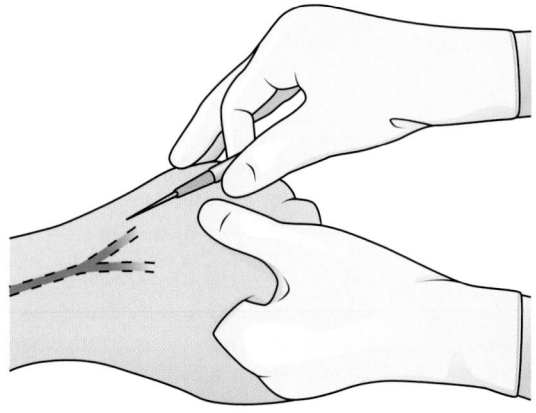

Figure 202-2   Insertion of the IV catheter into the skin.

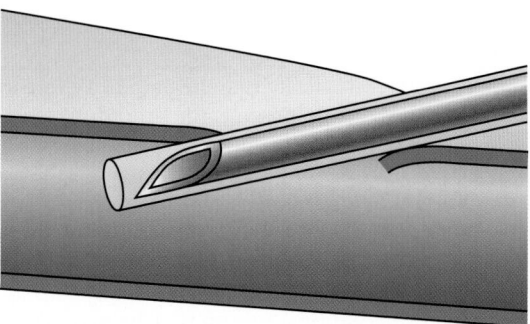

Figure 202-5   Withdraw the needle, leaving the catheter in place intravenously.

determines whether there will be local injury. Infection (phlebitis) can occur on occasion and is associated with the duration of placement. Thromboembolism is also possible if a clot forms on the catheter; catheter fragment embolism and air embolism are other possible complications. Severe complications are uncommon.

SUGGESTED READING

Bhende MS: Venipuncture and peripheral venous access. In Henretig F, King C (eds): Textbook of Pediatric Emergency Procedures. Baltimore, Williams & Wilkins, 1997, pp 797–810.

CHAPTER 203

Intraosseous Catheters

Eron Y. Friedlaender

Intraosseous (IO) cannulation is an effective and reliable means of rapidly accessing the central circulation for the administration of fluids, medications, and blood products. The noncollapsible intramedullary venous sinuses of the long bones offer great stability during states of shock and arrest characterized by profound vasoconstriction and circulatory failure, as seen with severe trauma, extensive burns, profound dehydration, and status epilepticus.[1] Highly vascular marrow spaces are capable of absorbing a wide range and a large volume of infused materials, with timely distribution to the rest of the body.[2] The procedure requires minimal training and can be safely performed by prehospital providers as well as by staff skilled in pediatric hospitalist, emergency, and critical care medicine.[1,3-6]

INDICATIONS

IO access is appropriate for young pediatric patients requiring resuscitative efforts in whom placement of a peripheral intravenous cannula is unsuccessful after two to three attempts or 90 seconds.[1,7] For patients in cardiac arrest, IO placement should be performed before all other means of securing access; it is generally successful in 30 to 60 seconds.[1,3,6-8] IO catheters have traditionally been recommended for children younger than 6 years; however, the procedure can be attempted in any person in whom peripheral access is unsuccessful.[9,10] Importantly, IO use must be limited to immediate resuscitative efforts and discontinued once peripheral or central access has been secured, to avoid complications. In addition, IO infusion rates under pressure are no greater than 11 to 29 mL/minute,[11] making this an impractical method for continuous and rapid administration of the high volume of fluids frequently required in patients in extremis.

IO lines can be used to deliver any medication, fluid, or blood product prepared for intravenous administration. There is a strong evidence base supporting IO use for anesthetic induction with atropine and neuromuscular blocking agents, as well as for resuscitative agents such as catecholamines (bolus preparations and continuous infusions), lidocaine, calcium, and sodium bicarbonate.[12-15] Additional reports document the safe IO administration of antibiotics, heparin, digitalis, and phenytoin.[1] In general, the onset of action and drug levels in the central circulation following IO delivery are comparable to those achieved with intravenous administration.[1,16] Boluses of crystalloids, colloids, blood products, and viscous medications must be delivered under pressure, either manually with a large-caliber syringe or with the assistance of a pressure bag, to overcome the resistance of the emissary veins running through the bony cortex, which are responsible for transporting materials from the intramedullary space to the central circulation.[1]

CONTRAINDICATIONS

Few contraindications to the use of IO catheters exist. Absolute contraindications include a recent fracture in the bone to be used for the procedure, osteogenesis imperfecta, and osteoporosis.[17] In addition, cellulitis and infected burns at a potential site of IO insertion are considered relative contraindications to the procedure.

EQUIPMENT

Several catheters can be used to establish IO access: a Jamshidi bone aspiration-infusion needle, a Cook IO infusion needle, or a wide-gauge spinal needle with an internal stylet. All function effectively, but the literature suggests that the Jamshidi needle may be the easiest to place.[17,18] Table 203-1 lists the other equipment needed for IO placement.

ANATOMY

IO needles can be placed into any intramedullary space, but the distal lower extremities are preferred, given their large marrow cavities, distance from the airway and site of potential chest compressions, and low potential for injury to surrounding tissues.[17] Recent evidence suggests that IO infusion may be successful in bones without medullary cavities as well, including the calcaneus and radial styloid.[19] The proximal tibia, just inferior to the tibial plateau, has been identified as the most appropriate initial site for placement. If this is not possible, the distal femur (1 cm proximal to the femoral plateau) has been recommended as an insertion site in infants; the distal tibia (proximal to the medial malleolus) can be used in older children.[17]

PROCEDURE

Preparation

Place the patient in the supine position, and identify an accessible lower extremity site for placement. Because the most common location for insertion is the proximal tibia, the following discussion relates to placement at this site. Prop the knee over a rolled towel or blanket at 30 degrees of flexion, allowing the patient's heel to rest on the stretcher.

Palpate along the anteromedial surface of the bone, 1 to 3 cm (or approximately 1 finger breadth) below the tibial tubercle, to find a smooth, flat surface for needle placement.

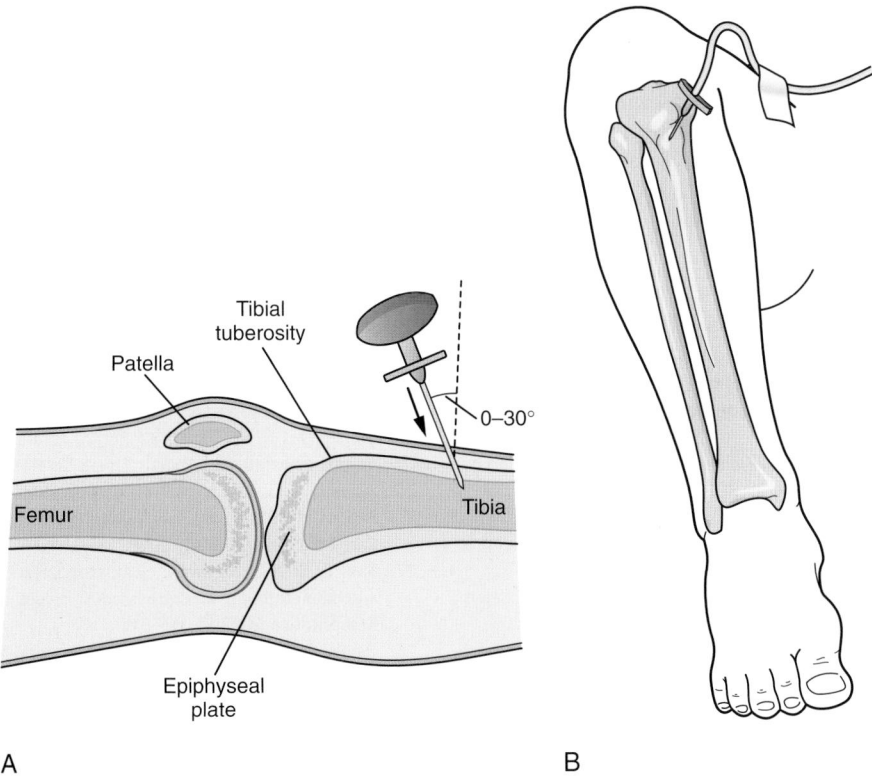

Figure 203-1 Intraosseous needle placement in the proximal tibia.

Table 203-1 **Equipment Needed for Intraosseous Catheter Placement**

Antiseptic solution (e.g., povidone-iodine [Betadine])
3- or 5-mL syringe
Saline flush
1% lidocaine for topical anesthesia (conscious or awake patients)

Using sterile technique, clean and drape the area. In conscious or awake patients, infiltrate the skin and underlying periosteum with local anesthetic.

Technique[19-24]

Firmly grasp the patient's lower extremity over the distal anterior thigh with one hand, and introduce the IO needle with the other hand, directing the bevel distally at a 90-degree angle through the skin. The operator should avoid placing his or her fingers behind the site of insertion, to prevent inadvertent puncture should the needle pass through the bone and posterior soft tissues. Hold the hub of the IO catheter in the palm of the hand, and grasp the IO needle close to the tip with the thumb and index finger. Use continuous rotary motion with steady, firm downward pressure at a 45- to 60-degree angle away from the growth plate to enter the cortex (Fig. 203-1). Successful penetration of the marrow space occurs with a significant drop in resistance.

To confirm placement, remove the stylet and attempt to aspirate bone marrow contents with a 3- or 5-mL syringe. If this is unsuccessful, test for correct positioning with an infusion of saline through the needle; there should be no evidence of extravasation into the surrounding subcutaneous tissues. Extravasation results in an increased circumference of the extremity proximate to the infusion site, an increased resistance to product infusion through the needle, or tense soft tissues in the area surrounding the needle. In addition, a correctly placed IO needle should remain upright without support. Once appropriate placement of the IO needle has been demonstrated, secure it in place, taking care to facilitate direct visualization of the insertion site to monitor for dislodgment, subcutaneous infiltration, and local skin reactions. Connect the IO needle to a syringe or to intravenous tubing, and begin use. Follow all medication infusions with a saline flush.

Blood aspirated from the IO needle can be used for all blood gas analyses, blood chemistries, type and crossmatching of blood products, and cultures; it does not, however, reflect an accurate peripheral complete blood count and differential.

COMPLICATIONS

There are relatively low complication rates with IO catheter use. Perhaps most significant is through-and-through penetration of the bone or failure to perform the procedure satisfactorily.[25,26] Less than 1% of patients experience a true complication from successful IO catheter placement. Infection has been associated with the procedure, including osteomyelitis, furunculosis, osteochrondritis, septicemia, bacteremia, cellulitis, and subcutaneous abscess.[1,7,27] Additional complications include subcutaneous or periosteal infiltration, pressure necrosis of the skin surrounding the needle insertion site, physeal plate injury, fracture, local hematoma formation, arterial thrombosis, and compartment syndrome.[1,7,25,26,28-32] Investigators have also demonstrated evidence of universal bone marrow and fat emboli in patients after IO catheter placement; however, this has had no clinical significance.[33] IO catheter use has minimal effects on the long-term growth and health of the bone and bone marrow.[34-37]

REFERENCES

1. Pediatric Advanced Life Support. American Heart Association, 1997.
2. Cunningham F, Spivey W: Intraosseous infusion. In Roberts J, Hedges J (eds): Clinical Procedures in Emergency Medicine, 3rd ed. Philadelphia, WB Saunders, 1998.
3. Seigler R, Tecklenburg F, Shealy R: Prehospital intraosseous infusion by emergency medical services personnel: A prospective study. Pediatrics 1989;84:173-177.
4. Miner W, Corneli H, Bolte R, et al: Prehospital use of intraosseous infusion by paramedics. Pediatr Emerg Care 1989;5:5-7.
5. Fuchs S, LaCovey D, Paris P, et al: A prehospital model of intraosseous infusion. Ann Emerg Med 1991;20:371-374.
6. Smith R, Keseg D, Manley L, et al: Intraosseous infusions by prehospital personnel in critically ill pediatric patients. Ann Emerg Med 1988;17:491-495.
7. Advanced Trauma Life Support for Doctors, 6th ed. Chicago, American College of Surgeons, 1999.
8. Glaeser P, Losek J, Nelson D, et al: Pediatric intraosseous infusions: Impact on vascular access time. Am J Emerg Med 1988;6:330-332.
9. Chadwick V, Arrowsmith J: Recent advances in pediatric resuscitation. Pediatr Anesth 2004;14:417-420.
10. American Heart Association, International Liaison Committee on Resuscitation: Guidelines 2000 for cardiopulmonary resuscitation and emergency cardiovascular care. Part 9. Pediatric basic life support. Part 10. Pediatric advanced life support. Circulation 2000;102(Suppl I):253-342.
11. Hodge D 3rd, Delgado-Paredes C, Fleisher G: Intraosseous infusion flow rates in hypovolemic "pediatric" dogs. Ann Emerg Med 1987;16:305-307.
12. Berg R: Emergency infusion of catechoalmines into bone marrow. Am J Dis Child 1984;138:810-811.
13. Tobias J, Nichols D: Intraosseous succinylcholine for orotracheal intubation. Pediatr Emerg Care 1990;6:108-109.
14. Sacchetti A, Linkenheimer R, Lieberman M, et al: Intraosseous drug administration: Successful resuscitation from asystole. Pediatr Emerg Care 1989;5:97-98.
15. Katan B, Olshaker J, Dickerson S: Intraosseous infusion of muscle relaxants. Am J Emerg Med 1988;6:353-354.
16. Cameron J, Fontanarosa P, Passalaqua A: A comparative study of peripheral to central circulation delivery times between intraosseous and intravenous injection using a radionuclide technique in normovolemic and hypovolemic canines. J Emerg Med 1989;7:123-127.
17. Halm B, Yamamoto L: Comparing ease of intraosseous needle placement: Jamshidi versus Cook. Am J Emerg Med 1998;16:420-421.
18. Glaeser P, Losek J: Intraosseous needles: New and improved. Pediatr Emerg Care 1988;4:135-136.
19. McCarthy G, O'Donnell C, O'Brien M: Successful intraosseous infusion in the critically ill patient does not require a medullary cavity. Resuscitation 2002;56:183-186.
20. Hodge D: Intraosseous infusion. In Henretig F, King C (eds): Textbook of Pediatric Emergency Procedures. Baltimore, Williams & Wilkins, 1997.
21. Hodge D III: Intraosseous infusions: A review. Pediatr Emerg Care 1985;1:215-218.
22. Fiser D: Intraosseous infusion. N Engl J Med 1990;322:1579-1581.
23. Stovroff M, Teague W: Intravenous access in infants and children. Pediatr Clin North Am 1998;45:1373-1393.
24. Spivey W: Intraosseous infusions. J Pediatr 1987;111:639-643.
25. Christensen D, Vernon D, Banner W, et al: Skin necrosis complicating intraosseous infusion. Pediatr Emerg Care 1991;7:289-290.
26. LaSpada J, Kissoon N, Melker R, et al: Extravasation rates and complications of intraosseous needles during gravity and pressure infusion. Crit Care Med 1995;23:2023-2028.
27. Stoll E, Golej J, Burda M, et al: Osteomyelitis at the injection site of adrenalin through an intraosseous needle in a 3-month-old infant. Resuscitation 2002;53:315-318.
28. Galpin R, Kronick J, Willis R, et al: Bilateral lower extremity compartment syndromes secondary to intraosseous fluid resuscitation. J Pediatr Orthop 1991;11:773-776.
29. Vidal R, Kissoon N, Gayle M: Compartment syndrome following intraosseous infusion. Pediatrics 1993;91:1201-1202.
30. Moscati R, Moore G: Compartment syndrome with resultant amputation following intraosseous infusion. Am J Emerg Med 1990;8:470-471.
31. Bowley D, Loveland J, Pitcher G: Tibial fracture as a complication of intraosseous infusion during pediatric resuscitation. J Trauma 2003;55:786-787.
32. Launay F, Paut O, Katchburian M, et al: Leg amputation after intraosseous infusion in a 7-month-old infant: A case report. J Trauma 2003;55:788-790.
33. Orlowski J, Julius C, Petras R, et al: The safety of intraosseous infusions: Risks of fat and bone marrow emboli to the lungs. Ann Emerg Med 1989;18:1062-1067.
34. Pollack C, Pender E, Woodall B, et al: Long-term local effects of intraosseous infusion on tibial bone marrow in the weanling pig model. Am J Emerg Med 1992;10:27-31.
35. Fiser R, Walker W, Seibert J, et al: Tibial length following intraosseous infusion: A prospective, radiographic analysis. Pediatr Emerg Care 1997;13:186-188.
36. Brickman K, Rega P, Schoolfield L, et al: Investigation of bone developmental and histopathologic changes from intraosseous infusion. Ann Emerg Med 1996;28:430-435.
37. Claudet I, Baunin C, Laporte-Turpin E, et al: Long-term effects on tibial growth after intraosseous infusion: A prospective, radiographic analysis. Pediatr Emerg Care 2003;19:397-401.

CHAPTER 204

Central Venous Access

Suzanne Beno and Frances Nadel

Central venous cannulation (CVC) involves percutaneously placing a vascular catheter into a high-flow vein located in either the thorax or the abdomen. It is an essential skill for the resuscitation and stabilization of critically ill children. The main sites of access include the femoral, internal and external jugular, and subclavian veins.

INDICATIONS

There is risk with any procedure, and the operator must be knowledgeable about the indications for CVC. CVC should be considered for patients needing the following:

- Vascular access for circulatory failure if peripheral access is unobtainable.
- Infusion of vasoactive medications, blood products, or large volumes of fluid when rapid distribution and onset of therapy are vital.
- Insertion of devices such as transvenous pacemakers or Swan-Ganz catheters.
- Ongoing measurements of venous pressures or mixed venous blood gases.
- Delivery of hypertonic fluids such as total parenteral nutrition and chemotherapy.
- Long-term vascular access for repeated medication administration or frequent blood sampling.

CONTRAINDICATIONS

CVC should not be attempted at sites with abnormal vasculature. Relative contraindications include a bleeding diathesis or hypercoagulable state, as well as overlying cellulitis, acute inflammation, or skin injury at the planned site of entry. Other contraindications specific to the different sites are discussed with each approach.

EQUIPMENT

Table 204-1 lists the equipment needed for central venous catheter placement. Virtually all hospitals use commercially available, prepackaged kits that contain most of the necessary equipment; however, they usually do not contain local anesthetic, antiseptic solution, or heparinized saline.

It is important to note that the equipment in each kit is size specific. If one has opened more than one kit of different sizes, it is extremely important to ensure that the equipment is not mixed up. For example, a guidewire from one kit may not be long enough to accommodate a catheter from another.

PROCEDURE

Four different catheters have been used for percutaneous CVC, each involving a slightly different technique. By far the most common is the Seldinger technique, which is based on passing a catheter over a guidewire; that is the technique discussed here.

It is important to recognize that different patients need varying amounts of sedation and analgesia for this procedure, based on their clinical condition (see Chapter 197). The success of the procedure can be greatly enhanced by immobilization and proper positioning, as well as ensuring that all necessary equipment is available and ready.

The first step, after the chosen site is sterilely prepared, draped, and anesthetized with local anesthetic, is to puncture the skin and blood vessel with a small-gauge needle attached to a syringe while applying gentle negative suction until there is free flow of blood. The syringe is then removed, the operator's thumb is placed over the hub, and the guidewire is threaded through the needle into the vein. The needle used for entry is removed, with the wire left in place. A small incision, using a number 11 scalpel, is usually made at the entry site to facilitate insertion of a larger catheter. The catheter of choice (Table 204-2) is then advanced over the guidewire into the desired vessel, and the wire is removed. It is vital to hold the end of the wire to prevent inadvertently losing it in the vessel. Different kits have different sizes of catheters, some of which require dilation of the vessel before insertion. When dilation is necessary, a dilator is inserted over the wire after the skin incision has been made. Once the dilator is removed, the catheter can be easily advanced over the wire into the vessel. The catheter is then sutured, and the site is dressed with a transparent occlusive dressing.[1]

SITE-SPECIFIC CONSIDERATIONS

Femoral Vein

The femoral vein is the most popular approach for pediatric central venous access (Fig. 204-1). Advantages include its distance from the head and chest, and thus minimal interference with the evaluation and treatment of critically ill children; the requirement of less technical expertise; and the exposed anatomy. Disadvantages include contamination risk, difficulty securing the line, and difficulty in obese patients. Relative contraindications include abnormal vascular anatomy; abdominal trauma, tumor, or ascites; femoral hernia; and future need for cardiac catheterization.

The entry point is identified 1 to 2 cm medial to the femoral artery and 1 to 2 cm below the inguinal ligament. If

Table 204-1   Equipment Needed for Central Venous Catheter Placement
Catheter
Flexible guidewire
Finder needle
Sterile gloves, gowns, masks, and drapes
Sterile gauze
Antiseptic solution
Syringes
Heparinized saline
Silk suture on straight needle, needle holder
Transparent dressing
Tissue dilator
Number 11 scalpel
Topical anesthetic

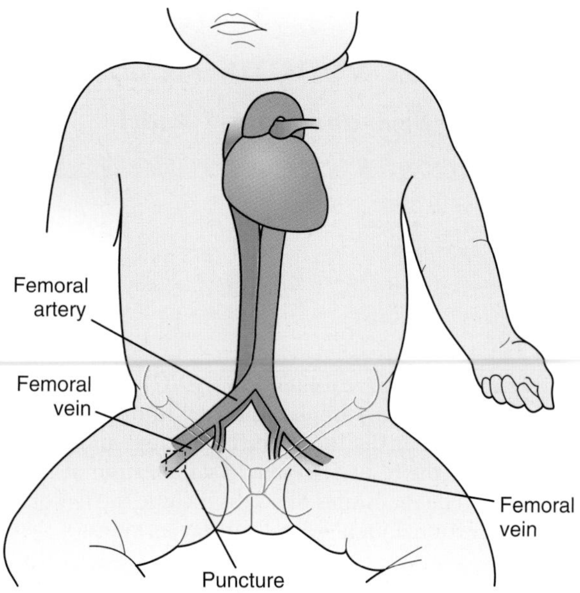

Figure 204-1   Femoral venous anatomy.

Table 204-2 Catheter Choice for Pediatric Patients						
	AVERAGE CATHETER DIAMETER (FRENCH) AND LENGTH (cm)					
Age	Femoral		Internal Jugular		Subclavian	
1 mo	3	15.7	3	6.0	3	5.5
3 mo	3	17.3	3	6.6	3	6.0
6 mo	3/4	19.1	3	7.3	3	6.6
9 mo	3/4	20.1	3	7.6	3	6.9
12 mo	3/4	21.1	3	8.0	3	7.3
18 mo	3/4	22.9	3	8.7	3	7.9
2 yr	3/4	24.2	3	9.2	3	8.3
4 yr	4	28.1	4	10.6	4	9.6
6 yr	4	31.4	4	11.8	4	10.7
8 yr	4/5	34.2	4/5	12.9	4/5	11.7
10 yr	4/5	36.8	4/5	13.8	4/5	12.5
12 yr	4/5	39.9	4/5	15.0	4/5	13.5
14 yr	5	44.0	5	16.5	5	14.9
16 yr	5	46.3	5	17.3	5	15.7

Adapted from Lavelle J, Costarino A Jr: Central venous access and central venous pressure monitoring. In Henretig FM, King C (eds): Textbook of Pediatric Emergency Procedures. Baltimore, Williams & Wilkins, 1997, p 261.

pulses are weak or absent, the site can be estimated to be halfway between the pubic symphysis and the anterior iliac spine, still 1 to 2 cm below the inguinal ligament. Optimal patient positioning requires abduction and external rotation of the hip, often facilitated by placing a towel beneath the ipsilateral buttock. Needle entry is performed at a 45-degree angle, and care is taken not to puncture the inguinal ligament and thus place the patient at risk for bowel perforation or development of a retroperitoneal hematoma.

Internal Jugular Vein

Internal jugular venous access is less common than the femoral approach but is considered the entry site of choice by many experienced physicians because of the inherent advantages of increased stability, patient comfort, and more accurate central venous pressure measurements. The complication rate is somewhat higher than with a femoral line and includes inadvertent laceration of the carotid artery, thoracic duct, or stellate ganglion and pneumothorax. Of the three approaches (median, anterior, lateral) used in cannulating the internal jugular vein, the median approach is the most popular. All methods require the patient's head to be turned 30 degrees away from the puncture site while in the Trendelenburg position. Landmarking for the median approach involves locating the midpoint between the sternal notch and the mastoid process at the apex of the triangle formed by both heads of the sternocleidomastoid muscle. The internal jugular vein is lateral to the carotid artery. The needle is inserted at a 30-degree angle and aimed toward the ipsilateral nipple.

External Jugular Vein

Although the external jugular vein can be readily identified most of the time, the chance of successful CVC is low; however, complications such as pneumothorax, carotid artery puncture and hematoma, and injury to the sympathetic chain are much less likely than with an internal jugular vein site. The patient should be in 15 to 30 degrees of Trendelenburg, with the head turned 45 degrees to the contralateral side. Needle entry occurs where the external jugular vein crosses over the sternocleidomastoid muscle.

Subclavian Vein

The subclavian vein is the least common site for percutaneous CVC in children. Identification of landmarks is difficult in children because of their small size and increased chest wall compliance. Complications such as pneumothorax and subclavian artery puncture are highest with this approach. The subclavian vein can be accessed from either a supraclavicular or infraclavicular site. The patient should be supine in 10 to 25 degrees of Trendelenburg. The entry site for the supraclavicular approach is one finger width lateral to the clavicular head of the sternocleidomastoid muscle superior to the clavicle. The needle direction should bisect the angle formed by the clavicle and the sternocleidomastoid, be aimed toward the contralateral nipple, and be advanced two to three times the width of the clavicle. The entry site for the infraclavicular approach is just lateral to the midclavicular line below the clavicle. The needle should be advanced 2 to 4 cm toward the sternal notch parallel to the chest wall.

COMPLICATIONS

In addition to the site-specific complications already addressed, general complications include thrombosis, infection (cellulitis, bacteremia), air embolus, vascular or cardiac perforation, and cardiac arrhythmia. Guidewires have been lost in the central circulation, requiring surgical removal. This can be prevented by always securing the proximal end of the wire. Sterile technique can minimize the risk of infection.

A new technique is now employed using a Doppler ultrasound probe to enhance successful cannulation and decrease complications.[3] The probe allows the identification and visualization of the major vessels involved, can be used under sterile conditions, and has been validated in both infants and children.[3]

REFERENCES

1. Lavelle J, Costarino A Jr: Central venous access and central venous pressure monitoring. In Henretig FM, King C (eds): Textbook of Pediatric Emergency Procedures. Baltimore, Williams & Wilkins, 1997, pp 251-278.
2. Andropoulos DB, Bent ST, Skjonsky B, Stayer SA: The optimal length of insertion of central venous catheters for pediatric patients. Anesth Analg 2001;93:883-886.
3. Asheim P, Mostad U, Aadahl P: Ultrasound-guided central venous cannulation in infants and children. Acta Anaesthesiol Scand 2002;46:390-392.

CHAPTER 205

Umbilical Artery and Vein Catheterization

Bryan Upham

Unique to the neonate, lifesaving central access can be achieved through catheterization of the umbilical vessels. Umbilical artery catheterization can routinely be performed in newborns up to 24 hours old and occasionally in those up to 1 week old. Umbilical vein catheterization is feasible up to 2 weeks of age.[1]

INDICATIONS

Indications for central access include volume expansion, blood transfusion, infusion of resuscitative medications, administration of hypertonic solutions, and frequent laboratory draws. Peripheral access should be attempted first but should not delay central access in a critically ill infant.

Peripheral or central arterial catheters are indicated in newborns with cardiopulmonary insufficiency requiring mechanical ventilation or invasive blood pressure monitoring. An umbilical artery catheter has the advantages of rapid insertion and the ability to deliver fluids, medications, and blood products.

CONTRAINDICATIONS

Overlying soft tissue infection (e.g., omphalitis) is a contraindication to placing an umbilical vessel catheter. One should avoid placement of an umbilical catheter when the possibility of necrotizing enterocolitis exists. Known thrombotic complications limit the appeal of umbilical artery catheterization, and placement is rarely indicated in neonates weighing more than 1000 g.[2] Finally, one must remember that these are central lines and are not placed for routine blood sampling or administration of fluids or medications.

EQUIPMENT

Nonsterile

Radiant warmer with light source
Cardiorespiratory monitor
Pulse oximeter
Measuring tape
Surgical mask with face shield, surgical cap
D5W, D10W, or normal saline infusion setup (with heparin 1 unit/mL, unless medications are incompatible with heparin)
Soft infant restraints
Adhesive tape

Sterile

Povidone-iodine solution
Sterile drapes, gauze, gloves, gown
Scalpel (number 11 or 15)

Curved hemostats (2)
Straight forceps
3-0 silk suture
Needle driver
Scissors
Umbilical tape
Umbilical catheters (3.5, 5, or 8 French with end hole)
Three-way stopcock
Curved, toothless forceps or pointed, solid metal dilator
10-mL syringe filled with sterile normal saline (with heparin 1 unit/mL if available)

PROCEDURE

Preparation

Arrange the materials and warmer before the patient's arrival, if feasible. Address any cardiorespiratory issues before the procedure. Determine the length of the catheter by measuring the shoulder to umbilicus length in centimeters (Fig. 205-1). Venous catheter diameters are either 5 or 8 French. Arterial catheters are 5 French for infants weighing more than 2 kg and 3.5 to 4 French for smaller infants.

Place the infant in a radiant warmer with the arms and legs restrained in the supine, frog-leg position (see Fig. 205-1). Attach cardiorespiratory, temperature, and oxygen saturation monitors, and don appropriate surgical wear. Attach the three-way stopcock to the umbilical catheter, and flush both ports and the catheter with sterile solution. Turn off the stopcock to all ports.

Scrub the infant's abdomen with povidone-iodine from the xiphoid process to the symphysis pubis, including the umbilical stump. Have an assistant hold the umbilical clamp or nonsterile distal umbilicus away from the patient and sterile field while prepping the area. Drape the umbilical region in a sterile manner, but leave the infant's face uncovered. Apply either umbilical tape with a loose overhand tie or a pursestring suture around the base of the umbilicus. Use forceps to grasp the full-thickness cord between 0.5 and 2 cm from its base. Cut the cord transversely at the top of the forceps using the scalpel (Fig. 205-2A). Replace the scalpel, and slowly release the forceps to watch for bleeding. Adjust the umbilical tape or pursestring suture if necessary. Use two hemostats to grasp and evert the edges of the umbilicus and expose the umbilical vessels (Fig. 205-2B).

Umbilical Vein Catheter Placement
Emergent

Prepare the cord as described, and identify the umbilical vein. Remove any visible clot. Gently insert a 5- or 8-French flushed catheter into the vein lumen until blood return is noted, but no more than 4 to 5 cm (see Fig. 205-2B). This allows blood draws and infusion of high-osmolar solutions

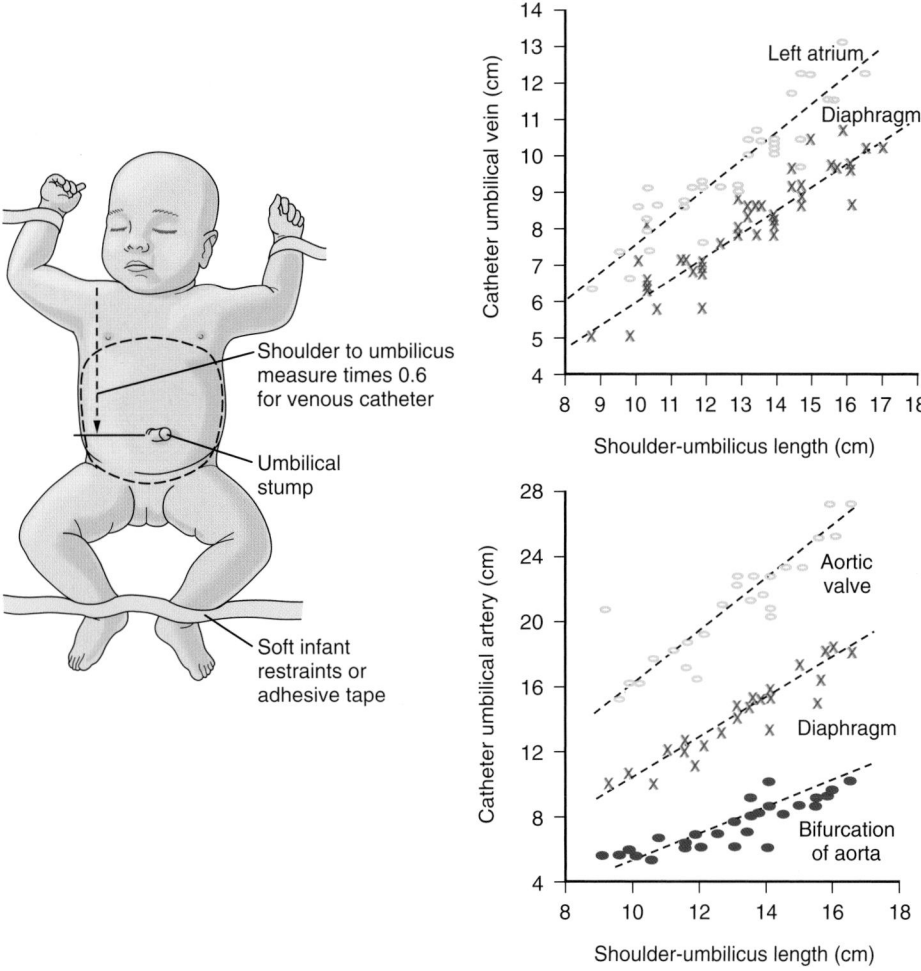

Figure 205-1 Infant placement and catheter lengths.

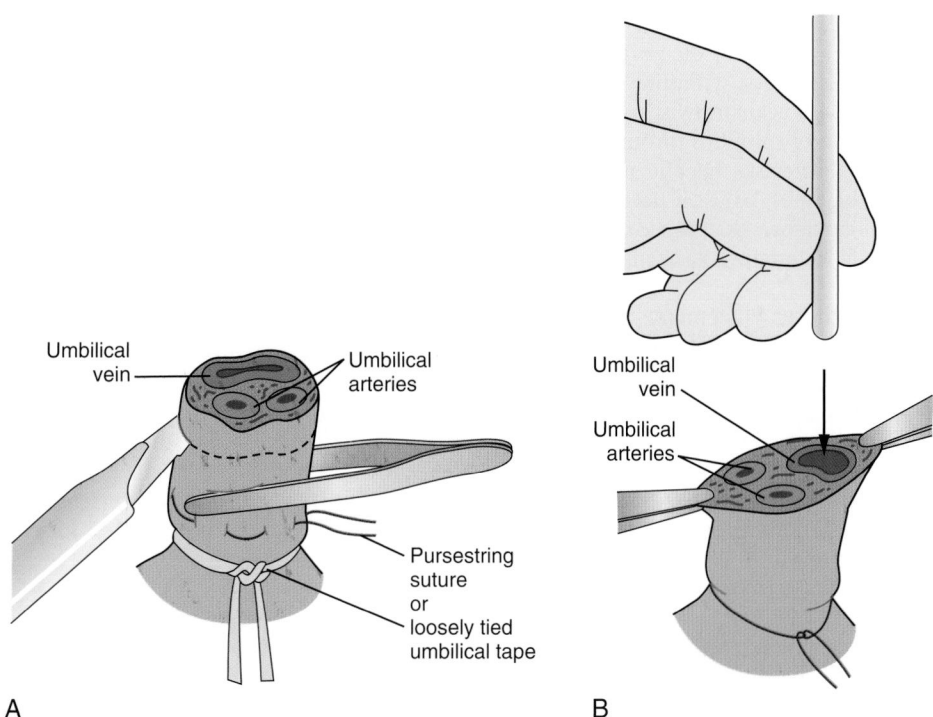

A

B

Figure 205-2 Preparing the umbilical cord. A, Cutting the cord. B, Exposing the vessels and inserting the umbilical vein catheter.

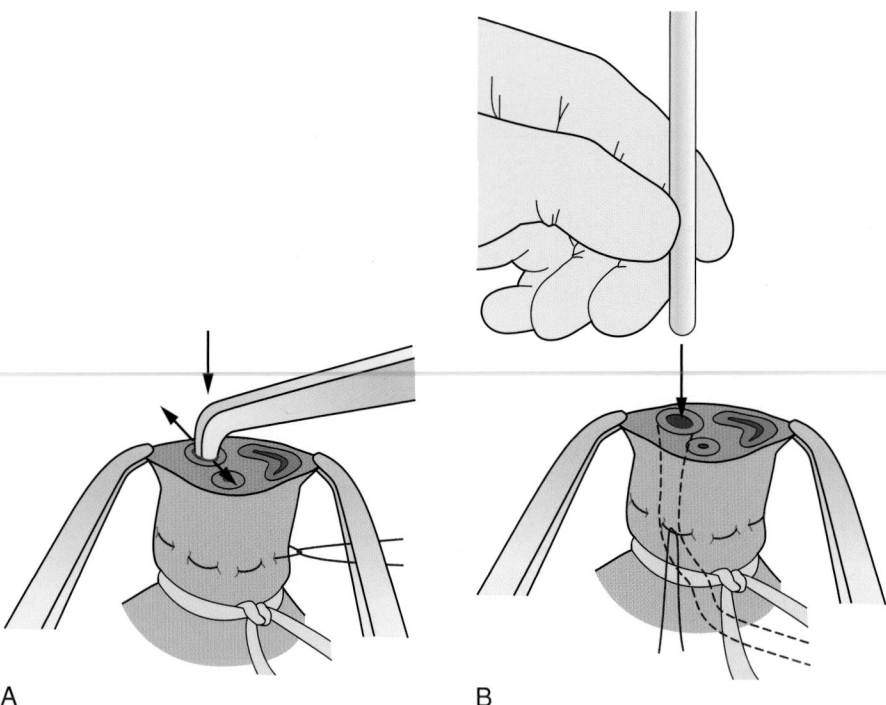

Figure 205-3   Umbilical artery catheter insertion. *A,* Artery dilation. *B,* Catheter insertion.

while minimizing the risk of hepatic injury. Remove the catheter once fluid resuscitation is achieved, and replace the umbilical clamp.

Nonemergent

Determine the appropriate catheter length (see Fig. 205-1). Ideal placement is above the diaphragm at the junction of the inferior vena cava and right atrium. Proceed as described earlier, but continue to advance the catheter to the desired length. If resistance is felt at 5 to 10 cm, the catheter may have passed into a branch of the portal vein and must be repositioned. If this occurs, withdraw the catheter to a depth of 1 to 2 cm and try again. A twisting motion can help avoid the liver. Infusion of solutions through a catheter suspected to be in the liver risks hepatic necrosis. Confirm placement with radiographs, adjust if necessary, and secure as detailed later. Remember that the catheter cannot be advanced once sterile technique is broken.

Umbilical Artery Catheter Placement

Ideal placement is above the diaphragm between the ductus arteriosus and the celiac root (thoracic spine level T6-T10). A recent meta-analysis advises against the use of low-placed umbilical artery catheters because of possible vascular complications.[3] If the catheter is initially placed too low, it can be withdrawn to the level between the inferior mesenteric artery and the aortic bifurcation (lumbar spine level L3-L4) and used temporarily.

Identify the umbilical artery as described earlier, and dilate the lumen gently by repeatedly inserting a closed, curved forceps and opening the tips in the lumen (Fig. 205-3A). The artery should be dilated to a depth of approximately 1 cm. Many catheter setups contain a pointed metal dilator that can be used for this purpose. Grasp the flushed

catheter 1 cm from the tip with the index finger and thumb or forceps. Gently introduce the tip into the lumen of the artery and apply countertraction to the cord in the cephalad direction so that the catheter is directed inferiorly along the natural course of the artery (Fig. 205-3B). Resistance may be felt at 1 to 2 cm as the artery courses inferiorly and at 5 to 6 cm at the junction with the internal iliac artery. A twisting motion can help overcome this resistance. If resistance is felt at 4 to 5 cm, strongly consider the creation of a false tract and try the other artery. Once the catheter has been advanced to the desired location, obtain radiographs to confirm its placement. If sterile technique is broken, the line cannot be advanced. If the line is too high, it can be withdrawn an appropriate amount. If it is too low, it can be withdrawn temporarily to the low-placed position.

Securing the Catheter

Secure the catheter with the ends of the previously tied pursestring suture or the ends of another suture placed at the skin margin of the umbilical stump. Be careful to avoid the umbilical vessels when suturing. Wrap each end of the suture in opposite directions one or two times around the catheter, and tie a square knot. For added security, repeat the knot 2 cm from the stump. Secure the catheter, and suture it to the body using a tape bridge (Fig. 205-4). Fluid should be run through the catheter continuously at a low rate to minimize the risk of thrombus formation and extend the life of the catheter.

COMPLICATIONS

Common complications include thrombosis (2% to 95%), bacterial colonization (14% to 60%), sepsis (3% to 5%), and peripheral vasospasm.[2,4-10] Thrombosis may

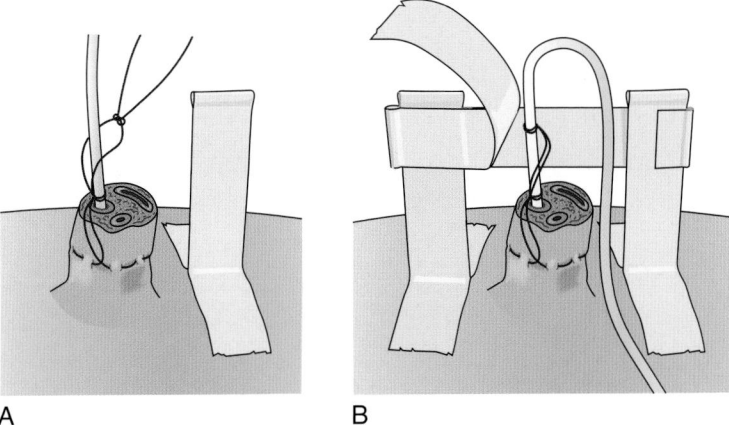

Figure 205-4 Securing the catheter. *A*, Suture anchor. *B*, Tape bridge.

present as limb ischemia, renal infarct, bowel ischemia, pulmonary embolus, or stroke and may result in septic emboli. Infusion of high-osmolar solutions into an improperly placed umbilical vein catheter in the liver can cause hepatic necrosis. Rare complications include pericardial, peritoneal, vessel, or organ perforation; aneurysm formation; air embolus; arrhythmias; significant blood loss; and portal hypertension.

Ischemia to the limbs or organs can result from improper catheter positioning. Lower extremity and buttocks ischemia can also be caused by vasospasm. If buttocks or lower extremity ischemia is suspected, apply warm compresses to the contralateral lower extremity; this results in reflex vasodilation of the ipsilateral extremity. If no improvement in limb color or pulse is seen within 15 minutes, remove the catheter.

Renal or bowel ischemia can result from improper placement of the catheter; this may respond to repositioning of the catheter. The risk of significant blood loss or air embolism is reduced by flushing all catheters before insertion, using a three-way stopcock, and taking care to secure the catheter with sutures and tape.

Cardiac arrhythmias should alert the practitioner to the possibility of inadvertent catheter placement in the right atrium. The catheter should be withdrawn immediately until the heart returns to its previous rhythm. Organ, vessel, pericardial, and peritoneal perforation are rare complications but require emergent surgical consultation.

REFERENCES

1. Lipton JD, Schafermeyer RW: Umbilical vessel catheterization. In Henretig FM, King C (eds): Textbook of Pediatric Emergency Procedures. Baltimore, Williams & Wilkins, 1997, pp 515-523.
2. Hodson WA, Truog WE: Principles of management of respiratory problems. In Avery GB, Fletcher MA, MacDonald MG (eds): Neonatology: Pathophysiology and Management of the Newborn, 5th ed. Philadelphia, Lippincott Williams & Wilkins, 1999, pp 535-537.
3. Barrington KJ: Umbilical artery catheters in the newborn: Effects of position of the catheter tip. Cochrane Database Syst Rev 2004;3.
4. Coleman MM, Spear ML, Finkelstein M, et al: Short-term use of umbilical artery catheters may not be associated with increased risk for thrombosis. Pediatrics 2004;113:770-774.
5. Boo N, Wong N, Zulkifli S, Lye M: Risk factors associated with umbilical vascular catheter-associated thrombosis in newborn infants. J Paediatr Child Health 1999;35:460-465.
6. Goetzman BW, Stadolink RC, Borgren HG: Thrombotic complications of umbilical arterial catheters: A clinical and radiographic study. Pediatrics 1975;56:374-379.
7. Neal WH, Reynolds JW, Jarvis CW: Umbilical artery catheterization: Demonstration of arterial thrombus by aortography. Pediatrics 1972;81: 814.
8. Wesstrom G, Finnstrom O, Stenport G: Umbilical artery catheterization in newborns: Thrombosis in relation to catheter type and position. Acta Paediatr Scand 1979;68:575-581.
9. Cronin W, Germanson TP, Donowitz LG: Intravascular catheter colonization and related bloodstream infection in critically ill neonates. Infect Control Hosp Epidemiol 1990;11:301-308.
10. Landers S, et al: Factors associated with umbilical catheter-related sepsis in neonates. Am J Dis Child 1991;145:675-680.

CHAPTER 206

Phlebotomy

Christine S. Cho and Jill C. Posner

Phlebotomy is the removal of blood through the puncture of a vein. The history of phlebotomy has its roots in bloodletting to cure multiple ailments. Today, the removal of blood as a therapeutic intervention is limited to a few conditions, but phlebotomy is widely performed to obtain blood for laboratory tests.

INDICATIONS

The most common indication for phlebotomy is to obtain a blood sample for laboratory testing. In pediatrics, the most common therapeutic reasons for phlebotomy are to reduce the hematocrit in infants with polycythemia and to perform exchange transfusions in patients with sickle cell disease and hemolytic disease of the newborn.

CONTRAINDICATIONS

There are virtually no absolute contraindications to phlebotomy. Relative contraindications are the existence of a bleeding disorder and severe anemia, but even in those circumstances, blood studies are needed for the evaluation of the patient. One should avoid drawing blood in areas where trauma or infection is a concern and from surgically placed fistulas for dialysis.

EQUIPMENT

Table 206-1 lists the equipment needed for phlebotomy.

PROCEDURE

There are two common collection methods when phlebotomy is used to obtain samples for laboratory testing. Blood can be collected into a syringe attached to the needle or directly into evacuated laboratory tubes if the needle is attached to a plastic evacuated tube adapter. In pediatric patients, 21-, 23-, or 25-gauge butterfly winged infusion needles (also called butterfly needles) are most frequently used.

After obtaining all the equipment, one should wash one's hands and put on gloves. Position the patient so that he or she is comfortably sitting or lying down, with the arm extended on a flat, sturdy surface. Some patients may need to be physically restrained by support staff or with a papoose; however, children often benefit from nonpharmacologic relaxation techniques or other distraction methods. The use of a child life therapist can be particularly helpful. In infants, orally administered glucose-containing solutions can reduce pain.

Tie a tourniquet on the upper arm, and inspect the antecubital fossa for a visible or palpable vein suitable for venipuncture. Repeat on the contralateral arm if needed. The dorsal surface of the hands is another location to search for veins (Fig. 206-1). In infants, it may be difficult to visualize or palpate veins, and one can consider using the lower extremities or scalp veins to obtain blood samples.

Cleanse the venipuncture site with an alcohol swab. When obtaining blood for culture, the area should also be cleansed with povidone-iodine solution; this should be allowed to dry completely before performing venipuncture.

Attach a syringe or evacuated tube adapter to the needle. With the nondominant hand, secure the patient's arm at the elbow, and use the thumb to apply downward traction to the skin below the venipuncture site (Fig. 206-2). Position the needle at a 15-degree angle to the skin with the bevel up, and insert the needle.

Remove the amount of blood indicated with a syringe, or fill the evacuated tubes directly from the needle with the adapter. Untie the tourniquet, hold gauze at the venipuncture site, and remove the needle. Apply pressure to the venipuncture site. Dispose of the needle in an appropriate sharps container. Check for hemostasis at the puncture site. Tape gauze to the skin once active bleeding has stopped.

Be sure to properly label each specimen.

COMPLICATIONS

Complications from phlebotomy include bleeding, hematoma, and, rarely, infection at the site of injection. Prolonged bleeding can be avoided if adequate pressure is applied to the venipuncture site once the needle is removed.

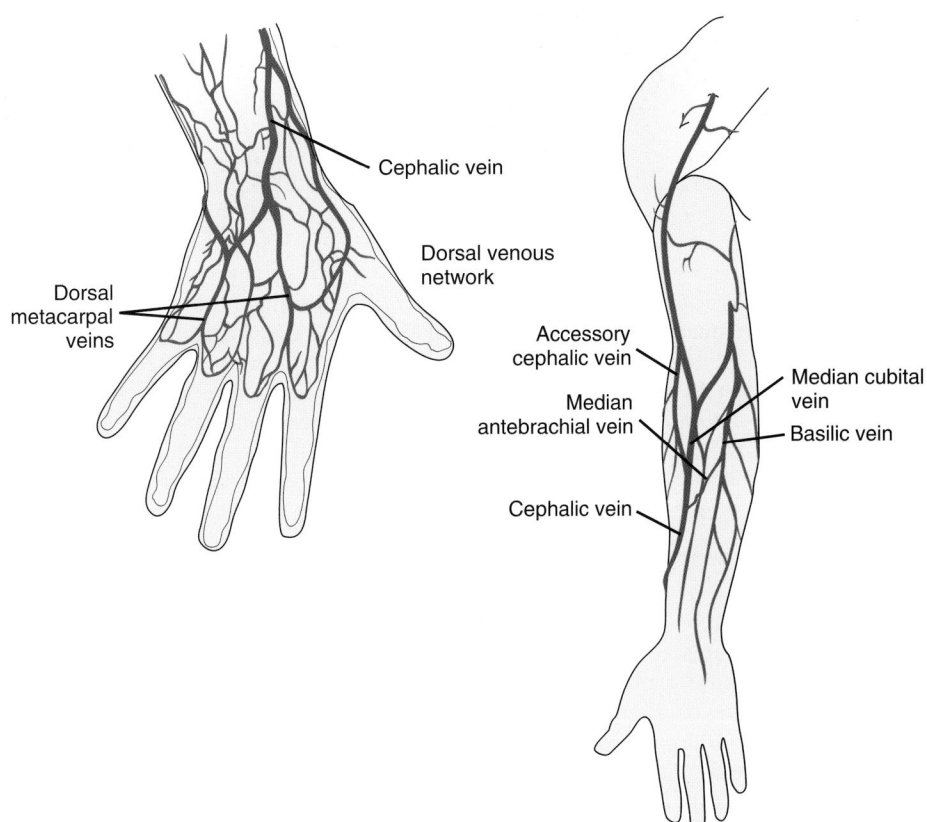

Figure 206-1   Common sites for venipuncture. (Adapted from Williams PL: Gray's Anatomy: The Anatomical Basis of Medicine and Surgery, 38th ed. New York, Churchill Livingstone, 1996.)

Table 206-1   Equipment Needed for Phlebotomy
Gloves
Tourniquet
Alcohol swab
Povidone-iodine solution (if drawing blood culture)
Butterfly needle (21, 23, or 25 gauge)
Syringe or evacuated tube adapter
Evacuated laboratory tubes
Gauze
Tape
Sharps disposal container

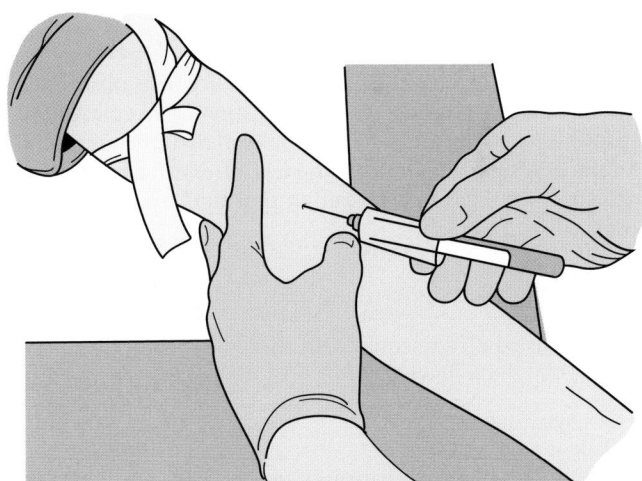

Figure 206-2   Venipuncture technique. (Adapted from Flynn JC: Procedures in Phlebotomy. Philadelphia, WB Saunders, 1994.)

Unless there is a coexistent bleeding disorder, hematomas are of little clinical significance to the patient and will resolve with time. Other complications include petechiae (where the tourniquet was tied) and anemia from frequent or excessive blood sampling.

SUGGESTED READING

Flynn JC: Procedures in Phlebotomy, 1st ed. Philadelphia, WB Saunders, 1994.

Garza D, Becan-McBride K: Phlebotomy Handbook, 1st ed. Upper Saddle River, NJ, Prentice Hall, 2002.

Pendergraph GE: Handbook of Phlebotomy, 1st ed. Philadelphia, Lea & Febiger, 1984.

CHAPTER 207

Replacing a Tracheostomy Tube

Kate Cronan

Tracheostomy tubes are changed at home by parents on a regular basis. This procedure is infrequently performed by hospital-based health care providers. However, when the procedure is indicated, it is often carried out under urgent circumstances. Thus, practitioners should acquire the skills to facilitate efficient replacement. Reinsertion is generally performed in patients with established tracheostomies, and this is easier to accomplish.

INDICATIONS

A tracheostomy tube requires changing in several scenarios. If a tube accidentally dislodges, a replacement tube must be inserted immediately. At times, respiratory distress caused by clogging from thickened secretions develops in a child with a tracheostomy tube in place. If suctioning fails to clear the blockage, the tracheostomy tube must be rapidly removed and a new tube inserted by a trained practitioner. These circumstances occur more often in infants. If a patient with a tracheostomy is in the hospital on a long-term basis, routine tracheal tube changes may be indicated. A hospital-based physician may be involved in these nonurgent changes.

CONTRAINDICATIONS

If a tracheostomy tube dislodges or becomes obstructed, there are no absolute contraindications to replacement. However, extreme caution must be exercised when replacing a tracheal tube in a patient who has a fresh tracheotomy. In this scenario it is best to call on otorhinolaryngology subspecialists if available.

EQUIPMENT

The usual airway equipment should be readily available, including the following:

Laryngoscope
Blade
Endotracheal tubes in various sizes
Suction equipment with catheters
High-flow oxygen
Bag-valve-mask device with several mask sizes
Additional equipment may be needed, including

Several sizes of tracheostomy cannulas
Tracheostomy twill tape
A pair of scissors
Surgical lubricant gel
Saline bullets
Towel for under the neck

Current tracheostomy tubes are made of polyvinyl chloride, which conforms to the shape and size of the trachea.

The tracheostomy tube size is determined by the inner diameter, the outer diameter, and the length. The internal diameter is routinely printed on the flange. There are a number of manufacturers of tracheostomy tubes. If the exact size replacement tube cannot be located rapidly, one should refer to charts designed to compare the various tube types and sizes. A tracheostomy tube may be cuffed or uncuffed. Cuffed tubes are especially beneficial in patients with tracheomegaly.

PROCEDURE

Dislodged Tracheostomy Tube

If a patient presents with a history of accidental decannulation and is dependent on the tracheostomy tube, the stoma should be recannulated immediately. First, supplemental oxygen should be administered via the nose, mouth, or tracheal stoma. Next, the tracheostomy ties should be cut. The patient should be placed in a supine position with a towel roll under the shoulders to allow hyperextension of the head and neck. This permits the best access to the tracheostomy site. If the replacement tracheal tube is cuffed, the balloon's integrity should be confirmed. If available, the same size and type of tracheostomy cannula should be inserted. However, if a clean tube is not accessible, one should reinsert the same tube if it is thought to be patent.

Before reinserting the new cannula, the obturator is inserted into the outer cannula and is used as a stylet. The cannula is then lubricated with a surgical lubricant gel and inserted into the stoma. The technique involves posterior and caudal insertion in one swift movement. It should be done gently to avoid trauma. The obturator is then removed immediately, and if indicated, the internal cannula is inserted. Some tracheostomy tubes have an inner cannula, whereas others do not. High-flow oxygen should then be administered via bag so that tube patency can be assessed. Breath sounds should be evaluated. To secure the airway, the flanges of the cannula must be tied around the neck with twill tracheostomy ties or a Velcro strap. Respiratory therapists are often available to assist with this portion of the procedure.

If the stoma is constricted, it may be difficult to pass the tracheal tube and resistance may be encountered. To avoid the creation of a false tract, one should not force the cannula into the stoma. Instead, it is recommended that one attempt to insert a smaller tracheal cannula or endotracheal tube to allow ventilation and oxygenation. If this fails, insertion of an oxygen catheter into the stoma is advised. It can serve as a stylet on which to place the new tracheal cannula. If successful recannulation is not possible, it may be necessary to provide bag-valve-mask ventilation via the mouth and nose and cover the stoma with a gloved finger. At this point the practitioner should call for assistance.

Obstructed Tracheostomy Tube

If the tracheostomy tube is still in the stoma but its patency is in question, the tube should be suctioned. If obstruction is still present, it should be removed gently. First, one should deflate the cuff if it is a cuffed tube. Next, the tracheostomy ties should be cut with scissors before removal. One should then proceed with the procedure as described earlier.

COMPLICATIONS

Changing a tracheostomy tube rarely results in complications. If there is difficulty replacing the tracheostomy tube, hypoxemia may result. Difficult reinsertion may result in the creation of a false tract, and pneumomediastinum or pneumothorax can develop. Rarely, bleeding related to reinsertion may occur.

SUGGESTED READING

Adirim T: Children with special health care needs: The technologically dependent child. In Fuchs S, Yamamoto L (eds): APLS: The Pediatric Emergency Medicine Resource. Sudbury, MA, Jones & Bartlett, 2004, pp 595-598.

Adirim T, Smith E: Tracheostomies and home ventilation. In Adirim T, Smith E (eds): SCOPE: Special Children's Outreach and Prehospital Education. Sudbury, MA, Jones & Bartlett, 2006, pp 56-60.

Fein J, Cronan K, Posner J: Approach to the care of the technology-assisted child. In Fleisher G, Ludwig S, Henretig F (eds): Textbook of Pediatric Emergency Medicine. Philadelphia, Lippincott Williams & Wilkins, 2006, pp 1738-1739.

Fein J, Cronan K, Posner J: Illustrated techniques of pediatric emergency procedures. In Fleisher G, Ludwig S, Henretig F (eds): Textbook of Pediatric Emergency Medicine. Philadelphia, Lippincott Williams & Wilkins, 2006, pp 1901-1904.

Kallis JM: Replacement of a tracheostomy cannula. In Henretig F, King C (eds): Textbook of Pediatric Emergency Procedures. Baltimore, Williams & Wilkins, 1997, pp 871-875.

CHAPTER 208

Intubation

Timothy Gibson

Emergent endotracheal intubation is one of the central elements of pediatric resuscitation. It often falls to the pediatric hospitalist to both determine the need for intubation and supervise (if not perform) the insertion of the endotracheal tube (ETT).

Pediatric patients require airway support for a variety of reasons, from a neonate who is apneic in the first seconds of life to an adolescent in respiratory failure due to status asthmaticus. These patients and their airway dimensions run the gamut. For some patients, only brief intervention with effective bag-mask ventilation is required. In fact, recent Pediatric Advanced Life Support protocols have placed an increased emphasis on the teaching of bag-mask ventilation, especially if an airway intervention must be performed by a practitioner who is inexperienced with ETT placement in children. For a patient who needs prolonged ventilatory support, however, an ETT is the definitive airway.

INDICATIONS

Numerous diseases and clinical scenarios require emergent endotracheal intubation. Common scenarios encountered by the pediatric hospitalist include the following:

- Apnea (e.g., related to respiratory syncytial virus)
- Loss of protective airway reflexes (e.g., obtundation from drug overdose)
- Respiratory failure (e.g., severe asthma with hypercarbia)
- Current or impending airway obstruction (e.g., epiglottitis)
- Reduction of intracranial pressure (e.g., head trauma)
- Overwhelming systemic illness (e.g., during cardiopulmonary resuscitation)

CONTRAINDICATIONS

There are no absolute contraindications to securing a definitive airway. Because the pediatric hospitalist is typically performing this procedure in an emergent (as opposed to elective) setting, one should assume that the patient may have a full stomach and is at risk for aspiration of gastric contents. In any patient in whom trauma is a consideration, the procedure should be performed with cervical spine stabilization. Finally, there are a number of factors that might cause a patient to have a difficult airway, including congenital anomalies, face or neck trauma, significant airway obstruction (e.g., epiglottitis), and any patient in extremis. If possible, an anesthesiologist should be consulted emergently and should be present to assist with or take over airway management in these patients.

EQUIPMENT

Once the decision has been made to intubate a patient, the importance of preparation cannot be overstated. Any piece of equipment that could potentially be necessary should be within reach (Table 208-1). There should be several assistants present to perform peripheral tasks (e.g., handing the physician the ETT for insertion, attaching a carbon dioxide detector, taping the ETT after placement).

ANATOMY

Clearly, the pediatric airway differs based on the patient's age. In a newborn, the tongue is large relative to the other airway structures, and the epiglottis has a more vertical orientation that often requires it to be retracted manually with the laryngoscope blade. The occiput is also relatively large, and it is usually not necessary to place a towel roll under the head, as is required with adolescents and adults. In contrast to adolescents and adults, the narrowest portion of the airway is just below the vocal cords, so younger children are often intubated with an uncuffed ETT.

PROCEDURE

Preparation

If possible, intravenous access should be in place before any emergent intubation. Many practitioners prefer to give a fluid bolus before intubation, if conditions permit, because the shift from negative- to positive-pressure ventilation impedes venous return to the right side of the heart, potentially compromising cardiac output.

Most, if not all, patients who require ETT placement also require medications to achieve a condition amenable to intubation. A full discussion of rapid-sequence intubation is outside the scope of this chapter, but briefly, medication considerations include preparatory agents (e.g., atropine, lidocaine), sedatives and analgesics (e.g., barbiturates, benzodiazepines, opioids, ketamine, etomidate, propofol), and neuromuscular blocking agents (e.g., succinylcholine, rocuronium). Cricoid pressure should be maintained once the process of sedation is initiated until tube placement is confirmed. One caveat is that the practitioner must be absolutely sure that an airway can be appropriately placed before administering a paralytic agent.

The patient must be preoxygenated, with bag-mask ventilation if necessary. The head should be placed in the so-called sniffing position in an attempt to align the oropharynx with the trachea.

Table 208-1 Equipment Needed for Endotracheal Intubation
Airway equipment
Laryngoscope handles and blades
Appropriate size endotracheal tubes (cuffed or uncuffed, with or without stylets)
Oral or nasal airways
Tape to secure tube in position
Oxygen
Positive-pressure delivery system
Tubing
Equipment for bag-mask ventilation
Suction
Flexible catheter or Yankauer suction device
Orogastric tube to decompress the stomach
Medications
Intravenous access
Sedatives, analgesics
Neuromuscular blocking agents
Other medications (e.g., atropine, lidocaine) as clinically warranted
Monitoring
Cardiac monitor
Pulse oximeter
Carbon dioxide monitor

Technique

Once the patient is appropriately sedated, the practitioner stands at the head of the bed and opens the patient's mouth by gently pressing the chin with the right index finger. The laryngoscope is always grasped with the left hand. In general, a straight blade is preferred over a curved blade in all but the oldest pediatric patients. The blade is inserted along the contour of the tongue, with a sweeping motion from the patient's right to left to allow visualization past the tongue. Once past the tongue, the blade is in the vallecula, and there are two options. One is to pull the laryngoscope at a 45-degree angle anteriorly and inferiorly, with the hope that the tension on the connective tissue will raise the epiglottis off the larynx, allowing visualization of the vocal cords. The second option, which is usually necessary in younger patients, is to manually elevate the epiglottis with the blade once it is visualized. Care should be taken not to lever the blade on the teeth or gums. Cricoid pressure applied by an assistant during insertion of the laryngoscope blade can be helpful in visualizing the airway.

Once the cords are visualized, the practitioner is ready to insert the ETT. The assistant places the ETT in the practitioner's right hand so that he or she can remain focused on the cords. The use of a stylet to stiffen the ETT during insertion may be helpful. Attempting to pass the tube down the barrel of the laryngoscope blade obscures the view of the cords. Rather, the tube should come in from the right side of the mouth at an angle, allowing the practitioner to visualize the tube passing through the cords. The ETT has three markings on its distal end, and the tube should be inserted so that the second of these lines is at the level of the cords. At this point, appropriate tube placement should be confirmed. The practitioner or assistant should look for a rising chest with bagged ventilations, auscultate over both right and left lung fields to ascertain that there are symmetrical breath sounds, and auscultate the stomach to determine whether inadvertent esophageal intubation may have occurred. All patients should have a carbon dioxide detector attached to the ETT, and return of carbon dioxide with respirations is the best way to confirm that the tube is in fact in the airway. Confirmation of appropriate depth in the trachea is obtained with a chest radiograph.

COMPLICATIONS

If at any time the patient has significant oxygen desaturation or bradycardia, the procedure should be aborted and the patient supported by bag-mask ventilation with 100% oxygen. It should be noted that a vagal response to manipulation of the upper airway is common. If at any point bag-mask ventilation becomes difficult, fiberoptic intubation or creation of a surgical airway may be required.

Other complications of endotracheal intubation include aspiration, inadequate oxygenation (e.g., inability to provide airway support, prolonged intubation attempt, esophageal or right main-stem intubation, tube obstruction), mechanical trauma, and barotrauma.

SUGGESTED READING

King C, Stayer S: Emergent endotracheal intubation. In Henretig F, King C (eds): Textbook of Pediatric Emergency Procedures. Baltimore, Williams & Wilkins, 1997, pp 161-238.

McAllister JD, Gnauck KA: Rapid sequence intubation of the pediatric patient: Fundamentals of practice. Pediatr Clin North Am 1999;46:1249-1284.

Todres ID, Frassica JJ: Tracheal intubation. In Todres ID, Fugate J (eds): Critical Care of Infants and Children. Philadelphia, Lippincott Williams & Wilkins, 1996, pp 31-38.

CHAPTER 209

Noninvasive Positive-Pressure Ventilation

K. Keilty, I. B. MacLusky, and R. Padman

Noninvasive ventilation refers to strategies that augment alveolar ventilation without indwelling artificial airways. Mechanical ventilation evolved first with negative-pressure ventilation devices, such as the iron lung, back in the 1920s. Positive-pressure ventilation via endotracheal tube or tracheostomy was developed in the 1960s and led the way to further mechanical advances, including positive-pressure administration via face or nasal mask devices. Over the last 15 years new technologies have become available that allow both short- and long-term noninvasive airway support in selected children. These devices, grouped together under the heading of noninvasive positive-pressure ventilation (NPPV), allow delivery of air, with or without supplementary oxygen, under pressure for respiratory support, usually through the nose or the nose and mouth. With the increased levels of acuity seen in many pediatric hospitals, as well as the increase in technology-dependent children in the community, the hospitalist may be required to initiate or maintain these ventilatory therapies in the emergency department, hospital ward, or other setting.

CONDITIONS REQUIRING NONINVASIVE POSITIVE-PRESSURE VENTILATION

The most common reasons for initiating NPPV are obstructive sleep apnea (OSA) syndrome and hypoventilatory states.

During sleep there is relative hypotonia of the upper airway muscles and hence an increase in upper airway resistance. Partial collapse of the upper airway results in vibration of the pharynx (snoring), whereas complete obstruction results in apnea. OSA syndrome comprises a spectrum of disorders ranging from partial obstruction, with snoring associated with hypoventilation and hypoxemia (obstructive hypopnea), to complete obstruction of the upper airway resulting in no airflow (obstructive apnea) (see Chapter 74).

Despite medical advances, chronic respiratory failure will eventually develop in a number of children with progressive diseases such as severe chronic lung disease or respiratory muscle wall weakness secondary to neuromotor disease. Hypoventilation occurs initially during sleep but, with progression of disease, ultimately becomes present throughout the day. Sleep fragmentation can be significant, with repeated or persistent nocturnal desaturation before any alteration in daytime blood gas parameters. Respiratory failure typically develops insidiously, usually with only subtle symptoms such as morning headaches and tiredness. Growth failure is also common, but it is often attributed to the underlying disease. Pulmonary function testing can be a helpful, but not always reliable tool in predicting which children may be at risk for significant nocturnal hypoventilation. In children with neuromotor disease, forced vital capacity less than 40% of predicted has been associated with sleep-disordered breathing and may be an ideal time to consider initiating NPPV.[1,2]

In patients with neuromotor disease, repeated admission to the hospital for pneumonia and atelectasis may indicate the onset of chronic respiratory failure. In children with severe restrictive lung disease or chest wall disease, such as secondary to kyphoscoliosis, the insidious onset of hypoxia may indicate progressive hypercapnia as a result of failure of the patient's compensatory efforts. In the absence of definitive therapy for the underlying condition, nocturnal ventilatory failure will commonly progress to daytime failure and eventually death. Well before then, increasing daytime symptoms with deteriorating quality of life will usually develop. Treatment of progressive hypoventilation with assisted ventilation, either noninvasive (via face mask or nasal pillows) or invasive (usually via a permanent tracheostomy), should therefore be considered.

Hypoventilation may also occur with acute illness, especially in patients with underlying chronic respiratory compromise. A common example would be a premature infant with chronic lung disease in whom severe bronchiolitis develops. In such a setting, the need for ventilatory support is short term, and return to respiratory sufficiency is expected as recovery from the acute illness progresses.

TECHNOLOGY AND MODES

A number of different devices can be chosen, each with their own advantages and disadvantages.[3] In general, most devices for noninvasive ventilation are pressure (rather than volume) controlled, with limited adjustment options.

Continuous Positive Airway Pressure

Devices for continuous positive airway pressure (CPAP) provide a high flow of delivered air at a preset pressure throughout the respiratory cycle (Fig. 209-1). A "ramping" feature may allow the patient to fall asleep with the device set at a low pressure, and then, over a preset period, the machine incrementally ramps up to full therapeutic pressure. This feature is useful in patients unable to fall asleep with the full pressure already in place. Devices contain leak alarms that may warn of disconnection or detachment of the mask. CPAP devices increase end-expiratory volume and prevent airway collapse during inspiration, but they do not directly increase tidal volume and hence provide respiratory support rather than true ventilation.

Bilevel Positive Airway Pressure Ventilation

Bilevel positive airway pressure devices (e.g., BiPAP) can provide different pressures during inspiration and expiration.[4] Expired positive airway pressure (EPAP) helps maintain end-expiratory lung volume and airway patency, similar

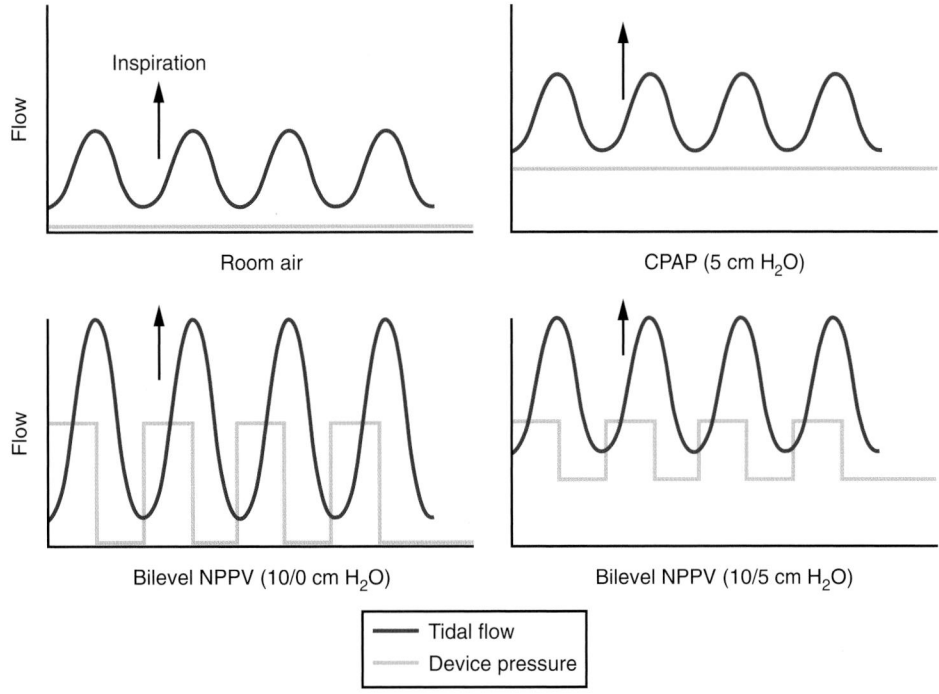

Figure 209-1   Respiratory air flow with various modes of noninvasive ventilation. Bilevel NPPV, bilevel positive airway pressure; CPAP, continuous positive airway pressure.

to CPAP. The pressure difference between EPAP and inspired positive airway pressure (IPAP) serves to increase tidal volume and hence minute ventilation (see Fig. 209-1).

Bilevel NPPV is commonly delivered in either the spontaneous (S) or spontaneous-timed (S/T) mode. In S-mode each patient breath is assisted by machine-delivered IPAP when the machine senses the change in airflow triggered by the inspiratory effort of the patient. Because there is no background respiratory rate set on the machine, children have to initiate each breath on their own. However, tidal volume is enhanced by the machine delivering a preset IPAP level.

In S/T-mode a respiratory rate can be set to provide a backup rate in the event that the child slows or ceases respiratory efforts. In this mode, the device responds to inspiratory and expiratory flow rates to cycle machine-initiated breaths between the patient's inhalation and exhalation. It reliably senses a patient's breathing efforts even when moderate air leaks are present in the circuit. Earlier bilevel NPPV units were designed for adults. Children with small tidal volumes were therefore frequently unable to develop sufficient inspiratory flow to trigger the respiratory cycle on such devices. Many newer units consequently have an adjustable sensitivity feature to accommodate patients with small tidal volumes. The downside of such units is that the presence of a significant leak may trigger IPAP and result in autocycling of the ventilator.[4]

Because they have limited alarm capabilities and are designed to function with an ongoing air leak, NPPV cannot guarantee delivered minute ventilation. These units should therefore be used with significant caution in ventilator-dependent patients, who require guaranteed mechanical ventilation. For these patients, ventilation via tracheotomy or endotracheal tube may be preferred for survival. Bilevel NPPV machines are, however, able to compensate for significant leaks without loss of tidal volume. Nonetheless, the tidal volumes delivered by pressure modes of ventilation will still fall in the presence of increasing airway resistance or reduced lung compliance.

TREATMENT OUTCOMES

By providing a constant distending pressure, CPAP is useful in preventing airway collapse, such as occurs with OSA or tracheomalacia. By increasing intrathoracic pressure, it also acts to effectively reduce left ventricular afterload and can therefore be useful in treating left ventricular failure unresponsive to other therapies. CPAP does, however, increase right ventricular preload and should thus be used with caution in children with right ventricular dysfunction.[5] In the majority of children with OSA, surgical revision of enlarged adenoids or tonsils (or both) is curative in approximately 85% of cases,[6] nasal CPAP generally being used only in patients for whom there is no surgical option for long-term cure (i.e., those with obesity or facial anomalies). On occasion, bilevel nasal ventilation is indicated in patients with severe OSA to provide inspiratory pressure in excess of that usually tolerated with CPAP alone (usually in excess of 12 cm H_2O).

By improving both minute ventilation and the work of breathing, bilevel NPPV improves gas exchange, decreases respiratory effort, and reduces sleep fragmentation. In selected populations, long-term bilevel NPPV has demonstrated improvement in nocturnal respiratory parameters and daytime functioning, as well as significant improvement in nutritional status.[7] Bilevel NPPV also seems to improve perceived quality of life, reduce the frequency and duration of health care utilization, and be associated with significant cost savings in the year after initiation of bilevel NPPV in comparison to the preceding year. The incidence of admission for recurring pneumonia in the neuromuscular

Table 209-1 Indications for Noninvasive Positive-Pressure Ventilation

Tachypnea
Use of accessory muscles of ventilation
Reduced tidal volume and/or subjective complaints of fatigue (often associated with a rise in $PaCO_2$)
Obstructive sleep apnea
Diaphragm and phrenic nerve weakness or malfunction
Respiratory failure secondary to pulmonary edema (to prevent alveolar filling) and disorders associated with recurrent atelectasis
Neuromuscular disorders resulting in hypoventilation
Malformation/damage to the respiratory center or spinal cord
Chronic depressed left ventricular function

Table 209-2 Conditions Requiring Close Monitoring When Initiating Noninvasive Positive-Pressure Ventilation

Known or suspected gastroesophageal reflux, particularly in the presence of oropharyngeal dyscoordination
Excessive secretions
Gastrostomy tube or gastrojejunostomy tube feeding
Abdominal distention
Struggling or refusal of the patient to cooperate with the device
Latex hypersensitivity (use a latex-free mask)
Pneumothorax with a chest tube in place
Bullous lung disease
Oxygen need in excess of 40% FiO_2

disease population may also decrease after the initiation of bilevel NPPV.[8] When compared with invasive ventilation via tracheostomy, bilevel NPPV is associated with less morbidity, including a reduction in lung infections and a reduced negative impact on lifestyle.

There is increased use of long-term bilevel NPPV in palliative care, both in the hospital and at home, for patients with progressive neuromotor or respiratory disease. Bilevel NPPV is generally preferred over invasive ventilation and is better tolerated by patients.[9] Many pediatric patients are living longer and at home with progressive respiratory failure. On a short-term basis, bilevel NPPV is now considered a potential alternative to invasive ventilation for the acute management of infants and children with impending respiratory failure for whatever reason.

INDICATIONS

NPPV is considered for use on the inpatient unit for physiologically stable chronic patients or palliative patients with respiratory muscular weakness or malfunction, including but not limited to the indications listed in Table 209-1.

Additionally, NPPV can be instituted in some patients with acute or subacute respiratory decompensation, although this therapy is often initiated in an intensive care setting. Once respiratory stability has been established with the new technology, many institutions allow its use outside an intensive care unit.

SPECIAL CONSIDERATIONS

Although generally well tolerated, care must be taken in patients in whom NPPV may be associated with increased risks that require close observation for optimal safety, especially when initiating the device for the first time (Table 209-2).

It is also imperative to ensure adequate mask venting. In smaller children with low tidal volumes, particularly if full face masks are used, the volume of the mask may approach or even exceed the patient's tidal volume. Rebreathing may

then occur, with increasing hypercapnia. Most masks have a port on the mask itself to allow supplementary oxygen to be blown directly into the mask. If used in small patients, one of these ports should be left open in addition to the application of a leak adjunct (i.e., whisper swivel) to allow the escape of exhaled gas.

In the presence of gastroesophageal reflux it is advised that children remain without oral intake for 2 hours before bedtime or the initiation of bilevel NPPV. If a gastrostomy tube is in place, it should be vented when NPPV is initiated to relieve gastric distention caused by any air forced down the esophagus. Once the child and caregivers have gained experience with the device, some children can tolerate being fed overnight while using NPPV.

CONTRAINDICATIONS

As noted, bilevel NPPV is not capable of providing guaranteed ventilation and is therefore contraindicated when guaranteed ventilation is required. There are other clinical scenarios in which NPPV may be contraindicated (Table 209-3).

For these patients, NPPV should either be used in a highly monitored setting or may not be the best option for respiratory support; in such cases, conventional invasive ventilation is the preferred method.

INITIATION AND MONITORING

With the increasing use of these devices, a pediatric hospitalist can expect at some time to be responsible for the inpatient management of a child who is either already on NPPV at home or has been transitioned from the intensive care unit. Parents of children already on NPPV are usually expert in the specifics of their child's care because they have gained extensive experience using the technology at home. For many families, admission to the hospital will occur despite the use of sophisticated equipment and skilled, vigilant caregiving provided at home.

There are no clear guidelines regarding the precise indications and timing for initiation of NPPV.[3] If initiated too

Table 209-3   Absolute and Relative Contraindications to Noninvasive Positive-Pressure Ventilation

Absolute Contraindications
Acute ventilatory failure ($PaCO_2$ >60 mm Hg and pH ≤7.25)
Unevacuated pneumothorax
Anatomic anomalies prohibiting effective application of a
   nasal/facial interface (e.g., choanal atresia, cleft palate,
   unrepaired tracheoesophageal fistula)
Hemodynamically unstable cardiac failure
Absent airway protective reflexes

Relative Contraindications
Decreased airway reflexes
Inability to tolerate a nasal/face mask
Massive epistaxis or history thereof
Acute sinusitis, otitis media, or perforated ear drum
Requiring a full face mask for initiation of therapy if the
   patient is unable to independently remove it (because of the
   risk of vomiting and aspiration)
Refractory hypoxemia

early, for example, when the patient still has adequate spontaneous ventilation as demonstrated by normal blood gas parameters, it may be poorly tolerated, with resulting poor compliance with therapy.

The actual NPPV settings required for any specific patient are highly idiosyncratic. Pressure settings range from 2 to 25 cm H_2O for IPAP and from 2 to 20 cm H_2O for EPAP. Initial IPAP and EPAP settings are based on known patient respiratory system compliance and the presence of respiratory muscle weakness or airway collapse (or both). Patients with poor respiratory system compliance, such as restrictive lung disease or scoliosis, usually require high ventilator pressures, for example, IPAP greater than 15 cm H_2O. Patients with high compliance, such as infants with neuromotor disease, may require relatively low pressures to achieve adequate ventilation, for example, IPAP/EPAP of 10/4 cm H_2O. Initial settings are therefore empirical, usually starting at low pressures and then increasing once the patient has acclimatized up until pressures have been reached that produce optimal ventilation and patient comfort. The initial setup is ideally performed when continuous observation is possible, such as in the intensive care unit or a properly supervised sleep laboratory. A trained observer can adjust the pressure throughout the night in response to the effect of NPPV on respiration as demonstrated by changes in the respiratory rate, the use of accessory muscles, the heart rate, and sleep. Once NPPV has been established, pressures frequently have to be readjusted after a period of use as the patient adjusts to the equipment, the condition changes, or the patient experiences significant changes with respect to growth.

Oxygen saturation monitoring is another helpful tool, but care must be taken to not assume that adequate saturation represents normal blood gases when supplemental oxygen is being used. Many children with central blunting of their respiratory drive will appear comfortable with supplemental oxygen in place that masks an elevated or climbing PCO_2. Care must also be taken in the use of any sedating drugs (including some over-the-counter cough medicines), which may, by reducing respiratory drive, interfere with a child's

ability to trigger the NPPV machine. Formal blood gases or continuous carbon dioxide monitoring (transcutaneous capnography) is therefore frequently required to assess the adequacy of ventilation.

LIMITATIONS AND COMPLICATIONS

NPPV has significant practical limitations that limit its clinical use:

1. The connection at the nasal mask interface is insecure. Leaks may be both uncomfortable (especially into the eyes) and make control of ventilation parameters unreliable and unsafe in certain circumstances.
2. There are limitations in the maximal pressure that can be delivered, particularly in hypotonic children, who may have difficulty keeping their mouth closed. Although this problem can be overcome with full face masks, with increasing pressure there is a risk of distention of the esophagus and, at least in theory, a risk of gastric distention and gastroesophageal reflux. There is also a risk of aspiration if the child vomits into a full face mask, particularly in children lacking adequate upper limb control.
3. NPPV is predominantly a nocturnal therapy. Although it can be used on a continuous (24 hr/day) basis for short periods, it limits patient mobility, and skin breakdown is a significant concern. With long-term use, both bilevel NPPV and nasal CPAP have been associated with facial remodeling, particularly in smaller children.[10]
4. Nasal obstruction, such as occurs with viral upper respiratory tract infections, can make it difficult or impossible to use NPPV for several days. During the acute illness, attempts to clear the nasal passages with saline sprays and intermittent nasal suctioning can be of some help, but it is frequently necessary to temporarily discontinue NPPV until secretions diminish and it can again be tolerated.
5. NPPV may fail to be tolerated if there is a sudden change in pulmonary resistance, as in the case of partial or total collapse of a lung. If clinically aware, children will demonstrate agitation or discomfort with the NPPV interface because of their sense of impending respiratory failure.
6. Certain patient populations may not ever tolerate the interface well. Some patients with trisomy 21 would benefit from NPPV, but in practice, it is extremely difficult to achieve adherence so that children leave the mask in place, even with elaborate behavior modification programs.
7. The risks associated with positive expiratory pressure in children with right ventricular dysfunction need to be remembered.[5]
8. Skin breakdown from pressure of the face mask, especially common at the nasal bridge, can occur and limit use of the device for a period.
9. Barotrauma such as pneumothorax can occur, especially with increased pressure settings and in patients with high lung compliance.

IN A NUTSHELL

- Noninvasive ventilation is a technique of augmenting alveolar ventilation without requiring an artificial airway. It is a safe and viable alternative for management of acute and chronic respiratory failure in select pediatric patients.

- CPAP provides a high flow of delivered air at a preset pressure throughout the respiratory cycle.
- Bilevel NPPV can provide different pressures during inspiration and expiration and serves to increase tidal volume and minute ventilation.
- Bilevel NPPV can be used in the spontaneous mode to support patient-initiated breaths. Alternatively, it can be used in the spontaneous-timed mode to supply machine-initiated breaths in addition to support of patient-initiated breaths.
- NPPV has a highly individualized response and therefore requires application by skilled and knowledgeable staff on a pediatric inpatient unit; it can also be established for long-term use safely in the home.
- For infants and children in chronic respiratory failure, NPPV has been associated with significant improvement in quality of life and growth parameters and reduction in morbidity, including the need for intubation and hospitalization.
- NPPV is recognized as having a growing role in the supportive care of infants and children with life-limiting illnesses and can provide relief of both acute and long-term symptoms, as well as prolong life while avoiding invasive ventilation.

SUGGESTED READING

Padman R, Lawless ST, Kettrick RG: Noninvasive ventilation via bilevel positive airway pressure support in pediatric practice. Crit Care Med 1998;26:169-173.

Padman R, Nadkarni V: Noninvasive ventilation: Past, present and future: A focus on pediatric applications. Clin Pulm Med 2000;7:199-207.

Teague WG, Fortenberry JD: Noninvasive ventilatory support in pediatric respiratory failure. Respir Care 1995;40:86-96.

REFERENCES

1. Phillips MF, Quinlivan RC, Edwards RH, Calverley PM: Changes in spirometry over time as a prognostic marker in patients with Duchenne muscular dystrophy. Am J Respir Crit Care Med 2001;164:2191-2194.
2. Lyager S, Steffensen B, Juhl B: Indicators of need for mechanical ventilation in Duchenne muscular dystrophy and spinal muscular atrophy. Chest 1995;108:779-785.
3. Make BJ, Hill NS, Goldberg AI, et al: Mechanical ventilation beyond the intensive care unit. Report of a consensus conference of the American College of Chest Physicians. Chest 1998;113:289S-344S.
4. Marcus CL: Ventilator management of abnormal breathing during sleep. In Loughlin GM, Carroll JL, Marcus CL (eds): Sleep and Breathing in Children. New York, Marcel Dekker, 2000, pp 797-812.
5. Huemer G, Kolev N, Kurz A, Zimpfer M: Influence of positive end-expiratory pressure on right and left ventricular performance assessed by Doppler two-dimensional echocardiography. Chest 1994;106:67-73.
6. Guilleminault C, Li KK, Khramtsov A, et al: Sleep disordered breathing: Surgical outcomes in prepubertal children. Laryngoscope 2004;114:132-137.
7. Khan Y, Heckmatt JZ, Dubowitz V: Sleep studies and supportive ventilatory treatment in patients with congenital muscle disorders. Arch Dis Child 1996;74:195-200.
8. Katz S, Selvadurai H, Keilty K, et al: Outcome of non-invasive positive pressure ventilation in paediatric neuromuscular disease. Arch Dis Child 2004;89:121-124.
9. Bach JR: A comparison of long-term ventilatory support alternatives from the perspective of the patient and care giver. Chest 1993;104:1702-1706.
10. Li KK, Riley RW, Guilleminault C: An unreported risk in the use of home nasal continuous positive airway pressure and home nasal ventilation in children: Mid-face hypoplasia. Chest 2000;117:916-918.

CHAPTER 210

Thoracentesis

Manoj K. Mittal and Jill Baren

Thoracentesis is the evacuation of fluid or air from the pleural space. This discussion is limited to the evacuation of fluid (effusion) from the pleural space.

INDICATIONS

The indications for thoracentesis can be either therapeutic, to remove fluid that is causing pain or respiratory distress, or diagnostic, to determine the cause of the pleural effusion. The diagnosis of pleural effusion should be established by clinical examination and chest radiograph. A lateral decubitus film or ultrasonography is useful in identifying small effusions and determining whether the pleural fluid is free flowing or loculated.

CONTRAINDICATIONS

The following are relative contraindications to thoracentesis:

- Uncooperative patient (consider procedural sedation).
- Skin infection at the site of needle or catheter insertion.
- Bleeding disorder, disseminated intravascular coagulation.
- Small collection of fluid or pleural adhesions (increased danger of causing iatrogenic pneumothorax; consider doing the procedure under ultrasound guidance).

EQUIPMENT

Virtually all hospitals carry a commercially or locally made kit that contains most of the equipment needed for thoracentesis (Table 210-1).

ANATOMY AND PHYSIOLOGY

The pleural space is the potential space that exists between the visceral and parietal pleura in the lung. Normally, there is only a small amount (15 mL) of fluid in this space. Pleural fluid can accumulate when there is a systemic change in the forces that govern fluid production and drainage. The effusions can be classified as transudative (ultrafiltrates of plasma with a low protein concentration) or exudative (due to increased capillary permeability and the resulting accumulation of larger molecules). Common causes of transudative effusions in children are congestive heart failure, nephrotic syndrome, cirrhosis, and hypoalbuminemia. Exudative pleural effusions are usually caused by pneumonia (parapneumonic effusion), empyema, connective tissue disease, malignancy, pancreatitis, trauma, or pulmonary infarction.

PROCEDURE

The following method is recommended when there is a significant amount of free-flowing pleural fluid. In the case of a small or loculated effusion, it is better to perform the procedure with ultrasound guidance.

Preparation

- Explain the procedure to the child in an age-appropriate manner.
- Place an intravenous line if not already established; draw blood for protein, lactate dehydrogenase (LDH), glucose, and other studies as indicated.
- Continuously monitor heart rate, respiratory rate, oxygen saturation, and blood pressure.
- Administer supplemental oxygen as needed.
- Use procedural sedation as needed.

Thoracentesis is best performed with the child in the sitting position. The upright position ensures that the diaphragm is dependent and facilitates the removal of fluid that localizes at the base of the chest. Have the child lean over a pillow placed on a bedside table or over the back of a chair (Fig. 210-1). The patient's arms should be abducted and resting on the table. If the child is unable to sit, the procedure can be done with the child lying with the affected side down.

The thoracentesis site is determined on the basis of the chest radiograph and physical findings, with attention to the site of maximal dullness on percussion. A reasonable site is in the midscapular line in the intercostal space immediately below the tip of the scapula. This usually corresponds to the seventh intercostal space.

Technique

The area is prepared with povidone-iodine solution and draped with sterile towels. Raise a wheal of local anesthetic with a 25-gauge needle over the rib below the desired intercostal space. Remove the 25-gauge needle and substitute a 22-gauge needle. Enter perpendicular to the skin, injecting lidocaine into the periosteum. Slowly walk the needle above the rib and toward the pleural space while aspirating and injecting lidocaine (Fig. 210-2). Avoid the inferior rib area to prevent injury to the neurovascular bundle (intercostal artery, vein, and nerve), which runs in the groove in this location. Once pleural fluid is aspirated, mark the needle at the skin surface by clamping with a hemostat. Withdraw the needle and syringe.

Connect the 30-mL syringe to a 16- to 18-gauge angiocatheter using a three-way stopcock. Determine the depth of

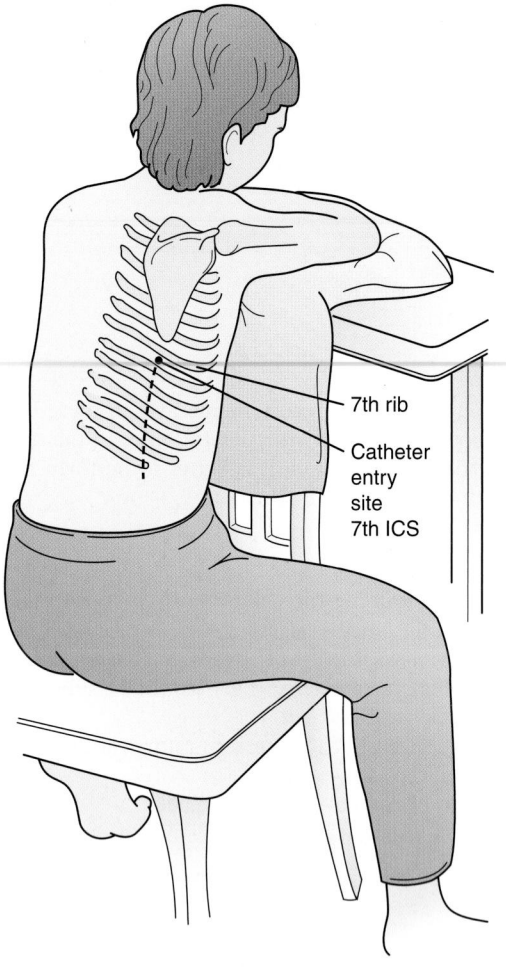

Figure 210-1 Patient position for thoracentesis. ICS, intercostal space.

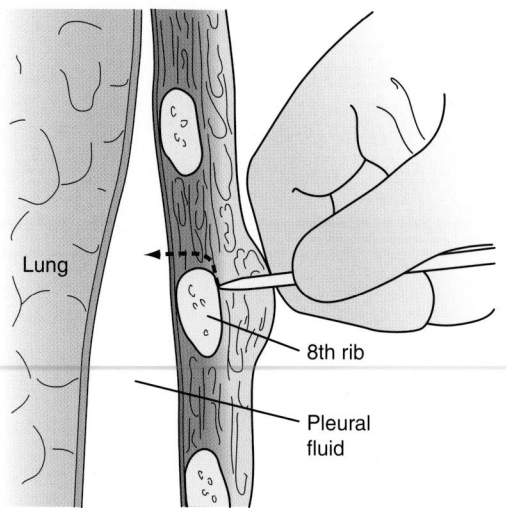

Figure 210-2 Technique of thoracentesis.

Table 210-1 Equipment Needed for Thoracentesis
Sterile gloves
Povidone-iodine solution
Sterile gauze, sterile dressing, tape to secure bandage
Sterile towels and drapes
Syringes—5 mL, 15-30 mL
25-, 22-gauge needles
14- to 22-gauge angiocatheter
1%-2% lidocaine
Three-way stopcock
Intravenous tubing, vacuum bottle (optional)
Sterile specimen collection bottles, blood gas syringe

insertion from the hemostat mark on the previously used needle, and enter the pleural space through the anesthetized area of the skin, with gentle negative pressure on the syringe. Once fluid is obtained, advance the needle by 1 to 2 mm to ensure that the catheter is in the pleural space, withdraw the needle, advance the catheter into the pleural space, and occlude the catheter with a fingertip. Attach the syringe with the stopcock to the catheter, and withdraw about 20 to 30 mL of fluid for diagnostic testing. A larger volume can be drained if the patient is in respiratory distress, using tubing attached to a vacuum bottle.

Once the appropriate amount of fluid is withdrawn, remove the catheter and apply a sterile dressing. Perform an upright chest radiograph immediately after the procedure to assess for possible pneumothorax.

PLEURAL FLUID TESTING

If pleural fluid is obtained for diagnostic purposes, the most important step is to decide whether the effusion is exudative or transudative. Pleural fluid analysis should include measurement of the following:

- Protein level (pleural-plasma protein ratio >0.5 implies exudate).
- LDH level (pleural-plasma LDH ratio >0.6 implies exudate).

Treatment of a transudative pleural effusion is directed at the underlying cause. If the fluid is exudative, additional tests must be considered based on the history and physical examination findings. The pH, glucose level, and Gram stain of the pleural fluid can help determine whether a parapneumonic effusion should be drained by tube thoracostomy. The differential diagnosis of a pleural effusion includes other diseases that may be apparent with additional testing such as cell count with differential, culture and sensitivity, cytology for malignant cells, and amylase, antinuclear antibody, and complement levels.

COMPLICATIONS

The most common major complication of thoracentesis is pneumothorax. Other potential complications include laceration of an intercostal neurovascular bundle and subsequent hemothorax, inadvertent puncture of subdiaphragmatic organs (e.g., liver, spleen), and local infection or pain.

Patients may also experience transient hypoxia associated with thoracentesis. Finally, hypotension or pulmonary edema can occur if too much fluid is removed too quickly. In an adult-sized patient, no more than 1000 to 1500 mL of fluid should be removed at a time. In children, one should avoid taking off more than a few hundred milliliters at one time.

SUGGESTED READING

DiGiulio GA: Thoracentesis. In Henretig FM, King C (eds): Textbook of Pediatric Emergency Procedures. Baltimore, Williams & Wilkins, 1997, pp 829-887.

CHAPTER 211

Paracentesis

Karen J. O'Connell

Paracentesis, also known as a peritoneal tap, is a procedure that involves aspiration of peritoneal fluid by entering the peritoneal cavity. In the early 1900s it was a popular diagnostic and therapeutic tool. Although its diagnostic capabilities remained strong, its therapeutic benefits fell out of favor from the mid-1900s until the late 1980s because of the increasing trend of medical management with diuretics. More recent studies have revitalized the use of paracentesis as a safe and effective means of diagnosing causes and controlling symptoms associated with ascites, the abnormal accumulation of fluid within the peritoneal cavity.

INDICATIONS

Abdominal paracentesis has both diagnostic and therapeutic usefulness. Diagnostic paracentesis is indicated in any patient with a new onset of ascites or in a patient with known ascites when there is concern for infection. Therapeutic paracentesis is directed at stabilizing any respiratory compromise caused by considerable collections of fluid. Large amounts of peritoneal fluid elevate the diaphragm and compromise lung capacity. Paracentesis is also indicated in the relief of abdominal pain caused by tense ascites.

CONTRAINDICATIONS

There are very few contraindications to paracentesis. Coagulopathy is a potential risk, but one that should not preclude the decision to perform this procedure. Given that many patients who require paracentesis will have a coagulopathy, bleeding complications are rare. In the only prospective study that evaluated complications of paracentesis, there was less than a 2% incidence of abdominal wall hematomas reported, even though 71% of the patients had an abnormal prothrombin time.[1] Routine administration of prophylactic blood products is not supported; instead, blood products should be reserved for patients who have clinical evidence of fibrinolysis and disseminated intravascular coagulation.[2] Patients who have undergone previous abdominal surgeries should be treated cautiously. Ultrasound guidance should be used in cases of suspected adhesions or bowel obstruction. Visible areas of engorged abdominal veins, surgical scars, and areas of cellulitis or infection should be avoided when performing paracentesis.

EQUIPMENT

Gown and face shield
Sterile gloves
Sterile drapes
Antiseptic solution
5- and 20-mL syringes
16- to 22-gauge standard metal or spinal needle—3 cm or longer, up to 8.9 cm in length (depending on patient size)
1% lidocaine (with or without epinephrine)
Sterile specimen tubes

PATHOPHYSIOLOGY

Several pathologic mechanisms can lead to the development of ascites, including alterations in hydrostatic pressure (e.g., congestive heart failure or hepatic venous obstruction), decreased colloid osmotic pressure (e.g., hypoproteinemia secondary to liver damage), disturbances in membrane permeability (e.g., inflammatory, genetic, metabolic, or neoplastic causes), lymphatic obstruction (e.g., congenital anomalies or trauma), genitourinary obstruction, and a ruptured viscus. A list of potential causes is presented in Table 211-1.

CLINICAL PRESENTATION

Patients who present with ascites may have symptoms as subtle as an increase in abdominal girth to the more severe symptoms associated with end-stage liver disease, which include but are not limited to gastrointestinal bleeding associated with portal hypertension, coagulopathies, hepatic encephalopathy, and nutritional deficiencies. Small amounts of ascites may be asymptomatic. With larger collections, an infant or child may present with a history of having abdominal distention or an increase in abdominal girth, an inverted umbilicus, a new hernia, or scrotal edema. They may have symptoms of abdominal fullness, nausea, abdominal pain, anorexia, and even respiratory distress with considerable collections of fluid. The diagnosis of ascites is often made by physical examination. The child may have bulging flanks in the supine position, shifting dullness to percussion when the child moves from supine to the lateral decubitus position, a positive fluid wave when the opposite flank is palpated, or peripheral edema. Abdominal radiographs and ultrasound may help with the diagnosis. Abdominal radiographs are helpful when larger amounts of fluid are present. The abdominal flat plate may have a ground-glass appearance with opacification of the flank margins or obscuring of the definition of the psoas muscle. Ultrasound is more sensitive at identifying free fluid in the abdominal cavity and can detect as little as 50 to 100 mL of free fluid. One study reported endoscopic ultrasonography to be more sensitive than computed tomography in detecting small amounts of ascites.[3] With small or loculated collections, ultrasound can

Table 211-1 Differential Diagnosis of Pediatric Ascites

Genitourinary
Bladder outlet obstruction
Ureteropelvic junction obstruction
Nephrotic syndrome

Gastrointestinal
Meconium peritonitis
Midgut volvulus
Congenital diaphragmatic hernia

Hepatobiliary
Portal hypertension
Biliary tract abnormalities/atresia
Primary biliary cirrhosis
Secondary cirrhosis/hepatic fibrosis
Autoimmune hepatitis
Tumors

Infectious
Peritonitis
    Spontaneous bacterial peritonitis
    Bacterial peritonitis secondary to perforations of the
        gastrointestinal tract
    Tuberculosis
    Fungal
    Hardware-associated peritonitis: peritoneal dialysis
        catheters, ventriculoperitoneal shunts
Hepatitis
    Hepatitis B, C, and D
    Cytomegalovirus
    Parvovirus
    Toxoplasmosis
    Syphilis
Chlamydia, *Neisseria gonorrhoeae* through the fallopian tubes

Cardiac
Congestive heart failure
    Arrhythmias
    Congenital heart disease
    Arteriovenous malformations

Metabolic
Galactosemia
Fructosemia
Tyrosinemia
Cystic fibrosis
Wilson disease
α_1-Antitrypsin deficiency
Gaucher disease
GM gangliosidosis

Chromosomal
Trisomy 21
Turner syndrome

Lymphatic
Thoracic duct obstruction

Other
Neoplasia
Malnutrition

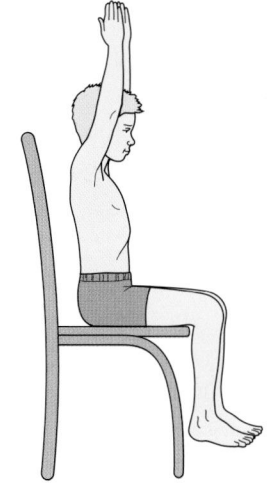

A   "Sitting" position

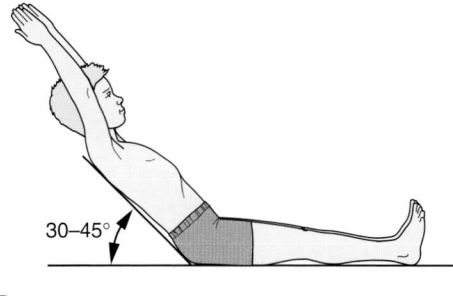

B   "Semi-supine" position

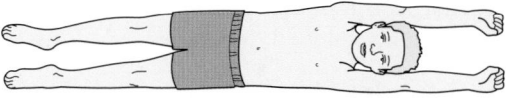

C   "Lateral decubitus" position

Figure 211-1 Drawing of a child seated in a 90-degree position on a chair with the arms held over the head (A), in the semireclined position with the arms held over the head (B), and lying on the left side with the arms held over the head (C).

be used to guide needle insertion during diagnostic or therapeutic paracentesis.

PREPARATION

First, to avoid potential bladder perforation, the bladder should be emptied (with a Foley catheter if necessary). If applicable, gastric distention should be ameliorated by insertion of a gastric tube. When choosing the optimal patient position, the goal is to make the tap location as dependent as possible. The patient should be placed in one of three recommended positions: semisupine with the head of the bed elevated at 30 to 45 degrees, supine with left lateral decubitus positioning, or sitting (Fig. 211-1). Patients in respiratory distress are most comfortable in the semisupine or sitting position. Patients with large volumes of ascites can be successfully tapped in the semisupine or sitting positions.

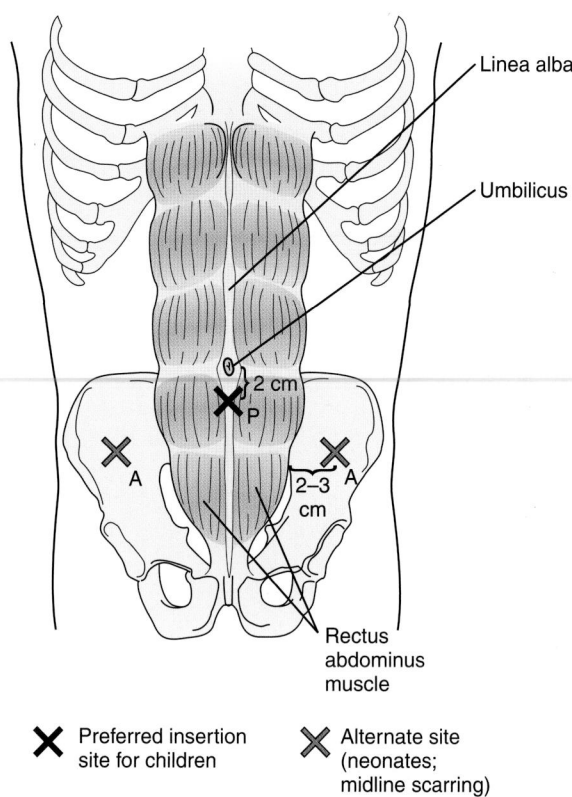

Figure 211-2 Paracentesis—needle insertion sites.

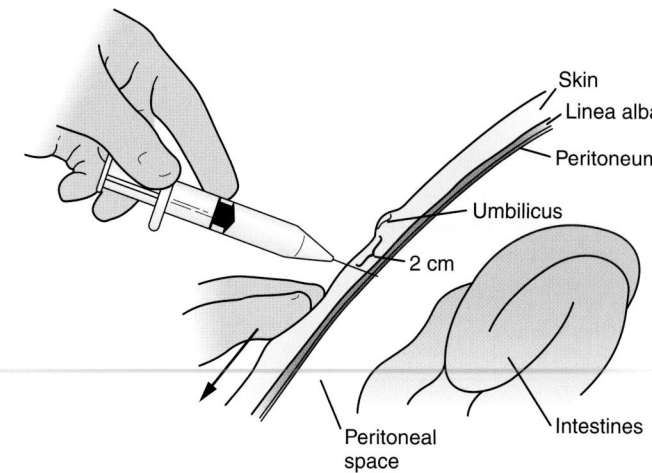

Figure 211-3 Two-tract formation. The skin is pulled approximately 2 cm caudally by the non–needle-bearing hand while the paracentesis needle is slowly inserted directly perpendicular to the skin.

Those with less fluid should be placed in the lateral decubitus position, with the lower left quadrant being the most dependent. Ultrasound guidance should be used for very small amounts of fluid.

SITE OF ENTRY

The paracentesis needle can be inserted at various sites (Fig. 211-2). In the semisupine and sitting positions, the preferred and most common site used in children is midline, approximately 2 cm below the umbilicus. In neonates and in patients with midline scarring, the needle should be inserted below the umbilicus and 2 to 3 cm lateral to the rectus abdominis muscle border (approximately 2 fingerbreadths cephalad and 2 fingerbreadths medial to the anterior superior iliac spine). This location should also be used for obese patients because their abdominal wall is thicker in the midline than in the lower quadrants. With the lateral decubitus approach, the needle should be introduced midline and below the umbilicus or into the dependent lower quadrant. Care should be taken to insert the needle lateral to the rectus sheath to avoid the inferior epigastric artery. Needle insertion in a pregnant patient should be above the umbilicus and lateral to the midline to avoid the uterus and major abdominal vessels.

PROCEDURE

Persons performing this procedure should comply with regulations for body fluid precautions. The patient should be draped and an area from above the umbilicus to the

symphysis pubis prepared in sterile fashion. Anesthetize the needle insertion site down to the peritoneum with 1% lidocaine (maximum infiltration dose, 7 mg/kg per dose for lidocaine with epinephrine, 4 mg/kg per dose for lidocaine without epinephrine, doses not to be repeated within 2 hours). A standard 3-cm (or longer 8.9-cm), 20- to 22-gauge metal needle with a 5-mL syringe attached is appropriate for diagnostic taps. For therapeutic taps, larger-bore needles allow better outflow. The use of smaller syringes (5 mL) with the initial insertion allows better control of the speed of fluid flow and the volume extracted. Larger syringes can then be attached for fluid collection. Plastic sheathed cannulas should be avoided because of their tendency to kink and obstruct flow once the needle is removed and because there is a risk of the plastic sheath being sheared off into the peritoneal cavity. The needle can be inserted directly perpendicular to the chosen site; however, the "Z-tract" method is more commonly used (Fig. 211-3). With this technique, the skin is pulled downward approximately 2 cm with the non–needle-bearing hand while the paracentesis needle is slowly inserted at a 30- to 45-degree angle. Slowly advance the needle in 5-mm increments to allow detection of blood if a vessel is entered. Manual suction should be applied intermittently to the syringe while advancing the needle. A slight "pop" may be felt, and fluid should enter the syringe freely when the peritoneum is entered. Do not release the skin until the needle has penetrated the peritoneum and fluid flow is established. Approximately 20 to 50 mL of peritoneal fluid should be sent for diagnostic evaluation, including cell count and differential, Gram stain, cultures (bacterial, fungal, viral as clinically indicated), total protein, glucose, albumin, lactate dehydrogenase, amylase, triglycerides, cytology, acid-fast bacillus smear, specific gravity, and other clinically appropriate tests. Interpretation of ascitic fluid is beyond the scope of this procedural review but can be found in the suggested references. When fluid aspiration is complete, remove the needle. The "Z-tract" insertion approach will allow the skin to return to its original position and seal the needle tract, thereby preventing peritoneal fluid leak. Dress the entry site with clean gauze and an adhesive bandage.

Unsuccessful peritoneal taps are often caused by incorrect patient positioning, technique, or needle size. If fluid is not obtained, reposition the patient and attempt the same approach or choose an alternative approach. The most common cause of unsuccessful paracentesis is technique. The needle is often inserted too rapidly with continuous aspiration applied. This can cause omentum or bowel to occlude the needle when the peritoneal cavity is pierced. Persons performing paracentesis may also try to aspirate from the needle too early, before the peritoneum is entered. The needle should be inserted slowly with intermittent aspiration until a "pop" is heard or a change in resistance is felt. If this "pop" or change in resistance does not occur, consider a longer needle. If paracentesis is still unsuccessful, use ultrasound guidance.

COMPLICATIONS

Complications from paracentesis are rare. With large amounts of peritoneal fluid removed, there is a risk of rapid fluid shifts with hypotension and hypovolemia. Close attention should be paid to fluid and electrolyte status during and after paracentesis. Administration of albumin intravenously at a replacement ratio of 6 to 8 g of albumin per liter of peritoneal fluid removed can help prevent these effects. Albumin replacement is considered optional for paracentesis of volumes greater than 5 L and is not recommended for lesser volumes. Other potential complications include intraperitoneal hemorrhage from perforation of the inferior epigastric artery, abdominal wall hematomas,[1] bowel perforation,[1,2] persistent leakage of fluid, infection at the entry site, and peritonitis.

SUGGESTED READING

Lane NE, Paul RI: Paracentesis. In Henretig FM, King C (eds): Textbook of Pediatric Emergency Procedures. Philadelphia, Williams & Wilkins, 1997, pp 921-926.

Marx JA: Peritoneal procedures. In Roberts JR, Hedges JR (eds): Clinical Procedures in Emergency Medicine, 4th ed. Philadelphia, WB Saunders, 2004, pp 851-856.

McVay PA, Toy PT: Lack of increased bleeding after paracentesis and thoracentesis in patients with mild coagulation abnormalities. Transfusion 1991;31:164-171.

Nguyen PT, Chang KJ: EUS in the detection of ascites and EUS-guided paracentesis. Gastrointest Endosc 2001;54:336-339.

Runyan BA: Paracentesis of ascitic fluid: A safe procedure. Arch Intern Med 1986;146:2259-2261.

Runyon BA: Ascites and spontaneous bacterial peritonitis. In Feldman M, Friedman LS, Sleisenger MH (eds): Feldman, Sleisenger and Fordtran's Gastrointestinal and Liver Disease: Pathophysiology/Diagnosis/Management, 7th ed. Philadelphia, WB Saunders, 2002, pp 1519-1527.

Yu AS, Hu K: Management of ascites. Clin Liver Dis 2001;5:541-568.

REFERENCES

1. Runyan BA: Paracentesis of ascitic fluid: A safe procedure. Arch Intern Med 1986;146:2259-2261.
2. McVay PA, Toy PT: Lack of increased bleeding after paracentesis and thoracentesis in patients with mild coagulation abnormalities. Transfusion 1991;31:164-171.
3. Nguyen PT, Chang KJ: EUS in the detection of ascites and EUS-guided paracentesis. Gastrointest Endosc 2001;54:336-339.

CHAPTER 212

Arthrocentesis

Eron Y. Friedlaender

Arthrocentesis, the puncture and aspiration of a joint, can be both a diagnostic and a therapeutic tool in the assessment of musculoskeletal disease and trauma. Often this procedure can be done at the bedside using local anesthesia, without radiographic guidance or significant risk to the patient.

INDICATIONS

The diagnostic indications for arthrocentesis include confirmation of either nontraumatic joint disease or ligamentous or bony injury. The former includes the identification of infectious or immunologic markers in the synovial fluid. In contrast, the presence of blood in the joint space affirms traumatic injury; more specifically, the finding of blood and fat globules may be used to identify an intra-articular fracture.

The therapeutic indications for arthrocentesis include pain relief secondary to a tense effusion or hemarthrosis and the direct instillation of anti-inflammatory medications for the management of severe rheumatic arthritides.

CONTRAINDICATIONS

The only absolute contraindication to arthrocentesis is infection in tissues overlying the puncture site—that is, a skin abscess or cellulitis. Relative contraindications to the procedure include bacteremia, because it may facilitate the spread of infection to the joint space; active anticoagulation; and joint prostheses. In addition, bleeding diatheses should be corrected with appropriate factor or blood product replacement before arthrocentesis to prevent a significant hemarthrosis.[1-4]

EQUIPMENT

Table 212-1 lists the equipment needed to perform arthrocentesis.

ANATOMY

Successful arthrocentesis begins with a careful examination of the affected joint and familiarity with the local anatomy. Palpable bony landmarks are most often used to identify the insertion site, and knowledge of the location of tendons, nerves, and blood vessels is essential to avoid potential complications. As a rule, arthrocentesis of any joint is more safely done on extensor surfaces to avoid the majority of neurovascular and tendinous structures. In addition, the synovial membrane tends to lie more superficially on extensor surfaces compared with flexor surfaces.

PROCEDURE

Preparation

Sterile technique is mandatory to reduce the risk of iatrogenic joint infection. Prepare the site using an antiseptic surgical scrub followed by alcohol. Avoid introducing povidone-iodine (Betadine) into the joint space, because it may precipitate an inflammatory reaction. Next, position the joint such that the opening to the joint space is maximized.

Anesthetize the skin at the needle insertion site with either a vapor coolant or application of a topical lidocaine preparation. Infiltrate the skin and subcutaneous tissues with 1% or 2% lidocaine using a small-gauge needle, taking care not to introduce anesthetic into the joint space, which might affect subsequent synovial fluid analysis.

Technique

Insert an 18- or 20-gauge needle attached to an empty sterile syringe into the joint space at 10 to 20 degrees above the horizontal. Enter the joint in one fluid motion along a straight line; side to side manipulation of the needle risks

Table 212-1 Equipment Needed for Arthrocentesis
Antiseptic solution (iodine, povidone-iodine [Betadine])
Sterile drapes
Sterile gloves
Alcohol wipes
Sterile gauze dressings (2 × 2 inch)
Sterile tubes for fluid collection
Test tubes (red top and lavender top)
18- or 20- gauge, 1.5-inch needles
Topical anesthetic
1% lidocaine solution
Bandage and dressing

Study	Normal	Septic Arthritis	Inflammatory Arthritis	Traumatic Arthritis	Lyme Disease
Appearance					
Color	Clear-yellow	White-gray	Xanthochromic-white	Gross blood	Xanthochromic-white
Clarity	Translucent	Turbid	Translucent-opaque	Opaque	Translucent-opaque
WBC count					
Total (mm^3)	0-200	50,000-300,000	3000-50,000		<1000-300,000
Differential	<25% PMNs	>90% PMNs	>70% PMNs		>60% PMNs
Gram stain	No bacteria	50% with bacteria	No bacteria	No bacteria	No bacteria
Culture	No growth	65% bacterial growth	No growth	No growth	No growth

Table 212-2   Synovial Fluid Evaluation

PMN, polymorphonuclear lymphocyte; WBC, white blood cell.

permanent damage to the articular cartilage. Draw back on the syringe plunger as the needle is advanced until fluid flows easily into the syringe. Synovial fluid collected for culture must be placed in a sterile vial, fluid collected for a cell count requires a specimen tube containing EDTA, and fluid sent for crystal analysis requires a tube prepared with sodium heparin. Table 212-2 highlights synovial fluid analysis for the most common causes of joint effusions in the pediatric population.[3,5-10]

Once the procedure is completed, dress the needle site and wrap the joint to prevent reaccumulation of intra-articular fluid.

COMPLICATIONS

There are few complications associated with arthrocentesis; however, there is a small risk of joint infection, bleeding into the joint space, hypersensitivity reaction to the local anesthetic, and permanent cartilage damage if the articular surface is nicked or scraped by the needle.

REFERENCES

1. Benjamin G: Arthrocentesis. In Roberts J, Hedges J (eds): Clinical Procedures in Emergency Medicine. Philadelphia, WB Saunders, 1998, pp 919-932.
2. Clark M, Rothrack S: Athrocentesis. In Henretig F, King C (eds): Textbook of Pediatric Emergency Procedures. Baltimore, Williams & Wilkins, 1997, pp 1063-1074.
3. Staheli L: Fundamentals of Pediatric Orthopedics. Philadelphia, Lippincott-Raven, 1998, p 17.
4. Fleisher G, Henretig F (eds): Textbook of Pediatric Emergency Medicine. Philadelphia, Lippincott Williams & Wilkins, 2000, pp 1872-1873.
5. McCarty D: Synovial fluid. In Koopman WJ (ed): Arthritis and Allied Conditions. Baltimore, Williams & Wilkins, 1997, pp 81-102.
6. Eichenfield AH, Goldsmith DP, Benach JL, et al: Childhood Lyme arthritis: Experience in an endemic area. J Pediatr 1986;109:753-758.
7. Culp RW, Eichenfield AH, Davidson RS, et al: Lyme arthritis in children. J Bone Joint Surg 1987;69:96-99.
8. Gerber MA, Zemel LS, Shapiro ED: Lyme arthritis in children: Clinical epidemiology and long-term outcomes. Pediatrics 1998;102:905-908.
9. Bachman DT, Srivastava G: Emergency department presentations of Lyme disease in children. Pediatr Emerg Care 1998;14:356-361.
10. Willis AA, Widman RF, Flynn JM, et al: Lyme arthritis presenting as acute septic arthritis in children. J Pediatr Surg 2003;23:114-118.

CHAPTER 213

Cerebrospinal Fluid Shunt Assessment

Christine S. Cho and Jill C. Posner

Cerebrospinal fluid (CSF) shunt systems are used to treat hydrocephalus by draining excess CSF to an alternative location in the body. A shunt has three segments: a proximal catheter, a valve and reservoir or reservoirs, and a distal catheter. The proximal catheter is commonly placed in a ventricle of the brain, but it may also be placed in a cyst. The valve of the shunt system controls the drainage of CSF. Some examples of valve mechanisms include regulation by differential pressure, siphon resistance (which prevents overdrainage in the upright position), flow regulation (in which different flow rates change the regulation mechanism), and external adjustment. Shunt systems often have one or two reservoirs (sometimes referred to as bubbles) that can be either part of or separate from the valve. CSF can be accessed from the reservoir to help diagnose shunt infection or malfunction (see Chapter 214). The distal catheter is commonly inserted into the peritoneal cavity, but it can also be placed in the right atrium, pleural cavity, and rarely the gallbladder or ureters.

INDICATIONS

Evaluation of a CSF shunt is indicated when the clinical history and physical examination suggest the diagnosis of shunt malfunction or shunt infection, or both. Because the symptoms of shunt malfunction may be subtle or nonspecific, the clinician should always keep malfunction in the differential when evaluating a child with a CSF shunt. In infants and preverbal children, the symptoms (Table 213-1) may be difficult to differentiate from those of other diseases. The parental history is valuable for giving the practitioner an understanding of the patient's baseline, as well as perspective on how shunt malfunction normally manifests in the child.

Shunt infection is most common in the first few months after placement or revision of a shunt. CSF shunts that end in the peritoneal cavity can also become infected from a primary abdominal infection. Symptoms of shunt infection include those of shunt malfunction, as well as fever and erythema or edema of the skin along the shunt site. Please see Chapter 71 for further discussion of device-related infections.

CONTRAINDICATIONS

There are no contraindications to evaluation of a CSF shunt.

PROCEDURE

The majority of CSF shunt assessment is done through the history, physical examination, and radiologic studies. The history should include an assessment of the type and location of the shunt and its reservoir or reservoirs. Common signs on physical examination that suggest shunt malfunction are listed in Table 213-2. The shunt can also be evaluated by pumping the reservoir (Table 213-3). This procedure should be interpreted cautiously because it is not a sensitive method of detecting shunt malfunction.

To pump a single-reservoir shunt, compress the reservoir bubble and note the refilling time. Difficulty in compression of the bubble suggests distal obstruction, whereas delay of more than 1 second in refilling suggests proximal obstruction. In a double-reservoir shunt, first compress and hold the proximal bubble and then compress the distal bubble. Difficulty compressing the distal reservoir suggests distal shunt obstruction. Then release the proximal bubble while holding pressure on the distal one. Sluggish refilling of the proximal reservoir suggests proximal obstruction.

If patients are clinically stable, radiologic studies are useful adjuncts to the clinical history and physical examination in diagnosing shunt malfunction. A shunt series is a series of radiographs that follow the course of the shunt from the skull to its distal end. The tubing is visualized by these radiographs and inspected for disconnection or kinks. In addition to the shunt series, a computed tomography (CT) scan of the head will evaluate ventricular size. To assess whether the ventricles are enlarged, compare them with a previous baseline CT. Rarely, shunt systems can be evaluated with radionuclide studies. Radioactive material is injected and followed as it flows through the shunt system.

After these initial steps in the assessment of CSF shunt systems, if necessary, the shunt can be punctured to measure pressure and obtain a sample of CSF for laboratory testing (see Chapter 214).

COMPLICATIONS

Pumping the reservoir may cause obstruction of the shunt by trapping choroid plexus or debris in the shunt tubing.

Failure to recognize the signs and symptoms of shunt malfunction may lead to progressive deterioration of a patient's clinical status. Patients with signs of impending herniation need immediate intervention.

Table 213-1 Symptoms of Shunt Malfunction
Headache
Change in vision
Nausea
Vomiting
Behavioral or personality change
Sleepiness
Irritability
Change in mental status
Abnormal gait
Seizures

Table 213-2 Physical Examination Findings in Patients with Shunt Malfunction
Sleepiness or lethargy
Hypotonia
Macrocephaly
Split sutures
Bulging fontanelle
Sunsetting
Sixth cranial nerve palsy
Papilledema (late finding)
Decreased visual acuity
Palpable kinks, fluid collections, or disconnections along the shunt
Abdominal mass or tenderness (suggesting distal CSF fluid collection that impedes resorption)

Table 213-3 Manual Assessment of Ventriculoperitoneal Shunt Function	Distal Obstruction	Proximal Obstruction
Single reservoir	Resistance felt when pressure is applied to the reservoir during attempt to compress it	Delayed filling of reservoir when pressure is released after compression of this reservoir*
Double reservoir	Resistance felt when pressure is applied to the distal reservoir during attempt to compress it after the proximal reservoir is compressed and held down	Delayed filling of proximal reservoir when pressure is released while still holding down the distal reservoir*

*Delayed filling would also occur when the ventricle is well drained and therefore cerebrospinal fluid would not be flowing into the shunt.

SPECIAL CONSIDERATIONS

Slit-ventricle syndrome may decrease the utility of CT in evaluating shunt malfunction. Because of chronic overdrainage, these patients will have normal or small ventricles despite shunt malfunction.

SUGGESTED READING

Albright AL, Pollack IF, Adelson PD: Principles and Practice of Pediatric Neurosurgery. New York, Thieme, 1999.

Raimondi AJ: Pediatric Neurosurgery: Theoretical Principles—Art of Surgical Technique, 2nd ed. New York, Springer, 1998.

CHAPTER 214

Cerebrospinal Fluid Shunt Puncture

Christine S. Cho and Jill C. Posner

The first steps in evaluating the function of a cerebrospinal fluid (CSF) shunt are a careful history, physical examination, and radiologic evaluation of the shunt system (see Chapter 213). Shunt infection and malfunction can also be assessed by puncture of the shunt reservoir with a needle to measure pressure and obtain CSF for laboratory testing.

INDICATIONS

Indications for CSF shunt puncture include (1) direct measurement of CSF pressure, (2) drainage of excess CSF, (3) obtaining a sample of CSF for laboratory evaluation, and (4) infusion of antibiotic or chemotherapeutic drugs. Obtaining CSF is especially useful when a culture is needed to evaluate for shunt infection.

CONTRAINDICATIONS

Infection of the skin overlying the reservoir is a contraindication to CSF shunt puncture.

PROCEDURE

1. Assemble the equipment (Table 214-1).
2. Identify the type of shunt, location of the reservoir or reservoirs, and preferred tapping site. Shunt reservoirs

Table 214–1 Equipment for CSF Shunt Puncture

Scissors
Povidone-iodine solution
Sterile gloves
Sterile gown
Mask
Sterile drapes or towels
Butterfly needle (23 or 25 gauge)
Pressure manometer (optional)
Syringe
Sterile tubes for CSF
Sterile dressing

may be located on the ventricular catheter, on the valve, or both (see Chapter 213).

3. If necessary, cut the hair over the area of the reservoir to be tapped.
4. Prepare the skin over the reservoir with povidone-iodine solution.
5. Wash your hands and put on a mask, sterile gown, and sterile gloves.
6. Lay sterile drapes to create a sterile field in which to perform the puncture.
7. Puncture the reservoir with the butterfly needle. Dome-shaped bubble reservoirs should be punctured at approximately a 45-degree angle to the skin. Reservoirs on the ventricular catheter should be punctured at a 90-degree angle to the skin.
8. Hold the butterfly tubing perpendicular to the floor at the level of the ear. The pressure in cm H_2O is the height of the CSF fluid column in the tubing. Alternatively, a manometer can also be attached.
9. Observe the flow of CSF and whether it is absent, slow, or fast.
10. Brisk flow and/or high opening pressure indicates distal obstruction. Slow or absent flow and/or decreased opening pressure indicates proximal obstruction in the setting of dilated ventricles on computed tomography.
11. Remove fluid into sterile tubes for culture and laboratory assessment.
12. If needed, continue to drain CSF by using the measured pressure as a guide.
13. Remove the butterfly needle and apply dressing.

COMPLICATIONS

Puncture of a CSF shunt can cause local infection of the skin or introduce infection into CSF. Complications also include bleeding, hematoma, CSF leakage at the site of puncture, and possible damage to the reservoir or valve, or both.

SPECIAL CONSIDERATIONS

No special considerations need be taken with CSF shunt puncture.

CHAPTER 215

Child Development for Inpatient Medicine

Deirdre Caplin and Maura Cooper

Childhood is by definition a time of continuous growth and change. Child development proceeds along complex but predictable pathways, and there is great variability within the normal range.[1,2] Just as constant cognitive, social, emotional, and physical changes reflect the growing child, so does the forward process of development demand an educated flexibility in the physician's approach to each child. Children's health needs change with development, and the care delivered is better when medical assessment and treatment are considered within the context of the general developmental stage.[3,4]

Early life experience is tremendously important in shaping children's intellectual, emotional, and social development.[1,2] Many children treated in hospitals are socioeconomically disadvantaged and therefore more vulnerable to developmental delay. Because as many as a third of parents of young children report never having discussed key developmental issues with their child's physician or health care professional, rapid but accurate developmental assessment of hospitalized children is an excellent means of identifying those in need of early intervention.[3]

Human development is a highly dynamic process. By school starting age there is great individual variation in the behavior and cognitive function considered normal.[2,5] Just as expectations of children change with their age, so should the care they receive. The developmental stages of childhood generally considered include

- Infancy—1 to 12 months
- Early childhood—1 to 5 years
- Middle childhood—6 to 10 years
- Adolescence—11 to 17 years

MAKING DEVELOPMENTAL SURVEILLANCE EASY IN MEDICAL SETTINGS

Typically, children are monitored in the domains of cognitive, language, social/emotional, and physical (gross and fine motor) development. Within the context of the clinical encounter, there are numerous ways to screen developmental status.[4]

Play is a natural form of communication for children and can provide a wealth of information to any observant clinician. A few "play props" such as a small box of 1-inch cubes will provide an easy method for obtaining "data" about developmental status. Coloring/drawing activities and stethoscope play (see Table 215-1) are other readily accessible methods of gathering developmental physical data.[5]

Observation of a child's normal activity can assist you in tracking motor status. Allowing a child free movement provides an easy opportunity to observe motor skills.[4,5] Observing parent-child interactions also provides a great deal of information about how the child is developing socially, how well the parent can read a child's signals, and where a child's communication skills are. For example, in the average 8-month-old, physician presence is likely to create some initial distress. Try to observe how the child responds to stress and how the parent responds to the child.

When working with older children, asking "benign" questions about interests, getting them to tell jokes, or asking them to explain things are all easy ways to assess cognitive understanding of a child's life, hospitalization, and health status.

Cognitive Development

Cognitive development is a significant factor shaping a child's attitudes, beliefs, and behavior, as well as overall adjustment to disease, injury, and illness.[6] A basic understanding of cognitive developmental processes provides the necessary context to consider how children formulate ideas about their own health and illness. In fact, it has been shown that cognitive developmental status predicts childhood understanding of disease and medical procedures better than age or other variables do.[6]

According to Piaget's theory, children form and alter *schemas* to meet the ever-changing needs of environmental demands and new experiences. In Piaget's theory, children progress through stages of development, each with tasks necessary for cognitive progression to the next stage. Table 215-2 summarizes the Piagetan progression of cognition and the impact that it has on understanding illness.

Assessing a child's gross cognitive status is relatively easy if you are a good observer. Sometimes, having children explain their disease or asking them to define words will give you a window into their understanding. Table 215-3 provides some basic guidelines for assessing cognitive abilities without the formal information provided by psychological or educational assessment.

Social and Emotional Development

The development of adequate social and emotional skills is one of the most complex and critical tasks of childhood. Children with poor social or emotional regulation struggle with daily tasks, as well as with acute events such as illness or hospitalization. In addition, social development is interdependent on other streams of development and may be inhibited because of delay in another area, such as language skill. Conversely, children who are articulate and advanced might have social skills that make them stand out when compared with same-age peers.[7]

In the medical setting, adherence, adjustment to disease and illness, and family adaptation are all correlated to the social and emotional abilities of a chronically ill child.[6,8] Social and emotional strength, when present, makes children resilient to the stress of acute and chronic disease manage-

Table 215-1 Developmental Progression of Stethoscope Play

Action	Age
Regards at midline	Birth-1 month
Follows to at least 90 degrees	2-6 weeks
Swipes at it	2-4 months
Reaches for it	4-5 months
Brings it to the mouth	5-8 months
Reaches across midline	6-8 months
Pivots to get it while seated	8-11 months
Unilateral reach	9-11 months
Examines parts of it	12-15 months
Imitates use	15-19 months
Pretends with others	2 years
Knows where the heart is and perhaps what it does	3-5 years

Adapted from Dixon S, Stein M: Encounters with Children: Pediatric Behavior and Development, 4th ed. St Louis, CV Mosby, 2006, p 314.

ment.[8,9] Social and emotional difficulties often interfere with good disease management practices and may sabotage physician efforts at managing medical difficulties in both acute and chronic care.[10-12]

To be aware of what children are capable of emotionally and what they can expect from children in the clinical setting, physicians should be familiar with the basic social and emotional milestones in development.[4] Table 215-4 provides a brief overview of the major developmental tasks associated with various ages.

Language and Speech Development

Language is one of the more awesome human achievements, and it universally develops at an astonishing rate with little apparent effort. Language is part of a broader set of *communication* skills that involve a complex combination of speech content and character (e.g., intonation), nonverbal gestures, attention, and comprehension skills. These skills are thought to be the building blocks for socialization, memory formation, achievement, and learning. Table 215-5 outlines what can be expected in terms of speech development at various ages.

In medicine, patient-provider communication involves understanding the level at which your patient can communicate effectively to you and is vital to quality patient care.[3] Asking children about their symptoms plus explaining regimens in ways that are understandable requires a fundamental understanding of the basic developmental milestones of expressive and receptive communication.

Motor Development

Beginning with neonatal reflexes, the development of gross and fine motor skills is a process of extreme variability, both in the *rate* of maturation and in the *way* that skills

are achieved.[13] The range of what is normal development is wide, especially in early childhood.

Despite this variability, there are constants in motor development that are predictable and largely universal. For example, reflexive movement always precedes voluntary movement, proximal control always precedes distal control, and pronation always precedes supination.[14] In addition, children will develop the ability for a particular action before they are able to inhibit it; if they begin to run, it may take a few falls before they learn how to stop.

Monitoring plus awareness of motor development is important for early detection of problems such as developmental delays, as well as physical or neurosensory disorders.[13] These tasks are easily contrived in most settings and are observable and recordable. Tables 215-6 and 215-7 outline expected motor milestones for both fine and gross motor skills, with special attention paid to age "at risk" for a developmental problem.[5,15-17]

ASSESSING DEVELOPMENT

Sensitivity and understanding of development are helpful in treatment but are not typically the focus of inpatient care. A developmentally appropriate approach to care will strengthen the physician-patient relationship and the quality of care delivered. However, formal developmental assessment is often not reasonable in a busy inpatient setting.

Despite its complexity, development may be rapidly and rather easily evaluated as part of every examination with the tools presented in this chapter. Parents are an excellent source of information about development because most know what their child can do if asked. In addition to parents, Dixon and Stein note that "children will [often] do their own developmental assessment" if given the opportunity.[5] Presenting pediatric patients with a means of communication (i.e., a toy, a crayon, a tongue blade or stethoscope, a challenge) will facilitate children letting practitioners know what they are capable of and how they think. The key to success is often knowing what to look for and knowing how to interpret one's observations. As one developmental expert stated, "A knowledge of child development allows us to be efficient and even downright lazy as we get the child and family to do all the work."[5]

DEVELOPMENTAL REGRESSION DURING HOSPITALIZATION

Hospitalization is a major stressor for children of every age. With admission, the child's familiar and typically nurturing environment is suddenly lost. Parents are, at least partially, replaced by strange new caregivers. The attachments to parents that every child depends on in times of stress are altered. Moreover, no matter how welcoming, the hospital is a supremely foreign environment: a different bed, room, and routine from what is regular for the child. Children often communicate their stress through changes in behavior, sometimes dramatically.

Developmental regression is a common response to hospitalization. It involves the loss of developmental milestones during and after hospitalization. There are a variety of factors that determine each child's regression in response to hospitalization:

Table 215–2 Piagetan Understanding of Illness and Pain

Piagetan Stage	Age Range	Developmental Tasks/Status	Understanding of Illness	Concept of Pain
Sensorimotor period	0-2 years	**Status:** Developing schemas to integrate and organize motor movements with sensory input from the environment **Task:** Intentional goal-directed behavior	No real understanding of illness	Expressions of pain show little variability (cry/whimper) Little or no understanding of what pain is
Preoperational period	2-7 years	**Status:** Concrete thinking, irreversibility of experiences, fantasy-reality confusion, egocentrism, no ability to generalize **Task:** Generation of a hierarchic internal cognitive structure based on permanence and conservation	Illness is a sensory experience Cause is magical and illogical (often co-occurs temporally with onset) Illness is a unique (egocentric) and particular experience (not generalizable)	Pain is an uncontrollable physical, external entity Appear unaware of the affective aspects of pain or the concept of internal pain Pain relief is magical and not controllable
Concrete operational period	7-11 years	**Status:** Temporal and spatial understanding, reversibility, conservation all present. This allows for distinction between fantasy and reality and ability for rule orientation **Task:** Ability for logical thinking but still in concrete and experiential context	Only 6% of 7- to 9-year-olds have an accurate understanding of their illnesses The source of illness is seen as external and concrete, and control is related to avoidance Able to describe causes in terms of body processes such as inhalation and swallowing Understand that these processes directly affect internal systems Appreciate the reversibility of illness and healing	Understanding includes physical and affective awareness of pain Develop understanding of reversibility of pain (can do things to make it go away) Develop awareness of qualitative and quantitative variability of pain Begin to understand the unpredictability of onset and duration of pain Pain as something you *feel* rather than *have*
Formal operational period	11+ years	**Status:** Thinking reflects logical causality with the ability for both inductive and deductive reasoning **Task:** Understanding of hypothetical and abstract events	Define illness in terms of internal organs and functions that are not visible Able to perceive multiple causes and cures Understand that their own actions can influence the disease process Able to differentiate between physical and psychological domains of self Aware that thoughts and feelings can affect how the body functions	Concept of pain reflects capacity for abstraction and introspection Subjective nature of pain becomes prominent Decreased emphasis on the physical aspects of pain Descriptions of pain increase in complexity with age

- The child's level of development before hospitalization
- The child's ability to separate from parents before the hospitalization
- The length of separation
- The child's unique, inborn temperament
- The child's coping style
- The characteristics of the illness or injury
- The child's own imagination and perspective with regard to the illness
- Family interaction style
- Responsiveness of hospital staff

Developmental regression is an expected and self-protective response to hospitalization across all age groups.

Table 215-3 Major Cognitive Milestones

Average Developmental Age	Cognitive Tasks	Age at Which Absence of Skill Is a "Red Flag"
1.5 months	Notices own hands	2.5 months
2 months	Tracks moving objects with eyes	3 months
3 months	Brings objects to mouth	4 months
8 months	Searches for hidden object	12 months
9 months	Uses gestures to indicate thoughts (pointing, shaking "no," waving)	12 months
12 months	Imitates correct use of objects (cup, brush, etc.)	15 months
12 months	Explores new object uses (shake, throw, pull, etc.)	18 months
20 months	Can give you "one" of something if asked	24 months
24 months	Begins make-believe play	36 months
30 months	Knows own full name	5 years
36 months	Sorting by shapes and colors	4 years
36 months	Pick shorter or longer of 2 lines	4 years
36 months	Can follow 2-step directions	4 years
4 years	Count sequentially from 1 to 10	5 years
4.5 years	Knows colors and at least 5 letters	5 years
4.5 years	Can fully dress self	5 years
5 years	Knows own birthday or address	6 years
5 years	Does simple addition	6 years
5.5 years	Reads 4 or more words	7 years
6 years	Understands common jokes/humor	7 years
7 years	Able to provide directions	11 years
12 years	Able to use deductive reasoning in problem solving	16 years
12 years	Uses abstraction as method of communication and logical reasoning	16 years

It is a healthy way for many children to cope with the hospital experience and typically resolves when daily patterns and activities return to normal. An age-related approach to the behavioral changes associated with hospitalization highlights the continuum of development.

The Infant

Infants younger than 6 months may actually recognize their primary caregiver or caregivers as distinguished from the strangers typically caring for them in the hospital. However, few behavioral changes are noted with hospitalization at this age, and young infants generally reestablish relationships with parents quickly after hospital discharge.

The Toddler

In a toddler, behavioral changes associated with hospitalization are both more pronounced and more prolonged than in younger infants. A toddler is both wary of strangers and anxious about the separation from parents. Toddlers are acutely aware of the new hospital environment. The entire process of hospitalization is threatening and difficult. There is a predictable progression of behavioral change in hospitalized toddlers:

Stage I—Protest reaction (tantrums, regression)
Stage II—Despair (quiet, sad, withdrawn)
Stage III—Denial (outgoing, but with a flat affect and constricted emotional range)

The Preschooler

Preschool-aged children may tolerate separation from parents for longer periods than toddlers might. At this age children have a broader cognitive repertoire and can grasp the idea that an absent parent will return. However, their more highly developed memory and imagination may lead to magical thinking regarding their illness. Children at this age may develop their own causal hypotheses for their illness and their role in it: "I was bad, so I got sick. If I am good, I will get better."

Table 215-4   Major Social and Emotional Milestones

Average Developmental Age	Social and Emotional Tasks	Age at Which Absence of Skill Is a "Red Flag"
Birth	Shows interest, disgust, and distress	Birth
4-6 weeks	Shows recognition of familiar people	2 months
6-8 weeks	Displays social smile	3 months
2 months	Stops crying with anticipation	4 months
3.5 months	Experiences anger, surprise, sadness	4 months
3 months	Shows a variety of facial expressions	4 months
3 months	Engages in interactive "play," laughing	7 months
6 months	Shows fear, shame, shyness	8 months
8 months	Appears wary of strangers	12 months
8 months	Distressed with caregiver, leaving/excited at return	12 months
9 months	Waves bye-bye or hello	12 months
10 months	Tests parent responses to new behavior	15 months
18 months	Reappearance of stranger anxiety	24 months
18 months	Shows defiance and need for independent behavior	24 months
24 months	Spontaneously expresses affection for family and others	4 years
24 months	Imitates adults and playmates	36 months
30 months	Can take turns in games	4 years
30 months	Objects to changes in routine	4 years
3 years	Fantasy and role-play: "I'm the mom"	4 years
3 years	Responds to people with wide range of emotions	5 years
3 years	Friendships based on convenience	6 years
3.5 years	Aware of own gender/sexuality	5 years
3.5 years	Able to separate from parents easily	5 years
3.5 years	Negotiates solutions to conflicts (makes deals)	4.5 years
4 years	Wants to please and be like friends	5 years
4 years	Tells stories, lies; relates day's events	5 years
6 years	Friendships based on common interests	8 years
7 years	Worries focus on school, health, and personal harm	9 years
8 years	Focus on rule-oriented games, competition	11 years
8 years	Friendship preference for same sex	12 years
8 years	Worries focus on friends and acceptance	11 years
11 years	Friendships based on companionship, understanding	14 years
11 years	Preference for friends over family members	15 years
12 years	Social awareness is more abstract than personal	16 years

Table 215-5   Major Speech and Language Milestones

Average Developmental Age	Speech and Language Tasks	Age at Which Absence of Skill Is a "Red Flag"
3 months	Vocalizes when hears speech	5 months
4 months	Babbling	6 months
7 months	Imitates syllables of language	9 months
7 months	Says "dada" or "baba"	10 months
8 months	Responds to his/her name	10 months
9 months	Points to indicate interest or desire	12 months
10 months	Repeats sounds/gestures for attention	12 months
12 months	Knows 1 word of meaning	14 months
14 months	Has at least 3 words of meaning	16 months
15 months	Attends to simple commands/gestures	18 months
20 months	Points to simple body parts	24 months
21 months	Uses 2-word phrases	24 months
24 months	Asks for common objects, food by name	30 months
24 months	Uses at least 1 personal pronoun	30 months
3.5 years	All speech is intelligible	4 years
3.5 years	Understands prepositions	4 years
4.5 years	Follows 3-step commands	5 years
4.5 years	Understands time sequences	5 years
4.8 years	Uses future, past, present tense correctly	5.3 years
5.5 years	Uses irregular nouns correctly	6 years
6 years	Can articulate things that have not yet happened	7.5 years
7 years	Appreciates multiple meanings of words, puns, metaphors	9 years
10 years	Can articulate logical sequence of abstract events (more effective arguing)	13 years
11 years	Understands irony and sarcasm	14 years
12 years	Refined grammatical structures such as the passive voice	15 years

The School-Aged Child

Fewer behavior problems are expected in school-aged children because they have acquired many cognitive skills that help them process the stress of hospitalization. They are capable of comprehending the cause of their illness. They may be able to participate constructively in the process of treatment and healing. Finally, children at this stage have emerging internal control over their behavior. The stresses of hospitalization can challenge this self-control and result in anxiety, depression, and even behavioral regression.

The Adolescent

In adolescence, illness may challenge the child's quest for identity with loss of the idealized self. Hospitalization and the external structure that it imposes may hinder the adolescent quest for independence. The somatic invasion associated with treatment may create a distortion of body image.

Although children in this age group possess the cognitive skills needed to understand the cause of their illness and the need for hospitalization and treatment, the disruption of present and perhaps future life may cause much psychic distress.

SUPPORTING THE HOSPITALIZED CHILD

- Before elective admission, have children tour the pediatric unit to acquaint them with the new environment. Anticipate the experience and encourage age-appropriate medical play and role-playing.
- Allow and encourage parents to room-in, as well as to visit liberally.
- Explain the need for hospitalization in an age-appropriate manner. Ask children why they think they are in the hospital.

Table 215-6 Gross Motor Development

Average Developmental Age	Gross Motor Tasks	Age at Which Absence of Skill Is a "Red Flag"
3 months	Pulls to sit Rolls over	5 months
6 months	Sits without support	7 months
7 months	Stands while holding on	9 months
12 months	Walking	14 months
17 months	Walking up stairs	21 months
24 months	Jumping with both feet	28 months
30 months	Standing on one foot momentarily	36 months
3.5 years	Hopping	4 years
4.5 years	Able to walk a straight line back and forth Able to balance on 1 foot for 5-10 seconds	5.5 years
5.5 years	Able to ride a 2-wheeled bike with training wheels Able to skip	6 years
6.5 years	Able to perform a "jumping jack" Able to repeat a physical sequence of movements	7 years
7.5 years	Able to engage in rhythmic hopping and movement Able to throw a ball >25 feet	8 years
9.5 years	Intercepts path of objects thrown from a distance Able to wash and dry own hair	11 years

Table 215-7 Fine Motor Development

Average Developmental Age	Fine Motor Tasks	Age at Which Absence of Skill Is a "Red Flag"
3 months	Holds rattle	4 months
6 months	Rakes food Passes object from one hand to the other	7 months
8 months	Has pincer grasp	10 months
12 months	Able to put object in/take out from a jar Scribbles	15 months
17 months	Removes socks or gloves alone	20 months
20 months	Stacks 5 blocks	24 months
22 months	Washes and dries hands Brushes teeth with help	30 months
30 months	Stacks 8 blocks Draws a straight line	36 months
3.5 years	Stacks 10 blocks Cuts with scissors Copies a circle	4 years
3.5 years	Copies a cross	4.5 years
4.5 years	Copies a square if demonstrated Picks longer of 2 lines	5 years
4.5 years	Builds a staircase of blocks Draws a picture of a person with at least 6 body parts	5.5 years
5.5 years	Copies a triangle Colors within the lines in a coloring book	6 years
6.5 years	Copies a diamond Shows good control and grasp of pencil, comb Able to use a knife to spread and cut	7 years
7 years	Able to use common household tools/utensils	8 years
9 years	Smoothing of perceptual motor coordination	12 years

- Tell the truth about painful procedures. "It will hurt for a moment," stated just before a painful procedure provides helpful preparation for a verbal child.
- Give the child as much control as possible. For example, allow the child to choose the site to draw blood from.
- Describe sensory information that the child will encounter as part of the procedure, such as the smell of the alcohol or the prick of the needle.
- Help the child develop effective coping strategies such as visualization, self-relaxation, and self-distraction. Develop an alliance with the child.

The goal of hospitalization is to promote healing of the body, as well as rapid recovery from the psychological impact of the admission. Careful attention to the developmental needs of the hospitalized child, as well as age-appropriate support, will optimize the outcome. Ideally, an ill and hospitalized child will emerge from the experience with accelerated development and increased self-esteem.

CONCLUSION

Child development is a complex process in which the domains of cognitive, language, social-emotional, and physical development are critically interrelated. Understanding this relationship and accurately assessing each child's developmental level are crucial to grasping the impact of hospitalization and illness on each child. Accurate developmental information facilitates children participating at an age-appropriate level in their own care, coping with hospitalization and illness, and developing mastery of an often stressful experience.[5]

SUGGESTED READING

Dixon S, Stein M: Encounters with Children: Pediatric Behavior and Development, 4th ed. St Louis, Mosby, 2006.
Frankenburg WK, Dodds J, Archer P, et al: The Denver II: A major revision and restandardization of the Denver Developmental Screening Test. Pediatrics 1992;89:91-97.

REFERENCES

1. Brazelton TB: Infants and Mothers: Differences in Development. New York, Dell, 1983.
2. Brazelton TB: Toddlers and Parents: A Declaration of Independence. New York, Dell, 1989.
3. Leatherman S, McCarthy D: Quality of Health Care for Children and Adolescents: A Chartbook. Chapel Hill, NC, University of North Carolina Program on Health Outcomes, 2004.
4. Green M (ed): Bright Futures: Guidelines for Health Supervision of Infants, Children, and Adolescents. Arlington, VA, National Center for Education in Maternal and Child Health, 1994.
5. Dixon S, Stein M: Encounters with Children: Pediatric Behavior and Development, 4th ed. St Louis, CV Mosby, 2006.
6. Thompson R, Gustafson K: Developmental Changes. Adaptation to Chronic Childhood Illness. Washington, DC, American Psychological Association, 1996, pp 177-224.
7. Timler GR: Reading emotion cues: Social communication difficulties in pediatric populations. Semin Speech Lang 2003;24:121-130.
8. De Civita M, Dobkin PL: Pediatric adherence as a multidimensional and dynamic construct, involving a triadic partnership. J Pediatr Psychol 2004;29:157-169.
9. Melnyk BM, Alpert-Gillis L, Feinstein NF, et al: Creating opportunities for parent empowerment: Program effects on the mental health/coping outcomes of critically ill young children and their mothers. Pediatrics 2004;113:e597-e607.
10. Alonso EM, Neighbors K, Mattson C, et al: Functional outcomes of pediatric liver transplantation. J Pediatr Gastroenterol Nutr 2003;37:155-160.
11. Phadke SM: Post-transplant complications. Pediatr Pulmonol Suppl 2004;26:119-120.
12. Mackner LM, Sisson DP, Crandall WV: Review: Psychosocial issues in pediatric inflammatory bowel disease. J Pediatr Psychol 2004;29:243-257.
13. American Academy of Pediatrics: Developmental competency. In Wolraich M, Felice M, Drotar D (eds): The Classification of Child and Adolescent Mental Diagnoses in Primary Care: Diagnostic and Statistical Manual for Primary Care (DSM-PC): Child and Adolescent Version. Elk Grove Village, IL, American Academy of Pediatrics, 1996, pp 59-89.
14. Touwen BC: The neurological development of prehension: A developmental neurologist's view. Int J Psychophysiol 1995;19:115-127.
15. Ireton HR: Child Development Inventory Manual. Minneapolis, MN, Behavior Science Systems, 1992.
16. Frankenburg WK, Dodds J, Archer P, et al: The Denver II: A major revision and restandardization of the Denver Developmental Screening Test. Pediatrics 1992;89:91-97.
17. von Hofsten C: Motor development as the development of systems. Comments on the special issue of developmental psychology on motor development. Dev Psychol 1989;25:950-953.

Index

Page numbers followed by f indicate figure(s); t, table(s); b, box(es).

Research—cont'd
   in pediatric hospital medicine, 107
   planning of project in, 96-98, 97b
Research networks, 17. *See also* Pediatric
      Research in Inpatient Settings
      (PRIS).
Reservoir nebulizer, 185t
Residents. *See also* Medical education.
   families' fear of, 89
   follow-up with discharged patients by, 94
   in hospitalist systems, 8, 49
   hospitalists as educators of, 105-106, 106t,
      113
   pursuing hospitalist careers, 107
   quality of care with, vs. hospitalists, 87
   reprimanded in front of family, 88
   staffing levels and, 76
   teaching evidence-based medicine to, 34-35
   transfers of patient to or from, 62t
   work-hour restrictions for, 4, 106
Residual volume, 507, 508f
Resource utilization. *See* Efficiency.
Resource-Based Relative Value System
      (RBRVS), 74-75
Respiratory. *See also* Breathing; Lung *entries*;
      Pulmonary *entries*.
Respiratory acidosis, 125, 126f, 131-132, 131t.
      See also Acidosis.
   in asthma, 465
   in bronchiolitis, 371
   regulatory impairment and, 218
Respiratory alkalosis, 126f
   in asthma, 465
   in chest pain with tachypnea or hyperpnea,
      144
   in hyperammonemia, 835, 839
Respiratory distress, 218-222. *See also*
      Choking.
   in croup, 375
   diagnostic studies in, 222
   differential diagnosis of, 218, 219t, 220t
   emergency department visits for, 218
   history in, 220, 221b
   initial stabilization in, 220
   in medically complex child, 1193, 1193t
   in newborn, 265-267
      clinical features of, 265
      with congenital diaphragmatic hernia,
         260-261
      differential diagnosis of, 266, 266t
      with peripheral nerve injury, 256
      with pneumothorax, 259
      vs. total anomalous pulmonary venous
         return, 537t, 543
      transfer to NICU in, 244, 267
   noisy breathing with, in infant, 902-903
   oxygen delivery for, 220, 220t
   paradoxical thoracoabdominal movement
      in, 465
   pathophysiology of, 218
   physical examination in, 220-222, 221b
   treatment of, 222
Respiratory distress syndrome
   acute, in near drowning, 1158, 1159, 1160
   persistent pulmonary hypertension in, 265
   surfactant deficiency in, 265
Respiratory droplets, pathogen transmission
      by, 28

Respiratory failure, 218
   chronic, positive-pressure ventilation in,
      1268, 1270
   in cystic fibrosis, 495, 496
   impending
      in asthma, 464, 465, 466t, 470, 472
      positive-pressure ventilation in, 1270
Respiratory infections. *See also* Bronchiolitis;
      Croup; Epiglottitis; Pharyngitis;
      Pneumonia.
   otitis media secondary to, 352
   sinusitis secondary to, 352, 359
Respiratory insufficiency, 218
Respiratory muscle strength, 508
Respiratory physiology, 218
Respiratory protection, 29, 30
Respiratory quotient, 181
Respiratory rate. *See also* Tachypnea.
   age and, 182t
   altitude and, 182t
   in cardiac examination, 514
   fever and, 220
   in newborn
      Apgar score and, 245t
      full-term, 248t
   ventilation and, 218
Respiratory syncytial virus (RSV)
   apparent life-threatening event with, 454,
      456, 459
   bacterial infection risk and, 317, 371
   bronchiolitis caused by. *See* Bronchiolitis.
   bronchopulmonary dysplasia and, 487, 489
   congenital heart disease and, 545-546
   croup caused by, 375
   immunoprophylaxis against, 373-374, 374t
   infection control for, 29t, 30, 373
   laboratory testing for, 370
   in organ transplant recipient, 446
Respiratory therapist, medically complex
      child and, 1190t
Restraining order, in suspected child abuse,
      89
Restraint of patient, 1056, 1057
   legal issues in, 92-93
   mechanical, 1056, 1059
   sedation for, 1056, 1057-1059, 1057f, 1058t
Restrictive cardiomyopathy, 564
Resuscitation. *See also* Advanced Life Support,
      Pediatric; Do-not-resuscitate
      (DNR) orders.
   ABCDs of
      in altered mental status, 133-136, 134f,
         135t
      in drug-of-abuse patient, 1137, 1138t
      in near drowning, 1159
      in poisoned patient, 1106t
   family presence at, 1201
   in hypothermia, 1155
   in near drowning, 1159
   of neonate. *See* Delivery room medicine,
      resuscitation in.
   of poisoned patient, 1105, 1106t
   religious beliefs and, 53
   research on outcomes of, 1200, 1201
   in shock, 178-179
   in trauma, 892
Reticular activating system, 133, 136, 137
Reticular dysgenesis, 739

Reticulocyte count, 723t
Reticulocytosis, on peripheral smear, 723f,
      724t
Retinal hemorrhage
   in birth trauma, 1088
   examination for, 136
   in infective endocarditis, 549
   in shaken baby syndrome, 1087, 1088,
      1091
Retinoblastoma, 778
Retrograde urethrography, 1218, 1219, 1219f
Retroperitoneal mass, palpation of, 117
Retropharyngeal abscess, 209-210, 222, 310t,
      363-364, 364f, 1228f
Reverse transcriptase inhibitors, 436
Reviews, systematic, 97
Reye syndrome
   aspirin and, 198
   vomiting in, 230
Rhabdomyolysis
   in heatstroke, 1149, 1150
   in hypothermia, 1154
   in malignant hyperthermia, 1149, 1150
   in near drowning, 1161
Rhabdomyosarcoma, 778
   cutaneous, 778, 951f
   gallium 67 scintigraphy of, 1222
Rh$_0$D. *See* Anti-Rh$_0$D immune globulin.
Rheumatic disorders, primary
      immunodeficiency diseases and,
      864-865
Rheumatic fever, acute, 573-577
   antibiotic prophylaxis of, 573, 575t, 576,
      576t, 577
   arthritis associated with, 573, 574, 575, 576,
      676, 677, 677t
   diagnosis of, 574-575, 574t, 577
   new developments on horizon, 577
   recurrent, 576
   treatment of, 575-576, 575t
Rheumatoid arthritis. *See* Arthritis, juvenile
      idiopathic/rheumatoid.
Rheumatoid factor, 197, 670, 672
   in systemic lupus erythematosus, 684t
Rhinitis
   allergic, atopic dermatitis with, 981
   syphilitic, 268
Rib fractures, 894, 895
   in abused child, 1090, 1091f, 1212, 1212f-
      1213f, 1214
   pain associated with, 142-143
Ribavirin, for bronchiolitis, 373
   in transplant recipient, 446
Richter hernia, 890
Rickets, chronic renal failure with, 693, 694
Rickettsial infections, 329, 336-337
   septic shock in, 179t
Riley-Day syndrome, 809
Riot control agents, 1181t
Risperidone, 1060, 1064, 1065t, 1066
Ristocetin cofactor activity assay, 754
Rituximab
   for autoimmune hemolytic anemia, 729
   for idiopathic thrombocytopenic purpura,
      744, 745, 746, 746t, 748
   for juvenile dermatomyositis, 669
   for juvenile idiopathic/rheumatoid
      arthritis, 674

V